WITH 1368 ILLUSTRATIONS ON 720 FIGURES

Ninth Edition

Christopher's
Textbook
of
SURGERY

Edited by
LOYAL DAVIS, M.D.
PROFESSOR OF SURGERY, EMERITUS,
NORTHWESTERN UNIVERSITY MEDICAL SCHOOL

W. B. SAUNDERS COMPANY · Philadelphia · London · Toronto

W. B. Saunders Company: West Washington Square
Philadelphia, Pa. 19105

12 Dyott Street
London W.C. 1

1835 Yonge Street
Toronto 7, Ontario

Reprinted October, 1968

Christopher's Textbook of Surgery

Preface

In the ninth edition of this textbook of surgery, the primary aim of the contributors, all authoritative teachers, is to emphasize the basic principles of the surgical treatment of disease.

The education of a surgeon includes the acquisition of many skills and a particular kind of art. This art, an application of understanding the basic fundamentals to the surgical care of sick patients, receives renewed emphasis in this ninth edition. The authors, both the new and the continuing ones, have been asked to concentrate on presentation of these basic considerations rather than on the technical details of operations.

Not less than four years of *postgraduate* work are needed to complete a surgeon's education — with extensive training and practice in special skills included. Such a program is entered upon voluntarily and has as its aim and purpose the development of a thoroughly competent and capable surgeon.

The *undergraduate* course, on the other hand, needs to include only the fundamentals and the principles of their application. We have designed this textbook to satisfy the requirements of the undergraduate and to provide at the same time an up-to-date and thorough review of basic materials for graduate students and practicing surgeons.

Many surgical diseases involve more than one part of the body. It therefore seemed appropriate to add new chapters which integrate knowledge of these disorders. Thus we have new sections on Oncology, Diseases of Degeneration, Congenital Diseases, and Trauma. There are also exciting new chapters on Artificial Organs and on Transplantation of Tissues and Organs. A further addition, a chapter entitled The Surgeon, gives deserved attention to education, ethics, and social and economic factors in surgical practice.

It is impossible that every student in a surgical graduate program can be by choice, personality, or talent, a potential member of a medical school surgical faculty. There are a great many very excellent surgeons who prefer to practice in community hospitals not affiliated with a university. Therefore, graduate residency education and training programs should provide teaching and experience in the entire broad field of surgery instead of being confined to a narrow and specialized area. Many will, of course, choose to specialize, but the surgeon, whether he be general or special, who has had a broadly based education is prepared to recognize his limitations and to visualize the necessity for other special surgical care. The caliber of care he would desire for himself is what he must see that his patients receive.

LOYAL DAVIS

Contributors

J. WESLEY ALEXANDER, M.D.

Assistant Professor, Department of Surgery, University of Cincinnati College of Medicine, Cincinnati.

WILLIAM A. ALTEMEIER, M.D.

Professor and Chairman, Department of Surgery, University of Cincinnati College of Medicine, Cincinnati.

ARJAN D. AMAR, M.B.

Chief, Department of Urology, Kaiser Foundation Hospital, Walnut Creek, California.

CURTIS P. ARTZ, M.D.

Professor and Chairman of Department of Surgery, Medical College of South Carolina, Charleston.

ROBERT K. AUSMAN, M.D.

Associate Professor of Pharmacology, State University of New York at Buffalo; Executive Director of Health Research, Inc., Roswell Park Memorial Institute.

JOEL W. BAKER, M.D.

Chief of Surgery, Virginia Mason Hospital and the Mason Clinic, Seattle.

JOHN L. BELL, M.D.

Associate Professor of Surgery, Northwestern University Medical School, Chicago.

LAWRENCE BRETTSCHNEIDER, M.D.

Assistant Professor of Surgery, University of Colorado School of Medicine, Denver.

JAMES BARRETT BROWN, M.D.

Professor of Clinical Surgery, Washington University School of Medicine, St. Louis.

EDWARD A. BRUNNER, M.D.

Assistant Professor of Anesthesia, Northwestern University Medical School, Chicago.

LARRY C. CAREY, M.D.

Assistant Professor of Surgery, Marquette University School of Medicine, Milwaukee.

WALTER W. CARROLL, M.D.

Professor of Surgery, Northwestern University Medical School, Chicago.

JAMES R. CHANDLER, M.D.

Professor of Surgery (Otolaryngology), University of Miami School of Medicine, Coral Gables, Florida.

CLARENCE DENNIS, M.D.

Professor and Chairman, Department of Surgery, State University of New York Downstate Medical Center, Brooklyn, New York.

JAMES E. ECKENHOFF, M.D.

Professor and Chairman of Department of Anesthesia, Northwestern University Medical School, Chicago.

F. HENRY ELLIS, JR., M.D.

Professor of Surgery, Mayo Graduate School of Medicine (University of Minnesota), Rochester, Minnesota.

EDWIN H. ELLISON, M.D.

Professor and Chairman of Department of Surgery, Marquette University School of Medicine, Milwaukee.

IRVING F. ENQUIST, M.D.

Professor of Surgery, State University of New York Downstate Medical Center, Brooklyn, New York.

WILLIAM J. ERDMAN, II, M.D.

Professor and Chairman of Department of Physical Medicine and Rehabilitation, University of Pennsylvania School of Medicine, Philadelphia.

MINOT P. FRYER, M.D.

Professor of Clinical Surgery, Washington University School of Medicine, St. Louis.

JOHN T. GRAYHACK, M.D.

Professor and Chairman, Department of Urology, Northwestern University Medical School, Chicago.

E. S. GURDJIAN, M.D.

Professor and Chairman, Department of Neurosurgery, Wayne State University School of Medicine, Detroit.

R. CAMERON HARRISON, M.D.

Professor and Head, Department of Surgery, Faculty of Medicine, University of British Columbia, Vancouver, British Columbia.

COLIN T. HOWE, B.M., B.Ch.

Senior Lecturer in Surgery, King's College Hospital Medical School, London, England.

JAMES R. JUDE, M.D.

Professor of Surgery, University of Miami School of Medicine, Coral Gables, Florida.

KARL E. KARLSON, M.D.

Professor of Surgery, State University of New York Downstate Medical Center, Brooklyn, New York.

C. EVERETT KOOP, M.D.

Professor of Pediatric Surgery, University of Pennsylvania School of Medicine, Philadelphia.

HIRAM T. LANGSTON, M.D.

Clinical Professor of Surgery, University of Illinois College of Medicine, Chicago.

WILLIAM A. LARMON, M.D.

Associate Professor of Orthopaedic Surgery, Northwestern University Medical School, Chicago.

HAROLD LAUFMAN, M.D.

Professor of Surgery, Albert Einstein College of Medicine, Bronx, New York.

ROBERT A. MACBETH, M.D.

Professor and Chairman, Department of Surgery, Faculty of Medicine, University of Alberta, Edmonton, Alberta.

IAN MACDONALD, M.D.

Late Clinical Professor of Surgery, School of Medicine, University of Southern California.

WALTER C. MacKENZIE, M.D.

Professor of Surgery and Dean of Medicine, University of Alberta, Faculty of Medicine, Edmonton, Alberta.

CHESTER B. McVAY, M.D.

Clinical Professor of Surgery, School of Medicine, State University of South Dakota, Vermillion, South Dakota.

GEORGE E. MOORE, M.D.

Clinical Professor of Surgery, State University of New York at Buffalo; Director of Public Health Research, New York State Department of Health.

MARSHALL J. ORLOFF, M.D.

Professor and Chairman, Department of Surgery, School of Medicine, University of California, San Diego.

LANGDON PARSONS, M.D.

Clinical Professor of Gynecology (Emeritus), Harvard Medical School, Boston.

JOHN F. PERRY, JR., M.D.

Professor of Surgery, University of Minnesota Medical School, St. Paul.

GERALD H. PRATT, M.D.

Associate Clinical Professor of Surgery, New York University School of Medicine, New York.

BRONSON S. RAY, M.D.

Professor of Surgery (Neurosurgery), Cornell University Medical School, New York.

ROBERT K. RHAMY, M.D.

Professor of Urology and Chairman of the Division, Vanderbilt University School of Medicine, Nashville.

H. WILLIAM SCOTT, JR., M.D.

Professor of Surgery and Chairman of the Department, Vanderbilt University School of Medicine, Nashville.

NORMAN E. SHUMWAY, M.D.

Professor of Surgery, Stanford University School of Medicine, Palo Alto.

F. A. SIMEONE, M.D.

Professor of Medical Science, Brown University, Providence.

PRENTISS E. SMITH, M.D.

Instructor in Surgery, University of Miami School of Medicine, Coral Gables, Florida.

THOMAS E. STARZL, M.D.

Professor of Surgery, University of Colorado School of Medicine, Denver.

EMERY K. STONER, M.D.

Associate Professor, Department of Physical Medicine and Rehabilitation, University of Pennsylvania School of Medicine, Philadelphia.

BRADLEY R. STRAATSMA, M.D.

Professor of Surgery/Ophthalmology, University of California School of Medicine, Los Angeles.

ORVAR SWENSON, M.D.

Professor of Surgery, Northwestern University Medical School, Chicago.

L. M. THOMAS, M.D.

Associate Professor and Assistant Chairman, Department of Neurosurgery, Wayne State University School of Medicine, Detroit.

RICHARD L. VARCO, M.D.

Professor of Surgery, University of Minnesota Medical School, Minneapolis.

C. STUART WELCH, M.D.

Professor of Surgery, Albany Medical College of Union University, Albany.

HENRY M. WEYRAUCH, M.D.

Late Clinical Professor of Surgery and Chief of Division of Urology, Stanford University School of Medicine, Palo Alto.

ROGER D. WILLIAMS, M.D.

Professor of Surgery, University of Texas Medical Branch, Galveston.

BERNARD ZIMMERMANN, M.D.

Professor and Chairman, Department of Surgery, West Virginia University School of Medicine, Morgantown.

ROBERT M. ZOLLINGER, M.D.

Professor and Chairman of the Department of Surgery, Ohio State University College of Medicine, Columbus.

Contents

Chapter *1*

THE HISTORY OF SURGERY

by
C. STUART WELCH, M.D.

Born in Newburyport, Massachusetts, C. STUART WELCH received his education at Tufts College and Tufts University Medical School. After an internship at the Boston City Hospital, he completed a Fellowship in Surgery at the Mayo Clinic. He earned Master of Science and Doctor of Philosophy degrees in surgery at the University of Minnesota. He is Professor of Surgery at Albany Medical College of Union University. His interest in medical history and books has brought him acclaim and recognition from the surgical profession.

DEFINITION AND SCOPE OF SURGERY

The third-year medical student is thrown somewhat precipitously into clinical work and often does not have the opportunity to form a proper concept of surgery. One misconception is that surgery is concerned largely, if not solely, with operating and technical considerations. The present-day surgeon must be a good technician, it is true, but he is much more than an artisan. There was a time when the surgeon or his predecessor, the barber, was told when and where to operate by the physician. The surgeon at one time had little or no medical education and no status. A gradual evolution brought surgery into medical education. There is, therefore, a historical background for a misconception of surgery. There is also a general feeling among men that he who works with his hands has less time for thinking and is less intellectual.

Today, surgeons make important scientific contributions to medicine by their clinical and laboratory research, which have no technical aspects whatsoever. Indeed, their interests may be entirely nontechnical, concerned with body metabolism, genetics or chemistry. Education and training in surgery today put special emphasis on collateral reading and instruction in the basic medical sciences. Many surgical residents spend time not only in the surgical research laboratory but in basic science laboratories.

Perhaps the great difference between the practice of surgery and internal medicine is found in the responsibility which the surgeon takes in transgressing the human body by an elective type of operation, one calculated to improve the patient's health but not a critically needed one. Since there is always some risk to operation and anesthesia, the responsibility in recommending certain elective operations is great. Surgery requires its disciples to have high principles, personal integrity and compassion for their fellow men.

The Oxford University Dictionary defines surgery as "the art or practice of treating injuries, deformities, and other disorders by manual operation or instrumental appliances. . . ." The definition is archaic in that it fails to mention the great nonoperative labor of surgery which is concerned with the restoration and maintenance of optimal body function before, during and after the operation. This latter aspect of surgical knowledge and practice is the surgery of modern times.

There are but three basic injuries with which the surgeon deals either separately or in combination. These are the treatment of wounds, the loss of body fluids and the invasion of the body by pathogenic microorganisms.

Historically, operative surgery can be divided into three basic types. These are the

1

repair of wounds, the extirpation of diseased organs or tissue and reconstructive surgery. These categories have more fundamental significance than the division of surgery on a regional or systemic basis, as is seen in surgical practice with its many specialties. To these three categories two more developments of the twentieth century must be added: physiologic surgery and replacement surgery.

The treatment and repair of wounds is a part of every operation. Every day the surgeon treats wounds as he closes the incisions he has made or repairs accidental injuries. Theodor Billroth said, "The proper treatment of wounds is to be regarded as the first and most requisite qualification for the surgeon." The operation must be executed properly, making a proper incision, attaining good exposure, effecting good hemostasis and repairing the wound with minimal trauma and bacterial contamination.

Extirpative surgery needs little explanation in its simple form. A diseased gallbladder, uterus or appendix is removed, entirely alleviating the patient's illness, exemplifying the principle of excisional or extirpative surgery. Refinements of extirpative surgery have evolved, particularly in surgery for cancer. Radical excision for cancer of the breast removes not only the tumor in the breast but the breast itself and tissue in the axilla containing lymph nodes to which the cancer may have metastasized.

Reconstructive surgery is practiced extensively in orthopedics and the specialty of plastic surgery, but this basic surgical category is commonly applied to a greater or lesser extent in all operations. In gynecology, for example, the procedure of anterior and posterior colporrhaphy for the repair of childbirth injuries is reconstructive.

Physiologic surgery requires knowledge of the functions of the systems of the body and their interrelations, because its beneficial results depend upon altering normal physiologic mechanisms for the general good of body function. The disease is not attacked directly by a physiologic operation, either because the etiology of the disease is not known or because the lesion cannot be operated upon directly. Physiologic operations are usually palliative but often they are curative from the practical standpoint. Sympathectomy for certain types of vascular disease and vascular shunts for heart disease and portal hypertension are operations in this category. Operations for duodenal ulcer are of the type that take advantage of altering bodily function for its effect. Obviously, present-day operations for duodenal ulcer do not attack the cause of the disease but suffice to control gastric acidity. The field of physiologic surgery is an ever-increasing one, fed by knowledge gained in the experimental surgical laboratory.

Replacement surgery is a unique field not only because worn or diseased organs or parts can be reconditioned or replaced by living human tissue or by inserting plastic, metal or fabrics but more important because in this field the surgeon defies basic surgical principles. Replacement of the abdominal aorta by plastic fabrics after aneurysmectomy is a good example of this type of surgery. More fascinating and somewhat promising is tissue and organ transplantation.

The surgical specialties gradually evolved from what is still known as general surgery. General surgery remains the mainstay of surgical teaching and research. It is difficult to define general surgery, since its practice varies greatly, depending upon where it is practiced.

There are now ten recognized surgical specialties. Their inception was initiated by the increasing scope of surgery, wherein it became difficult for one man to be the complete master of diagnostic and operative work all over the body. This cause, coupled with the interest, taste and predilection of surgeons, has helped to build each field. In the present era, there has arisen a tendency to overspecialization. Movements to establish new specialties are not always justified; divisiveness does not always serve the interest of surgical practice and teaching.

The history of surgery may be divided for convenience into prehistoric surgery and the surgery of antiquity, surgery of the Middle Ages to the Renaissance, surgery from the Renaissance to modern times, and modern surgery. It can be read and studied profitably in relation to political and social eras or dynasties.

PREHISTORIC TIMES AND ANTIQUITY

Operative surgery of a primitive type is as old as mankind. Much of it was done instinctively and without special training. A loose tooth begs for extraction; an abscess wants to be opened.

In Babylonian society of two or three thousand years before Christ, Montaigne says,

"The whole people was the physician." It was their custom to bring the sick and wounded into a public place where they could be seen and examined by anyone, with the purpose of finding someone of the population who might help them. It was the duty of the healthy to look the sick over and give such advice as their experience offered. The usual practice was for the well to advise on diseases or injuries which they had had themselves. In the course of time there developed a medical system of sorts in which there was a specialist for every disease.

From the beginning of history, one finds medicine in the hands of those who dealt with the supernatural and religious needs of the community. Medicine has a long history of this association. It exists today among our Christian medical missionaries, although to a much less extent and upon a different basis. In ancient times any operation that was done was often supplemented by appeals to the gods, and various forms of exorcism played a large part in the treatment.

Trephining of the skull was used in prehistoric times for treating fits and insanity. Mutilating operations of a senseless nature were done electively, and much of this kind of surgery was harmful, although it represented the first gropings of man in surgical therapy based on a kind of physiologic knowledge, correct or incorrect. Antiquarians of medicine have studied most interesting archeologic specimens of bones from which they have made conjectures that operations had been performed at very early periods. Inscriptions on tombs and on walls of sepulchers in Egypt which date from 2500 B.C. to even earlier times have given unequivocal evidence of the proper treatment of fractures by splinting, or the operation of circumcision, and suggestions of more advanced surgery.

One must keep in mind the fact that societies were isolated in antiquity. A relatively high degree of civilized behavior, accompanied by an interest in learning and investigation of man's nature, might be found at not a great distance from places in which men were living in the stone age. Communication is the foundation for the dissemination of knowledge, and communication is a complex business involving spoken and written language, travel and a peaceful intercourse among men. Advances in medicine were, therefore, intermittent and independently made. Too often progress was lost with the destruction of a people and their civilization.

Among those ancient peoples of whose medical practices we have some knowledge, the Sumerians, Egyptians, Hindus, Chinese and Jews, the Egyptians and Hindus stand out as surgeons. The Jews excelled in hygiene and preventive medicine but not surgery. The Hindus recorded innumerable operative procedures which they did, but their influence on Western society was small. Evidence of the superiority of Hindu surgery is recorded in the *Susruta*, in which an operative manual describing vesicolithotomy and rhinoplasty is found. Incisions and surgical instruments are also described.

The long period of Egyptian civilization produced a worthy medicine in which surgery had a respectable place. Two papyri, the *Edwin Smith* (circa 1700 B.C.) and the *Ebers* (1500 B.C.), document the sophisticated surgery of our oldest historic phase of medicine. The treatment of accidental wounds, fractures, dislocations, head injuries, operations for circumcision and superficial surgery of the extremities are mentioned in these fragments. There is no evidence, however, that the Egyptians opened the body cavities. Egyptian civilization ultimately declined and with it medical and surgical practice. The importance of Egyptian medicine is in its contributions to Greek medicine.

The next two great schools of medicine existed in Greece and Alexandria from 500 B.C. to just before the birth and the rise of the Western Roman Empire. Best of all is the medicine of the Classical Period of Greece (460–130 B.C.) as found in the Hippocratic School. This medical era was the precursor of European medicine. Hippocrates (460–370 B.C.) wrote and taught extensively on surgery, and his treatment of fractures, dislocations and wounds was especially good in light of what we know today. But most of all, his emphasis on rational conduct based on studied conclusions as opposed to prejudicial and emotional ones elevated medicine to a higher level than ever before and set the stage for its place as a science. One of the greatest medical aphorisms, *vis medicatrix naturae*, comes from Hippocrates. The healing power of nature is great; it must be conserved; the methods which nature uses to heal are to be imitated and improved upon, he taught. This respect for the *vis medicatrix naturae* which Hippocrates had was later appreciated by John Hunter (1728–1793) when he said: "What does the wound signify to the organism? By what mechanism does the organism safeguard itself against the effect of the wound immediate and remote?" Later, Hilton in his beautiful essays on "Rest and Pain" given before the Royal College of Surgeons in 1860 to 1862, repeated the essence of Hippocrates' teaching:

> Entertaining, as I do, the most exalted admiration of Nature's powers of repair, the thought has not unfrequently occurred to my mind, when watching cases of extensive injury, "What would have been the condition of man on earth, had it pleased the Creator to withhold from him this power of repairing his injured tissues?"
>
> In my reflections on the subject of rest as a curative agent, my mind naturally reverted to that period of man's existence when it was the sole curative means of which he could avail himself. I could but picture to myself the timorous awe which must have been engendered in his mind by the first accident which happened to him. Let us imagine our first parents suddenly thrust out of the Garden of Eden, and doomed to toil for their daily bread; with hands unused to labour, inexperienced in the substitutes for unnecessary exertion and in the avoidance of local injury, and exposed to all the accidents of a precarious existence. Let us try to realize the awe-stricken dismay which must have oppressed man's mind on the infliction of his first wound, his first experience of pain; the breach of surface disclosing to his sight his blood flowing unceasingly, or leaping, at sustained intervals, from its opened chambers; his sense of fainting and his ultimately sinking on the earth under the foretaste of death; this, too, with the recent denunciation "Thou shall surely die," still ringing in his ears. Can words depict the hopeless anguish which he must have endured? But what follows? See him awakening to life again, the stream of blood stayed, the chasm plugged, his strength revived, and day by day that wound—which he regarded as the badge of death, the vengeance of the Creator's wrath—narrowing and healing till it could hardly be seen.
>
> I have made these observations for the purpose of showing the original promptings of Nature to man, for the alleviation of what must have necessarily befallen him in his altered condition. Pain was made the prime agent. Under injury, pain suggested the necessity of, and indeed, compelled him to seek for, rest. Every deviation from this necessary state of rest brought with it, through pain, the admonition that he was straying from the condition essential to his restoration. He must have observed with astonishment the breaking asunder of the newly-formed tissue or the steady development into normal structure, which occurred in exact accordance with the disturbance or rest to the parts, which the sense of pain had enabled him to regulate so accurately, and to enjoy so beneficially for his own personal relief and comfort.
>
> That the Lord of all should have implanted in man, beyond the endowments which enable him to sustain his existence under the punishment of labour and the vicissitudes of his daily life, a recuperative power from the accidents and mischances of his previous existence, appears to me to supply an evidence of His merciful and unspeakable love, too lightly considered.

These teachings are the fundamental concepts which ultimately developed into the concept of homeostasis, as Cannon expressed it in his book, *The Wisdom of the Body.*

The decline of Attic Greece after the Peloponnesian Wars initiated a shift of medical pre-eminence. Medicine rises and falls with the fate of empires and dynasties. Good medicine is practiced only in rich societies. The great city of Alexandria, founded in 332 B.C., was next to forward medicine and particularly anatomy and surgery. It was here that the ligature was used to arrest hemorrhage and a substantial number of elective operations performed.

The period from 150 B.C. until the Middle Ages is the long period of Greco-Roman medicine. A continuity of Greek medicine to Roman is understandable in the political and social circumstances of the time. Alexandrian medicine was also transitional. The great recorder of medical practice of these times was Celsus, who was probably not a physician.

The great name of the period was Galen. Galen's writings were on anatomy, pathology, physiology, pharmacology, medicine and surgery. In fact, he wrote authoritatively upon all medical subjects. His dogmatic pronouncements and teachings suited well the generations to follow him in a period of intellectual stagnation. Galen's early descriptions of wound treatment were good; he used wine for lavage, followed by primary suture with linen thread with good results in clean, contaminated wounds. Later his obsession with wound medicaments and applications supplanted his first technique and was to prevail as a heritage from him during several centuries. So influential was Galen that his medical writings stifled progress and dominated medicine in the Western world during the period of the Middle Ages in which scholastic dogmatism was prevalent.

THE MIDDLE AGES TO THE RENAISSANCE

Greco-Roman medicine in its best form flourished during the early centuries after the birth of Christ, but deteriorated with the decline of the Western Roman Empire (500 A.D.). The Byzantine Empire was to endure 1000 years longer, but its medicine, which was inherited from Greece, showed no progress. Alexandria was an important repository of medicine and was especially noted for its progress in surgery at the beginning of our times.

The writings of Paul of Ægina, seventh century A.D., give testimony to an advanced surgical practice of that period, which might be called the beginning of the end of the best in Greco-Roman medicine.

The rise of Islamic culture and supremacy of the Mohammedan Empire produced a period known as the Arabic period of medicine, which lasted from the seventh to the eleventh centuries. It can be fairly stated that the Islamic people contributed little to medicine in an original manner. They obtained their knowledge of medicine principally from the Nestorians, a persecuted Christian sect which sought refuge in the desert and brought with them their medical knowledge. Their medical practice was of Greek origin from Constantinople. Translations were made of Greek and Roman texts into Arabic at this time. These Arabic texts were read and used in Western Europe at a much later period.

Surgery cannot be said to have advanced in Arabic medicine. The names of several teachers stand out, especially Rasis (865–925 A.D.) and Avicenna (980–1037 A.D.). The latter wrote *The Cannon*, but neither of these teachers added anything to surgery. In the eleventh century Albucasis, a Moslem born in Spain, wrote a much-used surgical treatise of little originality. Most of his writing was a reiteration of Paul (Alexandrian School) and Galen (Roman). He did, however, include in his writing personal, practical experience, and in many instances he proved to be very wise in the management of surgical patients.

It is to the Arabic School of medicine and surgery that the harmful use of the actual cautery in wounds can be attributed. There was much evidence in the earlier writings of Hippocrates, Celsus, Paul, and even some of Galen's work that gentle cleansing, minimal trauma, irrigation with nonirritating solutions, and even primary suture, offered a chance of healing. The ligature introduced in the Alexandrian School was to take second or third place to cauterization in Arabic medicine and for a long time in the surgery of Western Europe. Good methods of hemostasis were to wait out the period in which Arabic medicine was practiced. Suppuration, secondary hemorrhage and poor healing with huge tissue defects were to be the fruits of the influence of this school for many years to come. Unfortunately, Latin translations of Arabic works were to be the principal books for medical knowledge during medieval times in the Western world.

Actually, there was no real progress in surgery from about 500 to 1000 or 1200 A.D. In Western Europe, this time was characterized by a separation of surgery from medicine. But more significant in retarding medical progress was the rapid spread of Christianity, with its emphasis on moral philosophy to the neglect of science.

The development of medical knowledge, along with that of letters, art and science, lagged because of the overpowering religious interest which engaged the minds of all scholars. The custodians of medical information and its practitioners were primarily priests who were only secondarily interested in medicine. Nevertheless, the ancient medical literature of the Greek, Arab, Chinese and other societies was preserved during these centuries. The monks of the Middle Ages constituted the sole body of scholars, and their function in saving and copying manuscripts of the past, during the period when the general education of laymen was at a low ebb, was extremely important for the future.

Monte Cassino, so well remembered because of its devastation during World War II, was a particular repository of medical knowledge, and, indeed, Saint Benedict and the order of the monks which he founded became the best physicians of their time. In the late Middle Ages, the Benedictine Order also established cathedral schools in several European centers in which medicine was taught. The decline of ecclesiastic medicine began in about the year 900 A.D., but active lay participation in the field had already begun.

The reason for the shift from clerical to lay practitioners is easily understood. In the beginning of this period, priests were the only scholars. They alone could read and write, and thus, of necessity, had command of the only sources of medical knowledge. With the foundation of universities in the form of cathedral schools, the laity commenced to have access to this knowledge. Then, too, the church decided during the twelfth and thirteenth centuries to restrict the practice of medicine by monastic orders and secular priests on the grounds that it did not represent a true function of religious life. In some instances, monks had been taken entirely away from their religious duties; they were no longer priests preaching for the salvation of souls, but had become physicians attending bodily illnesses. Finally, at the end of the twelfth century, all priests were forbidden to practice either law or medicine, a rule which is in effect today in the Roman Church.

Secular education at the University of Salerno, beginning in the ninth century, resulted in the first great school of medicine in the Middle Ages. In this school was collected and integrated the best of Greco-Roman, Oriental and Arabic medicine. In the Italian schools, the art along with the science of medicine was practiced, and it remained in the structure of surgical education. Roger of Salerno's famous *Fabrica* became the standard textbook of surgery and remained so for 300 years. Together with Roland of Parma, one of his pupils, Roger made a departure from Arabic medicine and surgery. In the writings of these men, suture ligature for hemostasis is described. Circular suture of the intestine and a description of second intention wound healing are among the important items of these writings. The treatment of wounds at this period, however, left much to be desired in that the adherence to the Galenic principle that suppuration was a necessary forerunner of healing was strict.

The University of Salerno was at the height of its glory between the twelfth and fourteenth centuries. The Universities of Padua and Bologna rose in prestige as Salerno declined, but the light of medicine burned brightly in the Italian universities during the latter days of the Middle Ages. By this time, the teaching of medicine to laymen had begun in the northern universities as well. At Bologna, the study of anatomy, particularly, was pursued, and the Galenic texts which had been accepted as gospel without inquiry for many years were criticized and repudiated in many instances. No great advances were made over previous knowledge in surgical technique and practice, but the teaching of surgery was put on a better basis by Saliceto, Theodoric and others of the Bologna School.

Theodoric is especially important as a teacher of surgery during the Middle Ages because his teaching on the treatment of wounds was so good in the light of present-day treatment. His surgery was a departure from the time-honored Galenic and Arabic teachings. Theodoric was a pupil of Hugh of Lucca, from whom he undoubtedly inherited considerable knowledge about wounds. Lucca's methods of wound treatment were simple and kind to tissues.

Although Theodoric was addicted to the use of unguents and poultices in certain wounds, it is probable that he used these only in the open treatment of contaminated and infected wounds. He certainly was an advocate of free drainage in contaminated wounds and in those in which moderate hemorrhage or seep-

age was an uncontrollable factor. In his writings, he advocated mild medication, cleansing and lavage with wine as the best and most innocuous measure for procuring a dry wound with primary healing. In Chapter II of his book he says:

In whatever part of the body a cut may have occurred, let everything be done in order, according to the rules laid down for wounds in the scalp and face. Indeed, above all else a wound must be made clean. Secondly, having brought the lips of the wound together, they should be replaced accurately in the position which they had in their natural state; if necessary, they should be held there by stitches taken in accordance with the size of the wound. Let the size and depth of the wound determine the closeness and depth of the stitches. For let the physician make no mistake; as has already been said many times, he should be prudent and attentive to every detail. After the suturing has been properly done and the dressings have been carefully arranged, let the wound be bound up skillfully as the position and condition of the part require, that is to say, so that neither the stitches nor the dressings can be disturbed at all. And, just as we have often said before, do not undo the dressing until the third or fourth or fifth day if no pain occurs. Afterwards, let the dressings be changed every day, observing the aforementioned directions. And always, whenever the dressing is changed, by pressing gently upon the wound with a little wine-soaked tow you may express any retained bloody matter. Afterwards, let it be kept thus until the patient has completely recovered. And if proud flesh should become excessive on a wound, as has been said before, put on the green ointment or something similar, for as long as you see that it is necessary.

Next in order of progress in Western European medicine came France, particularly the school at Montpellier which was important during the beginning of the twelfth century. Montpellier reached its eminence in the thirteenth century. Lanfranc of Milan, who worked also at Lyon and finally Paris, where he became a teacher at the College de Saint Côme, completed his notable *Chirurgia Magna* in 1296. Besides his original surgical contributions, he stands out as a staunch opponent of the schism between medicine and surgery, which he found so marked in France. He was not, however, an advocate of the dry treatment of wounds, as was his contemporary, Henry de Mondeville. De Mondeville castigated the Galenic principles of wound therapy as well as Galenic medicine in general. He is credited with saying, "Many more surgeons know how to cause suppuration than to heal a wound."

The most famous product of the French School, Guy de Chauliac, became the mentor of surgical practice for many years to come in his *La Grande Chirurgie*, written in 1363, the vade mecum of surgery through the sixteenth century. Chauliac, educated at Bologna, Montpellier and Paris, was in holy orders. He taught some at Montpellier, but his principal function was that of physician and chaplain to the Avignon Popes. For the most part he was a good observer and a sound surgeon, but in the treatment of wounds he was a proponent of interference, somewhat of the nature of Galen's, in which the teaching was concentrated on the application of medications, powder, salves and poultices. In fact, he denounced Theodoric's teachings. Thus, the great respect and authority in which he was held, perpetuated by his textbook which became standard for several centuries, ensured the continuation of the Galenic and Arabic principles of wound treatment to the detriment of surgery in general. The efficacy of minimal interference and major dependence on the healing power of nature in wound management, a teaching of the Hippocratic School and later of Theodoric and de Mondeville, was given a great setback for 400 years by Chauliac's influence.

The important advances in the art and science of medicine during the Middle Ages were the establishment of secular education and the divorce of the practice of medicine from the church, and church sanction to scientific investigation in medicine.

Dissection of the human body was permitted officially by Pope Sixtus IV toward the end of the fifteenth century. The fact that the treatment of bodily illness was not, per se, dependent upon or necessarily influenced by religious intervention, also became recognized. Also in the late Middle Ages, the best of ancient medicine was studied and correlated. The faculty of Salerno and other Italian universities had Jews, Arabs and a generally free society of teachers contributing to the medical education of the time. There was a distillation of the best of past medical knowledge going on in these universities, which created a firm basis upon which to build the medical future. In addition to universities for lay education, hospitals for the care of the sick were also established in Italy and had become fairly well organized by the end of the fifteenth century. A great deterrent to continued advance was the trend, developing in the late Middle Ages, toward the transfer of responsibility for surgery from the hands of physicians, where it had been in ancient Greece and in the Physician's School at Salerno, to the hands of illiterate barbers.

As the Middle Ages closed, surgeons no longer had university rank; rarely did they read Latin, and rarely did they come from the educated medical group. Since much of the operative work was done by this semi-ignorant class of persons, little progress occurred. Surgery regressed as an art, and its scientific development ceased. In England, the inferior education and status of surgeons was particularly pronounced. Here and throughout the European continent, barbers and quacks were the surgeons of the time and for a few centuries to come. It is understandable, therefore, that little original work in surgery was produced.

THE RENAISSANCE AND EARLY MODERN TIMES

The end of the Middle Ages and the beginning of the Renaissance cannot be fixed with an exact date, since changes are always gradual. At the end of the Middle Ages, the stage was set for progress by the turn of events which left medicine entirely in lay hands. The early Christian point of view, which looked on illness as a punishment for sin, had by now been completely abandoned by ecclesiastic scholars and churchmen. The fifteenth and sixteenth centuries, the period now known as the Renaissance, represented a transitional phase of our civilization which bridged the gap between medieval and modern times. The sixteenth century saw the Protestant Reformation. Investigators, scholars and teachers then determined to abandon the great yoke of the past which, in scholastic life and thought, required an acceptance of past teachings without inquiry into their essential truth. While it is true that the Middle Ages saw some progress in this regard in the science of anatomy, as exemplified by the anatomic studies of the Italian schools which shook Galenic teachings, the Renaissance spirit of search for truth had much more vitality. Re-examination of the anatomy of the body and a study of the physiologic concepts prevalent up to that time were carried out with much less regard for the established dogmatic writings of the great teachers of the past.

The name of Vesalius and his great work, *De Humani Corporis Fabrica*, published in 1543, defied Galenic anatomy and furnished a solid basis for accurate surgery. Vesalius was only 28 years of age when he wrote his *Fabrica*. Vesalius practiced military and civilian surgery and was Imperial Physician to Charles V until the abdication of that monarch in 1555.

The Renaissance in Germany and England brought forth a new and progressive medicine. Paracelsus, the great German surgeon (1493–1541), appreciated the healing power of nature when he said:

You should know what it is which heals a wound because without this knowledge you cannot use any medicine correctly. You should know that it is the nature of flesh, of the body, of the blood vessels, of the limbs to have within themselves an inborn balsam that heals all wounds, stab wounds or any other sort. It is the balsam in the limb that heals a fracture, the balsam that resides naturally in the flesh that heals flesh. So with every limb it should be understood that it carries its own healing in itself which heals it when it is wounded. Every surgeon therefore should know that it is not he who heals the wound but the balsam in the part that heals it. If he thinks he heals it, he fools himself, and does not know his art.

It cannot be said, however, that operative surgery advanced a great deal during the Renaissance, although the advance in general medical scientific knowledge pushed forward tremendously. The rigid structure of Galenic scholasticism in medicine was broken by investigation that found much of the older medical dogma to be false. There were, perhaps, so many fundamental facts to be established that the best minds in medicine of that period could not concern themselves with mere operative surgery. The educational status of surgeons in the period was still very low; the art was still in disrepute and separated from established medicine.

Ambroïse Paré, a gifted but poorly educated barber-surgeon, emerged as the great figure of Renaissance surgery. His contributions were important, and as a teacher his mark was felt, yet it cannot be said that he had uncovered any new concept—all his best observations and practices were known to the ancients. Most significant of his work was his use of the ligature on blood vessels and the abolition of the old Arabic treatment of wounds by cautery and hot oil instillation in favor of the more sound practice of gentle cleansing and milder medication. A profoundly religious man, a Huguenot who was the surgeon and adviser to the kings of France, Paré recognized the importance of the healing power of nature.

Toward the end of the sixteenth century, progress in surgery finally came about through the improvement of the educational status of surgeons. The organization of the Company of Barbers with the Surgeons of London, under a charter of Henry VIII in 1540, started in that country the important

control of surgery by a responsible group. This guild lasted for two centuries and controlled the requirements for the practice of surgery. It may be looked upon as the precursor of the present Royal College of Surgeons of England. The inclusion of surgery in the curricula of medical schools began again in the late sixteenth and early seventeenth centuries, and surgery resumed a place it had formerly held in the Italian Schools of the twelfth century.

The seventeenth and eighteenth centuries saw continued scientific progress in the Western world, and, with this progress, definite changes in medical practice and teaching. Basic investigations in anatomy, pathology and physiology brought forth the new science of medicine. We have only to recall the names of William Harvey, John Hunter and Morgagni from among the many contributors of this period to recognize that these two centuries were extremely productive. In most places in Europe, however, the practice of surgery was still considered inferior to medicine, principally because adequate education of surgeons was not general throughout the seventeenth century and a good part of the eighteenth century. Barbers were still the principal surgeons in the middle of the eighteenth century in some parts of Europe, although a change was in the making. It is not strange, then, that there were few outstanding contributions coming from surgical practitioners, since most of these men were not university trained. They lacked the basic applicable medical knowledge with which to make progress in their art.

The study and practice of surgery were taken over by the medical profession during the seventeenth and eighteenth centuries, and there was a great development in manual skill and surgical technique. Operations were more skillfully performed by men who had accurate anatomic knowledge and who had, at the same time, as good an understanding of the diseases with which they dealt as could then be obtained. Better instruments were evolved. Speed in the performance of operative procedures was particularly developed because the avoidance of shock became recognized as necessary for survival of the unanesthetized patient.

The art of operative surgery became highly developed in England during the eighteenth century by Cheselden, Pott, John Hunter and Cooper. Hemostasis by ligature, as the better means of controlling hemorrhage, became firmly established by the end of the eighteenth century. Such advances were important and should not be minimized; yet, in the light of our knowledge of the more distant history of surgery, it cannot be said that many new principles evolved during these two hundred years. The period may be looked upon rather as a time in which surgery was catching up with the higher standard of internal medicine, by consolidating past knowledge and applying it to the care of the patient at a higher level and with more skill than ever before. The stage was set for the birth of modern surgery in the nineteenth century, when Americans were for the first time to play their part.

The end of the eighteenth and the beginning of the nineteenth century was a time of great political and social upheaval. The French and American Revolutions occurred. The period was one of uprising of the common man in the Western world. Although these changes impeded the progress of scientific achievement and of medicine for a time, they ultimately resulted in a new stimulus to their development. The lower classes of society found it possible to enter the universities. The main force that motivated these revolutions was materialistic — the seeking for all of a larger share of the world's wealth. This political and social revolution created a climate congenial to advance in scientific investigation. The decidedly objective approach toward settling the affairs of men carried over into medicine. This way of thinking brought an end to any sovereignty which dogmatic scholasticism might still have over the interpretation of biologic phenomena. The American Revolution brought with it the birth of medical education and improved practice in the United States.

In the battle before Moscow at Borodino, which has been so vividly portrayed by Tolstoy in *War and Peace*, Larrey, the celebrated surgeon of Napoleon's army, is said to have performed more than 200 amputations during the day's fighting. His rapid surgery on the field prevented serious infection and achieved a low mortality rate. Another important innovation of Larrey's was the field ambulance and field operating facilities, a forerunner of our modern military surgical system. At the same time, however, the mortality from wounds and from military surgery in general was still frightful. The conditions under which operations on the battlefield were done were appalling, and sepsis killed many of those who survived operation in most armies. A good picture of the Russian military

surgeon and the operating tent of these times is given also by Tolstoy as he follows the severely wounded Prince Bolkonski through his operation during the Battle of Borodino.

The Operating Tent. Portion of Prince Andrew's Thighbone Extracted. Anatole's Leg Amputated. Prince Andrew Pities Him.

One of the doctors came out of the tent in a blood-stained apron, holding a cigar between the thumb and little finger of one of his small bloodstained hands, so as not to smear it. He raised his head and looked about him, but above the level of the wounded men. He evidently wanted a little respite. After turning his head from right to left for some time, he sighed and looked down.

"All right, immediately," he replied to a dresser who pointed Prince Andrew out to him, and he told them to carry him into the tent.

Murmurs arose among the wounded who were waiting.

"It seems that even in the next world only the gentry are to have a chance!" remarked one.

Prince Andrew was carried in and laid on a table that had only just been cleared and which a dresser was washing down. Prince Andrew could not make out distinctly what was in that tent. The pitiful groans from all sides and the torturing pain in his thigh, stomach, and back distracted him. All he saw about him merged into a general impression of naked, bleeding human bodies that seemed to fill the whole of the low tent, as a few weeks previously, on that hot August day, such bodies had filled the dirty pond besides the Smolensk road. Yet it was the same flesh, the same *chair à canon*, the sight of which had even then filled him with horror, as by a presentiment.

There were three operating tables in the tent. Two were occupied, and on the third they placed Prince Andrew. For a little while he was left alone and involuntarily witnessed what was taking place on the other two tables. On the nearest one sat a Tartar, probably a Cossack, judging by the uniform thrown down beside him. Four soldiers were holding him, and a spectacled doctor was cutting into his muscular brown back.

"Ooh, ooh, ooh!" grunted the Tartar, and suddenly lifting up his swarthy snub-nosed face with its high cheekbones, and baring his white teeth, he began to wriggle and twitch his body and utter piercing, ringing, and prolonged yells. On the other table, round which many people were crowding, a tall well-fed man lay on his back with his head thrown back. His curly hair, its color, and the shape of his head seemed strangely familiar to Prince Andrew. Several dressers were pressing on his chest to hold him down. One large, white, plump leg twitched rapidly all the time with a feverish tremor. The man was sobbing and choking convulsively. Two doctors — one of whom was pale and trembling — were silently doing something to this man's other, gory leg. When he had finished with the Tartar, whom they covered with an overcoat, the spectacled doctor came up to Prince Andrew, wiping his hands.

He glanced at Prince Andrew's face and quickly turned away.

"Undress him! What are you waiting for?" he cried angrily to the dressers.

His very first, remotest recollections of childhood

came back to Prince Andrew's mind when the dresser with sleeves rolled up began hastily to undo the buttons of his clothes and undressed him. The doctor bent down over the wound, felt it, and sighed deeply. Then he made a sign to someone, and the torturing pain in his abdomen caused Prince Andrew to lose consciousness. When he came to himself the splintered portions of his thighbone had been extracted, the torn flesh cut away, and the wound bandaged. Water was being sprinkled on his face. As soon as Prince Andrew opened his eyes, the doctor bent over, kissed him silently on the lips, and hurried away.

The last part of the eighteenth century and beginning of the nineteenth century was characterized by surgical advancement through individual prowess. The preanesthesia, preantiseptic surgical period of the nineteenth century ended with a high development of technical skill. It was hindered by a lack of these two boons to surgery, but was firm in anatomic and pathologic knowledge. Most of all, the surgeon was at last the surgeon-physician and held a respectable place in medicine. If the surgeons of the early part of the nineteenth century could have lived to its end and have seen the addition of anesthesia and asepsis to the surgical armamentarium, they would have had their greatest dreams fulfilled. In the United States, the name of Ephraim McDowell stands out for his first successful ovariotomy performed without anesthesia in 1809.

MODERN SURGERY: 1846 TO PRESENT

BEGINNINGS. The great era of scientific achievement began with the close of the eighteenth century and the beginning of the nineteenth century. Advances in the natural sciences, physics and chemistry were made rapidly, and it is not surprising that there were parallel gains in medicine. In 1859, Charles Robert Darwin published his monumental treatise representing 20 years of work: *On the Origin of Species by Means of Natural Selection*. A great period of clinical development in medicine began in France and England, noteworthy for the study of specific diseases and their accurate description. It was the period of Virchow with his *omnis cellula e cellula* theory.

Anesthesia, the development of the science of microbiology, the discovery of x-rays, the discovery of blood types and the development of safe blood transfusion methods, and finally the discovery of penicillin and subsequent manufacture of other antibiotics are the five great scientific achievements which made modern surgery possible. All of these were developed during the last 100 years, beginning in 1846, the date of the first public demonstration of ether anesthesia. When one adds to these acquirements the better education of the surgeon, particularly in the area of basic medical scientific knowledge, the result is surgical practice today which has accomplished feats beyond the imagination of preceding generations of surgeons.

Anesthesia. The credit for the discovery of the value of sulfuric ether as an anesthetic agent goes to an American physician, Crawford W. Long, who first used it in a surgical operation in 1842. In 1844, Horace Wells, a dentist of Hartford, Connecticut, used nitrous oxide for a tooth extraction. It remained, however, for W. T. G. Morton, also a dentist of Hartford, Connecticut, together with John Collins Warren of the Massachusetts General Hospital, to give anesthesia by ether the publicity necessary to establish its place in surgery. The demonstration of a successful surgical operation under ether anesthesia at the Massachusetts General Hospital in 1846 was followed by a rapid and successful trial of this new adjunct to surgery throughout the world within a few months.

In 1847, chloroform was introduced by Sir James Simpson of Edinburgh. The tremendous difference which anesthesia has made in the practice of surgery cannot be appreciated today by those who have never operated without it. Since Morton and Warren's ether demonstration on October 16, 1846, just a little more than 100 years ago, the art and science of anesthesia has continued to progress and has added greatly to the results which surgery is now attaining.

From the beginnings of open inhalation of ether and chloroform, anesthesia has developed rapidly, particularly in the last 50 years. Of primary importance has been the development of intratracheal anesthesia with respiration controlled by intermittent positive pressure. In 1878, Macewen first described the use of an intratracheal tube introduced via the mouth. The intratracheal catheter has proved to be one of the greatest boons to anesthesia technique and has been of particular value in open chest surgery. In 1904, Sauerbach of Berlin demonstrated the use of a low pressure chamber for operating within the thoracic cavity in order to avoid the bad effects of pneumothorax. His early experiments paved the way for successful thoracic surgery by applying physiologic principles to surgical practice. The much more practical method of intratracheal anesthesia with a closed system and intermittent positive pressure soon became universally used and solved the problem of open thoracic surgery in a more practical way. In 1909, Meltzer and Auer demonstrated the insufflation technique of administering oxygen without continuous respirations. In 1915, Dennis Jackson of Cincinnati added the carbon dioxide absorption technique to the closed-system method.

In the last part of the nineteenth century spinal anesthesia, local infiltration and nerve blocking were first introduced. In 1884, Koller first used cocaine for ophthalmic surgery. At the same time, Halsted carried out his experiments with the use of cocaine in nerve blocking. The first spinal anesthetic was obtained inadvertently by Corning in 1884 by the accidental injection of cocaine in the subarachnoid space. Rudolph Matas introduced spinal anesthesia in the United States in 1899. It was not until procaine hydrochloride was discovered by Einhorn in 1905 that regional anesthesia became practical.

Most important of all in the recent history of anesthesia has been the birth of anesthesia as a specialty. Thirty years ago, there were only a few specialists in anesthesia. In teaching hospitals and large centers, the anesthetic was given by an intern, usually the most junior man, with little supervision except for the operator's suggestions and complaints. In private practice, younger surgeons usually "poured ether" for their seniors. In small hospitals, general practitioners usually were the anesthetists. While some of these men developed great skill in this avocation, it was not until the specialty of anesthesiology came into being that surgery and surgeons could safely perform the feats they do today. Resident training programs specifically in anesthesia have produced a group of physicians who are physiologists and pharmacologists of a high order. This specialization was much needed to better what is a right arm of surgery.

Antisepsis and asepsis.   When one considers that only slightly more than 100 years ago surgeons were operating without anesthesia and with poor preparation of the operating room, instruments and hands, it is not surprising in the light of our present knowledge that elective surgery was not accepted by patients with much enthusiasm, and that conservative physicians were slow to recommend any but the most necessary procedures

designed to save life in an emergency. In the last part of the eighteenth century and early nineteenth century, it was necessary to restrain patients on the operating table. Sometimes they were made drunk with alcohol and drugs. The use of alcohol as an aid in performing operations is mentioned in the ancient Hindu *Susruta*.

The importance of cleanliness has been stressed as important to good results by many ancient surgical teachers, but the true nature of the relation of microorganisms to wound sepsis was not really appreciated, accepted and established until the last half of the nineteenth century. The names of Pasteur, Lister, Koch and to a lesser extent, von Bergmann, are associated with the development of the science of bacteriology and the applied practices of antisepsis and asepsis in surgery. While we can date Pasteur's publications from 1857 and Lister's writings from the 1860's, the acceptance of the work of these men and their teaching cannot be said to have become universal until 30 or 40 years later. Ether and chloroform were immediately adopted for use in surgery, since their value was so obvious and could be easily demonstrated. In contrast, there was a large literature and theory on wound putrefaction prejudicial to accepting environmental bacteria as the cause of infection. The most widely held concept of wound inflammation was that a chemical reaction produced the inflammation and the pus. The demonstration of bacteria in pus was explained by a theory that these particles or germs were products of a physicochemical reaction, rather than the cause of wound suppuration. The great German teacher, Theodor Billroth, a contemporary of Lister, believed this concept and did not accept or employ antiseptic methods in his clinic for a considerable length of time.

The term "laudable pus" is replete in the historic literature on wounds, and indeed the design of surgery in some eras was the production of pus. Pus was considered laudable since patients who lived to produce it in their wounds represented the group who contained their infection through host resistance and natural means, whereas those who died had rapidly spreading cellulitis and massive types of disseminating infection. These latter died without the formation and ejection of purulent fluid from their wounds.

How well Pasteur's words, "Chance observation favors only the receptive mind," applied to Lister. Lister's simple observation that closed wounds do not generate suppura-

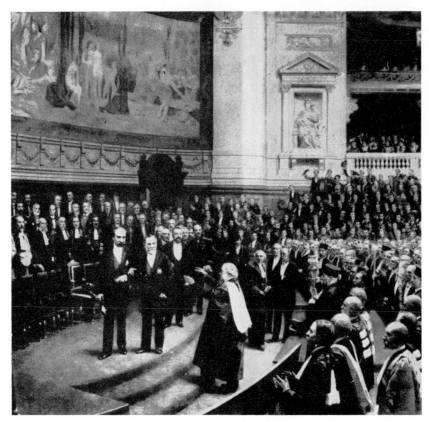

Figure 1.   Lister, on the steps, greets Pasteur when they meet for the first time at the Jubilé de Pasteur, University of Lyon, 1892. This scene is from the painting which hangs in the Grand Salon of the Sorbonne. (Courtesy of l'Institut Pasteur, Paris.)

tion, whereas compound wounds invariably do, convinced him that there existed in the environment noxious agents which cause suppuration. In his search along these lines, he read Pasteur's work a considerable time after the epochal paper, "Mémoire Sur La Fermentation Apelée Lactique," which contained Pasteur's manifesto of the germ theory. Pasteur's most important paper for Lister appeared in *Comtes Rendus Hebdomadaires des Seances de l'Académie des Sciences* in 1863 and was entitled "Reserches Sur La Putréfaction."

It was about 20 years after the discovery of ether that Joseph Lister, Professor of Surgery at Glasgow, introduced his theory and practice of antisepsis. This was to revolutionize surgical practice and ultimately to control introduced infection. It is hard for us to appreciate the appalling loss of life on the surgical wards of hospitals before Lister's and Pasteur's work made its impression. Hospital gangrene and fever were the rule, and in many institutions a surgical operation meant certain death from infection. Since surgeons had no correct appreciation of the cause of

wound infection by contamination, the infected wounds of one patient contaminated each successive new patient on the unhygienic hospital wards of the times. The carriers of infection were surgeons, nurses and other assistants who performed dressings and took care of patients. So bad was the situation that at Halle, in Germany, surgical operations were interdicted for as long as a quarter of the year. In many institutions, even small operations meant certain death as late as 1860 and until Lister's principles became recognized by the surgical world.

Lister appreciated and taught that wound infection came from outside the body, and was introduced by contamination of accidental or incised wounds by direct contact with the air or physical objects. It remained for Pasteur to corroborate Lister's theories by his discovery of specific microorganisms and his proof of their relation to disease and infection. Lister first began his antiseptic treatment in dealing with compound fractures, on which he used carbolic acid dressings. After publishing this work, in 1867 he gave his great paper, "On the Antiseptic Principle in the Practice of Surgery," before the British Medical Association meeting in Dublin. He followed this work with the elimination of cross-infections on the hospital wards by avoidance of contamination. Carrying the theory of the relation of microorganisms to infection into the operating theater, he devised his famous carbolic acid spray. By keeping the operating field permeated with this powerful antiseptic vapor, which destroyed microorganisms, he was able to demonstrate that primary closure of wounds was possible without infection. Since surgeons before Lister's time were generally of the opinion that infection of wounds resulted from chemical factors or substances which were produced in the tissues as a reaction to injury and disintegration, it was difficult to convince them that the principles of antisepsis had a correct basis. The continental surgeons were particularly slow to accept Lister's ideas. For as long as 25 years after his first publication, many clinics had not adopted his methods, in spite of the fact that he constantly published his continued good results and made convincing animal and human experiments to prove his points. His technique was quite elaborate for the times, and in many places in which it was tried, there was inadequate attention to details. When these imperfect trials failed to fulfill expectations, the method was discarded.

In Germany, von Volkmann of Halle became the greatest advocate of Lister's antiseptic treatment, and by the middle of the 1870's had conclusively demonstrated its effectiveness in reducing infection in his clinic. Conditions at the Munich Hospital, however, were still poor as late as 1875, and it was not until Nussbaum adopted Lister's methods in that institution that the appalling rate of 80 per cent incidence of hospital gangrene was controlled.

At the Allgemeine Krankenhaus in Vienna, under the direction of Theodor Billroth, the "open treatment" of wounds was continued for a long period after Lister's work. Leaving incised wounds open after operation is a better policy than primary closure when antiseptic or aseptic methods are not used, but the results from this treatment of clean, noncontaminated wounds alone cannot be compared favorably with those in which antiseptic methods have been employed. Varying degrees of suppuration sometimes occurred, and when drainage was adequate, the flow of "laudable pus" was considered a good sign. Certainly, drainage of such pus was better for

the recovery of the patient than its retention in the wound, but the avoidance of suppuration in the first place gave far superior final surgical results. Unfortunately, Billroth did not accept in principle Lister's ideas, largely because of his own studies on the subject of wound healing, which tended to refute the fact that bacteria or cocci were pathogenic. This is a classic example of a blind spot in a man whose vision was otherwise great. It is probable that his great influence as a teacher in the German medical world retarded the acceptance of antiseptic surgery in Austria and Germany.

It remained for the epoch-making work of Pasteur and Koch and the rapid growth of the science of bacteriology to establish with finality the value of Lister's principles, and to place the responsibility for infection in surgery definitely at the door of introduced microorganisms. It is not strange that the techniques of bacteriology were then applied to surgical operations and that the aseptic preparation and management of instruments, hands and other materials coming into contact with open wounds supplanted the less certain and more injurious method of antisepsis with carbolic acid products.

Aseptic technique was developed by von Bergmann in Berlin. He considered antisepsis but a transitional stage in the control of infection at operation. It was not, however, until 1892 that Schimmelbusch, one of von Bergmann's pupils, formalized and described in detail the aseptic technique as practiced by his preceptor. This brought the method of asepsis definitely to the forefront and effected the replacement of antiseptic methods in all clinics of the world. Nevertheless, Lister's principles were correct, and to him must go credit for being the great crusader in surgery, teaching as he did, in advance of the knowledge of bacteriology, the fundamentals which were later to be found so valuable in the control of surgical infections.

In some regards, the replacement of the term antisepsis by asepsis is unfortunate since the latter state cannot be obtained in surgical practice. It can only be approached. Therefore, the term asepsis is misleading, and it lacks the quality of vigilance and constant warfare against sepsis that the word antisepsis does. In an address given before the Clinical Society of Maryland in 1891 on "Some Considerations of Antiseptic Surgery," William Henry Welch said, "Permit me to say in this connection that I fail to see the advantage of using the term aseptic surgery in the sense in which it is generally employed at the present time, as something distinct from antiseptic surgery." He went on to say that it would seem that antisepsis refers to nothing but chemical disinfection, whereas the substitution of heat for chemicals in the disinfection of instruments, sutures and operative materials capable of being subjected to the required heat is but another antiseptic method. "The object of antiseptic surgery is to secure an aseptic condition of a wound, and here it may well be remarked that this rarely is equivalent to the condition generally understood in a bacteriological laboratory, namely, freedom from bacteria." There is no such thing as aseptic surgery; therefore, the term antiseptic or perhaps contraseptic surgery is much more descriptive of our total effort to reduce bacterial contamination of the operative wound to a minimum. The wound is always subject to contamination from the goods, persons and air which surround it. Reducing such contamination to a minimum and treating the patient and the wound in such a way that minimal bacterial contamination shall not result in clinical infection is the end to which the surgeon strives.

The work of Ignaz Philipp Semmelweis, on the etiology of puerperal sepsis, stands out as a singularly important contribution not only to obstetrics but also to knowledge of the fundamental principles of surgery. Beginning in the middle of the nineteenth century, Semmelweis made continued observations on the importance of cleanliness and asepsis in delivering children. His advices were not heeded for many years, and in fact were severely criticized by his fellow obstetricians. He made the important observation of the similarity between the pathology in patients dying with puerperal sepsis and in those with infected wounds. The rate of infection in some institutions of his time was exceedingly high, so much so that delivery of the mother at home was far preferable to delivery in the hospital. He noted that when medical students came directly from laboratories of pathology and from septic wards, the incidence of puerperal sepsis increased. He also showed that careful washing of the obstetrician's hands before delivery and the introduction of measures approaching present-day aseptic technique could greatly reduce the incidence of this feared complication of childbirth. It is a sad commentary on his times that his views were not well received by his medical colleagues. He was a zealous teacher of his principles, but he was forced to resign his position at Vienna, and during the course of his relatively short life, the criticism and disappointments which he received weighed heavily upon him, although he later became Professor of Obstetrics in Budapest. He died before the age of 50 in an insane asylum. In 1842, Oliver Wendell Holmes published in the *New England Quarterly Journal of Medicine* his famous paper, "On the Contagiousness of Puerperal Fever," antedating Semmelweis, although the total work and effort of Semmelweis in proving that puerperal fever was a septicemia gives him one of the first places in the history of surgery after Lister in establishing the importance of "aseptic technique."

Finally, in the late part of the nineteenth century, the Swiss surgeon Theodor Kocher crystallized the best of surgical thought on the treatment of wounds, and his techniques became the heritage of American surgeons through the teachings of William Stewart Halsted. But it is not America alone which owes a debt to Halsted by way of his instituting long-term hospital training in surgery in this country. His contributions to surgical technique are of even more importance and had universal application. His introduction of the use of rubber gloves in operating represented a very important innovation.

The importance of hemostasis in surgery should be emphasized. The use of pressure, cautery, the ligature, the tourniquet and, finally, the invention of the artery forceps for the grasping of vessels and ligating them evolved over a long time to reach the modern system of dealing with hemorrhage. Péan popularized a forceps in 1867 which is still used. Halsted taught and insisted on maintaining a dry operative field at all times. He also put particular emphasis on securing the least amount of tissue in the hemostatic forceps so as to leave the least amount of dead tissue in the wound. Before blood transfusion was safe and blood replacement facilities were available, the ligation of even small bleeding vessels and strict hemostasis was mandatory for avoiding shock. Halsted also showed the importance of using fine silk sutures because of their properties of nonreactivity, as opposed to using the inferior catgut available in his time. He recognized, however, that nonabsorbable silk was undesirable in infected wound sites.

Halsted's remarks in Samuel C. Harvey's book, *The History of Hemostasis*, about his observations of operations in Billroth's Vienna clinic in 1877 are interesting: "Clamps had

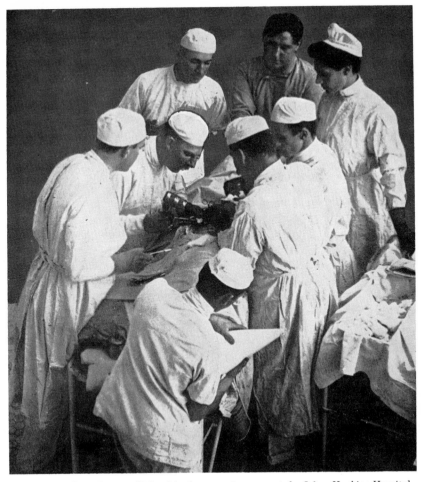

Figure 2. William Stewart Halsted in the operating room at the Johns Hopkins Hospital.

come into use and Billroth was evidently learning some of the various purposes which they were to serve; for example, he divided tissues containing vessels between two of them and would leave a number hanging in the wound." The development of the modern hemostat is best given in Halsted's own words:

On my return from Germany in 1881, I was impressed with the fact that our surgeons were greatly handicapped in most of their operations by lack of proper instruments, particularly of artery clamps. These were insufficient in number and faulty in design. In most of the New York Hospitals the only artery clamps were of the fenestrated, mouse-toothed, spring forceps variety (Liston's and Wakley's), indeed, these were about the only ones procurable either in this country or England. In the elaborate catalogue for 1882 of S. Maw, Son and Thompson, London, no other artery forceps, torsion forceps excepted, is mentioned.

In a catalogue of Collins et Cie, Paris, undated, but evidently of about the same period, the little artery clamps of Koeberle and of Pean are the only ones figured; "pinces à arteres à ressorts" are cata-logued, the latter probably being the mouse-toothed forceps given in the London catalogue (Maw and Son) and quite universally employed in America until 1880 or a little later. In Gunther's Surgery (vol. i, Plate 5, opp. p. 36) is a remarkable litho-graph which indicates the part played by the tenac-ulum in hemostasis in 1859. The divided artery, open-mouthed, is hooked up on the point of the instrument, the handle of which is held in the mouth of the operator who, evidently, was short-handed. Until about 1890, the tenaculum was a favorite instrument in America for checking hem-orrhage, especially with some of the senior sur-geons, and until about 1880 was quite universally employed here, its only rivals being the inadequate mouse-toothed, spring forceps and the Pean or Koeberle clamps. Then almost simultaneously came the clamps of Spencer Wells and (1879) of the writer, of which the Pean-Koeberle clamp was the prototype. The point of my clamp was snub-nosed originally, but the length and spread of the handles, the essentially new features, were the same as at present. With the development of the transfixion method with milliner's needles and use of the fine black silk, the nose of the clamp was made finer (1889). Two or three years later it assumed its present form. Rarely had I seen in our country, prior to my first visit to Europe (1879), more than one artery clamp at a time left hanging in a wound. Clamps were too few for this—four to three or even two being considered ample for an operation. Few hospitals, in New York at least, possessed as many as six artery clamps in 1880. I recall vividly an operation in Vienna performed by Mikulicz in 1879 in Billroth's clinic. Americans, newly arrived in Austria, we were greatly amused at seeing perhaps a dozen clamps (Schieber) left hanging in a wound of the neck while the operator proceeded with his dissection, and were inclined to ridicule the method as being untidy or uncouth. Slowly it dawned upon us that we in America were novices in the art as well as the science of surgery. The artery forceps, adequate in number and design, undoubtedly played a very important role in the strikingly rapid progress in the art of operating made by surgeons, the world over, in the final quarter of the past century. The value of the artery clamps is not likely to be overestimated. They determine methods and effect results impossible without them. They tranquilize the operator. In a wound that is perfectly dry, and in tissues never permitted to become even stained by blood, the operator, unperturbed, may work for hours without fatigue. The confidence gradually acquired from masterfulness in controlling hemorrhage gives to the surgeon the calm which is so essential for clear thinking and orderly procedure at the operating table.

POST-LISTERIAN SURGERY. Following the discovery of anesthesia and the control of infection, surgeons must have found their fields of usefulness and exploration expanding so rapidly that they had little time for all that demanded doing and that had been impossible to accomplish. In the latter part of the nineteenth century, new operations were being devised, new boundaries constantly exceeded, and a wealth of operative experience being obtained by the master surgeons of the time. There is scarcely a single extirpative operative procedure now performed that had not been tried by surgeons before the beginning of the twentieth century.

Surgeons throughout the world found that the abdominal cavity could be entered almost with impunity by following the simple rules of antiseptic technique. In 1883, Theodor Billroth of Vienna performed a successful resection of the stomach for cancer. The first successful resection of the colon for cancer was reported. There was scarcely a single expendable part or organ of the human body that was not subjected to surgical attack. It was the great period of trial for surgery with its new wings, and while accomplishment showed that these new daring operations were possible, the experience gained soon indicated that many were still risky.

The German surgical clinics were foremost in excellence at the turn of the century. Billroth as a teacher was unexcelled. He was also an investigator, performing surgery on dogs before applying new operations on human beings. Billroth was Professor of Surgery at the University of Vienna and Chief of the Second Surgical Service of the Allgemeine Krankenhaus. His most important work, *General Surgical Pathology and Therapeutics*, appeared first in 1863 and went through almost a score of editions.

Art was still the master of surgery, but science was advancing. While a group of great master surgeons developed in this era, there was no great increase in the number of trained men, nor had the modern concept of a surgical team developed. Many operative procedures, which the imagination of intrepid men had conceived, had to be abandoned because of high mortality rates in the absence of good ancillary and supportive therapy. Still, progress continued steadily. Among the outstanding pioneers of this time was Sir Victor Horsley (1857–1916), who did a great deal to enlarge the scope of neurosurgery.

In 1886, Fitz of Boston described the pathology of appendicitis, and the early surgical treatment of this disease which had caused so many deaths from peritonitis soon followed on a large scale. The advent of the operation of appendectomy for acute appendicitis is an important milestone in modern surgery. Resection of the colon by the two-stage exteriorization procedure came into general use at the turn of the century—because of the work of Block and, perhaps more importantly, because of the wide influence he exerted, of Mikulicz. The high mortality rate which resulted from immediate resection of colonic cancer and anastomosis of the bowel was reduced by the use of the exteriorization principle with delayed excision of the intestine. Modifications of this exteriorization technique were used up until the antibiotic period of surgery after World War II. Such outstanding accomplishments are, to mention a few, among many which were made in the immediate post-Listerian period when surgeons had finally obtained a true appreciation of bacteriology and the control of infection.

It soon became apparent that anesthesia and asepsis were not enough to extend the field of surgery to desirable limits. As late as 1913, Osler stated that the mortality of operations for the removal of cancer of the stomach was so great that surgery was not justified. What disappointments there must have been for the surgeons of the early part of the twentieth century to be denied the chance of saving lives by well-conceived operations which would leave the patient in a normal or reasonably normal physiologic state, but which could not be justifiably performed because there still remained barriers against the safe conduct of the patient through the whole ordeal.

In the twentieth century, and particularly in the past 25 years, every operation planned and executed by the post-Listerian surgeons of the nineteenth century has been refined to the point where it can be carried out with safety and reasonable ease. In addition, the boundaries of the most fertile surgical imaginations have been exceeded in the present decade, as the most recent additions to the lists of successfully performed operations show. Review of a typical hospital record of a patient who has undergone an extensive and long operation performed to remove a cancer involving several organs and lymphatic metastatic regions reveals that a host of ancillary services has made the procedure successful.

Among the most important developments in medicine which have affected surgery in the twentieth century are the diagnostic techniques by roentgen rays, the development of safe methods for the transfusion of blood, the orientation of the surgeon toward an interest in physiology and chemistry, the new chemotherapeutic and antibiotic discoveries of present times, and the expanded system for educating and training surgeons in the United States so that the best of surgical therapy can be made available to the mass of citizenry.

Roentgenology. The discovery of x-rays by Roentgen in 1895 was soon followed by the use of the diagnostic technique now known by his name. X-ray examination of fractures and localization of foreign bodies, by the plain film technique, came first and were followed by the tremendous elaborations of roentgenology which are in common use today. Cannon's application of roentgen rays to the study of the physiology of the gastrointestinal tract, and the later application of this technique to diagnosis, ranks as one of the great additions to medical practice and, particularly, to surgery. His original studies of the gastrointestinal tract were made using bismuth meals and, incidentally, were done by him while still a medical student in 1898. This roentgenologic technique, using a radiopaque meal, important as it has come to be in the diagnosis of disease of the gastrointestinal tract, has proved to be equally important in the development of other diagnostic techniques using contrast methods. There is no cavity or system in the body that has not been subjected to special examination by roentgenologists, and there are many instances in which diagnosis by x-rays is more accurate than inspection by the naked eye. Therapy by radiation, either emanating from radioactive substances or generated by large machines, has followed the diagnostic application of x-rays. While radiation therapy has not reached its peak of application and usefulness, it has been a great boon to countless sufferers who could not otherwise be helped.

Blood transfusion. That there were certain basic blood groups was discovered by Landsteiner in 1900. In 1902, he published his first paper on this discovery, for which he received the Nobel Prize in Medicine. To say that this scientific advance has been the greatest contribution to surgical practice made in this century might not be wrong. The refinements of blood transfusion methods which have developed since World War I have made operative surgery of great magnitude safe beyond all previous hope. Surgeons in front-line hospitals during World War II had available an almost unlimited supply of blood, which very often had been drawn less than ten days previously in the United States. This blood had been carefully processed and preserved and was safe to use three weeks after it had been taken from the donor. Scarcely a major procedure in surgery is done today without replacement of blood loss which exceeds 500 cc.

The availability of blood for transfusion, its preservation and distribution are routine today, but were beyond conception 25 years ago. At that time, although direct and indirect methods of transfusion were used, preservation, storage, and having a large quantity available were not possible. At that time a blood transfusion was a "major operation." Techniques were elaborate up until 1930. Replacement therapy was, therefore, always inadequate. Crile's cannula, developed during World War I, first replaced direct artery-to-vein transfusion and was followed by the use of the paraffin tube and other methods of direct transfusion. Finally, the use of citrated blood and indirect transfusion came into general use. At the present time, preoperative and postoperative transfusions, as well as blood replacement during surgery, are quantitatively managed.

Antibiotics. The discovery of penicillin in 1929, by Alexander Fleming, and the subsequent development of other antibiotics must be regarded as one of the great steps toward realizing surgical successes hitherto impossible. It is not to be denied that antibiotic therapy has brought certain new problems into medicine; antibiotics have been overused, unnecessarily used, and therefore abused. Nevertheless, the antibiotic surgical period is without a peer in the past in the control of surgical infections and pulmonary complications of operation.

CONTEMPORARY SURGERY. In all but the most modern times, the surgeon has been oriented toward the basic sciences of anatomy and pathology in his search for new truths which might advance his science. Almost all teachers of surgery served their apprenticeships in the dissecting laboratories, or made researches on the pathology of disease as it was related to concepts of operative technique which needed improvement. Today these two subjects, anatomy and pathology, are still basic to surgery and must be thoroughly learned. To say that they are counterparts of the Latin and Greek of a liberal education is to give them the deference due them, but it should not imply that they are dead subjects.

Physiology and chemistry, the living sciences, so to speak, are the companions of present surgical progress. Preoperative preparation over a short period of time has greatly reduced mortality rates for patients. Furthermore, the number of patients who can withstand a surgical procedure has been multiplied by this orientation toward restoring a depleted patient to as near normal a physiologic state as possible. Also, dividing major surgical accomplishments into two or more operations, has been a great contribution to surgical safety, especially so in the recent period when reparative preoperative therapy was not so highly developed as at present.

In 1929, Cannon first presented his concept of homeostatis in *Physiological Reviews* under the title "Organization for Physiologic Homeostasis." His work represented an extension of the ideas of the nineteenth century French physiologist, Claude Bernard. In 1932 appeared his popular book, *The Wisdom of the Body*, written for general readers. His elucidation of the importance of observing, studying and understanding the interrelation of various physiologic mechanisms has had tremendous impact on the conduct of all therapy in medicine. The understanding of

bodily mechanisms has developed a new surgical field, which, for want of a more descriptive term, can be called physiologic surgery. The modus operandi of this new surgical field is the production of such alterations in the function of the body that the end result favorably affects the general state of a patient with a disease which cannot be directly benefited by surgery.

Finally, the twentieth century saw the United States emerging as the giant among the countries of the Western world. This growth in stature came about as a result of numerous factors. Essentially, however, the natural wealth of the country and the incentive of its immigrant population, now freed from prejudices and abnormal restraints and anxious to apply an unlimited energy, were two great contributors to our advancement. Progress in the economic and social spheres was paralleled by improvement in education, which was reflected in the medical field by better standards. While formal education and training for surgeons was not universal, it was begun by Halsted at the Johns Hopkins School at the turn of the century. His model was the German school of surgery. Apprenticeship surgical training, however, was still the common practice with the United States until after World War I.

THE INFLUENCE OF MILITARY SURGERY. The War Between the States was horrendous for the poor soldier, not only because of the inadequacy of the Army Medical Department in numbers of surgeons and the surgical limitations of the time, but also because of the high death rate from contagious diseases. This great war resulted in 620,000 deaths and 10,000,000 cases of sickness; it was by far the worst war of our country and of the times.

Organization of facilities is extremely important in the handling of mass casualties of any kind. Mobility of surgical units and efficient evacuation are essential. Out of the Civil War came one great medical contribution made by Johnathan Letterman in the form of a system of evacuation through units of surgical care graded in their extent of service from first aid to definitive care. This included medical facilities beginning with a regimental medical detachment and progressing to field and base hospitals in a retrograde manner.

The proportion of fatal casualties was high in World War I, especially with the multiple involvement of body cavities. Chemotherapeutic agents were not available to combat virulent infections associated with extensive soft tissue injuries, and controlled operations were found difficult under field conditions.

However, certain specialties profited by this war experience, especially neurosurgery and reconstructive surgery. Before the war, cranial surgery was limited to the treatment of closed trauma and to the treatment of diseases involving the cranial nerves and the coverings of the brain. In the great anatomic range of injuries produced by small arms and shrapnel, Harvey Cushing found counterparts of many neurologic deficits produced by selective ablation of brain tissue in the animal. This experience served as a stepping stone for the rapid extension of neurosurgery to lesions involving the human brain. The scholarliness of Cushing's work and the accuracy of his records are a lasting tribute to his genius. Cushing was one of Halsted's residents, and his greatest contribution to surgery was his application of Halsted's teachings and techniques of hemostasis to neurosurgery.

The debridement of wounds, first practiced extensively in modern times by Napoleon's great surgeon-in-chief, Larrey, was carried out to a fairly high degree of efficiency in World War I. Advances were made in the chemical treatment of infected wounds by the use of the Carrel-Dakin technique. This rather tedious and meticulous method of cleansing and preparing contaminated and infected wounds was not entirely suited to the treatment of mass casualties. Wounds treated in this fashion are not closed immediately, but only after a varying period of delay. Despite its disadvantages, this system did reduce the length of hospitalization and loss of limb as compared with results obtained from earlier methods. Careful debridement and toilet of wounds, which include removal of all dead tissue and foreign bodies, using the open technique and followed by secondary closure at the proper time, must be looked upon as the important contribution to surgery of both World Wars.

A by-product of World War I was realized in the group of men who became surgeons by on-the-job training, so to speak. Upon their return to civilian life, they brought surgery to the medium and small-sized cities which had never had this service. The greatly increased population of the country could now be better taken care of as far as trauma and uncomplicated surgery were concerned. Another by-product of World War I was the realization that the United States needed better

educated and trained surgeons. America had a nucleus of experienced surgeons in the larger centers who could begin more formal educational and training programs. Gradually, short-term surgical residencies were established throughout the country, meeting important needs for community surgeons. Standards for surgical practice were established by the American College of Surgeons. Finally, in 1937, the American Board of Surgery was formed. Standard qualifications for education, training and practice now had come to stay. The country found itself better medically prepared for World War II by virtue of a remarkable growth of surgical educational and training programs in the 1930's.

Regrettable as wars are, they provide the surgeon with his great opportunity for service to his fellow men. The surgeon's life is never quite complete without the experience of warfare. If he is advantageously situated, he can do more good in the course of two or three years of military service in the saving of life and limb than he can in a score of years in civilian practice, for he has the opportunity of serving the young rather than the aged. The surgeon is the only victor in war. A life saved at 20 years has great expectations. The experiences of young, qualified surgeons in World War II brought to present-day surgery a wealth that cannot be assessed.

The great achievement of American surgery in World War II was in the area of wound healing. The universal adoption of the open wound technique after debridement in contaminated wounds of the battlefield, followed by delayed closure, resulted in earlier rehabilitation and less loss of tissue and function. The use of this old technique was new to most civilian surgeons thrown into war. Their entire previous training sought for primary wound healing by prompt wound closure. This technique of elective surgery in the civilian operating room was doomed to failure when applied to contaminated and infected wounds of the battlefield.

Except for the introduction of chemotherapy and antibiotics, there were no really new scientific and purely medical armaments available to make the great record in the care of the wounded which was attained in this war. Debridement and open wound technique had been used in other wars and fairly extensively in World War I. It was rather the organization of personnel and the mobilization of ancillary surgical services in the most effective manner which made possible the results obtained. The best young surgeons, the best equipment and materials, the best consultants and surgical teachers were at the strategic spots. The treatment of wounds was standardized and the period of disability decreased. The lessons of American industry were applied to surgery, and the concept of teamwork was developed to a degree impossible in civil life. The remarkable record in wound healing accomplished by the application of the open treatment of contaminated wounds resulted in 85 to 90 per cent healing of all wounds within three to five weeks in the Mediterranean Theater of Operations.

On the technical side of surgery, an extension of the magnitude of operative procedures followed World War II. Old boundaries delineating the normal extent of extirpative surgery were discarded. This was the natural outcome of a wide experience in trauma and a greater facility for control during operation and the subsequent period of repair.

TEAM SURGERY. The importance of the institution in contrast to the individual or master surgeon is a late twentieth century development. Many factors have brought about this change. The complexity of techniques, the need for concentration of trained personnel and the evolution which has shown the effectiveness of team surgery have been the principal forces in the socialization of surgery. Great surgical or medical discoveries do not come from the team or group, however. The latter's function is in application. The individual is still important because of his ideas, and there is no substitute for the mind with originality.

The large and small clinic has been an American development of this century. The oldest of these institutions, the Mayo Clinic, was begun by an ex-Civil War surgeon in rural Minnesota at the turn of the century. Smaller clinics of five to 20 doctors in group practice abound in this country, especially in the Middle West, Southwest and Far West. Clinics have become popular with patients and referring physicians because of the ready availability under one roof, so to speak, of an excellent staff, laboratory facilities and operational methods which get the patient to the right physician or surgeon for treatment without delay. Some university hospitals have followed the clinic design for private patient work.

SURGICAL SPECIALIZATION. After World War II, surgeons returned to a life in which they were to find regulation, organization and standardization the rule of surgical practice. For this stage, they were well prepared psy-chologically. The controls of surgical practice now in effect are good. They are safeguards of the public and of the reputation of medicine in general. At the same time, however, there has arisen a strong trend toward specialization in surgery which has been partly initiated by the need to qualify in some field in order to practice. In fact, it might be said that specialization in surgery has created important difficulties for surgery. While it is to be expected that a complete general surgeon cannot be made today, the time has been reached when further specialization will make it difficult to train any sort of generalist in surgery. The general surgeon is still needed in some communities for wide service. He is essential to the medical schools and medical centers for teaching and direction. Specialization in surgery is a dilemma of our times.

EXPERIMENTAL SURGERY. Experimental surgery has developed enormously in the United States. William Stewart Halsted, Professor of Surgery at the Johns Hopkins Medical School, established his department of surgery as a prototype of what a surgical teaching unit should be. As early as 1895, it included a laboratory for operating upon animals, which later became what is now the Hunterian Laboratory of that institution. Both students and teachers were encouraged to bring their ideas to the laboratory, where they could be tried and proved. This represents the scientific approach to surgery, and it has been a fruitful source of advancement. In the course of time, the contribution of surgeons to our knowledge of anatomy, pathology, physiology and biologic chemistry has been so considerable as to offer a challenge to the accomplishments of specialists in these fields of basic medical research. Today thousands of animals are put through carefully planned experiments, which may prove that ideas are not sound and, therefore, not to be used on the human patient. This aspect of research is an important one, along with the happier circumstance of working out a feasible technique for a hitherto unapproachable problem.

Finally, it can be said without apology or exaggeration that a science of surgery has evolved in the twentieth century. This science has basic principles upon which all fields and specialties in surgery depend. From time to time criticisms have been made about the extent of certain operations. That is to say, while certain operations are technically possible, are they always justifiable? This has brought up moral questions about how great the surgeon's effort should be to maintain life when it may be life alone, devoid of individuality and personality. For the most part, these questions have resolved themselves in time, and some experimental, "super-radical" operations have been abandoned. That new operations are conceived and undertaken with good will toward the sufferings and illnesses of mankind cannot be denied. This is the important consideration.

SOCIAL, ECONOMIC AND INTELLECTUAL ASPECTS OF MEDICINE. The present time finds medicine deeply involved in a social contract which seems bound to evolve rapidly into what is commonly referred to as socialized medicine. Mankind has been captivated by certain ideas expressed by Marx in his *Das Kapital*. The motivating force behind this acceptance of socialism is the growth of scientific knowledge and education of the masses. Today's man wants to live the good life now; he is biologically oriented and does not have the spirituality of his forebears, who to a considerable extent were schooled to the idea of a reward after death. Medicine, therefore, is extremely important to man today and, therefore, must be available readily to all. Americans speak of themselves as capitalists in contrast to socialists, whereas at the same time they have traveled a long way on the road of socialism.

Tocqueville says something to the effect that men claim to believe things long after they have ceased to believe them. It would seem from recent legislation that Americans are pragmatic toward socialism. The doctor will soon find himself in a system of prescribed service, rather than in the role of dispensing largesse according to the old code of freely given services on request with the aid of charity. This will change the life in medicine somewhat but it need not thwart all of our feeling of freedom.

The idea that medicine is a service profession only is as old as Hippocrates. But to have been satisfied during all these years with the service alone as our highest attainment was folly as a teaching and as a standard to which we called our recruits. In fact, it was not a true picture of medicine. Medicine is an intellectual pursuit of a high order which can bring great happiness to its disciples. It has a catholicity of interests and an educational structure far greater than those of the other two learned professions of law and holy orders. It is the greatest of all cultural pursuits.

A life of service alone leads only into a void as far as medicine is concerned, for it is ordained that man shall die. Yet within the power of medicinal knowledge lies help for mankind far greater than the immediate concern for his body. It is, therefore, now time that the profession take greater leadership in the total affairs of mankind.

READING REFERENCES

Brooks, S.: Civil War Medicine. Springfield, Illinois, Charles C Thomas, 1966.

Campbell, E., and Colton, J.: The Surgery of Theodoric. New York, Appleton-Century-Crofts, Inc., 1955.

Castiglioni, A.: A History of Medicine. (Krumbhaan, E. B., Ed.) New York, Alfred A. Knopf, 1941.

Cushing, H.: The Life of Sir William Osler. Oxford, Clarendon Press, 1925.

Garrison, F. H.: An Introduction to the History of Medicine. 4th ed. Philadelphia, W. B. Saunders Company, 1929.

Harvey, S. C.: The History of Hemostasis. New York, Paul B. Hoeber, Inc., 1929.

Lee, A. J.: A Synopsis of Anesthesia. Baltimore, The Williams & Wilkins Company, 1959.

MacCallum, W. G.: William Stewart Halsted, Surgeon. Baltimore, The Johns Hopkins Press, 1930.

Musil, R.: The Man Without Qualities. New York, Capricorn Books, 1965.

The Pasteur Fermentation Centennial, 1857–1957. Scientific Symposium, New York, Charles Pfizer Company, 1957.

Schonbauer, L.: Das Medizinsche Wien. Berlin and Vienna, Urban and Schwarzenberg, 1944.

Vallery-Radot, R.: The Life of Pasteur. New York, Dover Publications, Inc., 1961.

Welch, C. S., and Powers, S. R., Jr.: The Essence of Surgery. Philadelphia, W. B. Saunders Company, 1959.

Wrench, G. T.: Lord Lister, His Life and Work. New York, Frederick A. Stokes Company, 1913.

Zimmerman, L. M., and Veith, I.: Great Ideas in the History of Surgery. Baltimore, The Williams & Wilkins Company, 1961.

Chapter 2

THE PRINCIPLES OF WOUND HEALING

by
IRVING F. ENQUIST, M.D.

IRVING ENQUIST was born in Wisconsin but considers Minnesota his home. His elementary and high school education was obtained in the Duluth public schools. His college and medical school education was received at the University of Minnesota. His wife and he are incurable devotees of antique American furniture, which he restores and refinishes during the winter indoor hours. Dr. Enquist is Professor of Surgery, State University of New York College of Medicine and Director of Surgical Services, Methodist Hospital of Brooklyn.

"The urge to heal is as strong as the urge to grow." All surgeons are convinced of this urge after observing Nature's efforts to close large skin defects in otherwise healthy patients. The urge is there, and usually the result is good, but problems still develop in the healing of many wounds. All doctors, particularly surgeons, are constantly looking for methods to make wounds heal better. Much of the surgeon's activity involves the caring for wounds, whether they are the result of accident or disease, or are created by the scalpel. Although in many patients the healing of the wound is less important than the patient's more serious medical problems, in a large percentage of the surgeon's patients the proper healing of a wound or wounds might dictate the patient's outcome. Therefore, the surgeon is constantly devoting much of his interest to his patients' wounds and in many instances coddles the wound to protect it from evil forces—motion, infection and trauma. It is his responsibility to know and apply all of the newly gleaned knowledge of the fundamental processes involved in wound healing.

Wound healing is more than just an interesting phenomenon. Impaired healing of a crucial suture line might well result in a calamitous complication or even death of a patient. The surgeon's interest in the sutured skin incision does not hide his more serious concern about the repairs which have gone on in the patient's depths—the suture of fascia to fascia, the intestinal anastomosis and the arterial repair. A wound disruption at

any of these sites could have drastic consequences. Impaired, delayed or angry healing of the skin wound might concern the patient, but results only in a slight blemish on the surgeon's reputation.

Healing is commonly categorized into three main types: primary, secondary and tertiary. In *primary* healing, a clean incised wound, elective or traumatic, is closed carefully and anatomically by sutures. There is no gap between the wound margins and the ensuing scar, in whatever tissue, is expected to be hairline. In *secondary* healing, there is a gap or defect which fills in from the sides and bottom, and the resulting scar is not hairline. Secondary healing, or healing by second intention, involves significant contraction of the surrounding tissues to make the ultimate scar much smaller than the original defect. Because most healing by second intention is seen in surface wounds, epithelization, whereby new cells grow into the defect from the edges of the wound, is an important counterpart of contraction. Both processes are necessary for the ultimate healing of open wounds. *Tertiary* healing, or healing by third intention, refers to the late repair of an open, granulating wound by approximation of the edges in order to hasten the healing process; this term is rarely used.

The fundamental processes which result in the healing of primary and secondary wounds may be quite different; it is not correct to think of them as identical processes. This difference has been shown clearly in ex-

22

perimental studies in scurvy and in alloxan diabetes. Although in both studies there was serious impairment of primary healing, the secondary healing of open skin defects was not affected.

HISTORICAL REVIEW

Man has been fascinated by the healing of wounds since ancient times. This fascination led naturally to the use of favored medicaments to speed up the healing process, and through the ages the number and variety of substances used are legion. That some wounds healed at all after treatment by any number of weird concoctions is a tribute to man's natural indestructibility. However, many early surgeons brought shrewd scientific knowledge to their handling of wounds, particularly war wounds, and they include such illustrious names as Ambroïse Paré, John Hunter and Sir James Paget. Even the famous Halsted was intensely interested in the wound healing phenomenon and devoted much of his research to this problem.

The first large-scale, wide-based, truly scientific approach to wound healing was made by Alexis Carrel and his associates at the Rockefeller Institute in the early 1900's. Working primarily with surface wounds they studied patients as well as laboratory animals. Careful observation and original methods of mensuration permitted them to find that surface wounds healed at a predictable rate, if the animals and patients were healthy. Optimal or standard healing curves could be drawn for wounds of different sizes and shapes, and if the healing of a particular

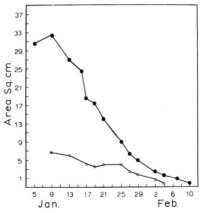

Figure 2. Healing curves of two open shell wounds in a 31-year-old male. Note the more rapid cicatrization of the larger wound. (Redrawn from Carrel and Hartman: J. Exper. Med. 24:429, 1916, with permission.)

wound did not fit the curve, something was interfering with healing (Figs. 1 and 2). These workers demonstrated the effects of age, temperature, infection, avitaminosis and other conditions on wound healing. Some of their conclusions are today not acceptable, but their work represented a milestone in the application of the scientific approach to wound healing.

Not long after the studies by Carrel, Harvey and Howes provided another important contribution to wound healing by their studies of incised wounds. Using the gain in breaking strength as an index of the rate of healing, they were able to use this method in the study of wounds in skin, fascia and stomach and to study the effects of infection, diet and various suture materials on the healing rate. Their method has been widely used in innumerable would healing studies since that time, and has proved to be an extremely simple and effective tool.

With much data available about the healing patterns in open and closed wounds it remained for Dunphy to encourage surgeons and basic scientists as well to probe more deeply into the fundamental biochemical phenomena of wound healing. Dunphy and several collaborators first showed the reproducible chemical changes that occur in wounds, and related these changes to the rate of healing in the same or similar wounds. They also showed the patterns of abnormal healing resulting from dietary deficiencies. All their methods have been adopted and used freely by other investigators and have proved indispensable in modern wound healing studies.

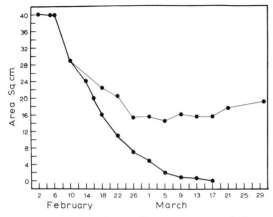

Figure 1. Area of granulating open wound (lower curve) and of wound plus cicatrix in a 21-year-old soldier injured by a shell fragment. (Redrawn from Carrel and Hartman: J. Exper. Med. 24:429, 1916, with permission.)

EXPERIMENTAL WOUND HEALING

In any area of surgery or medicine, it is difficult to prove the effectiveness of a new drug or a new method of therapy by studies on patients; it is much easier, and usually more accurate, to prove the effectiveness in a scientifically sound experiment using laboratory animals. Fortunately, it is quite a simple matter to pursue wound healing studies in small animals, and to translate these results into clinical application. However, a few safeguards must be maintained. Optimal healing in small animals is easily altered by such trivial factors as cage size, amount of sunlight, room temperature, character and the size of chunks of food and the shape of the water dispenser. In our laboratory, it was learned that any young animal which was not gaining weight at the normal rate was not in optimal condition and would not show optimal healing. Sandblom found that the differences occasioned by the position of the surgeon at the operating table affected the healing of the wounds created. If one observes the many precautions, however, wound healing can be studied readily in the laboratory, for it is a simple matter to compare small wounds in animals in which only one parameter has been altered.

Most present-day studies are concerned with the observation of sutured, incised wounds, or open skin defects. The method of Howes, Sooy and Harvey is most often used to measure the rate of healing in incisions, and the results are accurate and quite reproducible (Fig. 3). More than simple observation is necessary to obtain scientifically accurate data on the healing of open wounds. Carrel and his co-workers traced the shape of wounds on clear paper at regular intervals following wounding, and calculated by planimetry the area at each observation. When they plotted these data the resulting healing curves were smooth and parabolic (Fig. 1). Many other methods of mensuration are available; the present choice in our laboratory is to photograph the wound through a metal grid at regular intervals after wounding, to count the number of grid squares described by the wound and to calculate the area of the wound at each observation. The plotted data result in smooth, exponential curves (Fig. 4). From these and other curves, it is apparent that the process of contraction results in an exceptional decrease in the total size of the wound. Billingham and Russell found that rabbit skin wounds of 12 sq. cm. reduced in size to a mean of 0.5 sq. cm. – only one twenty-fourth of the original size. In their studies, the shape of the wound was also very important, for square skin defects healed more rapidly than round defects of the same area (Fig. 5). The actual site of the stimulus for the contraction process is not presently known, although the granulation tissue, the wound margin and the fibroblasts have all been implicated and studied. Whatever the source, the stimulus for contraction is an extremely powerful force which results in marked diminution in the ultimate size of the wound.

CHEMISTRY OF WOUND HEALING

Although chemists and other biologists had studied the chemistry of any number of wounds over many years, the first true exposure of surgeons to the chemistry of wound healing occurred in 1955 when Dunphy and Udupa published their report. Although they studied the rate of healing, tensile strength, in sutured incisions and measured various biochemical parameters in open wounds, the relationship was consistent and striking (Fig. 6). Their studies pinpointed the early wound accumulation of ground substance which contained large amounts of sulfated mucopolysaccharides detectable as hexosamines. In the first three to four days of wound healing in normal animals, the concentration of these substances increased rapidly, reached a short plateau and then decreased just as rapidly. As the hexosamine level fell off, collagen-rich material detectable as hydroxyproline was found in rapidly increasing amounts, and the rate of this increase paralleled the increase in tensile strength of healing incisions. The parallelism between collagen concentration and tensile strength of wounds has been demonstrated repeatedly

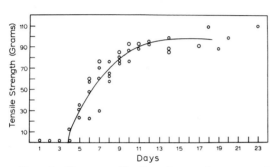

Figure 3. The curve of healing of a wound as expressed by its tensile strength. (Redrawn from Howes, Sooy and Harvey: J.A.M.A. 92:42, 1929, with permission.)

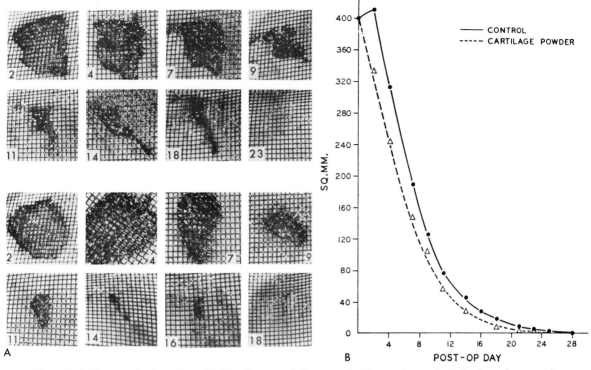

A

B   POST-OP DAY

Figure 4. *A*, Photographs through a grid of healing granulating wounds. The numbers refer to the days after wounding. The upper wound was a control, the lower was treated with local cartilage powder. *B*, Curves of the mean areas of healing open wounds—control and cartilage treated. (Reprinted from Sabo, Oberlander and Enquist: Surg. Gyn. & Obst. *119*:559, 1964, with permission.)

since it was first noted by Dunphy. Present opinion favors the view that collagen fibers are formed outside the fibroblasts to which they are adjacent, after some gel-like precursor substance has been extruded through the cell wall. Collagen will precipitate in vitro, when no ground substance is present, but most investigators feel that the latter is in some way essential to proper collagen fiber production.

Collagen is a quite insoluble material of molecular weight 340,000, with mature fibers having a size of 3000 Å by 14 Å and cross banding at a periodicity of 640 Å. The linkages occurring at these cross bandings are necessary for maximal strength. Because hydroxyproline is an amino acid found only in collagen, analysis for hydroxyproline can be used to determine the amount of collagen present. Many workers have confirmed

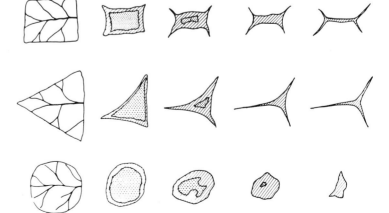

Figure 5. The shapes of healing in rectangular, triangular and circular skin defects in healthy rabbits. (Reprinted from Billingham and Russell: Ann. Surg. *144*:961, 1956, with permission.)

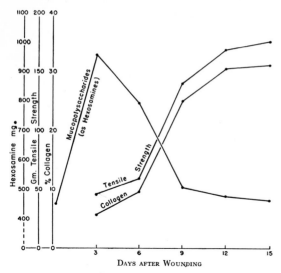

Figure 6. Normal chemical pattern of wound healing. Note the relationship between collagen and tensile strength. (Reprinted from Dunphy and Udupa: New England J. Med. 253:847, 1955, with permission.)

Dunphy's findings and have expanded his methods to the study of other healing problems. It has also been shown that the chemical pattern of incised wounds is nearly identical to that of open, granulating wounds.

When the clinician is concerned about, or has evidence of healing problems in his patient, he tends to categorize the possible etiological factors into those which are local and those which are systemic.

LOCAL FACTORS

A surgeon accepts the importance of his technique to the healing of his patients' wounds. After a planned operation, healing will progress more favorably if the tissues are handled gently, if they have not been dried, if fine rather than large suture materials are used, if the tissues are approximated with just the right amount of tension, if no dead space remains in the wound and if near-perfect hemostasis has been achieved. These are the surgeon's responsibilities.

There is controversy about whether wounds heal more favorably if sutured with nonabsorbable materials, rather than with catgut, which is absorbable. Although this controversy has waged for many decades and is still not settled, in several definitive experimental studies catgut and silk closed wounds healed equally well. The absorbability of catgut, however, must certainly be considered an advantage, for the presence of foreign

bodies of any type in the wound increases the risk of infection. This risk is increased 10,000 times by the mere presence of one silk suture, according to the study of Elek and Conen. Alexander, Kaplan and Altemeier proved that not only the size, but also the character of the suture material is an important factor. Monofilament sutures are preferable to loosely woven threads because the interstices in the latter allow for the collection of protein-rich tissue juices in and around the suture—a perfect culture medium. In this age of modern surgery, when all sizes and shapes of prosthetic materials are inserted into any and all organs and tissues, the surgeon must remember that the prosthesis is a foreign body, and that it increases the risk of infection. It is still a good rule to avoid foreign bodies in the wound if at all possible.

When the patient's wound is not healing properly, the surgeon should first be critical of his own technique; if the technique was perfect, other local factors may be responsible.

BLOOD SUPPLY. All wounds represent areas of inflammation; the necessary nutrients must be provided, and the resulting waste, dead cells, local toxins and bacteria, must be removed. This demands an adequate arterial and venous blood supply. Areas with borderline arterial supply may run into difficulty only after a wound or another form of inflammation demands increased cellular and acellular elements which the impaired blood supply cannot provide. The result is a local area of tissue death, often with superimposed infection. Common examples of impaired healing from inadequate arterial supply are loss of mobilized pedicled skin flaps in plastic surgery; delayed or absent healing in amputation stumps; local infection or gangrene in injured toes of patients with arteriosclerotic vascular disease; breakdown of intestinal anastomoses because vascular arcades were improperly divided or became thrombosed, and aseptic necrosis of the femoral head following a subcapital fracture which destroys the blood supply to the head. Another classic example is the impaired arterial supply in skin following radiation therapy. Radiation destroys or causes thrombosis in small arterioles and leaves the local tissues with borderline nutrition; inflammation in these areas often results in necrosis.

For proper healing, venous drainage of the wound should be unimpaired. From Starling's law, it can be calculated that there will be decreased perfusion of oxygenated blood and increased local edema if the local venous pressure is elevated. Although it has not been proved experimentally, edema is felt to be a common and important cause of impaired healing. By way of contrast, the results of Findlay and Howes in a study of wounds in rabbit ears suggested that edema resulted in improved healing. However, their study was done in too few animals to give truly significant results. It is important to keep injured extremities elevated in order to take advantage of the gravitational effect for reducing edema.

MOTION. Bony fractures heal best when completely immobilized. Most surgeons believe that soft tissue wounds also do better with immobilization. Certain wounds, such as pedicled skin flaps and free grafts of skin and cartilage, require complete rest, but this may not be true for many other wounds. Practically, it is nearly impossible to immobilize soft tissue wounds completely, although a well-applied plaster cast often achieves this goal. It is obvious that wounds in the heart, lung, chest wall and arteries cannot be immobilized. A common surgical problem is the upper abdominal laparotomy incision; the surgeon would like it kept relatively immobile postoperatively, but knows that there is constant push and pull on the incision from respiratory movements, coughing and straining. In spite of this, nearly all these incisions heal well, although the patient who coughs excessively may subject his incision to intolerable motion and stresses which result in a wound dehiscence.

INNERVATION. One would expect that intact innervation would be necessary for optimal healing, but this is not true. In a simple, convincing study, Localio, Lowman and Gibson found that wounds made in the denervated skin of paraplegic patients healed just as well as comparable wounds made more cephalad and in skin with intact innervation. Also, Muren removed the innervation of the lower extremities in rabbits and then compared the healing of wounds in these extremities with wounds in normal extremities. There was no difference.

INFECTION. The most common and important factor resulting in healing problems in clinical surgical practice is local wound infection. All surgeons are aware of the iniquitous effect of infection, and each has his favorite untested method for preventing infection in clean wounds. The healing impairment in infected open wounds was well shown by Carrel (Fig. 7), and in our laboratory

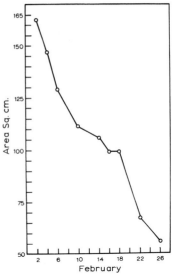

Figure 7. Healing curve of a granulating open abdominal wall wound in a 21-year-old male. Horizontal portion of curve represents a period of infection. (Reprinted from Carrel and Hartman: J. Exper. Med. 24:429, 1916, with permission.)

the impairment in healing by staphylococcal infection was recently shown in laparotomy wounds (Fig. 8). One is justified in applying antibacterial agents locally to ward off infections in contaminated wounds. Their use in clean wounds is to be decried, but it is widespread nonetheless. Systemic antibiotic therapy as a prophylaxis against local wound infection is a point of controversy even today, but it is totally unnecessary. To be effective at all, the antibiotics must be given prior to wounding.

DRUGS. The drugs used upon open wounds

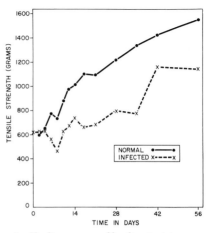

Figure 8. Healing curves of healing incisions, one clean and the other infected with Staphylococcus aureus. (Reprinted from Smith and Enquist: Surg. Gyn. & Obst. 125: 965, 1967, with permission.)

or incisions for the purpose of promoting healing may, in fact, be exerting an opposite effect. Many of these drugs are irritating and cytotoxic. Carrel showed that a slightly irritating cover for wounds was better than a bland and innocuous one, because there was more rapid healing. This may not be acceptable to modern surgeons, and a more recent study by Randall and Randall showed that many compounds used by plastic surgeons for their healing properties actually interfered with healing. These included scarlet red, tannic acid, silver nitrate and balsam of Peru, among others.

SYSTEMIC FACTORS

PROTEIN. The two nutritional factors shown to be most directly related to healing are dietary protein and vitamin C. The deleterious effect of hypoproteinemia on healing has been well documented. Clinicians are so well steeped in this knowledge that elective operations are no longer performed upon patients with hypoproteinemia. Rhoads, Fliegelmen and Panzer attributed the healing effect of protein to its oncotic pressure, and claimed to correct deficient healing in hypoproteinemic animals by giving acacia. However, they and others could not confirm these observations, and it is presently felt that only biological proteins are effectively metabolized by patients and return plasma protein levels to normal. Although Harvey and Howes found slightly improved healing in animals receiving a superabundance of dietary protein, others have not been able to confirm this. The essentiality of amino acids containing sulfhydryl groups has been shown clearly and often; cysteine or methionine alone will correct the healing defect in hypoproteinemic animals.

VITAMIN C. The healing defect in scurvy is unchallengeable. This defect represents, according to Dunphy, "a failure of fibroblast differentiation and impaired synthesis of collagen and sulfated mucopolysaccharides." All cellular and biochemical activity is hindered. In true scurvy, the wound is profoundly altered and reveals an almost total lack of any repair or healing. Serious vitamin C deficiency is rarely encountered in healthy Americans today, but the problem is important in seriously ill hospital patients with medical or surgical problems. Modern surgeons have been thoroughly indoctrinated about the importance of vitamin C and use

this vitamin indiscriminately in surgical practice. Fortunately, no difficulties from hypervitaminosis C have been reported. It is also fortunate that the patient with depleted stores of vitamin C, probably not frank scurvy, can be operated upon in an emergency, for the administration of the vitamin during and following operation will immediately correct the situation and will result in normal healing. This assumes, of course, that hemoglobin and other protein stores are not depleted; their correction takes much more time. Although no direct effect on wound healing has been found in avitaminosis A, B, D, E or K, common sense dictates the addition of these vitamins to the patient's intake, dietary or otherwise. Vitamins B, C and K can easily be given parenterally, because they are water soluble, but vitamins A, D and E must be eaten or given into the gastrointestinal tract.

ANEMIA. Anemia should be expected to give wound healing problems, but experimental studies to document this yield conflicting results. Chronic anemia is often associated with hypoproteinemia so that the specific effects of the two cannot be separated. No elective operation should be performed in an anemic patient, but emergency procedures are often performed upon patients with acute anemia, usually from hemorrhage. Whether these patients heal normally is not known.

INFECTION. The infected wound also has systemic effects. Smith has shown the significant and prolonged changes in hexosamines and hydroxyproline in muscle far removed from a laparotomy incision infected with *Staphylococcus aureus*. Carrel also found that healing of clean wounds was delayed in animals with infections elsewhere in the body. Today's surgeon will not perform an elective operation upon a patient with a significant superficial or deep-seated infection anywhere. The risk is not only that of impaired healing in the clean wound; there may be embolization of bacteria from the original infection to the wound. The stress of anesthesia and major operation may also affect adversely the body's handling of the original infection. Even the lowly pimple has deterred bold surgeons from performing elective herniorrhaphies.

AGE. "The young heal better than the old" is a well accepted axiom, and there is good experimental evidence supporting it. DuNouy and Howes and Harvey showed beyond a doubt that wound healing proceeded more rapidly in the young and Carrel even claimed to have extracted a "wound hormone" from the blood of old animals which would delay healing in younger animals. Scientists today believe that young, growing animals heal better than older ones, but do not accept the wound hormone thesis.

TEMPERATURE. Healthy animals respond to infection and other types of inflammation by increasing the body temperature. Although a fever may be injurious to the elderly patient, it may be innocuous and even beneficial in a young patient, for the increased cardiac output, circulatory rate and local tissue metabolism result in more rapid removal of dead cells, bacteria, toxins and cellular debris, and more rapid healing of the infection. Because of the acceleration in all bodily processes, wound healing should be increased. Ebeling claimed that increased body temperature did result in more rapid healing. However, his data are at best skimpy, for he studied the healing of only two incisions, one in each of two alligators kept at different environmental temperatures. With the increasing use of local and general body hypothermia in the management of many difficult clinical problems, there should be some concern about the effect of decreased body temperature on healing. There is no experimental evidence to show that it has any effect.

DRUGS. If all the drugs purported to achieve improved healing actually worked, there would be no clinical problem in wound healing. Only one substance has been shown by repeated, scientifically sound experiments to increase the rate of healing in open and closed wounds; this substance is acid–pepsin-digested bovine cartilage powder, and it exerts its effect on many types of wounds in several animal species (Fig. 9). To date, no other substance has been shown to have this healing-promoting effect.

The powerful chemotherapeutic agents used to treat cancer might be expected to interfere with healing, and this has been shown experimentally for some of them. However, the healing wounds in skin, fascia, bronchus, stomach and intestine appear unaffected by these drugs, although there are other adverse effects of these compounds in patients undergoing resection for cancer.

HORMONES. Cortisone, thyroxin, androgens and estrogens have definite effects on wound healing, but other hormones have not been shown to exert any effect. In countless experimental studies, cortisone has been shown to offer a serious impairment to heal-

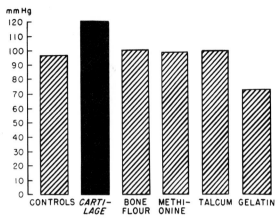

Figure 9. Bursting strength of rat laparotomy incisions. The increased strength resulting from cartilage treatment is significant. (Reprinted from Prudden et al.: Surg. Gyn. & Obst. *105*:283, 1957, with permission.)

ing. However, the clinical experience with cortisone, and other adrenal cortical hormones, is contrary to this. Most surgeons are pleasantly surprised at the dearth of wound complications in postoperative patients receiving cortisone or related steroids. There are two possible explanations. Many patients receiving cortisone have no endogenous adrenocortical activity, and Chassin and others have shown that the cortisone effect is present only in patients with intact adrenals. Also, that which pertains to the experimental animal may not pertain to patients, because several studies have shown that guinea pigs, monkeys, apes and presumably man are not cortisone sensitive.

Although the mechanism is poorly understood, thyroxin inhibits healing in experimental wounds; Moltke has shown that l-thyroxin has this effect whereas r-thyroxin does not. The racemic mixture apparently contains more of the levorotatory form because it also provokes the inhibitory effect on healing. Healing problems in patients receiving thyroxin have not been described. In the study of Jorgensen and Schmidt, androgens and estrogens stimulated healing. Douglas found that hypophysectomy, adrenalectomy and thyroidectomy in rabbits did not alter wound healing; however, the number of animals studied was too small to give significant results.

OTHER DISEASES. The patient requiring operation may be suffering from another disease which may have a profound effect on his ability to heal. Patients with diabetes mellitus, uremia, Parkinson's disease, multiple sclerosis, jaundice and Cushing's disease seem to have undue healing problems.

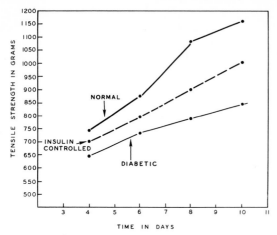

Figure 10. Tensile strength of healing incisions in normal alloxan-diabetic and insulin-controlled diabetic rats. (Reprinted from Rosen and Enquist: Surgery 50:525, 1961, with permission.)

That diabetics are very susceptible to infections, including wound infections, is recognized, but there is no proof that clean wounds in areas of good blood supply cannot heal normally in diabetics. Most clinicians believe that clean wounds in well-controlled diabetics heal well. In alloxan-diabetic rats, uncontrolled diabetes results in marked healing impairment in primary incisions; this is partially or completely corrected by insulin control (Fig. 10).

The healing problems in patients with Cushing's disease are obvious, serious and well documented. An excess of circulating adrenal cortical hormones, or abnormal hormones, is felt to be responsible, but the true mechanism is unknown. Patients with Parkinson's disease, cerebrovascular accidents and multiple sclerosis appear to have healing problems, but this clinical impression has not been confirmed by scientific study. Perhaps in all these patients inadequate stores of proteins or vitamin C are the true causes of the healing difficulties.

THE FUTURE

Will the surgeon of 2000 A.D. encounter the same healing problems as the present-day surgeon? Let us hope not. Prudden's studies with cartilage have shown unquestioned stimulation of the healing process in a number of different healing situations; surely a purification and chemical dissection of this crude product can result in a sterile, more potent compound which can be used paren-

terally as well as locally. There may be no need to use such a compound in normal patients, but it could prove invaluable in patients in whom impaired healing is to be expected.

Wound healing can be stimulated by other chemical compounds, including metals. In the study of Wu et al., it was shown that various metal sutures resulted in an increased gain of tensile strength in healing wounds. Aluminum was the best (Fig. 11). This effect of metals appeared to be related to their position in the electromotive series, and is a lead demanding exploration. It should be relatively easy to incorporate a strand of aluminum, another metal or an alloy into all sutures, if warranted. This property of aluminum could also be exploited in the creation of any number of prostheses implanted by surgeons in the heart, arteries and bones.

It will be important in the near future to determine the magnitude of collagen lysis in healing wounds. Lapiere and Gross identified

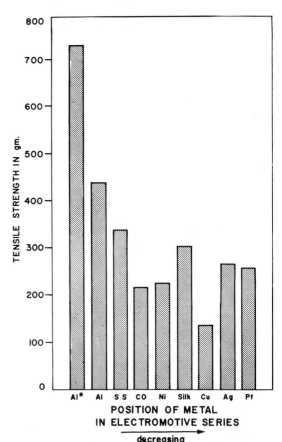

Figure 11. Tensile strength of wounds sutured with various metals. Al* indicates the tensile strength of wounds sutured with aluminum paired with contralateral incisions sutured with stainless steel. (Reprinted from Wu et al.: Surg. Forum *16*:90, 1965, with permission.)

a collagenolytic factor in the decreasing tadpole tail, and differentiated it from other proteolytic enzymes. Schaub found collagenolytic activity in rat uteri, and Peacock felt that selective lysis and remodeling of wound collagen was necessary for restoration of gliding function in tendon grafts. In our laboratory, it is believed that collagen lysis also occurs regularly in healthy, musculofascial incisions. Wound breakdowns may be the result of unusual lysis from a collagenase. Proper identification of these enzymes and the discovery of antagonists may help to prevent such breakdowns.

READING REFERENCES

Adamsons, R. J., and Enquist, I. F.: The relative importance of sutures to the strength of healing wounds under normal and abnormal conditions. Surg. Gyn. & Obst. 117:396, 1963.

Adamsons, R. J., Musco, F., and Enquist, I. F.: The relationship of collagen content to wound strength in normal and scorbutic animals. Surg. Gyn. & Obst. 119:323, 1964.

Adamsons, R. J., Musco, F., and Enquist, I. F.: The comparative effects of silk and catgut on collagen lysis during the lag phase of primary healing. Surg. Gyn. & Obst. 121:1028, 1965.

Alexander, J. W., Kaplan, J. Z., and Altemeier, W. A.: Role of suture materials in the development of wound infection. Ann. Surg. 165:192, 1967.

Billingham, R. E., and Russell, P. S.: Studies on wound healing, with special reference to the phenomenon of contracture in experimental wounds in rabbits' skin. Ann. Surg. 144:961, 1956.

Carrel, A., and Hartmann, H.: Cicatrization of wounds. The relation between the size of a wound and the rate of its cicatrization. J. Exper. Med. 24:429, 1916.

Chassin, J. L., McDougall, H. A., Mackay, M. I., and Localio, S. A.: Is the stress-induced inhibition of wound healing due to an excessive endogenous secretion of the adrenal glands? Surg. Forum 4:608, 1953.

Chassin, J. L., McDougall, H. A., Stahl, W., Mackay, M., and Localio, S. A.: Effect of adrenalectomy on wound healing in normal and in stressed rats. Proc. Soc. Exper. Biol. & Med. 86:446, 1954.

Douglas, D. M.: The tensile strength of healing wounds in aponeurosis. In Wound Healing, D. Slome (ed.). Oxford, Pergamon Press, 1961.

DuNouy, P. L.: Cicatrization of wounds. The relation between the age of the patient, the area of the wound and the index of cicatrization. J. Exper. Med. 24:461, 1916.

Dunphy, J. E.: On the nature and care of wounds. Ann. Royal Coll. Surgeons England 26:69, 1960.

Dunphy, J. E., and Udupa, K. N.: Chemical and histochemical sequences in the normal healing of wounds. New England J. Med. 253:847, 1955.

Dunphy, J. E., Udupa, K. N., and Edwards, L.: Wound healing. A new perspective with particular reference to ascorbic acid deficiency. Ann. Surg. 144:304, 1956.

Ebeling, A. H.: Cicatrization of wounds. Temperature coefficient. J. Exper. Med. 35:657, 1922.

Edwards, L. C., and Dunphy, J. E.: Wound healing. I. Injury and normal repair. New England J. Med. 259:224, 1958.

Edwards, L. C., and Dunphy, J. E.: Wound healing. II. Injury and abnormal repair. New England J. Med. 259:275, 1958.

Elek, S. D., and Conen, P. E.: The virulence of Staphylococcus pyogenes for man. A study of the problems of wound infection. Brit. J. Exper. Path. 38:573, 1957.

Findlay, C. W., Jr., and Howes, E. L.: The effect of edema on the tensile strength of the incised wound. Surg. Gyn. & Obst. 90:666, 1950.

Grillo, H., Watts, G. T., and Gross, J.: Studies in wound healing. I. Contraction and the wound contents. Ann. Surg. 148:145, 1958.

Harvey, S. C., and Howes, E. L.: Effect of high protein diet on the velocity of growth of fibroblasts in the healing wound. Ann. Surg. 91:641, 1930.

Howes, E. L.: The strength of wounds sutured with catgut and with silk. Surg. Gyn. & Obst. 57:309, 1933.

Howes, E. L., and Harvey, S. C.: The age factor in the velocity of the growth of fibroblasts in the healing wound. J. Exper. Med. 55:577, 1932.

Howes, E. L., Plotz, C. M., Blunt, J. W., and Ragan, C.: Retardation of wound healing by cortisone. Surgery 28:177, 1950.

Howes, E. L., Sooy, J. W., and Harvey, S. C.: The healing of wounds as determined by their tensile strength. J.A.M.A. 92:42, 1929.

Jackson, D. S.: Some biochemical aspects of fibrogenesis and wound healing. New England J. Med. 259:814, 1958.

Jorgensen, O., and Schmidt, A.: Influence of sex hormones on granulation tissue formation and on healing of linear wounds. Acta Chir. Scandinav. 124:1, 1962.

Kobak, M. W., Benditt, E. P., Wissler, R. W., and Steffee, C. H.: The relation of protein deficiency to experimental wound healing. Surg. Gyn. & Obst. 85:751, 1947.

Lanman, T. H., and Ingalls, T. H.: Vitamin C deficiency and wound healing. An experimental and clinical study. Ann. Surg. 105:616, 1937.

Lapierre, M., and Gross, J.: Animal collagenase and collagen metabolism. Publ. Am. Assoc. Adv. Sci. 75:663, 1963.

Lattes, R., Martin, J. R., Meyer, K., and Ragan, C.: Effect of cartilage and other tissue suspensions on reparative processes of cortisone-treated animals. Am. J. Path. 32:979, 1956.

Lattes, R., Martin, J. R., and Ragan, C.: Suppression of cortisone effect on repair in the presence of local bacterial infection. Am. J. Path. 30:901, 1954.

Levenson, S. M., Birkhill, F. R., and Waterman, D. F.: The healing of soft tissue wounds. The effects of nutrition, anemia and age. Surgery 28:905, 1950.

Localio, S. A., Lowman, E. W., and Gibson, J.: Wound healing in the paraplegic patient. Surgery 44:625, 1958.

Moltke, E.: Wound healing influenced by thyroxine and thyrotropic hormone. A tensiometric study. Proc. Soc. Exper. Biol. & Med. 88:596, 1955.

Muren, A.: Wound healing after denervation. Acta Physiol. Scandinav. (Suppl. 111) 1953.

Nelson, C. A., and Dennis, C.: Wound healing. Technical factors in the gain of strength in sutured abdominal wall wounds in rabbits. Surg. Gyn. & Obst. 93:461, 1951.

Peacock, E. E., Jr.: Some aspects of fibrogenesis during the healing of primary and secondary wounds. Surg. Gyn. & Obst. 115:408, 1962.

Peacock, E. E., Jr.: Fundamental aspects of wound healing relating to the restoration of gliding function after tendon repair. Surg. Gyn. & Obst. 119:241, 1964.

Prudden, J. F., Nishihara, G., and Baker, L.: The acceleration of wound healing with cartilage. Surg. Gyn. & Obst. 105:283, 1957.

Randall, P., and Randall, R. J.: The effects of various methods of treatment on wound healing. Plast. & Reconstruct. Surg. 14:105, 1954.

Rhoads, J. E., Fliegelman, M. T., and Panzer, L. M.: The mechanism of delayed wound healing in the presence of hypoproteinemia. J.A.M.A. 118:21, 1942.

Rosen, R. G., and Enquist, I. F.: The healing wound in experimental diabetes. Surgery 50:525, 1961.

Sandberg, N., and Zederfeldt, B.: The tensile strength of healing wounds and collagen formation in rats and rabbits. Acta Chir. Scandinav. 126:187, 1963.

Sandblom, P.: The tensile strength of healing wounds. An experimental study. Acta Chir. Scandinav. 90 (Suppl. 89), 1944.

Schaub, M. C.: Abban von Kollagen durch Factor im Uterus, Helv. Physiol. Pharm. Acta 22:(1) C38, 1964.

Shewell, J., and Long, D. A.: A species difference with regard to the effect of cortisone acetate on body weight, gamma globulin and circulating antitoxin levels. J. Hyg. 54:542, 1956.

Slome, D. (ed.): Wound Healing. Oxford, Pergamon Press, 1961.

Smith, M., and Enquist, I. F.: A quantitative study of the impaired healing resulting from infection. Surg. Gyn. & Obst. 125:965, 1967.

Thompson, W. D., Ravdin, I. S., and Frank, I. L.: Effect of hypoproteinemia on wound disruption. Arch. Surg. 36:500, 1938.

Williamson, M. B., and Fromm, H. J.: The incorporation of sulfur amino acids into the proteins of regenerating wound tissue. J. Biol. Chem. 212:705, 1955.

Wolfer, J. A., Farmer, C. J., Carroll, W. W., and Manshardt, D. O.: An experimental study in wound healing in vitamin C depleted human subjects. Surg. Gyn. & Obst. 84:1, 1947.

Wu, K., Enquist, I. F., Dennis, C., and Sawyer, P. N.: Effect of various metal electrode sutures in the production of increased tensile strength of wounds. Surg. Forum 16:89, 1965.

Chapter 3

THE INFECTIONS

by
WILLIAM A. ALTEMEIER, M.D.
and
J. WESLEY ALEXANDER, M.D.

WILLIAM ARTHUR ALTEMEIER, a Cincinnatian by birth, is a product of his home city's educational institutions. He progressed through the ranks of the department of surgery of the University of Cincinnati College of Medicine to become professor and chairman of the department. He was director of the surgical bacteriologic laboratory and his interests in the area of infections has continued as evidenced by his investigative and clinical contributions which have been fundamental.

J. WESLEY ALEXANDER, a Kansan, was educated in college and medicine in Texas. He received his postgraduate education in surgery at the University of Cincinnati and the Cincinnati General Hospital where he has been associated with Dr. Altemeier in the study of surgical infections and their control. He is an Assistant Professor of Surgery at the University of Cincinnati College of Medicine.

The infections which occur in the practice of surgery continue to present major problems in their prevention, diagnosis, and management. Approximately one-third of the patients on a busy ward in a general hospital have infections of various types and degrees of severity. Some infections develop spontaneously and require the patient's hospitalization for effective treatment. Some may develop in or adjacent to wounds resulting from surgical operations, accidental trauma, or violence. Others may occur postoperatively in areas remote from the operative wound, such as pneumonia or cystitis.

In modern hospital practice increasing numbers of infections are being encountered as the result of iatrogenic factors. The past generation of surgeons has seen the emergence of increasing numbers of serious, sometimes lethal, infections related to a complex combination of factors, including the performance of more complicated and lengthier operations, an increase in the number of geriatric patients with accompanying chronic or debilitating diseases, and an increased utilization of treatment modalities which result in greater bacterial exposures and suppress normal host resistance. Unfortunately, a number of infections have resulted from laxity in aseptic technique, disregard for established surgical principles, and unwarranted reliance upon prophylactic antibiotic therapy. For these and other reasons, the physician must keep in mind that the modern general hospital is a complex community in which people are concentrated who have been admitted with a variety of infections, as well as many others who are unusually susceptible to secondary or hospital-acquired infections.

With the introduction of antibiotic therapy in 1942, it was hoped that serious infections complicating surgical practice would be eliminated. Unfortunately, this has not occurred. Not only has the problem of hospital infection continued, but widespread antibiotic therapy has undoubtedly increased the complexities of problems related to the prevention and control of surgical infection.

The outcome of bacterial contamination in the soft tissues of the body continues to be of primary concern to the surgeon. Open wounds, whether accidentally or surgically induced, provide the possibility of bacterial colonization and disturbances in the normal relationship between host and microorganism which may result in clinical infection. The interrelationship between the bacterial invaders and the human host seemingly rests upon a delicate balance, but closer examination will show that the balance is rarely tipped in favor of the pathogen unless there has been a gross disturbance of the normal defense mechanisms of the host.

HOST RESISTANCE AND DEFENSE MECHANISMS

All higher animals live in a sea of bacteria, viruses, and fungi which exist in a symbiotic or parasitic relationship, although most of these microorganisms may become pathogenic providing that proper conditions develop. Examples are widespread and include a myriad of species which find their home on epithelial surfaces such as the skin and mucous membranes of the oropharynx, nasal passages, vagina, and gastrointestinal tract. The vast majority of bacteria in contact with the host are denied entrance into the body by these epithelial surfaces. Epithelial function is by no means perfect, however, and viable microbes which are normally destroyed or excreted by the host occasionally gain entrance to the physiologic interior. Such minuscule invasion is usually of little consequence but may become of marked significance if the host's defenses are depressed, or when abnormally large numbers of highly pathogenic bacteria gain entrance. The host-parasite interaction may also vary considerably owing to differences between microbial species, but the defense mechanisms against different species are generally similar and should be studied as a whole to establish principles upon which modifications may be made as necessary (Fig. 1). This is particularly applicable to the surgeon, because the principles involving wound healing and patient care closely coincide with the principles of treatment relevant to the prevention and control of infection.

VASCULAR RESPONSE.   An inflammatory response is an essential part of defense against bacterial invasion. The development of an inflammatory focus depends upon a vascular response which may be elicited by bacterial products or tissue injury. Mediators of the vascular response include endotoxin, histamine, bradykinin, serotonin, slow-reacting substance, permeability producing globulin, and other vasoactive substances derived from tissue extracts. These chemical stimuli initiate a vascular response which is usually characterized by constriction of the venular sphincters at the junction of the venules and small veins, venular and capillary dilatation, slowing of flow, and resulting hypoxia. The endothelial surfaces become sticky so that

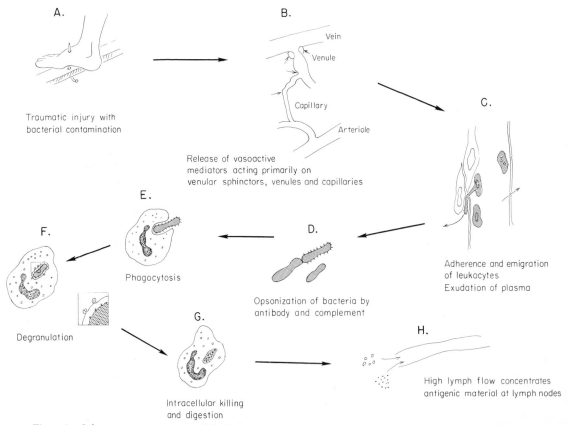

A.
Traumatic injury with bacterial contamination

B.
Vein
Venule
Capillary
Arteriole
Release of vasoactive mediators acting primarily on venular sphinctors, venules and capillaries

C.
Adherence and emigration of leukocytes
Exudation of plasma

D.
Opsonization of bacteria by antibody and complement

E.
Phagocytosis

F.
Degranulation

G.
Intracellular killing and digestion

H.
High lymph flow concentrates antigenic material at lymph nodes

Figure 1.   Schematic representation of the basic physiological events necessary for host antimicrobial defense.

granulocytes and monocytes marginate over the endothelium, and emigration of leukocytes through the intercellular junctions occurs by the process of diapedesis. Unless phagocytic cells can be delivered to sites of bacterial contamination, the organisms usually grow with minimal inhibition. An increased permeability to plasma proteins is also an important characteristic of the vascular response.

HUMORAL RESPONSE. Among the exuded plasma proteins at a new inflammatory focus are several which play an important role in the body's defense. Specific antibody directed toward a given microbe is frequently present because of past experience of the host with that organism. The so-called natural antibodies, exemplified by those directed against the enteric bacilli, probably represent no more than a result of this past exposure. Specific antibody directed against a microbe combines with surface antigens, and this union serves as a specific activation site for complement. In this system, the primary function of antibody is to serve as a binding site and activator for complement which otherwise has no specific activity against bacteria. Complement is an inclusive term for 11 chemically distinct serum constituents which, acting together, serve as a biological amplification system for the interaction between antigen and antibody. When complement is activated by antigen-antibody complex, a series of enzymatic reactions are produced which in their fullest expression damage or lyse the cell wall of the bacterium, prepare it for phagocytosis, release chemotactic substances, and produce immune adherence. Neither complement nor specific antibody has bactericidal capabilities, but acting together they may kill many species of gram-negative bacteria and a few species of gram-positive bacteria. The presence of antibody and complement is relatively unimportant *in vivo* in the absence of an adequate cellular response, however, and the primary function of antibody and complement in defense against microbial invasion is to prepare the microbe for phagocytosis and intracellular destruction. Other humoral factors have been found to be relatively unimportant, although lysozyme occasionally has a synergistic action with antibody and complement.

CELLULAR RESPONSE. As a result of the vascular response, leukocytes invade an inflammatory focus by emigration through the intercellular spaces in the capillaries and venules. The nature of the stimulus determines somewhat the characteristics of the inflammatory cellular exudate, but granulocytes are the predominant cells of the early lesion. Unless the vascular response is perpetrated, mononuclear cellular infiltration tends to dominate the later picture because the survival of mononuclear cells is considerably longer than that of neutrophils. Both monocytes and granulocytes are capable of phagocytosis and intracellular destruction of bacteria, but it is the neutrophil that plays the dominant role. It is the essential phagocytic cell of the body which protects from overwhelming microbial invasion. An estimated 20 to 50 billion neutrophils are circulating in the normal human adult at any given time, and an equal number are sequestered or marginated on vascular walls. These neutrophils, however, represent only a fraction of the number held in the bone marrow reserve. Vast numbers of neutrophils are lost into the gastrointestinal, respiratory, and genitourinary tracts daily, and the half-life of a neutrophil has been estimated to be only 24 hours.

Once in the extravascular tissues, phagocytes move about randomly until they come within a relatively short distance of an attractive particle, at which time they may be affected by chemotactic forces and abandon their random motion to proceed directly to that particle, a phenomenon which apparently involves a chemical concentration gradient affecting the gel-sol state of the cell membrane. There is very little evidence, if any, to support the concept that leukocytes are brought from other portions of the body to an inflammatory focus by chemotactic or leukotactic agents. Although such substances do exist, they are effective for only short distances, and the deposition of leukocytes at an inflammatory focus appears to be solely a function of the vascular response.

PHAGOCYTOSIS. After a phagocyte has made contact with a microbe, phagocytosis will follow, providing that the conditions for it are satisfactory. Organisms may be phagocytized and killed to a limited extent in the absence of detectable antibody and complement, but, in general, particle uptake by phagocytes is strikingly dependent upon the presence of antibody and complement. The process of preparing an organism for phagocytosis by antibody and complement is referred to as opsonization. Specific antibody in the absence of complement will act as an opsonizing agent. However, the bulk of evidence at present indicates that antibody serves primarily as an activation site for the complement system and that it is complement which has the greater influence upon the opsonization of bacteria. Complement has also been found to influence the phagocytosis of inert particles such as starch.

Other evidence for the importance of complement in opsonization is the observation that phagocytosis can be largely blocked by antibody specifically directed to complement, even in the presence of specific antibody to bacteria. It is also noteworthy that a variety of substances which have anticomplement activity, such as mucin and hemoglobin, inhibit phagocytosis. Inhibition of phagocytosis by capsules of certain organisms is also mediated through an anticomplement action of the capsule. Because it is the specific union of antigen and antibody which activates complement and directs its site of action, it must be concluded that both antibody and complement are vitally important for opsonization.

INTRACELLULAR DIGESTION. Once phagocytosis has occurred, the opportunity for destruction of the bacterium is finally at hand. For many years, the mechanism of bacterial killing by phagocytic cells was largely unexplained. Although some of the questions remain unanswered, the following sequence of events has been shown to be an extremely important pathway in the intracellular destruction of bacteria by phagocytes, particularly the neutrophils. After ingestion of a bacterium, fusion of the membrane confining the granules (*lysosomes*) occurs with the membrane surrounding the ingested bacterium (*phagosome*) with emptying of hydrolytic enzymes into the phagosome. A large number of hydrolytic enzymes are present in the lysosomes which may have an antibacterial action. Among these are lysozyme, phagocytin, catalases, lipases, proteases, ribonucleases, and deoxyribonucleases. In addition, there is a lowering of the pH to levels as low as 4 or 5, which in itself tends to have a destructive effect on the bacterium as well as providing the range of pH optimum for activity of the lysosomal enzymes. The emptying of lysosomal enzymes into the phagosome represents degranulation. Certain bacteria such as Mycobacterium, Salmonella, and Brucella often successfully resist intracellular digestion by these enzymes and may remain viable intracellularly for long periods of time.

TRANSFER TO IMMUNE COMPETENT CELL. The production of specific antibody follows an initial experience of the host with the offending organism. Following phagocytosis and digestion of microorganisms, material remains which may act as an antigenic stimulus after processing by the leukocyte. The exact processes involved in the transfer of antigenic information to immune competent cells are still poorly understood, but it has been shown that ribonucleic acid, with or without the antigen derived from degraded bacteria, may be transferred to immune competent cells which are felt to be small lymphocytes or their precursors. Once the antigen or directing nucleic acid has been obtained by the lymphocyte, antibody synthesis is stimulated and specific antibodies are produced. Other antigens degraded by intracellular digestion may be released in a soluble form at the time of the death and disintegration of leukocytes.

This is obviously a brief, somewhat oversimplified presentation of a complex subject, but it provides a foundation upon which better understanding of the nature of surgical infections can be built. The various components of normal host resistance are strongly interrelated and interdependent. Like blood coagulation or complement activity, a defect or abnormality in any one of the steps may lead to malfunction of the entire system.

CAUSES OF INFECTION

The pathogenesis of infections resulting from surgical treatment may be related either to a breakdown in host defense or to an overloading of the normal capabilities of the system. In surgical practice, both of these may occur frequently.

BACTERIAL FACTORS. The deposition and growth of bacteria within wounds are obvious prerequisites for the development of infection. The kind and numbers of bacteria contribute significantly to the establishment of overt infection, or the lack of it.

Several bacterial species have surface components which contribute to their pathogenicity by inhibiting phagocytosis, such as the capsule of Klebsiella and the M protein of Streptococcus. Other bacteria, notably the Enterobacteria, have surface components which are toxic, and still others produce powerful exotoxins. The development of infection is thus somewhat dependent upon the virulence of the organism and its ability to resist phagocytosis and intracellular destruction. With highly virulent and pathogenic organisms, relatively few may be required to establish an infection.

Careful studies of the bacterial flora of clean surgical wounds taken at the time of closure have shown that many, and perhaps most, of these wounds have one or more types of organisms which can be cultured from them. Far fewer organisms are necessary to cause an infection in a wound than in normal tissues, but, nevertheless, overt infection develops infrequently in such instances if cardinal surgical principles have not been violated, and if the number of organisms introduced into the wound does not exceed the capability of the phagocytic cells to remove them. Once this capability has been overcome, infection will occur.

DECREASED DELIVERY OF PHAGOCYTES. Virtually any condition which contributes to a decreased delivery of phagocytes to an area of bacterial contamination will promote the development of infection. These conditions include a diminution in blood flow such as may be found in vascular occlusive states, hypovolemic shock, or following the use of vasopressors. The presence of devitalized tissue, foreign bodies, hematomas, and seromas produces ideal opportunities for the development of infection largely because of the physiologic state of the wound favorable for bacterial growth, and the inhibited or abolished delivery of phagocytes to these areas.

A decreased vascular reactivity, such as may be found in uremic conditions or in patients receiving high doses of steroids, may promote the development of infection by preventing the development of a normal inflammatory response. Even when vascular reactivity and flow are normal and there is no foreign body or dead space, decreased delivery of phagocytes may accompany a decreased production, such as is found during nitrogen mustard therapy, irradiation, or granulocytopenic states.

ABNORMAL PHAGOCYTOSIS. Defects in phagocytosis may result either from a deficiency of serum opsonins or from an abnormality of the phagocyte itself. Defects in ingestion have been implicated in uremia, diabetes mellitus, prematurity, and certain malignancies, notably leukemias.

INTRACELLULAR KILLING. Even when the process of ingestion of bacteria is normal, intracellular killing may occur at a decreased rate. Two categories of defects are found: those involving an abnormality of the lysosomal membrane, and those in which there is a deficient amount of enzyme. Recently, an intracellular killing defect has been demonstrated in the leukocytes of patients with severe thermal injury. In these patients, phagocytosis by peripheral leukocytes occurs at a normal or increased rate, but intracellular killing is deficient. The total content of lysosomal hydrolytic enzymes has been found to be severely decreased, with the greatest deficiency being present six to ten days after burn injury, the time when clinical infection occurs most frequently. The pronounced deficiency in lysosomal enzymes is reason enough to explain an increased susceptibility to bacterial infections in severely burned patients.

The acute starvation associated with traumatic injury or surgical therapy does not adversely affect phagocyte function, nor is the production of specific antibody altered to any significant degree unless severe inanition and vitamin depletion occur.

ABNORMAL SERUM FACTORS. At any site of injury, there is an exudation of plasma protein into the area. The specific antibody and complement contained therein may act as strong opsonizing agents for phagocytosis of contaminating bacteria. If the host has had no prior experience with the offending organism, he will have no specific antibody, and the rate of phagocytosis by competent leukocytes will be considerably diminished. Specific immunization might help in specific instances in which the species of contaminating organism could be anticipated far in advance, but one seldom has this opportunity. The level of titer of complement components is amazingly similar between individuals, and with the exception of certain hereditary and consumptive conditions, complement levels are usually normal. Individuals who produce little or no gamma globulin or respond to an antigenic stimulus with an abnormal type of gamma globulin are occasionally encountered. In such cases, the end result is similar to those in which the host has had no prior experience with the offending organism.

There are several substances which promote the development of infection through an anticomplement activity. Among these are heparin, mucin, hemoglobin, and sodium polyanethol sulfonate. Each of these, when administered locally with bacteria, contributes to an increase in susceptibility to infection.

PREVENTION OF INFECTION

Prevention of septic complications is far more practical than their treatment once they have become established. Strict adherence to the principles of wound care and application of knowledge concerning the pathogenesis of wound infections will prevent the vast majority of complicative infections in surgical practice.

AVOIDANCE OF PREDISPOSING CONDITIONS; BACTERIAL CONTAMINATION. The most obvious means for controlling the bacterial population of clean surgical incisions is avoidance of undue contamination during operation. Even in well-ventilated operating rooms, occasional bacteria from the air settle in the wound, but by far the greatest sources of contamination are from the patient's skin, the hands of the operating team, and breaks in sterile operative technique. Organisms reaching the wound from the patient's skin may be kept to a minimum by adherence to a ten-minute surgical scrub of the operative area, using sterile gloves and painting the region with a germicidal agent such as tincture of Ceepryn or iodine and alcohol. Once the skin incision is made, the wound edges should be covered with towels held in position with towel clips or suture. An alternative method currently in general use is the application of sterile plastic film to the entire operative area and making the incision through the plastic.

As many as 90 per cent of the members of an operative team develop punctures or tears in their gloves at some time during an operation. These must be changed immediately to avoid bacterial contamination of the wound because the hands can never be sterilized by scrubbing. Even though the numbers of organisms present after a surgical scrub are low, they increase progressively with the length of the operation, and the numbers of organisms inside the glove often increase remarkably at puncture sites when blood has gained entrance. Laxity in aseptic technique can be prevented only by constant awareness on the part of the operating team. So-called minor infringements must not go unnoticed and should receive immediate attention just as major breaks in technique.

Laxity in isolation procedures or indifference for patients having open infections, burns, and tracheostomies is a frequent basis of nosocomial infections. Air-borne infections of wounds occur infrequently in hospitals, and person-to-person transfer is the major culprit. The use of aseptic techniques for tracheostomy care and wound care is an essential prerequisite for the prevention of hospital-acquired infections.

WOUND CARE. Prevention of infection in wounds resulting from either injury or planned operative procedures may have a profound effect on the morbidity and mortality resulting from that injury or operation. Every patient deserves meticulous wound care, but this is particularly true in those instances in which there may be an impairment of the overall defense. The surgeon must realize that every wound transecting epithelial surfaces and a large percentage of so-called "clean surgical wounds" are contaminated by viable and potentially pathogenic bacteria. When the numbers of these bacteria are kept to a minimum, infection will not occur. All devitalized tissues and foreign bodies should be removed. When complete debridement is not possible, the wound should not be closed because foreign bodies left in a wound may decrease the minimal infective dose of a bacterial inoculum by as much as 10,000-fold or more. Nearly a million viable Staphylococci are necessary to produce a clinical infection when injected subcutaneously or intradermally, but when these same organisms are introduced on a piece of suture material, as few as 100 can produce a significant infection. Similar results have been shown with the enhancement of clostridial infections by devitalized muscle and sterile foreign bodies. It is easy to see that in grossly contaminated wounds, not only must debridement be complete but careful consideration must be given to the introduction of the new foreign bodies such as prostheses, grafts, and suture materials. In contaminated wounds, experimental investigation indicates that monofilament types of suture materials are preferable to multifilament types, all other things being equal.

The presence of hematomas or dead spaces acts like foreign bodies and also prevents the delivery of phagocytic cells to bacterial foci. One mistake frequently encountered in closing contaminated wounds is leaving a dead space between the layers rather than obliterating all potential dead spaces either by suture or suction drainage. Insertion of a catheter through a separate stab wound into a dead space and application of continuous or intermittent suction to remove fluid collections have been shown to be effective means of accomplishing this purpose. The bacterial population in contaminated wounds can be controlled somewhat by washing the wound prior to closure, but only a relative decrease in numbers can be accomplished.

In heavily contaminated wounds, or in wounds in which all of the foreign bodies or devitalized tissue cannot be satisfactorily removed, the use of a delayed primary closure will, in most instances, minimize the development of serious infection. With this technique, the subcutaneous and skin wounds are left open and packed loosely with gauze after fascial closure. The number of phagocytic cells at the wound edges progressively increases to reach a peak four or five days after the injury. Capillary budding is intense at this time, and closure may often be successfully accomplished even in the face of heavy bacterial contamination. It has been shown experimentally that the number of organisms required to initiate an infection in a surgical incision progressively increases as the interval of healing increases up to the fifth postoperative day.

SYSTEMIC FACTORS. Leukocyte function has been found to be abnormal in a variety of systemic diseases, including leukemia, diabetes mellitus, prematurity, and several hereditary conditions. Any disease or treatment associated with a significant neutropenia adversely affects the host defense against bacterial infection. When treating surgical patients with these or similar problems, extraordinary precautions should be taken to prevent the development of wound infection. These should include correction or control of the underlying defect whenever possible. The administration of many drugs, including steroids, antimetabolites, and anticancer agents, has been found to be associated with an increased incidence of septic complications. Unnecessary use of these drugs is to be avoided in the surgical patient.

INCREASED DELIVERY OR FUNCTION OF PHAGOCYTE. If impairment of the delivery or a diminution of the function of phagocytic cells occurs at sites of bacterial contamination and adversely influences the development of wound infections, it would follow that the opposite should also be true.

A number of chemicals and biological agents stimulate the activity of the reticuloendothelial system when administered to experimental animals and increase their resistance to controlled or graded bacterial challenge. However, there has been surprisingly little investigation concerning the use of such agents in humans. It has been shown that the administration of vitamin A to individuals with an abnormal stability of their lysosomal membranes partially corrects the deficient intracellular killing capacity of their leukocytes. The administration of estrogenic substances to experimental animals increases their resistance to infection. This observation has been utilized in clinical practice to some degree in the treatment of acne. Transfusions with leukocytes in leukopenic individuals with septicemia has been beneficial in selected instances.

IMMUNOTHERAPY. Active and passive immunization procedures for the prevention of surgical infections have merit only in specific instances. Tetanus is one condition in which the use of immunotherapy has had outstanding success in prevention of the disease. Individuals who have had a full course of active immunization are protected against the development of tetanus for years in most cases and for a lifetime in many. Once a patient has had a full course of basic immunization with tetanus toxoid, a booster injection of toxoid invariably elicits protective levels of antibody in all individuals tested for periods of as long as 20 years, and the administration of antitoxin for the prophylaxis of tetanus in these patients is not indicated except under unusual circumstances. For those persons who have not been actively immunized against tetanus before the time of their injury, it is important that they receive tetanus antitoxin.

In recent years, the use of antitoxin obtained from human donors has antiquated the administration of antitoxin obtained from animals, and by comparison represents an extremely safe therapeutic measure. At the time of injury, 250 to 500 units of human tetanus antitoxin should be administered intramuscularly, depending on the severity of the injury. If the patient is seen more than 24 hours after injury, the dose should be increased. Simultaneous administration of the initial injection of tetanus toxoid for active immunization is indicated in every case. A careful follow-up should be obtained to ensure completion of the course of active immunization. Tetanus antitoxin does not prevent infection with *Clostridium tetani*, but it does inactivate the toxin produced. Careful surgical debridement with removal of all devitalized tissue is also an important means of prevention. The administration of systemic antibiotics has been recommended in the past for the prevention of tetanus, but it is felt that this is of secondary importance and usually unnecessary.

Gas gangrene antitoxin and toxoid have been utilized prophylactically for clostridial infections, but they are generally considered to be without benefit. The best prophylaxis for gas gangrene is adequate surgical management of the local wound. Vaccination against rabies is effective, but the vaccination procedure can be complicated by an allergic encephalitis. Specific bacterial vaccines may be of benefit in selected situations in which other treatment modalities have failed. The use of pooled human gamma globulin for the prevention of bacterial infections should be limited to those individuals who have agammaglobulinemia or a dysgammaglobulinemia.

CHEMOTHERAPY. The use of prophylactic antibiotic therapy has continued to be a controversial subject among surgeons, mostly because of a lack of understanding of the basic principles involved. There is little doubt that the administration of therapeutic doses of antimicrobial agents is capable of preventing infection in wounds contaminated by specific and highly sensitive bacteria. There is some evidence that it can attenuate a developing infection in others. The decision for the use of prophylactic antibiotic therapy must be based upon the weight of evidence for possible benefit against the weight of evidence for possible adverse effects. Indiscriminate or blind use of antibiotics is to be thoroughly discouraged because this may lead to infection with secondary or superimposed antibiotic-resistant strains of organisms, serious hypersensitivity reactions and postponement of indicated surgical treatment. The indiscriminate use of antibiotics may also mask the signs and symptoms of established infections, making diagnosis more difficult.

USE OF PROPHYLACTIC ANTIBIOTIC THERAPY. Prophylactic antibiotics are clearly contraindicated for the performance of clean surgical operations in which no obvious bacterial contamination has occurred. The incidence of wound infections in elective clean operations such as herniorrhaphies and thyroidectomies is less than 1 per cent when careful, meticulous aseptic technique is practiced. When infections do occur, they can usually be traced to poor surgical technique. Prophylactic antibiotic therapy is not a substitute for careful surgical technique or established surgical principles, and its indiscriminate or general use is to be discouraged. A more discriminating, limited, purposeful, and intelligent use of antibiotic therapy should be adopted. Experience has emphasized the fact that antibiotic agents are used more effectively as adjuvants to adequate surgery.

There are several clinical situations, however, in which the administration of prophylactic antibiotic therapy is usually of benefit. It is, therefore, generally recommended in the following:

Open anastomosis of the unprepared colon.

Penetrating injuries to a hollow intra-abdominal viscus.

Accidental wounds contaminated with large amounts of foreign material.

Accidental wounds requiring surgery in which treatment is unavoidably delayed.

Injuries in which adequate debridement cannot be accomplished, and contaminated or devitalized tissue must of necessity remain.

When known, gross bacterial contamination has occurred.

When emergency operation is indicated in patients with pre-existing or recently active infections.

When pre-existing valvular heart damage is present in a patient in order to prevent the development of bacterial endocarditis.

The prophylactic use of antibiotics may also be useful under certain other conditions, and the decision for their use should be made after careful consideration.

The early administration of penicillin in burn patients has been effective in preventing invasive infections of the wound by the beta *Streptococcus hemolyticus* and the Pneumococcus. Many surgeons continue to use this as part of the initial therapy and at the time of skin grafting. The indications have become less clear with the recent widespread use of topical antimicrobial agents such as Sulfamylon and silver nitrate, because rapidly advancing hemolytic streptococcal and pneumococcal infections are seen infrequently with this type of therapy.

In operative procedures categorized as "clean-contaminated," in which there is transection or resection of hollow viscera such as the gastrointestinal tract, biliary tract, respiratory tract, or genitourinary tract, varying degrees of bacterial contamination may occur. It is in this group of patients that the decision for use of antibiotic therapy must be based upon careful consideration of the evidence for and against its effectiveness. Evaluation should include an estimate of the degree of contamination, the status of nonspecific host resistance, the age of the patient, underlying disease conditions, drug therapy, and the length and severity of operation. Each patient should be evaluated independently.

The administration of oral nonabsorbable antibiotics for the suppression of growth of intestinal bacteria has been successful in some hands and detrimental in others. One serious consequence of their administration has been shown to be the emergence and overgrowth of virulent and antibiotic resistant bacteria, particularly the *Staphylococcus aureus*, UC/18. Staphylococcal enterocolitis following antibiotic bowel preparation may develop as a consequence of a serious nosocomial infection. Staphylococcal wound infection may also occur. Mechanical cleansing of the intestinal tract is more important than prophylactic antibiotic bowel preparation, and is preferable providing that systemically administered antibiotic therapy is given immediately before, during and for two to four days after the operation.

For this purpose, a combination of aqueous penicillin and tetracycline has been employed effectively. Therapeutic doses should be given from the very beginning and continued for the first three or four days postoperatively, at which time they should be discontinued. For the average adult, this means 2.5 to 3 million units of aqueous penicillin and 1.0 gm. of tetracycline daily given intravenously in three or four divided doses. Intermittent intravenous therapy is probably preferable to continuous intravenous therapy.

Prophylactic antibiotic therapy is generally more effective when started preoperatively and continued through the intraoperative period by a continuous intravenous drip. This procedure produces therapeutic levels of the antibiotic agents at the operative site and in any seromas and hematomas which may develop subsequently. Antibiotics started as late as six to 12 hours after bacterial contamination are relatively less effective. Failure of the effectiveness of prophylactic antibiotic agents has resulted in part from a lack of appreciation of the importance of the timing and dosage of these agents which are critical determinants.

DIAGNOSIS OF SURGICAL INFECTIONS

The diagnosis of established surgical infections is usually not difficult, but several types, such as abscesses of the retroperitoneal tissues, subphrenic space, liver, or pancreas, and deep-seated wound infections, may tax the ingenuity of the most astute clinician. Accurate and prompt diagnosis with evaluation of the patient is a necessary prerequisite for adequate treatment, and in many instances for survival.

By far the most important part of the survey of a patient suspected of having a surgical infection is a careful history and physical examination. Many times the lesion is characterized by the cardinal signs of inflammation, but this is not always the case, especially when infection is deep seated or has been attenuated by intensive antibiotic therapy. In the latter instance, massive pyogenic abscesses may occur in the absence of fever, tenderness, or leukocytosis. The most important physical finding in localizing an infection is the presence of a tender mass.

Urinalysis and complete blood count should be done on all patients suspected of having a surgical infection because these measures may aid greatly in the diagnosis. Intra-abdominal infections are frequently mimicked by pyelonephritis, and the presence of diabetes mellitus is usually detected by urinalysis. This is particularly important because both infection and diabetes are difficult to control when they occur together. Occasionally, infections caused by hemolytic bacteria such as *Streptococcus hemolyticus* and *Clostridium welchii* may cause a profound anemia. An elevation of the leukocyte count may or may not be helpful in the diagnosis of surgical infections. With most infections it is elevated, but in many conditions such as typhoid fever, overwhelming infection, concomitant antibiotic therapy, and immunosuppressive drug treatment, the leukocyte count may be within the normal range. In overwhelming infections, and infections developing in the face of antibiotic therapy, there is often a shift to the left and toxic granulation of the cells even though the total leukocyte count is not elevated. Blood cultures may help to establish the etiologic agent in a surgical infection but do not help to pinpoint its location. In patients with chills, several blood cultures should be obtained at frequent intervals of two to four hours, because one culture often is negative. Roentgenographic examinations may aid in localizing deep-seated abscesses.

Whenever possible, pus or infectious exudate from the area of the infection should be examined to establish an etiological diagnosis because this may be a significant aid in selecting the correct method of therapy. In deep-seated abscesses, pus can be obtained by needle aspiration or at the time of definitive drainage. Surface infections can be examined directly. To the experienced observer, gross examination of the pus with notation of its odor, color, and consistency will give important diagnostic suggestions. Microscopic examination of a smear of the material after Gram's stain, Ziehl-Neelsen stain, or other techniques often yields immediate information regarding the etiologic agent.

In many types of infection, however, the etiologic agent may not be apparent on direct smear, and therefore immediate culture of the purulent material using aerobic and anaerobic techniques should always be made. Cultures, particularly anaerobic cultures, must be placed immediately into the appropriate media and incubated. Material kept in the refrigerator or at room temperature frequently yields inconclusive or even false results, particularly when mixed infections are present. A direct smear of the pus onto a blood agar plate will often yield characteristic colonies within a few hours. Definitive antibiotic sensitivity tests can be obtained within 24 hours in most instances when this information may be critical to the management of the patient.

Biopsy of the lesion in granulomatous infections may provide valuable information in establishing the definitive diagnosis. Utilization of the fluorescent antibody technique for identifying organisms in tissue sections has added significantly to the value of biopsy. Other tests such as skin tests and examination of the patient's serum for specific antibody may be of additional help when indicated.

TREATMENT

Prevention is obviously the best form of therapy, but postoperative infections occur occasionally under even the best means of preventive management. Other types of surgical infections arise spontaneously, and these require surgical management, as indicated earlier.

SURGICAL INTERVENTION. The backbone of surgical treatment for infection is incision and drainage of localized collections of purulent material. In considering surgical intervention, one must take into account the location of the infection, the presence or absence of complicating cellulitis, the duration of the lesion, and the presence or absence of complicating disease. Surgical drainage permits the removal of bacteria, dead leukocytes, and necrotic tissues, and permits access of new phagocytes, antibiotic agents and plasma proteins to the remaining infecting bacteria. When incision and drainage is employed as a method of treatment, it is essential that complete decompression be obtained. The incision must be large enough to accomplish free drainage with the use of mechanical drains whenever these are indicated. Walls between loculations must be broken down or these areas drained separately. Dependent drainage is a cardinal principle to be practiced

whenever possible. Needle aspiration of abscesses does not provide free drainage, and should not be done except for the purpose of establishing a diagnosis or localizing the site of an abscess. Surgical drainage of an abscess, like any other operation, should be accomplished under controlled and otherwise aseptic conditions to prevent the introduction of additional types of microbes into an already infected area. Synergistic or superinfections may occasionally develop under these conditions, becoming considerably more recalcitrant to treatment.

A thorough search should always be made for the underlying cause of the infection as a part of therapy. Other systemic and local diseases may be contributory. Surgeons should not neglect evaluation or considerations of local complications of systemic diseases such as malignancies, diabetes mellitus, Cushing's disease, hypogammaglobulinemia and fatal granulomatous disease of childhood, to name only a few.

Occasionally, surgical decompression of a rapidly progressing and fulminating infection becomes necessary by radical incision and drainage or amputation when other means of controlling a life-threatening infection fail. Examples of this include gas gangrene, anaerobic crepitant cellulitis, and acute hemolytic streptococcal gangrene. Excision of specific chronic or indolent infections may also become necessary in rare instances.

CHEMOTHERAPY AND ANTIBIOTIC THERAPY. In treatment of infections when there is a localized collection of pus, antibiotic agents serve only as adjuncts to incision and drainage. Their widespread use in the treatment of abscesses has contributed little to any increase in survival, and their primary beneficial effect is brought forth by decreasing the incidence of complications and shortening convalescence.

When certain infections are manifested by diffuse cellulitis, antibiotic therapy may have a primary role in the management of the patient. In such instances, early and effective therapy usually results in resolution of the infection with minimal complications. Antibiotic therapy for diffuse cellulitis should be aggressive, but close observation of the patient must be made for signs and symptoms of any associated abscess which develops. Failure of the systemic signs and symptoms of infection to recede within 48 to 72 hours after the beginning of specific antibiotic therapy often indicates the development of a collection of purulent material or metastatic complications.

Selection of antibiotic agents. Because of the widely varying spectrum of sensitivity to the presently available antibiotic agents, early identification of the offending organism and antibiotic sensitivity testing are essential for the most effective use of these agents. So-called "shotgun" therapy is to be discouraged, except possibly in established infections in which death of the patient appears certain in the absence of effective therapy. Even in these instances, it is far more acceptable to use one or two antibiotics covering a broad spectrum of activity rather than many anti-bacterial agents. A knowledge of bacterial sensitivity patterns associated with an edu-cated guess as to the offending organism fre-quently leads to selection of the proper anti-biotic. Direct examination of stained smears of the pus obtained by incision and drainage or needle aspiration of the lesion often re-veals the nature of the infecting organism, as previously noted. In critical situations when there is an immediate need for information concerning antibiotic sensitivity of the organ-ism, direct sensitivity tests may be done by plating the purulent exudate directly on a blood agar plate and simultaneously testing with sensitivity discs. Definitive information can thus be obtained usually within 12 hours.

The results of culture and sensitivity tests in many laboratories are unnecessarily de-layed, and the report may not be available to the attending physician for several days. Se-lection of antibiotic agents for therapy should be based upon sensitivity studies whenever possible. These may be done by the serial dilution technique or the disc method, using commercially prepared discs. The latter is considerably easier to perform but is not as sensitive or as reliable. Its usefulness, how-ever, can be increased when consideration is given to the size of the zone of inhibition, the completeness of the inhibition, and the con-trolled concentration of antibiotic in the disc. Under the circumstances, the disc method provides valuable information, and experi-ence has shown a strong correlation between the results obtained by *in vitro* sensitivity tests by the disc method and the clinical response obtained.

Administration of antibiotic agents. In minor infections, antibiotic therapy is often unnecessary and may even be contraindi-cated. In patients with severe systemic in-fections, however, antibiotics should be administered as soon as possible after a defin-itive diagnosis has been made. In severe in-fections, the agents are preferably admin-istered intravenously or intramuscularly. When the intravenous route is used, injection of the antibiotic agent at intermittent inter-vals is preferable to continuous infusions, because higher levels are obtained in the blood and extracellular fluids with intermit-tent therapy. It is important to recognize that antibiotic agents have their greatest effect upon actively growing bacteria but little or no effect on phagocytized organisms. Bacteria may remain viable intracellularly for pro-longed periods of time even in the presence of very high concentrations of antibiotics in the extracellular fluid. Microbes damaged by antibiotics before phagocytosis, however, have been shown to be more readily killed by the phagocytic cells.

Complications of antibiotic therapy. Treatment with antibiotic agents is not with-out danger. In addition to a false sense of security and inappropriate reliance upon their effectiveness, complications during or following their use may occur. Untoward re-actions may be toxic in nature, associated with hypersensitivity reactions, or caused by idiosyncrasies. All the antibiotics commonly used have at one time or another produced one or more of these types of adverse reac-tions.

Toxic reactions are related to overdosage and can be easily managed by decreasing the dosage of the drug or discontinuing it. When sensitization occurs, severe allergic reac-tions may accompany administration of the drug. Penicillin sensitivity is the classic ex-ample of this type of reaction, and too many patients still die in this country from this cause each year. Although often unreliable, the clinical history of past sensitivities is the only source of information available to the clinician treating acute infections. Recently developed *in vitro* lymphocyte stimulation tests and skin sensitivity tests may be of value in determining drug sensitivities after re-covery, but the time requirement for their performance precludes their usefulness in patients with acute, severe infections. Several antimicrobial agents such as chloramphenicol and the sulfonamides are capable of pro-ducing agranulocytosis or aplastic anemia. Regularly repeated blood counts should be used to monitor the bone marrow response when these agents are used. Other drugs such as kanamycin, gentamycin, polymyxin, and colistin can produce renal damage and uremia, particularly in individuals having previously existing renal disease. Streptomycin, dihydrostreptomycin, kanamycin, and gentamycin may all produce ototoxicity when given in large doses or for a prolonged period. Tetracycline may cause severe yellow staining and deformity of the teeth when given to infants; this may also occur in infants born to mothers given tetracycline therapy in the prenatal period. Individuals who have developed a hypersensitivity reaction to one drug are more prone to develop hypersensitivity reactions to other therapeutic agents. Other antibiotics such as erythromycin, tetracycline, and ampicillin may produce diarrhea.

The administration of any antibacterial agent may produce a suppression of susceptible microbes with the emergence and overgrowth of those strains resistant to the antibiotic administered. The development of diarrhea in most instances is related to a change in the bacterial flora of the intestine. An overgrowth with strains of *Staphylococcus aureus* may occur in the intestine during systemic antibiotic therapy, but it is seen most frequently when nonabsorbable antibiotics have been administered orally for intestinal antisepsis. Staphylococcal enterocolitis in its severest form is a dire emergency and must be treated by immediate fluid replacement and antistaphylococcal drugs. The emergence of resistant organisms is particularly prone to occur when antibiotics are administered for the treatment of lesions subject to contamination from external sources such as open wounds, leg ulcers, burns, and avulsion injuries. Superinfections with fungi have become increasingly more frequent and are especially difficult to treat. Systemic fungal infections are usually associated with diminished host resistance, and they almost invariably occur subsequent to antibiotic therapy.

IMMUNOTHERAPY. At present, the usefulness of specific immune therapy in the practice of surgery is limited primarily to the administration of antitoxins against tetanus, rabies, and poisonous snakes. Polyvalent gas gangrene antitoxin may be of some value in the treatment of severe cases of gas gangrene with marked toxemia. An intensive re-evaluation of the possible use of immunotherapy for problematical gram-negative infection is now being undertaken but insufficient data have accumulated to warrant widespread clinical use. Occasionally, specifically directed vaccines may be of value in the management of infections resistant to all other forms of therapy.

CLASSIFICATION OF SURGICAL INFECTIONS

The anatomical location of a lesion often provides valuable clues concerning the etiologic agent. The majority of wound infections are caused by *Staphylococcus aureus* or a mixed bacterial flora. Intra-abdominal infections associated with perforation of the gastrointestinal tract are usually polymicrobial and involve gram-negative enteric bacteria. Infections arising in the genitourinary tract are predominantly from gram-negative organisms, and the most common of these is *Escherichia coli*. A spreading subcutaneous cellulitis most frequently results from infection with *Streptococcus pyogenes* but may be caused by *Staphylococcus aureus*.

STAPHYLOCOCCAL INFECTIONS. A large number of infections encountered in surgical practice are caused by *Staphylococcus aureus* (Fig. 2). It is an important pathogen in postoperative wound infection and in infections following penetrating wounds. The lesions produced by *Staphylococcus aureus* are characteristically localized with an indurated area of cellulitis which undergoes central necrosis and abscess formation with a thick, creamy, odorless, and yellow or cream-colored pus. Bacteremia may occur with the development of metastatic abscesses. Fever and leukocytosis are usually present in staphylococcal infections. Staphylococcal infections acquired during the course of hospitalization are often caused by antibiotic-resistant bacteria of increased virulence.

The treatment of established infections caused by *Staphylococcus aureus* includes adequate surgical drainage in those infections which have progressed to abscess formation and active supportive therapy with heat, rest, and elevation of the affected part. A spreading cellulitis is occasionally seen with staphylococcal infections and should be treated vigorously with appropriate antibiotic therapy. When staphylococcal infections occur in postoperative incisions, the wound should be opened widely to facilitate free drainage of the purulent material. Drainage is promoted by loosely packing the abscess cavity with fine mesh or iodoform gauze at the time of drainage. Antibiotic therapy in all cases

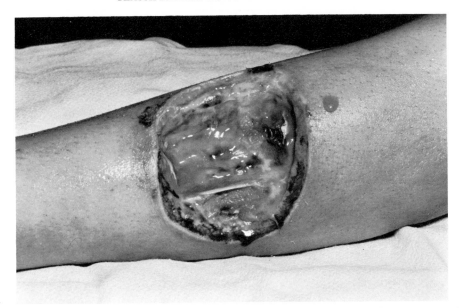

Figure 2. Acute postoperative localized wound infection caused by the hemolytic *Staphylococcus aureus*. Note thick creamy pus.

should be started at or before the time of operation for the establishment of drainage. The preferred route of administration depends upon the clinical circumstance.

STREPTOCOCCAL INFECTIONS. A variety of streptococcal organisms produce infections seen in surgical practice. The most frequent of these is *Streptococcus pyogenes* (Group A, beta hemolytic), although others such as *Streptococcus viridans* (alpha hemolytic), *Streptococcus anaerobicus*, microaerophilic Streptococcus and *Streptococcus faecalis* (Group D enterococci) may be encountered.

The lesions caused by *Streptococcus pyogenes* are characteristically invasive with a rapid course (Fig. 3). Full-blown infections are often seen within 12 to 24 hours after the time of contamination, but may occur as late

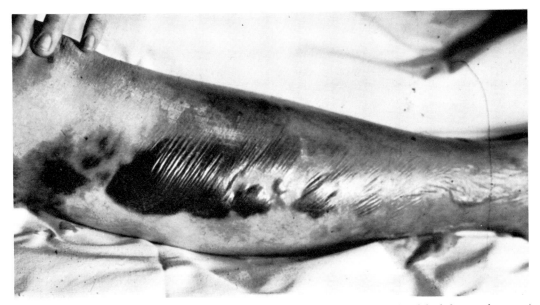

Figure 3. Acute far-advanced hemolytic streptococcal cellulitis of lower leg associated with high fever and prostration. Note patchy necrosis of skin and bullae.

as one or two weeks. The infections are characterized by diffuse cellulitis, lymphangitis, lymphadenitis, and extension of the inflammation along fascial planes. A thin watery pus may develop, but frank abscess formation rarely occurs. Gangrenous processes may be caused by thrombosis of small vessels. Bacteremia occurs rather frequently, and is usually heralded by the development of chills, high fever, a rapid, thready pulse, and general signs of toxemia.

Several specific disease syndromes are related to streptococcal infection. Among these are erysipelas, which is most often produced by *Streptococcus hemolyticus*. It usually occurs in the epifascial tissues and skin, although it may develop at other sites of trauma or surgical incision. After an incubation period of one to three days, fever, chills, rapid pulse, and severe toxemia develop, associated with a spreading superficial cellulitis which has a characteristic appearance with an indurated, raised, and irregular margin. These are often self-limited and improvement is seen within a period of four to eight days.

Acute, recurrent lymphangitis may also result from infection with *Streptococcus pyogenes*, which usually has its portal of entry through small cracks in the skin. This syndrome is characterized by a sudden onset of high fever, chills, and painful swelling of the leg with regional adenopathy.

Surgical scarlet fever occurs with a typical scarlatiniform erruption two to four days after injury or operation, and results from local wound infection by the hemolytic Streptococcus which produces the erythrogenic toxin.

Streptococcal gangrene is a spreading, invasive, epifascial, and subcutaneous infection which usually occurs in the lower extremities, and is associated with thrombosis of nutrient vessels and slough of the overlying skin. The development of clear, bullous lesions which later coalesce and become filled with hemorrhagic fluid is typical. Necrotizing fasciitis caused by the Streptococcus is occasionally associated with cutaneous gangrene. Treatment of this condition is dependent upon wide surgical incision and drainage in association with adjuvant antibiotic therapy. A chronic type of infection may develop with multiple draining sinuses intercommunicating with areas of underlying necrotic fascia.

The microaerophilic Streptococcus causes infections which develop and progress relatively slowly. Chronic burrowing ulcer and chronic progressive cutaneous gangrene are both results of infection by this type of organism. The former is characterized by surface ulcerations and communicating and burrowing sinus tracts. In both conditions, there are minimal signs of systemic toxicity, but marked pain at the site of infection is characteristic. Radical incision and drainage or excision is almost invariably necessary for eradication of the infection. Without surgical treatment, antibiotic therapy is inadequate.

INFECTIONS CAUSED BY GRAM-NEGATIVE BACILLI. A variety of gram-negative bacteria indigenous to the genitourinary and gastrointestinal tracts of humans may cause surgical infection. Wound infection by these organisms usually results from operative contamination of spilled gastrointestinal content and may be related to improper surgical technique. In other instances of wound infection or invasive systemic infection, these organisms act as opportunistic invaders, and most frequently cause infection when there is impairment of the host defense mechanism as previously discussed. They are frequent pathogens when there has been bacterial contamination from exogenous sources of incompletely removed devitalized tissue in burns, and in infections associated with perforations of the gastrointestinal or genitourinary tract (Fig. 4). Gram-negative infections are often polymicrobic, with both anaerobic and aerobic organisms, but are often not recognized as such because anaerobic cultures are infrequently done on a routine basis in clinical practice. Postoperative wound infections caused by enteric bacilli usually have a longer incubation period than those caused by the Staphylococcus or Streptococcus. Surgical treatment of these infections, like those caused by gram-positive organisms, includes the establishment of free drainage with the administration of antibiotic agents as indicated.

Infections with a species of Bacteroides may be associated with thrombophlebitis developing in regional veins adjacent to areas of infection or in systemic veins such as the iliofemoral, and are thought to be related to the heparinase activity of the organism. Occasionally, there is no other local clinical or pathological change to suggest infection by this organism, and it is discovered only by blood culture or culture of the thrombus. Treatment should include the administration of anticoagulants and tetracycline and surgical removel of the thrombi. When only protoplastic or L-forms of the organism are present, bacterial diagnosis is particularly difficult.

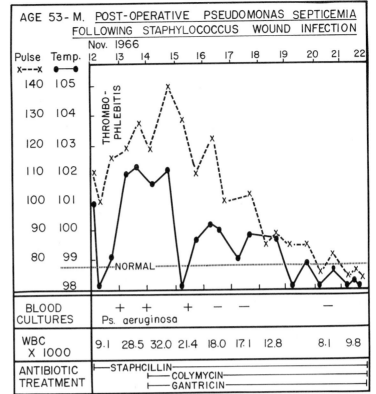

Figure 4. Chart showing course of 53-year-old diabetic male with *Pseudomonas aeruginosa* septicemia complicating acute thrombophlebitis of arm related to continuous intravenous infusion. Recovery followed appropriate antibiotic therapy.

CLOSTRIDIAL INFECTIONS. Infections with anaerobic clostridial organisms may cause three diseases of major consequence in surgical practice. These are gas gangrene, or clostridial myositis, clostridial cellulitis, and tetanus.

Clostridial cellulitis is a serious septic process of areolar tissues caused by one or more of the Clostridia, most commonly *Clostridium welchii*. The infection is characterized by a crepitant cellulitis which spreads rapidly along fascial planes. Eventually, necrosis and sloughing of aerolar tissues, fascia, and skin may occur as a result of thrombosis of neighboring blood vessels (Fig. 5). Pain about the wound is characteristic, as is a gray or reddish-brown discharge. The symptoms associated with clostridial cellulitis are similar to those of clostridial myositis but occur to a lesser degree. Treatment should include extensive surgical decompression with elevation of skin flaps superficial to the fascia and the administration of systemic antibiotic agents, usually penicillin and one of the tetracyclines.

Clostridial myositis primarily involves muscle with a spreading gangrene and profound toxemia. A rapidly fatal course may be followed in the absence of prompt therapy. This lesion is usually associated with delayed or inadequate surgical care. The chief etiologic agents are *Clostridium welchii*, *Clostridium novyi*, *Clostridium septicum*, and *Clostridium sordellii*. Gas formation with crepitation

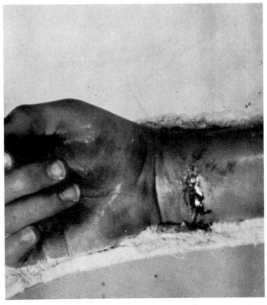

Figure 5. Gas gangrene of forearm and arm secondary to compound fracture-dislocation of the right wrist. Crepitation was evident.

within the muscles is characteristic, but may be absent. Swelling and pain occur early, usually within the first 24 hours after injury. The infected muscle becomes soft, swollen, and dark red. There is frequently a foul-smelling, brown, watery exudate. Early diagnosis is facilitated by examination of the discharge which usually contains many large gram-positive rods and usually without spores. Prostration is often far out of proportion to the fever. The patient may develop listlessness, profuse sweating, and a grayish pallor. Stupor and delirium occur as the disease progresses. Marked anemia may develop. Surgical treatment should be prompt with extensive decompression of all involved muscle compartments by incision and fasciotomy, or amputation of the part if irreversible gangrenous changes have developed in the extremity. The toxemia associated with gas gangrene is related primarily to the exotoxins produced by the Clostridia, but antitoxin therapy directed toward neutralizing these toxins in clinical practice has been relatively ineffective. Although antibiotic therapy cannot be depended upon to prevent gas gangrene or to cure an established infection, its use is recommended as an adjunctive measure to surgical operation.

Tetanus, caused by the *Clostridium tetani*, is another serious anaerobic infection. It is unusual in that the entire clinical disease is caused by a powerful exotoxin released by the growing bacteria, the toxin being one of the most potent known to man. The incubation period varies from four to 21 or more days. A prodromal period is often seen at the onset of the illness, being characterized by restlessness, yawning, headache, stiffness of the jaw muscles, and tetanic intermittent contractions in the region of the wound. Tonic spasm of the skeletal muscles with generalized tetanus usually follows within 12 to 24 hours and causes the classic facial distortion, opisthotonos and rigidity. Clonic contractions may result from the slightest stimulation, and respiratory arrest may occur suddenly in association with these convulsive seizures. A rapid pulse, sweating, and salivation are accompanying symptoms. There is seldom depression of mental acuity, making it a particularly agonizing disease to the patient. Death usually results from respiratory arrest.

Treatment is best directed toward prevention, both by proper surgical therapy of wounds and through a program of active or passive immunization as previously indicated. The established disease is treated by local and intravenous administration of tetanus antitoxin and local excision or debridement of the wound as soon as possible. Since the availability of human tetanus antitoxin, treatment as well as prophylaxis has been more effective. External stimuli must be kept to a minimum, and medical personnel must be in constant attendance so that respiratory arrest may be immediately treated when it develops. The convulsive seizures may be difficult to control, but pentobarbital sodium used carefully as a continuous intravenous drip has proven to be most useful. Nasotracheal intubation and tracheostomy are to be done as indicated to preserve the airway and support artificial or assisted respiration. Curare-like drugs may be of benefit. Antibiotic therapy is of no value in the treatment of established tetanus per se,. but may be helpful in preventing or controlling associated or complicating infections.

MIXED BACTERIAL INFECTIONS. The human bite is an example of a serious infection of mixed bacterial etiology.

The introduction of human saliva into a puncture wound which contains crushed tissue, either as a result of a cut on the fist by the teeth of an intended victim or by deliberate biting, may be followed by the development of an unusually severe infection involving the skin and underlying subcutaneous tissues, fascia, tendon, joint, and bone. These infections are almost always polymicrobic, and oral spirochetes usually participate with other aerobic and anaerobic mouth bacteria to produce a synergistic lesion. Prevention is again the most effective treatment. The recent bite wound should be left open after its thorough debridement, the part immobilized with a dressing incorporating a splint, and antibiotic therapy instituted. Primary tenorrhaphy or neurorrhaphy should not be attempted. If a human bite infection develops, it is usually characterized by high fever, marked swelling and tenderness, and a thick, foul-smelling, purulent exudate associated with necrosis of the underlying areolar and fibrous tissues. Radical surgical decompression, systemic antibiotic therapy, and purposeful splinting of the parts are necessary for treatment.

NONCLOSTRIDIAL CREPITANT CELLULITIS. This mixed infection usually is found as a complication of wounds which have been contaminated by gastrointestinal or genitourinary discharges. A wide variety of etiologic agents have been associated with this condition, including the anaerobic Bacteroides, the anaerobic Streptococcus, and many strains of the coliform group. The infection is characterized by necrosis of the areolar and fascial tissues with progressive gangrenous

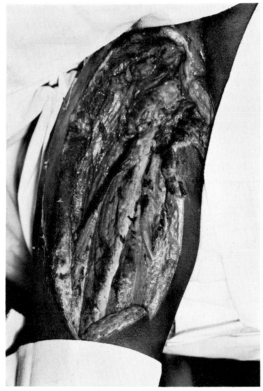

Figure 6. Mixed aerobic and anaerobic infection of medial posterior aspect of thigh complicating rectal injury. The bacterial flora included the anaerobic *Streptococcus* and the *Bacteroides melanigenicum* which contributed to the grayish-black discoloration of the infected tissues.

changes in the skin secondary to thrombosis of nutrient vessels. Crepitation of the wound results from the formation of gas by the bacteria. Surgical decompression with extensive surgical incisions, combined with intensive antibiotic therapy, is recommended for control of this condition (Fig. 6).

SYNERGISTIC GANGRENE. The chronic progressive cutaneous gangrene first described by Meleney is an infrequent but important type of infection caused by the synergistic action of the aerobic hemolytic *Staphylococcus aureus* and a microaerophilic nonhemolytic Streptococcus. It usually complicates wounds or incisions after an incubation period of one to two weeks. It is characterized by a wide area of bright red cellulitis with a purplish central area which finally becomes gangrenous and ulcerates. The ulceration gradually enlarges as its purplish-black and very painful margin extends peripherally. Treatment depends upon correct diagnosis and should include radical excision of the ulcerated lesion, systemic antibiotic therapy with penicillin or erythromycin, and delayed skin grafting. Local bacitracin therapy may be of some value before or following excision.

Similar lesions may be caused by the synergistic action of a microaerophilic Streptococcus with other strains of bacteria such as Proteus.

PERITONITIS AND ABSCESS. Infections which follow perforation of the gastrointestinal or genitourinary tract or from contamination of their contents are frequently polymicrobic, and many combinations of etiologic agents have been found. As many as four, five, or more different types of aerobic and anaerobic bacteria have been cultured simultaneously from the same wound. The synergistic action between an anaerobic Streptococcus and a Bacteroides species occurs with considerable frequency. This may not be appreciated because the Bacteroides are anaerobic organisms which are difficult to culture and identify.

MYCOTIC INFECTIONS. **Actinomycosis.** Infections caused by *Actinomyces bovis* occur infrequently but may present particularly challenging diagnostic and therapeutic problems. The lesion is typically a burrowing infection characterized by suppuration and discharge of pus through multiple sinus tracts (Fig. 7). Sulfur granules are characteristically found in the purulent discharge and their identification may be a valuable aid in diagnosis. Three principal forms of infection are recognized clinically: the cervicofacial, thoracic, and abdominal. All may be associated with extensive burrowing sinuses and cutaneous fistulae. Treatment involves incision and drainage of abscesses and pro-

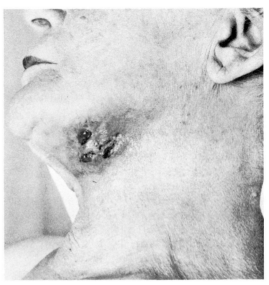

Figure 7. Cervicofacial actinomycosis with granuloma and multiple draining sinus tracts. Diagnosis established by demonstration of sulfur granules in hanging drop preparation and by anaerobic cultivation of *Actinomyces bovis*.

longed therapy with penicillin and sulfadiazine or another antibiotic regimen.

Blastomycosis. Blastomycosis is usually a progressive, indolent, cutaneous infection with ulceration caused by yeast-like organisms, the Blastomycetes. It is characterized by a chronic ulceration with multiple small daughter abscesses along the advancing margin and a tendency for central healing of the lesions as the margins progress. Systemic spread with distant metastases may occur, giving a grave prognosis. Radical excision with skin grafting of the cutaneous lesion is recommended. In systemic lesions stilbamidine or large doses of sodium or potassium iodine may be of benefit.

Moniliasis. Primary infections by *Monilia albicans* are encountered infrequently in normal and diabetic individuals, but this pathogen is being seen in recent years with increasing frequency as an opportunistic invader. Secondary infections with this organism are particularly prone to occur in patients receiving intensive or prolonged broad-spectrum antibiotic therapy, especially in patients already debilitated by their underlying disease. Control of the diabetes, if present, is essential. Amphotericin B is used in treatment of systemic infections, and topical application of gentian violet or nystatin may be useful for local infections.

Other fungi. Infections caused by other fungi are occasionally encountered in the practice of surgery, such as coccidioidomycosis and sporotrichosis. Coccidioidomycosis, caused by *Coccidioides immitis* usually occurs as a pulmonary infection resembling pulmonary tuberculosis. Diagnosis is usually possible through recognition of the organisms in smears of sputum or local discharges and in biopsied material. Skin sensitivity tests may be helpful.

Sporotrichosis, caused by *Sporotrichum schenckii*, is a rare disease which follows contamination of a wound, usually on the extremities. It is characterized by a primary area of ulceration, regional nodular lymphangitis, and secondary ulcerations along the course of the involved lymphatic. Systemic invasion is very rare. Treatment with large doses of potassium iodide solution is usually effective. Systemic infections with Asperigillus as an opportunistic invader are also seen occasionally in debilitated patients.

Viral infections. The most important viral infection of surgical significance is rabies. Rabies is a fatal encephalitis caused by a neurotropic virus which is inoculated by means of a bite from another animal. It has been reported after bites from a variety of domestic as well as wild animals. The incubation period varies between two weeks and several months, and is related to the distance between the site of injury and the brain. The established disease is characterized by maniacal excitement and paralysis of the muscles of deglutition, followed by agitation and finally stupor. Established rabies is invariably fatal and the only means of treatment is through prophylaxis. Wounds caused from the bite of any suspected animal should be cleansed and debrided thoroughly. Whenever possible, the animal responsible for the bite should be impounded and observed for at least 14 days. If it has been killed, the brain should be examined for the presence of rabies virus particles. When the animal cannot be impounded or examined, a series of rabies vaccinations should be administered to the patient.

READING REFERENCES

Alexander, J. W.: Immune mechanisms of gram-negative infections. S. Clin. North America 47:1235, 1967.

Altemeier, W. A., and Culbertson, W. R.: Acute non-clostridial crepitant cellulitis. Surg. Gyn. & Obst. 87:206, 1948.

Altemeier, W. A., and Furste, W. L.: Gas gangrene. Internat. Abstr. Surg.; in Surg. Gyn. & Obst. 84:507, 1947.

Altemeier, W. A., and Wulsin, J. H.: Antimicrobial therapy in injured patients. J.A.M.A. 173:527, 1960.

Dowling, H. F., Lepper, M. H., and Jackson, G. G.: The clinical significance of antimicrobial resistant bacteria. J.A.M.A. 157:327, 1955.

Edsall, G.: Current status of tetanus immunization. Arch. Environ. Health 8:731, 1964.

Hill, E. O., Altemeier, W. A., and Culbertson, W. R.: An appraisal of methods of testing bacterial sensitivity to antibiotics. Ann. Surg. 148:410, 1958.

Mulholland, J. H. (ed.): Postoperative wound infection: the influence of ultraviolet irradiation of the operating room and of various other factors. Report of an Ad Hoc Committee of the Committee on Trauma, Division of Medical Sciences, National Academy of Sciences, National Research Council. Ann. Surg. 160, 1964, Supplement, pp. 1-192.

Pulaski, E. J.: Surgical Infections. Springfield, Illinois, Charles C Thomas, 1954.

Suter, E., and Ramseier, H.: Cellular reactions in infection. In, Dixon, F. J., Jr., and Humphrey, J. H. (eds.): Advances in Immunology. New York, Academic Press, 1964, pp. 117-173.

Wilson, G. S., and Miles, A. A.: Topley and Wilson's Principles of Bacteriology and Immunity. 5th ed. Baltimore, Williams & Wilkins Co., 1964.

Zweifach, B. W., Grant, L., and McCluskey, R. T. (eds.): The Inflammatory Process. New York, Academic Press, 1965, pp. 161-353, 449-463.

Chapter 4

ONCOLOGY

by
GEORGE E. MOORE, M.D.
and
ROBERT K. AUSMAN, M.D.

GEORGE EUGENE MOORE was born in Minneapolis. He received his premedical, medical and postgraduate surgical education at the University of Minnesota. As Director and Chief of Surgery at Roswell Park Memorial Institute in Buffalo, New York, he heads one of the first, and now one of the largest, groups to focus on the study of tumors. His present research includes the culture of human hematopoietic cells, chemotherapy and tobacco-product carcinogenesis. During his directorship, a dull state institution has become an active health center with a widespread reputation for leadership in cancer research and treatment. Dr. Moore flies airplanes and plays touch football and volley ball to balance his output of concentrated energy in the operating room and research.

ROBERT K. AUSMAN was educated at Marquette University in his native city, Milwaukee, Wisconsin. He was a research assistant during his last two years in medical school. He received his postgraduate education at the University of Minnesota, where he was a medical fellow in the Department of Surgery. He is engaged in cancer research at the Roswell Park Memorial Institute and is an Associate Professor of Pharmacology, University of Buffalo.

INTRODUCTION

The malignant diseases have some unique characteristics which affect the diagnosis and treatment of these illnesses.

Cancer can be considered as one disease with protean manifestations depending on the tissue of origin, or as a group of diseases with many factors playing an etiological role. The spectrum of malignancies is broader than that of infectious diseases. Cancers may grow very slowly or be as rapidly lethal as many bacteria, remaining dormant for decades like *Mycobacterium tuberculosis*, or appearing as growths similar to local or spreading infections in the blood and lymphatics, even with inflammatory changes mimicking the hemolytic streptococcus.

The varied and unpredictable behavior of cancers makes it difficult to give a succinct and accurate definition. Ambrose and Roc have offered the following description which has the virtue of utility: "Cancer is a disease of multicellular organisms which is characterized by the seemingly uncontrolled multiplication and spread within the organism of apparently abnormal forms of the organism's own cells."

Autonomy, atypical morphology, invasiveness and abnormal cellular multiplication are common properties of malignant diseases. An accelerated growth rate alone does not identify a cell as malignant. Elements of the bone marrow and the lining of the gastrointestinal tract may multiply faster than a cancer, but the progeny is subject to both inherent and host controls. Epithelial cells adjacent to a skin laceration are stimulated to divide rapidly and migrate long distances from the normal epithelium, but as soon as the wound is covered, mitotic activity slows and normal activity returns. Malignant cells, however, may overgrow normal tissue structures, form huge amorphous masses of undifferentiated cells, parasitize the local blood supply and stimulate new vessel formation, and invade blood and lymphatic vessels and the serous cavities.

Features of malignant cells which permit unbridled growth include modified growth inhibition when contact is made with neighboring cells, ameboid movement, short mitotic cycles, and nutritional and environmental adaptability. Host resistance may be defective. There are many other aspects which have been studied for decades without full clarification, such as "toxic substances," which may cause debilitation of the host disproportionate to the size and site of the tumor.

A host can defend itself against cancer cells. For example, some thyroid cancers may produce enough thyroxine to inhibit the production of pituitary thyrotropic hormone. Other cancer cells appear to change to benign forms. There is evidence for host resistance to malignant cells. In a different way, the host mediates some control over hormone-dependent tumors. The physician may use the same mechanism for effective therapy in certain human tumors (Table 1).

Table 1. *Frequent Tumors Subject to Hormone Therapy*

PRIMARY TUMOR	HORMONE THERAPY
Breast	Estrogen, androgen
Prostate	Estrogen
Endometrium	Progesterone
Thyroid	Thyroid hormone

ETIOLOGY OF THE MALIGNANT DISEASES

There is a substantial body of information concerning the environmental and genetic causes of human cancers. Just as one cannot expect a single kind of bacterium to produce all infectious diseases, it is not reasonable to anticipate a single cause of cancer. It is possible that a common pathway exists through which all malignant transformation occurs, although this theory is not supported by current evidence. Actually, the major theories of etiology overlap considerably, an observation which is immediately apparent to everyone but the sponsors of these concepts.

One of the oldest theories postulated that undifferentiated cells or "embryonic rests" retained the ability to proliferate as cancers at any time during life. Portions of this theory are considered valid; for example, Wilms' tumor. The teratomas and teratocarcinomas, examples which were used as initial support, are interesting but unique phenomena. Many cells in the body do retain the ability to divide rapidly and differentiate into cells with various functions, just like embryonic cells. There is, however, no correlation between the incidence of malignancy and the number of such cells. For example, malignancies of myeloid cells are relatively rare, despite their rapid and continuous differentiation and proliferation into mature blood cells. Malignancies also develop in tissues in which cellular proliferation is relatively slow, such as the brain and the breast.

GENETIC FACTORS. There are numerous major and minor theses concerned with aber-

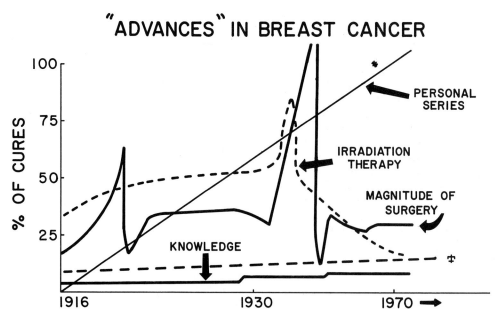

"ADVANCES" IN BREAST CANCER

% OF CURES

PERSONAL SERIES

IRRADIATION THERAPY

MAGNITUDE OF SURGERY

KNOWLEDGE

1916   1930   1970 →

* CURES / PATIENTS SEEN / MINUS UNCOOPERATIVE, LOST AND "UNSUITABLE" ONES

☩ VALID CLINICAL STUDIES

rant genetic alterations or mutations of cells, or the inheritance of gene-associated causal factors and cancer susceptibility. Epidemiological studies of the role of heredity are extremely difficult because of the heterogeneity of human populations. Only several rare types of cancer, or precursors such as retinoblastoma, neurofibromatosis, and familial polyposis of the colon, follow simple mendelian laws; these cancers are probably related to a single dominant gene. Other kinds of cancer can be traced directly to a unique inherited susceptibility of an organ system, such as the predilection to skin cancers in youngsters with albinism and xeroderma pigmentosum if they are exposed to ultraviolet light.

There are many studies in which the incidence of cancers of the breast, stomach, colon, prostate, and uterine cervix has been reported to be higher in close relatives. It is difficult to assess these data in view of the finding that a disproportionate incidence of the same cancer rarely occurs in identical twins. However, in most instances, these increases in incidence probably represent an enhancement in susceptibility and, perhaps, exposure to similar environmental factors such as diet and viruses.

There are many other significant differences in incidence figures among various countries, which probably reflect environmental factors rather than a national susceptibility. For example, the Japanese experience breast cancer infrequently but have a very high incidence of cervical and gastric cancer.

Unfortunately, environmental causes or genetic factors often are not considered as causal because the genetic theories are cited without substantial supportive evidence; therefore, preventive measures are not sought. Gastric cancer was thought by many to be an example of an inevitable kind of malignancy which accompanied old age. No cause, or causes, of stomach cancer could be found, although there was disturbing evidence that the incidence of this disease varied widely among countries. In the last few decades, however, the incidence rates for gastric cancer have been dropping rapidly. Thus, it is clear that this kind of cancer was not directly associated with aging but was the result of environmental factors.

The development of aberrant cells with malignant properties is a result of somatic mutations, the loss of control genes, gene depletion, chromosome abnormalities, and faulty duplication of chromosomes, which have been suggested as major causes of malignant transformation. In support is the finding of Moorhead that almost all chronic myelogenous leukemia cells had an abnormally small autosome, the so-called Philadelphia chromosome. Hungerford and Nowell have observed this abnormally small autosome only in the bone marrow of three-fourths of patients with chronic myelogenous leukemia. A French scientist discovered that trisomy of one of the smallest chromosomes was associated with mongolism or Down's disease. Children thus afflicted have an incidence of leukemia 18 times that of other children.

No definite causal relationship has been established between chromosomal defects and solid tumors. Because each chromosome may contain 25,000 to 75,000 genes, it is understandable that significant deletions, alterations, or additions of genetic material might take place without detectable structural changes.*

INFECTIOUS AGENTS. There are many varied theories concerning the premise that infectious agents transmit abnormal genetic material into susceptible cells and alter the genome of the cells, thereby conferring the property of malignancy upon them, and either remain part of the genome of the daughter cells or disappear.

In the past, suspected agents included other cells, bacteria, parasites, mycoplasma, and viruses. The first virus-induced malignant tumor of animals was reported by Ellerman and Bang in 1908. Subsequent classic studies have followed.

1908 — chicken — leukosis — Ellerman and Bang
1911 — chicken — sarcoma — Rous
1932 — rabbit — fibroma — Shope
1936 — mouse — mammary — Bittner
1951 — mouse — leukemia — Gross
1958 — hamster — multiple tumors — Stewart-Eddy polyoma virus
1962 — man — lymphoma — Burkitt-Epstein
1962-1966 — 70 species — 150 tumors — many authors

---

* The concept of the role of nucleic acids in cancer biology has been further complicated by the finding of deoxyribonucleic acid in various cell organelles, such as mitochondria. Clarification of the involvement of extrachromosomal genetic aberrations and cytoplasmic influences on protein metabolism in malignant cells will require new methodology.

Many important discoveries of methods, assays, and biochemical relationships made these findings possible. Since 1962, there has been a pandemic of tumor-virus research. Studies of the possible viral etiology of human malignancies have been focused on the leukemias and lymphomas. Following Burkitt's description of an unusual lympho-sarcoma principally affecting children in certain regions of Africa, and the suggestion that the disease occurred principally in hot, humid areas at low altitudes, a search for an insect vector was begun. Subsequently, similar lymphomas were recognized in other countries, including the United States. Epstein established cell lines from the Burkitt tumors which contained a herpes-type virus particle. In 1964, Iwakata and Grace successfully cultured myelogenous leukemia cells which had a similar or identical virus. Since then, cultured cells obtained from other human leukemias and lymphomas, and even from normal persons, have been found to contain a morphologically similar virus.

Nonetheless, the basic mechanisms involved in virus-induced malignant transformations are still unknown. No human cancer definitely can be said to be caused by a virus, and those viruses which have been isolated from human tumors may be merely passengers. Despite these facts, we personally have the opinion that viruses will be found to cause a few kinds of human cancers.

It is noteworthy that some of the key studies have been made by surgeons.

PHYSICAL AND CHEMICAL CARCINOGENIC AGENTS. In 1775, a London surgeon, Percival Potts, made the observation that chimney sweeps had an unusual form of malignancy, cancer of the scrotum, and that it was probably the result of constant exposure to soot.

In 1917, two Japanese scientists, Yamagiwa and Ichikawa, induced squamous carcinomas on the ears of rabbits by painting them with coal tar over a period of many months. Kensaway isolated benzopyrene from coal tar in 1930 and demonstrated that it was a powerful carcinogenic agent. At the time, it was felt that the synthesis and assay of related hydrocarbons would prove extremely valuable in relation to carcinogenesis. Unfortunately, the prospect has not come to fruition.

During this period, clinical observations revealed a growing number of other cancer-producing agents, some of which are listed in Table 2.

Table 2. *Significant Human Carcinogens*

AGENT	IMPORTANT SITE OF DISEASE
Social	
Cigarette smoking	Lung, bladder, larynx
Pipe smoking	Lip, oral cavity
Snuff chewing	Oral cavity
Occupational	
Arsenic compounds	Skin
Asbestos	Lung
Benzene	Bone marrow
Coal tar and related tars and oils	Skin
Chromium compounds	Nasal passages
2-Napthylamine and related aromatic amines	Bladder
Nickel compounds	Nasal passages
Radioactive ores	Lung
X-rays	Bone marrow, skin
Medical	
Arsenic compounds	Skin
X-ray, radioactive isotopes	Thyroid, bone marrow, skin
Geographic	
Ultraviolet light (sun)	Skin

One of the agents studied most thoroughly is radiation. The first x-ray-caused cancer was a squamous carcinoma on the hand of a research physicist seven years after the remarkable discovery of radium by the Curies. Subsequently, many pioneer scientists and radiologists died from irradiation injuries and malignancies. Even the tragic deaths of the women who painted watch dials with radium, using their lips to point the brushes, were not believed by all to be caused by radioactivity. Radiologists continued to protect themselves and their patients inadequately, and scientists operating radon plants and handling other therapeutic devices, such as radium packs, continued to die of leukemia or lymphomas, and sustain damages and cancers to the hands and hematopoietic system.

The development of nuclear devices for warfare and industrial use revitalized studies of radiation biology. From a scientific standpoint, much has been learned about the injury to various cells—increased mutation rates, fragmentation of chromosomes, and physical alterations in the nucleic acids as a consequence of direct hits with ionizing energy. Even more perplexing and amazing is the ability of cells to recover and effect repairs following sporadic exposure to irradiation.

In recent years, the use of tobacco and its relationship to several malignant diseases have been the subject of widespread discussion and controversy. A majority of the estimated 300,000 premature deaths each year among heavy smokers are the result of cardiovascular and pulmonary diseases. However, it is well established that over 40,000 men who are heavy cigarette smokers die each year from lung cancer. In addition, there is an increased incidence of cancer of the urinary bladder and cancer of the intrinsic larynx among heavy cigarette smokers. The smoking of pipes and cigars is less dangerous because of the usual inability of smokers to inhale the smoke into the bronchi.

In 1936, Ochsner observed that many lung cancer patients were heavy cigarette smokers. In 1950, two independent reports, by Wynder and Graham and by Levin, provided valid evidence of an association between cigarette smoking and lung cancer. Over 100 additional clinical studies from various countries have verified these observations. This problem also has important public health aspects. As a matter of clinical importance, most lung lesions in a heavy cigarette smoker, revealed by x-ray, are bronchogenic cancers.

From a biological standpoint, the occurrence of premalignant and malignant changes in the mucosal surfaces exposed repeatedly to tobacco or smoke is interesting. Tobacco chewers develop lesions of the lips, mouth and extrinsic larynx. These cancers are a predominant cause of death in India, Ceylon and other parts of the world where the chewing of tobacco, betel nut, and other similar substances begins during childhood.

The carcinogenic activity of tobacco smoke has been confirmed by inducing cancerous lesions in mice, rats, hamsters, rabbits, and dogs. Approximately one-third of mice painted daily with tobacco smoke develop skin cancers and over one-half develop papillomas and other precancerous changes.

PATHOGENESIS

Great harm may be done by clinicians who generalize about tumor development, growth rates, and interaction with the host. It is true that a surgeon must decide whether a lesion is a slow-growing, circumscribed cancer or a tumor which is often systemically distributed by the time it is diagnosed. Through the years, most tests of the degree of malignancy of a tumor have proved inadequate. Surgeons should plan therapy accordingly, always regarding tumors as being more malignant than

they appear. Further, the surgeon who treats cancer patients must have some knowledge of cancer pathogenesis.

THE SPREAD OF CANCER

Various cancers spread into adjacent tissues, displace normal structures by their growth, or infiltrate nerves, lymphatics, blood vessels, and body cavities. The predominant kind of invasion depends upon the site of the lesion and the characteristics of the tumor cells. The plural form "cells" was used purposely, because most cancers are made up of cells with many different characteristics despite their identification as a uniform kind of cancer. Some cells may divide rapidly, as often as every 20 hours, whereas others may have generation times of several days. Some cancer cells are dependent for survival upon their attachment to the primary growth, whereas others are autonomous units capable of independent maturation and further dissemination. The slow-growing and dependent cells generally have more differentiated characteristics of the related normal cell, whereas the rapidly growing cell frequently is undifferentiated, with a large nucleus and nucleoli and little cytoplasm.

Many malignant cells retain the primitive ability of ameboid movement which aids the invasion of tissue spaces. Cell culture techniques have been used to demonstrate the migration of cancerous cells. In both experimental and clinical specimens, cancer cells penetrating the walls of blood vessels have been detected.

Another characteristic of many cancer cells is the lessening of mutual cohesiveness, permitting detachment of individual cells. A related characteristic is the lack of growth inhibition when two cancer cells contact each other. This lack of inherent control is one of the qualitative aspects of cancer cells which has not yet been clarified. In cultures, the multiplication of benign cells slows when they touch adjacent cellular membranes, whereas cancer cells continue to multiply and build up layers and clusters.

Various hormones can promote, as well as inhibit, the growth of some tumors. For example, thyroid cancer cells which have retained some of the characteristics of normal thyroid cells can be stimulated by the thyrotropic hormone and conversely inhibited by excessive amounts of thyroxine and related analogues. Androgens and estrogens also play a role in the treatment of breast cancer and prostatic cancer.

Finally, there are systemic host factors and presumably immunological factors and local factors, such as selective antagonism to cancer cells by normal cells, which have not been identified clearly. Although clinical observations provide evidences of such defenses, it must be remembered that nearly all cancers in most hosts are progressive diseases.

On occasion, established cancers undergo spontaneous cures; the number of these cures is extremely small, but important.

Certain seemingly malignant tumors change to benign growths by maturation, as is seen in some neuroblastomas.

Cancer cells can remain viable in the body for years and then develop with explosive growth at many sites. Cancer of the breast provides examples of the dormancy of cancer cells; the longest recorded interval before recurrence of breast cancer is 46 years. Certainly, some general factor seems to be involved, because literally hundreds of metastases may start to grow at the same time in various parts of the body. Instances have been seen in which regrowth at multiple metastatic sites followed therapy with cortisone and irradiation, but no satisfactory experimental models for these provocative observations have been developed.

Regrettably, instances have been noted in which the use of toxic and relatively ineffective chemotherapeutic agents has been followed by rapid growth of the malignancy. The effects of chemotherapy furnish one of the best examples of the balance of forces between the growth potential of the cancer cells and the resisting factors of the host, both local and systemic.

Rarely do metastases undergo an actual decrease in size when a large primary lesion is excised. This observation has been made most consistently for hypernephroma.

Partial remissions of malignant growths have sometimes been associated with concomitant infections by viruses or bacteria. Although such occurrences have been few in number, they are of theoretical importance.

The number of cancer cells recovered from the blood and lymph vessels is ordinarily far greater than the number of metastases that actually develop. This finding reflects the interdigitated relationship between cell viability and host resistance. Similar observations of tumor cell survival in body cavities have been made.

Cancerous tissue reimplanted in the host often fails to survive, even though other areas of the body are being overwhelmed by the same malignant growth.

Certain experimental tumors possess tumor-specific antigens capable of conferring resistance against transplantation of genetically compatible malignant cells. Some of these tumors grow progressively, despite the protective immune response. The balance of power rests with the tumor.

There must be relatively potent defense mechanisms for destroying the millions of aberrant cells that are formed daily. Surely, failure of all of these cells to survive is not due to an inherent lack of viability.

Pathologists have provided histological evidence of increased numbers and activity of histiocytic, lymphocytic, and plasmacytic cells at tumor sites and in the associated lymph nodes. These observations have been supported by experimental work in which aggressor lymphoblasts destroy tumor cells.

ROUTES OF SPREAD

LYMPHATIC.　Many epithelial cancers have a predilection to invade the lymphatics and be retained temporarily in the afferent subcapsular sinuses of the regional lymph nodes. As the capacity of one or more nodes is filled by embolic cancer cells or growth lodged in the nodes, additional lymphatic channels may dilate and divert the cells being shed from the primary site to adjacent nodes or into channels circumventing the first lymph node chain. For example, squamous carcinomas of the hand may be arrested temporarily in the epitrochlear nodes, but often they will by-pass these few nodes at the elbow and involve the axillary nodes. Less frequently, tumor cells attach themselves to walls of lymphatic channels, and the surgeon may see a chain of metastases along a major lymph vessel. This phenomenon is more common with certain kinds of aggressive cancers, such as malignant melanomas. Abnormal sites of metastases may develop distal to lymphatics blocked by tumor, or as the result of a previous operative procedure which interrupted the proximal lymphatics—for example, a groin dissection. In such instances, hundreds of metastases may develop, probably because of the stasis and perhaps more optimal environmental conditions.

As a result, several principles should govern the surgical treatments of malignant tumors.

The farther a primary cancer is situated from the regional nodes, the less worthwhile it will be to perform excisions of the tumor, lymphatic channels, and nodes in continuity.

If the nearest set of nodes is enlarged with metastatic tumor, the next set of nodes should be included in the primary treatment, if feasible.

Many tumors invade both blood vessels and lymphatics, but if there are no distant metastases evident, it is often worthwhile to perform a lymph node dissection.

If a tumor is excised at a distance from the proximal lymph nodes, a separate excision of the lymph nodes may be performed at the same time. There is no valid evidence favoring the choice of simultaneous or delayed excision of the nodes under such circumstances.

Vascular metastases. Tumors of mesenchymal origin are more apt to invade blood vessels, usually veins; again, lymphatics may also be involved. Actually a considerable number of tumor cells, from lung and stomach, for example, enter the blood by way of the thoracic duct. Pathologists often detect intravascular invasion in an excised specimen, and when present, the prognosis for the patient is usually poor.

Various investigators at the turn of the century reported an occasional tumor cell in a smear of peripheral blood; until the report of Engell in 1955, no attempts to isolate tumor cells from the blood were made. As might be expected, the largest concentration of tumor cells and cell clumps was found in the veins directly draining a tumor site. Large numbers were identified in peripheral blood samples, thus confirming clinical observations that the cells must be able to pass through or circumvent the capillary networks of the liver and lung. Undoubtedly, many of the cells traverse venous-venous and arteriovenous shunts.

Manipulation of a tumor site increases the number of tumor cells collected from regional veins. Fortunately, only a few tumor cells, or cell clumps, released into the blood survive, attach to the vascular wall, penetrate into the tissues, and establish a growing metastasis.

Invasion and growth inside nerve sheaths, in distinction to growth in the perineural lymphatics, is relatively rare, but of importance in the spread of certain tumors of the head and neck.

Body cavities. Cancers of the bronchi, or of various abdominal organs, may penetrate the serosa and exfoliate throughout the pleural or abdominal cavities. The most frequent cause of death from ovarian carcinomas is the widespread implantation of tumor cells on the surfaces of the intestines and on the parietal peritoneum. Because of the effect of gravity, metastatic growths often develop in the rectal, vaginal, and rectovesical pouches; hence, a rectal examination of any patient suspected of having an abdominal malignancy is important.

A variation of the implantation of tumor cells in the serous cavities is the spread of tumor cells in cerebrospinal fluid from tumors of the brain, meninges, and metastatic sites.

Another kind of implant occurs on the epithelial lining of the respiratory tree, intestinal tract, and urogenital system. Intact epithelial surfaces are very resistant to tumor implantation; however, if there is a denuded defect, an area of inflammation, or a mechanical break in the epithelial surface, such as a surgical wound, growth can occur.

Examples of these phenomena include the frequent recurrence of cancer at the site of anastomoses of the large bowel and in hemorrhoidectomy wounds, implants distal to oral lesions, and implants from carcinomas of the renal pelvis along the ureter and in the bladder. Unfortunately, these types of recurrence, as well as implants in wounds following radical mastectomy and biopsy excisions, all have been attributed to direct implantation, whereas many of these recurrences are probably the result of hematogenous spread of tumor cells to the injured site. For this reason, surface application of anticancer agents is not totally effective. Evidence of the hematogenous and lymphatic transportation of tumor cells to wound sites can be found in some patients who, owing to irradiation therapy, have developed hundreds of superficial skin recurrences within the confines of the area irradiated.

Much pertinent literature concerning animal experimentation in regard to the spread of tumor cells is available, but it must be remembered that tumor-host relationships are often altered drastically by various immunological incompatibilities, such as the transplantation antigens.

Factors Affecting Metastases

The distribution of metastases has been related to the mechanical trapping of tumor cells and cell clumps in lymph nodes and capillary beds and to the environment, or soil, which is particularly suited to survival and growth of tumor cells. These and many other factors determine which few of many thousands or millions of tumor cells shed daily from the primary site will survive and grow. Thus, routes of distribution are important, but even more significant are those local conditions which determine why some epithelial organs have disproportionately more metastases than, for instance, the spleen or the skeletal muscle. Many additional examples of peculiar distributions of tumor growth can be given, such as the rarity of metastases in the bones and soft tissues distal to the elbows and knees and the frequency of malignant melanoma metastases in cardiac muscle in comparison to skeletal muscle. Unfortunately, no unique property of a given tissue has been correlated with the ability to support metastases.

It appears that most cancer cells fail to survive or are actually destroyed while they are still confined to the vascular system. Highly significant for most cancer cells, perhaps even including leukemia cells, is a successful exit through the vascular endothelium. The blood is not an optimal environment, and if a method or methods could be devised to avert the penetration of these cells through the endothelium, metastases from single tumor cells would be greatly reduced. The effectiveness of anticoagulants in preventing and reducing certain experimental metastases has been demonstrated. The problem is not an easy one, because of the heterogeneous types of tumor cells and blood vessels. This aspect of cancer research has not received as much attention as it deserves.

The next challenges to survival of the invading cancer cells are humoral factors, and local, systemic, and cellular elements with the capacity to recognize and destroy the aggressor cells. This area of research has lagged until recently. Attempts are presently being made to sensitize lymphoid cells against the host's cancer in order to increase the killing power of the cells. No adequate studies of the similar or related functions of nonhematopoietic cells have been made.

SURGICAL PRINCIPLES FOR THE THERAPY OF MALIGNANCIES

Probably the single most important aspect of surgery for malignant diseases is the understanding of the probable biologic nature of the tumor and management of the diagnostic and treatment modalities in a manner which will provide a maximal chance of cure, maximal length of comfortable, useful life and minimal chance of erroneous diagnosis, useless procrastination, and purposeless therapy. An outline for the development of such a management plan is shown in Table 3.

Diagnostic Procedures

Indirect diagnostic procedures, such as physical examinations, x-ray examination, angiography, isotope scanning, and biochemical tests, may be nearly 100 per cent accurate. There are instances in which these tests, used as direct evidence of malignancy, have resulted in serious errors. Similarly, the tests should rarely be used as sole evidence of incurability. However, when these tests are used in association with a pertinent clinical history, presumptive evidence can be obtained and one can proceed efficiently toward establishing a definitive diagnosis.

We have seen intestinal abscesses (one caused by a chicken bone), gastrocolic fistulas, perforated diverticula, and many similar conditions with severe weight loss and abdominal masses, all of which simulated malignant processes threatening the patients' lives. In many instances, conservative errors were made by specialists about lesions which normally would not be handled by them.

"Rules of thumb" which were applicable before the advent of more sophisticated diagnostic procedures were often lethal to a patient. Physicians too frequently concluded, before obtaining pathological proof, that shadows, masses, and undefined acute illnesses were recurrent cancer.

PATHOLOGICAL DIAGNOSES. A most important and sensitive area of professional collaboration in a clinic or hospital in which cancer patients are treated is that between the pathologist and surgeon. There should be no clear separation of responsibility; unless members of these two departments share a great deal of overlapping responsibility, ineffective and dangerous practices will develop. Each must maintain an interest and participate actively in joint professional services. The pathologist should scrub and gown for the operating room, so that he is prepared to see and feel lesions which are puzzling and actually observe the performance of crucial biopsies, so that there is no question about the site and orientation of the

Table 3

DECISION PATTERNS IN MANAGEMENT OF MALIGNANT DISEASES

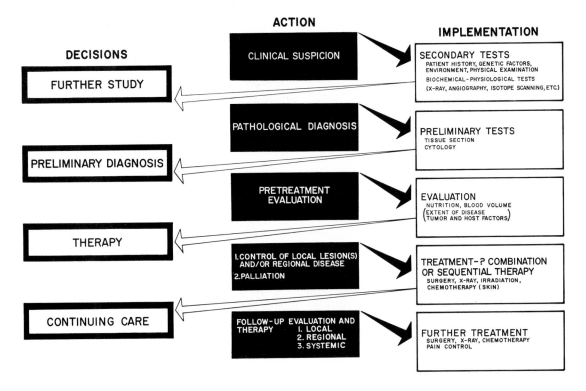

tissue. He should be acquainted with all major clinical aspects of the patients' problems.

The surgeon should continue his training in macroscopic and microscopic pathology and be able to prepare and stain imprint preparations and frozen sections. He should not unequivocally accept reports that seem incompatible with the clinical situation. The surgeon is in a far better position to plan future therapy for his patient after he reviews with his residents and pathologist the sections of tumors and related tissues which have been removed.

BIOPSIES. The procedure for obtaining sufficient tissue for a pathological diagnosis is not complicated. First, a biopsy should always be obtained if doubt exists concerning the nature of a lesion; second, a biopsy should be obtained before beginning any therapy even if there is no doubt as to the nature of the lesion. Grievous errors, which have occurred because of failure to obtain a biopsy, include radical mastectomy for fat necrosis, radical gastropancreaticoduodenectomy for localized pancreatitis, x-ray therapy for renal cysts, and amputation of feet for recurrent hypertrophy of the plantar fascia. There are

dangers associated with biopsies, but the dangers of omission are infinitely greater.

From a biological standpoint, one must realize that a biopsy of a carcinoma may spread the tumor by opening lymphatic and vascular channels leading to the escape of cancer cells. However, there is little if any valid evidence that the prognosis of a significant group of patients has been worsened in this way. Repetitive normal body movements, bumps, and self-palpation are probably even more dangerous. The dangers of hemorrhage, the spread of an associated infection, and the spillage of tumor cells can be minimized by proper planning, such as the preplacement of retention sutures, consideration of the displacement of vital structures by the tumor mass, and proper isolation of the biopsy site.

TECHNIQUES AND SPECIAL PROCEDURES. The pathologist is at a disadvantage if the tissue sample is dried out, crushed, burned, necrotic or does not include the base or junction of the tumor and normal tissue. Grasping forceps, such as the Gaylord or the Allis clamp, are helpful in avoiding crushing the specimen. Specimen bottles of various sizes should be available. Nothing is more annoying than searching for a small crumb of tissue rubbed on the side of a one-gallon container. Biopsy bottles and Silverman needles should be included in a standard surgical pack. The pathologist may not want the specimens placed in fixatives, in which instance it is important that they be sent promptly to the laboratory.

Highly recommended are routine requests for immediate diagnosis from smear or imprint preparations and stained sections which are sliced with the freezing microtome. The advantages include confirmation of the diagnosis, adequacy of the biopsy, and extent of the disease. Too many patients undergo abdominal surgery without a sufficient biopsy having been obtained. Such patients should be explored to confirm the diagnosis. The surgeon may feel a nodule in the liver and assume incorrectly that the patient is incurable. It is unorthodox to suggest that the surgeon, if he has adequate assistants, leave the operating room and view the slides himself, but such a practice has considerable value.

When possible, a questionable lesion should be excised, but if impractical, incision biopsy and, in limited instances, aspiration biopsy, should be performed. Aspiration biopsy of an enlarged liver in an elderly patient may be a better choice than a surgical procedure.

Cytological techniques are valuable for the diagnosis of malignancy, but they occupy a variable region labeled tentative on one side and confirmed on the other. Often, pathologists have been reluctant, and rightly so, to make a definite diagnosis of malignancy on the basis of individual cells rather than cells which are a part of a tissue structure. Nevertheless, the examination of vaginal smears, bronchoscopic washings, pleural and peritoneal fluid, and urine specimens for diagnostic purposes is an established practice. The surgeon must know what the pathologist means when he reports a "negative," "inadequate," "suspicious," or "positive" sample. The desirability of a confirmatory biopsy is evident.

In the future, more specific ways of determining the malignancy of cells, other than by cytology and morphology, will be found. Biochemical methods and cell culture techniques may become useful for diagnostic purposes. If certain indirect diagnostic methods, such as x-ray, could be replaced with systemic detection and screening procedures, the effect on the treatment of some cancers would be enormous.

THE CANCER PATIENT

Surgical procedures cannot be separated from planned total therapy for the patient. Nevertheless, major surgery for the control of malignancy has several special features. The surgeon must include in his excision the entire gross lesion and a margin of normal tissue in an attempt to circumscribe microscopic extension of the tumor. The operation, in certain instances, must be designed to include adjacent lymph node bearing areas in continuity, if possible. The surgeon may be forced to alter, or even withdraw from, his initial operative plan once or perhaps several times, depending upon his judgment and the diagnosis by frozen section of the extent of the tumor. At present, there is a wave of popularity for conservative surgery. In general, surgeons must remember that it is far better to proceed with a curative procedure, unless there is absolute proof, usually histological proof, that the lesion has extended or metastasized beyond resection boundaries.

Often the physical condition of cancer patients is relatively poor. Many malignancies seem to have a toxic effect on the host disproportionate to the size of the lesion(s). A patient may have an adverse nutritional status because of interference with normal functions of the oral pharynx, esophagus, and intestinal tract and associated glandular organs. Pain may contribute to anorexia and severe electrolyte disorders. Anemia, vitamin deficiencies, and defects in the coagulation mechanisms must be corrected before an operation can be safely performed.

As in other types of surgery, impaired cardiovascular, pulmonary, renal, and hepatic functions may require modification of planned surgical therapy.

A major consideration, and one that is most likely to be overlooked or misjudged, is the mental status of the patient. This factor is particularly critical with aged persons. The physiological age of elderly persons is more important during the postoperative period than at the time of operation. A patient who is physically active, independent, and alert is a far better surgical risk than a passive person who spends his days reading the paper and watching television.

PREOPERATIVE CARE

Every effort should be made to correct nutritional deficiencies, anemia, infection, and avitaminosis. Depleted serum proteins and blood volume, prolonged prothrombin time, and stasis of bronchial secretions must be remedied. Special diets can be given, but it is not always possible for the patient to tolerate high calorie intake. In this case, operation should not be delayed in the hope of reversing existing deterioration. The parenteral administration of special protein hydrolysates has not been particularly helpful. Cessation of smoking will decrease bronchial secretions and improve ventilation. Multiple whole blood or red cell transfusions may be necessary to restore the blood volume and ensure adequate oxygenation. Partial relief of the effects of bowel obstruction by intestinal intubation or a preliminary operation, such as a colostomy proximal to carcinoma of the colon, may be indicated.

Some years ago, it was fashionable to perform many major operations in two steps. Unfortunately, the stress of the preliminary operation was often more severe than the beneficial effects of various by-pass procedures in improving the cancer patient's condition. These techniques have decreased in popularity.

Antibiotics to reduce the bacterial content of the colon in preparation for surgery have been valuable. The reduction in stool volume is as helpful as reduction in bacteria. The techniques for bowel preparation and the associated complications have been reviewed many times. Several surgeons have reported that recurrences at a suture line in the bowel of experimental animals were more frequent if the bowel had been prepared by antibiotics. This thesis is reasonable and may be of clinical importance, even though valid proof is not available. It has not been considered necessary or desirable to use systemic antibiotics either before or after operation unless there is a specific indication.

Unique Aspects of Cancer Surgery

There are several unique aspects of the surgical care of malignancies, in addition to the importance of obtaining biopsies during the course of an operation, which deserve emphasis.

All cancerous lesions should be handled by the surgeon as carefully as if these masses contained deadly bacteria. The tissues should be manipulated as gently as possible. Every attempt should be made to interrupt the vessels draining the malignancy as quickly as possible. Similarly, the lumen of hollow organs should be separated from the normal areas which are to be repaired. Unfortunately, these simple suggestions, which constitute good sense, even though absolutely convincing studies of them have not been made, are not used in many operations. Surgeons must plan ahead as they are operating, for example, remembering to insert catheters if postoperative perfusion with chemotherapeutic agents is contemplated. The outline of a lesion and involved lymph nodes with silver clips is of great value to the radiotherapist. Modern x-ray devices provide adequate depth doses with less scatter; therefore, it is important to localize the beam accurately.

The insertion of radium needles, radon seeds, and radioisotopes at the time of surgery has decreased in popularity because it is extremely difficult to provide an evenly distributed cancericidal dose of irradiation without danger to normal structures. A few skilled surgeons have demonstrated the usefulness of these techniques, but too often these substances, which are dangerous to both patient and surgeon, have been used carelessly and without proper knowledge.

Chemosurgery, which consists of the application of locally acting fixatives, has been developed by Mohs and his students as a useful therapy for slow-growing cancers of the face and a few other areas. This technique is particularly useful for the treatment of recurrent basal cell carcinomas which have spread near vital structures. The fact that serial biopsies of the treated areas can be examined microscopically and fresh fixatives applied only to those sections containing tumor cells makes this method desirable. Much practice is needed in order to learn this method. Most often, the cooperation of a pathologist is essential. The treatments, which can be administered in the outpatient department, are especially useful in elderly patients who are not good candidates for regular surgical procedures.

Cryosurgery is the application to a tumor of a probe cooled to $-195°$ C. with liquid nitrogen. This technique has not been used long enough for proper evaluation, but it shows promise for the treatment of a limited number of locally invasive malignancies and some benign tumors.

The laser beam provides a high energy source which appears to be differentially absorbed by pigmented areas. It destroys experimental melanomas and has been used successfully to repair detached retinas. Unless a specific kind of differential absorption of the beam in tumor tissue can be enhanced by pigments or similar materials, it is doubtful that the laser will be a practical therapeutic agent.

PSYCHOLOGICAL CARE OF THE CANCER PATIENT

One of the most crucial decisions that the surgeon must make is whether or not to tell the patient that he or she has a malignancy. We believe the patient should usually be told the truth, but not the whole truth. A responsible member of the immediate family should always be told the full implications of the patient's condition and prognosis. The surgeon should help members of the family to accept the tragic news and ask them to use the same words and phrases which he thinks will be acceptable to and believed by the patient. The most difficult situations for the patient and the surgeon arise when the patient, doctor, and relatives all lie to each other; the family insists that the patient not be informed of his condition, despite the need for further therapy; and the patient is not told of his condition and is unable to help his spouse or family arrange personal affairs.

The physician need not provide specific details about the patient's disease and should never remove all hope of survival. Patients with a rapidly advancing disease are far easier to care for than those with a chronic terminal illness complicated by pain. After the first few weeks, visits by doctors and relatives become less frequent, and the patient begins to feel deserted. The surgeon can help the patient by warning him that he may lose weight before he gets better, trying to focus attention on diet and exercise, even if he is confined to bed.

False hopes may be helpful, if the timing is commensurate with the patient's condition, and may be offered just before the patient becomes semicomatose. The surgeon should never depart from his usual mannerisms and speech. A blunt, forceful personality may be as effective as a mild, respectful, and sympathetic manner. A gentle surgeon who assumes a bluff, hearty demeanor, or the reverse situation, will render any message useless, because its false presentation can be detected easily.

Much has been written about the use of modern medical techniques to prolong the life of a dying patient. If a patient is conscious and alert enough to converse with his family, he should be maintained. On the other hand, a patient who has become comatose is already dead from a humanistic point of view, and if there is no possible chance of survival, extraordinary measures should be discontinued.

Contrary to belief, a majority of cancer patients do not require narcotics for the control of pain. In employing other drugs, the surgeon should make every effort to postpone and minimize the use of narcotics, so that they will be effective if required later.

Finally, there is an extraordinarily low incidence of suicides among patients who are maintained in a follow-up program. Over the past ten years, there have been only three recognized suicides among patients at Roswell Park Memorial Institute, although some additional incidents undoubtedly have taken place. This record is remarkable when one considers that approximately 75,000 patient visits are made to the Institute each year, including many persons with advanced disease.

PATIENT PARTICIPATION IN CLINICAL STUDIES

The need for good clinical studies is great. Many of the diagnostic and therapeutic procedures considered to be effective probably would not withstand a valid evaluation. Medical testimonies by academicians are no longer acceptable means of testing clinical methods, despite the fact that such papers constitute over 90 per cent of the literature. Classification schemes, to aid in obtaining a favorable group of patients for the writer's purpose, may be very misleading. Cooperative clinical investigations have been helpful in studying accepted medical practices and new therapeutic agents. This type of study is not a panacea. There continues to be a need for original and unique observations by the individual clinician, but proper evaluation of a procedure can best be done by a group of clinicians studying their patients according to a protocol, so that the results will be meaningful and a broad test of various circumstances will have been performed.

Protection of the patient's rights, informed consent, and suitable control or comparison studies pose problems which have been magnified by the use of controlled clinical trials. Philosophical discussions and guiding precepts of these problems are undergoing continuing change; therefore, only a few basic rules are offered.

All clinical studies should be specifically described in a written protocol, and the protocol should be approved by a committee of colleagues possessing knowledge of the procedures and drugs, if any, to be used.

The patient must be fully informed of the nature, purpose, and risks of the study and exercise his free choice to participate.

The responsibility to protect the life and well-being of the individual must be retained by the investigator, even after formal consent is obtained.

The subject, or his guardian, must be able to exercise his free consent to withdraw from the study at any time.

Written consent is desirable, but it is not and should not be considered absolute protection from litigation. It will always be possible for a skillful lawyer to explain that the patient did not recognize completely the nature of the study, the meaning of technical words, and the possibility of unforeseen complications.

Despite the heavy burden of all of these responsibilities and the frustrations associated with working according to strict protocols, often with large groups, departments, and institutions, clinicians must continue valid human studies. Reports of small series of personal observations are no longer acceptable as definitive evaluations of therapy.

THE SURGEON'S ROLE IN CANCER RESEARCH

It is important that the physician treating cancer patients maintain an interest in all aspects of cancer research, because principles which affect patient care evolve from such work. For example, a considerable delay occurred before clinicians recognized that most, if not all, chemotherapeutic agents could produce serious adverse effects and, in fact, depress the host's defense mechanisms, if their anticancer potency was limited. All researchers tend to be enthusiastic about new treatments; however, before application, the biological rationale of these proposals should be considered.

Surgeons have provided, by necessity, most of the care and almost all of the curative procedures for malignant diseases. They have an excellent opportunity to participate in clin-ical research and utilize investigative techniques to search for new ways of preventing, diagnosing, seeking causes of, and treating malignant diseases. Unless surgeons participate in cancer research, they will be less able to understand, evaluate, and improve new types of diagnosis and therapy which will be used as adjuvants to surgery.

The role of the surgeon in advancing our knowledge of the malignant diseases has become a distinguished tradition which should be continued.

READING REFERENCES

Ackerman, L. V., and del Regato, J. A.: Cancer: Diagnosis, Treatment, and Prognosis. 3rd ed. St. Louis, C. V. Mosby Company, 1962.

Bittner, J. J., and Little, C. C.: Transmission of breast and lung cancer in mice. J. Hered. 23:117, 1937.

Bock, F. G., Moore, G. E., and Clark, P. C.: Carcinogenic activity of cigarette smoke condensate. 3. Biological activity of refined tar from several types of cigarettes. J. Nat. Cancer Inst. 34:481, 1965.

Cole, W. H.: Dissemination of Cancer: Prevention and Therapy. New York, Appleton-Century-Crofts, Inc., 1961.

Dowling, H. F.: Human experimentation in infectious diseases. J.A.M.A. 198:133, 1966.

Eddy, B. E., Stewart, S. E., Young, R., and Mider, G. B.: Neoplasms in hamsters induced by mouse tumor agent passed in tissue culture. J. Nat. Cancer Inst. 20:747, 1958.

Ellerman, V., and Bang, O.: Experimentelle Leukämie bei Hühnern. Centralbl. f. Bakteriol. 46:595, 1908.

Engell, H. C.: Cancer cells in the circulating blood; a clinical study on the occurrence of cancer cells in the peripheral blood and in venous blood draining the tumour area. Acta. Chir. Scandinav. (Suppl.) 201:1, 1955.

Epstein, M. A., and Barr, Y. M.: Characteristics and mode of growth of a tissue culture strain EG-I of human lymphoblasts from Burkitt's lymphoma. J. Nat. Cancer Inst. 34:231, 1965.

Fine, S., and Klein, E.: Biological effects of laser radiation. Advances Biol. Med. Phys. 10:149, 1965.

Gross, L.: Pathogenic properties and "vertical" transmission of mouse leukemia agent. Proc. Soc. Exper. Biol. & Med. 78:342, 1951.

Haddow, A., and Greenstein, J. P. (eds.): Advances in Cancer Research. Vols. 1-9. New York, Academic Press, 1965.

Hiatt, H. H.: Cancer chemotherapy—present status and prospects. New England J. Med. 276:157, 1967.

Iwakata, S., and Grace, J. T.: Cultivation in vitro of myeloblasts from human leukemia. New York J. Med. 64:2279, 1964.

James, S., and Rosenthal, T. (eds.): Tobacco and Health. Springfield, Illinois, Charles C Thomas, 1962.

Ladimer, I., and Newman, R. W. (eds.): Clinical Investigation in Medicine: Legal, Ethical, and Moral Aspects. Law-Medicine Research Institute, Boston University, 1963.

Levin, M. L., Goldstein, H., and Gerhardt, P. R.: Cancer and tobacco smoking; preliminary report. J.A.M.A. 143:336, 1950.

M. D. Anderson Hospital and Tumor Institute: Cancer Chemotherapy. Springfield, Illinois, Charles C Thomas, 1961.

Mohs, F. E.: Chemosurgery in Cancer, Gangrene, and Infections, Featuring a New Method for the Microscopically Controlled Excision of Cancer. Springfield, Illinois, Charles C Thomas, 1956.

Nadel, E. M.: Symposium on tumor cells in the peripheral blood. Acta Cytologica 9:1, 1965.

Nadler, S. H., and Moore, G. E.: Evaluation of the effectiveness of immunologically activated lymphoid cells against cancer cells. Surg. Forum 16:229, 1965.

Nadler, S. H., and Moore, G. E.: Clinical immunologic study of malignant disease: response to tumor transplants and transfer of leukocytes. Ann. Surg. 164:482, 1966.

Nowell, P. C., and Hungerford, D. A.: A minute chromosome in human granulocytic leukemia. Science 132:1497, 1960.

Pack, G. T., and Ariel, I. M.: Treatment of Cancer and Allied Diseases. 2nd ed. Vol. I. New York, Paul B. Hoeber, Inc., 1958.

Recent Advances in Diagnosis of Cancer. A Collection of Papers Presented at the Ninth Annual Clinical Conference on Cancer. Chicago, Year Book Publishers, 1964.

Rous, P.: A sarcoma of the fowl transmissible by an agent separable from the tumor cells. J. Exper. Med. 13:397, 1911.

Shope, R. E.: Transmissible tumor-like condition in rabbits. J. Exper. Med. 56:793, 1932.

Shope, R. E.: Filtrable virus causing tumor-like condition in rabbits and its relationship to virus myxomatosum. J. Exper. Med. 56:803, 1932.

Smoking and Health; Report of the Advisory Committee to the Surgeon General of the Public Health Service. Public Health Service Publication No. 1103, 1964.

Willis, R. A.: Pathology of Tumours. 3rd ed. Washington, Butterworth, 1960.

Wynder, E. L., and Graham, E. A.: Tobacco smoking as possible etiologic factor in bronchogenic carcinoma; study of 684 proved cases. J.A.M.A. 143:329, 1950.

Wynder, E. L., and Hoffman, D.: Experimental tobacco carcinogenesis. Advances Cancer Res. 8:249, 1964.

Chapter 5

DISEASES OF DEGENERATION

by
JAMES R. JUDE, M.D.
and
PRENTISS E. SMITH, Jr., M.D.

Born in Minnesota and educated in the grade and high schools of a small town; graduated from the College of Saint Thomas and the University of Minnesota Medical School, JAMES R. JUDE continued his surgical education at The Johns Hopkins Hospital. His scholarly attainments and investigative imagination and talents have been recognized consistently since his high school days. His surgical interests have been directed toward thoracic and cardiovascular surgery and the improvement of cardiopulmonary resuscitation methods. He is Professor of Surgery at the University of Miami School of Medicine and Chief of the Division of Thoracic and Cardiovascular Surgery at the Jackson Memorial Hospital.

PRENTISS SMITH is a Mississippian by birth and an alumnus of Tulane University, its School of Medicine and the Charity Hospital of Louisiana at New Orleans. He was an Instructor in Surgery at the University of Miami School of Medicine, and now is in the U.S. Army Medical Corps.

Diseases of degeneration produce a diminution of the functional capacity of a tissue or organ system. All organs and tissues degenerate to a greater or lesser degree with aging of the organism. In addition, there are certain conditions that accelerate the degenerative processes. The processes are relentless and progress at a greater or lesser speed, depending on augmenting function, toward complete cessation of function. If the organ or system is one that is necessary to sustain life, the organism dies when reduction in functional capacity reaches a critical level. During the process of degeneration, varying degrees of symptomatic disability are produced.

The causes of degeneration are numerous. The more common degenerative conditions and their symptom complexes may affect the decision regarding the necessity or desirability of an operation.

Many patients who require surgical correction of an anatomical or functional defect have one or more degenerative conditions. The surgeon has the responsibility to evaluate properly the functional capacity of organ systems affected with diseases of degeneration. Diseases of degeneration of organ systems vital to life often produce a fairly predictable reduction in life expectancy and this must be taken into account when surgical therapy is considered.

AGING

Aging is a degenerative condition that affects all people at a greater or lesser rate. Aging begins before birth and continues until death. It proceeds at different rates in different parts of the body, at different rates for different people, and is governed by the balance between concomitant growth and atrophy. In the early years growth and evolution predominate, whereas in later years atrophy and involution are the predominant processes.

There are many anatomic changes, characterizing aging of organs or organ systems, that are not synonymous with any disease process. Aging, in all organs, results in an increase in connective tissue and a gradual loss of its elastic properties. A reduction of the number of normally functioning cells all over the body and an increased amount of fat are also seen. A decreased cardiac output under resting conditions and a decrease in muscular strength accompany a diminished use of oxygen and result in a decreased metabolic rate. Endocrine secretion is decreased.

There is an alteration of the connective tissue of the dermis and a reduction of its elastic properties. In the older person, there is a gradual thinning of the epidermis and a loss of the rete pegs despite an increase in mitotic activity. There is a gradual atrophy of the nails, hair and cutaneous glands and a loss of pigment in the hair shaft. The sweat glands diminish in number but sebaceous secretion is increased. The skin of the older person does not respond to injury as well as the skin of a young person. Scar tissue formation is not as exuberant and firm healing is sometimes delayed. Atrophic and seborrheic dermatitis, common in older people, may make preparation of the operative site difficult and increase the infection rate.

There is a gradual decrease in muscle mass and muscular strength which may progress to extreme feebleness. In muscle, there is an increase in the collagenous and elastic interstitial connective tissue. In the heart, there is a decrease in the size of the muscle fibers, an increase in elastic tissue and an increase in pigment content of the cells. This seems to be relatively constant regardless of the status of the coronary arteries and reduces the functional capacity of the heart. The heart of senescence characteristically is decreased in size, although coexisting coronary artery disease, hypertension or valvular dysfunction may cause enlargement.

Demineralization and a loss of elasticity of the bony skeleton occur. The bones are more likely to fracture and do not heal as well as in a young person. The hematopoietic capacity is reduced significantly, the marrow becoming more fatty. Older people do not respond as well to acute or chronic reduction of the circulating red cell mass.

There is a generalized loss of elasticity of large and small arteries. Ectopic foci of atypical lymphoid tissue are deposited in the walls of the blood vessels and lipoid deposition has been noted in the media. These structural changes diminish the ability of the vascular tree to contract and compensate for rapid changes in blood volume.

There is atrophy of lymphoid tissue and replacement of the cellular elements with fat. One might infer from this that the natural defense mechanisms and immune mechanisms of the older individual are not as active.

In the gastrointestinal tract, in contrast, there is lymphoid hyperplasia.

A decrease in the mucosal thickness of the stomach accompanies a metaplasia of the glandular elements. The muscle and mucosa of the intestinal tract are generally atrophic, particularly in the colon. The appendix may be reduced to a fibrous cord even in the absence of previous inflammatory disease. Fatty degeneration of the salivary glands and pancreas has been noted and results in an overall diminution of secretion. Concomitant squamous metaplasia of the ducts is noted.

There is generalized atrophy of the mucous glands in the upper and lower respiratory mucosa. The resulting dryness of the mucosa causes a reduction of sensitivity and an increased viscosity of secretions, and makes aspiration and dysphagia common problems in the older person. The aged person may have a markedly attenuated cough reflex. This is particularly important after operation and makes the older person prone to develop pulmonary complications.

Stooped posture from muscle weakness and degeneration of the bony and cartilaginous portions of the thoracic spine alter the shape of the thorax. It becomes narrow in its lateral dimension and increased in the arterior-posterior diameter. The ribs become flat and less elastic and respiratory excursion is diminished. There is a concomitant decrease in elasticity and compliance of the pulmonary tissue and dilation of the alveoli. The vital capacity and the residual capacity are slightly decreased and there is a moderate decrease in total lung capacity. The maximum breathing capacity decreases slightly and oxygen saturation of the arterial blood usually drops to 92 to 93 per cent. Grossly, this produces the classic deformity of senile emphysema. All these changes make the older person a higher risk for operations of any type, but in particular for operations upon the chest and upper abdomen.

In the kidney, hyalin and fibrous transformation produce a gradual decrease in the number of functional glomeruli. Tubular atrophy and an increase in fibrous connective tissue are also seen. Even though no biochemical evidence of renal failure is demonstrable, there may be a marked decrease in the functional reserve of the kidneys, making them particularly susceptible to any alteration in blood volume, or use of nephrotoxic drugs. It should be remembered that renal excretion of some drugs and electrolytes may be markedly retarded and toxic blood levels may result at normal doses. The aging process is usually associated with a decrease in metabolic rate and degenerative changes in the organs which detoxify and excrete drugs. Dosage of drugs should be reduced accordingly.

In the brain, there is an atrophy or narrowing of the cerebral gyri and a widening and deepening of the sulci. The lateral ventricles are increased in size and the meninges become thickened and adherent to the surface of the brain. In the substance of the cerebrum, there is usually an accumulation of excess pigment and fat. This causes a reduction in reactive ability and sensory capacity of the older person.

It is obvious from the foregoing statements that advanced age increases the risk of an operation. Even though many surgical successes are recorded in people of advanced age, the mortality and morbidity rate is unquestionably higher than in younger patients. In general, healing of tissues is not as good, resistance to infection is diminished and because of changes in the blood vessels, the response to acute hemorrhage is less effective. The blood volume may be low in old people and circulation of blood is not as brisk as in the young. Hypotension or immobilization increases the likelihood of intravascular thrombosis and results in an increased incidence of thromboembolic complications. In addition, because of decreased muscular strength, the older patient cannot be expected to perform rigorous early ambulation necessary to prevent thrombosis in the veins of the legs.

It is important, before operation, that the patient be adequately hydrated and that the blood volume be restored to normal or nearly normal. Older patients have less cardiac and renal reserve and maintenance of adequate circulating blood volume is important. During operation, hypotension should be avoided as even slight reduction in blood pressure may produce severe impairment in cerebral, coronary and renal blood flow.

Although the average life expectancy of man has increased over the past half century, the maximum life span has not increased. The age of the patient can give the physician some indication of how long a healthy person might be expected to survive without his disease process. The prognosis for survival at any given age is indicated in Table 1. If a person survives to an advanced age, his prognosis for survival without his disease process is fairly good. With these statistics in mind, the surgeon might want to modify his therapeutic approach in an older person. From these statistics probably comes the often-quoted remark, "Age is no contraindication to surgery."

Table 1. *Life Table for the Total Population of the United States 1959–61, Ages 60 to 99 Years**

AGE (YEARS)	AVERAGE REMAINING LIFETIME IN YEARS	AGE (YEARS)	AVERAGE REMAINING LIFETIME IN YEARS
60	17.7	80	6.4
61	17.0	81	6.0
62	16.3	82	5.6
63	15.7	83	5.3
64	15.0	84	4.9
65	14.4	85	4.6
66	13.8	86	4.3
67	13.2	87	4.0
68	12.6	88	3.7
69	12.0	89	3.5
70	11.4	90	3.2
71	10.8	91	3.0
72	10.3	92	2.9
73	9.7	93	2.7
74	9.2	94	2.6
75	8.7	95	2.4
76	8.2	96	2.3
77	7.7	97	2.2
78	7.3	98	2.1
79	6.8	99	2.0

* From the Vital Statistics of the United States 1959–61.

SPECIFIC DEGENERATIVE CONDITIONS

ARTERIAL SYSTEM

In an aging population, the most common cause of symptomatic disease is arterial degeneration. The gradual occlusive, degenerative process may involve large or small vessels or both to a greater or lesser degree. Patients with generalized atherosclerosis have a decidedly shortened life expectancy. Some investigators report only a 50 per cent three-year survival in patients admitted to the hospital with the diagnosis of generalized atherosclerosis, the most common single cause of death being myocardial infarction. Other causes are cerebral thrombosis or hemorrhage, pulmonary embolism, mesenteric thrombosis or complications of arterial aneurysm.

One of the more common degenerative conditions affecting the arterial system is aortic aneurysm. Before major surgery for extirpation of an aneurysm is undertaken, it is important to weigh operative mortality against prognosis for survival if the aneurysm remains untreated.

For untreated abdominal aortic aneurysm the prognosis is rather grim. Approximately 30 per cent of patients with this type of aneurysm will die within one year; from 50 to 70 per cent are dead in three years; by five years, approximately 80 per cent of patients are dead. In an equivalent population of the same age, approximately 80 per cent would be alive in five years. About 75 per cent of patients die from rupture of the aneurysm, the remainder dying from causes related to atherosclerotic occlusive cardiovascular or cerebral vascular disease. Approximately 30 per cent of patients with abdominal aortic aneurysms are asymptomatic at the time of diagnosis. One series indicated that the average duration of life following the onset of symptoms of abdominal aortic aneurysm was six months, and the duration of symptoms before death was less than 12 months in almost 90 per cent of patients.

From this, it may be concluded that if a person has an abdominal aneurysm his prognosis for survival, simply because he has the aneurysm, is considerably less than the average population. If the aneurysm is symptomatic, life expectancy is measured in months unless the aneurysm is excised. Any decision to subject a patient to any operation other than aneurysm excision should be influenced by a person's prognosis for survival.

Kampmeier, in his classic article about thoracic aortic aneurysms, showed that the survival of patients with this disease, from the onset of symptoms, rarely exceeded eight months and that most patients died because of the aneurysm. This suggests that in the absence of other disease, once a thoracic aneurysm becomes symptomatic, it should be repaired.

Aneurysms of the vessels of the extremities, although causing some risk to the extremity, are not generally considered lethal. Excision with graft replacement does not entail a great risk when the operation is performed by an experienced vascular surgeon. Most can be repaired under local anesthesia.

The other great degenerative condition affecting the vascular system is atherosclerotic occlusive disease. The most common site of symptomatic atherosclerotic occlusive disease of the peripheral arteries is in the vessels of the lower extremities. The most common symptom complex causing the patient to seek medical attention is intermittent claudication. Statistics are available regarding life expectancy and prognosis for limb survival when a patient presents complaining of intermittent claudication.

Large series of patients indicate a grim prognosis even when a patient presents with only intermittent claudication and a good femoral pulse on that side. Approximately 25 to 30 per cent of these patients will be dead within five years and 50 to 60 per cent will die in 10 years. Eighty-five per cent of the deaths will be due directly to complications of occlusive vascular disease and only 15 per cent will be from unrelated causes.

Other factors that have come to light in statistical analysis of these patients require some consideration. If a patient survives longer than five years, there is a 20 per cent chance that he will have had, in addition to claudication, a nonfatal coronary artery occlusion or a cerebral infarction that will add significantly to his disability and decrease the necessity for use of his lower extremities.

The amputation rate is surprisingly low. There is only a 7 per cent chance that amputation of the lower extremity will be required when claudication is the presenting symptom. Deterioration in limb symptoms leading to gangrenous or pregangrenous changes occurs in only about 30 per cent of those suffering with intermittent claudication. In actual fact, survival longer than five years is associated with improvement in symptoms in approximately 65 per cent of cases. In general, it should be remembered that the older the patient is, when he presents with intermittent claudication, the shorter his life expectancy.

Information is also available on large series of patients who have suffered occlusion of a major coronary vessel with resultant myocardial infarction. Analysis of over 1400 patients shows that from the time the pain of an acute myocardial infarct strikes, a patient has approximately a 50 to 60 per cent chance of surviving two years. By the end of five years 70 to 80 per cent of patients who have had a myocardial infarction will have succumbed to the process. The average survival for a patient who has had an acute myocardial infarction varies with the series reported but averages slightly less than five years. One should consider this prognosis before subjecting a patient to extensive surgery. If he has survived longer than three years after his infarct, however, he is a better operative risk.

Angina pectoris is perhaps a slightly less severe manifestation of occlusive disease of the coronary arteries. Statistical analysis of several thousand patients who complained of exertional chest pain showed that 40 per cent had died in five years and 60 per cent had died in ten years. This provided a 30 per cent decrease in chance for survival in any given age. Angina pectoris, although not incompatible with a long life, provides for an average survival only slightly longer than five years from the time of onset of symptoms.

Degeneration of the conduction system of the myocardium is worthy of consideration. Complete heart block resulting from ischemic fibrosis of the myocardial conduction system carries an extremely high mortality if untreated or if treated only by medical means. The average life expectancy of all patients with heart block is two and one-half to four years. With frank Stokes-Adams attacks, however, even under good medical treatment, 30 per cent of patients will be dead in six months and 50 per cent of patients will be dead in one year. Only 20 per cent will survive four years. Permanent artificial electrical pacing of the heart provides for immediate relief of symptoms and an increase in longevity when compared to the mortality rate of the general population in that age group.

In a patient with heart block, treatment of the heart block should be begun before other surgical therapy is undertaken. In a patient with heart block requiring emergency surgery, it would be wise first to insert a temporary intravenous pacemaker for electrical pacing of the heart. This can be left in place for weeks if necessary.

Occlusive arterial disease affecting the extracranial and cranial cerebral vessels produces a definite reduction in life expectancy. It has been noted that 75 to 80 per cent of patients who sustain a cerebral vascular occlusion will survive the initial attack but a large number of the survivors will die in the ensuing year. Most of the survivors will be severely disabled.

Imminent strokes are usually preceded by prodromal symptoms in 25 to 30 per cent of the patients. These consist of transient attacks of dizziness, loss of vision, fainting, focal weakness or sensory change. In considering the patient for surgery, the presence of these symptoms should alert one to the possibility of imminent occlusion of a major cerebral vessel and should prompt angiographic study of the cerebral circulation prior to any operative procedure. Correction of any significant extracranial vascular lesion before other major surgery is probably indicated. The presence of these symptoms with the past history of a neurologically significant stroke should suggest that the prognosis for longevity should be extremely guarded. In general, it might be stated that rarely is any extensive surgery indicated in one who has had a significant cerebral vascular accident. Circumstances may, however, alter a decision to subject the patient to surgical therapy.

URINARY SYSTEM

As a person ages, the kidney undergoes degenerative fibrosis or hyalinization of the glomeruli. Coexistent vascular disease or hypertension results in more rapid glomerular degeneration. It is estimated that degenerative diseases can affect as many as two-thirds of the glomeruli before there is biochemical evidence of renal decompensation, as evidenced by elevation of the blood urea nitrogen or serum creatinine. In the absence of obstructive uropathy or dietary factors which increase the blood urea nitrogen, an elevation of the blood urea nitrogen above 15 mg. per 100 ml. should be interpreted as severe depletion of the renal reserve. A more precise test, less influenced by dietary factors and fluid intake and more indicative of pure renal function, is the concentration of the serum creatinine. Normally, this is below 2 mg. per

100 ml. and usually is below 1.5 mg. per 100 ml. Elevation above 2 mg. per 100 ml. is evidence of severe renal disease.

When evidence of renal decompensation is present, all efforts should be made, during a surgical procedure, to prevent hypotension that might further damage renal tissue. All nephrotoxic drugs should be avoided and extreme caution should be exercised in recommending operations which involve temporary interruption of the blood supply or manipulation of the kidney. In the face of biochemical evidence of impaired renal function, it might be wise to undertake any surgery involving temporary interruption of the renal blood supply under moderate hypothermia.

Impairment of renal function may also be indicated by a fixed specific gravity of urine, even in the presence of a normal blood urea nitrogen and serum creatinine. A fixed specific gravity should also be regarded as evidence of severe impairment of renal tubular function.

Severe impairment of renal function is, however, not incompatible with a long life. Good medical management of fluid and electrolyte intake, dietary regulation and avoidance of nephrotoxic drugs may allow a patient a comfortable existence for a long period of time. A blood urea nitrogen in excess of 50 mg. per 100 ml. may be tolerated quite well. For these reasons, less precise data are available about longevity of patients with renal disease.

RESPIRATORY SYSTEM

A common degenerative condition that affects many people past 40 years of age is pulmonary emphysema. The so-called senile emphysema is largely a physical and roentgenologic finding and rarely produces other than minimal reduction in life expectancy. In contrast, pulmonary emphysema caused by allergic asthma or asthmatic bronchitis associated with chronic irritation from cigarette smoking pursues a relentless downhill course. Even successful therapy rarely maintains the status quo and merely retards inevitable respiratory decompensation.

When a patient exhibits exertional dyspnea, it is unusual for him to survive more than five to ten years, even with good, continuous medical management. When hypercapnia or decreased arterial oxygen saturation appears after exercise or at rest, the prognosis is particularly grave. From the onset of dyspnea, 50 per cent of patients are dead in seven years if smoking is not avoided. Even if the patient does give up smoking and is well managed, there is a 50 per cent chance that he will die within ten years from his pulmonary disease. In selecting treatment, the surgeon should be cognizant of this reduced life expectancy.

It would be inadvisable to subject such a patient to any ablative pulmonary surgery or thoracic surgery of any type except under a condition which poses an immediate threat to his life. If such surgery becomes necessary, it is wise to avoid completely allergens or pulmonary irritants and use intermittent positive pressure breathing, bronchodilators, broncholytic agents and antibiotics before operation. If this therapy is unsatisfactory or inadequate, or if hypoxemia at rest exists, prophylactic tracheostomy with a cuffed tube and assisted respiration for several days after operation may be indicated. Complete removal of secretions, as aseptically as possible, from the tracheobronchial tree is essential, for accumulation may cause pulmonary infection or atelectasis. The same principles hold true for the patient upon whom abdominal surgery of any type is contemplated. It should be remembered that an abdominal incision can produce as much immediate diminution of pulmonary function as a thoracic incision.

ENDOCRINE SYSTEM

The only disease of degeneration of major importance affecting the endocrine system is diabetes mellitus. Although widespread use of parenteral insulin has reduced the immediate mortality of diabetes mellitus, patients with this disease have a shorter life expectancy than the general population. This is particularly true when diabetes has its onset at a young age. Although insulin has reduced the number of deaths from diabetic coma and antibiotics have reduced markedly the deaths from infection, renal disease and atherosclerosis associated with prolonged diabetes mellitus continue to reduce the life expectancy of the diabetic.

The average life expectancy for diabetics of all ages after the onset of the disease is approximately 18 years. Most people who acquire diabetes at an early age can be expected to live only about 25 years after the onset. During operation, therapeutic efforts should be directed toward prevention of metabolic acidosis and the osmotic diuresis associated with an excessively high blood sugar.

With aging there is a gradual diminution in function of the other organs of internal secretion. Gradual loss of the cellular elements, fibrosis, and nodular hyperplasia affect all of them, but this usually presents no problem in surgical therapy. The diminished secretion of thyroid hormone and adrenal cortical steroids makes the aged patient more sensitive to drug therapy; however, by proportionately diminishing drug dosage, most difficulties can be avoided.

Many series of statistics could perhaps be selected that do not exactly agree with the ones presented here. These were selected as representative. The data selected are calculated to emphasize the possible effects of disease processes. Such an approach is not unreasonable when it is remembered that the physician in practice usually encounters symptomatic disease. Minimally symptomatic diseases of degeneration are usually less significant prognostically, more likely to be overlooked by the doctor and, more important, more likely to be overlooked by the patient.

Certainly no dogmatic claims for exact survival can ever be made for any particular person in a given situation, as many tangible and intangible factors will affect the prognosis of any person with a disease of degeneration. The point made is that disease of degeneration usually causes a reduction in life expectancy; the greater the intensity of symptoms and number of degenerative conditions affecting a patient, the poorer his prognosis for survival. It is important in selecting surgical treatment to realize whether one is palliating or correcting a condition which threatens life, or alleviating symptoms which could easily and without added risk be controlled by something less than an operation.

Often an experienced surgeon will look at a patient and state that he does not think that the person will tolerate an operation. Not infrequently, a proper evaluation may be made in this manner. As increasing information becomes available about the natural history of disease, such intangible evaluation of a patient will be less frequently necessary.

The surgeon should not necessarily be concerned with complete cure of a particular degenerative condition but rather achievement of the maximal number of comfortable, productive months of survival. In general, surgery specifically for diseases of degeneration is palliative and coexisting degenerative diseases should probably make the surgeon less aggressive. Selection of surgical therapy should take into account the disease process causing the presenting symptoms, the prognosis with and without treatment, concomitant diseases, age and the general health of the patient.

READING REFERENCES

Begg, T. B., and Richards, R. L.: The prognosis of intermittent claudication. Scottish M. J. 7:341, 1962.

Block, W. J., Crumpacker, E. L., Dry, T. J., and Gage, R. P.: Prognosis of angina pectoris. J.A.M.A. 150:259, 1952.

Bloor, K.: Natural history of the atherosclerosis of the lower extremities. Ann. Roy. Coll. Surgeons England 28:36, 1961.

Blumenthal, H. T.: Medical and Clinical Aspects of Aging. New York, Columbia University Press, 1962.

Campbell, M. F.: Urology. 2nd ed. Philadelphia, W. B. Saunders Company, 1963.

DeBakey, M. E.: Report to the President: A National Program to Conquer Heart Disease, Cancer, and Stroke. Vol. 1. 1964.

Ebert, R.: The natural history of emphysema in man. Am. Rev. Resp. Dis. 80:169, 1959.

Estes, J. E.: Abdominal aortic aneurysm: a study of one hundred and two cases. Circulation 2:258, 1950.

Friedberg, C. K.: Diseases of the Heart. 3rd ed. Philadelphia, W. B. Saunders Company, 1966.

Hines, E. A., and Barker, N. W.: Arteriosclerosis obliterans. A clinical and pathologic study. Am. J. M. Sc. 200:717, 1940.

Hinshaw, H. C., and Garland, L. H.: Diseases of the Chest. 2nd ed. Philadelphia, W. B. Saunders Company, 1963.

Johnson, W. M.: The Older Patient. New York, Paul B. Hoeber, Inc., 1963.

Joslin, E. P., Root, H. F., White, P., and Marble, A.: The Treatment of Diabetes Mellitus. Philadelphia, Lea & Febiger, 1959.

Kampmeier, R. H.: Aneurysm of the abdominal aorta: A study of 73 cases. Am. J. M. Sc. 192:97, 1936.

Kampmeier, R. H.: Saccular Aneurysm of the Thoracic Aorta: A clinical study of 633 cases of thoracic aneurysm. Ann. Int. Med. 12:624, 1938.

Katz, L. N., Mills, G. Y., and Cisneros, F.: Survival after recent myocardial infarction. Arch. Int. Med. 84:305, 1949.

Levine, S. A., and Rosenbaum, F. I.: Prognostic value of various clinical and electrocardiographic features of acute myocardial infarction. Arch. Int. Med. 68:913, 1941.

Orie, N. G. M., and Sluiter, H. J.: Bronchitis, an International Symposium. Springfield, Illinois, Charles C Thomas, 1964.

Pratt-Thomas, H. R.: Aneurysm of the abdominal aorta. An analysis of 17 cases. J. South Carolina M. A. 40:251, 1944.

Scott, V.: Abdominal aneurysms: report of 96 cases. Am. J. Syph. Gonor. & Ven. Dis. 28:682, 1944.

Sigler, L. H.: Prognosis of angina pectoris and coronary occlusion. J.A.M.A. 146:1000, 1951.

Taylor, G. W., and Calo, A. R.: Atherosclerosis of arteries of the lower limbs. Brit. M. J. 1:507, 1962.

Thygesen, P., et al.: Cerebral apoplexy. Dan. M. Bull. 11:233, 1964.

Wedd, A. M., and Smith, Z. E.: Observations on prognosis in angina pectoris. Am. J. M. Sc. 189:690, 1935.

White, P. D., and Bland, E. F.: A further report on the prognosis of angina pectoris and of coronary thrombosis. A study of 500 cases of the former condition and of 200 cases of the latter. Am. Heart J. 7:1, 1931.

Wolff, K.: The Biological, Sociological and Psychological Aspects of Aging. Springfield, Illinois, Charles C Thomas, 1959.

Chapter 6

CONGENITAL DISEASES

by
C. EVERETT KOOP, M.D.

Early in his professional career, C. EVERETT KOOP became interested in the surgical problems of children. He is an educational product of Flatbush School in Brooklyn, Dartmouth College, Cornell University Medical School, Pennsylvania Hospital and was Harrison Fellow in Surgical Research at the University of Pennsylvania School of Medicine for five years. Dr. Koop was an early advocate of pediatric surgery as a special field. He is Professor, Pediatric Surgery, University of Pennsylvania School of Medicine and Surgeon-in-Chief of The Children's Hospital of Philadelphia.

A classification by causes is a logical approach to congenital malformations. Some malformations, few in number, are caused by single genes, whereas others are caused by chromosomal abnormalities. Environmental factors are known to produce some birth defects. However, the largest group of congenital anomalies is of unknown etiology and contains not only the most common but also the most severe deformities, such as those of the central nervous system and cardiovascular system. The etiology of such defects as cleft lip and palate, congenital dislocation of the hip and clubbed foot is likewise unknown.

The chromosome breakthrough really began in 1959 when three boys with mongolism were found to have a small extra chromosome. In spite of the tremendous amount of literature concerning chromosome studies, the investigation of chromosomal relationships to lesions of surgical significance is barely under way.

Teratogenic agents in man include drugs, viruses and radiation. Such agents must affect a specific metabolic process in the developing embryo and experimental models have been established to prove teratogenicity. The timing of embryologic development is so precise that the application of a teratogen must also be extremely precise and many experimental teratogens are known to exert their effect over a very limited time period during embryonal organogenesis. The effect of rubella infection illustrates this well, for it has been shown that major birth defects in infants following maternal rubella infection in pregnancy vary from 50 per cent if the virus infection takes place in the first four weeks of pregnancy to 17 per cent if the infection occurs in the third month of pregnancy, after which time the incidence of anomalies approaches zero.

At least in experimental animals, in addition to the teratogen, the genotype of the embryo is also important in relation to the susceptibility of the embryo to a given malformation-producing agent. The rubella virus has been associated with congenital heart disease, cataracts and deafness in infants born to mothers infected during pregnancy. The cytomegalovirus has been implicated in microcephaly and psychomotor retardation. The occurrence of what would be an institution's entire years' experience with esophageal atresia in a period of several weeks, half of the patients coming from one community, lends support to the thought that other teratogenic viruses will eventually be identified.

Radiation effects have been implicated in the development of microcephaly and congenital dislocation of the hip. Sporadic instances of multiple congenital defects occurring in the offspring of individuals exposed to excessive radiation are impressive but difficult to prove.

The effect of drugs such as thalidomide in producing multiple congenital anomalies, of which phocomelia is the most common, is now well known. Hormone therapy in pregnant women has linked progestin with masculinization of female fetuses.

Other factors such as sex, geography, sea-

72

son and parity must be taken into account in reference to some malfunctions. In anencephaly, for example, which has no surgical management, the incidence is 50 times as common in Belfast as in Lyons; the sex ratio is one male to two females; there is a higher frequency in the winter; and first-born children appear to be more susceptible than those born later.

CLASSIFICATION

Congenital anomalies defy simple or satisfactory classification. To clarify the approach to these problems, those of surgical importance can be divided into several loose groups.

LESIONS INCOMPATIBLE WITH LIFE BUT AMENABLE TO SURGICAL CORRECTION

Except for the rare lesion producing respiratory obstruction such as a teratoma of the mediastinum, or a cystic hygroma involving the trachea, almost all anomalies in this category are comprised of five diagnostic entities. These five conditions account for 95 per cent of those lesions demanding immediate surgical treatment.

Omphaloceles, large defects which represent failure of extruded abdominal viscera into the base of the umbilical cord to return to the coelomic cavity during the twelfth week of fetal life, are diagnosed by inspection. These may be large or small, ruptured or unruptured, contain most of the liver or only a small portion of that viscus, and may be associated with other intra-abdominal anomalies, of which intestinal obstruction is the most common. Surgical correction is dictated by the size of the defect and the variety of associated lesions, and not infrequently repair must be staged by first covering the defect with abdominal skin, converting the omphalocele into a ventral hernia, and later performing an anatomical closure of the abdominal wall. Some success has been achieved with the use of artificial membranes which are reduced in area every few days until anatomical closure of the abdominal wall is possible. With the use of muscle relaxants the temptation to achieve initial anatomical repair at the expense of too tight an abdominal closure must be resisted, because of the subsequent respiratory difficulty caused by elevation of the leaves of the diaphragm. Particular care must be taken to identify the small omphalocele containing one loop of small intestine, or perhaps the appendix, which may be caught in the clamp or ligature applied to the umbilical cord.

Imperforate anus seldom exists without an accompanying fistula to the urinary tract in the male, to the genital tract in the female or to the perineum in either sex. The surgeon may temporize with perineal fistulas in either sex or with the genital fistulas in the female, but the other varieties demand immediate surgery. When the colon has penetrated the puborectalis portion of the levator ani sling, and has descended below a line drawn from the coccyx to the pubis, the defect is repaired immediately from a perineal approach. Some surgeons perform a definitive operative repair on the high varieties of imperforate anus with rectourethral or rectovesical fistulas as a neonatal procedure. More commonly, a colostomy is constructed and a definitive operation postponed in view of the fact that continence is dependent upon proper placement of the colon in the levator sphincter mechanism.

Esophageal atresia is associated with a tracheoesophageal fistula between the lower segment of esophagus and the trachea usually just above the carina in 85 per cent of patients. A variety of other anatomical situations have been reported, ranging from a common tracheoesophagus to absence of the distal esophagus without fistula. Diagnosis should be suspected in the newborn with an excessive accumulation of mucus in the nose and mouth and can be proved by the inability to pass a small, flexible opaque catheter which coils in the proximal esophagus above the obstruction. The introduction of radiopaque media into the upper esophagus is not necessary and invariably results in tracheobronchial aspiration and attendant chemical pneumonitis, which in turn is associated with increased morbidity and a higher mortality. Pure tracheoesophageal fistulas without atresia are not commonly diagnosed in the neonatal period but are lethal lesions when uncorrected.

Diaphragmatic hernias produce symptoms in accordance with the amount of abdominal viscera compressing the ipsilateral lung in the pleural cavity and displacing the mediastinum to the contralateral side. Of the five conditions in this category, symptomatic diaphragmatic hernias represent the most urgent of neonatal surgical emergencies. The ipsilateral lung is commonly hypoplastic and should not be subjected to excessive intra-pulmonary pressures for expansion and after diaphragmatic repair should be allowed to fill the pleural space gradually in the presence of one of several varieties of thoracic drainage.

Intestinal obstruction in a newborn produces vomiting and frequently distention and failure to pass a meconium stool. The specific lesions causing neonatal intestinal obstruction are malrotation of the colon with duodenal compression or midgut volvulus; atresia of the small or large intestine; meconium ileus due to absence of pancreatic enzymes in association with cystic fibrosis of the pancreas; internal hernias, and aganglionic megacolon. A variety of less common defects are also encountered.

Highest survival rates are reported in those patients operated upon within the first 48 hours of life. Diagnosis frequently is delayed beyond this time because the symptoms of cyanosis, excessive mucus, vomiting, abdominal distention and failure to pass a meconium stool which lead to diagnosis are also common physiologic variants in newborn infants. For this reason a simple screening procedure, which can be done by a nurse or delivery room attendant, is recommended. Such an examination consists of inspection of the base of the cord for abdominal viscera, insertion of a fifth finger into the infant's rectum, passage of a catheter into the esophagus to rule out atresia and aspiration of the gastric contents through the same catheter. More than 50 cc. of gastric fluid is indicative of probable intestinal obstruction. Although passage of a copious normal meconium stool following the rectal examination does not absolutely exclude intestinal obstruction, the diagnosis is quite uncommon if the infant evacuates after such an examination. Such screening procedures are frequently neglected because the yield of positive diagnoses is small, yet several states have laws requiring screening for phenylketonuria, a diagnosis much less common than these surgical lesions and one for which therapy is not nearly as satisfactory. Prematurity is a common finding in association with these surgical lesions and two or three of these anomalies may be found in the same patient. Reports of surgical success and failure should be evaluated in the light of prematurity, associated pneumonitis and the presence of more than one major congenital anomaly.

LESIONS INITIALLY COMPATIBLE WITH LIFE BUT WHICH CARRY A POTENTIAL EARLY HAZARD TO LIFE

This category includes such congenital defects as sacrococcygeal teratoma, which can produce intestinal obstruction or obstructive uropathy and which may undergo malignant change. Other examples are duplications of the esophagus, which encroach upon the pleural space or mediastinum to produce respiratory distress, dysphagia or vascular compression, and duplications of the small or large intestines, which produce incomplete or intermittent intestinal obstruction or which may result in volvulus or intussusception.

DEFECTS NOT IMMEDIATELY RECOGNIZED BUT RESPONSIBLE FOR PROGRESSIVE DETERIORATION

Atresia of the bile ducts is a notable example of such defects. This condition is difficult to diagnose because of its confusion with neonatal hepatitis, which is not readily separated from the surgical lesion by laboratory examinations or even by liver biopsy in some circumstances. Most pediatric surgeons favor liver biopsy and operative cholangiography at six to eight weeks of life followed by any indicated surgical procedure if the cholangiogram is abnormal. The number of patients with biliary atresia amenable to surgical correction is extremely small, leading some surgeons to postpone early operative exploration rather than expose the infant with neonatal hepatitis to the hazards of anesthesia and surgery. Some authors, however, recommend a more aggressive approach.

Another classic example of this category of congenital defects is the posterior urethral valve which produces far-reaching obstructive changes in bladder, ureters and kidneys. Early recognition and decompression permits regression of the effects of obstruction and permits eventual safe definitive surgery.

LESIONS COMPATIBLE WITH LIFE BUT ALTERING FUNCTION

The number of such lesions is almost legion and representative defects include major orthopedic anomalies such as phocomelia, the absence or deformity of major bones, clubbed feet and congenital dislocation of the hip. Webbed fingers, absence or deformity of the pinna of the ear with or without accompanying abnormalities of the external auditory canal, and defects in the orbit or globe of the eye are other examples. Hamartomas such as hemangiomas or lymphangiomas are extremely common.

Neurological anomalies are not uncommon and the successful management of internal hydrocephalus by shunting procedures has kept alive many myelomeningocele patients who would otherwise have died. As a result the associated defects of the lower extremities, bladder and bowel demand surgical attention.

Congenital heart lesions may be of the cyanotic or acyanotic variety. Many of these are not evident at birth but become apparent shortly thereafter as fetal circulatory dynamics are altered and exist either as isolated cardiac lesions or complicate other of the congenital defects previously enumerated. Most of these cardiac anomalies are now subjected to surgical correction but operation is usually postponed to beyond the neonatal period when possible. The mortality is still unfortunately extremely high with or without attempts at surgical repair or palliation. Early definitive diagnosis will allow the correct decision to be made when dealing with multiple anomalies.

PRINCIPLES OF SURGICAL MANAGEMENT

Although the neonate with a surgical lesion requiring immediate attention may have some electrolyte imbalance and dehydration requiring correction, a point of diminishing returns is soon reached in prolonged preoperative preparation. Relatively rapid correction of fluid and electrolyte deficits, the correction of acidosis based on blood gas analyses, the administration of appropriate antibiotics and vitamin K, intestinal decompression and the preparation of plasma or blood to replace operative loss are usually all that need be done in view of the urgency of the surgical procedure at hand. Early diagnosis and the performance of only the essential diagnostic procedures are the factors that contribute to a lower mortality in this group.

When the neonatal surgical patient is jaundiced and may later require an exchange transfusion, blood used during operation should be of the same type that would be used for the exchange, and preferably from the same donor unit. It may be preferable to use only plasma if the initial hematocrit and operative losses allow. When the abdominal wall is incised, the umbilical vein should be preserved for later exchange transfusion if it should prove necessary.

Nowhere in medicine is the concept of the team approach more applicable than in pediatric surgery. From the initial newborn examination by the pediatrician to the final words of instruction to the mother from the neonatal surgical nurse on discharge, many interests must work together to provide the infant with his best chance for survival. The radiologist must be familiar with the conditions seen in the newborn and must be prepared to perform only the essential studies with efficiency, and the anesthesiologist must be experienced with the special problems of the newborn patient. When one keeps in mind the special problems of these patients, such as temperature regulation and the possibility of aspiration, it becomes apparent that postoperative care by the resident staff and nursery personnel contributes immensely to survival. The surgical procedure itself should be brief, gentle and corrective, and postoperative care must be meticulous.

One exception to the principle of immediate surgery for the five conditions incompatible with life is the staging of the operative procedures in the correction of atresia of esophagus with tracheoesophageal fistula. A quick transthoracic or extrapleural procedure to ligate or divide the tracheoesophageal fistula, followed by gastrostomy for feeding purposes, will lower mortality. When definitive esophageal reconstruction is performed, the patient is no longer premature, and the pneumonia and associated anomalies have been treated. During the interim a sump catheter placed in the upper pouch prevents aspiration of accumulating mucus.

There are advantages to early operation in lesions such as sacrococcygeal teratoma even though there is no pressing need for surgery on pathologic grounds. Because newborn tissues tolerate anoxia and minimal blood supply better than the tissues of older children and because the tissue planes are readily defined, one should consider immediate surgery rather than postponement. The facts that the bacterial flora of the gut has not yet become established and that the physiologic fall in the hemoglobin has not yet occurred are additional reasons for early intervention.

In obstructive uropathy, the most simple operative procedure likely to produce improved physiology is the procedure of choice. After that the planning of multiple procedures can be carried out at relative leisure once renal function has been stabilized.

Although in general one would like to wait until hands, feet, ears, lips and palates grow to maximal size, there are other considerations. Operation should be undertaken before functional disuse becomes apparent or before the deformity necessitates improper use of a limb or produces faulty speech. In planning a series of operations on patients in this category, one is always confronted with the psychological needs of the patient. In a well-run pediatric unit the child usually adjusts well to separation from his parents and in general does better if the decision to operate is based upon his physiological needs rather than his psychological requirements. There are occasions when the psychological reactions of parents may influence the hastening or postponement of a surgical procedure which might be done with equal functional results at another time.

READING REFERENCES

Apgar, V.: Infant resuscitation. Postgrad. Med. *19*:447, 1956.

Danks, A. M., and Campbell, P. E.: Extrahepatic biliary atresia: comments on the frequency of potentially operable cases. J. Pediat. *69*:21, 1966.

Holder, T. M., McDonald, V. E., Jr., and Wooley, M. M.: The premature or critically ill infant with esophageal atresia: increased success with a staged approach. J. Thorac. & Cardiovasc. Surg. *44*:344, 1962.

Kasai, M., Yakovac, W. C., and Koop, C. E.: Liver in congenital biliary atresia and neonatal hepatitis. A histopathologic study. Arch. Path. *74*:152, 1962.

Koop, C. E., and Hamilton, J. P.: Increased survival with staged procedure in the poor risk patient. Ann. Surg. *162*:389, 1965.

Lejeune, J., Gautier, M., and Turpin, R.: Les chromosomes humains en culture de tissus. C. Rend. Acad. Sc., *248*:1721, 1959.

McKusick, V. A.: Mendelian Inheritance in Man. Baltimore, The Johns Hopkins Press, 1967.

Rhodes, A. J.: Virus infection and congenital malformations. *In*, Congenital Malformations: Papers and Discussions presented at the First International Conference on Congenital Malformations. Philadelphia, J. B. Lippincott Company, 1962, pp. 106-116.

Thompson, J. S., and Thompson, M. W.: Genetics in Medicine. Philadelphia, W. B. Saunders Company, 1966.

Chapter 7

SURGICAL METABOLISM AND ELECTROLYTE BALANCE

by
BERNARD ZIMMERMANN, M.D.

BERNARD ZIMMERMANN was born in Minnesota and received his education at Harvard College and Medical School. He spent time in research in endocrinology and metabolism before beginning his surgical education and training, which he received at the University of Minnesota. He is Professor and Chairman of the Department of Surgery at West Virginia University Medical School. He has retained his interest in investigations of the relation between endocrinology and electrolyte and fluid balance in surgical patients.

Most of the ventures which have resulted in present-day surgery would not have been successful, or perhaps even attempted, had it not been for the concomitant development of an extensive body of information pertaining to the support of the physiologic needs of patients following extensive surgery. The emergence of radical visceral cancer surgery, modern thoracic surgery and cardiovascular surgery exemplify the significance of such fundamental knowledge.

Effective methods for management of surgical patients require recognition of profound physiological alterations caused by injury. Adequate support is based on realization that the operative experience is more than merely a period of alimentary deprivation, and requires respect for the biological responses to the operation. Some of these responses are the result of local effects of the procedures. Others are in the nature of conservative and protective reactions mobilized for defense against the lethal effects of injury. As a result of these changes the postoperative patient's need for some substances is far greater and his tolerance for others is less than that of normal individuals. The problem has become much more complicated than the simple calculation of requirements from the difference between what goes into the body and what comes out.

PHYSIOLOGIC CHARACTERISTICS OF POST-OPERATIVE PATIENTS. Trauma of a degree comparable to that represented by major surgical operations results not only in rather characteristic alterations in metabolism, but also in gross changes in such tissues as the formed elements of the blood and the lymphatic system, the thymus and the adrenal glands. Nitrogen and carbohydrate balance are altered so that blood sugar tends to be elevated, glucose tolerance is decreased, glycosuria is not uncommon and, in instances in which marginal glucose tolerance exists, transient or even permanent diabetes may be precipitated by a major surgical procedure. Along with this, the balance of nitrogen becomes negative as measured by an increase in its output in the urine, and a relative inability of the organism to utilize exogenous amino acids for the synthesis of structural body proteins. Sodium and chloride tend to be withheld from the urine and, in the immediate postoperative phase, urinary concentrations of these two ions may drop to almost zero even when the amounts given are greater than that normally necessary for daily replacement. Urinary potassium concentrations, on the other hand, are regularly elevated. Potassium balance becomes negative. That this urinary excretion of potassium is not entirely the result of tissue breakdown can be proved by demonstrating that the potassium-to-nitrogen ratio of the urine is greater than that which characterizes the interior of the cell.

The postoperative patient is frequently oliguric, even in the absence of preceding shock or other factors which might be expected to predispose to disturbances of renal function. More consistently than this, however, postoperative patients display intolerance to water. This implies that their diuretic response to a water load is impaired, so that they excrete excess water sluggishly and may suffer the consequences of dilution or hydremia before the kidneys are able to respond to an excess of administered fluid.

These metabolic alterations are associated in patients following operation, and in experimental animals following trauma, with certrain morphologic changes including depression of the number of lymphocytes and the eosinophils in the blood, involution of the lymphoid tissues such as the thymus and enlargement of the adrenal cortices. The underlying factor in these morphologic changes and certain of the metabolic effects is the production of an increased amount of hormones by the adrenal cortex.

ANTERIOR PITUITARY–ADRENAL FUNCTION. The pituitary rapidly secretes increased amounts of adrenocorticotropic hormone with the inception of an operation or accidental injury, and this is responsible for the production of one or more steroid hormones with potent metabolic activity. The work of Hume and Egdahl has helped elucidate the pathways by which even minor somatic injury activates the hypophysial system. It is apparent that peripheral nerves play a dominant role in transmitting the impulses of injury to the central nervous system, since corticotropic activity is greatly reduced by section of these nerves or their tracts in the spinal cord. Similarly, afferents may also transmit pressure stimuli from blood vessels and activate corticotropic activity in response to hemorrhage. The relationship of centers in the brain to corticotropic function is more complex. There is evidence that areas in the hypothalamus and, perhaps, also in the hindbrain, act directly upon the anterior pituitary. It is presumed that the relationship between these centers and the hypophysis is a humoral rather than a neural one. Such a humoral substance, called corticotropin-releasing factor, has been isolated from the hypothalamus. It is probably secreted by nerve fibers in the hypothalamus into the portal-hypophyseal vessels, a system of vessels which carry blood from the ventral hypothalamus to the anterior pituitary.

The adrenal product which is elaborated in greatest amounts under the influence of pituitary stimulation is 11-oxy-17-hydroxycorticosterone which is known as cortisol, compound F, or hydrocortisone. This is largely responsible for changes in organic metabolism which result in increased nitrogen excretion and decreased glucose tolerance, as well as the alterations in the formed elements of the blood and regression of lymphoid tissue. It also has a mild effect on mineral metabolism, causing sodium retention and potassium excretion, but is obviously not a dominant mediator of changes in inorganic metabolism. Aldosterone is produced by the adrenal in much smaller quantities, but has a vastly more powerful effect on mineral balance. It is subject to a type of control which is in part separate from that of cortisol. The question whether there is a third adrenal hormone, which has the characteristics of an androgen, remains debatable. Following castration, the adrenal does secrete a substance which is capable of maintaining secondary sexual characteristics, promotes nitrogen anabolism and is excreted like testosterone as a 17-ketosteroid. The function of such a substance under normal circumstances, however, is problematic.

Although the relationship of 11-oxy-17-hydroxycorticoids to alterations in organic metabolism had been recognized for a long time, the endocrine substance responsible for regulation of sodium and potassium balance was not known until the recent discovery of aldosterone and the demonstration of its presence in various pathologic states associated with sodium retention.

The finding of increased amounts of this hormone in the urine of postoperative patients leaves no doubt that it is mobilized by surgery. The intermediate mechanism, however, which results in the stimulation of aldosterone production by the adrenal is of considerable interest. It is known that, unlike cortisol, aldosterone does not require the presence of the pituitary for its mobilization. Nevertheless, under appropriate circumstances adrenocorticotropic hormone can cause aldosterone to be secreted, so that the action of adrenocorticotropic hormone can be described as a sufficient but not necessary factor for the release of salt-regulating hormones. Sodium restriction causes a greatly increased output of aldosterone, but it is probable that the effect of sodium restriction is mediated through changes in circulatory volume rather than reduction in the sodium levels. Reduction of sodium concentration by itself apparently has nothing to do with aldosterone release.

The work of Bartter would indicate that for normal day-to-day homeostasis, the most important single mechanism is reduction in extracellular volume and, more specifically, the volume of blood which is perfusing the arterial circulation. Aldosterone, therefore, acts as a mechanism for preserving the circulating volume by controlling the balance of sodium ion. Although the question of the anatomic location of "volume receptors" is not completely answered, the work of Davis and of Mulrough indicates that the circulation of the kidney itself fulfills this role. The renal pressor substance, angiotensin, is the tropic hormone which, having been released into the circulation, acts upon the adrenal to stimulate the secretion of aldosterone.

There is reason for believing that the stimulus of a surgical operation, or major systemic trauma, involves mechanisms for the production of excessive amounts of aldosterone which are separate from those involved in the day-to-day regulation of sodium and potassium balance. Blood volume maintenance is, obviously, an important factor in the circumstances of injury, but all patients who respond to operations with the output of this steroid do not suffer significant losses in circulating volume. Potassium infusion has been shown to be a potent mechanism for stimulating aldosterone output and, like the volume stimulus, apparently acts independently of the anterior pituitary. Since a major function of aldosterone release following tissue damage would appear to be that of clearing the circulation of potentially toxic concentrations of potassium, it is reasonable that the serum concentration of this ion would be a factor involved in stimulating the release of aldosterone.

Adrenocorticotropic hormone is known to be released immediately after operation in quantities adequate to produce aldosterone output. All these factors have been studied in detail following surgical procedures, and as can be seen in Figure 1, there is a quantitative and chronologic relationship between the secretion of cortisol and aldosterone after operation, which does not obtain during control periods nor in the later phases of convalescence. This and evidence obtained from

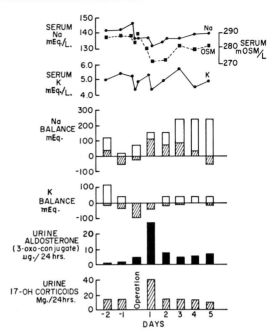

Figure 1. The course of the blood levels and balance of electrolytes as related to the urinary excretion of aldosterone and 17-hydroxycorticoids following a typical operation.

patients with pituitary insufficiency undergoing surgical procedures suggest that in the immediately postoperative period, adrenocorticotropic hormone represents the dominant mechanism for aldosterone release.

Although it appears that the role of aldosterone must be of great importance in the regulation of mineral balance immediately following operations, it is by no means clear that this substance is totally responsible for the overall change in mineral metabolism which occurs. Aldosterone, as measured in the urine of these patients, appears early in the postoperative course and almost uniformly returns to basal levels in two to three days. Positive sodium balance, on the other hand, may persist for six or seven days and almost regularly obtains after the aldosterone levels are normal. Even in the immediate postoperative period, detailed studies correlating sodium-potassium ratio with steroid output suggest that the excretion of these ions is related not to the concentration of this steroid alone, but to the summation of its effect and the relatively weak electrolyte-mobilizing properties of cortisol.

It is likely that none of the metabolic responses to operation is exclusively regulated by the endocrine system, and it must be remembered in this connection that hormones, in general, only catalyze and do not originate metabolic and membrane-transfer phenomena. There is a considerable body of evidence suggesting that, in both man and animals devoid of adrenal glands but maintained on constant amounts of cortical replacement, nitrogen excretion, sodium retention and potassium loss can all be induced by the imposition of nonspecific stress. This strengthens the notion that the underlying pathways for these reactions exist in the basic enzymatic machinery, and do not depend exclusively on an acceleration in endocrine function. Nevertheless, the importance of the endocrines for preservation of life under circumstances of systemic stress is adequately demonstrated by the almost uniformly fatal results of even minor operations inadvertently carried out on patients with adrenal insufficiency.

ANTIDIURESIS: ROLE OF POSTERIOR PITUITARY. A seeming paradox exists in the fact that during the period following extensive surgery, when sodium and chloride tend to be withheld from the urine, plasma levels of these ions are commonly reduced. The question whether this reduction of plasma levels represents only the addition of salt-free water which is not excreted, or must be explained in part by some presently undefined sequestration of sodium and chloride ions, remains debatable. A more significant fact is that in postoperative patients, the administration of salt-free solutions, such as 5 per cent glucose, is followed by only sluggish diuresis and by reduction of plasma electrolyte concentrations. Administration of the same amount of glucose solution to normal individuals, or preoperative patients, results in almost no change in the plasma concentrations. Various lines of evidence suggest that this diminution of urine output in the early postoperative course is related to antidiuretic activity of posterior pituitary origin.

In the normally hydrated patient, the surgical operation produces physiologic effects similar to those of Pitressin. Urine flow decreases, urine osmolality increases and serum osmolality decreases. The "free" water clearance (C_{H_2O}), which is defined as the difference between urine flow (V) and the osmolar clearance $\left(\dfrac{U_{osm}}{P_{osm}} \cdot V\right)$, decreases. Thus,

$$C_{H_2O} = V - \frac{U_{osm}}{P_{osm}} \cdot V.$$

This value is negative when water is being conserved at the expense of solute.

It is important to realize that these observations regarding water and solute output following operation are not by themselves unequivocal evidence of antidiuretic activity. They can only be so interpreted if glomerular filtration is shown to be either constant or increasing, a circumstance which has not been met in most studies of the subject. Recent experiments have shown, for example, that even in the animal with experimental diabetes insipidus, a hypertonic urine can be produced by restriction of renal blood flow and glomerular filtration. The importance of serious alterations in renal blood flow following major surgical procedures cannot be disregarded.

More direct evidence concerning the role of antidiuretic hormone in postoperative water balance has been made available by the development of a very sensitive method for the determination of arginine vasopressin, the human antidiuretic octapeptide. Because this assay is capable of measuring concentrations in peripheral blood, it has been possible to follow antidiuretic hormone during the course of surgical operations and to demonstrate that operations are accompanied by output of large amounts of antidiuretic hormone by the posterior pituitary. Also, it has been demonstrated that the blood level is related to details of the surgical procedure such as blood loss and stimulation of visceral afferent autonomic nerves by dissection and manipulation of viscera. Elevated levels persist as long as three to four days after major surgical procedures.

The development of a precise assay method has also made possible experiments to determine the mechanisms for regulation of anti-

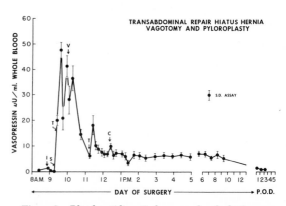

Figure 2. Blood antidiuretic hormone levels during surgical procedure illustrating changes during induction of anesthesia (I), skin and soft tissue incision (S), traction on viscera (T), vagotomy (V) and closure (C). (From Zimmermann: Curr. Probl. Surg. Chicago, Year Book Publishers, 1965.

diuretic hormone output and the pathways through which injury and surgical operations increase the circulating levels. The painstaking studies of Verney demonstrated that antidiuresis was produced following injury of even trivial magnitude, pain, hemorrhage, fear and other emotional stimuli, and elevation of plasma osmolality. Verney studied the last of these mechanisms by injecting concentrated solutions into exteriorized arterial loops in dogs, by which method he was able to show that antidiuresis followed the introduction of sodium chloride and other substances into the carotid system. He postulated that osmoreceptors were situated within the ramifications of the internal carotid system. The concept that circulating volume, in addition to tonicity, was important in the regulation of antidiuretic hormone output began with the work of Henry and Gauer. Their experiments, in which diuresis was produced by distention of balloons in the left atrium of dogs, suggested that there were volume receptors in the region of the left atrium and pulmonary veins. Studies in which arginine vasopressin was actually measured have confirmed this. High levels of circulating antidiuretic hormone can also be produced by traction on the abdominal viscera and experiments in animals demonstrate that these impulses are carried over afferent nerves following both sympathetic and parasympathetic pathways. Sensory nerves are also capable of transmitting stimuli which result in increased antidiuretic hormone output. Thus, there are a variety of sources of stimulation to the supraoptic and paraventricular nuclei of the hypothalamus which transmit stimuli to the posterior pituitary. It is believed that the octapeptide is actually produced in the hypothalamic nuclei and carried in connection with a neurosecretory carrier substance down to the capillary plexus which surrounds the neurohypophysis. These stimuli are much more potent than those related to the osmoreceptors and hence the effects of operative stress and hemorrhage readily overwhelm those of changes in tonicity. Therefore, antidiuresis occurs even in the face of lowered serum sodium and osmolality.

OXIDATIVE METABOLISM. Surgical injury results in an increase in oxygen consumption, which varies with the extent of the procedure and is greatly enhanced by the presence of infection and inflammation. This increase in metabolism involves the body stores of fat and protein. Much remains to be learned about the basis for this accelera-tion of oxygen utilization. There is no evidence for a consistent increase in thyroid activity. The studies of Kinney suggest that the pituitary may be involved, in that the metabolic rate in hypophysectomized individuals declines rather than increases after operation, although such individuals can still respond to the appropriate caloric expenditure through the stimuli of late surgical complications.

SIGNIFICANCE OF ENDOCRINE AND METABOLIC CHANGES ASSOCIATED WITH OPERATIONS. It is possible, as Moore has done, to divide the metabolic changes associated with surgical convalescence into a number of phases. The first, or injury, phase is dominated by the rapid secretion of adrenal steroids, vasopressin, vasoactive amines and associated changes in nitrogen, water and mineral balance. The second, or turning point, phase is characterized by a return toward a normal level of endocrine activity, diuresis of water and sodium, and reduction in the initially elevated rate of urinary nitrogen excretion. The third phase consists of protein anabolism and the restoration of substance and strength to the muscle mass. The last stage of convalescence involves the restoration of stores of body fat. A great deal of controversy and misunderstanding surrounds the implication of the early metabolic changes following injury with respect to treatment. A teleologic argument exists as to whether these are harmful effects which should be combated, or beneficial ones to be encouraged.

The negative balance of nitrogen and catabolism of tissue protein would appear to be an inevitable consequence of trauma. Despite the fact that a positive paper balance of nitrogen can be achieved by the rapid administration of protein hydrolysate, or other protein units, at a rate temporarily higher than nitrogen excretion, there is little evidence that a true net positive balance can be attained during the initial catabolic phase. This in no way denies the importance of making adequate amounts of protein and calories available during the period of recovery and anabolism.

A similar question of interpretation concerns alterations in fluid and electrolyte metabolism. There appears to be no question that, in the injured organism, the preservation of circulating volume by the conservation of sodium and water is of critical survival value. The mobilization of an endocrine mechanism to accelerate the excretion of potassium may also be of great importance. Destruction of cells can liberate this ion into the extracellular space in amounts sufficient to produce lethal concentrations. Mechanisms which are basically conservative become hazardous only in the presence of therapy. They are designed to protect the organism, which, because of circumstances of injury, does not have access to the major constituents which are necessary for maintaining the extracellular fluid volume and composition. The importance of these patterns of response is that they greatly modify the tolerance of patients to administered fluids and solutes, and create the background for a group of electrolyte anomalies which are seen with considerable frequency in surgical patients.

FLUID COMPARTMENTS; THEIR BOUNDARIES AND CONSTITUENTS. The tendency of clinicians to describe abnormalities of fluid and electrolyte physiology in terms of plasma values results only from the relative simplicity with which a sample can be drawn from the circulating blood. Although blood values are obviously of great importance, any rational consideration of abnormalities of fluid and electrolyte physiology must take into account all the major fluid spaces, and the nature of the boundaries which separate them.

It is important to consider the dynamics which maintain the separate characteristics of the fluid spaces of the body. For convenience reference is made to anatomically discrete spaces, but in truth there are no compartments. There are phases which can be defined only arbitrarily in terms of the methods by which they are measured. There are no rigid boundaries but only gradients of concentrations which are maintained by active metabolic processes. Although our present knowledge of the volume and composition of these phases has been greatly enhanced by the use of tracer techniques, deductions made from such dilution measurements require assumptions regarding the manner in which tracers are distributed, and even greater ones regarding the consistency of such distribution under circumstances of disease. Total body water is measured most frequently by the use of deuterium oxide (D_2O) or tritiated water (THO) and surprisingly varies widely depending on the proportion of adipose tissue which is almost anhydrous. Average values in young adults are 63 per cent of the total body weight in males and 52 per cent in females. The most difficult phase to define is the extracellular space. In fact, there is no real agreement as to what it should include. Opinion differs regarding the classification of the water of bone and intraluminal secretion of glands and viscera. The tracers used are substances which behave like halogens, bromide, radiobromide, radiochloride and thiocyanate, nonmetabolizable sugars such as inulin and most recently thiosulfate and radiosulfate ($S^{35}O_4$). Conventionally, the extracellular fluid includes the blood plasma, which is 4.5 per cent of the body weight, the interstitial fluid, which is approximately 16 per cent, and the lymph, which is approximately 2 per cent. The intracellular volume is obtained by subtracting the extracellular volume from the total body water and represents the sum total of all the water in all the cells of the body. It is obviously, therefore, not a continuous phase, but an average of the content of cells which vary enormously in their individual composition. The intracellular water comprises more than half the total body water, and in an average individual constitutes 30 to 40 per cent of the body weight. Transcellular water is a portion of the extracellular fluid which deserves special consideration in relationship to disease and injury. It includes the cerebrospinal fluid, the intraocular and pleural and peritoneal contents, the secretion of salivary and digestive glands and the contents of the alimentary tract. Although in a sense they do not contribute to the normal circulation, these spaces have been shown to be in active equilibrium with the extracellular phase. Whereas this volume is normally less than 3 per cent of body weight, in some surgical conditions the transcellular space can be greatly enlarged with concomitant depletion of the active circulating extracellular volume. The *plasma volume* is approximately 4.5 per cent of the body weight. It can be calculated either by the administration of labeled substances such as Evans Blue (T-1824) or radioiodinated serum albumin. An alternative method involves the use of determining the red cell mass with cells labeled with radioactive phosphorus (P^{32}) or chromium (Cr^{51}) from which, when the hematocrit is known, the plasma volume can be calculated.

The blood plasma and interstitial fluid are essentially the same in composition except for the difference in protein concentration which results from the relative impermeability of the capillaries to these large molecules. The relative volumes of the plasma and the interstitial space are regulated by the forces which govern the equilibrium of fluid and solute movement across the capillary membrane. This relationship, which was described by Starling in 1896, implies that the pressure at any point in the capillary is balanced by the sum of the tissue turgor pressure and the net intravascular colloid osmotic pressure. Thus, shifts between these two spaces are caused by changes in either plasma protein concentration or intravascular pressure. The composition of the cell fluid differs radically from that of the extracellular environment. Whereas sodium is the major extracellular cation, potassium occupies this position in the cell, where phosphate is the predominant anion. Despite this, it is not true, as was once believed, that sodium is completely excluded from the cell. A definite amount of sodium ion constitutes a portion of the intracellular ionic structure and there is a great deal of evidence that this quantity may be increased under circumstances of injury and disease. It must also be recognized that the relative exclusion of sodium from the cell is not a matter of permeability of the cell wall. Individual sodium ions have been shown by tracer techniques readily to permeate the cell membrane, showing that maintenance of an unequal gradient is not a matter of permeability but an active process requiring the expenditure of metabolic energy. The perpetuation of these unequal concentrations is, therefore, a function of normal cells and a characteristic of life as significant as the utilization of oxygen and the production of carbon dioxide. It is typical, moreover, of sick cells that these gradients tend to break down and the intracellular concentrations approach those of the surrounding medium.

The values for the volumes of the intracellular and extracellular compartments describe the situation in the normal individual. It is of some importance to consider the factors which regulate these volume relationships. The critical quantity in this regard is the extracellular sodium, for the intracellular volume does not depend on the available water of the extracellular space but rather its total ionic concentration. Since sodium exists in largest concentration, the level of this ion is the most important controlling factor. A decrease in sodium ion concentration results in a movement of water into the cells, with consequent enlargement of the intracellular volume, and similarly, an increase in sodium concentration results in cellular dehydration. Therefore, just as intravascular protein is largely responsible for the maintenance of equilibrium between the plasma volume and the interstitial space, extracellular sodium serves this function in regulating the relationship between extracellular and intracellular water. Changes in cell water have profound functional implications and the central nervous system is particularly sensitive to them. Consequently, changes in tonicity underlie many of the clinical manifestations for which deviations of water and electrolyte balance are responsible.

REQUIREMENTS OF SURGICAL PATIENTS. The initial consideration for fluid replacement is the basal requirement for the human being who, for reasons of disease or surgery, is denied the oral route of alimentation. The minimal quota for an adult must take account of an insensible loss through the skin and lungs ranging from 600 to 1000 ml. and an anticipated urine output of 1000 to 1500 ml. Insensible losses may, of course, be far greater than this, particularly in the circumstances of fever, which raises metabolic requirements about 10 per cent for each degree, or a prolonged operation under heavy cloth draping.

It must also be appreciated that exogenous water is not the sole source of fluid for extracellular hydration in seriously ill patients. Moore has pointed out that in severe injury or chronic illness as much as 1000 ml. of water can be mobilized daily from endogenous sources. This is made up of cell water (about 700 ml. per kg. of lean tissue), oxidation of protein (about 150 ml. per kg.) and of fat (1080 ml. per kg.). Accurate studies on patients with anuria, in whom the control of water administration must be extremely precise, have shown that as little as 400 to 500 ml. of exogenous water may sometimes be required. In providing fluid for surgical patients, body size is obviously important and a provision of 1400 to 1500 ml. per square meter of body area (70 kg. = 1.76 sq. ml.) will approximately meet the minimal requirements in the absence of abnormal losses, internal translocations or excess metabolic demands.

The factors of insensible loss and endogenous water are not only variable but highly unpredictable, and this is the reason for the unique value of the body weight in assessing states of hydration. In addition, therefore, for accurate measurement of the fluid intake and output, surgical patients should be weighed daily on a balance which is accurate to 0.1 kg. The weight should be recorded on the chart along with the fluid balance data. In patients too ill to stand on a scale, this can be accomplished by a balance which utilizes a litter upon which the patient is lifted from his bed.

The use of body weight in assessing fluid balance is based on the assumption that significant changes over short periods are largely the result of changes in hydration. This assumption is not valid over periods of many days in chronically ill patients in whom cumulative decrements in tissue mass are occurring. It should be kept in mind that large amounts of fluid may be sequestered temporarily in areas of the body which play no role in the maintenance of circulation or the state of hydration. This so-called "third space" effect occurs to some extent following any operation or injury. It assumes significant proportions when there are extensive areas of tissue damage, localized edema peripheral to sites of venous or lymphatic obstruction, or intestinal ileus. It would be absurd, for example, to calculate the fluid requirements for a patient with a major burn on the basis of the changes in body weight, when his fluid losses are almost entirely within his own body.

Large amounts of sodium chloride are not required for basal maintenance of patients who do not suffer from external losses, blood loss, or major internal translocations. The normal kidney can restrict sodium excretion to less than that contained in 1 gm. of sodium chloride (17 mEq.), and the insensible water loss excluding palpable sweat contains only traces of sodium salt.

POTASSIUM REQUIREMENTS. The ability of the kidney to conserve in the absence of intake does not hold for potassium ion, since 30 to 40 mEq. of potassium may be excreted by patients receiving none by oral or parenteral route. It is necessary, therefore, to include in a parenteral regimen at least 2 to 3 gm. of a salt such as potassium chloride for routine maintenance. This, however, should not be given immediately after operation, or until normal renal function has been adequately established. The losses of potassium may, of course, be much greater following the stress of major surgery, burns and trauma.

EFFECTS OF SHOCK, HEMORRHAGE, TRAUMA AND EXTENSIVE SURGERY. There is a great deal of evidence that in contrast to the individual who has not sustained injury, the patient who has suffered hemorrhage, injury, or undergone extensive surgical operations cannot be optimally managed with quantities of sodium and extracellular-type electrolyte solutions which are limited to the requirement predicted on the basis of external balance. There are a number of reasons why, under the latter circumstances, more sodium-containing solution should be given than is required to make up for external losses. The first of these has to do with factors controlling water excretion in the presence of a strong antidiuretic stimulus. The definitions outlined in relationship to the regulation of urine osmolality imply that the total urine output is equal to the algebraic sum of the osmolar clearance and the free water clearance. Because the latter is controlled by antidiuretic hormones, it is apparent that an increase in total urine volume can only be accomplished by addition of a solute load for excretion. It has actually been demonstrated in patients following major surgical procedures that urine output and weight loss are enhanced by administration of modest amounts of sodium chloride as compared with regimens in which no sodium is included. There is good reason for assuming that this state of water balance which more closely approximates that of the relatively fasting normal individual is desirable.

The second consideration has to do with recent observations on changes in the extracellular fluid during hemorrhage. It has been recognized since the time of Starling's work that transcapillary refilling of the circulation from the interstitial space takes place when the capillary pressure is temporarily reduced by bleeding. The recent studies of Shires in which plasma volume, red cell volume and extracellular space were separately measured suggest that during hemorrhage a greater depletion of the interstitial space occurs than can be accounted for by the blood loss alone, and that this is neither prevented nor restored by the administration of whole blood. The significance of this has been confirmed by the demonstration in both animals and patients that administration of lactated Ringer's solution concomitantly with blood transfusion replaced the extracellular fluid deficit and increased survival after hemorrhage.

Thirdly, it must be recognized that tissues which have been subjected to trauma or surgical dissection are responsible for sequestration of more edema fluid than is apparent to the eye of the surgeon, and that the necessity for replacement of this has been judged on the basis of the type of tissue and extent of injury. It is likely, for example, that a radical pancreatoduodenectomy requires the replacement during the intraoperative and postoperative period of 2000 to 3000 ml. of extracellular-type fluid in excess of that necessitated by a cholecystectomy. Recognition of all these factors and appropriate administration of sodium-containing solutions have virtually eliminated postoperative oliguria in the absence of renal damage. Administration of Ringer's solution during operations has resulted in continuous urine flow under circumstances in which patients were virtually anuric when salt-free glucose solutions alone were used.

EXTERNAL LOSSES. In addition to the basal amounts of fluid to provide for urine output and to replace insensible losses, parenteral administration must include volume-for-volume replacement of water lost through the abnormal routes of tubes and fistulae. The replacement of solutes lost through these channels must take into account the origin of the secretions, for the ratio of sodium to chloride in various gastrointestinal fluids differs greatly from that of plasma. Their loss will produce not only overall electrolyte depletion but also profound disturbances in acid-base equilibrium. Thus, withdrawal of normal gastric juice, which contains more chloride than plasma and very little sodium, rapidly produces alkalosis. Conversely, pancreatic juice, which possesses a sodium concentration comparable to that of plasma but relatively little chloride, causes acidosis when lost from the body in significant amounts.

Bile is more alkaline than plasma though its sodium-to-chloride ratio is not nearly so high as that of pancreatic juice. Intestinal fistulae, except for high ones, tend also to produce acidosis because of relatively greater sodium losses. Most aspirates from tubes and fistulae are of mixed, and frequently of undetermined, origin. It may be occasionally necessary to make actual measurements of solutes in the secretions in order effectively to provide for their replacement.

A very special type of intestinal fluid loss is occasionally seen in connection with villous adenomata of the colon and rectum. This rare manifestation is characterized by copious watery rectal discharge associated with severe fluid and electrolyte loss, which if untreated leads to dehydration, hyponatremia, hypokalemia, prerenal azotemia, circulatory collapse and death. Potassium loss is particularly striking and levels in the rectal discharge of 12 to 15 times that of plasma have been measured.

For common situations, average values for gastrointestinal fluids based on previous experience are adequate. Table 1 and Table 2 from the work of Lockwood and Randall present some mean concentrations of sodium, potassium and chloride for typical secretions. Reference to these tables is useful in approximating the requirements in average situations. To replace the acid secretion from a normal stomach, it is usually only necessary to use sodium chloride solutions even though this may entail giving an excess of sodium

Table 1. *Values for Content of Sodium, Potassium and Chloride in Gastrointestinal Tract Losses (Milliequivalents per Liter)**

		NA	K	CL
Gastric (Fasting) 130 specimens	Average	59.0	9.3	89.0
	Range	6.0–157	0.5–65.0	13.2–167.2
	2/3 Cases	31.0–90.0	4.3–12.0	52–124
Small bowel (Miller-Abbott suction) 89 specimens	Average	104.9	5.1	98.9
	Range	20.1–157.0	1.0–11.0	43.0–156.1
	2/3 Cases	72–128	3.5–6,8	69–127
Ileum (Miller-Abbott suction) 17 specimens 7 patients	Average	116.7	· 5.0	105.8
	Range	82–147	2.3–8.0	60.7–137.0
	2/3 Cases	91–140	3.0–7.5	82–125
Ileostomy (Recent) 25 specimens 7 patients	Average	129.5	16.2	109.7
	Range	92–146	3.8–98.0	66–136
	2/3 Cases	112–142	4.5–14.0	93–122
Cecostomy 20 specimens 9 patients	Average	79.6	20.6	48.2
	Range	45–135	3.7–47.3	18–88.5
	2/3 Cases	48–116	11.1–28.3	35–70

* From Randall, H. T.: Water and electrolyte balance in surgery. S. Clin. North America 32:457, 1952.

Table 2.   *Sodium, Potassium and Chloride Concentration of Bile and Pancreatic Juice (Milliequivalents per Liter)**

		NA	K	CL
Bile				
22 specimens	Average	145.3	5.2	99.9
12 patients	Range	122–164	3.2–9.7	77–127
	2/3 Cases	134–156	3.9–6.3	83–110
Pancreas				
3 patients	Average	141.1	4.6	76.6
	Range	113–153	2.6–7.4	54.1–95.2

* From Randall, H. T.: Water and electrolyte balance in surgery. S. Clin. North America 32:458, 1952.

ion. Since a normal kidney excretes the sodium, acid salts such as ammonium chloride are rarely necessary, except when serious distortions of body chemistry have become established. However, in the management of pancreatic, biliary and intestinal fistulae when sodium loss predominates, replacement cannot be achieved by the use of sodium chloride alone. Alkaline solutions, such as sodium bicarbonate or lactate, are necessary. In this connection, it will be recalled that the plasma is normally alkaline. The administration of sodium chloride alone is an acidosis-producing procedure and lactated Ringer's solution is, therefore, much more appropriate than neutral saline in the replacement of extracellular fluid losses.

The question of replacement of magnesium ion and the rare occurrence of magnesium deficiency syndromes are matters of considerable current interest. Although the intake of magnesium in the average diet is said to be around 300 mg. per day, the normal individual appears able to conserve this ion effectively in the presence of deficient intake. Studies of Barnes and Cope suggest that as little as 1 mEq. per day would maintain a normal adult in magnesium balance, that a magnesium-deficient diet can be tolerated for as long as 38 days and that there is no significant obligatory loss by normal kidneys and gastrointestinal tract over that period of time. Nevertheless, the magnesium content of gastric aspiration fluid is about 2 mEq. per liter and there is some evidence that magnesium behaves partly like potassium with respect to adrenal function in that mineral-regulating corticoids accelerate its excretion. One would expect, therefore, that major operations, particularly gastrointestinal operations, would present a threat to the magnesium stores. This occurs most frequently in patients who have diarrhea, gastrointestinal drainage or defunctionalization of large portions of the intestinal tract for protracted periods, in addition to parenteral maintenance without inclusion of magnesium ion. Clinically and chemically proved instances of magnesium deficiency are characterized by neuromuscular irritability, disorientation, fibrillary twitchings, tremor and even convulsions, which respond to magnesium therapy. If these clinical signs appear following long periods of parenteral maintenance, and are associated with blood levels below the normal range of 1.5 to 2.5 mEq. per liter or urinary excretion of less than 3 mEq. per day, parenteral administration of magnesium ion is indicated.

DISTURBANCES OF ACID-BASE EQUILIBRIUM. Clinical disturbances of acid-base balance may be either metabolic or respiratory. Whereas, in the past, metabolic disturbances were considered to be vastly more frequent, the recent growth of thoracic surgery and the more intensive study of inhalation anesthesia have served to emphasize the comparative frequency with which respiratory disturbances of acid-base regulation actually occur in surgical patients. Consequently, it is of great importance in evaluating acidosis or alkalosis that the necessary data be available to demonstrate clearly what the underlying basis for the clinical disturbance in pH is. In most institutions, a measurement approximating the plasma bicarbonate, such as the carbon dioxide combining power, is used for clinical purposes. Reliance on this value alone is frequently adequate. It must be kept in mind that this quantity is by itself no index of the direction of the pH change. The pH maintained by the buffering system of the plasma is related to the bicarbonate of the blood and the dissolved carbon dioxide, or carbonic acid, by the familiar Henderson-Hasselbalch equation:

$$pH = pK + \log \frac{BHCO_3}{H_2CO_3}.$$

When numerical values are introduced for the dissociation constant and the solubility constant of CO_2, it becomes:

$$pH = 6.1 + \log \frac{BHCO_3}{0.03pCO_2}.$$

The bicarbonate of the plasma can be altered by changes in its rate of renal excretion. The carbonic acid concentration depends on the rate at which carbon dioxide is removed by the lungs. By their individual control of these two quantities, the lungs and kidneys are the organs primarily responsible for the preservation of normal pH in the face of circumstances tending to disturb it. In deviations of a primary metabolic nature, the initial effect is on the bicarbonate, which is decreased in acidosis and increased in alkalosis. The respiratory apparatus responds to shift the carbonic acid in the same direction,

so that the ratio $\frac{BHCO_3}{H_2CO_3}$, which is normally

20:1, is minimally altered. Respiration is, therefore, accelerated in acidosis and depressed in alkalosis although the latter adjustment is minimal and frequently not clinically apparent. In disturbances of a primary respiratory nature, however, the initial effect involves the carbonic acid. Compensations must be made by the kidneys which retain or excrete bicarbonate. They retain bicarbonate when carbonic acid has been inadequately removed by the lungs, and they excrete an excess of bicarbonate to compensate for the alkalosis which follows hyperventilation. Since the final bicarbonate value, which is the most commonly used index for acid-base disturbances, is elevated in metabolic alkalosis and respiratory acidosis and depressed in respiratory alkalosis and metabolic acidosis, it is not possible to distinguish between acidosis and alkalosis on the basis of the carbon dioxide combining or the total CO_2 content. In most instances, the clinical information points to a disturbance which is primarily of metabolic or of respiratory origin. Occasionally, however, the situation is not clinically obvious and the complete acid-base picture must be obtained by establishing a value of a second of the three possible variables in the Henderson-Hasselbalch equation. This is done ordinarily by determination of the blood pH and preferably with the simultaneous measurement of the pCO_2 of the arterial blood.

Metabolic alkalosis is most commonly seen in surgical patients as a result of the loss of large amounts of gastric secretion, a material which has high chloride content with relatively low concentrations of sodium. It is ordinarily lost either through vomiting or continuous inlying gastric suction. Alkalosis can develop in as brief a time as 24 hours in the face of total diversion of gastric content. Figure 3 illustrates the ionic pattern in such a situation compared with the normal concentration.

POTASSIUM DEFICIENCY. The relationship between metabolic alkalosis and potassium deficiency is an important one. Initially, in the face of a deficit of chloride ion for reabsorption by the kidney along with sodium, the latter remains in the renal tubule and is excreted in the urine in large amounts. Alkalosis of chloride loss is initially compensated by the accumulation of a sodium deficit but because a mounting sodium deficiency cannot be tolerated for long, the normal renal and adrenal mechanisms for sodium conservation come into play to allow exchange of potassium and hydrogen ion for sodium in the distal tubule. Thus, the urine which was initially alkaline becomes acid ("paradoxical aciduria"), and in addition there is accumulative potassium deficiency superimposed on the depletion of chloride and sodium. As alkalosis persists, particularly in the absence of

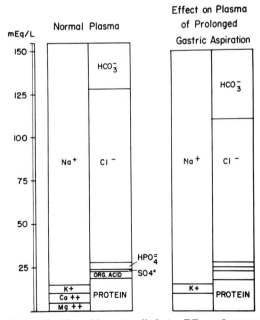

Figure 3. Hypochloremic alkalosis. Effect of several days of nasal tube suction, without adequate chloride replacement, on the composition of plasma. Note reduction of chloride with expansion of bicarbonate and essentially normal sodium.

exogenous potassium ion, the potassium deficit increases. It is necessary, therefore, that replacement therapy include sodium, potassium and chloride, and the patient probably cannot be restored completely to health without administration of potassium solution as well as sodium. The key to the situation is the replacement of the anion, chloride, because its deficiency is initially responsible for the derangement. The replacement of chloride is usually accomplished by the administration of both sodium chloride and potassium chloride in replacement solutions.

It is unfortunate that for several years the known reciprocal relationship between potassium and hydrogen ion in tubular urine, and the association of potassium deficiency without alkalosis, led some clinicians to assume that it was potassium deficiency rather than anion deficiency which precipitated alkalotic states. This fallacy persisted despite the repeated demonstration of failure to reverse acid-base imbalance with potassium salts other than potassium chloride. It is now clear, however, that hypokalemic alkalosis only occurs when there has been excessive chloride loss, when excessive amounts of alkaline solutions have been given, or in the presence of large quantities of steroid hormones possessing electrolyte activity. The last circumstance does exist following surgical operations, and there is no doubt that formidable operations with protracted convalescence can lead to hypokalemia and hypokalemic alkalosis if adequate amounts of potassium are not included in the parenteral regimen (Fig. 4). The likelihood of this complication is greatly increased if more than one operation is required within a few days, such as reopening the abdomen following a previous laparotomy, repair of wound dehiscence and similar situations. The signs of potassium deficiency are those of failure of normal contractility of smooth, skeletal and cardiac muscle. Ileus and weakness are seen in addition to alkalotic tetany and Trousseau's sign.

The diagnosis is usually suspected in the presence of relatively refractory alkalosis. Serum levels of potassium are usually low, although they need not always be. The characteristic electrocardiographic findings — prolongation of the Q-T interval, depression of the RS-T segment and eventually inverted T waves — are valuable confirmatory signs. The response to treatment is frequently best followed by measurement of the bicarbonate. In profound alkalotic states, the simultaneous

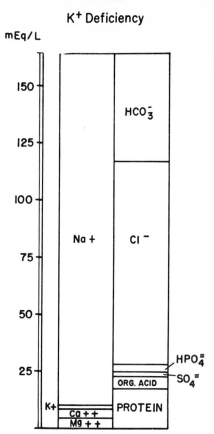

Figure 4. Hypochloremic alkalosis associated with potassium deficiency in a patient following prolonged parenteral therapy without potassium replacement.

administration of solutions containing sodium chloride, potassium chloride and ammonium chloride is useful.

Table 1 indicates the amounts of potassium in milliequivalents per liter of drainage which may be lost from the body through gastrointestinal siphonage. Even when gastrointestinal siphonage is employed, the loss through the gastrointestinal tract is usually not the largest source of negative potassium balance. Even under normal circumstances, an individual receiving no potassium by mouth may put out large amounts of urinary potassium. Under circumstances of stress, imposed by a major surgical procedure or acute intestinal obstruction, these urinary losses are greatly increased.

With the rapid recent increase of interest in surgery of the cardiovascular system, the relationship of the potassium ion to cardiac function has assumed great importance. Potassium deficiency enhances the effect of digitalis glycosides and can be responsible for the clinical and electrocardiographic evidence of digitalis toxicity. Adequate potassium replacement is, therefore, of particular importance in digitalis-treated patients who may be depleted of this ion by operations or by preoperative treatment with chlorothiazide diuretics.

Metabolic acidosis is frequently seen following the loss from the body of secretions possessing high sodium concentration. The typical case is that of pancreatic fistula. Pancreatic juice, which possesses a sodium concentration comparable to that of plasma but very little chloride, is almost an isotonic solution of sodium bicarbonate. Diversion of this solution from a normal path of being secreted and reabsorbed from the intestine results very rapidly in profound acidosis with a blood picture of low sodium and low bicarbonate values. The electrolyte picture resulting from a chronic pancreatic fistula is illustrated in Figure 5. A similar situation is, of course,

produced by sodium loss through fistulae from the lower intestine where the sodium-to-chloride ratio is also high. Reversal of the blood electrolyte values in these situations cannot be ordinarily accomplished with sodium chloride, and the use of sodium solutions with labile or metabolizable anions, such as sodium lactate or sodium bicarbonate, is ordinarily required.

These examples of acidosis result from the loss of the extracellular cation, or what was referred to in the older clinical terminology as "fixed base." Another type, "addition acidosis," is the result not of loss of base but of accumulation of abnormal acids, which results in displacement of bicarbonate. An example of this is the acidosis which accompanies uremia with accumulation of phosphate, sulfate and organic acids. Another type results from the excessive reabsorption of chloride from the intestine following surgical procedures in which the ureters are transplanted into the intestinal tract. This so-called chloride acidosis frequently follows such procedures but is more likely to exist when drainage of the intestinal segment is inadequate, or when poor renal function exists in addition to discharge of urine into the intestine. It is also occasionally present in abnormal communication between the urinary and intestinal tracts resulting from neoplastic and inflammatory diseases and congenital anomalies.

Respiratory acidosis associated with anesthesia and thoracic surgery has become a matter of increasing significance in recent years. It is important to recognize that the administration of oxygen to individuals with respiratory impairment resulting from pulmonary disease, inadequate pulmonary tissue or impairment of motor respiratory activity will maintain oxygen saturation of the blood but may not achieve adequate removal of carbon dioxide. The greatly enhanced opportunity for management of respiratory disturbances of acid-base balance by the development of modern respirators and methods for control of ventilation require that complete assessment of the acid-base status be made in a large number of patients in whom such disturbances are suspected.

DISTURBANCES OF FLUID VOLUME. A consideration of daily importance in the management of postoperative patients is the maintenance of normal extracellular fluid volume. This quantity, which is very sensitively regulated in the normal individual, is readily sub-

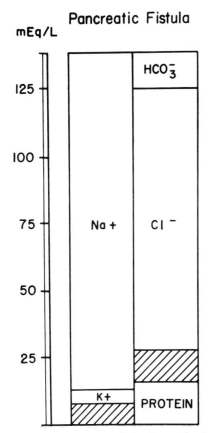

Pancreatic Fistula

Figure 5. Hyponatremic acidosis; the result of chronic sodium loss through a pancreatic fistula. Note reduction of sodium with corresponding contraction of bicarbonate. Cross-hatch indicates normal values assumed (cations) or determined by subtraction (anions).

ject to distortion when the oral intake, or the effect of thirst, is removed and when renal regulation of fluid volume may be impaired. Dehydration in the strict sense refers to the effects on the body of water loss alone. It most frequently is used to describe the deficiency of water in combination with electrolytes. Pure water dehydration is actually rare. The familiar signs of combined extracellular fluid deficiency include loss of turgor of the skin, sunken eyes and dryness of the mucous membranes. Change in body weight is the best index of the development of dehydration. Serum electrolyte concentrations can be elevated, depressed or normal, and give no indication of the overall deficit of ionic components. If a patient admitted to the hospital has been vomiting, or has suffered other perceptible fluid losses, it must be remembered that if he has not been drinking, water loss almost invariably exceeds electrolyte loss so that it is best to begin hydration with solutions which are dilute with respect to ionic constituents. Subsequent blood chemical determinations frequently reveal the presence of electrolyte deficit as a more normal state of hydration is approached.

Edema in association with surgery was frequently seen in earlier days when "physiologic saline" was used routinely as a hydrating solution. After the recognition by Coller and his associates of the tendency for patients to retain sodium in the period after operation, excessive use of sodium chloride was almost universally discontinued. Postoperative edema became far less common and today is most frequently seen in combination with protein depletion. In this situation, as with dehydration, the serum levels of ions do not, of course, give any index of the overall excess of extracellular electrolytes which may be present. The familiar clinical signs of pulmonary and peripheral edema are obviously of the greatest importance, and serial body weight determinations will demonstrate incipient fluid retention long before clinical edema is apparent. It should be emphasized that the central venous pressure, though useful in detecting acute hypervolemia precipitated by administration of blood and colloid-containing solutions, is of no value in assessing overall extracellular fluid excess and that massive expansion of the interstitial space occurs without elevation of the venous pressure.

DISTURBANCES OF CONCENTRATION. Because of the importance of the sodium concentration of the extracellular fluid and its critical role in the distribution of water between the cells and the fluid which surrounds them, it is not surprising that the normal sodium level is maintained within rather narrow limits. Nevertheless, following operation and in the absence of oral intake, elimination of the factor of thirst and with certain impairments in renal function, disturbances in the regulation of sodium concentration do occur. Such a deviation represents in effect an abnormality in the overall effective osmotic properties of extracellular fluid.

HYPONATREMIA. Following major operations, the sodium concentration of the plasma tends to drop despite the fact that sodium balance inclines to be positive. This situation results from an intolerance of the postoperative patient to administered water with subsequent dilution, and possibly also from factors having to do with translocation of the sodium ion possibly into other reservoirs, which are at present poorly understood. Although this frequent depression of sodium concentration is not ordinarily accompanied by symptoms, it occasionally is severe enough to cause profound functional disturbances. The most dramatic of these involve the central nervous system, which reflects the depression of sodium concentration and reacts to intracellular shift of water by the physical signs of stupor, irrationality, neuromuscular phenomena and sometimes convulsions. Depending on the circumstances leading to such clinical symptoms, they are referred to as "water intoxication" or "low sodium syndrome." The most profound effects are produced when an injudicious amount of water is given to a patient within the first two to three days after surgery. Nevertheless, instances of so-called water intoxication have been observed under circumstances in which entirely appropriate amounts of water have been administered (Fig. 6).

The low sodium syndrome has been particularly observed following the operation of valvuloplasty for mitral stenosis. The cardiac impairment in these individuals prior to operation creates an even greater intolerance to administered water than the usual surgical patient exhibits. The total measurable sodium in such patients actually tends to be high as does their total extracellular space. This further emphasizes the fact that it is the concentration of the sodium in the plasma which is of the greatest importance in regard to the cellular content of water.

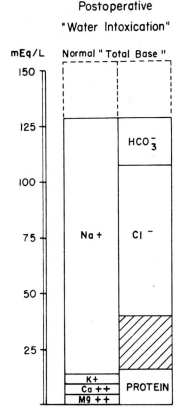

Figure 6. Water intoxication occurring 30 hours after colectomy in an elderly woman with cardiac disease who had been maintained on a low sodium regimen prior to surgery.

POSTCOMMISSUROTOMY SYNDROME. Most patients with mitral stenosis have been prepared for operation with low sodium diets and mercurial diuretics. Nevertheless, it does appear that they have an even greater susceptibility to postsurgical complications of dilution and hyponatremia than other patients so prepared. These patients appear to be under the influence of an unusually potent antidiuretic stimulus and the basis for this has been elucidated to a considerable extent by studies which were designed to identify the locus of volume receptors in regulation of antidiuretic hormone release. When balloons were distended in the left atrium, antidiuretic hormone secretion decreased, but when the distention was released, there was a striking overshoot resulting in blood antidiuretic hormone of several times the baseline. It would appear that sudden release of atrial pressure causes hypersecretion of antidiuretic hormone and that this may well be the cause of hyponatremia following surgical relief of mitral stenosis. The practical fact is that the intolerance of these individuals to even slight excesses of water be recognized and fluid administration, during and after operation, rigorously limited.

HYPERNATREMIA. Of theoretical value and occasional practical importance is the clinical effect which results when the serum sodium is forced above its normal level. This situation is fortunately rare, since the normal mechanisms for regulation of the extracellular fluid concentration rather strongly resist any elevation of the serum sodium. There are surgical situations, however, wherein such hypernatremia may occasionally be observed. One is in certain types of central nervous system damage involving hypothalamus and the frontal lobes. The second follows varieties of injury to the kidneys. Although the latter was originally described in connection with sulfathiazole poisoning, it is now recognized that it can follow almost any type of acute renal damage. An important factor underlying the development of hypernatremia in the phase of diuresis may be the excretion of a large load of crystalloid materials, such as urea, which act as osmotic diuretics.

A third mechanism which may either produce hypernatremia in the obtunded surgical patient, or contribute to its development in other situations, is the use of hyperosmolar tube feedings for purposes of alimentation. Highly concentrated solutions of carbohydrate and protein fragments, so administered, produce osmotic diuresis. Urea and mannitol given deliberately for osmotic diuresis may produce a similar result. The consequence is hyperconcentration of plasma electrolytes.

The underlying mechanism responsible for clinical signs of hypernatremia and hyperosmolality is clearly a movement of water from the intracellular to the extracellular compartment in response to elevation of the serum sodium. The cells of the central nervous system are particularly sensitive. The signs which result are those of profound stupor, central nervous system depression, hyperpyrexia and, occasionally, athetoid and choreiform movements of the extremities. Although little is known of the treatment of this disorder, it is apparent that, whenever feasible, complete avoidance of parenteral salt administration must be enforced with administrations of as large amounts of salt-free glucose solution as the patient can tolerate.

ELECTROLYTES IN ACUTE RENAL INSUFFICIENCY. Acute renal shutdown, being a rather common complication of surgery, is one that every surgeon must be prepared to meet. In most situations, gross departures from the ideal fluid and electrolyte management are compensated for by the kidneys, whose regulatory powers are normally able to correct the errors of the clinician. In the absence of renal function, however, fluid therapy must be extraordinarily precise. Every measure that is taken is reflected in the actual composition of the interior of the body.

Although the reactions caused by incompatible transfusion and prolonged periods of shock appear to be the cause of many occurrences of postsurgical or posttraumatic anuria, it must be admitted that many instances of such acute renal failure are ascribable to no single cause. It would appear that in renal shutdown which does not result clearly from transfusion reactions or other toxic agents, the common factor is reduction of effective blood supply to the kidney. This may occur even when reduction of the systemic blood pressure does not take place. Ischemia, resulting in varying degrees of necrosis of renal cells, is histologically most frequently demonstrable in the distal tubular epithelium. It is not at all clear, however, that those cells which can be seen to be damaged under a microscope are the only ones which are functionally impaired. The important fact is that if one follows the changes in the damaged tubular epithelium, regeneration begins to occur within eight to 14 days and, if the patients can be maintained in adequate fluid and metabolic equilibrium until that time, the majority can survive such periods of severe reduction in renal function. Many instances of survival from periods of prolonged anuria have been recorded with little specific therapy. Unfortunately, when the use of parenteral fluids and electrolytes became widespread, the overzealous use of these agents resulted in the death of many such patients. Precise quantitative fluid therapy is the mainstay of management in acute renal insufficiency with early recourse to one of the presently highly successful methods of artificial dialysis when clinical deterioration or otherwise irreversible chemical imbalance occurs.

Anuria is arbitrarily defined as a urine output of less than 100 ml. in 24 hours. Characteristically, anuric patients have certain electrolyte deviations. Both sodium and chloride in the extracellular fluid tend to be low (Fig. 7). The main reason is that no matter how early the condition is recognized, the patient will have been given, or have ingested, water which has not been excreted. Consequently, a certain amount of overhydration exists from the start. In chronic renal insufficiency, the inability of the kidney to conserve sodium may play a role in the genesis of this diluted state, but is of no importance in the completely anuric individual. In addition to the alterations in sodium and chloride, bicarbonate is almost uniformly reduced. This indicates metabolic acidosis resulting from a combination of the depressed serum sodium level, and an abnormal accumulation of anionic metabolites, such as sulfate, phosphate and organic acids.

Fluid administration must be limited to that which is required to replace insensible losses. In addition to accurate recording of intake and output, daily determination of the body weight is absolutely necessary because of the great variation in insensible water loss among individuals. The body weight should be allowed to fall 0.2 to 0.3 kg. per day, and to accomplish this, the restriction of fluid in-

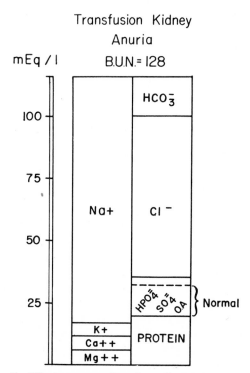

Figure 7. Effect on serum electrolytes of acute anuria. Note reduction in total base as well as chloride and bicarbonate and extension of phosphate, sulfate and organic acids normally excreted by the kidney.

take to 500 to 700 ml. daily to replace water loss and frequently to as little as 300 to 400 ml. is required. If suction tubes or fistulae are present, the loss through these channels must be added to these amounts. Within reason, it appears definitely valuable to take what measures are necessary to maintain as normal as possible a composition of the extracellular fluid. This should be done only when it is possible to add the necessary components without exceeding the rigid quota of fluid established by the insensible water loss. Therefore, particularly when the sodium level is low, it is advantageous to use small amounts of sodium bicarbonate or sodium lactate to correct the metabolic acidosis. Similarly, when sodium and chloride deficiencies clearly exist and are not the result of overhydration, appropriate amounts of these ions should be given. Frequently, this must be done by resorting to hypertonic solutions in order not to increase overall fluid intake. The only deviation which cannot be dealt with in this manner is a mounting potassium level, the most hazardous and frequent complication of prolonged anuria. Within limits, this can be prevented by the avoidance of oral and parenteral administration of potassium ion and omitting blood transfusions when they are not absolutely necessary.

Since reduction of extracellular pH favors movement of potassium out of the cell, it is important to treat acidosis when possible by administration of sodium bicarbonate or lactate. Although this may require use of hypertonic solutions, and occasionally the administration of more sodium ion than would otherwise be desirable, reduction of extracellular potassium to below critical levels can frequently be effected. When potassium levels rise above 6 mEq. per liter, exchange resin such as polystyrene sulfonate, a cation exchange resin in the sodium cycle, should be used. This is best administered by mouth with glucose and sorbitol, but is also effectively given by enema when the oral route is denied. Transitory reduction in serum potassium level can be achieved by giving glucose intravenously, with or without insulin, which causes a small amount of the plasma potassium to be transferred to the interior of the cell in association with glycogen. Persistent increase in potassium level over the level of 7 mEq. per liter must be specifically dealt with by extracorporeal dialysis.

With appropriate treatment, many instances of anuria will be carried to spontaneous diuresis within seven to ten days. At this point, careful scrutiny of the blood chemistry values is also required, for all modalities of renal function do not recover simultaneously. In some instances, the initial diuresis will include large amounts of all the extracellular electrolytes. In the absence of complete tubular regeneration, the urine may very closely approximate glomerular filtrate. Under the latter circumstances, very large amounts of water and electrolytes may be required to avoid the creation of overwhelming extracellular fluid deficiency or serious hypochloremia and hyponatremia. Under other circumstances, sodium and chloride may not be excreted at all in the urine, but only large amounts of water may be put out during the period of diuresis. Hypernatremia may develop with its attendant effects on the central nervous system. When this situation is recognized, only salt-free fluids should be given, frequently in very large amounts. It is necessary, therefore, to follow patients carefully not only during the period of anuria but through the phase of diuresis.

READING REFERENCES

Albright, F.: "Cushing syndrome," its pathological physiology, its relationship to the adreno-genital syndrome and its connection with the problem of the reaction of the body to injurious agents. Harvey Lect. 38:123, 1942-43.

Barnes, B. A., Cope, O., and Gordon, E. B.: Magnesium requirements and deficits. Ann. Surg. 152:518, 1960.

Casey, J. H., Bickel, E. Y., and Zimmermann, B.: The pattern and significance of aldosterone excretion by the postoperative surgical patient. Surg. Gyn. & Obst. 105:179, 1957.

Coller, F. A., and others: Postoperative salt intolerance. Ann. Surg. 119:533, 1944.

Cuthbertson, D. P.: Post-shock metabolic response. Lancet 1:433, 1942.

Darrow, D. C.: Body fluid physiology; the role of potassium in clinical disturbances of body water and electrolyte. New England J. Med. 242:978, 1950.

Darrow, D. C., and Yannet, H.: The changes in the distribution of body water accompanying increase and decrease in extracellular electrolyte. J. Clin. Invest. 14:266, 1935.

Davenport, H.: ABC of Acid-Base Chemistry. 4th ed. Chicago, University of Chicago Press, 1958.

Davis, J. E., Seavey, P. W., and Sessions, J. T., Jr.: Villous adenomas of the rectum and sigmoid colon with severe electrolyte depletion. Ann. Surg. 155:806, 1962.

Davis, J. O.: Mechanisms regulating secretion and metabolism of aldosterone. Rec. Prog. Hormone Research 17:293, 1961.

Elkington, J. R., and Danowski, T. S.: The body fluids: basic physiology and practical therapeutics. Baltimore, The Williams & Wilkins Company, 1955.

Gamble, J. L.: Extracellular Fluid – Chemical Anatomy, Physiology, and Pathology. Cambridge, Massachusetts, Harvard University Press, 1954.

Hayes, M. A., Williamson, R. J., and Heidenreich, W. F.: Endocrine mechanisms involved in water and sodium metabolism during operation and convalescence. Surgery *41*:353, 1957.

Howard, J. E., and Bigham, R. S., Jr.: Transactions of Tenth Conference on Metabolic Aspects of Convalescence. New York, Josiah Macy, Jr., Foundation, 1945.

Howe, C. T., and LeQuesne, L. P.: Pyloric stenosis: the metabolic effects. Brit. J. Surg. *51*:923, 1964.

Hume, D. M., Bell, C. C., and Bartter, F.: Direct measurement of adrenal secretion during operative trauma and convalescence. Surgery *52*:174, 1962.

Kinney, J. M., and Roe, C. F.: The caloric equivalent of fever. I. Patterns of postoperative response. Ann. Surg. *156*:610, 1962.

Moore, F. D.: Common patterns of water and electrolyte change in injury, surgery, and disease. New England J. Med. *258*:277, 325, 377, 427, 1958.

Moore, F. D.: Metabolic Care of the Surgical Patient. Philadelphia, W. B. Saunders Company, 1959.

Moore, F. D.: Volume and tonicity in body water. Surg. Gyn. & Obst. *114*:276, 1962.

Moran, W. H., Jr., Miltenberger, F. W., Shu'ayb, W. A., and Zimmermann, B.: The relationship of antidiuretic hormone secretion to surgical stress. Surgery *56*:99, 1964.

Moyer, C. A.: Fluid Balance, A Clinical Manual. Chicago, Year Book Publishers, 1952.

Randall, H. T.: Water and electrolyte balance in surgery. S. Clin. North America *32*:445, 1952.

Roe, C. F., and Kinney, J. M.: The caloric equivalent of fever. II. The influence of major trauma. Ann. Surg. *161*:141, 1965.

Schloerb, P. R., and Grantham, J. J.: Intracellular pH and muscle electrolytes in metabolic alkalosis from loss of gastric juice. Surgery *56*:144, 1964.

Selye, H.: Stress. Montreal, Acta, 1950.

Shires, T.: The role of sodium-containing solutions in the treatment of oligemic shock. S. Clin. North America *45*:365, 1965.

Shu'ayb, W. A., Moran, W. H., Jr., and Zimmermann, B.: Studies of the mechanism of antidiuretic hormone secretion and the postcommissurotomy dilutional syndrome. Ann. Surg. *162*:690, 1965.

Smith, H. W.: Salt and water volume receptors—an exercise in physiologic apologetics. Am. J. Med. *23*:623, 1957.

Strauss, M. B.: Body Water in Man. Boston, Little, Brown & Co., 1957.

Verney, E. B.: Some aspects of water and electrolyte excretion. Surg. Gyn. & Obst. *106*:441, 1958.

Wacker, W. E. C., and Vallee, B. L.: Magnesium metabolism. New England J. Med. *259*:431, 475, 1958.

Wangensteen, O. H.: Controlled administration of fluid to surgical patients including description of gravimetric methods of determining status of hydration and blood loss during operation. Minnesota Med. *25*:783, 1942.

Zimmermann, B.: Pituitary and adrenal function in relation to surgery. S. Clin. North America *45*:299, 1965.

Zimmermann, B.: Postoperative Management of Fluid Volumes and Electrolytes (Monograph). Current Problems in Surgery. Chicago, Year Book Medical Publishers, 1965.

Zimmermann, B., Casey, J. H., and Bloch, H. S.: Mechanisms of sodium regulation in the surgical patient. Surgery *39*:161, 1956.

Zimmermann, B., and Wangensteen, O. H.: Observations on water intoxication in surgical patients. Surgery *31*:654, 1952.

Chapter 8

SHOCK

by
F. A. SIMEONE, M.D.

FIORINDO ANTHONY SIMEONE was born in St. Ambrose, Italy, and was raised in Rhode Island, a state with a prominent Italian population. After graduating from the Classical High School of Providence, he received Bachelor of Arts and Master of Science degrees from Brown University. He received the Doctor of Medicine degree, with honors in physiology, from Harvard Medical School. In World War II, Dr. Simeone was detached from the United States Fifth General Hospital and placed in charge of a unit to study severe combat wounds. After the war, he returned to the Massachusetts General Hospital and the Harvard Medical School. In 1950, he was appointed Professor of Surgery at Western Reserve University School of Medicine and Director of Surgery at the Cleveland Metropolitan General Hospital. Presently, he is Professor of Medical Science, Brown University, and Surgeon-in-Chief of the Miriam Hospital, Providence, Rhode Island.

Shock is common among the seriously ill and the severely injured. When it appears, it is an ominous sign and demands aggressive, but careful, therapy. A study of the pathogenesis and physiology of shock will provide the necessary background for the appropriate management of patients who develop the condition. At the same time, it will serve as an example of the evolution of thought in a fascinating chapter of surgical history.

HISTORICAL CONSIDERATIONS

Shock is among the oldest of clinical conditions. However, very little of note was known about the nature of its manifestations until recent years. In fact, even now next to nothing is known regarding the nature of the changes which convert the readily correctable, hemodynamic abnormality of certain early forms of shock into the unfortunate state which is intractable to the best available therapeutic measures.

Early Roman mention of the condition used the descriptive word "conlapsus," from which is derived the English "collapse." This remained a convenient term for many years, and as late as 1879, Savory's chapter on this subject in a standard textbook of the time was entitled "Collapse; and the General Effects of Shock upon the System." In the days of John Hunter and well into the nineteenth century, the irritation caused by trauma was thought to require a certain "reaction" on the part of the patient in order to effect healing. Fever would result. Patients who became apathetic after injury and showed the signs and symptoms now recognized as shock were thought to have failed in developing this reaction and the condition was referred to as "irritation without reaction."

The first use of the word "shock" in the English language is credited to the translator of the second edition of LeDran's *Traité ou Réflexions Tirés de la Pratique sur les Playes d'armes à feu*. However, the translator used the word not for the French "choc," but rather for such terms as "saisissement," "secousse" and similar words meaning a jolt, commotion or shock in the sense of a sudden impact. Woolcomb and John Hunter used the word in this same sense of a sudden impact, and not in the sense of circulatory failure. James Latta first used the word "shock" in an English treatise on surgery. However, he, too, used it in the sense of a sudden deceleration or jarring, and not to indicate the clinical state now implied by the term.

The first monograph on shock was written by Morris in 1867. He ascribed to Guthrie the use of the word shock in the sense in which it is employed today. In subsequent years, the term was used very loosely and, anticipating the present situation, Cooper complained in 1838: "Surgeons were in the habit of saying men died of shock without asking themselves very strictly what they meant by the term. It is, however, a convenient name, although not perhaps a philosophical one." By the end of the nineteenth century, excellent clinical descriptions of shock had been written, and Morris had suggested a classification of the condition into two major categories: "Shock following surgical operations and injuries, and shock arising from mental causes." While incomplete, this classification at least implied that the clinical symptoms of shock can result from different causes.

The beginning of the twentieth century saw the discovery of blood groups by Landsteiner, and Crile demonstrated the feasibility of blood transfusion. The modern complex testing of blood to assure its safety, and modern techniques for banking and administering blood, have stemmed from these discoveries. They have paved the way to sound treatment for most forms of shock.

The nature of the phenomena observed in clinical shock remained obscure until the establishment of experimental physiology as a science. Numerous theories concerning the causative mechanisms of shock were discussed, tested and found wanting. With the advent of World War I came the first objective systematic study of man in shock resulting from wounds. The data obtained by such observers as Dale, Richards, Bayliss, Cannon, Keith, Bock, Robertson and Cowell were interpreted and published in a classic monograph on *Traumatic Shock* in 1923. In this monograph, Cannon stated: "The reader should understand from the beginning that the mystery of the onset of shock has not been definitely cleared away despite a considerable increase in our knowledge of it, and that there still remains much work to be done before we shall have elucidated all the factors which play a role in its establishment." The data were interpreted as suggesting that a toxemia, possibly involving a histamine-like substance produced in the wound, played the decisive role in the development of shock. The observations of Keith and of Robertson and Bock, which related the presence or absence and the severity of shock to deficits in circulating blood volume, were recognized but unfortunately were relegated to secondary importance.

Phemister and Blalock, in 1928 and 1930 respectively, reported their classic observations on shock following trauma in animals.

Thereby, they provided background for the unprecedented amount of work which has been done during the past three decades. They showed that after trauma to the limbs in animals, enough fluid is lost into and about the injured areas to account for the development of oligemia and shock. This demonstration countered the suggestion that a histamine-like toxin could arise from traumatized tissue and could cause shock from the toxemia. The toxin had been thought to cause a general, as well as a local, increased capillary permeability, loss of plasma-like fluid through the capillaries, hemoconcentration and oligemia. While toxemias do cause certain types of shock, they do not play a fundamental role in shock which follows trauma.

Observations of severely wounded casualties of World War II added considerably to the available information bearing on the problem of shock. The close relationship between the manifestations of shock and the degree of oligemia was strengthened. Finally, Grant and Reeve, in their objections to the use of the word "shock," stressed the fact that clinical shock can result from a variety of causes which for correction may require quite different approaches. Thus, they emphasized the necessity of defining the nature of the defect which has resulted in shock, since the term, while connoting a well-recognized group of clinical symptoms, is nondiscriminative as to etiologic mechanism. Indeed, abandonment of the term has been urged, but its convenience and time-honored place in the surgical vocabulary will undoubtedly protect its status.

DEFINITION

To be useful a definition should be brief, concise and informative. A definition of shock is difficult to fit to these requirements because of the complexity of the syndrome. There are multiple inciting causes and several signs and symptoms, and the condition itself produces complex metabolic changes which sustain it and set up a vicious circle. A definition of shock in terms of these several aspects would require a long description and would be useless as such. Nevertheless, within the limits of these considerations, shock can be defined as a clinical condition in which because of insufficient effective circulating blood volume or because of abnormal partitioning of the cardiac output the capillary blood flow in vital tissues, or in all tissues, is reduced to levels below the minimal requirements for normal oxidative metabolism. Some of the signs and symptoms are referable to the oligemia and insufficient cardiac output, but others reflect the activity of physiologic mechanisms which normally act to compensate for oligemia, reduced cardiac output, and low arterial blood pressure.

This definition may be considered deficient because it makes no mention of what the signs and symptoms are, does not make reference to the several different causative mechanisms, and does not define the physiologic abnormalities or the metabolic disturbances caused by the inadequate perfusion. On the other hand, this definition has many advantages as it stands. The symptoms and signs are well known and need not be mentioned individually. The definition relates the findings in any patient in shock to an arterial oligemia, absolute or relative, which results in a diminution of the rate of blood flow in the various tissues and organs. The volume of blood pumped by the heart into the arterial tree is inadequate for maintaining the normal blood pressure—flow relationships. The cardiac output can become inadequate because blood is not brought to the heart, as in the oligemia of hemorrhage and plasma loss; because the heart fails as a pump, as in coronary thrombosis and cardiac tamponade; or because of excessive demand for blood flow, as in large acute arteriovenous fistula, and extensive inflammation or overwhelming sepsis.

The definition emphasizes the cardinal features of shock: insufficient cardiac output and deficient perfusion of organs and tissues with blood. The patient's welfare is in jeopardy when the rate of perfusion drops sufficiently to cause anoxia, and living cells turn to anaerobic metabolism. Experiences with artificial perfusion in man suggest that the lower limit for adequate overall perfusion is 50 ml. of blood per minute per kilogram of body weight.

TERMINOLOGY AND CLASSIFICATION

A great number of qualifying terms have been used to define the kind of shock encountered in any particular patient. The terms employed are descriptive with reference either to the clinical type, to the etiology or to the temporal relation of the condition to its cause. Many of the terms used are repetitive and analogous, adding little additional discriminative information. Therefore, a single classification is proposed, combining clinical and etiologic categories with an attempt to reconcile different terms commonly encountered in the literature.

OLIGEMIC SHOCK. This is the most common kind of shock likely to be encountered by the surgeon, the causative abnormality being a deficit of effective circulating blood volume. In Table 1 are noted the several conditions which result in a reduction of the circulating blood volume in oligemic shock. Cowell first introduced the term "wound shock" to characterize the circulatory failure observed among battle casualties in World War I, and to emphasize the fact that, clinically, this condition differed from shock secondary to other causes. The very presence of a wound and the treatment for it, as well as the physiologic and psychologic state of the fighting man, modified the clinical findings. "Traumatic" and "wound" shock are similar.

Primary wound shock, according to Cowell, became manifest almost immediately upon wounding; *secondary wound shock* developed more slowly. "Surgical shock," developing sometime after operation, is comparable to secondary wound shock and is seldom used as a term. In his etiologic classification, Blalock included hemorrhagic shock and wound shock under "hematogenic shock" in which the abnormality was caused by loss

Table 1. *A Classification of Shock*

Oligemic (hypovolemic) *shock*
  Hemorrhage
  Wounding (with bleeding)
  Burns
  Crush syndrome
  Dehydration

Cardiac (cardiogenic) *shock*
  Pulmonary embolus
  Cardiac tamponade
  Tension pneumothorax
  Myocardial infarction
  Myocarditis
  High-output myocardial failure
  Arteriovenous fistula
  Severe inflammation

Neurogenic shock
  "Vasovagal effects"
  Vasoconstrictor paralysis

Septic shock
  Inflammation (vasogenic shock)
  Endotoxin
  Exotoxin

of whole blood. He left unclassified oligemic shock, such as burn shock and similar forms, in which a diminution in circulating blood volume resulted from a loss of plasma-like fluid instead of whole blood, and in which there is a high hematocrit reading instead of a low one as is found when whole blood has been lost. The elevated hematocrit value in itself may so increase the vascular resistance to blood flow as to exaggerate the impedance to circulation through the tissue capillaries caused by vascular constriction.

Dehydration, or loss of water and salts from the body, may result in oligemia and shock when the homeostatic mechanisms responsible for maintaining the circulating blood volume are overpowered. However, the metabolic disturbance in dehydration complicates the effects of the oligemia, and the mechanism of shock which results under these circumstances is complex.

CARDIAC OR CARDIOGENIC SHOCK. This is found among patients with heart disease in whom the heart intrinsically fails as a pump, or in whom conditions other than lesions of the heart itself interfere with its action. Among them may be listed pulmonary embolus, cardiac tamponade and tension pneumothorax. Some have referred to the circulatory collapse which follows coronary heart disease as "coronary shock." Blalock grouped these all together in the category of cardiogenic shock.

NEUROGENIC SHOCK. Circulatory failure may result from affections of the nervous system. In his studies of vagal effects upon the heart in the frog, Goltz was probably the first to observe vasovagal shock. He reflexly activated the vagus nerve by tapping upon the abdomen. The condition is not uncommon in man. In this category is included the kind of collapse which follows receipt of ill tidings, viewing of blood, anticipation of venipuncture or arterial puncture and mild injury associated with intense fear or worry. There is a reduction of cardiac output with slowing of the heart, vasodilation in skeletal muscle, nausea and vomiting, and cold perspiration. There may be overventilation and respiratory alkalosis.

Very early in wound shock, one may detect a vasovagal component: normal or slow pulse, cold sweat, nausea and vomiting, and respiratory alkalosis if the acid base balance of the blood is examined. Cowell called this "primary wound shock," occurring especially among high-strung, nervous individuals whose recovery was rapid unless superseded by secondary wound shock which developed slowly over the ensuing hours. The use of the expression "primary" wound shock has created confusion because the term may refer to a trivial circulatory problem or to a very serious one, such as a massive wound resulting in immediate exsanguination, or destruction of a vital organ from which recovery might be impossible. Cowell used the term for both. If used at all, it would be preferable to use the term to indicate neurogenic shock resulting from reflex nervous effects. As a matter of fact, neurogenic shock, even when defined in this restricted sense and although usually of little consequence, can be lethal in patients with pre-existent serious obliterative arterial disease. The decreased blood flow to brain and heart may result in thrombosis of arteries in these organs.

In the category of neurogenic shock should also be included those patients in whom there is paralysis of sympathetic vasoconstrictor activity, as occurs in high spinal anesthesia. The concept that in these patients the fall in blood pressure is secondary to arteriolar paralysis with a fall in the peripheral vascular resistance is an oversimplification. When the blood pressure falls below mean pressures of approximately 50 mm. of mercury, the hemodynamics become very complex, there being a great fall in cardiac stroke volume and output.

In his classification, Blalock included the category of "vasogenic shock," in which vasodilation resulted in circulatory failure. Although this reaction could be the result of local or systemic vasodilation resulting from infections, vasoconstrictor nerve paralysis from spinal anesthesia or from neurogenic disturbances also could cause a comparable reduction in vascular resistance and fall in blood pressure. It is better to avoid the term "vasogenic" shock and to refer to a patient in shock with vascular paralysis by the category descriptive of the cause of the decreased vascular resistance and increased volume of the capacitance vessels.

Shock secondary to overwhelming infection was once referred to, along with cardiogenic shock, as "medical shock." This terminology no longer applies because surgeons have become as cognizant as internists of the systemic effects of severe infections and of failure of the heart. The gram-negative bacteria are the common causative agents in septic shock, although equally severe circulatory failure can be caused by gram-positive organisms liberating exotoxin. Although most of the gram-negative organisms liberate an endotoxin, some of them exert their effects by forming an exotoxin as well. Students of this problem have insisted on positive blood-culture before making a diagnosis of septic shock. Although desirable, this is not always possible, and circulatory failure not infrequently is observed in the presence of surgical infections with negative blood cultures.

When large endothelial-lined cavities are involved, hemoconcentration and oligemia are often demonstrable. However, usually as the result of treatment, the circulating blood volume may be found normal or sometimes increased to well beyond the normal despite the presence of clinical shock. One kind of experimental shock is produced by the injection of effective doses of endoxin or exotoxin variously purified, and is referred to as "endotoxin shock" or "exotoxin shock." Although much information can be and is gained by such experiments, the models are not strictly comparable to septic shock as seen clinically and produced by overwhelming bacterial infection.

As opposed to oligemic or hemorrhagic shock, septic shock is likely to be normovolemic and even hypervolemic because of the volumes of parenteral fluids generally administered to such patients. Similarly, the cardiac output in septic shock is frequently normal and sometimes greater than normal. Presumably because of the direct effects of infection upon the myocardium, some element of impaired cardiac function and varying degrees of elevation of the central venous pressure are found in septic shock.

"Irreversible," "intractable" or "refractory" shock is commonly used to refer to any type of shock which is not responding to therapy. It is thought to develop when subliminal tissue perfusion with blood has lasted beyond a critical period of time, two to six hours in patients whose mean arterial pressures have fallen below 50 mm. Hg. The terms should never be used until the physician is certain of the causative mechanism for the circulatory failure, is certain that all possible complicating factors have been excluded and is certain that the therapy being employed is appropriate both qualitatively and quantitatively. Indeed, the terms are of questionable semantic propriety, because what is irreversible and intractable is not the shock or

circulatory failure, but the virtual death of cells and tissues responsible for the integrity of the biologic mechanisms which normally protect and assure adequate circulation for living tissues.

SIGNS AND SYMPTOMS OF SHOCK

The signs and symptoms of shock are those of peripheral circulatory failure, and are easily recognized. Those observed in wound shock, as a prototype, include the important findings in patients with other types of shock and have been documented by many observers. Typical are the tired, wan expression; the cold, pale mottled skin; the thin, rapid, thready pulse; and the low blood pressure. The capillary circulation is slow. The eyes are sunken and relatively soft. In many clinical descriptions of the signs and symptoms of shock, the skin is described as cold and clammy. The clammy skin is a manifestation of sudomotor sympathetic activity; while it sometimes is seen in wound shock or in hemorrhagic shock, it is not common. It is almost always observed among patients in septic shock, among those who are about to develop syncope in neurogenic shock, and in cardiogenic shock.

Characteristically, the pulse rate is increased in shock. In neurogenic shock the pulse rate is normal or decreased. Occasionally, and in particular among elderly patients, the pulse rate may not be increased despite considerable blood loss in wound shock or hemorrhagic shock.

The state of the sensorium is of particular interest. Early after wounding or gross visible bleeding, a patient may show anxiety and restlessness because of the excitement and emotional impact of the event. He may complain of weakness and fear of impending death. Occasionally, restlessness becomes a prominent feature of the condition, as happens especially in the presence of infection or central nervous system injury. Pain is seldom a major complaint, except in patients with unsplinted fractures and with intra-abdominal wounds of the gastrointestinal tract. As shock progresses, overactivity diminishes and the patient becomes apathetic. He may complain of weakness and of being cold. He becomes increasingly more difficult to arouse, and lapses into a coma. It is well to emphasize that in wound shock without infection coma develops only in the severest

Table 2. *Signs and Symptoms of Wound Shock in Man, According to Overall Severity*

DEGREE OF CLINICAL SHOCK	BLOOD PRESSURE	PULSE QUALITY	PULSE RATE	TEMPER-ATURE	SKIN COLOR	CIRCULA-TION IN NAIL BED	THIRST	MENTAL STATE
None	Normal	Normal	Normal or rapid	Normal or cool	Normal or pale	Normal	Normal	Clear, excited
Slight	20% below normal	Normal	Rapid	Cool	Pale	Slow	Normal or mild	Clear, dis-tressed, anxious
Moderate	40% below normal	Decreased volume	Rapid	Cool	Pale	Slow	Definite	Clear, some apathy
Severe	40% or more below nor-mal, some-times not recordable	Thready, weak or imper-ceptible	Very rapid, until slowed in extremis	Cold	Ashen gray to mottled and cya-notic	Very sluggish	Severe	Apathy to coma

degrees of shock, when the patient is mori-bund. When the associated findings do not indicate an excessive degree of blood loss, or when the deficit is corrected by transfu-sion and coma persists, the strong likelihood of intracranial injury must be considered. On the other hand in septic shock, stupor and coma are commonly observed.

A most annoying symptom for the patient in shock is thirst. This is attributed to a great diminution or cessation of function of the salivary glands in response to only moderate decreases in the circulating blood volume, which may be so slight as to cause no de-tectable decrease in blood pressure. This is of practical importance for the management of wound shock in particular. The surgeon must curb his desire to comply with the pa-tient's demand for water to drink, until he is convinced that the gastrointestinal tract is intact and early operative intervention is not indicated.

In the case of wound or hemorrhagic shock, in which the fundamental cause of the decreased cardiac output is a deficit in the volume of circulating blood, the symp-toms and signs vary widely in degree and can be tabulated according to severity (Table 2). The degree of shock, as evaluated clinically, has been found to correlate extremely well with the deficit in blood volume and with the biochemical findings in the circulating blood. Having made such a clinical appraisal, the surgeon can estimate the volume of blood needed for replacement therapy and can anticipate the likelihood of serious renal dam-age (Tables 3 and 4).

Respiration is variable in wound shock, and depends upon the location and severity of the wound. Splinting of the diaphragm in thoracic and upper abdominal wounds re-sults in shallow, rapid respiration. Fear and excitement may result in similar respiration, and occasionally the respiratory minute vol-ume is increased to the extent that respira-tory alkalosis develops. Ordinarily, at least in the early stages of shock, the oxygen sat-uration of the arterial blood is normal. When respiratory minute volume is decreased, pul-monary ventilation is hampered and arterial oxygen saturation may be decreased. Carbon dioxide retention occurs only in the very severe degrees of respiratory embarrassment, as in direct injury to the organs of respiration themselves.

Shock is characterized by a fall in body temperature. This may be attributed partly to the lowered metabolic rate and oxygen consumption, and partly to the decreased circulation of active organs such as the liver. In keeping with the latter observation is the fact that in the liver the internal temperature of the organ rises during hemorrhagic hypo-

Table 3. *Degree of Wound Shock in Relation to Deficit of Circulating Blood Volume*

DEGREE OF CLINICAL SHOCK	DEFICIT OF CIRCULATING BLOOD VOLUME* Per cent	DEFICIT OF CIRCULATING BLOOD VOLUME* Milliliters
None	15	750
Mild or slight	20	1000
Moderately severe	35	1800
Severe	45	2400

* Estimated average for young man weighing 70 kg.

Table 4. *Concentration of Glucose and Nonprotein Nitrogen in Plasma, and Distribution of Renal Insufficiency by Clinical Degree of Shock Among Battle Casualties*

DEGREE OF CLINICAL SHOCK	DEFICIT IN CIRCULATING BLOOD VOLUME*	GLUCOSE CONCENTRATION (mg. per 100 ml.)	NONPROTEIN NITROGEN (mg. per 100 ml.)	RENAL INSUFFICIENCY, EXCLUSIVE OF CRUSH SYNDROME (per cent of group)
None	15	134	34	9.0
Mild or slight	20	149	35	18.4
Moderately severe	35	178	37	51.8
Severe	45	202	44	66.7

* Percentage of decrease from normal in round figures.

tension, while the core temperature of the body falls. In septic shock with hypotension and a rapid thready pulse, a fall in body temperature is an ominous sign when not accompanied by obvious clinical improvement. In clostridial myositis, the body temperature may be normal or below normal, to values of 95° F., when the arterial blood pressure is too low to measure clinically, and the pulse rate may be 140 per minute.

Most of the signs and symptoms of wound shock and hemorrhagic shock are, in fact, the clinical manifestations of the activation of corrective physiologic mechanisms. The adjustments which take place result in a normal, or nearly normal, blood pressure despite the contracted blood volume. In fact, on occasion, there is an overadjustment. For a time, the blood pressure of a wounded patient may be abnormally high. The blood pressure falls when the combined organization for circulatory homeostasis is overtaxed by excessive loss of blood or plasma. Thus, tachycardia, pallor and cyanotic mottling of the skin, decreased rate of peripheral blood flow, sweating and thirst are obvious marks of sympathicoadrenal activity.

While certain of the signs and symptoms of shock are comparable for the various forms of the condition, there are some differences. The color of the skin differs on careful inspection. The pallor is not as blanched in any kind of shock as it is in patients in whom hemorrhage is the cause of the arterial oligemia. The pallor due to ventricular failure from coronary thrombosis is characterized by its grayish hue. Even more striking is the cyanosis of massive pulmonary embolism. The livid mottling of patients in shock from causes which lead to hemoconcentration is distinctive.

In wound shock, or after severe hemorrhage, the venous pressure is low and the right atrial pressure, usually lowered to 1 or 2 mm. of mercury, may actually be negative. The veins of the extremities are constricted or collapsed. In cardiogenic shock, in which there is redistribution of blood, the venous pressure is high and the veins of the extremities are prominent.

Sweating is not common in wound shock or after uncomplicated hemorrhage, except when there is a considerable emotional reaction or when infection is present in addition. Sweating and the "cold clammy skin" are common in septic shock and in neurogenic shock. Nausea and vomiting frequently are observed after wounds and hemorrhage, but may be due to injuries and perforations of the gastrointestinal tract in the absence of shock. These symptoms are common in neurogenic and cardiogenic shock as well.

CLASSIFICATION OF SHOCK WITH REFERENCE TO THE CARDIAC OUTPUT

The cardiac output can serve as a point of departure for discussions of hemodynamics in shock, and a classification of shock on the basis of factors which influence the cardiac output is reasonable. In most instances of clinical shock, the cardiac output is lower than the expected normal; but in some, especially in septic shock, the cardiac output is normal and may be even greater than normal. Thus, an etiologic classification may be proposed which defines the conditions causing a decrease in the cardiac output and those which place demands upon the cardiac output which the heart cannot meet and shock therefore develops (Table 5).

The history and the physical examination are usually adequate for classifying the patient in shock into one or another of the cate-

Table 5.   *Classification of Shock Based on the Cardiac Output*

I. *Decreased cardiac output*
  A. Decreased venous return of blood to the heart
    1. Loss of whole blood from the circulation (olige-mia, exemia of Cannon)
      a. Hemorrhage, internal or external, secondary to disease or injury
    2. Loss of plasma or water from the circulation (oligemia)
      a. Burns, the crush syndrome, severe peritonitis, or pleuritis
      b. Heat exposure and severe dehydration
    3. Redistribution of blood within the vascular system (other than that owing to interference with the heart as a pump)
      a. Severe infections
      b. Late stages of shock
      c. High spinal anesthesia
    4. Mediastinal venous obstruction
      a. Tension pneumothorax
      b. Acute mediastinal shift
  B. Failure of the heart as a pump
    1. Coronary thrombosis, infectious or toxic myo-carditis
    2. Cardiac arrhythmias
    3. Cardiac tamponade
      a. Trauma
      b. Disease, aneurysms (dissecting, other)
  C. Miscellaneous mechanisms and combinations
    1. Intestinal strangulation obstruction, ischemic or congestive necrosis
    2. Reflex and other nervous effects upon the cardiac output
II. *Inadequate, although increased, cardiac output*
  A. Arteriovenous fistula
  B. Inflammation

gories in Table 5. The pallor and the collapsed, or constricted, veins of the oligemic patient are characteristic. The hematocrit of the blood slowly falls in man when whole blood is lost from the circulation; it rapidly rises when plasma and water are lost. Severe infections and the late or normovolemic stages of shock from other causes often present clinical appearances which are very similar. In these patients, blood is not lacking from the body as a whole, but is redistributed in such a manner as to fill the relaxed venous system, which serves as a reservoir of increased capacity. A grayish, dusky or livid pallor is observed in the skin of these patients; and their cutaneous veins, while not distended, are not nearly as collapsed as they are in hypovolemic wound shock.

Under high spinal anesthesia, patients do not appear to be in shock as long as the skin remains warm and of normal color, despite the fall in blood pressure. However, when the mean arterial pressures fall below 50 mm. of mercury, the color of the skin begins to lose its pink hue, and becomes pale and rather cool. The clinician should now consider the patient to be in shock.

Studies of this kind of hypotension have revealed interesting facts. The pulse rate remains unchanged or low despite the hypotension. Particularly important is the fact that, despite the obviously increased flow of blood in the skin, the fall in blood pressure is associated with a decreased ventricular stroke volume and output, and a decreased right atrial pressure. This can mean only that, despite the good color and warmth of the skin, there must be serious diminution of blood flow elsewhere in the body. In fact, the blood flow in the liver and kidneys does decrease under such circumstances, as it does in other kinds of shock.

The hemodynamic changes of high spinal anesthesia imply a decreased venous return of blood to the heart. The mechanism for this is not known, but may be secondary to a paralysis of venomotor nervous activity. The actions of such nerves have been demonstrated for systemic and splanchnic veins, but not for the vena cava itself. With increased capacity of the paralyzed venous bed, the volume of blood available for return to the heart is decreased. Some similarities are apparent between this and the circulatory failure of septic shock and normovolemic shock.

It is understood that while hemorrhagic and wound shock do have diminution of the circulating blood volume as the dominant abnormality in common, the terms are not synonymous. In wound shock, the effects of oligemia are complicated by the general and specific effects of the wound itself. Often the injury to certain organs obscures the effects of blood loss, as in wounds of the brain and spinal cord, the lungs, the liver and the gastrointestinal tract. It is essential to separate, insofar as possible, these specific effects from those of the oligemia. Failure to respond to therapy should not be designated irreversible shock when death is inevitable because vital organs have been injured beyond repair.

Paradoxical as it would seem, certain patients in shock have been found to have a high cardiac output to twice or more the normal basal value for the patient. This has been observed especially among patients in septic shock with generalized infection and toxemia, or with localized severe infection and its systemic effects. Because these patients are commonly found to have a low arterial-venous oxygen difference and low peripheral vascular resistance, they can be assumed to have developed innumerable arteriovenous communications. The effect is similar to that of large traumatic arteriovenous fistula. Shock does not develop so long as the cardiac output can be increased sufficiently to provide an adequate blood flow for the body while meeting the demands of the low-resistance arteriovenous communications. The heart itself becomes a limiting element. Heart failure before the abnormal hemodynamics are corrected by healing and despite the employment of inotropic agents, spells defeat. It is in this situation that artificial assistance to the failing heart may play a role.

THE ADAPTIVE OR HOMEOSTATIC RESPONSE

The reaction to wounding and hemorrhage is immediate. Within seconds, the signs of sympathicoadrenal activation are clinically apparent. Examination of the blood reveals not only the prompt elevation of catecholamine levels, indicative of adrenal medullary activity, but of adrenal cortical and pituitary hormones as well: 17-hydroxysteroids, aldosterone and the antidiuretic hormone. Hemorrhage is believed to be the most effective stimulus for the prompt liberation of antidiuretic hormone and of aldosterone. In addition to the pituitary-adrenal-cortical effects, certain other responses take place that appear to be of immediate survival value. These reactions are referable primarily to activation of the sympathetic division of the autonomic nervous system, including the adrenal medulla.

BLOOD PRESSURE. The normal arterial blood pressure is maintained by the cardiac output and the peripheral vascular resistance, and is directly proportional to the product of these two. Thus, the blood pressure can remain unchanged when the cardiac output drops because of hemorrhage, so long as the total vascular resistance can be increased to compensate for it. High spinal anesthesia and sympathetic blockade, by means of chemical agents, interfere with the compensatory mechanisms which evoke increased vascular resistance, and the blood pressure is determined almost entirely by the cardiac output and the viscosity of the blood. Under such circumstances, very small drops in cardiac output have a marked effect upon the blood pressure.

From the surgical physiologic standpoint, the function of the blood pressure within an artery is to provide force for overcoming the resistance offered to flow by the combined vascular beds supplied by the artery. The vascular resistance varies for different organs and in different parts of the same vascular bed, depending upon local conditions which determine the state of vasoconstriction or vasodilation.

Neurogenic and humoral vasoconstrictor activity can modify the vascular resistance to different degrees in different vascular beds. In response to wounding and hemorrhage, the resistance is greatly increased in some vascular beds, such as the skin and the kidney. In others, the resistance is not affected at all; or, as in the case of the myocardium, it is actually decreased.

Fortunately, in the blood vessels of organs such as the heart and brain alpha receptors are not abundant; and consequently active vasoconstriction does not occur in these organs when sympathicoadrenal activity is excited by hemorrhage and hypotension. The increased resistance in other vascular beds, therefore, causes a relative diversion of blood to the heart and brain, which are more immediately essential for survival than are most other organs. In wound shock, as much as 25 per cent of the cardiac output may go to the myocardium, instead of the normal 5 per cent; and as much as 70 or 80 per cent of the output may go to the heart and brain together, instead of the normal 20 per cent.

The physiologic organization for homeostasis of the circulation is set to protect the perfusion of essential organs with blood. Since this is achieved in large measure by increasing the vascular resistance in some organs, the blood pressure indirectly is also protected. Thus, the blood pressure does not fall appreciably when blood is lost from the circulation until the deficit is so great that the homeostatic mechanisms can no longer compensate for it.

Since the systolic component of the blood pressure is more closely dependent upon the systolic ventricular output than is the diastolic pressure, the systolic blood pressure falls sooner and more rapidly than the diastolic pressure, as the cardiac output decreases. The pulse pressure, therefore, is decreased and the pulse is said to be "contracted." This, combined with the decreased mean pressure and the tachycardia, results in the clinical "rapid, weak thready pulse" of wound shock and hemorrhagic shock. Occasionally, the pulse pressure is so reduced that the pulse is not palpable at the wrist, and Korotkoff's sounds are not audible. The auscultatory blood pressure is not measurable, despite the fact that a damped pressure as high as 80 or 90 mm. of mercury can be recorded through an intra-arterial needle.

PULSE RATE. The sinoauricular node, by its spontaneous rhythmic activity, is responsible for initiating the normal rhythmic contractions of the chambers of the heart. The activity of the node is modulated by nervous and humoral influences. The vagus nerves and the sympathetic nerves act synchronously and reciprocally. The former decreases the rate of the heart beat, the latter increases it. This functional organization facilitates a delicate control of the rate at which the heart contracts. The sinoauricular node is also influenced by humoral agents, such as adrenaline and noradrenaline and the parasympathetic mediator acetylcholine.

A century ago, Marey recognized an inverse relationship between the tension in the great vessels and the rate of the heart, an observation now known as Marey's law, or Marey's reflex. The reflex is afferently mediated through pressor receptors in the aortic arch, the carotid sinuses and other great vessels, and efferently through the vagus nerves and the sympathicoadrenal system, comprising the cardioaccelerator nerves, the vasoconstrictors and the adrenal medullary innervation. Thus, the slightest fall in pressure within the vessels bearing pressor receptors results in excitation of the sympathicoadrenal division of the autonomic nervous system and reciprocal inhibition of the vagal medullary center.

Therefore, with hemorrhage and other conditions which reduce the cardiac output, the resulting fall in systemic arterial pressure, however slight, causes an increase in the heart rate. Teleologically, this would increase the cardiac output and restore the blood pressure to normal. Obviously, this is possible only insofar as the venous return, ventricular filling pressures and ventricular distensibility are capable of permitting satisfactory filling of the ventricles.

Despite Marey's law, the rate of the pulse, except under conditions of continued observation, has not been a dependable index of the presence or absence of shock, or of its severity, for two reasons:

First, acceleration of the heart is caused by many conditions other than fall of pressure in the aorta and great vessels. Excitement, fear and anxiety are among the other causes. Thus, in shock after wounding or hemorrhage, the pulse rate becomes signifi-

cant if observed over a period of time during which the emotional reaction has subsided.

Second, in elderly individuals, considerable degrees of oligemia may develop, with or without a fall in blood pressure, without a demonstrable effect upon the heart rate. Possibly, aging decreases the responsiveness of the sinoauricular node. Whatever the cause, when caring for elderly patients, the surgeon cannot depend upon the pulse rate to detect shock or to follow its progress. During operative procedures, careful accounting of blood loss must be kept. Occasionally, even in young patients, tachycardia may fail to develop early after wounding when a vasovagal effect predominates.

VASCULAR RESISTANCE AND ARTERIOLAR CONSTRICTION. Considerations of the blood pressure and of the vascular resistance to flow bear directly upon the all-important problem of blood flow in shock. The rate at which a tissue is perfused with blood is directly proportional to the blood pressure in the vessels supplying the tissue, and inversely proportional to the resistance which the vessels offer against the flow of blood:

$$F \backsim \frac{P}{R}$$

F represents flow, *P* the differential pressure between the entrance and exit to a vascular bed, and *R* the resistance. Appreciation of this relationship is useful in considerations of therapeutic measures which concomitantly affect the arterial pressure and the vascular resistance.

Vascular resistances are not measured directly in man or in experimental animals. They are calculated from ratios of pressure and flow. Most simply, the vascular resistance can be expressed as resistance units by dividing the pressure gradient by the flow, the pressure being in millimeters of mercury and the flow in milliliters per second. The pressure may be converted to dynes by multiplying by the factor 1332, and the vascular resistance is then expressed in centimeter-gram-second units by the fraction:

$$\frac{P \times 1332}{F}$$

P is the pressure gradient in millimeters of mercury at 0° C. and *F* is the blood flow in milliliters per second.

The normal total systemic vascular resistance in man is about 1200 dynes sec. cm.$^{-5}$. Total resistances of 3000 dynes sec.

cm.$^{-5}$ are not uncommon in wound shock or after severe hemorrhage. In a patient recently studied, the total vascular resistance reached 4200, while the blood pressure remained normal and the cardiac index fell by 40 per cent. Of particular interest is the fact that the vascular resistance does not increase to the same degree in all organs and tissues. It is maximally increased in the skin and, in decreasing order, in the kidneys, the liver and the brain. In the heart, the vascular resistance actually decreases. This difference in the degree to which the vascular resistance in various organs is increased in shock has obvious protective value. Those vascular beds which develop less vascular resistance receive a greater proportion of the circulating blood volume than those which develop greater resistance.

VENOCONSTRICTION. There is a generalized constriction of the veins with sympathicoadrenal activity. This is of definite value because the veins and venules normally contain a large share of the organism's blood volume, possibly as much as 70 per cent, and with loss of venomotor tone can accommodate the entire blood volume or more. A decrease in capacity of the venous system can divert a considerable volume of blood to the circulation. While venoconstrictor activity can be demonstrated in visceral and other veins, it has not been shown to exist for the vena cava, the largest single reservoir of all. Contraction of the reservoir capacity of the venous system is one of the reactions which permits a normal cardiac output despite loss of 10 per cent of the normal blood volume.

MOVEMENT OF FLUID. The common types of wound shock and hemorrhagic shock are characterized by the entrance of a plasma-like, erythrocyte-free fluid into the circulation, resulting in hemodilution. Contraction of the spleen does occur as the result of sympathicoadrenal activity, but this cannot account for the entrance of more than 100 to 150 ml. of high-hematocrit blood into the circulation of man, and could elevate the hematocrit by 2 to 5 per cent, depending upon the degree of oligemia. Any possible effect of this reaction in the direction of hemoconcentration is masked by the forces which lead to hemodilution.

Hemoconcentration occurs in shock caused by, or associated with, the crush syndrome or with inflammatory reactions in large vascular areas, permitting increased capillary permeability. In the crush syndrome, large vascular beds in muscle masses, having been ischemic for some hours, are returned to the circulation. As a consequence of the prolonged ischemia, a reactive hyperemia with arteriolar dilation occurs when the obstruction to the circulation is released. The capillaries, already injured by the ischemia along with other components of the tissue, are subjected to abnormally high pressures, and plasma crosses the capillary membrane to enter the tissue spaces. Marked edema develops in the affected part, and the blood remaining in the circulation becomes concentrated. Insofar as the protein content of the plasma which crosses the capillary membrane is less than that of blood plasma, there will be a concentration of protein as well as of erythrocytes. Similar reactions leading to hemoconcentration occur in instances of extensive thermal injury, and in peritonitis and pleuritis with accumulation of large volumes of erythrocyte-free fluid in the peritoneal and pleural cavities. The highest reported hematocrit after trauma is in the crush syndrome. One such patient was recorded as having a hematocrit percentage of 80, and three others with hematocrit values between 60 and 70. At these levels, the viscosity of the blood seriously increases the vascular resistance to blood flow. In the report cited, the only casualties of this kind who survived had initial hematocrit values below 50 per cent.

The wound of the average patient in wound shock contains open lymphatics as well as arteries and veins, and there may be extensive damage to capillaries, muscle, skin and subcutaneous tissue. Plasma-like fluid can be lost in variable quantities across the capillaries in such wounds. The amount lost, other characteristics of the wound being equal, is proportional to the size of the wound. However, in the usual patient in wound shock, the hemodiluting influence of the deficit of whole blood in the circulation overpowers the hemoconcentrating effects of contractions of the spleen and loss of plasma-like fluid from and into the wound itself. The characteristic finding is hemodilution (Table 6).

The mechanism of hemodilution after severe trauma and hemorrhage is still debatable. The experiments of Hardaway and his associates suggest that dilution of the hematocrit of circulating blood may occur through removal of erythrocytes from the circulation, as the result of the aggregation

Table 6. *Plasma Protein and Hematocrit Values Among Battle Casualties with Wounds of the Extremities or of the Thorax and Abdomen**

DEFICIT OF CIRCULATING BLOOD	WOUNDS OF EXTREMITIES		THORACIC AND ABDOMINAL WOUNDS	
	PLASMA PROTEINS *(normal: 6.5)*	HEMATOCRIT VALUE *(normal: 47)*	PLASMA PROTEINS *(normal: 6.5)*	HEMATOCRIT VALUE *(normal: 47)*
Less than 30% below normal	6.4 ± 0.1 (10 patients)	39.0 ± 1.7 (10 patients)	6.5 ± 0.1 (17 patients)	43.0 ± 1.0 (17 patients)
More than 30% below normal	6.0 (8 patients)	35.0 ± 1.3 (8 patients)	6.4 (only 4 patients)	37.8 (only 4 patients)

* Patients received 0 to 1 unit of plasma before determinations were made.

of red blood cells or of intravascular clotting. While this does occur, the evidence is that the largest element in hemodilution after blood loss is the entrance into the circulation of plasma-like fluid from the extravascular space. On the basis of the Starling hypothesis, the reduced hydrostatic pressure in the capillary loop because of hypotension and vasoconstriction results in a shift of the pressure gradients favoring the passage of fluid from the tissue spaces into the capillaries. While this has been a satisfactory working theory, it was challenged from the very beginning, and recently the importance of lymphatic channels has been emphasized for the return of plasma-like fluid to the circulation. More study is needed, however, before the Starling hypothesis should be discarded.

From the teleologic standpoint of survival after injury, hemodilution is a protective response on the part of the organism. Thereby, the blood volume is increased by adding extracellular fluid to the circulating plasma volume. The ability of animals to survive hemorrhage has been related, among other variables, to their ability to effect a significant degree of hemodilution.

HORMONAL EFFECTS. Catecholamines are produced and enter the circulation in large amounts during the early stage of shock after wounding and hemorrhage. Produced, for the most part, by the adrenal medulla, and complementing the autonomic neural response, they promote several reactions which are protective in nature. They cause a reduction of the vascular resistance in the myocardium while increasing the resistance in most other vascular beds. They promote glycolysis and oxygen utilization, and they serve as cardiotonic agents to improve the efficiency of myocardial contraction.

The adrenal cortex also releases hormones, the corticosteroids, into the circulation in response to the stresses of injury and hemorrhage. The effects of these very active hormones upon carbohydrate and mineral metabolism as well as many other poorly understood physiologic effects must have important influence upon recovery and convalescence from trauma. The secretion of aldosterone by the adrenal cortex results in sodium retention and loss of potassium by the renal tubules in addition to a cardiotonic effect. Complementing this action is the secretion of the octapeptide antidiuretic hormone by the neurohypophysis. This hormone renders the distal tubules of Henle's loop and the renal collecting tubules permeable to water, and the loss of body water is counteracted. These hormonal effects upon water and salt metabolism have a bearing on cellular reactivity and many other phenomena. A better understanding of them would help answer some of the questions raised by the problems of shock.

METABOLIC EFFECTS OF SHOCK

Trauma and other stresses evoke a well-known metabolic response characterized by a negative nitrogen balance, retention of sodium and water, and negative potassium balance. This response begins immediately, but is recognized clinically only by the positive water balance, an antidiuretic effect, which is apparent during the first 48 or 72 hours after the stress. It occurs whether or not the clinical signs and symptoms of shock develop.

The metabolic effects of shock are superimposed upon the general metabolic reaction to injury. The increased production of catecholamines affects some of the biochemical findings in shock, but for the most part, the metabolic derangement attributed to shock is brought about by the reduction of the rate at which living tissues are perfused with blood. A low rate of blood flow may fail to provide tissues with necessary substrates, and may fail to remove the products of metabolism from the internal environment of the cells. However, the outstanding immediate result of a decreased blood flow, or low rate of perfusion, is a reduction in oxygen consumption per unit of time and a turn from normal aerobic to anaerobic metabolism. Thus, the energy made available by the oxidation of dextrose is reduced to 4 or 5 per cent of that provided by the aerobic process. Furthermore, an acidosis develops, since the end product of the anaerobic process is not carbon dioxide but lactic acid, which cannot be degraded further and combines with the available base in blood and other body fluids. This is recognized as a compensated acidosis by the decrease in carbon dioxide combining power of the blood. As the amount of available buffer base is progressively decreased, the respiratory compensation which maintains the normal 1:20 ratio of carbonic acid to bicarbonate begins to fail and the pH of the blood and body fluids falls.

Since renal function is usually impaired or absent in severe shock, the respiratory elimination of carbon dioxide is about the only compensatory mechanism left for maintaining normal acid-base balance. In fact, the ability of an animal to increase its respiratory tidal volume and, thereby, its minute ventilatory volume has been found related to survival from experimental hemorrhagic shock.

The increased production of lactic acid and the decrease in the alkali reserve of the blood under conditions of hypoxia and in experimental shock have been well established. In World War I, the degree of acidosis, or decrease of the alkali reserve of the blood, was correlated with the degree of shock as indicated by the blood pressure. In World War II, battle casualties were found to have about twice the normal concentration of lactic acid in the blood. The failure of renal function in shock contributes to the acidosis, but the accumulation of lactic acid is the principal cause.

Huckabee has quantitatively related lactic acid production to the extent of anaerobic metabolism. The formation of lactate from pyruvate results in the conversion of reduced nicotinamide adenine dinucleotide (NADH$_2$) to NAD.

The proportion of the conversion achieved by the formation of lactic acid can serve as an indirect measure of the degree of hypoxia.

The normal ratio of lactate to pyruvate in blood is about 5:1. Greater ratios indicate corresponding degrees of anaerobic metabolism. Huckabee considers the calculation of excess lactate, over and above the increased lactate expected from the increased pyruvate concentration, as a more sensitive index than the ratio of the concentration of the two substances. Excess lactate is calculated from the formula:

$$\text{Excess lactate} = (Ln - Lo) - (Pn - Po)\left(\frac{Lo}{Po}\right)$$

Ln and Pn represent the values for lactate and pyruvate concentrations after a period of shock, or hypoxia; Lo and Po represent control values. In examinations of man in shock, the control values for L and P usually are not available, and excess lactate may be approximated by using the 5:1 ratio as a reasonable assumption for the preinjury value.

A circulation which is inadequate to meet the requirements of oxidative aerobic metabolism can be said to be subliminal. As long as cells continue to live and the circulation remains subliminal, the metabolic derangement can be expected to worsen. Guyton and Crowell observed in their experiments on hemorrhagic shock that animals failed to survive periods of hemorrhagic hypotension when they had accumulated an oxygen debt of 100 ml. of oxygen per kilogram of body weight, as calculated from the difference in oxygen consumption between control and experimental periods. One may criticize the concept of oxygen debt during the experimental period, since the debt is conditioned by the requirement, but the fact remains that the more severe and the longer the period of poor tissue perfusion, the greater becomes the metabolic derangement, and the less likely are the affected cells to recover.

It is not surprising that the acidosis resulting from anaerobic metabolism has profound effects upon the biology of living cells. The nature of the effect is not known. Enzyme systems may be poisoned by the abnormal hydrogen ion concentration. Intra-cellular cytoplasmic proteins may be altered, or the membranes enclosing the cells, or those lining the mitochondria within the cells, may be irrevocably altered. Morphologic changes have been described in mitochondria obtained from myocardial and hepatic cells of animals which had been in severe hemor-

Table 7. *Distribution of Plasma Glucose Concentrations, Level of Nonprotein Nitrogen in the Plasma and Prevalence of Azotemia According to Deficit of Blood Volume Among Battle Casualties*

DEFICIT OF WHOLE BLOOD (per cent below expected normal)	CONCENTRATION OF GLUCOSE IN PLASMA BEFORE INITIAL SURGERY (mg. per 100 ml.)	LEVEL OF NONPROTEIN NITROGEN IN PLASMA BEFORE INITIAL SURGERY (mg. per 100 ml.)	PER CENT DEVELOPED AZOTEMIA (NPN > 65, exclusive of crush syndrome)
0– 5	143	31	0
5–15	159	36	10
15–25	153	37	18
25–40	177	38	20
40 +	194	41	37

rhagic shock. The significance of these findings remains obscure.

A characteristic finding in wound shock, is an elevation of the blood sugar related to the degree of blood loss and to the severity of clinical shock. This was observed among the casualties studied in World War I, and since then has been thoroughly confirmed. Although hyperglycemia is common among casualties in shock, glycosuria is rare despite glucose concentrations in the blood approaching 300 mg. per 100 ml. Recent experiments suggest that hepatic glycolysis resulting from increased circulating epinephrine is responsible at least in part for the hyperglycemia. The diabetogenic effects of trauma also play a part.

The nonprotein nitrogen content of the blood increases with shock. The exaggerated catabolism of tissue protein after trauma may be important in this connection, but the reduced renal function is also significant. Creatinuria has been found among battle casualties who had been in shock. This could result from tissue destruction caused by the wound, or a gross disturbance in energy metabolism. The concentrations of potassium and of magnesium in the blood also increase with shock beyond what one would expect from the disturbance of renal function.

Much remains to be learned about the abnormal products of tissue metabolism in wound shock. They may well play an important role in the development of post-traumatic anuria. Two factors appear essential for the development of this kind of renal failure in man: a prolonged period of shock and diminished renal blood flow, and the urinary excretion of abnormal pigments showing a positive benzidine reaction. The pigments could be only bystanders, and the actual injurious agents could be abnormal products of metabolism which as yet have not been recognized.

LABORATORY FINDINGS IN SHOCK

The diagnosis of shock is clinical and ordinarily does not require laboratory aids. Occasionally, the blood pressure of a patient, as measured clinically, may be normal or actually elevated after trauma and hemorrhage. Sympathicoadrenal activity compensates for the hypovolemia. A clinical suspicion of shock, or impending shock, would be supported by the finding of excess lactate in the blood and a decreased alkali reserve. Characteristically, eosinopenia and lymphocytopenia are found in the blood, but these are nonspecific. Together with thrombocytopenia, which is commonly observed early in shock, the disappearance of eosinophils and lymphocytes reflects the pituitary-adrenal cortical response to stress. The reduced platelet count, however, could also be attributed to the utilization of platelets in the formation of erythrocyte aggregates or thrombi. The urinary findings are of some interest. In general, the urine is acid and concentrated. However, if oligemia or anuria develops, the urine becomes less acid, reaching a pH of 6.0 or more, and the specific gravity approaches 1.010.

Since the fundamental defect in wound shock is an absolute oligemia, measurements of the circulating blood volume are of special interest but are rarely necessary for diagnosis. The several available methods depend upon the dilution of a substance which remains in adequate concentration in the circulation after injection long enough to be measured. Measurements of the hematocrit, after injections of plasma or of erythrocytes, have served this purpose. Various dyes have been used, including vital red, in the studies of casualties in World War I, and Evans blue (T-1824) developed prior to World War II. This dye was used for determining blood volumes among casualties in World War II. Employing the same principle of indicator dilution, albumin or erythrocytes tagged respectively with radioactive iodine (I^{131}) or iron (Fe^{59}) and chromium (Cr^{51}), are now more commonly used for this purpose.

One instrument, the Volemetron, has become popular for easily measuring the blood volume under clinical conditions, employing isotope-tagged albumin or erythrocytes. It is easy to use and extremely accurate, so long as it is provided with a proper sample. The principle of indicator dilution is the same as with other instrumentation, but a great advantage is a built-in computer, which spares the observer the task of cumbersome arithmetic.

All instruments are subject to three important variables: the injection of the indicator into the circulation without losing any around the vessel, the proper recovery of a sample of blood for measuring, and the complete mixing of the indicator with the circulating blood whose volume is to be measured. The first two are matters of technical experience and care; the third variable depends upon the hemodynamic situation and is outside the control of the investigator, except insofar as he determines the time for mixing. A single specimen allowing ten minutes for mixing is recommended for counting with the Volemetron, and is satisfactory in normal subjects. In shock, however, mixing is not as rapid, and under some circumstances the indicator injected will equilibrate with extravascular fluid more rapidly than normally. This error may be overcome by counting three or more specimens during a period of 30 to 60 minutes, constructing the standard semilogarithmic disappearance curve and extrapolating to zero time.

In wound shock, a reasonable estimate can be made of the degree of blood loss by the clinical evaluation of the patient. In shock which develops from blood loss during operation, the deficits of circulating blood can be estimated by taking count of the blood on sponges and in suction bottles. There are occasions, however, when a reasonably accurate determination of the circulating blood volume in a patient in shock may be of de-

cisive value. Thus, continued bleeding can be detected when the blood volume fails to increase despite transfusion. Wound shock similarly may be distinguished from septic shock when other criteria are equivocal. The blood volume often is normal or above normal in septic shock. For practical purposes, useful though less discriminative information can be obtained from measurements of the right atrial pressure, which is low in wound shock and remains low as long as the patient is significantly hypovolemic. In septic shock, the right atrial or central venous pressure more commonly is normal or elevated.

The application of objective data to the management of patients in shock requires an estimate of the patient's normal blood volume. On the basis of an extensive experience, Moore recommends estimating the blood volume as 7.0 and 6.5 per cent of body weight for normal men and women respectively. The estimate is decreased by 1.0 per cent for obese individuals and increased by 0.5 per cent for especially muscular men and women. Recently, with the aid of statistical regression analysis, formulas have been developed which take both weight and cubed height into account for calculating the predicted blood volume (PBV) in liters. Thus, for men and boys:

$$PBV = 0.3669 \ H^3 + 0.03219W + 0.6041$$

and for women:

$$PBV = 0.3561 \ H^3 + 0.03308W + 0.1833$$

H represents the height of the patient in meters; W is the body weight in kilograms. Practically, the estimates obtained by this and by the factors suggested by Moore are not significantly different.

FAILURE OF CIRCULATORY HOMEOSTASIS

Early in shock, a vigorous neuroendocrine response results in maintenance of an effective circulation in the heart and in the brain by selectively increasing the arteriolar resistance in organs such as the skin, the kidneys and the liver. Experimentally, the vascular resistance in the heart is actually decreased by this response, so that considerable fall in aortic pressure may occur before the myocardial circulation is seriously affected. The circulation in the brain is not greatly below normal until a mean arterial pressure of 60 mm. of mercury is approached. However, if the oligemia is allowed to persist unduly long, the neuroendocrine response gradually subsides, the preferential circulation to the vital organs is no longer effectively maintained, and the organism progressively deteriorates. This process of homeostatic failure can be reversed if the oligemia is corrected before the causes of failure have advanced too far. Later, restoration of normal blood volume and other supportive measures are no longer effective, shock progresses and death ensues. In this problem, one of the most important questions is what development is responsible for the failure of homeostatic mechanisms when shock has been severe and prolonged. Recognition of the crucial change would facilitate its management and prevention.

The possible sites of failure are many within the complex organization for maintaining normal circulatory function. The theories of nervous exhaustion, exhaustion of the medullary centers, hypocapnia, generalized capillary transudation and fat embolism have been found wanting. The theory of a toxemia as the principal abnormality in wound shock, the wound serving as the source of the toxin, has been replaced by the demonstration of hypovolemia as the fundamental abnormality caused by bleeding and oozing into and from the wound. In connection with the toxin theory of Cannon and Bayliss, implicating histamine or a histamine-like substance, it is of particular interest that Schayer recently has demonstrated increased histidine-decarboxylase activity and increased histamine synthesis in mice after stress and endotoxin. He suggests that a proper balance between histamine and catecholamines is necessary in tissues to meet the injurious effects of endotoxin and other stresses. The eventual depletion of catecholamines and the continued rapid production of histamine would lead to an injurious imbalance that could be lethal. Whether these studies are reproducible in wound shock and in animals other than the rodent, remains to be seen.

A deficit of circulating blood volume is the most important of the factors which initiate the clinically recognized reactions of wound shock. These subside if the cause of the oligemia is corrected and the deficit replaced. If not, the reactions continue and the metabolic defect which they cause increases. Eventually, a vicious circle is established, Guyton's "positive feedback," which results in progressive worsening of the physiologic status of the organism and which is not reversed, despite correction of the oligemia and its cause. Through the years, various local products of tissue metabolism have been implicated, but their respective roles have not been defined. Other causes have been sought for the progressive deterioration, among them failure of the reticuloendothelial system, potassium intoxication, failure of the adrenal glands, failure of the heart, pooling in the splanchnic vascular bed and failure of the mechanisms for venous return of blood to the heart.

RETICULOENDOTHELIAL SYSTEM. The reticuloendothelial system, widely distributed throughout the body, is known to be responsible for the immunologic adaptation that affords protection of the organism against injurious agents. It can be conditioned so as to render the animal more resistant than normally to various stresses. On the other hand, its activity can be inhibited or blocked in many ways, to the point that the animal succumbs to normally nonlethal injury. Severe hemorrhagic hypotension has been found experimentally to depress the functional capacity of the reticuloendothelial system. Consequently, the blood might not be freed of such substances as abnormal products of protein catabolism, ferritin, vasodepressor material, endotoxins and other humoral substances which conceivably could be produced in anoxic living tissue.

While the effectiveness of the protective reticuloendothelial system may be seriously diminished as the result of hemorrhage or wound shock, the role of the suggested accumulation of toxins and other vasoactive substances in fatal shock has not been demonstrated. The causal relationship of ferritin to the downhill course late in wound shock, or in hemorrhagic shock, has not been supported by recent experiments. Similarly, the mass of evidence interpreted in support of the theory that an accumulation of circulating endotoxins is the lethal factor when the reticuloendothelial system is depressed by hemorrhagic shock has not been confirmed. While endotoxins can be lethal to man and to animals, the evidence is lacking that in late hemorrhagic shock they are responsible for the unrelenting deterioration.

ROLE OF POTASSIUM. The general metabolic response to trauma is characterized by retention of sodium and loss of potassium.

In the presence of shock, renal function may be totally suppressed. Potassium is not excreted and it may accumulate in the blood. Thus, high values for blood potassium have been found in hemorrhagic and other forms of shock, and a causative relation has been suggested. The concentration of potassium is elevated in severe dehydration with depressed or absent renal function, as in cholera, strangulation intestinal obstruction, and similar conditions which also exhibit circulatory failure. However, hyperkalemia is not a constant finding in shock, is rarely observed early in shock and is no longer believed to play an important role either as an initiating or a sustaining cause of shock.

ADRENAL GLANDS. In 1934, Swingle, having observed that animals from which the adrenal glands had been removed developed hemoconcentration, depressed vascular reactivity and circulatory failure, compared these findings with those of traumatic shock and concluded that adrenal cortical failure may be an important factor in the progressive deterioration of certain forms of shock. Patients with Addison's disease, and with depressed adrenal cortical function as the result of steroid administration, do develop circulatory failure when subjected to the slightest stress. However, in hemorrhagic shock and in wound shock, there is no evidence that the adrenal cortex fails. If anything, its activity is increased. Shock has been induced by exaggerating sympathicoadrenal activity. Circulatory collapse also results from suddenly increased liberation of adrenal medullary hormones, epinephrine and norepinephrine, into the circulation, as in pheochromocytoma.

The effects of stress when the adrenal glands have been removed or have atrophied, and the effects of the sudden entrance of catecholamines into the circulation, are dramatic and of great clinical importance in their own right. However, previously normal adrenal glands probably play no part in the development of refractoriness to therapy in the usual patient in the late stages of wound shock.

HEART. Since the heart is such an important component of the cardiovascular system, it is not surprising that it has been held suspect for over a century with regard to eventual deterioration in wound shock. It was temporarily exonerated by observations made in World War I. However, the question again has been raised and remains unsettled.

It is true that in hemorrhagic shock the circulation of the myocardium is decreased, myocardial metabolism is altered, focal histologic changes may be demonstrated in the myocardium and its contractile force is decreased. However, using right atrial pressure as a monitor, heart failure does not occur until the very end. General deterioration is well advanced before there is evidence of ventricular failure. Furthermore, while the experimental animal is generally failing, any increase in the venous return to the heart by transfusion of blood results in temporary restoration of cardiac function to normal or near-normal, only to deteriorate again. Especially pertinent is the fact that the mean blood pressure drops before the myocardial contractile force begins to fall. Central venous pressure does not rise during this recurrent deterioration, but rises only at the very end when the animal is agonal. These observations suggest that, starting with a normal heart, the lethal progression of hemorrhagic shock is attributable to inadequate venous return and not to heart failure.

POOLING OF BLOOD IN SPLANCHNIC AREA. For many years, a sequestration or detention of blood in the splanchnic area was suspected to occur in shock which had become unresponsive to therapy. The likelihood of increased vascular resistance in the liver as an explanation for the progressive accumulation of blood in this area was strengthened by the description of a "sphincteric mechanism" in the hepatic venous outflow from the liver. Such a mechanism which would increase the resistance to venous outflow from the liver in late shock, and would thereby selectively retain more blood within the liver and splanchnic area, has not been observed in man.

Venous congestion in the splanchnic bed, without elevated portal pressure, such as one would expect with pooling of blood in this area, has not been seen at operation in man. However, the submucosal vessels of the stomach and intestine can contain large volumes of blood in man without being visible on the surface. Recent experiments in the dog failed to show anything but a temporary increase above normal portal vein pressure when the reservoir blood was returned to the animal after a period of hemorrhagic hypotension sufficient to cause irreversibility. The temporary increase in portal pressure to above normal control pressures with reinfusion was attributed to a return of splanchnic blood flow toward normal and to the critical opening pressure in the portal bed, to be overcome after a period of hypotension. Regardless of cause, this temporary elevation of portal pressure was actually too short-lived to be a determining factor in the development of irreversibility. Studies of pooling in the splanchnic bed after reinfusion of blood in the dog have not pointed to this area as a sufficient reservoir by itself to account for decreased venous return and progressive deterioration of the animal in normovolemic and hypervolemic shock.

FAILURE OF MECHANISMS OF VENOUS RE-TURN. The venous return of blood to the right side of the heart depends upon skeletal muscular compression of valve-bearing veins, the respiratory changes of intrathoracic pressure, the capacity of the venous system as a reservoir, and the "vis a tergo" of pressure transmitted through the capillaries or the arteriovenous communications in the microcirculation. The greater part of the blood volume is contained within the large and small veins. If these dilated to any considerable extent, they could easily accommodate the entire blood volume. This venous dilation could occur, especially in nonmuscular areas of the body, and this has been suggested as the primary reason for the progressive circulatory failure leading eventually to death. Thus, there is a return to Henderson's proposal of venomotor paralysis of over half a century ago, modified by the elimination of acapnia as the cause of the venous paralysis.

Obviously, the assignment of the continued deterioration of the circulation in shock to a progressive decrease in the venous return of blood to the heart answers little, if anything. The decreasing venous return could be due to obstruction of the microcirculation by erythrocyte and platelet aggregates or thrombi, or to the progressive loss of plasma from the circulation in the late stages of shock, as occurs to some extent in the experimental animal, but has not been demonstrated in man except in severe infection. The suggested paralysis of the muscular coats of the veins could result in the accommodation of much more blood than normal, and this would decrease the volume available for return to the heart. This theory is attractive but remains to be proved.

Wherever may be the site or sites of failure, it is reasonable to attribute the failure to the drastic changes in the internal environment of living cells caused by the progressive anoxia and associated metabolic disturbance. Free energy, already curtailed by the shift to anaerobic metabolism, may become totally lost when NAD is no longer re-formed from $NADH_2$. The integrity of cells is lost and physiologic mechanisms fail.

PATHOLOGIC FINDINGS. The failure to distinguish between cause and effect in the past has led to confusion with regard to the pathologic findings in shock. It is generally agreed that shock produces its injurious effects by the reduction in the rate of perfusion of tissues with blood to the point that the circulation becomes subliminal and incapable of sustaining normal metabolism. Therefore, to be characteristic of shock, the pathologic findings should be related to the effects of inadequate perfusion of tissues during the period of circulatory depression. One would expect that such parenchymatous changes would take time to develop and would heal if the patient survived the period of shock long enough. Mallory studied the histologic findings in a large number of battle casualties and found changes which could be attributed to shock among those who survived at least 18 hours. Further evidence that these were attributable to shock came from the observation that these particular histologic abnormalities persisted among casualties who survived for three days, and began to clear among those who lived four days and longer.

Employing these criteria, Mallory described two types of parenchymatous changes as characteristic of shock in man: fat vacuolation in the heart, liver and kidney, and depletion of doubly refractile lipid in the zona fasciculata of the adrenal cortex. Mallory acknowledged that none of these changes individually could be considered pathognomonic of shock, but the pattern of change in the four organs could be.

In the myocardium, the lipid vacuoles are very small, seldom larger than 2 microns, and are found throughout the cell. The muscle fibers are affected singly or in groups, but not evenly throughout the myocardium. The extent and intensity of vacuolation was related to the severity of shock. In the liver, fat vacuolation affected primarily the central cells of the lobule, and extended peripherally with increasing severity. The vacuoles are distinctive by their small size and their failure to coalesce within a cell. The severity of these changes, too, was related to the degree of shock. Fat vacuolation was found in the ascending limb of Henle's loop in the kidney in 85 per cent of patients who developed shock and survived one to four days after wounding. This kind of vacuolation in the kidney normally does not occur.

The pathology of the kidney has been extensively studied in relation to trauma because of the frequent persistence of renal failure after recovery from wound shock. The gross and microscopic findings are consistently found among such patients who have been in wound shock, have renal functional impairment, and survive longer than 24 hours.

The kidney may look normal on the surface. The degree of swelling of the kidney depends upon the degree of excessive hydration employed during the period of oligemia and anuria. When the kidney is incised, the capsule rolls away from the edge when there is appreciable edema. On cut surface, the most striking feature is the contrast in color between the cortical and medullary layers of the kidney. The pale yellowish cortex contrasts strikingly with the dark mahogany color of the medulla. The histologic findings differ according to the interval between injury and examination. As described by Mallory, they are fat vacuolation of the ascending limb of Henle's loop, 18 to 72 hours after injury; precipitation of pigment as casts, hemoglobin or myohemoglobin, in the distal convoluted and collecting tubules, 24 or more hours after injury; moderate dilation of the proximal convoluted tubules, 24 or more hours after injury; interstitial inflammation, 72 hours or more after injury; degeneration of cells of ascending limb of Henle's loop, 72 hours or longer after injury; tubular rupture with extrusion of nonpigmented casts, four or more days after injury; formation of granulomas about areas of tubular necrosis, four or more days after injury; and thrombophlebitis in renal parenchyma, five or more days after wounding.

Since the preponderance of the changes are in the distal segments of the nephron, the lesion was originally referred to as "lower nephron nephrosis." Though minor, however, some changes do occur in the more proximal portions of the nephron and, at the present time, most pathologists prefer the term "acute tubular nephrosis." It is noteworthy that of the several findings described for the kidney, only the fat vacuolation of the ascending limb of Henle's loop can be considered as specifically secondary to a period of shock. The other abnormalities are found in a great variety of conditions which cause oligemia and anuria.

After the administration of endotoxin, bleeding and reinfusion, the dog, but not certain other animals such as the cat and spider monkey, develops dramatic hemorrhagic necrosis of the intestinal mucosa and hemorrhage into the intestinal wall largely limited to the small intestine. Gurd and his associates have been able to prevent this reaction after hemorrhage by protecting the intestine from the actions of pancreatic secretion and by providing an elemental diet. This kind of intestinal pathologic change does not occur in man.

Other pathologic findings are common among patients who die after shock and severe trauma. Pulmonary edema, once thought to be characteristic of shock and to be causally related to it, is present when heart failure has supervened, renal insufficiency has developed, and severe overhydration has resulted from therapy. Pulmonary edema could not be related to the wound shock itself. Fat embolism has also been suspected of a causal relation with wound shock. In fact, it is found in varying degree in the majority of casualties after trauma and is always demonstrable in patients who have been in severe wound shock. From the information available, fat embolism cannot be considered a result of wound shock, but when severe it sometimes can cause shock.

MANAGEMENT OF THE PATIENT IN SHOCK

GENERAL. The clinical signs and symptoms which collectively lead to a diagnosis of shock represent a final common path taken by a variety of derangements leading to circulatory failure. Successful therapy depends upon detection and correction of the causative mechanisms and support of the circulation while recovery is taking place. Under some circumstances, as in the course of posttraumatic anuria, therapy may need to be directed toward the support of individual organs, in this case, the kidneys. When shock develops during the course of a severe infection, the source of the bacteria, or the site of the toxin-producing infection, must be eradicated or exteriorized by drainage. Appropriate parenteral antibiotics must be used in large doses to curtail the invasive properties of the organisms involved. In wound shock, the

many factors which the wound and its circumstances contribute to the clinical symptoms should be eliminated. As observed in
World War I, improvement is sometimes
dramatic when a casualty is removed from
cold wet ground, splinted as needed, comforted and reassured.

The treatment of the causative wound is
an essential part of the management of the
patient in shock following injury. Appropriate
treatment for the wound is mandatory, and
is usually started in the form of first-aid
measures before it is possible to begin resuscitation. Naturally, since the fundamental
abnormality in wound shock is a deficit in
circulating blood volume, the early surgical
management of a severe wound should be
directed toward the stemming of further
blood loss, and protection against increasing
bacterial contamination by means of appropriate dressings. Until a definitive operation
can be performed, bleeding is best controlled
by means of pressure dressings. The use of
tourniquets is a last resort. Once applied, the
tourniquet is not released again until an
operation can be done to control the bleeding.
Antibiotics or chemotherapeutic agents are
administered in the case of open wounds to
forestall the development of advancing infection from the contamination.

As soon as resuscitation has proceeded to
the point of compensation, that is, the pulse
rate has begun to fall, the blood pressure is
rising, the skin is warming and the capillary
circulation is improving, and while resuscitation is still continuing, the wound is treated
definitively. The control of continued oozing
of blood and plasma, the application of an
appropriate protective covering for the
wound, and the reassurance of the patient
that a corrective program has been initiated
are important factors in recovery.

The same principles apply to the treatment
of shock in severe burns. However, these
comprise a special situation in that the wound
continues to be a source of serious fluid loss
from the circulation for 48 to 72 hours.

In all patients in shock, adequate pulmonary function must be ensured. A normal
airway must be maintained, with the help of
tracheostomy if necessary; normal pulmonary aeration must be maintained. Such
lesions as "flail chest" from multiple rib fractures, massive atelectasis, simple pneumothorax, tension pneumothorax, open pneumothorax and hemothorax, all of which
interfere with adequate pulmonary aeration,
must be sought and corrected when found.

TREATMENT OF PAIN. The observations
which Beecher made among wounded men
in World War II have served as a guide for
the treatment of pain among the injured. He
emphasized the fact that, with the exception
of casualties with such lesions as unsplinted
fractures and chemical peritonitis as seen
with wounds of the gastrointestinal tract,
pain is not a serious complaint. More important among recent casualties are the anxiety,
fear and uncertainty of the future which
beset them. After reassurance, a mild sedative if needed, and surprisingly little analgesic, the injured patient whose wounds are
dressed and fractures splinted no longer complains of pain.

When a narcotic analgesic is needed, it is
important that the drug be administered
intravenously. In shock, the dose is likely to
be ineffective when given subcutaneously or
intramuscularly, and it may, therefore, be
repeated one or more times. When the circulation is restored, the absorption of the total
amount can prove catastrophic. The use in
adults of as little as 8 or 10 mg. of morphine
sulfate (4 or 5 mg. intravenously) is as effective and less deranging than the usually administered 15 mg.

GUIDES TO TREATMENT OF SHOCK. The
diagnosis of clinical shock is made on the
basis of circulatory abnormalities detected
directly or indirectly, low arterial blood pressure, rapid pulse rate, pallor and coldness of
exposed skin, slow filling of blanched venules
of the skin, thirst, oliguria or anuria and
changes in the sensorium. By definition, a
patient may be in shock without hypotension,
such as may occur after hemorrhage insufficient to overwhelm the physiologic mechanisms which normally protect the blood
pressure. Also, very early after injury, a patient with exaggerated vagal activity may
show bradycardia instead of tachycardia.
Nevertheless, the experienced clinician can
judge the severity and the progress of clinical
shock without more complicated observations.

However, objective physiological and biochemical data serve not only to support the
clinical findings, but also to guide therapy
with a precision that is not possible by clinical
observation alone.

Hematocrit value. The hematocrit is a
graduated tube which permits the estimation
of the proportions of erythrocytes and plasma
in centrifuged blood. The normal hematocrit
value for erythrocytes is 45 per cent among
men and 40 per cent among women. When

blood is lost by bleeding, hemodilution takes place, but unlike the dog the process is slow in man. A spontaneous lowering of the hematocrit, therefore, cannot be awaited as a guide to continued bleeding or resumption of bleeding because the change would not be apparent until some hours later. However, an increase in hematocrit value after a severe burn or after release of a crushing injury is very prompt and the hematocrit value can serve as a guide for fluid replacement therapy or, preferably, as a check on fluid replaced in anticipation of loss.

Urinary output. The urinary output is a sensitive indicator of effective circulating blood and, in the early stage of shock, can serve as a guide for adequate correction of oligemia. A urinary output of 50 to 75 ml. per hour may be considered adequate. The urinary volume alone, however, is not an index of renal function. When, in the late stage of shock or during convalescence from shock, the kidneys have suffered damage, evaluation of renal function requires determination of urinary osmolality or, at least, specific gravity in order to be certain that the observed urinary volume is more than just glomerular filtrate.

Acid-base balance. Patients in shock characteristically develop a metabolic acidosis. Normally, the acidosis is corrected by respiratory loss of carbon dioxide. The lowered buffer base of the blood is thus compensated for by a fall in the CO_2 or carbonic acid content of the blood. The increase in hydrogen ion concentration is thereby prevented or tempered. A metabolic acidosis, however, is not invariable. Sometimes, alkalosis is found, as in the occasional patient who develops shock after having been on prolonged treatment for peptic ulcer; and sometimes early after trauma or severe infection hyperventilation results in a respiratory alkalosis, later superseded by metabolic acidosis. Furthermore, patients in shock may have respiratory difficulties which impair the acid-base regulatory function of the lungs. They may be incapable of compensating for metabolic acidosis or may actually superimpose upon it a respiratory acidosis by carbon dioxide retention.

These biochemical relationships are not discernible by clinical observation alone. The values for hydrogen ion concentration and for partial pressures and contents of carbon dioxide and oxygen in the arterial blood must be determined. Advances in instrumentation have made it possible for determinations such as these to be made at the bedside within five minutes after taking a specimen of blood. The data so obtained are invaluable for the choice of appropriate therapy.

Arteriovenous oxygen difference. The arterial oxygen saturation is usually normal in shock, at least in the early stages. The venous oxygen saturation, however, is reduced, and in proportion to the severity of shock. The reduction in oxygen saturation of venous blood is attributable to the decreased rate of capillary blood flow and therefore greater than normal extraction of oxygen from capillary and possibly venular blood as well. Improved cardiac output and improved circulation in tissues results in a decrease in the elevated arteriovenous oxygen difference. This interpretation, of course, depends upon the assumption that the rate of oxygen consumption remains constant and that arteriovenous shunting does not change. Ideally, pulmonary arterial or right ventricular blood should be obtained in order for it to be representative of the average venous oxygen saturation throughout the body. Specimens of right atrial blood obtained through a central venous catheter are quite adequate.

The arteriovenous oxygen difference can be useful for documenting improvement or worsening of the patient in shock and serves to alert the physician. However, the information does not prescribe the treatment needed except insofar as a low arterial oxygen tension would suggest the need for improvement in the pulmonary ventilatory function.

Blood lactate, pyruvate and buffer base. The determination of the concentrations of these substances in the blood has become standard practice in the management of patients in shock. Much can be learned from the absolute individual values of these substances as determined in arterial blood. The calculation of excess lactate over and above the amount of lactate one would expect on the basis of the concentration of pyruvate is a refinement which relates the lactate increase to subliminal perfusion of tissues with blood rather than to overventilation or to hypoxia. A decrease in the buffer base indicates a metabolic acidosis with or without compensatory hypocarbia.

The data are useful especially for determining the severity and course of the condition and the prognosis of the patient.

Central venous pressure. Measurement of the pressure within the superior and inferior venae cavae within the thorax, or within the right atrium, is indicative of the adequacy of the venous return to the right atrium and of right ventricular function. When venous return is inadequate, as in hypovolemia, the central venous or right atrial pressure is low or approaches zero. When more blood is returned to the right atrium than it or the right ventricle can pump forward, the central venous pressure rises. This usually reflects varying degrees of failure of the right ventricle. For dependability, the central venous pressure should be measured with the zero point at the level of the right atrium, and the observer should be cognizant of the increased central venous pressure caused by the open chest and by positive-pressure artificial respiration.

In the course of management of shock, the physician may not know the status of the circulating blood volume, may not have means for measuring it or may have evidence that the blood volume has been restored to normal and the patient continues in shock. Knowledge of the central venous pressure can tell him whether the venous return is or is not adequate to maintain a normal filling pressure for the right ventricle without overwhelming it, that the filling pressure is normal or that the pressure is well above normal (over 15 mm. Hg) and indicates right ventricular failure. Certainly, when the central venous pressure is low or normal and the patient continues in shock, more fluid may be introduced into the circulation in the hope of increasing the cardiac output. When the venous pressure is high, over 15 mm. Hg, the administration of more fluid by vein, without improving myocardial function, can only make matters worse.

It is important to note that the central venous pressure is not a measure of circulating blood volume or of cardiac output. It represents no more than the pressure with which blood is presented to the right ventricle, the filling pressure. Because a patient in shock may require above normal circulating blood volume and cardiac output, the limiting factor being the ability of the heart to pump the needed increased volume, knowledge of the central venous pressure can be the most useful single datum available to the physician. Measurements of the circulating blood volume and of the cardiac output are very valuable for diagnostic and prognostic purposes, but a normal blood volume and cardiac output should not be interpreted as contraindicating the administration of additional appropriate intravenous fluid.

SPECIFIC THERAPY FOR SHOCK. The objectives of specific therapy for shock are to correct the fundamental abnormality after having removed its cause, and to provide ancillary support for recovery from the earlier effects of the inadequate circulation.

While true that shock can be caused by a great variety of abnormalities, most patients seen by the surgeon have a deficit in circulating blood volume. In wounds of some magnitude involving soft tissues and bone, most of the fluid lost from the circulation is whole blood. The ideal fluid for replacement, therefore, is properly matched type-specific whole blood. When this is not immediately available, Rh-negative universal donor (group O) blood with low anti-A titer can be administered until type-specific blood is available. In the absence of whole blood, plasma has been a very serviceable substitute. Unpooled plasma carries with its administration the same risk of viral hepatitis as is carried by whole blood. On the other hand, pooled plasma is far more likely than single units of unpooled plasma to carry the infective agent. Freshly pooled plasma, or dried pooled plasma, should not be used in man except under dire circumstances. Storage of liquid plasma at warm room temperature improves its safety.

In burns and in the crush syndrome, the fluid lost from the circulation is not primarily whole blood, but for the most part is a plasma-like fluid containing electrolytes comparable in concentration with those of blood plasma, and proteins in approximately half the concentration of those in plasma. A solution of equal parts of blood plasma and of balanced salt solution is the appropriate fluid for replacement of such losses.

There is no substitute for blood or for plasma in the strict sense of the word, for none of the substitutes can provide the biologic and metabolic properties of blood and plasma. The volemic functions of blood and plasma can be fulfilled by substitutes, including solutions of crystalloids, for brief periods of time.

A number of substances have been proposed for transfusion in wound shock since the experimental observations on solutions of acacia in World War I (Table 8). Among other materials tested are polyvinylpyrrolidone, various gelatins of animal origin, and dextran. Macromolecular dextran, macrodex, consists of large molecules of high molecular weights, about 75,000. This has found considerable application in pa-

Table 8. Blood Substitutes

Colloidal solutions of human or other animal origin
    Plasma and concentrated albumin prepared from blood
       plasma
    Globin prepared from human erythrocytes
    Gelatin (nonantigenic; prepared from beef bone, fish
       and hog skin)
Colloidal solutions of vegetable origin
    Gum acacia
    Methyl cellulose
    Pectin, a polygalacturonic acid
    Polysaccharide from okra
    Dextran, molecular weight 70,000 or more, 6 per cent
       solution in isotonic sodium chloride; produced by
       fermentative action of *Leuconostoc mesenteroides*
       on sucrose
    Rheomacrodex, low molecular weight dextran, molecu-
       lar weight 40,000
    Hydroxyethyl starch (experimental)

Colloidal solutions, synthetic
    Polyvinylpyrrolidone (Kollidon, Periston), synthesized
       from acetylene, ammonia and formaldehyde

Solutions of crystalloids
    Nonelectrolytes: dextrose, sucrose, mannitol, urea
    Electrolytes: sodium chloride with or without sodium
       lactate dextrose, lactated Ringer's solution

---

tients in shock until blood or suitably prepared plasma is available. It should be used with caution, however, because occasional antigen-antibody reactions are produced and because of defects in blood clotting when, as shown in volunteers, amounts greater than 20 per cent of the normal blood volume have been injected. The effect of dextran in maintaining an expanded plasma volume lasts for 24 to 48 hours.

The recent introduction of dextran of low molecular weight has received considerable attention because of its ability to lower the viscosity of blood when administered intravenously, and to prevent sludging or aggregation of erythrocytes under various conditions, including shock. These are attractive properties, in view of the importance of maintaining an open microcirculation for the perfusion of tissues with blood.

Hydroxyethyl starch has recently been introduced for experimental purposes. It appears to have many of the advantages and disadvantages of dextran, but much more work is needed before its usefulness can be established.

The work of Shires and of others has emphasized the usefulness of balanced solutions of electrolytes, such as lactated Ringer's solution with pH adjusted to 8.0 or 8.5 for the treatment of shock. Experimentally, such electrolyte solutions have proved effective when used alone for treating experimental

shock from hemorrhage or from tumbling. Clinical tests among patients with severe burns have revealed no advantages of plasma over solutions of electrolytes except in children. Experiences among patients in shock from severe hemorrhage have demonstrated significant benefit from the administration of balanced solutions of electrolytes in volumes up to 25 or 30 per cent of the estimated normal blood volume in conjunction with whole blood given in volumes approximating the blood loss.

The administration of isotonic dextrose in water and of solutions of electrolytes is essential for maintaining renal function and for meeting losses of body fluids other than blood, normal or abnormal. It is well to remember, however, that insofar as these substances are retained within the circulation they dilute the hematocrit value of the blood. In exceptional acute situations, a hematocrit value of 15 per cent can be tolerated, but, in general, it is well not to permit the proportion of erythrocytes in circulating blood to fall below 30 per cent, ideally not below 40 per cent, especially among patients who are likely to require operative intervention under general anesthesia.

Renal tubular necrosis is a serious complication of shock. Evidence has accumulated through the years since World War II that the renal tubules are obstructed by the formation and impaction of pigment casts within them. The resulting increased intratubular and parenchymal pressures at least contribute to the tubular necrosis. This can be prevented by maintaining a satisfactory diuresis so that casts will not form within the tubules and obstruction is prevented. Diuresis can be maintained by the administration of isotonic solutions of crystalloids and of electrolytes. Recently, solutions of mannitol have become popular for establishing and maintaining an osmotic diuresis for this purpose. They must be used with care to avoid overtaxing the pulmonary circulation. Although probably useful for preventing renal tubular necrosis, mannitol has not been helpful when renal tubular function already has become seriously impaired.

It is common practice to place patients who are in shock and individuals who experience syncope or collapse in the headdown, or Trendelenburg position. Although it is generally accepted that syncope corrects itself when the patient falls into a horizontal position or is tilted head-down, and that syncope can be induced by tilting a normal subject from a horizontal to a head-up position on a tilt-table, the effect of posture on the cerebral circulation remains in debate, both in normal persons and in individuals after blood loss.

Clinically, most patients in shock improve when placed in the Trendelenburg position. The beneficial effects of this position are probably related to autotransfusion with blood from the elevated lower extremities and can be achieved by elevation of the limbs alone. Lowering of the head below the level of the heart does not improve cerebral circulation, and, in fact, may embarrass it. The Trendelenburg position is contraindicated in patients with generalized peritonitis and in casualties with injuries or other lesions of the chest in whom the weight of the abdominal viscera pressing on the diaphragm may further interfere with pulmonary ventilation.

The inhalation of 100 per cent oxygen has always had considerable lay appeal. Physicians have viewed this form of therapy with skepticism on the basis that the blood is nearly maximally saturated with oxygen in one passage by alveoli containing modified atmospheric air in which the oxygen concentration is about 15 volumes per cent and its partial pressure is about 140 mm. of mercury. It has been argued that on the basis of the peculiarities of the oxygen dissociation curve of hemoglobin, the saturation of this pigment with oxygen would not significantly be improved by breathing oxygen. However, the inhalation of 100 per cent oxygen, while increasing the oxygen content of blood only by as little as 3 per cent, can at least theoretically increase the partial pressure of oxygen at the venous end of the capillary by more than 50 per cent (Table 9). Furthermore, while true that in the early phase of wound shock the oxygen saturation of blood is normal, in the late stage some degree of desaturation commonly exists and this can be im-

proved by inhaling high concentrations of oxygen.

The mode of administration of oxygen for patients in shock, or recovering from shock, must be dictated by the special circumstances in any particular instance. The airtight mask permits the inhalation of oxygen in nearly the concentration supplied. The nasal catheter, passed to the level of the nasopharynx, provides oxygen in approximately 50 per cent concentration when supplied from a source of 100 per cent oxygen. The oxygen tent generally is less efficient than either of these two methods, but in most cases is better tolerated by the patient.

The use of oxygen under higher than atmospheric pressures is now under examination. In view of the possible risks of employing 100 per cent oxygen under such high pressures, this form of therapy is still experimental and its general application should await confirmation of data to support the present enthusiasm.

When, in 1895, a pressor agent was found in extracts of the adrenal medulla, physicians foresaw the solution of the problem of shock. Disillusioned by observations which have been recorded, but stimulated by the development of sympathomimetic agents possessing only the positive actions of epinephrine, the employment of vasopressor drugs for various kinds of shock continues as a popular form of therapy. The evidence regarding the effects of these drugs on corrective hemodilution is contradictory. Nevertheless, they are warranted only under very exceptional circumstances, so exceptional, indeed, that they hardly merit consideration. In high spinal anesthesia, in which there is increased blood flow to the skin at the expense of visceral circulation, a constrictor agent may be indicated to re-establish normal proportionate blood flow.

One is tempted to apply the same argument to certain patients in whom shock is

Table 9. *Oxygen Tension of Blood in Venous End of Capillary in Failure of Peripheral Circulation (After Boothby)*

OXYGEN TENSION IN ALVEOLAR AIR (mm. mercury)	OXYGEN IN BLOOD IN VENOUS END OF CAPILLARY		
	CONTENT (vol. per cent)	SATURATION (per cent)	TENSION
100	5	25	16
673	8	40	25

associated with widespread vasodilation in some unusual kinds of infection. As a matter of fact, the problem is different from that of neurogenic or vasogenic shock as seen in high spinal anesthesia, in which the cardiac output may reach unusually low levels and vasodilation results from interruption of nervous vasoconstrictor activity. In vasogenic shock of sepsis with vasodilation, the vessels may be affected directly by the toxin. The large amounts of vasoconstrictors needed to constrict such dilated vessels could cause overpowering vasoconstriction and ischemia in essential vascular beds. Moreover, it is well to bear in mind that even in septic shock the skin is pale, cold and moist, not pink, warm and dry.

Thus, for nearly all patients in shock, agents which cause an improvement in the blood pressure by their vasoconstrictor action are contraindicated. This thought is not new. It was clearly expressed by Cannon in 1923. In the management of shock, the physician is interested in the blood pressure only as a means to an end, the end being the perfusion of tissues with blood. If the blood pressure is raised by increasing the peripheral vascular resistance by arteriolar constriction, that end is thwarted. Unless for a particular vascular bed the blood pressure is raised to a proportionately equal or greater degree than is the vascular resistance, the perfusion of tissues with blood is further decreased and the metabolic derangement, the injurious effect of shock, is worsened.

Adrenergic drugs do not constrict all vascular beds. While constricting the small vessels of the skin, l-norepinephrine causes a dilation of those of the myocardium and of skeletal muscle. In acute severe hypotension because of massive hemorrhage, the circulation of the heart and of the brain can fall to dangerous levels. Since cerebral vascular constriction is minimal when l-norepinephrine is administered, the rise in blood pressure can improve the circulation of both the myocardium and the brain. However, it must be emphasized that, while momentarily protecting the heart and the brain, this form of therapy, if continued for more than a very few minutes, sets the stage for normovolemic shock and death. It increases the rate of progress of the metabolic acidosis of inadequate blood flow and the accompanying biochemical changes. These are the changes which, despite the heart and the brain, lead to the well-known state of dis-organization of the mechanisms which maintain circulatory homeostasis, commonly referred to as irreversibility. The first objective in the specific therapy of wound shock must be to restore the circulating blood volume to near-normal levels.

Catecholamines are known to exert an inotropic effect upon the heart. When administered in small doses, they could have a cardiotonic action without causing vasoconstriction and tissue ischemia, and this could be beneficial. Objective evidence that this is the case is lacking. Furthermore, until very shortly before death, the otherwise normal heart functions reasonably well and is hampered principally by a failure of the mechanisms which return blood to it for pumping.

Recently, angiotensin has become available as an arteriolar constrictor and powerful hypertensive agent. Formed naturally by the enzymatic action of renin on a polypeptide precursor in the plasma, it has been produced synthetically as an octapeptide. Unlike noradrenaline and similar catecholamines, it does not cause venular constriction, a property of doubtful value especially in late shock. Angiotensin has less to recommend it than the constrictor catecholamines, since it does not increase renal or myocardial blood flow and has no inotropic effect upon the heart.

Late in wound shock which has become refractory to treatment, and in shock secondary to infection, the cardiac output may be seriously impaired by failure of venous return attributed to increased capacity of venous channels in particular. Blood is diverted to fill those channels and is unavailable for a satisfactory cardiac output. If such reservoirs could be constricted by catecholamines, then their use might improve the cardiac output. Whether this occurs with certainty is not known. It is clear, however, that the administration of pressor agents has not altered significantly the mortality of animals and patients in normovolemic shock or in shock secondary to the administration of endotoxin.

A drug which would have no vasoconstrictor action but would serve to improve cardiac function and decrease vascular resistance could be valuable in the treatment of shock. The actions of isoproterenol, a catecholamine derivative, approach these requirements. Isoproterenol experimentally has chronotropic and inotropic effects upon the heart and reduces the peripheral vascular resistance by causing vasodilation in skeletal muscles and in the splanchnic area. Encouraging results have been obtained by some with the use of this drug in the treatment of septic and other forms of shock.

Weil reported a beneficial effect of a vasopressor in shock secondary to endotoxin, but Spink and Vick could detect improvement in survival only if metaraminol was used in combination with hydrocortisone. Corticosteroids can increase the responsiveness of depressed smooth muscle to catecholamines, and possibly this mechanism accounts for the positive results obtained by Spink and Vick. In addition, hydrocortisone, prednisone and dexamethasone inhibit the activity of plasma kinins and may maintain stability of the lysosomal membrane, thereby preventing the suicidal disruption of enzyme-laden lysosomes which is thought to occur in shock and other conditions of cellular injury.

Objective evidence in man is difficult to obtain with regard to the effectiveness of the corticosteroids. When the patient in shock is known to be normovolemic and, indeed, hypervolemic to the point of a rising central venous pressure toward 10 mm. of mercury, and when correctable causes for shock have been excluded, it may be reasonable to resort to the use of these drugs as ancillary measures. When indicated on this basis, corticosteroids should be administered in large doses, of about 4 or more gm. of hydrocortisone in divided doses during a 24-hour period. Recently, aldosterone has been found to be effective in animals in endotoxic shock as well as in hemorrhagic shock. This hormone has many actions, including an inotropic effect upon the myocardium, but the nature of its effect in experimental shock remains to be clarified.

In recent years, experimental evidence has accumulated to indicate that blockade of sympathetic vasoconstrictor activity can improve the rate of survival of animals in shock from a variety of causes. Application of this principle to the treatment of shock in man has not been widespread. All who have been interested in this approach to the problem emphasize that the drug must not be used unless the patient has been transfused at least to normovolemia. Some degree of hypervolemia is preferable. The most commonly advocated drug at this time is dibenzyline (phenoxybenzamine hydrochloride, 1 mg. per kg. body weight). As the drug is administered, concomitant falls in blood pressure

Table 10.   *Reversible Causes of "Irreversibility"*

I. *Inadequate replacement of blood volume*
  1. Failure to appreciate extent or rate of blood loss
     a. Transfusion inadequate as to volume and rate
  2. Failure to detect continued bleeding
     a. Bleeding inconspicuous
        1. From principal wound
        2. From other, less dramatic wounds
     b. Bleeding occult
        1. Into pleural cavity
        2. Into peritoneal cavity
        3. Into injured extremities
        4. Into tissue planes (retroperitoneal space)
II. *Failure to detect primary mechanism of shock or contributing causes*
  1. Cardiopulmonary causes
     a. Massive atelectasis
     b. Tension pneumothorax
     c. Open pneumothorax
     d. Fat embolism
     e. Cardiac tamponade
     f. Myocardial infarction
  2. Infections
     a. Peritonitis, retroperitoneal infection or subdiaphragmatic infection
     b. Clostridial myositis (gas gangrene)
     c. Cerebrospinal infection
     d. Intracranial injury

are countered by transfusion. A fall in blood pressure caused by tilting toward the upright position indicates a need for more transfusion.

The rationale for the use of autonomic blocking agents for their vasodilator effects in shock is that, so long as the patient is adequately transfused, release of vasoconstriction should improve the perfusion of tissues and organs with blood. This would reverse the progressive anoxia of tissues, correct the metabolic acidosis and restore normal function. The theory needs further testing.

A variety of other drugs have been advocated from time to time, including such substances as cytochrome, vitamins and chlorpromazine, a metabolic depressant. Some have merit, in particular chlorpromazine, and have been tried in man. The results of their use have not been convincing.

The significance of adequate perfusion of the microcirculation for normal metabolism has repeatedly been emphasized. It would seem reasonable that reduction of the metabolic requirements of tissue would convert a less than adequate rate of perfusion to one which would deliver oxygen and substrates, and would remove products of metabolism at a rate sufficient to meet the lowered demands. In fact, this has been demonstrated experimentally.

Reports of the use of hypothermia in man have been concerned primarily with the treatment of septic shock. Although suggestive, and bolstered by the thought that with improved techniques for the care of the patient under prolonged hypothermia the results would be better, the available data for man are not really convincing.

To be sure, one would expect that the establishment of a lower metabolic requirement for circulation, as soon as trauma is incurred, would prevent or delay the development of the changes which eventually lead to death when the circulation is depressed below minimal essential levels. But once these changes have already developed, hypothermia might be expected to delay the course of reparative processes as well as the accumulation of products of anaerobic metabolism. The net result would be at least debatable.

While the induction of hypothermia is still experimental, it is generally agreed that the application of external heat is contraindicated. The heated shock table which frequently caused serious burns has been abandoned. Instead, the patient is separated from any cold, wet clothing and protected by an appropriate dry, comfortable cover.

"Irreversibility" is the descriptive term applied to the stage of shock, whatever its initiating mechanism, in which improvement fails to take place despite active therapy. It is a dangerous term and is better not used. It is a misnomer, because it is the cellular death which results from prolonged cumulative anoxia which is irreversible, and not the overall condition of shock. Death of the organism results when enough vital cells have died so that the deficit is incompatible with life. Thus, a patient may die of uremia and anuria many days after all signs of shock have been reversed, or he may die of irreparable brain damage despite adequate treatment of shock. Criticism of the term "irreversible shock" emphasizes the fact that shock is a dynamic process which can be reversed by aggressive therapy; if reversal is too long delayed, however, biochemical changes take place which cause the death of cells. Emphasis is placed upon prompt and aggressive therapy.

Use of the term encourages the establishment of a state of helplessness which permits errors of omission. Before reaching the conclusion that one is dealing with irreversibility, the several correctable causes for the failure to respond to therapy should be thoroughly examined and ruled out. A successful outcome often rewards this kind of diligence.

READING REFERENCES

Allen, J. G., Inouye, H. S., and Sykes, C.: Homologous serum jaundice and pooled plasma-attenuating effect of room temperature storage on its virus agent. Ann. Surg. 138:476, 1953.

Beecher, H. K.: Preparation of battle casualties for surgery. Ann. Surg. 121:769, 1945.

Blalock, A.: Acute circulatory failure as exemplified by shock and hemorrhage. Surg. Gyn. & Obst. 58:551, 1934.

Blalock, A.: Experimental shock. The cause of the low blood pressure produced by muscle injury. Arch. Surg. 20:959, 1930.

Blattberg, B., and Levy, M. N.: A humoral reticuloendothelial depressing substance in shock. Am. J. Physiol. 203:409, 1962.

Board for the Study of the Severely Wounded: Surgery in World War II. The Physiologic Effects of Wounds. Medical Department, U. S. Army. Washington, D.C., Government Printing Office, 1952.

Bondoc, C. C., Beskid, G., Wolferth, C. C., Jr., Howard, J. M., and O'Malley, J. F.: Cardiovascular and antitoxic effects of aldosterone on cats in endotoxic shock. Surg. Gyn. & Obst. 114:43, 1962.

Bounous, G., Cronin, R. E. P., and Gurd, F. N.: Dietary prevention of experimental shock lesions. A.M.A. Arch. Surg. 94:46, 1967.

Cannon, W. B.: Traumatic Shock. New York and London, D. Appleton & Company, 1923.

Catchpole, B. N., Hackel, D. B., and Simeone, F. A.: Coronary and peripheral blood flow in experimental hemorrhagic hypotension treated with l-nor-epinephrine. Ann. Surg. 142:372, 1955.

Chien, S.: Role of sympathetic nervous system in hemorrhage. Physiol. Rev. 47:214, 1967.

Cooley, J. C., and McIntosh, C. L.: Myocardial contractile force in experimental hemorrhagic shock. Arch. Surg. 87:330, 1963.

Cope, O., and Litwin, M. S.: Contribution of the lymphatic system to the replenishment of the plasma following a hemorrhage. Ann. Surg. 156:655, 1962.

Cowell, E. M.: The initiation of wound shock. J.A.M.A. 70:607, 1918.

Dillon, J., Lynch, L. J., Jr., Myers, R., and Butcher, H. R.: The treatment of hemorrhagic shock. Surg. Gyn. & Obst. 122:967, 1966.

Fine, J.: Endotoxins in traumatic shock. Fed. Proc. Supplement No. 9, 1961, pp. 166-170.

Fine, J., and Seligman, A. M.: Traumatic shock. An experimental study including evidence against the capillary leakage hypothesis. Ann. Surg. 118:238, 1943.

Finnerty, F. A., Jr.: Hemodynamics of angiotensin in man. Circulation 25:255, 1962.

Giannelli, S., Jr., Navarre, J. R., Mahajan, D. R., and Pratt, G. H.: Use of vasopressor agents in hemorrhagic shock. Effect on post-hemorrhagic hemodilution. Ann. Surg. 156:41, 1962.

Grant, R. T., and Reeve, E. B.: Observations on the general effects of injury in man. Medical Research Council, Special Report Series No. 277. London. His Majesty's Stationery Office, 1951.

Guntheroth, W. G., Abel, F. L., and Mullins, G. L.: Blood pressure and cerebral flow in shock: the case against the Trendelenburg position. Circulation 26:725, 1962.

Guthrie, C. J.: On Gunshot Wounds of the Extremities. London, Longman, 1815.

Guyton, A. C., and Crowell, J. W.: Dynamics of the heart in shock. Fed. Proc. Supplement No. 9, 1961, pp. 51-60.

Haddy, F. G., Molnar, J. I., Borden, C. W., and Texter, E. C., Jr.: Comparison of direct effects of angiotensin and other vasoactive agents on small and large blood vessels in several vascular beds. Circulation 25:239, 1962.

Hardaway, R. M., Brune, W. H., Geever, I. F., Burns, J. W., and Mock, H. P.: Studies on the role of intravascular coagulation in irreversible hemorrhagic shock. Ann. Surg. 155:241, 1962.

Hardaway, R. M., James, P. M., Jr., Anderson, R. W.,

Bredenberg, C. E., and West, R. L.: Intensive study and treatment of shock in man. J.A.M.A. *199*:779, 1967.

Henderson, Y.: Acapnia in shock—on carbon dioxide as a factor in the regulation of the heart rate. Am. J. Physiol. *21*:126, 1908.

Henderson, Y., and Haggard, H. W.: Circulation in man in head-down position, and the method for measuring venous return to the heart. J. Pharm. & Exp. Therapy *11*:189, 1918.

Hift, H., and Strawitz, J. G.: Irreversible hemorrhagic shock in dogs: structure and function of liver mitochondria. Am. J. Physiol. *200*:264, 1961.

Hift, H., and Strawitz, J. G.: Irreversible hemorrhagic shock in dogs: problem of onset of irreversibility. Am. J. Physiol. *200*:269, 1961.

Hopkins, R. W., Sabga, G., Bernardo, P., Penn, I., and Simeone, F. A.: Significance of post-traumatic and postoperative oliguria. Arch. Surg. *87*:320, 1963.

Huckabee, W. E.: Relationships of pyruvate and lactate during anaerobic metabolism. I. Effects of infusion of pyruvate on glucose and of hyperventilation. J. Clin. Invest. *37*:244, 1958.

Hume, D.: Discussion of some neurohumoral and endocrine aspects of shock. Fed. Proc. Supplement No. 9, 1961, pp. 87-97.

Hunter, J.: Observations on Certain Parts of the Animal Oeconomy. Philadelphia, Haswell, Barrington & Haswell, 1841.

Keith, N. M.: IX. Blood volume changes in wound shock and primary hemorrhage. Med. Research Committee, Special Report Series No. 27. London, His Majesty's Stationery Office, 1919, pp. 3-16.

Kety, S. S.: Circulation and metabolism of human brain in health and disease. Am. J. Med. *8*:205, 1950.

Lassen, N. A.: Cerebral blood flow and oxygen consumption in man. Physiol. Rev. *39*:183, 1959.

LeDran, H.-F.: A Treatise or Reflections Drawn from Practice on Gunshot Wounds. Printed for John Clarke under the Royal Exchange Cornbill, London, 1743.

Lynn, R. B., Sancetta, S. M., Simeone, F. A., and Scott, R. W.: Observations on the circulation in high spinal anesthesia. Surgery *32*:195, 1952.

MacLean, L. D., Duff, J. H., Scott, H. M., and Peretz, D. I.: Treatment of shock in man based on hemodynamic diagnosis. Surg. Gyn. & Obst. *120*:1, 1965.

Mallory, T. B., Sullivan, E. R. Burnett, C. H., Simeone, F. A., Shapiro, S. L., and Beecher, H. K.: VII. The general pathology of traumatic shock. Surgery *27*:629, 1950.

Marey, E. J.: Physiologie Médicale de la Circulation du Sang. Paris, A. Delahaye, 1863.

Moore, F. D.: Metabolic Care of the Surgical Patient. Philadelphia, W. B. Saunders Company, 1959.

Nadler, S. B., Hidalgo, J. V., and Bloch, T.: Prediction of blood volume in normal human adults. Surgery *51*:224, 1962.

Nickerson, N., and Gourzis, J. T.: Blockade of sympathetic vasoconstriction in the treatment of shock. J. Trauma *2*:399, 1962.

Noble, R. P., and Gregersen, M. I.: Blood volume in clinical shock. I. Mixing time and disappearance rate of T-1824 in normal subjects and in patients in shock; determination of plasma volume in man from 10-minute sample. J. Clin. Invest. *25*:158, 1946.

Parsons, E., and Phemister, D. B.: Haemorrhage and "shock" in traumatized limbs, and experimental study. Surg. Gyn. & Obst. *51*:196, 1930.

Phemister, D. B.: The vascular properties of traumatized and laked bloods and of blood from traumatized limbs. Ann. Surg. *87*:806, 1928.

Roberts, B. E., and Smith, P. H.: Hazards of mannitol infusions. Lancet *2*:421, 1966.

Robertson, O. H., and Bock, A. V.: VI. Memorandum on blood volume after hemorrhage. Special Reports. Medical Research Committee. Series No. 25, His Majesty's Stationery Office, 1918, pp. 213-244.

Rose, J. C., Kot, P. A., Cohn, J. N., Freis, E. D., and Eckert, G. E.: Comparison of effects of angiotensin and norepinephrine on pulmonary circulation, systemic arteries and veins, and systemic vascular capacity in the dog. Circulation 25:247, 1962.

Rosenblueth, A., and Simeone, F. A.: The interrelations of vagal and accelerator effects on the cardiac rate. Am. J. Physiol. *110*:42, 1934.

Rothstein, D. A., Rosen, S., Markowitz, A., and Fuller, J. B.: Ferritin and antiferritin serum treatment of dogs in irreversible hemorrhagic shock. Am. J. Physiol. *198*:844, 1960.

Sapirstein, L. A.: Regional blood flow by fractional distribution of indicators. Am. J. Physiol. *193*:161, 1958.

Schayer, R. W.: Relationship of induced histidine decarboxylase activity and histamine synthesis to shock from stress and from endotoxin. Am. J. Physiol. *198*:1187, 1960.

Schmutzer, K. J., Raschke, E., and Maloney, J. V., Jr.: Intravenous l-norepinephrine as a cause of reduced plasma volume. Ann. Surg. *156*:49, 1962.

Shires, T., Coln, D., Carrico, J., and Lightfoot, S.: Fluid therapy in hemorrhagic shock. A.M.A. Arch. Surg. *88*:688, 1964.

Shoemaker, W. C., Walker, W. F., and Turk, L. M.: The role of the liver in the development of hemorrhagic shock. Surg. Gyn. & Obst. *112*:327, 1961.

Shorr, E., Zweifach, B. W., and Furchgott, R. F.: Hepatorenal factors in circulatory homeostasis. I. On the occurrence, sites, and modes of origin and destruction of principles affecting the compensating vascular mechanism in experimental shock. Science *102*:489, 1945.

Simeone, F. A.: Some issues in the problem of shock. Fed. Proc. Supplement No. 9, 1961, pp. 3-11.

Simeone, F. A.: Shock and blood pressure. Surg. Gyn. & Obst. *108*:740, 1959.

Simeone, F. A., Husni, E. A., and Weidner, M. G., Jr.: The effect of 1-norepinephrine upon the myocardial oxygen tension and survival in acute hemorrhagic hypotension. Surgery *44*:168, 1958.

Simeone, F. A., Mallory, T. B., Burnett, C. H., Shapiro, S. A., Beecher, H. K., Sullivan, E. R., and Smith, L. D.: The crush syndrome in battle casualties. Surgery *27*:300, 1950.

Spink, W. W.: The Dilemma of Bacterial Shock: With Special Reference to Endotoxin Shock. Royal College of Physicians of Edinburgh, Publication No. 29. London, T. and A. Constable, Ltd., 1964.

Spink, W. W., and Vick, J.: Evaluation of plasma, metaraminol, and hydrocortisone in experimental endotoxin shock. Circulat. Res. *9*:184, 1961.

Starling, E. H.: On the absorption of fluids from the connective tissue spaces. J. Physiol. *19*:312, 1896.

Swingle, W. W.: Function of adrenal cortical hormone and cause of death from adrenal insufficiency. Science *77*:58, 1933.

Takaori, M., and Safar, P.: Treatment of massive hemorrhage with colloid and crystalloid solutions. J.A.M.A. *199*:297, 1967.

Teschan, P. E.: Acute renal failure: the cycle of military medical research from combat zone laboratory and return. Milit. Med. *130*:1165, 1965.

Walker, W. F., Zileli, M. S., Reutter, F. W., Shoemaker, W. C., Friend, D., and Moore, F. D.: Adrenal medullary secretion in hemorrhagic shock. Am. J. Physiol. *197*:773, 1959.

Weidner, M. G., and Simeone, F. A.: Physiology of prolonged oligemic hypotension: investigation of pulmonary function. Ann. Surg. *156*:493, 1962.

Wiggers, H. C., Goldberg, H., Roemhild, F., and Ingraham, R. C.: Impending hemorrhagic shock and the course of events following administration of Dibenamine. Circulation *2*:179, 1950.

Williams, J. A., Grable, E., Frank, H. A., and Fine, J.: Blood losses and plasma volume shifts during and following major surgical operations. Ann. Surg. *156*:648, 1962.

Wilson, J. N.: Rational approach to management of clinical shock. A.M.A. Arch. Surg. *91*:92, 1965.

Chapter 9

TRAUMA

by
JOHN F. PERRY, JR., M.D.

JOHN FRANCIS PERRY, JR., is Texan born and educated. He received his post-graduate surgical education at the University of Minnesota, where his major interest was in gastrointestinal physiology. His contributions to the surgical literature reveal his wide interests which have provided him a broad base for his valuable additions to the surgical treatment of trauma. He spends his infrequent free time fishing and camping in the north woods of Minnesota. He is a Professor of Surgery at the University of Minnesota.

Injuries are surpassed only by cardiovascular and malignant diseases as a cause of death in the United States. Among persons one through 34 years of age, accidents are the leading cause of death. More than half of all fatalities in the group between 15 and 24 years of age result from accidents. In this country each year 50 million persons are injured, or approximately one person of four. Forty-five million receive medical care, ten million are bed disabled and two million are hospitalized. In addition to the mortality and morbidity from this cause, trauma is responsible for staggering economic losses because the majority of injured persons are young and in the productive years of life. Injuries cause 500 million days of restricted activity, 130 million days of bed disability and 90 million days lost from work each year in the United States.

Although the treatment of injuries is commonly given little emphasis in the undergraduate medical curriculum, it is a problem which occupies a significant portion of the surgeon's time. Management of the injured patient includes resuscitation, evaluation, initial treatment and priorities for the treatment of specific injuries.

TYPES OF INJURY

Proper treatment of trauma requires a knowledge of types of injury encountered and the agents responsible for wounding. A broad spectrum of bodily damage is produced by numerous physical forces and chemical agents. Trauma includes penetrating and incised wounds, blunt injuries, damage from excessive cold or heat, bites of animals and man and stings of venomous insects and snakes.

Penetrating wounds involve any part of the body and are a result of injury by knife, gunshot or other flying missiles such as shrapnel or glass fragments. Penetrating wounds are also caused by wooden splinters, nails and the countless other common sharp objects encountered in everyday life. The wound of entrance is usually, but not necessarily, small in comparison to the length or depth of the tract through underlying tissues. Wounds with a site of exit of the agent from the body are termed perforating wounds, but such a subclassification of penetrating wounds serves no really useful purpose.

The damage resulting from a penetrating wound depends upon the tissues traversed by the wounding agent and the physical characteristics of the agent itself. In gunshot wounds, the effects produced depend on velocity of the wounding agent and in some instances upon blast effect. The degree of tissue injury by gunshot is a function of kinetic energy of the missile which varies as the square of its velocity ($E = 1/2\ MV^2$). The shock wave generated in tissues by a high velocity rifle slug produces damage which extends well beyond the confines of the tract of the missile itself, and the injury resulting is far greater than that which follows entrance of a low velocity missile of comparable size, weight and composition. Fragments of the missile or bone splinters to which it imparts kinetic energy in its passage through the body become secondary missiles which extend the area of injury. Shotgun wounds suffered at close range show not only the effects of entering pellets but direct damage from the blast effect which propelled them. Wadding may also be carried into the wound by a shotgun blast at close range. Injury caused by a shotgun at longer range is confined to that caused by the pellets themselves. In penetrating wounds caused by knives or other sharp objects which enter the body at low velocity, the damage is confined largely to the tract of the wounding agent. If vital structures are severed, the wound may assume life-threatening proportions.

Incised wounds are produced by sharp objects such as knives or glass which divide the skin and variable amounts of underlying tissue. Damage is confined principally to structures directly in the path of wounding agent, although indirectly other organs or tissues may be affected as a result of neural or vascular injury at the wound site.

Injury caused by blunt trauma may or may not be associated with disruption of the skin. Lacerations or lacerated wounds result from tearing of skin and underlying soft tissues when force is applied by blunt objects. There is usually more damage to adjacent tissues in the lacerated wound than in the case of the incised wound. Contusion, tearing, squeezing, crushing, fracture or bursting of tissue and organs occurs from blunt trauma. Injury may be produced by rapid deceleration of a moving patient who strikes a fixed object, or of a moving object as it strikes the patient. The resultant damage is related to the surface area of the body over which the kinetic energy is dissipated, whether the affected tissues are young or old, tough or friable, healthy or diseased, and the rate at which deceleration occurs. In crushing injuries, which are a specific type of blunt trauma, force is usually applied over a longer period of time than in the case of deceleration injury and the mass of the wounding object is more important than its velocity or rate of deceleration.

Blunt trauma occurs from a variety of causes. Auto occupants involved in traffic accidents and pedestrians struck by moving vehicles account for the largest number of major injuries in this category. Falls from heights, farm and industrial accidents, altercations and motorcycle crashes occur less frequently. Crushing injuries occur in industrial, mining and construction accidents.

Bruises and other minor blunt injuries occur as a result of a variety of accidents at home, in sports, in school and at work.

LOCALIZED VERSUS MORE EXTENSIVE INJURY

Trauma includes minor localized damage associated with slight systemic effects as well as major injuries which result rapidly in death. The first requirement in management of injuries is separation of those patients who need hospital care from patients who require only outpatient treatment. When the history and initial evaluation clearly indicate that the victim has suffered a minor injury localized to an extremity or part of the body, examination and treatment are confined to the involved area. There is usually no need for complete examination of the patient to determine if other injury is present. In such circumstances, the prime consideration is the proper definitive surgical treatment of the injury itself. If systemic treatment is required, it will usually be analgesic or prophylactic in character.

When the history of the accident indicates a more complex situation wherein the victim has or may have suffered one or more injuries, the approach must be totally different. While necessary resuscitation from the systemic effects of trauma is accomplished, examination is carried out to determine the presence and extent of injury of each organ system and part of the body. Because the possible combinations of injuries which can result from major accidents are practically unlimited, a systematic examination is necessary if all trauma is to be recognized. Because the time involved from accident to treatment may be crucial, it is often necessary to accept a much less precise diagnosis than is possible in other disease states. For example, it may be apparent that massive hemorrhage is occurring into the peritoneal or pleural cavity, but the injured organ or organs which are the exact source of such bleeding will be determined only at laparotomy or thoracotomy.

RESUSCITATION

Resuscitation includes those procedures and techniques designed to restore effective pulmonary alveolar ventilation, to restore effective circulating blood volume and blood pressure, and to ameliorate the deleterious effects of injury otherwise.

Major trauma often produces respiratory and cardiovascular derangements of great severity. Under such life-threatening circumstances, pulmonary ventilation which is adequate to supply oxygen needs of the injured patient must be rapidly restored and steps taken to assure effective circulating blood volume. The majority of severely injured patients respond to measures designed to restore cardiovascular and pulmonary function; it is then possible to proceed with the examination to determine extent of trauma. Subsequently, definitive surgical treatment of all injuries can be accomplished. In some circumstances, the restoration of cardiovascular or pulmonary function may be possible only by definitive treatment of the injury itself or of some physiologic derangement which it has produced.

RESTORATION AND STABILIZATION OF CARDIOVASCULAR FUNCTION. Cardiovascular resuscitation has as its goal the restoration of normal circulating blood volume and normal tissue perfusion. The resuscitative measures to be employed depend upon the degree of deterioration of cardiovascular function which has occurred. The injured patient may reach the hospital with normal pulse and blood pressure and good tissue perfusion as evidenced by pink lips, warm skin and clear sensorium. Likewise, he may arrive pulseless and apparently moribund with or without audible heart tones. Intermediate between these extremes, all degrees of compromise of cardiovascular function are seen. It is usually not too difficult to determine that a patient is in poor condition at the time of hospital arrival—the lips are blue, face is pale, extremities are cold and pulse is small. There may be nausea and vomiting, obscured vision and syncope. It is much more difficult to recognize the patient whose condition initially appears good but who is deteriorating rapidly even while the extent of his injuries is being determined.

Profound derangements which are potentially reversible are seen in the apparently moribund patient. If evidence suggests that the patient has been without effective cardiac action for only a few minutes, efforts to restore heart action by external cardiac massage are in order. Simultaneously, endotracheal intubation is carried out, artificial ventilation is begun and the patient is connected to an electrocardiographic monitor.

Intravenous replacement of blood and fluids is begun. If resuscitation is successful under these circumstances, it will soon be apparent. There will be electrocardiographic evidence of return of cardiac activity, either spontaneous beats or vigorous fibrillation which will respond to electric shock. Spontaneous respiration ensues and pupils return from a dilated fixed state to one of constriction. Blood pressure rises and can be sustained by transfusions and fluids. Ultimate salvage of most injured patients arriving in such a moribund state depends upon the length of time that effective cardiac action has been absent and whether the underlying cause can be recognized and corrected without delay. When arrest has been precipitated by anoxia due to inadequate alveolar ventilation, improvement may occur rapidly once the airway is re-established and cardiac resuscitation begun. When arrest has been precipitated by massive hemorrhage and shock, successful resuscitation depends upon whether it is possible to restore and maintain effective circulating blood volume and perfusion of vital organs by transfusion of blood, infusion of fluids and correction of acidosis until definitive surgical treatment can be carried out to arrest the source of hemorrhage. Successful resuscitation also depends in part upon the duration of the state of impaired circulation, whether it is due primarily to anoxia from inadequate ventilation or to blood loss. The anoxia which causes cardiac arrest is also responsible for varying degrees of brain damage. Dilatation of pupils and persistent apnea despite resuscitative efforts indicate increasing cerebral edema and irreversible changes in the brain. Although cardiac action may be transiently restored, patients with such evidences of cerebral damage usually are not retrievable.

The majority of seriously injured patients when first seen are suffering from lesser degrees of cardiovascular collapse. Restoration of cardiovascular function to normal is dependent primarily upon repletion of circulating blood volume by administration of whole blood and fluid. Although balanced salt solution administered intravenously may be adequate replacement when only 10 to 20 per cent of circulating blood volume has been lost, whole blood is essential for resuscitation when there is a volume deficit of 25 to 35 per cent or more.

Blood for typing and crossmatch should be obtained as soon as possible after arrival while intravenous therapy with balanced salt solution is begun. When the response to the infusion of salt solution is favorable, transfusion can be delayed until crossmatched blood is available. If it is apparent that the condition is deteriorating as evidenced by increasing pulse rate and falling blood pressure, type specific blood can be given even while the crossmatch is being carried out. The transfusion of O-negative uncrossmatched blood is not ordinarily recommended. However, there is a group of patients who are essentially moribund on arrival at the emergency room because of blood loss. Internal hemorrhage may be continuing at a rapid rate even while resuscitative efforts are underway. Under these circumstances, transfusion of O-negative, uncrossmatched blood is a life-saving measure until type specific blood is available and while the patient is being prepared for an operation to control hemorrhage.

A large bore polyethylene tubing is placed in an extremity vein for administration of blood, fluids and drugs. At a separate site, a second large bore tubing is placed in another vein and its tip advanced into the superior vena cava for monitoring of central venous pressure. Intravenous catheters should not be introduced in extremities which are the site of fracture or other injury. When there is abdominal injury or severe pelvic fracture, cutdowns should not be placed in the lower extremities because the administered blood or fluids may be lost into retroperitoneal tissue or the peritoneal cavity if injury of iliac veins or vena cava is present.

Restoration of circulating blood volume usually is followed by decrease in the pulse rate, elevation of blood pressure, improvement in color and clearing of sensorium. A rise in central venous pressure usually indicates adequate volume replacement unless cardiac failure is present. Changes in vascular tone, cardiac action and blood volume all influence central venous pressure. When cardiovascular dynamics are stable, central venous pressure reflects changes in blood volume. However, central venous pressure serves only as an index of blood volume relative to cardiovascular capacity. When estimated blood deficits and metabolic derangements incident to shock have been corrected and the arterial blood pressure and central venous pressure remain low, this constitutes presumptive evidence of continuing hemorrhage either into fracture sites, retroperitoneal tissues, peritoneal cavity or pleural cavity. A rapid examination to determine if one of these sites is responsible for the continued hemorrhage is necessary, because definitive surgical treatment may be the only means of controlling blood loss. Low blood pressure is not ordinarily a manifestation of intracranial hemorrhage and occurs with head injury only as a terminal event.

VENTILATION AND RESPIRATION. Injury is associated with increase in tissue oxygen consumption and CO_2 excretion. Although these increases are not large, they occur at a time when the ability to increase pulmonary ventilation may be compromised. Dyspnea, tachycardia, cyanosis and change in mental status may indicate oxygen lack. In other circumstances, tissue needs for oxygen may not be so accurately reflected in symptoms and signs, but from the type of injury present it may be obvious that interference with pulmonary ventilation has occurred.

Effective pulmonary alveolar ventilation depends upon a patent airway from lips or nostrils to the alveoli of the lungs. Obstruction of the airway of the injured patient occurs at several sites and from a number of causes. The supine unconscious patient, or the patient with an unstable fracture of the mandible, develops occlusion of the airway because the tongue falls back into the pharynx. Severe facial injuries may produce such distortion of soft tissue and bone that unaided ventilation is not possible. Blood, mucus, vomitus and foreign bodies such as dentures can occlude the pharynx. Blunt or penetrating injury of the neck ruptures the larynx or trachea with resultant airway occlusion. The trachea and bronchi may also be obstructed by aspirated blood, vomitus or foreign bodies. Rupture of the tracheobronchial tree in the thorax resulting from either blunt or penetrating injury can effectively occlude the airway. Rarely, hemorrhage into the parenchyma of the lung may be extensive, occluding sufficient alveoli so that effective ventilation is not possible.

Thoracic injuries which interfere with the bellows action of the chest also prevent effective alveolar ventilation. Open and closed pneumothorax, hemothorax, ruptured diaphragm with abdominal viscera herniated into pleural cavity, and crushing injuries of chest wall all compromise this function. Although there is no obvious mechanical obstruction to ventilation, it is necessary to establish an airway and provide a high concentration of oxygen for the patient with severe blood loss because pulmonary ventilation is often not adequate under these circumstances.

Restoration of the airway is accomplished by determining the sites of obstruction and relieving them. The airway can be re-established by position, traction on tongue, endotracheal tube or tracheostomy. Oxygen delivered from a gas machine through a mask may be useful to supplement ventilation when the airway is patent but respiratory exchange is not adequate. Lifting the mandible of the unconscious patient forward causes the tongue to be lifted away from the pharynx, allowing air to enter the laryngeal aperture. Grasping the tongue and pulling it forward accomplishes the same purpose. Either of these methods provides an adequate airway if the patient needs only transient help or either technique suffices until more permanent means for securing the airway are available. Blood, mucus, vomitus and foreign bodies are removed from the mouth and pharynx by a finger, gauze sponge, or catheter suction.

Tracheal intubation is the best means to provide an airway for the gravely injured patient on his arrival at the hospital. House officers and practicing physicians who are likely to treat accident victims must be proficient in intubation of the trachea by the oral route using a laryngoscope and endotracheal tube. Passage of an endotracheal tube provides an immediate assured airway through which spontaneous or assisted ventilation can occur. Blood or vomitus can be suctioned or washed from the tracheobronchial tree. The tube can be left in place for hours or days until the need for an artificial airway has passed. If the type of injury dictates that long-term respiratory support will be necessary, tracheostomy is carried out. In unconscious patients, the possibility of cervical spine injury is always present and this injury can be made worse by the manipulation of the head and neck incident to intubation. This possibility must be borne in mind in intubation of the trachea of the unconscious subject.

Tracheostomy is usually not the most rapid emergency means to establish an airway. When indicated, it is much easier to carry out tracheostomy after orotracheal intubation has been accomplished and an airway secured. However, some injuries render the passage of an endotracheal tube virtually impossible and immediate tracheostomy is necessary as a life-saving measure. Patients with head and neck injuries with gross de-formity and hemorrhage, patients with a crushed chest injury or pneumothorax associated with hypoxic agitation, unconscious patients with tightly clenched teeth, and patients with respiratory obstruction from any cause who are awake but unable to cooperate all fall into this category. It is preferable to establish the tracheal stoma at the level of the upper tracheal rings below the isthmus of the thyroid. In extreme emergency, it can be made much more rapidly through the cricothyroid membrane.

Severe upper respiratory tract injury may produce complete or nearly complete airway obstruction and at the same time may make orotracheal intubation impossible. Patients with such airway obstruction who reach a hospital alive are in desperate straits; they are intensely cyanotic and in immediate danger of hypoxic cardiac arrest. In this circumstance, it may be possible to prolong survival long enough for tracheostomy to be carried out by the insufflation of oxygen into the tracheobronchial tree. A large bore (No. 15 to 18) needle inserted through the cricothyroid membrane into the trachea is attached by tubing to an oxygen source. Although oxygen insufflation through such a small aperture will not sustain life for a prolonged period, it may be possible to provide enough oxygen by this route to prevent cardiac arrest or cerebral damage while tracheostomy is accomplished. It should be emphasized that this is only an interim measure which is carried out while a tracheal stoma is being created. It does not substitute for tracheostomy and should not delay its performance.

Establishment of an airway into the upper trachea will not provide alveolar ventilation if trachea and bronchi are occluded by retained secretions, aspirated blood, vomitus or foreign bodies. Tracheobronchial suction with a catheter and suction source can be utilized to remove such foreign matter. When the catheter is introduced through endotracheal tube or tracheostomy, suction is usually adequate to remove most secretions or small amounts of blood. When aspiration of large quantities of blood or vomitus into the tracheobronchial tree has occurred, tracheobronchial lavage is utilized in addition to suction. Increments of 50 ml. of warm physiological saline are instilled into the trachea by endotracheal tube or tracheostomy. Most of this amount will be expelled by cough and the rest is removed immediately by catheter suction. The lungs must be carefully ventilated with

100 per cent oxygen after the suction removal of each increment of instilled saline to prevent hypoxia. If this is carefully done, total volumes of 350 to 500 ml. can be safely utilized in adults for this purpose. In emergency situations in which aspiration of large amounts of blood or vomitus has occurred, tracheobronchial lavage has proved to be a life-saving measure.

The bellows action of the thorax must be restored if it has been compromised by injury. The crushed chest with multiple rib fractures, flail chest, open and closed pneumothorax, massive hemothorax and diaphragmatic rupture with herniated abdominal viscera all interfere with this function. When the integrity of the chest wall has been destroyed by a crushing injury, endotracheal intubation or tracheostomy, combined with manually controlled intermittent positive pressure ventilation with oxygen delivered by gas machine, is necessary to assure an adequate exchange of air. Control of ventilation by this means is one of the first steps in resuscitation of the patient with a severe crush injury of the thorax. Because crushed chest injury usually produces prolonged interference with respiration, a mechanical respirator to provide support on a long-term basis is necessary once definitive treatment of other injuries has been accomplished.

Open chest wounds are covered with a thick layer of sterile vaseline gauze and a dressing. This converts the open pneumothorax into a closed one. Closure of the chest wall defect prevents mediastinal flapping with each respiratory effort and the lung on the uninjured side can once again effectively participate in gas exchange. Ventilation should be aided by oxygen delivered by mask or through an endotracheal tube after the open chest wound has been closed by dressing. Following resuscitation surgical closure of the chest wall defect is required.

The interference with ventilation produced by closed pneumothorax depends upon the degree of pulmonary collapse and pulmonary reserve. The deleterious effects of closed pneumothorax on respiration are much less than are those of an open pneumothorax unless associated with positive pressure in the pleural space. With a lesser degree of collapse there may be few or no symptoms. With greater collapse there may be severe dyspnea and other respiratory symptoms, especially if the pulmonary reserve is limited. Traumatic pneumothorax with few exceptions should be treated by re-expansion of the lung as soon as the pneumothorax is recognized. This is best accomplished by the insertion of a catheter into the pleural space and suction drainage of the pleural cavity thereafter.

Tension pneumothorax interferes not only with gas exchange by the lung on the affected side, but as pressure increases in the one hemithorax, the mediastinum is pushed toward the unaffected side and ventilation of the contralateral lung is compromised as well. As the intrathoracic pressure increases, venous return to the heart is also reduced. The patient with tension pneumothorax presents cyanosis, agitation, extreme air hunger, dyspnea, tachypnea, arterial hypotension and at times impaired cerebration because of hypoxia. The involved side of the chest appears fixed in inspiration and moves poorly with respiration. Resonance over the involved hemithorax is increased and breath sounds decreased, neck veins are distended and the trachea is shifted toward the uninvolved side of the chest. Because this condition poses an immediate threat to life, it must be diagnosed without delay. Thoracentesis utilizing a 50 ml. syringe and large bore needle demonstrates air under pressure in the pleural cavity. As the pleural space is entered, the plunger is driven back by a rush of air into the syringe. The syringe can be removed and the needle taped in place to prevent a reaccumulation of air under positive pressure until closed thoracotomy and placement of a chest tube are accomplished. Usually dramatic improvement follows decompression of tension pneumothorax.

Massive accumulation of blood in the pleural cavity may interfere with ventilation by compression of the lung on the affected side and by shift of the mediastinum to the opposite side. Usually, initially the cardiovascular effects of such massive blood loss overshadow the mechanical interference with ventilation. However, restoration of normal cardiorespiratory dynamics requires both the restoration of blood volume and evacuation of blood from the chest.

Traumatic rupture of the diaphragm may be associated with dislocation of abdominal viscera into the thorax sufficient to produce pulmonary collapse and interference with adequate ventilation. Respiratory support can be provided by oxygen delivered under positive pressure by mask or endotracheal tube but ultimate correction of this problem requires surgical treatment to replace the viscera in the peritoneal cavity and repair the torn diaphragm.

OTHER PROCEDURES. On arrival at the hospital, the seriously injured patient should be transferred to a litter where all necessary treatment is carried out without moving him again until his condition is stabilized. An injured patient whose blood pressure is precariously maintained can become rapidly hypotensive if roughly handled in transportation. Multiple transfers of the injured patient increase shock and blood loss from fracture sites and may be responsible for increasing the degree of injury already present. To avoid these complications, a 3/4-inch plywood litter covered with foam rubber padding and plastic sheeting is utilized for the patient if serious injury is suspected. This litter can be placed on an operating table if surgical treatment is necessary. X-rays can be made without moving the patient by positioning the cassettes under the litter because the litter is radiolucent. The litter can also be placed in a hospital bed if the patient is to be observed.

Obvious external hemorrhage from wounds is controlled by a dressing held in place with elastic bandages or with manual pressure if necessary until the patient can be taken to the operating room. Pressure dressings are much more satisfactory, equally effective and less damaging than attempts to clamp vessels in a bleeding wound in the emergency room. Blind attempts to control bleeding by hemostats applied under such conditions are liable to result both in further injury to the vessels themselves complicating repair and in injury to other vital structures such as nerves. Manual pressure over a dressing held against a wound controls bleeding from almost any site. The tourniquet is probably necessary only for traumatic extremity amputations. When applied at all, the tourniquet is placed just above the amputation site and not removed until the patient is in the operating room prepared for definitive surgical treatment.

The accidental wound, unlike the operative wound, is almost uniformly contaminated. It is imperative that it not be subjected to further contamination and increased risk of infection in the hospital before surgical repair. All external wounds requiring debridement and suture in the operating room are covered by sterile dressings which are not removed until proper light, equipment and anesthesia are available.

Pain, contrary to popular thought, is frequently not a major problem for the patient who has suffered a major injury. Thirst is much more likely to be a complaint than pain. In circumstances such as abdominal injury in which pain may be severe and there may be some delay before surgical treatment, an opiate can be given in small doses intravenously and repeated if necessary. This is to be preferred to administration of narcotics by the subcutaneous or intramuscular route when the drug is likely to be poorly absorbed during the phase of shock and poor tissue perfusion.

Splinting of fractures is an essential part of resuscitation because immobilization decreases both hemorrhage at the fracture site and the injury to soft tissues caused by bone fragments. Splinting should be accomplished in such a manner that the extremity is stabilized but the splinting process itself must not contribute to damage at the fracture site. The fracture is preferably immobilized in the position in which it presented and attempts at manipulation are avoided until proper roentgenograms and other accessories for treatment are available.

Gastric emptying by the normal route does not occur following severe trauma. A gastric tube should be placed and suction employed to empty the stomach. In the unconscious patient whose reflexes do not prevent aspiration into the tracheobronchial tree if vomiting occurs, an endotracheal tube or tracheostomy tube with an inflated rubber cuff should be utilized to protect the respiratory system.

HISTORY OF INJURY

Once the procedure of resuscitation has been set in motion and it is apparent that stabilization of the patient's condition can be achieved, a more detailed history of the injury is obtained from the patient, if possible, or from others present at the time of injury. In the case of penetrating injuries the wounding agent, the time of injury and the position of the patient at the time that injury occurred are determined. The latter may indicate the course of the penetrating wound and the organs or body cavities which may have been injured. The composition of the last meal eaten before injury and the time it was eaten are recorded.

Following blunt trauma knowledge of recent intake of food, time of injury and mechanism of injury are likewise sought. The latter is especially important because it may give some clue to the injuries which may be present. Despite the infinite numbers of combinations of blunt injuries which can and do occur, certain multiple injury patterns are more likely to occur with one type of blunt trauma than with others. Pedestrians struck by moving vehicles are more likely to have certain fractures and soft tissue injuries than are persons who are riding in automobiles at the time of accident or persons who are injured by falling. These latter in turn often show characteristic injury patterns also. It must be emphasized, however, that knowledge of such patterns of injury is of help only in that it suggests that specific injuries may have occurred; it in no way excludes the possibility that other, less characteristic damage may be present.

The history of alcohol ingestion is important not only in interpretation of changes in sensorium but also because acute and chronic alcohol ingestion is associated with special problems in the injured patient. Acute intoxication renders both the experimental animal and man more liable to profound hypotension and shock from trauma and blood loss. There is also an increased risk for anesthesia and surgical procedures with acute intoxication. Chronic alcoholic intake produces nutritional deficits, liver damage and central nervous system changes which likewise compromise the injured patient's chances for recovery from a given injury. Knowledge of chronic ingestion of alcohol also helps in interpretation of changes in mental status during the injured patient's hospital course.

History should include a search for other diseases. Pulmonary emphysema, epilepsy, cardiac disease, hypertension, endocrine derangements, steroid therapy and diabetes all require special consideration in the injured patient. A history of allergy to drugs or medications is important. It is important to discover which medications are being taken by the trauma victim because failure to provide them may prove deleterious or even fatal.

As soon as possible, a record should be started including the patient's name, if known, his history of injury with as much detail as is practicable, a statement of his condition on admission and a record of vital signs including pulse, respiration, blood pressure and temperature. Mental status should be evaluated as accurately as possible because subsequent changes are of importance in diagnosis of intracranial hemorrhage. The state of consciousness immediately following the injury is recorded, if known, as well as that upon arrival at the hospital. The patient's complaints of pain, loss of function, thirst, nausea or other symptoms are recorded also.

EXAMINATION

Because one or more major injuries has occurred or is likely, it is necessary that a systematic physical examination be carried out as in other disease states. Although the signs and manifestations of injury are distinct, the approach in physical diagnosis is different only in that there is a greater degree of urgency. Obviously, there are injuries of such life-threatening proportions that patients must be subjected to major surgical procedures for their correction with only a fragmentary history and limited examination being carried out beforehand. A wound of the heart or one of the great vessels with profound shock and massive hemothorax creates such a situation. Thoracotomy for suture of the bleeding vessel or heart as soon as the intrathoracic bleeding has been recognized is mandatory. A concomitant pelvic fracture, or even an abdominal injury of less threatening proportions, might not be diagnosed until after such a procedure had been accomplished. If such a therapeutic procedure is necessary as an immediate life-saving measure, the examination for other injury then proceeds in orderly fashion as soon as this problem has been solved.

An obvious injury with little immediate life-threatening potential must not absorb the attention and energy of the attending physicians while other more serious but less obvious injury is ignored. A patient with an open fracture of the femur with protrusion of bone and gross deformity of the extremity and a crushed thorax with an unstable segment of chest wall is not in immediate danger of losing his life from the lower extremity injury. To treat the open fracture of the femur before establishment of adequate pulmonary ventilation by endotracheal tube or tracheostomy and manually controlled positive pressure ventilation is to risk death from hypoxia and pulmonary edema. Resuscitation and examination of the injured patient proceed hand in hand and there is no clear-cut end of the one phase and beginning of the other. Urgency may demand that either be replaced by a definitive therapeutic maneuver. Nevertheless, the ultimate aim remains the same: to assure that no injuries are overlooked. Complete examination cannot be accomplished unless the patient's clothing is completely removed. This must be done by cutting the clothes away if necessary.

HEAD AND FACIAL INJURIES. Examination of the head includes an inspection of the scalp for lacerations and hematomas. Palpation of the scalp aids in locating such lesions if the patient has a thick growth of hair on the head. The amount of blood loss from scalp lacerations can be large and should be noted. The face is examined for lacerations, contusions and evidences of asymmetry. Pain, swelling, change in vision and alteration of bite or jaw function also suggest facial injury. Palpation may reveal depressions of areas of facial skeleton, the result of fractures. Facial lacerations often bleed profusely initially but bleeding is usually easily controlled by pressure. With facial lacerations, the integrity of the facial nerve and Stensen's duct must be determined. The eyes are examined to determine if there are evidences of laceration or other injury of cornea, conjunctiva or sclera. Subconjunctival or palpebral hemorrhage may indicate basilar fracture of the anterior cranial fossa. Pupillary size and reaction to light are noted and any deviations suggesting cranial nerve palsies are sought. If the patient is conscious, it is possible to determine extraoccular motion. Blood in the anterior chamber may be seen. Funduscopic examination is carried out if there is head injury or injury to the eye itself.

The nose is inspected for deformity and patency of the air passages. Bleeding from the nose or cerebrospinal rhinorrhea may occur, the latter indicating a fracture through the cribriform plate. The external ears are examined for lacerations. Blood behind the tympanic membrane or blood and cerebrospinal fluid draining from the external auditory meatus are evidences of basilar skull fracture. A hematoma or hemorrhage beneath the skin overlying the mastoid process also indicates such a fracture.

Head injury may or may not be associated with signs of injury to the brain. A decrease in or progressive worsening of the level of consciousness, focal neurological deficits, decerebration, dilatation of the pupils and respiratory irregularities indicate injury to the nervous system.

INJURIES OF THE CERVICAL REGION. In the conscious patient who has suffered nonpenetrating trauma of severe degree, evaluation of the neck includes a search for tenderness, guarding or pain on motion which suggest fractures or dislocation of the cervical spine. If there is neck pain or limitation of motion, the head and neck are immobilized with sandbags until roentgenograms of the cervical spine have been obtained to rule out or confirm existence of cervical fracture or dislocation. When cervical spine injury is suspected, a neurological evaluation is carried out before x-rays are made. The neck is protected from motion and cervical spine films are made in all unconscious patients to rule out cerebral spine injury. Fracture of the odontoid process of the second cervical vertebra and other cervical fractures occur fairly commonly in association with head injuries. This is especially true in children.

Cervical subcutaneous emphysema may indicate rupture of the respiratory tract or alimentary canal in the neck or in the mediastinum. Distended neck veins occur with both pericardial tamponade and tension pneumothorax. Penetrating wounds of the neck are injuries of great potential seriousness. Such wounds may or may not be associated with significant hematomas or other abnormalities. The absence of hematoma, pain on swallowing, subcutaneous emphysema, tenderness or swelling does not rule out major injury to vascular, respiratory or alimentary structures in penetrating cervical wounds or following blunt trauma to the neck.

CHEST INJURIES. Signs and symptoms which may be indicative of thoracic injury include subcutaneous emphysema over the chest wall, dyspnea, tachypnea, decreased movement of the hemithorax with respiration, paradoxical motion of a segment of chest wall, bloody sputum, tracheal displacement and venous distention. Chest injury may also be suspected from the location of a penetrating wound or when otherwise unexplained hemorrhagic shock is present.

The thorax is involved in both penetrating and nonpenetrating injury. Penetrating chest injuries vary from simple wounds to those which involve loss of extensive areas of the chest wall. Penetrating injury may result in a sucking chest wound with consequent open pneumothorax and its deleterious effects. Such injuries are more likely to be encountered in war. In civilian chest wounds, the wounds of entrance and exit, if present, are likely to be small and most of the derangements produced are from injury to the intra-thoracic viscera.

Hemothorax, pneumothorax or a combination of the two occurs following both penetrating and blunt chest trauma. Pneumothorax may be manifest by subcutaneous emphysema over the thoracic wall, increased resonance and decreased or absent breath sounds on the side of injury. Hemothorax can be diagnosed if signs of fluid in the pleural cavity are elicited by examination of the chest. Because the severely injured patient is usually lying supine, blood in the posterior gutter may not be readily apparent from the limited physical examination which can be conducted with the patient in this position. In the supine subject, decreased breath sounds over the posterior chest wall may suggest intrathoracic bleeding. Radiographic examination is the most accurate method for documenting air or blood in the pleural cavity when there is no great urgency. However, if massive bleeding into the chest is suspected as the cause of arterial hypotension which is unresponsive to blood replacement, diagnostic thoracentesis can be employed to demonstrate blood in the pleural cavity.

Penetrating wounds which enter the mediastinum may produce hemorrhage of alarming proportions when the heart or great vessels of the thorax are injured. If free bleeding into the pleural cavity occurs, the systemic manifestations are those of massive hemorrhage and hemothorax will be present. The important diagnostic consideration is recognition that the hemorrhagic shock is caused by blood loss into the pleural cavity. If hemorrhage into the mediastinum is impeded from free rupture into the pleural cavity, signs of blood loss may be less apparent and the first indication of great vessel damage will be a widened, indistinct mediastinal shadow apparent in the chest radiograph. Free bleeding into the pericardial sac produces pericardial tamponade and the consequent interference with cardiac function; distended neck veins, distant heart sounds, reduced blood pressure and pulse pressure and paradoxical pulse result from pericardial tamponade. Pericardiocentesis is both diagnostic and in some patients therapeutic in this condition.

Blunt trauma produces damage to the chest wall and any of the thoracic viscera. Rib fracture or costochondral separation results in pain at the site of injury which is accentuated by breathing, coughing or motion. There is point tenderness and often crepitus over the fracture site. Sternal fracture is also charac-terized by tenderness and crepitus on palpation over the fracture site. Multiple rib fractures lead to decrease in respiratory movements on the involved side of the chest because of pain. If several ribs are each fractured in two locations, a segment of chest wall may become unstable and demonstrate paradoxical motion with respiration. Paradoxical motion is usually apparent on inspection of the chest.

Blunt chest injuries and occasionally penetrating wounds lacerate the diaphragm and extrusion of abdominal viscera into the pleural cavity occurs. This condition is seen more commonly on the left than on the right and is usually the result of severe blunt trauma such as traffic accidents. Patients with this injury commonly have multiple other severe injuries and the diaphragmatic rupture is often overlooked. The presence of abdominal viscera in the thorax not only interferes with the function of the lung on the involved side but the blood supply to the herniated abdominal viscera may be severely compromised. Although the condition may be suspected from physical examination, if breath sounds are decreased or absent and intestinal borborygmi are heard instead on the involved side, the diagnosis primarily depends on an awareness of this possibility and appropriate x-ray study of the chest and abdomen.

ABDOMINAL INJURIES. Penetrating wounds of the trunk which enter the peritoneal cavity can produce injury to any of the abdominal viscera. Thus, not only wounds of the anterior abdominal wall but also those of the lower thorax, lumbar areas, groin, perineum and buttocks may have entered the abdominal cavity. This is especially true when the wound has been produced by gunshot, but wounds from knives and other penetrating objects can enter the abdominal cavity by unusual routes as well. Abdominal visceral injury will not be overlooked in penetrating abdominal trauma if abdominal exploration is carried out when entrance of the wounding object into the abdomen is suspected from its path or if signs and symptoms of peritoneal irritation are present.

Blunt abdominal trauma poses more difficult diagnostic problems. If the patient is alert and not otherwise injured, the diagnosis of intraperitoneal hemorrhage or intraperitoneal spillage of intestinal content is not too difficult because signs of blood loss and peritoneal irritation are present. Abdominal pain, tenderness, rebound tenderness and rigidity occur with blood or intestinal contents in the peritoneal cavity. Thus, the diagnosis of visceral injury is usually possible on the basis of physical signs with isolated abdominal trauma. However, even under optimal circumstances the signs are not always reliable and bleeding or intestinal perforation may go undetected. This is especially true if bleeding is small in amount or if secretions or intestinal contents do not leak into the general peritoneal cavity. With pancreatic injuries, there may be bleeding and leakage of pancreatic secretions into the lesser bursa only. Retroperitoneal rupture of the duodenum is not associated with general peritoneal contamination. Both these injuries are diagnosed with difficulty because signs of peritoneal irritation are often not impressive.

The situation becomes even less clear in the patient who has suffered multiple injuries or who is unconscious from a head injury. Not only are signs and symptoms of abdominal injury obscured but other injuries can mimic abdominal injury. Acute gastric dilatation, the result of air swallowing in children, may lead to abdominal tenderness, pain, distention and even rigidity, suggesting abdominal visceral injury when none in fact is present. Passage of a nasogastric tube relieves gastric distention and symptoms disappear. Fractures of the lower ribs often cause rigidity of upper abdominal muscles which lasts for several hours. Contusion of the abdominal wall sometimes causes pain and tenderness when no underlying visceral injury is present.

In the unconscious patient, the signs of peritoneal irritation cannot be elicited and it may be extremely difficult to determine if visceral rupture or intraperitoneal hemorrhage has occurred. Rigidity of abdominal musculature may be present but there often is reluctance to explore the abdomen of an extremely ill patient on the basis of this sign alone. It is not surprising, therefore, that undiagnosed abdominal visceral injury is not infrequently the cause of death of unconscious patients or patients with multiple injuries.

Because of the inability to rely on symptoms and physical findings in patients with blunt trauma, other means of supporting a diagnosis of visceral injury have been utilized with varying degrees of success. Hemoglobin levels in peripheral blood, if reduced, are suggestive of hemorrhage. If bleeding occurs rapidly, dilution will not have had time to occur and hemoglobin levels will be within the normal range even in the presence of profound shock. Leukocytosis with levels above 15,000 white blood cells per cubic millimeter also is suggestive of visceral injury or intraperitoneal hemorrhage. Other injuries may produce leukocytosis, however, and visceral injuries do occur without elevation of the leukocyte count. Hemoglobin levels and white cell counts cannot therefore be relied upon for the diagnosis of visceral injury.

Diagnostic peritoneal tap can be utilized in patients with blunt trauma in whom abdominal visceral injury is suspected. An 18-gauge needle attached to 20-ml. syringe is used to explore the peritoneal cavity by puncture of each of the four quadrants of the abdomen or the flanks. Recovery of at least 0.1 ml. of nonclotting blood is evidence of a positive tap. Recovery of blood which clots in the syringe is presumed evidence that a mesenteric vessel has been entered with the needle. The technique is innocuous because puncture of the bowel with an 18-gauge needle leads to no significant spillage. Success rates of 85 to 95 per cent are reported with this method. The chief drawback to the peritoneal tap is that failure to recover nonclotting blood from the peritoneal cavity does not exclude visceral injury. Taps can be repeated at intervals of a few hours if the diagnosis remains in doubt.

Diagnostic peritoneal lavage is a test designed to extend the sensitivity of peritoneal tap. Under local infiltration anesthesia, a small incision is made just below the umbilicus in the midline and a small catheter with multiple side holes is introduced into the peritoneal cavity. Peritoneal dialysis catheters work well for this purpose. If gross blood returns through the catheter, the diagnosis of intraperitoneal hemorrhage is confirmed. If not, in adults 1 liter of balanced salt solution is introduced into the peritoneal cavity and the fluid is then withdrawn. Smaller volumes are used in children. Return of grossly bloody fluid or fluid containing particulate matter comparable to intestinal content constitutes a positive tap. If the fluid is grossly clear or only pink in color, it is analyzed for amylase content and white blood cells. High white blood cell counts or high amylase levels indicate visceral injury. Diagnostic peritoneal lavage has proved very accurate for recognizing abdominal visceral injury in patients in whom the diagnosis is obscured by multiple injuries or head injury with coma.

INJURIES OF THE GENITOURINARY TRACT. Although genitourinary injury is suspected from the type and location of other injuries and from symptoms and signs, more precise diagnosis is dependent upon radiographic examination. Renal injury is suspected if there is injury to the lumbar area, abdomen or lower chest with pain and hematuria. A mass in the flank owing to retroperitoneal hemorrhage from renal injury occurs but is uncommon. Bladder injury is suspected with hematuria, inability to void and especially with pelvic fractures. Recovery of grossly clear urine from the bladder does not rule out rupture of the bladder. Rupture of the urethra is suspected in perineal injuries and pelvic fractures if the patient cannot void and a catheter cannot be passed into the bladder. Intravenous pyelography, cystography and urethrography are utilized for more specific delineation of the injury.

INJURIES OF THE PELVIS AND SPINE. Fractures of the pelvis usually produce major disability. Careful compression over the crests of the ilium, pubic rami, ischia and sacrum demonstrates tenderness and suspected fractures. Displaced pelvic fractures can be associated with massive blood loss into retroperitoneal tissues or the peritoneal cavity and hemorrhagic shock may result.

Fractures or dislocation of the bony spine may or may not involve the spinal cord. Pain in the back suggests the possibility of spinal injury. The neck and back are palpated to seek areas of tenderness or deformity. This can be done in the supine patient by slipping the examiner's hand under the patient's back. A neurological evaluation for symptoms of numbness, tingling and loss of function of extremities, signs of motor or sensory loss, and change in reflexes is carried out as soon as possible. This provides a baseline for comparison in subsequent examinations, because changes in neurological status may influence treatment of spinal cord injuries.

INJURIES OF THE EXTREMITIES. Examination of the extremities provides information regarding damage to the nervous system as well as injury of the extremities themselves. Lacerations, penetrating wounds, loss of function and deformity are sought. Fractures are suggested by swelling, shortening, angulation, crepitation or false motion of the extremity. Dislocations are suggested by gross deformity at articulations. Closed fractures are covered at least by intact skin; in open fractures the fracture hematoma is in communication with the external environment. Innervation and circulatory status are evaluated in all fractures and dislocations of ex-

tremities. Radiographs are necessary to delineate the extent and character of bony injuries.

Penetrating wounds of the extremity often produce more injury than is apparent on physical examination. Peripheral pulses, sensation, motor function and skin temperature distal to the injury may give some indication of involvement of neurovascular bundles by penetrating wounds. A hematoma may indicate major blood vessel damage but its absence does not exclude such injury. Palpable pulses distal to penetrating wounds likewise do not exclude vascular injury. Lacerated or incised wounds or wounds complicating fractures of extremities are covered with sterile dressings and not explored to determine extent of injury until definitive treatment in the operating room is carried out.

RADIOGRAPHIC EXAMINATION OF THE INJURED PATIENT

X-ray studies provide information of much value in assessment of some injuries. The urgency to obtain radiographic studies in a particular injury depends upon the information to be gained thereby, how it will influence the treatment, and the priority for treatment of the injury.

Skull x-rays are primarily useful to demonstrate fractures of the cranium. It is to be emphasized, however, that the decision for or against surgical treatment of a head injury, with the exception of depressed skull fractures, is not usually made on the basis of findings in plain radiographs of the skull. Although skull x-rays are an important part of the diagnostic evaluation of an injured patient, they should be made when the patient is in condition to tolerate the examination, because depressed skull fractures, unless associated with open scalp lacerations, are usually not high priority emergencies.

X-rays of facial bones are necessary for proper delineation of the extent and character of bony injury. Because these injuries usually are not life-threatening, they are treated only after more serious damage has been repaired. Radiographs to demonstrate fractures of the facial skeleton are obtained only after all injuries which pose any threat to life have been adequately treated.

X-rays of the spine are necessary to determine if bony injury has occurred and what type of definitive treatment will be employed. Patients with symptoms or physical findings suggesting injury to the bony spine or spinal cord should, therefore, have radiographs of the spine as soon as resuscitation has been carried out and cardiorespiratory stability achieved. The patient is moved only with a physician in attendance until it has been determined whether or not a fracture or dislocation of the spine exists. All patients who are unconscious from head injury should have x-rays of the cervical spine to rule out fractures and dislocations.

X-rays of the chest provide a great amount of information of importance in diagnosis of both thoracic and abdominal injury. Upright chest films or lateral decubitus views are of most value in delineating blood or fluid in the chest. Total opacification of one side of the chest with mediastinal shift indicates a massive hemothorax. Pneumothorax will also be more likely to be apparent on these views than on films taken with the patient supine. Mediastinal shift associated with air in the pleural cavity and collapse of the lung indicates a tension pneumothorax. Subcutaneous emphysema usually is caused by a laceration of lung; an associated pneumothorax is usually present. Mediastinal air apparent soon after injury may arise from injury to the intrathoracic trachea, bronchus or esophagus. Widening of the mediastinum is caused by hemorrhage contained in the mediastinum by the pleura and indicates great vessel injury. Rib fractures are indications of injury to the chest itself and the location of fractures may lead one to suspect other injury. Lower rib fractures on the left are commonly associated with a ruptured spleen. On the right, lower rib fractures may be associated with rupture of the liver. A globular, gas-filled structure in the lower thorax may be mistaken for eventration of the diaphragm or a high paralyzed diaphragm with gas-filled viscera lying beneath it. Following a major injury, this appearance is usually caused by gas-filled abdominal viscera which have herniated through a ruptured diaphragm and are actually lying above the diaphragm within the pleural cavity. Fractures or dislocations of the thoracic spine may be visible in the chest film. Chest x-rays are usually obtained as soon as cardiorespiratory stability has been achieved if chest injury is suspected. Massive hemothorax, tension pneumothorax and pericardial tamponade may have to be diagnosed and treated on the basis of clinical signs alone and without the benefit of radiographic examination.

Abdominal x-rays provide a few clues to visceral injury. The abdominal radiograph is much less likely to be of help than is the chest film in deciding if an injury has occurred. In most abdominal injuries, films of the abdomen are not the factor in deciding upon abdominal exploration. Free intraperitoneal air demonstrated by upright or lateral decubitus x-rays is evidence of possible perforation of abdominal hollow viscera in penetrating wounds and absolute evidence of such injury following blunt trauma to the abdomen. Air outlining the right kidney and bubbles of air in the region of the descending duodenum indicate retroperitoneal rupture of the duodenum. A ground-glass appearance on the abdominal radiograph with obliteration of the psoas and renal shadows occurs with massive retroperitoneal or intraperitoneal hemorrhage. Intraperitoneal exudate secondary to peritonitis following injury may also produce this appearance. Injury to bony structures may also be apparent on the abdominal films and may suggest visceral injury. Fractures of the spine may be seen and fractures of transverse processes lead one to suspect renal injury. Pelvic fractures are visible on the abdominal film. Pelvic fracture suggests that bladder rupture, laceration of iliac vessels and, less frequently, injury to mesentery and small bowel may have occurred.

The extent of genitourinary injury is determined primarily by contrast medium when renal rupture involves the calyceal system or if ureteral injury is present. Failure to visualize a functioning kidney on the side of injury suggests possible renal pedicle injury. The delineation of the functioning kidney on the opposite side is important when contralateral renal injury is present. Cystograms properly performed demonstrate both intraperitoneal and extraperitoneal rupture of the bladder. A urethrogram shows extravasation of contrast medium when urethral rupture has occurred.

X-ray of the extremities is principally of value to demonstrate the extent and character of injury to bones and joints.

Radiopaque foreign bodies are demonstrable by radiographs of any part of the body. The path of a missile can be deduced from the location of the wound of entrance and the location of the missile. This information may suggest unsuspected visceral or other injury.

PRIORITY FOR SURGICAL TREATMENT
OF INJURIES

When a patient has more than a single injury, the priority for surgical treatment of each injury is determined by the rapidity with which it compromises his chances for survival. An old adage of trauma surgery is that life comes first, then limb. Thus, it is necessary to delay for a while the surgical treatment of some injuries which, though severe, pose no immediate threat to life if other conditions are present which, left untreated, will rapidly cause death.

An immediate operation is required when the deleterious effects leading to death can be reversed only by surgical treatment. Injuries requiring immediate operation are in three groups:

Rapid external or internal bleeding which leads to progressively more severe hypovolemic shock despite nonoperative resuscitative measures and the rapid replacement of blood volume.

Intra-abdominal hemorrhage caused by hepatic rupture, vena caval laceration, mesenteric vascular injury or, rarely, extensive pelvic fracture may produce these clinical symptoms. Intrapleural bleeding requires immediate thoractomy in a few patients. Usually, hemorrhage in these circumstances is caused by injury of the heart or one of the great vessels. Rarely, extensive external wounds, or wounds with major vessel injury, may fall into this category if bleeding cannot be controlled by nonoperative measures.

Airway obstruction which cannot be relieved by endotracheal intubation.

This may occur with maxillofacial injuries, cervical trauma and occasionally with chest injuries. Tracheostomy is the surgical treatment usually required.

Rapidly expanding intracranial hematomas which may require immediate decompression for survival. If such intracranial bleeding occurs at the same time as life-threatening hemorrhage into one of the body cavities, the two conditions may require surgical correction simultaneously.

Urgent surgical treatment is required when initial stabilization of cardiorespiratory function has been achieved by resuscitative measures but the injury continues to produce derangements which will lead to death or ultimate severe disability. Included in this category are most abdominal injuries with moderate to severe intraperitoneal hemor-

rhage, most renal pedicle injuries, abdominal trauma with peritoneal soiling from the intraperitoneal rupture of gastrointestinal tract or genitourinary system, continued intrathoracic hemorrhage requiring transfusion to keep up with significant blood loss through chest tubes, external wounds when severe hemorrhage has initially been controlled by pressure bandages, most vascular injuries of the extremities and most brain and spinal cord injuries.

Less urgent are injuries of the bladder and urethra without intraperitoneal contamination, extensive soft tissue wounds, open fractures and most eye injuries.

Least urgent are maxillofacial injuries, closed fractures and external wounds not associated with severe hemorrhage.

Emergency services of hospitals which handle more than an occasional accident victim must be organized to carry out the resuscitation, examination and surgical treatment of the injured patient without delay or confusion. The treatment of trauma requires a team approach by surgical specialists because multiple organ systems are often involved. However, there must always be one surgeon who has overall responsibility for the patient. Most often this will be the general surgeon who is charged initially with resuscitation and examination of the injured subject. He is responsible for surgical treatment of those injuries which fall within his domain and coordinates with the neurosurgeon, urologist, orthopedist, otolaryngologist and ophthalmologist the treatment of the specific injuries for which each is responsible.

The emergency facility must be established in such a manner that the patient with major injury is not taken care of in the same geographic area as those patients who require only outpatient treatment. The confusion, traffic and generally contaminated environment of a busy emergency room are far from ideal circumstances for the initial handling of severely injured persons. In some hospitals, this problem has been solved by the policy that all patients who may be severely injured are taken directly to the operating suite for resuscitation. This policy has many advantages. The emergency room is relieved of a responsibility which could absorb the energies of most of its personnel for a prolonged period, totally disrupting its normal operations. The injured patient can be observed under optimal circumstances in the operating room and if a surgical procedure is necessary, it can be accomplished without delay. If operation is not necessary, the patient can be taken to a ward for further observation and care as soon as his condition is stable. This is probably the best method for handling victims of major accidents.

READING REFERENCES

Altemeier, W. A., and Wulsin, J. H.: Antimicrobial therapy in injured patients. J.A.M.A. *173*:527, 1960.

Clark, K.: The incidence and mechanisms of shock in head injury. South M. J. *55*:513, 1962.

Conn, J. H., Hardy, J. D., Fain, W. R., and Netterville, R. E.: Thoracic trauma. Analysis of 1022 cases. J. Trauma *3*:22, 1963.

Crenshaw, C. A., Canizaro, P. C., Shires, G. T., and Allsman, A.: Changes in extracellular fluid during acute hemorrhagic shock in man. Surg. Forum *13*:6, 1962.

Dzieman, A. J., Mendelson, J. A., and Lindsey, D.: Comparison of the wounding characteristics of some commonly encountered bullets. J. Trauma *1*:341, 1961.

Fogelman, M. J., and Stewart, R. D.: Penetrating wounds of the neck. Am. J. Surg. *91*:581, 1956.

Gettler, D. T., and Allbritten, F. F., Jr.: Effect of alcohol intoxication on the respiratory exchange and mortality rate associated with acute hemorrhage in anesthetized dogs. Ann. Surg. *158*:151, 1963.

Injury Control Program—Epidemiology and Surveillance. United States Public Health Service, January 1967 statistics.

Jacoby, J. J., Hamelberg, W., Ziegler, C. H., Flory, F. A., and Jones, J. R.: Transtracheal resuscitation. J.A.M.A. *162*:625, 1956.

Kinney, J. M., and Wells, R. E., Jr.: Problems of ventilation after injury and shock. J. Trauma *2*:370, 1962.

Lumpkin, M. B., Logan, W. D., Couves, C. M., and Howard, J. M.: Arteriography as an aid in the diagnosis and localization of acute arterial injuries. Ann. Surg. *147*:353, 1958.

McLaurin, R. L., and Ford, L. E.: Extradural hematoma. Statistical survey of forty-seven cases. J. Neurosurg. *21*:364, 1964.

McLaurin, R. L., and Tutor, F. T.: Acute subdural hematoma. Review of ninety cases. J. Neurosurg. *18*:61, 1961.

Murphy, J. J., Iozzi, L., and Schoenberg, H. W.: Principles of management of renal trauma. J. Trauma *2*:327, 1962.

Nahum, A. M.: Early Management of Acute Trauma. St. Louis, C. V. Mosby Company, 1966.

Noer, R. J.: Emergency care of critically injured. J. Trauma *3*:331, 1963.

Raaf, J.: Treatment of the patient with acute head injury. J. Trauma *4*:168, 1964.

Reed, C. R. W.: Trauma to the pelvis and hip. Arch. Surg. *75*:736, 1957.

Root, H. D., Hauser, C. W., McKinley, C. R., LaFave, J. W., and Mendiola, R.: Diagnostic peritoneal lavage. Surgery *57*:633, 1965.

Schramel, R. J., Tyler, J., Kilpatrick, J. L., Ziskind, M. M., and Creech, O., Jr.: Studies of respiratory function after thoracic injuries. J. Trauma *3*:206, 1963.

Shires, G. T.: Care of the Trauma Patient. New York, McGraw-Hill Book Company, 1966.

Simenstad, J. O., Galway, C. F., and MacLean, L. D.: The treatment of aspiration and atelectasis by tracheobronchial lavage. Surg. Gyn. & Obst. *115*:721, 1962.

Teabeaut, J. R.: Aspiration of gastric contents. An experimental study. Am. J. Path. 28:51, 1952.

Vandenbas, K. Q.: Wound shock and debridement. Arch. Surg. 75:707, 1957.

Wilson, J. N., Grow, J. B., Demong, C. V., Prevedel, A. E., and Owens, J. C.: Central venous pressure in optimal blood volume maintenance. Arch. Surg. *85*:563, 1962.

Chapter 10

THERMAL AND RADIATION INJURIES

by
CURTIS P. ARTZ, M.D.

CURTIS PRICE ARTZ was reared in a farming community near Jerome, Ohio and received his undergraduate and medical education at Ohio State University, to which he returned for his surgical education and training. Dr. Artz practiced medicine in West Virginia for four years and then entered the army medical service. At the Brooke Army Medical Center, where he served as Director of the United States Army Surgical Research Unit, he began fundamental investigations on the systemic response to burns and their management. As Director of the United States Army Surgical Research Team in Korea, he pursued other surgical scientific investigations. Dr. Artz is Professor of Surgery and Chairman of the Department at the Medical College of South Carolina.

BURNS

The clinician faced with a severely burned patient should have an understanding of the current information concerning pathophysiology of the burn injury to make necessary day-to-day decisions concerning treatment. No two burned patients are alike. A burn may vary from a very minor first-degree wound to the most severe form of injury to which man is liable. The significant burn evokes a myriad of systemic responses. The magnitude of the injury determines the extent of the physiologic changes. Unlike other wounds that can usually be closed either immediately or in a few days, the deep burn requires time for removal of the dead eschar before closure. The persistence of this dead tissue furthers the injury and additional systemic derangements occur.

The variety of recommendations for treatment make it clear that there is still no single best treatment for burns. To make the maximal use of modern materials and techniques, the surgeon must be able to choose a method of management which is most suitable under the particular circumstances for each individual patient. The care of all phases of an extensive burn injury taxes the skill and knowledge of the surgeon to the utmost. The difference between success and failure may depend as much upon minute details as it does upon the execution of major operative procedures.

In general, there is no injury that is treated less expertly by the medical profession at large than a burn. Attention to the numerous details so necessary in ideal burn care is often not appreciated by the physician, nor does he always have the time or team of assistants to execute them. Progress in burn therapy during the past 20 years has been slow but steady.

Burns are an ever present problem. An extensive burn is a catastrophic illness—catastrophic in the overwhelming insult to the patient, catastrophic in its psychologic aspects and catastrophic in cost and suffering to the family involved. Data from the National Health Survey for the years 1957 to 1961 show that the average number of burn injuries annually is 1,973,000. Of these 937,000 are activity-restricting injuries and 268,000 are classed as bed-disabling injuries. Each year in the United States about 7.5 persons per 1000 population are injured by coming in contact with hot objects or open flames. More than 7000 deaths annually in the United States are due to accidents caused by fire and explosion.

Moyer states that in the year 1940, accidents destroyed 17.04 years of human life for every 1000 inhabitants in the United States. Cancer was less destructive; it took 15.5 years of life per 1000 persons during the same year. The total working years of life lost to accidents during 1940 was 1,769,000 years, and thermal injuries accounted for 7.7 per cent of this loss or 135,000 working years. Nearly 6000 hospital beds are occupied the year around by burned patients.

From the foregoing statistics, it is obvious that burns are a major disease entity in the United States. Although the number of deaths is small in comparison to the number caused by the great killers heart disease, cancer and stroke, the number of working years lost is appreciable because of the younger age group in which burns take their toll.

HISTORY. Interest in injuries caused by fire reaches back to the early days of mankind. Aristotle was interested in the pathogenesis of burns, and believed that burns caused by hot ore showed a tendency to heal more rapidly. Hippocrates used pork lard and white wax. He proposed the use of warm vinegar-soaked dressings to relieve the burn pain, and later treated burns by tanning with solutions of oak bark. Fabricius Hildanus, in Switzerland, gave the first printed extensive description of burns, their classification and treatment, in his book *De Combustionibus* in 1607.

In 1832, Dupuytren classified burn lesions according to depth into six degrees of injury. The effect of the burn insult was taken into consideration for the first time about 100 years ago. Baraduc, in 1863, maintained that the decrease of the circulating blood volume in burns was the most probable cause of death, and that the viscosity of the blood was increased in burns. A major advance in burn care was made in 1870, when Reverdin introduced his method of skin grafting for the closure of the burn wound. Many types of local treatment have been used. Oils and waxes have been placed on burns since Roman times. Tannic acid was used with the idea of coagulating the wound as early as 1858. Lizfrank, in 1835, recommended wet dressings containing sodium and calcium chloride. Syme, in 1833, proposed the use of dry cotton wool dressings applied with a firm degree of pressure, later known as the so-called pressure dressing.

The earliest American reference to exposure of burn wounds was in a publication by Copeland in 1887. Sneve, in 1905, gave an excellent detailed description of the exposure of burns, and recorded much that is in accord with the present-day concept of the method.

Underhill, in 1923, studied fluid requirements in burns and tried to outline necessary replacement solutions according to the size of the burn surface, and the age and general condition of the patient. Interest in the escharotics was renewed by Davidson in 1925, who made great claims for spraying tannic acid on the burn wound. It was believed that this technique decreased the fluid loss, relieved pain and produced a better eschar. This technique was finally abandoned in 1942, when McClure pointed out that it was toxic to the liver and produced an eschar that enclosed the infection.

The modern era of local burn care was initiated by Allen and Koch in 1942, who advocated and popularized the use of petrolatum gauze, bulky, occlusive dressings and strict immobilization. This technique of local care was the one in vogue until Wallace, in 1949, reintroduced the exposure method in Great Britain. Pulaski and Artz, and Blocker evaluated the exposure method in the United States and outlined its indications and contraindications.

One of the greatest disasters from fire was the Cocoanut Grove fire in Boston in 1942. This stimulated fundamental research on the systemic response to burning by Cope and Moore. They demonstrated that the fluid loss of burns was inside the patient and not exclusively outside, which provided an explanation for the hidden fluid loss in burns. Cope, in 1947, emphasized the early aggressive attack on the removal of eschar and early closure of the burn wound.

A real advance in burn management was the introduction of the Brown electric dermatome in 1949. This instrument permitted almost any physician to obtain skin easily for early wound closure. It was not until 1953 that septicemia was emphasized as a common cause of death in burns by Liedberg, Reiss and Artz.

CAUSES. In children under three years of age, most burns are due to scalds. From three to 14 years flame burns, due to clothing catching on fire, predominate; from 15 to 60 years, industrial accidents account for a large number of burns; over 60 years of age, accidents associated with momentary blackouts, smoking in bed, or houses catching on fire are the most common. About 80 per cent of burn accidents occur in the home. Home accidents are 15 times more common than burns in industry. Many burns in infants result from boiling water or hot coffee. The common burn in the southern part of the United States is seen in the little girl who, clothed only in a housecoat, backs up against an open fire. The housecoat catches on fire, the child runs, fans the flames and becomes the victim of a severe burn.

In young children, scalds are more common in boys, probably because they are more curious. Clothing burns are more common in girls because their clothing is more vulnerable to the risk of fire. More children's deaths occur in girls because of the large number of clothing burns in this group.

A high percentage of burns in the military service is caused by airplane accidents. In time of war, the incidence of burns in combat zones and in the rear areas from gasoline explosions, flame throwers, incendiary bombs or simple accidents creates large numbers of long-term casualties. In industrial accidents, electrical injuries and chemical injuries constitute a moderate group in addition to thermal burns.

At least half of all burning accidents could be prevented. One of the great needs in the United States is a more active program for the prevention of burns.

CLASSES OF BURN INJURY. Several classifications have been used to differentiate various depths of burns. In recent years, it has been common practice to divide burns into three categories: first degree, second degree and third degree. First-degree and second-degree burns are known collectively as partial-thickness burns, and third-degree burns as full-thickness burns.

Since the systemic and local changes are directly related to the amount of tissue destroyed, this classification is probably an oversimplification. Greater clarity might result if second-degree burns were further divided into superficial second-degree and deep dermal burns. Third-degree burns should be classified as full-thickness skin loss and as deep third-degree burns in which the injury involves the underlying subcutaneous tissue, muscle or bone.

A *first-degree burn* involves only the epidermis. It is characterized by erythema that appears after a variable latent period. A first-degree burn may follow prolonged exposure to bright sunlight or instantaneous exposure to more intense heat. Because tissue damage is so superficial, minimal systemic derangements occur. Pain and a slight amount of edema are the chief problems. The uncomfortable burning sensation and pain usually subside after 48 hours unless the first-degree

burn is quite extensive, as in a severe sunburn. Since this is only a superficial injury, the capacity of the skin to prevent infection is retained. Healing usually takes place uneventfully. Within five to ten days the epidermis peels off in small scales. There may be residual redness for a few days, but no scarring results.

A *second-degree burn* is a deeper injury than a first-degree burn. It involves all the epidermis and much of the corium. Most second-degree burns are characterized by blisters, and are usually accompanied by considerable subcutaneous edema. The rate of healing is dependent upon the depth of skin destruction and on whether or not infection occurs. In superficial partial-thickness burns, healing usually occurs uneventfully within a period of ten to 14 days unless infection supervenes. Deep dermal burns are injuries that extend down deep into the corium. Epithelial regeneration takes place principally from the epithelial lining of the sweat glands and hair follicles. In the event of infection, deep dermal burns are readily converted to full-thickness injury. If the wound is properly protected, however, it will be covered with a thin layer of epithelium in 25 to 35 days. There may be thick scarring. Not infrequently, this thin epithelium is injured, giving rise to denuded areas and further scar formation. When the thin epithelial covering of deep dermal burn is stretched by motion, blister formation may occur.

The deep dermal burn is of significant clinical importance. It is difficult to diagnose. It causes physiologic derangements that are more severe than those following superficial second-degree injury. It heals spontaneously if kept free from mechanical and bacterial trauma. If infection occurs, it becomes converted into full-thickness injury and grafting is necessary. Many areas commonly diagnosed as third-degree burns are really only deep dermal burns. By newer methods of local chemotherapy such as Sulfamylon and silver nitrate, bacterial growth is controlled and epithelization occurs.

A *third-degree burn* is a very severe form of injury. The entire dermis down to the subcutaneous fat is destroyed by coagulation necrosis. Thrombosis occurs in the small vessels of the underlying tissue. Increased capillary permeability and edema are greater than in the second-degree burn. In two or three weeks, the full-thickness dead skin liquefies, partially by autolysis and partially by leukocytic digestion. This process is accompanied by suppuration. Capillary tufts and fibroblasts organized into granulating tissue are found beneath the eschar. Deep third-degree burns are considerably different from the third-degree burns that involve only full-thickness skin loss. If the burn extends into the subcutaneous fat, liquefaction occurs in that area. Burns deep into the muscle cause increased destruction of red blood cells. The physiologic derangements which occur in deep third-degree burns may be severe even when the injury is of limited extent.

Full-thickness burns are treated by the removal of the eschar and the application of a skin graft to cover the wound. If grafting is not performed, a thick layer of granulating tissue will form, followed by severe contracture. The only method of epithelization in this type of burn is slow proliferation from the wound edges that occurs at the rate of about 1/8 inch per week. The granulations become soft, overgrown and infected, thus hindering epithelization. After months and even years, the wound might heal but not without considerable scarring and disfigurement.

DETERMINATION OF DEPTH OF BURN. Even in the most experienced hands, the diagnosis of the depth of burn is not too accurate because there are no definite clinical criteria for the depth of burn. This difficulty might be expected because there are various gradations of injury in the extensive burn. In addition, thickness of the skin varies with age and body location. The central area of the burn surface may be full thickness with a surrounding zone of deep dermal and superficial second-degree burn and first-degree burn at the periphery. One depth of injury seems to fade into the other in such a way that definite demarcation and gradation are almost impossible.

First-degree burns usually occur after gas explosions, brief contact with hot liquids or prolonged exposure to sunlight. They appear as a simple erythematous flush. First-degree burns are dry and quite painful; blistering seldom occurs.

Second-degree burns are caused by short periods of exposure to intense flash heat or contact with hot liquids, or they may form the peripheral zone of a deeper flame burn. They are frequently characterized by the formation of blisters. The surface is mottled red or pink in appearance and it is usually moist because a plasma-like fluid exudes

from the injured area. A second-degree burn is quite painful and sensitive to the air. In a deep dermal burn, the surface may be moist, but the exudate that forms is not as profuse as in the superficial second-degree burn. The surface has a mottled appearance with a predominance of white rather than red or pink areas.

Third-degree burns are generally caused by flames or contact with hot objects. Because the outer layer of the skin is involved in the coagulation necrosis, the third-degree burn is usually dry and dead white or charred in appearance. The skin feels leathery in contrast to the moist, soft surface of a partial-thickness burn. Third-degree burns are not very painful; in fact, the area is almost insensible because the terminal nerve endings are inactivated by the deep injury. The impairment in sensation has been used clinically as a test for depth of skin loss. A hypodermic needle may be used to test pain sensation in the injured area. This so-called pin prick test may show greatly reduced pain sensibility which is indicative of full-thickness injury. If there is increased sensitivity to pain or only slightly diminished pain sensibility, most likely the burn is partial thickness. One of the best ways of differentiating between second- and third-degree areas is by pulling on a hair. If the hair pulls out easily and painlessly, it is a third-degree burn.

EXTENT OF BURN INJURY. The extent of a burn is usually expressed as a percentage of the total area of body surface. In 1924, Berkow presented data concerning percentage surface area of various parts of the body. Lund and Browder found that Berkow tables were not applicable to all ages; they determined the changes in percentage of body surface of various parts that occur during different stages of development from infancy through childhood and devised a special chart. The most accurate method for determining percentage of body surface burn is to map out the areas of injury on a Lund and Browder chart (Fig. 1). This is best done after the burn wound has been cleaned and all the loose, devitalized epithelium removed.

A rapid and popular method for estimating per cent of body surface burn is by the use of the *Rule of Nines* (Fig. 2). This rule, first devised by Pulaski and Tennison, divides the body surface into areas representing 9 per cent or multiples of 9 per cent. The head and neck are graded as 9 per cent; the anterior trunk, twice 9, or 18 per cent; the poste-

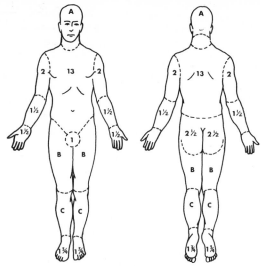

Figure 1. Classic Lund and Browder chart. The best method for determining percentage of body surface burn is to mark the areas of injury on a chart, then compute total percentage according to the patient's age. Every emergency room should have such a chart for the plotting of the burned area soon after the patient is admitted.

Relative Percentages of Areas Affected by Growth
(AGE IN YEARS)

	0	1	5	10	15	ADULT
A: ½ of head	9½	8½	6½	5½	4½	3½
B: ½ of thigh	2¾	3¼	4	4¼	4½	4¾
C: ½ of leg	2½	2½	2¾	3	3¼	3½

Total Per Cent Burned_____2° +_____3° =_____

rior trunk, 18 per cent; each lower extremity, 18 per cent; each upper extremity, 9 per cent; and the perineum, 1 per cent. This is a good, rapid method of estimating the percentage of a body surface burn, but is not nearly so accurate as the use of the Lund and Browder chart.

PROGNOSIS. It is extremely difficult to determine prognosis with any degree of accuracy in any specific burn. Mortality increases with the severity of burning and with advancing age. At one time, few patients survived burns involving more than one-third of their body surface, but this is no longer true. With modern treatment for many patients with burns up to 50 or 60 per cent of the body surface and for those more extensively burned, the outlook is not entirely hopeless. The prognosis of the burned patient should be guarded if the percentage of second- and third-degree burn is more than 40. It may be several days or weeks before the ultimate outcome can be predicted. Frequently, extensively burned patients survive the initial few weeks after the injury only to succumb later to complications. In severe

injuries, prediction of survival should be withheld until about 30 days after the burn.

Pruitt and others published an excellent study of 1100 burned patients treated at the U.S. Army Surgical Research Unit at the Brooke Army Medical Center from 1950 to 1960. He constructed a mortality contour plot from the data in this series for ease in approximating expected mortality. This graphic illustration of mortality trends according to age in years and percentage of burns is reproduced in Figure 3.

PATHOPHYSIOLOGY. The pathologic changes which occur within the skin and subcutaneous tissue, or the deeper structures, depend naturally upon the intensity of the heat and the length of time that it has been applied. At the surface of the burn, a greater or lesser depth of the skin is actually destroyed by heat. Immediately underneath this dead tissue, the deeper layers of the skin and subcutaneous tissue are severely affected by the heat but are still viable. The capillaries become widely dilated, with greatly increased permeability. This increased permeability causes a disturbance in the normal exchange of fluid between the plasma and the interstitial space. As fluid is lost into the skin, it appears as blisters. When fluid is lost into the subcutaneous tissue, it causes edema. The fluid which escapes into the burned area

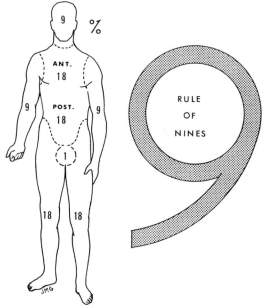

Figure 2. Schematic outline of the *Rule of Nines*. The use of this rule provides a rapid method for determining percentage of body surface burned, but it is of limited accuracy.

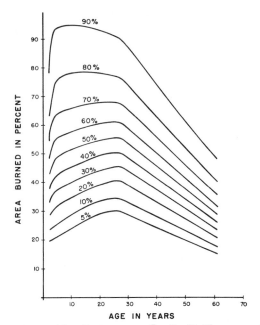

Figure 3. Mortality contours after Pruitt. The per cent mortality that can be expected at varying age with different areas of body surface burn is shown by three contours.

deep burn. If the quantity destroyed is sufficient, this will become manifest as hemoglobinemia and hemoglobinuria. A number of red cells not destroyed by heat at the time of the burn are rendered abnormally fragile, and these are removed in the first few hours by the reticuloendothelial system. Thrombosis of vessels beneath the burned area occurs and may contribute to the decrease in red cell mass. The phenomenon of sludging has been well demonstrated in burns. The importance of sludging in the diminution of the functional red cell mass is not known but it may be considerable. In deep third-degree burns, the red cell destruction during the first 48 hours is approximately 10 to 15 per cent of the total red cell mass.

The local changes which occur in a third-degree burn produce an ideal environment for infection. There is dead tissue covering the wound. The bacteria that remain viable in the deeper crypts of the skin tend to proliferate rapidly on the dead, burned tissue because the thrombosis and edema beneath the burn inhibit the movement of the usual defense mechanisms into the area (Fig. 4).

FIRST AID. A person whose clothes are on fire should not run, as this only fans the flames. He should not remain standing since this position may cause him to inhale flames

is carried away by the lymphatic drainage from the local site, but soon the amount of fluid exceeds the ability of the lymph channels to withdraw it. It accumulates in the interstitial spaces and produces edema, not only of the wound, but also of the area surrounding the wound. A large amount of fluid can be hidden when it is sequestered deep in the soft tissue and about the burned areas.

The loss of fluid from the circulation continues at a rapid rate for several hours, but gradually decreases over the course of 48 hours as the capillaries recover their tone and permeability. After this period, reabsorption of the edema fluid slowly takes place. The loss of this protein-rich fluid from the plasma at the site of the burn results in a fall in plasma volume. Fluid loss may be so great that it represents a high percentage of the total circulating fluid volume of the body, and the patient may go into shock. In some instances, the edema may become so intense as to jeopardize the vascular supply of an extremity.

In addition to the losses of plasma, there is a diminution in red cell mass. This loss is associated primarily with deep burns and is not very great with superficial burns. The diminution in red cell volume is usually gradual and not so severe as was originally thought. Many of the red blood cells are actually destroyed by heat at the time of the

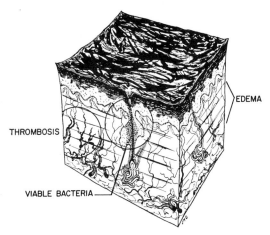

Figure 4. Diagrammatic outline of changes occurring in the subcutaneous tissue beneath a full-thickness burn. Although the surface and all layers of the skin may be burned, viable bacteria remain in the crypts and hair follicles. Thrombosis occurs in the small vessels beneath the burned surface. An outpouring of fluid in and around burned areas produces a massive edema. Thrombosis and edema prevent the transport by way of the blood of host defense mechanisms to the area. With this limitation of the defense mechanisms and the excellent pabulum of the burned tissue, viable bacteria proliferate rapidly. The local pathologic changes in a third-degree burn provide an ideal environment for infection.

or cause the hair to be ignited. A burned person should be placed in a horizontal position, and then rolled in a blanket or rug to smother the flames. Coats or other garments may be used for this purpose.

The initial step in the care of the burned patient is to cover the wound. This minimizes contamination and inhibits pain by preventing the air from coming in contact with the injured surface. The use of towels soaked in ice water will bring almost immediate relief from burn pain. The cold may also have some value in arresting the effect of the heat on the tissue. Any burn involving more than 10 per cent of the body surface should be seen by a physician. Medicaments or home remedies should not be applied to the burn. A clean sheet or cloth may be used as an emergency dressing. The patient suffering from respiratory arrest due to smoke inhalation should receive artificial respiration by positive pressure breathing using the mouth-to-mouth technique.

MINOR BURNS. Minor burns include those partial-thickness burns of less than 10 per cent of the body surface and full-thickness burns of less than 2 per cent of the body surface. These do not usually require fluid replacement, and should be treated with local cleansing and the appropriate type of wound care. Usually, a grease gauze dressing is applied. In burns of 10 to 20 per cent of the body surface, intravenous fluids are occasionally required, particularly in children. During the first 24 hours, lactated Ringer's solution may be given intravenously in the amount of 2 ml. per kg. of body weight for each per cent of burn.

The chief aim of the local care of minor burns is to make the patient as comfortable as possible. Although exposure is a good method of local care, most patients with minor burns treated on an outpatient basis should receive a well-applied, occlusive dressing that will permit them to continue their activities. They should return for redressing three to five days later. Antibiotics are rarely necessary.

EARLY SYSTEMIC MANAGEMENT. The emergency room care of a patient with a major burn should be the orderly execution of several established routine procedures. These include a quick history, estimation of the extent and depth of burn, drawing a sample of blood for cross-matching and baseline laboratory determinations, insertion of a cutdown cannula and an indwelling urinary catheter, determination of the need for tracheostomy, administration of antibiotics and tetanus immunization, and planning of fluid therapy.

History. A brief history should include when, where and how the accident happened, and something concerning the status of the patient's health prior to the injury. When the accident may have legal implications, a color photograph should be taken of the injured areas for record purposes.

Initial venipuncture. As soon as the patient has been examined, a large bore needle should be inserted into an accessible vein and a blood sample drawn for cross-matching, hematocrit, blood urea nitrogen and other specific laboratory determinations. Dextran or lactated Ringer's solution should be administered through this needle until a cutdown cannula is in place. To make the patient more comfortable, eliminate apprehension and alleviate pain associated with cleansing the burn wound, morphine may be given through the venipuncture needle. Narcotics should always be given intravenously; when given subcutaneously to burned patients with circulatory deficiency, the narcotic is poorly absorbed, and therefore ineffective.

Tracheostomy. A mechanically clear airway must be assured from the beginning. The need for a tracheostomy can usually be determined while the history is being obtained. A tracheostomy must be performed if there is severe respiratory obstruction. It is also indicated in the initial management when respiratory tract injury is suspected. The presence of established pulmonary damage may be diagnosed by hoarseness, coughing, rapid respirations or cyanosis. A history of the patient being burned in a closed space, or the appearance of redness in the posterior pharynx, may suggest respiratory damage. Singeing of the nasal hairs, stridor or rales in the chest may give indication of pulmonary irritation. Although some deep burns of the face and neck may require a tracheostomy later, it is usually not indicated in the first 24 hours. Addition of a tracheostomy to the already complicated condition of the burned patient frequently gives rise to many complications. Patients with burns about the head and neck may do very well without a tracheostomy which is always associated with increases in water loss and infection, and requires additional nursing care.

Intravenous administration. Since the

life of a burned patient frequently depends upon the infusion of replacement solutions, it is wise to plan initially the utilization of various routes of administration. A cutdown cannula should be inserted in adult patients with greater than 20 per cent burn injury, and in children with greater than 10 per cent. Intravenous fluids may be required for as long as 12 days. During this time, thrombosis may occur in several veins and necessitate a change in infusion site from one vein to another. Good veins for intravenous infusion may be difficult to find; therefore, a plan for saving veins should be worked out before therapy is started.

When cutdown cannulas are inserted into the saphenous vein, superficial phlebitis is common after four or five days. If available, one of the best areas for the cannula is the cephalic vein in the shoulder area. Although it is more difficult to perform a cutdown in this area, it is the best site for prolonged administration of intravenous fluids because less phlebitis is seen in this area.

When a cannula has to be inserted into a leg vein, it is wise to start as far distally as possible. If thrombosis of the vein occurs, the cannula may be moved proximally. Considerable interest has arisen recently in the use of femoral vein catheters. Using this route initially, however, might well preclude subsequent use of the saphenous vein. This route is not void of complications, such as edema of the lower extremity, septic thrombophlebitis, deep venous thrombosis, erosion of the vein wall and lost tubing. The use of a femoral catheter should be reserved for the time when no other veins are available. It should not be left in place longer than seven days because complications are frequent after this period.

Indwelling urinary catheter. In all burns involving more than 25 per cent of the body surface, the most reliable method for determining the adequacy of fluid therapy is by the insertion of an indwelling catheter into the bladder and the hourly measurement of the urinary output. As soon as the catheter is not absolutely necessary, it should be removed. In most instances, it can be discontinued after 72 hours. While it is in place, the patient should receive the appropriate antibacterial therapy to prevent urinary tract infections.

Fluid therapy. Burns differ from most conditions characterized by losses of water and electrolytes in that the rate, volume and composition of fluid losses can be anticipated. Clinical shock is a preventable syndrome, providing adequate therapy can be initiated soon after injury. Several factors influence the amount and type of fluid therapy. These include extent and depth of burn, weight, age and general physical status of the patient, and degree of respiratory tract involvement.

No mathematical formula exists by which all burns can be treated. A given formula should be regarded only as a means of providing an order of magnitude of fluid requirements, and not as outlining a course of action which should be followed blindly. Without a predetermined estimate, gross errors are often made, usually in the direction of overtreatment. Because the volume and rate of fluid losses are predictable, several fluid formulas for estimating the types and amounts of therapy have been devised. These include the Evans formula, Moore's budget, the Massachusetts General Hospital formula, the Parkland Hospital regimen and the Brooke formula. The Moore budget and the Massachusetts General Hospital formula favor larger quantities of colloids and less electrolyte solution. The Parkland regimen uses no colloids and accomplishes the entire replacement therapy with a balanced salt solution. The Brooke formula is a middle of the road one. At the present time, it is the most popular. In accordance with current knowledge of fluids in burns, however, this formula requires certain specific adjustments. It seems most adequate for a burn of up to 40 per cent in an adult. In more extensive burns, it is probably wise to increase the colloid estimate at the expense of the electrolyte requirement. Certainly, in infants a larger proportion of the replacement solution should be given as colloids than is estimated in the Brooke formula. Each individual clinician should use the formula with which he is most familiar. There is an advantage to selecting one method of estimated fluid requirements in burns and gaining as much experience as possible with it. The Brooke formula estimates the following for the first 24 hours following injury:

Colloids (plasma, Plasmanate or dextran):
  0.5 ml./kg./per cent of body surface burn
Electrolyte solution (lactated Ringer's):
  1.5 ml./kg./per cent of body surface burn
Water requirement (dextrose in water):
  2000 ml. for adults, children correspondingly less

Water requirements in children vary. The following is a rough guide to daily water requirements in infants and children: during the first two years, 120 ml. per kg.; second to fifth year, 100 ml. per kg.; fifth to eighth year, 80 ml. per kg.; eighth to twelfth year, 50 ml. per kg.

It is important that burns of more than 50 per cent of the body surface be calculated as 50 per cent burns, or excess quantities of fluid will be given. In the second 24 hours after injury, about one-half the colloid and electrolyte requirements of the first 24 hours is needed.

After having estimated the requirements, a number of factors must be considered before proceeding with therapy. Young children and elderly adults will not tolerate excessive fluids, and, therefore, should receive minimal amounts. Patients with pre-existing cardiovascular or renal disease should be treated similarly. When there has been respiratory tract irritation, pulmonary edema is a threat. In patients with severe burns around the head, cerebral edema may develop if excessive fluids are administered.

Most of the calculated colloid requirement should be given early. Relatively more colloids should be given to burns of greater magnitude. Plasma, Plasmanate, dextran, albumin and blood have been used as colloid therapy in burns. In recent years, it has become evident that less blood is required in the first 48 hours than was formerly believed. It is doubtful that any blood should be used in a second-degree burn. Occasionally, in deep burns of more than 50 per cent of the body surface and in burns associated with electrical injury, one unit of blood is advisable in the first 48 hours. Thereafter, the blood requirements should be determined by the hematocrit.

Plasma is the preferred colloid for use in burns. When plasma is not available, Plasmanate or albumin may be used. Clinical dextran with an average molecular weight of 75,000 in saline is also an acceptable plasma volume expander. It has been used abundantly in the treatment of burns with rewarding benefits. Because of its protein content, plasma is preferred as a colloid solution by most clinicians.

Because of the tendency of metabolic acidosis to develop in the early period after injury, lactated Ringer's solution, a balanced salt solution, is preferred to normal saline for fulfilling the electrolyte requirement.

A profound paralytic ileus not infrequently accompanies severe burns. Because of this, oral fluids should be withheld for two days in patients treated by intravenous infusion. Although most well-treated burned patients are thirsty during the first 48 hours, withholding oral fluids is indicated because of the fear of gastric distention and dilatation followed by vomiting and aspiration.

Clinical appraisal of therapy. After an approximation of fluid requirements has been made, some thought must be given to the order in which the various solutions should be administered. The first eight-hour period is the most important because the most rapid fluid losses occur soon after thermal injury. Generally, one-half of the first 24-hour fluid requirement is given in the first eight hours, one-fourth in the second eight-hour period and one-fourth in the third eight-hour period. Fluid therapy so planned should be calculated for the period following injury rather than the period following admission to the hospital. If the patient's treatment has been delayed, initial fluid therapy should be given as colloid. Sometimes, it is advisable to give the colloid solution in one vein and lactated Ringer's in another. The initial fluids should be given rather rapidly, at least 1 liter in the first hour. Thereafter, the rate of administration should be determined by the rate of urinary flow. Unfortunately, there are no laboratory determinations that serve as adequate guides to therapy. Sometimes in the first 48 hours, observations of the hematocrit are helpful. Severe thirst, collapsed veins and hypotension obviously denote a fluid deficiency. The best guide to the rate of fluid infusion is the urinary output which should be measured and recorded hourly. The ideal output in an adult is 30 ml. per hour. The rate of infusion should be increased if the urinary volume falls below 15 ml. per hour and decreased if it exceeds 50 ml. per hour. Excess water and electrolytes in amounts which will produce a urinary output of more than 50 ml. per hour may lead to overexpansion of the interstitial space. Too often, the clinician feels that the patient must be doing well if he is excreting 100 ml. of urine per hour. With such an output the intake must be more than is necessary, and additional troublesome edema may develop. Excessive fluid administration is a more common error than inadequate fluid therapy. A decreasing blood pressure and decreasing urinary output mean that colloids should be given. A decreasing urinary output with a normal blood pressure indicates that additional electrolyte solution or water is required. Gross hemoglobin in the urine is an indication that the burn is quite deep. In such instances, a high renal output should be forced to flush the kidney tubules. This may be accomplished with a high intake; sometimes mannitol is used.

Regular auscultation of the lungs and chest roentgenograms to detect the early signs of pulmonary edema should be routine. In patients with burns about the head, cerebral edema may occur during the course of treatment. This is more common in children. It is usually heralded by a sudden rise in temperature in a patient who otherwise is doing well.

Determination of the venous pressure is one of the best techniques in avoiding over-infusion. It should be used routinely in all severe burns. It is of little value in determining adequacy of fluid therapy, but when the venous pressure rises above normal there is positive evidence that fluid therapy should be temporarily curtailed. A venous pressure above normal means that the right side of the heart is being overloaded. Either too much fluid is being given or there is impending heart failure.

Laboratory determinations. Electrolyte determinations are of little value in guiding fluid therapy during the initial 48 hours. Hematocrit determinations during this period offer some guide to the clinical evaluation of fluid replacement, but should not be the sole determinant for the types and amounts of therapy. After 48 hours, the serum sodium concentration should be determined daily. In extensively burned patients, the serum sodium, potassium, chloride and carbon dioxide combining power should be followed each day or every other day. The nonprotein nitrogen frequently is a guide to prognosis; few patients survive with a persistent level above 100 mg. per 100 ml.

Therapy after 48 hours. After 48 hours, most of the fluids given should be electrolyte-free water and blood. A hematocrit of less than 36 is an indication for additional blood. Hyponatremia is usually present in spite of the large sodium load in the interstitial space. A low serum sodium in burned patients is associated with a good clinical response and is desirable. The insensible water loss after the first 48 hours may be quite marked, as much as 5000 or 6000 ml. per day in an adult.

After the acute stress of the burn injury, the body has a tendency to hold on to sodium, and very little is excreted by the kidneys. The loss of water by the insensible route and by the urine may be relatively greater than the loss of sodium. This means that the water load is diminishing more rapidly than the sodium load and, therefore, a rise in serum sodium may occur. A serum sodium concentration of 135 mEq. per liter is usually ideal in the first few days after injury (Fig. 5). When the serum sodium rises to 145 mEq. per liter or more, additional electrolyte-free water must be given. When insufficient water is infused, the serum sodium may rise rapidly and lead to severe hypernatremia.

After the first 48 hours, many burned patients will take oral fluids and regulate their own intake. When food cannot be taken orally, after 72 hours it may be necessary to give 40 or 80 mEq. of potassium each day.

Special problems in children. The successful management of fluid replacement in severely burned infants and small children is based on a constant critical evaluation of the patient's clinical course, always remembering to stay on the conservative side. Intravenous fluid therapy may be disregarded in the child with less than 6 per cent of the body surface burned, but is mandatory in the child with more than 12 per cent. The safe limit for total volume of electrolyte and colloid infused over the first 24-hour period is equal to 10 per cent of the preburn body weight. Infants do not utilize sodium-containing solutions as well as adults; therefore, until two years of age the calculated electrolyte requirement should be given as one-half electrolyte solution and one-half 5 per cent dextrose in water. The hourly urinary output should be kept in a range of 5 to 10 ml. per hour in infants under one year; 10 to 20 ml. per hour in children from one to ten years of age; and 15 to 30 ml. per hour in children over ten years. As long as a child is excreting small quantities of clear urine regularly, there is evidence that fluid intake is adequate. A large urinary output is frequently associated with overloading of fluids.

Kefalides has pointed out the value of gamma globulin in the prevention of septicemia in young children. The use of this material is recommended in infants up to four years of age. The usual dosage is 1 ml. per kg. intramuscularly on the day of injury, repeated on the third and fifth postburn days.

Antibiotics and tetanus immunization.

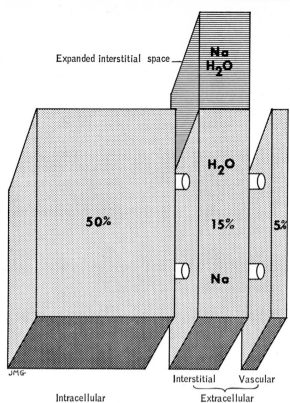

Figure 5. Body water compartments and changes that occur after burning. There is a shift of water from the vascular and intracellular spaces into the interstitial space. With additional replacement therapy this interstitial space expands. This expanded interstitial space contains sodium and water. This means that the body of a well-treated burned patient has an excess of water and sodium. As the interstitial space returns to normal after 48 hours, the loss of water is relatively greater than the loss of sodium because of the high insensible water loss. During this period the serum sodium concentration is an excellent guide to fluid therapy. A serum sodium level of about 135 mEq. per liter seems to be ideal.

Although there are different opinions concerning the use of antibiotics initially in burns, it is doubtful that such therapy is indicated. Some surgeons routinely give penicillin and streptomycin to all hospitalized burned patients. Others believe that penicillin therapy for the first five days prevents infection by the beta hemolytic streptococcus. It is doubtful that prophylactic antibiotics are necessary in a clean hospital environment. If a streptococcal infection does develop, and this is rare, it is easily abated by the use of penicillin. Routine antibiotic therapy in burns only permits the growth of resistant organisms. Except in certain instances, antibiotics should be withheld until there is some evidence of infection. A concentrated effort should be made to determine the offending organism and the appropriate antibiotic administered. When patients have a concomitant disease or injury indicating antibiotics, they should be used.

Since tetanus may be a complication of burns, appropriate immunization against tetanus must be given to all patients with full-thickness burn injury.

WOUND MANAGEMENT. The chief problem in the management of large burn wounds is the control of infection. This emphasizes the importance of local care. The aim in the treatment of first- and second-degree burns is to provide an environment of cleanliness so that the areas will heal free from infection. The aim in the local management of third-degree burns is the early removal of dead tissue and closure of the wound with a skin graft as soon as possible. Every effort should be aimed at minimizing further contamination and achieving a surgically clean wound. All personnel who come in contact with the patient must be masked. The patient should be taken to a clean dressing room or operating room where aseptic technique can be followed in the initial management of the wound. In the extensively burned patient, fluid and electrolyte replacement should take precedence over local care. Intravenous morphine provides adequate analgesia for cleansing the wound, and a general anesthetic is contraindicated.

The burned area should be cleansed thoroughly. All debris and detached epidermis must be removed. Some type of bland soap and warm water may be used for initial cleansing. The blisters and detached epidermis can usually be pulled away by grasping the loose tissue with a dry gauze pad. Occasionally, it is necessary to use forceps and scissors. All blisters should be removed except those very thick blisters which form on the palm of the hand. They need not be broken. After the first cleansing procedure, a second washing, followed by rinsing with large quantities of water, prepares the surface for definitive local care.

There are many acceptable methods of local care. These may be classified primarily as occlusive dressings, exposure, initial excision, Sulfamylon cream or silver nitrate soaks. Most surgeons use all methods. The type selected varies with each individual patient. In many instances, some areas will be treated by one method and other areas by another in the same patient. At times, treatment of a burn may be started by one method of local care and then changed to another during the course of therapy. It is impossible to dictate any particular method. All are acceptable, and it is up to the physician to select the one most desirable for a particular patient at a particular time. The choice of method is determined by the location of the burn, size of the injury, depth of the burn, type of patient, facilities available, and the patient's response. Only certain small full-thickness burns lend themselves to initial excision. Most patients treated on an outpatient basis

do better when the wounds are dressed. Exposure, Sulfamylon cream and silver nitrate soaks require more nursing care than other methods.

Occlusive dressings. The aim of a good dressing is to cover the open wound to protect it from infection. It should not necessarily be a pressure dressing because pressure does not really inhibit the loss of fluid.

The material placed next to the wound must not macerate the tissue or damage the remaining viable epithelium. Several types of fabric are available; commercially prepared nylon fabric, Carbowax gauze, dry fine-mesh gauze and lightly impregnated petrolatum gauze are satisfactory.

The dressing must be occlusive to prevent the invasion of bacteria. It should be absorptive to keep the wound surface dry and thereby inhibit the growth of bacteria. It should be bulky and applied with an even, resilient compression so that it eliminates dead space, gives vascular support and produces a splinting effect (Fig. 6). Many hospitals prepare thick, one-piece dressings of various sizes. Such burn pads are useful and practical, as they save a great deal of time during dressing changes. The initial dressing

A burn dressing should be:

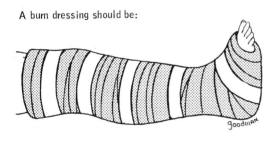

A. Occlusive

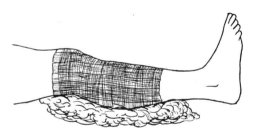

B. Absorptive

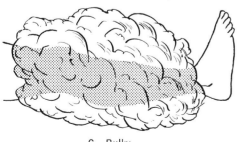

C. Bulky

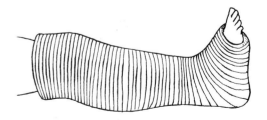

D. Put on with even, resilient compression

Figure 6.   Important aspects of a satisfactory burn dressing. *A,* It should be applied in such a way that it occludes the entire injury from outside invasion by bacteria. *B,* The dressing should be absorptive, so that the wound surface will be kept dry and thereby inhibit the growth of bacteria. *C,* It is important that the dressing be bulky, so that it provides a splint for the part and does not soak through within a short period. *D,* It should be put on with even, resilient compression to be comfortable and provide support to the vascular system.

frequently can be left in place for five days. In general, burn dressings should be changed every four or five days.

Exposure. The accepted technique for the exposure method includes initial cleansing of the burn wound and placing the patient in bed on clean sheets in the position that best exposes the affected areas. Sterile sheets are unnecessary. The exudate of a partial-thickness burn dries in 48 to 72 hours and forms a hard crust that serves as a natural protective cover for the wound. Epithelial regeneration proceeds beneath this crust unless impeded by infection. In 14 to 21 days, the crust falls off spontaneously, leaving an unscarred, well-healed surface (Fig. 7). The evolution of a full-thickness burn treated by exposure is different. Surface exudation is minimal and crust formation does not occur. The dead tissue of the full-thickness burn becomes dehydrated and is converted to a thick, tough eschar after about 72 hours of exposure.

The technique of exposure may be different in every patient because different configurations of the burned surface pose individual problems. Much of the success of exposure depends upon the ingenuity of the surgeon and nursing staff in achieving a good protective cover. This protective cover must be managed in such a way as to minimize softening, maceration and cracking.

Burns of the face are easily exposed. In full-thickness burns, removal of eschar may be hastened by application of saline soaks beginning on the eighth to the tenth day. Burns of the anterior aspect of the neck should be positioned with the neck in extension; this minimizes maceration. In almost every instance, cracks will occur in the region of the thyroid cartilage because of deglutition. Fortunately, these cracks are rarely troublesome because the excellent blood supply of the neck promotes rapid healing.

Burns that are circumferential are difficult to position. In a circumferential burn of the upper extremity, the part may be tied to an intravenous pole. This provides elevation and reasonably comfortable exposure. Circumferential burns of other areas of the body must be exposed on one side and then turned and exposed on the other. This is usually accomplished by the use of a turning frame; probably the best is the circo-electric bed. By turning the patient every four hours a fairly good protective covering will form.

One of the chief problems in exposure of circumferential burns is the adherence of the bed clothing or dressing to an exposed area. It is always painful when the patient is turned because he is stuck to the dressing. A new nonadherent plastic dressing (Microdon) is now available. It is truly a nonstick comfortable dressing. This smooth material does not adhere to the wound surface and is easily pulled away when the patient is turned.

Burns of the perineum are difficult to expose properly and drying is rarely seen. Some suppuration is almost inevitable, but for-

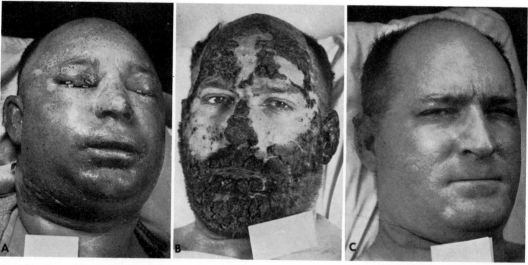

Figure 7. Second-degree burn of the face treated by exposure. *A*, The burned face has been cleansed and all detached epithelium removed. Massive edema was present when this photograph was taken at 48 hours. *B*, At eight days post burn, the edema has disappeared and the entire burned surface is covered by a crust. Part of this crust has separated. *C*, Appearance of the face 19 days post burn. There is very little evidence of scarring. All the crust has desquamated except a little on the right ear. Second-degree burns of the face do extremely well when treated by exposure.

tunately the skin of the perineum possesses a great capacity for regeneration and spontaneous healing occurs even in the presence of minimal infection.

Clinically, all patients who are exposed complain of being cold. Some type of tent made by sheets and blankets should be placed over the exposed burned patient. A portable hair dryer used to blow heated air underneath this tent increases patient comfort.

One of the most important facets in the conduction of the exposure method is the constant daily observations of the integrity of the crust or eschar. Frequently, small cracks develop in the crust and fluid or pus collects beneath. The success of exposure depends upon the integrity of the crust. When there is a crack, the edges of the crust should be cut away and the area covered with a small piece of fine-mesh gauze.

One of the problems in the exposure of full-thickness circumferential burns is the tight or constricting eschar. As the burned skin dries, it contracts and the coagulated protein forms a stiff inelastic eschar. A tight constricting eschar after a circumferential burn of the chest will greatly limit respiratory exchange and can result in fatal hypoxia. Similarly, a circumferential full-thickness burn of the extremity unyielding to the pressure of edema fluid within it forces pressure occlusion of the arterial supply to distal tissues. Both problems can be solved by escharotomy of the burned skin down to the deep fascia.

Exposure ends in partial-thickness burns when the crust desquamates and falls off. Exposure ends in full-thickness burns when the eschar begins to soften and is ready for removal.

Initial excision. Initial excision during the first day or two post burn is a desirable procedure because it permits removal of all dead tissue soon after injury and encourages early closure of the wound. It has two distinct disadvantages; in the first few hours or even days, it is difficult to determine accurately the extent of the full-thickness injury, and surgical excision of extensive areas may compound the initial injury. Although extensive initial excision has been tried, it is not recommended. In patients with burns not exceeding 15 per cent of the body surface, however, in whom there is definite evidence that the injury is of the full-thickness variety, initial excision followed by grafting four days later is a highly desirable procedure.

Sulfamylon cream. Abundant laboratory and clinical experience attests to the fact that Sulfamylon cream locally applied is an effective method of minimizing infection in burn wounds. This chemotherapeutic agent has the unique property of penetrating the thick heavy eschar and thereby diminishes the growth of bacteria beneath the burned skin. Sulfamylon cream is prepared as a 10 per cent concentration of Sulfamylon acetate (para-aminomethylbenzene sulfonamide acetate) in a water-soluble base. It is effective against a wide range of organisms, both gram-positive and gram-negative, and is particularly effective against anaerobes. Sulfamylon is soluble in water, actively diffuses into avascular tissue, is locally nontoxic and is broken down in the blood to produce p-carboxybenzene sulfonamide, an acid salt. Application of Sulfamylon in a water-soluble base, which itself is 43 per cent water, has resulted in a significant decrease in the evaporative water loss from the burned surface.

Although the application of this material is simple, definite procedures and close observation of the patient are required. After the burn wound has been cleansed, the Sulfamylon cream is applied with a gloved hand to a thickness of 5 mm. over the entire wound (Fig. 8). During the first 48 hours after injury, the exudate from the wound may cause the cream to slip off, and reapplication may be necessary two or three times a day. The cream should be washed from the wound surface at least once daily and the entire wound examined. This can be done most conveniently in a Hubbard tank. The cream is easily removed with water, movement is encouraged and the patient has an increased sense of well-being. The usual procedure is to place the patient in a Hubbard tank each morning, wash off the cream and reapply shortly thereafter. There is occasionally a local burning sensation for 15 to 20 minutes after the material has been applied, but this is usually not severe and does not require analgesia. The eschar remains on the burn wound longer than usual. It may be necessary after 30 days to excise the eschar in the operating room. The use of Sulfamylon has markedly decreased the conversion of deep partial-thickness burns to full-thickness wounds.

Sulfamylon is a strong carbonic anhydrase inhibitor and thus impairs the effectiveness of the renal tubular buffering mechanism in maintaining normal body pH. In extensively burned patients, the continuous use of Sul-

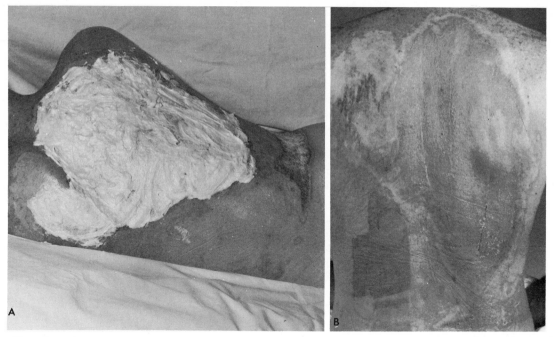

Figure 8. *A*, Sulfamylon acetate cream applied to a second- and third-degree burn of the back. *B*, After grafting, complete healing has taken place.

famylon acetate with its Diamox-like effect may lead to rapid respirations as the pulmonary mechanism attempts to compensate for the lack of buffering by the renal tubules. If the pulmonary tree fails to compensate, acidosis may occur. When Sulfamylon is used in extensively burned patients, the respiratory rate should be observed carefully. Should it become rapid and labored, Sulfamylon treatment should be discontinued for two or three days irrespective of whether or not the patient's blood studies show an acidosis. As soon as the respiratory rate returns to normal, daily Sulfamylon application may be reinstituted.

Silver nitrate soaks. Another effective topical antibacterial compound for use in burns is 0.5 per cent silver nitrate. Like Sulfamylon cream, this type of treatment diminishes infection in and around the burn wound. Its indications for use are similar to those for Sulfamylon. It prevents the growth of bacteria and does not interfere with epidermal proliferation.

The application of silver nitrate soaks is more involved than the Sulfamylon treatment, and requires more nursing personnel. The wound is cleansed and then the aqueous solution is applied in a large dressing directly to the burn wound. Approximately 40 layers of 4-ply, 9-inch dressing gauze are soaked with the solution of 0.5 per cent silver nitrate and closely applied to the wound surface with

elastic wrappings of gauze or stockinette. This dressing complex is kept dripping wet by the addition of silver nitrate solution every three or four hours between daily changes of the dressing. A patient treated by wet dressings must be covered with a layer or two of dry cotton sheeting or a blanket to minimize evaporation and the loss of heat through the dressing. Each day as the dressing is changed any loose eschar is gently pulled away.

There are several disadvantages with this technique, although in burn centers with sufficient personnel and facilities these problems are well managed. Silver nitrate stains black when it is exposed to light; therefore, bed clothing, nurses' and physicians' clothing and the materials on the ward must be segregated for the laundry. The sodium and chloride ions are rapidly diluted in the serum and they are also depleted with the use of these dressings. In children with large burns, this may occur within a matter of a few hours. Potassium deficiency is also seen, although it usually does not occur as rapidly. Calcium deficits have been noted. Electrolyte determinations must be done frequently in extensively burned patients. It is absolutely essential that supplementary sodium chloride, potassium and calcium be given. These supplements may be administered intravenously at first and later orally. Calcium lactate, 4 to

8 gm., should be given each day. If the serum calcium falls below 9 mg. per 100 ml., supplementary calcium gluconate should be given. After the fourth postburn day, 40 to 80 mEq. of potassium is necessary. Ten grams of sodium chloride and 30 to 50 ml. of molar sodium lactate are orally administered daily for burns covering 50 per cent of the body surface. This dosage is increased if the burns are of greater extent. These dosage schedules are for adults; correspondingly smaller doses are indicated for infants and children.

Removal of eschar. The ultimate aim in the treatment of full-thickness burns is to remove the eschar and apply a skin graft as soon as feasible. The technique for removal of eschar depends upon the extent of the burn and the type of local care employed. When occlusive dressings are used, the eschar softens and comes off earlier because of bacterial proliferation and autolysis beneath the eschar. When antibacterial agents such as Sulfamylon and silver nitrate are used, the eschar remains tightly adherent for a much longer period of time because bacterial growth is minimized.

If exposure or dressings are used, the eschar will usually begin to soften about the fourteenth day. Wet soaks may hasten its removal. When topical antibacterial therapy is used the eschar may remain firmly attached for 25 to 40 days. If the patient is burned over more than 40 per cent of the body surface, the eschar should be allowed to remain intact until all the surrounding deep dermal burn has healed. It may be necessary then to take the patient to the operating room and as gently as possible under anesthesia remove the dead, leathery eschar. In burns of lesser extent, removal of the eschar under anesthesia should be accomplished between the twenty-fifth and the thirtieth days.

WOUND COVERAGE. A split-thickness skin graft should be applied to the third-degree burned area as soon as the eschar is removed and the recipient site is prepared.

Preparation of recipient site. The aim in preparing a recipient site is to obtain a wound surface on which an excellent graft take may be expected. It is almost impossible, and certainly unnecessary, to sterilize a granulating surface for a good graft take. If the amount of purulent material and bacterial contamination are minimal, a graft will usually take unless the surface is colonized by Group A beta hemolytic streptococci.

Several methods may be employed to prepare the recipient site for grafting. In some instances frequent changes of dry dressings will achieve the desired result. Soaking the patient in a Hubbard tank daily cleanses the wound and removes debris. Wet dressings changed every four hours provide a good technique for preparing the recipient site. If homografts are available, their application every four or five days is an excellent method of treating the recipient site. The homografts must not be allowed to stay on the wound longer than five days or they will cause bleeding when they are removed.

When grafting has been delayed, soft, pale, heaping granulations are often present. Skin grafts do not take well on such granulations. They must be shaved down to the base and a dressing applied for two days. In old burns with a considerable amount of fibrous tissue beneath old granulations, it is advisable to excise the entire area down to the subcutaneous tissue or underlying fascia and graft two days later.

Grafting. Certain sites have priority for skin coverage. Areas around joints are covered before large flat surfaces, except in the extensively burned patient in whom rapid wound coverage must be obtained to save life. In most instances, skin should be placed first around the eyes, on the hands and other areas of motion such as the knees, elbows and axillae. When only the lower extremity is burned, priority should be given to the area around the knee, then the lower part of the leg, with the larger surface on the thigh being grafted later.

In extensive burns, flat surfaces should be covered with thin skin, approximately 0.010 to 0.012 of an inch in thickness. Skin for areas over joints should be somewhat thicker, about 0.015 of an inch.

The donor site should be the most accessible area from which skin can be taken and the site then properly exposed. This exposure is both effective and desirable. In extensively burned patients, every available area of skin should be used as a donor site. As soon as the wound is ready for grafting as much as possible of the area should be covered at the first grafting procedure. It may be necessary to take skin from the dorsum of the foot, the arms and unburned areas between granulating surfaces. It is frequently possible to graft anterior wounds from donor sites on the anterior surface at the first grafting procedure; then ten to 14 days later the patient can be turned on his abdomen, and skin removed from the posterior aspect of the body to cover recipient sites in that area.

Dermatomes. A variety of instruments is available for obtaining a split-thickness skin graft. The use of the electric dermatome is one of the outstanding advances in the care of burns in the past several years. Recently, this instrument has been equipped with an air-driven motor in place of the electric one. This new air-driven dermatome is much easier to use and cuts more evenly. With this instrument, large sheets of split-thickness skin can be obtained rapidly. When skin must be taken from irregular areas, infiltration of the subcutaneous tissue with saline provides an even, firm surface for cutting the grafts.

The drum-type dermatomes are useful over certain areas of the body, particularly the chest and abdomen. The wide sheets of skin available with the drum dermatome are particularly useful around joints, in the popliteal areas, and especially on the dorsum of the hand. In many grafting procedures, both types of dermatomes may be advantageous.

Some surgeons like to use the mesh dermatome when skin is in short supply. This dermatome permits a small piece of skin to be stretched to cover a larger surface. It has been of most value in treating children with extensive injuries.

Application of skin. There are many methods for the application of a skin graft. If the area is small, it is usually wise to apply a sheet of skin and suture it in place. When large flat surfaces are to be covered, the skin may be placed in lay-on fashion. Sheets of skin are placed on the wound and then pushed into position so that there is little space between the sheets. In areas of motion, especially on the hands and around joints, it is usually wise to suture large sheets of skin in place.

The best graft take is achieved when a skin graft is exposed. The skin is merely placed over the recipient site and no dressing is applied (Fig. 9). It usually begins to adhere within a matter of a few hours. Once or twice each day any serum that collects beneath the graft is rolled out by the use of a cotton-tipped applicator. When the patient is cooperative and the surface is one that lends itself to exposure of graft, this technique should be used. Unfortunately, many areas are not suitable for exposure and a dressing must be applied. The application of the dressing is most important because it maintains the graft in place. A large bulky dressing applied with even, resilient compression should be used. In some instances, it is wise to use a

stent dressing which is particularly useful on uneven surfaces or areas of motion. The dressing should be changed about four or five days after grafting.

Treatment of donor sites. For many years, the accepted method of treatment of donor sites has been the application of a large, bulky dressing. Infection frequently occurs on the moist surfaces underneath this dressing. In more recent years, it has been found advantageous to treat donor sites in the burned patients by the exposure method. Immediately after the skin has been removed, the donor area is covered by fine-mesh gauze. A moist gauze pad is applied for hemostasis. At the end of the operation, the gauze pad is removed but the fine-mesh gauze is left over the wound. Sometimes it is wise to apply a light dressing over the gauze and remove it 24 hours later. Blood will clot in the interstices of the gauze and form a firm coagulum. This coagulum dries, hardens in 48 hours and serves as a good protective covering. Epithelization proceeds beneath the coagulum, and the area usually heals within 14 days.

Homografts. In severely burned patients, providing temporary skin cover with homografts may be lifesaving. Homografts persist for 15 to 30 days and serve as a biologic skin dressing, preventing infection and the loss of body fluids. In some patients, autografts may be available to cover a portion of the wound and homografts may be used for the remainder. The decision to use homografts is always determined by the size of the wound and the general condition of the patient. In seriously ill patients, it is wise to apply homografts to close the wound until the nutritional status improves and autografts may be obtained. If it seems impossible to obtain autografts to close the wound in a reasonable period, the use of homografts as biologic skin covering is indicated. Homografts may be taken from live donors or recently deceased bodies.

NUTRITIONAL SUPPORT. The maintenance of blood volume of extensively burned patients during the grafting period is important. It is sometimes necessary to give transfusions as often as every other day. The hematocrit must be determined twice weekly and sufficient blood given to maintain it at about 40. Large quantities of blood are required for three reasons: the life of the red blood cell in the burned patient is not as long as in a normal patient; considerable blood is lost

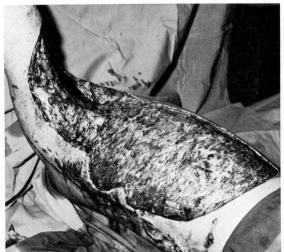

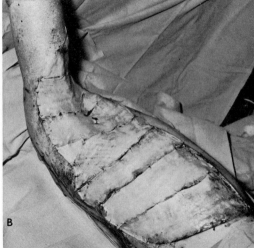

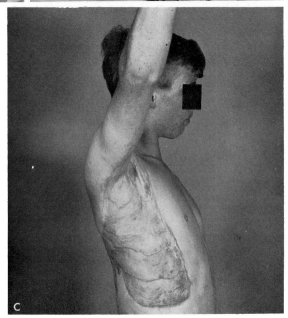

Figure 9. A, Area on arm, axilla and right chest of electrical injury has been excised. This has left a large open wound. A dressing was applied for three days. B, On the large open wound sheets of split-thickness skin have been placed in lay-on fashion. A few sutures of 4–0 silk are used to hold the grafts in place. This grafted area was completely exposed; no dressing was applied; the right arm was suspended by tying it to an intravenous standard. C, Complete healing of area after grafted area was treated by exposure. There is no evidence of contracture in the axilla.

from the oozing, granulating surfaces, particularly at the time of dressing changes; and infection in burn wounds depresses erythrocyte formation by the bone marrow.

In the early postburn period, a strongly negative nitrogen balance is characteristic of the severely burned patient because of large nitrogen losses and low nitrogen intake. The duration and magnitude of negative nitrogen balance is influenced by the severity of the burn as well as by the nutritional regimen used (Fig. 10). Negative nitrogen balance is more intense and persists longer in extensive burns than in small ones.

An energetic nutritional regimen, instituted seven to ten days after burning, is desirable.

It should be comprised of a high protein, high caloric diet with supplemental high protein liquid nourishment given as between-meal feedings. A daily protein intake of 2 to 3 gm. per kg. of body weight is desirable. In most adults, the daily intake should range from 150 to 220 gm. of protein. The caloric intake should be 50 to 75 calories per kg. per day. Routine vitamin supplements are recommended as follows: ascorbic acid, 1500 mg.; thiamine, 50 mg.; riboflavin, 50 mg.; and nicotinamide, 500 mg. Oral feeding is preferred; occasionally, however, when a patient will not voluntarily consume an adequate intake, it may be necessary to provide nutritional support by nasogastric tube feeding.

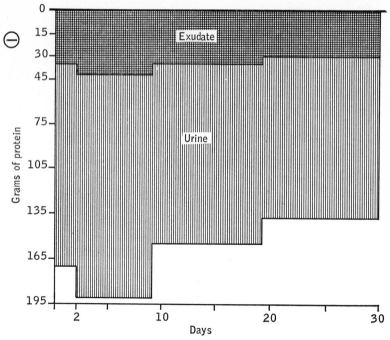

Figure 10. Composite protein losses typical of a 25 per cent second- and third-degree burn in an average adult male. The losses in grams of protein are plotted from the zero line down. During the first eight days, the loss of protein approximates 190 gm. per day. Extensive losses continue for the first 30 days and then diminish as wound coverage is achieved. Most of the protein is lost in the urine, but the exudate is usually responsible for 15 to 20 per cent of the loss.

Severely burned patients may lose as much as 1 pound a day fof the first 30 days post burn. As soon ás the wound is closed, positive nitrogen balance can be achieved and a weight gain program started. One of the most important factors in the recovery of an extensively burned patient is his acceptance of a large intake of protein and calories each day. The use of narcotics after the first day or two should be discouraged because they have a tendency to interfere with the patient's nutritional intake.

COMPLICATIONS. An extensively burned patient has suffered a severe form of trauma and, therefore, is prone to a variety of complications. Many of these complications are the immediate result of thermal tissue destruction or the natural concomitant of a serious and prolonged illness. Some are iatrogenic, however, and can be avoided with proper care.

Infection. Infection is the cardinal problem in the treatment of burns. Although appropriately treated second-degree burns usually heal without any evidence of infection, all third-degree burns become infected because the protective barrier, the skin, is destroyed. The newer methods of local care such as Sulfamylon cream and silver nitrate soaks aim at the control of this infection.

In second-degree burns and donor sites, local infection can usually be controlled by appropriate systemic antibiotic therapy and frequent changes of dressings. Infections caused by *Pseudomonas aeruginosa* in second-degree burns and donor sites can be brought under control by simple exposure of the wound.

Local invasive infection is manifested by clinical signs such as cellulitis, lymphangitis and general lymph adenopathy. A culture in or around the burned area usually determines the primary offending organism. The best treatment is the administration of the appropriate antibiotic systemically and warm, moist compresses to the area.

The source of systemic infection in the burned patient is usually the wound itself. The bacterial inoculum originates from the burn wound even in those instances in which the infection can be classified as iatrogenic. A common example is the thrombus which develops on the intimal surface of a vein at the site where a chronically indwelling intravenous catheter has damaged the wall. Many infections in burns can be attributed to this etiology. The most common offending organism associated with septic phlebitis is *Staphylococcus aureus*. Such a thrombus may be the source of bacteremia and septic emboli to various organs of the body. Therapy must be directed toward the removal of the catheter and the administration of an appropriate antibiotic in large doses. Other sites of iatrogenic sepsis are the genitourinary tract secondary to chronic indwelling urethral catheters and the upper respiratory system as the result of tracheostomy.

Overwhelming sepsis. The most common cause of overwhelming sepsis in burns is *Ps. aeruginosa*. Such sepsis is unique in that there are few organisms existing within the blood at any one time, but the involvement is primarily by way of the lymphatics. This embolic involvement is not particularly characteristic as is the case when such sepsis is caused by the staphylococcus.

The first symptom of overwhelming sepsis is an increase in the already febrile state, clouding of the sensorium and paralytic ileus. The intermittent disorientation rapidly becomes more profound and persistent; abdominal distention is a prominent feature. The wound then begins to deteriorate, and a relative hypothermia may supervene with hypotension and oliguria as the terminal events. The development of overwhelming sepsis is an insidious process usually becoming progressively more severe over a period of three or four days.

The use of topical chemotherapeutic agents from the first treatment of the burn injury is aimed at the prevention of sepsis. Once overwhelming sepsis has become established, therapy is very difficult. Treatment consists of massive doses of systemic antibiotic therapy on the basis of the predominant organisms cultured from the wound or blood. This may mean the simultaneous administration of two or three antibiotics. In addition, every effort is made to remove gently the devitalized tissue whenever possible. If the dead tissue can be removed, homografts should be applied. The homografts are ordinarily put on without dressing so that they can be inspected several times a day. When purulence develops beneath, the area is evacuated and the homograft reapplied. This usually means removal of the homograft and reapplication every day or two.

Every effort should be made to provide the best supportive therapy possible. Since the insensible water loss in patients with sepsis is quite high, careful attention must be given to providing an adequate quantity of water either orally or intravenously. The requirement for blood is greatly increased during septicemia and two or three transfusions a week may be necessary to maintain the hematocrit at about 40.

Acute dilatation of stomach. This complication is more common than is usually recognized and may occur during the first week after injury. It is characterized by regurgitation of fluid, upper abdominal distress and dyspnea. It is important to recognize this complication immediately; burned patients frequently aspirate after regurgitation of fluids, and aspiration in a critically ill patient may lead to death.

Curling's ulcer. An acute ulceration occurring in the stomach or duodenum associated with burns has come to be known as Curling's ulcer. It is almost invariably associated with extensive burns or moderate burns with significant sepsis. The cause of the acute ulceration is unknown. Clinical studies have failed to demonstrate any consistent relation with gastric acid or uropepsin secretion. The lesions are seen with more frequency in the stomach than in the duodenum. In the stomach, they are more frequently multiple, small, elongated and usually hidden within the mucosal folds. In the duodenum, the lesion is characteristically single, located on the posterior wall, large and deeply penetrating.

Symptoms other than epigastric discomfort or some distention are rarely present except when massive hemorrhage occurs. Frequently, the first symptom of Curling's ulcer is hemorrhage.

It is difficult to make a positive diagnosis of such an ulcer because the patient is usually too ill to withstand a satisfactory roentgenographic study of the upper gastrointestinal tract. Should hemorrhage occur, management should be similar to the treatment of bleeding from a chronic duodenal ulcer. A bleeding Curling's ulcer usually is a single ulcer in the duodenum or one or two large ulcers in the stomach. The same indications for surgical intervention that apply to a bleeding chronic duodenal ulcer should apply to Curling's ulcer. The surgeon usually determines the type of operative procedure after the abdomen is opened and the site of the bleeding is determined.

Miscellaneous complications. Fecal impaction is particularly common in the burned patient. Prolonged immobilization and dehydration lead to the development of impaction. Cystitis and urethritis are complications of prolonged indwelling catheters. Urinary catheters should be removed as early as possible. Pulmonary edema may follow excessive fluid therapy. Pneumonia is not uncommon in children and elderly patients. Burns about the face and neck are frequently complicated by respiratory tract injury and major lung pathology.

In deep circumferential injury of the extremities and of the chest, troublesome constriction may occur when the eschar dehydrates and contracts. Circumferential chest eschars must be incised to permit adequate expansion of the chest. Relaxing incisions should be made in constricting extremity eschars to prevent vascular insufficiency of the distal extremities.

Decubitus ulcers are prone to develop in the extensively burned patient. They may occur in the sacral region, over the anterior superior iliac spine, on the posterior aspect of the head and on the back of the heel.

Chemical burns. Most chemical burns occur in laboratories and industrial plants. In time of war, chemical burns are caused by phosphorus, magnesium and vesicant gases. Acute injury to the skin resulting from chemical agents is similar to that caused by heat. In fact, injurious effects of the chemical are sometimes due in part to the development of heat. The lesions produced by a chemical agent present a pathologic picture showing different degrees of destruction from a central zone of necrosis to a peripheral hyperemic zone.

Alkali burns are usually caused by sodium hydroxide, potassium hydroxide or calcium oxide. Alkalis exert their pathologic effect in three ways: by saponifying the fat; by extracting considerable water from the cells because of their hydroscopic nature and by dissolving and uniting with the proteins of the tissues to form alkaline proteinates. The initial treatment for burns caused by a strong alkaline solution is washing with large quantities of water. Pouring the water over the area permits the fluid to carry away excess alkaline agents as well as the heat of dissolution. In lime burns, the dry lime should be brushed away before washing so that the calcium oxide will not unite with water to form calcium hydroxide, a reaction which produces a tremendous amount of heat.

Concentrated acids withdraw water from cells and precipitate proteins to form acid proteinates. Sulfuric acid converts the corroded tissue into a greenish black or dark brown slough. Nitric acid causes a yellow color, which becomes a yellowish brown. Hydrochloric acid is a much more severe caustic than nitric or sulfuric acid and stains the skin yellowish brown. Trichloracetic acid is the most corrosive of all organic acids. It forms a white, soft slough. Phenol, a destructive and poisonous organic acid, causes an initial white slough which turns to a greenish

black or copper color. Acid burns should be treated by diluting or removing the acid as rapidly as possible, usually by irrigation with large quantities of water. After removing the maximum amount of acid by washing, the remainder may be neutralized by a weak solution of baking soda.

Phosphorus burns are extremely painful and a common injury of modern warfare. This substance melts at body temperature and penetrates deeply into the tissue. The particles of phosphorus continue to cause damage until washed or picked out of the wound. The wound can be seen to emit smoke if the phosphorus is exposed to air and in the dark the wounds glow with a blue-green color. When the injury is extensive, there may be hepatic and renal damage. For decades it has been advocated that copper sulfate is the optimal substance for the therapy of burns caused by organic phosphorus. The use of this agent is based on its reaction with phosphorus to produce an inert shell of cupric phosphide over the surface of the organic phosphorus. This inactivates the phosphorus and stops the tissue destruction. At the same time, it colors the particles black so that they can be identified and removed. There is some evidence that large doses of copper sulfate may lead to copper toxicity manifested primarily by massive hemolysis of red blood cells and subsequent acute renal tubular necrosis. When copper sulfate is used great care must be taken to wash it from the wound and to maintain adequate urinary flow either by the use of an appropriate fluid load or mannitol.

Magnesium burns produce ulcers which are small at first but gradually enlarge to form an extensive lesion. Magnesium may be a rapid or slow-burning ember depending upon the size of the particles involved. If the slow-burning embers penetrate deeper than the outer layers of the skin, they must be excised completely and the resulting wound closed by skin grafting.

Mustard gas and lewisite are war gases which cause severe blister formation. Early care consists of washing with large amounts of water. Later definitive care is the same as that for other second-degree burns.

ELECTRICAL INJURY. Damage after electrical injury is frequently referred to as an electrical burn. Because there is usually damage to the deeper tissues by the electricity, an electrical injury more nearly simulates crush injury than it does a thermal burn (Fig. 11).

ELECTRICAL INJURY IS :

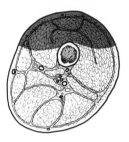 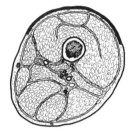

more   *than*

CRUSH INJURY   BURN

Figure 11.   Schematic outlines emphasizing that electrical injury is a deep injury and is more like a crush injury than a thermal burn.

Damage associated with electricity may be divided into three categories:

Electric contact injury caused by an electric current passing through the skin pro-duces damage to the skin's subcutaneous tissue, muscle and other deeper structures. It is well known that the current follows blood vessels and that thrombosis even at some distance from the original injury is common. This thrombosis is at least partly responsible for the fact that more tissue is always destroyed by an electrical injury than is apparent at first inspection. Necrosis of blood vessel walls frequently leads to secondary hemorrhage. The histologic appearance of the dead muscle varies. Immediate heat coagulative changes add a pale appearance to the muscle. As time progresses, some muscle becomes soft. The death of muscle bundles is usually very uneven. It is not infrequent after the first five or six days to find nonviable muscle present where there is a good nutrient artery in normal conditions supplying the muscle bundle. One of the delayed effects of electrical injury, especially about the head, is the development of cataracts.

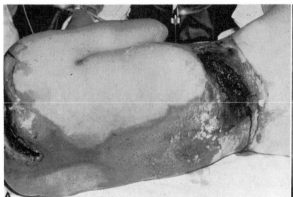 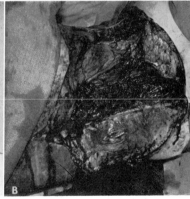

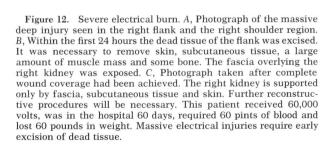 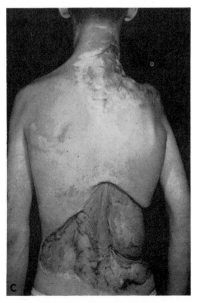

Figure 12.   Severe electrical burn. *A*, Photograph of the massive deep injury seen in the right flank and the right shoulder region. *B*, Within the first 24 hours the dead tissue of the flank was excised. It was necessary to remove skin, subcutaneous tissue, a large amount of muscle mass and some bone. The fascia overlying the right kidney was exposed. *C*, Photograph taken after complete wound coverage had been achieved. The right kidney is supported only by fascia, subcutaneous tissue and skin. Further reconstructive procedures will be necessary. This patient received 60,000 volts, was in the hospital 60 days, required 60 pints of blood and lost 60 pounds in weight. Massive electrical injuries require early excision of dead tissue.

Electrothermal burns which result from the electrical generation of heat outside the skin, such as flash or arc burns, occur by the leaping of an electric arc from the conductor to the skin. These are mainly associated with high tension current. They are severe burns of the skin caused by high intensity heat of short duration.

Flame burns resulting from the ignition of clothing by electrical sparks or arcing are associated with electrical injury, the lesion varying according to the type of accident. Many times all three types of injury may be evident in the same patient.

The treatment of electrothermal burns and flame burns associated with ignition of clothing is the same as for any similar thermal injury. The management of a true electrical injury is entirely different. Such an injury must be treated more like a crush injury. Renal damage is more common and, therefore, massive replacement therapy is essential. In many instances, the use of an osmotic diuretic is indicated. Electrical injury frequently requires the use of whole blood in the first 24 hours. If there is a massive amount of dead tissue, an emergency operation to amputate the part or remove the dead tissue may be necessary.

One of the most important factors in the management of the local wound is the incision of the overlying damaged skin to ascertain whether or not there is deeper injury such as dead muscle. If dead muscle is present, it must be excised. Failure to remove extensively damaged muscle may lead to clostridial myositis and death. After excision, a dressing should be applied and the wound reinspected with possible further debridement four days later (Fig. 12).

With small, low intensity electrical injuries the areas should be kept clean and observed for several days. Many of these heal without too much difficulty. Other areas, with moderate electrical injury, may be observed until they are well demarcated at seven or eight days after injury and then excised.

COLD INJURY

Cold injury is trauma produced by exposure to cold and includes such entities as chilblains, frostbite, immersion foot and trench foot. The type of injury produced is dependent upon the degree of cold to which the body is exposed, the duration of the exposure and environmental factors which intensify the effect of the low temperatures.

Chilblains result from exposure to temperatures above freezing associated with high humidity. The term immersion foot implies a cold injury of the feet resulting from prolonged exposure, usually in excess of 12 hours, in water at temperatures below 50° F. Trench foot results from prolonged exposure to cold at temperatures from just above freezing to 50° F. and wetness of the feet. The term frostbite is applied when crystallization of tissue fluids occurs in the skin or subcutaneous tissue. It is produced by exposure at temperatures of freezing or below. High altitude frostbite results from exposure at high altitudes to temperatures usually varying from −20 to −80° F. The areas most commonly affected are the feet and toes, hands and fingers, and ears and nose.

Cold injury occurs sporadically in the civilian population, but is of primary concern in the military service. It has been recognized as a problem of military importance since the days of Alexander of Macedonia. Napoleon's famous surgeon, Baron Larrey, classically described the role which cold injury played in the defeat of Napoleon's army in Poland in 1812. It was of considerable military significance in World War II, in aerial battles, in the Battle of Ardennes Forest during December, 1944, and at the Chosen Reservoir during the Korean conflict in 1951. Among United States troops, there were approximately 92,000 cases of cold injury during World War II and more than 9000 during the Korean War.

PATHOGENESIS.   There are two main theories concerning the pathogenesis of frostbite. The first postulates that the tissue injury is secondary to vasoconstriction, vasodilatation, edema, sludging of erythrocytes in capillaries, and thrombosis with subsequent necrosis of tissue. The second theory postulates that the tissue injury is due to the direct action of the cold on tissue cells, a true thermal injury.

Exposure to cold causes vasoconstriction of the arterioles and small arteries. This vasoconstriction contributes to local tissue anoxia. When frozen tissue is placed in a warm environment, thawing occurs first along the course of the blood vessels. Vasodilatation subsequently occurs with an outpouring of protein-rich fluid through capillary walls rendered hyperpermeable by the effects of cold or anoxia. Edema and capillary stasis then develop. Tissue necrosis can be attributed to vascular occlusion from conversion of sludged blood to agglutinative thrombi and thrombosis.

This vascular theory appeared to be adequate in explaining entirely the pathogenesis of cold injury until it was experimentally demonstrated that cold causes direct tissue injury. Degenerative changes in muscle fibers have been noted as early as 15 minutes after exposure to cold. Marked changes occur in four to six hours and gross necrosis has been noted after 72 hours. Most surgeons favor the vascular theory in the pathogenesis of cold injury in man.

Tissues do not show the same degree of susceptibility to cold injury. Nerves and striated muscle are highly sensitive; skin, fascia and connective tissue are quite resistant, but not as resistant as compact bone or tendon. Blood vessels are highly susceptible to injury, resulting in leakage of plasma into the surrounding tissue. This difference in resistance has resulted in the observation of muscle gangrene in humans and animals, without necrosis of the overlying skin following exposure to cold.

SYMPTOMS AND SIGNS. Usually, there is an uncomfortable sensation of coldness followed by numbness. There may be a tingling, stinging or aching sensation. The skin is first red, but later becomes pale or waxy white.

The clinical manifestations and course subsequent to rewarming vary with the severity of the cold injury, which may be classified into four degrees: first degree, hyperemia and edema; second degree, hyperemia with blister formation; third degree, necrosis of skin and subcutaneous tissue; and fourth degree, complete necrosis and loss of tissue.

In *first-degree frostbite,* the skin becomes mottled blue or purple, then red. Swelling begins within three hours; the edema persists for ten days or more. Desquamation of the superficial layers of the skin begins five to ten days after injury. Hyperhidrosis and coldness of the injured part may appear two to three weeks after injury, and may persist for many months.

Second-degree frostbite is characterized by hyperemia and edema with vesicle formation appearing 12 to 24 hours after rewarming. The edema is usually not marked and disappears within five days. The blisters dry and form black eschars within 11 to 24 days. Throbbing and aching pain are noted three to 20 days after injury. The eschar gradually desquamates, revealing an intact skin which is thin, soft and easily injured (Figs. 13 and 14).

Third-degree frostbite involves the full thickness of the skin and extends into the subcutaneous tissue, leading to ulceration. Vesicles may be present at the periphery of the area of damage. Edema of the entire part may occur. This usually disappears in about six days. Most patients have burning, aching, throbbing or shooting pains which may persist for five weeks. The skin overlying the area of third-degree frostbite forms a black, hard, dry eschar. This eschar finally desquamates and the remaining ulcer epithelizes. Healing occurs in about two and one-half months.

Fourth-degree frostbite is characterized

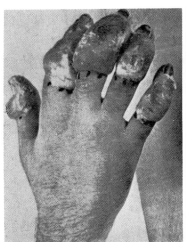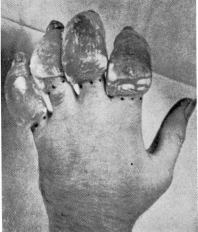

Figure 13.   Photograph of severe blistering which occurs with high altitude frostbite 24 hours after injury.

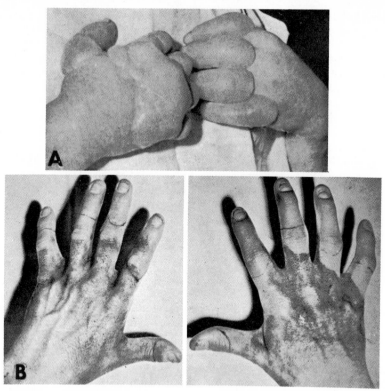

Figure 14.   *A*, Photograph of severe blistering following high altitude frostbite 24 hours after injury. *B*, Appearance of hands two months later. The lost nails show regeneration and the skin is beginning to recover its normal surface markings. Sensory disturbances and loss of sweating persisted for many months.

by destruction of the entire part including the bone. Edema may extend far beyond the area of frostbite. There may be severe paresthesia, which appears three to 13 days after rewarming. The injured tissues become black, dry, shriveled and mummified. Usually, the area appears as dry gangrene. The line of demarcation becomes apparent in about one month, and extends down to the bone in two months or more.

PRODUCTION OF COLD INJURY.   Cold is the specific agent in cold injury and is the immediate cause of tissue damage. A variety of environmental and host factors influence the incidence, type and severity of the injury. Weather is a predominant influence in the causation of cold injury. Low temperatures and low relative humidity favor frostbite, whereas higher temperatures together with moisture are usually associated with trench foot.

Wind chill is considered to be one of the important factors in the production of cold injuries. Wind velocity greatly increases wind chill. For example, a temperature of 38° F., with a wind velocity of 10 miles an hour, has the same effect on exposed flesh as a temperature of 0° F. at a wind velocity of 1 mile an hour.

Increasing tissue heat loss is a most important factor in cold injury. Wind blast was a prominent feature leading to the development of cold injuries in high-altitude bomber crew members during the early part of World War II. On the ground, lesser cold breezes favor the development of cold injury. The movement of cold air removes the warm layer of insulating air from around the exposed parts. When water or metal replaces air as the medium surrounding cold-exposed parts, cold injury is more apt to occur than when air is the medium, since water and metal conduct heat better than does air. Persons with wet feet develop injury at considerably higher temperatures than those exposed in cold, dry air. Contact of the skin with cold metal can produce almost instantaneous freezing of tissue.

Conditions which decrease the internal heat supply include those which mechanically obstruct blood flow to the extremities, such as constrictive clothing or other pressure-producing objects. Tight or stiff clothing is especially harmful if individuals must remain in cramped quarters with arms and legs flexed. Wet clothing is especially dangerous. Environmental protection, including shelter and the quality and quantity of clothing has a profound effect upon the development of cold injuries.

The fact that freezing and nonfreezing injuries are the same pathologically, and that both may or may not result in gangrene, emphasizes that it is not the attained tissue temperature which will determine the final injury, but the product of the temperature, the conducting medium and the exposure time.

It has been shown experimentally, by covering exposed parts with rubber boots during immersion, that water merely acts as a thermal conductor in the production of immersion type injuries. Maceration of the skin, commonly observed in immersion injuries, is not due to cold but is a local effect of moisture.

The majority of cold injuries are of the nonfreezing type and are generally associated with wetness with the ambient temperatures several degrees above freezing. Immersion of extremities in the South Atlantic Ocean at temperatures of 60 to 70° F. for days or even weeks produced serious cold injuries, often with gangrene, during World War II. Actual solidification of tissue from freezing has been observed relatively rarely. Probably, in most persons with frostbite incurred during exposure to dry air at below-freezing temperatures, actual freezing has not occurred. Under such conditions of exposure, the body can defend against cold effectively in spite of steep temperature gradients existing between the body and the surrounding atmosphere, because air is a good thermal insulator. Prolonged exposure may be endured without tissue solidification, although sufficiently severe chilling does occur to produce damage.

TREATMENT. The treatment of cold injury remains somewhat controversial. Anticoagulant therapy would appear to be the treatment of choice if the vascular theory of pathogenesis is correct. A few investigators believe heparin is of value, the majority do not. Although the early use of heparin may be of value, its efficacy was not proved in the treatment of frostbite in Korea. Sympathetic nerve interruption, like other methods of increasing the blood supply to a frozen extremity, was for a long time condemned without trial. Several investigators believe

that lumbar blocks, sympathectomy or the use of vasodilators such as Priscoline are of value, but extensive use of vasodilators in the treatment of frostbite in Korea did not prove to be of significant value. Lumbar blocks and early sympathectomy were also of little or no value. The trial of unilateral sympathectomy in bilateral cold injury of the feet resulted in no significant difference in the amount of tissue loss and the residuals in the two feet.

The treatment of cold injury may be divided into the emergency management and later hospital management. Initially, all constricting items of clothing such as boots, gloves and socks should be removed. The injured parts, if still frozen, should be rapidly rewarmed by immersion in warm water at 90 to 104° F., and the general body warmth is maintained. Large vesicles or bullae are covered with a loose, dry dressing. Petrolatum dressings must not be applied. A booster dose of tetanus toxoid and penicillin should be administered.

Definitive treatment includes absolute bed rest for those with cold injury of the feet. The patient should be kept in bed until subsidence of edema or complete drying of vesicles has occurred. Patients with third-degree injury remain in bed longer, until areas of ulceration have been epithelized; those with fourth-degree injury, until treated surgically.

All lesions are exposed to the air, and a ward temperature of 70 to 74° F. should be maintained. Smoking is discouraged. Active physical therapy is instituted at the bedside as soon as possible. Attention is directed toward the position of the feet and movement of the fingers, toes and other major joints to prevent ankylosis. Second-, third- and fourth-degree lesions are cleansed daily with a mild antiseptic solution such as aqueous Zephiran solution. Superficial debridement of broken vesicles or necrotic tissue must be accomplished frequently. Suppurative eschars and partially detached toenails should be removed. Lesions must first be cleansed with hydrogen peroxide solution, then soaked in normal saline for 30 minutes before starting debridement. The necrotic eschar on digits is bivalved early to prevent contraction and further tissue damage. Patients with third- and fourth-degree injuries remain on antibiotic therapy until their lesions have dried.

Buerger's exercises may be started as soon as the lesions show signs of healing. As soon as the eschar has desquamated, whirlpool therapy should be started and continued for two weeks. Emergency amputations are seldom indicated except in unusual cases with extensive wet gangrene and general sepsis. The part is not ready for amputation until the edge of the eschar has separated from the normal tissues by the ingrowth of epithelium. There is no specific therapy for cold injury; prevention is the only cure.

RADIATION INJURY

One of the outstanding features of twentieth century medicine is the increasing role played by radiation. Radiation serves the physician as an indispensable tool in diagnosis and therapy. The widespread industrial use of radiation, however, has created a problem in public health, and the application of radiation in warfare has made radiation effects a major subject of military medicine.

Radiation may be divided into two major groups. *Electromagnetic radiation* comprises, in addition to visible light, the infrared, ultraviolet, x- and gamma rays. These electromagnetic oscillations have different wavelengths, but all travel with the speed of light (3×10^{10} cm. per sec.). *Corpuscular radiation* comprises alpha and beta particles, neutrons, protons and positrons. All these radiations are characterized by a mass and, with the exception of the neutron, by an electrical charge.

DEFINITIONS. For a clear understanding of radiation injury, it is necessary that there be proper definition of terms. *Alpha particles* are nonpenetrating rays bearing a positive charge. They are stopped by the thickness of a single sheet of paper and travel in air a distance of 2.7 to 8.6 cm., depending upon their energy. Because of their inability to penetrate tissue, they are essentially harmless as external sources of irradiation.

Beta particles are actually electron particles of small mass and carry a negative charge. They are ejected from their parent atoms at much higher speeds than alpha particles, some with velocities approximating that of light. Most of them do not penetrate 1 mm. thickness of lead. In body tissue, they penetrate only thin layers and are therapeutically of value only when they can be employed under circumstances where this characteristic can be of advantage. The

measurement of beta emitters within the body is made possible with the Geiger counter or sensitive scintillation detectors, which detect the soft x-rays resulting from beta energy absorption in tissue.

Gamma rays travel with the speed of light, are electromagnetic but are not electrically charged. They are capable of penetrating several centimeters of lead. Because gamma rays usually have a shorter wavelength than x-rays, their penetrating power is generally greater. X-rays are also electromagnetic and uncharged, and are considered identical with gamma radiation of other sources.

Technical developments in physics and radiology have been enormous during the past 20 years. X-ray machines currently employed in treatment include the 10 kv. grenzray machine used by the dermatologists and the 100 and 400 kv. machines employed by the radiologists for superficial and deep therapy. X-ray generators of the two million volt variety are currently in use in many hospitals. Betatrons of various designs for x-ray and electron generation range upward from 30 million volts. Recently, the proton beam of the cyclotron has been under test in the treatment of malignant disease.

A number of units for biologic measurement of radiation have been devised to determine radiation exposure in biologic tissue. The basic unit of dosimetry of ionizing radiations is represented by the roentgen (*r*). Its form was adopted by the International Commission of Radiological Units in Chicago in 1937, and confirmed in London in 1950: "The roentgen shall be the quantity of x- or gamma radiation such that the associated corpuscular emission per 0.001293 gm. of air produces in air, ions carrying one electrostatic unit of quantity of electricity of either sign." The roentgen-equivalent physical (*rep*) is defined as 1 rep, the energy absorption dose in irradiated tissue of 93 ergs per gm. The roentgen-equivalent man (*rem*) is the estimated amount of energy absorbed in tissue which is biologically equivalent in man to 1 r of gamma or x-rays. The radiation absorbed dose (*rad*) is used to define the absorbed dose of any ionizing radiation. One rad is 100 ergs per gram.

ACUTE RADIATION INJURY

An understanding that not all tissues and cells are equally sensitive to radiation injury must be reached to appreciate the different clinical responses to varying doses. Certain tissues and cells, including the lymphoid tissue, bone marrow and blood cells are especially sensitive. Other tissues and organs are moderately sensitive to such injury. These include gastrointestinal mucosa, adrenal and thyroid tissue. In higher doses, injury to these predominates the clinical symptoms. Resistant or relatively resistant cells and tissues include nerve cells, bone, the eyes and muscles. With large doses, injury to these structures becomes manifest before injury to the more sensitive parts has time to reveal itself.

SOURCES OF INFORMATION ON HUMAN INJURY. In addition to animal experimentation and experiences with x-ray, radium and radioisotopes in clinical therapy, information on acute radiation injury in man is limited to a few disasters.

The Japanese bomb casualties represent the greatest number of human beings ever exposed to large doses of penetrating ionizing radiation. Although the Atomic Bomb Casualty Commission has derived and continues to derive much useful information about the late and long-term effects of radiation, poor recording of the early findings gives little information about the acute and immediate effect. The clinical course of radiation injury, as it appeared following the bombings at Hiroshima and Nagasaki, is now known to have been influenced by confusion generated by the use of the weapon. There is disagreement among qualified physicists concerning the dose and energy of radiations received at various points from ground zero. Many useful data, however, have come from the careful study of this group of patients.

The Marshall Islands fallout radiation victims, injured as a consequence of an unpredicted wind change following the detonation of a thermonuclear device on Bikini Atoll in March, 1954, comprise a large group of patients with radiation injury from which abundant useful information has been derived. Included with the natives of the island were 28 American servicemen and 23 Japanese fishermen, a total of 290 persons. Unlike the Japanese victims after atomic detonation, the patients from the Marshall Islands were very carefully documented. A close approximation of the whole body exposure dose was available. The fact that the maximum dose received by a relatively small number of the victims was in the vicinity of 175 r is the major limiting factor on the data from this group.

Laboratory and industrial accidents involving approximately 30 individuals in the United States, Russia and Yugoslavia constitute a small but extremely valuable group from the viewpoint of medical data. The small number of injuries over nearly 20 years of research and military application of radioactive matter is profound testimony to the care and control exercised by those governing the use of such materials. In these accidents, the dose is well documented and encompasses a range from trivial levels to many thousand roentgens.

Although each of the categories of radiation victims has limitations imposed on the data provided, the information from each group reinforced or complemented by findings from the other groups and from animal research provides sufficient material from which to extract typical clinical symptoms to describe a wide range of dose-effect relationships.

CLINICAL DESCRIPTION. The acute radiation syndrome follows total body receipt of gamma rays, neutrons, or both. The type and severity of response in man is especially dose-dependent. In describing the syndrome, it is presumed that all doses are received in a short period, up to 48 hours; that the body is uniformly irradiated; that no significant prior or concomitant injury exists; that the dose is known; and that the individual is neither excessively resistant nor excessively sensitive to radiation. The injury which follows may be described for clinical purposes in four categories: no obvious disease; the hematopoietic form, manifested by injury to the blood and blood-forming organs; the gastrointestinal form, manifested by injury to organs of the gastrointestinal tract, and the cerebral form, manifested by injury to the central nervous system.

No obvious disease. The state of no obvious disease implies there is no apparent clinical symptomatology or disability, even though there may be demonstrable alterations of the blood and tissues on laboratory analysis. The range of absorbed dose for this effect is perhaps up to 100 r. Victims of this amount of radiation require no treatment and certainly no hospitalization.

Hematopoietic form. The hematopoietic form of acute radiation injury occurs when the total dose absorbed is in the range of 100 to 1000 r. The clinical severity and mortality is directly related to the severity of the dose. The hematopoietic form of the disease is the type that is of greatest concern for it represents the radiation injury in which proper treatment may exert considerable influence on its course. The type of response is usually uniform and, for the most part, predictable. The typical hematopoietic form of the syndrome, which occurs in an average individual after receiving 300 to 350 r, provides a basis for understanding the clinical nature of the injury and the alterations that different doses and treatments may make.

The typical hematopoietic form is characterized by four phases: a prodromal phase, a latent phase, a bone marrow depression phase and a recovery phase.

The *prodromal phase* is a two- or three-day period characterized by signs and symptoms similar to those of motion sickness. The laboratory findings are those of nonspecific mild leukocytosis with a relative and absolute lymphopenia. True diarrhea is not characteristic of the hematopoietic form of the disease. Immediately after receiving 300 to 350 r, there may be no subjective sensations or objective findings. Within a few hours listlessness, fatigue, disinterest and sometimes lethargy appear. When the victim knows or suspects he has been exposed to an appreciable radiation injury, his psychogenic reaction may produce symptoms which confuse or obscure the true sequence of changes caused by radiation. The initial symptoms become increasingly more severe and are associated with headache, anorexia, nausea and vomiting. Maximum severity of symptoms is reached by the fifth to the eighth hour. Some authorities feel that the severity of nausea and vomiting in the prodromal phase may be directly proportional to the amount of food in the stomach at the time of injury, and may be prolonged by attempts to feed the patient. By the end of the second day, a state of comparative well-being is regained with mild cyclic fatigue as the only residual symptom. Vomiting during the prodromal phase may be the only symptom of value in estimating the degree of injury if psychogenic overlay can be discounted. Vomiting which occurs late and is of short duration suggests a lower dose than that which occurs early and is severe and prolonged. In doses below 100 r, vomiting rarely occurs. The laboratory findings during the prodromal phase are limited to alterations in the peripheral blood. Although serial bone marrow studies, mitotic indices, thymidine uptake determinations, complicated enzyme studies, examination of hair roots and determination of changes in platelet structure give an indication of severity of injury, they are difficult laboratory maneuvers and may be of little practical value. The earlier changes in the peripheral blood involve a decrease in the lymphocyte count, which occurs within hours, and fluctuation in the total white cell count, showing a mild overall increase during the first few days. Since a baseline white cell count prior to the injury is never available, changes in this parameter may be of little diagnostic or prognostic value. The early lymphopenia, however, is suggestive of radiation damage; it is appreciable with high doses and less definite with low doses. A rising lymphocyte count after the first few days is usually associated with a good prognosis.

The *latent phase* begins on the third or fourth day, depending upon the severity of the initial reaction. It persists for about three weeks from the time of exposure and is characterized by a remarkable freedom from symptoms. In some individuals, mild recurrent fatigue may occur. The laboratory findings in the early part of this phase fail to suggest the severity of the disturbances to come. There is a progressive decrease in the total white cell count, which is moderate for granulocytes and quite pronounced for lymphocytes. Near the end of the second week after exposure, epilation occurs. Since epilation occurs with exposure to more than 300 r, the loss of hair is of significance only insofar as it attests to the probability that the dose was at least that high to the parts that epilate. All body and head hair is subject to loss following a large enough dose of radiation, but the hair of the eyebrows and lashes is apparently less sensitive than that of other parts of the body. During this phase, the victim continues to feel well and is able to perform his normal duties.

The *bone marrow depression phase* beginning during the third week starts with the return of signs and symptoms suggesting the onset of an acute infectious process. Chills, fever, malaise, increased fatigability and pharyngitis may occur. Within the next few days, the clinical status deteriorates rapidly, causing the patient to be hospitalized. The oropharynx becomes swollen; the gums and tonsillar areas show a marked reaction and early ulceration. As the disease progresses, a tendency to bruise easily or to bleed slightly from the gums appears. Coincident with these findings in the mouth and on the skin, the general condition of the patient reflects the compromise that has affected his blood-forming organs. Steplike fever suggests septicemia. Petechiae and ecchymosis may involve broad zones of the skin. In very severe forms of the disease, the hemorrhagic phenomenon may involve the lining and covering of internal organs. Despite earlier predictions based on bomb casualty data in Japan, gross hemorrhage from the orifices and into the hollow organs is usually not massive and continuous, but is generally self-limiting. The return of illness and the signs, symptoms and laboratory findings associated with it produce a classic picture of acute aplastic anemia. A continuous fall in white blood cells and platelets, ulceration of the mucous membranes, septicemia and bacteremia following absorption of organisms from the damaged gastrointestinal tract present serious clinical symptoms associated with severe bone marrow injury. In the typical patient, the symptoms and findings reach maximum severity between the fourth and fifth weeks. Thereafter, if the patient is to survive, recovery begins. This is manifested by gradual return of the temperature to normal, healing of the ulceration of the mucous membrane and beginning regrowth of hair. These improvements signify the return of bone marrow function with increase in the white cell components of the blood toward normal levels. Return of the lymphocytes, however, is very slow and many months may be required before the count reaches normal. Although it can be anticipated, at this level of radiation, that sperm production in the male and ovulation in the female will have ceased, return of these functions will not occur for a period of months. The clinical course during this phase is serious to fatal depending upon the dose, susceptibility of the patient and treatment. When death occurs, it is usually due to uncontrolled, overwhelming infection at about the second month after injury.

The *recovery phase* is that period during which the clinical and laboratory alterations, having reached their maximum severity during the bone marrow depression phase, continue to improve until a state of relative normality is reached. The period is of varying length, from three to six months, depending upon the degree and duration of dose, individual response of the patient and the presence or absence of associated injury. Major complications, such as pneumonia,

multiple abscess formation and bacterial resistance to available antibiotics can be expected to occur in a significant number of individuals.

In the whole body dose range from 200 to 400 r, the prognosis for recovery is generally good. Treatment in this range, especially at the upper extreme, may play the determining role in recovery. At the range 400 to 600 r, the LD_{50} for man is approached according to many authorities. Others feel that 600 r represents the near LD_{100} for man and that 450 r or even lower is the appropriate LD_{50}.

In the dose range from 600 to 1400 r, the prognosis must be guarded. Treatment may considerably improve the chances for survival in the lower part of this range, but as the upper limits are reached almost all patients can be expected to die. The area of immediate interest lies in a dose between 200 and 800 r. Above this range treatment has no effect, and under this range recovery almost invariably occurs without treatment.

Gastrointestinal form. The gastrointestinal form of the acute radiation syndrome occurs when the acute dose is between 1000 and 5000 r, and is invariably associated with a fatal outcome. At 800 r, the bone marrow injury will predominate the clinical symptoms, but evidence of injury to the gastrointestinal tract may begin to appear. The prodromal phase is more abrupt in onset, more violent in character and more prolonged in duration than in the hematopoietic form. Diarrhea is characteristic of the prodromal phase in the gastrointestinal form. The early signs and symptoms finally subside after several days, and a short latent period follows. Soon after, the symptoms of nausea, vomiting, diarrhea and fever recur. Death, as a result of gross electrolyte and fluid imbalance, may result within two weeks. Frank hemorrhage and epilation do not occur because the course of the disease is too short to permit these events to develop. The blood changes parallel those found in the high dose range of the hematopoietic form. Treatment is palliative. With time and increased knowledge, beneficial therapeutic measures may become available which will improve the present hopeless prognosis for this form of the disease.

Cerebral form. The cerebral form of the acute radiation syndrome may occur when the dose exceeds 5000 r. Death within hours can be anticipated. Symptoms suggesting an overwhelming insult to the brain and spinal cord are predominant. They include explosive transient nausea, vomiting and diarrhea. Except for a prompt fall in lymphocytes, the findings of leukopenia, bleeding, epilation and infection characteristic of the other forms do not have time to appear. Irrational behavior, circulatory collapse and neuromuscular discoordination occur within minutes. Irrational behavior follows a temporary recovery period; convulsions and coma precede death, which usually occurs within two hours.

TREATMENT. Since there is no specific acute major pathology and no clearly understood reversible physiologic, biochemical and biophysical series of events in acute radiation injury, there is no specific therapy for it. Time and the accumulation of knowledge may eventually invalidate this statement, but it is currently true. It is in the range of 250 to 800 r that intensive treatment can be expected to exert the greatest beneficial influence. Below 500 r, treatment will ordinarily be conservative and will be directed primarily toward the complications, mainly infection. Above 500 r, where the prognosis becomes more and more unfavorable, a more radical approach is indicated wherein therapeutic procedures must be given in anticipation of signs and symptoms which have not yet become manifest. During the first few hours, patients estimated to have received more than 250 r should be hospitalized. Early severe vomiting and skin erythema suggest high doses. Sedation and the use of antiemetic drugs should be of value. Fluid and electrolyte replacement may be necessary in patients with severe vomiting. Probably, the most important therapeutic procedure which can be performed during the first few hours is to resist the temptation to load the patient with blood, drugs and synthetic metabolic poisons.

During the first few days, a definite pattern develops which should provide differentiation between high dose and low dose victims, and make appropriate determinations possible, insofar as further supportive measures are concerned. In those patients who have received high doses, bone marrow replacement, if such is feasible, should be considered. Most authorities feel that bone marrow should be given early in the first few days following injury. The procedure is neither simple nor innocuous. Whether it represents a practical therapeutic measure, except in very limited circumstances, is debatable.

In the latent stage, no special therapy is indicated. Patients should remain in the hospital. The bone marrow depression phase is managed by the judicious use of fresh whole blood. Broad-spectrum antibiotics are given when indicated, but not prophylactically. The desirability of giving only platelets and white cell extract of whole blood to patients with an adequate red cell count is obvious, but techniques for this type of therapy may not always be available.

Nothing specific is available to reverse or minimize radiation effect. Bed rest, good nursing care and a nourishing, easily digested diet provide the basic therapy. Complications should be anticipated, and the best available forms of treatment used when they occur. Research on preventive drugs has not yet provided an effective and safe substance, although several avenues of approach are being explored.

LOCAL RADIATION INJURY

The effects of ionizing radiation on the skin belong to the earliest observations of the biologic effects of this type of radiant energy. It was in December, 1895, that C. W. Roentgen published information on his fundamental discovery of x-ray. Three months later, in March, 1896, John Daniel at Vanderbilt University described the depilatory action of x-rays; in July, 1896, a German physician, W. Marceuse, described the occurrence of dermatitis and alopecia subsequent to fluoroscopy with x-rays. Codman, in 1902, collected 172 instances of x-ray burns.

Irrespective of the nature of ionizing radiation, it produces reversible changes consisting of an inflammatory reaction of the skin, the so-called skin erythema; conditional reversible changes made up by the pigmentation of the irradiated skin, which may last from weeks to months and even years; and irreversible changes consisting of acute or chronic dermatitis with atrophic or hypertrophic skin changes and formation of telangiectases, ulcers and cancers.

CAUSES OF IRRADIATION INJURY. Irradiation injuries may be caused by almost any source of radiation, such as x-rays, radium, radon or radioactive isotopes. Overexposure beyond tissue tolerance may be caused by a single massive dose of radiation or by the cumulative effect of frequently repeated small exposures. Usually, acute irradiation burns are caused by a single, massive overdose such as might occur with a prolonged fluoroscopic procedure. The chronic irradiation injuries occur more commonly after smaller but frequently repeated radiation exposures in excess of tissue tolerance. Physicians, dentists and technicians may be exposed unwittingly to small doses of radiation over a prolonged period of time, and develop pathologic changes in the skin of the hands after a lapse of many years.

Repeated dosages of irradiation for the treatment of skin diseases, usually of the dermatitis group, may be followed occasionally by irradiation damage requiring excision and skin grafting. Growing bone and cartilage are extremely vulnerable to radiation, and treatment of overlying skin lesions with improperly applied irradiation has caused injury to these structures.

The tissue-sparing effects of irradiation dose fractionation and protraction were reported by Strandquist in 1944. A working knowledge of this together with properly calibrated, collimated and filtered diagnostic and therapeutic irradiation devices in the hands of trained radiologists have eliminated many unnecessary instances of irradiation injury. The dermal changes described as reversible are often necessary sequelae to an adequate carcinocidal or carcinostatic dose applied to a deep body organ. Prolonged ulcerations and dermal neoplasms are now largely avoidable because of appropriate irradiation methods.

ACUTE IRRADIATION INJURY. The course of skin reactions after an acute single exposure to x- or gamma radiation is largely determined by the radiation dose. After exposure of the skin to radiation doses which do not destroy the epidermis completely, the exposed skin area will show a reddening, the so-called skin erythema which proceeds in waves. The irradiated skin appears slightly red a few hours after exposure. The intensity of the red color increases for about 24 hours. Having reached a peak, the color intensity decreases again until about the third day, when the irradiated skin appears normal. About the tenth day, there will be reddening of the exposed skin again. This is called the main erythema phase. The color intensity of the main erythema is usually stronger than that of the more fleeting early erythema. This main erythema phase usually ends about the twenty-eighth day.

It appears that during the first erythema, changes in the cutis outweigh those in the epidermis. The cutis blood vessels are congested, and there are paravascular infiltrations indicating an inflammatory process. From the second to the sixth day, pathologic figures are noted in the epidermal cells. With larger doses, the occurrence of multinuclear cells is seen during the second week. Keratinization proceeds unchanged, and finally leads to a thinning of the epithelium to two or three layers. At this point, the basal cells may resume their regenerative activity and restore the normal epidermal structures.

With larger doses of irradiation, roentgen or radium pigmentation of the skin may occur. Repetition of irradiation with a full erythema or even a smaller dose may lead to irreversible skin changes. The phenomenon of roentgen pigmentation results from increased pigment formation in basal cells of the epidermis as well as in the chromatophores of the dermis. The long-lasting pigmentation due to chromatophores is considered a characteristic feature of x-radiated skin.

With larger doses of irradiation, *radiodermatitis bullosa* may occur. The latent period between exposure and the occurrence of the main erythema is shortened. About the tenth day, the skin assumes an intense bluish red color followed by the formation of blisters containing a serous fluid. The condition is extremely painful. Many of the bullae burst and become secondarily infected. Healing is slow and may require months.

Sometimes radiodermatitis bullosa is very severe and radiodermatitis ulcerosa, or the so-called roentgen ulcer, develops. This takes place about six weeks after a single, large exposure. In some instances, ulceration may occur after many years in telangiectatic skin, due to additional thermal or mechanical injury. The ulcer is characterized by marked pain, a punched-out appearance, undermining growth, and inclination to recur. The process may remain stationary for months or even years and then spontaneous healing, with severely deforming scar tissue, may take place.

Treatment consists of the use of a bland ointment and protection of the lesion from further trauma and infection. Local anesthetic ointments are rarely effective. Sedation and pain-relieving drugs are usually necessary. Exclusion of the air from the burned surfaces is of definite value in alleviating pain. Immobilization of the part with a large bulky dressing aids in the process of repair and the control of pain.

When a single large dose of irradiation has caused a fairly well delineated burn which does not appear to have a chance of healing spontaneously, the area may be excised and a split-thickness skin graft applied. This is not always successful on the first attempt because it is difficult to determine the depth of injury, and the take of the graft may be jeopardized by inadequate excision of the burn.

CHRONIC IRRADIATION INJURY.   Chronic exposure of the skin to ionizing radiation leads to two groups of lesions: the chronic roentgen or radium dermatitis, and roentgen carcinoma of the skin. These two groups of skin lesions, if resulting from chronic exposure, usually represent professional or industrial diseases.

The first indication of a chronic radiation dermatitis is a change in the epidermal ridges of the fingers, which may be of atrophic or hypertrophic character. The typical "roentgen hand" shows deepened creases. The epidermis is thickened and the hair is scanty. The skin is dry due to atrophy of the sweat glands. Numerous warts are characteristic. Hyperkeratoses dominate the picture. In general, the skin shows certain features of senile atrophy. The nails become cracked and brittle, and eventually the skin becomes hyperesthetic.

Areas of atrophy with loss of rete pegs may alternate with those of hypertrophy, showing marked acanthosis and hyperkeratosis which may be of tremendous extent. The changes of the corium consist of marked fibrosis and hyalinization. Changes in the blood vessels of the skin include advanced fibrosis of the adventitia and the media, resulting in endarteritis obliterans.

Wound healing is delayed when sufficient irradiation has been administered. In acute but comparatively low doses, 400 r or less, little change from the normal pattern of events is noted. More commonly encountered in surgical patients are the large carcinocidal exposures. Under these circumstances, the healing process is impaired. Surgical incisions heal poorly, if for no reason other than that the blood supply in irradiated tissue is markedly impaired. Necrosis often follows incisions in the irradiated skin and necessitates grafting or excision with closure by full-thickness skin flaps.

The surgical treatment of chronic irradiation injuries should be instituted before malignant changes, ulcerations and intractable pain occur. Surgical therapy for chronic irradiation burns is too often necessary because of malignant changes. The combination of atrophy, telangiectases and keratoses is a forewarning sign of the development of a malignancy. Adequate excision and repair are the essentials of the proper surgical management for chronic irradiation burns.

Atrophy and faint telangiectases may not require treatment if there is no progress in clinical or pathologic changes, but some patients will seek surgical therapy to improve appearance. In areas of abundant telangiectases, which are exposed to the possibilities of repeated trauma or to sunlight, early surgical excision is advisable because of the likelihood of detrimental pathologic changes. Surgical excision and repair by skin grafting should be performed while the areas are still in relatively good condition.

The local application of various drugs has no lasting beneficial effect on the pathologic course of chronic irradiation burns.

Chronic irradiation injury is a complex problem in that it is difficult to determine the severity of the injury by clinical appearance. The surface lesion is not indicative of the degree of deeper involvement. Although most superficial irradiation injuries may be surgically excised and repaired by the application of a split-thickness skin graft, excision leaves avascular structures exposed which require more adequate coverage for restoration of function and appearance. When bone, tendon and cartilage are uncovered by excision, flaps of whole-thickness skin and subcutaneous tissue are necessary to cover the area.

Roentgen carcinoma of skin.   Roentgen carcinoma of the skin is more frequently seen as a late sequela of professional exposure to ionizing radiation. Occasionally, it may be a complication of irradiation therapy. The lesion develops either from chronic roentgen dermatitis or from persistent ulcers. The latent period between irradiation and the appearance of carcinoma is very long, varying from four to 39 years. The carcinoma may develop as a solitary lesion or as multiple ones. It metastasizes in about one-fourth of the cases by way of the lymphatic channels. This type of malignancy metastasizes late and its growth is slow.

The majority of the tumors are of the squamous cell type, but basal cell tumors have occasionally been described. Rather extensive surgical procedures are indicated. In spite of this, the prognosis is not good.

READING REFERENCES

Artz, C. P. (ed.): Research in Burns. Philadelphia, F. A. Davis Company, 1962.

Artz, C. P., and Gaston, B. H.: A reappraisal of the exposure method in the treatment of burns, donor sites and skin grafts. Ann. Surg. *151*:939, 1960.

Artz, C. P., and Reiss, E.: The Treatment of Burns. Philadelphia, W. B. Saunders Company, 1957.

Brown, J. B., McDowell, F., and Fryer, M. P.: Radiation burns, including vocational and atomic exposures. Ann. Surg. *130*:593, 1949.

Bull, J. P., and Fisher, A. J.: Study of mortality in a burns unit: a revised estimate. Ann. Surg. *139*:269, 1954.

Cope, O., and Moore, F. D.: The redistribution of body water and fluid therapy of the burned patient. Ann. Surg. *126*:1010, 1947.

Cronkite, E. P., and Bond, V. P.: Diagnosis of radiation injury and analysis of the human lethal dose of radiation. U.S. Armed Forces Med. J. *11*:249, 1960.

Davis, L., Scarff, J. E., Rogers, N., and Dickinson, M.: High altitude frostbite; preliminary report. Surg. Gyn. & Obst. 77:561, 1943.

Departments of the Army and the Air Force: Cold Injury. TB MED 81, AFP 160-5-10. Washington, D.C., U.S. Government Printing Office, 1954.

Ellinger, F.: Medical Radiation Biology. Springfield, Illinois, Charles C Thomas, 1957.

Harrison, H. N., Moncrief, J. A., Duckett, J. W., Jr., and Mason, A. D., Jr.: The relationship between energy metabolism and water loss from vaporization in severely burned patients. Surgery 56:203, 1964.

Hedblom, E. E.: Polar Manual. Bethesda, Maryland, United States Naval Medical School, National Naval Medical Center, 1962.

Hollingsworth, J. W.: Delayed radiation effects in survivors of the atomic bombings. New England J. Med. *263*:481, 1960.

Liedberg, N. C.-F., Reiss, E., and Artz, C. P.: Infection in burns. III. Septicemia, a common cause of death. Surg. Gyn. & Obst. *99*:151, 1954.

Moncrief, J. A.: Complications of burns. Ann. Surg. *147*:443, 1958.

Moncrief, J. A., Lindberg, R. B., Switzer, W. E., and Pruitt, B. A., Jr.: Use of topical antibacterial therapy in the treatment of the burn wound. A.M.A. Arch. Surg. *92*:558, 1966.

Moncrief, J. A., and Mason, A. D., Jr.: Evaporative water loss in the burned patient. J. Trauma *4*:180, 1964.

Moyer, C. A., Brentano, L., Gravens, D. L., Margraf, H. W., and Monafo, W. W., Jr.: Treatment of large human burns with 0.5 per cent silver nitrate solution. A.M.A. Arch. Surg. *90*:812, 1965.

Moyer, C. A., Margraf, H. W., and Monafo, W. W., Jr.: Burn shock and extravascular sodium deficiency; treatment with Ringer's solution with lactate. A.M.A. Arch. Surg. *90*:799, 1965.

Muir, I. F. K., and Barclay, T. L.: Burns and Their Treatment. Chicago, Year Book Medical Publishers, Inc., 1962.

Order, S. E., and Moncrief, J. A.: The Burn Wound. Springfield, Illinois, Charles C Thomas, 1965.

Orr, K. D., and Fainer, D. C.: Cold injuries in Korea during winter of 1950-51. Medicine *31*:177, 1952.

Oughterson, A. W., and Warren, S. (eds.): Medical Effects of the Atomic Bomb in Japan. New York, McGraw-Hill Book Company, Inc., 1956.

Pruitt, B. A., Jr., Tumbusch, W. T., Mason, A. D., Jr., and Pearson, E.: Mortality in 1,100 consecutive burns treated at a burn unit. Ann. Surg. *159*:396, 1964.

Sevitt, S.: Burns, Pathology and Therapeutic Applications. London, Butterworth & Company, Ltd., 1957.

Soroff, H. S., Pearson, E., Reiss, E., and Artz, C. P.: The relationship between plasma sodium concentration and the state of hydration of burned patients. Surg. Gyn. & Obst. *102*:472, 1956.

Topley, E., and Jackson, D. MacG.: The clinical control of red cell loss in burns. J. Clin. Path. *10*:1, 1957.

Washburn, B.: Frostbite: what it is—how to prevent it—emergency treatment. New England J. Med. *266*:974, 1962.

Chapter *11*

PRINCIPLES OF PREOPERATIVE AND POSTOPERATIVE CARE

by
RICHARD L. VARCO, M.D.

RICHARD LYNN VARCO, born in Montana, was educated at the University of Minnesota, and has had teaching and research experience in the Departments of Medicine, Physiology and Surgery during his surgical education. He is a Professor of Surgery at Minnesota. His investigative work exemplifies the rewards to the patient which can result from practical application of the principles of the basic sciences to the art of surgery.

INTRODUCTION

Medical students often freely concede that the numerous, at times intricate, and perhaps tedious, problems of preoperative and post-operative care fail to capture their interest quite as readily as do the more glamorous operative aspects of surgical practice. With experience, however, they are more willing to acknowledge that efforts devoted to these less dramatic activities are necessary to ensure a smooth or even successful convalescence. In fact, during recent years, the steady decline in the mortality and morbidity rates for surgical procedures has depended in a fair measure on this wider recognition and practice of the principles of preoperative and postoperative care. Besides making any procedure safer, this knowledge has eased the restrictions against operating on both elderly persons and the very young. Now these patients need rarely be refused the most formidable type of operation solely because of age. Finally, through careful attention to these details, it has become possible to broaden, generously, without incurring an unreasonable hazard, the magnitude of surgery undertaken to meet the most complex therapeutic problems.

PREOPERATIVE CARE

EMERGENCY CONSIDERATIONS. An orderly plan for questioning and examining each surgical patient, even in an emergency, is of fundamental importance. In this situation the prime considerations are to ascertain that cardiac arrest has not occurred, to ensure that ventilation is unimpaired and to locate and control gross sites of external bleeding. If internal bleeding is a possibility, diligent search to confirm or disprove this possibility is in order. Intra-abdominal hemorrhage can be identified by a tap of the peritoneal cavity. Root has made this good suggestion: add several hundred cubic centimeters of saline to the peritoneal cavity by means of a small catheter inserted below the umbilicus and in the midline. For patients the percentage of false negative aspirations thereafter is lower than for a four-quadrant needling. If the blood loss is intrapleural and of sufficient volume to cause concern about the amount being sequestered from the circulation, an intercostal catheter is best for both diagnostic and therapeutic purposes. Additional contamination to all significant external wounds should be minimized. Fractures or dislocations should be protected against additional displacement including inadvertent conversion of a closed to an open fracture.

In the event that cardiac action has ceased and ventilation is at a standstill, prompt effective correction of both of these life-threatening events should proceed. Ideally, these problems are solved with the cooperation of an anesthesiologist equipped to insert an endotracheal tube, suction the air passages of any blood, mucus, gastrointestinal contents or foreign material, and provide the lungs with a free flow of an oxygen-enriched mixture. He can temporarily stablize a flail chest wall, when the lung is capable of being ventilated, and thereby overcome any paradoxical movement which had made voluntary breathing inefficient.

Tension pneumothorax can be suspected from the history of a combination of typical events and the physical findings of collapsed lung. The "scratch test" is helpful. This consists of auscultation of corresponding areas on the chest wall while scratching the adjacent skin on one side and then the other. There will be a hollow resonance on the side of a significant pneumothorax. Its existence should be confirmed by x-ray studies and prompt relief provided by decompression of the pleural space with intercostal catheter siphonage.

Underlying pulmonary injury is frequently revealed by the appearance of subcutaneous emphysema. This produces crepitus on palpation and signifies the presence of a torn lung usually in association with a tension pneumothorax and not uncommonly coexisting with a hemothorax. An expedient widely available and effective for limited to modest-sized air leaks relies on insertion of an Intracath or a Rochester needle attached to an underwater seal or some controllable suction source. A tracheostomy or inlying endotracheal tube, preferably of the minimally reactive Portex type, by eliminating glottic resistance further decreases the tendency toward progressive subcutaneous emphysema arising on the basis of torn pulmonary substance. Each of these two techniques reduces airway obstruction, and thus peak expiratory pressures, thereby limiting the progression of gaseous dissection.

Internal hemorrhage of traumatic origin usually requires an operating room and the paraphernalia available to ensure its successful management. For visible blood loss, firm compression usually stanches the flow, even when this is caused by brisk arterial bleeding. Should a tourniquet be required, or if one is already in place, careful notation of time of application is important to record the duration of the ischemia produced.

In all patients who are clearly the victims of severe trauma, provision should be made for continuing measurement of urine output. This allows early recognition of the effectiveness of resuscitative techniques. Failure to establish a urine output of greater than 25 cc. per hour requires prompt attention to ascertain that the urinary tract is intact. On the other hand, an estimate of functional ability of the kidney reserve can readily be derived from a comparison of the serum and urine osmolalities. Appropriate therapy for partial immediate restoration of circulating blood volume through the use of lactated Ringer's solution and, ultimately, with plasma and whole blood are appropriate techniques. Their precise quantities depend on the severity of the injury and the time lapse since the traumatic episode, as well as the physical condition of the individual, his age, the ambient temperature of the environment and a host of considerations unique to the particular event.

When adequate ventilation is established, with means to maintain it, as well as control of external hemorrhage, blood should be secured for cross-matching, and urine for analysis. If necessary, the patient should be catheterized.

PREOPERATIVE ROUTINES. It is important to learn to listen well in order to secure a maximum of information from the patient. To avoid grave and embarrassing oversights, a precise method of history taking and physical examination should be followed. Information and findings should be recorded accurately just as a protocol for an experiment is established. Background facts thus obtained are an important preamble to the intelligent care of each patient.

After the patient's history and physical data have been precisely recorded, laboratory tests and roentgenographic studies should be obtained.

The urine should be analyzed for specific gravity, albumin, sugar, acetone or diacetic acid, and microscopic sediment.

There should be a hemoglobin estimation and a red blood cell count, or both; total white blood cell and differential counts; and blood typing. A carefully taken history, with emphasis on past traumatic or surgical events, usually proves to be a reliable guide to the detection of abnormal bleeding states. Whenever there is evidence to suggest, on the basis of alcoholic intake or a history of hepatitis, a possibility that liver damage might be present, a prothrombin time is indicated. In fact, reliance on the following three tests, in addition to the history, provides a safe basis for decision making about an elective procedure or, in the event that an abnormality is revealed, suggests the need for more sophisticated studies capable of revealing the precise coagulopathy: partial thromboplastin time, normal (kaolin) 35 to 45 seconds; prothrombin time, normal (Quick), 12 seconds; platelets, normal 150,000 to 300,000 per cubic millimeter.

During the menstrual phase in some women, and very frequently in patients with cyanotic congenital heart disease, markedly abnormal bleeding times are encountered. This situation need not preclude an emergency operation or even a carefully evaluated elective procedure, if painstaking attention to meticulous hemostasis is achieved during the operation. Under these circumstances, the operative risk can be maintained at a reasonable level. Furthermore, the availability of fresh whole blood and platelet transfusions provides additional safeguards under such circumstances.

A chest roentgenogram should be taken and reviewed by the surgeon. This procedure should be practiced with all roentgenographic studies. It is by such day-to-day comparison of the patient's status that the surgeon develops a keener ability to analyze even the most complicated problems.

A careful appraisal and correlation of the history, physical findings and laboratory data will serve as a guide to initiating care for the usual patient. In many surgical patients, it will represent an adequate preoperative preparation. The pathologic-physiologic alterations of starvation, dehydration, salt loss, anemia, diabetes, cardiovascular, hepatic, renal or pulmonary disease, and potential immunological deficits, may be recognized in other patients. In some, the situation may prove to be so intricate that a variety of complex laboratory, roentgenographic and diagnostic procedures are required. Each patient's needs will have to be decided upon and these will sometimes require consultation to determine the best use of the more complicated and costly diagnostic tools. It is advantageous, whenever an excretory cholecystogram or urogram is likely to be included along with roentgen studies, using barium as the contrast agent, to schedule the former first so as to avoid difficulties in interpretation occasioned by the residual blobs of opaque. For all laboratory tests, forethought should be given as to their discriminative value, cost, urgency and scheduling so as to minimize delays in initiating treatment or purposeless prolongation of hospitalization. Abuse of an emergency service by requests which are not genuine but rather are a substitute for reasonable anticipation will dull even the most cooperative technologist's ardor for service.

BEHAVIORAL ANALYSIS. It is incumbent in each surgeon to assess the patients' emotional makeup. Tactfully phrased questions in an atmosphere of understanding and interest in the individual's problems as well as appropriate, and discreet, inquiry into relevant aspects of the patient's family and social history can, and should, provide fundamental data about the personality under study. Decision making should take into account excessive somatization on the part of the complainant. Similarly, and only to a slightly lesser degree, destructive hostilities and deep-rooted insecurities should not be disregarded in the preoperative evaluation with particular reference to the extent and nature of the operation contemplated, especially when it is an elective procedure.

NUTRITION. The person who has been eating well and has lost little or no weight will require no special preoperative dietary management. On the other hand, the patient who is cachectic from a recent serious weight loss, in the range of 35 to 50 per cent, represents a substandard operative risk. Major operations performed on these individuals, without regard for the advisability of preoperative preparation, carry increased mortality and morbidity rates. The patient may react unfavorably from the outset, with an instability of blood pressure out of proportion to the actual blood loss. Numerous transfusions at the time of operation perhaps will provide only transient support to the blood pressure. Convalescence can be slower than normal and disturbed by a greater incidence of complications such as ileus, impaired wound healing and disruptions, or stomal obstruction. This patient, already enervated by starvation, lacks the vitality to overcome such hazards and the surgical risks are greater than for a properly nourished patient. Fortunately, examples of such severe nutritional deficit are becoming less frequent with broader extensions of identifiably comprehensive community health services. These gains are bolstered also by an improved public awareness of the widespread availability of community medical resources.

Those bodily derangements likely to be produced by severe starvation are hepatic dysfunction, impaired wound healing, hypoproteinemia and a contracted blood volume. These pathologic changes are reversible when appropriate dietary management is possible. The return to normal is slow, and it requires many days or weeks of therapy to achieve recognizable nutritional restitution. Sudden and dramatic benefits are rarely obtained.

The clinical problem is complicated by a dearth of simple, accurate methods for precisely measuring the various effects of starvation. Likewise, there is no test to indicate the quantity of nourishment required for the re-establishment of sufficient health to allow major surgery without excessive risk. Fortunately, the restoration of the bodily economy to less than ideal performance usually suffices. After an adequate, albeit partial nutritional restoration of the patient, the surgeon can operate and anticipate a convalescence as free from complications as in a standard-risk individual.

During periods of relative starvation, the patient becomes autocannibalistic. His energy requirements are derived principally from body protein and fat. He subsists on a low calorie, low protein, high fat diet. Logic suggests, and experience confirms, the characteristics of a diet most likely to correct the consequences of such starvation. In the laboratory and from clinical studies, it has been found that this diet should be rich in protein and carbohydrate, high in calories and low in fat content. Of all these constituents, protein plays the leading role. The principal sources of protein in natural foods are meat, fish, eggs, certain dairy products and cereals. Yet in each of these, the protein contributes but a small fraction of the total bulk. It becomes necessary, therefore, to give an enormous quantity of food when a large protein intake is desired. To achieve a protein intake of 300 gm. when beef is the source, about 1400 gm. of lean meat would have to be eaten. This gargantuan feat is usually beyond the capacity of a patient who is weakened and anorexic from prolonged starvation. However, reasonable quantities of tastily prepared and attractively served foods will foster the acceptance of a relatively high protein diet.

The stimulus of a freshly devised daily menu and the cooperative appeal from bedside consultations among the surgeon, dietitian and nursing staff will add vitality to this nutritional program. In analyzing the effectiveness of the regimen, reasonably accurate calculations of the caloric intake can only be made from reappraising those quantities which the patient does not eat of a diet with known composition of protein, carbohydrate and fat. An erroneous judgment is almost certain if reliance is placed on equating a prescription for a high protein and caloric diet with its consumption. Certainly, every patient who willingly consumes the necessary quota from the available hospital fare should be encouraged to continue.

Physical factors will, however, tend to limit the accomplishments possible by this means. In such patients, liquid feedings provide a useful means of supplementing the protein intake. Milk is an excellent vehicle for such mixtures and will hold substantial quantities of protein concentrate and carbohydrate. A wide variety of protein concentrates or digests are available. Skimmed milk powder, about 38 per cent protein, is among these. It is inexpensive, widely available and stores well in bulk form. Its natural taste can be disguised to enhance its palatability. Also, it contains complete proteins which possess a better than average capacity for inducing plasma protein regeneration.

The use of a liquid diet to supplement the hospital fare, or as the sole source of calories, is sound practice. It finds frequent application in patients with lesions of the esophagus, stomach and duodenum. When mild to severe degrees of alimentary tract obstruction complicate the preoperative status, a liquid diet is particularly beneficial. Commonly, incomplete mastication of solid, high fiber content food results in even greater degrees of obstruction. When this occurs, one should lavage the chunks of swallowed food by means of a large-bore gastric tube, and thereafter a satisfactory amount of a liquid diet may be able to pass the stenotic area each 24 hours.

Several diets have been tried at the University of Minnesota Hospitals, but the one shown on page 176, with minor variations, has proved most useful.

This mixture passes readily through a 16 Fr. nasogastric catheter or a small Penrose drain. A plastic tube is less irritating to the patient than a red rubber tube, particularly when it must be in place for several days. The liquid diet can be dispensed through a drip-feeding apparatus. For this arrange-

Liquid Diet (2446 Calories)
(About 1.6 calories per cc.)

	CARBO-HYDRATES (GM.)	PRO-TEIN (GM.)	FAT (GM.)
Whole eggs, 6		36.0	36.0
Egg whites, 2		8.0	
Skimmed milk powder, 4 oz.	58.8	40.4	1.2
Lactose, 300 gm. (beet or cane sugar may be substituted)	300.0		
Skimmed milk, 1000 cc.	50.0	36.0	
Salt, 5 gm.*			
	408.8	120.4	37.2

* When omitted, the formula serves as a relatively low sodium diet for patients with heart disease requiring salt restriction and a high protein preoperative diet.

ment, the best functioning containers have been adapted from intravenous flasks with dependent air vents. This permits the entering bubbles, as they rise, to agitate the mixture gently, reducing the tendency toward sedimentation and plugging. A Murphy drip apparatus is inserted into the connecting tubing and the visible rate of flow can be regulated by the patient with a thumb screw attachment. Particularly in the case of a feeble person, it is a wise precaution to have the head of the bed elevated while the patient is being drip fed. Excessive sedation should be avoided to reduce the likelihood of overfilling the patient's stomach, which may result in regurgitation, aspiration and pneumonia.

For those who prefer to drink the mixture, the taste is similar to an eggnog. This flavor can be readily modified with chocolate, vanilla or other obvious choices. The diet can be used by outpatients also. Simple mimeographed directions about its preparation, the volume to be consumed daily and the refrigeration requirements should be given to the outpatient, together with instructions covering the importance of regular consumption of the prescribed amount. Whenever this liquid diet constitutes the sole source of food for the patient, he should be urged to take daily, if possible, about 5000 calories, i.e., 3 liters. When it is used as a supplement to ordinary fare, the consumption of 1 liter may suffice.

Diarrhea will sporadically occur in persons receiving this diet, but it can largely be avoided by keeping unused portions of each feshly prepared batch under refrigeration and by the use of clean or sterilized

dispensing equipment. If diarrhea occurs despite these precautions, small doses of paregoric or Amphojel, or both, together with temporarily decreasing the dietary supplement, will ordinarily correct the situation. Patients with regional enteritis or ulcerative colitis are rather consistent exceptions to this rule and should be tested with small amounts to determine their individual tolerance. In patients with severe impairment of renal function, care must be taken not to impose an intolerable nitrogen load through utilization of this high protein diet. These patients may require additional fluid, with a low residual urinary solute content, to compensate for the limited renal functional capacity.

For a hospitalized patient, the use of this liquid with a fixed caloric value per cubic centimeter simplifies the calculation of the daily caloric intake on the basis of the volume consumed. The amount is charted, preferably as calories, along with the temperature, pulse, respiratory rate, fluid intake, output volumes and body weight. The nutritional status is thus brought into focus at the bedside while work rounds are being held. This close contact with dietary management through a day-to-day accounting of progress, or lack of it, is of fundamental importance for the consistently effective preoperative care of nutritionally substandard risk patients.

Currently, precise, tailored mixtures of essential amino acids are procurable for such individuals as those who have undergone extensive resection of the small, and perhaps large, intestine. The amount absorbed—a function of intestinal transit time—from these components is demonstrably superior to the yield derived from the intestinal enzymatic breakdown of orally ingested native protein, under these abnormal circumstances. In fact, provision of these elemental units permits a reduction in the parenteral protein load.

When dietary preparation is required, it is important that it take place in the preoperative phase. The weight of investigative evidence indicates a greater percentage of nitrogen retention from protein ingested preoperatively. The establishment of any large nitrogen gain after an operation offers considerable difficulty because of the catabolic phase present in that period. The problem becomes even more trying when the enteral route is no longer available, as is likely in this stage of convalescence, because of ileus or vomiting.

Objective measurements of the accomplishments of this hyperalimentation regimen are virtually nonexistent. Until more critical tests are available, the method to be presented offers a reasonably reliable means of calculating the duration of the special dietary regimen. First, it is important to find out the approximate amount of weight the patient has recently lost. This figure should regularly be made available and recorded in the admission history. Ill persons often do not know the exact amount of weight recently lost, but nearly always are able to recall a maximum weight determined for some time during the previous three to six months. Any change assumes more significance if expressed as a percentage of the total body weight. When this value represents a loss of 25 per cent or more, a period of at least two weeks of dietary preparation is desirable. A portion of this period can frequently be spent outside the hospital, or in a nursing unit less intensively staffed than regular hospital facilities.

Each day the patient should try to consume about 4500 to 5000 calories. If this total is obtained solely from consumption of a mixed diet, the proportions of protein, carbohydrate and fat should approximate those indicated in the liquid diet mixture. These estimates for the duration and amount of augmented caloric intake have been tested by trial and error for many patients having nutritional problems and probably are maximal rather than minimal. However, if such a patient has had an adequate nutritional preoperative preparation, he can usually leave the hospital after about the same postoperative period that a standard-risk patient requires.

In some nutritional problem patients, the oral route is not available for protein and caloric replenishment because of alimentary tract obstruction or such factors as intractable diarrhea or complicated fistulas. Ulcerative and neoplastic disease of the esophagus, stomach or duodenum are common obstructive mechanisms and sites. Ultimately, a surgical procedure of considerable magnitude may be required to correct the specific pathologic condition. Two alternative methods are available for nutritional preparation. A jejunostomy can be made and the feeding mixtures then dripped into the intestine at this level. In many of these patients, diarrhea develops before the quantity of material fed daily reaches the required caloric intake. This diarrhea often fails to respond despite recourse to a wide variety of dietary formulas. Certain of the patient's limited reserves are depleted in the volumes of liquid stool lost.

The alternative is the establishment of a comprehensive parenteral feeding program, which strives to attain a dual goal of meeting the daily caloric requirements and acquiring the maximum possible nitrogen retention.

A 5 to 20 per cent intravenous solution of glucose, in volumes sufficient to provide 200 to 250 gm. of carbohydrate to the body, is the principal exogenous source for energy requirements. If fructose is substituted, less may be lost in the urine even when higher concentrations are administered. Unless this, or fat, is available, substantial quantities of body protein or of infused nitrogenous material will continue to be catabolized for fuel. Hence, the more complete the provision for protein sparing by adequate carbohydrate intake, the greater will be the conservation of potentially critical protein resources.

Intravenous fat emulsions can also provide energy units which thus reduce the drain on exogenous and endogenous protein expenditure as calories. A good feature of fat emulsions is their higher caloric value. Two limiting factors in their use are instability problems under varied climatic conditions and toxic systemic reactions with fever, chills, nausea, vomiting and headaches. In addition, knowledge to date is incomplete concerning the late consequences of prolonged use of these infusions. Instances of hepatomegaly, a hemorrhagic tendency, and lowering of the plasma albumin fraction have been reported. The frequency of these side effects appears roughly proportional to the number of bottles of intravenous fat given to the patient during one period of treatment. Therefore, prevailing opinion favors the tendency to limit this amount to 10 to 12 separate half-liter infusions. Meanwhile, its use for a specific need which cannot otherwise be met has considerable justification and reasonable safety. For instance, this material may yield some temporary benefits in the nutritional care of severely burned patients requiring higher caloric intakes than can be achieved without such supplementation.

For the severely burned patient, far greater gains in energy conservation can be achieved through a reduction in the considerable evaporative heat loss associated with this type of injury to the tegument, if provision is made for elimination of this "heat sink" by early allo- or autografting. Other techniques designed to minimize water vaporization from the highly permeable burned area can make an equivalent contribution to reduction in the extra caloric drain produced by this type of trauma.

The other major control of the state of the nitrogen balance comes through the kind and amount of the nitrogenous compounds administered parenterally. The nitrogen-containing compounds available for parenteral use are pure amino acid mixtures, gelatin, protein hydrolysates, albumin, plasma and whole blood.

Gelatin has some application in the emergency restoration of blood volume of hypovolemia, if plasma and whole blood are not immediately available, as have also the other plasma volume expanders. The contribution of gelatin to parenteral nitrogen replacement therapy is dubious.

Protein hydrolysate mixtures are obtained from the acid or enzymatic hydrolysis of a variety of substrates. The resultant commercial preparations, usually after tryptophan enrichment, are widely available. Casein has frequently furnished the source of protein in these digests. The hydrolysates are readily infused as 5 per cent solutions, with an equal or lesser concentration of glucose. A rate of infusion up to 400 cc. per hour is well tolerated by most patients during waking hours. If the injection is much faster, the incidence of unpleasant systemic reactions increases. The total nitrogen intake from parenteral use of hydrolysate mixtures is, therefore, limited to a smaller value than when the oral route is available. In addition, the total urinary nitrogen loss in 24 hours following venoclysis of hydrolysates and glucose is greater than after the feeding of equivalent amounts of skimmed milk powder protein. Hence, nitrogen replenishment by parenteral hydrolysate mixtures is doubly handicapped when compared with oral protein achievements. Despite these limitations, the hydrolysates occupy an important role in nitrogen replacement therapy. Through their agency, it is possible to retard the steady protein losses from starvation and allied depleting mechanisms such as ulceration, sepsis and hemorrhage. Testosterone, in the Depo form as cyclopentylpropionate, has some anabolic effect and could also curb the nitrogen losses. Use of this hormone, or the similarly effec-

tive, nonvirilizing methandrostenolone, unfortunately induces sodium retention. Therefore, intake of this electrolyte should be restricted to 75 mEq. per day, particularly for the malnourished person or the individual with an associated cardiac problem. The theoretically attractive concept of providing exogenous human growth hormone for its tissue anabolic action awaits further practical confirmation.

The daily nitrogen intake is most effectively augmented by repeated transfusions of plasma or whole blood, a regimen which is not followed by a prompt neutralizing increase in the urinary nitrogen losses. Blood transfusions are preferable in the anemic patient. Blood volume determinations, calculated for the usual weight prior to the current illness, provide a fair analysis of these requirements. The current availability of a portable, rapidly accurate, relatively inexpensive and simple to operate electronic instrument has made this important technique more practical in many hospitals. Daily infusions of 500 to 1000 cc. of whole blood should continue until the hemoglobin and hematocrit values reach and remain in the normal range. As a corollary, it can be expected that until the patient's normal blood volume has been reached, successive transfusions will not bring the hematocrit above a normal value in the absence of dehydration or other causes of plasma volume loss. For the poorly nourished patient, as much as 2500 cc. or more of blood may be required. Clearly, a patient suffering from such a contracted blood volume is a poorer operative risk until the normal vascular space has been appropriately filled. Adequate correction of these defects involving hypovolemia and reduced red cell mass can be customarily realized by this plan.

The associated hypoproteinemia is less regularly and predictably restored to normal because slight changes in plasma protein values are in dynamic equilibrium with quantitatively large debits in the total body protein. The plasma protein value can be raised additionally by the injection of albumin; however, it is not always available and is relatively costly. After this phase of blood volume replenishment, a daily transfusion of plasma, whole blood or packed red blood cells, plus as much as 3 liters of nitrogen enriched-glucose mixture, can be relied upon to provide the soundest possible parenterally induced positive nitrogen balance. At least a partial restoration of these various depots is essential in order to fulfill the aggressive protein demands of the healing tissues, the countless maturing phagocytes and the reticuloendothelial elements creating immune bodies in response to infectious processes. Gamma globulin supplements given intramuscularly can be beneficial in special circumstances of demonstrated need. With great emphasis on careful selection of donors free of even a suggestion of a positive history of hepatitis and long-term storage of plasma at room temperature, the incidence of serum hepatitis can be kept acceptably low.

Parenteral preparation is complicated and requires the services of a conscientious, tactful and patient house officer with sufficient skill to minimize the development of thromboses in all the cutaneous veins available to and essential for a prolonged period of intravenous therapy. Use of a forearm vessel away from the antecubital fossa avoids the distress of hyperextension at that joint. Also, it permits some latitude of movement without the danger of dislodging the needle and burying it into adjacent tissue, thereby causing a painful perivenous injection.

In anticipation of a prolonged intravenous therapy program, sterile, small-bore polyethylene tubing can be inserted through, or over, a large intravenous needle and into the blood stream. The inserting cannula can then be withdrawn and the plastic tube fastened with a dressing and left in place for several days. This conduit can be connected to the drip apparatus and avoids the need for frequent punctures of the patient's arm veins. At the conclusion of each day's infusion schedule, the tubing should be flushed with a few cubic centimeters of isotonic saline solution containing heparin, and then plugged with a sterile intravenous needle of appropriate size to which has been attached a 2-cc. syringe containing a dilute solution of this anticoagulant. It then remains patulous and ready for the next injection. When there is a paucity of superficial veins, this method will help resolve that dilemma. Caution is offered against routine use of the saphenous venous system lest one thereby provoke a high incidence of thrombophlebitis and phlebothrombosis. The saphenous vein is quite prone to those complications when it has been used for prolonged intravenous therapy. Veins of the upper extremity seem distinctly less likely to become the sites of future pulmonary emboli.

The preparation of this group of patients by parenteral feeding should be compressed into as short a period as possible. This applies even to those with marked weight loss, anemia, hypoproteinemia, edema and other stigmata of starvation. They are prone to develop regurgitation and aspiration due to the prolonged use of an inlying feeding tube. While enduring the tedium of parenteral alimentation, they are more liable to the concomitant adverse effects of prolonged postural immobilization. Usually, from seven to ten days can safely be devoted to achieving maximum nutritional benefits. Even less time will need to be spent in rehabilitating those patients who are only moderately malnourished from this same type of partial, high alimentary tract obstruction.

OBESITY. The obese patient requiring an elective operation presents a substantial nutritional problem. Reference to standard tables of age, sex and body build for various heights and weights serves as an approximate basis for identifying the magnitude of the problem in any particular patient. Skin fold thickness calipered over the triceps is perhaps a more reliable index of obesity. To accept an obese patient for a major surgical procedure, without due preparation, is to accept an increased incidence of pulmonary cardiovascular problems and wound complications. Technical difficulties during the course of the operation are enhanced, perhaps even beyond remedy. The excessively fat person should earnestly, and with firm patience, be advised to lose weight before any elective major procedure. The surgeon who fails to so advise is remiss in the discharge of his obligation. The patient should be given a diet to follow, and his adherence to it must be closely supervised. The early establishment of a physician-patient rapport, based upon mutual understanding of agreed upon weight-losing objectives, will contribute much to success in this phase of preoperative dietary preparation. In fact, if he is to undergo the safest operation, his wholehearted participation will have to be enlisted by reasoning with him, and by pointing out the life-endangering consequences of rashly disregarding this advice to lose weight.

Any balanced, weight-reduction diet adhered to by the patient can prove satisfactory because the most important factors are low calorie content, a suitable protein and vitamin intake and patient cooperation. For this purpose, a simple yet effective plan allows the patient about two quarts of skimmed milk per day, along with medical supplements as needed to meet adequately the vitamin requirements. A built-in advantage of the skim milk plan lies in the lack of numerous calorie-riddled choices to confuse and weaken the resolve of the patient at each meal. This program will have a tendency to produce constipation unless provision is made for stool softening medication or the addition of reasonable quantities of vegetable cellulose low in calories. Finally, when the lower poundage desired has been reached, based on standard weight and height tables, primarily at the expense of body fat deposits, the individual represents a far better surgical risk. His state should not be thought analogous to the malnourished state encountered in starvation. The physiologic mechanisms and consequences differ in important characteristics.

VITAMINS. The chronically malnourished patient may have either occult or manifest hypovitaminosis. If the clinical symptoms or laboratory tests suggest the diagnosis, specific vitamin therapy is indicated and, whenever the oral route is available, it is preferable. Intravenous preparations should be reserved for those patients in whom the enteral route is unavailable because of obstruction, vomiting, diarrhea or other mechanisms interfering with absorption. In the absence of a deficiency requiring specific therapy, only vitamins B_1, C and K are important in the routine surgical care of patients.

Thiamine (vitamin B_1) participates in those enzyme systems which regulate carbohydrate metabolism and maintain normal gastrointestinal activity. In any nutritional preparation involving large quantities of carbohydrate, liberal amounts of thiamine (10 to 20 mg. daily) are advised. Intravenous infusions of glucose rapidly deplete the existing stores of vitamin B_1, thus aggravating any latent deficiency. Carbohydrate metabolism itself is impaired, further hampering the nutritional rehabilitation. Sulfasuxidine given orally will increase the thiamine requirements in the diet. When excess quantities of thiamine have been provided, they are either lost in the urine or stored and appear to cause no deleterious effects. The preferred route for administration is the oral one, because of the slower absorption and hence more prolonged systemic action. If thiamine is given intravenously with glucose solutions, the daily dosage should be divided, lest an unnecessary excess of the vitamin be lost by diuresis.

The contribution of *vitamin C* to wound healing is clearly established. A low tissue vitamin C content is correlated with an increased incidence of wound disruption, the edges of which would reveal a collagen-formation deficit. The plasma ascorbic acid content can be readily measured. Vitamin C deficiencies result from an inadequate intake, faulty intestinal absorption or an excess loss from, or sequestration by, the tissues. In the instance of burns, abscesses or large ulcerating areas, this mechanism can increase the daily requirements to at least 1000 mg. Tissue saturation is easily attained by means of oral preparations, and parenteral solutions are available when that route cannot be used. Probably, no large-scale, long-term storage exists in man. Any superfluous intake is lost in the urine, causing no harmful reaction. A daily dose of 500 mg. is ample for most contingencies met with in the preparation of surgical patients.

A prolonged deficiency of *vitamin K*, a fat-soluble vitamin, disrupts the clotting mechanism by preventing the formation of prothrombin by the liver. The resultant hypoprothrombinemia interferes with blood clotting at the thrombin-conversion stage. The common antecedent to vitamin K deficiency is any mechanism which prevents its formation in, and absorption from, the intestinal tract. Prolonged oral use of poorly absorbed antibiotics can so reduce the bacterial flora of the intestine as to inhibit vitamin K synthesis sufficiently to cause serious hypoprothrombinemia. In some types of biliary obstruction, or with an external biliary fistula, the emulsifying action of bile is lost and, consequently, this naturally fat-soluble vitamin cannot be absorbed. Persons taking large amounts of cholestyramine can also lose substantial amounts of bile salts from the intestinal tract through the sequestering influence of this compound. Vitamin K should be given parenterally in these patients. Hypoprothrombinemia occurs also in association with severe hepatic disease, and if the plasma prothrombin value is not correctable to around 80 per cent of normal with therapeutic amounts of parenteral vitamin K, it becomes of grave prognostic significance.

Essential hypoprothrombinemia, a rare disease and conceivably a congenital metabolic defect, is an exception since other evidence of hepatic disease may be lacking in these patients. For those persons with hypoprothrombinemia which is not benefited by vitamin K therapy, massive transfusions of freshly drawn plasma or whole blood will temporarily elevate the plasma prothrombin content. The bleeding tendency can usually be controlled sufficiently to permit an operation. In any emergency, minor defects of circulating prothrombin concentration can be so managed. With the availability of vitamin K_1 oxide for intravenous use, a more prompt restoration of prothrombin content to circulating blood is now possible, even in persons who have been receiving Dicumarol-like compounds.

All patients suspected of being hypoprothrombinemic should have a test for prothrombin concentration. This result is usually checked by determining the prothrombin time of a normal patient's plasma, used as a control for the materials and methods. Also, this function can be charted as the percentage of normal prothrombin activity: the normal patient's plasma prothrombin time divided by the patient's plasma prothrombin time multiplied by 100.

The prothrombin percentage can be calculated from a curve derived by plotting prothrombin times against serial dilutions of normal plasma. The curve is accurate as a standard only when the same potency of thromboplastin used in obtaining the curve is used for testing the unknowns. Prolonged bleeding is unlikely to occur unless the patient's prothrombin time is more than twice that of the control, or until the percentage of activity is lower than 50 per cent. In most instances of vitamin K deficiency, considerable response is seen within 24 to 36 hours after therapy is started. A daily oral dose of 5 to 10 mg. of vitamin K customarily will suffice for this purpose, unless intestinal absorption is impaired, as may occur in severe jaundice, profuse diarrhea or pronounced "short bowel" syndrome. Quantities of the vitamin in excess are well tolerated and apparently do no harm. Water-soluble preparations for parenteral use are available whenever medication cannot be given orally or would be ineffective.

ANEMIA AND HYPOPROTEINEMIA. Chronically ill patients regularly exhibit some degree of anemia and protein depletion. The total extent of these defects is masked to a a greater or lesser degree by contractions of the blood volume, red cell mass or plasma volume, and protein reservoirs. As a consequence of this decrease in the red cell mass and in the total amount of circulating plasma protein, these patients are less tolerant of additional blood loss during operation. They may display evidence of impaired wound healing and decreased resistance to infection.

HEART DISEASE. The patient with heart disease may require a major operation as urgently as does his healthier contemporary. With careful attention to certain details, his chances of successfully undergoing an abdominal or thoracic operation of magnitude can be greatly improved. An individual with historical or physical evidence of heart disease deserves to have any necessary additional studies carried out. Electrocardiography, cardiac fluoroscopy, central venous pressure determination, circulation time, and a functional test of exercise capacity will furnish worthwhile preoperative data. The normal value for pressure in a cubital vein is less than 13 cm. of saline above a baseline measured 10 cm. dorsal to the spine and with the patient recumbent. Whether the findings are nearly normal or grossly altered, they represent significant baselines for comparison with later values. In the event of a complicated convalescence, a suspicion of incipient trouble gains greater credence and is easier to verify with such information available.

When frank heart failure is detectable on the basis of pulmonary congestion or effusion, hepatomegaly, ascites or peripheral edema, preoperative management which includes sodium intake restriction, fluids if necessary, diuresis and digitalization is advisable.

Hypoxia, hypercarbia, hyperthermia, metabolic acidosis, shock, overhydration with an excessive salt intake and hyper- or hypokalemia are the more common surgically induced mechanisms functioning as potential or real precipitants of cardiac disaster. It is important also to recognize the magnitude of work requirements imposed on the heart by labored, tachypneic breathing in particular or even that occurring in the postoperative period in general. As much as 25 per cent of the cardiac output may be required to meet these energy needs. For the heart with limited reserves this can prove intolerable, and therefore judicious use of a respirator under such circumstances provides an extracorporeal power source that may be lifesaving.

Shock can readily precipitate a cardiac complication in the organ which is already diseased. When the surgeon has been warned by the admission history, the physical examination and special tests, he should take certain precautions. Among these is provision for accurate volumetric replacement of the measured blood loss during the operation. The reliability of this mensuration will be enhanced by meticulous operative hemostasis. Attention to painstaking hemostasis avoids the mystery of concealed bleeding into the operative field taking place after wound closure.

This is particularly important because the prevention of shock is much more successful than its treatment. The duration of the hypotension and the mechanism producing it are critical considerations in arriving at the prognosis for any specific situation. The longer the period with a profoundly low blood pressure, less than 60 mm. Hg, the poorer the outlook, as in endotoxin shock produced by a gram-negative bacteremia. This predicament is in contrast to the usually benign situation in a patient suffering from brief hypotension due to acute hypovolemia, which promptly responds to adequate transfusion.

On the other hand, a second, even moderate, bout of hypotension can produce widespread multiple organ damage of a serious degree. These consequences are probably synergized by the initial modest insult to cellular metabolism. Another insult occurring during the vulnerable period of impaired transport activity can prove intolerable.

The injudicious employment of inappropriate volumes of sodium-containing parenteral fluids is capable of imposing a serious overload in persons with cardiopathy. Unless careful attention is focused on this issue, heart failure will develop in many patients with a low cardiac reserve. This sodium-retained accumulation of fluid can delay the operation or, remaining unrecognized and untreated, complicate the convalescence or even be fatal. As a corollary of this, attempts at abrupt restoration of low sodium values to normal levels, by giving intravenous normal saline, may also have lethal consequences in a patient previously maintained on a low sodium diet for the control of his heart disease and who already exhibits marked water retention. This patient must be dehydrated in order to raise his serum sodium.

Potassium deficits, and their capacity for triggering serious, even intractable cardiac arrhythmias, must be considered in patients who require an operation. Those circumstances associated with abnormal potassium losses can create significant states of intracellular depletion. The magnitude of this withdrawal is imperfectly revealed by the plasma level of potassium at any given moment. Replenishment therapy, therefore, must always be guided as well by any residual ion depletion effects on cardiac function after apparently satisfactory restorative therapy. Unfortunately, during repletion the heart is distressingly intolerant of potassium overloading.

PULMONARY DISEASE.   The presence of any substantial amount of pulmonary disease is ordinarily ascertainable from the history, physical examination and admission chest roentgenogram, with an assist at times from electrocardiographic findings of cor pulmonale. Routine preoperative measurement of the timed vital capacity is desirable before every major operation. Any serious reduction is particularly important if the patient is asthmatic, chronically bronchitic, emphysematous or has advanced pulmonary hypertension. The use of the one-second vital capacity test provides a valuable index of functional capacity in these crippled people. The first second volume should be at least 80 per cent of the total expiratory volume. A simple, but functionally useful, test of the patient's respiratory reserve is to walk up a few flights of stairs with him and note his tolerance to this amount of physical activity, observing whether he is still able to converse naturally without labored breathing.

In any potential problem situation blood gas analyses and arterial pH values are essential for proper evaluation of the patient. Furthermore, in a difficult diagnostic problem they can provide fundamental differential data leading to the need for confirmatory pulmonary angiograms or scans.

Patients with excessive tracheobronchial secretions benefit from preoperative postural drainage of the respiratory tract; the use of surface tension-lowering and smooth muscle-relaxing drugs added to inhalants; avoidance of a very low environmental humidity, and differential ventilatory instructions, if a pulmonary resection is contemplated. Patients with frankly purulent sputum should receive appropriate antibiotic therapy based on gram stains, cultures and sensitivity tests for the predominant organism. Until this condition has been essentially cleared up, the patient is not a candidate for an elective operation. The prophylactic use of penicillin for several days preoperatively in such patients, as well as in those with related disorders, appears to lower the incidence of postoperative pulmonary complications from atelectasis and pneumonia.

Tobacco smokers, especially those addicted to the heavy consumption of cigarettes, should interrupt this habit for at least ten to 14 days prior to an elective major procedure. Those patients awaiting a hernia repair, an extensive pulmonary resection, or an abdominal operation likely to require a long midline incision are particularly benefited by the consequences of this action. Cigarette smokers are more likely to develop respiratory complications in the postoperative period than are nonsmokers. Even temporary preoperative discontinuance of this habit has a beneficial effect on restoring ciliary motility within the tracheobronchial tree.

RENAL DISEASE. In the absence of historical evidence either for renal disease or symptomatic involvement, a urinalysis that includes microscopic characteristics, specific gravity and testing for carbohydrate, along with the blood values for urea nitrogen and creatinine, suffices for the usual renal study for an elective operation. However, when chronic uropathy is a likely probability more detailed procedures are required. Fortunately, urinary tract disease can usually be diagnosed with considerable accuracy when suitable procedures are requested. The 24-hour endogenous creatinine clearance test provides very useful data about glomerular functional reserve. Values secured longitudinally in the management of a particular problem serve to guide the continuing therapy and quantify clinical prognostications. Cultures should regularly be made for any specific organisms whenever pyuria or bacteriuria has been demonstrated. With sensitivity studies to follow, the correct antibacterial program can confidently be initiated. Excretory or retrograde urography, in conjunction with selective angiography when necessary, reveals significant aspects of many uropathies, ranging from obstructive processes through degenerative lesions and including a variety of indigenous tumors. The value of determining renal reserve is real, for severe functional impairment poses serious additional burdens on the traumatized patient. The invalid may have a uremia-induced anemia and certain immunological capacities may be depressed. Positive nitrogen balance is likely to be more difficult to restore, especially if there is a significant albuminuria. Gastrointestinal bleeding is not uncommon and hiccoughs may compli-cate the convalescence as well as threaten the wound with dehiscence. Fever and fatigue are constant threats and both place abnormal demands in energy costs at a time when the balance may be precarious at best.

For those patients requiring a surgical procedure despite marked renal disease, for example, a person with a leaking abdominal aneurysm, particular precautions are essential in order to avoid further compromise of function. The routine should include particular care to avoid renal ischemia, as from a period of systemic hypotension. Dehydration magnifies the consequences of such a low flow state. Therefore, both fluid and solute for obligatory diuresis should be available to the body. The patient should also be protected against hypotension by suitable volume expansion with plasma or blood. Proper hydration and blood pressure stabilization are the key measures; exclusive reliance on or routine use of osmotic diuretics is not necessary. Rather, the entire pattern of salt and fluid management must be kept in exquisite order while titrating the patient's needs and his tolerance to parenteral therapy.

GASTROINTESTINAL PREPARATION. Insertion of a nine-holed gastric tube and the application of continuous, gentle suction to it on the evening before a major intra-abdominal operation permits the surgeon to work with a collapsed bowel and can facilitate procedures thereon. This is especially effective in combination with a thorough cleansing bowel preparation in a patient requiring repair for a pendulous ventral hernia. Another type of patient who will benefit from prophylactic use of gastric siphonage is the abnormally apprehensive, air-swallowing individual.

For operations upon the stomach and esophagus in the presence of obstruction, extra care should be taken to remove food debris, which can be a rich medium for pathogenic bacteria, particularly in an achlorhydric environment. Repeated washings with a large-bore tube are required upon these occasions to remove partially digested material. This precaution effectively decreases the potential for regurgitation and aspiration of material which upon reaching the bronchioles and air sacs inflames, obstructs and necrotizes these tissues. Such a complication, assisted by any bacteria present, produces diffuse, even life-endangering, pneumonitis. The use of neomycin or kanamycin orally will effectively reduce the gastric bacterial flora. All persons undergoing major abdominal operations do not require gastric suction to ensure a safe convalescence. It should neither be routinely used nor routinely banned.

In patients having incomplete or potential obstruction of the colon, it is highly desirable to prevent this from becoming complete. Otherwise, a preliminary decompression operation may be necessary in addition to the resection procedure later. Therefore, care should be taken to alert the radiologist to avoid forcing any substantial amount of barium proximal to a narrowed area in a patient in whom an x-ray examination seems necessary to confirm the nature of the large bowel obstruction. In persons so threatened, the diet should be selected for its low residual content. The bulk and consistency of the stool can be effectively reduced also by giving kanamycin or a combination of poorly absorbed sulfa preparations and neomycin by mouth. Rarely, this regimen so disrupts the intestinal flora that an overgrowth of staphylococcal organisms takes place. The individual may then develop pseudomembranous enterocolitis. The process is characterized by diarrhea, evidence of sepsis and prompt patient deterioration unless it is treated. The objectives of therapy are restoration of a normal colonic bacterial population by means of a fecal enema or Lactobacillus organisms by mouth and, equally important, antibacterial therapy to control the staphylococcal sepsis problem. Additional fluids, including plasma and whole blood transfusions, may be required in some to combat any hypotension or low flow state. Mineral oil given orally several times a day will further counteract a tendency to impaction above the lesion. If these measures prove ineffectual and some degree of obstruction persists, although it is still incomplete, the temporary use of continuous gastric suction may obviate the necessity of a colostomy. Any final nutritional preparation can then be accomplished through parenteral alimentation.

For any major abdominal procedure, the administration of 2 to 3 ounces of mineral oil by mouth the night before an operation, and again when the nasal tube is removed, will minimize the distress of passing the first postoperative, often inspissated, stool.

FINAL PREPARATORY STEPS. When an operation is likely to be started late, it is wise to begin to meet the patient's fluid requirements earlier in the day with an intravenous injection of 1000 to 1500 cc. of a 5 to 10 per cent glucose solution containing 77 to 115 mEq. (4.5 to 7 gm.) of sodium chloride together with any vitamin supplements. In addition to fulfilling some of the body's energy requirements, any tendency to preoperative dehydration is controlled. In fact, for certain operations associated with a greater tendency toward postoperative oliguria or anuria, preoperative hydration by means of a "water load" is an effective means for avoiding that complication. The patient can be given approximately one-third of his calculated daily fluid requirements as 5 per cent glucose in half-strength saline (77 mEq. per liter) during the two or three hours prior to anesthetization. The resultant preoperative diuresis will substantially reduce the likelihood of postoperative renal shutdown, in the absence of contributing complications additionally interfering with renal function. Unless the patient voids or is catheterized before going to the operating room, serious vesical overdistention may develop before the patient can micturate or be catheterized postoperatively.

Whenever nasogastric suction is started the night before the operation, intravenous fluids with sodium chloride are particularly desirable in order to avoid any possibility of lowering the volume of the extracellular fluid compartment. Extracellular fluid depletion just prior to anesthesia, among other adverse consequences, is a strong stimulus to aldosterone formation.

The availability of prepared preoperative order sheets on the surgical stations simplifies this stage of readying the patient for his operation. It also serves as a useful check list of the customary things to be done.

SKIN PREPARATION. Vexing difficulties with wound infections, unfortunately often of a staphylococcal nature, may stem from multiple sources. One is from organisms within the patient's own dermal crypts. Some protection against this locus can be realized by repeated lathering of the patient's entire body with soapsuds containing hexachlorophene. For the ambulatory individual, this need involve no more than thorough sessions in the shower, with attention directed especially to the cleansing of scalp, face, axillae, groin and anogenital areas. The action of this surface-acting germicide requires time. Therefore, this program should be carried out in elective surgical procedures on two or three occasions prior to the day of the opera-

Preoperative Order Sheet

1. Scrub   a. Entire patient with G-11 soap
              b. _____ area

2. Fluids today

         _____ cc. 5% glucose
               with _____ mEq. NaCl
               with _____ mEq. KCl
         _____ cc. 10% glucose
               with _____ mEq. NaCl
               with _____ mEq. KCl
            Rate _____ cc./hr.

3. Tap water enema _____ tonight
                           _____ A.M.

4. Draw blood and cross-match _____ bottles

5. Pentobarbital, mg. _____ h.s.
                           _____ A.M.

6. Weigh patient before going to O.R. in A.M.

7. Nothing by mouth after _____ A.M.
                           _____ P.M.

8. Insert nine-holed nasogastric tube____ P.M.
    (connect and check function of it)

9. Insert urinary catheter (connect and
    check function of it) _____ P.M.
    (Have patient void before being taken to
    O. R. if not catheterized) _____ A.M.

10. Wrap both limbs (toes to groin)
     with elastic bandages   _____ A.M.
                                _____ P.M.

11. On call from O.R. sedation_____

tion. A final similar cleansing of the area adjacent to the incision is recommended just prior to application of the skin antiseptic in the operating room except when that area overlies a soft tissue malignancy. Finally, the application of an adhering plastic sheet to the isolated operative field effectively separates the line of incision made through it from the adjacent cuts. Thereafter, moist packs, which are applied to wound edges for protection of the soft tissues against drying, do not accumulate bacteria that would be flushed thereby from dermal recesses. In theory, the patient should not be shaved the day or evening before an operation because any scratches or abrasions of the skin thus created can become infected. If the operative incision crosses such an area, these multiplying bacteria will be seeded into the depths.

DISCUSSION OF OPERATION WITH PATIENT AND RELATIVES. The preoperative preparation has not been completed until the surgeon has described carefully, in language which the patient should be able to understand, the procedure contemplated. A discussion of the operation should include clear-cut explanations as to why it is necessary. It is particularly important to describe the consequences of that operation to a person about to acquire a permanent colostomy, an ampu-

tation, a visibly deforming procedure, or an endocrine removal certain to require substitution therapy or to alter the patient's life-giving powers. This discourse must be carefully balanced so as to be informative but not anxiety inducing, and is always to be couched in terms of interest in the person and with sympathy for his problem. When the patient is a child, this dialogue will usually be with the parents. Nevertheless, it is both humane and sound psychologically to enlist the youngster's cooperative understanding by conversations phrased in respect for limited vocabulary and tender emotions.

The principle of informed consent is more emphatically before us today than in the past. Although the boundaries vary within reasonable latitudes, the fundamental theme resides in the precise phrase "informed consent." Therefore, stress on communication achieved by means of a viable dialogue between patient, parent or guardian and the surgeon is critical to achieving this objective. Specifically, the surgeon's role in this significant life episode should be both personal and identifiable. Relatives, or friends, should be specifically informed about the place where the surgeon will converse with them. Some explanation for the necessary paraphernalia cluttered about the postoperative patient is desirable. Such briefing will contribute to basic understanding, meanwhile partially allaying overstrained anxieties.

After ascertaining that the patient is doing satisfactorily in the immediate postanesthetic phase, the thoughtful surgeon communicates with the relatives. He should devote as much time as may be required to a forthright discussion of the problems encountered and how they are being solved. He should appraise the likelihood for a successful outcome. This can be reassuring, for those in waiting are naturally anxious. If the news is bleak, a few moments' warning provides some emotional cushion against this impact.

OPERATIVE CARE

The induction of anesthesia disadvantages the inductee. For those individuals with a less resilient psyche it must be quite traumatic. On the other hand, an induction room apart from the hubbub of operating room traffic can provide greater privacy in a generally more relaxed environment. In addition, the surgeon should make a distinct effort to strengthen the patient's emotional base by his personal presence and a few thoughtful words of reassurance just prior to beginning the anesthetic manipulations.

During an operation, attention should continue to be focused on the same physiologic factors which were of concern preoperatively: any blood, electrolyte or fluid deficiencies, together with attention to cardiorenal and pulmonary dysfunction. The employment of a scale for accurately weighing the blood lost during the operation is of value. Throughout the dissection dry fluffs and packs are used to collect the blood and, in addition, all blood suctioned from the field is collected into a calibrated trap system. With practice, reasonable estimates can be made of that volume of blood absorbed by drapes in the field. If these tabulations are kept current by an attendant, a running account of the estimated blood loss is available to the surgeon. The resultant figure is uniformly on the low side of the actual volume of blood lost, and should be so interpreted when the amount and rate of blood for replacement are ordered.

Exposed viscera should be protected against dehydration by covering with packs moistened in saline or Ringer's solution. Otherwise, various types and sizes of dry sponges are employed. When these become blood-stained and have been passed out of the sterile field to be counted by a circulating nurse, their gain in weight can be tabulated. This gravimetric determination of the blood loss onto sponges compares reliably with either colorimetric or isotopic estimates. The wisdom of shock prevention as opposed to shock therapy is endorsed by providing the patient with an amount rather in excess of those volumes which have been measured.

For children up to 20 kg. in weight, use of a scale in the operating room is a highly accurate means of measuring the total blood loss during an operation. If the child has been precisely balanced just before the operation begins, the only change at the termination of the surgical procedure must be from blood loss and any specimens removed.

The fluid losses through sweating during a prolonged operation can be considerable in an adult if the weather is hot and the operating room is not air conditioned. These fluid requirements should be met by replacement of water and electrolytes during the operation. Maintenance of adequate hydration will reduce the number of mechanisms provoking postoperative oliguria. The routine inclusion of a well-functioning intravenous apparatus among the operating room facilities is, therefore, strongly recommended for all major procedures. This equipment should be so adaptable as to permit the ready infusion of a variety of solutions and should include a plastic cannula, or needle, suitable for rapid transfusions. Preferably, an upper extremity vein is used. The needle must be shielded from possible dislodgment and the tubing from kinking during operative manipulations.

For surgical procedures of any duration, some protection should be provided for all the patient's bony prominences. A sponge rubber or air mattress is best, but air-filled rings will suffice. A scrawny individual, in particular, can readily acquire areas of pressure necrosis, particularly on the heels and sacrum, unless protected. The unrelieved weight of the patient, the drapes, sundry equipment and a tired, leaning assistant have undoubtedly caused some bedsores customarily ascribed to negligent nursing care. Enough padding around the patient's elbow to prevent pressure palsy of the ulnar and radial nerves or the brachial plexus, particularly if a deep Trendelenburg position is to be used, is always a wise precaution. Constrictive wrappings about the legs, especially in the elderly person with arteriosclerotic vascular insufficiency who is positioned for long periods in stirrups, can have a serious aftermath. A mattress type device capable of use either as a warming or cooling unit is likely to be advantageous in maintaining body temperature near normal during operations on neonates, or the enfeebled elderly individual. In both instances, significant degrees of hypo- or hyperthermia can create serious problems including ventricular fibrillation for the former and convulsions for the latter temperature deviation. Whenever the possibility of widely abnormal temperature drifts is real, monitoring by a rectal or esophageal thermistor will provide a handy periodic reference device. To avoid the at times catastrophic infusion of large volumes of cold blood, equipment is now available which promptly raises the temperature of injected units taken directly from cold storage. One hundred cubic centimeters per minute at normal body temperature can thereby be introduced.

HYPOXIA. Avoidance of hypoxia is largely in the province of the anesthesiologist. It is his obligation to ensure that there is an open airway at all times from the moment of induction through the recovery of consciousness and until the patient is fully self-sufficient for breathing. Therefore, it is important that the patient have an empty stomach at the time of inducing anesthesia, so as to minimize the opportunity for vomiting material that can be aspirated. If the gastric pouch cannot be emptied safely by alimentary intubation, the anesthesiologist should introduce an occlusive endotracheal tube after abolishing the gag reflex with a local anesthetic. With the cough reflex thus preserved, until the possibility of aspiration has been controlled, the substantial hazard in an unconscious patient of disseminating gastrointestinal vomitus throughout the tracheobronchial tree is materially lessened. Aspiration under such circumstances is a not uncommon harbinger of cardiac arrest. During attempts to treat the situation, particularly in the more seriously ill, calamity can progress to disaster. The next commitment is to provide for adequate pulmonary ventilation with an appropriate concentration of an oxygen-enriched gas mixture. Whenever the patient fails to, or cannot, voluntarily respire deeply enough, the prevention of hypoxia is incumbent on the anesthesiologist. The surgeon in turn should learn to adjust his techniques and accept any inconveniences of motion or patient position necessary to the attainment of this goal.

HYPERCARBIA. Far more insidious than hypoxia, and at least as detrimental to the patient's welfare, is hypercarbia. The gradual accumulation of significant volumes of carbon dioxide in the anesthetized patient's blood, due to inadequate ventilation, produces profound metabolic consequences when allowed to persist for any substantial time. This treacherous situation has few overt manifestations likely to alert the anesthesiologist. Direct measurements of pH or pCO_2, either in the circulating arterial blood or appropriate analyses of the expired breath, are revealing of the problem's magnitude. It is surprising that a rapid carbon dioxide analyzer is not routinely used, despite the fact that this instrument is readily available, clinically important and has an acceptable accuracy over a reasonable range. In the absence of such precautionary devices, the only protection against hypercarbia is an unflagging attention to the maintenance of effective manual or mechanical ventilation. Failure to recognize the accumulation of carbon dioxide, until it is able to produce severe acidosis, may well be an initiating factor in triggering abnormal vagal reflexes and cardiac arrhythmias, including ventricular fibrillation and cardiac arrest. Moreover, hypercarbia through its vasopressor effect may mask coexisting hypovolemia, and become disastrously apparent only in the postanesthetic recovery period when the carbon dioxide tension in the blood has been reduced toward normal.

Hypoxia and hypercarbia place additional and adverse demands on the entire organism. The sum total of these effects is likely to be particularly onerous for the elderly patient. They relate directly to the lung and kidney, sites of frequent reduction in functional reserve. Upon these specific organs we depend for compensatory control over all those events stemming from low tissue oxygen tension as well as associated subnormal oxyhemoglobin saturation values. Inevitably, under these conditions there is anerobic glycolysis and intracellular acidosis. The superimposition of respiratory acidosis potentiates the seriousness of the already threatened integrity of cellular metabolism.

CARDIAC ARREST AND RESUSCITATIVE MEASURES. The term "cardiac arrest" is meant to include all forms of cardiac standstill in asystole or ventricular fibrillation, wherein the heart is no longer able to propel a sufficient volume of blood through the circulatory system to produce a detectable blood pressure. With either cardiac standstill or the ineffectual motions of ventricular fibrillation, no more than a few minutes must be allowed to intervene before the circulation is restored at normal or elevated body temperature, if death or irreparable brain damage is to be prevented.

The cells of the cerebrum are particularly vulnerable to the metabolic consequences of circulatory stagnation associated with cardiac arrest. After an interval of no more than five minutes, their destruction progresses rapidly and so, even though other major organ systems may ultimately be restored, including effective cardiac activity, the individual may have been made decerebrate during this period of inadequate cerebral blood flow.

The suggestion to reduce the self-destructive metabolic demands of the brain, in the early postarrest period, by prompt utilization of general hypothermia (30 to 32° C.) has much to recommend it, once an effective cardiac beat has been restored. Any tendency to shivering or convulsions must then be eliminated with muscle-paralyzing drugs, to avoid inducing an increase in body temperature. It may be necessary to maintain the lowered body temperature for 24 to 72 hours before restoration to a euthermic state is safe.

There are many methods of preventing this grave complication. It is to be emphasized that a definite number of such instances in the immediate postoperative period can clearly be identified as arising from improper anesthetic techniques, with particular reference to the management of high levels of carbon dioxide accumulation in the blood during the anesthetic interval. Hyperventilation, even with air, under these circumstances can trigger a bout of ventricular fibrillation.

Likewise, relentless persistence during pharyngotracheal aspiration in the acidotic patient can contribute to the onset of cardiac arrest. Another susceptible group can be identified by a tendency to runs of premature ventricular contractions.

It is crucial to the success of resuscitative measures that provision be made in advance. The equipment required must be available and the principles involved in surgical technique must be clearly understood. An airway must be promptly established and adequate ventilation achieved. A tank, valve and conduction system capable of delivering oxygen in high concentration to a tight-fitting mask, or even better into an endotracheal tube, should be regularly and immediately available; mouth-to-mouth insufflation should be tried. Any arrangement selected must permit satisfactory ventilation of the lung. A prolonged search for a mask, oxygen tank and other special instruments converts an outlook which is grim, at best, into a hopeless cause.

Fortunately for the patient, the prospects of a successful restoration of an effective cardiac action have been improved by the introduction of closed chest cardiopulmonary resuscitation by Jude and Kouvenhoven. The procedure is simple and in many instances will avoid the necessity of a thoracotomy and internal cardiac massage. Certainly, this closed technique should be tried first, even when the event occurs in the operating room, unless the thorax is already open. In fact, the method can be used outside a hospital and by suitably trained nonmedical personnel. Whenever it is thus employed for cardiac resuscitation, mouth-to-mouth respiration should be established simultaneously with initiation of external massage. It is preferable to position the patient on a firm flat surface. The resuscitor tries to locate himself higher than the patient, places the heel of one hand on the lower sternum, with fingers extended. The second hand is then put down on the back of the first and both elbows are extended. Thus reinforced, he thrusts with firmness posteriorly seeking thereby to compress the myocardium with the sternal components and so force blood through the pulmonary and systemic circuits. With vigor, particularly in younger persons, it is possible to depress the sternum at least 4 to 5 cm. When this force is relaxed, the thoracic cage returns to its original shape. With the resultant intrathoracic expansion, the heart fills and awaits the next thrust. At a compression rate of 60 per minute, an induced systolic pressure of at least 125 mm. Hg can frequently be measured.

Having re-established both ventilation and circulation, attention can be directed in a more leisurely fashion to the electrical restoration of cardiac rhythm. External cardiac defibrillation should be attempted if spontaneous conversion has not already occurred in response to improved perfusion pressure and myocardial oxygenation. For this purpose, commercially available square wave, direct current instruments are both more effective and less damaging to the myocardium when tested at the voltage-amperage and impulse duration required to shock the heart into sinus rhythm. Myocardial damage from excessive electrical heat can also be reduced through improved transmission of the defibrillatory impulse by coating the contact surfaces on the paddles with electrocardiographic electrode jelly. Use of this, or a similarly suitable conductor, will avoid varying degrees of electrical burn prone to appear when the electrodes are positioned on dry skin.

The use of certain drugs may be helpful in restoring better cardiac function during one of these episodes. These medications can be given intravenously, if the circulation justifies that route, or if a more direct and concentrated action is required, a fourth left interspace, parasternal intracardiac injection should be tried. An intracardiac injection of M/7 sodium lactate, or a solution of 7 per cent sodium bicarbonate, in 10 to 50 cc. increments will at times facilitate subsequent electrical defibrillation of a heart recalcitrant to the establishment of a normal rhythm despite massage and previous electroshocks. It should be recalled also that until the tissue pH has been restored to normal values from the state of metabolic acidosis present in hypoxia, the pharmacologic effectiveness of pressor amines is materially reduced.

After correction of the pH, the heart, if still flabby in tone, will derive appreciable benefit from the judicious use of dilute solutions of epinephrine (0.5 to 1.0 cc. of 1:10,000) or equal volumes of Isuprel (isoproterenol) 1:50,000 introduced into the blood and perfusing the myocardium. Caution is urged against injection of calcium solutions into a venoclysis system which is in use simultaneously for transfusions of citrated blood, without flushing the tubing first. It is even more important to avoid direct intracardiac injections of calcium salts during the resuscitation of a person receiving large volumes of citrated blood, perhaps because of associated blood loss, and in whom the circulation is slowed. Abrupt recalcification of the transfused blood can occur and promptly thereafter lead to fatal intravascular clotting.

Digitalization may be required during or shortly after such a testing episode of cardiac arrest. If so, preference should be given the shorter acting compounds. If the serum and cellular potassium might conceivably be low, one should be reluctant to order full therapeutic amounts of any digitalizing compound, because of increased toxicity under such circumstances.

Whenever adequate additional assistance becomes available at any stage of this rapidly moving sequence of events, to someone should be delegated the responsibility of placing a wide-bore cannula of metal or polythene into an acceptable peripheral vein. The availability of this route for infusion is always helpful and may prove of considerable importance at any given moment. The ability to establish deftly a cut-down type venous cannulation, leading to a smooth-working infusion, is a modest skill, yet one to be admired and cherished by the surgeon regardless of his stage of development. In other words, the venous anatomy adjacent to the medial malleolus, in the groin or the forearm should be common knowledge.

If a catheter is not already in the bladder, one should be inserted in order to secure hourly information about urine volume and specific gravity. Unless urine formation is restored promptly, serious consideration should be given to the infusion of mannitol (50 cc. of 25 per cent solution) or low molecular weight dextran (500 cc. of 10 per cent solution). The former can induce protective osmolar diuresis in the temporarily hypofunctioning kidney that develops secondary to cardiac arrest, followed by hypotension of such reasonable duration and degree that it can be corrected without repeated recourse to exogenous sources of vasospastic drugs. Rheomacrodex protects against the sludging tendency present and evokes a diuresis on this basis as well. Since each preparation performs best the earlier its therapeutic contribution is made, prompt diagnosis of their need is essential. In other patients, central nervous system injury may be apparent. If kidney function is adequate, intravenous urea, dexamethasone and a few degrees of systemic hypothermia may benefit any cerebral edema present.

Despite reasonable precaution during the performance of closed chest cardiopulmonary resuscitation, injury to the heart, lung, liver, spleen and sternum, costal cartilages and ribs can occur. In untrained and unskilled hands, the frequency of these events is certain to be higher. Therefore, it clearly behooves each person likely to encounter the problem of cardiac arrest to familiarize himself with the basic aspects of treatment by the potentially lifesaving Jude technique. The ultimate prognosis in any given case of cardiac arrest will depend upon a host of factors, but the most important items probably are the duration and degree of cerebral hypoxia. Underlying myocardial disease will inevitably prejudice the end result. With attention to details, dozens of patients every year can now be saved who would have previously been lost because of this abrupt and rarely anticipatable disaster.

DRAINS. The use of drains after surgical procedures remains a controversial subject. Advantages can be cited on both sides of the question. The blood, plasma, bile, pancreatic juice or intestinal contents which drain denote the presence of this problem and suggest its need for treatment. Those who prefer not to use drains cite a lower incidence of such complications, and suggest that these events are produced in part by the presence of these foreign materials.

Several types of simple drains can be used.

Penrose tubing, soft-rubber catheters, rubber wicks and cigarette drains rely on capillarity, gravity or slight pressure differences to effect the removal of fluid. Intra-abdominal drains customarily seal off from the adjacent viscera within 48 hours. However, if one continues to ooze fluid, such as bile, from a site of leakage for many days, there should be no haste about removing it.

The other common type of drain is usually a more complex apparatus. It may have the form of a sump pump, a double-lumen catheter, air-vent suction, or a multiple-holed catheter. All of these are open-circulation suction drains. They require mechanical suction to supplement the other forces of drainage and keep the selected area dry. They eventually become walled off, but serve to keep a site of leakage or a pocket drier, and thereby facilitate local healing. However, they draw air-borne bacteria into the wound, thereby adding pathogenic contaminants to the problem. Continuous, low pressure suction applied to a multiple-holed catheter, positioned under the skin flaps in a neck dissection or a radical mastectomy, is a particularly effective technique for coapting widely reflected surfaces. Intrapleural catheter suction assures lung expansion and controls air leaks.

The principal purposes of drainage are to prevent pocketing by revealing the existence and volume of internal accumulations, and to provide for external fistulation at the site of any leak. Once the drain has ceased doing either or both of these functions, it should be eased out gradually, a few centimeters at a time. In this way, the tract can fill in from the depths. If all the tubing is pulled away at one time, the skin can seal before the depths are firmly united by healthy tissue. Pocketing and suppuration can still develop inside and complicate the later convalescence. Pain and localized tenderness will be noticeable in that area and may require subsequent reopening of this channel, or some form of dependent drainage.

Drains, particularly the firmer types, have been accused of abetting, or even causing, fistula formation when alongside an intestinal anastomosis. It is felt by those opposed to using them that the suture line is weakened by its proximity to a foreign body. Those in favor suggest that, if provision for such drainage had not been supplied when the suture line gave way, subsequent leakage and contamination would have dissected more widely while seeking a path to the outside. Drains serve a necessary purpose when used to maintain an evacuation track from an abscess pocket; their prophylactic, routine employment has little to recommend it.

OPERATIVE AND PROGRESS NOTES. An accurate and informative operative report should be promptly dictated by the surgeon for insertion upon the patient's chart, while the details are fresh in his mind. The first surgical assistant should write a note immediately and place it upon the chart to help in guiding the postoperative care. Such a summary is not designed to replace, but rather to supplement the formal operative report prepared by the surgeon. This precis should mention the kind of anesthetic, type and location of the incision, pertinent and unusual details of the operative findings, principles of the operation carried out, amount of blood lost and transfused, the nature and volume of fluids given while patient was in the operating room, type and location of drains, whether a T-tube or catheter was used and method as well as kind of suture materials used in the closure. Finally there should be a realistic description of any complications developing during the transoperative period. Simple line drawings are frequently helpful, out of proportion to the artist's skill. Any unusual technical problems or maneuvers should be appropriately identified. Progress notes should be regularly added to this report, particularly during the first few days and always whenever any new problem arises to mar the convalescence. Any significant changes in therapy should be cited. A specific note should be made when any drain is removed or allowed to remain in place at the time of the patient's leaving the hospital.

Finally, the notes should include a tabulation of the discharge instructions regarding diet, medications and recommendations for outpatient follow-up visits. In all these reports, the emphasis should be upon clarity and brevity without sacrificing relevant information but with minimal reliance on use of eponyms, colloquialisms, initial-type abbreviations and other pet symbols indecipherable to future generations seeking knowledge from these charts.

COMMUNICATION WITH PATIENT AND RELATIVES. Those moments right after the operation are particularly propitious for creating a charismatic bond with relatives and friends of the patient. Even a brief, warmly informative dialogue emphasizing the positive features of the overall situation reveals empathy and creates a stronger family-physician alliance. It will be appreciated by all. Should complications mar the patient's surgical experiences, all interpersonal relationships will weather this storm more certainly when such communion prevails.

Any colleague who may have shared in the diagnostic preambles will appreciate the courtesy of a telephone, or brief typewritten, report on the findings and treatment provided during the operation. At the time of discharge, a concise letter is in order. In fact, if the recovery is protracted or does not proceed smoothly, he deserves to be so informed, for you have been given his vote of approval by the referral of the patient for surgical treatment.

POSTOPERATIVE CARE

POSTANESTHETIC CARE. The unconscious or semicomatose patient should be returned from the operating room positioned on his side, with the dependent thigh and knee flexed and the upper one extended to provide some rotational stability. The head then lolls from the shoulder, allowing secretions to drain away. Whatever the position or method of transport, a clear airway is the first consideration. Periodic checks should be made even while the patient is en route from the operating room to his bed. The principal object of any position is to prevent regurgitation and aspiration. Certainly, saliva or gastrointestinal contents which are allowed to accumulate in the tracheobronchial tree postoperatively are a major cause of atelectasis, pneumonitis and pneumonia. When aspiration occurs, the tracheobronchial tree should be thoroughly cleansed at once of all foreign material and then washed with generous amounts of saline. This latter procedure will contribute to the thoroughness of the toilet and also be beneficial through its dilution of damaging proteolytic gastrointestinal secretions. Dexamethasone, if given immediately after the insult to the tracheobronchial tree, seems to reduce the serious inflammatory aspects of the bronchitis and pneumonitis which frequently prove hazardous after such an event. An effective prophylaxis against this occurrence is the routine use of gastric siphonage during operation. This arrangement also minimizes the development of distention secondary to the anesthesiologist's

pumping gas into the intestinal tract while he is forcefully ventilating the patient by means of a face mask. In the early postoperative phase, repeated nasopharyngeal aspirations are frequently required to care for the gathering saliva when the volume exceeds the patient's capacity to handle it.

The use of a recovery ward in proximity to the operating room represents a widespread modern trend which has understandably earned general acceptance. When this helpful arrangement exists, all anesthetized patients should be kept in the recovery area during the immediate postoperative phase, until the vital signs are stable and the individual responds to inquiry.

The management of postoperative emergencies is also improved because responsibility for the patient's nursing care during the important first few hours is met by a trained organization. The training of a few specialized individuals for a postanesthetic care unit is more effective than equivalent efforts spread throughout the surgical nursing service.

Oxygen therapy equipment, tracheostomy trays, transfusion apparatus, motor-driven suction and other resuscitative equipment and drugs should be kept on hand for prompt use. Customarily, a standard monitoring device for the electrocardiogram should be available. More sophisticated intensive care units contain apparatus capable of translating appropriately derived signals into oscilloscopic images or digitized values for such variables as cardiac output, changing myocardial power requirements, and work of breathing. A well trained group of nurses and doctors staffing a recovery ward can demonstrate teamwork in the management of an individual with cardiac arrest. This is as emergent a situation as can confront any doctor and must be handled promptly, decisively and effectively in order to provide that patient with the best opportunity for survival despite this catastrophe.

After the patient reaches the recovery ward, or his own room, it is best to elevate the foot of the bed slightly unless he is fully conscious and active. The slope promotes evacuation of tracheobronchial secretions, discourages venous stagnation in the lower limbs and contributes to stabilization of the blood pressure. Until the patient has resumed control of his faculties, it is important to remove excess mucous secretions regularly by the use of suction, which is applied intermittently through a catheter passed via the nose into the upper portion of the trachea. Pulmonary ventilation is promoted by turning the patient at intervals, urging him to cough and breathe deeply, or through periodic utilization of intermittent positive pressure breathing by means of a respirator. These measures will contribute to a substantial lowering of the incidence of atelectasis and postoperative pneumonia.

Until the patient's orientation returns, someone should remain in close attendance and side rails are advisable lest an inadvertent turn lead to a tumble onto the floor. This bad bump or even a fracture can be avoided. Beds low to the floor, although perhaps a bane to those giving nursing care, do provide a safety factor for the patient.

Transfusions are given to balance losses noted in the operating room or recovery area. They are continued until the blood pressure and pulse rate remain stabilized well outside any shock range. Sufficient fluids and electrolytes are supplied to meet the total daily requirements. It is unwise to follow unqualifyingly the practice of giving only glucose in distilled water on the premise that sodium retention exists in the early postoperative period. Water intoxication, as manifest by weakness, paralysis, twitchings or even convulsions, can develop. This syndrome may appear abruptly on the first or second postoperative day, particularly if it is a child receiving parenteral fluids totally lacking in sodium.

INTENSIVE CARE UNIT.   All patients should be kept in the recovery room until fully conscious and free from certain of the immediate effects of the operation. Some hospitals provide recovery room convalescent care until the patient is ambulatory and has little demand for specialized nursing. Other institutions have developed a subrecovery, or intensive care unit, in which specialized nursing is given to the patient after transfer from the recovery room. Patients remain there until they are out of bed and become minimal care problems.

The availability in these areas of mimeographed postoperative order sheets for the doctors ensures use of this list and will simplify the nursing routine and avoid overlooking important measures in this phase of postoperative care. A workable example of this arrangement is listed.

ATELECTASIS.   Atelectasis can arise either from pulmonary compression by intratho-

Doctor's Postoperative Order Sheet

1. Vital signs q. 15 min. x 4
   q. ½ hr. until stable then
   q. 2 hr. x 24 hr.
2. Position
   _____ Low Trendelenburg
   _____ Semi-Fowler's
   _____ Flat
3. Hemoglobin stat. and in A.M.
4. Turn, cough, hyperventilate q. 2 hr. x 24 then q. 4 hr. until up and about.
5. Suction trachea and aspirate pharynx p.r.n.
6. Continuous gastric suction. Check p.r.n. (at least q. 4 hr.) and irrigate as necessary with _____ cc. of _____ solution.
7. Straight drainage to urinary catheter. Irrigate p.r.n. with sterile water.
8. Chart urine specific gravity b.i.d. 8–6 or q. 2 hr.
9. Weight daily: litter_____ standing_____
10. Sedation _____
11. Antibiotic _____
12. Fluids
    _____ cc. 5% glucose
       with _____ mEq. NaCl
       with _____ mEq. KCl
    _____ cc. 10% glucose
       with _____ mEq. NaCl
       with _____ mEq. KCl
       Rate _____ cc./hr.
13. Catheterize (if unable to void) at _____ A.M.
    _____ P.M.
14. Transfuse _____ cc. blood
    _____ cc. plasma
15. Blood loss _____ (chart on face sheet)
16. Privileges _____
17. Diet _____
18. Chest x-ray stat. _____ A.M. _____
19. Oxygen therapy:
    Tent _____ Nasal _____
    IPPB _____

racic accumulations of air, blood clot, fluid or tumor, or from obstruction of a portion of the bronchial tree by a mucous plug. The former mechanism rarely causes systemic symptoms other than a decrease in maximum ventilatory capacity and, occasionally, osteoarthropathy. The latter invariably provokes a clinical picture characterized by fever and some tachycardia. Imperfect expansion of the lung, whether massive, patchy or platelike, occurring in the postoperative phase, is invariably due to obstruction of a bronchus or its distal ramifications by a mucous plug. A unique form of atelectasis, termed congestive, occurs at times in patients undergoing open heart surgery with a pump oxygenator and a cardiopulmonary by-pass technique.

This lesion probably arises on the basis of interference with surfactant (dipalmitoyl lecithin) metabolism induced by the decreased pulmonary perfusion during the by-pass. High concentration of oxygen above

60 per cent, maintained for several days by means of a respirator system, has also been associated with progressive loss of pulmonary compliance, hypoxia and an inability to wean the patient from this assisting device. Death with "heavy lungs," weighing greater than 1800 gm., has followed usually in such patients. The respirator complex has been falsely charged with creating these developments. Rather, the best evidence to date indicates that the fault appears to be with the high oxygen concentrations. Certainly, the loss of sufficient surface tension lowering substance at the alveolar level eliminates full participation in each breathing cycle for these involved sites. Atelectatic foci promptly develop.

Secondary factors which may contribute to the development of obstructive atelectasis include:

Hypoventilation can result from too profound sedation but is more commonly secondary to pain in the operative site. This tends to limit the usual costal activity. A vertical upper-abdominal incision can contribute to this mechanism. As the ribs flare out with each breath, lateral tension pulls painfully on the wound edges. When pain is a restricting factor in the patient's ventilation, administration of a suitably effective anodyne, or providing a local anesthetic block of the area, will often increase the depth of voluntary respiration.

An operation which weakens, paralyzes or elevates the diaphragm is commonly followed by some ventilatory impairment. After biliary tract surgery, atelectasis is not uncommon and may be related to enthusiastic displacement of the hepatic attachments of the diaphragm while seeking better exposure of the biliary situation. Marked abdominal distention also interferes with normal diaphragmatic activity.

Aspiration of intestinal contents irritates the tracheobronchial mucosa chemically and bacteriologically, and provokes an inflammatory reaction which may progress in many instances to pneumonia. In milder cases, an increase occurs in the volume of local secretions, including mucus, and this too contributes to the high incidence of atelectasis after the accidental aspiration of intestinal contents. The aspiration of coagulable fresh blood is likewise provocative of atelectasis and pneumonitis. Its removal, even by bronchoscopy, can be troublesome.

The administration of large doses of atropine inspissates the mucus and makes it more tenacious, thereby increasing the difficulty in bringing up these sticky plugs.

Certain anesthetic gases are more rapidly absorbed from the lungs than is air. Failure to wash out these mixtures at the end of an operation may contribute to an early appearance of atelectasis.

In the presence of bronchiectasis or a lung abscess, pus, excess mucus and other secretions are already present and available. Loss of the cough reflex during anesthesia fosters retention of secretions and their spillage into either adjacent or contralateral pulmonary segments. This is even more likely to occur during the operative manipulations unless provision is made to prevent such flooding. The patient with pulmonary suppuration should spend a period several times each day before his operation in the head-down position, and try to cough out as much as possible of the accumulated material. Bronchoscopy should also be done before and after the operation in order to ensure thorough evacuation of the tracheobronchial tree, thereby minimizing the chances of postoperative atelectasis. The preoperative use of an appropriate antibiotic, on the basis of smear or culture, for a few days in any patient requiring an operation despite the presence of coexisting, bacterially induced tracheobronchial disease will usually alter the tracheobronchial flora favorably and likewise reduce the volume of secretions. The likelihood of postoperative atelectasis and bronchopneumonia will thereby be reduced.

Cigarette smokers, particularly the heavy users, should be urged to stop this habit for at least ten to 14 days before any elective major surgical procedure. This interval will permit the tracheobronchial tree to recover, at least partially, from the irritation and excess mucus formation frequently associated with "smoker's cough." Ciliary activity of the mucous membrane may partially recover from the depressed state associated with pronounced cigarette addiction.

Dehydration, both systemic and topical, can play a role in the genesis of atelectasis through inspissation of mucous secretions.

Usually, a diagnosis of obstructive atelectasis serious enough to cause clinical symptoms is readily made from examination of the chart and the physical findings. Its presence can be confirmed by a chest film. Though the pulse is rapid, the temperature is elevated often out of proportion both to the heart rate and to the apparent illness of the patient. The onset of fever is sudden, and commonly a temperature of 102° F. or higher is reached. On palpation of the trachea in the neck, a deviation to the affected side can often be noted. The respiratory excursion is more limited over one side than over the other. On auscultation, a few sticky rales can be heard, but either the usual breath sounds are absent or bronchial breathing is noted in the area of involvement. Cyanosis and dyspnea may be present. The roentgenogram shows an area of increased density on the involved side, with a lobar, mottled or platelike distribution, in association with elevation of the diaphragm, narrow rib spaces and variable degrees of displacement of the trachea, mediastinum and heart to the affected side.

The treatment of atelectasis begins with attention to the predisposing and contributing factors. A lowered incidence and milder examples of this complication will result from such prophylaxis. Early ambulation probably helps avoid this complication by increasing the patient's ventilatory efforts. Once the process has developed, it is essential to treat it until it is cured. Failure to reinflate an atelectatic lung is likely to lead to chronic pulmonary changes and irreparable damage. Recurrent atelectasis or pneumonitis in any patient indicates the possibility of intrinsic bronchial obstruction from an adenoma, carcinoma or nonopaque foreign body. Inducing the patient to cough, turning him in bed, hyperventilation with 5 to 10 per cent carbon dioxide in oxygen, and a sharp blow over the side of involvement are often effective means of dislodging a plug and expanding a collapsed segment. Auscultation of the chest should confirm the efficacy of the treatment or indicate the need for further active therapy. Endobronchial aspiration with a catheter attached to suction will make the patient cough and may pull out the offending mucus. In a particularly uncooperative or lethargic patient, translaryngeal suctioning of the trachea and bronchi can be facilitated by using a laryngoscope and an appropriately curved, open-tipped catheter. For the tenaciously adherent plugs, lavaging of the tracheobronchial regions with saline can be helpful. If these measures fail, bronchoscopic management is indicated. The end results of treatment are uniformly good when the disorder is corrected at an early stage of the process. If atelectasis proves intractable, or has been neglected for many days, re-expansion is slower and chronic, irreversible pulmonary changes are more likely to occur.

TRACHEOSTOMY. Tracheostomy can provide lifesaving advantages in the management of the postoperative patient. The problem of excessive or retained secretions, a recurrent tendency toward aspiration, and depressed or impaired ventilation may require this procedure. However, a growing awareness of associated disadvantages necessitate careful evaluation prior to committing any patient to it. For some, the needs can be met by use of an oral or nasal endotracheal tube. The Portex type works well, and creates minimal reaction despite being in place for several days. In the case of infants, it is particularly well tolerated, molds to the airway and hence does not need a cuffed segment, has less tendency to erode adjacent tissues and can be quickly inserted. There must be precise fixation to avoid extubation or migration down a bronchus. Subglottic stenosis is a definite but uncommon complication of these endotracheal tubes. Just as for tracheostomy cannulae, regular, thorough, aseptic cleansing of all inspissated mucus or accumulating secretions is essential for sound function. Disposable sterilized catheters, saline cotton-tipped applicators, and wearing of autoclaved rubber or plastic gloves are mandatory precautions in order to protect the patient's tracheobronchial tree from the ubiquitous and pathogenic bacterial flora of the hospital. Induced gram-negative tracheal contamination leading to pulmonary sepsis is a grave complication with which to burden the convalescent. Painstaking attention to aseptic technique of the tracheostomy toilet can minimize its incidence and severity.

Tracheostomy is at times a wise prophylactic step; on other occasions, it is a well chosen supplemental method of retrieving a deteriorating situation. It may complement the patient's convalescence when extensive surgery about the head and neck has temporarily abolished full control of the swallowing reflexes, so that saliva or liquids are prone to trickle into the trachea. A cuffed tracheostomy tube permits easy and effective aspiration of this airway-clogging, mucoid drainage before it can reach the pulmonary terminals. After deglutition has been recovered, this accessory vent for saliva can be abandoned. For other individuals, whose prolonged efforts to rid themselves of excess secretions have led to exhaustion and a weakened coughing power, the addition of a tracheostomy is of considerable benefit. Its establishment can prevent drowning, by aspiration of secretions, in a patient who is comatose, or profoundly debilitated, and insensitive to the healthy cough-provoking mechanisms of foreign material in the respiratory tract. Moreover, when a tracheostomy opening is available, it simplifies the technique of bronchoscopy. It ensures more ready use of this means to achieve the most complete and thorough removal of all retained secretions. The ease of handling this problem afterward and the minimal disturbance to the patient are certain to encourage more frequent recourse to endoscopy. Whenever the eventual need for a tracheostomy appears likely, it is best to establish one electively a few days prior to the major surgical procedure. A technically neater operation can then be done and the patient's respiratory tract will have had adequate time to adapt to the altered humidity of the air, which now by-passes the oronasopharynx. During this interval, it is particularly important to add moisture to the ambient air, preferably through humidifiers. If oxygen is piped directly into the tracheostomy opening, it should first be dispersed through water in an attempt to saturate it. This is more thoroughly accomplished by heating the pot of water to be vaporized into the tracheal atmosphere. The naturally low environmental humidity of northern winters makes this especially important in tracheostomized patients during that season. Otherwise, desiccation and excessive tracheitis are likely to complicate and needlessly prolong the recovery from a tracheostomy.

Another major benefit associated with tracheostomy derives from the handy and functionally simple attachment of a respirator. Known concentrations of oxygen can be delivered to the patient with confidence that the augmented mixture is washing the tracheobronchial alveolar network. However, it is incumbent on those responsible for the management of respiratory care that high (greater than 60 per cent) concentrations of oxygen are not used for more than a few hours. Assisted respiration with compressed air is best whenever this suffices to maintain the arterial pO_2 near normal values. Intermittent positive pressure ventilation, including a negative phase if advantageous, is also readily included in this system for managing better the more troublesome pulmonary problems. These instruments can be altered to function over b____ad ranges of timed inspiratory and expiratory phases, each cycle of which is self-initiated or automatically predetermined.

Many persons otherwise well versed in postoperative problems exhibit a surprising reluctance to do a tracheostomy. They overlook, or reject, the possible contributions of this simple procedure until terminal and irreversible states of pulmonary congestion and pneumonia prevail. The patient is then being destroyed by infection, hypoxia and hypercapnia. Unless last-minute efforts at removing the occluding plugs and pools are successful, he is doomed.

OLIGURIA-ANURIA REGIMEN. Acute hypovolemia, cardiac arrest, endotoxin shock and certain operative procedures may be followed by oliguria, less than 400 cc. per 24 hours for adults, or anuria, less than 100 cc. urine per 24 hours. This state is both quantitatively and qualitatively distinct from urinary output reduction secondary to the antidiuretic hormone effect induced by operative trauma, blood loss and anesthesia. It needs no special treatment because the latter is a self-limited event.

It is important to recognize promptly this manifest state of functional renal insufficiency. Mere dehydration as a cause of oliguria can usually be suspected from the higher than normal specific gravity, in the absence of other factors. Moreover, a trial response to an hour or so of "water loading" will tend to verify or disprove that tentative diagnosis. Any question of obstructive uropathy should be resolved by pyelography or ureteral catheterization.

For the other and more serious causes of oliguria, a regimen designed to avoid overhydration, control hyperkalemia and minimize acidosis is necessary. An intake-output record is kept for all fluids given and their composition, as well as fluid losses in urine, stools, vomitus and gastrointestinal drainage. The aim is to keep the daily volume intake about equal to output. Insensible losses plus sweating will tend to balance out fluid formed through metabolism of protein and fat for bodily energy. These latter processes add to the fluid compartments and can make a significant contribution to overhydration in the starving and oliguric patient. Specifically, these patients should lose weight daily or serious fluid retention subtly occurs.

To control this accumulation, in part, such patients are maintained on a high carbohydrate diet, when the oral route becomes available. For this eventuality, 50 per cent glucose flavored with orange, lemon or lime is provided either as frozen popsicles or ice cold nectar. Besides sparing body protein breakdown just for energy, the high sugar intake also helps control a tendency toward hyperkalemia through any conversion of carbohydrate to glycogen containing potassium. This process and the subsequent storage of the latter in the liver can be aided by the exogenous administration of insulin. Fifty per cent glucose by mouth has some tendency to produce liquid stools. This sequence may also remove excess potassium. Once the oliguria improves, or after successful treatment with the artificial kidney, considerable skill and painstaking attention are required to assure a smoothly progressing recovery. During the diuretic phase that follows, with its rapid shifts in fluid and electrolyte balance, serious deficits can quickly create new problems. Frequent blood and urine electrolyte determinations, plus accurate recordings of intake-output volumes and composition, are basic to successful management of this stage.

A more subtle form of functional renal insufficiency may occur, characterized by an apparently adequate or even generous urine output. The solitary clue may be a rather fixed specific gravity, near 1.010. When this appears in a patient without previously revealed renal disease, the presumption is strong that a substantial renal insult has occurred. Comparative analysis of the serum and urine osmolarity will reveal that little concentration is being done by the kidney tubules. Customarily, the damage is reversible and the consequences transient. Until recovery, however, attention must be directed toward avoiding a potentially disastrous, additional renal insult. The fluid and electrolyte administration for this patient must be con-

trolled accurately because unusually large urinary volumes may be required in order to avoid progressive azotemia.

NUTRITIONAL REQUIREMENTS. Granted that a reasonably satisfactory preoperative dietary preparation has been possible, the total caloric needs of the postoperative patient are of small concern if no serious complications arise to prolong this period. As soon as peristalsis has been re-established and after removal of the gastrointestinal tube, some patients can be permitted a full liquid or soft diet. Others will do better if food and fluids are withheld for 24 to 48 hours until intestinal motility is more nearly normal. By the fifth to seventh day, the convalescent often accepts with gusto the solid fare which is offered, and is soon ready for hospital discharge. Those persons of a leaner habitus, after gastric resection, may feel the need of several small meals daily until the residual pouch and jejunum have become accommodated to the new status. Since some of these patients tire easily from a moderate work load and are handicapped by their limited gastric capacity, if they will drink 1 or 2 ounces of salad oil, topped with fruit juice for increased palatability, two or three times daily, energy units will be provided with but little bulk.

Certain annoying postgastrectomy sequelae can be minimized, or even avoided, if the convalescent will not indulge in eating to satiety during each meal. Rather, he should fill his stomach incompletely upon seven or eight occasions daily, taking care to select a diet high in calories per unit volume. Fluids should be consumed mostly between meals. If the food is kept on the dry side, this arrangement will decrease any tendency toward "dumping."

WOUND HEALING AND WOUND INFECTION. The avoidance of wound complications begins with the patient's preoperative preparation. Especially important are the nutritional aspects, including establishment of near-normal plasma albumin and hemoglobin values. A reduction in skin bacterial flora and sterilization of intestinal contents when the bowel is to be opened are also major safeguards. Failure to meet these several requirements can result in wound infection, disruption or evisceration.

Wound infections occurring despite careful attention to sound practices usually develop from unrecognized, gross contamination. Strict adherence to aseptic techniques by the operating personnel is essential, but it alone will not suffice. The more effective the precautions taken to control air-borne, bacteria-laden dust, the lower the incidence of infected wounds.

The use in the operating suite of conditioned air, under slightly positive pressure, which has been filtered or passed over either an electrostatic particle collector or a wet sorbent technique, and is exchanged at least 20 times per hour during occupancy by a reasonable number of persons, contributes to further reduction in wound seeding from air-borne bacteria. Freshly laundered canvas boots with nonporous soles should be placed over the street shoes of every person who enters each operating room.

Requiring students, nurses, anesthesiologists and surgeons to provide extra foot gear to be worn only in the operating rooms will serve to decrease the amount of contamination introduced from other areas. Whenever architectural arrangements permit, the normal ebb and flow of hospital traffic should be routed so as to by-pass the operating rooms. There should be posted, and enforced, simply worded but reasonably stringent rules designed to discourage congregation of curiosity seekers and others without genuine purpose in the operating room. Unnecessary talking should be prohibited.

Operations upon clearly infected patients should be so scheduled. Then specific precautions will be instituted which are designed both to reduce contamination of the operating room and to ensure a bactericidal cleanup of all potentially polluted regions.

During an operation, the wound edges can be protected against excessive air-borne contamination, as well as against drying, by packs moistened with saline or Ringer's solution. Prior to closure, all wound layers should have a generous washing with this solution to free them from the rich bacterial nutrient present in clot and tissue debris.

Careful hemostasis throughout the operation, gentle handling of tissues, routine use of fine suture material, avoidance of mass ligation with its secondary necrosis, elimination of tissue dead spaces, anatomic dissections and repair guided by a profound respect for maximal preservation of the blood supply, all contribute to primary wound healing.

A wound hematoma usually arises from careless hemostasis, and a seroma from failure to obliterate dead space. Therefore, all incisions through a deep panniculus adiposus should be carefully approximated side to side as well as to the suture line of deeper fascia, from which fibrous layer it should not have been scraped. Continuous closed suction to the wound depths is a useful alternative in this type of problem. It is probably the only sound procedure for dealing with widely undermined flaps and pockets necessarily developed in the course of certain operations. The widespread availability of various sized, multiply perforated, siliconized, shape retaining polyethylene catheters has contributed to more general acceptance of this concept. Either homemade low pressure, manometrically regulated devices actuated by a Stedman pump, or the Hemo-Vac will serve as suitable suction devices. An appropriately sized catheter is positioned at operation in the potential dead space to be obliterated. A partial vacuum is maintained postoperatively until the plasma aspirate is minimal for 24 hours, and the catheter is then withdrawn.

Rarely, a hematoma is found to be secondary to excessive postoperative anticoagulation therapy, or due to an unrecognized preoperative bleeding tendency. When one does develop for any cause, the area of involvement should be opened widely and the clot evacuated, lest it become secondarily infected. If liquefaction has occurred, and if the volume of liquid is small, aspiration under sterile precautions followed by a compression dressing will sometimes suffice.

The routine use of retention sutures is a matter of individual choice. Often, they are inserted under so much tension, however, that considerable loss of effectiveness soon occurs from subsequent necrosis and shearing of the tissue inside each loop.

Various materials are used in skin closures. If metal clips are employed, their removal in two or four days is wise in order to avoid local necrosis and unsightly postoperative blemishes. Broadly placed, coapting skin stitches may remain five to seven days. The smallest cutaneous sutures, catching merely the epithelial elements, cause no disfigurement when left 14 to 16 days. They support the edges during the later stages of healing.

A strong case can be made for using only the finest nonabsorbable sutures, foregoing all forms of catgut during most operations, if one is to obtain both the highest freedom from wound difficulties and the least discernible wound reaction. A monofilament material, such as stainless steel wire, is superior to braided sutures particularly whenever the contamination has been unavoidably gross.

CONTAMINATED WOUND. Certain wounds are unavoidably and heavily contaminated during operation and may become seriously infected, if closed primarily. Delayed closure is advantageous. In this technique, the deeper fascial planes are approximated in the usual manner, after a particularly thorough flushing with Ringer's or saline solution. Stainless steel monofilament, 34-gauge wire sutures are placed in the superficial structures, but with a bite into the depths so that when tightened potential pockets will be obliterated. They are not tightened, however.

After closing the depths, a dry gauze pack is inserted loosely into the incision to hold the wound edges apart and the entire area is covered with a dressing. At 48 to 72 hours, the pack can be removed. If the drainage is purulent or voluminous, the wound should be packed open until the acute invasive process subsides. In the absence of any serious reaction, the previously placed sutures can be gently approximated and the edges united with tape strips. A fresh external dressing is then applied. Provision for the interval of drainage and the walling-off process that is initiated by the inflammatory phase of wound healing, averts any tendency to destructive burrowing by pocketed infection. Satisfactory healing will be assured both in the depths and at the skin edges.

WOUND DISRUPTION AND EVISCERATION. Wound disruption is a serious sequel to impaired healing, frequently arising on a technical basis. It occurs most commonly in vertical abdominal incisions. Many factors can predispose to this grave complication, and several may contribute in any one instance. A knowledge of the more common mechanisms and how to avoid or overcome these hazards should help to reduce the incidence of this dangerous complication. The more common factors contributing to wound disruption and evisceration are the following:

Preoperative
  (a) malnutrition
  (b) hypoproteinemia
  (c) chronic anemia
  (d) massive recurrent hemorrhage with or without shock
  (e) vitamin C deficiency
  (f) prolonged adrenal steroid medication

Operative
  (a) improper selection of suture material, and poor suturing technique
  (b) careless hemostasis
  (c) idiosyncrasy to absorbable suture material
  (d) midline or long vertical incision
  (e) disregard of blood supply to incision
Postoperative
  (a) unusual abdominal wall strain from retching, coughing, hiccoughing, sneezing or uncontrolled movement
  (b) distention
  (c) uremia
  (d) ascites
  (e) infection

Evisceration may occur through any type of incision. It may occur whether the wound is closed with absorbable or nonabsorbable sutures. However, much of the experimental and clinical evidence suggests, although it does not conclusively prove, that an oblique or transverse incision, closed with some form of nonabsorbable material, is less likely to be followed by wound disruption.

Whenever, despite precautions to the contrary, the possibilities of wound disruption become real, a tightly applied spica arrangement of tape to the abdomen, extending from each groin to opposite costal margins, will lessen this likelihood. That advantage is somewhat counterbalanced by the concomitant interference of such tight strapping with normal ventilation and venous return from the lower extremities.

Violent straining or retching is likely to occur at times just as the patient is recovering from the anesthetic. During such episodes, if the sutures give way, an audible though muffled sound can sometimes be heard, and this requires investigation.

When wound disruption is suspected, most surgeons advise a prompt return of the patient to the operating room, where he can be reanesthetized, prepared and draped. The wound is then opened and the damage corrected with suture material having greater holding power. If knots have become untied, particular attention should be given to "squaring" their replacements. Any subsequent postoperative episodes of struggling should be controlled with a small dose of Pentothal given intravenously. With awakening thus cushioned, it can be made less violent; any unusual pain should be obtunded with narcotics. Persistent coughing may be controlled with ample sedation, bearing in mind the greater likelihood of atelectasis during periods of prolonged suppression of the cough reflex.

Unremitting, protracted hiccoughing exerts a severe strain on any abdominal wound. It may develop from a variety of harmless and inexplicable mechanisms but should suggest the possibility of such complications as gastric dilatation, peritonitis with subphrenic abscess, or uremia. In the absence of any specifically treatable etiologic mechanism, brief, periodic inhalations of 5 to 10 per cent carbon dioxide in oxygen will frequently interrupt the cyclic diaphragmatic spasm. Occasionally, it may be necessary to block the phrenic nerve on the side involved.

Wound disruption and evisceration may occur at any time in the postoperative period, but customarily this regrettable event takes place about the seventh day. The patient occasionally volunteers that "something gave away inside." Loss of a palpable "healing ridge" in the wound depths argues in favor of wound breakdown.

If the skin remains intact, the condition is called wound disruption or dehiscence; if abdominal viscera are extruded, it is called evisceration. In cases of disruption, loops of bowel can sometimes be palpated under the cutaneous layers. Intestinal obstruction may occur from knuckling of a bowel segment into the separation. This may be the first recognized sign of wound disruption if the character of the initial wound drainage has been ignored. Severe localized pain in an incision, if accompanied by other evidence of mechanical bowel obstruction, should also suggest this possibility. In fact, refractory ileus of otherwise unexplained origin may portend the development of this condition. Shock may be present or develop rapidly in patients with evisceration. Appropriate measures must be taken to provide transfusions promptly.

Any sudden staining of the dressings with a profuse, pink, serous drainage is virtually diagnostic of wound disruption or worse, and makes it mandatory to remove all dressings and examine the incision. Before doing this, however, one should anticipate the probable need for special dressings and equipment. The surgeon should don sterile rubber gloves, a cap and a mask in order to avoid adding contamination to the wound. A sterile covering should be at hand to lay over any protruding loops of bowel. In the event no viscera are visible or palpable, and uncertainty persists about the diagnosis of wound disruption, a few sutures should be removed with an aseptic technique. The depths of the wound should then be examined to confirm or disprove the fact that dissolution has taken place. It is unusual not to find some area of disruption after the staining produced by a profuse, typically serosanguineous discharge.

Treatment of wound disruption. Two methods are used to treat disruption or evisceration. In the case of disruption of an abdominal wound, before either method is used, the passage of a nasal tube into the stomach to evacuate its contents will reduce the likelihood of regurgitation under anesthesia, followed by endotracheal aspiration and probably pneumonia. Several preliminary applications of a topical anesthetic to the nasopharynx will minimize retching and further disruption of the wound during passage of the intestinal catheter.

The patient, who is already a poor surgical risk, may have a tenuous parietal fascia, and perhaps is in profound shock, can be benefited by a more conservative technique which can even be carried out at the bedside, if necessary. After the adjoining skin and wound edges have been prepared with an antiseptic, visible loops of bowel or other viscera should be cleansed thoroughly with liberal amounts of sterile, warm, isotonic saline solution and then returned to the peritoneal cavity. They should next be held in place temporarily with a sterile towel or wide gauze packing. If cooperation or relaxation is unsatisfactory, the patient can be lightly anesthetized and given intravenously a muscle-paralyzing drug. Soft rubber drains, one inch wide, are positioned full length between the upper and lower extremities of the wound. The skin of the entire abdomen, flank and lower part of the chest is then cleansed with ether-dampened sponges and painted with compound tincture of benzoin. Long adhesive strips, which have been flamed for bactericidal purposes and to enhance their grip to the skin, are used to draw the wound edges together. These strips, stretching diagonally from gluteal fold to axilla, overlap each other from below upward. The defect is closed by developing traction each time toward the wound edges as each strip is alternately applied from side to side. With each inferior tape end stuck firmly, any tendency to retraction of the gaping incision is countered by sliding the lateral tissues medially. When the imbrication of the adhesive strips has been completed, the rubber drain should jut enough beyond the upper and lower extent of the wound so as to carry away those discharges which might otherwise loosen the effectiveness of the tape's holding power. Care is required to prevent a bowel knuckle from becoming incarcerated in the wound during this type of closure. The appearance of signs of mechanical intestinal obstruction and localized pain would point to this possibility. Some inhibitory ileus is liable to develop in most patients, and may require prolonged nasogastric siphonage in others. The dressing, if properly functioning as a binder, should remain in place for at least two weeks, or longer if the patient has been poorly nourished. Although most of these patients will recover, a ventral hernia in the line of closure is likely.

A healthier patient with wound disruption will tolerate a return to the operating room, where formal repair can be carried out. After a nasogastric tube has been inserted and connected to suction, and arrangements made for whole blood transfusions, the patient is anesthetized and the abdominal wall can be resutured under aseptic conditions. With the patient under a general anesthesia, decompression by means of a long tube may be quite advantageous whenever generalized intestinal distention is present. It may be essential to be able to reduce a marked degree of distention in order to close the abdomen without pushing the diaphragm so high that respiration is seriously interfered with. After the small bowel loops have been emptied by threading the balloon-tipped tube down to the cecal area, the resultant gentle curves create an excellent arrangement for the adhesions certain to develop. For the actual wall closure, steel wire tension sutures tied down over a dental roll work well. A delayed closure of the superficial aspects of the wound is advisable whenever contamination has been heavy. It is believed by those who favor the reoperation method that convalescence is shorter, intestinal obstruction less likely to occur and ventral hernia formation less common.

INTESTINAL FISTULA. The treatment of an intestinal fistula is usually easier the more distal the segment of bowel from which it arises. When the fistula develops from the colon, as after its resection or at an appendectomy site, healing is slow but steady if no obstruction is present. The more proximal the fistula in the small intestine, the greater the difficulties with water and electrolyte loss and the more destructive to other tissues in the vicinity of the fistula are the bowel contents. Those from a high intestinal fistula will rapidly digest all types of tissue of the abdominal wall. These structures can be partially protected by the following plans:

Proximal control of the volume of intestinal contents by limiting the oral intake; passage of a long type intestinal tube down to the fistula site, with continuous suction and sufficient inflation of the distal balloon to obstruct the lumen and thereby reduce the amount of discharge.

Control at the external opening by means of motor- or water-driven suction delivered through a multiple-holed catheter to the proximal limb of the fistula, thereby aspirating these accumulations.

Protection of the skin and adjacent tissues. Many kinds of paste are available for this purpose. While the dermis is intact, powdered aluminum rubbed into the area periodically will give considerable protection. Ladd's paste, brewer's yeast and tannic acid in lanolin also are sometimes effective in controlling tissue digestion.

Relief of any intestinal obstruction distal to the fistula which would otherwise perpetuate this complication. As soon as the patient's condition permits, the obstruction should be corrected by lysis of the adhesive bands, by a short-circuiting procedure, an intestinal resection or by some other means of intestinal deviation.

Better drainage for the intra-abdominal abscessed ramifications associated with a fistula-forming episode can be obtained by placing the patient face down on a Foster or Stryker frame for specified intervals, as tolerated, several times each day.

The amount and kind of fluids and electrolytes necessary in these patients can tax the judgment of an experienced clinician; overall nutritional care is an equally difficult problem. Both must be judged on an individual basis.

DISTENTION. Distention may develop during the postoperative period in either of two forms: acute gastric dilatation or mechanical or inhibitory paralysis of the large or small bowel.

Acute gastric dilatation can appear after almost any operation, including thoracic and cardiac procedures. At times, the procedure may seem almost too inconsequential to have caused this complication. Acute gastric dilatation appears also in patients with diabetes, during uremia and after vertebral fractures. Persons with compression fractures of the spine treated with a hyperextension frame or a cast are particularly likely to have this complication. The superior mesenteric artery-duodenal compression syndrome may also play a role in these circumstances. After a variety of thoracic operations, patients at times exhibit mild to moderate gastric dilatation.

The inexperienced house officer can hardly be condemned for thinking first of hemorrhage or embolism when called to see a patient who, a few days after a major operation, is obviously in a grave condition, appears slightly cyanotic, is dyspneic, has a rapid, thready pulse and cool extremities covered with perspiration. However, if percussion of the upper abdomen elicits tympanitic sounds over a wide area, the presumptive diagnosis can be established by passing a gastric tube and releasing an initial gush of air, and then a considerable volume of fluid-containing material that resembles coffee-grounds. Copious vomiting may never occur as a warning sign for this complication. Rather, the patient repeatedly regurgitates small amounts of hematin-tinged fluid. Meanwhile, liters of fluid can accumulate in the stomach and yet the underlying problem remain unrecognized. In fact, enough gastric juice may already have become sequestered in the stomach to leave the patient hypochloremic. With decompressive relief from the gaseous distention of the stomach and restitution of adequate quantities of salt and water, and occasionally after a transfusion of plasma or blood, the patient usually makes a prompt convalescence. In a few hours, it may be difficult to realize that only a short time before the patient's condition was critical.

Failure to recognize and treat acute gastric dilatation can, on the other hand, lead to a fatal outcome. Prophylaxis is as effective as therapy, and has the added advantage of reducing the opportunity for a missed diagnosis. The routine use of a continuous indwelling gastric siphonage system, following major surgical operations, will virtually abolish postoperative dilatation of the stomach. When the patient becomes ambulatory, or intestinal activity is restored, the possibility of this complication developing becomes minimal and suction should be discontinued.

After intra-abdominal manipulation, normal peristalsis is inhibited for periods of up to several days. Any extensive degree of traumatic, chemical or bacterial peritonitis will contribute to the duration of this effect. For instance, a mass ligation technique which leaves behind clumps of necrotic omentum is liable to curtail intestinal activity. Local inhibitory effects are aggravated further by any marked increase in bowel diameter. Therefore, food and fluids by mouth should be withheld pending restoration of a satisfactory state of intestinal activity. Other accumulations contributing to distention are gaseous material, of which at least 70 per cent is swallowed air; the unabsorbed residue from the oral intake; saliva; gastric and pancreatic juices; bile; succus entericus; and bacteria and their end products.

Apparently, the predisposing mechanisms for some degree of ileus are present in every abdominal procedure. A nine-holed gastric catheter should be positioned so that a few holes are in the lower gullet and the remaining tube lies unkinked in the stomach and at times the duodenum. The tube should be attached to continuous suction equipment and function for a few hours before the operation. It should continue to serve throughout the procedure and until intestinal activity is restored two to four days afterward.

It is easier to prevent ileus than to overcome it. In the treatment of adynamic ileus, the Miller-Abbott tube, or, preferably, the Leonard modification, becomes really effective only after having been passed through the duodenum, a maneuver requiring patience, skill and experience. However, in some patients it may be impossible, for all practical purposes, to intubate the small intestine. Still another drawback occurs once distention is permitted to develop. The differentiation between inhibitory, or adynamic, and mechanical ileus must be made. If localized pain, a mass, rebound tenderness and leukocytosis are present, a strangulating obstruction may be the cause. A sudden onset of pain referred to the lumbar area favors this diagnosis.

It can be observed that marked abdominal distention immobilizes and elevates the diaphragm, contributing thereby to a greater incidence of atelectasis and other pulmonary complications. The development of marked abdominal distention also favors venous stasis in the lower extremities. It is a reasonable presumption, therefore, that this state increases the likelihood of phlebothrombosis and, hence, embolic phenomena.

A few cases of postoperative ileus are well-nigh intractable, but most will eventually respond to one or more procedures, including intestinal siphonage, splanchnic block, spinal anesthesia and the use of Pituitrin or Mecholyl. Hypokalemia will induce intestinal atony and hence contribute to the development and perpetuation of ileus. Ambulation, when feasible, is one of the best means of inducing peristaltic activity, and will usually prove helpful unless mechanical ileus, or chemical or bacterial peritonitis exists. When no systemic contraindication to an augmented salt intake is present, an enema of 100 to 200 cc. of a 10 per cent sodium chloride solution will often induce peristalsis.

However, in any patient with persistent intestinal atony, it is imperative to exclude an intra-abdominal abscess before fruitless efforts are expended on the management of associated ileus. If a leak at a suture line is suspected, or an extraenteric accumulation with a fluid level is discernible on an upright x-ray film of the abdomen, the first step required to relieve the ileus is to drain effectively this pocket of infection. Then if Congo red by mouth stains the wound dressings, the existence of an intestinal communication has been confirmed.

The concept of electrically induced peristalsis, initiated by a pacemaker implanted in the pyloric area, has not proved to be an effective device for hastening the restoration of natural intestinal peristalsis.

SUBPHRENIC OR SUBHEPATIC ABSCESS. Abscess in these areas should be an uncommon complication after standard abdominal operations. On the other hand, a perforated ulcer or a ruptured appendix is the usual cause when there has been no antecedent procedure. On the other hand, after abdominal trauma in which the liver has been torn, bile leakage secondary to incomplete decompression of the biliary tract readily creates subhepatic or phrenic accumulations. The onset may be insidious. Exploration of one or both subdiaphragmatic, or the subhepatic, areas is frequently postponed. When the abscess is sought, it may be anterior or posterior and on the left or right side. Combinations of these sites are possible, and rarely all spaces can be infected simultaneously.

In a patient who has recently undergone a gastrointestinal operation, or has had another type of intraperitoneal insult, fever of unexplained origin should arouse a suspicion of subphrenic abscess. The physical findings may be surprisingly meager, slow to appear or even inconsistent. To wait until all consultants agree upon the diagnosis is often to delay too long. X-ray and fluoroscopic study can contribute considerable information and support for a tentative diagnosis. At fluoroscopy, the diaphragm may be found to be elevated, sluggish or paralyzed. A fluid level pocketed under this leaf, and in a specific area outside the intestine, is virtually diagnostic. A small quantity of barium in the stomach, with the patient in the head-down position, will help demonstrate an abnormal separation between the diaphragm and the gastric pouch. The presence of pleural effusion with obscuration of the costophrenic sinus is also a helpful sign pointing at subdiaphragmatic inflammation. This finding has many times erroneously been construed as having arisen from a pneumonic process. Plain and overexposed Bucky films in anteroposterior and lateral projections are useful to identify the true nature of this complication and to locate the abscess as accurately as possible.

Recognition of a subphrenic abscess is at times difficult in the early postoperative period after abdominal surgery. Air is invariably present under the diaphragm following such operations, and may remain easily identifiable for two weeks. Persistence, a tendency toward encapsulation, any increase in size, and the appearance of a fluid level are significant signs pointing more to an infection than toward some benign residuum of the operation. Tomography can help in localizing the process. However, a subphrenic or subhepatic infection need never show a fluid level and may merely remain as a smoldering granulomatous process. The patient may be febrile from causes other than the abscess. At times, it may be impossible to make the categorical diagnosis. Exploration is often justifiable then on the basis that further delay fosters the complications of diaphragmatic perforation, empyema, lung abscess, bronchial fistula, rupture and generalized peritonitis, all capable of elevating the mortality rate and prolonging the morbidity.

The principal purpose of operative treatment for a subphrenic abscess is to achieve continuous dependent drainage, whether the patient is reclining or standing. Except in the case of infection in the right posterior space, this goal is rarely realized. When the pocket has been definitely localized there, the best approach is through the bed of the twelfth rib. For an anterior accumulation, and after an anterior drainage procedure, some residual puddling in the depths is almost inevitable whenever the patient is supine. The prone position will, therefore, provide better drainage. It should be sought by maintaining the patient on a Foster or Stryker frame for periods as long as tolerated, several times daily. Occasionally, a secondary posterior opening will be required to complete the drainage process. The preferred approach to an anterior encapsulation is through a subcostal incision. Extraperitoneal dissection is carried down to the area of involvement and the pocket is then entered. Aspiration through a large-bore needle can be of help in finding the abscess.

In both the anterior and the posterior approaches, extraperitoneal dissection should be utilized to reach the abscess and to evacuate it. The overlying surfaces tend to become agglutinated around the pocket, and the free peritoneal cavity sealed off by the adjacent inflammatory reaction. Drainage across the free peritoneal cavity, on the other hand, is much more likely to contaminate uninvolved visceral and parietal surfaces, thereby increasing the morbidity. With care, only infrequently is it necessary to use this less desirable route to a subphrenic abscess. Subhepatic processes are usually sealed by adjacent viscera from the uncontaminated residual abdominal cavity. A safe anterior access route is thus often available.

A fact about the subphrenic abscess problem which has become increasingly evident is the relatively small contribution that antibiotics have made to a reduction in the mortality. The pace of the disease may be slowed and the onset masked to some extent, but few abscesses are cured by chemotherapy alone. It is questionable that the patient's recovery is materially hastened by antibiotics, once ample drainage has been secured.

In general, convalescence remains protracted, while the body slowly absorbs the inflammatory residue and heals the abscess cavity.

The energy costs of sepsis cannot be ignored, particularly when limited cardiac or pulmonary reserves are available. The demands imposed by an infection can easily double the basal cardiac output (about 3 liters per minute per square meter). Inevitably, for some, this is an intolerable burden.

Mechanically assisted circulation decreases the work load up to 50 per cent under circumstances of heightened respiratory effort. In addition, use of an antipyretic and a cooling blanket to return the core body temperature to euthermic levels, likewise reduces the abnormal demands on the heart. Judiciously applied, these techniques can be lifesaving.

STRESS ULCER. The term "stress ulcer" has been applied to that complication characterized by upper gastrointestinal bleeding presumed to arise on the basis of acid-peptic digestion of mucosa in these areas. The term has little to recommend its use. Circumstances creating demonstrably greater physical, and probably emotional, stress in nontraumatized persons are quite unlikely to produce an ulcer de novo. Stress alone, with some special exceptions, does not produce gastrointestinal ulceration in experimental animals. Nor is the exhibition in these preparations of excessive amounts as adrenal steroids likely to do so either when given as individual components or in the aggregate. Nevertheless, the term has won popular acceptance.

In reality, the syndrome is nothing more or less than either erosive gastritis or a bona fide ulceration in the stomach or duodenum. It is a response to the totality of emotional, physiological, and biochemical changes evoked by trauma, and its complications, together with the treatment imposed upon the individual. Recognition of the event is usually easy and is characterized by the appearance of bloody vomitus or the presence of similar material in the gastric siphonage or a melanotic stool. The rate of bleeding under such circumstances may be mild, episodic and nonthreatening. On the other hand, the initial manifestation may be a massive, exsanguinating hemorrhage. If the patient can tolerate a continuous, slow cold skim milk drip without producing gastric or intestinal overdistention, this treatment is likely to control most instances of mild to moderate degrees of bleeding. For the more serious cases, operation with a vagotomy and pyloroplasty as well as oversewing any actual bleeding ulcer sites may prove necessary. The balloon technique for gastric hypothermia and for gastric freezing has not proved predictably beneficial in the management of these problems.

THROMBOPHLEBITIS. All forms of thrombophlebitis produce fever. There are three principal types. Inflammatory changes develop after prolonged perfusion into superficial limb veins, particularly when the solution is strongly hypertonic. This lesion is characterized by a painful, often red and tender linear extension over the proximal distribution of that particular venous channel. In time the process abates; the lumen is obliterated by contracting scar tissue and becomes a painless thrombosed knot or cord.

Venous thrombosis may occur as spontaneous, idiopathic, post-traumatic phlebothrombosis or deep venous thromboses. It is always treacherous when present, but carries an even graver outlook when there is a history of previous pulmonary emboli; in the presence of heart disease; with a limited pulmonary reserve, and obesity. Furthermore, it has a tendency to spread progressively through more and more venular branches. The appearance of pain when the foot is dorsiflexed on the ankle with the knee bent, or deep calf pain on palpation, especially if associated with prominent antetibial veins in a recumbent patient, strongly suggests this diagnosis. Pulmonary embolization is a genuine threat; residual serious damage to vein wall and valvar mechanisms leading to late circulatory difficulties is a common aftermath.

Septic thrombophlebitis with inflammatory change and thrombus formation developing in association with a septic focus can produce septic emboli. These fragments lodging in the lung produce infarcts which progress rapidly through abscess formation with considerable parenchymal destruction. The patient can die either from the massive nature of the circulatory insult or the late complications induced by infection. Therapy should be initiated promptly even on suspicion of such an event. The treatment for each of these venous lesions is different.

Chemical phlebitis rarely requires more than symptomatic relief by hot packs or medications. The process is self-limited; it is scarcely more than an annoying incident.

Venous thrombosis always carries the potential threat of embolization. Prompt treatment is indicated. For the usual case, particularly when the degree of actual involvement of the deep venous system may be uncertain, if no systemic contraindication exists, systemic heparinization is the treatment of choice. The plan should be to maintain the Lee-White clotting time at two to two and one-half times the control value. First, the patient is given a loading dose of 1 mg. per kg. of heparin intravenously. A microdrip apparatus is established in conjunction with an intravenous catheter. Five per cent glucose containing 100 to 200 mg. of heparin per liter is infused continuously at a rate which will maintain the Lee-White values in the desired range. This should be checked every four hours night and day. This regimen should be maintained for at least 24 to 48 hours after the patient has become asymptomatic. Five to seven days prior to discontinuing heparin therapy, Coumadin is started and the prothrombin time, or per cent, should be reduced to a therapeutic range. A helpful adjunct to therapy for this type of thrombophlebitis consists of using 75,000 molecular weight dextran. Moncrief has shown that this material prevents the propagation of experimental thrombi when given intravenously (600 mg. per kg. 6 per cent solution on day one and one-half that dose daily for three to four days). This regimen has been associated with the disappearence of pain, tenderness, local heat and swelling in the involved limb for 90 per cent of the patients. When the lower limb has been the site of involvement, elastic stocking support will reduce the tendency toward late venous difficulties if this garment is worn regularly, for at least three months, during all waking hours.

Venous thrombosis involving the iliofemoral area can produce a dramatic syndrome. This may require emergency treatment if the patient's limb or even if his life is to be saved. When seen within the first day or so after onset, thrombectomy is indicated. In brief, the clots are massaged from the distal vein through the opened common femoral and extracted from the proximal regions by means of Fogarty catheters positioned so as to preclude the proximal migration of any clots as pulmonary emboli. Use of the Valsalva maneuver also protects against centripetal movement of the thrombus. The patient should be heparinized as soon as possible after the thrombectomy. For those patients who cannot be treated with heparin and other forms of anticoagulation therapy, inferior vena caval suture plication or fenestration with a serrated clip is the treatment of choice. Any large ovarian veins should be interrupted at the same procedure. Pulmonary embolectomy using cardiopulmonary by-pass should be reserved for selected patients suffering from massive pulmonary embolization and who clearly reveal cor pulmonale. If circumstances permit, the presence of the embolus should be confirmed by angiography prior to operation.

Superficial femoral vein ligation has no place in the management of suspected distal venous thrombosis.

Septic thrombophlebitis occurs most often after uterine infection induced at the time of a criminal abortion. Second only to the treatment of life-threatening pelvic sepsis is the need for ligation of the vena cava upon first evidence, or reasonable suspicion by a positive scan, that pulmonary embolization has occurred. Following caval ligation, venous congestion of the lower extremity is a likely complication. The patient should be protected against edema of the lower extremities by wearing a well-tailored, firm elastic support continuously during the months thereafter.

GOUT. Gout, at times a bit atypical in the symptoms produced and the sites involved, may be manifest for the first time in the early postoperative period. Both the distress induced by this lesion, which can be quite annoying, and the importance of applying specific therapy rather than mere anodynes, plead for an early, correct diagnosis. The individual with uricacidemia is clearly benefited by prompt recognition and treatment of this latent metabolic error which has been unmasked by protein catabolic events surrounding the operation.

POST-TRAUMATIC PSYCHOSES. Major mind disorders can develop after any traumatic event. Yet a much higher incidence has become apparent after open heart operations, as compared to other types of major abdominal or thoracic procedures. Perhaps the concept of living, even briefly, without a beating heart is emotionally cataclysmic. In other instances, restoration of health after prolonged periods of invalidism uproots dependency relationships and imposes responsibilities for which that particular patient has made no realistic preparation. Fortunately, in most circumstances regardless of the cause, or the form of the psychiatric abnormality, the prognosis for recovery is good when there has been no previous history of psychotic episodes. Psychiatric consultation should always be sought promptly whenever a psychotic episode is even suspected.

PAROTITIS. Acute inflammation of the parotid gland, except in association with mumps or secondary to sialolithiasis, was much more commonly seen in early times as a postoperative complication than it is now. The current liberal use of antibiotics, the giving of fluids orally after an operation and the avoidance of dehydration through better attention to the fluid and electrolyte requirements all combine to reduce the incidence of parotitis.

The most likely candidate for parotitis is the elderly, debilitated patient undergoing a febrile convalescence, poor in oral hygiene and exhibiting a parched mucous membrane. The parotid lesion is more often initially unilateral, with a subsequent occasional appearance on the opposite side. It is characterized by local tenderness and swelling, some trismus and expressible pus from a swollen, inflamed Stensen's duct. Fluctuation is difficult to elicit because of the gland's fibrous septa and tense capsule, and the infection's deep location in the gland.

As a rule, early parotitis will respond to antibiotics and to correction of the predisposing mechanisms. Deep x-ray or radium therapy to the area gives satisfactory results if abscess formation has not occurred. Early treatment is particularly effective. The development of portable deep x-ray therapy units which can be brought to the bedside has increased the usefulness of x-ray management. If abscess formation is suspected, incision and drainage parallel to the main fibers of the facial nerve should be performed. In a few patients, the condition is fulminant and progresses rapidly unless actively treated. The high mortality ascribed to this condition in the past may well be related to the appearance of this complication as a terminal incident in very poor risk patients.

AMBULATION. Renewed interest has developed in Ries' recommendation, made a half-century ago, of early ambulation. At the time, his idea evoked no widespread acceptance and it was only tardily submitted to a limited practical trial by a few clinicians. Now, many subscribe to a program for early ambulation. In cases of sepsis, however, conservatism is probably still indicated. In the presence of purulent foci, or of widespread infection, any undue activity is more apt to disseminate the process. Rest rather than exercise is indicated until the inflammatory process is under control. Otherwise, many leaders in obstetrics, gynecology, neurosurgery, thoracic and cardiovascular surgery, orthopedics and general surgery now urge their patients to be up and about soon after major operations.

Although there has been a growing acceptance of this idea, it remains difficult to identify precisely the various contributions of early ambulation to better patient care. Some of the apparently good effects are unquestionably obscured by the concomitant benefits from antibiotics, superior anesthetic agents, more liberal transfusions, better nutritional preparation, the more physiologic management of water and electrolyte problems, and other factors.

Over and above any ambiguous contributions of early ambulation, several considerations appear to have merit. Pain disappears more promptly from the operative site and is usually less exquisite. Inhibitory ileus, voiding difficulties and other postoperative sequelae occur less frequently and in a milder form. The patient's morale is better and his psychologic reaction following the operation is healthier. This is of special concern and benefit in care of the elderly patient, for once he is up and about, it is easier to rouse him from self-pity and discouragement. The incidence of serious complications is not increased. For example, the recurrence rate seems no greater if early ambulation is practiced after herniorrhaphy. Early ambulation shortens the duration of hospitalization after a major operation. Convalescence at home is hastened and, hence, the overall economic loss to the patient is reduced.

The incidence and severity of thrombophlebitis and phlebothrombosis remain approximately the same, unfortunately. Wrapping the patient's legs from foot to midthigh, with elastic bandages before surgery, and rewrapping them at least twice daily until the discharge date is the best simple method for routine prophylaxis against these complications. Just why early ambulation appears to be of such little value in preventing venous complications is puzzling, but that this is the case has been concluded from various collected studies.

Ambulation is most effective when started within the first 24 hours after an operation, but this schedule should not be inflexible.

Those patients who are too ill or enfeebled to get out of bed before a major operation can hardly be expected to do so shortly afterward. It is wisest to modify the regimen so that, as the patient assumes an upright position, he experiences no serious blood pressure change. A preliminary trial of dangling the feet for a few minutes may indicate the individual's tolerance to resumption of the vertical habitus. Any tendency toward syncope is cause for temporizing and returning the patient to bed; then gradually, after recovery from that episode, he may again attempt an erect posture. Once he is up, he should be encouraged to exercise and then return to bed. If this exercise is tolerated, he can try to walk more often and farther each day. At first, he may be unable to attempt more than a few steps in the morning and again in the afternoon.

"Ambulate" is a term meaning "to walk." It is the surgeon's responsibility to confirm the fact that nurses so interpret this order to the patient. It is an error to consider early ambulation as synonymous with getting the patient out of bed and into a chair as soon as possible after an operation. An elderly patient who falls asleep in the sitting position is prone to orthostatic hypotension. Confusion, disorientation and syncope, followed by a fall, a concussion, fracture or other forms of severe trauma may result.

Early ambulation, properly supervised, is decidedly beneficial and should be an integral part of any comprehensive program for postoperative management.

FEVER. Although fever in the postoperative patient may arise from a variety of individual factors, certain probabilities are more frequently causative and also more likely to exhibit revealing clues. The febrile patient deserves a careful evaluation for these significant signs. In the instance of a sharp rise of the temperature line, it should not be construed as ample treatment by the house officer merely to order double the dosage and variety of antibiotics. In a postoperative patient with an elevated temperature, probable reasons for it will be found in the lungs, urinary tract, operative area and veins of extremities, including the sites of intravenous therapy, and in an abnormal systemic reaction to drugs. However, the actual mechanism can remain perplexingly obscure. For instance, the patient with pseudomembranous enterocolitis can also exhibit fever even before the stage of diarrhea.

Particular sources of febrogenic complications are more apt to attract attention at certain periods in the postoperative phase. Pulmonary problems are more often noticed within the first 24 to 48 hours. Later, urinary tract infection becomes manifest, particularly if the catheter has just been removed or had to be reinserted. Because the incidence of urinary tract infections associated with indwelling catheter is a function of time, removal at an early date, consistent with the patient's problem, is in order. Gantrisin or Furadantin provides reasonable protection during the period it is in place.

Leakage from a suture line is rarely apparent before the fourth or fifth postoperative day. Wound infection and disruption begin to attract notice on the sixth to tenth day; thrombophlebitis tends to come about then or slightly later. Drug idiosyncrasies can be the reason for a febrile course at any time, including well into the recovery interval.

A history of burning on urination, frequency and urgency with voiding, and renal tenderness points strongly to involvement in the urinary tract. Microscopic examination of a centrifuged fresh specimen is then indicated. A positive urine culture from a catheterized, or midvoided, specimen will prove that consideration. Any male patient who is either repeatedly catheterized, or wearing an inlying tube, should have a careful genitorectal examination to identify the presence of epididymitis or prostatitis as a cause of fever.

Complete examination of the operative area is awkward sometimes, but this should not serve as an excuse for failing to uncover and carefully inspect the wound itself. The practice of removing all dressings from clean wounds after the edges seal, and leaving them open, encourages their regular examination during ward rounds. No harmful aftermath is readily apparent, and certainly an increased incidence of wound infection does not occur. Clean surgical incisions should be free of the usual signs of an acute inflammatory reaction. On the contrary, an incision which shows signs of inflammation probably is infected. Elective incisions should heal kindly and remain free of exquisite tenderness to the carefully palpating finger. If in doubt, a responsible person should antiseptically prepare the skin, don sterile rubber gloves, remove a few sutures aseptically and gently part the superficial tissues so as to reveal any purulent loculus. If an abscess is present, generous drainage must be established promptly. This will ease the pain in the patient's incision, will save valuable time and will shorten the morbidity. Should the area prove clean on inspection of the outer layers, the convalescence will not have been materially prolonged. The gaping wound edges can either be snugged together with flames, or Steritape, or resutured, using a local anesthetic. Deeper-seated purulent accumulations may reveal themselves in the pelvis upon rectal or bimanual examination. Abnormal aggregates of air and fluid lying just beneath the diaphragm are quite recognizable on upright films of the abdomen. An unusually high diaphragm and pleural effusion may be clues to the existence of this process.

A bizarre, poorly understood and aggravatingly enduring febrile state arises in some patients after heart operations. It has inappropriately been termed "commissurotomy syndrome," although it can appear after a wide variety of cardiac procedures, including heart catheterization. This febrile state is resistant to nearly all forms of treatment and is probably of viral origin; the temperature returns to normal by lysis.

Displaced loops of bowel about a constant area of opacification, in association with a partial small bowel obstruction or clinical ileus, are strongly suggestive signs of an intra-abdominal abscess. Localized and abnormal degrees of tenderness over this suspect area will influence one's decision to explore and drain that locus extraperitoneally, if at all feasible.

Abnormal drug reactions, although uncommon, work their consequences onto the temperature chart with sufficient frequency to disrupt even the smoothest running service. Whenever the magnitude of the rise in the patient's fever is quite out of proportion to the pulse response and other more likely causes have been excluded, a medication reaction moves from the realm of a remote possibility to a realistic probability.

FOLLOW-UP. The suggestion has been made at some institutions that prospective programs for regular long term follow-up are unnecessary, that new longitudinal studies should not be instituted and those in existence be curtailed. On the contrary, this area of clinical medical research continues to produce new and, in certain instances, the only factual knowledge there is for certain controversial problems. In fact, studies of this type are an obligation of the profession. Therefore, procedures for facilitating and improving follow-up observations should be strengthened and modernized.

The use of punch card systems of various types is but an initial step in that direction. One of these techniques permits the collection on a few 7½ by 3½-inch cards of literally hundreds of comparable facts about a particular disease. Any or all of these data under collation can rapidly be retrieved subsequently. Or, these facts can be stored in an even more accessible and compact fashion on magnetic tape. In the latter case, the print-out of myriads of correlative items can be performed by machines in a few minutes. To achieve a comparable result by the tedious fashion of chart reviewing manually could require hundreds of hours.

For those persons dedicated to studies in extenso of the natural history and treatment of breast and stomach cancer, gastrointestinal and biliary tract surgical diseases, and metabolic problems, among many others, the evidence is clear that greater utilization of modern computer techniques is essential for future contributions to surgical practice.

It is true that traditionally surgeons have not always clearly identified themselves with the rigorous scientific community of medicine. In fact, in the recent past it was indicated that the four essential components of an effective surgeon were technology, humanism, empiricism and science. It may have been symbolic that the analytical techniques were relegated to fourth place. However, if that concept of first order qualifications identified the superior surgeon of another era, one can currently state that those composite characteristics of a contemporary surgeon are substantially different, with scientific competence no worse than second to acknowledged clinical skills. Thus, many in this discipline are now understandably restive at traditional techniques which continue to seek for biological solutions through unimaginative applications of glacially paced trial and error methods.

Even less acceptable working arrangements depend on doctrinaire prejudices which masquerade as the ultimate in senior surgical judgments but which under penetrating scrutiny are frequently revealed to be opinions largely untested by rigorous logic and hence with all of the shortcomings intrinsic to ritual.

This hierarchal approach is all the more distressing when one contemplates the incredible power of the scientific method. Nature cannot deny an honest answer to any inquirer once the question has been properly constructed and appropriately posed. Thereafter, granted the proper coincidence of a keenly motivated mind, well-trained in the appropriate disciplines coming to grips with a specific problem, we can confidently predict that an audacious capacity for delivering new knowledge to the benefit of mankind will be unleashed.

READING REFERENCES

Arhelger, S. W.: The advantages of tracheotomy and the use of a new tracheal tube in the management of intratracheal aspiration. Surgery 29:260, 1951.

Cannon, P. R., Wissler, R. W., Woolridge, R. L., and Benditt, E. P.: The relationship of protein deficiency to surgical infection. Ann. Surg. 120:514, 1944.

Clark, J. H., Nelson, W., Lyons, C., and Mayerson, H. S.: Chronic shock: the problem of reduced blood volume in the chronically ill patient. Ann. Surg. 125:610, 1947.

Crandon, J. H., and others: Ascorbic acid economy in surgical patients as indicated by blood ascorbic acid levels. New England J. Med. 258:105, 1958.

Cuthbertson, D. P.: Post-shock metabolic response. Lancet 1:433, 1942.

Dietzman, R. H., Lyons, G. W., Bloch, J. H., and Lillehei, R. C.: Relation of cardiac work to survival in cardiogenic shock in dogs. J.A.M.A. 199:825, 1967.

Edwards, L. C., and Dunphy, J. E.: Wound healing: injury and normal repair. New England J. Med. 259:224, 1958.

Eiseman, B., Silen, W., Bascom, G. S., and Kouwan, A. J.: Fecal enema as an adjunct in the treatment of pseudomembranous enterocolitis. Surgery 44:854, 1958.

Elman, R.: Parenteral Alimentation in Surgery. New York, Paul B. Hoeber, 1947.

Gamble, J. L.: Chemical Anatomy, Physiology, and Pathology of Extracellular Fluid. 6th ed. Cambridge, Massachusetts, Harvard University Press, 1954.

Hampton, O. P., Jr., Furste, W., and Skudder, P. A.: Prophylaxis against tetanus in wound management. Committee on Trauma. American College of Surgeons, September, 1965.

Harrison, H. N., Moncrief, J. A., Duckett, J. W., Jr., and Mason, A. D.: The relationship between energy metabolism and water loss from vaporization in severely burned patients. Surgery 56:203, 1964.

Houle, D. B., Weil, M. H., Brown, E. G., and Campbell, G. S.: The influence of respiratory acidosis on ECG and pressor responses to epinephrine, norepinephrine, metaraminol. Proc. Soc. Exp. Biol. & Med. 94:561, 1957.

Jude, J. R., Kouwenhoven, W. B., and Knickerbocker, G. G.: Advantages of external cardiac massage. Ann. Surg. 154:311, 1961.

Leonard, A. S., Nicoloff, D. M., Griffen, W. O., Peter, E. T., and Wangensteen, O. H.: Long coiled spring tube for operative intestinal decompression. Am. J. Surg. 104:427, 1962.

Leonard, A. S., and Wangensteen, O. H.: Operative intestinal decompression by means of a long coiled-spring intestinal tube. Surgery 57:491, 1965.

Lillehei, R. C., Dietzman, R. H., Movsas, S., and Bloch, J. H.: Treatment of septic shock. Mod. Treatm. 4:2, 1967.

Lown, B., Neumann, J., Amarasingham, R., and Berkovits, B. V.: Comparison of alternating current with direct current electroshock across the closed chest. Am. J. Cardiol. 10:223, 1962.

Lyons, C., and Mayerson, H. S.: The surgical significance of hemoglobin deficiency in protein depletion. J.A.M.A. *135*:910, 1947.

Machella, T. E.: The mechanism of the post-gastrectomy dumping syndrome. Ann. Surg. *130*:145, 1949.

Madden, S. D., and Whipple, G. H.: Plasma proteins; their source, production and utilization. Physiol. Rev. *20*:194, 1940.

Mayer, J.: Obesity: physiological considerations. J. Clin. Nutrition *9*:530, 1961.

McKittrick, L. S.: The Shattuck Lecture: The patient. New England J. Med. *256*:1211, 1957.

Miller, F. A., and others: Respiratory acidosis: its relationship to cardiac function and other physiologic mechanisms. Surgery *32*:171, 1952.

Miller, W. F., Johnson, R. L., Jr., and Wu, N.: Half-second expiratory capacity test: convenient means of evaluating nature and extent of pulmonary ventilatory insufficiency. Dis. Chest *30*:33, 1956.

Moore, F. D.: Metabolic Care of the Surgical Patient. Philadelphia, W. B. Saunders Company, 1959.

Moore, F. D., et al.: The Body Cell Mass and Its Supporting Environment. Philadelphia, W. B. Saunders Company, 1963.

Pontoppidan, H., Hedley-White, J., Bendixen, H. H., Laver, M. B., and Radford, E. P., Jr.: Ventilation and oxygen requirements during prolonged artificial ventilation in patients with respiratory failure. New England J. Med. *273*:401, 1965.

Price, P. B.: Stress, strain, and sutures. Ann. Surg. *128*:408, 1948.

Randall, H. T., Hardy, J. D., and Moore, F. D.: Manual of Preoperative and Postoperative Care. American College of Surgeons. Philadelphia, W. B. Saunders Company, 1967.

Reifenstein, E. C., Jr.: The rationale for the use of anabolic steroids in controlling the adverse effects of corticoid hormones upon protein and osseous tissues. Southern Med. J. *49*:933, 1956.

Root, H. D., Hauser, C. W., McKinley, C., LaFave, J. W., and Mendiola, R. P.: Diagnostic peritoneal blood lavage. Surgery *57*:633, 1965.

Sawyer, R. B., Moncrief, J. A., and Canizaro, P. C.: Dextran therapy in thrombophlebitis. J.A.M.A. *191*:740, 1965.

Schoenheimer, R.: Dynamic State of Body Constituents. Cambridge, Massachusetts, Harvard University Press, 1942.

Thompson, W. D., Ravdin, I. S., and Frank, I. L.: The effect of hypoproteinemia on wound disruption. Arch. Surg. *36*:500, 1938.

Varco, R. L.: Preoperative dietary management for surgical patients; with special reference to lesions of stomach and duodenum. Surgery *19*:303, 1946.

Wangensteen, O. H.: Care of patient before and after operation. New England J. Med. *236*:121, 1947.

Wangensteen, O. H.: Controlled administration of fluid to surgical patients, including description of gravimetric methods of determining status of hydration and blood loss during operation. Minnesota Med. *25*:783, 1942.

Wangensteen, O. H.: Intestinal Obstructions; A Physiological and Clinical Consideration with Emphasis on Therapy, Including Description of Operative Procedures. 2nd ed. Springfield, Illinois, Charles C Thomas, 1942.

White, R. J., and Terry, H. R., Jr.: The difficult venous cutdown in the small neurosurgical patient. Proc. Staff Meet. Mayo Clin. *35*:467, 1960.

Williams, G. R., Jr., and Spencer, F. C.: Clinical use of hypothermia following cardiac arrest. Ann. Surg. *148*:468, 1958.

Chapter *12*

ANESTHESIA

by
JAMES E. ECKENHOFF, M.D.
and
EDWARD A. BRUNNER, M.D.

It is said that those who are born in Maryland on the eastern shore of Chesapeake Bay lay claim to a particular inheritance of independent thinking and action. JAMES EDWARD ECKENHOFF was born in Easton, Maryland. He is a graduate of the University of Kentucky and the University of Pennsylvania School of Medicine. He served an internship in Lexington, Kentucky, and received his post-graduate education in anesthesia at the University of Pennsylvania. His investigative activities have been in the field of physiology and he has had teaching experience in pharmacology. He is Professor and Chairman of the first Department of Anesthesia at Northwestern University.

EDWARD BRUNNER, a Pennsylvanian by birth and education, received a Doctor of Philosophy degree in pharmacology in preparation for his post-graduate education in Anesthesia at the University of Pennsylvania. He is an Assistant Professor of Anesthesia at Northwestern University.

INTRODUCTION

The usual concept of anesthesiology relates only to the prevention of pain perception·during an operation. Initially, such a concept was appropriate and perhaps for as long as six decades after the introduction of ether, this was the only concern of the anesthetist. Because the hazards associated with anesthesia became apparent early, the British entrusted the administration of ether or chloroform to physicians. The American philosophy of training nurses as anesthetists materialized during the late nineteenth century and many years passed before physician anesthetists appeared in this country. It is likely that the early reliance of the British on the more dangerous chloroform and the preference of Americans for the safety of ether was responsible for this divergent development.

As surgical procedures became more complex, the demands upon anesthesia and anesthetists increased. The physiologic and pharmacologic effects of old and new anesthetic agents had to be thoroughly understood. Profound muscle relaxation had to be provided safely and because this often led to respiratory insufficiency, a background knowledge of pulmonary physiology and the control of ventilation became a necessity. As the critically ill and those at the extremes

of life began to be operated upon, a sound foundation in medicine became mandatory to prepare these patients successfully for operation, and to care for them during the procedure. More recently, it became apparent that the expertise gained by the anesthetist should be utilized into the postoperative period; hence the modern participation of anesthetists in intensive care units.

GENERAL CONSIDERATIONS. A classification of the methods by which anesthesia may be provided should be preceded by an outline of the mechanisms by which a patient interacts with his environment because anesthesia is a modification of such interaction. Sensory perception requires a stimulus to excite a receptor. This sets into motion events leading to awareness of the stimulus and ultimately to action by the organism. This is represented schematically in Figure 1. A stimulus excites a receptor (a). The response of the receptor is to initiate a nerve impulse (b) which is conducted to the central nervous system at the level of the spinal cord or brain stem (c). In the spinal cord, the impulse may be transferred to motor pathways which initiate an involuntary response (i), thereby completing a reflex arc; or the impulse may be transmitted to higher centers in the central nervous system (d), where perception of the sensation (e) combines with a psychological reaction to that

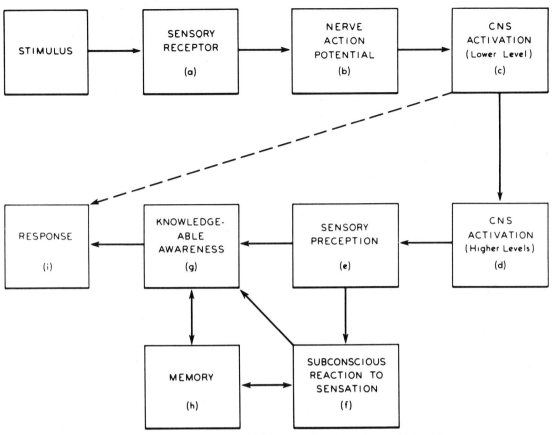

Figure 1.   Schematic representation of the interaction of a patient and his environment.

sensation (f) to produce knowledgeable awareness (g), which may be stored in memory (h) subject to recall. Knowledgeable awareness may initiate a voluntary response (i), thus completing the interaction of the organism and its environment. Some of these events are physical, such as the stimulus, some physiological, the nerve action potential, and some psychological, perception. Some of the mechanisms have been studied extensively and are well understood whereas others defy investigation.

The pathways outlined in this schema may be interrupted at different points to alter environmental interaction seemingly to provide the same result. For example, a blindfold placed over the eyes prevents light from exciting the retinal receptors and blocks visual awareness of the environment; local anesthetic agents injected into the retrobulbar space block the transmission of the nerve action potential from the retina to the brain; a general anesthetic agent affects the brain but just as surely blocks knowledgeable awareness of the environment; a neuromuscular blocking agent on the other hand leaves the receptors intact, transmission unimpeded and perceptive areas of the brain active, but response to the stimulus becomes impossible. Following this pattern, one or more anesthetics, acting at known sites in the pathway, can be chosen to provide desirable and acceptable conditions for a surgical procedure, or for the relief of painful states.

CLASSIFICATION OF ANESTHETIC TECHNIQUES.   In a broad sense, all types of anesthesia may be classified as either regional or general. Regional anesthesia is more discreet in that the sensorium remains clear and pain relief follows a block of the sensory receptor or of peripheral nerve conduction. Other modes of sensory perception remain intact and sight, sound, taste or smell may evoke an undesirable response during an operative procedure. General anesthesia is produced by agents which act primarily on the brain and interfere with normal neuronal activation, sensory perception or knowledgeable awareness. Some drugs can influence many pathways; for example, narcotic analgesics may alter reaction to pain as well as diminish perception of the stimulus. Pain may be perceived but it does not cause discomfort. Psychological support from a physician, family or religious counselor can mimic this effect. Drugs such as scopolamine are capable of blocking memory and are sometimes employed for their amnesic qualities. The neuromuscular and ganglionic blocking agents and the belladonna alkaloids are examples of drugs which act at the terminal portions of nerve pathways to prevent activation of peripheral end organs.

REGIONAL ANESTHESIA

Regional anesthesia implies reversible blockade of pain perception or transmission by local anesthetic drugs, although physical agents such as cold or pressure can act similarly. In appropriate concentrations, these drugs prevent activation of pain receptors and block the transmission of nerve action potentials along all types of nerve fibers. The area influenced by the agent is governed by the anatomic site of application.

Regional anesthesia is classified into seven types on an anatomic basis. The first two types, topical anesthesia and local infiltration, involve principally sensory receptors. The next four, field block, peripheral nerve block, epidural anesthesia and spinal anesthesia, involve nerve conduction; therefore, the use of the term conduction anesthesia. The mechanism of action of the last type, intravenous regional anesthesia, is unclear.

Topical anesthesia results from the application of certain local anesthetics to skin or mucous membranes. The technique is ineffective if the skin is intact and healthy, because aqueous solutions of the salts of local anesthetics lack penetrability of normal epidermis. When applied to inflamed or diseased skin, an anesthetic action will result. Ointments containing local anesthetic bases are effective on normal skin. Aqueous solutions of the salts of cocaine, lidocaine or tetracaine will block the sensory receptors of mucous membranes. Good surface anesthesia of the conjunctiva and cornea, of oral, nasal and pharyngeal cavities, of esophagus, larynx and trachea and of urethra and anus will result from application of these agents. Because the blood supply to mucous membranes is rich, absorption of the drug is rapid. The amount of local anesthetic used topically must be reduced to one-fourth to one-half of the maximum allowable by infiltration.

Local infiltration involves the injection of the anesthetic directly into the operative field so that the sensory receptors that would be stimulated by the surgical procedures are rendered insensitive. Obviously, some of the most distal segments of the conduction system will be blocked.

Field block is produced by circumscribing the operative field with a continuous wall of local anesthetic. Nerve fibers supplying the site of operation and traversing this barrier are blocked and the operative area is rendered insensitive. Large volumes of anesthetic agents are usually required so the most dilute effective concentrations must be injected to minimize the possibility of overdosage and toxic reactions.

Peripheral nerve block is performed by depositing a local anesthetic in proximity to major nerve trunks. Combinations of several nerve blocks, or injection of a nerve plexus, will render a large area of the body anesthetic. Nerve blocks may be combined with local infiltration to provide anesthesia for a particular surgical procedure. Examples include brachial plexus block to provide regional anesthesia for operations on the hand, forearm or arm; femoral, sciatic and obturator nerve block to anesthetize the entire lower extremity, and a combination of intercostal nerve blocks with celiac plexus block to provide anesthesia for laparotomy.

Epidural anesthesia follows the deposition of a local anesthetic agent into the extradural space within the vertebral canal. When anesthesia of caudal, sacral or low lumbar dermatomes is indicated, the sacrococcygeal hiatus is a convenient approach to the epidural space. This is called caudal anesthesia, a technique particularly useful in perineal and rectal operations and for pain relief in the terminal stages of labor and delivery. The epidural space extends cephalad to the foramen magnum and may be penetrated at any level, although the lumbar area is most frequently used because of the ease of approach and the minimal danger of trauma to the spinal cord. Thoracic and cervical epidural blocks are not used as often because the epidural space is narrow and the risk of injury to the cord is greater. The site of action of local anesthetics injected into the epidural space is in doubt but in all likelihood they act at the point where the nerves lose their dural sleeves at the intervertebral foramina. Some contend that the site of action is central to the pia arachnoid because an appreciable concentration of local anesthetic is detectable in cerebrospinal fluid after epidural block.

The physiological changes associated with epidural anesthesia are similar to those observed with spinal anesthesia. However, larger volumes of local anesthetic drugs are required for epidural anesthesia and systemic reactions are more likely to occur. Catheters can be placed into the epidural space with relative ease, thus permitting the intermittent injection of local anesthetics for prolonged operations or for nonsurgical applications. The latter include control of pain due to operation, pancreatitis or malignancy; vasodilation of the lower extremities in acute vascular occlusion; sympathetic blockade to allow for the evaluation of effects of sympathectomy prior to operation, and use as a differential diagnostic measure in chronic pain states. The major advantage of the epidural technique compared to spinal anesthesia is that it produces extensive regional anesthesia without the hazards of dural puncture and injection of foreign substances into the cerebrospinal fluid.

Spinal anesthesia results from the injection of a local anesthetic into the cerebrospinal fluid so that the drug bathes the origin of the peripheral nerve roots. The term "saddle block" designates spinal anesthesia limited to the sacral and caudal dermatomes and is obtained by injection of a small volume of anesthetic solution usually with the patient in the sitting position.

Puncture of the dural sac in the low lumbar area can be performed easily. In this area the sac is about 15 mm. in diameter, narrowing as it extends caudally to terminate at the level of the second lumbar vertebra. The area between L2 and L4 is nearly always chosen for lumbar puncture.

The choice of drugs and technique depends upon the level and duration of anesthesia desired, the position and height of the patient and the presence or absence of factors which modify cerebrospinal fluid dynamics. The duration of anesthesia is largely determined by the local anesthetic used. Procaine produces a block lasting less than an hour, tetracaine acts for one and one-half to two hours and dibucaine, about three hours. The addition of 0.3 to 0.5 mg. of epinephrine increases the duration by 50 per cent or more, the block tending to last longer in the elderly. The level of sensory and motor block obtained is a function of the length of the dural sac

and the volume and baricity of the drug mixture injected. As the volume becomes larger, the spread of the anesthetic increases and the level of anesthesia rises. In conditions associated with increased intra-abdominal pressure, the epidural venous plexus is usually engorged, constricting the dural sac and reducing the volume of spinal fluid. The volume of drug injected intrathecally should be reduced under these circumstances to prevent inordinately high levels of spinal anesthesia.

The specific gravity of cerebrospinal fluid is 1.006. Drug mixtures with greater specific gravity are called hyperbaric and tend to settle by gravity to the lowest point of the dural sac. Those which are lighter are hypobaric and rise in the cerebrospinal fluid; those of similar specific gravity are isobaric and are inclined to layer without rising or falling. About 90 per cent of spinal anesthetics are performed using hyperbaric techniques with 10 per cent dextrose providing the hyperbaricity.

Local anesthetics injected into the subarachnoid space block autonomic preganglionic fibers as well as motor and sensory nerves. The sympathetic blockade results in peripheral arterial and venous dilation and pooling of blood in the peripheral vascular system. This effectively reduces venous return to the heart. If the anesthetic extends high enough, sympathetic fibers innervating the heart may be blocked. Both factors combine to reduce cardiac output and blood pressure during spinal anesthesia. This can be overcome by the prophylactic intramuscular injection of sympathomimetic drugs five minutes before administration of a spinal anesthetic. An intravenous infusion of pressor agent may be required in some patients.

Spinal anesthesia has advantages other than simplicity. Complete anesthesia is readily obtained for operations on the lower extremities, the perineal area and the lower abdominal wall. Good conditions for intra-abdominal operations can be provided, accompanied by profound muscular relaxation, quiet breathing, constricted bowel and lack of venous congestion. Spinal anesthesia is an excellent choice for patients who have eaten recently because the protective pharyngeal reflexes are intact in case vomiting should occur. It is also a good choice in the alcoholic who might otherwise require large quantities of general anesthesia. There is no danger of systemic toxicity from local anesthetic agents, as is potentially true of epidural anesthesia, because little drug is needed for the desired effect.

The disadvantages of the technique include the lack of patient acceptance of a method which does not provide sleep; fear of permanent neurological impairment, and its limitation to operations below the diaphragm. The incompleteness of autonomic blockade during operations in the abdominal cavity, particularly in the upper abdomen, may at times be bothersome because visceral traction may cause discomfort, nausea or vomiting. Supplementation with light levels of general anesthesia may overcome some of these disadvantages. Despite impressions to the contrary, high spinal anesthesia has little effect upon pulmonary ventilation, presumably because the diaphragm compensates for the paralyzed abdominal and thoracic muscles.

The presence of disease of the central nervous system, whether neoplastic, infectious, traumatic or degenerative, is a contraindication to the use of spinal anesthesia. Peripheral neuropathies, such as those associated with diabetes or syphilis, represent relative contraindications to subarachnoid block. A history of frequent severe headache warrants careful consideration before choosing the technique. Skin disease, or infection of the area chosen for lumbar puncture, and fear of spinal anesthesia will exclude some patients. The administration of spinal anesthesia to patients with marked hypovolemia will often result in precipitous hypotension. The technique should be avoided in this circumstance.

Despite the ease with which it can be performed and the excellence of the operating conditions offered, spinal anesthesia has been associated with controversy and emotionalism. Reports of major neurologic sequelae have caused concern about the safety of the technique. A wide variation in the incidence of neurological complications has been reported. Although one study reported six instances of residual paralysis following 1200 spinal anesthetics, another study of 11,000 patients in whom this technique was employed with careful follow-up failed to uncover a single major neurological sequela.

Puncture of the dural sac and injection of foreign substances into the cerebrospinal fluid can be dangerous. Even without injection, lumbar puncture produces local trauma, changes cerebrospinal fluid dynamics and may lead to the introduction of infection into the subarachnoid space. With attention to detail, the risk of lumbar puncture can be minimized. The injection of toxic substances into the intrathecal space must be avoided. In the past, carelessness in this respect has undoubtedly contributed to the complications reported. By use of meticulous technique, beginning with the proper cleansing and sterilization of equipment, choice of reputable drugs, use of safe concentrations and careful selection of patients, this pitfall can be avoided. Minor neurologic sequelae related to spinal anesthesia may occur, but are usually transient. These often relate to poor technique and improper positioning of the patient on the operating table. The mortality rate following spinal anesthesia is similar to that recorded in comparable series after general anesthesia.

Intravenous regional anesthesia follows the injection of a large volume of dilute local anesthetic solution into a vein of a bloodless extremity. The injected solution is confined to the extremity by a tourniquet. The anatomic site of action of the anesthetic is not clear. This technique may represent either a massive transvascular infiltration blockade of the extremity, or a conduction blockade resulting from the anesthetic agent leaking extravascularly near major nerve trunks. Anesthesia obtained by this means is effective only as long as the tourniquet remains inflated. With deflation of the cuff, the blood level of the local anesthetic drug rises rapidly, creating the risk of systemic toxic reaction. This is a problem only if the operation requires less than 30 minutes. Intermittent release of the tourniquet minimizes this danger. Operations of or below the elbow require 25 to 40 ml. of 0.5 per cent procaine or lidocaine, whereas procedures below the knee require 40 to 60 ml. of solution. The technique is most suitable for superficial procedures.

USEFUL LOCAL ANESTHETICS

A variety of unrelated chemical compounds are capable of reversibly blocking neural transmission. To be clinically useful, an agent must be nonirritating, must not produce local tissue destruction in therapeutic concentrations and must have low systemic toxicity in relation to nerve-blocking potency. Most of the currently used local anesthetics are relatively simple synthetic chemical compounds, but cocaine is a natural alkaloid. Procaine, the synthetic prototype, characterizes the fundamental chemical structure common to most drugs of this type (Fig. 2). The common components of this structure are a secondary or tertiary amino group (1); an aromatic group, often an acid (2); an aliphatic chain joining the two (3), and an ester, amide or ether linkage (4). A large number of local anesthetics are modifications of this basic chemical structure (Table 1).

Cocaine is used exclusively as a topical anesthetic and is the only one to possess a prominent vasoconstrictor action. This makes it particularly valuable for operations in the nasal cavity. It is used in concentrations ranging from 4 to 10 per cent. The maximum safe dosage is 200 mg., although toxic effects from as little as 20 mg. have been witnessed. It may be applied by droplet, spray, pledget or pack. At one time, it was used extensively in the eye, but now has been almost abandoned in favor of safer agents. The ability of cocaine to produce mild central nervous system excitation has led to problems of addiction, so its use is controlled by federal narcotics regulations. Toxic symptoms from central nervous system stimulation may appear abruptly and run a rapid course. A high index of suspicion must be maintained because early manifestations are often mistaken for apprehension.

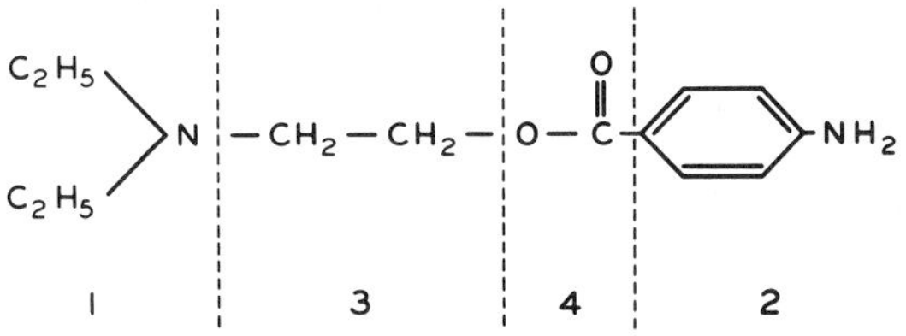

Figure 2. Chemical structure of procaine as a prototype of the synthetic local anesthetic agents, illustrating common features of chemical structure often found in these drugs.

Procaine (Novocain) is an efficient local anesthetic which has had extensive clinical use since its introduction in 1905. It is not effective topically but has been used by all other methods. It is one-fourth as toxic as cocaine and amounts of up to 1 gm. may be administered by infiltration in the average adult. Concentrations of 0.5 per cent are suitable for infiltration anesthesia but 2 per cent may be needed for major nerve blocks. Procaine acts relatively rapidly but has a short duration of action. Vasoconstrictors are often added to slow absorption and prolong the duration of block. Plasma contains procaine esterase which rapidly hydrolyzes the drug once it reaches the circulation.

Lidocaine (Xylocaine) is a widely used drug, effective by topical application or by injection. Solutions of 2 to 4 per cent strength are used topically, 0.5 per cent for local in-

Table 1. *Commonly Used Local Anesthetic Agents*

TECHNIQUE	LOCAL ANESTHETIC	CONCENTRATION RANGE	DURATION OF ACTION	MAXIMUM SAFE DOSE*
Topical anesthesia	Lidocaine	2-4 %	15 minutes	100 mg.
(mucous membranes)	Cocaine	4-10%	30 minutes	100-200 mg.
	Tetracaine	1-2 %	45 minutes	40 mg.
	Benzocaine†	2-10%	Several hours	—
Local infiltration	Procaine	0.5 %	1/4-1/2 hour	1000 mg.‡
	Lidocaine	0.5-1 %	1/2- 1 hour	500 mg.‡
	Mepivacaine	0.5-1 %	1/2- 1 hour	500 mg.‡
	Tetracaine	0.025-0.1%	2- 3 hours	75 mg.‡
Major nerve block	Lidocaine	1-2 %	1- 2 hours	500 mg.‡
	Mepivacaine	1-2 %	1-2¼ hours	500 mg.‡
	Tetracaine	0.1-0.25%	2- 3 hours	75 mg.‡
Epidural anesthesia	Procaine	1-2 %	1/2- 1 hour	1000 mg.‡
	Lidocaine	1-2 %	3/4-1½ hours	500 mg.‡
	Mepivacaine	1-2 %	1-2¼ hours	500 mg.‡
	Tetracaine	0.1-0.25%	2- 3 hours	75 mg.‡
Spinal anesthesia	Procaine	5 %	1/2- 1 hour	—
	Lidocaine	5 %	3/4-1½ hours	—
	Tetracaine	0.5 %	1- 2 hours	—
Intravenous regional anesthesia	Lidocaine	0.25-0.5%	Varies	100-150 mg.

* The maximum safe dose listed is that dose most widely accepted as safe for administration to an average adult. Lower doses may produce toxic symptoms if inadvertent intravascular injection occurs. The safe dose must be reduced if disease, small patient size and other factors might act to produce high blood levels of local anesthetic.
† As the base.
‡ With epinephrine, 1:200,000 added.

filtration and 1 to 2 per cent for conduction anesthesia. A maximum injected dose of 500 mg. should not be exceeded in the average adult. The chemical structure of lidocaine is characterized by its amide linkage which resists hydrolysis by plasma esterase. It produces a more prompt and longer lasting anesthesia than equal concentrations of procaine, and appears to spread better in the tissues. Mild sedation often accompanies its use. It depresses the myocardium and the cardiac conduction system and can be used intravenously as an antiarrhythmic agent.

Mepivacaine (Carbocaine), like lidocaine, is an amide. Its onset of action is slightly more rapid, duration longer, and sedative effect less. The two drugs are similar in other respects.

Tetracaine (Pontocaine) is about ten times more potent and toxic than procaine. It is effective by all methods of application and is widely used, especially for spinal anesthesia. One to 2 per cent concentrations produce adequate topical anesthesia of the respiratory tract and concentrations of 0.1 to 0.25 per cent are enough for infiltration and nerve block. The maximal allowable dosage is about 75 mg. in the average adult. Its chief disadvantage is its slow onset of action, although its duration of effect is twice that of procaine.

Benzocaine typifies the local anesthetics that are poorly soluble in water. It is effective when applied to mucous membranes or open wounds, and remains localized for long periods, accounting for its sustained action and relatively low toxicity. It is the active ingredient in many analgesic ointments, but is not useful for injection procedures.

General Rules for Use of Local Anesthetics

Toxicity. The total dose should be limited to the smallest amount that will serve the purpose. Local anesthetics are toxic drugs which produce dangerous side effects on the cardiovascular and central nervous systems.

Latency. There is a characteristic period of latency between application of drug and onset of block. It is essential to wait for the full effect before evaluating the response to the drug and before beginning the operation or administering additional drug.

Concentration. For each agent there is a minimum effective concentration below which adequate block will not appear. Higher concentrations often produce more rapid onset but also increase the possibility of toxic reactions. The concentration used should be appropriately selected and should be the least that will provide the desired effect.

Maximum dose. A maximum dose for each local anesthetic is recommended in Table 1 but symptoms of toxicity may occur below that dose level if inadvertent intravascular injection occurs. Doses must be reduced by one-half to one-third when topical or intravenous techniques are used.

Use of vasoconstrictors. The addition of epinephrine to local anesthetic solutions produces vasoconstriction and slows absorption from the injection site, prolongs duration of anesthesia and reduces the total dosage of drug required. The optimal concentration of epinephrine to be used in this manner is 1:200,000. Stronger concentrations may lead to symptoms that mimic reactions to a local anesthetic.

Toxic Reactions to Local Anesthetics

Acute systemic toxicity from local anesthetics is caused by high blood levels of these agents. This is avoided by using techniques which prevent rapid absorption. Symptoms arise from the central nervous, cardiovascular and respiratory systems. Central nervous system stimulation occurs, followed by depression. Garrulousness sometimes precedes other symptoms and should be regarded as an early warning. Restlessness, anxiety, confusion and twitching may precede convulsions followed by coma. Cardiovascular depression may be prominent. Arterial hypotension results from vasodilation and cardiac depression. Cardiac action may cease or become ineffective owing to depression of the myocardium or of the myocardial conducting system. Inadequate ventilation occurs during the convulsion or following depression of the central respiratory center.

Therapy must support the cardiovascular and respiratory systems and control convulsions, if present. Currently, there are two different therapeutic approaches to control convulsions. The first considers the increased electrical activity of the cortex during convulsions to be detrimental and attempts to abolish this with small doses of rapidly acting barbiturates. Thiopental is preferable because of its ability to penetrate brain tissue most rapidly. This method recognizes that postictal depression will occur and can summate with the barbiturate-induced depression. By the use of small doses of drug, prolonged depression is avoided. The newer approach treats the peripheral manifestations of the convulsion. Succinylcholine is injected to suppress convulsive muscular motions, thereby permitting artificial ventilation of lungs. With either form of therapy, the administration of oxygen, maintenance of adequate ventilation and support of the cardiovascular system with intravenous fluids and pressor drugs are indicated.

GENERAL ANESTHESIA

General anesthesia is defined as a reversible state of insensibility with loss of consciousness. It can be produced by a variety of chemical agents which act on the brain. Neither the mechanism nor the exact site of action of the general anesthetic agents has been classified, probably because the structural and functional complexity of the central nervous system has escaped full definition. It is known, however, that there are two afferent systems which carry information to the brain (Table 2). The lateral ascending sensory pathways rapidly conduct

afferent impulses to primary receiving areas in the brain by means of fibers which are specific with respect to modality and topography. The medial multisynaptic ascending pathways in the core of the brain stem serve as a second and nonspecific sensory system which is important in the regulation of consciousness and is valuable in the integration of central nervous system function. Collaterals from the primary lateral pathways carry impulses to this system, called the ascending reticular activating system, in which conduction is slow and transmission diffuse. Peripheral and cortical impulses converge and interact and modalities lose their individuality. This system projects to wide areas of the cortex and promotes wakefulness and alertness. Experimental interruption of the ascending reticular activating system results in somnolence or unconsciousness, although sensory conduction via the classic sensory pathways remains intact. General anesthetic agents produce similar changes in a reversible manner. This has led Brazier to conclude that, "It is the ascending activating influence of the brain stem reticular system on cortical excitability that is impaired by most anesthetics."

The site of anesthetic action may be anywhere in the ascending reticular activating system between the peripheral afferents and the outflow to the cortex, with location dif-

Table 2. Ascending Pathways to the Brain

LONG ASCENDING SENSORY PATHWAYS	ASCENDING RETICULAR PATHWAYS
I. *Somatotopical Organization* (a) Point for point projection from periphery to thalamus to cortex (b) Modality-specific fiber pathways	I. *No Somatotopical Organization* (a) Single reticular unit responds to afferent stimulation from widely separated peripheral areas (b) Single unit responds to a variety of sensory modalities
II. *Discrete Well Defined Pathways* Usually a three neuron pathway: neuron I with axon extending from sensory receptor to central nervous system, where synapse occurs with neuron II whose axon joins modality-specific fiber pathways to thalamus; neuron III projects from thalamus to specific area of cortex	II. *Diffuse Pathways* A multineuron pathway: input to ascending reticular system from (a) ascending sensory pathways of cord, (b) sensory nuclei of brain stem, (c) cerebral cortex, (d) cerebellum, (e) basal ganglia; neurons of medial reticular formation of brain stem are of small (12 microns) to large (90 microns) size, with short to long axons, ascending and descending in direction; conduction in short or long steps with multiple collateral synapses; there is lack of modality-specific pathways; reticulofugal projections via thalamic relay or directly to widespread areas of cortex
III. *Discrete Electrophysiological Response Pattern* A single peripheral stimulus produces a discrete response in the thalamus and a discrete projection to a specific location in the cortex	III. *Widespread Response Pattern with Long Time Course* Single peripheral stimulus evokes a bombardment of impulses over a considerable period of time in intralaminar nuclei of thalamus; this in turn projects to entire cortex by diffuse thalamocortical circuits to produce electrical desynchronization of resting EEG

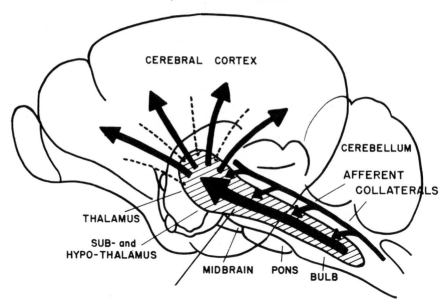

Figure 3. Outline of brain of cat showing extent of medially placed ascending reticular activating system of the brain stem (cross-lining) and distribution of collaterals to it from laterally situated long ascending sensory pathways. Diffuse projection to cortex from ascending reticular activating system is also shown. (From Starzl et al.: J. Neurophysiol. *14*:479, 1951.)

fering among agents and dose. Stimulation of the anesthetized animal leads to recordable activity in the reticular formation; therefore, the collateral input from the primary sensory pathways is not blocked. Anesthetic agents do block synaptic transmission at lower concentrations than those which influence conduction in nerve fibers. Comparison of the multisynaptic character of the reticular pathways with the paucisynaptic lateral pathways suggests greater susceptibility of the former to anesthetic depression and supports the concept that a primary mechanism of anesthetic action may be suppression of synaptic transmission in the ascending reticular activating system.

Anesthetic agents influence portions of the central nervous system other than the ascending reticular activating system. Primary sensory pathways can be depressed as anesthetic concentrations increase. Amnesia prior to loss of consciousness may indicate synaptic blockade in the hippocampus by anesthetic agents at concentrations too low to affect the ascending reticular activating system. The analgesic effects of subanesthetic doses of diethyl ether, methoxyflurane and nitrous oxide may indicate a site of action in the limbic system or in the rhinencephalon at doses insufficient to affect the reticular system.

Body systems other than the central nervous system are also susceptible to the effects of general anesthetic agents. Before the introduction of curare into clinical medicine, muscular relaxation was produced by deep anesthesia, probably through a direct depression of muscle. Hypotension, cardiac arrhythmias and prolonged postoperative ileus bear witness to other extraneural effects of anesthetics.

Neurophysiological studies continue to disclose previously unrecognized effects of anesthetics upon the central nervous system; however, these studies are hampered by the imprecise methods available for measuring and controlling the depth of general anesthesia. The electroencephalograph has been disappointing as a clinically useful instrument to document varying levels of anesthesia. The depth of anesthesia in animals or man is as accurately determined by clinical signs as by any other means. This aspect of anesthesiology is much the same today as it was decades ago. In short, an agent known to produce unconsciousness, analgesia, and sometimes relaxation safely and reversibly is administered to a patient; its pharmacologic effects are evaluated on the basis of the anesthetist's experience; adjustments in concentration are made, and the patient is again observed. The cycle is repeated again and again. The practice of anesthesia, despite modern knowledge, is still an art.

The Depth of Anesthesia

Anesthetists have attempted to define a method for assessing the degree of anesthetic-induced depression ever since ether was introduced. Guedel's guide to the levels of ether anesthesia stands today as the classic. This requires assessment of muscle function, respiratory and eye motions, pupillary size and presence or absence of certain reflexes, without consideration of the degree of surgical stimulation taking place. Despite its reliability, the system is little used today because ether has largely been replaced by modern anesthetic agents. An equally acceptable system to assess the levels of today's agents is not available. There are several reasons for this void. Guedel's schema was developed when anesthesia was produced almost exclusively by ether. Today, amnesia, analgesia, unconsciousness, reflex blockade and muscle relaxation each can be achieved by separate drugs. Guedel's guide required a patient who breathed spontaneously, albeit often inadequately. Studies have now shown that nearly every central nervous system depressant used by the anesthetist is a respiratory depressant. Anesthetization of a patient, therefore, carries with it the obligation to assess and often control pulmonary ventilation. Furthermore, the use of muscle relaxants has added to this obligation and completely removes respiratory motions and voluntary muscle action as a means for evaluating anesthetic depth.

A change in assessment of levels of anesthesia has become mandatory. The patient is now viewed as a living organism, responding to stimulation. The characteristics of the response depend on the stimulus and on the presence of modifying factors which in this sense are anesthetic drugs. A concept of too light, or too deep, or adequately anesthetized has replaced the more static classification of Stage 3, plane 2 in which the character of the surgical stimulus was ignored. Obviously, the patient adequately anesthetized for excision of a superficial lipoma is too lightly anesthetized to allow removal of the gallbladder. Current estimates of anesthetic depth, therefore, are made on a dynamic scale, and depend upon surgical activities (Fig. 4). To use this scale effectively, the anesthetist must observe the surgical field as well as the patient so that he can evaluate both stimulus and response. He must infer from these observations the adequacy

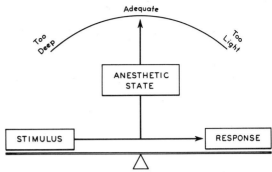

Figure 4. The interaction of strength of surgical stimulation and patient response in determining depth of anesthesia. If response to stimulus is excessive, the pointer swings to the "Too Light" side. If the response is too small for the strength of stimulation, the pointer swings to the "Too Deep" side. The anesthetic state is modified to balance stimulus and resultant response at the "Just Right" point. This requires assessment of both stimulus and response.

of the anesthesia. He must appreciate the period of latency between administration of a drug and manifestation of its action and be sufficiently familiar with surgical technique to anticipate changes in the level of anesthesia before they are required.

The clinical concept of the anesthetic state itself has also undergone evolution. Woodbridge suggested that general anesthesia is composed of four components: sensory, motor and mental block, and prevention of noxious reflexes. Each drug administered during an anesthetic produces a characteristic spectrum of action when viewed in this light. For instance, the barbiturate produces sleep without sensory blockade; spinal anesthesia results in sensory and motor block without sleep, and nitrous oxide can produce sleep and sensory block without motor or reflex obtundity. Muscle relaxants inhibit motor activity only. By considering the action of anesthetic drugs and the surgical demands, an anesthetic technique can be selected by which adequate conditions in each of these four categories are produced for surgical procedures (Table 3). Only in this way will a properly balanced anesthesia result.

One other factor demands recognition. The patient's preoperative physiological and psychological status may significantly influence his response to anesthesia. The debilitated require only small doses of drugs to provide anesthesia for a major surgical procedure. A healthy, muscular individual requires vastly larger doses and the alcoholic may have increased tolerance to depressant drugs. The apprehensive or excited patient often

Table 3. *Signs of Depth of the Four Components of Anesthesia**

	SENSORY	MOTOR	MENTAL	REFLEX CIRCULATORY	RESPIRATORY	GASTROINTESTINAL
Insufficient depth of anesthesia	Breath holding Deep breathing Phonation Laryngospasm Tachycardia Rise or fall of blood pressure Movement with painful stimulus Coughing	Movement Insufficient muscle relaxation for surgical procedure	Motor response to stimulation Delirium Uninhibited speech or actions	Bradycardia and hypotension Tachycardia and hypertension Arrhythmias	Mucus Spasm: laryngeal bronchiolar chest wall Sucking	Nausea and retching Salivation Swallowing
Sufficient depth of anesthesia	Minimal response to painful stimulus followed by accommodation Stability of cardiovascular and respiratory systems	Quiet surgical field Adequate muscle relaxation when needed	Amnesia Ataraxia Sleep	Absence of troublesome reflexes from cardiovascular, respiratory or gastrointestinal systems		
Excessive depth of anesthesia	No response	Muscular flaccidity Inability to reestablish normal ventilatory function at termination of anesthesia	Prolonged obtundation in pre- or postanesthetic period	Bradycardia or tachycardia Hypotension Arrhythmias Intolerance to change of position	Respiratory arrest†	Intestinal atony during surgery Postoperative ileus

* Adapted from Woodbridge, P.D.: Anesthesiology *18*:536, 1957.
† In absence of muscle relaxants or hyperventilation.

needs appreciably larger quantities of medication. The response of the living system to stimulation serves as a guide to a proper titration of drug-induced depression.

GENERAL ANESTHETIC AGENTS

There are nearly 20 general anesthetic agents available for clinical use, yet a recent study shows an increasing preference for halothane, usually in combination with thiopental and nitrous oxide, and a corresponding decrease in the use of all others (Table 4).

In 1962, nearly 85 per cent of all anesthetics administered were one of four agents or combinations of agents: ether, cyclopropane, nitrous oxide and a barbiturate, or halothane with or without nitrous oxide and a barbiturate. Halothane was given in nearly 50 per cent of all anesthetics and in all probability is now used in 70 per cent. Agents such as ethylene, chloroform, divinyl ether and ethyl chloride are rarely used except by the occasional enthusiast. Others, such as ether and cyclopropane are diminishing in popularity, and ether is used mostly in teaching institutions.

Table 4. *Percentage Distribution of Anesthetic Practice, by Year**

YEAR	HALOTHANE	N–B†	CYCLOPROPANE	ETHER	OTHER	ESTIMATED NUMBER OF ADMINISTRATIONS
1959	11.0	35.5	20.5	17.3	15.7	207,261
1960	22.7	28.4	18.8	14.3	15.8	211,421
1961	35.1	23.4	16.4	9.6	15.5	210,728
1962	48.5	15.5	13.4	6.9	15.7	227,105
Total %	29.8	25.5	17.2	11.9	15.6	
Number	254,896	218,221	147,358	102,014	134,026	856,515

* Numbers vary slightly or may not add to the exact total due to rounding.
† N–B = nitrous oxide–barbiturate.
Data from Committee on Anesthesia, National Academy of Sciences – National Research Council: J.A.M.A. *197*:775, 1966.

Inhalation Agents

GASES. *Nitrous oxide* was the first anesthetic gas described and today is probably the most widely used anesthetic agent. Many operating rooms have nitrous oxide as well as oxygen supplied to wall outlets from remote bulk storage areas. The gas comes in steel cylinders painted blue, as a liquid under pressure and when released from the cylinder is colorless with a sweet odor. The possibility of contamination of nitrous oxide with toxic, higher oxides of nitrogen has been noted recently. This is the least potent of the anesthetic gases and its effectiveness is further reduced by the necessity that it be administered with at least 20 per cent oxygen. Seldom used alone because of its inability to produce surgical anesthesia, it is most often combined with a narcotic or barbiturate, a muscle relaxant or a volatile agent such as halothane. In the absence of hypoxia, there is little effect on the circulation, respiration, liver or kidney. It is nonexplosive and does not provide muscle relaxation. It is an analgesic. A balanced technique has gained favor in some areas; this consists of a thiopental induction to anesthesia, followed by maintenance of unconsciousness and analgesia with nitrous oxide and total paralysis with large doses of muscle relaxants. More widely accepted, however, is the use of nitrous oxide with potent inhalational agents such as halothane which decreases the need for muscle relaxants. If inhaled in subanesthetic concentrations of 20 to 50 per cent, analgesia sufficient to allay the discomfort of uterine contractions during labor will result.

Cyclopropane is a potent, flammable anesthetic agent capable of producing deep anesthesia, muscle relaxation and cardiovascular and respiratory depression. The gas is supplied in orange tanks as a pressurized liquid. Because of its potency, alveolar concentrations of 1 to 3 per cent lead to analgesia without loss of consciousness and those of 10 to 30 per cent produce surgical anesthesia. Induction of anesthesia is usually accomplished quickly. Maintenance is associated with a mild elevation of blood pressure and a slow pulse during stable periods whereas emergence occurs within a few minutes after the anesthetic is discontinued, depending upon depth and duration. There is a progressive diminution of respiratory tidal volume as anesthesia deepens and assisted or controlled ventilation is mandatory if respiratory acidosis is to be avoided. Narcotic premedication hastens the onset of respiratory depression. Pharyngeal and airway reflexes are enhanced. Bronchiolar constriction sometimes appears. Narcotics given preoperatively predispose to bradycardia during cyclopropane anesthesia.

Cardiac arrhythmias may appear as increasing concentrations of cyclopropane are given or as respiratory acidosis appears. This agent enhances the ability of catecholamines to cause cardiac arrhythmias, an effect termed myocardial sensitization and probably most prominent with cyclopropane. However, in the absence of exogenous catecholamines, the agent is unlikely to cause ventricular fibrillation. Arrhythmias during anesthesia generally respond readily to conservative therapy, such as pulmonary ventilation and decreasing the cyclopropane concentrations. All general anesthetic agents are cardiovascular depressants but cyclopropane masks this by stimulating the sympathetic nervous system and elevating the blood levels of catecholamines. This results in maintenance of cardiac contractility, increased total peripheral resistance and mild elevation in blood pressure. In deeper levels of anesthesia, the depressant effects of cyclopropane may supervene and cardiac depression and hypotension may appear. Although muscle relaxation for most surgical procedures can be obtained with deep cyclopropane anesthesia, the more common practice is to use neuromuscular blocking agents and less cyclopropane. The incidence of postoperative nausea and vomiting is high after use of this agent.

In considering the use of cyclopropane, the physician weighs the disadvantages of flammability, the possibility of cardiac arrhythmias and the high incidence of postanesthetic nausea and vomiting against the advantages of rapid induction, high oxygen concentration and well-maintained levels of blood pressure.

Ethylene is a flammable anesthetic agent, lighter than air and with the least pleasant odor of all gaseous agents. It is only slightly more potent than nitrous oxide and must be administered in the same concentrations. It is supplied as a compressed gas in red, steel cylinders. The disadvantage of flammability does not outweigh the slightly higher potency. Few find the agent of significant value.

VOLATILE LIQUIDS. *Halothane* (Fluothane) is a potent, nonflammable, halogenated hydrocarbon with which anesthesia may be induced smoothly although relatively slowly. It is supplied in 125- or 250-ml. brown bottles and is usually given with 50 to 60 per cent nitrous oxide, although many use it with oxygen alone. With the latter technique, higher concentrations of the agent are required. Because of its potency, special vaporizers such as the Fluotec or copper kettle are usually indicated. Recovery from anesthesia is rapid, although this probably relates to the low 1 to 2 per cent concentration usually inhaled and the duration of administration. The incidence of nausea and vomiting with recovery is small.

Halothane causes depression of normal ventilatory responses to carbon dioxide and respiratory acidosis develops if ventilation is not supported. Laryngeal and pharyngeal reflexes are obtunded early in the course of anesthesia. Respiratory tract secretions are minimal and bronchodilation occurs, making halothane the anesthetic of choice for patients with bronchial asthma. Halothane, like cyclopropane, is a cardiovascular depressant but does not cause stimulation of the sympathetic nervous system and blood levels of catecholamines are not increased. The direct myocardial and vascular smooth muscle depressant effects of halothane are, therefore, unopposed and anesthesia is characterized by a decrease in both cardiac output and total peripheral resistance, resulting in hypotension. Arrhythmias are less common with halothane than with cyclopropane, although the myocardium is sensitized to catecholamines. The heart rate slows in deep levels of anesthesia. Some degree of muscle relaxation is characteristic with halothane but supplemental relaxant drugs are usually required for abdominal surgery.

The role of halothane in producing postoperative hepatic damage has been studied extensively after suspicion was raised that it was hazardous in this respect. Although the rare occurrence of hepatic damage could not be excluded, the harmful effect, if any, was found to be small and not to differ in incidence from that of other agents. Halothane has a record of safety comparable with any other agent.

The smoothness of induction of anesthesia, ease of maintenance, lack of flammability and pleasantness of recovery have led to wide acceptance of halothane. It is the most extensively used of all volatile liquid anesthetic agents.

Diethyl ether is a highly volatile liquid with a pungent, flammable vapor which is capable of producing all depths of surgical anesthesia to respiratory arrest. It is usually supplied in copper-lined metal cans. Induction is prolonged, respiratory secretions are copious, and struggling and vomiting may occur before an adequate level of anesthesia is obtained. The signs of anesthetic depth are well demarcated and muscle relaxation is present for most surgical procedures without the need for supplementary neuromuscular blocking drugs. Ether enhances the neuromuscular blocking effect of curare and if both drugs are used concomitantly the dose of curare must be reduced. The irritation of ether vapor reflexly stimulates respiration and respiratory alkalosis appears early, although this may be superseded subsequently with a metabolic acidosis. Blood pressure, pulse and cardiac rhythm are normal in lighter levels and hypotension may occur at deep stages. Direct myocardial depression by the anesthetic is counterbalanced by stimulation of the sympathetic nervous system. However, the myocardium is not sensitized to catecholamines.

The flammability of ether, the prolonged induction, emergence and the frequency of nausea and vomiting during recovery have led to a decreasing acceptance of this agent in clinical anesthesia, although some still find it useful, especially because of its respiratory stimulating properties.

Methoxyflurane (Penthrane) is another potent, nonflammable, liquid ether with a low vapor pressure. Because of the low volatility and high fat solubility, induction of anesthesia is very slow and most often is aided by use of an intravenous thiobarbiturate. With surgical anesthesia, respiratory depression, hypotension and muscle relaxation may be prominent. Although some degree of myocardial sensitization occurs, it is not important and cardiac arrhythmias are uncommon. Recovery is slow and may be accompanied by prolonged analgesia. Nausea and vomiting are infrequent.

Methoxyflurane has obtained a measure of popularity because of its lack of flammability, good muscle relaxation, prominent analgesia and minimal nausea and vomiting. However, the slow induction and emergence are decided disadvantages.

Other volatile anesthetics are available but are not widely used clinically. *Divinyl ether* and *ethyl chloride*, once used for the rapid induction of inhalation anesthesia by the open drop technique, are now seldom employed. *Trichlorethylene* is a halogenated hydrocarbon, nonflammable, and useful to supplement nitrous oxide for minor surgical procedures or manipulations, or for use alone as an inhalational analgesic. However, it is not potent and reacts with soda lime to form toxic products. It must, therefore, be administered by techniques which do not rely on soda lime for carbon dioxide disposal. During surgical anesthesia, tachypnea and cardiac arrhythmias may occur; the drug sensitizes the heart to the arrhythmic actions of injected epinephrine. Trichlorethylene does not damage the liver or the kidneys, nor does it produce muscle relaxation. It is useful in providing analgesia for labor and delivery.

Techniques of Administration of Inhalation Agents

The original technique of administering volatile anesthetic agents was to pour them on a folded towel or gauze placed over the patient's nose and mouth. This provided a vaporizing surface and as air was breathed through the mask, the vapor was drawn into the lungs. There were disadvantages such as poorly controlled anesthetic concentration, inability to assist ventilation, and increased dead space leading to hypoxia and hypercarbia. Although this technique was popular in America for nearly a century, it has largely been abandoned in the operating room. It still proves useful in certain circumstances.

Current techniques employ sophisticated equipment to administer anesthesia. This is relatively simple to understand and operate if one understands its basic components (Fig. 5).

Gas sources (A) of oxygen and other anesthetic gases are supplied in tanks as pressurized liquids or gases. Machines are equipped with a pin index system to prevent improper placement of cylinders. These cylinders are painted in distinctive colors so that their gas content is easily recognized, although the same color code is not used universally. Anesthetic machines often incorporate gauges so that the gas pressure in the tanks can be observed. Usually two tanks each of oxygen and nitrous oxide are available. These gases are sometimes supplied from remote sources to the anesthetic machine by high pressure hoses.

Reducing valves (B) or pressure regulators

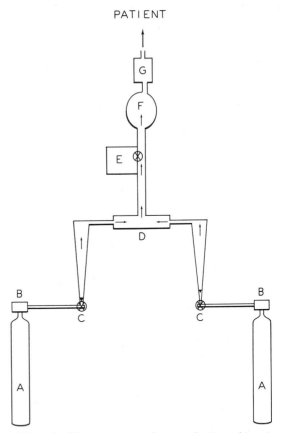

Figure 5. The components of an anesthetic machine. *A,* Source of anesthetic gases and oxygen. *B,* Reducing valves. *C,* Needle valves and flowmeters. *D,* Mixing manifold. *E,* Vaporizer for volatile anesthetic liquids. *F,* Reservoir bag. *G,* Delivery apparatus.

are built into most anesthetic machines. Frequently pressure reduction is accomplished in several stages, so that the high pressures within the tanks are reduced to safe levels within the machines.

Metering devices (C) are calibrated, tapered glass tubes in which light weight bobbins float in the flowing gas streams. The most common metering devices incorporated in modern anesthetic machines are Rotometers. The rate of gas flow is regulated by a needle valve at the bottom of the meter. As the aperture becomes wider, the flow of gas increases and the bobbin rises in the tube. Gas flow rates are read directly from the calibrated tube.

The mixing manifold (D) acts as a collecting and mixing space for the gases at the outflow end of the meter.

Vaporizers (E) of various designs may be included in the equipment. The simplest of these is the draw-over type, in which variable amounts of inspired air are drawn through a bottle containing a volatile anesthetic and in which a wick is placed to increase the volatilizing surface. More sophisticated devices are flow and temperature compensated. Many factors govern the efficiency of a vaporizer, including ambient temperature and pressure, the liquid agent being used, the rate of gas flow through the vaporizer and the surface area of the gas-liquid interface. Modern vaporizers are commonly constructed of copper because of the efficiency with which this metal conducts heat and keeps the volatile anesthetic at a reasonably constant temperature.

A reservoir bag (F) is usually necessary so that the rate of gas flow demanded by the patient at any phase of respiration need not be matched throughout the respiratory cycle by that supplied from the meters. Respiratory gas flow in the patient's airway is intermittent and bidirectional. Anesthetic machines are available which provide intermittent gas flow on demand by the patient but most modern machines provide for constant flow of anesthetic agents into a reservoir bag. With these machines the bag fills when the flow from the machine exceeds the inspiratory demands of the patient, and provides a ready supply of anesthetic gases at all times. In addition, the bag furnishes a means of applying pressure to the airway to assist or control ventilation. The reservoir is most often a part of the delivery apparatus.

The delivery apparatus (G) may be one of many arrangements to control the inspired atmosphere of the anesthetized patient and to provide for the elimination of expired carbon dioxide. These can be designated by two systems of nomenclature, one describing the pathway of respiratory gases in the anesthetic apparatus, the other the method of dealing with expired gases. According to the latter, the apparatus is either open, semi-open, semi-closed or closed. In an open system, expired gases are completely vented to the atmosphere and carbon dioxide is thus eliminated. In a closed system, expired gas is retained within the system and is rebreathed during subsequent respiratory cycles. This requires inclusion of a chemical method for the removal of carbon dioxide. Semi-open and semi-closed systems incorporate intermediate degrees of rebreathing.

The pathway of gas flow in nearly all anesthetic systems can be described by one of three terms: to and fro, non-rebreathing or circle (Fig. 6). If the inspiratory and expiratory gases use a common pathway, the apparatus is named to and fro (A). This does not require valves to direct gas flow, although a spring-loaded valve to allow venting of excess gas may be included. If directional valves separate inspiratory and expiratory pathways, the system is called either non-rebreathing or circle. In a non-rebreathing system (B) the inspiratory pathway is unidirectional, from the reservoir to the patient, and the expiratory pathway vents expired gases to the atmosphere. All non-rebreathing systems are open systems as well and demand a fresh gas supply in excess of the patient's respiratory minute volume. In circle systems (C), which are commonly used in this country, valves direct expired gas completely or partially to a reservoir bag or to a spring-loaded vent, depending largely upon the rate of fresh gas flow being provided to the apparatus. Circle systems are either closed or semi-closed and usually depend on the chemical removal of carbon dioxide within the circuit.

All anesthetic apparatus must provide for the disposal of expired carbon dioxide. In open systems, because expired gases are vented to atmosphere, the patient inspires only fresh anesthetic mixtures. Systems in which both fresh and expired gases pass together into the reservoir usually include a carbon dioxide absorption canister charged with soda lime, which is a mixture of soda hydroxide and calcium hydroxide, or baralyme, a mixture of hydroxides of barium and calcium. Both mixtures contain sufficient moisture to allow formation of carbonic acid from exhaled carbon dioxide. The acid is then chemically neutralized. In this manner, expired carbon dioxide is eliminated. Alternately, if fresh gases are added to the system at a rate equal to twice the minute volume of ventilation, the expired carbon dioxide is usually flushed from the apparatus.

Each of these delivery systems has advantages and disadvantages which determine the selection for a particular clinical situation. Circle systems, because of the use of directional valves, add significantly to ventilatory resistance and the work of breathing but they are convenient to use. Respiratory resistance can be overcome by assisting or controlling ventilation. To and fro systems, on the other hand, incorporate the advantage of low respiratory resistance because directional valves are not needed, but when used with soda lime canisters they are cumber-

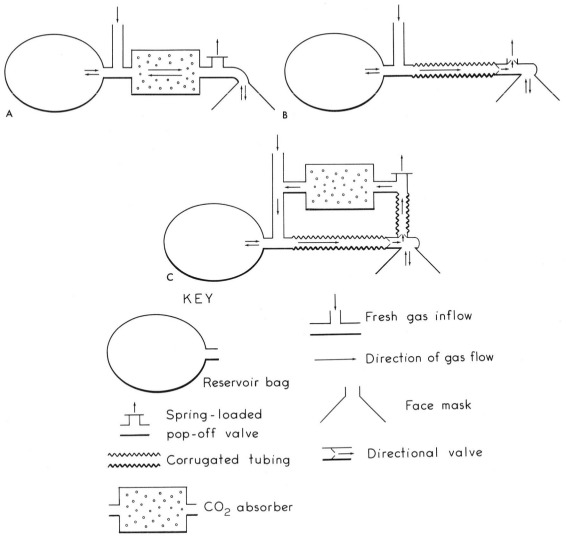

Figure 6. The to and fro (*A*), non-rebreathing (*B*) and circle (*C*) systems for delivering anesthesia. There is a common pathway for inspiratory and expiratory gases in the to and fro system, and a separation of these pathways by valves in the non-rebreathing and circle systems. The circle system provides for return of expired gas to the system by way of a carbon dioxide absorber.

some. Open systems allow loss of heat and moisture from the respiratory tract, a factor of importance particularly in small children. Closed systems require the use of soda lime or baralyme and, therefore, cannot be used with trichlorethylene, but they are particularly indicated when explosive agents are being administered. Circle systems represent considerable initial cost but offer the versatility of either high or low flow techniques. Open systems are relatively inexpensive but require high flows of anesthetic gases, adding to the cost of each procedure. The simple equipment used for a to and fro system is easily sterilized, making it an ideal choice in patients with a pulmonary infection. In-

crease in respiratory dead space and in resistance to respiration occurs with the best anesthetic equipment but is generally of little consequence in the adult. In children, this consideration is important and special equipment is required.

Uptake and Distribution of Anesthetic Agents

The depth of anesthesia produced by inhalation agents varies according to the partial pressure of the anesthetic in the brain. This can only be controlled indirectly. Altering the composition of the inspired atmosphere leads to successive pressure gradients from inspired atmosphere to alveolus, arterial blood and brain. The partial pressure of agents in the brain always attempts to reach equilibrium with that in arterial blood. If blood gas tension is higher than that in the brain, anesthetic agents enter the brain and depth of anesthesia increases; if arterial tension is lower than that of brain, the reverse occurs. A similar relationship occurs in the lung where alveolar tension determines the arterial tension. The uptake and transport of anesthetic agent from the external environment to its site of action in the brain is affected by inspired concentration of the agent; ventilatory factors, such as minute volume of ventilation, functional residual capacity, respiratory dead space and distribution of inspired gas within the lung; circulatory factors, such as cardiac output and its distribution in lung and body tissues; physical factors, such as a solubility of the agent in blood, partition of the agent between blood and body tissues, particularly brain, and partial pressure gradients of the agent within the body.

During induction of inhalational anesthesia, the higher the partial pressure of anesthetic inhaled, the faster the anesthetic tension rises in the lung and the faster the arterial tension rises. Large minute volumes of ventilation also hasten the buildup of anesthetic in the lung. When there is an abnormally great functional residual capacity, as in pulmonary emphysema, the rise in alveolar tension of the agent is slowed and induction prolonged.

If the anesthetic is highly soluble in blood, for example, methoxyflurane or ether, it is removed from the lung rapidly. This impedes the rate at which the partial pressure in the lung approaches that in the inspired air. Similarly, a high cardiac output, such as is present in hyperthyroidism, causes a fast removal of anesthetic agent from the lung and a slow rise of pulmonary partial pressure of the agent. On the other hand, nitrous oxide is of low solubility and is sparingly removed from the lung; the alveolar tension rapidly reflects the inspired tension. If abnormalities exist in the distribution of inspired gas within the lungs, or of pulmonary blood flow, or if ventilation-perfusion ratios are abnormal, then gradients in alveolar and arterial anesthetic tensions may occur and slow the rate of induction.

The delivery of anesthetic agent from the lung to tissues is dependent on the distribution of the cardiac output throughout the body. Hemorrhage, vascular shunts, or other factors which alter the proportion of cardiac output delivered to the brain may significantly influence the clinical management of an anesthetic. The solubility of an anesthetic agent in body tissues influences its uptake. This is most often expressed as the blood-tissue partition coefficient and for most anesthetics and tissues is near 1.0, indicating that the agent is equally soluble in blood and tissue. Fat has a greater affinity for anesthetic agents than do other body tissues. This is particularly true of ether, halothane and methoxyflurane. When anesthesia is prolonged, enough anesthetic agent may be sequestered in fat depots to impede normal recovery significantly.

Intravenous Anesthetic Agents

Although a wide variety of drugs, ranging from diethyl ether to a nonhormonal steroid, have been administered intravenously to produce general anesthesia, only the ultrashort-acting barbiturates have gained wide support for use by this route. Of all anesthetic agents available, none approaches the popularity of the thiobarbiturates, or has the patient appeal for induction of anesthesia.

Thiopental (Pentothal) or *thiamylal* (Surital) is administered intravenously in a 2.5 per cent or more dilute solution, care being taken to avoid intra-arterial injection which can lead to arterial occlusion, or subcutaneous injection which may cause tissue slough. These drugs are useful because of two characteristics of the anesthetic state which they produce: rapid onset and short duration. Their high fat solubility allows them to penetrate all tissues of the body without delay, the tissue uptake being a function of local blood flow and arterial concentration of the drug. Because the brain receives a high proportion of the cardiac output, a large percentage of the injected dose reaches the brain rapidly and causes unconsciousness. Excitement is rare. The duration of the central depression is dependent upon the redistribution of the drug from the brain to viscera and other well perfused body tissues.

After a single dose, the concentration of barbiturate at the neural site of action declines rapidly and progressively and central depression is reversed. The duration of the initial effect is dependent upon the size of the initial dose and the adequacy of the circulation. Anesthesia induced by these drugs is associated with respiratory depression or apnea if the dose given is large. Little analgesia or muscle relaxation is provided. Cardiovascular depression is dependent upon the dose but may be profound in hypovolemic or debilitated patients. By using fractional doses which are carefully administered, this can be avoided. Large amounts of the agent, even though injected over periods of several hours, slowly saturate fatty depots, leading to maintained blood levels and prolonged unconsciousness. For this reason, the thiobarbiturates are seldom given as the sole anesthetic for other than very brief operations.

Thiopental and similar drugs provide a rapid and pleasant induction of anesthesia which can later be maintained by inhalational agents. They may be administered intermittently or continuously by intravenous infusion to potentiate nitrous oxide and muscle relaxants, thus producing a balanced anesthesia. When used sparingly with regional techniques, they cause sedation. They are also effective when administered rectally to produce a basal narcosis in children.

Neuromuscular Blocking Agents

Prior to 1945, the muscle relaxation required for abdominal operations was provided either by deep general anesthesia or by spinal anesthesia. This was unsatisfactory because many patients were too ill to tolerate either technique and spinal anesthesia was often insufficient for extensive upper abdominal procedures. The introduction of muscle relaxants solved this problem and changed the concepts of general anesthesia. Now deep general anesthesia is rarely required; only first or second plane anesthesia need be provided and if relaxation is needed, the appropriate relaxant drug can be administered intravenously. Some have even advocated techniques which combine the minimal anesthesia of nitrous oxide with complete flaccidity provided by muscle relaxants.

Clinically, muscle relaxants act postsynaptically at the neuromuscular junction. They are divided into two classes according to their mode of action. The non-depolarizing competitive blocking agents prevent combination of normally liberated acetylcholine with the muscle endplate receptors, thereby blocking normal neuromuscular transmission. d-Tubocurarine, gallamine (Flaxedil)

and dimethyl tubocurarine (Metubine) belong to this group. The depolarizing agents combine with the endplate receptor to cause an initial but prolonged depolarization of of the postjunctional membrane, resulting in blockade of normal neuromuscular transmission. Succinylcholine (Anectine, Scoline, Quelicin) and decamethonium (Syncurine) belong to this group. There are other pharmacologic and pathologic causes of neuromuscular blockade. Some diseases and drugs decrease the mobilization or release of acetylcholine upon nerve stimulation. These include magnesium ion excess, calcium ion deficit, botulinus toxin, antibiotics, quinine and procaine. A postjunctional desensitization action has been described which explains, in part, the muscle relaxation caused by ether and halothane, as well as the otherwise ill-defined, occasional persistent effect of depolarizing agents.

The neuromuscular block produced by the competitive agents can be antagonized by substances which increase the concentration of acetylcholine at the motor endplate. An anticholinesterase drug, neostigmine (Prostigmin), is used for this purpose if preceded by a large dose of atropine to block muscarinic actions such as excessive airway secretions and bradycardia. Antagonists to the action of depolarizing blocking agents are not available. The usefulness of the depolarizers is dependent upon dissipation of the pharmacologically induced paralysis which, with succinylcholine, usually occurs within five minutes. Prolonged blockade is occasionally seen after use of these drugs in two groups of patients. In the first, relative overdosage occurs because of the presence of an atypical plasma pseudocholinesterase. This enzyme normally metabolizes and inactivates succinylcholine. The atypical enzyme is unable to hydrolyze the drug in a normal manner and succinylcholine remains in the plasma until slower nonenzymatic hydrolysis occurs, usually within an hour or two depending on the dose given. This condition can be recognized early and treated with respiratory support without risk to the patient. In the second group, prolonged paralysis results from a change in the character of the block produced by depolarizing agents. When relaxation has been prolonged by repeated injections or infusions of depolarizing drugs, the blocking effect sometimes outlasts the depolarizing action. In this situation, there is a return of membrane potential toward normal but a persistence of blockade. This has been called "desensitization blockade." It is similar in some respects, but different in others, to the blockade produced by the competitive blocking agents.

The treatment of prolonged paralysis in both these groups is maintenance of pulmonary ventilation until spontaneous respiration becomes adequate. Attempts at pharmacologic therapy under these circumstances may confuse the issue and prolong the block.

The muscle relaxants are usually given intravenously and the paralyzing effect follows promptly. There is a question as to whether or not the various muscle groups are affected equally but it should be assumed that the respiratory muscles are affected early and respiratory support will be required. These drugs should never be administered unless the means for artificial ventilation are immediately available and assembled for use. The dose of drug required to produce a given effect is dependent on many factors. These include physical fitness, muscular development, age, body temperature, concomitant diseases, anesthetic agent and depth of general anesthesia. It is always wise to give a small dose first, 6 mg. d-tubocurarine, observe the effect and repeat or increase the dose as indicated. The ease with which muscle relaxation can be produced with these agents has deluded many into believing their use is innocuous. Complications from muscle relaxants are more common after completion of the operation when normal ventilation cannot be re-established. It is a foolish surgeon who badgers his anesthetist to give more relaxant to provide better exposure. He and the patient will be safer to exploit the surgical means available to obtain the same effect.

THE PREANESTHETIC EVALUATION

The objectives of the preanesthetic evaluation are to identify abnormalities that are likely to affect the anesthetic and surgical risk; to ensure that, when possible, action has been taken to correct or improve abnormalities; to help prepare the patient emotionally as well as physiologically for the stress of anesthesia and operation; to assess the need for special intraoperative monitoring devices or anesthetic techniques and to plan for special postoperative care, and to determine the patient's concurrent and past experience with drugs and anesthetics. It is well to determine the frequency with which alcohol or barbiturates are used because either may affect the tolerance to anesthetics. Many drugs may influence the course of an anesthetic. Included among these are antibiotics, digitalis, adrenal steroids, phenothiazines, rauwolfia, and monamine oxidase inhibitors.

Ideally, all patients should be evaluated preoperatively by an anesthesiologist. This is not possible at present because of an acute shortage of physician anesthetists. Of necessity, therefore, a surgeon or internist sometimes assumes responsibility for preanesthetic evaluation and preparation. Because these physicians lack extensive experience with the physiologic changes which occur during anesthesia and with the pharmacologic idiosyncrasies of the anesthetized patient, this must be regarded as a temporary necessity which is less than ideal. If a physician anesthetist is available and fails to assume his responsibility in this respect, he is not giving his patients the care due them and he risks being considered a technician rather than a physician.

The examination, evaluation and preoperatreatment of most surgical patients take place after their admission to the hospital. Before the anesthesiologist sees the patient, the results of the history and physical examination should be written on the chart, and a hemoglobin determination and a urinalysis report appended. The need for further laboratory information must relate to the history and physical examination. The Committee on Pre- and Postoperative Care of the American College of Surgeons suggests a routine chest x-ray for all preoperative patients and for those over 50 years of age, an electrocardiogram, fasting blood sugar and blood urea nitrogen determination. If a history of cardiovascular, pulmonary, renal or hepatic disease exists, further evaluation may be necessary. Patients with heart disease should be classified as to type of disease, functional capacity of the heart and evidence for or against decompensation. If this has not been done by the referring physician, it should be done by a cardiologist. Patients with pulmonary disease are especially prone to postoperative lung complications and deserve careful preoperative attention. Chest physiotherapy and intermittent positive pressure treatments with bronchodilator and mucolytic agents are helpful in improving the ventilatory status. More ex-

Table 5. *Anesthetic Mortality Related to Physical Status**

PHYSICAL STATUS	NUMBER OF PATIENTS	NUMBER OF DEATHS	RATIO: DEATHS/PATIENTS
I	16,192	0	0/16,000
II	12,154	7	1/1740
III	4070	11	1/370
IV	720	17	1/40
V	87	4	1/20

* Data from Dripps, R. D., Lamont, A., and Eckenhoff, J. E.: J.A.M.A. *178*:261, 1961.

tensive use of pulmonary function tests in evaluation of these patients is encouraged. The availability of equipment for blood gas analysis and acid-base balance determinations leads to better preparation of surgical patients. It is unrealistic to believe that this type of preparation or these studies can be completed overnight.

In the case of an emergency operation, the same considerations apply but may be superseded by the urgency of the situation. Emergencies vary in degree and fixed rules for rapid evaluation cannot be given. However, the patient must be examined by an anesthesiologist under even the most dire circumstances. In an emergency situation, each physician tends to view the patient in the light of his own specialty. For instance, recent food intake is often ignored in the patient with an acute surgical emergency, until an anesthesiologist's examination, although the risk of vomiting and aspiration is well known.

PHYSICAL STATUS. The preoperative status of the patient often dictates his response to anesthetic drugs. The risk associated with anesthesia and operation is directly related to the patient's physical condition. Because of this the American Society of Anesthesiologists has adopted the following *Classification of Physical Status:*

Class I. Patients with no organic, physiologic, biochemical or psychological disturbance. The pathological process for which the operation is to be performed is localized and not related to a systemic disturbance. Examples are the physically fit for elective inguinal herniorrhaphy or hysterectomy.

Class II. Patients with mild to moderate systemic disturbance caused by the condition to be treated surgically or by other pathophysiological processes. Examples are mild diabetes or mild hypertension.

Class III. Patients with systemic disturbance from whatever the cause even though it may not be possible to define the degree of disability with finality. Examples are recent myocardial infarction or severe thyrotoxicosis.

Class IV. Patients with severe systemic disorder already life threatening and not always correctable by the operative procedure. Examples are cardiac insufficiency or advanced pulmonary disease.

Class V. Moribund patients with little chance for survival who are subjected to operation in desperation. Examples are the moribund patient with a ruptured aortic aneurysm or a mesenteric thrombosis.

The significance of the assignment of physical status to a patient should not be lost to the anesthesiologist nor to the patient's surgeon and internist. Experience has shown that as the physical condition of the patient worsens, the possibility of mortality from anesthesia increases. In a study of the causes of death in 33,224 surgical patients, the figures reproduced in Table 5 were obtained. Only those deaths thought definitely related to the anesthesia were included.

THE CHOICE OF ANESTHESIA

For nearly 90 years after the introduction of surgical anesthesia, a choice among anesthetic agents or techniques was negligible. During this period, interest lay only in providing oblivion and freedom from pain during operations. The last several decades have seen a change in this attitude. There is now available a wide variety of anesthetic agents and adjuvants with pharmacologic activities reasonably well-defined. The wide scope of modern surgical procedures has also individualized anesthetic requirements. Nonetheless, although choices do exist, they are for the most part relative. Few contraindications to any specific agent or technique have been accepted by most anesthetists. Among these might be listed the administration of spinal anesthesia to patients with pre-existing central nervous system disease, the use of muscle relaxants in patients with myasthenia gravis, and the administration of thiobarbiturates to patients with porphyria. An anesthetist skilled in a variety of anesthetic techniques can usually so apply them that a patient can be anesthetized in several ways. The final selection of agents and techniques is often a matter of individual preference or experience.

Although indications and contraindications are admittedly few, the skilled anesthetist has several ways of choosing agents and techniques for individual patients. The following are some guide-lines:

PREOPERATIVE DISEASE. This can justify exclusion of certain agents or techniques. Some agents are poorly tolerated by patients with certain diseases; for example, muscle relaxants in post-poliomyelitis patients with thoracic muscle involvement. Similarly, fear of confusing the natural progress of disease with a possible late postanesthetic complication may interdict the use of spinal anesthesia in patients with diabetic neuropathy or central nervous system syphilis.

THE BODILY HABITUS OF THE PATIENT. The asthenic, frail, elderly or chronically ill generally require minimal amounts of anesthetics. They do best with inhalational agents. The robust often require larger concentrations of anesthetics and metabolize injected substances quickly. Weak anesthetics are ineffectual. The obese patient absorbs large amounts of volatile anesthetic and presents the problem of respiratory obstruction soon after induction of general anesthesia. Spinal anesthesia is often a better choice.

PREOPERATIVE EMOTIONAL STATE. The emotionally unstable and very apprehensive require heavy premedication and rapid induction of anesthesia. They do poorly with regional techniques or those which provide a slow induction of general anesthesia.

REQUIREMENTS OF THE SURGEON. Important considerations that help dictate the choice of anesthetic agents and techniques include intended use of electrocautery, the need for muscle relaxation in an abdominal operation, the duration of the operation and the position of the patient during the operation.

REQUIREMENTS OF THE RECOVERY PERIOD. The postanesthetic disposition of the patient may influence the choice of anesthesia. Rapid recovery of consciousness is important in outpatients or in those who do not receive recovery room care. If postoperative straining must be especially avoided, as in removal of cataract, agents associated with a high incidence of vomiting, such as ether or cyclopropane, are contraindicated.

THE EXPERIENCE OF THE ANESTHETIST. At times this may be a most important consideration. Physician specialists should be familiar with all agents and techniques, but even the busiest may not have enough personal experience to be expert with all. Nurse anesthetists have a more limited spectrum of experience which wholly excludes regional techniques.

These judgments are best made by the anesthesiologist, not by the internist or the surgeon. Few internists or surgeons have made a study of anesthesia and its problems. Few have knowledge of the detailed pharmacology of anesthetic agents. Lacking such experience and training, they are not equipped to make a choice of anesthetics in the presence of a more qualified person, the anesthesiologist. As in other branches of medicine, the final decision should follow consideration and discussion and should not be accomplished by mandate.

ADMINISTRATION OF THE ANESTHETIC

An anesthetic begins with the administration of the premedication. After this has been given, the patient should be confined to bed. Ideally, after all has been prepared, the patient should be moved directly to the room where his operation will be performed, although modern operating suites have a holding area in which patients wait their turn for operation. These areas should be quiet, or have soft music. They should be apart from the sights and sounds of an operating room and an attendant should be assigned to observe the occupants.

The patient should be moved from the transportation cart to the operating table with assistance because of the effects of the premedication. The table should be slightly flexed for the patient's comfort. At this point, the need for fluids is considered. When there is a possibility that a large blood loss may occur, it may be wise to provide several intravenous routes. A large reserve supply of blood serves little purpose if it cannot be given quickly when it is needed. For minor procedures in healthy patients, an indwelling needle or scalp vein needle should suffice. There is a growing tendency to use intravenous catheters or short plastic cannulae for all operations. The technical difficulties of insertion and the high incidence of thrombophlebitis postoperatively should limit their use to major operations when fluids or blood must be given for several days postoperatively.

MONITORING EQUIPMENT. Equipment to monitor many vital functions is now available. Periodic determinations of arterial blood pressure and heart rate are traditional. However, the practice of counting respiratory rate during anesthesia has lost its significance because of the employment of muscle relaxants as well as the use of assisted or controlled respiration. Little refuge can be taken in counting the rate of respiration, either spontaneous, assisted or controlled, because it signifies so little in reference to pulmonary ventilation. Several ventilation meters are available but these are expensive, often inaccurate and may give false security because, as commonly used, they measure gas flows within the anesthetic system and not into or out of the patient's lungs. Improvement is needed in monitoring equipment in this area. Breath and heart sounds are often monitored continuously, either by affixing a stethoscope to the chest wall, or by the use of an esophageal stethoscope. Auscultatory monitoring is especially common in pediatric patients.

Monitors are available for the electrocardiogram, end-expired oxygen and carbon dioxide tensions, the venous pressure and the muscular response to nerve stimulation. Although the electroencephalogram is seldom used today to assess depth of anesthetic, it is useful to detect cerebral hypoxia in specific circumstances, such as during extracorporeal circulation or operations upon the carotid artery. Monitors for carbon dioxide and oxygen tensions of respired gases are still chiefly research techniques. Those for nerve-muscle stimulation are not in wide clinical use, although they are gaining in popularity for diagnosing the cause of persistent neuromuscular blockade. Central venous pressure is frequently monitored in those operations in which blood loss may be excessive or hypovolemia is feared. The interpretation of the data requires careful standardization as well as an understanding of circulatory physiology. The electrocardiogram is most frequently monitored and a surfeit of equipment is available for this purpose. If, however, the anes-

thetist's attention becomes centered on this type of device to the exclusion of an overall observation, the patient's condition may be jeopardized.

PREPARATION FOR THE ANESTHETIC. There is no substitute for prior planning in conducting an anesthetic. The anesthesia machine must be checked to see that it functions properly and is adequately supplied with gases, volatile agents and drugs. This is true whether a general or regional technique is to be employed. Equipment must be available for supporting the patient's ventilation and for intubating the trachea. Fluids and drugs should be readily accessible for the support of the cardiovascular system and treatment of unexpected cardiac arrhythmias and arrest.

If a regional technique has been chosen, it should be performed in advance of the projected operating time to allow establishment of sensory anesthesia. If the patient is to remain awake during the operation, personnel should be instructed to speak quietly. Some patients may require heavy sedation or light general anesthesia for supplementation of regional blocks and preparation must be made for this. When local anesthetic agents are injected or applied topically, treatment of toxic reactions should be anticipated. When spinal anesthesia is chosen, hypotension or a total spinal paralysis may result. Preparation for treatment should be made before the intrathecal injection. Only in this way will these complications be readily and successfully treated.

When general anesthesia has been chosen, additional preparations are indicated. A functioning suction apparatus must be at hand to clear airway secretions and vomitus. Induction of anesthesia produces relaxation of the jaw and soft tissues and results in airway obstruction. Anesthesia must not be induced unless an adequate airway can be guaranteed. In most situations, extension of the head upon the neck, elevation of the jaw or insertion of an oropharyngeal airway suffices to maintain airway patency. For most upper abdominal operations and all intracranial and intrathoracic procedures, endotracheal anesthesia and control of ventilation are indicated. In rare instances, the surgeon may be required to perform a tracheostomy under local anesthesia before general anesthesia is induced.

TRACHEAL INTUBATION. There are advantages to the intubation of the trachea. The airway is likely to remain patent. The respiratory dead space is reduced and the removal of secretions is facilitated. Control of respiration is made easier and the danger of inflation of the stomach from pressure applied to a face mask is removed. By the use of cuffed tracheal tubes, the danger of aspirating gastric contents is minimized. The patient can be placed in any position and the anesthetist can be situated away from the patient's face and yet retain control of ventilation. There are also disadvantages and these must always be weighed against the advantages. The trachea in some patients is difficult or impossible to intubate under any circumstances. A variety of technical difficulties can lead to trauma from the laryngoscope to the lips, teeth, gums and oral or pharyngeal structures. The use of a tube of improper size may lead to increased resistance to respiration if too small, and laryngeal or tracheal damage if too large. The use of long tubes may result in bronchial intubation and contralateral pulmonary collapse. Contaminated equipment or mechanical trauma to the larynx may precipitate laryngeal edema in children. This is a valuable technique but it should not be taken lightly and not used if not needed.

MAINTENANCE. The anesthesiologist should observe the patient constantly throughout the anesthesia and operation, making frequent assessment of the vital signs and paying attention to the progress of the operation. He should stand to observe the surgical field or sit so that he can see over the screen. Among the things he should watch are the color of the blood, the degree of muscle relaxation and the stage of the surgical procedure. An anesthetist unable or unwilling to watch the surgical field can be compared with an individual driving a car in a fog and being unable to see the road clearly. Legible, accurate and up-to-the-minute records should be kept during the anesthesia and operation. The medical reasons for this do not require amplification but the medicolegal reasons have assumed increasing importance in recent years. Most malpractice suits involving anesthesiologists are notable for the poor records kept by the defendant.

TERMINATION OF THE OPERATION. By the end of the operation, the patient should be breathing spontaneously with a good respiratory exchange. He should have regained normal muscle tone as well as his protective airway reflexes. Little is gained, however, by having him wide awake before being moved from the operating table, particularly if the operation was a major one. Under these circumstances, the patient would as soon be oblivious to his surroundings for a few hours. The anesthetist must use good judgment in this matter. Transfer from the operating table to bed or litter must be made with care and at least four people should participate. The blood pressure should be checked immediately after the move because hypotension is common at this moment. Having satisfied himself that the blood pressure and respiration are satisfactory, the anesthesiologist may move the patient to the recovery room but should not leave until he has rechecked the vital signs and assigned supervision to another competent person.

THE RECOVERY ROOM

The purpose of the recovery room is to provide close observation and patient care during a period when normal protective mechanisms may be obtunded and the sensorium clouded. The unit should be immediately adjacent to the operating rooms. Because the patients in this unit are usually under the influence of an anesthetic, it is logical for the anesthesiologist to continue his supervision. Because of the interaction of anesthetic agents with other drugs, therapy should not be administered in the recovery room without his express approval. He knows better than others what the patient has had in the way of depressants. He knows, for instance, that because of general anesthesia, narcotic analgesics must be injected in sharply reduced doses to avoid respiratory and circulatory catastrophe.

The heart of the recovery room is its professional staff. An anesthesiologist must always be available. Nursing personnel should be permanently assigned and specially trained for their work. Private duty nurses have no place either in a recovery room or in an intensive care unit. A supervisor, responsible to the chief of anesthesia, should be in charge during all hours the unit is open. A suggested ratio of one nurse to three patients with a minimum of two nurses always available in the unit is appropriate.

Maximum observation of unconscious patients is the primary consideration of a recovery room. It is essential that the room be well-lighted and of open construction to allow for constant surveillance of the patients.

Each bed area should be provided with wall oxygen and suction, adequate electrical outlets, supports for intravenous solutions and a supply of disposable suction and oxygen catheters, syringes, needles and the like. In addition, emergency equipment must be available to provide for intubation of the trachea, treatment of cardiac arrest, cardiac defibrillation, mechanical ventilation, thoracentesis and electrocardiographic monitoring. A supply of intravenous fluids, plasma expanders and resuscitative and supportive drugs must be at hand. Ideally, type O, Rh negative blood should be stored in a refrigerator and replaced if unused each week. Patients should not be discharged from the unit until an anesthesiologist has signed their release.

POSTOPERATIVE COMPLICATIONS

Those complications which are most likely to occur during the immediate postanesthetic period fall into two groups, respiratory and circulatory.

RESPIRATORY COMPLICATIONS

ASPIRATION. Vomiting may occur in any patient awakening from anesthesia, particularly in the patient whose abdomen has been opened. The inhalation of gastric contents into the tracheobronchial tract may be disastrous. Aspiration of large volumes, as may follow gastric dilation, can result in death from drowning; smaller volumes induce laryngospasm or bronchospasm and produce acute hypoxia. Aspiration of acid liquid gastric contents leads to chemical pneumonitis, whereas particulate matter may cause atelectasis, pneumonia or lung abscess. Prophylaxis is best achieved by placing the patient in the lateral recumbent position with a pillow against the abdomen to prevent his rolling face downward. If regurgitation occurs, the head should be kept low and the mouth and pharynx cleared by suction. Once an airway has been obtained, ventilation and oxygenation are afforded if necessary. If aspiration has occurred, treatment should consist of suctioning the trachea, washing it with 10-ml. volumes of saline followed immediately by suctioning and administering hydrocortisone, 100 mg. three times a day for three days.

AIRWAY OBSTRUCTION. This can sometimes be anticipated before leaving the operating room and transportation delayed, an endotracheal tube left in place, or rarely a tracheostomy performed. Such patients require close supervision and should never be left in the care of the less experienced until the concern has subsided. The most common site of airway obstruction in the postanesthetic period is the upper airway. This is most easily treated by inserting an oropharyngeal airway if tolerated or by hyperextension of the head on the neck with elevation of the jaw. It may be necessary to free the airway of secretions by frequent use of a suction device. If a patent airway cannot be maintained by these simple procedures, an endotracheal tube can be reinserted. Airway obstruction may not be recognized in the obtunded patient and may lead to inadequate ventilation.

HYPOVENTILATION. This may occur because of the action of anesthetics, narcotic analgesics and muscle relaxants, along with or superimposed on underlying medical disease. Abdominal or thoracic incisions markedly reduce maximum breathing capacity and many patients develop some degree of hypoxia and hypercapnia after these procedures. Treatment of respiratory insufficiency, regardless of cause, requires two simple steps: establishment of a clear airway and maintenance of adequate pulmonary ventilation. The latter can be accomplished by mouth-to-mouth ventilation, use of a self-inflation bag and mask, manual compression of a breathing bag or ventilation with a mechanical respirator. All recovery room personnel should be trained in the use of each of these methods. Even a brief period of hypoventilation can induce hypoxia sufficient to precipitate cardiac arrest. The administration of oxygen by a disposable face mask has much to recommend it during the early postanesthetic period.

CIRCULATORY COMPLICATIONS

These occur because of the effects of anesthesia, operation or antecedent respiratory insufficiency. All patients in the recovery room should have blood pressure, pulse and respiratory rate recorded at least every five minutes. At the same time, the patient should be evaluated for respiratory adequacy, changes in level of consciousness and skin color. Moderate elevation or depression of blood pressure and pulse sometimes occurs because of awakening and perception of pain. Marked changes in blood pressure or pulse are not to be expected. Blood pressures below 90 mm. Hg and above 180 mm. Hg systolic in previously normotensive patients are to be viewed with concern. Pulse rates below 60 per minute or above 110 are likewise unusual in the recovery period. A persistent brady-cardia from continuing action of drugs used during anesthesia may reduce cardiac out-put and cause hypotension. Atropine is some-times helpful in this situation. Tachycardia may result from pain, apprehension, hypo-ventilation or hypovolemia. If the tachycardia is caused by hypoxia, administration of oxy-gen by mask decreases the heart rate promptly by at least 20 beats per minute. If caused by hypercarbia, assisted ventilation is required.

Hypotension with or without tachycardia may indicate hypovolemia which must be appropri-ately treated. The use of Trendelenburg's posi-tion, which has been traditional in the treat-ment of hypovolemia, is no longer accepted because of associated diaphragmatic eleva-tion and decreased vital capacity. Elevation of the legs mobilizes blood from the periphery but the body should remain horizontal. Oc-casionally, a severe hypertension may require small doses of short-acting ganglionic block-ing agents for adequate control. This must al-ways be combined with respiratory support.

CARDIAC ARREST. This is the most demand-ing complication that can occur in a hospital. Immediate recognition is the most important

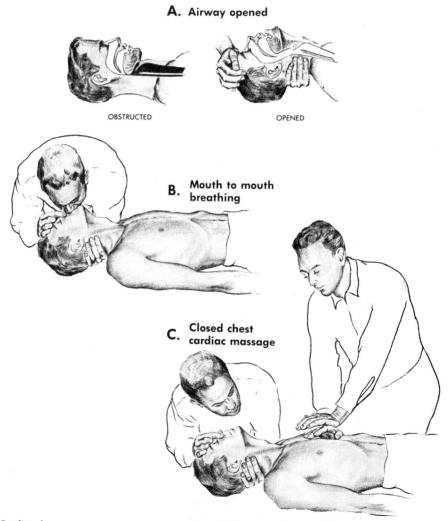

A. Airway opened

OBSTRUCTED OPENED

B. Mouth to mouth breathing

C. Closed chest cardiac massage

Figure 7. Cardiopulmonary resuscitation—the essentials. *A*, The airway is opened by cleaning the pharynx of foreign material and hyperextending the head. *B*, Breathing is instituted by the mouth-to-mouth method at a rate of about 15 per minute. *C*, Circulation is restored by application of firm downward pressure sufficient to move the sternum 3 to 4 cm. toward the spine 60 times per minute. Breathing and cardiac compression are often coordinated at a 1:4 ratio. Definitive therapy is established after the adequacy of the first three steps is determined. (From National Academy of Sciences—National Research Council.)

factor if recovery is to be expected. The term "cardiac arrest" as commonly used describes any situation in which the circulation is inadequate to perfuse the myocardium and brain. It includes severe hypotension with apparent but not definitely diagnosed arrest, cardiac standstill and ventricular fibrillation. It may be accompanied by pallor or grayish cyanosis of the skin, absence of palpable pulses over the carotid or femoral arteries, respiratory arrest and rapidly dilating pupils. Cardiopulmonary resuscitation involves, in order, opening of the airway; restoration of breathing; restoration of circulation, and establishment of definitive therapy. Therapy should be instituted as quickly as possible (Fig. 7).

The patient should be placed on a firm surface such as the floor or on a bed board. If two operators are available, one should be responsible for ventilation, hyperextending the head on the neck, clearing the mouth and pharynx of foreign material, elevating the jaw and applying either mouth-to-mouth or mouth-to-nose ventilation. By placing one hand behind the neck and the other on the forehead, maximum backward tilt of the head can be maintained. Adequacy of ventilation can be assessed by visually evaluating movement of the chest, feeling resistance of the lungs to inflation and estimating passive exhalation. Inadequate chest movement indicates airway obstruction which may be overcome by improving the position of the head. Ventilation should be maintained in this manner at the rate of about 15 per minute, alternating one breath with four to five cardiac impulses until proper equipment becomes available, at which time the trachea may be intubated and respiration continued with oxygen. If only one operator is available, each inflation of the lungs should be followed by five or six cardiac impulses.

The second operator should be responsible for external cardiac compression. The heel of one hand should be placed at the xiphisternal junction with the fingers pointed cephalad, the second hand placed on top of the first, and the sternum depressed sharply at a rate of 60 to 70 per minute. Adequacy of circulation should be checked by a third person by palpation of a femoral pulse. External cardiac compression must always be accompanied by artificial ventilation; chest compression is not adequate to ventilate the lungs simultaneously,

Once ventilation and circulation have been restored, intravenous solutions should be started, sodium bicarbonate injected and cardiac monitoring established. Once a diagnosis has been established, decisions for the use of vasopressors, antiarrhythmics, cardiac stimulants or electrical defibrillation can be made.

SPECIAL ANESTHETIC TECHNIQUES

There are some diseases which can be treated surgically but for which the usual methods of anesthesia are inadequate. In such situations, special techniques such as induced hypothermia, deliberate hypotension, or cardiopulmonary bypass may allow the performance of operations which otherwise would be associated with undue risk or might be impossible to perform.

Induced hypothermia involves a deliberate reduction of body temperature. It is used to lower the rate of body metabolism and reduce the danger of hypoxic cellular damage which might result from temporary interruption of circulation to major organs. The metabolic processes of the body involve chemical reactions and as such are governed by physical laws. The rate at which chemical reactions proceed is directly related to the temperature at which they occur. The utilization of oxygen by tissues is also a chemical reaction and by lowering body temperature, the rate of oxygen uptake and the need for its delivery to the tissues is diminished. Hyperpyrexia is associated with increased oxygen utilization and the same methods used to produce hypothermia return elevated body temperatures to normal and reduce tissue oxygen demands.

There are three methods of producing hypothermia: surface cooling, internal or body cavity cooling and extracorporeal cooling. Surface cooling is most commonly employed for those operations in which extracorporeal circuits are not indicated. It is accomplished by immersion in iced water or by use of refrigerated blankets. The rapid evaporation of highly volatile agents such as rubbing alcohol from the surface of the body also has been employed to induce mild hypothermia. The fastest surface method is the immersion technique, although refrigerated blankets are more widely used. The patient must be anesthetized, the trachea intubated, and anesthetic agents or adjuvants used to produce peripheral vasodilation and to prevent shivering. The time required to reduce body temperature from 37° to 28° C. is largely dependent upon size and body structure of the patient, but varies between one and three hours. Surface cooling is associated with a continuing reduction of body temperature of 1 to 3° C. after active cooling has been discontinued.

Internal or body cavity cooling is little used for total body hypothermia, but has been used for localized hypothermia of the stomach and bladder. It carries with it the risk of inducing generalized body hypothermia. Extracorporeal methods pass blood through a heat exchanger whose temperature is regulated by circulating hot or cold water and are frequently used in conjunction with open heart operations. Cooling of the body core is more rapid than is possible with surface cooling. Because of the temperature differentials created in various tissues, metabolic acidosis often occurs. Hypothermia below 28° C. is associated with risk of ventricular fibrillation. When using a heat exchanger with cardiopulmonary by-pass, this is relatively unimportant and the body temperature is often reduced to 10 to 15° C. Provision for surface rewarming is made no matter what method is employed. This must be undertaken with care because the skin of the hypothermic patient is sensitive to burning. The temperatures of the rewarming surfaces should not exceed 40° C. A posthypothermic overshoot of body temperature is common and may require control by the use of antipyretics or mild surface cooling. Cardiopulmonary by-pass is normally used for open heart procedures or in other operations in which circulatory arrest for periods longer than five minutes is anticipated.

Deliberate hypotension involves the reduction of arterial pressure to reduce operative blood loss, shorten operating time, allow for more accurate tissue dissection and minimize the local effects of surgical manipulation. The physiology associated with deliberate hypotension differs markedly from that of shock. With the former, blood volume is normal, peripheral vascular beds are dilated, cardiac work is decreased and blood pH is relatively normal. In shock, blood volume is reduced, vascular beds in the main are constricted, cardiac work is increased because of elevated peripheral resistance and increased blood levels of catecholamines and metabolic acidosis are present. Moreover, deliberate hypotension is used in anesthetized patients in whom cerebral metabolism is likely to be reduced and in whom pulmonary ventilation is controlled with high inspired oxygen content. The opposite situation is likely to obtain in shock.

Hypotension may be induced by the use of high spinal anesthesia, deep general anesthesia or a combination of anesthesia and ganglioplegics. The first method is too uncontrollable, the second is likely to be associated with a major degree of cardiac depression and the third produces a situation akin to shock. The more common technique involves use of a general anesthetic agent, usually halothane, which produces vasodilation, a ganglionic blocking agent to block peripheral sympathetic pathways and interfere with normal vasomotor tone, usually trimethaphan or pentolinium, the utilization of body position to allow blood to pool in dependent dilated vascular beds and, if needed, positive airway pressure to reduce venous return and lower cardiac output. Various combinations of those four factors can be employed to control the level of blood pressure. Studies in normal man have shown that vascular beds of both the myocardium and the brain can compensate for systolic pressures of 40 to 60 mm. Hg in the head-up tilt position. The blood pressure should be lowered only to that point at which bleeding ceases to be a problem in the operative field. In some patients, this is obtained at levels between 80 and 90 mm. Hg systolic, whereas in the young and healthy, systolic pressures below 60 mm. Hg usually are required. It is incumbent upon the anesthetist using this technique to assure accurate minute-to-minute determinations of blood pressure. An oscillometric technique has proved most reliable for this purpose. Pulmonary ventilation and oxygenation must be well maintained at all times. It is also necessary that the surgeon obtain meticulous hemostasis. Failure to accomplish this during hypotension may lead to postoperative bleeding when blood pressure returns to normotensive levels. This technique has had its most promising application in radical operations about the upper chest, neck and head.

SURGEON-ANESTHETIST RELATIONSHIPS

Surgeons and anesthetists form a team of physicians striving for the welfare of the patient. The discipline of each is different but the common meeting ground is the patient. Each member of the team must recognize his own responsibilities and yet be aware of the difficulties faced by the other. The anesthetist must be aware of the patient's medical history, the proposed surgical procedure and the risk involved from both the surgical and anesthetic points of view. He should confer with the surgeons, the internist or other consultants about vague aspects of the patient's disease. He must keep the surgeon informed of the patient's condition during the operation by transmission of important details, and continue the care of the patient during the immediate postoperative period when the attention of the surgeon may be elsewhere.

The surgeon should inform the anesthetist of any unusual aspect of the patient's disease or of the surgical procedure. He should not insist upon one anesthetic agent or technique, although he should convey the patient's wishes. He should not promise the patient one anesthetic or another but leave this to the discretion of the anesthesiologist. Rapid induction, prompt awakening or profound relaxation should not be demanded or expected with every procedure. It should be understood that anesthetists as well as surgeons sometimes have difficulties and complications.

At one time, the surgeon was medicolegally responsible for all that took place in the operating room. Today, each member of the surgical team being specifically trained for his task is likely to be responsible for his own acts, although the tendency is to name all physicians involved with a patient's care in case of suit. The surgeon should not assume that the ultimate responsibility for the anesthetic rests on his shoulders. This may be true if the anesthetic were administered by a technician but is unlikely if given by a physician.

The best relationships between anesthesiologists and surgeons are based upon and promoted by mutual professional confidence, respect and an awareness of each other's problems.

THE ANESTHESIOLOGIST OUTSIDE THE OPERATING ROOM

Daily experience in managing anesthetized individuals under a variety of stressful situations has made the anesthesiologist a specialist in the care of critically ill and comatose patients. Skill in supporting normal pulmonary and circulatory function, in managing fluid therapy and in using vasopressors, narcotics, local anesthetics, antiarrhythmics

and other drugs is equally applicable to the nonanesthetized. This has led to the current participation of the anesthetist in surgical, cardiac and respiratory intensive care units and in inhalation therapy. This interest is not confined to the postsurgical patient. It extends to the care of any critically ill patient, including those with strokes, shock, head injuries, drug intoxication, crushed chest, chronic cardiac or pulmonary failure and certain advanced neurologic diseases. The anesthesiologist is also active in the resuscitation field and in many hospitals he directs the cardiopulmonary resuscitation team.

The anesthesiologist has also made significant contributions in the management of patients with acute or chronic pain. Proficiency in the application of spinal, epidural and caudal anesthesia, regional nerve blocks, local anesthetics and narcotic analgesics is useful in both diagnosis and treatment of pain. Work in this field may be useful in helping to establish a diagnosis to permit a more definitive surgical operation or to provide optimal conditions while a patient recovers from an operation such as continued sympathetic blockade after embolectomy or arterial graft. Therapy must also be directed toward the relief of acute pain, chronic pain or intractable pain of terminal cancer. In some institutions, pain clinics have been established and are jointly managed by anesthesiologists, surgeons, neurosurgeons, neurologists and psychiatrists. The current daily activities of the staff of an anesthesia department range beyond the confines of the operating room.

READING REFERENCES

Adriani, J., and Campbell, D.: Fatalities following the topical application of local anesthetics to mucous membranes. J.A.M.A. *162*:1527, 1956.

Adriani, J., Zepernick, R., Arens, J., and Authement, G.: The comparative potency and effectiveness of topical anesthetics in man. Clin. Pharmacol. & Ther. 5:49, 1964.

Bowsher, D.: The reticular formation and ascending reticular system. Brit. J. Anaesth. 33:174, 1961.

Brain, W. R.: Perception: trialogue. Brain 88:697, 1965.

Brazier, M. A.: Some effects of anaesthesia on the brain. Brit. J. Anaesth. 33:194, 1961.

Campbell, D., and Adriani, J.: Absorption of local anesthetics. J.A.M.A. *168*:873, 1958.

Committee on Anesthesia, National Academy of Sciences, National Research Council: Summary of the national halothane study. J.A.M.A. *197*:775, 1966.

Committee on Cardiopulmonary Resuscitation of Division of Medical Sciences, National Academy of Sciences–National Research Council: Cardiopulmonary resuscitation. J.A.M.A. *198*:372, 1966.

Committee on Pre- and Postoperative Care of the American College of Surgeons: Manual of Preoperative and

Postoperative Care. Philadelphia, W. B. Saunders Company, 1967.

Cotev, S., and Robin, G. C.: Experimental studies in intravenous regional anesthesia using radioactive lignocaine. Brit. J. Anaesth. 38:936, 1966.

Crul, J. F., Long, G. J., Brunner, E. A., and Coolen, J. M.: The changing pattern of neuromuscular blockade caused by succinylcholine in man. Anesthesiology 27: 729, 1966.

Dripps, R. D.: Signs and stages of anesthesia. *In*, Goodman, L. S., and Gilman, A. (eds.): The Pharmacological Basis of Therapeutics. 3rd ed. New York, The Macmillan Company, 1965.

Dripps, R. D., Eckenhoff, J. E., and Vandam, L. D.: Introduction to Anesthesia. 3rd ed. Philadelphia, W. B. Saunders Company, 1967.

Dripps, R. D., Lamont, A., and Eckenhoff, J. E.: The role of anesthesia in surgical mortality. J.A.M.A. *178*:261, 1961.

Dripps, R. D., and Vandam, L. D.: Long term follow-up of patients who received 10,098 spinal anesthetics. I. Failure to discover major neurological sequelae. J.A.M.A. *156*:1486, 1954.

Dripps, R. D., and Vandam, L. D.: Long term follow-up of patients who received 10,098 spinal anesthetics. II. Incidence and analysis of minor sensory neurological defects. Surgery *38*:463, 1955.

Eckenhoff, J. E.: Circulatory control in the surgical patient. Ann. Royal Coll. Surg. *39*:67, 1966.

Eckenhoff, J. E.: The care of the unconscious patient. J.A.M.A. *186*:541, 1963.

Eckenhoff, J. E., and Helrich, M.: A study of narcotics and sedatives for use in preanesthetic medications. J.A.M.A. *167*:415, 1958.

Editorial: Higher oxides of nitrogen as an impurity in nitrous oxide. Brit. J. Anaesth. *39*:343, 1967.

Egbert, L. D., Battil, G. E., Turndorf, H., and Beecher, H. K.: The value of the preoperative visit by the anesthetist. J.A.M.A. *185*:553, 1963.

Egbert, L. D., Battil, G. E., Welch, C. E., and Bartlett, M. K.: Reduction of postoperative pain by encouragement and instruction of patients: study of doctor-patient rapport. New England J. Med. *270*:825, 1964.

Goodman, L. S., and Gilman, A. (eds.): The Pharmacologic Basis of Therapeutics. 3rd ed. New York, The Macmillan Company, 1965.

Hamilton, W. K.: Nomenclature of inhalation anesthetic systems. Anesthesiology *25*:3, 1964.

Harris, L. C., Kirimli, B., and Safar, P.: Ventilation-cardiac compression rates and ratios in cardiopulmonary resuscitation. Anesthesiology *28*:806, 1967.

Larabee, M. G., and Posternak, J. M.: Selective action of anesthetics on synapses and axons in mammalian sympathetic ganglia. J. Neurophysiol. *15*:91, 1952.

Linssen, A.: Curariform Drugs. Nijmegan, The Netherlands, Thoben, 1961.

Magoun, H. W.: Brain mechanisms for wakefulness. Brit. J. Anaesth. *33*:183, 1961.

Mark, L. C., and Papper, E. M.: Advances in Anesthesiology: Muscle Relaxants. New York, Hoeber Medical Division, Harper and Row Publishers, 1967.

Moore, D. C., and Bridenbaugh, D.: Oxygen: the antidote for systemic toxic reaction from local anesthetic drugs. J.A.M.A. *174*:842, 1960.

Norris, W. and Campbell, D.: Anaesthetics, Resuscitation and Intensive Care. Baltimore, Williams & Wilkins Company, 1965.

Rosenbaum, H. E., Long, F. B., Hinchey, T. R., and Trufant, S. A.: Paralysis with saddle-block anesthesia in obstetrics. Arch. Neurol. & Psychiat. *68*:783, 1953.

Thesleff, S.: Effects of acetylcholine, decamethonium, and succinylcholine on neuromuscular transmission in the rat. Acta Physiol. Scand. *34*:386, 1955.

Woodbridge, P. D.: Changing concepts concerning depth of anesthesia. Anesthesiology *18*:536, 1957.

Wylie, W. D., and Churchill-Davidson, H. C.: A Practice of Anaesthesia. 2nd ed. Chicago, Year Book Medical Publishers, 1966.

Chapter 13

THE DISEASES AND INJURIES OF THE SCALP AND SKULL

by
E. S. GURDJIAN, M.D.
and
L. M. THOMAS, M.D.

ELISHA STEPHENS GURDJIAN was born in Smyrna, Asia Minor, now Turkey, and received his Doctor of Philosophy degree and medical education at the University of Michigan. He has combined experimental and clinical investigation upon the forces of stress and strain produced in craniocerebral injuries in such a successful way that he has added considerable knowledge to the understanding of the many factors involved in these injuries. His concentration on these problems has shed light upon a hackneyed, categorized subject in surgery. Dr. Gurdjian is Professor and Chairman of the Department of Neurosurgery, College of Medicine, Wayne University, Detroit.

LLYWELLYN MURRAY THOMAS is a native of Detroit and received all of his education there, graduating from Wayne State University College of Medicine. He is Associate Professor of Neurosurgery at his alma mater.

In the United States over 100,000 deaths may be directly attributed to head injury each year. More than 2,500,000 people have injuries to the head which necessitate some form of medical attention. The head may be injured by a variety of forces, the most common of which result from low velocity impacts such as falls and car accidents. Many accidents producing injury to the head occur in and about the home as the result of falls down steps, from ladders or porches. The energies acting upon the head result in deformation, linear acceleration and angular acceleration. These forces result in combinations of compressive, tensile and shear stresses which fluctuate rapidly in magnitude, time and location during the few milliseconds in which they act. The linear and angular acceleration components, together with deformation of the skull, produce intracranial pressure gradients and relative movements of the brain in relation to its bony covering. It is through these mechanisms that external forces damage the brain in the common case of closed head injury.

THE SCALP

Increasing mechanization in industry and the ever-growing number of automobile accidents have resulted in an increased incidence of scalp trauma. In addition to trauma, the scalp may be the site of tumors and infections. Infections may result in osteomyelitis of the skull, meningitis or brain abscess. Certain tumors and cysts have a predilection for scalp. Hematomas of the scalp occur frequently.

ANATOMIC CONSIDERATIONS. The scalp is a 5-mm. thick structure consisting of five layers. The outer three layers are closely connected and move as a unit.

The skin of the scalp is thick. Connecting the skin and galea aponeurotica is a layer of close subcutaneous tissue. This subcutaneous tissue may be divided into a superficial, fatty, avascular layer and a deep, membranous, vascular portion which contains the larger vessels and nerves. Many fibrous septa traverse the subcutaneous tissue and restrict the elasticity of this layer. As a result, the scalp gapes when cut and the blood vessels do not retract, which causes profuse bleeding.

The third layer consists of the epicranial aponeurosis or galea aponeurotica and the occipitofrontalis muscle. It is attached to the external occipital protuberance, the higher nuchal line and the zygomatic arch. It is sensitive to pain.

Loose subaponeurotic connective tissue comprises the fourth layer and contains the emissary veins. This loose subaponeurotic space is responsible for the mobility of the scalp. Collections of blood and pus may spread throughout this space, and infection may spread through the emissary veins to the intracranial structures.

Pericranium, the external periosteum of the skull, is the fifth layer. It is relatively insensitive to pain. It has poor osteogenic properties, and bone regeneration seldom occurs if a segment of bone is not replaced. The pericranium is fixed to the connective tissue between the bones of the skull, and later to the sutures after the fontanelles have been obliterated. This mechanically restricts subpericranial effusion to one bone of the calvarium.

The nerves and blood vessels of the scalp enter from below and ascend in the second or close connective tissue layer. The arterial blood supply is abundant and has many anastomoses. The major supply is from branches of the external carotid, although the supratrochlear and supraorbital arteries are branches of the internal carotid. The nerves parallel the arteries.

SCALP WOUNDS. Scalp wounds vary widely in type, but usually are related to the physical properties of the injuring object. Every scalp wound may be a penetrating wound, causing injury to the skull and brain. Even the most innocent-appearing wound may be related to intracranial damage, and if not properly treated may serve as an avenue of infection to deeper tissues.

Careful cleansing and debridement are essential in the repair of any scalp wound. This must include careful shaving of the hair in a wide area around the wound. Hemorrhage is controlled best by pressure and hemostats on the galea. Suture should be performed in two layers, the innermost closing the aponeurosis and close connective tissue, and the outer layer closing the skin. If the laceration involves underlying muscle such as the temporalis, two additional layers

of sutures in the muscle and muscle fascia should be used.

A portion of the scalp may be avulsed or sheared off completely. This portion should be carefully cleansed, replaced and sutured. Many such portions of avulsed scalp may remain vital, even when used as a free graft in this manner.

Usually, a scalp wound which is associated with more serious underlying damage, such as depressed fracture, is repaired at the time of fracture debridement. Occasionally, however, it may be expedient to clean and close the scalp overlying a compound wound for control of hemorrhage until the patient can be readied for more complete care in the operating room.

HEMATOMAS. Hematoma of the scalp results from an extravasation of blood in the subcutaneous tissue about a point of impact. The skin may become detached from the galea at this point, permitting an effusion or collection of blood surrounded by a zone of hemorrhagic infiltration in the intact subcutaneum. Such a hematoma has a soft, compressible center surrounded by a hard peripheral zone, and may mimic a depressed skull fracture. It should be remembered that depressed fractures rarely occur in adults in the absence of an open wound.

Hematoma in the subaponeurotic tissue may result from tear or rupture of the emissary vessels. Such a hematoma may extend from one temporal crest and zygoma to the other, and from the eyelids in front to the superior nuchal line behind. Fortunately, infection in this space is rare. When it occurs, pus may extend in all directions. It may destroy the pericranium and cause necrosis of the skull. Infections and infected thrombi may enter the dural sinuses through the emissary veins. Incision for drainage of such an abscess is made parallel to the large vessels, usually in the temporal area.

Cephalhematoma, or subpericranial hematoma, occurs in infants and is usually due to molding of the head during labor. Such hematoma is limited by the suture lines. It is usually unilateral, and is most common in the parietal region. Like most hematomas, it is rapidly absorbed and may completely disappear in two to three months. Occasionally, the hematoma may ossify entirely or in part.

EPITHELIAL CYSTS (WENS). Epithelial or sebaceous cysts result from occlusion of the duct of a sebaceous gland, causing accumulation of sebum. As the cyst enlarges, the secretory epithelium flattens. The contents consist of castoff epithelium, keratin and cholesterol crystals. Wens are slow-growing, raised and soft, and are in, or attached to, the dermis. They are more frequent on the scalp, face and back. Malignant degeneration has been reported, but it is rare.

Excision is performed, usually under local anesthesia, after careful sterile preparation of the skin, including adequate shaving. An elliptical incision including the area of cyst attachment to the skin is used. The entire cyst and wall are removed, preferably without rupture. Complete removal of the wall is necessary to avoid recurrence.

CIRSOID ANEURYSMS. Arteriovenous communications may be congenital in origin, or may occur as a result of rupture of an arterial aneurysm, trauma or infection. Occasionally, such an abnormal tortuous mass of vessels is referred to as a cirsoid aneurysm, or it may be related to intracranial vascular anomalies. At times, these varixlike masses may consist of dilated venous channels without associated arterial involvement, and may deserve excision. Prior to surgical intervention, study of the vascular supply should be carried out, including careful angiographic evaluation.

MALIGNANT TUMORS. Malignant new growths of the scalp are not common. The basal cell epithelioma is the most frequent. Included in this group are various tumors often classified as specific tumors of the skin appendages, such as sweat gland carcinoma and cylindroma. The basal cell epithelioma grows by direct extension and invasion, and is frequently most aggressive.

The truly malignant squamous cell carcinoma is next in frequency. These tend to grow rapidly and are subject to regional and distant metastases.

THE SKULL

The skull serves as a complicated bony protective container for the brain, and provides passageways for the special sense organs of sight, hearing, smell and taste. It is composed of a series of bones united for the most part by immovable joints. The cranial bones consist of an inner and outer table of compact bone separated by a spongy layer, the diploë. The word cranium commonly refers to the skull exclusive of the mandible; calvarium is used to designate the skull cap or vault, not including the facial bones.

TUMORS OF THE VAULT. *Metastatic carcinoma* of the skull is fairly frequent, although primary tumors are rare. Carcinoma of the breast is the most common source of metastatic disease involving the skull. It may frequently present as multiple, small, sharply punched-out osteolytic foci somewhat similar in appearance on roentgenograms to multiple myeloma. Occasionally, metastatic carcinoma may appear as a diffuse area of demineralization.

Osteoma, the most benign tumor of the skull, grows slowly and presents as a well circumscribed, moundlike swelling of bony hardness which is fixed and usually painless. These are usually first noted in childhood or early adult life. They most commonly occur in the frontal or temporoparietal bones and are rarely seen in the occipital bone. The x-ray appearance of osteoma is characteristic: a well circumscribed mass of dense new bone with a sharp line of demarcation and no evidence of bony structure.

Hyperostosis frontalis interna, an excessive deposition of bone on the internal table of the skull, usually in the frontal area, is most common in women of the fifth decade of life. It is usually asymptomatic, but may be associated with endocrine and metabolic disturbances.

Angioma of bone frequently involves the skull. It may remain stationary for years. Roentgen examination reveals a sharply delineated area of fine, mottled osteoporosis described as "foam rubber" in appearance. Projecting striations of bony spicules radiate from the tumor.

Fibrous dysplasia may affect many bones, but on occasion may be monostotic. This frequently occurs in the skull. Roentgenograms show areas of decreased density, although increased densities may be seen occasionally.

Multiple myeloma may involve the skull. Multiple, usually discrete, 1 to 2 cm., punched-out lesions may be identified by roentgenograms. Rarely, a myeloma may show a diffuse honeycombed area of decreased density similar to metastatic carcinoma (Fig. 1, *C*).

Dermoid and *epidermoid tumors* usually arise between the tables of the skull. In tangential roentgenograms, they appear as localized lozenge-shaped thickenings with gradual erosion of the inner and outer tables. A scalloped edge is said to be characteristic (Fig. 1, *B*).

Meningioma of the hyperostosing variety involves the skull. On occasion, skull x-ray

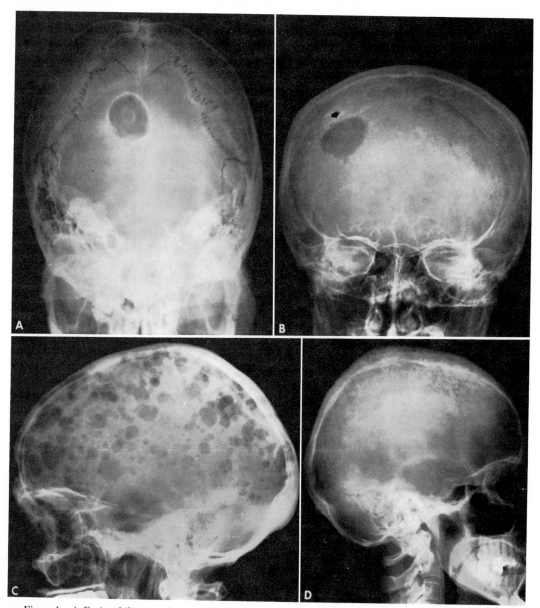

Figure 1.   *A*, Eosinophilic granuloma. *B*, Epidermoid. *C*, Multiple myeloma. *D*, Hyperostosing meningioma.

films may permit the diagnosis of this disease. Some surgeons believe that characteristic bony changes may be seen in 50 per cent of meningiomas, including increased vascularity of the bone, thinning of the bone, thickening of both tables of the skull, dense eburnation of the outer table and hyperostosis with vertical striations (Fig. 1, *D*).

Osteogenic sarcoma and *Ewing's sarcoma* occur primarily in the skull, but are quite rare. Ewing's sarcoma may metastasize to the skull from another primary area.

NONNEOPLASTIC DISEASE. *Osteitis deformans* (Paget's disease) is a disorder of the entire skeletal system, more commonly seen in the male than in the female. Histologically, this disease is characterized by the simultaneous formation and absorption of bone. This gives rise to the characteristic "cotton wool" appearance of the skull on roentgenograms. So-called "osteoporosis circumscripta" may be an early manifestation of Paget's disease of the skull. This is characterized by demineralization of bone bounded by a sharply defined line of slightly increased density. Sarcomatous changes may be superimposed upon Paget's disease.

Hand-Schüller-Christian disease, eosinophilic granuloma and *Letterer-Siwe disease* are granulomatous lesions involving the skull, resulting from proliferation of reticulo-endothelial cells which may become collagenized. Letterer-Siwe disease occurs in infancy and early childhood and is always fatal. Hand-Schüller-Christian disease is more chronic and may be seen in children or adults. It may take a benign course or may be more malignant. X-ray examination may reveal single or multiple rarefying lesions of varying size. The defects are irregular or serpiginous in configuration, with smooth margins. Eosinophilic granuloma is considered a relatively benign disease. It occurs mainly in young people and offers a good prognosis after surgery or irradiation. The bony lesion of the eosinophilic granuloma is usually a well circumscribed, rarefied lesion (Fig. 1, *A*).

Osteitis fibrosis cystica, or primary hyperparathyroidism, results in decalcification of bone with accompanying hypercalcemia and hypophosphatemia. Roentgen ray films of the skull may reveal diffuse granular osteoporosis, which is occasionally similar to the osteoporosis circumscripta of early Paget's disease.

Rickets, or vitamin D deficiency, results in defective calcification of osteoid tissue and abnormalities of the epiphysial cartilage. In the active stage, the skull may be demineralized, soft and easily indented. In the first year of life this results in so-called craniotabes.

CONGENITAL ABNORMALITIES. A skull abnormally long in relation to its breadth is usually referred to as dolichocephalic, while the converse state is described as brachycephalic. As the result of premature fusion of the cranial sutures, other deformities of skull shape, such as oxycephaly and scaphocephaly, may occur.

Platybasia, or basilar impression, may occur as a congenital anomaly or may be associated with rickets, osteomalacia or Paget's disease. There is an invagination of the base of the skull and a change in the basilar angle so that the odontoid process lies above a line from the tip of the hard palate to the posterior lip of the foramen magnum. Platybasia may be asymptomatic or may be associated with a varying neurologic defect resulting from abnormal pressures upon the brain stem, medulla and spinal cord. There may be associated hydrocephalus.

Cleidocranial dysostosis is a congenital disease consisting of dystrophic changes of the skeleton associated with an absence of part or all of the clavicles. The anterior fontanelle of the skull persists. The facial bones are small and there is maldevelopment of the teeth. There is frequently a basilar impression and wormian bones are present in the skull.

INFECTIONS. Osteomyelitis of the skull may result from introduction of infection through an open wound, or from extension from an infectious process in the sinus or mastoid regions. Osteomyelitis of the skull may occasionally be blood-borne. Roentgenograms show an area of diminished density with irregular or frayed margins. Relatively denser islands of bony tissue within the area represent sequestra of bone. Aseptic necrosis may produce the same appearance.

MECHANISM OF SKULL FRACTURE

The velocity of the injuring object and the force applied to the head govern the type of fracture which occurs in the skull. Within limits, the faster the blow, the greater the likelihood of depression or perforation. The slower the blow, providing the force is ade-

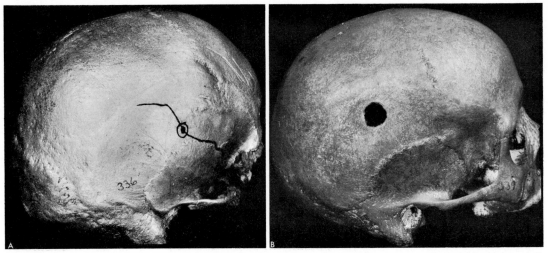

Figure 2.   Impact with a ¾-inch steel ball. *A*, Impact velocity 50 feet per second. *B*, Impact velocity 90 feet per second.

quate, the greater the likelihood of generalized skull deformation resulting in linear fracture. A simple experiment consists of having a steel pellet, ¾ inch in diameter, traveling at 50 feet per second, strike an exposed cadaver skull. A linear fracture is produced (Fig. 2, *A*). The same pellet traveling at 90 feet per second causes a perforation of the skull (Fig. 2, *B*).

With very high velocities, the missile may impart radial acceleration to the tissues it contacts. As a bullet or shell fragment traverses the skull, shattering may occur owing to the radial acceleration imparted to the pieces of bone.

LINEAR SKULL FRACTURE

About 70 per cent of skull fractures are single linear breaks. A low velocity impact causes an area of inbending around the point of the blow. Simultaneously, areas of outbending occur in the skull adjacent to the inbended portion. The tensile stress causes initiation of the fracture line. The fracture extends toward the point of impact and in the opposite direction toward the base of the skull. In order to cause linear fracture, it is necessary to expend 450 to 750 inch-pounds upon the head if the scalp and cranial contents are intact. A linear fracture is an index of the severity of the blow but it should be emphasized that in some skulls more energy may be expended without resulting in a fracture.

Simple linear fractures of the skull require

no specific treatment but should alert the examining physician to the severity of the blow received. Occasionally, such linear fractures may involve the petrous portion of the temporal bone with resultant cerebrospinal otorrhea and damage to the seventh and eighth nerves. Linear fractures similarly may involve the paranasal air sinuses and result in cerebrospinal rhinorrhea. If there is a laceration overlying the linear fracture, the fracture site should be meticulously inspected for contamination and the presence of foreign material. It may be necessary, in these circumstances, to debride the bony fracture line.

DEPRESSED SKULL FRACTURE

Depressed skull fractures usually result from moderate velocity impacts by blunt objects, although slow moving objects with a high kinetic energy may likewise cause depression. The management of a closed depressed skull fracture without complicating intracranial damage or hematoma is not a surgical emergency. Virtually all depressed fractures should be elevated. It is essential to remember that the area of inner table involvement will be much greater than that visualized in the outer table and greater than suggested by x-ray examination.

The management of an open depressed skull fracture requires early debridement and wound closure to prevent infection. It is well to follow the dictum that an open depressed skull fracture should be repaired as soon as the patient's general condition permits. Occasionally, such a fracture may be attended by severe generalized brain injury with marked swelling and contusion. Under these circumstances, it is advisable to delay operative intervention for 24 to 48 hours in an effort to avoid the complications resulting from progressive brain swelling at the time of operation.

Surgical debridement requires an adequate exposure, best obtained through the development of a skin flap. Occasionally, an S-shaped incision may permit adequate exposure. The presence of an open wound frequently dictates the most suitable incision. The bony fragments must be removed carefully, avoiding damage to the underlying dura and vascular sinuses. Frequently, a trephine opening in the normal bone adjacent to the fracture provides a starting point for bony removal or elevation. If the bony depression lies over one of the major dural vascular sinuses, special care is necessary. The depressed fragment of bone may have torn into the sinus, preventing bleeding by tamponade. If this fragment is pulled from the sinus, brisk hemorrhage develops. Adequate bony excision prior to removing the offending piece makes control of hemorrhage easier.

Injuries to the dura and brain beneath the depression must also be debrided. The dural defect should be carefully repaired. A graft of fascia taken from the temporal muscle or from the fascia lata of the thigh may be utilized if needed.

In a closed depressed skull fracture, the bony fragments may be saved and utilized as an autogenous cranioplasty. If the bony fragments do not seem suitable, a primary methyl methacrylate cranioplasty can be carried out. In open depressions, cranioplasty should be delayed for four to six months. Prophylactic antibiotics should be administered to all patients with open depressed skull fracture.

PERFORATING AND PENETRATING WOUNDS OF THE SKULL

Perforating and penetrating wounds of the skull usually result from high velocity missiles and are common in military neurosurgical practice and uncommon in civilian practice. The treatment of penetrating injuries includes early meticulous debridement with excision of devitalized and contaminated tissue and antibiotic therapy. One must be ready at any moment to revise a treatment plan should the patient's condition change for the worse. After initial treatment, such worsening occurs mainly from intracranial hemorrhage or infection.

INTRACRANIAL INJURIES

The brain may be damaged by direct injury as in the case of depressed or penetrating wounds of the skull. Shearing injuries may remove portions of the scalp, skull and underlying brain without producing unconsciousness. More frequently, however, brain damage results from the forces of acceleration and from the forces producing deformation of the skull. Linear acceleration and deformation of the skull institute a pressure gradient across the cranial cavity. The resulting flow toward foramen magnum develops shear stress in the area of the brain stem. The degree of injury is directly proportional to the time over which the forces last. Angular acceleration may result in mass movements of the brain in relation to its bony coverings, causing tears of the connecting vessels with resultant intracranial hemorrhage. Mass movements may also cause the brain to strike against the irregular bony contour of the frontal fossa or the anterior portion of the middle fossa, resulting in contusions and lacerations.

The management of closed head injury depends upon the injuring mechanisms and the presence or absence of intracranial hematoma. The interpretation of signs and symptoms must be cautious. Good surgical judgment requires an understanding of the underlying pathology and its effects upon cerebral physiology. It demands frequent observation of the patient along with the judicious use of adequate diagnostic studies.

X-ray evaluation is essential and should be performed at the earliest practical opportunity. Extradural hematomas are almost invariably accompanied by a linear fracture crossing the middle meningeal groove. A calcified pineal gland may indicate a shift in the presence of intracranial hematoma. Angiography is an important x-ray aid in the management of intracranial mass lesions, much more effective than diagnostic trephination. Angiography, like all diagnostic studies, entails a certain risk but there are few absolute contraindications. The diatrizoate compounds appear most effective and least harmful. The common carotid artery may be punctured percutaneously under local anesthesia. X-rays should be obtained in the anteroposterior Towne projection and in a true lateral projection, each taken at the end of an injection of 10 cc. of 50 per cent Hypaque. Properly done, angiography in acute head injury should be carried out bilaterally.

The presence of edema without an appreciable amount of bleeding into the tissues is difficult to explain. Many years ago, vasomotor paralysis of cerebral vessels by trauma, with subsequent venous stasis and tissue waterlogging due to increased permeability of the capillaries, was thought to be a cause for the brain swelling. Recently, the same opinion has been restated by neuropathologists.

Other explanations of increased intracranial pressure are increased activity of the choroid plexus due to irritation and stimulation by the injury, resulting in increased cerebrospinal fluid formation; and lowering of the rate of absorption of the cerebrospinal fluid due to venous stasis, with venous pressure elevated well above that of the cerebrospinal fluid. Increased protein content in the cerebrospinal fluid due to blood retards its absorption and, since bloody cerebrospinal fluid is quite common in head injury, in-

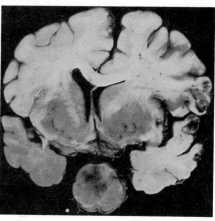

Figure 4. Left temporofrontal contusion and swelling of the left hemisphere. Note cingulate gyrus herniation from left to right over the corpus callosum, hemorrhages in the brain stem due to incisural herniation and the ventricular shift from left to right in the absence of a mass lesion. Uncal herniation has resulted in brain stem hemorrhage.

creased intracranial pressure may then be due in part to a deficient absorption of the cerebrospinal fluid. That edema and swelling of the brain occur is unquestioned. That this can take place in the absence of large mass lesions in the cranial cavity is also well substantiated (Figs. 3 and 4).

CLINICAL MANIFESTATIONS. The clinical manifestations of acute head injuries depend mainly upon the degree of involvement of the brain. The gravity is indicated, in part, by the length of unconsciousness following trauma. However, a certain number of apparently serious open wounds of the cranial cavity may be unassociated with initial unconsciousness, or a very short period of unconsciousness. On the other hand, many closed injuries of the head may be associated with severe derangement of the conscious state for many days.

The older classifications of patients with head injury have emphasized the terms concussion, contusion and laceration.

Cerebral concussion may be defined as an immediate posttraumatic unconscious state resulting from a head injury and is considered the result of damage in the brain stem. Such an injury may or may not be reversible.

Contusions and *lacerations* of the brain may accompany concussion but need not do so. Lacerations and contusions may occur without associated involvement of brain stem centers (Figs. 5 and 6).

Present-day classification of head injury recognizes the fact that patients who have

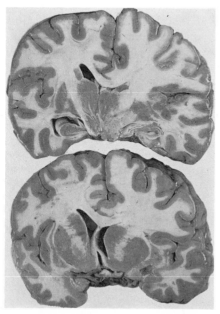

Figure 3. *Above,* Cross section of brain, showing compression of the upper brain stem by a left-sided uncal herniation. *Below,* Marked swelling of the centrum ovale on the left side is seen. Such swelling of the white matter extends all the way into the brain stem.

initial unconsciousness following the trauma have brain stem involvement. However, patients without initial unconsciousness may have extensive brain damage without involvement of the brain stem. Patients with brain stem syndromes present posttraumatic unconsciousness, their pulse is slow and the pallor of their skin suggests a shocklike state. The brain stem dysfunction may be of varying intensity involving both reversible and irreversible states. The reversible state may result in complete recovery.

Another group consists of patients having a combination of a brain stem syndrome with a severe wound of the nervous system. A patient who may begin with no evidences of brain stem dysfunction may, through edema of the brain or intracranial hemorrhage, develop evidences of involvement in this region. These secondary manifestations of brain stem derangement are, of course, quite common in head injury. If we are to use the term "concussion," it should be defined as posttraumatic unconsciousness following impact, due to functional or anatomic derangement of the upper brain stem. Concussion may occur with or without brain contusion or laceration, or with or without a skull fracture and vice versa.

The management of head injury is based on the clinical manifestations (Table 1) and is best considered under the groups of conscious state, neurologic deficit, vital signs, associated injuries and later complaints and complications.

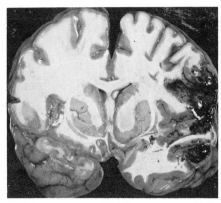

Figure 6. Deep contusion of the left frontotemporal region with petechial hemorrhages surrounding the area of contusion. If the patient survives for several days, such an area will soften and become infarcted, and may constitute an intracerebral hematoma with severe tissue loss.

State of consciousness. The level of consciousness and changes in this level provide one of the most important and sensitive clinical methods of appraising acute head injury. A normal state of consciousness, or a rapid progression toward normal, is a favorable sign and almost always favors an excellent prognosis. It should be pointed out that major perforating or penetrating wounds of the brain can take place without loss of consciousness. Many bullets traversing the frontal or occipital lobes and missing vital centers may produce extensive damage without alteration in conscious state. In general, however, one may grade the severity of the head injury by a careful appraisal of the level of awareness. The attending physician must be constantly alert for changes in the conscious state. A decreasing alertness signifies an increase in intracranial pressure and should alert those concerned to the possibility of an intracranial mass hemorrhage.

A lucid interval—that period of consciousness between an initial unconsciousness and the subsequent lapse into coma—is an important sign usually, but not always, signifying an expanding intracranial mass lesion. It has been considered pathognomonic of epidural hematoma. It may also be seen in acute subdural collections of blood and, occasionally, may be mimicked by brain swelling.

In order to avoid confusion, it is best to disregard terms such as semicoma, stupor and semistupor. The patient's ability to respond to command or to noxious stimuli should be recorded. It is then a simple matter

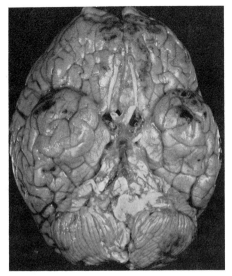

Figure 5. Contusions of the temporal and frontal tips in a patient with an occipital fracture.

Table 1. *Clinical Manifestations of Acute Craniocerebral Trauma*

Scalp
  Contusion
  Laceration
  Hematoma

Skull
  Fracture: open or closed
    Linear
    Comminuted
    Depressed
    Expressed
    Penetrating

Intracranial contents
  Brain
    Concussion
    Contusion
    Laceration
    Edema and increased intracranial pressure
    Subdural accumulation of cerebrospinal fluid
    Hemorrhage
      Epidural
      Subdural
        Acute
        Subacute
        Chronic
      Subarachnoid: localized or generalized
      Intraparenchymatous
        Petechial
        Massive

Discharge of blood, cerebrospinal fluid, or brain tissue from:
  Ear
  Nose
  Open head and brain wound

Infection
  Osteomyelitis
  Meningitis
  Cerebritis and cortical ulceration
  Brain abscess
    Epidural
    Subdural
    Intraparenchymatous

Complications
  Pneumocephalus
  Spurious meningocele

Associated injuries elsewhere
  Fractures
  Spinal injuries
  Chest injuries
  Abdominal injuries

to gauge an improvement or worsening of the conscious state.

In a certain number of head injury patients, extreme disorientation alternating with periods of semiconsciousness and psychotic manifestations is seen. An injury to the temporal tip frequently results in this state. Area 44, which is at the junction of the frontal and temporal lobes, may be injured in severe craniocerebral trauma, the result of mass movements of the brain. Unilateral or bilateral contusions of this region may occur. Acute psychotic states usually tend to resolve, but personality derangements may exist for a long time.

In general, patients who remain unconscious for many days return to consciousness through a transitional state of semi-consciousness with disorientation and confusion. Occasionally, the return to normality is quite prompt, but more often it is prolonged. Neurotic and psychotic manifestations associated with head injury are difficult to evaluate in respect to cause-and-effect relationship. Psychoneurotic manifestations seen several months or years after a head injury from which the patient apparently has made a satisfactory physical recovery are probably not related to the head injury per se, but to the experience of stress upon an abnormal pretraumatic personality. A proper evaluation should include a careful consideration of the patient's psychiatric background, his ability to tolerate stress and his reactions to environmental experiences. In some patients, mental deterioration following a severe head injury with no improvement in the intellect can undoubtedly be ascribed to the total devastating effect of the trauma upon the central nervous system. Among the patients with this class of injury, adolescents and children rehabilitate better than do adults. The latter may remain in a vegetative state for weeks or months following a severe head injury. In these patients, the condition appears to be related to cortical brain damage with or without a major degree of brain stem injury.

Amnesia following head injury is quite common. Usually, the patient remembers neither the accident nor activities immediately preceding the accident. Sometimes, the amnesic state may be present in patients who appear normal. Such patients may have a short period of posttraumatic unconsciousness or may be merely dazed for several seconds. Nearly 80 per cent have complete amnesia for the experience of the injury itself and the period just before the impact. According to some observers, prolonged posttraumatic amnesia increases the likelihood of posttraumatic epilepsy, but at the same time suggests that the interval between trauma and the development of epilepsy is going to be longer.

Vital functions. Vital functions are judged by the heart or pulse rate, the respirations, the body temperature and the blood pressure. In general, these may be altered from the normal at the time of injury and as the results of the injury become evident.

In the seriously injured patient, the pulse may initially be full, slow and bounding. As improvement takes place, the pulse may become somewhat faster, less full and bounding. If the patient fails to improve, it may first become slower. A pulse rate of 40 to 55 per minute is quite common in the patient with an acute, severe head injury. Eventually, in the fatally injured patient, the pulse may suddenly increase in rhythm with lowering of the amplitude. It may become elevated to 120 to 180 or higher, becoming thready in the patient who is failing. These changes occur in the course of ten to 24 hours or longer following the injury.

A pulse rate of 40 to 50, unassociated with abnormalities of the heart, occurs in some patients who are conscious following head injury and are feeling quite well. A cause for such a low rate may be a period of vagal stimulation with resultant bradycardia. In other patients, the pulse may be within the range of normal to start with, but over a period of several days may show a lowering in rate. Such a decrease should be carefully evaluated in conjunction with other signs of increase in intracranial pressure due to a dynamic lesion in the cranial cavity. In patients having fatal lesions, such a pulse will eventually increase in rate and become thready. A fast, thready pulse may be seen from the beginning and may be associated with a shocklike state, particularly if injuries to other parts of the body are also present.

Depending upon the degree of the injury, respirations may be normal or variously altered. In a lethal injury, the patient may take gasping breaths. In the less seriously injured individual, there may be deep, stertorous breathing which may become accelerated. The hyperpnea may be associated with atony of the bronchiolar and bronchial epithelium with collections of excretions in the upper respiratory passages resulting in typical noisy hyperpnea. In other patients, the respirations may be slow and labored with evidence of difficulty in obtaining a satisfactory exchange. In some, following a normal respiratory rhythm there may be a lowering of the rate. Under these circumstances, the presence of a dynamic lesion may be considered likely. Rapid respirations associated with a high temperature and un-

consciousness indicate a poor prognosis. Rapid respirations in a conscious patient usually result from other than intracranial abnormalities; a chest lesion may be present.

Hyperpnea in patients with severe head injury is common. Its association with obstructive collections of tracheobronchial secretions is also common. The reason for this collection may be a poor exchange of air in the establishment of the vicious cycle with pulmonary edema; improper activity of the ciliated epithelium of the bronchial tree due to the severity of the injury, or improper activity of the muscular layers of the smaller bronchioles resulting in poorer excretion. These abnormalities of the muscular activity and the ciliated epithelium may result from a central mechanism with paralysis of parasympathetic and sympathetic impulses. Cheyne-Stokes respirations are also present occasionally in the head injury patient, although the slow, gasping respirations are much more common. Cheyne-Stokes respirations indicate a poor prognosis.

Respiratory embarrassment with poor exchange may be improved by careful toilet of the upper respiratory passages and employment of a tracheotomy. The latter may be likesaving in many patients by preventing obstruction. Less effort is required to ventilate the unobstructed lungs.

The temperature of the patient with an acute head injury may be subnormal or normal soon after trauma. It may be higher several hours or days after the accident. Particularly if there is associated injury elsewhere, early subnormal temperature, as a part of a shock state, may be noted. Associated with such a low temperature there may be a peculiar yellowish gray discoloration of the skin, the extremities being quite cold. In many patients with severe head injury, the blood pressure may be at a normal level. In this respect, the shock state in the craniocerebral trauma patient is different from shock in the patient having skeletal and bodily injury.

In the patient with severe contusions of the brain and with bloody spinal fluid, a slightly elevated temperature with a warm dry skin may continue for several hours. Then hyperthermia may develop with a temperature of 104 to 107° F., associated with hyperpnea, pulmonary edema and a rapid pulse rate. If such a state is not attended with unconsciousness, other causes for the hyperpnea and the elevated temperature should be found. In patients with moderately severe head injury, the temperature is elevated to 101 to 103° F. and it tends to lower as the patient shows improvement. Dehydration, absorption, repair processes and infection may cause some increase in temperature. A high level of temperature sustained for many days or weeks is unusual. Even though the craniocerebral trauma may have initiated some of the upward trend of the temperature, other factors such as pulmonary, genitourinary or meningeal infections should be sought. In the course of convalescence, a sudden rise of temperature should be carefully evaluated, particularly in patients upon whom an operative procedure has been performed. It may signify a complicating infection requiring reexploration of the wound.

In the emergency room, the blood pressure readings of most patients with head injury are near normal. The blood pressure is well sustained even though the patient may present the appearance of a shocked state. It has been shown experimentally that in the seriously injured animal there is a central vascular dilatation with peripheral vasoconstriction. In the human being, essentially the same changes probably take place with peripheral vasoconstriction, resulting in cold limbs and a pale, yellowish gray, sweating face.

Occasionally, the blood pressure may rise in association with increasing intracranial pressure produced by a massive intracerebral hematoma. Slowing of the pulse and respirations may accompany an increase in the blood pressure. In some patients, there may be an increase in blood pressure and a high level of systolic and diastolic pressures may be sustained for several days but become normal as the patient improves. Most often the blood pressure readings are not of much help in assessing the level of the increase in intracranial pressure. Except for the fact that the pressure level records the general functional competency of the vascular system, blood pressure readings are of minor help.

Vomiting. Vomiting is frequently associated with craniocerebral trauma. In a large series of patients having head injuries, it occurred in about 20 to 30 per cent. In the patient with a minor head injury, nausea and vomiting may be the result of a reflex stimulation of the vagoglosso-pharyngeal system. In some individuals, it may be due to the activation of this reflex through the presence of swallowed blood in the stomach. In the more seriously injured patient, nausea and vomiting may develop with recovery from an unconscious state. Sometimes, vomiting and nausea are associated with changing of the position of the patient. When this occurs, vestibular damage with nuclear and peripheral involvement of the vestibular system may be the cause. Usually, vomiting is a frequent manifestation in the less seriously injured individual. In the profoundly injured patient, it does not occur as frequently. The vomitus is usually bloody or coffee-ground color, either from the presence of swallowed blood from trauma to the oral cavity, or from gastric bleeding from an abdominal injury. In some instances, vomiting may be the result of hypothalamic abnormalities producing ulceration and hemorrhage of the gastric mucosa. Because of the possibility of aspiration of the vomitus, the management of patients with head injury may require washing out the stomach soon after admission to the hospital. Vomiting, along with dehydration and fluid imbalance, may result in chemical changes, including hypochloremia and hypokalemia, which delay or prevent recovery.

Neurologic manifestations. In acute craniocerebral injuries, neurologic manifestations may be disguised by abnormalities in the state of consciousness. Thus, an accurate evaluation of the patient's ability to cerebrate normally, his visual acuity, difficulties of hearing, abnormalities of the sense of smell, speech disturbances and sensory abnormalities may be impossible. Important conclusions may be drawn from the neurologic examination. Repeated examinations are valuable and often mandatory. Minor changes in the neurologic status of the patient may signify abnormalities not suspected previously. In the presence of extensive intracranial damage, certain abnormalities in the sensory sphere also become evident as the patient recovers consciousness. Visual defects, abnormalities in the power of thinking, sensory phenomena, and auditory, olfactory and speech disturbances may become evident.

In the early stages following an acute severe head injury, the examiner is often limited in his evaluation by the lack of cooperation of the patient. Under these circumstances, an examination of the pupils and fundi, search for bleeding from body orifices and an evaluation of gross abnormalities of motor function may be of value. In over 90 per cent of the patients having inequality of the pupils, the dilated pupil is on the side of the intracranial lesion. A dilated pupil may indicate partial or complete involvement of the oculomotor nerve. There may be divergent strabismus, or conjugate deviation of the eyes to one or the other side. Usually, in patients with cortical lesions, the eyes are turned toward the lesion. In those with nuclear lesions, the eyes are turned away from the lesion. Examination of the fundi may show the presence of hemorrhages in the aqueous or vitreous humor or in the retinas. Such hemorrhages, when present soon after injury, may indicate local forces acting directly on or about the globe. In other instances, there may be evidence of venous engorgement, diffuse retinal edema, blurring of the disks or choked disks.

Nuchal rigidity may be present in patients with blood in the subarachnoid space. Its absence does not preclude the presence of subarachnoid hemorrhage. There may be varying degrees of associated decerebrate rigidity. In some patients who are profoundly ill, there may be limpness or flaccidity with a generalized areflexia, which is an ominous sign.

Weakness or paralysis of an extremity, facial weakness and the presence of certain abnormal reflexes may be identified in the unconscious or semiconscious patient. It may be evident that the patient moves one upper extremity more frequently than the other. On stimulation, one may notice that one entire half of the body is paralyzed as compared with the other half. There may be facial distortion suggesting a weakness on one side of the face. Unilateral corneal reflex loss is probably due to the presence of central or peripheral facial weakness and consequently may be significant as a localizing finding.

Speech disturbances may occur in some patients with severe brain damage, but with little or no evidence of brain stem involvement. Open, depressed skull fractures in the left frontoparietal area may be associated with motor aphasia and, in some instances, with jargon speech. An inability to understand spoken language may be present. As a patient becomes more cooperative, evidences of sensory aphasia, alexia, agraphia and apraxia may be noted.

Visual disturbances, particularly involvement of the visual fields, may be noted in the convalescent patient, although suspected by the extent and location of damage sustained at the time of the accident. Homonymous hemianopsia with occipital lobe involvement is occasionally noted. In temporal lobe lesions due to open depressed skull fractures, there may be quadrant defects or homonymous defects. Some patients who are conscious on admission to the hospital may have a bilateral blindness which disappears after several minutes to hours. A history of a blow on the occiput may suggest the possibility of a contusion with edema of the calcarine area bilaterally with resultant blindness. Persisting unilateral blindness may occur in patients who are only briefly unconscious. The optic nerve of normal appearance at the first examination becomes atrophic in two or three weeks.

Sensory abnormalities of cortical origin are not common in patients with head injury. However, astereognosia may be noted. Some loss of tactile and vibratory sense on one side of the body as compared with the other may be found in some patients with extensive parietal damage. In the majority of patients, light touch and tactile sense are well preserved even though there may be known parietal lobe damage.

The syndrome of the superior longitudinal sinus was first described by Holmes and Sargent in patients with tangential fractures of the vault near the midline. Paresis of the lower limbs and one or both upper limbs occurs. The pathologic anatomy is either that of contusion of the lower extremity cortical area or a compression or thrombosis of the sagittal sinus.

Catatonic states in persons with head injuries almost always have left frontoparietal injuries with aphasia. The association of aphasia and catatonia was pointed out by Kleist, who thought that catatonia may be a pyramidal tract dysfunction. It is felt that a catatonic attitude suggests a left frontoparietal lesion in a right-handed individual. These patients may be conscious or semiconscious and frequently, they are aphasic. When a limb is placed in a certain position, this position is sustained until fatigue causes the limb to be lowered.

Contusions and lacerations of the frontotemporal junction may be associated with central facial weakness on the opposite side, and jacksonian seizures of the face and the mouth on the one or both sides. These may become generalized seizures. Frontotemporal junction contusions are common in serious head injuries. When there are circumoral twitchings associated with jacksonian or generalized seizures, the possibility of frontotemporal junction contusions should be considered.

Plegic states with pseudobulbar paralytic phenomena are common in the more seriously injured individuals with extensive brain damage. Bilateral spasticity eventually disappearing, but associated with some unsteadiness and ataxia, is seen. This may result from bilateral pyramidal tract involvement in the posterior thalamus or bilateral contusions and lacerations of the motor cortex. Associated with this condition is a change in the patient's voice to a nasal tone, as well as an early inability to swallow normally. Later, swallowing may become normal, but the abnormal pseudobulbar speech may continue for many years.

An intracranial mass lesion, such as an extradural or subdural hematoma, as well as severe swelling of the brain may result in a brain stem herniation through the incisura, or a temporal lobe herniation with the uncus extending into the posterior fossa through the incisura. Thus, the brain stem and certain cranial nerves, particularly the third cranial nerve, may be compressed. In some patients, involvement of the third cranial nerve, resulting in a dilated pupil, is due to hemorrhage from the middle meningeal artery in the middle cranial fossa. Pupillary inequality as a result of brain stem compression, bilateral pyramidal tract signs and decerebrate attitudes and rigidities are manifestations of temporal lobe or brain stem herniations. With compression of the brain stem, the vessels about the structure may become compressed with resultant congestion and ischemia. Hemorrhages in the upper brain stem may occur by diapedesis. Such hemorrhages occur in patients with fatal subdural and epidural hematomas, but similar lesions may occur as a result of the initial impact. An initial impact resulting in brain stem hemorrhage may cause death within a matter of a few minutes to several hours.

Diagnosis of this condition is made by the observation of abnormalities of the pupils, body tone, the reflexes and deterioration of the conscious state. Its management in most instances consists in removal of the initial cause of the herniation. An epidural, subdural or intracerebral hematoma should be removed with dispatch. Prompt surgical treatment may be lifesaving. On the other hand, if the temporal lobe or brain stem herniation has been present for too long a time, an irreversible state may be present.

Herniation of the medulla and cerebellar tonsils in acute head injury is uncommon but may occur in conjunction with a posterior fossa massive hemorrhage. Sudden stoppage of respirations, with heart action continuing, is the typical clinical result in the untreated patient.

The cranial nerves may be injured in craniocerebral trauma. The first cranial nerves are injured in association with anterior fossa fractures and injury in the neighborhood of the cribriform plates. Anosmia may result, with improvement in olfactory function in eight to 12 months. If of longer duration, anosmia usually becomes permanent. In anosmic patients, the sense of taste is fairly well preserved at least for basic flavors.

Injury to the optic nerves locally may occur by impact of the fracture and by hemorrhage into the vaginal sheath of the nerve. Usually, blindness is permanent and the nerve head atrophies.

The third, fourth and sixth cranial nerves are frequently injured in patients with extradural and subdural hematomas. The sixth nerve may be injured at the base because of distortion of the brain at impact. Occasionally, the third and fourth nerves are also injured in this manner. Diplopia due to paralysis of one or more ocular muscles is frequently the result of intraorbital damage. Third nerve paralysis on one side, with contralateral paralysis of the body, may suggest a midbrain injury, but it is also seen in association with subdural and epidural hematomas in a basilar location.

Paralysis of ocular movements may occur in patients with head injuries complicated by an arteriovenous fistula between the carotid artery and the cavernous sinus. Proptosis of the eyeball develops, often within 48 hours; chemosis occurs and a bruit may be heard over the globe. The ipsilateral common carotid artery should be promptly ligated in treating this condition.

The fifth cranial nerve may be injured in its supraorbital and infraorbital portions by fractures involving the foramina bearing the same names. Occasionally, the ganglion and the entire fifth nerve are involved with fractures of the middle fossa.

The seventh and eighth cranial nerves are

injured in transverse fractures of the petrous bone. Bleeding from the ear may accompany seventh nerve paralysis with longitudinal fractures invading the facial canal and the middle ear. Complete deafness with a dead labyrinth usually indicates a transverse fracture through the internal auditory meatus. Seventh nerve paralysis of the peripheral type involves paralysis of the forehead, orbicularis oculi and orbicularis oris as well as the platysma muscles. Seventh nerve paralysis may be due to injury of the nerve at the time of impact, or it may result from edema and hemorrhage in the facial canal neighborhood. In the latter instance, it makes a delayed appearance four to 12 days after the injury. In most of these patients, peripheral facial paralysis improves.

The ninth, tenth, eleventh and twelfth cranial nerves are injured in penetrating wounds of the head. They are almost never involved in the usual civilian type of head injuries.

Abnormal neurologic findings may be of value in localizing the lesion and, depending upon their pattern of appearance, may indicate the presence of a dynamic lesion. Weakness or paralysis of one-half the body seen soon after an injury may signify a laceration of the motor region. Weakness or paralysis of one-half the body developing over a period of 24 to 36 hours may indicate the presence of a subdural, epidural or intracerebral hematoma. The importance of repeated neurologic examinations cannot be overemphasized.

Convulsions. In patients with acute head injury, convulsive disorders are seen in less than 10 per cent. These include focal or jacksonian, generalized or grand mal, petit mal and psychomotor convulsions. Commonly noted are decerebrate rigidity patterns, particularly in patients with serious head injuries. Less common are generalized convulsive seizures of the grand mal variety. Least common are jacksonian manifestations which may become generalized.

Decerebrate spells are seen in the seriously injured. Almost always, these patients have bloody spinal fluid with elevated spinal fluid pressures. The patient may become rigid. At times, the rigidity may involve one-half of the body and change from one side to the other. Usually, both sides become rigid when the patient is moved or stimulated. The patient has bilateral pyramidal tract signs with Babinski reflexes present bilaterally. At times, particularly among the young, the Babinski signs may be continuous. Nuchal rigidity and opisthotonos may be present. Usually, there are no associated convulsive movements of the body, but occasionally decerebrate rigidity may be followed by a generalized convulsive seizure. The patient has a set, rigid jaw and at times there may be some foaming at the mouth. The attacks usually last from a few minutes to several hours. Frequently, short-lasting attacks may continue to occur. As the patient fails, he may be less rigid and more flaccid. Usually, decerebrate rigidity attacks in the adult mean a fatal outcome. In a child, such attacks may not be as serious and recovery often occurs. Particularly is this true when the decerebrate state is caused by a mass lesion which can be evacuated.

Decerebrate rigidity may be due to brain stem involvement from the initial impact, or it may result from brain stem or temporal lobe herniation resulting from brain swelling, or a large epidural or subdural collection. If such subdural or epidural collections are not promptly treated, an irreversible state due to brain stem herniation may occur.

Grand mal seizures occur less frequently. Occasionally, they are seen soon after injury as the patient recovers consciousness. They may be seen later in the course of a serious head injury. The spinal fluid is frequently bloody. The pressure may be high. There may or may not be a history of idiopathic epilepsy, and this should be noted carefully in all patients with generalized convulsive seizures following head trauma. No definite localizing signs may be present. However, in many instances, there may be bilateral Babinski signs soon after a generalized convulsive seizure. At times, generalized convulsive seizures occur as a sequel to jacksonian seizures or, in some instances, following decerebrate seizures. The attacks may become continuous, resulting in status epilepticus. This is not commonly seen in head injury patients since such individuals are energetically treated early. Patients of the younger age group, particularly infants and children, are more apt to develop convulsive seizures of a grand mal variety than are adults. At times, meningitis, traumatic cerebritis or a brain abscess may be initiated with a jacksonian or grand mal seizure.

Jacksonian seizures, or focal seizures, are important because they imply a discrete type of lesion of the brain, commonly a mass lesion. Jacksonian seizures of the mouth and upper extremity area may be followed by generalized seizures and may signify contusions of the frontotemporal junction. More frequently, localized compression of the motor areas by a subdural or epidural hematoma and contusions of the motor region may result in jacksonian seizures. These may eventuate in generalized convulsions in the untreated patient or the patient upon whom operation has not been performed.

The management of a patient with convulsive seizures requires a proper airway. In some instances, hypoxia may be the initiating factor and a good airway provided by an intratracheal tube or tracheostomy may be valuable. Focal signs may indicate the need for operative intervention. Epidural, subdural and intracerebral hematomas may be associated with focal seizures followed by focal neurologic signs.

Cerebrospinal fluid findings. Routine use of a lumbar puncture is not indicated. Early, a lumbar puncture may upset the hydrodynamics in the cranial cavity sufficiently to influence the signs and symptoms of a dynamic lesion. A forming epidural hematoma may be associated with lowering of the spinal fluid pressure even though the patient's mass lesion is expanding. If performed, the spinal fluid pressure should always be recorded. The blood content should be noted and this can be done by making a complete blood count of the cerebrospinal fluid. Cerebrospinal fluid which is bloody to start with may clear in eight to ten days. Within two days, bloody spinal fluid may be faintly xanthochromic in some patients. The red blood cells hemolyze and disappear much more rapidly than do the white blood cells. At the end of four or five days, a lumbar puncture may reveal xanthochromic fluid with a white cell count out of proportion to the red count in the same specimen. Usually, the white cells in such a count are divided between polymorphonuclears and lymphocytes.

In general, low spinal fluid pressure does not rule out the possibility of a massive lesion in the cranial cavity. However, most dynamic lesions in the cranial cavity are associated with fairly high cerebrospinal fluid pressures, over 250 to 300 mm. of water.

Hypotension of the cerebrospinal fluid is often a grave sign. A seriously ill patient having a cerebrospinal fluid pressure of 75 mm. or less may be in an extremely poor condition.

Brain swelling may be present, with or without high cerebrospinal fluid pressure. In some instances, the cerebrospinal fluid pressure gives an index of the degree of brain swelling. In other instances, because of the presence of hydrodynamic abnormalities, the level of cerebrospinal fluid pressure may not be high, even though edema of the brain is present either locally or generally.

Concomitant injuries. In the usual high velocity deceleration injuries, the possibility of damage not only to the head but to other parts of the body is great. Associated injury elsewhere in the body is often responsible for the morbidity as well as the fatal outcome. Particularly in the unconscious patient, consideration must be given to the possibility of injuries to the extremities, chest and abdomen.

Headache. Headache is a common symptom in patients with head trauma. As the seriously injured patient improves from the initial disturbed conscious state, he may complain of headaches. In other instances, headache may be the result of an increase in intracranial pressure in patients without unconsciousness. In still others, it is seen following minor head injuries unassociated with unconsciousness at the time of impact. These patients, nevertheless, complain bitterly of headaches which are caused neither by intracranial bleeding nor increased intracranial pressure.

The headaches are usually generalized, but they may be localized to one or the other side of the head and are frequently located in the vicinity of scalp lacerations and bruises. Some patients may have headaches only when in the upright position, noted upon getting up and about from bed. These headaches disappear when the patient is in the recumbent or semi-Fowler's position. It has been postulated that such headaches may be due to generalized hypotension with traction upon the intracranial blood vessels.

The mechanism of headache in the patient with a head injury may be related to several factors. Recent information suggests that headache is usually due to changes in the blood vessel tone and caliber of intracranial and extracranial vessels. The vessels at the base of the brain and those of extracerebral structures may become dilated or constricted. Pain resulting from dural vessel involvement also is possible. Abnormalities of tone in the blood vessel walls may result from both mechanical and hypothalamic disturbances.

Traction upon the larger vessels at the base

of the brain may develop from abnormal cerebrospinal fluid hydrodynamics related to the presence of blood in the subarachnoid space. In patients who obviously have no cerebrospinal fluid hypertension and yet complain of headaches, traction on the larger blood vessels of the circle of Willis may be a factor, particularly with change of the position of the patient's head.

An important cause for headaches in the posttraumatic patient involves an associated injury to neck structures, including muscles, ligaments and the cervical nerves. Since many deceleration and acceleration injuries result in traction of the head away from the neck, and compression of the head toward it and the trunk, damage to the second and third cervical vertebrae with associated involvement of muscles and nerves may result in head and neck pain. Particularly in injuries of the second cervical area, painful conditions in the back of the head and neck on one or both sides may result and eventually generalized headaches may develop.

When, in the less seriously injured individual, there is history of migraine or periodic headaches prior to the head injury, the patient may complain that the headaches following the injury are aggravated. Whether these complaints can be ascribed to a neurosis or a compensation syndrome is a question. In a few instances, patients have complained that migraine states which have been quiescent for three or four years have been reactivated following a head injury. It is difficult to evaluate such a relationship. The head injury in such patients probably is a precipitating factor. Other stresses involving psychic injury, such as a divorce or financial loss, may have the same effect.

Headaches observed in the posttraumatic syndrome usually improve in a period of three weeks to three or four months. Occasionally, a patient may continue to complain, but often this is found to involve compensation factors. These patients continue to benefit financially as long as their complaints are validated. Dizziness usually disappears before the attacks of headache subside. Occasionally, headaches are absent from the beginning while dizzy attacks predominate. In some, the attacks of dizziness are completely absent. In general, complaints of intermittent headache and dizziness favor an organic cause, while persistent headache or dizziness which never disappears completely suggests the presence of a neurosis or malingering.

Dizziness. Dizziness is a common complaint during the convalescent period. When the extremely ill individual recovers, attacks of dizziness are not quite as common as in patients with less severe craniocerebral trauma. Many patients with a minor head injury, with or without an initial period of unconsciousness at the time of impact, may have residual dizziness. Two types are noted: the vertiginous, an actual feeling of rotation or whirling of the body or surrounding objects, and a giddiness with a feeling of unsteadiness and lightheadedness which is unassociated with feeling of whirling or vertigo. A change in position frequently initiates the dizziness. In the vertiginous type, certain positions of the head and the direction of gaze may result in symptoms. The patient becomes giddy, may feel nauseated and may vomit. Patients learn to refrain from the undesirable posturing of their body and their eyes.

Changing the body position, such as from a supine to a standing position, or vice versa, or bending forward, may result in a feeling of losing balance and meeting the floor. Many patients learn to move more deliberately in order to prevent the feeling of giddiness. Patients frequently identify their spells by the term "blackout," but on questioning admit that unconsciousness does not accompany their spells. The giddiness or vertiginous attacks tend to disappear over a period of several weeks or a few months.

The cause for dizziness is not completely understood. Vertiginous attacks are due to an involvement of the vestibular nerves, the labyrinths peripherally or their central connections in the brain stem. Occasionally, true vertigo will occur as a temporal lobe irritative phenomenon. Although giddy attacks may be due to an involvement of the cerebrum, no definite area has been related to their production. The disturbance in the peripheral balancing mechanism seems a more likely cause.

The combination of headaches and dizziness as posttraumatic sequelae, particularly in minor head injuries, is known to both the physician and the layman. The protraction of such complaints may be due in part to functional factors, but that they have an organic basis in the early stages is unquestioned. In part, these complaints are on an organic level, but psychoneurotic influences alter, lengthen or reinforce these sequelae.

The study of the labyrinthian mechanism in patients with head injury has not been fruitful. Those who complain of giddiness have shown no unusual degree of abnormality of the labyrinthian structures, excepting possibly for some decrease in the reaction to stimuli. In patients who have severe vertigo, caloric tests have shown some impairment of the labyrinth function in association with nerve deafness. Many of the latter group also complain of tinnitus, usually on the one side. A ringing in the ear may be associated with a history of bleeding from one or both ears.

CLINICAL-PATHOLOGIC CORRELATIONS. When the patient with a head injury is first seen in the emergency department of a hospital, he may appear profoundly, moderately or slightly injured, as evidenced by the immediate clinical findings.

A patient with a closed head injury may be conscious or deeply comatose. Patients with open wounds of the head may have varying degrees of involvement from a minor-appearing laceration of the scalp to an extensive wound with extrusion of brain tissue. Patients with open wounds and with extensive damage of nervous tissue may have little or no evidence of brain stem involvement, no initial unconsciousness, or an unconscious state of a very short duration. In both types of closed and open head injuries, the condition of the patient may be influenced by later developments of the craniocerebral trauma, including swelling and edema of the brain, hemorrhages into the intracranial spaces and intracranial infection.

Contusions and lacerations of the scalp are the commonest types of head injury. Ecchymosis of the eyelids may rapidly develop with marked swelling, or there may be small hemorrhagic discolorations, manifest several days after an injury, surrounding the upper and lower eyelids as well as the conjunctiva. Ecchymosis of the mastoid area has long been recognized as indicating a fracture of the base of the skull; it is known as Battle's sign. This discoloration may be more apparent two or three days after injury than immediately after the initial trauma. Lacerations of the scalp may be single or multiple. In civilian injuries caused by repeated blows upon the head by a sharp instrument, multiple lacerations are common. Lacerations extending to the subgaleal region may be associated with varying degrees of avulsion of the scalp. Careful cleansing of the wound, which then should be meticu-

lously sutured, will frequently result in good healing.

In the depth of a scalp laceration, particles of bone and brain tissue may be seen on careful inspection, but in the final analysis a careful roentgen ray survey is much more accurate and dependable. Patients with extensive lacerations of the scalp may be conscious and may have had no period of unconsciousness following their trauma.

Hematomas of the scalp are frequent. At times, palpation of these may give the wrong impression of a depressed fracture. Hematomas occurring in the subgaleal region may extend to the limits bordering this space. This is particularly seen in young adults and children and may result in severe blood loss. In the infant, hemorrhage under the periosteal lining of the bones of the cranial vault may result in cephalhematoma. The characteristic feature of cephalhematoma is that it is within the confines of the periosteal attachment of the bone involved. Aspiration of the hematoma under aseptic conditions will enhance the healing and the absorption of blood. In cephalhematoma, aspiration or removal through a small incision will restore the scalp to its normal dimensions.

Open wounds of the head include linear fractures of the skull with an overlying laceration; depression of the skull with or without dural tear and with or without brain laceration; cerebrospinal fluid rhinorrhea and cerebrospinal fluid otorrhea resulting from cranionasal and cranioaural communications (Fig. 7).

Open fractures of the skull, with no depression, may be treated by closing the laceration overlying the fracture after careful cleansing and debridement of the wound. Open depressed fractures may be associated with dural lacerations in about 15 per cent of patients admitted to large head injury services. Many patients with open depressions may have had no initial unconsciousness, or may have been unconscious for a short time. The majority of depressions occur in the anterior half of the vault. Few occur in the posterior third, in the occipital and the posterior parietal areas. Such depressions occur in the forward portions of the head, since these portions are the most frequently injured. About 75 per cent of skull depressions have an overlying laceration, making them open wounds. At times, the laceration may be a small puncture wound not commu-

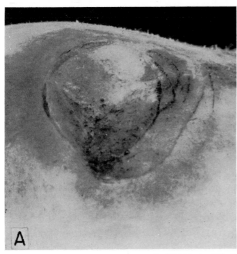 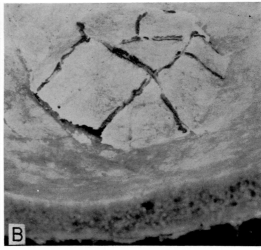

Figure 7. *A*, External appearance of experimental depressed fracture in cadaver head. *B*, Internal surface, showing extensive fragmentation of the inner table. Note the difference between the amount of involvement of the external and internal surfaces.

nicating with the underlying depression or comminution. The depression may be over functional centers of the brain so that the patient enters the hospital with weakness or paralysis of the opposite half of the body, aphasia or other clinical abnormalities. Depressions in the more forward portions of the head are attended with a low mortality. Depressions involving the frontal sinus may be associated with a high morbidity, in view of the possibility of cranionasal communications with complicating intracranial infection.

The site of the depression may determine the underlying damage. Depressions may overlie the larger venous sinuses, such as the sagittal and lateral sinuses, producing a tear of the sinus which bleeds as the fragments of bone are removed at operation. The patient's preoperative roentgen ray studies should be carefully evaluated so that the surgeon may be prepared to meet such complications. In some depressions, the middle meningeal vessels may be involved. Depressed fractures involving the temporal bone with a dynamic syndrome suggest the possibility of venous or arterial tears and a mass lesion in an epidural position.

A detailed roentgen ray delineation of depressed fractures is extremely important. When there is fragmentation of bone, the number of fragments should be noted so that at operation one can account for their removal. This is particularly true in war wounds where fragments of bone and other organic

matter left in the cranial cavity are of serious consequence in the causation of posttraumatic infection.

Open wounds over the frontal sinus neighborhood may be associated with cranionasal fistula. In many instances, such communications are established in closed injuries without evidence of a skull fracture. Such injuries have to be considered as open wounds. Linear fractures extending into the base of the anterior fossa may be associated with tears of the dural lining in the region of the cribriform plate with resultant infection many months or even years later. Only at postmortem examination may a short fracture be seen to extend into the anterior fossa and the cribriform plate. Sometimes, there may be a discrete and separate skull fracture with an unsuspected dural tear because the fracture is far removed from the region of the visible damage, such as in a bullet wound of the parietal or occipital region with cribriform plate fracture. Complicating meningeal infection may point to an injury in this region related to a patent cranionasal communication. However, the most important causes of cranionasal fistulae are compound depressions of the frontal sinus region.

With cranionasal and cranioaural communications, pneumocephalus may occur. When pneumocephalus is associated with an open depressed fracture and dural tear, repair of the latter usually suffices in curing the pneumocephalus. Pneumocephalus may appear several months or years after the acute injury, because of the presence of a patent cranionasal communication. In some instances, the patent cranionasal communication may exist even though cerebrospinal fluid rhinorrhea is not recognized, or the patient shows no air in the cranial cavity upon roentgen ray examination. Under these circumstances, the only basis for suspecting such a patent communication may be repeated attacks of meningitis.

Penetrating wounds of the head of the low velocity type, such as knife-blade and other sharp instrument wounds, are commonly seen in civilian practice. Frequently, there is no history of unconsciousness at the time of impact, and it is possible for the blade of the knife to break off so that on inspection only a small laceration of the scalp may be seen with the end of the blade embedded deeply in the scalp, skull or cranium. When such foreign bodies are left in the cranial cavity, there may be an inflammatory reaction surrounding the foreign body, and a brain abscess may form or meningitis may develop. When the patient has extensive involvement of the craniocerebral structures in open wounds, the diagnosis is usually made and prompt care of the wound results in a cure with little likelihood of infection.

High velocity wounds of the head present a different problem, particularly with bullets traveling over 1000 feet per second. The area of scalp penetration may be extensively devitalized so that incomplete debridement will result in breakdown of the wound. The passage of the missile through the cranial cavity results in forward as well as radial forces, causing pulping of brain tissue. An adequate debridement requires complete removal of the brain tissue so destroyed. Improper debridement will result in late infection, cerebritis and brain abscess.

Shell fragment wounds due to high velocity missiles cause more extensive damage because of the varying sizes and irregularity of the contour of the shell fragments. With wounds by shell fragments, complete removal of the fragments and foreign particles is mandatory for a good result. Brain stem involvement may be associated with both bullet and shell fragment injuries of the brain, so that these patients may be moribund soon after the injury. On the other hand, some of the patients may show little or no evidence of brain stem involvement, and consciousness may be retained until lost through factors other than the initial trauma. Secondary

involvement of the brain stem centers through brain edema or hemorrhage may occur. Hematomas in the track of the bullet, particularly of small firearms, are present in fully half of the patients and removal may be lifesaving.

In open wounds, the rationale of operative management is to prevent the introduction of infection into the intracranial spaces and structures. The sooner the wound is debrided and closed, the sooner protection from infection is secured. The possibility of associated hemorrhage causing compression should be considered.

Traumatic intracranial hemorrhage. Intracranial hemorrhage due to trauma may be epidural, subdural, subarachnoid or intraparenchymatous. Combinations of hemorrhagic collections in various locations in the cranial cavity are quite common. Particularly is this true with the usual type of deceleration injuries from falls and automobile accidents.

Epidural hemorrhage may be of middle meningeal, dural sinus or diploic origin (Fig. 8). It is located between the dura and the skull. At times, it forms a large mass; as much as 350 to 400 cc. of blood may collect in such an epidural position. Occasionally, the lesion is bilateral or it may cross the midline superiorly. The most common epidural hemorrhage is that of middle meningeal artery origin. Less common are epidural hematomas in the posterior fossa of lateral sinus tear origin, and hematomas resulting from sagittal sinus tears in vertex injuries.

A history of a fall or a low velocity impact, such as a bicycle-car accident, falling on the sidewalk and falling down steps, is usually present. The patient may or may not have an initial brain stem syndrome with immediate posttraumatic unconsciousness. The injury may be followed by a lucid interval of a few hours to several days. This is followed by a primary or secondary attack of unconsciousness with weakness of one-half the body and a dilated pupil on the same side as the lesion. The pupillary dilatation may not be marked in some instances. The more completely dilated the pupil, the greater the likelihood of the lesion being in a more basal position in the middle fossa. At times, there may not be an initial period of unconsciousness. The patient may reach the hospital conscious and eventually become unconscious, or he may be brought into the hospital in an unconscious state with a history that initially there was no unconsciousness. A weakness of one-

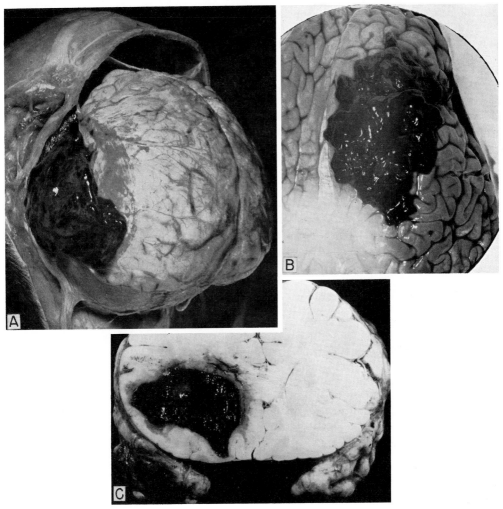

Figure 8. An epidural (*A*), an acute subdural (*B*) and an intracerebral hematoma (*C*) as seen in the autopsy room. Note the petechiae about the intracerebral hematoma in the right frontal lobe.

half of the body may not develop with a clot more posteriorly or more anteriorly located. In most of the patients, there is a linear fracture crossing the middle meningeal groove of the parietal and temporal bones. Particularly in those patients who have an initial period of unconsciousness, there may be associated evidences of other involvement of intracranial structures, such as pia arachnoid tears with bloody cerebrospinal fluid and bruises and lacerations of the temporal and frontal poles of the hemispheres. Massive intratemporal hematomas may occur. Occasionally, depressed fractures may be associated with an epidural hematoma.

Epidural hematoma is usually seen among adolescents and adults, although it has also been described in children and infants under the age of two years. In some patients, there

may be third nerve paralysis on the side of the lesion and weakness or paralysis of the opposite half of the body. If the patient's condition is not recognized and immediate operation is not carried out, he may rapidly deteriorate with irreversible changes ensuing. The vital functions at first are characterized by a slow pulse, slow respirations, a temperature of about 100 to 101° F. and a blood pressure which is usually within normal levels. In many instances, the spinal fluid may be bloody and its pressure is moderately elevated. In the untreated patient, the pulse becomes faster and eventually thready. The respirations increase in rhythm and the patient may eventually become hyperpneic, with pulmonary edema, or there may be slow gasping respirations as a final phase before death. In the untreated patient, late effects may be the result of brain stem herniation through the incisura with generalized rigidity, bilateral pyramidal tract signs, dilation and fixation of pupils, and loss of corneal reflexes.

The presence of an extradural hematoma of dural sinus origin in the posterior fossa should be suspected in association with an occipital fracture. The patient may have cerebellar hypotonia and weakness on the same side of the body as the hematoma. However, because of the associated injury to other parts of the nervous system, typical signs may not be found in the patient with a posterior fossa hematoma. Exploration along a fracture site in a patient whose condition is gradually deteriorating is justified and, under these circumstances, hematomas in the posterior fossa may be located.

Extradural hematoma from diploic and emissary veins is never of sufficient size to cause compression of the intracranial contents, although fairly large extradural hematomas in depressed fractures posterior and above the mastoid area have been seen.

Subdural hematoma is a collection of blood in the subdural area, a potential space between the dural lining and the arachnoid membrane. Mass movements of the brain may result in tear of connecting veins between the sagittal sinus and the surface of the brain as well as between the dura and the surface of the brain. Such tears result in hemorrhage into the subdural area. Depending upon the size of the torn vessels, the hemorrhage may be of proportions to result in signs of compression soon after its occurrence. On the other hand, a small amount of bleeding may occur into the subdural area and, as the subdural pressure increases, the bleeding from the venous channel may be stopped. Such a hemorrhage may be silent for varying periods.

Such hemorrhages may occur over one or both hemispheres. Depending upon the severity of the head injury, there may be clinical symptoms suggesting diffuse brain damage and masking a surface lesion. In the absence of brain stem involvement, if the hematoma is small enough so that the patient can tolerate its presence, the condition may be asymptomatic for several days or weeks. If, on the other hand, it is of larger size, there may be either immediate symptoms and signs or the symptoms and signs may be manifested within a period of several days to a week or ten days.

Thus, on the basis of the time of the appearance of clinical effects, a classification into *acute, subacute* or a *chronic* type, has been made. If the bleeding is severe and symptoms are manifested almost immediately, one is dealing with an acute and dangerous process. If the bleeding is somewhat smaller in amount, and if it is tolerated by the host for a week or ten days, one is dealing with a subacute form. Patients with the chronic variety may have associated severe craniocerebral injury and, therefore, may be ill following the trauma. These patients may improve for several weeks until evidence of a chronic subdural hematoma is noted. In other patients, the initial hemorrhage is silent for several weeks until signs of a chronic subdural hematoma supervene. The division of subdural hematomas into acute, subacute and chronic forms is of prognostic value. The earlier an acute subdural hematoma causes symptoms and signs necessitating intervention, the worse the prognosis; the longer the time before intervention is indicated, the better the prognosis.

The diagnostic features of acute subdural hematoma include a deteriorating conscious state with focal signs. The most common position is frontoparietal on one or both sides. However, subdural hematomas may be found between the hemispheres in an interhemispheric position, in the anterior fossa and in the parieto-occipital area. They may also occur between the brain stem and the hemispheres and extend into the posterior fossa about the cerebellar hemispheres, brain stem and medulla. The presence of a fracture of the skull is not of localizing value in most instances of acute subdural hemorrhage. In two-thirds of the patients, the fracture is on the opposite side or there may be no fracture demonstrated by roentgen ray examination or by autopsy. In only one-third is the fracture on the same side as the subdural hematoma. The clot in the subdural space may be liquid and easily drained, or it may be solid with some liquid and hemolyzed portions. The type of clot is important in the management of the patient and determines the type of operative treatment to be instituted. The mortality in the acute form is 50 to 75 per cent.

Subacute subdural hematomas are tolerated by the patient for several days before signs of compression supervene. After three to ten days of stabilizing clinical condition, the patient may show increasing drowsiness, evidences of localization not previously noted and, if untreated, may become comatose with increase in the respiratory rate, hyperpnea and pulmonary edema. Such patients may have a subdural hematoma on one or both sides. Prompt surgical intervention may be lifesaving. The mortality in this group is 30 to 40 per cent.

The chronic subdural hematoma may either accompany a severe craniocerebral injury, or it may occur without initial associated involvement of the brain stem centers (Fig. 9). Under the latter circumstance, the patient may be well for three to seven weeks and then may complain of headache which becomes progressively worse. The headaches are usually lateralized to the side of the hematoma, although in many instances subdural hematomas may be bilateral. In other patients, there may be signs of increased intracranial pressure, choked disks and weakness of one-half of the body. Diagnostic studies may show evidence of a mass lesion. In some instances, a brain tumor may be suspected when a history of trauma is not elicited from the patient or relatives, though usually such a history exists.

The chronic subdural hematoma is usually covered with a thick outer wall and a thin, almost single layer of cuboidal epithelium, inner wall. Within these walls is contained clotted and hemolyzed old blood. In other instances, the hematoma may be almost all liquid with a very thin wall surrounding the mass. Chronic subdural hematomas may be bilateral in 20 per cent of patients. Under any circumstance, both sides of the skull should be explored even though initial diagnostic studies may implicate only one side.

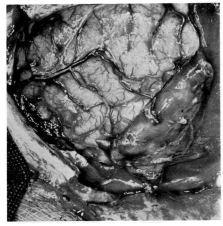

Figure 9. Chronic subdural hematoma seen in the operating room. The brain surface is exposed as the hematoma is removed through an osteoplastic flap.

If the initial subdural bleeding is severe and if the host cannot tolerate its pressure, signs and symptoms of acute subdural hemorrhage supervene. If the hematoma is smaller, the patient may tolerate its presence for three to ten days with gradually developing signs and symptoms of subacute subdural hemorrhage. If the clot is carried by the host without any symptoms for three or more weeks, an attempt at absorption and organization results in formation of an outer thick wall on the dural side and a very thin wall on the arachnoid side. Its size may increase by transference of tissue fluids and cerebrospinal fluid, because of its high osmotic pressure, with the arachnoid acting as a semipermeable membrane. The size may also increase from hemorrhages of blood vessels in its outer wall. With increase in size, eventually the mass causes symptoms.

There are exceptions to these mechanisms. The hematoma may cause little or no symptoms for many months or years. In some patients, it may calcify; in others, a solid unexpanding mass of clot with a consistency of hepatic tissue may result. Some small hematomas may absorb and never cause symptoms.

The prognosis in the chronic type of subdural hematoma is gratifying. Mortality is usually 10 per cent or less, and patients usually regain their faculties to return to their former occupations and live usefully.

Subdural collections of cerebrospinal fluid mimic subdural hematomas of the acute and subacute variety. They are almost never diagnosed until an operation is performed. At times, such collections are found in infants and they may or may not be traumatic in origin. There may or may not be a membrane surrounding the fluid. Occasionally, postinflammatory collections in the infant and the young child are described as subdural effusions.

Traumatic subdural accumulations of cerebrospinal fluid may be due to a tear of the arachnoid membrane with escape of cerebrospinal fluid into the subdural area, causing localized pressure against the brain. The presence of small amounts of bloody material in an extra-arachnoid position may attract cerebrospinal fluid and tissue fluids into the subdural area because of an increase in the osmotic pressure in this region. Contusions and tears of the brain over the convolutional peaks, with resultant increased osmotic pressure, may cause fluid accumulation in the subdural area in this neighborhood. Coughing and sneezing have been thought to cause tears of the arachnoid membrane in some patients with nontraumatic subdural accumulations of cerebrospinal fluid. Finally, certain inflammatory diseases involving the pia arachnoid may cause collections in the subdural area. Subdural collections may also be found in the posterior fossa, under the tentorium and about the cerebellar lobes.

The symptoms of a subdural accumulation of cerebrospinal fluid include a lucid interval in some patients, weakness or paralysis of one-half of the body, generalized or jacksonian seizures and a general deterioration of the patient's status. Subdural collections of cerebrospinal fluid may be found bilaterally. They may coexist with subdural and epidural hematomas.

Intracerebral hematomas are less common than subdural hematomas. Deep contusions of the brain with necrosis and bleeding from vessels may result in a large intracerebral hematoma. Actual tears of vessels in the substance of the brain may be associated with a hematoma of this type, or there may be areas of infarction with hemorrhage in the distribution of larger vessels. Frontal and temporal hematomas are most common. Parieto-occipital hematomas are occasionally seen. Parenchymatous hematomas also may occur in the posterior fossa in the cerebellar lobes.

The signs and symptoms of intracerebral hematoma depend upon the location of the lesion. In the temporal and frontal portions of the hemisphere, there may be pyramidal tract signs in the opposite half of the body and speech disturbances if the lesion is on the left side. An intracerebellar hematoma is difficult to diagnose, except when there is an open wound suggesting the presence of a lesion in this vicinity. If the patient can stand the initial effects of the intracerebellar hematoma, a diagnosis may be reached at the operating table by exploration of the posterior fossa as indicated by the ventriculographic studies. In several patients with intracerebellar hematomas, a marked psychotic state has been noted. This may possibly have been due to increased intracranial pressure brought about acutely by the compressing hematoma against the aqueductal area.

Infections. Infections complicating head injury include meningitis, osteomyelitis and brain abscess. Before antibiotic therapy and chemotherapy, otitis media and mastoiditis were fairly common following head injuries involving the middle fossa and temporal bone. At the present time, meningitis is seen occasionally. Osteomyelitis may occur, particularly in the improperly treated open injuries of the head. Cerebritis and brain abscess may develop in inadequately debrided open injuries of the brain.

Traumatic meningitis may be noted six to eight days after an injury. In the seriously ill patient, its presence may be detected only through the study of the cerebrospinal fluid. When it occurs six to eight days after the injury, it frequently is ushered in as a fulminating disease. In a patient who has improved from the initial effects of the accident, there may be severe headaches, disorientation and coma. Occasionally, the disease may be initiated with a convulsive seizure. A high fever with a delirium state is common. The patient presents nuchal rigidity and there may be a Kernig sign. The spinal fluid examination reveals a turbid fluid with large numbers of polymorphonuclear cells and, in some instances, organisms which can be seen in the smear. Occasionally, meningitic infection may follow upon the presence of a patent cranionasal or a cranioaural fistula. It may occur in conjunction with a brain abscess.

The prevention of meningitis is undoubtedly aided by the use of antibiotics and chemotherapy in patients who have open injuries of the head, or who have communications between the outside and the cranial cavity through the nose or through the ear. In such patients, the preventive use of penicillin may be effective.

When a diagnosis of meningitis is made, the drug dosage is increased. From 10 to 25 million units of aqueous penicillin are administered intramuscularly per day in divided doses for four or five days until the meningitis is controlled. Twenty-five to 35 million units may be injected intravenously in 3000 cc. of 5 per cent glucose solution. Daily, 200 to 400 grains of sulfonamides are given. In the meantime, the organisms are studied by smear and culture and their drug sensitivity is identified. As the results of these tests are available, the medicinal treatment is altered as indicated. The spinal fluid obtained after the fever and the leukocytosis have subsided should contain few or no pus cells.

Osteomyelitis of the skull is a rare complication of a craniocerebral injury. Almost always, it is the result of improper treatment of open fractures of the head. Osteomyelitis at the site of trauma may arise as a result of an open wound, or it may occur in the area of trauma with the overlying scalp intact.

The more common form of osteomyelitis, due to implantation of bacteria in an open wound, is preventable by careful excision of the wound soon after injury. In instances where this has not been done, an area of inflammation may supervene with purulent matter exuding from the compound wound. If improperly treated, the patient may enter the hospital with fever, leukocytosis, some rigidity of the neck and evidences of meningeal irritation. X-ray examination of the skull may show an area of bony destruction which is characteristic (Fig. 10).

At operation, involvement may be seen with foreign particles, hair and other dirt embedded between the fragments of bone with purulent matter and sequestration of bone. Complete excision of the area, and the use of local and systemic antibiotic therapy and chemotherapy usually result in a cure over a period of several weeks. The possibility that osteomyelitis of the skull may be associated with a subdural abscess should always be kept in mind and, if necessary, the dura should be opened to inspect the subdural area. The skull defect may be repaired later with an inanimate transplant. However, it is important to wait six to nine months after complete healing before such a repair of the skull defect is undertaken.

Cortical ulceration, cerebritis and brain abscess result from the implantation of organisms in open wounds involving the brain. Occasionally, a blow to the head with concussive effects may be associated later with a brain abscess which may be unsuspected until operative removal. This type of abscess may be due to a contusional involvement with a blood-borne infection of the area. Eventually, encapsulation and evidences of compression may develop.

Cerebritis due to an infection of the brain which follows improper debridement of a penetrating wound is a common occurrence in war but is seldom seen in civilian practice. The management of such early brain abscesses or cerebritis is by complete excision of the area of inflammation with removal of all foreign matter.

The diagnosis of cerebritis is based upon the occurrence of fever and leukocytosis, and the demonstration of bone particles and foreign matter in the roentgen ray film in a patient with an improperly treated open brain injury.

DIAGNOSTIC AIDS. In addition to the information obtained from the history and neurologic examination, various diagnostic aids are available in evaluating patients with craniocerebral trauma. These include survey roentgen ray studies of the skull, lumbar or cisternal puncture, air studies including ventriculography and encephalography, angiography and electroencephalography (Figs. 11, 12 and 13).

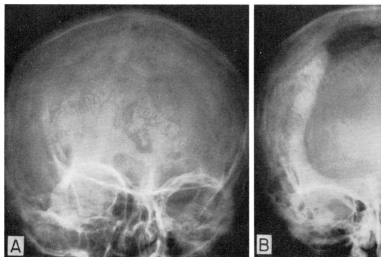
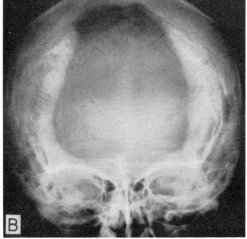

Figure 10. Trauma to the forehead in a patient with sinusitis, which resulted in extensive osteomyelitis of the skull associated with a subdural abscess over the left hemisphere and an intracerebral abscess in the left temporoparietal junction. Note the area of bone removal in B.

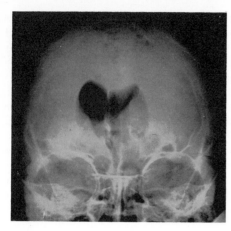

Figure 11. Air encephalogram in a patient with a left parietal epidural hematoma.

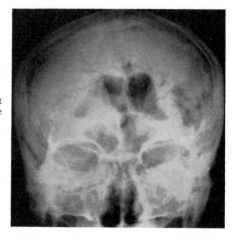

Figure 12. Air encephalogram in a patient with a right subacute subdural hematoma. Note the relative absence of subarachnoid pathways on the right.

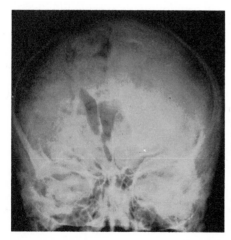

Figure 13. Air encephalogram in a patient with a left chronic subdural hematoma. Note the ventricular shift to the right and the absence of subarachnoid pathways on the left.

Figure 14. Pineal shift to the right showing the side of involvement. In bilateral lesions a pineal shift may be misleading, with the smaller lesion unsuspected. When a subdural hematoma is suspected, both sides should be explored in spite of lateralizing signs and diagnostic studies.

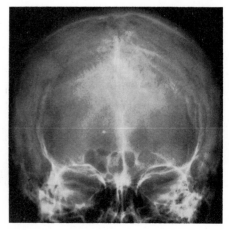

Survey roentgen ray studies are extremely valuable. The presence of a linear fracture, its position, the presence of comminution of fragments, depression, the number of fragments of bone in a depression and the presence of a foreign body in the cranial cavity may be detected by such studies. In those who have a calcified pineal gland, the presence of a pineal shift may aid in the diagnosis of a mass lesion (Fig. 14).

The concentration of blood in the cerebrospinal fluid may indicate the degree of subarachnoid hemorrhage and the severity of the intracranial involvement. The pressure of the cerebrospinal fluid in some instances may point to a mass lesion, although normal or low levels of cerebrospinal fluid pressure may be seen with mass lesions. The total protein content of the cerebrospinal fluid, if elevated, may indicate a poor prognosis. Glutamic oxalacetic transaminase determinations may show an increase in association with brain contusions and lacerations.

Air studies are valuable for localizing lesions or ruling out their presence. Ventriculography is preferable in the acute case. Encephalography may be used in the more chronic cases after the first two weeks. In the acute case, air studies may be dangerous. Such patients may have marked swelling of the brain and additional pressure caused by the injected air may be injurious.

Percutaneous angiography is the study of greatest value in acute craniocerebral trauma presenting a syndrome of increasing deterioration of the conscious state and focal manifestations. The diatrozoates are the contrast media of choice (Figs. 15 and 16).

Multiple exploratory trephinations are often unsatisfactory in many patients. Some surgeons feel that one may survey the intracranial conditions by means of four or more openings in the head, in the frontal, temporal, parietal and occipital regions on each side. The use of multiple trephinations without the additional use of diagnostic studies may lead to serious mistakes.

Electroencephalography in the patient with acute injury is of questionable diagnostic or prognostic value. In patients with the more chronic conditions, such as a chronic subdural hematoma, electroencephalography is valuable.

A radioactive brain scan has proved of value in the diagnosis of mass lesions as well as areas of intracerebral hematoma and infarction. With the use of technetium[99] the brain scan can be carried out in a short time on the unconscious patient and may give a great deal of information.

The use of echoencephalography permits the diagnosis of lateralized intracranial mass lesion based on a shift of the midline structures. This test is relatively simple and without danger. It does require some specific knowledge on the part of the individual performing the test. This is usually best done by a physician rather than a technician, although in some specialized institutions technicians may be trained well in this field. More sophisticated methods of echoencephalography may be utilized to determine, to some extent at least, the nature of the intracranial mass under study.

TREATMENT. The conservative management of craniocerebral injuries is determined

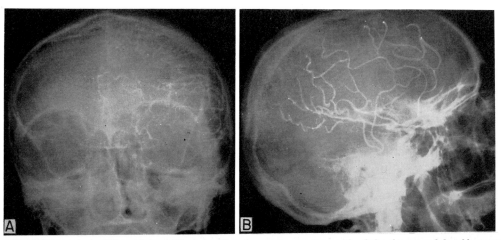

Figure 15. Anteroposterior (A) and lateral (B) views of angiogram in a patient with a left subacute subdural hematoma.

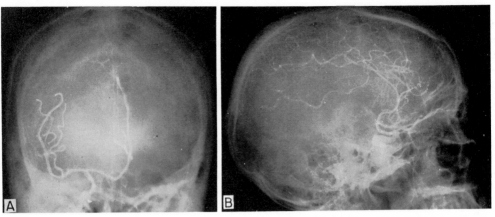

Figure 16. Angiograms in a patient with a right temporal intracerebral hematoma (*A*, anteroposterior view and *B*, lateral view). Note the elevation and bowing of the middle cerebral artery and branches.

by the degree of the injury. Patients with minimal injuries are treated by observation in the hospital for one to three days. They are seen later from time to time, since among this group a few will develop a subdural hematoma or subdural accumulation of cerebrospinal fluid. The patients with moderately severe injuries usually show improvement over a period of several hours to several days. These patients deserve careful neurologic observation, during their stay in the hospital, for the development of complications requiring surgical intervention. After the repair of small scalp lacerations, the patient is made comfortable with mild sedation and is placed in semi-Fowler's position in bed. There should be periodic observation of the pulse, blood pressure, respirations and temperature.

The patient with a serious injury deserves continuous attention. Many of these patients on entrance to the hospital have no need for surgical treatment. A few among them are moribund and a fatal outcome is evident. On the other hand, some patients in this group appearing near death may be resuscitated. Such patients may remain desperately sick for several days and their management involves meticulous nursing care. This includes keeping the air passages patent and clear, preventing the aspiration of vomitus, securing adequate fluid and food intake, temperature control, turning, bladder care and providing rest and comfort.

If there is continued respiratory distress, tracheostomy is imperative. Such a patient also should have a Levin tube passed into the stomach and the stomach contents removed to avoid aspiration during vomiting. The largest size tube should be used for tracheotomy intubation. Cuffed tubes allow the use of respirators and positive pressure breathing.

Frequent toilet of the upper respiratory passages by suction is essential. This is more important than the use of oxygen. The latter may be administered through a small catheter extending into the tracheostomy tube. Large tubes should not be used because they reduce the airway and consequently make breathing more difficult.

A small nasal tube passed into the stomach may be used for feeding the patient. The adult may be given 2000 calories of nutriment in 2500 cc. of fluid per day and proportional amounts may be used for the younger patient.

A higher temperature may quickly follow a cerebral injury, without sufficient evidence of infection to account for it. In these patients, the use of an automatically regulated blanket to reduce the temperature is valuable. The production of a hypothermic state of from 31 to 35° C. in these patients with damage to the central temperature control mechanism in the brain stem has been helpful.

In the patient who remains unconscious for several days, determination should be made of the output of sodium and nitrogenous products in the urine and of the levels of urea nitrogen, sodium, potassium and chlorides in the blood plasma. These values should be checked frequently in order to detect the development of a metabolic disorder of central origin. Such an abnormality may be more common than is suspected. If depletion states are noted, these should be adjusted over a period of several days by intravenous administration of adequate amounts of solutions. If a state of hyperosmolarity is noted, careful evaluation of the kidney function as well as the composition of the patient's feeding should be made. One may find that the patient is on a diet too high in protein which is resulting in derangement of kidney function not only for the protein, but also for sodium, thus causing hyperosmolarity of the blood. Lowering of the protein intake and administration of adequate amounts of carbohydrates and fats may suffice to correct the condition. Mercurial diuretics and forcing fluids may be of help in patients with hyperosmolarity caused by hypothalamic or frontobasilar brain involvement. A kidney shutdown syndrome associated with extensive injury to other parts of the body should be carefully evaluated and the patient's fluid intake should be restricted during this period of kidney dysfunction. In patients with severe head injury, the importance of proper blood matching when a transfusion is required cannot be overemphasized.

Specific measures. The use of certain drugs may be worth while to combat the effects of injury and prevent infection as well as for analgesia and sedation. Intravenous administration of hypertonic solutions and lumbar puncture for controlling cerebrospinal fluid pressure and brain swelling may be indicated.

Among the drugs used to help control the effects of a head injury are atropine, urea, mannitol and cortisone.

Cortisone, given in descending doses for a period of three to five days, has been employed with beneficial effects upon some of the patients. Dexamethasone and similar corticosteroids having less salt-retaining properties seem more effective. The stress of the injury may be in part responsible for the patient's serious condition and for such patients the use of cortisone has seemed valuable. In some instances, moribund patients have improved spectacularly. Patients unconscious for several days, and proved not to have an intracranial mass lesion, have seemed to become ambulatory sooner with the use of this drug than would otherwise be anticipated. However, cortisone, or any drug, should be discriminately employed. One must not overlook the presence of a mass lesion in the cranial cavity when utilizing drug therapy.

The drugs used to prevent infection in the cranial cavity or to control infection include the sulfonamides and antibiotics. In patients with open wounds of the head, these agents are given freely before and after operation. In patients who have cerebrospinal otorrhea or rhinorrhea and bleeding from the ear, these drugs should be employed routinely. When meningitis is manifest, the cerebrospinal fluid should be carefully studied for the organisms responsible and adequate doses should be administered of the drugs to which these organisms are sensitive.

The restless patient may be made comfortable with provision for good hygiene: a clean, dry bed, care of the distended bladder and attention to the bowels. By such measures restlessness may be reduced and the need for sedatives and narcotics minimized. A tracheostomy and clean respiratory passages relieve a patient's distress in breathing and promote comfort and rest. However, patients who fail to obtain satisfactory relief through these measures may need sedatives. Sedatives in head injury patients should be used with care. Morphine should not be employed except in patients with long bone fractures and excessive pain and only a mild craniocerebral injury. Codeine and phenobarbital, given by mouth or intramuscularly, have been found adequate to allay restlessness in most patients with head injuries. These drugs do not influence the conscious state or localizing signs in a dynamic lesion as does morphine.

The use of hypertonic solutions was in vogue for many years, but at the present time is seldom practiced. During a study of the effects of hypertonic solutions, it was noted that the seriously injured patient showed improvement as the pressure dropped, but became restless and stuporous again as the cerebrospinal fluid pressure rose. In the majority of clinics today, hypertonic solutions are used sparingly.

The intravenous administration of 30 gm. of urea dissolved in 300 cc. of invert sugar produces a significant and well-sustained decrease in intracranial pressure which is elevated following injury or the presence of space-occupying lesions. Hypertonic mannitol, 20 per cent solution, may be used for this purpose. One to 1.5 gm. per pound of body weight constitutes the usual dose.

The cautious use of a diagnostic lumbar puncture at any time in the course of the treatment of a patient with head injury may be indicated. When infection is suspected, lumbar puncture should be done with dispatch to determine whether evidences of infection exist in the cerebrospinal fluid. In some instances, intrathecal medication may be advisable.

INDICATIONS FOR SURGICAL TREATMENT. About 25 per cent of patients with craniocerebral injuries need operative intervention, including diagnostic operative procedures. Among those with skull fractures, the incidence of required operation is higher. About 15 per cent require debridement for compound or open wounds of the head. The rationale for the treatment is to prevent the introduction of infection into the cranial cavity. In the remaining 15 to 20 per cent, exploration is undertaken mainly for intracranial mass lesions.

Indications for operative intervention are clear-cut in open wounds of the head. As soon as the patient's condition permits, the wound is debrided and repair is carefully made. In closed depressions, the degree and area of the depression must be considered and the advisability of surgical treatment determined. The majority of patients with simple depressions should be operated upon except for those having slight depressions in the frontal area and small, simple depressions over the midline and the large venous sinuses.

Exploration for an intracranial hemorrhage is indicated when there is a deteriorating conscious state and when there are progressive focal localizing signs indicating a mass lesion.

Operative management. The operative treatment of patients with head injury includes the management of simple and open depressions, of penetrating wounds and of patent cranionasal and cranioaural communications manifested by cerebrospinal fluid discharge through these paths or pneumocephalus due to the introduction of air through the same pathways.

In patients with depressions, the large venous sinuses may be torn. They should be repaired either by the use of mattress sutures or the application of Gelfoam, which is held in place over the tear in the sinus by bridging stitches. Venous sinus injuries are more frequently seen in penetrating wounds of war than in civilian casualties. When torn, the lateral sinus may be doubly ligated. The anterior third of the sagittal sinus, if torn, may also be doubly ligated. The posterior two-thirds of the sagittal sinus and confluence of sinuses must be repaired to maintain the continuity of blood flow.

In the repair of a cranionasal fistula or a cranioaural fistula, the use of a fascial transplant is desirable. A complete watertight closure of the area of fistulous communication must be accomplished. Patients having repeated meningitis following a head injury should have an adequate exposure of the area of fistulous communication for repair. Closure may be made with either mattress sutures or a fascial transplant. When extensively torn areas are exposed, a piece of fascia lata, obtained from the thigh, may be sutured as a graft inside the dural opening. The use of muscle stamps or Gelfoam should not be depended upon when closure by suture or a graft can be effected. The opening in the bone may be closed with a methylmetacrylate prosthesis.

In the management of the patient with an epidural hematoma, an adequate craniotomy opening should be made over the clot, the clot removed and the bleeding vessel controlled. With a posterior fossa epidural hematoma, exploration in the vicinity of an occipital fracture may be followed by enlarging this opening to an adequate size for removal of the clot.

The use of multiple trephine openings to drain and counterdrain the liquid clot of a subdural hematoma is frequently successful. When the clotted material is solid, a small bone flap is indicated. Bilateral explorations should always be carried out. Subdural accumulation of cerebrospinal fluid is best treated by trephine openings on the affected side. Such collections are often bilateral.

Intracerebral hematomas may be identified through a trephine opening. They may be drained through a larger craniotomy opening after the area of hemorrhage is uncapped by applying suction to the overlying thin cortex if the clot is mostly fluid. When the clot is solid, an adequate bone flap, uncapping of the clot by suction, and removal are indicated.

READING REFERENCES

Brock, S.: Injuries of the Brain and Spinal Cord and Their Coverings. 4th ed. New York, Springer Publishing Co., Inc., 1960.
Cairns, H., Calvert, C. A., Daniel, P., and Northcroft, G. B.: Complications of head wounds with especial reference to infection. Brit. J. Surg., War Supplement No. 1. Bristol, J. Wright & Sons, 1947, p. 198.
Clinical Neurosurgery. Vol. 12. Baltimore, Williams & Wilkins Company, 1966.
Coley, B. L.: Neoplasms of Bone. New York, Paul B. Hoeber, Inc., 1960.
Davis, L., and Davis, R. A.: Principles of Neurological Surgery. Philadelphia, W. B. Saunders Company, 1963.

Denny-Brown, D.: Cerebral concussion. Physiol. Rev. 25:296, 1945.

Fremont-Smith, F., and Kubie, L. S.: The relation of vascular hydrostatic pressure and osmotic pressure to the cerebrospinal fluid pressure. Pro. Assn. Res. Nerv. & Ment. Dis. 8:114, 1929.

Galicich, J. H., and French, L. A.: Use of dexamethasone in the treatment of cerebral edema resulting from brain tumors and brain surgery. Am. Pract. Digest Treat. 12:169, 1961.

Gurdjian, E. S., and Webster, J. E.: Head Injuries—Mechanisms, Diagnosis and Management. Boston, Little, Brown & Company, 1958.

Head Injury Conference Proceedings. (Caveness, W. F., and Walker, A. E., eds.) Philadelphia, J. B. Lippincott Company, 1966.

Javid, M.: Urea in intracranial surgery—a new method. J. Neurosurg. 18:51, 1961.

Kennedy, F., and Wortis, H.: "Acute" subdural hematomas and epidural hemorrhage; study of 72 cases of hematoma and 17 cases of hemorrhage. Surg. Gyn. & Obst. 63:732, 1936.

Martin, J., and Campbell, E. H.: Early complications following penetrating wounds of the skull. J. Neurosurg. 3:58, 1946.

Putnam, T., and Cushing, H.: Chronic subdural hematoma, its pathology, its relation to pachymeningitis hemorrhagica and its surgical treatment. Arch. Surg. 11:329, 1925.

Rowbotham, G. F.: Injuries of the Head. 4th ed. Baltimore, Williams & Wilkins Company, 1964.

Shenkin, H. A., Goluboff, B., and Haft, H.: The use of mannitol for the reduction of intracranial pressure in intracranial surgery. J. Neurosurg. 19:897, 1962.

Surgery in World War II: Neurosurgery, Vol. 1. Office of the Surgeon General, Department of the Army, Washington, D.C., 1958.

Chapter 14

THE EYES, EYELIDS AND ORBITS

by

BRADLEY R. STRAATSMA, M.D.

After graduating with honors from Lawrenceville School, BRADLEY R. STRAATSMA returned to the University of Michigan in his native state. He received his doctor of medicine degree from Yale University School of Medicine. He continued to receive honors during his education in ophthalmology at the Institute of Ophthalmology of Presbyterian Hospital, New York, and Wilmer Institute of The Johns Hopkins University School of Medicine. In 1964, Dr. Straatsma became Professor of Surgery/Ophthalmology, Director, Jules Stein Eye Institute, and Chief, Division of Ophthalmology, Department of Surgery, University of California School of Medicine, Los Angeles.

Ophthalmology is the medical science that encompasses knowledge concerning the eyes, eyelids, orbits and other components of the visual system. For practical application, this knowledge, derived from many basic and clinical fields, must be carefully synthesized so that the patient may receive the best care. It is important that the physician have an understanding of the essential features of anatomy, the requirements of clinical examination, and the most important abnormalities of the visual system.

ANATOMY

EYELIDS. The eyelids extend from the brow to the cheek and from the medial margin of the orbit to the lateral orbital margin. In cross section, the principal layers of the lids are the skin, orbicularis oculi muscle, tarsus and septum orbitale and conjunctiva (Fig. 1). The levator palpebrae muscle inserts into the skin, tarsus and conjunctiva of the upper lid.

The blood supply of the lids is derived from the facial arterial system and the ophthalmic artery. Veins drain into a superficial system on the face and into a deep system joining the pterygoid plexus and cavernous sinus. Innervation of the orbicularis muscle is by the facial nerve and the levator muscle is supplied by the oculomotor nerve. The sensory nerve supply is from the first and second divi-

sions of the trigeminal nerve. Lymphatics drain into the preauricular and submaxillary nodes.

On each eyelid, the lacrimal drainage system begins at the punctum located on the lid margin near the inner canthus. From the punctum, this system extends through the canaliculus to the lacrimal sac and to the nasolacrimal duct which empties into the nasal cavity below the inferior turbinate.

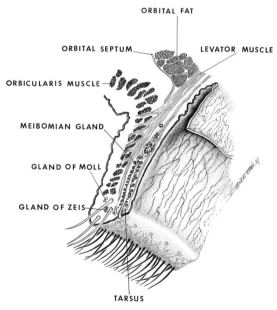

Figure 1.   The upper eyelid in cross section.

CONJUNCTIVA. The conjunctiva is the mucous membrane that lines the posterior surface of the eyelid, forms folds in the fornix and is reflected over the globe to the corneal margin. The lacrimal gland delivers fluid into the conjunctival sac through ten or 12 ducts which enter the temporal aspect of the superior fornix. Accessory lacrimal glands and goblet cells supply additional conjunctival moisture.

CORNEA AND SCLERA. Essentially, the adult eye is a sphere with an average diameter of approximately 24 mm. (Fig. 2). The outer layer of the eye is formed by the cornea and the sclera. The transparent avascular cornea has a diameter of about 12 mm. and a thickness of 0.6 to 1.0 mm. It is composed of five layers: the epithelium, Bowman's membrane, stroma, Descemet's membrane and endothelium. It obtains a sensory nerve supply from the first division of the trigeminal nerve. The eye contains no lymphatics. Forming the opaque posterior portion of the outer ocular layer is the sclera which is made up primarily of fibrous tissue and has blood vessels only in its superficial portion.

UVEA. Lying internal to the cornea and sclera, the uvea consists of the iris, the ciliary body and the choroid. The iris is a thin sheet of tissue arising from the ciliary body and extending into the eye anterior to the lens. This sheet forms the boundary between the anterior and posterior chambers of the eye and demarcates the pupil. By action of the sphincter muscle of the iris, innervated by the parasympathetic system, and the dilator muscle, which receives its nerve supply from the sympathetic system, the pupil may vary from a diameter of less than 2 mm. in bright light to a diameter of about 8 mm. in dim illumination.

The ciliary body forms a ring of tissue, measuring about 6 mm. in anteroposterior dimension. Anteriorly, it is attached to the iris and scleral spur and posteriorly, it joins the choroid. The thick anterior portion of the ciliary body contains the ciliary muscle which is active in accommodation. The internal portion consists of epithelial layers intimately related to the formation of aqueous humor.

The choroid is a pigmented, extremely vascular layer extending from the posterior border of the ciliary body to the margin of the optic nerve head. The external layers contain large blood vessels. Internal to these is a rich layer of capillaries and Bruch's membrane. From these choroidal vessels, the fovea and the external portion of the retina receive nourishment.

The blood supply of the uvea is derived from six to 20 short posterior ciliary arteries, two long posterior ciliary arteries, and seven or eight anterior ciliary arteries. Venous outflow is by way of four large vortex veins and several anterior ciliary veins.

RETINA. The retina is the thin neurosensory tissue of the eye. Located internal to the choroid, this structure originates at the optic disc, extends past the highly specialized macular region and terminates anteriorly at the ora serrata. The retina is composed of ten layers which are, from the external to the internal surface: the pigment epithelium, rod and cone layer, external limiting membrane, outer nuclear layer, outer plexiform layer, inner nuclear layer, inner plexiform layer, ganglion cell layer, nerve fiber layer and internal limiting membrane. The blood supply for the external retinal layers and the fovea is derived from the choroidal circulation. The internal portion of the retina is supplied by the central retinal artery, the central retinal vein and the intervening network of vessels and capillaries.

Closely related to the retina is the optic disc, which measures about 1.75 mm. in diameter and is round or vertically oval in shape. Visible on the optic disc are the optic nerve fibers, a physiologic cup and the central retinal vessels.

LENS AND VITREOUS. The crystalline lens

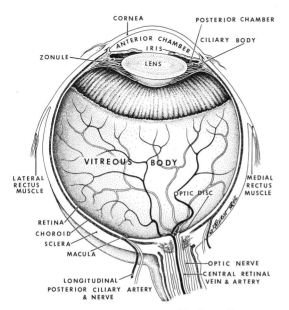

Figure 2. The eye sectioned horizontally.

is a transparent, avascular, biconvex structure located between the iris and the vitreous and suspended from the ciliary body by means of the zonule. Viewed from in front, the lens is a round structure with a diameter of about 9 mm., whereas it is approximately 4.0 mm. in thickness at the lens axis. The lens is made up of a clear and rather homogeneous lens capsule surrounding a single layer of cuboidal lens epithelium and a mass of elongated, regularly arranged lens fibers. The suspensory zonule of the lens is a sheet-like group of fibers that arises from the ciliary body and arches forward and centrally to insert into the lens capsule.

Immediately posterior to the lens and zonule and occupying about two-thirds of the volume of the eye is the vitreous. This is a transparent gel-like material of semisolid consistency containing water, a collagen type protein, hyaluronic acid and other components.

ORBIT. The orbit is the cavity that contains the eye and related tissues. Located just lateral to the nasal cavity and superior to the maxillary sinus, the orbit is shaped like a four-sided pyramid with its base anteriorly and its apex posteriorly situated. The bony orbit is formed by seven bones: three midline bones, the sphenoid, frontal and ethmoid, and four paired bones, the zygomatic, maxillary, lacrimal and palatine. Principal openings of the bony orbit include the anterior opening for exposure of the eye, the optic canal, the superior orbital fissure and the inferior orbital fissure.

Contents of the orbit include the eye, the optic nerve and its sheaths, the six extraocular muscles, the levator muscle, Müller's muscle, blood vessels and nerves. For the most part, these structures are surrounded by orbital fat and supported by an elaborate system of fascia.

EXTRAOCULAR MUSCLES. Six extraocular muscles control the movements of each eye. These muscles may be grouped in three pairs. The medial and lateral rectus muscles arise at the apex of the orbit and insert anterior to the equator of the eye in a horizontal plane. The superior and inferior rectus muscles arise at the apex of the orbit and insert anterior to the equator of the eye in a vertical plane that forms an angle of 23 degrees with the sagittal plane. The superior oblique arises at the apex of the orbit and is reflected about the trochlea in its course to the eye, whereas the inferior oblique arises in the

inferior portion of the anteromedial orbit. Both oblique muscles insert posterior to the equator of the eye in a vertical plane which forms an angle of 51 degrees with the sagittal plane. Richly supplied with nerve fibers, the lateral rectus is innervated by the abducens nerve, the superior oblique by the trochlear nerve and the other muscles by the oculomotor nerve.

With the eye in the primary or straight ahead position, the muscles have actions derived from their position of insertion on the eye and the plane of muscle action. These actions are: medial rectus – adduction; lateral rectus – abduction; superior rectus – elevation, adduction and intorsion; inferior rectus – depression, adduction and extorsion; superior oblique – depression, abduction and intorsion; and inferior oblique – elevation, abduction and extorsion.

OPHTHALMIC EXAMINATION

VISUAL ACUITY. The visual acuity of each eye is recorded for distance and near vision. Measurements of distance acuity use the Snellen system, which recognizes that the normal eye can distinguish letters or symbols subtending an angle of 5 minutes of arc when projected to the nodal point of the eye. Visual acuity is then recorded as a mathematical expression in which the numerator is the distance from the eye to the chart and the denominator is the distance at which the letters or symbols subtend 5 minutes of arc. For example, normal visual acuity is 20/20, whereas 20/40 is less than normal visual acuity.

Near vision is measured with various standard test types held at the conventional reading distance. For example, the normal eye of a young adult can distinguish size 0.37 mm. type, significantly smaller than newsprint, at 13 inches.

OCULAR MOTILITY. Ocular motility is evaluated by observing the alignment of the eyes in the primary position, the rotations of the eyes and the near point of convergence. In the primary position with the eyes straight ahead, alignment of the eyes may be determined grossly by general inspection and more accurately by noting the corneal light reflexes when the patient is looking directly at a light. Normally, the light reflexes are symmetrical and located just nasal to the center of the cornea. The cover-uncover test reveals even more precise information about alignment. The test is carried out while a patient with reasonably good vision in each eye is looking at a light or an object. An opaque cover is then placed over one eye. If the uncovered eye does not move, there is no evidence of tropia, a manifest deviation of alignment; but if the uncovered eye moves, a tropia is present. After the reaction is noted, the cover is removed completely and placed over the opposite eye while the response is again observed.

Rotations of the eyes are tested by requiring movement of the eyes into the cardinal positions of gaze. The near point of convergence is measured by noting the point on which both eyes can converge when an object is brought toward the patient.

EXTERNAL OCULAR EXAMINATION. The external ocular examination is designed to reveal characteristics of the facial area, the prominence of the eyes, and features of the eyelids, lacrimal apparatus, conjunctiva and cornea.

PUPIL REACTIONS, IRIS AND ANTERIOR CHAMBER. The pupils are observed for size, shape and equality. Reactions to light, direct and consensual, and to the near reflex are routinely tested. With oblique illumination, the iris is observed and the depth of the anterior chamber is estimated.

MEDIA AND FUNDI. Appraisal of media and fundi may be accomplished with direct and indirect ophthalmoscopy and with biomicroscopy. When direct ophthalmoscopy is used, the media are observed by directing the light into the patient's eye from a distance of 12 inches. Opacities interfere with the normal red reflex. Fundus examination is conducted with the instrument an inch or two from the eye while optic disc, retinal vessels, macula and general fundus areas are systematically observed.

INTRAOCULAR TENSION. Pressure within the eye may be estimated by palpation, indentation tonometry and applanation tonometry. Normally, intraocular pressure is maintained at 15 to 22 mm. of mercury above atmospheric pressure.

VISUAL FIELD. Visual field examination is used to determine the extent of the visual field of each eye and the relative sensitivity in various parts of the visual field. The field of vision may be evaluated by general confrontation methods, perimetry and tangent screen studies.

EYELIDS

ABNORMALITIES IN FORM AND POSITION. The principal abnormalities in form and position of the eyelids are epicanthus, ptosis, lagophthalmos, entropion and ectropion. Epicanthus is a fold of skin overlying the inner aspect of the palpebral fissure. The condition is normal in Orientals. It is also common in Caucasians during the early years of life, but as the face and features develop, the condition usually disappears and only rarely is surgical therapy indicated.

Ptosis of the upper lid is generally related to a defect in the levator muscle, an abnormality of the oculomotor nerve, myasthenia gravis, the mechanical effect of an eyelid mass or trauma. Treatment varies with the etiology and degree of the ptosis, but frequently the surgical procedure of choice is shortening or resection of the levator muscle.

The general converse of ptosis is lagophthalmos, or inability to close the palpebral fissure. This abnormality may result from many causes including paralysis of the orbicularis muscle, thyroid disease, exophthalmos, scarring of the lid or absence of the lid. When lagophthalmos is present, the cornea must be protected from excessive exposure and drying by the use of lubricants, protective dressings, a scleral type of contact lens, intermarginal eyelid adhesions and, if necessary, a reconstructive eyelid operation.

Entropion, or posterior turning of the eyelid margin, is classified as congenital, spastic, cicatricial or senile in type. In this condition, the cilia are apt to damage the cornea and this occurrence often warrants an eyelid operation.

An anterior turning of the eyelid margin, known as ectropion, may be of the congenital, spastic, paralytic, cicatricial or senile type. Usually, this condition affects the lower lid and permits tears to accumulate between the eye and the lid so that they overflow onto the cheek and irritate the skin. Therapy for this condition consists of surgical measures to correct the anterior turning of the eyelid and to restore normal relationship between the eyelid and the eye.

CIRCULATORY AND INFLAMMATORY DISORDERS. Circulatory and inflammatory disorders of the eyelids assume importance by virtue of their common occurrence. These disorders include edema of the lid, inflammation of the eyelid skin, inflammation of the lid margin and disorders of the eyelid glands. Because the skin is thin and loosely attached to underlying tissues, edema of the lid is often severe. Some of the generalized diseases responsible for eyelid edema are nephritis, trichinosis and angioneurotic reactions. Local causes include inflammation, allergy and injury. In all instances, treatment is related to the specific cause of the condition.

Inflammation of the eyelid skin, generally related to eczema, herpes zoster or vaccinia, is less common than inflammation of the eyelid margin. The latter presents in several forms. Squamous or seborrheic marginal blepharitis generally occurs in conjunction with seborrhea of the scalp or brow and is characterized by crusts and scales on the lid margin. Ulcerative blepharitis is usually caused by staphylococcal infection and associated with ulceration of the lid margin and loss of the eyelashes. Many patients have a mixture of seborrheic and ulcerative blepharitis. Angular blepharitis, caused by the diplobacillus of Morax-Axenfeld, typically causes inflammation of the lid margin near the lateral canthus. Treatment of marginal blepharitis combines therapy of scalp seborrhea with antibacterial measures, careful cleansing of the eyelid margin and, occasionally, topical corticosteroids.

The numerous glands of the eyelid may also become obstructed or inflamed. On the skin, subacute or acute inflammation may occur in the sebaceous or sweat glands, or develop in retention cysts derived from these glands. Affecting the lid margin, an external hordeolum, or stye, is a purulent infection of a sebaceous or sweat gland closely associated with the cilia. An internal hordeolum, or acute chalazion, is a comparable acute inflammatory process affecting a meibomian gland. Treatment of these inflammatory disorders consists of warm compresses, antibacterial agents and incision when the process is fully localized and spontaneous drainage is delayed.

Chalazion is a chronic inflammation of a meibomian gland which occurs when the gland is obstructed and infected. Chalazion is characterized by variable signs of inflammation and development of a firm nodule in the tarsal plate. The condition may drain spontaneously through conjunctiva, skin or the duct of the affected meibomian gland but frequently requires surgical treatment. This is aided by a clamp surrounding the

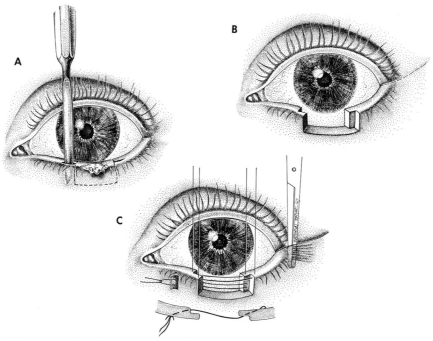

Figure 3.   Eyelid reconstruction. For reconstruction of one-third or less of the eyelid, tissue is sectioned in the pretarsal plane medial and lateral to the lesion (*A*). Tissue posterior to the split on the nasal side and anterior to the split on the temporal side is removed along with the lesion (*B*). A lateral canthotomy is performed to mobilize the remaining temporal portion of the lid. With a suture, the medial and lateral edges of the lid are overlapped (*C*). Redundant tissue adjacent to the repair and at the base of the canthotomy is excised to complete the reconstruction.

lesion which minimizes bleeding while the process is incised and the necrotic and inflamed tissue is removed.

TUMORS. Benign tumors of the eyelids include dermoids, nevi, hemangiomas, papillomas and neurofibromas. When these lesions are small and do not involve the lid margin, removal may often be effected by means of an elliptical excision oriented so that the axis is parallel to Langer's lines and the skin folds are related to habitual contraction of the facial muscles.

Basal cell carcinoma is the malignant tumor of the eyelid encountered most frequently. Other malignant tumors of the eyelid are squamous cell carcinoma and malignant melanoma. When excision of these tumors is indicated, various surgical procedures are feasible. For example, a method utilizing a sliding flap is suitable for reconstruction after removal of one-third or less of the lid (Fig. 3).

INJURIES. Eyelid injuries are capable of causing edema, erythema, ecchymosis, laceration, emphysema, if underlying fractures extend into the nasal cavity or sinuses, necrosis and loss of tissue. Management is based on the application of basic principles such as the prompt irrigation of chemical injuries, careful cleansing of contaminated wounds, preservation of as much tissue as possible and meticulous suturing of lacerations. In every instance of eyelid injury, the eye itself must be carefully examined and the cornea protected from exposure and drying.

LACRIMAL APPARATUS

LACRIMAL SECRETORY SYSTEM. Insufficient tear formation is a not uncommon consequence of inflammation, injury or involution of the lacrimal gland and the accessory structures of the lacrimal secretory system. This insufficiency may lead to corneal drying or ulceration and necessitate the use of artificial tear solutions. In contrast to this, an excess of tear formation is associated with many painful ocular disorders.

Although these conditions are important aberrations of the lacrimal secretory system, the principal indication for surgical therapy is enlargement of the gland, which may occur in conjunction with acute inflammation, chronic inflammation and tumors. As a result of this diverse etiology, patients with lacrimal gland enlargement should undergo careful general evaluation. When operation is indicated, a small and well localized lacrimal gland lesion of unknown cause should be removed by an excision of the entire abnormal process. When the enlargement is extensive or diffuse, the diagnosis should be established by biopsy before a more extensive operation is undertaken.

LACRIMAL DRAINAGE SYSTEM. Congenital obstruction, inflammation, acquired obstruction, tumors and injuries are the most important clinical conditions affecting the lacrimal drainage system. Congenital obstruction is usually caused by a persistent membrane at the lower end of the nasolacrimal duct. With conservative management, the obstruction generally corrects itself but probing of the lacrimal passages and rupture of the persistent membrane is occasionally necessary.

Inflammation of the canaliculus may be associated with a concretion of *Actinomyces israeli* (Streptothrix) and dacryocystitis may be either a cause or an effect of lacrimal passage obstruction. In any case, offending concretions should be removed and the infection controlled with appropriate agents.

Persistent acquired obstruction of the lacrimal passages causes epiphora, an abnormal overflow of tears onto the eyelid and cheek, or recurrent infections. When symptoms warrant, the exact site of obstruction should be determined by clinical and radiological studies of the lacrimal passages. Surgical procedures such as dacryocystorhinostomy can then be employed to restore the flow of tears from the eye to the nasal cavity.

Tumors of the lacrimal passages are rare and are treated by excision of the involved structures. Injuries may interfere with lacrimal passage integrity at any one of several sites. For example, a relatively minor appearing laceration on the eyelid between the lacrimal punctum and the inner canthus may sever the lacrimal canaliculus. Therefore, when an injury involves this area, the status of the lacrimal structures should be determined and a divided canaliculus should be repaired promptly. In the facial area, a severe injury may cause obstruction of the lacrimal duct and necessitate a dacryocystorhinostomy.

CONJUNCTIVA

CIRCULATORY AND INFLAMMATORY DISORDERS. The principal circulatory disorders of the conjunctiva are superficial congestion, deep congestion, subconjunctival hemorrhage and edema. Superficial congestion, a result of virtually any type of conjunctival irritation, is characterized by pink tortuous vessels that are more prominent near the fornix than the limbus. Irritation or inflammation of the anterior segment of the eye causes deep or ciliary congestion with dark red straight vessels that are most prominent near the limbus. Subconjunctival hemorrhage appears as a sharply outlined, bright red accumulation of blood beneath the conjunctiva. It may be related to straining, hemorrhagic tendency or injury but usually develops without known cause and generally absorbs spontaneously in a few days. Edema of the conjunctiva results from local irritation, or from inflammation due to generalized disorders such as nephritis and dysthyroid ophthalmopathy.

Conjunctival inflammation may be caused by bacterial, viral or fungal infection, allergy, or injury. All forms of conjunctivitis are characterized by itching, burning and a foreign body sensation associated with variable discharge, superficial conjunctival congestion, chemosis, conjunctival follicles and papules. Treatment includes measures appropriate for the etiologic agent, removal of discharge and symptomatic therapy.

DEGENERATIONS AND TUMORS. Pinguecula is a conjunctival degeneration which increases in incidence with age and is nearly universal in older people. It consists of a discrete, slightly elevated, cream-colored lesion located within the palpebral fissure medial and lateral to the cornea. No treatment is necessary, although the process may be excised for cosmetic reasons.

Benign tumors of the conjunctiva include dermoids, nevi, hemangiomas, papillomas and neurofibromas. Malignant neoplasms include squamous cell carcinomas and malignant melanomas. When excision of these conditions is carried out, epithelialization by growth from intact adjacent conjunctiva may be permitted, but small defects are usually closed with sutures and larger defects are reconstructed with conjunctival flaps or grafts.

INJURIES. Foreign bodies in the conjunctival sac often adhere to the tarsal conjunctiva of the upper lid but may also lodge at other sites. Usually, they can be removed with a sterile cotton applicator. If any dis-

comfort for the patient is anticipated, topical anesthesia is indicated.

Other forms of conjunctival injury are contusions, lacerations and burns. Chemical burns should be irrigated immediately with sterile saline or other appropriate solution. Copious irrigation should be continued for an extended period and care by a fully qualified physician is indicated. Many chemical burns of the eye are more serious than they appear initially.

CORNEA

CIRCULATORY AND INFLAMMATORY DISORDERS. Circulatory disorders of the cornea consist of deep or ciliary congestion, the growth of vessels into the cornea and corneal edema. Related to inflammation in the cornea or anterior segment of the eye, ciliary congestion is characterized by dilated, dark red vessels radiating from the corneal limbus. Persistent corneal inflammation may stimulate the growth of vessels into the cornea from the superficial conjunctival network or the deep ciliary arteries located in the limbal area. Edema of the cornea is associated with corneal inflammation but may also occur as a result of a disorder affecting the corneal endothelium or epithelium.

Corneal inflammation is caused by bacterial, viral or fungal infection; allergy; corneal exposure; trophic disorders; dermatologic disease, and systemic disease. This inflammation is usually accompanied by pain, photophobia and lacrimation in conjunction with variable signs such as ciliary congestion, corneal infiltration, discharge, iridocyclitis and hypopyon, a sterile collection of pus cells in the anterior chamber. As with all conditions, treatment is directed toward control of the etiologic factor whenever possible, and supplemented by appropriate measures to protect the cornea, alleviate any associated iridocyclitis and provide symptomatic relief.

DEGENERATIONS AND TUMORS. Arcus senilis, a common corneal degeneration, is present to some extent in most people over 50 years of age and rarely may be related to a metabolic disorder. It takes the form of a gray-white corneal band, concentric with the limbus but separated from it by a transparent zone. No treatment of this condition is indicated.

Pterygium is a degeneration of the cornea

which occurs most commonly in the nasal periphery and stimulates ingrowth of a wedge of vascularized conjunctiva. If the process is progressive, surgical removal of the abnormal vascularized tissue is necessary.

Keratoconus, a progressive thinning and bulging of the cornea, and the hereditary corneal dystrophies, progressive disorders affecting corneal transparency, are degenerations that frequently necessitate corneal transplantation. For these conditions, a full thickness or penetrating corneal transplant is used to replace the central portion of the patient's cornea. Donor material is obtained by the aseptic removal of eyes at autopsy. This material is carefully preserved and used as soon as possible. At the time of operation, the graft is cut from the donor cornea with a trephine. An opening of identical size is made in the patient's cornea and the graft secured in place with multiple, fine caliber, edge-to-edge sutures (Fig. 4). The operating microscope greatly facilitates this procedure.

Tumors of the cornea consist of dermoids, dyskeratosis of various types, squamous cell carcinomas and malignant melanomas. Excision of these growths is usually indicated and the resulting corneal defect often can be repaired with a lamellar or nonpenetrating corneal transplant.

INJURIES. A small, superficial corneal foreign body produces a localized ulceration which often becomes surrounded by a ring of rust, carbon or other material related to the composition of the foreign body. Removal of the foreign body along with the associated ring of altered cornea is performed under topical anesthesia with a sterile spud or knife blade held parallel to the surface of the cornea and used to lift the particle and associated necrotic material from the corneal ulcer. Magnification and oblique illumination greatly facilitate this procedure. After removal of the foreign body, topical antibiotics and a firm protective dressing over the closed lids facilitate healing of the corneal ulcer.

Corneal abrasions, burns and lacerations are additional forms of injury. Associated with pain, photophobia and lacrimation, corneal abrasions are detected by using a sterile solution of sodium fluorescein to stain the denuded area a bright green. Treatment with topical antibiotics and a firm bandage over the injured eye enhances healing. The blink reflex protects the cornea from most serious thermal burns, but chemical burns of very severe degree are not uncommon. They are always associated with conjunctival burns and are treated with irrigation.

Full thickness lacerations of the cornea are always serious. When detected, all unnecessary manipulation of the eyes and of the patient must be avoided and repair should be carried out by a fully qualified physician as soon as possible. Whenever the history or findings of clinical examination suggest the possibility of a retained intraocular foreign body, x-ray studies and measures such as ultrasonography and electronic foreign body detection should be employed to reveal the presence of intraocular foreign material.

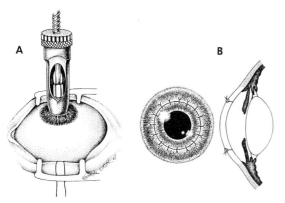

Figure 4. Penetrating corneal transplant. For penetrating keratoplasty, the graft is cut from the donor eye with a trephine. An opening of identical size is made in the patient's cornea with a trephine (A) and the graft is secured in place with multiple, fine caliber, edge-to-edge sutures (B).

SCLERA

INFLAMMATORY DISORDERS. Episcleritis is an inflammation of the superficial sclera associated with mild ocular irritation and deep red congestion of the episcleral vessels. Scleritis constitutes more extensive inflammation of the sclera with variable pain, episcleral congestion, scleral infiltration and uveal inflammation. The etiology of scleral inflammation includes rheumatoid and collagen diseases, granulomatous inflammatory diseases and allergic conditions; but in many patients, it is unknown. Treatment is directed to control of the cause whenever possible and to alleviation of the condition with symptomatic therapy and corticosteroids.

Inflammatory disorders, developmental

malformations and other conditions may be responsible for scleral thinning. Subjected to intraocular pressure, these thinned areas bulge and, because they are lined with pigmented uveal tissue, produce dark staphylomas. Scleral grafts may be used in the treatment of these staphylomas.

INJURIES. Burns, lacerations and other injuries of the sclera are comparable to corresponding corneal injuries. Therefore, management is the same as that for corneal trauma.

UVEA

DEVELOPMENTAL ABNORMALITIES. Typical coloboma of the uvea is a developmental defect resulting from faulty closure of the fetal, choroidal fissure. This defect, associated with virtual absence of the choroid and marked attenuation of the retina, presents as a white lesion possibly involving the optic disc, the retina and choroid inferior to the disc and a corresponding portion of the ciliary body and iris.

Atypical colobomas of the ciliary body and iris may occur in any meridian. Not related to the choroidal fissure, these defects occur where persistent blood vessels at the edge of the optic cup prevent normal development of the ciliary body and iris. There is no treatment for these developmental abnormalities.

INFLAMMATORY DISORDERS. Uveal inflammation is classified as suppurative and nonsuppurative and further considered as anterior iritis, cyclitis and iridocyclitis; posterior choroiditis and chorioretinitis, or diffuse uveitis.

Suppurative uveitis is usually related to an accidental wound, a perforated corneal ulcer or a surgical incision, but it may also be due to metastatic spread of a pyogenic infection. Arising from these causes, the purulent process may affect the anterior, posterior or entire uveal tract. Sometimes, it can be controlled with antibiotics, but all too frequently the inflammation produces severe damage or even total destruction of the eye.

Nonsuppurative uveitis is usually endogenous and of unknown etiology, but anterior uveitis of this type does occur in association with joint disease, such as ankylosing spondylitis, Still's disease and Reiter's syndrome, Boeck's sarcoid and infection. In addition, it may develop as an allergic reaction to focal infection or protein materials. Posterior non-suppurative uveitis is related to infection, protozoal disease and parasitic infestation. When diffuse, the process may be related to any of these conditions. Clinical forms of nonsuppurative endogenous uveitis have important distinguishing features.

Acute iridocyclitis is associated with a rather abrupt onset of pain, photophobia, lacrimation and some impairment of vision in addition to ciliary congestion, small keratic precipitates on the corneal endothelium, cells and flare in the anterior chamber and miosis. Adhesions between the iris and the lens may form and glaucoma can also develop. Prompt treatment with mydriatic-cycloplegics and topical corticosteroids is effective in preventing synechiae and the inflammation usually subsides in a few weeks. The pathology of acute iridocyclitis is a nongranulomatous inflammation.

Chronic iridocyclitis is accompanied by the insidious onset of mild pain, photophobia, lacrimation and vision impairment, in association with faint ciliary congestion, keratic precipitates on the corneal endothelium, cells and flare in the anterior chamber, miosis and extensive posterior synechiae. In some patients, glaucoma occurs and secondary cataract may develop. The insidious onset often delays discovery of the disorder, but treatment with mydriatic-cycloplegics and topical corticosteroids is indicated. Usually persisting for several months, chronic iridocyclitis is related to granulomatous inflammation.

Acute chorioretinitis is characterized by the rapid development of spots in the field of vision, a decrease in visual acuity and the accumulation of cells and fibrous material in the vitreous. Frequently, ophthalmoscopic examination reveals an acute chorioretinal lesion which initially appears yellowish and poorly demarcated but at a later stage is sharply outlined and associated with scarring and irregular pigmentation. Permanent vision loss is related to the size and location of this lesion. Treatment includes mydriatic-cycloplegics and in many instances systemic corticosteroids. Tissue studies reveal a nongranulomatous inflammatory process.

Chronic chorioretinitis is accompanied by the insidious onset of spots and cobwebs in the field of vision, a decrease in vision, cells and fibrous strands in the vitreous and in most instances one or more areas of visible chorioretinal inflammation. This inflammation progresses through active stages and terminates in a chorioretinal scar. The course is prolonged, and glaucoma, secondary cataract, macular degeneration, retinal detachment, degeneration of the eye and total loss of vision can occur. Treatment is directed toward the etiology, if known, and also includes mydriatic-cycloplegics and selective use of systemic corticosteroids. The pathologic process is a granulomatous inflammatory reaction.

Diffuse uveitis may be acute or chronic and assume various forms, but sympathetic ophthalmia is the most important entity in this group. Sympathetic ophthalmia is a bilateral, diffuse, granulomatous uveitis of unknown etiology that develops ten or more days after a perforating wound involving uveal tissue. Rarely, it follows a surgical wound, but after accidental corneoscleral perforation, 1 to 2 per cent of the injured eyes contract sympathetic ophthalmia. When this occurs, the signs and symptoms of chronic iridocyclitis and chronic chorioretinitis develop insidiously and vision may be seriously damaged or lost in one or both eyes. Treatment is prophylactic removal of hopelessly damaged eyes during the ten days after injury and, if sympathetic ophthalmia occurs, prolonged therapy with mydriatic-cycloplegics and corticosteroids.

DEGENERATIONS. Essential atrophy of the iris is a progressive degenerative disorder characterized by loss of iris substance, distortion of the pupil and development of secondary glaucoma. Treatment is directed toward control of the glaucoma. Choroidal degenerations usually involve the retina.

TUMORS. Of great clinical importance, uveal tumors include benign melanomas, malignant melanomas, hemangiomas and uveal manifestations of disseminated neoplastic disease.

Benign melanomas are surprisingly frequent in the uvea. In the iris, these tumors appear as localized, pigmented nodules which remain constant in size and shape throughout extended follow-up periods. Benign melanomas of the choroid present as small, flat, slate gray lesions; they do not interfere with vision and do not change in appearance over a prolonged period.

Malignant melanoma of the iris accounts for about 10 per cent of uveal melanomas. This condition usually occurs in Caucasians in the fourth or fifth decade of life, but may arise in any race and at virtually any age. It presents as a localized, dark lesion in the iris or as a diffuse iris tumor which causes glaucoma. Whenever possible, the tumor is excised by means of an iridectomy and only rarely is enucleation of the eye necessary. Five years after removal of the neoplasm more than 90 per cent of the patients are alive and apparently free of tumor.

Malignant melanoma of the ciliary body occurs more frequently than iris melanoma but is less common than choroidal melanoma. Ciliary body melanoma generally occurs in Caucasian adults and is often rather advanced before discovery. Characteristically, this tumor presents as a dark mass extending anteriorly into the chamber angle, medially to encroach on the lens, or posteriorly to invade the choroid. Treatment is by enucleation of the eye and, rarely, by local excision of the tumor. The prognosis is comparable to that for malignant melanoma of the choroid.

Malignant melanoma of the choroid is the most common intraocular malignant tumor. Although this tumor is discovered most commonly in Caucasians during the fifth and sixth decades of life, it can occur in all races and at any age. The lesion usually presents as a localized dark mass arising from the choroid. To a variable extent the retina is detached and visual field and acuity are impaired to a corresponding degree. When advanced, the melanoma may be responsible for inflammation, hemorrhage or glaucoma. Spread of the tumor may be by direct extension through the sclera or by blood-borne metastasis to distant organs, principally the liver, and the long bones.

Choroidal malignant melanoma is treated by enucleation of the eye (Fig. 5). Prognosis depends on the size and histologic characteristics of the tumor as well as the presence or absence of extension beyond the sclera but, five years after enucleation, somewhat more than 50 per cent of the patients with malignant melanoma are alive and apparently free of tumor.

Other uveal tumors are benign hemangiomas, often part of the Sturge-Weber syndrome, malignant disorders of the reticuloendothelial system and metastatic carcinomas. The latter are often bilateral, related to primary carcinoma of the breast or lung, located in the posterior choroid and responsive to radiation therapy.

INJURIES. Injuries of the anterior uvea may result in iridocyclitis, iridodialysis, lacerations of the iris or ciliary body, paralysis

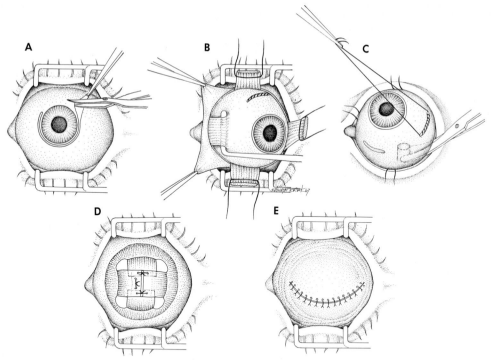

Figure 5. Enucleation. Enucleation is initiated with an incision of conjunctiva concentric with and adjacent to the cornea throughout 360 degrees (*A*). Extraocular muscles are divided near their scleral attachments (*B*) and the optic nerve is severed (*C*). After removal of the eye, an orbital implant is inserted and held in place by the extraocular muscles (*D*). Conjunctiva is then sutured over the implant and the extraocular muscles (*E*). After healing is complete, a cosmetic prosthesis is inserted in the conjunctival sac.

of the pupil or hemorrhage into the anterior chamber. Even a small hyphema may be complicated by additional and severe bleeding into the anterior chamber during the convalescent period. Therefore, the patient's activity should be severely curtailed and his treatment carefully supervised.

Injuries of the choroid may cause chorioretinitis, rupture of the choroid or choroidal hemorrhage. Treatment is guided by the extent and nature of the injury.

Following a perforating injury that involves any portion of the uvea, sympathetic ophthalmia may develop.

RETINA

CIRCULATORY DISORDERS. The most important retinal circulatory disorders are atherosclerosis, arteriolar sclerosis, arterial occlusion, venous occlusion, diabetic retinopathy and retrolental fibroplasia. Atherosclerosis is prone to develop in the central retinal artery where it penetrates the lamina cribrosa and at arteriovenous intersections in the adjacent retina. When visible ophthal-

moscopically, atheromas appear as irregular refractile lesions. Vessel occlusion is the principal adverse effect of atherosclerosis.

Arteriolar sclerosis is a rather diffuse disorder which produces alteration in arteriolar light reflex, changes at the artery-vein crossings and focal or generalized attenuation of the arteriolar lumen. This condition is frequently associated with hypertension.

Early or acute hypertension is characterized by a spastic focal or generalized attenuation of the arterioles. However, if hypertension persists for an extended period, arteriolar sclerosis develops. Therefore, in both acute and chronic hypertension, there is focal or generalized attenuation of the arteriolar blood column. Hypertension may also be responsible for retinal hemorrhages that are flame shaped if located in the nerve fiber layer, and round if located in the plexiform or nuclear layers of the retina; retinal edema and hard exudates which assume the pattern of a star in the macular region; small ischemic infarcts, appearing as cotton wool spots, and papilledema.

In appraising retinal changes associated with hypertension, it is important to evaluate signs of retinal vascular sclerosis and to evaluate, independently, alterations related to hypertension. In this way, the general duration of the disorder and probable response to blood pressure reduction, which would affect the manifestations of hypertension but not influence the features of sclerosis, can be estimated.

Occlusion of the central retinal artery or a branch usually occurs as a result of atherosclerosis, arteriolar sclerosis or embolism and produces sudden painless loss of vision. Following a central retinal artery occlusion, there is immediate segmentation of the blood column, retinal edema develops rapidly and a cherry-red spot becomes evident in the macula. Prompt treatment with massage of the eye to decrease intraocular pressure, paracentesis of the anterior chamber and vasodilators may be effective, but the usual result is permanent vision loss, attenuated retinal vessels and optic nerve degeneration.

Central retinal vein or branch occlusion, often secondary to sclerosis of the adjacent artery, is prone to occur at the lamina cribrosa or an artery-vein intersection. When vein occlusion occurs, the vision is decreased, vessels distal to the obstruction become dilated and tortuous and retinal hemorrhages and edema develop. Although treatment with anticoagulants may be effective, some degree of permanent vision impairment is customary and intractable hemorrhagic glaucoma may develop.

Diabetic retinopathy, one of the leading causes of blindness, may develop before the onset of abnormal carbohydrate metabolism but is usually associated with manifest diabetes mellitus of long duration. It is usually bilateral and characterized by angiopathy, exudates, proliferative processes and vitreous hemorrhages. Manifestations of angiopathy are microaneurysms, intraretinal or preretinal hemorrhages, retinal edema and venous dilatations. Exudates consist of hard, sharply demarcated, yellow-white deposits or soft cotton wool patches. Angiopathy and exudates may affect the macula and produce an impairment of vision.

Proliferative retinopathy is characterized by vasoproliferation and fibroproliferation on the inner surface of the retina and in the vitreous. All too frequently these proliferative processes are responsible for hemorrhages in the vitreous, traction on the retina and retinal detachment. Consequently, these proliferative and hemorrhagic alterations may produce vision impairment or total blindness. Treatment includes regulation of the diabetes mellitus and, in some instances of progressive retinopathy, photocoagulation of the retinal lesions, or pituitary stalk section.

Retrolental fibroplasia develops typically in the newborn premature infant exposed to excessive oxygen concentrations. It is usually bilateral and features retinal vascular abnormalities, retinal and vitreous hemorrhage, retinitis proliferans, retinal detachment and vision impairment or blindness. Treatment is preventive and related to the restriction of oxygen concentration during the neonatal period.

INFLAMMATORY DISORDERS. Other than chorioretinitis, retinal inflammation includes focal, infiltrative and hemorrhagic lesions associated with subacute bacterial endocarditis and retinal perivasculitis that may develop in the course of granulomatous infections, and other disorders. Whenever perivasculitis is related to a known granulomatous disease, treatment of the primary disorder is indicated. In other instances, retinal photocoagulation may be warranted in an effort to destroy areas of neovascularization and prevent recurrent intraocular hemorrhage.

DEGENERATIONS. Encompassing several significant conditions, degenerations of the retina and the closely related choroid include myopic degeneration, retinitis pigmentosa, drusen and macular degeneration. Myopic degeneration is associated with progressive deterioration of the retina and underlying choroid. This leads to formation of a temporal conus adjacent to the optic disc, degeneration of the macula and several types of peripheral fundus alteration. Surgical reinforcement of the sclera may be of value in selected patients with severe and progressive myopia, but there is no generally accepted method for arresting myopia or preventing the associated degeneration.

Retinitis pigmentosa is a condition of unknown etiology with a strong familial factor. Subjectively, the condition is associated with night blindness which may progress to tunnel vision and blindness. Objectively, there is scattered bone corpuscle pigmentation in the retina, attenuation of retinal vessels and waxy pallor of the optic disc. The primary process is degeneration of the retinal rods and cones and no effective treatment is known. Cataract, glaucoma, central nervous system disorders and systemic abnormalities are not infrequent in patients with retinitis pigmentosa.

Commonly present in the adult eye, drusen are excrescences on the external surface of the pigment epithelium and on the inner surface of the choroid. Appearing clinically as small yellow-white lesions, drusen do not cause any impairment of vision but are sometimes associated with macular degeneration.

Macular degeneration may occur at any age but senile macular degeneration affecting older individuals is most common. This disorder is characterized by painless loss of central vision, degeneration of the retina in the macula, alteration of the pigment epithelium in this area and, in some instances, choroidal hemorrhage which produces a disciform lesion in the posterior pole. Treatment is generally not effective.

DETACHMENT. Detachment of the sensory retina from the retinal pigment epithelium and choroid is a consequence of the normally weak anatomical union between these structures. When retinal detachment occurs, the retina is separated from its choroidal blood supply and a visual field defect corresponding to the involved section ensues. Moreover, once the process is initiated, there is no natural healing or delimiting process so the retinal detachment tends to become total.

Retinal detachment is generally related to an accumulation of material in the subretinal space, traction on the internal surface of the retina or holes and tears in the retina. The accumulation of material in the subretinal space may stem from hemorrhage, inflammatory diseases involving the choroid or retina or tumors such as malignant melanomas of the choroid.

Retinal detachment may also be caused by traction related to retinitis proliferans or organization in the vitreous body. In these circumstances, measures to reattach the retina are usually unsuccessful.

Retinal holes and tears caused by degeneration or trauma permit fluid from the vitreous to enter the subretinal space and separate the retina. Symptoms accompanying this condition include spots in the field of vision, light flashes and a fog or haze in the field of vision. Surgical therapy is designed to prevent retinal separation by the prophylactic treatment of appropriate retinal breaks and to reattach the retina when separation has occurred (Fig. 6). With operation, retinal

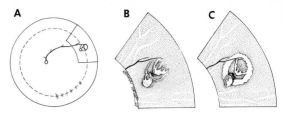

Figure 6.   Prophylaxis of retinal detachment. To prevent retinal detachment, a horseshoe-shaped retinal tear on the superior temporal quadrant of the fundus (*A* and *B*) is surrounded by a ring of chorioretinal reaction (*C*). In this case, photocoagulation was used to produce the reaction but diathermy and cryotherapy may also be employed to stimulate localized chorioretinal inflammation.

reattachment is achieved in about 75 per cent of the patients.

TUMORS. Arising from the retina, retinoblastoma is the most common malignant intraocular tumor in children. Significantly, there is a high incidence of this tumor in the offspring of retinoblastoma survivors and a lesser incidence in the siblings of retinoblastoma patients.

The condition affects both eyes in about half the patients and is usually discovered when an esotropia or an abnormal yellow-white appearance in the pupil prompts medical attention. Examination reveals a yellow-white neoplasm arising from the retina and extending into the vitreous cavity or the subretinal space. Spread from the eye is via the optic nerve or to distant bones and organs by way of blood-borne metastasis.

In almost all patients, treatment of unilateral retinoblastoma is enucleation of the involved eye. Bilateral disease is treated with enucleation of the eye containing the more advanced tumor and treatment of the opposite eye with radiation and chemotherapy, usually triethylenemelamine. About 80 per cent of patients with unilateral or bilateral disease are alive and apparently free of tumor five years after therapy. When the disease is bilateral, 50 per cent or more of the survivors retain some degree of useful vision in the eye treated with radiation and chemotherapy.

Gliomas and vascular tumors of the retina also occur but are relatively uncommon. Gliomas are slow-growing, white lesions, whereas angiomatosis retinae generally presents as one or more sharply demarcated pink-red tumors. Retinal photocoagulation has been of value in the therapy of retinal vascular tumors.

INJURIES. Retinal injuries include post-contusion retinal edema which appears as a diffuse white edema of the posterior retina with a cherry-red spot in the fovea, retinal hemorrhage, traumatic chorioretinitis, retinal breaks and retinal detachment. Management is in accordance with the nature of the retinal abnormality.

OPTIC NERVE

DEVELOPMENTAL ABNORMALITIES. Principal developmental anomalies of the visible intraocular portion of the optic nerve are medullated nerve fibers and pseudopapilledema. The former, related to anomalous myelination of the optic nerve fibers anterior to the lamina cribrosa, appears as one or more white patches with irregular, splayed ends on the optic disc or adjacent retina. Pseudopapilledema is characterized by indistinct or blurred margins and some elevation of the disc. Usually present in hyperopic eyes, pseudopapilledema is differentiated from papilledema by an appearance that does not change over an extended period and an absence of venous engorgement, hemorrhage or vision impairment.

Hypoplasia and other developmental abnormalities may affect the visible intraocular optic nerve or the more posterior portions located in the orbit, optic canal and cranium.

CIRCULATORY DISORDERS. Edema of the optic nerve head is called papilledema. In its early stages, blurring of the disc margin develops, the disc becomes hyperemic, the retinal veins become distended and the venous pulsation disappears. As the process continues, the physiologic cup is obliterated and the surrounding retina becomes edematous. Late in the course of papilledema, optic nerve degeneration may develop. Visual acuity is usually normal when papilledema is present but the visual field demonstrates enlargement of the physiologic blind spot.

Papilledema may occur as a result of several mechanisms which disrupt the circulation of the nerve head. These disruptions are interference with the venous outflow due to compression of the central retinal vein in the optic nerve; interference with the central retinal vein as it crosses the optic nerve sheaths in the presence of increased intracranial pressure; primary circulatory disease, and decreased intraocular pressure which permits passive edema of the nervehead to develop. Management of patients with papilledema includes complete general, neurologic and ocular examination with visual fields, x-rays and special diagnostic studies to determine the cause of the disorder. Treatment is, of course, guided by the etiology.

Vascular disease of the optic nerve may also occur in the course of arteriolar sclerosis or temporal arteritis and produce vision impairment or even total loss of vision.

INFLAMMATORY DISORDERS. Inflammation of the intraocular portion of the nerve is termed papillitis; inflammation involving the nerve posterior to the eye is designated retrobulbar neuritis. Papillitis produces an impairment of vision, a central scotoma, alteration of the pupillary light reflex, the signs of papilledema and frequently an accumulation of inflammatory cells in the posterior vitreous body. Recovery may be complete, or postneuritic atrophy with a variable amount of fibrosis, gliosis and pallor of the disc may ensue.

Retrobulbar neuritis is also generally associated with vision impairment, a central scotoma and a diminished pupillary light reflex; but there is pain on movement of the eye and the optic disc appears normal. Following retrobulbar neuritis, there may be complete recovery or postneuritic atrophy with pallor of the optic disc may develop.

The causes of optic nerve inflammation include an extension of intraocular, orbital, paranasal or intracranial inflammation; generalized infectious diseases; metabolic disorders; Leber's disease, a familial disorder of unknown etiology, and demyelinating disorders. Probably more than half of the cases of retrobulbar neuritis are caused by multiple sclerosis and other demyelinating diseases. Treatment of optic neuritis consists of correcting, when possible, any causative factor and, in some instances, vitamin supplements, vasodilators and systemic corticosteroids.

TOXIC REACTIONS. The optic nerve may be adversely affected by a number of toxic reactions. For example, methyl alcohol ingestion is followed by violent vomiting, acidosis, profound loss of vision and subsequent pallor of the optic disc, or blindness. There is marked individual variation in susceptibility to methyl alcohol poisoning and vigorous treatment of the acute acidosis may prevent or minimize the vision impairment. Lead, quinine and other substances are also capable of producing optic nerve degeneration.

DEGENERATION OR ATROPHY. The end result of many disease processes, optic atrophy or degeneration is characterized by loss of visual acuity, visual field defect, impairment of the pupillary light reflex and pallor of the optic disc. Following destruction of optic nerve fibers at any point between origin in the retinal ganglion cells and termination in the lateral geniculate body, pallor of the disc develops in from three weeks to two months.

TUMORS. Tumors of the intraocular portion of the optic nerve include gliomas and benign lesions associated with tuberous sclerosis, neurofibromatosis, and angiomatosis retinae. Posterior to the globe, the nerve is affected by gliomas and meningiomas.

INJURIES. Avulsion of the optic nerve is associated with severe trauma, usually eye gouging, that stretches the nerve. The nerve is torn at the lamina cribrosa and intraocular hemorrhage with severe or total loss of vision results. The optic nerve may be severed in the orbit by a penetrating stab or bullet wounds and, in the optic canal, nerve function may be destroyed by compression due to hemorrhage or fracture. When this occurs, surgical decompression of the nerve is not generally beneficial.

LENS AND ZONULE

As a highly specialized and unique structure without a blood supply or a connective tissue framework, the lens does not participate directly in circulatory diseases and is involved in inflammatory processes only when infectious organisms are introduced through a break in the lens capsule or proteins escape from the lens and incite a reaction. Related to these particular properties, developmental and acquired diseases of the lens are confined to abnormalities in lens transparency, shape or position.

CATARACT. Any opacification that interferes with transparency of the lens is by definition a cataract. On this basis, most young individuals and virtually all older people have cataract. However, the term cataract has such a widespread connotation of possible blindness that it is wise to use it only to designate significant or progressive loss of lens transparency and to refer to localized or minor areas of opacification as lens opacities.

The principal symptoms of cataract are painless loss of vision, monocular diplopia, change of color perception and progressive alteration in the refraction of the eye. The major sign associated with this process is white, yellow or brown opacification of the lens; this may be evident on external inspection but is usually revealed when the fundus reflex is studied during ophthalmoscopy or noted during slit lamp biomicroscopy of the lens.

The etiology of most forms of cataract is unknown. It is recognized, however, that progressive lens opacification is associated with diminished lens metabolism and significant biochemical abnormalities. With this limited basic etiologic knowledge, cataract is generally classified as developmental, senile, or associated with ocular disease, systemic disease, medication, trauma, radiation or electrical shock.

DEVELOPMENTAL CATARACT. Present at birth or evident early in life, developmental cataract is often familial and may be stationary or progressive and severe enough to require early therapy.

SENILE CATARACT. Senile cataract affects the lens nucleus, cortex, posterior subcapsular region or a combination of these areas. Nuclear cataract is associated with sclerosis of the central portion of the lens and deposition of a yellow or brown pigment. As the condition becomes more severe, myopia often develops and there is progressive impairment of vision.

Cortical cataract is characterized by spokes and wedges of opacification in the lens cortex. This form of cataract may cause total opacification and eventual liquefaction of the lens cortex.

With posterior subcapsular cataract, there is opacification of the lens in the axial portion of the posterior subcapsular region. This is a critical location near the nodal point of the eye; consequently, substantial vision impairment occurs at a relatively early stage.

CATARACT ASSOCIATED WITH OCULAR DISEASE. Secondary to longstanding uveitis, retinitis pigmentosa, retinal detachment and several other ocular disorders, cataract often develops. This generally begins as opacification in the axial portion of the posterior subcapsular cortex but may progress to total cataract.

CATARACT ASSOCIATED WITH SYSTEMIC DISEASE. A number of systemic diseases are associated with cataract. Interestingly, rubella contracted during the early phase of pregnancy is often followed by cataract in the offspring. In other instances, cataracts form in patients with galactosemia, mongolism, cretinism, myotonic dystrophy, tetany, atopic dermatitis and diabetes mellitus. These cataracts differ in age of onset, morphology of lens opacification and rate of progression.

CATARACT ASSOCIATED WITH MEDICATION. A number of medications are capable of producing cataracts in susceptible individuals and have been withdrawn from the market. In addition, long-term corticosteroid therapy has been related to the formation of posterior subcapsular cataracts.

CATARACT ASSOCIATED WITH TRAUMA, RADIATION AND ELECTRICAL SHOCK. Contusion of the eye without rupture of the lens capsule may cause localized or even total opacification of the lens. Moreover, rupture of the lens capsule may also be followed by a localized opacity, but total cataract is more likely to occur. Related to dosage, ionizing radiation produces equatorial lens opacities, posterior subcapsular opacities or total cataract. Electrical shock is also acknowledged as a cause of localized or total lens opacification.

CATARACT THERAPY. In general terms, the nonsurgical treatment of cataract consists of the alleviation of any specific cause, careful correction of any refractive error or optical defect and, occasionally, enlargement of the pupil. Surgical extraction of the lens is indicated when, despite nonsurgical methods, vision is significantly impaired by the cataract and inadequate for the needs of the particular patient. Cataract extraction is also warranted when the diseased lens is responsible for glaucoma or intraocular inflammation and, in some circumstances, when binocular vision is disrupted.

When a cataract operation is performed in the first two or three decades of life, the anterior lens capsule is opened, the lens substance is removed or allowed to absorb and the posterior lens capsule is left in place. In older people, the entire lens including its capsule is extracted (Fig. 7).

ABNORMAL LENS SHAPES. Abnormal lens

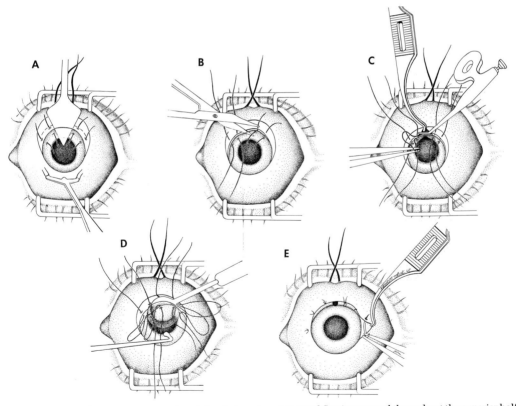

Figure 7. Intracapsular cataract extraction. A fornix-based conjunctival flap is prepared throughout the superior half of the corneal limbus, tract sutures are passed across the proposed line of incision and the anterior chamber is entered with a keratome (A). This incision is extended for 180 degrees with scissors and as each tract suture is divided it is rethreaded with a fine caliber suture (B). After an iridectomy is performed (C), an erisiphake (a small suction cup) is applied to the lens and used in conjunction with gentle pressure on the globe surface to rupture the zonule and permit removal of the lens (D). The corneoscleral incision is then closed with the preplaced sutures and reinforced by a conjunctival flap (E).

shapes are relatively rare. When they occur, the conditions are often familial and interfere with vision by disrupting the optical properties of the eyes. Included in this group of disorders are anterior and posterior lenticonus, conical projections of the anterior and posterior lens surfaces respectively.

LENS SUBLUXATION AND LUXATION. Lens subluxation may occur as an isolated developmental defect, present as a feature of arachnodactyly (Marfan's syndrome) or homocystinuria or arise as a consequence of trauma. Findings vary with the degree of lens displacement, but symptoms generally include impaired vision and decreased accommodation. Signs usually consist of tremulousness of the iris in the areas where the zonule is lacking, a visible equatorial edge of the displaced lens and a double ophthalmoscopic image of the fundus caused by the anomalous lens position. Treatment of lens subluxation is generally confined to optical correction and alteration of pupil size and shape. Lens extraction is carried out only when mandatory because of the likelihood of surgical and postoperative complications.

Lens luxation may follow a developmental subluxation but is usually the result of trauma. In most instances, luxation of the lens necessitates surgical lens extraction.

VITREOUS BODY

DEVELOPMENTAL ABNORMALITIES. Developmental abnormalities of the vitreous are related to persistence of the hyaloid artery, a vessel extending from the optic disc to the posterior surface of the lens, and the network of vessels normally surrounding the lens in fetal life. In most instances, these remnants do not interfere with vision; but in rare instances, they are responsible for cataract formation or vitreous hemorrhage.

OPACITIES. Vitreous opacities, capable of interfering with vision, are classified as acellular and cellular. Acellular opacities are caused by accumulation of calcium soaps, cholesterol crystals and protein.

Cellular opacities in the vitreous are related to red blood cells, white blood cells, tumor cells and parasites. If the process responsible for producing these opacities is controlled, the vitreous usually clears.

DEGENERATION. Vitreous degeneration occurs to some extent in all eyes during the normal process of aging and is increased by intraocular inflammation, tumor, injury or myopia. Manifestations of vitreous degeneration include liquefaction of the normally semisolid vitreous and separation of the vitreous from the retina. The latter is often accompanied by light flashes and a few spots in the field of vision, so it must be differentiated from retinal detachment. Vitreous degeneration and detachment do not interfere with vision and do not require treatment.

GLAUCOMA

The term glaucoma encompasses a group of ocular abnormalities in which intraocular pressure, normally maintained at a level of 15 to 22 mm. of mercury above atmospheric pressure, is increased and there is resultant damage to the eye. Elevated intraocular pressure can occur as a consequence of increased aqueous humor production, but this is uncommon; it usually stems from an impairment of aqueous outflow.

The symptoms and signs of glaucoma are related to the increased intraocular pressure. If intraocular pressure is abruptly raised to a high level, pain, photophobia, lacrimation, impaired vision and halos around lights occur in association with congestion of the eye, corneal edema and an elevated tonometric value. If intraocular pressure is raised insidiously, no symptoms or visible external signs are evident until vision impairment is noted and usually, at this stage, advanced damage to the field of vision is present.

Glaucoma is considered primary when the increased intraocular tension is unrelated to any other ocular disease and classified as secondary when elevated intraocular pressure occurs as a consequence of another ocular disease.

PRIMARY DEVELOPMENTAL GLAUCOMA. Usually, primary developmental glaucoma is genetically determined and characterized by an elevation in intraocular pressure at birth, or at some time during the first two or three decades of life. In general, infants affected with this form of glaucoma present photophobia and lacrimation. The cornea is either clear or cloudy and if the condition has been present for an extended period, the cornea and entire eye may be enlarged. An anomalous formation of the anterior chamber angle is often demonstrable and surgical incision of this abnormal tissue is the treatment ordinarily indicated.

As a rule, when developmental primary glaucoma presents in children or young adults, the onset is insidious, stretching of the globe is inconspicuous and visual field impairment is similar to adult primary open angle glaucoma. The usual treatment of these patients includes medications and surgical procedures comparable to the management of adult primary open angle glaucoma.

PRIMARY CLOSED ANGLE GLAUCOMA. Acute angle closure glaucoma develops in adults after a series of prodromal attacks, or as an initial acute episode precipitated by the use of medications to dilate the pupil, a long period in a dark room or other factors. Symptoms of the acute attack are severe pain in the involved eye, often associated with nausea and vomiting, blurred vision and colored halos surrounding lights. Signs include congestion of the eye, corneal edema, shallow anterior chamber, closed anterior chamber angle, dilated pupil and elevated intraocular pressure. Unless the condition is controlled promptly, permanent impairment of vision or blindness results from the elevated pressure.

The pathogenesis of acute angle closure glaucoma in eyes with shallow anterior chamber is related to a partial or complete block of aqueous humor flow from the posterior to the anterior chamber. As a result of this pupillary block, aqueous accumulates in the posterior chamber and forces the peripheral iris into contact with the trabecula. An abrupt rise in intraocular pressure follows obstruction of the aqueous outflow pathway.

Treatment of closed angle glaucoma involves the initial control of intraocular pressure with miotics, systemic medications which inhibit aqueous humor production and, if necessary, osmotic agents. After regulation of pressure, a peripheral iridectomy is performed to establish additional communication between the anterior and posterior chambers, eliminate the effect of pupillary block and prevent angle closure. Throughout the course of an episode of acute glaucoma, supportive and pain-relieving measures are appropriate and the opposite, uninvolved eye must be carefully observed. Prophylactic peripheral iridectomy on the uninvolved eye is often indicated.

Subacute and chronic angle closure glaucoma develop in similarly predisposed eyes and are characterized by prodromal episodes of partial angle closure and mild elevation of intraocular pressure. These recurrent episodes may result in permanent angle closure and severe glaucoma. Treatment is with miotics and peripheral iridectomy.

PRIMARY OPEN ANGLE GLAUCOMA. Open angle glaucoma is present in approximately 2 per cent of people over 40 years of age. Moreover, though it is a leading cause of blindness, most people with this type of glaucoma are unaware of their disease.

The onset of open angle glaucoma is insidious. In the early stages, there are no symptoms and by the time the patient notes vision impairment, the disease is generally far advanced in one or both eyes. Signs of chronic simple glaucoma include an elevated intraocular pressure, often subtle and demonstrated only with provocative tests and tonography, characteristic changes in the visual field and alterations of the optic disc. Visual field defects are the result of damage to the nerve fibers as they pass from the retina into the optic nerve. Because fibers at the upper and lower poles of the disc are most vulnerable, arcuate nerve fiber bundle defects are typical of open angle glaucoma. With destruction of the nerve fibers, the optic disc becomes pale and as pressure is maintained, a prominent excavation or cupping of the disc develops.

In open angle glaucoma, the iris does not interfere with aqueous exit; but the pathogenesis is related to an impairment of aqueous outflow in the trabecula, Schlemm's canal or the passages joining this structure to the venous circulation.

Treatment is designed to aid aqueous outflow with miotics and, when necessary, inhibit the production of aqueous humor with topical epinephrine compounds or systemic carbonic anhydrase inhibitors. When medical therapy is unsuccessful, ocular surgery, consisting usually of an external filtering operation, is employed. This type of operation enables aqueous humor to leave the eye and pass into the subconjunctival space.

SECONDARY GLAUCOMA. Secondary glaucoma may complicate many ocular diseases. It is usually unilateral and produces mild or severe elevation of intraocular pressure with symptoms and signs related to the rate of intraocular pressure increase and the level this pressure attains. Among the causes of secondary glaucoma are uveal disease, which causes glaucoma by obstructing the passage of aqueous from the posterior to the anterior chamber or by blocking the filtration meshwork with inflammatory debris or tumor cells; lens disease, which produces glaucoma by causing pupillary block or obstruction of the filtration meshwork; vascular disease, which stimulates neovascularization in the chamber angle and on the anterior iris surface to cause hemorrhagic glaucoma; and trauma, which is responsible for hyphema or damage to the filtration meshwork and ciliary body.

Treatment of secondary glaucoma varies greatly in accordance with the primary disease. However, carbonic anhydrase inhibitors are particularly helpful in the control of elevated intraocular pressure associated with secondary glaucoma.

OCULAR MOTILITY

Control of the complicated motor mechanism responsible for ocular motility is obtained by a coordinated system of voluntary and reflex movements. Voluntary movements are initiated in Brodmann's area 8 of the frontal cortex and, probably, in other areas of the cerebrum.

Reflex movements form the essential background on which voluntary movements are superimposed. The principal reflex movements are static reflexes derived from proprioceptive impulses and the otolith apparatus; statokinetic reflexes derived from the semicircular canals; optomotor reflexes, responsible for the fixation reflex and following movements, derived from the occipital cortex of the cerebrum, and fusion reflexes, responsible for the fine adjustment of eye position, probably derived from the cerebrum.

Eye movements that result from the actions of the control system are carried out by combinations of extraocular muscles. For every conjugate movement in which both eyes move in the same direction, an equal stimulus for contraction is sent to the muscle in each eye that is primarily responsible for the movement. The muscles are called synergists. In addition, an inhibition causing relaxation is sent to the muscle in each eye ordinarily opposing this movement. These muscles are called antagonists. For example, in eyes right, the contracting synergists are the right lateral rectus and the left medial rectus; the inhibited antagonists are the right medial rectus and the left lateral rectus. Every other position of gaze has comparable pairs of synergists and antagonists.

ORTHOPHORIA, HETEROPHORIA AND HETEROTROPIA. The system for control of ocular movements and the extraocular muscle mechanism combine, under normal circumstances, to direct the rotation of the eyes and to maintain the alignment of the two eyes. Orthophoria is the term used to describe the condition in which proper alignment of the two eyes is maintained even though a part of the control system, the fusion reflexes, is interrupted by the alternate occlusion of one eye and then the other. Though orthophoria may be considered the ideal, it is not usually present.

The usual condition is heterophoria, a state in which there is a tendency for misalignment of the two eyes. This tendency, however, is overcome by the fusion reflexes and demonstrable only when these reflexes are interrupted by the alternate cover test. Not usually responsible for any ocular symptoms, heterophoria may, uncommonly, cause discomfort associated with use of the eyes. When this occurs, treatment consists of the correction of any refractive error, orthoptic exercises, prism spectacles and, if necessary, operation on the extraocular muscles.

Heterotropia is a misalignment of the eyes that is not overcome by the fusion reflexes and, therefore, manifest. Heterotropia is classified as comitant or noncomitant.

Comitant heterotropia. Comitant heterotropia is tropia in which the amount of misalignment is constant in all directions of gaze. This type of heterotropia may be further described as esotropia, when there is an inward or nasal deviation of the eyes; exotropia, when the eyes possess an outward or temporal deviation, and hypertropia, when there is a vertical ocular misalignment.

Comitant esotropia, a rather common disorder of ocular motility, usually develops in children between two and four years of age and often demonstrates a familial tendency. It frequently occurs in a hyperopic child who must employ excessive accommodation to see objects clearly. Associated with this excessive accommodation is excessive convergence which causes an inward deviation of the eyes. In some instances, however, comitant esotropia is unrelated to accommodation and is caused by other factors.

Symptoms are usually absent because children with comitant esotropia promptly suppress the image from the deviating eye and diplopia is not experienced. For diagnosis, the manifest misalignment is revealed by observation of the corneal light reflex and by the cover-uncover test.

Treatment of comitant esotropia includes a complete ocular examination with cycloplegia, correction of any significant refractive error, treatment of suppression and amblyopia by occlusion of the fixing eye and, not infrequently, operation on the extraocular muscles. To overcome the nasal deviation, one or both medial recti are recessed (Fig. 8) and this may be combined with lateral rectus resection (Fig. 9).

Comitant exotropia, also a rather common disorder, is usually intermittent and, therefore, evident only under certain circumstances of fixation and attention. Presenting initially at the age of two or three years, it generally increases in frequency and degree as the patient grows older and is probably caused by an excessive divergence tonus. Comitant exotropia is constant in some patients and often stems from decreased or absent vision in the deviating eye. When one eye is blind, the lack of a stimulus for convergence permits divergence to develop.

Comitant exotropia is usually asymptomatic because suppression, or the limited acuity in the deviating eye, prevents diplopia. Therapy consists of a complete ocular examination, correction of any significant refractive error, measures to overcome suppression and amblyopia and, in some instances, extraocular muscle surgery. The temporal misalignment is corrected by recession of one or both lateral recti and, whenever appropriate, medial rectus resection.

Comitant hypertropia is uncommon and usually related to a developmental abnormality of structure or movement control. Symptoms, signs and treatment are variable.

Noncomitant heterotropia. Noncomitant heterotropia is tropia in which the amount of misalignment varies in different positions of gaze. This type of tropia may result from

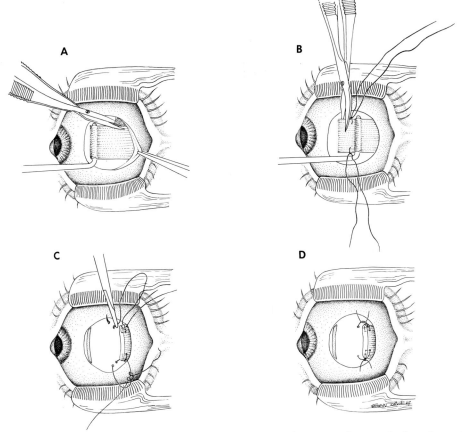

Figure 8. Extraocular muscle recession. Recession entails exposing the extraocular muscle through a conjunctival incision and freeing it from the intermuscular septum (A). Sutures are placed in the muscle very near its scleral attachment and the muscle is divided between these sutures and its insertion (B). The sutures are then used to reattach the muscle to the sclera (C) so that the muscle is recessed and separated from its original site of scleral insertion (D). The conjunctival incision is then closed.

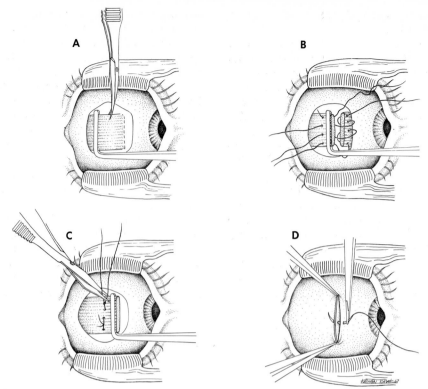

Figure 9. Extraocular muscle resection. The muscle is exposed, secured with a resection clamp and divided between the clamp and its scleral insertion (*A*). Sutures are passed through the scleral insertion and then through the body of the extraocular muscle (*B*). When these sutures are tied, the muscle is tightened and the redundant muscle tissue in the clamp is resected (*C*). The conjunctival incision is closed with sutures (*D*).

anomalies of muscle structure, paralysis of extraocular muscles and internuclear paralysis.

Anomalies of muscle structure produce various types of noncomitant tropia. An example is Duane's syndrome, a congenital disorder in which the lateral rectus appears to be replaced by an inelastic fibrous band. Clinically, this syndrome is usually characterized by normal alignment of the eyes in the primary position, inability to abduct the involved eye and retraction of the eye into the orbit when adduction is attempted.

Paralysis of one or more extraocular muscles causes a noncomitant tropia, usually sudden in onset and more frequent in adults than children. The etiology includes many disorders such as intracranial aneurysms, diabetes mellitus, inflammatory disease, degenerative disease, increased intracranial pressure and trauma.

Diplopia is the principal symptom of noncomitant tropia and the major sign is a tropia in the field of action of the involved muscles, greater when the eye with the paretic muscles is fixing than when the uninvolved eye is fixing. Therapy consists of a complete examination to determine the cause, occlusion of one eye to relieve the diplopia and, if the condition persists for an extended period, operation on the extraocular muscles.

Internuclear paralysis results from an interruption of the medial longitudinal bundle between the oculomotor and abducens nerve nuclei. In the usual form of this disorder, the medial rectus muscle does not act to adduct the eye and a tropia results, but the medial rectus muscle does contract in response to convergence stimuli. Multiple sclerosis is the most common cause of internuclear paralysis and there is no specific treatment other than occlusion to relieve diplopia.

ORBIT

DEVELOPMENTAL ABNORMALITIES. The most common developmental abnormalities of the orbit are related to craniostenosis and ocular hypertelorism. Craniostenosis encompasses a group of cranial and orbital deformities which have their origin in premature synostosis of the bones in the skull. As a result of this abnormal fusion, growth is inhibited in certain directions, enlargement occurs in other directions and the skull assumes characteristic forms. Oxycephaly, the most common form of craniostenosis, denotes a high-domed or pointed skull with a short anteroposterior diameter. Associated ocular abnormalities include shallow orbits causing exophthalmos, widely separated orbits producing exotropia and, frequently, optic atrophy with loss of vision. Craniofacial dysostosis is another abnormality in the shape of the skull associated with lateral enlargement, shallow orbits, exotropia and impaired vision.

Ocular hypertelorism is often familial and characterized by wide separation of the orbits and the not infrequent occurrence of exotropia.

CIRCULATORY DISORDERS. Carotid cavernous fistula is an abnormal communication between the carotid artery and the cavernous sinus. The disorder usually results from traumatic laceration of the carotid artery but may also be caused by rupture of a carotid aneurysm. Regardless of etiology, the fistula permits transmission of blood under pressure from the carotid arterial system to the cavernous sinus and its venous tributaries. There is subjective awareness of a swishing noise in the head and, frequently, diplopia or decreased vision. Signs include a bruit that is synchronous with the pulse, variable but often severe congestion of the orbit, impaired vision, paralysis of extraocular muscles and involvement of any of the cranial nerves one through eight. The diagnosis may be confirmed by angiography and treatment consists of carotid ligation, often combined with other vascular operations.

INFLAMMATORY DISORDERS. Orbital inflammation may result from accidental or surgical wounds, extension of intraocular inflammation, spread from an adjacent area, metastatic dissemination from a remote source and unknown causes. This inflammation may present as orbital periostitis, orbital cellulitis, cavernous sinus thrombosis or orbital granuloma. Orbital periostitis produces the symptoms and signs of localized infection. It may resolve on appropriate antibiotic therapy or progress to formation of an orbital abscess.

Orbital cellulitis is usually an acute process related to a bacterial or fungal agent. Symptoms are pain and the subjective indications of severe infection. Signs include swelling of the eyelids, exophthalmos, limitation of ocular motility, temperature elevation and leukocytosis. With intensive antibiotic and supportive treatment, the condition usually subsides.

Cavernous sinus thrombosis is a severe complication which may occur in association with periostitis, orbital cellulitis or a pyogenic infection of any type on the nose or eyelid. The initial symptoms and signs are identical with orbital cellulitis, but in a day or two proptosis becomes more severe, veins in the lid and in the eye show stasis, extraocular muscle paralysis develops and the condition may spread to involve the opposite eye and orbit. Cavernous sinus thrombosis is sometimes fatal but treatment with antibiotics and other measures to combat infection is usually followed by partial or complete recovery.

Orbital granuloma represents a chronic form of orbital inflammation that occurs with thyroid disease or as an isolated abnormality. Orbital granuloma produces exophthalmos and minimal, if any, indications of inflammation. Following diagnostic. studies, treatment with corticosteroids is sometimes beneficial, but surgical exploration of the orbit may be needed to rule out neoplasm.

ORBITAL MANIFESTATIONS OF GRAVES' DISEASE. Graves' disease is a clinical complex of signs and symptoms associated with hyperthyroidism. Patients with Graves' disease have ocular signs that vary greatly and range through a broad spectrum, extending from noninfiltrative dysthyroid ophthalmopathy to infiltrative dysthyroid ophthalmopathy.

Noninfiltrative dysthyroid ophthalmopathy, also known as thyrotoxic exophthalmos, is usually asymptomatic but signs include widening of the palpebral fissure, lid lag when the eyes are depressed, infrequent blinking and a mild degree of exophthalmos. Attributed to an overaction of the smooth muscle in the upper lid and an increase in water and fat in the orbit, these signs usually disappear after the hyperthyroidism is controlled.

Infiltrative dysthyroid ophthalmopathy, also known as thyrotropic exophthalmos, or malignant exophthalmos, may precede but usually follows the treatment of Graves' disease. Symptoms include lacrimation, a foreign body sensation, diplopia, impaired vision and pain. The usual signs consist of widening of the palpebral fissure, lid lag, infrequent blinking, exophthalmos which may be mild or very severe, lid edema and conjunctival chemosis, limitation of ocular motility and corneal exposure. These signs are due primarily to inflammation and round cell infiltration of the orbital tissues. The involved extraocular muscles are greatly enlarged, undergo degeneration and become fibrosed.

Infiltrative dysthyroid ophthalmopathy may be prevented in some patients by avoiding rapid correction of hyperthyroidism. If the condition develops, however, systemic corticosteroids may be beneficial. Corneal exposure is treated with protective ointments, intermarginal lid adhesions and orbital decompression.

TUMORS. Orbital tumors include lesions that are primary within the orbit, extend to the orbit from adjacent areas and develop in the orbit during the course of generalized diseases. Among the more common orbital tumors are hemangiomas, malignant lymphomas, lacrimal gland tumors, gliomas, meningiomas, muscle tumors, carcinomas and dermoid cysts. Exploration of the orbit through the lateral wall or roof may be necessary to establish the diagnosis, and benign tumor can often be excised with these surgical approaches. For malignant tumors, radiation, chemotherapy or orbital exenteration may be indicated.

INJURIES. Orbital injuries are related to penetrating wounds and the effects of blunt trauma. Stab and gunshot wounds involving the orbit often introduce infection and produce variable degrees of damage.

Blunt trauma may severely fracture the floor of the orbit so that orbital contents prolapse into the maxillary antrum and enophthalmos ensues. This type of blowout fracture is often masked initially by orbital edema and hemorrhage. However, early diagnosis facilitates reposition of the orbital tissues and repair of the bony defect.

READING REFERENCES

Adler, F. H.: Textbook of Ophthalmology. 7th ed. Philadelphia, W. B. Saunders Company, 1962.

Allen, J. H.: C. H. May's Manual of Diseases of the Eye. 23rd ed. Baltimore, Williams & Wilkins Company, 1963.

Arruga, H.: Ocular Surgery. 3rd English ed. J. H. Michael and L. E. Chaparro, translators. Barcelona, Salvat Editores S. A., and New York, McGraw-Hill Book Company, 1963.

Berens, C. and King, J. H.: An Atlas of Ophthalmological Surgery. Philadelphia, J. B. Lippincott Company, 1961.

Callahan, A.: Surgery of the Eye. Springfield, Illinois, Charles C Thomas, 1956.

Duke-Elder, W. S.: System of Ophthalmology. St. Louis, C. V. Mosby Company, 1958-1966. Vols. I, II, III, VII, VIII and IX.

Paton, R. T., et al.: Atlas of Eye Surgery. 2nd ed. New York, McGraw-Hill Book Company, 1962.

Vaughan, R., Cook, R., and Asbury, T.: General Ophthalmology. 4th ed. Los Altos, California, Lange Medical Publications, 1965.

Chapter 15

THE EARS, NOSE AND THROAT

by
JAMES R. CHANDLER, M.D.

The son of a physician, a South Carolinian by birth, JAMES R. CHANDLER received his elementary and secondary education in Florida. He graduated in medicine at Duke University and interned at the Protestant Episcopal Hospital in Philadelphia. He returned to his home in Daytona Beach and was in general practice for over two years. He entered the surgical residency in his specialty at the University of Michigan. He is chairman of the Division of Otolaryngology in the School of Medicine, University of Miami. He shares with many surgeons an enthusiastic participation in golf and fishing.

THE EARS

SURGICAL ANATOMY AND PHYSIOLOGY

The ear is conveniently divided into three parts: the external, middle and inner ears (Fig. 1). The external ear consists of the auricle and external auditory canal. The auricle is an appendage of yellow elastic cartilage covered by skin which is closely adherent to its lateral surface and loosely attached to its medial or posterior surface.

The external auditory canal is approximately 1 inch long and consists of an outer membranous portion comprising approximately one-third of this distance and containing ceruminous glands, and hair follicles. The inner two-thirds is the osseous external auditory canal and consists of the tympanic portion of the temporal bone lined by a very thin layer of squamous epithelium. No glands or accessory hair follicles are present in the osseous portion of the canal. The external auditory canal is separated from the middle ear by the tympanic membrane. The great auricular nerve from the second and third cervical nerves of the cervical plexus supplies the medial and posterior portions of the pinna and the mastoid process. The anterior or lateral portion of the ear and external auditory canal are supplied primarily by the auriculotemporal branches of the fifth cranial nerve. Small twigs from the seventh and tenth cranial nerves supply part of the canal and tympanic membrane.

The middle ear is bounded laterally by the tympanic membrane and medially by the promontory of the inner ear. The tympanic membrane consists of a thin, translucent, mobile membrane with three layers: an external layer consisting of squamous cell epithelium, a medial layer of thin cuboidal epithelium and a thin fibrous layer separating the two. The handle of the malleus is incorporated within its middle layer. Vibrations of the tympanic membrane are conducted to the inner ear through the malleus, incus and the stapes, the footplate of which closes the oval window. Anteriorly, the middle ear communicates with the nasopharynx through the eustachian tube superiorly and is in relationship to the carotid artery covered by a thin plate of bone inferiorly. Posteriorly, it is in communication with the pneumatized cell spaces of the mastoid process by means of the aditus ad antrum. Superiorly, it is in relationship to the middle cranial fossa and inferiorly to the dome of the jugular bulb. The seventh cranial nerve courses transversely across the superior portion of its medial wall and turns inferiorly at the pyramidal process to pass through the posterior osseous canal wall to exit at the stylomastoid foramen.

The inner ear consists of a convoluted osseous labyrinth consisting of three semicircular canals, the vestibule and the cochlea. Within the osseous labyrinth is the membranous labyrinth suspended in a fluid medium, the perilymph. The endings of the eighth

293

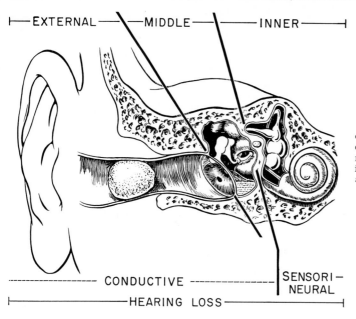

├─EXTERNAL─┤─MIDDLE─┤─INNER─┤

‑‑‑‑‑‑‑‑‑‑‑ CONDUCTIVE ‑‑‑‑‑‑‑‑‑‑ │ SENSORI‑NEURAL

├─────────HEARING LOSS──────────┤

Figure 1. Conductive hearing loss is caused by pathology in the external or middle ear: impacted cerumen, perforation or middle ear fluid. Sensorineural hearing loss is caused by pathology in the inner ear, acoustic nerve or brain.

cranial nerve terminate in the specialized sensory epithelium in the ampullated ends of the three semicircular canals, the maculae of the saccule and utricle, and in the cochlea. The former two portions are concerned with equilibrium and together with vision and the proprioceptive system serve to orient the individual in relation to space and his environment. The cochlea is the end organ of hearing.

DISEASES OF THE EXTERNAL EAR

Because of the ear's prominence, trauma in the form of contusions, lacerations and hematomas is quite frequent. Automobile accidents are by far the most common cause of trauma, although fisticuffs, either of the amateur or professional variety, account for many hematomas and their end result, the well known "cauliflower ear." Abrasions and lacerations should be cleansed thoroughly and sutured primarily, using fine interrupted sutures of nonabsorbable material. Hematomas of the auricle result from rupture of small vessels in the subcutaneous tissue and, when they extend beneath the perichondrium, elevate this layer from the cartilage and interfere with its nutrition. When the cartilage is fractured the hematoma may present itself on both sides of the auricle. If the hematoma is not evacuated and the skin approximated to the underlying cartilage, necrosis and subsequent scarring of the auricle produce the deformity. The treatment is evacuation of the clot by open incision on either or both sides of the auricle and the application of a tight conforming pressure dressing.

FOREIGN BODIES. Small stones, beads, beans and peas are frequently inserted into the ear canal by children and mentally deranged persons. They may result in hearing impairment and pain when infection occurs. Diagnosis can be made easily on inspection and the object removed by inserting a small cerumen spoon or right angle hook behind the foreign body and pulling it out. This must be done under direct vision. In children, attention must be paid that the child or infant is completely restrained. Occasionally, general anesthesia is necessary and even a postauricular or endaural incision and widening of the osseous canal may be required. Care should be taken to avoid perforating or injuring the tympanic membrane.

EXTERNAL OTITIS. Suppurative infections of the external auditory canal are occasionally surgical problems, particularly those which occur in the elderly diabetic individual. Such infections are usually caused by staphylococci or pseudomonas organisms and involve cartilage and bone of the external auditory canal. They may spread to involve the parotid gland, the soft tissues inferior to the temporal bone at the base of the skull and the tympanic and temporal bones themselves. These infections are uniformly unresponsive to antibiotic therapy and require wide surgical debridement and removal of all infected tissues followed by careful post-operative care.

DISEASES OF THE MIDDLE EAR AND MASTOID

SEROUS OTITIS MEDIA. This is a nonsuppurative collection of serous or mucoid material in the tympanic cavity. It results in a sense of stuffiness or pressure and causes a conductive hearing loss. It is most common in children and most often is secondary to eustachian tube obstruction as a result of hypertrophied or infected adenoid tissue in the nasopharynx. Diagnosis is frequently difficult, particularly in the child with unilateral disease, but is accomplished by careful history, inspection of the tympanic membrane with the aid of the pneumatic otoscope and evaluation of the hearing with tuning forks or audiometric means. The tympanic membrane may appear to be perfectly normal, but most commonly appears to be retracted and somewhat yellowish or bluish with some bubbles behind it. In older persons, it may be thick and opaque. Decreased

mobility to pneumatic otoscopy is a uniform and diagnostic finding. Tuning forks demonstrate a conductive hearing loss with the air-bone gap being decreased and the Weber test being referred to the involved ear.

If the effusion is part of a generalized upper respiratory tract infection, it may yield to conservative treatment consisting of vasoconstricting nosedrops such as 1 per cent ephedrine or ¼ to 1 per cent Neo-Synephrine, oral decongestive agents and clearing of the upper respiratory inflammatory process. An incision of the tympanic membrane and aspiration of the fluid are frequently necessary, particularly when the fluid is thick and mucoid in nature. These latter ears are given the descriptive term "glue ears."

The condition is frequently recurrent and taxes the resources and ingenuity of the physician. In former years, radium applications to the nasopharynx or low dose irradiation therapy to the lymphoid tissue of the nasopharynx was frequently utilized. More recently, treatment by incision into the tympanic membrane (Fig. 2), removal of the fluid and insertion of a drainage tube of various types has proved to be much more effec-

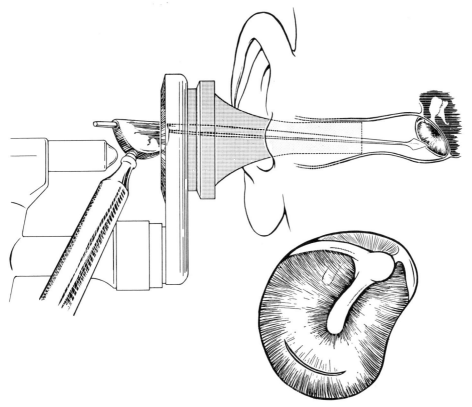

Figure 2. A myringotomy is performed in the posterior inferior quadrant of the tympanic membrane.

tive (Fig. 3). This technique should be uniformly preceded by a careful and meticulous adenoidectomy. The tubes tend to be extruded spontaneously, but should be left in place for three to six months. Frequently, unresponsive or refractory cases are found to be due to some type of allergy and yield only to appropriate management.

ACUTE SUPPURATIVE OTITIS MEDIA. One of the most frequent complications of upper respiratory tract infections, particularly in infants and children, is acute suppurative otitis media. It is most commonly a result of invasion of the middle ear by *Staphylococcus aureus*, the hemolytic streptococcus or the pneumococcus. They reach the middle ear space by means of the eustachian tube, peritubal lymphatics and venous channels or by hematogenous spread. The first route is the most common.

The initial stage of infection is one of hyperemia and is characterized by intense vasodilatation of the blood vessels of the mucous membrane in the middle ear. This is closely followed by actual suppuration and is accompanied by sharply localized pain, malaise, fever and chills. All symptoms are more marked in children and infants. The pain is frequently at its worst in the early morning or late evening hours. Pain is the most prominent symptom but a slight to moderate loss of hearing of the conductive type also occurs as a result of the impairment of conduction through the middle ear.

Examination during the initial stages may reveal only a hyperemic tympanic membrane with vascular engorgement of blood vessels, particularly in Shrapnell's membrane and along the handle of the malleus. The middle

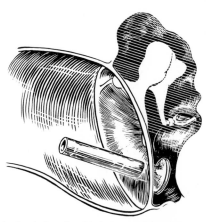

Figure 3. A flared polyethylene tube has been placed through a myringotomy to act as a pressure equalizer.

ear contains air at this point. If treatment with vasoconstricting nosedrops and appropriate antibiotic therapy is instituted immediately, this stage may resolve completely without suppuration. Frequently, this stage is difficult to differentiate from the hyperemia secondary to a viral infection of the upper respiratory tract or a simple inflammatory myringitis.

Examination during the stage of suppuration reveals an intense hyperemia of the tympanic membrane with bulging and obliteration of all normal landmarks. It is frequently difficult to delineate the junction of the bulging tympanic membrane and the posterior canal wall. A conductive hearing loss is uniformly present. Treatment consists of wide incision and drainage of the middle ear abscess by myringotomy and antibiotic therapy for at least seven days. Incision of the tympanic membrane is followed by immediate relief of pain and is the recommended treatment. If the tympanic membrane is not incised and treatment not begun promptly, spontaneous perforation of the tympanic membrane may occur. If this involves the flaccid membrane or a marginal area, the development of chronic suppurative ear disease and cholesteatoma and other complications may be the result. If antibiotic therapy is instituted promptly, the vast majority of acute infections resolve spontaneously without perforation. By and large, acute suppurative otitis media is a disease of infants and children, and such patients are uniformly seen by the pediatrician. Myringotomies are being performed less and less, and it is felt by some that this has been responsible for the increase of nonsuppurative serous otitis media. In addition, inadequate antibacterial therapy or resistant organisms in the presence of a severe infection may result in an aditus block and the development of "masked mastoiditis." This is the result of unabated mastoid infection in the presence of a resolving or healed otitis media and an intact tympanic membrane. A complete cortical mastoidectomy is then necessary.

Owing to inadequate treatment, or a nonresponsive infection caused by a virulent organism, spontaneous perforation of the tympanic membrane may occur. If the perforation occurs in the flaccid portion of the tympanic membrane, the development of a chronic suppurative otitis media and mastoiditis with probable formation of cholesteatoma is almost inevitable. If the perforation occurs in the pars tensa and the infection is treated adequately or subsequently resolves, the perforation may still persist.

ACUTE MASTOIDITIS. Acute mastoiditis usually develops as the result of inadequate treatment of the primary acute suppurative otitis media or as the result of a particularly virulent bacterial infection. As a result of inadequate treatment with antibiotics, occasionally granulation tissue blocks the communication between the middle ear and the pneumatized spaces of the mastoid process, thus resulting in a condition known as "masked mastoiditis." This condition is particularly difficult to diagnose and manage because the middle ear and tympanic membrane may frequently completely heal while the suppurative and destructive process continues in an indolent fashion in the pneumatized spaces of the temporal bone.

Most commonly, the disease is ushered in by the development of a deep pain in the ear which involves the mastoid process itself. The pain is more common in the late evening or early morning hours and is of a constant boring type. It is accompanied by general malaise and low grade fever in adults. Temperature may be quite high in infants and may be accompanied by nausea, vomiting and other intestinal symptoms. When the infection involves cells adjacent to the mastoid cortex, periosteal thickening and swelling of the tissue overlying the mastoid process tend to push the external ear down and out from the head. In children, it may rupture through the medial aspect of the temporal bone and dissect and present in the neck forming a Bezold abscess. If not treated adequately, it may rupture through the internal table of the skull, producing meningitis, brain abscess or extradural abscess. The same periosteal swelling overlying the mastoid cortex also causes edema of the posterior canal wall and the superior portion of the tympanic membrane, with the characteristic sagging of the posterosuperior canal wall. There may or may not be a perforation of the tympanic membrane with a purulent discharge. Roentgenograms reveal a diffuse opacity of the mastoid air cell system early with some definite bone destruction and coalescence of the septa in the later stages.

In addition to the physical signs, there is tenderness to deep pressure over the mastoid process. This may be most easily elicited directly posterosuperiorly to the meatus which is directly over the mastoid antrum, over the tip where the largest cells of the mastoid system are found, or more posteriorly over the emissary vein area.

Because the mucous membrane lining the pneumatic system of the temporal bone is continuous with that of the middle ear and is connected to it by the aditus, any suppurative infection of this latter space results in an infection of variable degree of the mastoid system. If mastoiditis is diagnosed early, is due to responsive organisms, and is treated with adequate doses of the proper antibiotic and a wide myringotomy, mastoiditis may respond to conservative treatment. On the other hand, "masked" mastoiditis and nonresponsive mastoiditis, particularly those which present with a dehiscence of the cortex, or those causing other complications of the disease, require a complete cortical mastoidectomy.

A complete mastoidectomy is a surgical procedure usually performed through a postauricular incision in which all the infected pneumatic spaces of the mastoid process are exenterated. The osseous posterior canal wall is left intact and the middle ear undisturbed. If an attic block exists, the granulation tissue must be removed from the aditus and free communication established between the antrum and the middle ear. A wide myringotomy is necessary. The tip of the mastoid process may or may not be removed. The mastoid cavity is packed with antibiotic-impregnated gauze for four to five days postoperatively and the patient treated with full doses of antibiotics. Upon removal of the pack, the postauricular wound heals primarily and usually the tympanic membrane does also as a result of the establishment of complete drainage and elimination of infected material.

CHRONIC SUPPURATIVE OTITIS MEDIA. Chronic suppurative otitis media may be the result of an inadequately treated acute suppurative otitis media, or may be due to hereditary or developmental abnormalities of the middle ear and the eustachian tube and its ventilating function. Perforations which occur early in Shrapnell's membrane tend not to heal and are associated with the migration of squamous epithelium into the epitympanum. When this occurs, the condition known as cholesteatoma develops. In its essentials, this is a cystic-like space occupying the middle ear, or the pneumatized spaces of the temporal bone, which is lined by squamous epithelium and filled with desquamated epithelial debris. The matrix of the cholesteatoma possesses a bone-destroying potential and if the neck of the cholesteatoma is small, the cholesteatoma may reach an extremely large size and erode important structures (Fig. 4). Cholesteatomas are usually accompanied by a purulent discharge with a peculiarly objectionable odor. The condition tends to erode ossicles and result in progressive loss of hearing, first of the conductive type and later of a sensorineural type. Pressure upon the facial nerve in its middle ear portion or even descending portion may erode the thin overlying bone and result in facial palsy. The cholesteatoma may erode the bone in the roof of the mastoid cavity and with the accompanying infection result in an extradural abscess, meningitis or brain abscess. Erosion of bone over the sigmoid sinus may result in an extradural abscess in the posterior cranial fossa or an abscess of the cerebellar lobe or thrombosis of the sigmoid sinus. This latter is accompanied by a septic temperature, chills and malaise. Practically all the complications of chronic suppurative otitis media and mastoiditis are the result of invasion and destruction of the bone by the associated cholesteatoma.

Occasionally, cholesteatomas develop in the absence of any previous suppurative middle ear disease and are believed to arise as the result of defects of aeration of the middle ear cavity due to faulty eustachian tube function. The thin tympanic membrane retracts as a result of the negative pressure

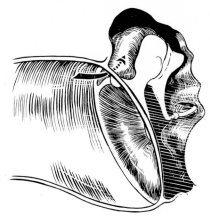

Figure 5.   Primary acquired cholesteatoma. The arrow passes through the neck of the sac, which resembles a pars flaccida perforation.

to form a narrow-necked epithelial-lined cyst which begins to desquamate and behave just as does a secondary acquired cholesteatoma (Fig. 5).

Depending upon the extent of the cholesteatoma, as determined by clinical and x-ray examination, a modified radical mastoidectomy with or without a tympanoplasty of some type is usually possible. In such a procedure, a complete mastoidectomy is accomplished which, because of the usual accompanying sclerosis of the temporal bone, results in a relatively small mastoid cavity. The posterior osseous canal wall may or may not be removed but in all instances the entire cholesteatomatous sac must be removed. Frequently, the incus, which is usually partly destroyed by the cholesteatoma, is removed as well as the head and neck of the malleus. The skin lining the posterior osseous canal wall may be preserved and used to line the medial wall of the modified mastoid cavity, or it may be applied in apposition to a pedicled muscle and soft tissue flap developed from the temporal muscle superiorly or from the soft tissues behind the ear. In the event that the osseous posterior canal wall is to be left in place, it is approached from an anterior direction by means of a transcanal procedure, from the rear by a postauricular incision, and is narrowed to a knife-like thinness. In this technique, all cholesteatoma must be completely removed from the antrum, periantral cells, aditus, epitympanum, about the ossicles and in the middle ear. Usually such a procedure is accompanied by repair of the tympanic membrane perforation and reconstruction of the disrupted ossicular chain by any of many appropriate

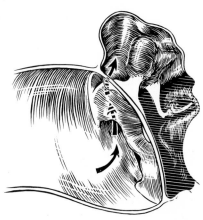

Figure 4.   Secondary acquired cholesteatoma. The arrow shows the path of invasion of squamous epithelium through a marginal perforation to the middle ear, attic and antrum.

techniques. A very successful technique is the removal of the incus from its normal position, the removal of any cholesteatoma which may be enveloping it and its repositioning in the middle ear in order to establish a communication between the reconstructed eardrum and the stapes. If the stapes is involved or has been destroyed by the destructive process, some connection must be made between the footplate and the remaining portions of the ossicular chain. An artifical incus may be constructed from cortical bone of the mastoid process; more commonly wire or polyethylene plastic is used to connect the neck or handle of the malleus to the footplate of the stapes. It is mandatory that all fragments of cholesteatoma be completely removed. This type of operation is usually performed under 16- to 25-power magnification of the operating microscope.

RECONSTRUCTIVE EAR SURGERY. The basic principles of reconstructive ear surgery were established by Zollner in 1951 and Wullstein in 1952. However, the fundamentals underlying such surgery were known previously and exemplified by the modified radical mastoidectomy described by Bondy. In its essentials, reconstructive ear surgery pertains to any surgical procedure designed to eradicate disease, repair the tympanic membrane and reestablish the sound-conducting mechanism of the middle ear. A tympanoplasty in its simplest form is a myringoplasty and implies the plastic repair of a perforation of the tympanic membrane without disturbing or otherwise altering the middle ear structures. Such an operation is absolutely dependent upon a functioning eustachian tube which must be thoroughly evaluated prior to any surgery. Infection of the middle ear and any associated suppuration or disease of the nasopharynx or paranasal sinuses must be controlled before operation. The patency and function of the eustachian tube may be evaluated by the passage of air through the tube from the nose by means of the Valsalva maneuver, politzerization or eustachian tube catheterization. Air may also be inflated through the tube in a retrograde fashion by means of radiopaque or fluorescein clearance studies. A nonfunctioning tube has not yet yielded to surgical attack and is a contraindication to extensive middle ear reconstructive operations.

Split thickness skin, full thickness skin, cartilage, perichondrium and banked tissues of all descriptions have been used with varying degrees of success. The most common tissues used at this time are autogenous vein, fascia or the skin from the posterior canal wall. Fascia is usually obtained from the nearby temporal muscle and is available in unlimited supply. It can be obtained through a postauricular incision through which the incidental mastoidectomy is performed, by means of an extension of an endaural incision or by a separate incision within the hairline above the ear. Vein is limited in amount but is easily procurable, usually from one of the veins of the antecubital fossa. Such tissue is smooth and nonadherent on one side and is thin, pliable and easy to manipulate. It is extremely useful for the repair of relatively small perforations. The skin of the osseous canal wall may be developed as a pedicled canal skin graft or may be removed and reinserted as a free graft, and because of its thinness and pliability is an excellent source of live grafting material. However, it is usually somewhat more technically difficult to develop this tissue and more and more frequent use is being made of fascia for larger perforations and vein for the smaller.

The grafting material may be placed on the external surface of the tympanic membrane, in which event it is necessary to remove the epithelium for several millimeters surrounding the perforation. If vein is used, the adventitia is placed down; if fascia is used, it makes no difference. If canal skin is used, the raw surface is placed on the perforation and may be further strengthened by the insertion of vein or fascia on the medial aspect of the drum. The osseous canal from which the skin is taken epithelializes spontaneously within a matter of ten to 14 days.

If the graft material is to be placed on the inner surface of the perforation, the mucous membrane from the medial aspect of the drum about the periphery of the perforation can be removed for several millimeters with appropriately shaped knives and curettes and the rolled epithelial margin of the perforation removed with cup forceps. If vein is used, the adventitia side must be placed against the denuded portion of the tympanic membrane with the endothelial surface directed towards the promontory. It is supported on a bed of Gelfoam or blood clot and may extend beneath the skin of the posterior or anterior canal wall and may be strengthened with skin from the external auditory canal. This type of myringoplasty is usually performed as an isolated surgical procedure in dry ears. If persistent suppuration or mucoid discharge does not respond to intensive preoperative care, a mastoidectomy of some type in association with the reconstructive surgery is indicated.

In patients with larger perforations, or those in whom the suppurative process has resulted in some destruction of the middle ear ossicles and disruption of ossicular continuity and transmission of sound from the tympanic membrane to the inner ear, a more extensive procedure is indicated. The graft or repositioned tympanic membrane may be approximated to a carious incus and draped directly over the superstructure of the stapes. If the long process of the incus fails to make contact with the stapes, the entire incus may be rotated out of its normal position and placed over the stapes and the graft or tympanic membrane placed upon the repositioned incus. This re-establishes a modified ossicular chain and permits the transmission of sound from the tympanic membrane to the inner ear via the normal stapes.

Total tympanic membrane reconstructions can be accomplished using either canal skin or fascia, though it is difficult to obtain adequate amounts of vein for this purpose. In the presence of cholesteatoma, all fragments of the cholesteatoma must be removed prior to carrying out any reconstructive phase of the surgical procedure. An intact and functioning eustachian tube is a prerequisite for such reconstructive surgery. Although the primary objective remains the removal of all diseased or infected tissue, the restoration of an intact tympanic membrane and the improvement of hearing are desired end results. If inner ear damage has been minimal and adequate provision for transmission of acoustic energy from the reconstructed tympanic membrane through the ossicular chain is accomplished, the prognosis for a hearing improvement is fair to good. Frequently, such an operation must be accomplished in two stages, with the first being directed toward the removal of all disease and the establishment of an intact tympanic membrane. The second stage consists of a tympanotomy and reconstruction of the sound-conducting mechanism in the middle ear. In addition, this provides a "second look" procedure in order to check on the completeness of cholesteatoma removal. It is generally performed from three to six months following a successful first stage.

Reconstructive ear surgery is frequently performed in conjunction with a mastoidectomy of some type. If the posterior osseous canal wall is removed, the mastoid cavity may be obliterated or filled in by soft tissue obtained from the temporal muscle, postauricular soft tissues or portions of the sternocleidomastoid and postauricular muscles. The meatal skin flap or posterior canal wall skin is placed upon the muscle and results in a small or no cavity. It is not yet certain whether or not the currently favored technique of leaving intact the osseous posterior canal wall in cholesteatoma will prove to be satisfactory. There are those who believe that the posterior canal wall should be sacrificed in order to facilitate removal of all disease. One of the benefits of leaving the osseous canal wall and avoiding a cavity is that following a successful operation the individual may engage in all normal activities, particularly swimming and other aquatic sports.

OTOSCLEROSIS. Closely allied to reconstructive ear operations for the sequelae of suppurative ear disease are procedures for the improvement or restoration of hearing following nonsuppurative diseases. By far the most common of these is otosclerosis, or more properly otospongiosis. This is a disease that involves the young adult and is more frequent in the female. It has been found to involve in varying degrees up to 10 per cent of all individuals as determined by unselected autopsy material. If the vascular disease and deposition of new bone involve the junction of the footplate with the rim of the oval window, limitation of motion of the footplate and eventual ankylosis are the results. When this occurs, a conductive hearing loss of up to 60 decibels may result. It was formerly thought that the pathological changes and disease process were confined to the otic capsule in the peristapedial area. However, it is now realized that the disease is occasionally responsible for purely sensorineural hearing losses.

The pathogenesis of the inner ear changes is not completely known. The cause of the disease is unknown and no medical treatment has proved beneficial. The fenestration procedure was devised as a one-stage practical operation in 1938 for the improvement of hearing in otosclerosis and ushered in a new era of modern otology. The procedure involved a modified mastoidectomy type of approach with a fenestration of the ampullated end of the horizontal semicircular canal. The tympanomeatal flap then covered the fenestra nov-ovalis and the ankylosed stapes was by-passed. This resulted in improvement of hearing up to the 25- or 30-decibel level.

Operative procedures directly upon the footplate have supplanted the fenestration procedure and generally involve the removal of all or a portion of the footplate of the stapes and the creation of a mobile soft tissue plug connected in some fashion to the incus (Fig. 6). The most common prostheses are preformed stainless steel wire and Gelfoam or a small segment of vein or compressed bits of Gelfoam placed over the oval window and connected to the incus by a wire crimped around the long process of the incus. This re-establishes the continuity of the ossicular chain and in individuals with normal inner ear function restores hearing to normal. Complications of stapes operations are few, but in 1 to 2 per cent of all patients in large series, a significant deterioration of the hearing occurs. Stapes operations have been perfected so that in 90 to 95 per cent of well-selected individuals a successful result can be expected.

BELL'S PALSY. Facial palsy not due to trauma, otitic infections or other known causes is called Bell's palsy. Its precise etiology is unknown, but it is most generally believed to be the result of ischemic changes in the descending portion of the nerve in the posterior osseous canal wall. Some recent studies have suggested the possibility of its resulting from an ascending viral infection of the chorda tympani gaining access to the nerve through the duct of the submaxillary gland. This disease afflicts individuals of all ages and is sudden in onset. It is lower motor neuron in type with paralysis of the frontalis and orbicularis oculi. Rolling upward of the eyes on attempted closure, known as Bell's phenomenon, is usually quite marked. There is decreased salivation on testing of the submaxillary gland secretions. Nerve excitability tests are variable but generally indicate some impairment of conductivity to complete absence of response.

Conservative treatment consists of vasodilating drugs such as nicotinic acid and anti-inflammatory steroid therapy for two to three weeks. In the presence of progressive decrease in excitability on serial testing, or failure of the facial muscles to respond at all to testing, serious consideration should be given to immediate decompression of the nerve. In any event, in any patient with Bell's palsy lasting longer than three months, the facial nerve should be decompressed.

The surgical procedure consists of a postauricular mastoidectomy approach with exposure of the descending and pyramidal portions of the facial nerve. The bony walls are removed from about the nerve and the perineurium is slit to release any pressure on the nerve. Although the prognosis for spontaneous return of facial function is variously estimated at up to 85 per cent, surgical decompression of the facial nerve in selected instances may increase this to 95 per cent or more.

DISEASES OF THE INNER EAR

Ménière's disease is by far the most common affliction of the inner ear for which surgical therapy is utilized. It is characterized by recurrent and intermittent episodes of vertigo, tinnitus and deafness. There is frequently a persistent pressure in the ear on the side of the disease. The hearing loss fluctuates and may precede the vertigo by months or many years. Its general course is one of progressive deterioration.

No known medical therapy is uniformly effective in relieving or preventing the vertiginous episodes characteristic of Ménière's disease and as a result many various types of surgical procedures have been devised in attempts to eliminate the episodes of vertigo while preserving residual hearing. Usually, patients who are considered for operation have developed essentially useless hearing in the diseased ear as a result of the disease. A phenomenon of Ménière's disease is recruitment, which consists of an abnormal growth of loudness in the diseased ear. This

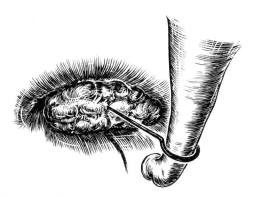

Figure 6. The stapes has been removed and replaced by a piece of soft tissue attached to the incus with stainless steel wire.

associated with poor discrimination often renders the ear useless and may even result in confusing what is heard in the good ear. For these reasons, the preservation of hearing in the diseased ear is not frequently a major surgical consideration. Because approximately 10 per cent of Ménière's disease patients develop symptoms in the second ear later on or concomitantly with the onset of the disease, it has seemed important in many instances to attempt to preserve hearing.

The standard surgical procedure for the relief of Ménière's disease is a labyrinthectomy which can be performed either through the mastoid or through the ear canal. If the former, a simple mastoidectomy is accomplished through a postauricular approach and the ampullated end of the horizontal canal opened, its contents, and that of the vestibule removed. The latter is performed by an incision made in the posterior canal wall, the elevation of the tympanomeatal flap, the extraction of the stapes and the removal of all contents of the vestibule. The vestibule is then packed with Gelfoam or bone dust. It is performed under 10- or 16-power magnification. These procedures uniformly result in complete relief of symptoms and loss of the residual hearing. Tinnitus usually persists.

Several other types of procedures are ultrasonic therapy, which is delivered to the ampullated end of the horizontal canal through a mastoidectomy approach; the decompression or shunting of the endolymphatic sac either into the subarachnoid space or into the mastoid cavity; and the sacculotomy operation of Fick. In this latter operation, an opening is made through the footplate into the dilated saccule directly beneath it. This is believed to result in a sheer membrane with the resultant decompression of endolymph into the perilymphatic spaces and submucosal tissues of the middle ear. With the exception of labyrinthectomy, all these procedures must be considered experimental at the present time.

NEOPLASMS

Basal cell and squamous cell epitheliomas of the external auricle are extremely common, particularly in older individuals. They are relatively simple to treat unless they involve the canal or cartilage and respond well to simple excision or radiation therapy. If they involve the membranous or osseous canals, wide surgical excision is necessary. On occasions, a mastoidectomy approach is necessary.

The most common tumor of the middle ear is the glomus jugulare tumor which arises from the glomus body in the dome of the jugular bulb or on the promontory along the branches of the nerve of Jacobson. They are very vascular neoplasms and cause tinnitus and hearing loss in their early stages and, upon rupturing through the tympanic membrane and the occurrence of secondary infection, result in a chronic purulent discharge. Those arising in the dome of the jugular bulb may involve the base of the skull and cause paralysis of the ninth, tenth and eleventh cranial nerves. When diagnosed early, small tumors in the middle ear may be removed by a tympanotomy approach. When larger, a radical mastoidectomy is required. Because they are extremely vascular tumors, they are frequently difficult to remove completely and post-surgical radiation therapy is frequently advised. They are relatively responsive and if not cured may be held in check for long periods of time.

Carcinoma occasionally arises in the middle ear or mastoid as a primary tumor and may suggest a glomus tumor, usually with decreased hearing acuity and a purulent discharge from the ear. Because of the bone involvement, such tumors respond poorly to irradiation therapy and more recently have been managed by a combination of preoperative radiation therapy and surgical excision. An en bloc subtotal resection of the temporal bone involves a combined intracranial and extracranial approach with sectioning of the temporal bone medial to the otic capsule and the en bloc resection of the inner, middle and usually the external ear as a single surgical specimen. The wound is closed by rotation scalp flaps or split thickness skin grafts. The operative morbidity and mortality is high, but salvage rates have increased to about 40 per cent.

With the exception of the glomus tumor, nonmalignant tumors are unusual. One of the most common consists of tumors arising from the bone of the external auditory canal. Osteomas, when large enough, result in complete obstruction of the canal and a significant hearing loss. They may be removed by a transcanal approach under microscopic control and visualization.

CONGENITAL MALFORMATIONS

These may occur isolated or in combination with congenital malformations elsewhere in the body. One of the most common causes is rubella occurring in the mother in the first trimester of pregnancy. The tragic outbreak of serious congenital deformities in Germany several years ago as a result of thalidomide's effect on the fetal development was accompanied by many abnormalities of the ear. The most common malformation is the "lop ear." This is an abnormality of the cartilage of the auricle in which the cartilage lacks its usual convolutions which form the superior and inferior crura of the anthelix and as a result the ear stands out from the head prominently. It may be unilateral. Surgical repair is simple and involves a postauricular approach with removal of redundant skin and the excision of small strips of cartilage along the line of the absent folds. Small external ears are common. They usually require no surgical treatment.

Some narrowing of the external auditory canal is extremely common and may vary from all degrees to complete atresia of the osseous canal. Such defects are usually associated with varying degrees of microtia. However, because of the separate development of the inner ear, the sensorineural component is usually normal. This allows reconstructive surgical procedures for the purpose of improving hearing. Surgery consists of a mastoidectomy type of approach, the creation of an air-containing cavity, various manipulations of the ossicular chain and the formation of a neotympanic membrane from a fascia graft. Hearing may be improved in such instances to a serviceable nonaided level. Operation is not usually indicated in unilateral afflictions. Total reconstruction of the absent or extremely malformed external ear has been one of the most challenging feats in plastic and reconstructive surgery and reliance is generally made upon a prosthetic appliance.

THE NOSE

In man, the chief function of the nose is respiratory rather than olfactory. The turbinates, the nasal septum and the anterior and posterior nares determine the size and shape of the nasal chambers and are directly concerned in regulating air currents and air flow during the respiratory cycle. Specialized respiratory ciliated columnar epithelium and its substratum cleanse and control the temperature and humidity of the inspired and expired air. Particulate particles within the inspired air are trapped by the mucus sheet and are swept into the nasopharynx. The pH of the mucus is 7.0. The average adult produces 600 to 800 ml. of mucus in the nose and paranasal sinuses during a 24-hour period.

NASAL SEPTUM

The nasal septum separates the two nasal chambers in the midline. The supporting structures of the nasal septum are the quadrilateral cartilage, the perpendicular plate of the ethmoid bone, the vomer and the palatine crest. It is covered by pseudostratified, ciliated columnar epithelium.

DEFORMITIES. Deformities of the nasal septum develop during growth and are often caused by trauma. During birth, the infant's nose and nasal septum may be twisted or bent as the head passes through the birth canal. This usually results in a greenstick fracture with the nose being displaced to one side. This injury is readily corrected by simple manual manipulation.

Nasal obstruction is the main symptom produced by septal deformities. If the ostium or one or more of the paranasal sinuses are blocked, particularly by spur formation, sinusitis may result. There is a wide variation in the type and extent of the deformity and the obstruction may be unilateral or bilateral (Fig. 7). Compensatory hypertrophy of the inferior turbinate of the opposite nasal chamber occurs, causing periodic nasal obstruction. Septal spurs impinging on one of the turbinates may cause headache. Drying and crusting of the septal mucosa caused by deviation are factors in producing ulceration.

Septal deformities may be corrected by submucous resection of the nasal septum. Classically, in this operation the obstructing bone and cartilage are removed. Recently, many rhinologists have preferred to reconstruct the nasal septum using the patient's own cartilage and bone. This procedure gives stability to the septum, restores the airway and supports the external nose. Compensatory hypertrophy of the inferior turbinate

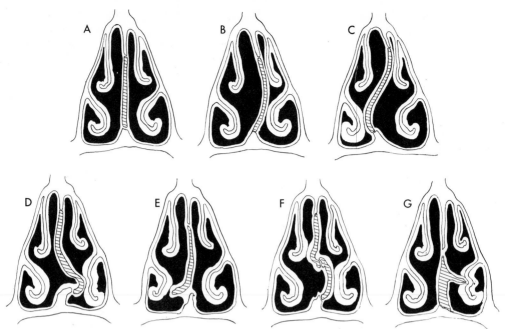

Figure 7. *A*, Normal nasal septum. *B*, Unilateral wide deflection of the cartilaginous septum. *C*, S-shaped deformity. *D* and *E*, Fracture-dislocations of the septum along the maxillary crest. *F*, Fracture-dislocation of the cartilaginous septum; these deformities often involve the bones of the nasal septum. *G*, Wide spur formation; such a spur in the middle meatus may block a sinus ostium.

bone and mucosa can be treated by submucous resection of the bony turbinate and judicious removal of redundant mucosa.

ABSCESS. Abscess of the nasal septum occurs spontaneously, and following operation and trauma. The infecting organisms are frequently streptococci, staphylococci or pneumococci. The nose becomes painful and swollen, and upon inspection, the septal mucosa is bulged and reddened bilaterally. There may be high temperature and chills. When the perichondrium is lifted off the cartilage, there is loss of blood supply to the cartilage. Necrosis of the cartilage may develop, causing a saddle deformity of the external nose.

Early unilateral incision and drainage are recommended. Full therapeutic doses of sulfonamide or antibiotic drugs are indicated. The patient must be observed for clinical signs of cavernous sinus thrombosis.

PERFORATION. Perforations of the nasal septum develop in the cartilaginous portion of the septum. They result from trauma, such as "nose picking," penetrating injuries and intranasal surgery. Other less common causes are syphilis, tuberculosis and neoplasm. If the perforation is large, crusting may result, causing repeated epistaxis. Bland ointments should be applied to the crusting areas of the perforation. Surgical correction

is usually successful only in patients with small perforations.

HEMATOMA. Hematomas occur following trauma and operative procedures on the nasal septum. The septal mucosa bulges bilaterally, and dark blood can be obtained by aspiration. Incision and drainage are indicated as well as nasal packing.

NASAL FRACTURES

The bony and cartilaginous framework of the external and internal nose is frequently fractured by blunt or penetrating types of trauma.

Fractures may be greenstick, linear, comminuted or compounded. Compounding may occur internally into the nasal chambers, into the cavities of the paranasal sinuses or externally. The cartilage and bones of the septum are frequently compounded. Nasal fracture may be associated with fractures of the facial bones as well. A common injury caused by blunt trauma is linear fracture of the nasal bones, wherein one is depressed and the opposite is displaced laterally, resulting in displacement of the nose.

Diagnosis is made by inspection and palpation. Crepitus may be present. The internal structures of the nose must be examined under satisfactory illumination. Roentgenographic studies are often unsatisfactory in patients with simple fractures because the normal vascular markings of the nasal bones may simulate fracture lines. However, x-ray examination should be carried out in patients sustaining nasal injuries to determine associated facial bone injuries.

The treatment of patients with nasal fractures may be delayed as long as seven to ten days, particularly if there is associated edema and hemorrhage within the soft tissues. Nasal fractures may be reduced by closed or open surgical techniques. Local or general anesthetics are used. Closed reduction consists of intranasal elevation of the displaced nasal bones and realignment of the nasal septum. Intranasal packing and external splinting are usually employed. Open reduction is indicated in compound comminuted fractures associated with hematomas. Incisions are placed within the vestibule of the nose and in the mucosa of the nasal septum. Hematomas are drained and bone and cartilage are accurately realigned. Fixation of bony and cartilaginous fragments may be accomplished by through-and-through wiring, direct wiring, septal sutures, intranasal packing and external splinting. Old traumatic deformities of the nasal septum and nasal bones must be corrected by refracture and reconstruction. Late saddle deformities of the dorsum are corrected by autogenous bone grafts.

EPISTAXIS

Bleeding from the nose can occur at any age and usually is spontaneous. Most commonly, it is the result of rupture of a superficial vessel in the mucosa of the nasal septum in Kiesselbach's area (Fig. 8). On the other hand, bleeding may be indicative of serious underlying disease within the nasal chambers, paranasal sinuses and nasopharynx, or constitutional disease such as a blood dyscrasia, a blood clotting defect, hypertension, arteriosclerotic heart disease or liver disease. In all patients, the etiologic factor must be sought.

During examination, the patient should be placed in an upright position to prevent

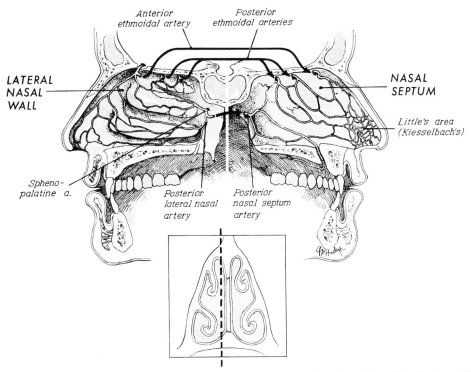

Figure 8. The dual blood supply of the nose is illustrated. A sagittal section to the right of the midline is shown. The nose is then "swung open." Note the external carotid system continues as the sphenopalatine artery. The sphenopalatine artery passes in the mucosa of the anterior wall and floor of the sphenoid sinus to the nasal septum. The anterior and posterior ethmoid arteries are derived from the ophthalmic artery (internal carotid). The ethmoid arteries cross the vault of the nose to reach the nasal septum. This third-dimensional concept is presented for clarity.

swallowing and aspiration of blood, providing that there are no signs of shock. Good illumination and suction must be available. If possible, the bleeding source should be located before any intranasal vasoconstricting medication is applied. If the source of bleeding is located, it can usually be stopped by local pressure, chemical cautery or electrocoagulation after topical application of 5 per cent cocaine hydrochloride.

The bleeding source, if behind septal spurs, beneath the turbinates, high in the vault or near the choanae, may be entirely inaccessible to cauterization techniques. In these instances, the nose must be topically anesthetized and the nasal chambers packed with ½-inch selvedged gauze impregnated with an antibiotic ointment. The gauze is then placed in laminated layers so that all areas within the nose are adequately compressed. All pieces of packing are anchored to the face by the use of strings or tape. It is permissible for nasal packing to remain in the nasal chambers five to eight days, providing that the patient is given antibiotic drugs to prevent suppuration of the sinuses or the middle ears.

Anterior packing may not control bleeding, particularly if the source is from the posterior recesses of the nasal chamber. In such instances, posterior nasopharyngeal packing must be used as well as anterior packing (Fig. 9). Packs are usually placed after local topical anesthesia of the intranasal and naso-pharyngeal structures. Posterior nasal packing may be left in place as long as five to seven days, providing that antibiotic therapy is used to prevent sinus and ear suppuration. It this fails to arrest nasal bleeding within a short period of time, the patient may be given a general anesthetic and the nose and nasopharynx may be repacked. If bleeding continues in spite of this treatment, submucous resection of the nasal septum may be indicated in selected patients.

Uncontrolled bleeding from high in the nose anteriorly may require ligation of the anterior ethmoid artery. Posterior bleeding may yield only to ligation of the internal maxillary artery or its parent vessel, the external carotid artery. The former is approached through the antrum and the latter in the neck. Any of these surgical procedures may be performed under local anesthesia.

In the treatment of patients with epistaxis one must be alert for evidences of shock. Blood loss, if excessive, must be replaced by transfusions. Constitutional disease must be treated as well as local disease.

Patients with recurring epistaxis from multiple hereditary telangiectasis may bleed repeatedly from one or both nasal chambers. Epistaxis may be so severe and prolonged that serious secondary anemia results. Repeated local therapy is difficult and frequently unsatisfactory. Septal dermatoplasty may be indicated. The telangiectatic mucosa is replaced by split-thickness dermal grafts.

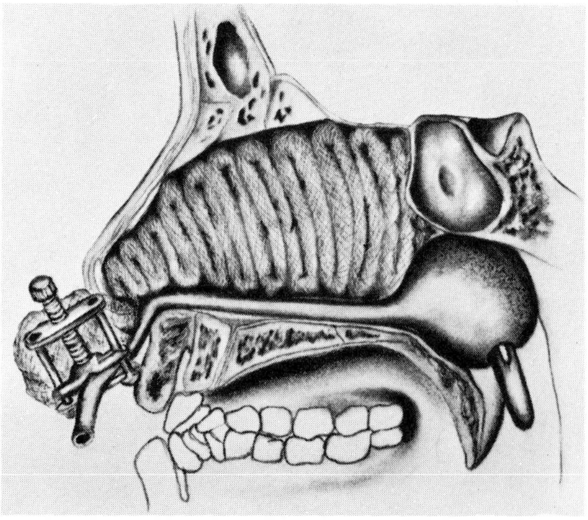

Figure 9. Postnasal packing. A 30 cc. Foley catheter has been passed through the nose, partially inflated with water and pulled up into the choana. The entire nasal cavity is tamponaded with gauze impregnated with antibiotic ointment.

DISEASES

NASAL POLYPS. Nasal polyps occur most often during adulthood and in patients with allergic rhinitis. Polyps form gradually from a localized swelling of the mucosa of the maxillary and ethmoid sinuses. As polyps accumulate fluid and become edematous, they protrude into the nasal cavity area and nasal obstruction results. The obstruction may also cause blockage of the paranasal sinus ostia, leading to stagnation and sinusitis. Polyps may be single or multiple; most frequently they originate in the middle meatus and ethmoid labyrinth. Large solitary polyps occasionally arise in the maxillary sinus and project from this site of origin by a stalk into the nasopharynx (Fig. 10). Intranasal surgical removal is the treatment of choice. Frequently, partial intranasal eth-

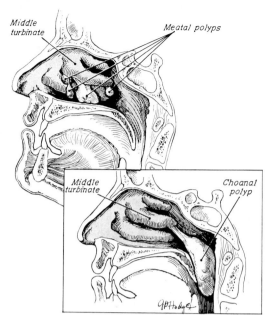

Middle turbinate   *Meatal polyps*

Middle turbinate   *Choanal polyp*

Figure 10. Polyps usually arise from the mucosa lining the ethmoid sinuses and present first in the middle meatus. Occasionally, a solitary polyp arises in the antrum, fills the nasal cavity and finally presents in the nasopharynx. Following simple removal, it is prone to recur and may require a radical antrum operation.

moidectomy is also indicated. In order to improve visualization, the operation is carried out with local anesthesia. In long-term treatment of patients with nasal polyposis, hyposensitization therapy is indicated.

Inflammatory nasal polyps may occur in patients with chronic suppuration of the paranasal sinuses. Operations designed to cure the suppurative sinusitis usually prevent further recurrences of this type of polyp.

CHOANAL ATRESIA. Choanal atresia may be unilateral or bilateral. Newborn infants must be examined carefully for bilateral choanal atresia if respiratory distress is present. The diagnosis can be made by attempting to pass a small soft rubber catheter through the nose into the pharynx. Methylene blue may be dropped in the nose and failure of the dye to appear in the oropharynx is also diagnostic. The instillation of Lipiodol into the nose and roentgenographic studies may further confirm the diagnosis (Fig. 11). An immediate airway must be established either by securing an oral airway or by the performance of a tracheotomy. The atresia is corrected by an intranasal surgical operation only after the airway and feeding prob-

lems are stabilized. If the choanal atresia is unilateral, the infant usually does not have difficulty in breathing or nursing. Unilateral mucoid nasal discharge develops and as a rule diagnosis is made later in childhood. In childhood and adulthood, surgical correction may be made by either transseptal or transpalatal approaches.

FOREIGN BODIES. Foreign bodies of the nose produce unilateral purulent discharge if not removed within a few days. The most common foreign bodies are pieces of paper, peas, beans, rubber erasers and buttons. All foreign bodies should be removed promptly after diagnosis. Care must be taken during removal that the foreign body does not slip from the grasping instrument, gravitate into the pharynx and be aspirated by the patient.

MALIGNANCIES. Unilateral nasal obstruction or bloody discharge from the nose may indicate malignancy in the older individual. Malignancies of the nasal chambers may be primary growths of the nasal fossa or secondary growths from primary neoplastic disease of the paranasal sinuses. Neoplasms of epithelial origin are more common than those of supporting tissues. Diagnosis is confirmed by microscopic examination of excised tissue. Roentgenograms may show bone destruction. When feasible, wide surgical ex-

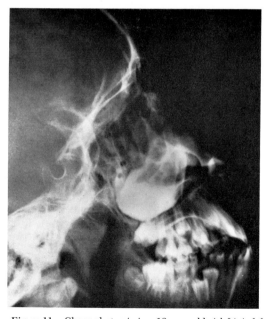

Figure 11. Choanal atresia in a 13-year-old girl. Lipiodol has been instilled into the nasal cavity. Complete choanal obstruction is evident.

cision is the treatment of choice. Radiation therapy may be combined with surgery.

PARANASAL SINUSES

The paranasal sinuses are paired. The maxillary and ethmoidal sinuses are present at birth, whereas the sphenoid and frontal sinuses develop during childhood. All groups are usually fully developed in early adulthood. They are lined with low cuboidal ciliated epithelium.

ACUTE SUPPURATIVE MAXILLARY SINUSITIS. Acute suppurative maxillary sinusitis seldom occurs as an isolated entity. When it does, apical tooth infections, septal spurs blocking the ostium, foreign bodies and neoplasms should be considered in the differential diagnosis. Most frequently, acute-suppurative maxillary sinusitis occurs in association with suppuration of the homolateral ethmoid, frontal and sphenoid sinuses. Predisposing factors are acute upper respiratory disease, allergic states, swimming and general debilitation. The symptoms are nasal stuffiness, purulent nasal discharge, pain over the affected sinuses, local tenderness and fever. Diagnosis can be made by intranasal inspection and by noting pus in the middle meatus. Roentgenographic studies show clouding of the affected sinuses. Streptococci, staphylococci and pneumococci are the most common infecting pyogenic organisms. Appropriate antibiotic therapy for seven to ten days and conservative treatment such as local heat, nasal vasoconstrictors and supportive measures should be carried out. Antral lavage by needle puncture through the inferior meatus or cannulation of the natural ostium should be performed only after the acute process has subsided, usually within five days.

Most patients with acute maxillary sinusitis are treated successfully by conservative management. If they prove refractory to such therapy, one should study the patient for unusual organisms, infected teeth, septal spurs, foreign bodies and neoplasms. Special bacterial smears and cultures, cytologic studies, biopsy and microscopic tissue examination, and repeated roentgenograms may be indicated. The results of such studies will guide the physician in further management, whether it be surgical or medical.

CHRONIC SUPPURATIVE MAXILLARY SINUSITIS. Chronic suppurative maxillary sinusitis may be manifested by persistent unilateral purulent rhinorrhea. Pain is usually absent. The mucous membrane becomes thickened and chronic changes may occur within the bony walls of the sinus. Organisms are of a mixed flora. Chronic maxillary sinusitis may be associated with tooth abscess or oral-antral fistula. The diagnosis is made by intranasal inspection, x-ray examinations, diagnostic antral irrigations and cultures (Fig. 12). The treatment should be conservative at the outset, consisting of antral lavages, local vasoconstrictors and the surgical removal of contributing causes such as septal spurs and polyps. If these measures fail, intranasal antrotomy may be indicated. In other patients with mucosal thickening, abscesses and osteitis, radical exenteration may be indicated. Because the ethmoidal labyrinth is usually infected also, transantral ethmoidectomy may also be indicated.

ACUTE SUPPURATIVE FRONTAL SINUSITIS. Acute suppurative frontal sinusitis occurs most frequently in patients with associated acute ethmoiditis and maxillary sinusitis of the homolateral side. It frequently develops following swimming or diving in the presence of an upper respiratory infection. There may be localized pain and fever. Upon intranasal inspection, pus will be found in the region of the nasofrontal duct. Roentgenograms may show clouding or a fluid level.

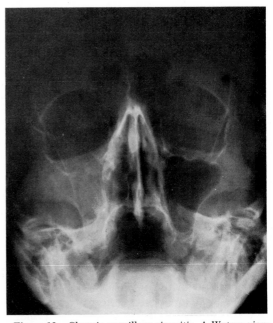

Figure 12. Chronic maxillary sinusitis. A Waters view reveals complete opacification of the right antrum in this 46-year-old man. Antral irrigation confirmed the diagnosis and a radical antrum operation cured his disease.

Conservative treatment in the form of hot packs, intranasal medication and systemic care should be instituted. Indiscriminate intranasal manipulation during the course of acute suppurative frontal sinusitis must be avoided. Contributing factors such as septal deviations and nasal polyps should be surgically removed after the subsidence of acute symptoms. Trephining of the floor of the frontal sinus during the course of a fulminating frontal sinusitis or empyema may be indicated in some patients. Antibiotic drug therapy should be administered in adequate doses for at least seven days.

CHRONIC SUPPURATIVE FRONTAL SINUSITIS. Chronic suppuration of the frontal sinuses is usually characterized by unilateral purulent nasal discharge. When present, pain is suggestive of an empyema caused by a blocked nasofrontal duct, or a complication such as extradural abscess, meningitis or osteomyelitis. Intranasal inspection shows unilateral purulent discharge from the region of the nasofrontal duct. Roentgenograms show a clouding of the frontal sinus or osteitis of the sinus margins (Fig. 13). A radical external operation is indicated only in refractory infections when conservative therapeutic measures have failed.

ACUTE SUPPURATIVE ETHMOIDITIS. Acute suppurative ethmoiditis usually results when a bacterial infection is superimposed on a viral upper respiratory infection. It is characterized by a stuffy nose and purulent nasal discharge, mild fever and malaise. It is ordinarily self-limited but yields readily to nasal vasoconstrictors and antibiotic therapy for five to seven days. Complications such as orbital cellulitis and cavernous sinus thrombosis may demand surgical drainage.

CHRONIC SUPPURATIVE ETHMOIDITIS. Chronic suppurative ethmoiditis usually accompanies chronic infections of the other homolateral sinuses and requires either an intranasal or external ethmoidectomy, usually in conjunction with surgical procedures directed to the other involved sinuses.

COMPLICATIONS OF ACUTE AND CHRONIC SUPPURATIVE SINUS DISEASE. Most complications of paranasal suppurative sinus disease occur in patients with allergic backgrounds and during the course of acute fulminating sinusitis or during an acute exacerbation of chronic suppurative disease. The complications occur either extracranially or intracranially or both. Soft tissue and bone may be affected. As a general rule, if there is a complication involving the soft tissues and bone, direct external drainage is indicated. In all patients, antibiotic agents should be administered in high doses. A direct external operative approach upon the infected sinus

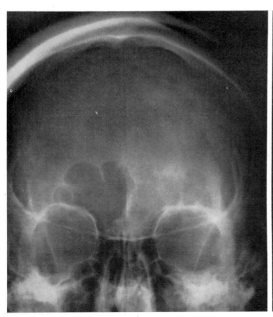
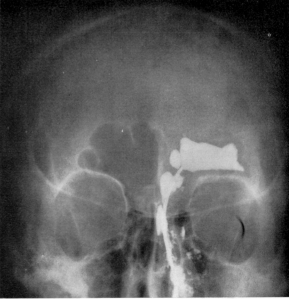

A   *B*

Figure 13. Chronic frontal sinusitis. *A*, The Caldwell view demonstrates clouding of the left frontal sinus. *B*, Lipiodol instilled through a canula in the nasofrontal duct clarifies the pathological changes. An external operation and obliteration with fat is indicated.

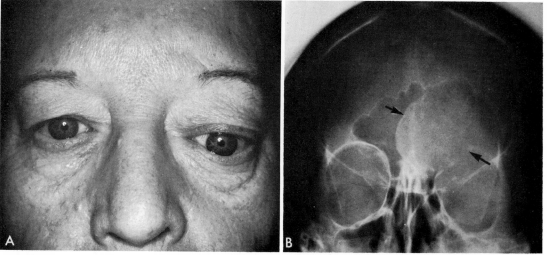

Figure 14.   Mucocele. *A*, The eye is displaced in a downward and outward direction. Diplopia is not usual because of its slow development. *B*, X-ray films show the rounded density of the left frontal sinus and erosion of the superomedial rim of the orbit.

or sinuses may be indicated later after the acuteness subsides. In patients with brain abscess, subdural and epidural abscess, in addition to chemotherapy and antibiotics, operation is indicated.

MUCOCELE.   Mucoceles develop as a result of blockage of sinus drainage. The cause of blockage may be congenital deformities of sinus ostia or scar formation following trauma or surgery. Mucoceles most frequently erode the floor of the frontal sinus and anterior ethmoid cells. There is an insidious development of proptosis; the orbital contents are displaced downward and outward. Diplopia may develop. The swelling is painless and without signs of inflammation (Fig. 14). If signs of inflammation develop, pain may be a dominant symptom. Infected mucoceles are known as pyoceles. Roentgenograms may show a smooth, cystic enlargement or be deceptively normal. Mucoceles must be exenterated by an external surgical approach and wide intranasal drainage established.

ORO-ANTRAL FISTULAE.   Oro-antral fistulae follow extraction of a tooth, penetrating wounds, surgical trauma or a neoplasm. Associated suppuration of the maxillary sinus tends to favor chronicity and persistence of the fistula. Patients complain of leakage of fluid and food into the nasal chamber. Early simple suture of the fistula may allow successful closure. When maxillary sinus suppuration is present, it must be cleared before closure of the fistula can be successful.

Sinusitis, as well as the oral fistula, may be treated by radical exenteration combined with the use of a palatal or buccal pedicle flap.

NEOPLASMS

OSTEOMAS.   Osteomas, although rare, occur most frequently in the frontal sinus. They produce varying degrees of pressure symptoms and pain. By expansion growth, intracranial complications may occur with secondary suppuration. Roentgenographic examination is usually diagnostic. Removal by an external operative approach is indicated only in patients with symptoms.

OSSIFYING FIBROMAS.   Ossifying fibromas are frequently located in the maxillary sinus. Symptoms are produced only by pressure from expansive growth and secondary suppuration. Because the fibromas are benign, radical excision is contraindicated. Cosmetic contouring and wide intranasal drainage are sufficient.

SQUAMOUS PAPILLOMAS.   Squamous papillomas are benign epithelial growths, arising most frequently in the nasal cavity. They do not metastasize but destroy adjacent structures by expansion. They are considered premalignant. The treatment is complete removal.

MALIGNANCIES.   Malignant neoplasms of the paranasal sinuses may be divided into those of epithelial and those of supporting tissue origin. Epithelial tumors are by far the most common. Metastatic malignancies from distant primary lesions occur rarely. Primary malignancy may arise in any of the paranasal sinuses, although the maxillary sinus is most frequently involved. Squamous cell carcinoma is the most commonly encountered single lesion of these areas. There may be direct growth into the ethmoid sinuses, orbit, nasal chamber, palate, buccal areas, pterygomaxillary fossa and soft tissues. Lymphatic metastases may occur to the cervical lymph nodes. Blood metastases can occur later in the course of the disease to the chest, abdominal viscera and brain. Unilateral purulent or bloody nasal discharge may be the presenting symptom. Later paresthesia and anesthesia may develop along the course of the infraorbital nerve. Teeth may be loosened. Masses are prone to develop in the orbit, soft tissues of the cheek, palate and buccal areas. The diagnosis of malignancy is made presumptively by direct inspection, palpation and roentgenograms. Diagnosis is confirmed by biopsy and microscopic tissue examination. Treatment is surgical or by x-ray therapy, or by a combination of both methods.

THROAT

The pharynx extends from the larynx upward to the base of the skull. The space is divided into the nasopharynx, or the space above the soft palate; the oropharynx, directly posterior to the oral cavity; and the hypopharynx, which extends from the base of the tongue inferiorly to the larynx and hypopharynx (Fig. 15). These cavities are enclosed in a muscular cone and mucosa. Their functions are for the passage of air, food and fluids.

OROPHARYNX

INFECTIONS. The structures in the oropharynx which may be involved in acute infections include the mucosa of the pharynx and lymphoid tissues of the lingual and faucial tonsils. Streptococci, staphylococci, pneumococci and Friedländer's bacilli are the most frequent causative organisms. Treatment is conservative, in the form of throat irrigations, systemic care, specific antibiotic therapy, as indicated, and local soothing medications.

Acute infections of the oropharynx may also develop as local manifestations of systemic disease in patients with such diseases as infectious mononucleosis, agranulocytosis and blood dyscrasias.

The most common chronic inflammation of the oropharynx is chronic tonsillitis. Other conditions such as tuberculosis, syphilis, drug irritations, viruses and fungous infections may also produce chronic inflammatory processes. Diagnosis may require special bacteriologic studies, biopsy and microscopic tissue examination.

PERITONSILLAR ABSCESS. Peritonsillar abscess usually occurs in patients with acute streptococcal or staphylococcal tonsillitis. Infection localizes in the peritonsillar tissues and the potential space between the tonsil capsule and the superior pharyngeal constrictor muscles. Symptoms are dysphagia, trismus and a muffled "hot potato in the mouth" voice. Fever and leukocytosis are present. Examination shows a bulging and protrusion of the affected tonsil toward the midline. The uvula is displaced and edematous (Fig. 16). Incision and drainage is the treatment of choice. Antibiotic drug therapy is indicated. The peritonsillar abscess cavity must be opened and spread with a hemostat daily in order to release residual pus during the period of aftercare.

RETROPHARYNGEAL ABSCESS. Retropharyngeal abscess occurs most frequently in young

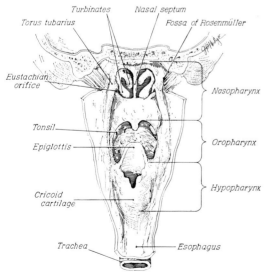

Turbinates   Nasal septum
Torus tubarius   Fossa of Rosenmüller
Eustachian orifice
Nasopharynx
Tonsil
Epiglottis
Oropharynx
Hypopharynx
Cricoid cartilage
Trachea   Esophagus

Figure 15. The pharynx as viewed from behind; its three anatomic divisions are clearly shown. These areas contain useful landmarks and should be learned by all physicians.

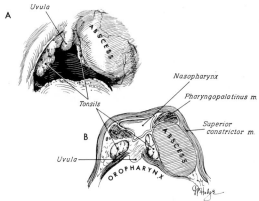

Figure 16. *A,* View of the oropharynx showing marked swelling of the left side of the soft palate. The tonsil and uvula are displaced to the patient's right. Fluctuation as determined by the palpating finger does not develop until 4 to 6 days have elapsed. *B,* Cross section showing abscess.

children. This is true because retropharyngeal lymph nodes are normally present only in the young child. These tend to atrophy in adult life. Retropharyngeal lymphadenitis and suppuration are usually secondary to acute tonsillitis or pharyngitis. Stridor, painful swallowing and obstruction to breathing are produced, depending upon whether the abscess is located in nasopharynx, oropharynx or hypopharynx. Fever and leukocytosis are present. There may be spasm of the neck musculature so that the head is held rigidly and tilted to the affected side. Finger palpation denotes a mass and even fluctuation, particularly during the fourth to sixth day of the disease. Roentgenograms show swelling of the retropharyngeal soft tissues. Incision and drainage are indicated when suppuration exists. The patient's head should be held in the headdown position when surgical drainage is performed. Full therapeutic antibiotic drug therapy is indicated.

LATERAL PHARYNGEAL SPACE ABSCESS. Lateral pharyngeal space abscess develops secondary to acute tonsillitis, peritonsillar abscess, dental infection or acute pharyngitis. This potential anatomic space lies in close relation to the superior and middle pharyngeal constrictor muscles, the stylopharyngeus and styloglossus muscles and the carotid sheath. Although infrequent, infection may gravitate along the carotid sheath to the mediastinum. There are symptoms and signs of sepsis, trismus and bulging of the lateral pharyngeal wall. The veins of the neck and scalp may be distended from jugular vein pressure. In more advanced suppurations of this space, brawny swelling, edema and red-

ness develop in the neck below the angle of the mandible.

Supportive measures such as hydration and antibiotics are indicated early. Incision and drainage is necessary and may be established either intraorally or externally.

MALIGNANCIES. Malignancies are almost exclusively of epithelial origin. They arise primarily in the mucosa of the posterior pharyngeal wall, soft palate, uvula, tonsil and tonsil pillars. The neoplasm usually reaches a large size before symptoms are produced which warrant medical examination. Cervical lymph node metastasis is frequent. Diagnosis is confirmed by microscopic tissue examination of excised tissue. Size, location and loss of function materially affect the prognosis by any form of treatment. Treatment may be carried out by x-ray therapy alone, by x-ray therapy combined with an operation or by an operation alone. Operation involves wide removal of tissues involved by the primary lesion in combination with an en bloc radical neck dissection. Excision of a part of the mandible is usually necessary.

TONSILS AND ADENOIDS. The indications for tonsillectomy and adenoidectomy in children are repeated attacks of tonsillitis, particularly with fever and leukocytosis; recurrent serous otitis media, acute and chronic suppurative otitis media and perforation of the tympanic membrane; enlarged tonsils and adenoids interfering with breathing and swallowing; diphtheria carrier status; persistent enlargement of cervical lymph nodes, and recurrent suppurative sinusitis.

The contraindications for tonsillectomy and adenoidectomy are blood dyscrasias, blood coagulation and clotting disorders, acute local inflammations and acute and chronic systemic diseases, including tuberculosis.

The preoperative measures should include a detailed history, physical examination, urine and blood examinations, chest x-ray, special blood studies and prior poliomyelitis immunization. It is most important that trained personnel be responsible for the patient's postoperative care to avoid serious complications and fatalities from hemorrhage. The surgeon should be familiar with the blood supply of the tonsils and use meticulous care in ligating all bleeding vessels.

Indications for tonsillectomy in the adult are similar. Tonsillectomy should also be performed following a peritonsillar abscess.

As a rule, adenoid tissue regresses by adulthood and adenoidectomy is rarely indicated. Tonsillectomy in the adult is frequently best performed under local anesthesia.

NASOPHARYNX

Because the nasopharynx is normally inaccessible by conventional methods of examination, primary nasopharyngeal disease may be far advanced before the patient seeks medical advice or before the examining physician recognizes its existence. Therefore, the following techniques of examination of the nasopharynx are emphasized: indirect mirror examination, direct examination by anterior rhinoscopy, palpation, nasopharyngoscopy and direct inspection through the oropharynx after elevation of the soft palate (Figs. 17, 18 and 19). Other than hypertrophied and infected adenoids, the nasopharynx is not subject to many diseases of surgical interest.

NEOPLASMS. Juvenile nasopharyngeal angiofibromas arise in the region of the occipital, sphenoid or ethmoidal bones. They occur principally in young males. Early symptoms of repeated epistaxis and nasal obstruction are frequent. Obstruction of the eustachian tube, producing ear symptoms, may be present. Epistaxis may be severe. Diagnosis is usually made by inspection and palpation (Fig. 20). Biopsy must be carefully performed to avoid undue hemorrhage. Because of its inaccessibility, operative approaches are many and varied. If possible, simple avulsion through an intraoral approach is favored. Combined attacks through the antrum, palate, external ethmoid sinuses or a lateral rhinotomy may be necessary. Hypotensive anesthesia and hypothermia have been helpful.

Malignancies of the nasopharynx include squamous cell, anaplastic and transitional cell carcinomas and lymphoepitheliomas. Symptoms produced are nasal obstruction, epistaxis, unilateral ear blockage associated with hearing loss and fluid in the middle ear. Intracranial extension may cause cranial nerve involvement. Unilateral lymph node metastases to the neck may be an early manifestation. In fact, such a lesion in the neck may be the first indication of the nasopharyngeal neoplasm. Distant blood-borne metastatic lesions can occur in the lungs, abdominal viscera and brain. Roentgenographic studies of the base of the skull are routinely obtained to aid the physician in determining local extension. Diagnosis is confirmed by biopsy and microscopic tissue examination. X-ray therapy is the treatment of choice for

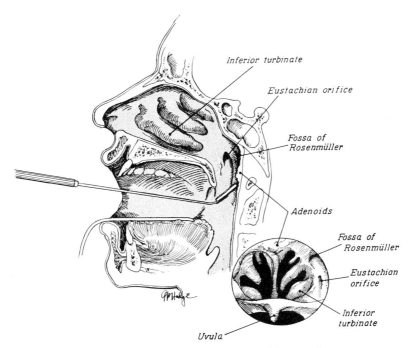

Inferior turbinate

Eustachian orifice

Fossa of Rosenmüller

Adenoids

Fossa of Rosenmüller

Eustachian orifice

Inferior turbinate

Uvula

Figure 17. Indirect mirror examination of the nasopharynx.

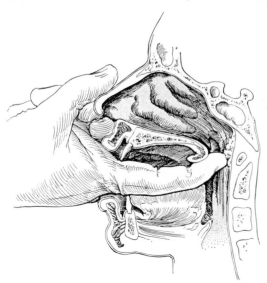

Figure 18.   Palpation of the nasopharynx may readily be accomplished in the child as well as the adult.

Figure 19.   The nasopharyngoscope is frequently used as an adjunct to complete the more detailed examination of the nasopharynx.

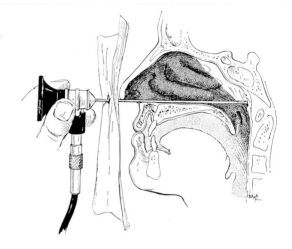

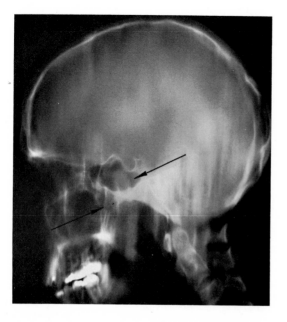

Figure 20.   A lateral soft tissue x-ray demonstrates a large nasopharyngeal tumor in this 15-year-old boy. It fills much of the sphenoid sinus. A nasopharyngeal fibroma was removed through the oropharynx.

the primary lesion. Persistent cervical lymph node metastases require a radical neck dissection.

Larynx

The important symptoms of laryngeal disease include hoarseness, dyspnea, dysphagia and pain. Voice disturbances may occur as a result of diffuse nonspecific inflammatory disease involving the vocal cords, weakness or paralysis of the vocal cords, or the presence of a localized specific inflammatory lesion, foreign body or neoplasm.

Laryngeal dyspnea may occur as a result of narrowing of the airway by edema, diffuse inflammatory disease, bilateral paralysis or benign or malignant tumor. Crushing injuries of the larynx, with displacement of cartilage or hematoma, may cause dyspnea with unexpected rapidity. Dysphagia is commonly observed in the presence of foreign body or acute inflammatory lesions of the laryngeal introitus, as well as in the presence of neoplasm or specific ulcerative lesions involving the supraglottic larynx or adjacent structures. Pain may frequently be referred to the ear.

Laryngeal obstruction. Although hoarseness is undoubtedly the most common symptom referable to the larynx, laryngeal obstruction constitutes the most urgent indication for treatment. The dyspnea of laryngeal obstruction is at first chiefly inspiratory, and is accompanied by a characteristic high-pitched stridor, as well as by "retraction" or "indrawing" of the suprasternal, supraclavicular, intercostal and infraclavicular spaces. Advanced degrees of laryngeal obstruction may be accompanied by a "two way" stridor and cyanosis, although in the presence of concomitant hypotension a grayish pallor may be observed instead of actual cyanosis. In the presence of increasing laryngeal obstruction, unless the cause can be quickly corrected, an adequate airway should be provided by endotracheal intubation, or tracheostomy, before the occurrence of hypoxia.

Methods of examination. In adults, the larynx is examined by indirect or mirror laryngoscopy, which in some instances is supplemented by direct laryngoscopic inspection, usually with topical anesthesia. In the presence of obstruction, direct laryngoscopy should not be attempted unless facilities are available for endotracheal intubation or tracheostomy. In the young child, direct laryngoscopy offers the only satisfactory method of examination. Obviously, in the patient with laryngeal complaints, the neck should be carefully inspected and palpated for evidence of cartilaginous deformity, enlargement of lymph nodes or thyroid gland and other abnormalities. Supplementary examinations of value in certain patients include roentgenographic study of the larynx and soft tissues of the neck, with and without contrast media laryngograms (Fig. 21), and coronal tomograms (Fig. 22).

Direct laryngoscopy is used in any patient in whom the indirect method of examination is unsatisfactory and is necessary for removal of small benign laryngeal lesions, taking of biopsy material and complete inspection of the laryngeal ventricles, subglottic region and pyriform sinuses. In the child, premedication alone is sufficient, but this should be avoided if laryngeal obstruction is present; no topical or general anesthesia is required. In the adult, premedication and topical anesthesia are adequate in most patients. Occasional patients with a short muscular neck, prominent upper teeth or narrow mandible may require general anesthesia, as will those who are temperamentally unsuited for manipulations under topical anesthetic.

The examination is usually performed with the patient supine, the head being elevated and somewhat extended. The laryngoscope is introduced along the right side of the tongue and beneath the epiglottis. The interior of the larynx is exposed by an upward lifting motion so that no undue pressure is exerted on the teeth or other structures.

Injuries. External injuries of the larynx may be the result of impact with blunt objects, penetrating wounds or incised wounds. Trauma by blunt objects may result in fracture of the thyroid or cricoid cartilage, usually the former. Following displacement of cartilaginous fragments, hemorrhage and edema of the tissues on the interior of the larynx are likely to occur, with respiratory obstruction of varying degree; tracheostomy may be required. Crushing injuries of the larynx may likewise be accompanied by forward dislocation of one or both arytenoid cartilages, due to compression of the larynx against the cervical spine.

Penetrating injuries due to missile or stab wounds may likewise damage the cartilaginous framework of the larynx and cause hemorrhage into the airway, intralaryngeal

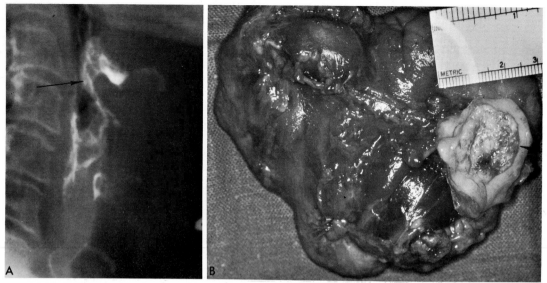

Figure 21. *A,* The contrast medium coats and outlines a large neoplasm confined to the laryngeal surface of the epiglottis. *B,* A neck dissection and supraglottic partial laryngectomy has been performed. The lesion involves most of the epiglottis. One large node was present in the neck of this 52-year-old woman.

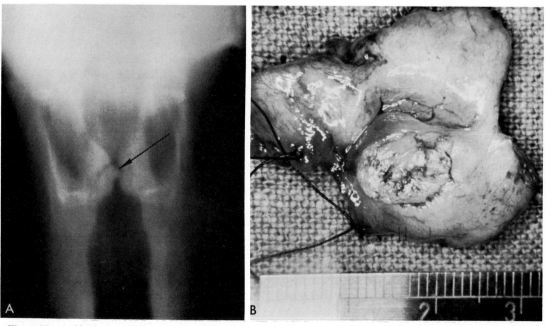

Figure 22. *A,* Glottic cancer. A tomogram taken on phonation demonstrates a mass lesion of the right vocal cord. *B,* A laryngofissure and partial laryngectomy cured this patient. The entire right cord, the right ventricular band and the anterior third of the opposite cord were removed.

hematoma or edema which requires tracheostomy. Incised wounds are most often the result of assault or attempted suicide; the degree of injury to the intrinsic structures depends on the level at which the larynx is incised. Concurrent infection of the cartilage or perichondrium will result in subsequent stenosis and voice impairment.

Fracture of laryngeal cartilages may be suspected by the occurrence of subcutaneous emphysema, or careful palpation may elicit crepitus of the fragments. Indirect and direct laryngoscopy will demonstrate the degree to which the laryngeal airway has been disturbed. Roentgenograms are of limited value in determining the presence or absence of fracture.

If no displacement of cartilaginous fragments is evident, no specific surgical treatment may be required except for the possibility of tracheostomy for laryngeal dyspnea. If sizable fragments of cartilage appear to be displaced, or if one or both arytenoids is dislocated, an attempt should be made to replace these and maintain proper position by insertion of an indwelling acrylic or polyethylene mold as an internal splint. It is rarely necessary or advisable to open the larynx for repair of the intrinsic structures. Penetrating injuries may require hemostasis or subsequent debridement and drainage, along with antibiotic treatment. Deep incised wounds may require surgical repair, using perichondrial sutures to maintain proper position of the divided cartilage.

TRAUMATIC MOTOR PARALYSIS. One or both recurrent laryngeal nerves may be injured or divided in penetrating or incised wounds, or during a thyroidectomy. A frequent cause is involvement of the nerve by carcinoma, either primary in the thyroid gland, esophagus or lung or by metastatic neck carcinoma from other primary sites in the oral cavity and upper respiratory tract.

Laryngoscopy shows a motionless cord, in or near the midline, with lack of tonus; dyspnea and stridor are unlikely if the contralateral cord has normal motion. Injury or division of both recurrent laryngeal nerves gives rise to inspiratory stridor and, on occasion, impending asphyxia. Although the voice is often not greatly impaired, laryngoscopy shows both cords in the midline position, so that the inspiratory airway is extremely narrow.

In trauma of the recurrent nerve without actual division, some return of function may occur within a few months. Attempts at nerve grafting or resuture in instances of division of the nerve have not been successful. However, the contour of the concave paralyzed cord may be improved and some voice improvement accomplished by intracordal injection of inert substances.

The occurrence of traumatic bilateral recurrent paralysis may require emergency tracheostomy. If, after one year, there is no return of motion of either cord, and if the passage remains inadequate, a satisfactory airway may be obtained by laryngoplasty, in which one arytenoid and the attached cord are mobilized and anchored in a position of permanent abduction, or by arytenoidectomy. As an alternative, in patients in whom the preservation of voice is important, a valved tracheostomy tube may be used to allow free inspiration, the expired air being directed through the larynx, by closure of the valve, for phonation.

LARYNGEAL EDEMA. Edema of the larynx may occur as a rapidly developing allergic response, as an accompaniment of laryngeal trauma or as a result of thermal injury. As an accompaniment of acute nonspecific inflammations of the larynx in childhood, and occasionally following bronchoscopy, subglottic edema may also occur rapidly and require tracheostomy.

Close observation is necessary in laryngeal edema, since obstruction may increase rapidly. Facilities for prompt intubation or tracheostomy should be available. The use of steroids has occasionally been found useful in diminishing the degree of laryngeal edema. In children, the use of high-humidity oxygen is helpful, provided undue dependence is not placed on this therapy as a substitute for tracheostomy when obstruction is increasing. In all patients with edema due to infection, antibiotic treatment, preferably based on culture and sensitivity determinations, is indicated. Lesser degrees of edema may occur in the chronic specific inflammatory diseases and in the presence of a foreign body.

CHRONIC STENOSIS. Chronic stenosis may occur as the healed result of trauma, or as a sequel of chondritis and perichondritis from other causes. Faulty tracheostomy, in which the cannula is allowed to remain through the cricothyroid membrane or cricoid cartilage, almost invariably results in a chronic fibrous subglottic stenosis. The tube should be inserted below the level of the first tracheal ring; otherwise chondritis and perichondritis of the cricoid cartilage is prone to occur. In instances of crushing or penetrating injury to the larynx, subsequent stenosis may be averted by tracheostomy and insertion of an indwelling "core mold" soon after the injury.

Chronic stenosis of mild degree may occasionally be treated by direct laryngoscopic dilatation, but more often the use of a core mold, with or without external operation to excise excess fibrous tissue and cartilage, at times with split thickness skin grafting, is required.

BENIGN TUMORS. Benign tumors and tumorlike lesions are commonly found on the vocal cords. The usual symptom is hoarseness. Removal is easily accomplished by direct laryngoscopy, which in most instances will restore a fairly normal voice. All tissues removed, no matter how benign in gross appearance, should be examined histologically.

Among the more common benign lesions are squamous papilloma and "vocal nodule" seen both in the child and in the adult, and the benign polyp and benign organizing hematoma, seen chiefly in the adult. The less common benign tumors include fibroma and angioma, myoblastoma and chondroma.

The so-called "contact ulcer granuloma," characteristically found on the medial surface of the posterior extremity of the vocal cord, may be a sequel of endotracheal intubation or the result of excessive, strenuous or faulty voice use. The excess granulomatous tissue should be removed by direct laryngoscopy, followed by a period of vocal rest and voice therapy. The granuloma accompanying laryngeal tuberculosis is diagnosed by the characteristic histologic appearance, and the almost invariable presence of an active pulmonary lesion with positive sputum. Granuloma due to luetic or mycotic infection is occasionally found.

MALIGNANT TUMORS. Squamous cell carcinoma accounts for more than 95 per cent of all malignant tumors of the larynx. The incidence is predominantly in the male sex, by about ten to one, and also in the later decades of life. More than half of the tumors appear to arise on the vocal cords, with hoarseness as the initial symptom. Subglottic carcinomas, however, may be manifested first by laryngeal dyspnea, and supraglottic lesions may reach a considerable size before giving rise to the characteristic symptoms of pain and dysphagia. Frequently, a lesion which has involved the vocal cord initially will have extended to the subglottic or supraglottic regions before the diagnosis is made.

Pathologic changes vary from the superficial "carcinoma in situ," often found in association with keratosis of the vocal cords, to instances in which there is deep invasion of the cartilage and extralaryngeal structures. Metastasis from cordal lesions is uncommon, but tumors involving other areas of the larynx, particularly those involving the arytenoids and aryepiglottic folds, are likely to be accompanied by metastases to the deep jugular nodes.

Although the nodular, proliferating or ulcerative gross appearance of the lesion is quite characteristic, reliance must be placed on biopsy for confirmation and differential diagnosis. This should usually be accomplished by direct laryngoscopy, which also allows an accurate estimate of the gross extent of the lesion. Supplementary roentgenographic studies including tomography, laryngography and contrast study of the hypopharynx, are useful in many instances.

Superficial cordal lesions, particularly those of carcinoma in situ, are amenable to irradiation and have an excellent prognosis. More infiltrative lesions of the vocal cord, in which cordal motion is not disturbed, may be treated by partial laryngectomy, the involved cord being removed in continuity with adjacent normal tissues and a portion of the underlying thyroid cartilage. An adequate airway can usually be preserved, and fair rehabilitation of the voice may be anticipated. Cordal lesions in which the cord is fixed, rather than mobile, require total laryngectomy.

Carcinoma involving the subglottic or supraglottic areas is most often treated by total laryngectomy and radical neck dissection, except that certain small superficial lesions of the epiglottis may be suitable for irradiation. In the presence of mobile palpable adenopathy, laryngectomy and therapeutic radical dissection in continuity is performed, including all tissues anterior to the scalene muscles on the involved side except for the carotid artery and its branches, the vagus and cervical sympathetic nerves, the phrenic nerve and the brachial plexus trunks. The spinal accessory nerve is usually sacrificed, but in most cases the lingual and hypoglossal nerves can be preserved.

Lesions confined to the expendable portions of the larynx, epiglottis, vallecula, aryepiglottic folds, ventricular bands and even one arytenoid, may be managed by a conservative operation upon the larynx with adequate excision of any part or all of these structures including a neck dissection (Fig. 23). Closure of the defect is made by approximating the base of the remaining tongue to the true vocal cords. Vocal function is preserved and deglutition can be managed with practice, even with sacrifice of one or both superior laryngeal nerves. Carcinoma of the laryngopharynx causes little or no hoarseness until late in the disease and frequently not until the appearance of metastatic neck nodes. Early symptoms consist only of a slight scratchiness or lump in the throat on swallowing. They are diagnosed and managed very much as large laryngeal cancers and require total laryngectomy almost always with a radical neck dissection.

In large lesions with bilateral palpable metastases, laryngectomy and simultaneous bilateral neck dissection is indicated. The internal jugular vein on the least involved side may be left intact.

Since the occurrence of secondary metastasis has been one of the important causes of failure following laryngectomy for extracordal lesions in the patient without palpable nodes at the time of initial operation, elective neck dissection in continuity with laryngectomy is now frequently performed in the absence of palpable nodes.

Increasing use is being made of planned preoperative radiation therapy in somewhat less than usual cancericidal amounts followed by extirpative surgery. Although morbidity and mortality are increased slightly, there is definite evidence that such combination therapy is increasing the cure rates.

Following partial laryngectomy, specific rehabilitative measures are rarely required, although voice therapy beginning a few weeks after operation may be helpful in ob-

taining the optimum voice. Following laryngectomy, instruction in esophageal voice should be provided; the use of an artificial larynx should not be advised until every effort has been made to develop the more useful and more natural esophageal voice.

TRACHEA

The symptoms of tracheal injury or disease include dyspnea, wheezing, hemoptysis and cough. Although little information regarding tracheal abnormalities, except for tracheal deviation, may be obtained by palpation of the neck, roentgenographic examination with and without contrast material, and planigraphic study may be informative. Direct inspection by tracheoscopy or bronchoscopy is invaluable. Premedication, topical anesthesia and position of the patient for this type of endoscopy is much the same as for direct laryngoscopy. The use of bronchoscopic telescopes allows detailed inspection, and specimens for laboratory study are taken by the use of aspirating tubes and biopsy forceps.

TRACHEAL OBSTRUCTION. Tracheal obstruction as a result of nonspecific inflammatory disease is uncommon. However, tuberculosis of the trachea is occasionally manifest by wheezing and dyspnea due to the occurrence of specific granuloma or healed cicatricial stenosis. The latter may require tracheostomy or plastic surgical correction.

The trachea may be narrowed by external compression due to neoplasms of the thyroid gland, mediastinum or esophagus, and malignant tumors of these structures may occasionally penetrate the tracheal wall to produce intraluminal obstruction. The deformities of the trachea resulting in association with these conditions, as well as in aortic aneurysm, may be demonstrated by appropriate roentgenographic studies, including planigraphy and tracheography, and bronchoscopy. However, in the presence of aneurysm, bronchoscopy should be avoided or done with extreme care. Tracheostomy may relieve dyspnea of high tracheal obstruction, but is of much less value if the obstruction is at or just above the carina level.

Primary tumors of the trachea are uncommon, although occasionally adenocarcinoma, usually of the cylindroma variety, or squamous cell carcinoma are observed. However,

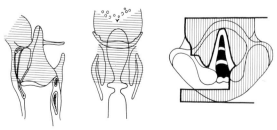

Figure 23. Any or all of the shaded areas of the tongue and supraglottic portion of the larynx may be excised with preservation of the essential laryngeal functions of speech and protection of the airway.

a bronchogenic carcinoma arising at or just below the tracheal bifurcation may extend upward to produce significant degrees of tracheal narrowing. Malignant tumors of the trachea may be amenable to palliative treatment by bronchoscopic electrocoagulation or removal of neoplastic tissue. Actual surgical resection and anastomosis can be accomplished only if the lesion is small, although progess is being made, both experimentally and clinically, in the various methods of tracheal replacement and reconstruction. Irradiation is helpful, but rarely curative.

TRACHEAL INJURIES. The upper trachea may be injured by crushing blows, penetrating or incised wounds. However, the mobility and elasticity of the trachea is such that it is resistant to damage by external violence. The intrathoracic portion of the trachea may be injured in severe crushing injuries of the chest, and rupture has been known to occur in violent torsion or extension of the neck or during instrumentation. In disruption of the tracheal wall, interstitial emphysema, palpable in the neck and visible on x-ray, occurs promptly and is usually of marked degree; intraluminal hemorrhage results in hemoptysis of varying severity. Dyspnea and wheezing may occur as a result of the tracheal distortion, accumulation of blood clots or secretions, or compression due to extraluminal emphysema.

Bronchoscopy is helpful in determining the location of the injury and its extent, and also provides an adequate airway and allows aspiration of blood and secretions. However, tracheostomy may be indicated, particularly if there is concomitant injury of the chest wall. Prompt surgical repair may be indicated if there has been disruption of the tracheal wall. The possibility of concomitant pneumothorax requiring aspiration or intrapleural suction must be kept in mind.

TRACHEOESOPHAGEAL FISTULA. Congenital tracheoesophageal fistula is a common accompaniment of congenital atresia of the esophagus, in which the lower segment of the thoracic esophagus may communicate with the trachea just above the carina level. In some patients, the patency of the esophagus is maintained and an "H" type of deformity, with a communication at the lower tracheal level, may be seen. These conditions must be quickly recognized in the neonatal period by the failure to take food properly, cough when feedings are given and demonstration of the deformity by small amounts of innocuous contrast material, so that surgical treatment may be carried out before the occurrence of aspiration pneumonitis. Tracheoesophageal fistula may also occur in later life as a result of erosion of calcified nodes, or penetration of both the tracheal and esophageal walls by malignant tumor.

FOREIGN BODIES

A history of coughing and choking with subsequent wheezing, dyspnea, hoarseness or aphonia is suggestive, although in children the initial episode may have not been witnessed. Persistence of such symptoms, and particularly the presence of wheeze audible at the open mouth, are suggestive. The presence of "audible slap" or "palpable thud" on forced expiration or cough are nearly diagnostic of tracheal foreign body.

Although roentgenographic examination may be helpful if the foreign body is opaque, undue reliance should not be placed on x-ray examination for excluding the possibility of foreign body. In the adult, indirect laryngoscopy, and in the child direct laryngoscopy should be done, along with bronchoscopy. Certain vegetable foreign bodies such as the bean, which increase in size with absorption of moisture, can be extremely dangerous and lead to asphyxia.

Tracheal foreign bodies are often freely movable and lodgment in a main or lobar bronchus may occur, with resultant obstructive emphysema or atelectasis. Such foreign bodies must be removed promptly if pneumonitis, pulmonary abscess, bronchiectasis and empyema are to be avoided.

TRACHEOSTOMY

Tracheostomy is frequently a lifesaving procedure in the presence of laryngeal or upper tracheal obstruction. In addition, tracheostomy has also been used increasingly in the prevention and management of retained tracheobronchial secretions which might otherwise result in pneumonitis and atelectasis, or both. The procedure is especially useful in debilitated patients, following thoracic or abdominal surgery, in conditions in which prolonged unconsciousness occurs and in poliomyelitis, tetanus and pulmonary emphysema. Tracheostomy is also frequently indicated in chest trauma.

Although tracheostomy may be performed

with a minimum of equipment under emergency conditions, an orderly procedure is much preferred. In the presence of dyspnea, preliminary insertion of an endotracheal tube or small bronchoscope will provide for comfortable breathing while the procedure is done. In certain conditions, positive pressure respiration by means of a cuffed tube may aid in the recovery of a desperately ill patient. The shoulders should be elevated so that the head and neck are somewhat extended.

The skin and subcutaneous tissues from the thyroid notch to the suprasternal notch are infiltrated with local anesthetic; anesthesia of the deeper layers is not required. Some favor the use of a transverse incision for the supposed optimum cosmetic result. This requires nicety of judgment in the relation between the level of the incision and the point at which the cannula is inserted into the trachea; otherwise, the midportion of the incision will later be displaced upward or downward. Most surgeons prefer a vertical incision from the cricoid to the suprasternal notch, which allows good access through an area in which bleeding is minimal (Fig. 24). The ribbon muscles are separated in the midline by blunt dissection and the thyroid isthmus identified. The position of the cricoid is verified by palpation and the cannula inserted below the level of the first tracheal ring following mobilization or division of the thyroid isthmus (Fig. 25). The incision should not be closed tightly, so that free drainage is provided around the tracheal cannula and the possibility of an undue degree of interstitial emphysema is avoided.

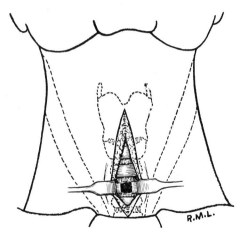

Figure 25. Tracheostomy. At least one intact tracheal ring should be left between the cricoid and the point of insertion of the tracheal cannula.

The most important item in postoperative care is thorough aspiration of secretions by means of a sterile soft rubber catheter whose lower end is smooth. Nursing personnel must be instructed to advance the catheter with inspiration into the depth of the bronchial tree on each side, rather than only a short distance beyond the end of the tracheal cannula. Nebulization of moisture by means of a plastic tracheostomy shield fitting over the outer portion of the tube is helpful in preventing drying or crusting of secretions.

Most complications of tracheostomy can be avoided by proper technique. The cannula should never be in contact with the cricoid cartilage, except in dire emergency. On the other hand, it is not advisable to insert the cannula too low in the neck, particularly in children, since undue degrees of mediastinal emphysema may result, occasionally followed by pneumothorax. The apices of the pleural spaces are avoided by an incision strictly in the midline. Thorough hemostasis is important. Although some degree of wound sepsis may be inevitable, this is minimized by frequent changing of the cannula, aseptic precautions when changing the tube and, occasionally, the use of topical antibacterial agents.

READING REFERENCES

EAR

Altman, F., Kornfeld, M., and Shea, J. J.: Inner ear changes in otosclerosis. Ann. Otol., Rhin. & Laryng. 75:5, 1966.

Armstrong, B. W.: Chronic secretory otitis media: diagnosis and treatment. Southern M. J. 50:540, 1957.

Arslan, M.: Ultrasonic destruction of the vestibular recep-

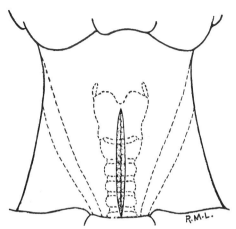

Figure 24. Vertical incision for tracheostomy. Ordinarily, a shorter incision from the cricoid to the suprasternal notch will suffice.

tors in severe Ménière's disease. Laryngoscope 74:1262, 1964.

Blatt, I. M.: Bell's palsy. I. Diagnosis and prognosis of idiopathic peripheral facial paralysis by submaxillary salivary flow—chorda tympani nerve testing: a study of 102 patients. Laryngoscope 75:1081, 1965.

Blatt, I. M., and Freeman, J. A.: Bell's palsy. II. Pathogenetic mechanism of idiopathic peripheral facial paralysis. Tr. Am. Acad. Ophth. 70:381, 1966.

Fick, J. A. van N.: Sacculotomy for hydrops. Laryngoscope 75:1539, 1965.

House, W. F.: Evolution of transtemporal bone removal of acoustic tumors. Arch. Otolaryng. 80:731, 1964.

House, W. F.: Subarachnoid shunt for drainage of hydrops: a report of 146 cases. Laryngoscope 75:1547, 1965.

Schuknecht, H. F., Chasin, W. D., and Kurkjan, J. M.: Stereoscopic Atlas of Mastoidotympanoplastic Surgery. St. Louis, C. V. Mosby Company, 1966.

Schuknecht, H. F., McGee, T. M., and Colman, B. H.: Stapedectomy. Ann. Otol., Rhin. & Laryng. 69:597, 1960.

Shambaugh, G. E., Jr.: Surgery of the Ear. Philadelphia, W. B. Saunders Company, 1967.

Sheehy, J. L.: Ossicular problems in tympanoplasty. Arch. Otolaryng. 81:115, 1965.

Sooy, F. A., Owens, E., and Theurer, D.: Air-bone closure and stability of hearing after stapedectomy. Ann. Otol., Rhin. & Laryng. 75:667, 1966.

Tabb, H. G.: Closure of perforations of tympanic membrane by vein grafts. Laryngoscope 70:271, 1960.

NOSE

Beinfeld, H. H.: Surgery for bilateral bony atresia of the posterior nares in the newborn. Arch. Otolaryng. 70:1, 1959.

Boies, L. R., Hilger, J. A., and Priest, R. E.: Fundamentals of Otology. 4th ed. Philadelphia, W. B. Saunders Company, 1964.

DeWeese, D. D., and Saunders, W. H.: Textbook of Otolaryngology. 2nd ed. St. Louis, C. V. Mosby Company, 1964.

Dingman, R. O., and Natvig, P.: Surgery of Facial Fractures. Philadelphia, W. B. Saunders Company, 1964.

Frazell, E. L.: Surgical treatment of cancer of paranasal sinuses. Laryngoscope 65:557, 1955.

Ireland, P. E., and Bryce, D. P.: Carcinoma of the accessory nasal sinuses. Ann. Otol., Rhin. and Laryng. 75:698, 1966.

Owens, H.: Observations in treating twenty-five cases of choanal atresia by the transpalatine approach. Laryngoscope 75:84, 1965.

Proetz, A.: Nasal Physiology. St. Louis, Annals Publishing Company, 1941.

Scott-Brown, W. G., Ballantyne, J., and Groves, J.: Diseases of the Ear, Nose and Throat. 2nd ed. London, Butterworth & Company, Ltd., 1965.

THROAT

Arnold, G. E.: Alleviation of aphonia or dysphonia through intracordal injection of teflon paste. Ann. Otol., Rhin. & Laryng. 72:385, 1963.

Conley, J. (ed.): Proceedings of the International Workshop on Cancer of the Head and Neck. London, Butterworth & Company, Ltd., 1967.

Goldman, J. L., Silverstone, S. M., Rosin, H. D., Cheren, R. V., and Zak, F. G.: Combined radiation and surgical therapy for cancer of the larynx and laryngopharynx. Laryngoscope 73:1111, 1964.

Jackson, C., and Jackson, C. L.: Bronchoesophagology. Philadelphia, W. B. Saunders Company, 1950.

Jackson, C., and Jackson, C. L.: Diseases of the Nose, Throat and Ear. 2nd ed. Philadelphia, W. B. Saunders Company, 1959.

Myerson, M. C.: The Human Larynx. Springfield, Illinois, Charles C Thomas, 1964.

Ogura, J. H., and Roper, C. L.: Surgical correction of traumatic stenosis of larynx and pharynx. Laryngoscope 72:468, 1962.

Scott-Brown, W. G., Ballantyne, J., and Groves, J.: Diseases of the Ear, Nose and Throat. 2nd ed. London, Butterworth & Company, Ltd., 1965.

Chapter 16

THE MOUTH, TONGUE, JAWS AND SALIVARY GLANDS

by
JAMES BARRETT BROWN, M.D.
and
MINOT P. FRYER, M.D.

JAMES BARRETT BROWN is a Mark Twain Missourian who became a pioneer in the specialty of plastic surgery. He was educated at Washington University in St. Louis, and has devoted his professional activities to that institution and Barnes Hospital. His surgical imagination has opened this field of surgery in many directions and his exacting, meticulous ideals have provided results of the highest standards. It was mainly through his efforts as consultant in plastic surgery to the Chief Surgeon of the European Theatre of Operations that emphasis was placed upon the care of American wounded with loss of tissue in hospital centers in this country.

MINOT PACKER FRYER, a pupil and colleague of Doctor Brown, is a product of Brown University and The Johns Hopkins Medical School. He is a disciple of the education and training in the school of plastic surgery developed at Washington University.

MOUTH

SOFT TISSUE INJURY. Injury in the region of the mouth does not respect arbitrary anatomic sites in its effect. Compound facial injury is used to describe the result of trauma of any severity, since there is injury to the soft parts, skin, subcutaneous tissue, fat, teeth and underlying bony support of the face and mouth.

Contusions, or bruises, can result from relatively mild soft tissue injury to the lips or elsewhere on the face without breaking the skin or mucosa.

Degree of swelling, ecchymosis and pain are in direct proportion to the extent of the injury. Treatment for the most part is symptomatic. Pain can usually be relieved by the usual analgesics, such as aspirin, and cold applications may help to control the swelling and the pain. Caution is indicated in the use of cold applications when the swelling is pronounced enough to cause tenseness of the skin, as a slough may result in the skin with the already compromised circulation. Ice or ice bags should not be used on a severely swollen area about the face or mouth because the added pressure may cause necrosis. Occasionally, a localized collection of blood may be present in a contused or undermined area, which may be evacuated by needle aspiration, and thereby hasten subsidence. Elastic or adhesive support of contused, swollen lips and undermined areas adds to the comfort of the patient, but should be changed frequently enough to be kept clean. The swelling in most contusions subsides in two weeks, but discoloration may persist considerably longer.

Lacerations and tears of the skin or mucosa may result from sharp cuts or from a blunt force. There are varying degrees of soft tissue contusion and explosion which may proceed to deep or superficial necrosis.

Simple lacerations of the lips and elsewhere about the face, resulting from sharp objects, will usually heal if further trauma is not added by the repair. Treatment of simple lacerations consists of adequate cleansing of the surrounding area, irrigation of the wound, minimal debridement, exploration for and removal of foreign bodies, ligation of individual bleeding points and careful approximation of the wound edges with deep sutures whenever possible. No viable tissue is cut away. Local anesthesia should be used. The injection may be made through the open wound after topical application has been made. Facial wounds are never packed open. Dirt blasted into wounds is completely removed to prevent permanent tattooing. Superficial sutures of the finest unabsorbable material practicable (3–0 to 7–0 silk) are placed close to the edges of the wound and a supporting pressure dressing is applied. Lacerations may be strapped with adhesive, or other prepared materials, when they occur in the forehead, over the prominence of the cheek or even on the chin. This is particularly useful in children because the ordeal of suturing is avoided. Strapping is always preferable to heavy sutures widely, hurriedly and painfully placed.

Repair of more complicated tears and trapdoor lacerations should be made as soon as the patient's general condition permits. General anesthesia may facilitate the repair and be to the patient's advantage. Known points are approximated first, such as lip, nose and eyelid border, and the remainder of the lacer-

ation is closed by successive bisection of the wound. Minimal debridement in facial wounds is of particular importance, as features are involved and cutting debridement may create deformities for which innumerable secondary operations cannot compensate (Fig. 1).

It is preferable to leave areas of questionable blood supply for later excision, in hope they may survive. Gas gangrene does not occur in the face and features may be lost by packing wounds open, or performing cutting debridement. The debridement is thorough as far as cleansing is concerned, but ragged, torn wounds which elsewhere would be excised are cleansed, sorted out and carefully put back together in their entirety.

Trapdoor lacerations tend to heal irregularly and require a most accurate approximation of all edges. Tears of the lips or lining of the mouth require careful closure of both skin and mucosal surfaces. Stay sutures should be put on the inside to try to convert the skin surfaces to the simplest possible closure. Mucosal surfaces should usually not be tightly closed, but only approximated.

Loss of tissue in facial wounds usually does

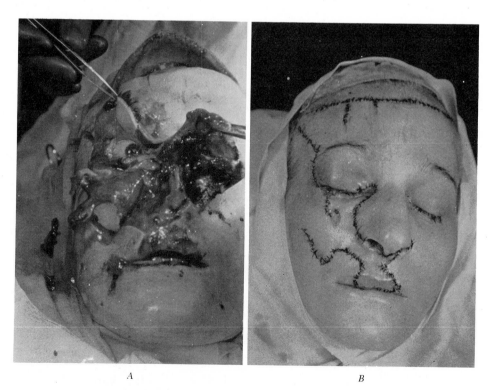

A   *B*

Figure 1.   *A*, Extensive soft tissue laceration and tearing exposing eye, extending into nose and mouth, with partial avulsion of scalp. *B*, Minimal debridement. Repair in one operation by careful closure with fine sutures placed close to edge of wound and approximating known points. Features saved, eye protected, secondary revision of resultant scars unnecessary.

not require immediate rotation of flaps for closure, because of the addition of scarring in the face and possible loss of motor and sensory nerve supply. Partial closure in areas of actual loss is usually preferable, healing is encouraged and secondary repair is done for a superior final result (Fig. 2). Free grafts may be used for coverage and distortion of features is avoided. Widely placed stay sutures are not used on the face, since it is impossible to eradicate their marks, which are known as a "ladder effect." If necessary, sutures at a distance from the edges of the wound can be tied over a fold of gauze to prevent permanent suture marks.

Lacerations resulting from a blunt force are usually accompanied by contusion, undermining and, in general, damage to all layers of soft tissue. Skin edges are ragged and may have questionable blood supply, but the same principles of treatment are employed in the repair. All areas which might not survive are left for secondary excision to avoid sacrificing a portion that would have lived.

Subcutaneous fat may be actually exploded from the tissues, and droplets will be seen scattered around the wound and over the clothing. This may occur when an individual is thrown forcefully from a car or suffers a similar accident. Deep cleansing of undermined areas by irrigation with normal saline solution is time consuming but invites early healing. Additional fixation may be secured by adhesive strapped across the wound. Steady even pressure is maintained, particularly over undermined areas, by fine-mesh gauze placed over the wound upon which surgical waste is held with a circumferentially wound soft gauze roll. The dressing is fixed in place with adhesive. This type of dressing is desirable over any area of repair.

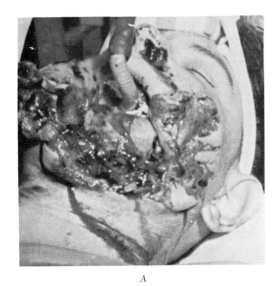

A

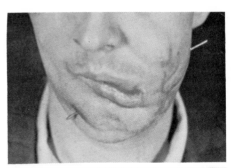

B

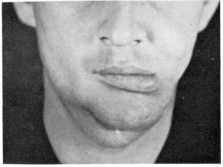

C

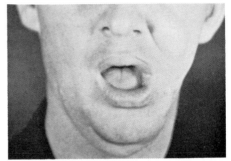

D

Figure 2. Soft tissue and bone damage resulting from shotgun wound. *A,* Soft tissue loss less than appears, as often occurs. Careful closure of lining of mouth and face after minimal debridement around comminuted fracture of the mandible. Features restored as well as possible. *B,* Segment of jaw blown out by close-range shotgun injury. Remainder of comminuted mandible fixed and collapse of soft tissue prevented by internal wire in jaw. *C* and *D,* Watertight mouth; good opening and closing action.

It is necessary over the site of more complicated injuries, but may not be practicable over simple lacerations. Sutures can be removed from most lacerations about the fifth day. Those in the mouth can be left longer. The wound may require support for an additional week.

Tetanus protection is routinely given. Prophylaxis against gas infection is given as indicated, but primary gas gangrene is extremely rare in the face. Antibiotics are administered as required.

Lacerations inside the mouth can be approximated to hasten healing but should not be tightly closed. Dependent drainage may be necessary. Repair of salivary ducts should be done primarily, if possible, using a lacrimal probe or small plastic tubing for a splint. When repair is not possible, the proximal end of the duct may be brought into the mouth as a separate opening and sutured to the lining of the mouth, or a local flap of mucosa approximated to this end.

Laceration of the tongue may not require suture, unless it extends through the edge of the tongue. The same is true of the soft palate, especially for puncture wounds. A general anesthetic is usually required in children, and the choice may be to do the suturing as a secondary procedure.

INFECTION OF SOFT TISSUES. Pustules are the simplest form of infection of the soft tissues, and may appear in crops. Cleanliness usually controls their spread.

Abscess of the lips, in the mouth or on the face is a localized collection of pus. There may be a mixture of organisms, but staphylococcus is usually present. Drainage is usually spontaneous, but conservative incision may hasten subsidence.

Cellulitis may follow abscess formation in the upper lip when a localized inflammatory process becomes diffuse and spreading. Drainage along the angular vein to the cavernous sinus with thrombosis is a potential danger. Treatment consists in local atraumatic management and large doses of antibiotics, to prevent intracranial extension and death.

Jaw abscess, or abscess in the soft tissue around the jaws, is usually related to the teeth as an extension or penetration of a gumboil or root abscess, or due to manipulation of an acutely ulcerated tooth. Acute pericoronitis, localized inflammation around a partially erupted third molar, is another common cause, as are improperly drained fractures. Bone necrosis and sequestrum formation from a variety of causes may be responsible for abscess formation. Extension from contiguous structures, such as obstructed salivary glands, or metastasis in the blood stream from an abscess elsewhere in the body is unusual. The inflammatory process from any of these causes may extend into the neck and cause respiratory difficulty.

Treatment consists of large doses of antibiotics and, whenever localization has occurred, drainage of the abscess. Localized collections, such as a gumboil, may be gently drained into the mouth. Otherwise, drainage is external through a small incision made below the jaw in a dependent position. Careful atraumatic exploration of the masseter and internal pterygoid regions is done, and a drainage tract is established by leaving a loose pack in the wound for 24 hours.

Ludwig's angina is a vague term applied to diffuse swelling of the neck, which may compromise the airway and is the result of an undrained abscess. It has become practically nonexistent since antibiotics have been employed.

Canker sore, or ulcerative stomatitis, is commonly recognized and may be due to a virus alone or in combination with mouth organisms. Treatment consists in attention to mouth cleanliness, the use of mercurial or methylene blue applications and improvement of the general health.

Stomatitis in many forms may occur and may be a manifestation of a general debility, such as anemia or vitamin deficiency. If Vincent's organism is the causative agent, control is achieved mainly by cleanliness and a soapy toothpaste. The fundamental deficiency in general health should be corrected.

Noma is a rapidly progressive gangrenous stomatitis, which is rarely seen, and is an expression of general debilitation or of some blood or metabolic dyscrasia (Fig. 3). Treatment is aimed at improving the general condition, and large doses of antibiotics are given. Local treatment is of little value.

Specific infections due to tuberculosis and syphilis are only rarely seen. Tuberculosis can cause deep, dirty, ragged ulcers in the mouth, most commonly on the central portion of the tongue, and treatment is that of the underlying disease combined with the use of the newer antibiotics. Syphilis or a gumma may be the primary lesion. This produces a foul, discharging, dirty ulcer without the surrounding characteristic hardness of

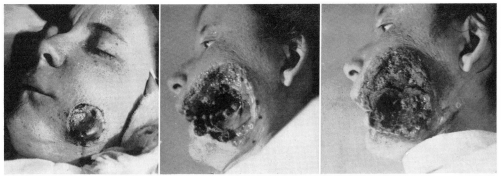

Figure 3. Noma: progressive gangrenous loss of entire cheek.

carcinoma. Systemic antisyphilitic therapy is indicated, but healing may be marked after the initial dose of the medication employed. Granuloma inguinale with involvement of the lips and mouth has been reported.

VITAMIN DEFICIENCIES. Vitamin A deficiency may be manifest as keratinization and hyperplasia of the gums and is treated by administering 25,000 units of the vitamin daily. However, absorption of the vitamin may be limited, particularly in the debilitated.

Deficiency in vitamin B complex can cause angular stomatitis and glossitis. Cheilosis is caused by lack of riboflavin and is manifest by superficial transverse fissures at the angle of the lips, with very little inflammatory reaction. Usually 3 to 5 mg. of riboflavin a day is sufficient for cure, but with difficulty of absorption 10 to 20 mg. of the crystalline riboflavin should be given by mouth.

Vitamin C deficiency is recognized in the mouth by the red, swollen appearance of the gums and interdental papillae; the manifestations may progress to actual scurvy, bleeding, ulceration and necrosis. Treatment is the administration of ascorbic acid by mouth or intravenously. Fresh citrus fruits and tomatoes are added to the diet, if tolerated.

CONGENITAL DEFORMITIES AND ANOMALIES. Cleft lip and cleft palate occur in some combination in one out of 600 to 1500 infants born alive. They may be accompanied by some other deformity. The cause is unknown, and though often present, there should be no parental feelings of guilt. In families, a tendency may follow recessive mendelian progression. Mental capacity of children with this deformity is the same as in the population as a whole.

Over-sympathetic parents, because of their own false feelings of guilt, hinder the child's progress to social adjustment more than does any single factor, except social agencies which brand him as "cleft palate" and thereby single him out from any other children. As in any child, a lifetime of productivity, happiness and acceptance by others more often stems from a home where there is love and a feeling of being wanted.

Embryologically, the lip and upper alveolus are a product of the fusion of two lateral maxillary processes and a central globular segment; this fusion occurs between the ninth and thirteenth week in the embryo. All varieties of clefts of the lip and palate—single or double, complete or incomplete cleft lip and palate or any combination thereof—can result from failure or incomplete fusions of these three elements. Single complete cleft lip and cleft palate is the most common type. Double cleft lip and palate is more common in males, but incomplete cleft of the palate alone, usually accompanied by an insufficiency or shortness of palate and a somewhat retruded lower jaw, is more common in girls.

Repair of single cleft lip can be done any time after birth if the infant is in otherwise good condition. Double cleft lips are repaired when the child is a month old, or has shown a real tendency to gain weight. Reconstruction of the nose at the initial operation is as important as repair of the lip. The excellence of the ultimate surgical result is dependent on the primary repair. No number of secondary procedures can compensate for the failure to construct initially the best possible lip and floor of the nose.

The palate is usually closed in the latter part of the second year. If done before, tooth buds located toward the midline of the palate are disrupted before they can migrate to the alveolus. There may be orthodontic reasons for postponing palate repair until the child is four years old, but these should be weighed

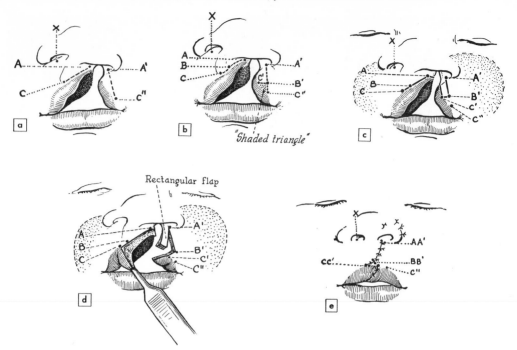

"Shaded triangle"

Rectangular flap

Figure 4.   Design for repair of single complete cleft lip.

a, The V-excision operation. While the columella is held over straight, A is marked at the junction of the skin and vermilion border at the level of the base of the columella. X is in the same relation to the columella on the sound side. A′ bears the same relation to the ala on the cleft side that X bears to the ala on the normal side. C is on the mucocutaneous junction at the point where the vermilion border first begins to thin out. C″ is on the mucocutaneous junction, the same distance from A′ that C is from A. To perform the V-excision operation, A′ is brought over to A and C″ to C, after excision of the edges of the cleft.

b, The flap operation. The V-excision operation is marked out first. C′ is on the mucocutaneous junction at the most medial point of good full vermilion border. B′ is on the line A′-C″, equidistant from C′ and C″. The incision is A′-B′-C′, saving the amount of lip indicated by the shaded isosceles triangle. B is on the mucocutaneous junction, the same distance from C that B′ is from C′.

c, The lines A-B-C and A′-B′-C′ are lightly incised with a knife. The incision is carried upward from C′ on the mucocutaneous junction to separate the vermilion border from the skin. This is also done on the other side at A, to keep any vermilion border out of the nostril floor. The triangle (see *b*) is to be undermined at the next step.

d, The lightly incised lines A-B-C and A′-B′-C′ are cut completely through the lip with a stab blade, with care to keep the knife exactly perpendicular to lip. All angles should be completely opened. The vermilion border is inspected and any attached skin removed with a stab blade. The rectangular flap freed from A′-B′-C′ must be loose enough to be rotated up 180 degrees into the nostril floor. Dotted stippling indicates areas of soft parts undermined.

e, C and C′ are united and the vermilion flaps are interdigitated in a zigzag fashion, fitting them so that they lie naturally together without any pull or stretching. Suturing is then continued on around the vermilion border and up the inside to the fornix. The little flap in the nostril is trimmed to fit with the one from the opposite side and they are sutured together to form the floor. A few key mattress sutures are placed through the ala to unite the lining and covering which were separated during the undermining. The mucosa inside the lip is then closed.

against the possibility of hearing loss from constant middle ear infection and the development of faulty speech habits. All-inclusive rules cannot be made as to time or type of closure, but decision must be made for each individual patient by a competent surgeon, with consultation as needed with the general dentist, speech trainer, otologist, orthodontist and prosthodontist.

Reconstruction of single cleft lip and nose deformity can be followed in Figure 4. The operative design is presented to demonstrate a proved method and means of repair. In general, a V-excision operation is first marked out and then a small triangular flap is de-

signed just above the vermilion border on the cleft side to save lip at this point, which is necessary for fullness and a normal relationship to the lower lip. A summary of the objectives of any operation for the repair of a cleft lip are a full upper lip in advance of the lower lip, with a flexion crease above the vermilion border (Fig. 5). The lip itself should be full, without notching, the floor of the nose should be closed at proper level, the ala should be symmetrical, of normal level and its direction should be with the curve toward a straight columella. The simplicity of the fundamental markings readily allows the repair to be fitted to the deformity. Variations

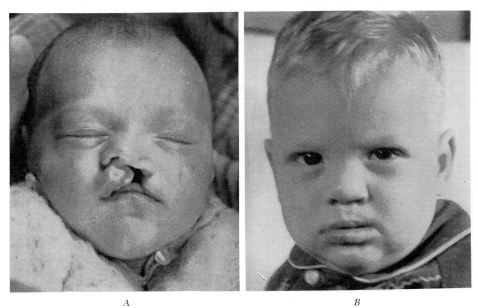

A   *B*

Figure 5. Complete single cleft lip. *A*, Wide defect of lip and usually associated marked deformity of nose. *B*, Repair of lip and nose done in one operation, as shown in Figure 4. Palate to be closed later.

found in each lip can be taken care of on an individual basis.

Repair of double cleft lips (Figs. 6 and 7) is usually not done until the infant weighs about 10 pounds, because of the technical difficulties of the repair and for the safety of the child. Repair of a double cleft lip is about twice as difficult as that of a single cleft lip and the result is, unfortunately, about one-half as good. The baby is held up at a 45-degree angle and fed by means of a syringe to which a short piece of rubber tubing has been attached. Gavage is rarely necessary, if nursing personnel or the family have the patience to use the syringe method.

Embryologically, the deformity is due to failure of fusion of the median globular and the two lateral processes of the maxilla. The degree of cleft on either or both sides is the result of the incompleteness of fusion. There can be double incomplete clefts; complete clefts on one side, incomplete on the other; or double complete clefts. The median globular process becomes the premaxilla-prolabium segment which is the central part of the lip and palate. This is an integral part of the lip and palate and is necessary for closure. If possible, the lip is closed without disturbing it unless it is too far out of position to allow for closure, or unless after closure the pressure of the closed lip will bend the septum and occlude the nasal airways. It is prefer-

able to set this segment back in a more optimal position, as shown in Figure 6, *a*.

Closure of the cleft palate is outlined and described in Figure 8. Adequate surgical repair is the only means by which normal physiologic relationship in the mouth and pharynx can be achieved. Dental prosthetics are an expensive supplement but are no substitute for direct muscle-controlled components of the palate.

Usually, the child with a cleft palate tries to talk at a later age than is considered normal. In addition to the cleft, there may be some unknown insufficiencies of development which might explain the inability of some children with a cleft palate to talk as well as others.

The time to close the cleft palate is usually during the latter part of the second year, before definitive speech habits have developed and after the tooth buds have migrated from the palate. Closure may be postponed until the fourth year because of the often cited observation that facial growth centers may be injured by operating before that time. This recommendation has been made on the basis of poorly executed surgical results and those operations which depend upon molding of the palate bone for closure.

Repair of the incomplete cleft palate which includes closure and elongation is illustrated and described in Figure 9. The incomplete

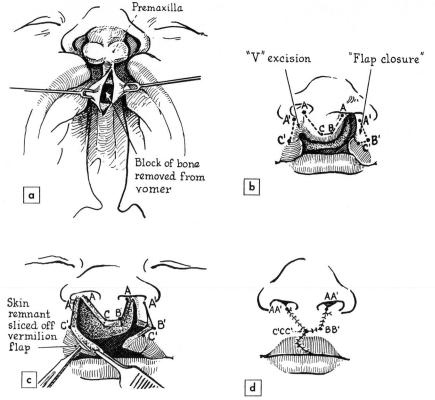

Figure 6. Design for closure of double cleft lip.

a, When the premaxilla is too far forward to permit closure of the lip, it may be set back by submucous excision of a block of bone from the vomer. This removal of a block, rather than a wedge, permits the pushing of the bone directly back like closing a drawer, rather than tilting it back. This factor is of some advantage, as the finished lip should slant forward in the profile view from above downward.

b, Flap closure is done on the total side and a V-excision operation on the partial side.

c, Both sides of the lip are opened up, going completely through the lip with a stab blade knife and using a perpendicular sawing motion. Any skin remnants are sliced off the vermilion flaps. The vermilion border of the prolabium is cut loose from the skin and turned back all around.

d, The closure is done with many fine silk sutures, put in not more than 1 to 2 mm. from the wound edges and about as far apart. Any stay sutures are put in from the inside and are not visible. The lip is closed by interdigitating small flaps.

cleft palate is usually shorter than the complete cleft and, unless adequate length is provided, speech may be poorer than expected in the complete cleft.

Ancillary requirements of the child with a cleft palate include general dentistry, which seems to be the most neglected. A child with a cleft palate needs the usual childhood dental care with the preservation of every available tooth. Orthodontia is necessary in some degree in most children with a cleft palate. Teeth in the line of the cleft are usually crooked and require straightening. Maintenance of the dental arch is important in some children. Speech training can best be carried out in the understanding privacy of the home after parent and child have had a few lessons, or even a single lesson, from a good speech trainer. Hearing measurements should be made if there have been repeated middle ear infections, and decision may be made for earliest possible palate closure. Prosthetic work is usually confined to tooth replacement and, rarely, it may be required when surgical closure has been improperly done. Most dentists can usually add a plug of some plastic material in any position on a partial or complete upper dental plate.

Pharyngeal flaps may be constructed and attached to the palate when there is insufficient length. Pharyngoplasty attempts surgically to duplicate the ridge in the posterior pharyngeal wall, called a Passavant's pad, seen in some patients with good speech. It is generally agreed that operations of this type should be secondary procedures. The

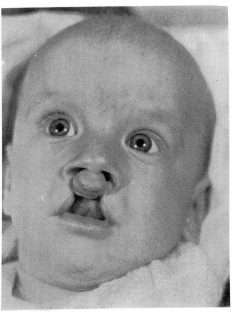 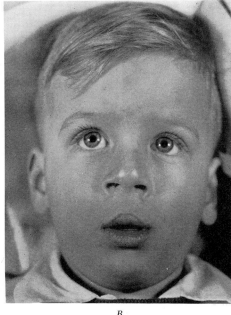

A   *B*

Figure 7.   *A*, Double complete cleft lip and palate. *B*, Lip and nose repaired on both sides in one operation as shown in Figure 6. Palate subsequently repaired.

primary target remains the deformed palate, which can usually be made to appear normal in one operation.

Efforts to improve any residual deformity in the lip and nose should be carried out until the best possible result is obtained with the tissue available, so that the patient may be as close to normal as is surgically possible. The best possible initial repair of a cleft lip may require some secondary operation and, although the change may be comparatively slight, it is worth while if it makes the patient look more normal. However, one operation each on the lip and on the palate, if properly done, is all that is usually required for the best possible result.

Irregularities in the lip or vermilion border may require smoothing out, or advancement of the upper lip on itself, or disproportion in the size or shape of the nostril may be improved. A cross-lip flap from the lower lip to the upper lip may be required for balance around the mouth because of disproportion of the lips, particularly in the profile (Figs. 10 and 11). The protruded lower lip and retracted upper one give the most noticeable deformity, more often in the double cleft lip than the single.

Orthodontia often is required to expand and maintain the upper dental arch and to bring the anterior forward. But if there is not sufficient success from orthodontia, ramisection, to set the lower jaw back into a more favorable occlusion, may be required to avoid the appearance of prognathism. This is especially true if the lower jaw happens to be large and forward.

Prognathism is protrusion of the lower jaw in relation to the upper jaw. Repair depends on the occlusion. The lower jaw may be placed in proper relationship with the upper by closed section of the ascending ramus of the mandible. If the occlusion is no problem, the bone in the symphysis region can be cut down surgically.

Micrognathia is a short underdeveloped mandible. This may be related to some disturbance in the growth centers of the jaw. Repair, as in prognathism, depends on the occlusion.

A short columella is a characteristic deformity of most complete double cleft lips, resulting in a snubbed-nose appearance, the tip of the nose being down on the lip. The columella can be elongated by a flap taken out of the upper lip and advanced upward along with the tip of the nose. The defect in the lip is carefully closed or covered with a full-thickness graft from behind the ear or neck to obtain the best color and character match of the skin.

Defects in the hard palate, alveolus and

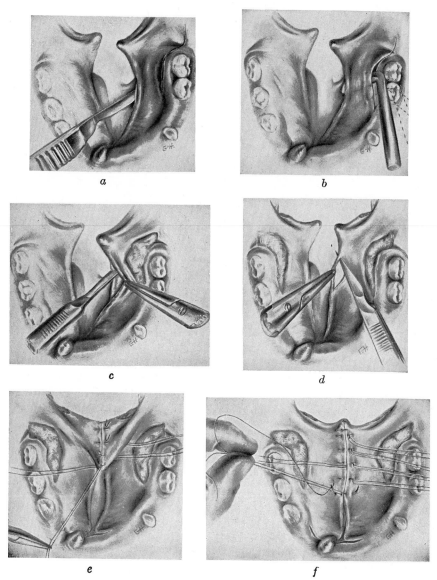

Figure 8.   *a*, Mobilization by Warren's approach. *b*, Mobilization by elevation of the mucoperiosteal flaps. The point of the angle elevator enters the lateral incision just in front of the postpalatine foramen, and then by working forward, the mucoperiosteum and with it the palatine artery can be freed from the underlying bone as far forward as the incisive foramen. *c*, Mobilization by division of the palate aponeurosis. *d*, Denudation of the cleft border by paring. *e*, Suturing the uvula and upper surface of the velum. *f*, Suturing the mucoperiosteal flaps. The mucoperiosteal palate flaps are united with vertical mattress sutures, bringing several millimeters of the raw upper surfaces into contact. It is at the junction of the velum with the mucoperiosteal flaps that one is most likely to have failure of union, either because of insufficient relaxation or a deficient blood supply, and it is to be remembered that tight suturing interferes with the blood supply. If there is any doubt of the integrity of the major palatine arteries, it is safer to suture as far forward as the original relaxation will permit without tension and to do the remainder at a subsequent stage, as failure of union is less catastrophic than a slough or a distorted flap.

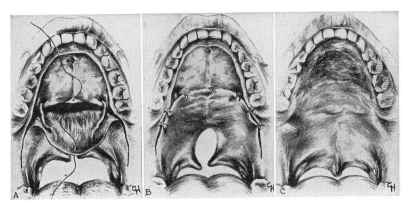

Figure 9. *A*, The whole palate has been loosened from the bony palate, the nasal mucosa opened, the major palatine arteries preserved and the suturing started to carry the palate back. *B*, The palate is held back with three to five sutures and the exposed bone in front is allowed to cover over. Healing is usually complete in one month. *C*, The elongated palate is shown, with the posterior opened space much smaller than it was originally.

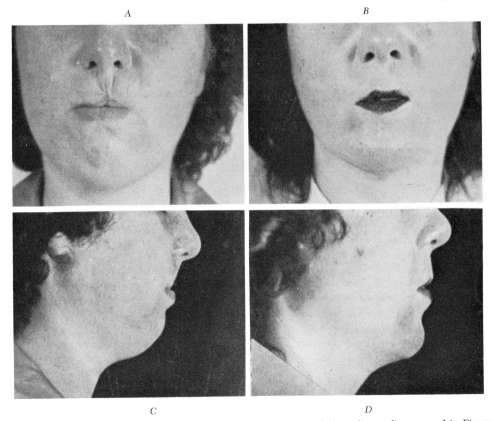

Figure 10. Cross-lip flap establishing proper balance between upper and lower lip, as diagrammed in Figure 11. *A*, Tight scarred upper lip previously repaired, with redundant lower lip. *B*, Balance created between lips by the addition of lower lip into upper lip. *C*, Profile emphasizes marked imbalance. *D*, After cross-lip flap which added bulk into upper lip from lower lip.

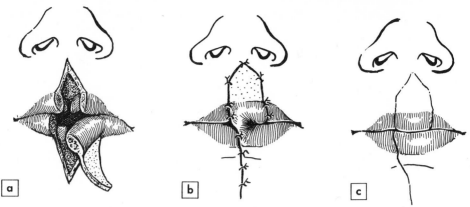

Figure 11. Diagram of lower lip flap adding bulk and creating proper proportion between lips. *a*, Flap removed from lower lip in triangular shape to allow for closure and, if necessary, it could be designed to fit into the floors of the nostrils. *b*, Lower lip flap in place sustained by inferior labial artery in the pedicle until flap can pick up its own blood supply from the upper lip. Lower lip closed. *c*, Pedicle has been cut and vermilion set into proper position.

fornix should be closed surgically whenever possible to stop leakage of air and food or accumulation of food in crevices and pockets. Dental prosthesis may be needed if there is no tissue available for closure. Repeated operations on the soft palate add scar with each procedure and this soft structure eventually approaches the character of an inert prosthesis.

BENIGN TUMORS OF LIPS AND MOUTH. Benign tumors can arise from any of the tissue elements in this location, as is true elsewhere in the body. That is, papillomas, fibromas, lipomas, myomas and nevi occur, as do benign tumors arising from any mixture of the basic histologic parts. They are usually easily recognized.

Treatment is usually surgical excision for cure and microscopic confirmation of the clinical diagnosis. This is not complicated except in the removal of large tumors located where features may be included or the airway is a problem. Closure of the defect may be possible following removal of large benign tumors, but coverage with a graft or substitution with a direct flap, or numerous secondary procedures, may be required for restitution of function and the best possible final appearance.

Nevi are divided into several different types, mostly on the basis of microscopic appearance. Intradermal nevi are often raised from the surface, may contain hair and, microscopically, show the majority of the nevus cells in the derma. Junctional nevi are usually flatter, do not contain hair and show nevus cells concentrated at the junction of the dermis and epidermis. Combined nevi show elements of both of the above. Intradermal nevi may never become malignant, but junctional nevi do and the combined variety may. Blue nevus contains characteristic cells and although it looks grossly very dangerous, it probably never becomes malignant. Sclerosing hemangioma and subepidermal nodular fibrosis may grossly be mistaken for nevi. Treatment is surgical excision with adequate margin of any nevus which is being irritated, bleeding, growing or otherwise changing in character. All junctional nevi should be removed if they can be recognized grossly, but final classification is usually dependent on microscopic appearance.

Cysts, ranulas, angiomas, lymphangiomas, keratoses, leukoplakias, epulides and mixed tumors are benign tumors, but their treatment may present particular problems.

Cysts are usually of the retention variety, readily recognized, and are seen in the lips or anywhere inside the mouth. If small, they are completely excised and the defect closed. Larger cysts may require staged removal or simple unroofing may suffice. It is apparent that there may be recurrence of swelling or obstruction to any of the many glands in the area of operation and the patient should be made aware of this possibility. Sebaceous cysts occur in the lips as elsewhere in the body and require excision for cure. Dermoid cysts, which are deep inclusion cysts, may occur in the lips and the floor of the mouth and require removal. They are more commonly seen about the face in early childhood.

Ranula is a more complicated type of cyst, as far as removal is concerned. It is recognized as a bluish swelling in the floor of the mouth, pushing up the tongue or even extending into the neck. It probably results from some anomaly of the accessory salivary glands and ducts. It may develop in a child or not become apparent until adult life. The fluid is usually clear and may be viscous. Ranulas have been controlled by developing permanent drainage with a seton, that is, a heavy silk or wire suture left in place until the lining of the cyst heals to the oral mucosa. Complete surgical removal may eventually be necessary, but this is often of such magnitude, because of the extent of involvement, that preliminary control with a seton or partial removal and packing may be safer.

Angiomas of different types occur in the mouth and may be an actual threat to life because of position. Growing hemangiomas, called arterial hemangiomas because of their bright red appearance, occur about the mouth or lips and are raised from the surrounding surface, but are in the skin (Fig. 12). These hemangiomas are seen in the newborn or infants, and the majority at any time cease to grow and eventually control themselves so that there may be some question as to whether they are true neoplasms, vessel anomalies or hypertrophies. Others of this same type, however, may proceed to

ulceration, recurrent bleeding and on occasion lead to death of the infant. They should be treated before destruction of a feature occurs. Microscopically, they are composed of growing small blood vessels and endothelial cells, but the microscopic picture has given no clue as to the eventual activity of the tumor.

Treatment should not be withheld if there is any question of progression of this type of angioma and usually a minimal dose of interstitial irradiation, i.e., radon seeds implanted directly into the tumor, will control the growth. Dry ice or injection of coagulants may be used as alternatives. Small growing hemangiomas can be excised or completely destroyed with the fine cautery, but if a feature is involved it can be saved with interstitial irradiation. Radon seeds of 0.05 millicurie or less implanted directly into each cubic centimeter of an extensive growing hemangioma in the tongue or spread out in the palate, for example, may avoid wide resection of the part and a serious operation for the infant.

Cavernous angiomas are beneath the skin, but may involve it. They are composed chiefly of larger vessels or blood spaces, appear bluish-red, are easily compressible and slow growing, may be first noticed at any age and

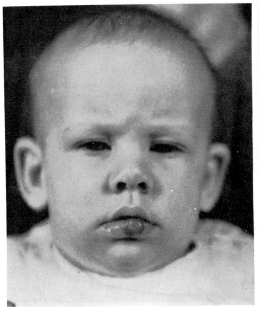
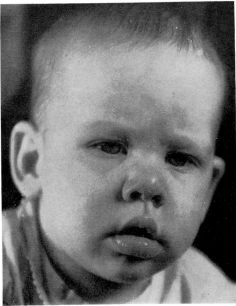

A   B

Figure 12. Growing, bright red, arterial hemangioma. A, Raised, red, growing hemangioma started as tiny red spot in lip. If allowed to progress, may destroy entire lip. B, Control of tumor by light dose of interstitial irradiation. One-twentieth millicurie gold radon seeds were used. Lip saved in one procedure.

markedly distend with dependency of the part. Microscopically, they are composed of thin-walled vessels or spaces, but they can be an extreme example of benignancy in respect to microscopic appearance and malignancy because of location. A large cavernous angioma of the palate, pharynx, tongue or floor of the mouth gradually enlarges with increasing age and, unless surgically controlled, can kill any time by rupture and drowning the patient. Sections of the tumor removed at postmortem examination show simple, enlarged vessels. Lip involvement with large vessel angioma presents a problem of increasing deformity with growth that necessitates control of the tumor with preservation of a feature.

Treatment of the small cavernous angioma may be by excision of the growth or cautery destruction. As features are involved, usually multiple stages are required for control. Multiple suture technique has been of real benefit in those angiomas involving the lip, tongue or elsewhere in the mouth by collapsing many of the vessels, yet preserving the feature or making subsequent excision easier. This consists of placing chromic catgut sutures directly into the growth from the surface and tying them on the surface to obliterate the spaces. The method depends on occlusion by healing of the thin collapsed wall. Total excision may later be possible and desirable. Interstitial irradiation has been helpful in those angiomas with a small vessel component in which eventual excision is indicated, since the caliber of the larger vessels is reduced by their collapse and scarring. The larger spaces are not much affected by irradiation unless a cauterizing dose is used, which should be avoided since the principle of treatment is to control the growth but leave the area intact.

Port-wine stains are the third most common types of angiomas. These are not tumors but rather congenital enlargements or excess of the small vessels in the skin. Mucosal involvement usually requires no treatment, but in the skin of the lip treatment may be indicated because of the appearance. Superficial abrasion has been of some limited value if this addition of scar is of no significance. Cosmetics may cover the redness. Excision and replacement with a graft is the alternative, but it should not be done until all possible spontaneous fading has occurred and until the patient is old enough

to understand the cumbersome process and the scarring that results.

The cavernous types tend to get worse with age from gradual destruction and form phleboliths that may be painful and become more prominent on the surface and cause increasing deformity. They may occur deep in the face, pharynx, tongue, parotid and pterygoid regions, extend into the temporal fossa and cause severe damage and trouble. There may be thrill and bruit from arterial leaks and, when these occur in the face and around the ear, they are very uncomfortable. Excision is necessary, but may be formidable and deforming. These lesions constitute a typical example of the microscopic pathologic appearance having no relation to the seriousness of the lesion. These angiomas may be malignant by position and extent.

Lymphangiomas can involve the lips or tongue, or be anywhere in the mouth. Usually, they extend into the neck and consist of multiple, flat, endothelial-lined spaces. They may be associated with a hemangioma, or the tumor may actually be a mixture of both. Sabin's theory of blood vessel development could explain this association. Lymphangiomas usually appear at an early age but may not become evident until later on in life. Small confirmed lymph tumors not involving features can best be surgically excised. Extensive involvement usually requires more than one operation for the safety of the patient. Aspiration and obliteration with escharotics are possible. Limited excision, breaking down the multiple septa, and packing with an escharotic pack are often the procedure of choice. Hygroma is a lymphangioma of the neck and may extend into the mouth, face or parotid region. Acute respiratory obstruction due to encroachment or pressure on the airway requires immediate relief.

Keratoses are rough, dry, raised areas which appear on the lips with advancing age. They are more commonly noticed in persons whose faces have been exposed to the out-of-doors. Certainly most keratoses never become malignant, but likewise most squamous cell carcinomas of the lips have developed on a pre-existing keratosis. Treatment is simple cautery destruction of the keratosis or, if there is any question of change to carcinoma, then excision for microscopic examination should be done. This simple surgical procedure is much more important in the control of cancer, and will save more patients than any extensive ablative procedures that can be done after cancer has developed.

Leukoplakia is readily recognized as flat or slightly raised white patches occurring anywhere in the mouth. It may be a small solitary spot or involve most of the mouth and tongue, and may be a response to some irritation. Progression to carcinoma is possible any time and the patient should be cognizant of the potentiality of this lesion. Initial treatment consists in the removal of any known irritant and mouth cleanliness. Smoking should be stopped, or at least cut to a minimum. The teeth should be cleaned, cavities filled and any sharp teeth or fillings removed or smoothed out. Small patches may be excised for microscopic examination. The more dangerous-appearing or piled-up areas in extensive involvement of the mouth or tongue may be excised and the remainder carefully followed in frequent examinations. If a large area requires total excision, it may be done in stages or a skin graft will be required for coverage of the defect. Irradiation seems to be of questionable permanent value in the treatment of leukoplakia.

Epulis is a benign tumor arising from the peridental membrane of a tooth and its character depends upon the predominance of fibrous tissue, blood vessels or giant cells in its make-up. It can be white or red, soft or hard, but is usually pedunculated. Treatment is excision of the tumor and usually removal of the associated tooth and its peridental membrane.

Mixed tumors occur in the mouth, palate, tongue and lips. Biopsy may be required for diagnosis of large mixed tumors, but small tumors can be completely removed for cure and for microscopic confirmation of clinical impression.

MALIGNANT TUMORS OF LIPS AND MOUTH.
Basal cell carcinoma is the most common malignant tumor occurring in the upper lip, as contrasted to the lower lip where squamous cell carcinoma is the most frequent. Basal cell carcinoma probably does not metastasize as such, but, contrary to the usual general impression and report of microscopic appearance, this tumor can kill as surely by local invasion and persistence as can squamous cell carcinoma. Failure to metastasize is no indication of benignancy. Prompt, aggressive treatment is necessary for control. These growths have been reported as metastasizing, but the metastatic lesions probably come from basal squamous growths (Figs. 13 to 17).

Basal cell carcinomas arise either from sebaceous glands or hair follicles in the skin, and do not occur in the mouth. They can more accurately be divided into three groups on the basis of gross appearance as to expected behavior, rather than by the microscopic picture.

Solid, raised basal cell carcinomas are slow-growing tumors with a tendency to grow up from the surface of the skin. They probably are the reason basal cell carcinoma is viewed with little concern by many. However, it can change character at any time, grow rapidly and become invasive, though previously dormant for years. These tumors are easily excised when small. Radiation may be effective. Later, when extension is wide, plastic surgery restoration of the area may be necessary following excision or radiation.

"Field-fire" basal cell carcinoma has a flat healed central area surrounded by a slightly raised smooth edge of actively growing tumor. Remnants of tumor may remain in the central healed section. Basal cell carcinoma

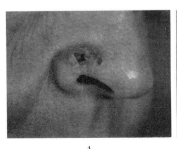 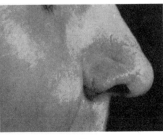 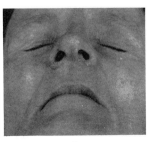

| A | B | C |

Figure 13. *A*, Basal cell carcinoma of the ala of the nose with involvement of the cartilage and lining. *B*, Excision and immediate repair with composite graft cut to pattern from the ear. Composite graft supplies lining for nose, skin for outside of the rim with cartilage contained between these two surfaces. *C*, View of nose from below showing support to graft by strut of contained cartilage in the composite graft. One operation. Staged flap repair avoided.

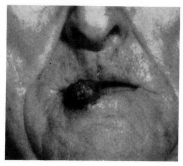

Figure 14. Carcinoma of lower lip. Outgrowing fungating epidermoid carcinoma of lip.

of multicentric origin is a term which has been used to describe this tumor. Treatment is excision of the entire area and replacement as necessary. Radiation may be used, but, if a biopsy is necessary, time and expense for the patient may be saved by one surgical procedure.

Invasive basal cell carcinoma was well named rodent ulcer by older clinicians because of its dangerous persistence. In the upper lip, it commonly arises or seeks the nasolabial fold where it eventually invades the pyriform recess and, unless stopped, proceeds to kill the patient over a long, painful debilitating course. Often, only a small portion of the tumor presents above the surface of the skin, while a solid, larger invasive component is located beneath the skin and is growing in all directions. The superficial part may or may not ulcerate. Treatment must be aggressive. Radical excision may be combined with irradiation. Interstitial irradiation with the use of 0.5 or 1 millicurie gold radon seeds may stop the deeper extension and avoid some secondary reconstruc-

tion. Composite grafts can be used for immediate total reconstruction, following removal of tumors involving full thickness of the nose, thereby avoiding complicated flaps and numerous operations. Thoughts of reconstruction are always secondary, however, to the most effective means for controlling the tumor.

Basosquamous carcinomas do occur in the upper lip but are more common in the upper part of the face. This classification is on the basis of microscopic appearance, in which elements of both basal and squamous growth are present. Grossly, they look like solid basal cell carcinomas which have a history of fairly rapid growth. They do metastasize, but do so as squamous cell carcinomas. Treatment is surgical excision of the local tumor and the regional nodes, as indicated. Irradiation may be effective in cancer dosage and wide application, but the tendency to recur is high.

Malignant melanomas occur in the lips and the possibility of effective control or cure is relatively high. The local lesion can be radically excised and the potential lymph-draining area resected, if necessary, en bloc. They can become uncontrollable, as elsewhere in the body, but in this area there often is better opportunity for radical cure, because of proximity of the primary and secondary spread. Chemotherapeutic means are probably less effective than when used on extremities.

Squamous cell carcinoma is more common in the lower lip than on the upper and is easily recognizable. There is no question of its potentialities. It usually occurs as a fissure, flat ulcer or chronic leukoplakia that

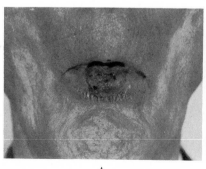
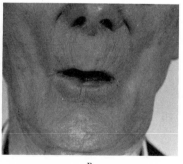

A   *B*

Figure 15. Carcinoma of lower lip. *A*, Widespread involvement of lip by epidermoid carcinoma. Carcinoma did not show invasive tendency. Oval cautery excision done. *B*, Defect in lip following excision of carcinoma allowed to heal and spontaneously reconstitute itself. One operation. No secondary reconstruction necessary in this patient.

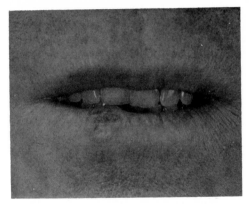

Figure 16. Carcinoma of the lower lip. Flat ulcer type, edges piled up. Oval excisional biopsy should be done, which may suffice locally or further excision or irradiation may be required. Decision as to time for bilateral upper neck dissection can be made any time.

finally becomes malignant or a fungating mass. Biopsy is required and removal of the entire tumor at this time is indicated if the extent is not too great. Complete excision for the biopsy may be the only treatment required. After a positive diagnosis has been made, decision as to the necessity for more radical excision of the lip, or some form of irradiation, can be made. V-excision of carcinoma of the lip is not planned for cure, but rather as a repair of a deformity.

Interstitial irradiation, with 0.5 millicurie of gold radon seeds and external x-ray and radium therapy, has repeatedly saved lip and reduced the necessity for secondary substitution operations.

It has often been stated that all carcinomas of the lip should be cured, and so they should. But they should also be prevented by early removal of suspicious lesions. If a lesion persists for two weeks and, at the outside, four weeks under usual treatment for infection, dyscrasia or irritation, then it should be removed entirely or as a specimen for microscopic diagnosis.

As to treatment of all malignant or potentially malignant tumors, cure depends on staying outside of the tumor field in the treatment, whether surgical or radiation. If the tumor field is entered, or some of it left behind in a small area, or if a small area has not been controlled by radiation, then a primary cure is not obtained.

For metastatic areas, the rule still applies. The ideal operation for any advanced malignant lesion is block resection of the growth and its regional lymphatics. Unfortunately, there are few such possibilities, but carcinoma of the buccal mucosa presents one of the best possibilities for this procedure.

Neck dissection, or removal of the lymph-bearing area in the neck which drains from the lip, may be the most important factor in the patient's cure. If neck metastases are palpable in a patient with carcinoma of the lip, a neck dissection should be done immediately or as soon as it can be determined that the local lesion can be controlled. No blanket rule can be made as to which patients without palpable metastases should have a neck dissection, except that all patients with a carcinoma of the lip are and remain candidates for a neck dissection as long as they live. This statement is substantiated by numerous long-term follow-ups. Statistics are available showing that 80 to 90 per cent of patients with carcinoma of the lip do not have neck metastases, but the physician in charge of the patient with a lip carcinoma should consider the patient in the 10 or 20 per cent group in which metastasis to the neck occurs.

Decision as to the necessity for neck dissection must be made on an individual basis. Various factors help with this decision, among which are: age—the young patient is more likely to have early metastasis than is an older one; duration—the longer the carcinoma has been in the lip the more likely it is that metastasis has occurred to the neck; the nature of the lesion—in the small ingrowing ulcer neck metastasis is more likely than in the more outgrowing type of carcinoma; availability for follow-up—some patients will be less faithful in returning for follow-up than others, for one reason or another, and in these it would be safer if a neck dissection were done; and the experience of

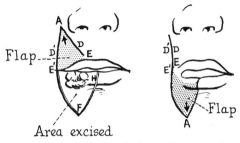

Figure 17. Cross-lip flap for immediate reconstruction of lip following excision of infiltrating, deep carcinoma. Area E'-F-H in the lower lip is excised and the defect replaced with E'-A-E (shaded area) from the upper lip and D'-D closed. Further revision at the corner of the mouth may be necessary.

the surgeon. The experience and ability of the surgeon probably comprise the most important single factor, since the usual bilateral upper neck dissection done for carcinoma of the lip should be associated with no mortality and require around a week's hospitalization.

A bilateral upper neck dissection is usually adequate for control of the area of spread from a carcinoma of the lip. Depending on the location of the primary tumor, metastasis can be to one or both sides of the neck. The operation can easily be varied to include all the lymph nodes on one side with the jugular vein, if necessary, and the upper part of the neck on the other. Again, selection of operation is made on an individual basis. A bilateral upper neck dissection includes all of the nodes to which carcinoma of the lip usually metastasizes first. This would embrace the region of the omohyoid muscle up to the jaw on both sides and the superior deep cervical chain of nodes with the contents of the submaxillary triangle en bloc. There is minimal scar and no actual disfigurement. The term "suprahyoid dissection" does not describe the operation, because in this procedure a serious potential area is left in the center of the neck. The term "upper or supraomohyoid dissection" is preferable.

Sarcoma of the mouth and lips is rare but may occur. Usually it appears as a solid, hard enlargement which does not tend to ulcerate. It has been seen arising from soft tissue elements following irradiation. Diagnosis is usually made on biopsy. Treatment is usually surgical excision because most types of sarcoma are resistant to irradiation.

Carcinomas of the cheek, alveolus and floor of the mouth are considered together as these regions are often involved by one carcinoma because of anatomic proximity and the treatment is often similar. Buccal carcinoma occurs more often in the older age group than in the younger, and may be slow growing and warty in appearance, even fungating out into the mouth. This latter type is called verrucous carcinoma. Deep invasion into the cheek may be late, but there may be extension down over the alveolus into the bone and into the floor of the mouth. Treatment of verrucous carcinoma can be local en bloc excision of the tumor. If bone involvement is suspected, the mandible may be included in the resection as may the floor of the mouth. When metastasis

or extension into the neck is present, the en bloc removal can be combined with or considered a part of a complete neck dissection on the involved side.

Carcinoma of the jaw is an extension of carcinoma of the buccal mucosa with early involvement of the bone. When the first lesion is on the gum, the extension is to the alveolus early and the lesion is sometimes called alveolar carcinoma. Alveolar carcinoma itself usually originates from a flat-type ulcer, but it may arise from leukoplakia as often do buccal carcinomas.

Carcinoma extending from the cheek or floor of the mouth, and secondarily involving the alveolus, invades the bone much later. Attention of the patient may be called to the carcinoma by a tooth socket that fails to heal. Bone involvement may be considerable when this type of carcinoma is first seen, and x-ray examination may not give a good indication of the actual wide extent. The best treatment is a combined operation in which the primary alveolar tumor and involved mandible are removed, and a complete neck dissection is executed in one block. This is the same type of complete radical neck dissection advised for carcinoma of the tongue.

Carcinoma of the floor of the mouth may start laterally or anteriorly to the tongue, and the bone is often involved very early. Therefore, a combined operation with removal of the primary tumor and involved mandible and complete neck dissection is necessary for control. Metastasis also occurs early in the course. If the mandible is not implicated, the primary tumor may be controlled with radon seeds and complete neck dissection on the involved side may be done.

Carcinoma of the hard palate and upper alveolus is similar to alveolar carcinoma. Recognition of possible extension of carcinoma of the upper alveolus to the antrum or pyriform recess or pterygoid region is of particular importance. Early bone involvement by the tumor is usual and cure necessitates its removal. The local area is usually left open for constant inspection, but food and saliva leak can be prevented by a dental plate made to fit into the defect. Later repair can be done with a local flap or, if this is not available, a distant flap, as from the arm. Neck dissection, as is done for carcinoma of the tongue, will eventually be required.

A low grade carcinoma such as that not infrequently seen covering a fairly extensive area of the hard palate may be locally excised and the lining to the nose and antra preserved.

TONGUE

Hypertrophied circumvallate papillae are frequently seen and often overtreated because of failure of proper diagnosis. The usual symptom is pain, and diffuse enlargement of the circumvallate papillae is seen, sometimes localized to one area or the other.

Irritation by strong chemical applications, cauterization or removal is contraindicated as the scar produced may make the process worse. At present, there is no known preventive or medical cure. Treatment consists of general mouth cleanliness, including no smoking, care of sharp teeth or fillings and, of course, close observation and the removal of any active lesions. Sometimes, the lesion may be widespread and thick and approach the process of verrucous carcinoma; the whole surface of a cheek or tongue may be involved.

Removal and repair with a free skin graft may be required. These widespread deep involvements require active treatment or removal, since they will frequently become cancerous.

CARCINOMA OF TONGUE. Carcinoma of the tongue is usually seen as a fissured ulcer with tissue piled up along the edges. The margins of the ulcer may be overhanging, bleed readily, may be sloughing and may be painful. The lesion may be a solid tumor, but usually ulceration has occurred. The most common location on the tongue is along the edge in the molar area, but the lesion may occur as a solid mass in the center of the tongue or anywhere else. The ulcer or solid component may extend to the floor of the mouth, over the alveolus, up the tonsillar pillar or backward to the epiglottis or pharynx. When it is located in the back of the tongue, there may be no pain until there is extensive development and even metastasis. This area may be practically a silent one as far as discomfort is concerned and the first symptom may be the appearance of a metastatic lump in the neck.

Lesions of the face, mouth, tongue and neck can be easily seen and palpated, biopsy is easily done and the presence and nature of none of them need be missed.

Any ulcer or area of growth in the mouth should be biopsied if present for three weeks, and if it has not responded to usual methods of treatment for inflammation, nonspecific or specific, or for lesions of dyscrasia, allergy or drug reactions. If there is no question as to the diagnosis or real evidence of growth, there is no reason to wait until the end of this arbitrary period. There also should be no further delay if the patient has waited this maximum period before being seen for the first time. Suspicion by the examining doctor or dentist that carcinoma may be present is as important in the control of cancer as encouraging the lay public to be on the lookout for such occurrence. Likewise, wishful thinking that a lesion is not cancer has no place in dealing with lesions that possibly are cancer. Progression to inoperability may be very rapid once the patient has noticed something wrong.

The method of taking the biopsy specimen is important. Small lesions may be totally excised since carcinoma may be present in a small area of leukoplakia or of an inflammatory reaction, and if carcinoma is not present total excision may effect a cure. Adequate sections should be taken from the most suspicious parts of larger tumors. Repetition of a biopsy is preferable to overlooking a carcinoma.

The cell type is usually that of the squamous variety with more or less pearl formation. In or around the tonsillar fossae, there may be little hornification of the cells. These tumors have been called transitional cell carcinoma or lymphocarcinoma since they contain small round cells. Tumors of this pathologic type, as would be suspected, are particularly sensitive to irradiation but tend to recur and metastasize readily. The more differentiated the individual tumor, the better the chances of control. Adenocarcinoma is infrequent but occurs usually in the body of the tongue. Sarcoma of the tongue is rare.

The farther forward on the tongue the carcinoma is located, other things being equal, except for involvement of the floor of the mouth, the better the chances of cure. This may be due in no small measure to the inescapable fact that the nearer the tip of the tongue the lesion is located, the sooner it will be noticed. Epidermoid carcinoma primary in the base of the tongue or pharynx may first be found after metastasis has occurred in the neck. This also is of particular importance as far as prognosis is concerned with carcinoma primary in this location.

Treatment of the primary tumor is usually

most successfully done with interstitial irradiation in the form of radon seeds. A calculated dosage is given to the tumor, usually by direct implantation of 1 millicurie of gold radon seeds, using one seed per cubic centimeter of tumor and tissue to be irradiated. Use of radium needles in the treatment of the primary tumors has been given up to a large extent because of the difficulty of maintaining accurate position in and around the tumor and the extreme discomfort to the patient during the period of application in this sensitive mobile structure. Use of external irradiation remains an alternative if radon is not available. In the employment of x-ray therapy on the primary tumor, there is apparently considerable difficulty in shielding the remainder of the mouth, and treatment is often followed by protracted painful dryness and other effects of irradiation directly on uninvolved mucous membrane.

Surgical excision of carcinoma of the tongue can be done adequately, but the magnitude of the operation itself, the mutilation resulting and the repeatedly superior results obtained with radon usually obviate the necessity for operation. Involvement of the jaw by extension of a carcinoma of the tongue or failure of radiation may require extirpation. Glossectomy or hemiglossectomy has been rarely necessary during the last 30 years.

Neck dissection is necessary for the cure of carcinoma of the tongue and is as much an integral part of the treatment as is treatment of the primary tumor. Over 60 per cent of carcinomas of the tongue metastasize to the neck, usually to the same side as that in which the primary lesion is located, and only occasionally to the opposite side. The time to do the neck dissection is the same as that of treatment of the primary tumor, un-

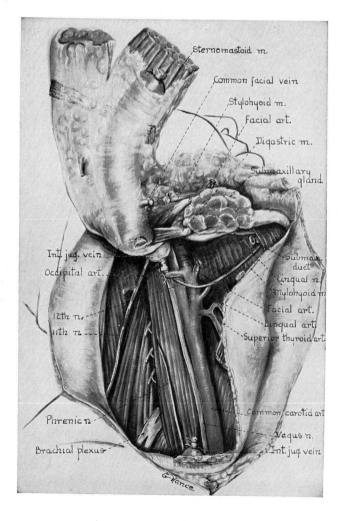

Figure 18. Complete unilateral neck dissection. Internal jugular bulb ligated and divided near the base of the skull. The submaxillary duct and chorda tympani branch of the lingual nerve are divided and the freed anterior segment is rotated out and up onto the external surface of the mandible. The mass containing the sternomastoid muscles, the contents of submaxillary triangle and the potential metastatic nodes from the clavicle to the base of the skull are ready for division at the jugular bulb, through the parotid gland and above the mandible. The remaining structures are indicated, any of which could be included with the block removed if necessary for cure of the cancer, yet compatible with life. Firm pressure dressing is applied with mechanics' waste held by gauze rolls after the flaps have been carefully approximated. The scar is minimal and the patient is usually discharged from hospital on seventh to tenth postoperative day.

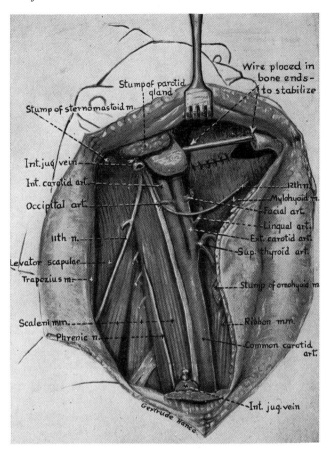

Figure 19. Combined operation for removal of carcinoma of the jaw and complete unilateral neck dissection. Complete removal of the potential metastatic nodes from the clavicle to the base of skull including the sternomastoid muscle, jugular vein and contents of the submaxillary triangle, with transection at the base of the skull and ligation of the jugular bulb. Primary tumor in the tongue, floor of the mouth or alveolus and involved bone removed in one block with the mass from the neck. The opening into the mouth is closed and jaw is stabilized with wire placed in the ends of the bone to prevent collapse. Tracheotomy is usually avoided. The structures remaining in neck are identified in Figure 18. The neck flaps are carefully closed and a firm pressure dressing is applied.

less it is felt that there is considerable doubt that the tongue lesion can be controlled. Postponement should not be longer than a month, particularly if metastases are already present in the neck. It should be common knowledge that removal of all the lymph-bearing area from the clavicle to the base of the skull, with preservation of vital structures, is necessary for cure. Adequate removal of the deep cervical chain is impossible without removing the internal jugular vein. Figure 18 shows the extent of removal and identifies the remaining structures. Figure 19 shows the combined operation for removal of carcinoma of the jaw and complete unilateral neck dissection. Deformity following this radical operation is minimal. Bilateral complete neck dissections have to be done at times, but it is safer if the jugular veins on both sides of the neck are not removed at the same operation.

JAWS

FRACTURE OF MANDIBLE. Because of the exposed position of the lower jaw, fractures of this structure are frequent. The type of fracture depends on the point of contact, the force of the trauma and the relative strength of various parts of the jaw. Displacement of the fragments also is the result of the type and force of the trauma with the addition of muscular pull.

Diagnosis of a fractured mandible is usually not difficult and can be made on examination. X-ray examination in the postero-anterior, right lateral and left lateral positions is routinely made. Special views of the condyle and temporomandibular joint may be necessary. The mandible is likely to be broken in more than one place. If one fracture is demonstrable, the presence of a second must be ruled out. The inferior alveolar nerve may be severed and if there is numbness of the lower lip, this should be recorded.

The time for reduction and fixation of a fractured jaw is as soon as possible, if the general condition permits. Swelling in itself is no contraindication to immediate repair. Postponement may make reduction more difficult and eventually fragments may be permanently fixed out of position or non-union of the bone will occur.

The airway may be of primary concern in patients with a fracture of the mandible. Bilateral fracture of the body of the lower jaw and the resultant loose central segment allow the tongue to drop back and occlude the airway. Immediate temporary fixation, positioning of the patient with the head down, traction on the tongue, or even tracheostomy may be necessary for survival, particularly in an individual with a shattered lower jaw. Blood in the mouth resulting from soft tissue tears, as is often found in persons with displaced mandible fractures, and secretions may actually drown a semi-conscious patient unless they are sucked out or allowed to drain out by putting the head down, or a tracheostomy opening is made. Accumulation of blood, or even air in the neck, may occlude the airway by compression and necessitate a tracheostomy.

Hemorrhage with a fractured mandible may require immediate control. Displacement of sharp fragments, which may cut major vessels in the neck, necessitates adequate exposure and individual ligation. Bleeding into the neck may be more dangerous by compression of the airway than is bleeding to the outside.

The general condition of the patient is of next consideration when the airway has been provided for and hemorrhage has been controlled. Complete physical examination is done to rule out the presence of intra-abdominal or chest injury and, if either is present, the necessity and the time for repair are decided. Fractures or injuries of the extremities may require treatment before, after or during jaw or facial repair. A careful, complete, neurologic examination is made in all patients having facial injuries or jaw fractures. For snap blows in which the head is forcefully flexed, cervical spine x-ray films should be studied, as fractures may occur in the spine and, when present, may be a serious complication.

Anesthesia for reduction and fixation of simple fractures of the jaw may be secured by procaine block of the dental nerves, or of the second and third divisions of the fifth cranial nerve as they leave the skull. General anesthesia may be preferable and decision is made as to whether general or local anesthesia would be better for each individual patient. An airway must, of course, be provided by a tube placed in the trachea, either through the nose or mouth, if general anesthesia is used.

Teeth may be involved in any fracture of the jaw or may in themselves be the extent of the injury. Chip fractures of the teeth can often be smoothed off by a dentist. Cracked teeth may be serviceable for years. If a tooth is loose, many times it will become solid again and stabilization with wires or an arch should be done. Single anterior teeth actually knocked out may be replaced in their sockets if available following the accident, as they may become serviceable again. However, this does not condone the practice of using another individual's teeth for reimplantation. Teeth in the fracture line of the jaw will probably eventually be lost, but they are usually retained to give aid in the fixation of the fracture. They may be removed later.

Reduction of fractures in the body of the mandible is accomplished when the teeth have been replaced in normal occlusion for the patient. Reduction of the edentulous jaw or positioning of the teeth may be done by palpation, under direct vision.

Fixation after reduction, if teeth are present in all fragments, is most simply done by interdental wiring. Steel wires, No. 24 or 26 gauge, are twisted around the necks of apposing teeth and the lower jaw is wired to the upper jaw, using the upper as a splint for the lower. The bicuspid or premolar teeth, if available, are the most satisfactory teeth for wiring. Loops may be made of the wires and rubber-band traction can be used for fixation or for gradual reduction. There are many forms of wiring and of bar appliances, but the basic procedure is to reduce the fracture so that the teeth will come into proper occlusion and be held there. Other means of fixation must be used if usable teeth are not present, even to wiring dentures in place with circumferential wires around the jaw and denture.

Internal wire-pin fixation has been found the most satisfactory supplement in fractures near the angle of the jaw or posterior to molar teeth; in fractures at the symphysis where nonunion can frequently occur without solid fixation; if there is extreme comminution of the mandible or widespread opening into the mouth; if there has been necessary delay in reduction and fixation, or in the edentulous jaw. Use of the wire-pin for fixation is not difficult but does take some practice. After the fracture has been reduced, a 0.05- to 0.08-inch steel wire is driven with a power drill through both fragments across the fracture site below the nerve canal. Multiple wire-pins may be needed in complicated fractures. Open mouth and some chewing are possible during the healing period. Circumferential wires have been used in conjunction with interdental and internal wire-pin fixation.

Direct wiring or using complicated, expensive external fixation or traction apparatus is usually unnecessary. Metal plates with screws have not proved consistently successful in fractures of the human jaw, as they tend to become loose and infected.

External drainage is considered in all mandible fractures. It is almost impossible to break the lower jaw and not have an opening into the mouth, particularly around the teeth. Drainage can be instituted simply by making a small incision beneath the jaw and carrying the opening up to the fracture site by blunt dissection and putting a small drain to this spot. Protracted healing and osteomyelitis can be avoided by this simple procedure. Obviously, with the aid and protection of antibiotics, this external drainage is omitted in many patients, but this is a deviation from the rule.

Condyle fractures are suspected if there is a history of trauma to the jaw followed by pain in the side of the face or near the temporomandibular joint and change of occlusion or bite. This is especially true in patients who have received blows to the chin in fights. Spontaneous fracture is rare. Condyle fractures are often associated with other fractures of the jaw and their presence must be ruled out if only one fracture is seen, as in the body. The condylar neck is one of the weaker areas of the jaw, and consequently is more likely to be broken even though the trauma be indirect. It is usually sufficient to wire the teeth in the patient's normal occlusion for three weeks, then to allow normal return of jaw action. Only very occasionally is open operation necessary and, even if thought necessary, a trial of wiring in occlusion may be done. Operation usually consists of exposure of the condyle, avoiding damaging branches of the facial nerve, and removal of the small upper fragment. Fixation, satisfactory for solid union in this location, is practically rarely possible and is unnecessary. Fracture of both condyles is an extremely serious situation and fixation in occlusion is especially indicated to try to prevent permanent deformity.

TEMPOROMANDIBULAR JOINT DISORDERS. The auriculotemporal pain syndrome is probably the result of erosion of the temporomandibular meniscus and joint and irritation of the auriculotemporal nerve. Diagnosis may be difficult, but the patient usually complains of severe pain about the ear and temporal region and radiation down into the tongue. Opposing molar support may be lacking and can be tested by seeing if relief is obtained by opening the mouth and swinging the jaw from side to side, or by building up the molar region with rubber mats or plugs. If relief is obtained by either maneuver, permanent build-up of the molars can be done by the dentist or, if the patient is edentulous, new teeth can be provided. X-ray examination of the joint may be helpful in making the diagnosis.

The temporomandibular meniscus syndrome results from derangement of the meniscus and may be acute following a difficult dental extraction or external trauma, or may appear suddenly in chronic progressive derangement. Cracking or popping, pain and blockage with the jaw open or closed are the usual symptoms, appearing often in that order as the disease progresses. Treatment consists in rest of the joint by avoiding wide opening, minimal chewing and wearing a chin-vertex bandage. Enforced rest with interdental wiring in occlusion may be necessary. Injection and joint operations have not been very successful.

Anterior dislocation of the jaw may be a part of the temporomandibular meniscus syndrome, or may result from trauma on the jaw while the mouth is open or from the pull-scar neck contracture. One or both sides of the jaw may be involved. Diagnosis is usually apparent, since the mouth is held open with the lower jaw forward, or pointing toward the unaffected side in unilateral dislocation. Inability to swallow or talk is usually present at first. X-ray films may be exposed to rule out the possibility of fracture of the neck of the condyle. Treatment, if there have been recurrent dislocations, may be carried out by the patient, since oftentimes the condyle slips back easily. Downward, backward pressure in the molar area may reduce the dislocation, but a general anesthesia may be necessary to accomplish this. If reduction is impossible, open operation may be necessary and the condyle may be removed. Trauma to the chin with the mouth open may drive the condyle up through the base of the skull into the brain and this dislocation may be called an antero-superior one. Treatment is usually directed toward the brain damage. Later, reduction can be done and occasionally repair of the glenoid fossa is necessary.

Posterior dislocation of the jaw usually results from a forceful smash on the chin when the mouth is closed. The condyle is driven back into and crushes the bony portion of the ear canal. Reduction is often spontaneous, but recognition of what has occurred is important so that steps may be taken to prevent permanent occlusion of the ear canal. Treatment usually consists of opening the ear canal and maintaining its patency. Reduction of condyle dislocation may require surgical exposure and possible removal of the condyle.

FRACTURE OF UPPER JAW. Fractures of the upper jaw are a part of middle-third facial fractures except for the occasional separate upper alveolar fracture.

The diagnosis of fractures of the upper jaw may be difficult because of swelling; however, palpation and suspicion that a fracture may be present following fairly severe trauma are of the most importance in making the diagnosis. X-ray examination may not give as good an indication of the type or severity of the fractures as will simple palpation because of superposition, but it is routinely made. Posteroanterior views of the facial bones showing the orbital borders or a modified Waters' film are the most valuable.

Upper alveolar fractures may involve any or all of the alveolus. Extension up into the pyriform recess or medially through the palate is common. The diagnosis is obvious on even cursory examination and palpation. Although minimal debridement in facial injuries is urged, removal of loose alveolar fragments may avoid troublesome drainage and future trouble. Reduction and fixation with interdental wires using the lower jaw as a splint are done if necessary and possible. Internal wire-pin fixation has been used as the only or supplementary means of fixation.

Transverse fractures of the upper jaw and face are frequently seen in persons involved in an automobile accident. These fractures usually result from striking the face on the dashboard, steering wheel or rear of the front seat. The diagnosis can be made on the basis of history of trauma, swelling and examination. Fracture lines may be palpated and movement of separate segments of the face or jaw can be seen. The line of fracture may start in the alveolus on one side, extend up into the pyriform recess and up into the orbit — a pyramidal fracture. If the main force is at a higher level, the nose will be crushed down into the face and the face will be completely detached from the skull. This separation can be demonstrated by grasping the teeth and moving them up and down, but this is not appreciated by the unanesthetized patient. The fracture line extends across both orbits. In severe facial crushes, there can be any combination of these transverse facial fractures and they are often associated with a fracture-dislocation of one or both zygomas. X-rays are routinely taken, but usually in no way indicate the extent of the actual damage. There may be multiple small chip fractures with fragments no larger than a fingernail, and these are not usually seen on the x-ray film. In a badly crushed face there may be 20 to 40 small fractures, like a broken egg or glass. Fracture lines through dense portions of bone may be seen, as may irregularities of the orbital borders and antral cloudiness. Reduction may involve pulling the face forward and the upper alveolus up or down, depending on the displacement. No preconceived routine is applicable; the reduction involves reversing the action and force of the trauma.

Fixation, particularly in severe facial crushes, requires all means of stabilization. The dental arch can be held, using the lower jaw as a splint, with interdental wires. Internal wire-pins anchored in any stable point, such as zygoma, can hold other loose points by cantilever action. Also, several loose sections of the face can be stabilized in one plane by internal wire-pins driven horizontally across the face. Needless to say, reduction or elevation to proper position is necessary before the permanent wire fixation is done. External and overhead traction apparatus is used by some surgeons.

Zygomatic arch fractures should be distinguished from displacements of the zygoma itself. Arch fractures usually result from direct trauma, such as that incurred by a fall on a curb or a blow with the fist. The deformity can be palpated through the swelling and x-ray pictures can be taken to compare the arches. Treatment consists in direct elevation of the depression in the arch with the hook through the skin (Fig. 20) or a large towel clip can be used. There is no scar. Impaction usually occurs and nothing further is needed. A more indirect approach may be

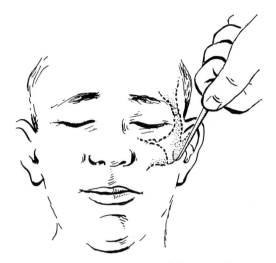

Figure 20. Method of reducing dislocation of zygoma. This is the simplest direct method applicable when fragments will impact in the reduced position. The position of the heavy hook beneath the flange of the zygoma after piercing the skin is shown. Reversing the direction through which the dislocated zygoma has passed by pulling on the hook, the zygoma is guided into impacted reduction with the fingers of the other hand on the upper border of the bone. This is the method of choice for the usual zygomatic arch fracture, avoiding an incision above the hairline. However, extreme care should be taken to keep the upward pull of the hook controlled at all times. Failure of the fragments to impact by this method or any other type of reduction necessitates changing to the approach through the fracture line above the canine fossa, which allows for fixation by the use of an internal splint in the form of a pack in the antrum.

made through an incision above the hairline and the depression may be elevated by sliding it down beneath the temporal fascia. Impaction is not dependent on the method of elevation. If impaction does not occur, open operation and wire fixation may be necessary.

Fracture-dislocation of the zygoma usually follows trauma to the cheek bone because of the prominent position of the zygoma and is often associated with fracture of other bones in the face or jaw. The zygoma itself is usually not fractured but is separated from all of its attachments and crushes the thinner surrounding bones, including the maxilla, with crumpling of the antrum and depression of the orbital border and floor. The effect of dislocating the zygoma might be compared to that of placing a marble on an egg and striking the marble with a hammer, the marble representing the zygoma and the egg the surrounding bones. As could be imagined, the marble would be broken if a strong enough blow were used, but crushing of the egg is inevitable.

Diagnosis of a fracture-dislocation of the

zygoma is usually easy to establish by palpation, particularly of the inferior orbital border. Swelling may be marked and may mask the flatness of the cheek, but the displacement can usually be felt. In addition to flatness of the cheek, which will be obvious when the swelling subsides, diplopia due to elongation of the orbital cavity with downward displacement of the zygoma, and with the eyeball following on down into the antral region, difficulty opening the mouth due to impaction of the zygoma on the coronoid, and infraorbital nerve paralysis due to crushing by the dislocated zygoma may be present. All of these signs or symptoms should be tested for and recorded, since only one may be elicited. Disability will be permanent unless the deformity is corrected. X-rays, made with the patient in the posteroanterior position or the modified Waters' position, showing the orbital borders of the facial bones, are of the most practical value and are taken routinely. Here again, an x-ray film many times does not give a very good indication of the extent of the damage.

Completely detached bits of bone may be removed, but if there is a chance of survival they are left, if necessary, for removal secondarily. Three weeks is about the limit of time at which the zygoma can be reduced from its displaced position.

Reduction should be done by the simplest possible method and will suffice if impaction occurs. A large jaw hook pushed through the soft tissue can elevate the zygoma by grasping the inferior border and probably provides the simplest direct approach to the zygoma. There are numerous other operations for reducing the zygoma, but if impaction in the normal position does not occur, a method of fixation is needed. Reduction and fixation are usually possible through entrance into the antrum through the fracture line in the buccal fornix. This requires only a short incision through the buccal mucosa. From inside the antrum, the displaced zygoma can be elevated with a palate elevator or Kelly clamp, the surgeon using his free hand for guidance as to proper position. The correct position can be maintained, until solid union occurs, with an iodoform pack incorporated with balsam of Peru lightly accordioned into the antrum. The pack acts as an internal splint and makes it possible to "mulch" into proper position the multiple comminuted fragments in the floor of the orbit and antral walls. This pack should be removed in ten to 20 days. Multiple internal wire-pins driven across the face using the opposite zygoma as a point for cantilever support have given sufficient fixation alone or may be used in conjunction with other methods. When both zygomas are loose, wire-pins have given enough fixation for solid union to occur and in severe facial crushes have even provided an initial point on which to base fixation of other shattered features.

So-called blowout fractures, a term applied to orbital floor displacement without orbital rim fracture, will not be overlooked if orbital levels are routinely checked at the original examination and daily subsequently. Early repair is done through the antrum; later an implant may be necessary.

JAW INFECTIONS. Osteomyelitis is most commonly caused by infections dependent on the teeth or by fractures of the jaw, but it may be associated with cysts in the jaw or follow injuries to the mucosa or infrequently result from infections elsewhere in the body such as in the paranasal sinuses. Other causes may be heat and irradiation.

The most common infecting organisms are staphylococci or streptococci, but others infrequently seen are the *Mycobacterium tuberculosis*, Actinomyces and *Treponema pallidum*.

Periapical abscess is really localized osteomyelitis and usually spreads by the extraction of an acutely abscessed tooth. Pericoronitis is soft tissue inflammation around a partially erupted third molar, which may spontaneously progress to osteomyelitis, but more commonly follows extraction performed when the tooth was acutely abscessed.

Fractures are the second most common cause of osteomyelitis. In all fractures of the jaw, drainage to the outside should be considered since it is almost impossible for the jaw to break and not lacerate the mucosa if teeth are present. An avenue to the bone for mouth organisms is opened up. Prevention by prophylactic drainage is the best treatment, although reliance is often placed on antibiotic protection.

Cysts are a potential pocket for infection and the avenue for mouth organisms may be via a nonvital tooth root.

Thermal necrosis of the jaw may follow cautery destruction of an overlying carcinoma, and is usually relatively localized.

Irradiation is not an infrequent cause of osteomyelitis, which is distinguished by the intense pain. It usually follows irradiation to carcinoma of the mouth near the bone. Involvement may be widespread, the healing slow and promise of secondary breakdown great.

In the acute stage of osteomyelitis, pain is the prominent symptom and it may be very severe. There may be a history of a recent extraction of an acutely inflamed tooth. Swelling may be diffuse about the face and extend down into the neck. Tenderness is marked and may be over the jaw or generalized over the swollen area. Trismus may be marked. There are also the general signs and symptoms of infection, such as fever and general malaise. X-ray films may show very little in this acute phase other than the cavity left by extraction of the tooth with slight bony erosion. In the chronic stage, there is local reaction to a foreign body and purulent drainage with acute exacerbations accompanied by general reaction. Multiple sinus tracts may be present, possibly with an oral fistula. X-ray examination in the chronic stage will show cavities, sequestra and, later, the developing involucrum.

Prevention is the best possible treatment and is worth while if one patient can be saved from osteomyelitis. Dentists have learned that an acutely inflamed tooth should not be extracted since, instead of allowing for drainage, new avenues for spread are opened up by this procedure. External drainage for fractures of the jaw will reduce the incidence of osteomyelitis.

Antibiotics in large doses are used and have prevented the local progress of the infection to extensive bone necrosis. Their use has also undoubtedly saved lives.

Upper alveolar or maxillary osteomyelitis is much less common than osteomyelitis in the mandible, and occurs most frequently in the region of the incisors, in the canines or at the tubercles. Infection may spread from the nose or paranasal sinuses in addition to that associated with the teeth. Often the most prominent symptom is periorbital edema. Treatment follows the same principles outlined for osteomyelitis of the mandible.

Gumboil, or alveolar abscess, should be drained by incising the mucosa and gently retracting the periosteum. The tooth can be extracted when the process has subsided.

Once an abscess has developed, it is usually opened externally; otherwise, the infection may spread and dissect all the closing muscles of the mouth, including the masseter, internal pyterygoid and the temporal. A short collar incision is made through the skin, followed by blunt dissection into the abscess and to the bone, care being taken to make the opening into the masseter space on the outside and into the internal pterygoid space on the inside.

The abscess is evacuated and a light iodoform pack is inserted to be left in place for 24 hours to establish the drainage tract.

No cutting of bone is done at this stage. The jaw sequestrates rapidly and to cut into it invites further spread of the osteomyelitis. Spontaneous separation of any fragments is awaited for up to 12 weeks and, during this time, secondary drainage may be necessary. Also during this time, the process changes from an acute to a chronic one and becomes less dangerous.

Maintenance of the arch of the jaw is the most important consideration when osteomyelitis has developed. Conservative management is indicated. Though antibiotics may hasten the development of an involucrum and save lives, the dental arch is a mechanical problem and the principles of handling potential sequestra are the same as those outlined 20 years ago. The involucrum must have formed before sequestra are removed and then they can be gently lifted out. If the jaw is allowed to collapse by radical debridement, it is almost impossible to reconstruct the arch.

Block necrosis of the mandible has been followed by regeneration of an essentially normal arch by conservative management of the sequestra.

Tooth buds in children should be conservatively drained.

Tuberculosis of the jaw is rare and is usually a more indolent process than is osteomyelitis. A large fluctuant area may be present over the jaw with multiple draining sinuses. X-ray examination may show spotty areas of necrosis. Identification of tubercle bacilli is necessary for the final diagnosis. Treatment may be more radical than for other forms of osteomyelitis. Sequestrectomy, excision of involved soft tissue and closure of the wound are done while an adequate streptomycin blood level is being maintained.

Infection of the jaw with Actinomyces should be strongly suspected from the history. Typically, a chronically infected lower molar is extracted and three weeks later a painless mass appears over the jaw, which increases in size and becomes painful and inflamed; trismus appears and there is the usual general response to infection. Drainage may be spontaneous and subsidence occurs, but the painful swelling appears recurrently. Later, there is widespread induration in the face and neck, multiple draining sinuses and scars, and inability to open the mouth. X-ray examination shows osteomyelitis. The diagnosis is established by finding sulfur granules in the drainage, but it may be necessary to open a new pocket to demonstrate them. Microscopic confirmation is advisable. Treatment consists in drainage of the multiple abscesses, x-ray therapy and prolonged systemic usage of antibiotics. Excision of the involved soft tissue may be necessary.

Syphilis involving the jaw bones is rarely seen. The usual involvement is of the hard palate and the supports to the nose. Treatment consists of the usual systemic therapy for syphilis, but later reconstruction and closing of the defects may be necessary.

Ankylosis may be true or false. True ankylosis results from bony union at or near the joint. It has been seen following mastoiditis, osteomyelitis elsewhere in the jaw, and fracture. Patients have been seen who were unable to open their mouths for years. One or both sides may be involved. When it occurs on one side, the body of the jaw appears more normal on the ankylosed side than it does on the uninvolved side. If any opening is possible, the jaw deviates to the ankylosed side, and the preangular notch is deepened on that side. X-rays may show the extent of damage and union at the joint. Also, involvement of the coronoid should be determined since it has been seen solidly fixed by bony union. A series of coronoid ankylosis alone, resulting from war wounds, has been reported. Treatment of true ankylosis consists in resection of enough bone for a false joint to develop. Bilateral true ankylosis is a particular problem, since forward support of the jaw may be lost and tracheostomy may be necessary. In such instances, the worse side should be operated on first and possibly enough opening may result following unilateral relief.

False ankylosis is due to scarred bands which prevent the jaw from opening, but may be difficult to distinguish from bony ankylosis; both may be present to some degree. The scar requires excision and some substitution with a graft or flap is required for relief of false ankylosis. The scar of a neck contracture may produce a type of false ankylosis by pulling on the chin and inducing an anterior dislocation of the jaw, as in Figure 21.

TUMORS OF JAW. Tumors, benign and malignant, which occur in other bones of the body also are found in the jaws. In addition, there are tumors in the jaw which are peculiar to it, owing chiefly to the presence of teeth.

Torus palatinus is an osteoma or exostosis which is more or less symmetrical and is found in the midline of the hard palate. Because of its size, which may affect the speech or prevent the proper fitting of dentures, or irritation, it may require removal. Excision is not difficult, but opening into the floor of the nose should be avoided. Torus mandibularis is a similar occurrence of an exostosis inside the lower jaw which may be in the midline or symmetrical on both sides. Removal is usually not required, but it may be necessary to allow for a lower dental plate.

Dental cysts, root cysts or radicular cysts are probably of infectious origin and are seen on x-ray films as a cyst in the bone surrounding a tooth root or a retained root. Cure requires removal of the root and the cyst. The bony defect is allowed to heal from the bottom.

Dentigerous cysts are lined by epithelia and contain a tooth bud or unerupted tooth. Bone is eroded as the cysts distend, but is not invaded by the cell. The cysts must be completely removed.

Adamantinomas, or ameloblastomas, are tumors which arise from the preameloblasts, or cells which later form the enamel of a tooth. They may be cystic or solid, but usually occur as a mixture of solid and cystic elements. X-ray films may show a multilocular arrangement with erosion of the bone by pressure. The more solid the tumor is, the more apt it is to invade bone. This may proceed so far as to make the tumor malignant by position or extension toward the base of the brain. Adamantinomas have been reported in the long bones. The benign character may change any time, and invasion of bone and soft tissue occurs. The change is usually to squamous cell carcinoma, though the original solid adamantinoma looks like a basal cell growth microscopically. Treatment, as long as the tumor is contained in the bone, may be intraoral as for dentigerous cysts. Invasion of the bone requires block excision, which has also been done intraorally and facial scars avoided. Extensive soft tissue involvement requires block removal through a neck approach.

Odontomas arise from odontoblasts. Small tumors of this type may be removed in the same way as are unerupted teeth, but larger

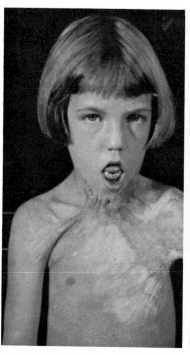

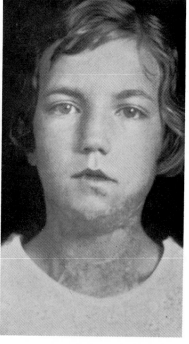

Figure 21. Contracture neck from old burn scar dislocating lower jaw. *A,* Repeated attempts by the body to heal the open flexion area have developed scar strong enough to actually dislocate the mandible. There is continual drainage of saliva onto the chest. *B,* The appearance of the patient following one operation. The deep scar has been excised, opening up the flexion area and releasing the jaw; defect has been covered with a free split-thickness graft. Watertight integrity of mouth has been restored.

A   *B*

ones may require removal of a segment of jaw.

Osteofibromas and giant cell tumors are probably the most common benign tumors found in the jaw which do not arise from dental elements, but they are seen only infrequently. In rare instances, giant cell tumors may occur as part of the picture of a parathyroid tumor.

Osteogenic sarcoma is infrequently seen, but is the most common malignant primary jaw tumor. Metastatic carcinoma, erosion or invasion by alveolar carcinoma, or that arising in salivary glands or by secondary invasion from metastatic lymph nodes, is of more common occurrence.

Chondrosarcoma usually occurs in the lower jaw about the joint and is perhaps one of the sarcomas most often controlled by operation.

Carcinoma of the jaw does not occur spontaneously, but by secondary invasion from buccal or alveolar carcinoma. There is, however, an exception in that adamantinomas may become malignant and form carcinomas in the jaw itself. The originating epithelial cell comes from the paradental debris left in the jaw following formation of the enamel organ.

BONE GRAFTS TO JAW. Bone grafts are necessary to bridge defects in the jaw following loss from any cause. They are often used to promote union where there previously has been failure and to fill out contours. Ribs are most useful for graft material because of their natural shape, and iliac crests may be well shaped to fit defects. Solid grafts may be wired in place to become their own splints. As these grafts may bridge defects and do not simply act as splints while union occurs, they are thought to be true grafts and to persist as such. Obviously, bone-bank nonviable material is not considered as applicable for this permanent bridging of defects as are fresh autografts.

The soft tissue pocket into which the graft is to be placed is most important for persistence of the bone graft and union to occur, because success of any deep repair is dependent on primary soft tissue healing over it.

SALIVARY GLANDS AND DUCTS

TRAUMA. Contusion of a salivary gland, duct or surrounding soft tissue may cause obstruction which is usually temporary and subsides spontaneously.

Laceration of a salivary gland may be associated with facial lacerations and will be evident on examination. Salivary drainage will be seen and is always looked for in the presence of laceration near the salivary glands. Tears of the parotid or submaxillary salivary glands may result from sharp fragments in jaw fractures. If the laceration is only in the substance of a salivary gland, no special consideration is necessary as healing will take place spontaneously.

Laceration of a duct can result from the same causes, and recognition is particularly important as drainage will continue or blockage develop unless it is repaired. All deep lacerations in the region of the salivary ducts should be carefully investigated, as should fractures of the mandible near the submaxillary duct, and immediately repaired. Late scarring may produce obstruction secondarily. Transplantation of the proximal duct opening farther back in the mouth may be done instead of anastomosis.

Salivary duct fistula to the outside persisting after injury is very annoying to the patient and requires operative closure, if drainage can be established through it. Changing of the fistula to the inside of the mouth may be necessary if the continuity of the duct cannot be re-established. X-ray treatment to shut off the salivary flow may result in the closure of some small fistulas but cannot be relied on for large ones.

OBSTRUCTION TO SALIVARY SYSTEM. Obstruction to the flow of saliva from any salivary gland may be due to compression or involvement by scar, infection or tumor or other mass near the duct; infection in the gland or duct; salivary calculus; tumor of the duct or gland; and scar or deformity of the duct. Obstruction without any demonstrable cause is not infrequent.

That obstruction is present is usually obvious as the affected salivary gland becomes enlarged and prominent. The swelling is usually worse on salivary stimulation, and may subside to some extent between meals. Swelling may appear suddenly or may develop gradually, depending on the cause. Pain is usually present and in degree related to the amount of swelling and its speed of development. Examination will reveal a swollen, tender gland and lack of salivary flow from the orifice of the duct in the mouth, even on tender pressure over the gland or milking of the duct. Purulent material may be draining from the duct. Fever and malaise may be evident, depending on the individual reaction to the particular obstruction. Careful examination of the duct with a lacrimal duct probe may determine the cause of obstruction. X-rays should be taken, but often they are of no or little aid in the diagnosis.

Extrinsic causes of obstruction, such as a constricting scar, infection or tumor, require relief of the primary condition. Care should be exercised in removal of tumors near the salivary ducts.

Infection in a salivary gland or duct is one of the most important causes of obstruction. It may be associated with a calculus and this should be established at the onset. Obstruction may result from the edema of infection or persist after removal of a stone. Although a single organism may initiate the infection, the usual mouth organisms can be cultured when symptoms begin. Swelling of both submaxillary and parotid glands may be noticed in severely debilitated subjects.

Treatment consists in the administration of systemic antibiotics and salivary stimulants; mouth cleanliness, including care of gum disease and carious teeth; and administration of sedatives or analgesics necessary for general comfort. Carefully probing the duct with a small lacrimal duct probe may reveal the presence of a stone. It is a part of the treatment, allowing draining and at least temporary relief from the swelling. Subsidence is usually fairly rapid unless there is some other fundamental reason for persistence, but recurrences are common and enlargement of the duct orifice may be necessary. Persistent infection in the gland may require its removal. Glandular elements by this time are pretty well destroyed. Use of irradiation to stop salivary secretion is considered in those patients in whom no cause for the obstruction is demonstrable.

Calculus in the duct or in the gland is the second most common cause of obstruction.

The signs and symptoms are those of obstruction and infection is usually present. Careful probing of the duct with a small lacrimal probe will establish the fact that obstruction is present, or a grating of the duct on the stone may be heard or felt. X-ray examination may help to determine the position of the stone (Fig. 22), but superposition of the jaw may prevent visualization. More than one stone is often present. Treatment consists in removal of the stone and relief is usually immediate. Enlargement of the duct orifice may prevent stone formation or permit passage of stones already formed. It may be impossible to remove stones in the gland or those which have migrated into the surrounding area, and it may be necessary to remove the affected gland and duct. Antibiotics and salivary stimulants are used.

Tumors arising from the salivary ducts are rare and obstruction is slower than that by stone or infection. Tumors in the gland itself are not usually present.

Scar or deformity of the duct from other causes resulting in obstruction is not uncommon. Scars following passage of a stone or resulting from excessive trauma in their removal are often not of sufficient severity to require operative correction. Repaired lacerations of ducts may be responsible for obstruction after healing is complete. Local revision of the scar may relieve the obstruction or a new opening may be made in the mouth proximal to the blocked area. Deformity of the duct may be due to atresia anywhere in the duct, but the commonest site seems to be at the orifice. The opening may be of sufficient size, but, in persons of any age, slight inflammation in the duct or around the opening into the mouth may cause obstruction to the salivary flow. Repeated careful dilation with a lacrimal probe may suffice, but the orifice may require enlarging.

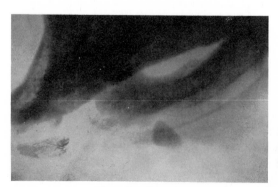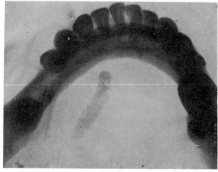

Figure 22.   X-ray appearance of salivary calculi in submaxillary duct.

Obstruction to any salivary gland may occur without any demonstrable cause being found. This may be recurrent. Three light doses of deep irradiation may be sufficient to shut off the gland, but, if not, actual removal may be necessary.

BENIGN TUMORS OF SALIVARY GLANDS. Benign tumors occurring in the major salivary glands are of the same types as those which are found in soft tissue elsewhere in the body, e.g., lymphangioma, angioma and lipoma.

Mixed tumors of anlage origin are usually thought of as being inherent in salivary glands, but they have been observed elsewhere in the body (Fig. 23). Papillary cystadenoma lymphomatosum is found in these salivary glands. One hundred and eighty-seven tumors were removed from the parotid gland over a 12-year period without evidence of recurrence or paralysis of the facial nerve. One hundred were benign mixed tumors. Papillary cystadenoma lymphomatosum comprised 3.4 per cent; lipoma, 0.6 per cent; angioma, 1.4 per cent; and 5.3 per cent proved to be lymphangioma.

Benign mixed tumors occurring in the salivary glands are thought to be of anlage origin, as postulated by Halpert, from nests of embryonal ectoderm which do not imitate salivary gland or distort the gland with growth. Similar tumors occur elsewhere in the body and the relationship between tumor and gland is incidental. Occurrence may be multiple. Eighty-nine per cent are found in the parotid, 10 per cent in the submaxillary and 1 per cent in the sublingual gland. They may be found in persons of any age, most commonly in those between 30 and 50 years. The characteristic microscopic appearance is that of epithelial cells in cords, lumps or stellate arrangement set in a stroma of collagen which may look like cartilage and which may be part of the tumor cells themselves.

The diagnosis is made on the history of a painless mass which appears in a salivary gland and slowly increases in size, but unrelated to salivary stimulation. A solid mass can be felt in the gland not attached to the skin. Facial nerve function remains unimpaired regardless of the ultimate size. Sialography usually does not help in making the diagnosis. Removal is recommended as soon as the diagnosis is made.

In the parotid gland, the closeness of the facial nerve and its frequent association with the tumor make the problem of complete tumor removal without damaging the nerve worthy of special consideration. Wide exposure to the entire surface of the gland is necessary to remove the tumor safely. A direct approach is made to the tumor and the mass is removed completely with careful, minute pressure on all surrounding gland elements, which might contain nerve filaments, before they are cut. Fortunately, the majority of tumors lie over the facial nerve. If the tumor is beneath the nerve, this will be evident. The major divisions of the facial nerve can be identified and protected from

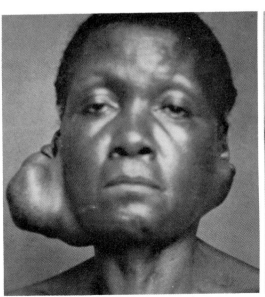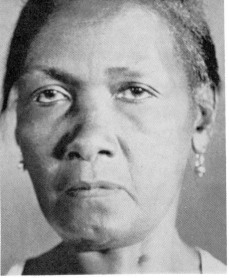

Figure 23. Bilateral benign mixed tumors of anlage origin; removed with preservation of the facial nerves.

injury by dissecting the tumor from these and smaller fibers. An individual observer of the face is part of the operating team, and he reports any movements or twitching of the face as the operation progresses. The skin is carefully closed and a comfortable, firm pressure dressing is applied. Healing takes place in five to seven days. The resultant scar is minimal, owing to the placement of the original incision.

Papillary cystadenoma lymphomatosum is removed in the same manner as are benign mixed tumors. It recurs less frequently than do the benign mixed tumors.

Lipomas are treated in a similar way as positive diagnosis often cannot be made until the tumor has been exposed.

Growing, solid hemangiomas which are found in infants usually do not require a biopsy for diagnosis and are very responsive to irradiation given in small doses. Surgical removal of this type of angioma is unnecessary and invites damage to the facial nerve. Cavernous angiomas, or a mixture of large and small vessel angiomas, are evident on examination and are treated by a combination of irradiation, packing and excision.

Lymphangioma is usually seen in infants but may be first noticed in individuals of any age. It occurs as a soft, compressible, painless tumor which is indefinite in outline. Change in character to an acutely swollen tender mass may be due to blood leak into one of the spaces. The tumor may extend into the mouth or into the neck, where it is called hygroma. The treatment is the same as that described for lymphangioma occurring in the mouth and it is sufficient to say that complete removal is often not possible or necessary. Making an opening into the area through the usual wide incision, partial excision of the mass and packing with gauze impregnated with a mild escharotic agent usually will result in destruction of the thin-walled flat endothelia-lined spaces and healing of the space may occur.

Other salivary glands may contain benign tumors. The easiest method for removal of these is usually total excision of the gland and the contained tumor.

MALIGNANT TUMORS OF SALIVARY GLANDS. Malignant tumors may occur in any salivary gland. The parotid is most frequently the seat of tumors, but the submaxillary tumors are most often malignant. Between 20 and 30 per cent of parotid tumors are malignant. Incidence of malignancy in the submaxillary gland is reported as high as 80 to 90 per cent.

The simplest microscopic classification of salivary gland tumors will be the most accurate because of the high incidence of a mixture of various types of carcinoma in the same tumor. Tissue resembling adenocarcinoma and squamous cell carcinoma has been seen on the same slide. In addition to these two types of carcinoma, a third, called malignant mixed tumor, is not infrequently seen. Evidence of benign mixed tumor may or may not be found in association with a malignant tumor. Carcinoma may originate as a benign mixed tumor.

Malignant tumors of the parotid gland can be accurately diagnosed by the history of a hard solid mass in the gland which has rapidly increased in size or has paralyzed part or all of the facial nerve, or if there is fixation of the mass to its surroundings or evidence of extension or metastasis. X-ray examination of the chest should be made. Biopsy is only occasionally necessary because of the high degree of accuracy of clinical diagnosis, and of the plan of procedure in which the original operation is considered as a biopsy if unsuspected malignant cells are discovered. Frozen sections of those tumors that are difficult to diagnose are not dependable in many instances. Microscopic interpretation is evidently so difficult that if biopsy is necessary, removal of adequate material is worth while. Tissue obtained by punch biopsy may show a benign tumor but, a few millimeters distant, there may be carcinoma which would be missed and the tumor can be spread. Biopsy, if necessary, has the same surgical requirements as does removal of a benign tumor.

Treatment of malignant parotid tumors may be by surgical excision, irradiation or a combination of both. Interstitial irradiation with radon seeds has been used very successfully to control the malignant tumor locally, and the facial nerve is saved if it is not already involved by the carcinoma. Cure of metastatic lesions, when present, requires surgical excision as do areas of potential spread. A radical operation for cure of carcinoma of the parotid includes removal of the entire gland, including the nerve, as indicated, and occasionally the overlying skin and mandible, combined with a complete neck dissection. En bloc excision of the primary tumor and area of lymph spread is possible; excision of the jaw and skin is carried out as necessary.

Malignant tumors of the submaxillary gland require removal of the entire gland and a neck dissection. The tissues can be removed in one block and as much of the mandible and skin is removed as is necessary. X-ray examination of the chest should be made.

PROSTHESES

Synthetic materials for subcutaneous prosthesis have been used for several years. Infections, trauma, ablative surgical operations and congenital deformities have created the need for hard and soft subcutaneous prosthetics. Fresh autogenous transplants are not always available or advisable, although they should be ideal.

Physical and chemical inertness is the chief requirement for a synthetic with persistence of form and consistency.

Laboratory investigations have been done including 600 implants in animals and followed through full life cycle observations with only one fibroma observed near a polyvinyl alcohol implant. No tumors have occurred following clinical use. We know of no report of tumor formation following the innumerable blood vessel transplants that have been done. It is recognized that no transplant has been followed for a full human life cycle, but animal experiments and the quantities of blood vessel replacements done mean safety for the patient requiring feature reconstruction. Preparation for all implants requires a proper sized pocket. Hemostasis is

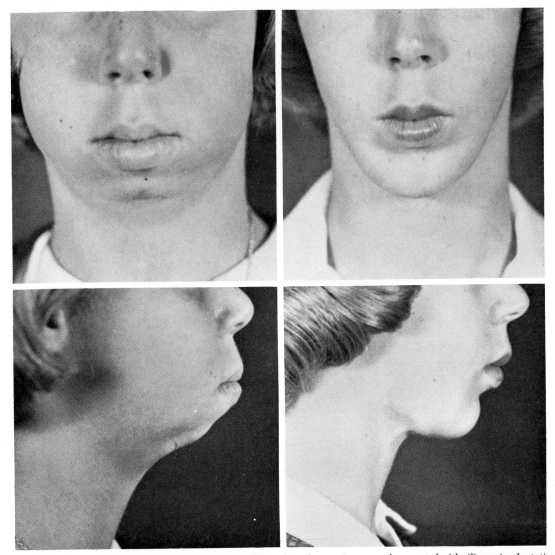

Figure 24.   Congenital absence of fourth function of face, that of appearing normal, corrected with silicone implantation from outside. Patient had had temporary construction with preserved cartilage during growing years.

obtained and the implant is shaped to the defect.

Polyvinyl alcohol is a soft subcutaneous prosthesis when wet or in the tissues. It is inert and its interstices are invaded by scar, giving fixation. Areas in the face and elsewhere in the body requiring building up with soft material have been filled with this synthetic. Polyvinyl alcohol is not perfect, however, since the invasion by scar tends to make the implant harder than is ideal and calcification may occur.

Silicones in their many forms and inertness hold promise of being the ideal synthetic prosthesis. Their value may only be limited by their absolute nonreactivity, since it is often necessary for the implant to cause enough fibrosis to fix itself. The dimethylsiloxane radical is the basic inert unit and may be polymerized thousands of times, from liquid to resins.

Silicone rubber has been produced for medical uses. This material is made from a viscous dimethylsiloxane by extracting one H molecule from a CH_3 group with benzoylperoxide, which is followed by cross linkages between the CH_2 groups and resulting in a soft, resilient material, difficult to distinguish from organic rubber. It can be cut with a knife and is shaped to size in the operating room for proper build-up. Figures 24 and 25 demonstrate the use of silicone rubber to construct the chin, and most importantly, the nose. Support of the skin envelope in these areas as it makes features completes the fourth function of the face: to look normal.

Teflon is one of the halogenated carbon polymers which are long chains of saturated fluorocarbons. It may be too inert to incite enough fibrosis for fixation in some areas; but where a hard subcutaneous prosthesis is necessary, as a substitute for cartilage or bone, Teflon is useful.

Etheron, diisocyanate, is being used clinically and in the laboratory. This is another soft sponge implant.

Difficulties of implantation include slipping, infection and extrusion. All have been encountered in earlier work and will continue, but are becoming less frequent. Abnormal final consistency of implants is a disadvantage, but lessens as improved synthetics become available. The search for the ideal subcutaneous prosthesis continues.

READING REFERENCES

Brown, J. B.: Double elongations of partially cleft palates and elongations of palates with complete clefts. Surg. Gyn. & Obst. 70:815, 1940.

Brown, J. B.: Preserved and fresh homotransplants of cartilage. Surg. Gyn. & Obst. 70:1079, 1940.

Brown, J. B.: The utilization of the temporal muscle and fascia in facial paralysis. Ann. Surg. *109*:1016, 1939.

Brown, J. B., and Cannon, B.: Composite free grafts of skin and cartilage from the ear. Surg. Gyn. & Obst. 82:253, 1946.

Brown, J. B., Cannon, B., and Lischer, C.: Ankylosis of coronoid process of mandible (and associated scar limitation of jaw function). Plast. Reconstr. Surg. 1:277, 1946.

Brown, J. B., and Fryer, M. P.: Plastic surgery for severe facial paralysis in elderly patients. J. Am. Geriatrics Soc. 2:820, 1954.

Brown, J. B., and Fryer, M. P.: Tumors in the parotid region. Am. Surgeon *18*:880, 1952.

Brown, J. B., and Fryer, M. P.: Inflammatory lesions of the jaw. *In*, The Cyclopedia of Medicine, Surgery, Specialties. Philadelphia, F. A. Davis Company, 1950, vol. 7, pp. 553-562.

Brown, J. B., Fryer, M. P., and Lu, M.: Polyvinyl and silicone compounds as subcutaneous prostheses. Arch. Surg. 68:744, 1954.

Brown, J. B., Fryer, M. P., and McDowell, F.: Internal wire-pin stabilization for middle third facial fractures. Surg. Gyn. & Obst. 93:676, 1951.

Brown, J. B., Fryer, M. P., and Ohlwiler, D. A.: Study and use of synthetic materials, such as silicones and Teflon, as subcutaneous prostheses. Plast. Reconstr. Surg. 26:264, 1960.

Brown, J. B., Fryer, M. P., Ohlwiler, D. A., and Kollias, P.: Dimethylsiloxane and halogenated carbons as subcutaneous prostheses. Amer. Surg. 28:146, 1962.

Brown, J. B., Fryer, M. P., Randall, P., and Lu, M.: Silicones in plastic surgery, laboratory and clinical investigations, a preliminary report. Plast. Reconstr. Surg. 12:374, 1953.

Brown, J. B., and McDowell, F.: Plastic Surgery of the

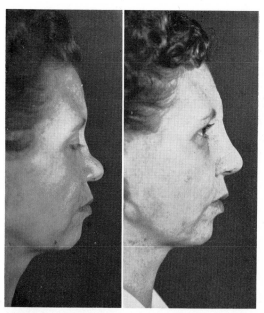

Figure 25.   Reconstruction of nasal support with silicone implant following traumatic loss.

Nose. St. Louis, The C. V. Mosby Company, 1952. Chapters XII, XV and XVI.

Brown, J. B., and McDowell, F.: Simplified design for repair of single cleft lips. Surg. Gyn. & Obst. 8:12, 1945.

Brown, J. B., and McDowell, F.: Neck dissections for metastatic carcinoma. Surg. Gyn. & Obst. 79:115, 1944.

Brown, J. B., and McDowell, F.: Field-fire and invasive basal cell carcinoma—baso-squamous type. Surg. Gyn. & Obst. 74:1128, 1942.

Brown, J. B., and McDowell, F.: Internal wire fixation for fractures of the jaw. Surg. Gyn. & Obst. 74:227, 1942.

Brown, J. B., McDowell, F., and Byars, L. T.: Double clefts of the lip. Surg. Gyn. & Obst. 85:20, 1947.

Brown, J. B., McDowell, F., and Fryer, M. P.: Direct operative removal of benign mixed tumors of anlage origin in the parotid region. Surg. Gyn. & Obst. 90:257, 1950.

Brown, J. B., McDowell, F., and Fryer, M. P.: Surgical treatment of irradiation burns. Surg. Gyn. & Obst. 88:609, 1949.

Fryer, M. P.: A simple direct method of reducing a fracture-dislocation of the zygoma. S. Clin. North America 30:1361, 1950.

Chapter 17

THE NECK

by
WALTER W. CARROLL, M.D.

WALTER WILLIAM CARROLL, Professor of Surgery at Northwestern University, received his surgical education and training at the University's School of Medicine. He is representative of the young surgeon in practice who devotes a large share of his time to teaching and research upon a wholly voluntary basis. His interest in surgery of the neck is manifested in his contributions to the literature. He has pioneered many of the innovations in utilizing closed circuit television in medical education.

Developmental Anomalies, Tumors, Infections and Wounds

DEVELOPMENTAL ANOMALIES OF THE NECK

Early in the course of intrauterine life, the embryo differentiates the anlage of adult neck structures. The jaws and neck are intimately related to the transient branchial arches which appear in the third and fourth weeks. The thyroglossal duct also appears at this time. During the course of the subsequent two to three weeks, these structures lose their identity as they form the more permanent organs of future life. Within the depths of these tissues, the paired jugular lymphatic anlage appears during the six- to eight-week period, and primary lymph nodes begin to differentiate shortly thereafter during the third month. Characteristic lateral and midline anomalies may result from slight alterations in these normal embryologic transitions. Defects in fusion or failure of normal obliterative processes results in formation of cysts, sinuses or even fistulae connecting with the pharynx. In the newborn, these may be of such size as seriously to interfere with vital functions. If respiratory or cardiovascular complications are minimal, they may remain only as cosmetic deformities or become the source of repeated episodes of infection.

LATERAL ANOMALIES

The majority of cysts, sinuses and fistulae located in the lateral portion of the neck are the result of faulty development. These lesions are found at any age, but for the most part are seen in the young. While in patients under 15 years of age more fistulae and sinuses than cysts will be found, in the age group over 15 years there will be a predominance of cysts. Of the fistulae which require surgical treatment, over half will have been present since birth, the majority of the remainder having appeared before the age of 15. On the other hand, cysts are found to arise more commonly as an insidious and painless swelling along the anterior border of the sternocleidomastoid muscle in the second and third decades.

While branchial cleft anomalies are usually thought to be developmental rather than genetic in origin, recent distribution studies of patients with bilateral defects have demonstrated a familial tendency, i.e., an inherited tendency which has been transmitted through the male as well as the female.

EMBRYOLOGY. Despite a high degree of consistency in the various locations, appearance and clinical courses of these anomalies, there are divergent views regarding their exact manner of origin. These entities have properly become known as branchial cysts and sinuses, because of the general agreement that those lesions found at or above the level of the hyoid bone arise from the second branchial cleft and pouch. Since some fistulae and sinuses are found below this level along the anterior border of the sternocleidomastoid muscle, some credence has been given to the consideration that their embryologic derivation may be the transient thymopharyngeal duct. The first view seems to be the more reasonable.

During the third week of intrauterine life, the human embryo presents rather clearly a series of five rounded branchial arches on either side of the neck. They are demarcated by four branchial clefts which run parallel to one another somewhat obliquely downward and anteromedially. Each external cleft is matched by an internal evagination called a pharyngeal pouch. Normally, the intervening membrane between each cleft and pouch does not rupture, so there is no communication between the pharyngeal pouch and the branchial cleft.

The first branchial cleft obliterates except at its dorsal part, which becomes the external auditory meatus. The remaining clefts disappear. Internally, the first pharyngeal pouch gives rise to the eustachian tube and the tympanic cavity; the second may be retained as the tonsillar and supratonsillar sinus; the third by entodermal outgrowth forms the thymus, by virtue of the thymopharyngeal diverticular duct, and the inferior parathyroids; and the fourth, the superior parathyroids. The tympanic membrane represents the dividing membrane between the first branchial cleft and the first pharyngeal pouch.

PATHOLOGY AND CLINICAL COURSE. Cysts and sinuses arising from the first branchial cleft are not common, less than 80 having ever been reported. These are usually very superficial and include the variable preauricular cutaneous cysts, dermoids and related sinuses. The classic example of the more complete first cleft anomaly consists of a high-lying lateral cyst or sinus just below the mandible with a tract leading upwards in relation to the parotid gland and facial nerve, opening into the anterior inferior portion of the ear canal near the outer third.

The more common branchiogenic cysts and sinuses arising from the second and third branchial arches are characteristically located anterior to the sternocleidomastoid muscle. The cyst usually will be found at the level of the hyoid, while the sinus openings may occur at any point from the ear to the suprasternal notch. Both the cysts and sinuses are lined with stratified squamous cells, but some will present columnar or ciliated epithelium. The walls are made up mostly of fibrous tissue interspersed with considerable amounts of lymphoid tissue in the form of scattered follicles. Squamous epithelium has been found by Ward lying deep in the lymphoid tissue and showing some degree of keratinization. This has been interpreted as a probable precancerous change in the same manner as one might consider leukoplakia in the mouth.

The contents of the cysts vary from clear serum to thick sebaceous material, according to the character of the lining. An opaque watery or milky fluid can be expected with squamous epithelium, whereas columnar epithelium produces a thick, sticky, mucoid material. Such cysts will not transilluminate on examination. If they become infected, the fluid content becomes frankly purulent and in some patients drains to the outside in a spontaneous manner. If this occurs, or if the cysts are drained surgically, a permanent sinus tract develops. The cysts are then converted into a sinus with cystlike pocketing above the opening.

These anomalous sinuses and fistulae may present three variations with respect to surface openings. The tract may be complete; that is, there may be a well-defined external cutaneous opening as well as an internal pharyngeal opening. In such instances, the external opening will be found anywhere along the anterior border of the sternocleidomastoid muscle, but most commonly along the lower third. Coursing upward, it is somewhat superficial but penetrates the platysma muscle and enveloping layer of the deep cervical fascia. It passes over the common carotid artery and, remaining anterior to the hypoglossal nerve, it turns medially to pass through the upper portion of the carotid bifurcation area to enter the pharynx at Rosenmüller's pouch (Fig. 1).

The sinus tract may be incomplete in one of two ways. The more common of this type are those in which there is a well-defined external orifice leading into a sinus tract which extends only a short distance into the neck but follows the general path upward as described for the complete fistula. The less

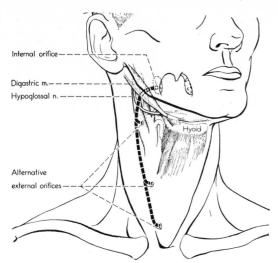

Internal orifice

Digastric m.

Hypoglossal n.

Hyoid

Alternative
external orifices

Figure 1. Course and relations of embryonic branchiogenic sinuses. All lateral cysts and sinuses follow this tract.

common variety is that in which there will be found only an internal opening into the pharynx which connects with a short sinus or flat cyst in the parapharyngeal region near the tonsil.

CORRELATION OF EMBRYOLOGY AND PATHOLOGY. It is significant to note that these complete fistulae extend from the tonsillar fossa downward under the angle of the mandible, passing under the midportion of the posterior belly of the digastric muscle, and anterior to the glossopharyngeal and hypoglossal nerves, eventually making their way to the cutaneous surface at some lower point. In an effort to substantiate the theory that these lesions arise from the branchial apparatus rather than from the thymic anlage, Gross pointed out that if a lateral cervical fistula were to develop from the second branchial cleft, it would have to lie between the internal and external carotid arteries and extend into the pharynx only in the area of the base of the tonsil or along the posterior tonsillar pillar. Since this is the common experience, it is concluded that the great majority of congenital fistulae of the neck originate from the second branchial pouch and cleft. The existence of this complete fistula presupposes the breaking through of the embryonic membrane separating the pouch from the cleft. This may come about through an embryonic perforation or post-natal infectious process.

DIAGNOSIS. Anomalies of the first branchial cleft are characteristically superficial and relate to the external ear and skin of the neck at or below the angle of the mandible. Very frequently, there is an associated discharge of the ear in the absence of otitis media. On the other hand, branchial cysts most commonly are found deeper, at the hyoid level. They tend to produce a superficial bulge which may displace the sternocleidomastoid muscle. They often can be moved slightly by the examiner and, on aspiration, yield a typical fluid which contains cholesterol crystals. The latter finding may be helpful since some of these contain fluid that bears a striking resemblance to tuberculous exudate. Injection of a radiopaque iodine solution into the cyst sometimes will confirm this differentiation. Branchial cysts are quite smooth-walled and thus will produce a sharp outline as compared with the ragged edges of tuberculous abscesses.

Branchial sinuses and fistulae can be recognized by their characteristic external opening along the anterior border of the sternocleidomastoid muscle. The only symptoms may be the annoying continuous or intermittent discharge. Occasionally, an episode of cellulitis may occur around the tract. Traction on the external opening may demonstrate the typical upward course of the fibrous-walled sinus. In children, x-ray visualization of the sinus tract is apt to suggest less extension than actually exists, but in adults the well-formed tract can be demonstrated by the injection of a suitable radiopaque solution. Under local anesthesia, a purse-string suture can be placed around the external opening to retain the dye, thus facilitating the making of x-ray films in various projections. If operation follows this examination immediately, the dye can be permitted to remain in order to add some bulk to the tract for identification during the excision. Demonstration of the internal opening can be accomplished by injection of methylene blue. This should be done about two days before a definitive operation is to be performed, because the dye is apt to diffuse into the tissues around the tract and be the source of confusion. After two days, it is sufficiently fixed to the tract tissues so that their identification can easily be made. In general, this dye is needed only to confirm location of the internal orifice and is not necessary to outline the tract for excision.

TREATMENT. Branchial cysts are treated entirely by surgical excision. The best approach is by means of a generous transverse incision parallel to the lines of skin cleavage

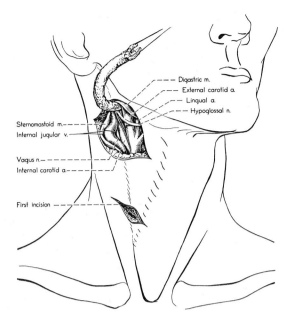

Figure 2. Dissection of branchiogenic sinus tract by means of stepladder incisions along skin creases. Typical relationship to digastric muscle and hypoglossal nerve.

and over the most prominent portion of the cyst. This will permit adequate mobilization of all surfaces, since these cysts often have numerous points of attachment. Particular care should be exercised to avoid any rupture, assuring complete removal of all epithelial elements. If there is a connection with the pharyngeal wall, careful closure of this should be done to facilitate primary healing.

Branchial sinuses and fistulae are best excised through the "stepladder" method developed by Hamilton Bailey, which is simple and practical (Fig. 2). It allows for entire excision, permitting adequate visualization of the critical uppermost parapharyngeal area. When the fistula is complete, the internal opening can be closed by direct suture of the pharyngeal wall. The skin closure produces a fine cosmetic result, since all incisions are parallel to the skin folds.

MIDLINE ANOMALIES

For the most part, midline cervical cysts and sinuses arise from remnants of the thyroglossal duct. They constitute the great majority of developmental anomalies located in the anterior portion of the neck. A few anteriorly located cysts, sublingual and submental, are classified as dermoid inclusion cysts since they stem from displaced epithelium. All these lesions produce some cosmetic deformity and, in addition, frequently produce considerable degrees of distress from repeated episodes of local infection. The rare teratomas of the neck occasionally present formidable pressure symptoms in the newborn, and therefore are significant.

Thyroglossal Cysts

EMBRYOLOGY. The thyroid anlage arises as a midline diverticulum from the first branchial pouch at a point marked in later life by the foramen caecum on the posterior portion of the dorsum of the tongue. This epithelial evagination is transformed into a stalked vesicle by the time the embryo has reached three weeks of age. It projects downward and backward from its point of origin as a tubular duct (Fig. 3). This thyroglossal duct bifurcates at its distal portion to form the thyroid lobes. During its transitory existence, the duct passes through an area which at a later date becomes the hyoid bone. Its distal end corresponds to the region which later becomes the pyramidal lobe of the thyroid. The duct usually atrophies during the sixth week of fetal life, but remnants of an epithelial cord persist for a short time. Rests of cells from this cord may remain anywhere along this tract and later can produce the cysts and sinus tracts found so characteristically in the anterior cervical midline.

PATHOLOGY AND CLINICAL COURSE. Thyroglossal cysts, sinuses and fistulae occur anywhere between the foramen caecum of the tongue and the region just above the suprasternal notch. They are most commonly found

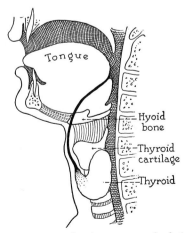

Figure 3. Diagram showing course and relations of the embryonic thyroglossal duct. Fistulae, cysts or thyroid remnants may involve any portion of this tract.

about halfway between these extremes, just below the hyoid bone. The majority can be found just beneath the enveloping layer of the cervical fascia, while a few will be deep to the pretracheal fascia. These locations are dependent upon the embryologic levels which the thyroglossal duct may take in relation to the hyoid bone and the fascia which attaches to its anterior and posterior surfaces. An occasional cyst can be found above the hyoid within the substance of the base of the tongue.

These cysts and tracts are lined by stratified squamous, columnar or, occasionally, transitional epithelium. The wall is composed almost entirely of fibrous tissue, the thickness being related to the amount of previous infection. Contrary to the characteristic finding in branchiogenic cysts, these do not have lymphoid elements in the walls. This correlates to some extent with similar findings in the preauricular cysts and sinuses of the branchial group which arise from the first arch and cleft areas. In about 80 per cent of the patients, the original lesion is a cyst, while in the remainder it is a sinus or fistula. The anomaly is discovered early in life, more than half being noted from soon after birth up until the patient is ten years of age. Since the lesions produce so few symptoms, there often is delay before patients in the remaining group report for treatment.

Thyroglossal cysts vary from 1 to 5 cm. in diameter, the average being about 2.5 cm. They are smooth, round and well defined. Because of their attachment to the hyoid bone, the cysts move directly with the act of swallowing but cannot be displaced by the examiner. Unless infection occurs, they are not attached to the skin. If drainage occurs, they immediately become attached to the skin with formation of a permanent sinus tract. Recurrent infection is the rule in such instances, even though the cyst has been surgically drained. Intermittent drainage then becomes an objectionable problem.

There have been rare instances of papillary thyroid carcinoma reported in thyroglossal cysts. Ward and Hendrick reported the finding of aberrant thyroid tissue within the wall of eight cysts from among 105 removed, and state, "In six of these cases, the aberrant tissue was embryological in structure." One might conjecture that this low instance of proved malignancy is related to the early removal of these cysts.

DIAGNOSIS. The salient feature in diagnosis of the average thyroglossal cyst consists in the finding of a smooth, well-rounded and well-demarcated mass lying anterior to the hyoid bone, which may transmit light and always moves easily with deglutition. In the absence of any sinus formation, three alternative lesions must be differentiated: submental dermoid inclusion cysts, sebaceous cysts and ectopic thyroid tissue.

TREATMENT. The majority of thyroglossal duct cysts and sinuses eventually require surgical excision. The smaller cysts may not seem significant, but the larger ones obviously are disfiguring. Both the large and the small cysts can be the site of bothersome local infection. When the cyst contents become suppurative, the abscess must be incised and drained as a preliminary procedure. After the induration in the surrounding tissue has resolved, the sinus tract and underlying cyst should be completely excised through a generous transverse elliptical incision. The tract or cyst will be found attached to the hyoid bone. In a few instances, there is no further upward extension, but a considerable number penetrate the hyoid. To prevent a recurrence, removal of the central portion of the hyoid should be included in the procedure. The persisting tract, or embryologic residue, above this level then can be cored out of the base of the tongue up to the foramen caecum. This type of block dissection, originally suggested by Sistrunk in 1928, reduces recurrence to a minimum. The hyoid bone need not be sutured in the midline, since this defect does not alter subsequent muscle action. The wound is closed primarily for the best healing.

Ectopic thyroid tissue occasionally will be found in the area usually occupied by thyroglossal duct cysts. This should be mentioned only as a warning, because such ectopic tissue may constitute the entire supply of thyroid for the whole body. The thyroid mass can be identified as solid reddish brown tissue rather than a substance of cystic nature. If no thyroid tissue is found beneath the strap muscles, this solid mass can be split in the middle and gently placed to each side of the trachea under the strap muscles without disrupting the blood supply.

Dermoid Inclusion Cysts

Submental dermoid inclusion cysts are the result of incomplete union of the first two branchial arch components. If the failure of union is external, the cyst will be more superficial and will be lined with epidermal elements, thus becoming known as a dermoid containing hair and various types of thick fluid. If the failure of union is internal, the cysts will be deeper in the floor of the mouth and may be lined with mucous membrane. The more common origin is faulty obliteration of the first and second clefts, so that the result is a simple inclusion cyst. The second cleft is the offender much more often than the first, the results being epithelial-lined cysts in the aural, submaxillary, sublingual and submental regions. They need not be attached to the overlying skin, as are the usual sebaceous cysts. Since they usually are larger than the latter and contain the mixed product of the sweat and sebaceous glands, the soft cheesy material may present a doughy sensation to the examiner and when found it is characteristic. Treatment is surgical excision.

Teratomas of the Neck

Teratomas of the neck are of rare occurrence, but when present are quite significant. They usually are noted immediately after birth. They consist of large, cystic, solitary masses in the anterior portion of the neck, often causing various degrees of tracheal obstruction. Their anterior or anterolateral location often suggests an origin from the thyroid gland, but in most instances this never is confirmed. They tend to be encapsulated and rarely, in patients of this early age, are found to be malignant. From the gross as well as the microscopic standpoint, these teratomas are the same as those found elsewhere in that all types of tissue are found, with cysts and solid material being freely interspersed.

Because of their size, they usually require early resection for relief of tracheal compression. In some instances, operation may have to be performed soon after birth in order to prevent further deterioration from respiratory obstruction or difficulties with swallowing. The prognosis in such children always is grave.

Cystic Hygroma Colli

Cystic hygroma is a benign multiloculated tumor of lymphatic origin. It is a well-recognized clinical entity which presents as an irregular endothelial-lined, fluid-containing tissue mass arising from the embryonic lymphatic buds. This lesion is encountered most often in infants and young children, but occasionally is seen in adults. Cystic hygromas have been found in the axilla, mediastinum, chest wall, groin and retroperitoneal tissues, but the cervical location is by far the most common.

ETIOLOGY. Prior to the embryologic studies of Sabin, the etiologic explanations for these growths were largely unsubstantiated. It is now appreciated that cystic hygromas occur in those areas in which the lymphatic sacs of the neck and of the iliac area were previously located. With respect to the cervical area, a capillary plexus is formed along each jugular vein, which eventually is cut off from the parent vein. The resultant isolated group of endothelial-lined spaces eventually forms primitive jugular sacs by virtue of dilatation and coalescence of these capillaries. The thoracic duct connects the pelvic and retroperitoneal sacs with the left jugular sac and joins the venous system at the jugular valve. An anomaly of development occurs in a few individuals so that portions of the jugular sacs fail to establish suitable communication but retain the growth factor. In addition, it has been demonstrated that hygroma cysts may extend from membranous sprouts derived from the walls of cystic spaces already present. This type of expansion produces a penetrating cystic growth which permeates surrounding tissue at a surprising rate and with a considerable degree of pressure, particularly in the newborn.

PATHOLOGY. Cystic hygroma consists of a benign multilocular cystic mass which is very thin walled. The contents are serous and straw colored, though sometimes they may be blood stained. Often, there is free communication of fluid between the many compartments so that the mass is not tense, but rather of a soft consistency. The cyst walls do not contain many vessels and those present are very small. Obvious lymph tissue or nodes can be found adherent to the cystic mass or as a part of the walls. On opening the specimen, the gray-white color of the lining endothelium is distinctive.

Microscopic examination of the hygroma reveals the wall to be made up of simple connective tissue, but of variable thickness and constitution. The youngest cyst will present scanty cellularity and have a myxomatous appearance. The lymphatic infiltrations will be variable. In older cysts, the collagen and fibrous components will be greater in proportion to the increased thickness of the wall.

CLINICAL COURSE. Two-thirds of these cystic masses will be found at birth, and 90 per cent of them will have developed by the end of the second year of life. Distribution between the sexes is equal. A few more are found on the left side than on the right, the ratio being about 3 to 2. They occur chiefly in the posterior triangle, behind the sternocleidomastoid muscle, and often occupy the whole supraclavicular area. A smaller number will be found in the submaxillary area of the anterior triangle, tending to infiltrate the floor of the mouth, producing macroglossia. While some may extend harmlessly into the axilla, others may present a serious mediastinal component, producing significant pressure symptoms. Dyspnea, wheezing, cyanosis, dysphagia and even obstruction of the superior vena cava have been known to occur with such severity as to require urgent surgical intervention.

The size of the mass does not bear any positive relationship to the age of the patient or to the duration of the lesion. Some of the largest specimens have been found in infants only a few weeks old. Since the symptomatology is minimal, there are instances in which many months, or even a year or two, may pass before definite treatment is considered. The cystic mass never is tense as are thyroglossal and branchiogenic cysts. The thin and fragile wall of the early cyst is such that the borders may be poorly defined. The lesion can easily be transilluminated in this phase. With the passage of time, some degree of infection may develop and a thicker-walled, more fibrotic cystic mass then develops with more extensive involvement through adhesion to the surrounding parts.

DIAGNOSIS. The characteristic presenting complaint is that of an asymptomatic mass in the neck, which produces some disfigurement and, occasionally, some limitation of motion because of its extremely large size. These cysts tend to lie in a superficial plane, despite the fact that they are known to infiltrate deeply even into the mediastinum. Since they do not interfere with the great vessels, trachea or esophagus, they do not present bothersome obstructive symptoms as a rule.

Considerable variation of opinion exists with regard to the value of roentgen ray examination in these patients because the full extent of the mass seldom can be determined by this method. Certainly, some of the cavities can be outlined by the instillation of an aqueous iodide solution. This may demonstrate more exactly any displacement of surrounding parts, as well as give further information concerning extension of the hygroma into the mediastinum. Such positive findings often are helpful to the surgeon, but negative results from such examinations should be recognized in advance as meaningless. On the other hand, roentgenologic examination of the thorax is helpful in demonstrating the presence of a mediastinal component associated with a soft tissue shadow in the neck. Variations in shape and size may be noted with changes in respiration.

TREATMENT. An expectant attitude once was advised in the hope that spontaneous regression might occur. Although temporary decrease in the size of such a cyst does occur, and even a spontaneous disappearance of the mass may take place, eventually it refills.

Radiation therapy is ineffective because hygromas are radioresistant.

Injection of sclerosing agents has been suggested and occasionally utilized, but this method of treatment is fraught with danger. Even though these thin-walled cysts appear to be ideal for this type of therapy, the complications of infection may be disastrous. On the other hand, sclerosing agents have been used most successfully by Ward, when followed within three to six weeks by surgical excision.

Surgical excision is the treatment of choice. To be curative it must include removal of all the endothelial-lined tissue. With the use of endotracheal anesthesia and extremely careful technique, the entire mass can be dissected from its multiple points of attachment. Some importance should be attached to early removal of these growths because, even though they are thin-walled at that time, they are more likely to be better confined to predictable fascial planes than they will later. Older growths tend to be more invasive and adhesive in character. This matter of delay may convert a relatively simple procedure into a long and hazardous operation. These wounds should be closed with suction drainage in order to prevent bothersome fluid accumulations. The recurrence rate following adequate excision is quite low.

PRIMARY TUMORS OF THE NECK

When one considers the diagnostic possibilities presented by a unilateral nonthyroid cervical mass in the adult patient, two-thirds of the time it will prove to be metastatic carcinoma arising from some primary site above the level of the clavicle. The most common locations are the oral cavity, the nasopharynx, the laryngopharynx or the thyroid gland itself. A nontender, discrete, hard and large lymph node, either movable or fixed to deeper structures, is the common physical finding in such instances. Tuberculosis, sarcoidosis and malignant lymphoma represent other possibilities, but these lesions are usually multiple. If all these entities can be excluded, including branchial cysts and salivary gland tumors, it is then logical to identify the mass tentatively as one of the primary soft-tissue tumors, such as lipoma, neurofibroma, neurilemmoma and uncapsulated fibrosarcoma. In such a differentiation, carotid body tumors and aneurysms should be included for the sake of thoroughness. Because these various lesions present such difficulties regarding diagnosis, it is not unusual that the real identity is not established until the mass in question has been surgically exposed and an adequate biopsy study made. In some instances, aspiration biopsy may be a helpful procedure preliminary to definitive therapy. This technique is especially useful when the surgeon wishes to avoid unnecessary incisions which might make later surgery more difficult.

Carotid Body Tumors

Although comparatively rare, carotid body tumors are of diagnostic and therapeutic importance. Full appreciation of all aspects of these lesions is most desirable for the best therapeutic results, because the integrity of the internal carotid artery is directly involved in the surgical excision. Definitive handling of the carotid artery has much to do with the postoperative course and, for this reason, this entity presents a real challenge when discovered.

EMBRYOLOGY. The carotid body is a small, ovoid, irregular mass of pinkish tan or gray tissue located within the bifurcation of the common carotid artery. At one time it was thought to be related to the so-called chromaffin system, but this does not seem to be the case since it actually is one of a group of discrete tissue masses found near ganglia of the cranial nerves or branchial arch arteries.

These organs and the tumors they produce are histologically similar. Though these tumors are recognized as paragangliomas, the term chemodectoma has been used more frequently in recent years, since they arise in chemoreceptor tissue. They do not give a true chromaffin reaction, contain no epinephrine and do not secrete a hormone. The nerve supply of these bodies is multiple, but mostly sensory; the carotid body, for example, being supplied by the glossopharyngeal nerve. These bodies have been described near the jugular bulb, the ganglion nodosum of the vagus nerve, the innominate artery, the tympanic membrane and the carotid bifurcation. The carotid body, in particular, is known to arise within the adventitial layer of the carotid artery early in embryologic development. Although it grows outward from this point as a discrete mass, it never loses this intimate anatomic relationship. In order to excise such a mass, dissection between the media and the outer adventitia is necessary.

PATHOLOGY AND CLINICAL FEATURES. Carotid body tumors are noted for their slow rate of growth. Estimation of malignancy from the histologic appearance has been difficult since mitotic figures are exceedingly rare in these tumors. They show a remarkable tendency to reproduce the normal architecture of the carotid body. Although they may vary from an epithelium-like appearance to that of an angioma-like type, the fundamental pattern of tissue origin can best be discovered by the use of reticulum silver-impregnation stains. The majority of them are somewhat adherent to their surroundings, especially to the arterial wall, but the latter point is of embryologic and not neoplastic significance.

Since it has been concluded that making the diagnosis of malignant versus nonmalignant carotid body tumors is a dubious venture by the pathologist, especially on a frozen section, the clinician can only recall that some of these tumors in the past have proved to be so invasive as to cause death. The remarkably slow rate of growth and the critical nature of the arteries involved may be the factors which confuse the issue. It is best to realize that the actual evidence of malignancy is lower than formerly was thought, but the growth potential of this particular tumor is such that, if given enough time, it acts much as a malignant lesion in the sense that it has the capacity to kill the host.

Carotid body tumors cause no subjective symptoms until they reach 5 to 6 cm. in size. Prior to this time, only the mass in the neck is noted and the average patient reports that it took five to seven years for the tumor to reach such size. Mild pain may be reported, but severe discomfort does not develop until other signs of nerve invasion have appeared.

External examination usually reveals a deeply situated tumor mass in the region of the carotid bifurcation, but the tumor never is attached to the skin. While these masses cannot be moved in the vertical plane, some will permit lateral displacement. Bimanual examination with one finger in the patient's mouth may outline the mass with considerable accuracy. When these tumors are of the more vascular type, firm squeezing pressure may temporarily reduce their size slightly by removal of some of the blood. Presence of a thrill and bruit can be elicited in a few. There may be a transmitted but not an expansile pulsation over these tumors.

DIAGNOSIS. Diagnosis is made on the history of a unilateral cervical tumor mass of some years' duration. Examination shows it to be in the carotid bifurcation area, as evidenced by its relationship to the two arteries, and by the fact that the mass may be moved only in the lateral plane. Carotid angiography may confirm the diagnosis by findings suggesting an intrinsic defect in the carotid wall, or demonstration of dye within the highly vascular tumor. Absolute diagnosis is accomplished by histologic study of either the biopsy material or the excised mass. If the study is made of biopsy material, the pathologist should not be required to rule on the question of malignancy since the diagnosis of carotid body tumor itself is difficult enough.

TREATMENT. In view of the fact that roentgenotherapy has proved to be of little if any value, surgical excision remains the only method by which these tumors can be eradicated. In the past, operative mortality has approximated 30 per cent when the internal carotid artery has been ligated under general anesthesia. In addition, among those patients who survived the procedure, numerous central nervous system sequelae have been noted. It is obvious that this is too

high a price to pay for the eradication of any neoplasm whose incidence of malignancy has been shown to be less than 10 per cent. On the other hand, Munro has reported that 30 per cent of the patients whose treatment was inadequate died as a direct result of their tumors. When the tumor was removed with preservation of the vessels, only 7.5 per cent of the patients died as a result of the tumor.

It must be concluded that early surgical removal is the treatment of choice. With care this can be achieved through the simple expedient of obtaining a plane of dissection in the artery wall between the media and the adventitia. Arterial continuity thus can be preserved, but, if this is impossible, definite efforts should be made immediately to restore arterial continuity by using a temporary arterial by-pass, followed by the insertion of an autogenous vein graft at the end of the procedure. Though this is a tedious and time-consuming operative procedure, such resections accompanied by carotid arterial preservation will be followed by minimal permanent disabling sequelae and a low incidence of tumor recurrence.

BRANCHIOGENIC CARCINOMA

The presence of a unilateral enlargement in the side of the neck most frequently is a sign of metastatic cancer. For practical purposes, no other diagnosis in the adult should be considered until this probability has been excluded. In addition to those primary tumors previously mentioned, carcinoma of the lung, breast, kidney, gastrointestinal tract and ovary can metastasize to this region. It is of interest to observe that when all of the primary malignant tumors peculiar to the neck are added up, the sum does not equal the incidence of involvement of cervical lymph nodes by metastatic disease.

The term "branchiogenic carcinoma" has been in medical literature since 1882, when it was suggested that malignant lesions found in the lateral neck might arise from the vestigia of branchial clefts. Prominent pathologists have refuted the existence of branchiogenic carcinoma as a real entity, pointing out that very few of the reported tumors could withstand strict scrutiny.

DIAGNOSIS. In order to make the diagnosis of branchiogenic carcinoma, the following criteria are necessary: the tumor must be located along a line drawn anterior to the ear, which passes downward along the anterior border of the sternocleidomastoid muscle; the histologic appearance of the tumor must suggest origin from epidermal branchial vestigia; the tumor should demonstrate some relationship to a cyst or sinus tract which might be considered branchial in origin; after removal of the tumor, the patient must survive five years without the development of any other primary malignant lesion which could possibly have produced, by metastasis, the previously excised lesion.

TREATMENT. If the mass strictly conforms to the first three criteria, a complete homolateral neck dissection would be the treatment of choice, especially if the presenting mass is quite large or if it proves to be radioresistant. Often, the solitary neck mass is reported only as "epidermoid carcinoma in lymph node." Because the primary site is not known, operation should be deferred. When the mass is located at the mid-level of the jugular chain, the undiscovered primary lesion might be in the pyriform sinus area, or the base of the tongue. By using a straight anterior port 6000 rads can be delivered to both areas from a cobalt source with considerable predictable effectiveness. When the mass is high and in the posterior triangle, the nasopharynx is always highly suspect as a primary source. For these patients, parallel apposing anterior and posterior ports should be used to deliver the same dose as primary treatment.

DEEP CERVICAL INFECTIONS

While at present not so common, deep cervical infections once were the cause of considerable morbidity and in the neglected state carried an unusually high mortality. Abscesses are particularly prone to occur in the deeper layers of the neck because the deeply situated lymphatics receive drainage of infected material from the oropharynx, dental structures, salivary glands, the esophagus and upper respiratory passages. The majority of the abscesses arise from dental infection or from infected tonsils. Continued improvement in the care of the teeth and overall oral hygiene combined with earlier correction of throat infections have done much to diminish these very troublesome and serious infections.

While, for many reasons, deep cervical abscesses previously were accompanied by a high mortality rate, one of the most significant reasons was the difficulty in accurate localization of the infection because of failure to appreciate the important relationships of the deep cervical fascia. Even though today we possess a chemotherapeutic and antibiotic armamentarium of considerable potency, early drainage of retained purulent exudate still is required for prompt recovery. The application of the principles of early surgical drainage is necessary in deep cervical infections and adequacy of such drainage often is dependent upon knowledge of these deep anatomic relationships.

The universal recognition of the importance of fascial planes in the diagnosis and treatment of neck infection has been a relatively recent development. The fascial planes of the neck form well-defined compartments and potential spaces. Infection confined within these compartments may be so hidden that the diagnosis of the presence of an abscess may often be seriously delayed. Extension into the mediastinum may take place while the patient is being observed. Moreover, cardiorespiratory complications may intervene before appropriate drainage has been instituted. Early diagnosis and appropriate treatment often are delayed because the signs usually associated with the accumulation of pus elsewhere in the body may not be manifest when there is a purulent pocket in the deeper structures of the neck.

ETIOLOGY. The great majority of these infections are due to some strain of streptococci, the latter frequently being obtained in a pure culture. It is not unusual to find a mixed infection, especially with both aerobic and anaerobic variants. While the fusospirochetal organisms of Vincent may be found in both the oral source and the abscess cavity, the blood stream invader may be only the hemolytic streptococcus. Accurate identification of these organisms is important from the therapeutic standpoint because specific sensitivities can be determined to assure the correct choice of antibiotic or chemotherapeutic agent.

Not only is the organism significant, but so are the portal of entrance of the bacterial invaders and the manner in which the infection has developed. Two mechanisms may be at work in the pathogenesis of these infections. There is the possibility of contiguous spread of the infection by direct extension or embolic spread may occur through the lymphatics to the collecting lymph nodes within certain compartments. For example, a peritonsillar infection can spread directly into the pharyngomaxillary space, or, more commonly, the submaxillary space will present a complication of dental infection without any break in mandibular continuity. In addition to these, there is a small group of infections which are secondary to a great variety of open and closed injuries in or about the mouth and neck.

APPLIED ANATOMY. **Cervical fascia.** The superficial cervical fascia consists of a layer of loose connective tissue located immediately superficial to the platysma muscle over the anterolateral aspects of the neck. It is the *tela subcutanea* which gives support to the skin and which carries a generous supply of nerves, vessels, fat and some muscle. The platysma is intimately attached to it. The superficial fascia encircles the neck as a single layer maintaining the same relationship to the skin throughout its distribution.

Immediately beneath the platysma, the deep layer of cervical fascia is clearly defined (Fig. 4). The outermost or anterior layer is an enveloping layer, surrounding the large neck muscles so as to invest and hold them to-gether. In the posterior half of the neck, the deep fascia functions entirely to support the heavy musculature, whereas in the anterior musculovisceral compartment, it consists of a number of layers, some ensheathing the long muscles, some covering the viscera and the deepest muscles lying over the vertebrae.

As the enveloping layer of the deep cervical fascia extends upward, it attaches anteriorly to the hyoid bone and, after splitting, it attaches to and extends upward over both surfaces of the mandible. It reaches inferiorly to the clavicle and sternum, attaching to the anterior and posterior surfaces to form in the midline the space of Burns. As it extends laterally, it divides to enclose the sternocleidomastoid muscle, crosses the posterior triangle and invests the trapezius. It continues around dorsalward to attach to the spines of the cervical vertebrae.

The middle layer of the deep cervical fascia is also known as the pretracheal fascia. It invests the sternohyoid, sternothyroid, thyrohyoid and omohyoid muscles. These split layers fuse laterally and attach to the carotid sheath for firm anchorage. This middle layer attaches superiorly to the hyoid and inferiorly to the posterior surface of the sternum and

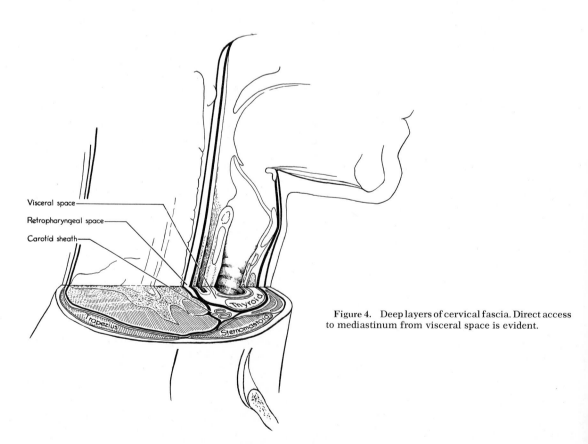

Visceral space
Retropharyngeal space
Carotid sheath

Figure 4.   Deep layers of cervical fascia. Direct access to mediastinum from visceral space is evident.

clavicle, fusing with the enveloping layer of the deep fascia.

The visceral layer of the deep cervical fascia encloses the hypopharynx, esophagus, trachea and thyroid gland. Known as the buccopharyngeal fascia, it covers and supports the outer wall of the pharyngoesophageal region, especially the constrictor musculature. The thyroid is covered by this layer by virtue of its embryologic descent through it, as it moved from the midline region to take up a position lateral to the trachea. This visceral fascial layer forms a definite compartment between the middle layer and the firm prevertebral fascia. It extends from the base of the skull to the thoracic mediastinum.

The prevertebral fascia is the deepest, or posterior, layer of the cervical fascia and as such covers the bodies of the cervical vertebrae, the longus colli and the scalene muscles, in the posterolateral neck area.

Fascial spaces (Fig. 5). MASTICATOR SPACE. The masticator, or submasseteric, space includes the area which contains the masseter, temporal and both pterygoid muscles and all the associated vessels and nerves. This compartment is the result of the upward splitting of the outer layer of the deep fascia as the latter comes into relation with the mandible. While this space is not primarily cervical in location, it has a direct bearing upon the dif-

ferential considerations of a deep cervical abscess.

Infection may reach the masticator space by direct extension from the second and, especially, the third lower molar teeth. Occasionally, this region may become indirectly involved by infection from the buccal area anterior to the body of the mandible, from the floor of the mouth or from the parapharyngeal region. Pain in the region of the masseter muscle with some swelling and tenderness accompanied by evident trismus indicates infection in the masticator space. An appropriate dental evaluation is necessary to confirm this diagnosis. Owing to the severe trismus, the patient may be unable to cooperate, so that examination must be limited to a roentgenogram of the jaw. A typical area of radiotranslucency will confirm the source of the infection as dental. If left untreated, this type of infection often spreads to the submaxillary compartment or posteromedially into the pharyngomaxillary space. Although accompanying cellulitis will be noted over the angle of the jaw area, a direct extension of the infection posteriorly into the parotid compartment is quite unlikely, owing to the thick fascial demarcation. Drainage of this space is accomplished by a small transverse incision over the lower portion of the body of the mandible just posterior to the facial ves-

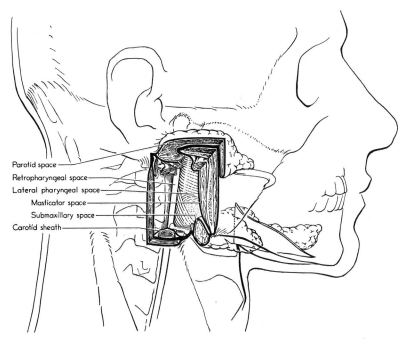

Parotid space
Retropharyngeal space
Lateral pharyngeal space
Masticator space
Submaxillary space
Carotid sheath

Figure 5. Cut-away diagram to show intimate relationships of fascial spaces in parapharyngeal regions.

sels as they lie in relationship to the anterior border of the masseter muscles. The muscle fibers can be divided by blunt dissection and an appropriate soft rubber drain inserted into the pocket. The superior extension of this cavity should be identified, since the temporal extension of this compartment may also require drainage near the zygoma.

PAROTID SPACE. This space contains the parotid salivary gland, a few significant lymph nodes, a major portion of the facial nerve and numerous vessels. The fascia which invests the masseter muscle thickens considerably at its posterior border and splits to surround the parotid gland. This thick parotid-masseteric fascia is firmly attached to the investing layer of the deep cervical fascia which covers the sternocleidomastoid muscle and, as a result, the gland is completely surrounded by heavy fascia except medially where the parotid tends to become retromandibular. At this point, the deeper layer of the fascia extends toward the pharynx in the region between the styloid process and the internal pterygoid muscle. This lack of covering permits free connection with the retropharyngeal and the pharyngomaxillary spaces at this point.

Infection originating within this space usually is directly related to the salivary gland itself. If it becomes secondarily involved from masticator or pharyngomaxillary space infection, the abscess can be drained by a small vertical incision made over the most prominent, dependent portion of the swollen gland. The thick capsule must be opened transversely to avoid injury to the facial nerve. More than one area may require incision. The gland then can be spread by blunt dissection to obtain drainage.

RETROPHARYNGEAL SPACE. The retropharyngeal space is that area found between the prevertebral fascia and the posterior wall of the pharynx. It contains rather loose connective tissue and a few lymph nodes. Inferiorly, this space is in direct contact with the mediastinum.

Retropharyngeal abscess most commonly is found in early childhood. At least two well-defined lymph nodes are located in this space at about the level of the second cervical vertebra. Infection in the nose, nasal sinuses or nasopharynx may spread to these nodes or infection may arise within the adenoid region of the posterior nasopharynx and thus extend directly into this area. This may easily become a serious infection since it lies upon the prevertebral fascia and thus it may extend downward into the mediastinum or laterally into the pharyngomaxillary space and eventually may involve the sheath of the great vessels. In neglected patients, this retropharyngeal swelling may protrude so far down the posterior pharyngeal wall as to involve eventually the larynx.

The symptoms may begin with fever and a cough and examination may not reveal the indistinct boggy swelling of the posterior pharyngeal wall. Dysphagia and dyspnea develop later. Lateral roentgenograms of the cervical spine area may be helpful in making the diagnosis inasmuch as the soft-tissue swelling displacing the pharynx forward may thus be identified. This abscess should be incised and drained orally before it extends into the lateral cervical region. It is most important in doing this to keep the patient's head low and to use suction to facilitate the immediate drainage.

PHARYNGOMAXILLARY SPACE. This is a cone-shaped potential space whose base is in relation to the skull around the jugular foramen and whose apex is at the greater cornu of the hyoid bone. Medially, it borders upon the superior constrictor of the pharynx and the tonsillar fossa. The posterior portion is in direct relationship with the retropharyngeal space, the prevertebral fascia actually forming its posterior border. The lateral surface anteriorly is in relation to the internal pterygoid muscle while, more posteriorly, it faces the retromandibular portion of the parotid gland which is not covered by fascia. At this level, as well as below the parotid, the space is in direct contact with the carotid sheath and its contained vessels.

There was a time when infections in this space accounted for over half the deep infections of the neck, but this number has been greatly reduced in the last decade owing to better control of infection in the usual portals of entrance. This space may be infected from the tonsillar fossa and peritonsillar region, more than half these infections coming from this source. Less common sources are mastoid infection, infected retropharyngeal nodes, molar teeth and invasion from the parotid and submaxillary spaces. The intimate relationship of the vessels which traverse this compartment is of extreme importance.

Purulent exudate in the pharyngomaxillary fossa may cause the lateral pharyngeal wall to bulge inward. Such change in contour may be mistaken for a simple peritonsillar abscess, but careful inspection will reveal that there is very little swelling of the tonsils themselves. The intimate relationship of the infection to the internal pterygoid muscle and the pterygomandibular ligament frequently results in trismus as an early sign. There also may be some swelling of the parotid gland because of involvement of the exposed retromandibular portion which is not covered by fascia and lies in direct relationship with the lateral aspect of the fossa. Internal pharyngeal swelling, trismus and parotid swelling are indicative of deep infection within the pharyngomaxillary space. Early diagnosis is of great importance because, if undetected, these infections may lead to serious deep jugular phlebitis.

Drainage of this space can be accomplished by a generous transverse incision in the lower submaxillary region anterior to the border of the sternocleidomastoid muscle. After the lower portion of the facial vein is divided, the submaxillary gland is elevated. To gain access to the latter, the outer layer of the deep fascia must be cleanly incised just above the level of the hyoid. Blunt dissection in the direction of the angle of the jaw and toward the styloid process deep to the mastoid tip will result in a free flow of pus as the pharyngomaxillary space is reached. Insertion of a soft rubber drain completes the procedure.

SUBMANDIBULAR SPACE. This is rather a large space located immediately beneath the body of the mandible. It is outlined by the peripheral borders of the submental and submaxillary triangles and its depth consists of all the tissues lying between the mucous membrane of the floor of the mouth and the outer layer of the deep cervical fascia (Fig. 6). This submandibular space contains the submaxillary and sublingual salivary glands, numerous related lymph nodes and the hypoglossal and lingual nerves and vessels. The anterior belly of the digastric, the mylohyoid, the geniohyoid and the genioglossus muscles add structure to the space.

It should be appreciated that there are three salient compartments within the submandibular space owing to the diaphragm-like arrangement produced by the mylohyoid muscle. The deepest compartment and actual floor of the mouth is the sublingual space. It contains those structures which lie superior to the mylohyoid and extends from the hyoid bone to the mandible. It connects at the

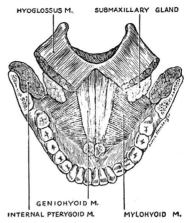

Figure 6. Semidiagrammatic sketch showing the diaphragm formed by the structures in the floor of the mouth.

midline with the contralateral sublingual space and with the ipsilateral submaxillary compartment by virtue of the course of the submaxillary salivary gland at the lateral edge of the mylohyoid. The submaxillary compartment contains the submaxillary gland and intimately related lymph nodes. It communicates posteromedially with the pharyngomaxillary and retropharyngeal spaces and thus indirectly with the mediastinum. The third, or submental, compartment consists of the superficial area between the median raphe and the submaxillary border deep to the outer layer of the deep cervical fascia but superficial to the mylohyoid muscle.

Infections in the submandibular spaces may vary from mild cellulitis to fatal phlegmon (Ludwig's angina). Since the different compartments of this space may participate in these infectious processes in varying degree, the anatomic relationships of the area must always be kept in mind (Fig. 7). While the right and left halves of this area may become confluent in the midline when serious infection is present, it is the deep and superficial sections of each half that must be separately evaluated. This is of specific importance in order that a correct diagnosis of Ludwig's infection be made in the event that it should occur. A submental abscess, submaxillary adenitis, cellulitis of the submaxillary gland or an infection limited to the floor of the mouth can be identified rather easily when this anatomic subdivision is kept in mind. On the other hand, a typical Ludwig's infection involves all three compartments, the sublingual, submaxillary and submental, on either one or both sides of the midline. This differential characteristic is

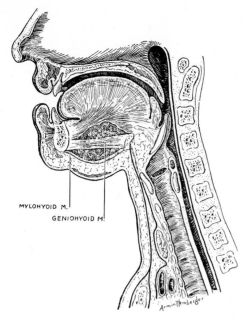

MYLOHYOID M.
GENIOHYOID M.

Figure 7. Semidiagrammatic sketch showing the location of infection in Ludwig's angina above and below the geniohyoid muscle. Note the boxlike compartment filled by the tongue and adjacent structures, and the ease with which inflammation may extend to the region of the larynx.

very important since only this latter type of infection carries with it any significant morbidity. When the objective findings of inflammatory involvement are such as to make the diagnosis of Ludwig's angina, early surgical drainage is required, while with the other infections some degree of temporization may be permitted.

The portal of entry of this infection may be a lesion anywhere about the tongue, floor of the mouth and teeth of the lower jaw. The role of dental infection is increasing and is reported to be as high as 90 per cent in some series. The infection may arise either by lymphatic spread or by contiguous extension from infection in the floor of the mouth. In either manner, the sublingual and submaxillary compartments eventually both become involved. The end result is the development of diffuse, edematous and rapidly spreading cellulitis beneath the outer layer of the deep cervical fascia.

Owing to the restraining capacity of the deep cervical fascia, and to a lesser extent of the mylohyoid muscle, inflammatory swelling within the submaxillary and sublingual compartments pushes the tongue upward and backward within the confines of the oral cavity. The patient will have difficulty with speech as well as swallowing. The

infection eventually may cause obstruction of the respiratory passages. In addition, a certain number of patients die from pulmonary infection because of extension if appropriate antibiotics are not used. Since the development of antibiotic therapy, not only has the incidence of this infection been greatly reduced, but also its mortality. Respiratory obstruction still remains the most feared complication despite these advances.

One should not wait for fluctuation as a sign of localization or it may be too late. The phlegmonous exudate always is quite deep, tends to expand and hardly ever is purulent. It is possible in some patients to abort the process by adequate drainage of a primary intraoral source, either through the mouth or through the submaxillary fossa as indicated. In the neglected individual, the need for maintenance of a satisfactory airway may take priority over plans for definitive drainage. Early tracheostomy under such circumstances will assure improved respiratory exchange so that the necessary drainage of the infection then may be accomplished with greater safety. Drainage is accomplished through a generous, transverse, curving incision below and parallel to the outline of the undersurface of the body of the mandible. The deep cervical fascia and the mylohyoid muscle are cleanly divided in order to open widely the submaxillary and sublingual compartments.

CAROTID SHEATH.   This space contains the great vessels of the neck and, in its more superior area, some of the emerging cranial nerves. It gives off fascial connections to the parotid, submandibular and pharyngomaxillary spaces. This relationship has been likened to a trifolium, the stem of which is the carotid sheath. The arterial and venous branches leave the sheath to enter these compartments invested with the fascia that composes the sheath and which is in direct continuity with the retentive and supportive layers of the deep cervical fascia. Inflammatory interrelationships between these spaces and the carotid sheath thus are quite real and often produce serious complications by virtue of such extension.

Because of its anatomic location, the carotid sheath can readily be infected from the parotid, submaxillary, retropharyngeal and, most commonly, from pharyngomaxillary space abscesses. It often has been pointed out that local signs are of little value in estimating the possibility of a carotid sheath infection or jugular phlebitis. The swelling and local tenderness in the region of the vessels usually arise from related jugular nodes involved by the prime infection. The only reliable data are those suggestive of severe sepsis: chills and fever, spiking temperature, leukocytosis and positive blood culture. Vigorous antibiotic therapy must be maintained. The importance of penicillin in particular should be stressed. Since an underlying deep abscess is the usual cause of carotid sheath infections, one must not forget the need for surgical drainage if the pocket can be found. Ligation of the deep jugular vein and drainage of the hidden deep abscess may quickly solve the problem.

VISCERAL SPACE INFECTIONS

Trauma from food, from foreign bodies, and from instrumentation may result in infection developing within the bounds of the pretracheal fascia, below the level of the superior constrictor muscle. This same space may be involved secondarily by extension from the prevertebral area, or the pharyngomaxillary fossa. Wounds and injuries of the neck also may result in infection along this enveloping fascia. Compound lacerations of the larynx, trachea or esophagus or tears and lacerations of the cartilage from blunt blows to the neck can be followed by this type of infection.

Visceral space infections always are serious, especially those following esophageal perforation. Mediastinitis is an almost immediate development, occurring within one to four days, before the usual protective barriers can be established by nature. Subcutaneous emphysema is diagnostic of the perforation and can be established either by the characteristic crepitus on physical examination or by roentgenograms. Soft tissue films may demonstrate air under the skin, in the anterior mediastinum or in the retropharyngeal space, under these circumstances. When appropriate early treatment has been omitted, the more fully developed infection will present signs and symptoms characteristic of the viscera involved. Dysphagia may occur when the infection borders upon the constrictors, while alterations in voice tone follow laryngeal edema. Dyspnea may result from either laryngeal obstruction or bronchopneumonia. A sustained febrile course will indicate the severity of the mediastinitis.

Once the presence of subcutaneous emphysema has been established, the treatment of choice for perforative infection of the visceral space is immediate surgical decompression. The deep fascia should be opened widely and the area drained to prevent further extension downward into the mediastinum. If visceral space infection is of the secondary type, treatment is aimed at correction of the source. This may mean simple intraoral drainage of a peritonsillar abscess or exploration and drainage of the pharyngomaxillary space. If obstructive dyspnea is present, a temporary tracheostomy may be required.

WOUNDS OF THE NECK

Injuries to the soft parts of the neck occur somewhat less often than might be expected in view of the extent of their surface in relation to other parts of the body. A portion of the anterior neck often is protected by a flexed jaw or raised shoulder. While such maneuvers often prevent or diminish the force of a blunt injury, they may compound or multiply the number of structures injured in instances of penetrating injuries. For example, fracture of the jaw is a common accompaniment of the deep neck wound. A stab wound at the base of the neck often involves the great vessels of the upper chest and even the heart.

Although obvious injury to deep structures of the neck may be self-evident, a small penetrating wound often may be very misleading. Preliminary evaluation and first-aid treatment should be as nonmanipulative as possible, the primary aim being to transport the patient to a hospital for more thorough examination and treatment. One should not tamper with the wound, or disturb blood clots, or try to remove foreign bodies at the scene of the injury. Sterile dressings of adequate size and volume should be applied to avoid further contamination. The amount of compression will be determined by the local situation. Constricting dressings should not be applied to control hemorrhage when the patient is unconscious unless he is constantly attended. If control of oral secretions is difficult, it is wise to transport the patient with the head slightly dependent in order to prevent fatal aspiration. Use of suction is very helpful under these circumstances. In civilian practice, correction of hypovolemia can usually be delayed until the patient has been transported, but when the injury is severe, plasma or blood substitutes should be administered while en route in order to combat shock.

While most blunt injuries can be correctly treated by conservative management, it has become increasingly evident that expectant therapy has been employed far too often in the care of penetrating wounds. Analysis of wartime statistics indicates that the great improvement in the care of such patients is directly related to the maintenance of an adequate airway by tracheostomy, the proper treatment of hypovolemia and early definitive surgical repair. Careful observation of patients with blunt neck injuries and the application of the same principles after minimal delay have saved lives that otherwise might have been lost.

SUPERFICIAL WOUNDS. Except for hemorrhage, superficial lacerations of the neck present no problems which differ from those in wounds of similar depth and extent found in other parts of the body. The external and anterior jugular veins, which are located immediately deep to the platysma muscle layer, may produce a startling amount of bleeding when divided. If the neck wound is uncomplicated by other injuries, appropriate first-aid care should be a simple but effective dressing until the patient can be transported to a point at which definitive surgical debridement and repair can be accomplished. The struggling behavior of an uncooperative or apprehensive patient will serve to increase the venous back pressure in the jugular system sufficiently to reactivate the venous bleeding to a distressing degree. Since some of this blood comes from the central side of the lacerated vein, a portion of this hemorrhage can be prevented by elevating the head 20 degrees during transportation.

DEEP WOUNDS. Wounds which penetrate the outer, or enveloping, layer of the deep cervical fascia usually are of considerable significance. The deep fascia surrounds the vascular and visceral compartments of the anterior neck in such a manner as to retain any extravasated blood or exudate. The major complications from such injuries, therefore, are hemorrhage, both internal and external, respiratory obstruction of varying degree and later infection.

A severe contusion on the side of the neck, such as that sustained in boxing when the chin is not flexed to protect the soft parts, may be very harmful. Varying degrees of damage to the wall of the larynx and trachea, as well as deep hematoma formation from ruptured veins, may result. Respiratory difficulties secondary to submucosal hemorrhage, and later edema, may first present as expectoration of blood-tinged sputum, hoarseness, dyspnea or even labored breathing with cyanosis. Severe respiratory difficulty may result from the pressure of a large expanding hematoma before it has been decompressed.

The most common incised wound of the neck is that inflicted in attempted suicide. This wound is more often made by the right hand and so extends more into the left than the right side of the neck. It may be located above the hyoid bone since the chin probably was extended upward. A deep wound at this level may reach the pharynx and even injure the epiglottis. At a lower level, the trachea may be severed by a similar transverse wound producing profuse bleeding from the anterior jugular veins as well as from the thyroid gland. It is quite possible that the large vessels of the carotid sheath will be protected by the sternocleidomastoid muscle or by their posterior position, as compared with those of the injured trachea and thyroid gland.

Anterior and anterolateral knife wounds from an assailant, commonly described as "cutthroat," present the immediate dangers of severe hemorrhage and asphyxia. Deep penetrating or stab wounds of the neck by knife or missile often are rapidly fatal, either as a result of immediate arterial hemorrhage or from extravasation of blood causing early respiratory obstruction by pressure. Hemorrhage may stop when the blood pressure falls to shock level, only to begin again when the patient strains or struggles or when the wound is manipulated. Sudden asphyxia may result from tracheal division, through either retraction of the cut edges or infolding of a part, or by inspiration of a clot of blood into the larynx or trachea. Division of the vagus or recurrent laryngeal nerve in the depths of such wounds causes further respiratory embarrassment through paralysis of the corresponding vocal cord.

Stab wounds in the supraclavicular region or injuries accompanied by forcible depression of the shoulder may result in severe and sometimes permanent damage to the brachial plexus by severance or by stretching. These lateral, incised wounds of the neck occur chiefly in fights or in attempted homicide. When the supraclavicular space is involved, the subclavian veins and their branches, and the thoracic duct and the lung may be injured. The possibility of a complicating pneumothorax or a delayed chylothorax must be kept in mind.

Bullet wounds, as well as the lacerations of war and civil life, are prone to infection. Perforated hollow neck viscera predispose to infection of the surrounding structures. Marked contamination of the deep tissue, involving directly the deep spaces, may occur. Foreign bodies may be driven into the area and nearby tissue damaged by the traumatic force. Anaerobic infection may be likely, especially when significant foreign bodies are not removed. Tetanus and gas-forming infection therefore should be feared.

Delayed or secondary effects within these deep wounds are edema of the larynx, varying degrees of tracheobronchitis, pneumonitis, infection along the prevertebral fascia with possible mediastinitis and secondary hemorrhage. If a suppurative process develops, not only mediastinitis, but also jugular septic phlebitis, must be feared. In all of these complications, glottic edema frequently may be the key to a chain of events leading to fatality. Maintenance of an adequate airway is essential and, therefore, early tracheostomy frequently will be necessary as a prophylactic lifesaving maneuver, either at the time of primary repair or later when dyspnea develops.

VASCULAR INJURIES. Fortunately, injuries to the great vessels in the neck and upper thorax occur rather infrequently. The significant vessels involved are the carotids, thyrocervical axis, vertebral, subclavian and innominate arteries, the jugular, subclavian and innominate veins and the arch of the aorta. Hemorrhage from these vessels can be so rapid and severe as to exsanguinate the patient before definite care can be attempted. In addition, strangulation by compression of the trachea may result from the effects of a massive, rapidly expanding, subfascial hematoma. Fatal cerebral thrombosis, or varying degrees of the hemiplegic state, may be late central complications of carotid injury in those who survive thrombosis. Late local effects consist in the formation of carotid aneurysms and arteriovenous fistulae.

Attention should be called to the fact that traumatic thrombosis of the internal carotid artery can take place in both penetrating as well as nonpenetrating injuries of the neck. In such patients, the symptoms may simulate those of an epidural or subdural hematoma. It is much more likely that this thrombosis will be recognized earlier following exploration of a penetrating injury and that there will be some expected delay in dealing with blunt injuries. Recent experience suggests that this diagnosis can be made earlier by means of percutaneous arteriography, and undoubtedly this procedure will be carried out more frequently in the future.

First aid for both arterial and venous hemorrhage should consist of direct packing of the wound reinforced by a gentle compressive dressing. While formidable bleeding may suggest the need for a more vigorous and more specific on-the-spot type of surgical first aid, one should withstand the temptation to perform such heroic attempts because hemostats, sutures and ligatures applied under adverse and contaminated circumstances add to infection and increase the possibility of intravascular thrombosis. Such a procedure merely complicates the later definitive surgical care. Immediate efforts should be directed toward proper transportation of the injured patient to a hospital where deliberate surgical repair can be accomplished.

VISCERAL INJURIES. Penetration of the oropharynx, esophagus, larynx and trachea, by the wounding mechanism permits bacterial invasion to take place along the fascial planes of the neck. Infection from these mucous-membrane-lined structures, especially from the pharynx and esophagus, is far more significant than infection into the wound from without. In a bullet or knife wound, the presence of subcutaneous emphysema, noted either by physical examination or by soft-tissue roentgenogram, indicates that one or more of these organs have been perforated. Wounds involving the floor of the mouth, pharynx or esophagus can be expected to heal quite well if appropriately repaired with adequate drainage of the visceral space. Small nasogastric tubes should be used for feeding purposes. On the other hand, if infection develops, these wounds are characterized by a foul exudate with considerable leakage of saliva. Edema of the glottis, mediastinitis or abscess formation with severe, secondary, venous hemorrhage may result. Although there may be difficulty with nutrition and healing is slow, the resultant orocutaneous fistula in some patients eventually may close spontaneously, but in others secondary closure will be required.

When the larynx or trachea has been cut across or severed by a bullet, there is a tendency for the parts to separate. A temporary tracheostomy may be required to facilitate good oxygen exchange and to permit safe transportation. If the division is complete, the lower end may retract beneath the sternum and be drawn downward with each inspiratory effort, especially if the distal opening is covered with soft tissue. When early repair is not possible, the lower cut end can be brought to the surface and a tracheostomy tube inserted as a temporary measure. Reconstruction can be done at a later time.

Blunt injury or minimal stab wounds sometimes produce tracheal fracture or puncture with little external evidence of serious trouble. In either instance, the soft tissues might temporarily occlude the tract. The appearance of subcutaneous emphysema and respiratory distress eventually leads to the correct diagnosis. The subcutaneous emphysema in such patients is first noted in the neck and then spreads rapidly to other areas, seemingly out of proportion to the injury. The extension into the mediastinum is responsible for the increasing dyspnea and cyanosis.

TREATMENT. The general principles of wound treatment in the neck are the same as those for any other part of the body, except that the local anatomy produces a few problems peculiar to the neck. Control of bleeding and maintenance of an adequate airway are of prime importance. In serious injuries, blood transfusion may be required to stabilize cardiovascular mechanics before surgical intervention can be attempted. A temporary tracheostomy performed under local anesthesia should be considered at this stage if respiratory obstruction is present. Atropine will help to diminish the bronchial secretions, but suction through the tracheostomy opening may be necessary to accomplish an adequate bronchial toilet.

After the general condition of the patient has improved, endoscopic and roentgen ray examination can be carried out with more care, in order to determine more fully the extent of the injury and to detect the presence of any hidden foreign bodies. If multiple injuries are present, all must be properly assessed and therapeutic priority established. With this information at hand, the wounds then can be repaired in proper order.

A general anesthetic should be administered, either by an endotracheal tube or in conjunction with the tracheostomy. Selection of the anesthetic for the patient with a serious neck injury is very important because a high oxygen content is absolutely essential. Although local anesthesia may be used for many elective surgical procedures in the neck, it is not suitable for these patients.

Following appropriate skin cleansing, the packing is removed from the depths of the wound. This is replaced by more specific pressure and each vessel is carefully ligated as fresh bleeding recurs. In knife or bullet wounds, a generous extension of the wound is mandatory to obtain satisfactory exposure and control of all bleeding points. Bleeding from large veins may be more troublesome to control than that from arteries, because vein walls are so fragile that they tear easily when handled. Ligation of a large vein requires good exposure and gentle technique. Debridement of devitalized tissue and removal of all foreign bodies are done as indicated. Clots are removed and the wound generously irrigated with saline solution.

While major veins and all the smaller arteries in the neck can be interrupted without fear of central complications, every effort should be made to restore vascular continuity when the carotid artery has been injured. Ligation of the common carotid artery involves the risk of hemiplegia or fatality when it is performed under general anesthesia and in the presence of shock. Suture of lacerations of the carotid wall or end-to-end anastomosis should be performed whenever possible.

When large defects are present, saphenous vein grafts or prosthetic replacement with flexible Dacron or Teflon grafts have proved to be successful on some occasions. When a graft is considered in gunshot injuries, the surgeon may be faced with a serious dilemma because of the extent of tissue damage in the surrounding soft parts. Local tissue necrosis may interfere with primary healing so that secondary fatal hemorrhage may be a strong possibility. One must weigh the risk of cerebral complications secondary to ligation against the risk of sudden hemorrhage from the infected anastomosis or graft. The age of the patient may be helpful in this decision, since younger individuals tolerate carotid ligation much better than older ones. The technique of primary anastomosis between the external and internal carotid arteries in the form of a loop, as suggested by Conley, should be considered when it is necessary for the common carotid to be ligated low in the neck.

A complete anatomic survey then is necessary in order to identify lacerations in the viscera and nerves. Small defects in the trachea can be sutured and covered with nearby thyroid or muscle. Sometimes, a two-layered closure of the pharynx can be obtained if the surrounding tissues are properly mobilized. Major defects in the larger muscles can be closed by loose suture. When viscera have been perforated, no attempt should be made to close the deep cervical fascia. A small, thin, rubber drain can be permitted to come to the outside from the visceral space, but it never should be left in direct contact with the sutured wall. These maneuvers serve to decompress the retropharyngeal and visceral spaces and diminish the potential of mediastinal infection. Gentle suction drainage will facilitate both wound healing and postoperative nursing care.

The apex of the lung or pleura can be perforated in any deep stab wound of the neck. When this occurs a tension pneumothorax is the common result. This should be anticipated and closed chest drainage under a water seal instituted. The thoracic lymphatic duct should always be ligated whenever found to be torn or lacerated. This will prevent the serious and troublesome complication of lymphorrhea and also the possibility of a delayed chylothorax.

Special mention should be made with regard to divided nerves in this area. The hypoglossal, spinal accessory, vagus, recurrent laryngeal and phrenic nerves and branches of the brachial plexus are to be considered. While there may be some debate about the value of primary or delayed repair of these nerves, it is generally held that it is possible to carry out a successful primary suture after early debridement, providing the wound heals without infection.

When dealing with deep blunt injuries, a period of observation is usually necessary before the need for active surgical intervention may become evident. Tracheal or laryngeal trauma due to a blunt instrument may take the form of a small rupture in which respiratory distress and subcutaneous emphysema may be delayed in their appearance. It is not unusual that four to six hours may be required before a small fracture or dislocation of the cartilaginous structures of the trachea may become evident. Prompt tracheostomy with decompression of the anterior mediastinum is necessary, and in most instances this procedure will control the life-endangering respiratory difficulties. The same time factor is to be noted when thrombosis develops within the bluntly injured common carotid artery. When arteriography confirms the diagnosis, immediate surgical extraction of the clot plus cervical sympathectomy and heparinization can be expected to produce good results in patients with an otherwise normal arterial tree.

The Thyroid and Parathyroid Glands

THYROID GLAND

The thyroid gets its name from the stem meaning "shield." This ductless gland has two lobes which are connected by an isthmus, which lies in front of the trachea just below the cricoid cartilage. Because of its numerous metabolic and neoplastic aberrations, this gland has been the target of surgical interest. Although considerable progress has been made in purely medical management of many of its disorders, the definitive surgical procedure is some form of thyroidectomy.

ANATOMY

The thyroid appears as an invagination of the midventral wall of the pharynx between the first and second branchial arches in the fourth week of fetal life. The resultant thyroglossal duct originates in the foramen cecum at the base of the tongue. When the gland reaches maturity, it is found to be located in front of the fifth, sixth and seventh cervical vertebrae. As it lies in relation to the anterior and lateral surfaces of the upper trachea and is invested by the cervical fascia which is attached to the thyroid cartilage, the gland characteristically moves upward with them on swallowing.

The normal thyroid weighs about 25 to 40 gm. in the adult and this can vary with sex, age and endemic factors. It is a very vascular organ, receiving its blood supply from the superior and inferior thyroid arteries, and often the thyreoidea ima from the aorta or innominate artery. There is a considerable amount of vascular anastomoses. The superior and inferior thyroid arteries communicate through an anastomosing trunk on the posterior aspect of the lateral lobes. This trunk is a guide to the parathyroid glands. There are three pairs of veins which drain the gland in addition to other accessory veins. The superior and middle thyroid veins empty into the internal jugular, whereas the inferior thyroid veins join as a trunk which empties into the left innominate. The veins cover the surface of the gland anteriorly and over the trachea and anastomose freely across the isthmus (Fig. 8).

The lymphatic drainage is very generous and especially significant when carcinoma is present. The intraglandular lymph vessels connect freely from one lobe to the other through the isthmus. External drainage is to the pretracheal nodes, often in association with the recurrent laryngeal nerve, to nodes in the deep jugular chain and related secondary triangles and, occasionally, into nodes located in the superior mediastinum.

The nerve supply to the thyroid comes from the middle and inferior cervical ganglia of the sympathetic chain and accompanies a blood vessel. In addition, the superior laryngeal and the recurrent laryngeals, both branches of the vagus, lie in such close approximation that they must be constantly considered during the operation of thyroidectomy.

Microscopically, the thyroid is made up of many spherical, small acini, supported by a connective tissue stroma which is in continuity with the capsule of the gland. The acini are lined with low, cuboidal epithelium and filled with a thick colloid containing a high percentage of iodine. This epithelium becomes enfolded and the cells enlarged, becoming columnar, when hypertrophy and hyperplasia occur. The nuclei can be found to occupy the middle of the cells and numerous mitoses are seen. Under these circumstances, the colloid is poorly stained and vacuolated, the vascularity of the gland increases and lymphocytic collections are to be found in the stroma. When glandular activity lessens, the hyperplasia is followed by a process of involution in which the acinar cells tend to flatten out and the colloid again accumulates. This accumulation within the alveoli, accompanied by the fibrous changes in the stroma, gives the gland a globular appearance.

PHYSIOLOGY AND STRUCTURE

It is well known that thyroxine and triiodothyronine directly stimulate tissue metabolism at all ages by acting as a catalyzing agent for oxidation enzyme systems. Thus, they promote growth and development of organs, relate directly to carbohydrate metabolism, relate also to calcium excretion from bones, directly relate to the flow of urine and participate in the regulation of the distribution of fluid within the body. These more distant endocrine effects have always been of great interest to thyroidologists; it is equally interesting to relate changes in the structure of the thyroid gland itself to changes in its own function. It has been known for some time that anything which depresses the production of thyroid hormone simultaneously initiates a compensatory mechanism with the result that the pituitary increases its

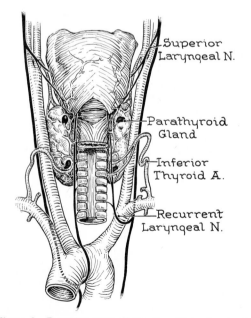

Figure 8. Posterior view of the thyroid trachea and esophagus. The laryngeal nerves and the parathyroid glands are emphasized.

output of thyroid-stimulating hormone (Fig. 9). This increase in thyroid-stimulating hormone produces intraglandular hyperplasia and hyperfunction of the thyroid itself. If this stimulation persists for a long period of time, the structural changes in the thyroid become more manifest.

It has been shown that a deficiency of dietary iodine is a significant factor in the production of endemic goiter. In the more civilized portions of the world, the intake of iodine is probably quite adequate by the utilization of iodized salt along with the more common availability of seafood. On the other hand, certain substances, such as vegetables of the rutabaga family, soybeans, cabbage and compounds such as thiouracil and some sulfonamides, are capable of decreasing the output of thyroid hormone. This block results in hypertrophy and hyperplasia of the thyroid gland from pituitary stimulation, so it must be concluded that there are factors other than iodine deficiency which cause intraglandular functional and structural change. The common anatomical changes following long-continued stimulation are areas of degenerating and regenerating epithelium which form nodules. The incidence of nodules is extremely low in children, but gradually increases throughout the life span, until one finds in certain areas of endemic goiter that the majority of the older age group present some form of nodular goiter.

Some of the compounds which block the enzymatic system within the thyroid do so by direct interference with thyroxine formation by preventing the oxidation of inorganic iodide to iodine. Thus, iodine remains as a central significant element in this hormonal interchange. From the therapeutic standpoint, iodine, when taken by mouth as Lugol's solution, inhibits both the synthesis of thyroxine and its release into the blood. From the practical standpoint, this usually permits the hyperthyroidism to decrease for about two weeks, following which there is a tendency for the glandular activity to return to a level about halfway between the original state of hyperfunction and the level of maximal improvement toward the euthyroid state. This is a critical time factor which has been known for years and utilized in preparing the hyperthyroid patient for operation. This therapeutic maneuver has been utilized both prior to and following the discovery of the depressant value of propylthiouracil. It is especially valuable because this reduces the vascularity and friability of the hyperplastic gland at the time of surgery.

For these same reasons, radioactive iodine (I^{131}) is concentrated in the thyroid gland and has the capacity to destroy the glandular tissue in such a selective manner as to control some forms of hyperthyroidism without injuring other tissues of the body.

GOITER

Not all enlargements of the thyroid gland are of the same nature, even though they are all called goiter. The term implies nothing more than an enlargement of the thyroid gland. The classification suggested by the American Society for the Study of Goiter is very practical: Diffuse nontoxic goiter, nodular nontoxic goiter, diffuse toxic goiter and nodular toxic goiter.

DIFFUSE NONTOXIC GOITER. This term refers to the situation often known as simple goiter, endemic goiter or adolescent goiter. This includes the enlargements of the thyroid which originally were seen in geographic areas deficient in iodine. Despite the frequent use of iodized salt, this entity has not completely disappeared. This seems to be explained by the possibility of hereditary factors, as well as the likelihood that a relative lack of iodine is still significant in the female at puberty or during pregnancy.

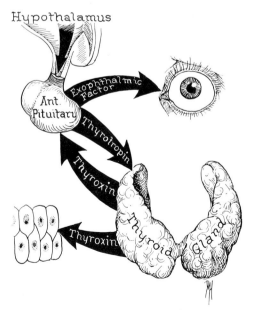

Figure 9. The pituitary-thyroid axis.

The thyroid gland is frequently called upon to secrete an increased amount of its hormone, and to do this it may undergo hypertrophy, hyperplasia or both. Having met the emergency, it may return to normal, or it may go into a resting stage in which the acini are filled with colloid. Later in life, it may undergo some incomplete involution or it may atrophy. Should it remain enlarged, with or without an excessive or perverted secretion, it forms a goiter. This smooth enlargement in the neck of adolescent girls is noted as a physiological enlargement. In some women during pregnancy, during the menopause or under any considerable mental or physical stress, the gland increases in size. There are no signs of toxicity or obstruction, and the metabolic rate is normal. Years ago, when such glands were more regularly surgically removed, the cut surface would be found somewhat translucent, in keeping with the excess of colloid, and microscopically, the alveoli would be lined with low epithelium and filled with densely staining colloid. In some sections, there would be alveoli with hyperplasia, lined by tall cells such as might indicate increased cellular activity.

There are no indications for operation for diffuse nontoxic goiter other than that relative to a demand for cosmetic improvement. Once recognized, the administration of iodine over a short period of time tends to decrease the size of the gland and small doses of dessicated thyroid control the tendency toward hypothyroidism. Occasionally, women with untreated diffuse nontoxic goiter may produce children with a severe degree of hypothyroidism and rarely, a true cretin may result. This can be prevented by proper dosage of dessicated thyroid during pregnancy.

NODULAR NONTOXIC GOITER. This condition is commonly referred to as adenomatous goiter and is most commonly found in areas where goiter is endemic. This is frequently a sequel to diffuse nontoxic goiter and is likely on the same basis. In approximately 15 per cent of all adult women, small nodules can be felt in the thyroid gland. This type of physiologic response is much more commonly found in women than in men. The gland may be considerably enlarged with palpable nodules of varying sizes and in various forms of degeneration. In some instances, these may represent large cavities distended by colloid, cystic areas containing a mixture of fluid or segments with mucinous transformation,

focal necrosis or areas of calcification. Spontaneous bleeding may also occur within the gland, followed by fibrous healing and the formation of very firm nodules. The end result is that of variegated degrees of pathologic change, best described as a degenerated goiter held together only by the usual fibrous capsule and network of blood vessels. Although areas of calcification may make sections of these glands extremely hard and presumably difficult to differentiate from chronic thyroiditis or malignancy, it is a well-known fact that calcification and malignancy in the same gland are extremely rare.

Usually, these goiters enlarge outwardly in the line of least resistance and produce remarkably little difficulty with breathing or swallowing. Upon occasion, the enlargement may become substernal or intrathoracic and under these circumstances, the pressure symptoms may be more significant.

The indications for an operation in nodular nontoxic goiter ordinarily relate either to cosmetic demand, fear of malignancy or the problem of unrelieved pressure. Subtotal thyroidectomy can easily be defended if there are symptoms of tracheal or esophageal compression. This is particularly significant when the goiter extends into the thorax and threatens to cause more serious trouble at a later date. On occasion, it is difficult to discriminate from a true single adenoma that is neoplastic in origin, and thus an operation is indicated for purposes of histologic identification. This is reasonable because there does occur a low but measurable incidence of carcinoma in patients with nodular nontoxic goiter.

DIFFUSE TOXIC GOITER. This disease process has frequently been referred to as exophthalmic goiter, primary hyperthyroidism, Graves' disease and Basedow's disease. An emotional crisis, or some illness no more unusual than an acute upper respiratory infection, has been known to be the inciting cause. It would appear that some kind of uncontrolled hypothalamic stimulation can produce an excess of thyroxine through the activities of the anterior pituitary gland. In addition to diffuse enlargement of the thyroid, the gland secretes something that makes the patient unusually ill. This form of hyperthyroidism is also referred to as thyrotoxicosis, a term which points not only to an overactive gland, but also to a perverted secretion from the thyroid gland. The word thyrotoxicosis implies that a toxemia exists, although no toxic substance has ever been actually identified. There is a low iodine content in the gland and an increase in blood iodine, but neither of these factors alone or in combination necessarily produces toxic goiter. Thyrotoxicosis has been induced by the ingestion of large amounts of thyroid extract. In such circumstances, the urinary excretion of radioactive iodine is high, whereas in the usual endogenous thyrotoxicosis it is low as compared with euthyroid persons.

Exophthalmos is often seen in true Graves' disease, but does not consistently parallel the severity of the hyperthyroidism. In some patients, this may also be more evident in one eye and may even antedate the clinical onset of hyperthyroidism. It is conjectured that some anterior pituitary product other than thyrotropic hormone may be involved in the etiology of this clinical finding.

Primary hyperthyroidism is usually found in young females of unstable temperament who present tachycardia, considerable agitation and other signs and symptoms of an increased metabolic rate. These patients demonstrate personality changes and are easily disturbed by minor behavioral problems. They complain of considerable weakness, fatigability, weight loss, palpitations, hand tremor, excessive perspiration, insomnia and intolerance to heat. Irregular gastrointestinal activity, such as diarrhea and vomiting, as well as menstrual disturbances, may also be observed. One of the most characteristic findings is the paradoxical loss of weight with a major increase in appetite. These patients also manifest some type of agitation characterized by intermittent useless movements of the extremities.

Because thyrotoxicosis influences the metabolic rate in all tissues, any system of the body may produce abnormal physical findings. Although the cardiovascular system may be most prominent in this regard, the nervous system, the gastrointestinal tract, the genitourinary system, the skin and the musculoskeletal system may be involved.

The first impression may be that of a patient who is very anxious, jittery and somewhat harassed. If there is exophthalmos, the sclerae are quite evident and there is significant lag in the motion of the upper lid when the eye looks to the floor. The hands are moist and warm and the skin may possess an exceedingly fine texture. A fine tremor of the fingers is accentuated when a single piece of paper is placed upon the unsupported extended hand. An elevated pulse rate is evident and rises sharply following mild exertion. Weakness in the quadriceps muscle parallels this phenomenon. A high pulse pressure is characteristic when the blood pressure is recorded.

On palpation of the neck, the thyroid gland is diffusely enlarged and smooth. In a slender individual, this may be grossly visible, though often not obvious in others. When the patient is asked to swallow a sip of water, the enlarged thyroid always becomes quite evident. The increased vascularity may be so impressive that a bruit can be heard over the gland.

The diagnosis of hyperthyroidism is not made entirely on the basis of symptoms and physical findings alone. This is an organic disease and it produces measurable biologic evidence of its activity and severity. Objective signs of increased metabolism can easily be verified by a simple basal metabolic rate determination. In the hands of well-trained technicians under basal conditions this is a very valuable laboratory test. It is especially helpful because the test can be easily repeated at intervals either to confirm the original diagnosis or to measure improvement in the clinical course. Symptoms of hyperthyroidism can be associated with readings only slightly above normal range. When moderately severe the rates may lie in the 40 to 60 range, whereas a very toxic patient may demonstrate a rate as high as 100. Among its limitations is the well-known fact that the basal metabolic rate may be elevated in some patients with severe hypertension, cardiac decompensation or leukemia.

Wherever its exacting technique has been perfected, the determination of protein-bound iodine has proved to be a reliable measure of thyroid function. Organic iodine constitutes approximately 90 per cent of the total iodine in the plasma. This protein-bound fraction reflects with reasonable accuracy the concentration of circulating thyroid hormone. In euthyroid individuals, the plasma values fluctuate within rather narrow limits between 4 and 8 gamma per 100 ml. The majority of patients with hyperthyroidism have an elevated protein-bound iodine just as most patients with hypothyroidism demonstrate levels below 4 gamma per 100 ml. Perhaps its greatest value is in the exclusion of hyperthyroidism in patients who have nonthyroid conditions producing hypermetabolism. A normal or low value practically always excludes hyperthyroidism from consideration, whereas slightly elevated values must be cautiously interpreted. Protein-bound iodine, for example, may be elevated in certain examples of nontoxic hyperplasia of the thyroid, and also when the patient has recently ingested iodine for either therapeutic or diagnostic purposes.

Historically, the use of I^{131} has contributed greatly to our knowledge of thyroid physiology. The measurement of radioactive iodine uptake by the thyroid has become a fairly common diagnostic maneuver, but its absolute value is open to considerable question. Progressive technical improvements now permit the use of very small test doses in the range of 5 to 10 microcuries. The accumulation of radioactivity within the gland is measured at fixed intervals up to 24 hours, at which time the uptake is maximum. In euthyroid individuals the uptake ranges from 15 to 45 per cent of the administered dose. In hyperthyroidism, these values range from 50 to 90 per cent, whereas values below 15 per cent usually denote the hypothyroid state. Scintigrams are often done at the same time to demonstrate the distribution of the I^{131} in the gland.

In recent years, the perfection of the triiodothyronine uptake test has eliminated the necessity of giving any radioactive iodine to the patient. This is becoming a frequently used test for thyroid function. It requires only a single visit to the laboratory for venipuncture. It can be used with complete safety in children and pregnant women and can be repeated as often as needed. Previous medication with iodine does not affect the results. Because there are a number of methods used in the actual performance of the test, each laboratory must establish its own standards based upon local experience.

In rare instances, the clinician may occasionally use antithyroid drugs as an aid in establishing the diagnosis. This may be somewhat complicated by the fact that the untreated patient with diffuse toxic goiter may spontaneously go into a remission. On the other hand, these remissions are almost always followed by an exacerbation which may be initiated by some minor functional or infectious problem. These normal variations should be understood because they must be correlated with both diagnostic and therapeutic courses of medical management. Certainly, no elective surgical procedure should be carried out until the patient is thoroughly controlled and returned to a euthyroid state. In some patients, this control may require considerable time and many vital organs, especially the heart, may suffer permanent damage during the process.

During the third and fourth decades of this century, the surgical approach to hyperthyroidism gradually evolved with the establishment of a reasonably standardized preparatory routine of medical management. This is characterized by the administration of Lugol's solution over a period of two to six weeks, combined with hyperalimentation, proper sedation and rest. When given enough time, the majority of patients approach a euthyroid level which makes them relatively safe surgical risks. This improvement is measured by weight gain and reduction in pulse and pulse pressure, along with suitable reduction in the basal metabolic rate. At the appropriate time the astute surgeon can submit his patient to some form of thyroidectomy, preferably subtotal. In the hands of better surgeons, more than 95 per cent of patients make a good recovery from this serious situation under such a program and with minimal morbidity.

During the last 15 years, the nonsurgical treatment for Graves' disease has become increasingly popular. With the advent of the antithyroid drugs, there occurred considerable interest in the short-term as well as the long-term medical management of hyperthyroidism. Although it has been recognized that propylthiouracil can render euthyroid a patient who has diffuse toxic goiter, the recurrence rate after withdrawal of treatment may be as high as 50 per cent, and even much higher in patients with toxic nodular goiter. When given in doses of approximately 600 mg. per day, it has been found that the basal metabolic rate will be reduced about 1 per cent for each day propylthiouracil is administered. When the patient becomes euthyroid, the maintenance dose may vary between 50 and 200 mg. per day. Even though continued for one to two years, only about half of these patients remain under control. The recurrence rate is always higher in the more toxic patients and there is always the danger of a drug reaction, particularly agranulocytosis. For these reasons, such drugs are now ordinarily best used only for the preparation of a toxic patient for definitive subtotal thyroidectomy. When the hyperthyroid patient has obtained full effect from such antithyroid drugs, in addition to proper sedation, rest and improved nutrition, the common practice is to administer Lugol's solution for two weeks leading up to the day of operation. The administration of iodine in this form reduces the size and vascularity of the gland and creates a better situation for the operation. In addition, propylthiouracil ordinarily is stopped approximately ten days before in order to prevent the possibility of creating an unfortunately severe hypothyroid state, coincident with the performance of the thyroidectomy.

Careful studies have shown that even in the hands of expert surgeons, conservative subtotal thyroidectomies may often be followed by a recurrence rate of 5 to 15 per cent if followed for as many as five years. This percentage is reduced according to the amount of thyroid gland removed. On the other hand, some degree of postoperative hypothyroidism, hypoparathyroidism, both transient and permanent, and damage to the recurrent laryngeal nerves must be noted as part of the anticipated possible morbidity. Although the recurrence rate of hyperthyroidism may be reduced to as low as 2 or 3 per cent, the morbidity may also rise to as high as 5 to 10 per cent when all these complications are grouped together.

While these statistics have been accumulating during the last two decades, considerable competitive therapeutic enthusiasm has developed in favor of the use of radioactive iodine as the ideal treatment for Graves' disease. It has been projected that radioactive iodine should be an effective, safe, economical and simple method for the treatment of this form of hyperthyroidism. Therefore, in recent years, the trend has been toward the primary use of radioactive iodine in the treatment of patients with Graves' disease. In the early phases of this development, treatment was limited to those patients in the older age groups, or for those with recurrent hyperthyroidism following subtotal thyroidectomy. As experience has increased, the age limits have been gradually lowered, and some physicians are treating people as young as 30 years of age with I^{131}. The agent is given by mouth in an amount determined by the estimated size of the toxic gland. Very often, a second and occasionally a third dose may be necessary before enough thyroid tissue is destroyed in order to control the disease.

There is no doubt that the oral administration of radioactive iodine is an attractive therapeutic maneuver aimed at avoiding an operative procedure. On the other hand, there are significant dangers and shortcomings in the administration of I^{131} which cannot be completely ignored. The administration of irradiation to children is a concern because of the possibility of eventual malignant change which might develop ten to 20 years in the future. This concern is based upon current recognition of the development of thyroid carcinoma in many adults who as children underwent irradiation of the thymus and nasopharyngeal lymphatic tissues many years ago. In addition, there is evidence in the literature indicating that children have developed carcinoma of the thyroid two to eight years following radioiodine treatment. Although the evidence has not been overwhelming, this experience, in addition to experimental studies in which thyroid carcinoma was induced in animals by the administration of radioiodine, should be a deterrent in using radioiodine for children with Graves' disease.

In addition, many individuals who were subjected to ionizing radiation at Hiroshima and Nagasaki are now demonstrating an increased incidence of thyroid carcinoma. From the genetic standpoint, there is the possibility of ovarian damage in women of child-bearing years. To date, this has not been significantly documented, but it remains a matter of concern. It is evident that this agent can easily pass the placental barrier and, therefore, should never be administered to a pregnant female who simultaneously is suffering from primary hyperthyroidism. The latter individual is best treated by the usual preoperative preparation followed by a subtotal thyroidectomy during the middle trimester of pregnancy. If such a procedure is not accepted, it is evident that the patient should at least be carried through her pregnancy with antithyroid drugs, but also should be given simultaneously adequate amounts of desiccated thyroid in order to prevent the birth of a cretin.

Over the long term, follow-up studies on patients treated with I^{131} have revealed that there is an unanticipated high incidence of delayed hypothyroidism. It has been reported that hypothyroidism occurs at an annual incidence of approximately 3 per cent after the first year, and that the cumulative incidence reaches approximately 40 per cent by ten years. Although hypothyroidism is readily treated by replacement therapy, the actual difficulty relates to the fact that this condition often goes unrecognized for an indefinite period of time for many different reasons. Untreated hypothyroidism can be a serious disease especially in older patients. The incidence of hypothyroidism following operation is very much the same as that following radioiodine therapy in the early post-therapy period, especially up to one year. Postsurgical hypothyroidism usually is immediately appreciated as a progressive problem and ordinarily is promptly treated as such. On the other hand, the insidious nature of the development of hypothyroidism following radioactive iodine is not appreciated and may become a severe problem when the patient is itinerant, when the responsible physician does not follow the patient long enough, and whenever the patient or the physician fails to appreciate the long-term potential of such a probability.

Another obvious disadvantage of radioiodine is that the nuclear therapist may require three to nine months or more in order to produce a euthyroid state. Bowers has recently reported a group of 81 medically treated patients in whom the average time needed to achieve euthyroidism was 453 days, compared with six weeks for a comparable group of surgical patients. In this same group, the obvious thyrocardiac patients became euthyroid in 695 days with medical therapy, and in 42 days with surgical treatment. Follow-up studies averaged eight years for the surgical patients, and four years for the medically treated patients. In the surgical group, there was recurrence in 5.8 per cent, whereas 19.7 per cent of the medically treated patients had persistent hyperthyroidism in half the time. Such comparisons obviously indicate that certain patients should be selected for classic subtotal thyroidectomy because of its therapeutic superiority.

The findings in general indicate that radioiodine therapy is superior to thyroidectomy in the patient with mild hyperthyroidism, the patient with recurrent thyrotoxicosis, the patient with malignant exophthalmos and, of course, the patient who does not desire, or whose associated conditions contraindicate operation. The thyrocardiac patients respond more favorably to operation than do the medically treated. Until radioiodine therapy improves, subtotal thyroidectomy appears to be superior for the more severe thyrotoxic goiters in young patients. All of this is based upon the assumption that the surgeon has the ability to leave a small thyroid remnant without interfering with the parathyroids or their blood supply, and without causing nerve injury of any degree, while performing an adequate subtotal thyroidectomy.

NODULAR TOXIC GOITER. This complication is often referred to as toxic adenoma and is a condition which occurs in older people. These adenomas have been referred to as the tombstones or indicators of a previous episode of significant hyperplasia. Perhaps, the disease started earlier in life as a diffuse hyperplasia and then, with subsequent involutional changes, a diffuse adenomatous goiter develops with some reactivated areas of hypertrophy and hyperplasia. Thyrotoxicosis in such glands may be due to hyperplasia and hypertrophy of residual normal areas of glandular parenchyma. Under such circumstances, therefore, the microscopic appearance may be that of both hyperplasia and abnormal adenosis such as is seen in the involution of fibrocystic mastitis. Because there is no evidence that the cells of these adenomas produce an abnormal secretion, it is concluded that the toxicity in a nodular goiter arises from activity in the thyroid tissue between the nodules. Only rarely do radioactive scintillation studies suggest the possibility of activity in these adenomas. As in most metabolic dysfunctions of the thyroid, the patient usually is a female and the enlarged nodular goiter may have been present for many years before the current symptoms became significant.

The toxic symptoms in these patients, although similar in general to those found in Graves' disease, are definitely of less severity and on the average the patients are about 20 years older. The local findings may be similar to those of nodular nontoxic goiter and on occasion these may be further complicated by the presence of mild obstructive pressure symptoms. There is a definite tendency for such patients to present cardiac symptoms, often accompanied by auricular fibrillation. From this, one can only conclude that other patients with cardiac decompensation and with an evident chronic nodular goiter should always be carefully studied for the possibility of hidden evidence of hyperthyroidism.

It has been agreed by most clinicians that patients with nodular toxic goiter are better treated by subtotal thyroidectomy in the accepted manner than with the use of radioactive iodine. The response to antithyroid drugs and iodine is not as prompt and high drug doses are required. With operation, the euthyroid state can usually be achieved within six weeks, whereas a comparable group of patients may require more than six months when treated with I^{131}. With prolonged periods of therapy, it is possible that some patients can be lost to follow-up while still hyperthyroid. This delay may be disadvantageous to the patient. Subtotal thyroidectomy has produced excellent results with prompt improvement in cardiac function and often with an early return to normal cardiac rhythm. The recurrence rate is low with subtotal thyroidectomy in such patients. It would appear that definite medical treatment should be reserved for only the most debilitated patients and those who have other serious diseases which might contraindicate thyroidectomy.

INDIVIDUALIZATION OF THERAPY. It is correct to conclude that there is a place for individualization in the treatment of hyperthyroidism. Excellence of results will depend to a great extent upon the skill of the individual physician, whether it be medical or surgical therapy that is chosen. Both the dosage of radioiodine therapy, on the part of the internist, and the skill of the surgeon are factors in the success of each plan of therapy.

In considering the individualization of treatment for hyperthyroidism, it is important to separate patients according to whether they have Graves' disease, toxic multinodular goiter or single toxic autonomous nodules. This can be accomplished on the basis of history, physical findings and the selective use of scintigrams of the thyroid before and after the administration of thyrotropic stimulating hormone. Radioactive iodine has become the standard therapy for Graves' disease in adults. On the other hand, the patient who is not likely to seek follow-up care and who cannot biologically afford to wait for correction by radioiodine is a prime candidate for a well-performed operation. The simplicity of radioiodine therapy and the fact that only a few patients are economically in serious difficulty because of Graves' disease will probably continue to make this the dominant therapy for adults. Individualization in patients who are pregnant is obvious. Similarly, recurrent hyperthyroidism following inadequate subtotal thyroidectomy is best treated by radioactive iodine.

An operation should be considered the treatment of choice for patients with toxic nodular goiter. The high incidence of a low uptake of radioactive iodine makes treatment with this substance more difficult, frequently inadequate, and may permit aggravation of cardiac influences of this disease during the months of waiting for the desired effects of therapy. On the other hand, surgical correction is prompt, reliable, requires little preparation with antithyroid drugs and rarely produces complications of hypothyroidism, recurrent laryngeal nerve damage or hypoparathyroidism, because removal of the thyroid tissue need not be so extensive.

A single toxic nodule, the least common cause of hyperthyroidism, is also best treated surgically. It should be noted that proper identification of this form of hyperthyroidism requires routine thyroid scintigrams, especially after the administration of thyrotropic stimulating hormones.

THYROIDECTOMY. In a few selected patients, local infiltration anesthesia combined with high cervical block technique may be the anesthesia of choice. On the other hand, general anesthesia administered through an endotracheal tube has become far more popular because this gives both the anesthetist and the surgeon better control of their respective areas of responsibility. The airway is easily maintained and extension of the neck improves exposure of the operative field. The standard approach by means of a low anterior cervical transverse incision is quite adequate and only in a few patients is it necessary to divide the strap muscles for greater exposure. There is no significant harm in this procedure, and it should be carried out whenever it facilitates the operation. Mobilization of each lobe is dependent upon the proper ligation of the superior and inferior thyroid vessels, as well as the middle thyroid vein. Preservation of the parathyroid glands and the recurrent laryngeal nerve depend upon their adequate exposure during the course of the dissection. Hemostasis must be as accurate as possible and the cut edges of the capsule should be closed over the raw surface of the residual gland when possible. No more than 3 to 4 gm. of tissue should be left behind when dealing with a diffuse toxic goiter. Greater amounts of tissue may be preserved when dealing with a nodular toxic or nontoxic goiter.

Postoperative bleeding is always the most immediate dangerous complication following thyroidectomy, but it is preventable. Despite all precautions, one must be aware that it may occur in any patient following thyroidectomy, no matter how much care has been used, or how dry the operative field may appear to be at the end of the operation. The necessary movements relating to swallowing and coughing may be sufficient to initiate bleeding. When this takes place, the trachea may become severely compressed by the developing blood clot which is held within the confines of the vertical strap muscles of the neck. Because this is a serious complication, one should be alert to the fact that it may be quite insidious in its onset, occurring anywhere between three and 12 hours after the completion of the operation. Whenever detected, the best procedure is to return the patient to the operating room to reopen the incision and control the bleeding under adequate anesthesia. If this is not feasible, the wound should be opened wherever the patient happens to be. Not all these patients require tracheostomy, but whenever in doubt, this should be a complementary procedure to prevent further serious tracheal obstruction from secondary edema. After evacuation of the clot, such a tracheostomy is easily performed because the trachea has already been skeletonized by the removal of the gland during the primary procedure.

Injury to the recurrent laryngeal nerve on one side results in homolateral paralysis with the vocal cord fixed near the midline. In the presence of edema, it may cause some respiratory difficulty as well as a temporary change in voice. In addition, when both nerves are injured, there is an early loss of voice and fixation of the cords in midline, with considerable difficulty in respiratory exchange. In some instances, this may create such a severe problem as to require temporary tracheostomy.

A thyroid crisis, or storm, is merely the acute accentuation of all of the symptomatology of hyperthyroidism. In previous years, before patients were properly rendered euthyroid before operation, this was a more common occurrence. It is thought to be due to the manipulation of the toxic gland, plus the hyperreactive response to be anticipated in any patient with a toxic goiter following any type of operative procedure. In its most severe form, the patient can develop extreme hyperthermia with major tachycardia, cardiac decompensation and death.

Whenever the post-thyroidectomy patient develops an immediate febrile reaction accompanied by rapid pulse, severe restlessness and cardiac irregularity, one should be deeply concerned regarding the possibility of this rather terrifying complication. One of the most recent explanations of this severe decompensation of such patients with thyrotoxicosis is the complete uncoupling of oxidative phosphorylation. With this in mind, vigorous methods should be used to bring the body temperature back to normal and to correct the cardiovascular abnormalities by the most direct means. Intravenous sodium iodide in doses of 1 gm. every six hours and propylthiouracil in doses of 600 to 800 mg. daily effectively block the synthesis and release of residual thyroid hormones. Reserpine should be given intramuscularly in doses of 2.5 mg. every six to eight hours. Hydrocortisone has also proved effective in such crises. Water, electrolyte and caloric balances must be carefully maintained and oxygen administered by nasal catheter. Whenever possible, hypothermia should also be used early in the course of this situation because the patients are unable to maintain their own cooling system, so necessary for survival.

Parathyroid insufficiency is a rare complication and the first manifestation is numbness of the hands, general weakness, difficulty in focusing the eyes and, occasionally, carpopedal spasm within 24 to 48 hours of the time of operation. In some instances, the voice may be altered by spasm of the vocal cords. When the circulation to the hand is reduced during the course of a routine blood pressure reading, there will be an obvious increase in the spasm of the forearm muscles. This produces the obstetrical position of the hand known as Trousseau's sign. Hyperexcitability of the facial nerve under such circumstances will be noted by contractions of the facial muscles when the examiner taps the facial nerve in the area of the parotid gland. This is referred to as Chvostek's sign.

The clinical symptoms of hypoparathyroidism seldom develop unless the blood calcium level falls below 8 mg. per 100 ml. Because most of these situations are transitory, it is thought that the tetany is the result of interference with the blood supply to the parathyroids, rather than their actual complete removal. The intravenous administration of calcium gluconate either reduces or completely eliminates these acute symptoms. Oral calcium administration can then be given until the parathyroid glands become more efficient. If symptoms persist, large doses of vitamin D should be added to the diet. If the symptoms are severe, dihydrotachysterol may be more effective. Although parathormone is known to be similarly effective, most investigators report that this only acts for a short period of time and unfortunately its effect is soon dissipated.

THYROID NEOPLASMS

There is probably no area in oncology wherein the pathologist is more important to the surgeon than in the field of thyroid neoplasms. Not only are there various shadings between normal and malignant tissue, but also there are innumerable confusing terms commonly used in describing the clinical situations which require definitive treatment. Superimposed upon this variegated classification are the well-intentioned subclassifications offered by many interested investigators.

BENIGN ADENOMA. The thyroid gland produces a localized neoplasm which can be identified as a benign adenoma. Both from the clinical and the pathologic standpoints, there is difficulty in distinguishing between the true adenoma of neoplastic origin and the nodules found in the adenomatous goiter which commonly results following the functional sequence of hyperplasia and involution. The ordinary benign neoplasm is often referred to as the follicular adenoma. Because the thyroid is a very active gland, there are histologic variations which result in a multiplicity of terms. Thus, one may be confronted with such terms as the embryonal adenoma, fetal adenoma, Hürthle cell adenoma or simple adenoma. The important point is that in none of these are there any indications of invasive malignancy.

Although much less common, there is another form known as papillary adenoma which is featured by the formation of papillary processes and cyst formation. Under these circumstances, the term papillary cystadenoma is used occasionally, and yet the same specimen may produce considerable concern in the pathologic laboratory because it may resemble papillary adenocarcinoma. This is particularly true when the patient presents evidence of metastatic papillary carcinoma in regional lymph nodes adjacent to the thyroid gland and no intralesional evidence of blood vessel invasion.

Thyroid adenomas are much more frequently found in females than in the male. They are usually well encapsulated and slow growing tumors, but microscopically, they all have a significant malignant potential. This particular characteristic may be detectable only on paraffin sections, a fact which renders frozen section identification techniques somewhat dubious. Most pathologists agree that they are willing to submit a positive diagnosis whenever this is quite obvious, but there are occasions on which the same technique may provide equivocal observations. Under such circumstances, one should be appreciative of this cooperative effort and withhold definitive surgical judgment until final histologic evidence is forthcoming. This means that definitive surgical treatment must be postponed for approximately 48 hours or longer. On the other hand, the experienced surgeon in the great majority of instances should be able to come to an appropriate conclusion in order to accomplish the best immediate therapeutic result for his patient.

Before the patient with a solitary nodule is submitted to operation, it should be realized that the expectancy of malignancy may vary somewhere between 5 and 20 per cent. The differences found within various clinical surveys relate only to the obvious factor of preselection. Any series of patients reported from a large general community hospital will indicate an incidence of malignancy between 5 and 10 per cent, depending upon how many patients with multinodular goiter are included. This may rise to a figure as high as 20 per cent when the clinical experience comes from institutions with a high referral rate relative to this problem and with more strict criteria for reporting their experience. The obvious conclusion from all this data is that a solitary nodule, or a firm or enlarging nodule in a diffusely nodulated goiter, should be removed in order to identify its true character.

Whenever an unidentified solitary mass in the thyroid is exposed, much consideration should be given to the method of excision. Because it is often difficult to be sure of the diagnosis of malignancy on frozen section, and because it has been proved that inept surgical intervention can disseminate cancer cells in the operative field, current best judgment dictates that thyroid lobectomy is probably the most efficacious operation. Thus, simple lobectomy may not only be diagnostic, but completely therapeutic.

INVASIVE ADENOMA OF THE THYROID. In previous years, malignant adenomas were formerly the commonest of the thyroid carcinomas. In recent years, the relative proportion of malignant adenomas appears to be decreasing whereas true invasive papillary adenocarcinoma is becoming more common. This may represent more of a change in the way pathologists apply terminology rather than a real change in incidence. From the gross standpoint, these malignant adenomas are usually well encapsulated tumors, and are significantly larger than the more common papillary adenocarcinomas. They vary in size as do the benign adenomas and on cut surface they have a more or less distinctive salmon-pink cast, in contrast to the brown or yellow-brown of benign adenomas. They are of softer consistency than the benign adenomas and frequently show both gross and microscopic evidence of neoplastic infiltration of the capsule.

When evaluated microscopically, it is often very difficult to differentiate the malignant adenoma from a benign lesion. Approximately 40 years ago, Graham concluded that this differentiation could probably be made in about 70 per cent of specimens, basing this upon the observation that the most consistent evidence of malignancy in such lesions is vascular invasion. Other pathologists, including Broders, have continued to depend upon cytologic differences to distinguish the benign from the malignant adenoma. Other investigators point out that invasion of the capsule constitutes a more convincing criterion and is easier to measure objectively. When both microscopic invasion of blood vessels and invasion of the capsule are present, there is little doubt but that the lesion must be classified as malignant. Invasion of the capsule alone is found in approximately 70 per cent of these patients, whereas both phenomena can be demonstrated in approximately 40 per cent.

A full microscopic evaluation of these adenomas is of practical significance. So long as the malignant adenoma remains within its capsule, there is no possibility of lymphatic spread because adenomas have no lymphatics. After capsular invasion, the malignant cells reach the thyroid parenchyma and metastatic invasion can take place. On the other hand, evident blood vessel invasion suggests the likelihood of blood-borne metastases and thus this criterion has, for many years, been the most significant in the minds of many pathologists. Permeation of veins and local thrombus formation, as well as tumor embolization, can be demonstrated in these lesions, though it must be realized that not all blood-borne metastases are capable of further growth. From this, it must be concluded that the prognosis for these tumors is excellent and clinical control can be accomplished by simple lobectomy. Because there is a low incidence of lymphatic invasion, radical neck dissection or supplementary radiotherapy is not routinely used for control of this lesion.

PRIMARY THYROID CARCINOMA. Amid the various reports relative to the clinical importance of thyroid cancer, there is clear evidence that the incidence of this disease is increasing every year. The cohort analysis done by Carroll indicates that in the state of New York the incidence has more than doubled from 1941 to 1962. This increase is noted in both sexes, but only in persons under the age of 55. It is believed that this is not due to any significant improvement in reporting, or diagnostic techniques, but rather that the data strongly support the hypothesis that irradiation in early childhood is a significant etiologic factor. The diversity of microscopic appearances of thyroid carcinoma and its variations in biologic behavior have made pathological classification somewhat difficult. Classifications have become greatly simplified as compared to the very complex and unusable categorizations available 30 and 40 years ago. By and large, the lesions of greatest significance are the independent carcinomas which arise from the thyroid as primary malignancies and demonstrate no pathogenetic relationship to any previous adenoma. In other words, these lesions are undoubtedly malignant tumors from their beginning and can be accurately described, histologically as well as biologically. These tumors are much more common in women than in men, but their rate of growth, their method of spread and their ability to destroy their host vary tremendously.

The simplest classification is *papillary adenocarcinoma, follicular adenocarcinoma* and *anaplastic adenocarcinoma*. Although these three categories ordinarily are sufficient, mixtures are often found such that the metastatic patterns relate more to one component than to the other. A fourth category of *sarcoma* probably should be included for the sake of thoroughness, though the lymphosarcomas and fibrosarcomas which are occasionally reported usually assume the clinical characteristics of anaplastic adenocarcinoma.

PAPILLARY ADENOCARCINOMA. Papillary adenocarcinoma accounts for at least 60 per cent of thyroid cancer. These lesions vary in size, but in general they tend to be small, varying between 1 and 3 cm. in diameter, and are usually associated with a fairly definite degree of desmoplastic reaction. This fibrosis is often rather evident and contributes to the local physical findings. These lesions are slow growing and are frequently found in patients under the age of 35. Microscopically, they are easily recognized by their papillary structure and cytologically, present the appearance of a low grade malignancy. Only one out of six such lesions is found to be a pure papillary tumor, whereas the remaining five will be found to contain varying amounts of follicular elements. As the follicular elements increase so do the degree of invasiveness and concomitant seriousness of the prognosis.

In keeping with their low grade of malignancy, the growth of papillary lesions is slow. These patients may often present a long-standing history without evidence of significant invasion of surrounding structures. In spite of their slow progression, these non-encapsulated tumors have a considerable tendency to metastasize to regional lymph nodes. Well over half of these patients present lymph node involvement in the jugular or mediastinal area. While the nodal involvement may be either considerable or limited, varying from patient to patient, it should be pointed out that these metastatic elements in lymph nodes do not tend to invade the capsule of the nodes and thus early in their course do not tend to involve the surrounding structures. As a result, these positively involved lymph nodes do not become fixed to surrounding tissues and are easily resectable. Following removal, these metastatic lesions do not tend to recur within the operative area from which they have been removed. This particular property is not shared by the primary lesion, which is definitely invasive by nature. If left alone, the primary lesion tends to invade the capsule of the thyroid and neighboring muscle, trachea and esophagus. Thus, local extension in some instances may be so great as to preclude the possibility of cure. This is far more significant in the life of the average patient than the possibility of distant metastases.

FOLLICULAR ADENOCARCINOMA. This neoplasm makes up about 20 per cent of the thyroid cancers. In its most characteristic form, it is found in patients slightly older than those with papillary lesions and there is a higher incidence of blood vessel invasion. In addition to significant regional lymph node involvement, there is a noteworthy incidence of metastases to bone and lungs. The metastases in follicular adenocarcinoma are so well differentiated that radioactive iodine often is assimilated with a detrimental effect on the growth pattern.

UNDIFFERENTIATED CARCINOMA. Undifferentiated carcinoma constitutes the residual 20 per cent of thyroid malignancies, occurs in growing lesions and shows considerable histological and cytological diversity. The follicular pattern is usually completely missing. The anaplastic cells may be round, spindle-shaped, small or large. Lesions made up of small round cells may resemble lymphosarcomas, whereas those composed chiefly of spindle cells suggest the possibility of fibrosarcoma. The undifferentiated adenocarcinomas develop in either a pre-existing goiter or within an otherwise normal gland. They have also been known to develop later in life after the patient has apparently been cured of an original slow-growing papillary lesion. These tumors infiltrate the capsule of the thyroid rather early and quickly become attached to the surrounding tissues as well as metastasizing by both the lymphatic and blood routes. The clinical course is usually rapid and almost invariably, regardless of treatment, the prognosis is hopeless. In a few instances, early local excision may be possible, but the lesion is ordinarily beyond the limits of surgical removal when first seen. Combined radiotherapy and tracheostomy may be the only palliative therapeutic aid of any value.

TREATMENT. Treatment of thyroid carcinoma is primarily surgical. The operative procedure is governed by the type and extent of the local involvement. The surgical approach to papillary follicular and mixed papillary adenocarcinoma is essentially the same for all lesions. The absolute minimal surgical procedure is unilateral thyroid lobectomy. Because these primary lesions are definitely invasive, the involved lobe must be removed as thoroughly as possible. Contralateral involvement in the opposite lobe can be demonstrated microscopically in as many as 30 per cent of these patients. In addition, there is always the likelihood of future necessity for the use of radioactive iodine in some of these patients. For these reasons, there is considerable justification in removing as much of the contralateral lobe as is compatible with the safety of the opposite pair of parathyroid glands, as well as the contralateral recurrent laryngeal nerve. Although total thyroidectomy has been occasionally advocated, this rarely seems to be practical, because of the distressing incidence of postoperative hypoparathyroidism. By preservation of a small sliver of thyroid tissue, simultaneous preservation of the contralateral parathyroids is usually assured. At a later time, this residue of thyroid tissue can be defunctionalized by the administration of a small amount of radioactive iodine if desired.

The question of dissection of cervical lymph nodes has been clouded by a variety of opinions. When one considers the fact that over 50 per cent of these patients suffer from metastatic involvement of the regional lymph nodes, the arguments relative to cosmetic results and the possibilities of residual disability seem quite minor. Fortunately, all these objections can be overcome and a logical homolateral neck dissection accomplished by following the technique developed by Marchetta and Sako. All triangles of the neck are included in the dissection, the function of the spinal accessory nerve is preserved and the contour of the neck relative to the sternocleidomastoid muscle remains unchanged. When there are palpably enlarged glands in the opposite side of the neck a similar dissection can be performed with preservation of the jugular vein.

Palliative surgical treatment also has an important place in the treatment of carcinoma of the thyroid. Because it is usually impossible to determine conclusively the resectability of any tumor prior to operation, all lesions must be explored. Although the surgical procedure may have to be limited to biopsy and some efforts to provide an airway, most surgeons are willing to make an extended effort on borderline patients in whom the lesion appears only to be attached to the trachea. An exceptional effort to free the trachea from a malignant lesion is warranted in practically all instances in which surgical removal is attempted. Although restoration of a small segment of the trachea is feasible when resection is otherwise possible, the same is not true regarding the thyroid cartilage or the larynx itself. Extensive resections which would include the adjoining larynx or esophagus at this time do not seem to be justified by current experience.

Tracheostomy should be strongly considered in any patient in whom an extensive dissection is carried out in the immediate vicinity of the larynx and trachea. This is particularly necessary when large masses of malignant tissue are left behind or when irradiation is contemplated. When the tracheostomy is established at the time of the original palliative procedure, postoperative care is made much easier and so also is the postsurgical radiotherapy better tolerated.

Adjunctive therapy. Carcinoma of the thyroid possesses certain biologic characteristics which facilitate the management of the disease when surgical treatment appears no longer to be beneficial. Although the value of cervical teleradiotherapy has been well documented, its value is largely limited to the anaplastic forms of the disease. Considerable palliation can be obtained and it is most useful when properly administered by those who are expert in this field. On the other hand, certain features of these carcinomas favor the use of thyroxine as well as radioactive iodine. In certain thyroid neoplasms, there is a definite dependency on the pituitary thyrotropic hormone for growth and progression. In addition, a sufficient number of these tumors retain the ability to trap and utilize iodides. Both these characteristics may be utilized in the management of some of the well-differentiated follicular adenocarcinomas and the mixed follicular-papillary lesions.

From the experimental standpoint, as well as clinical experience, thyrotropic hormone seems to be closely related to the evolution and progression of both benign and malignant thyroid tumors. The association of thyroid cancer with radiation during infancy and its increased incidence in areas of iodine deficiency, as well as its incidence in certain congenital goiters, would all be confirmatory of such a hypothesis. Although induced hypothyroidism permits thyroid cancer to grow at its own rate, it has been rather well proved that suppression of the thyrotropic stimulating hormone reduces the growth rate of thyroid cancer. The endogenous output of thyrotropin can be suppressed almost in its entirety by the administration of exogenous thyroid hormone. The administration of desiccated thyroid controls the growth of metastatic papillary adenocarcinoma of the thyroid for considerable periods of time.

It has become rather common practice to administer 3 or 4 grains daily of exogenous thyroid hormone to patients who have undergone operation for well-differentiated papillary-follicular or homogeneous follicular carcinomas, whether the thyroid is completely or incompletely removed. This certainly is particularly true when there is evidence that the disease has spread beyond the limits of surgical removal whether this be extensive local disease or distant metastatic involvement. Whether one uses desiccated thyroid, thyroxine, triiodothyronine or combinations of these, the medications ordinarily should be increased until there is some evidence of hyperthyroidism, as manifested by tachycardia, anxiety or nervousness. The dosage then can be reduced slightly until the side effects disappear.

Patients who have known residual malignant disease may also be candidates for therapy with radioactive iodine. Although treatment with both agents should not be considered mutually exclusive, only general principles can be offered as guides to appropriate therapy. Asymptomatic metastases are more commonly first treated with thyrotropic suppression. When regression or control of the metastatic lesions appears to be in progress, there is little need for supplementary radioiodine. Whenever this treatment fails to produce regression, the use of radioiodine is obviously justified. This also may be true when a tumor appears to regain its original autonomy and breaks through the previous thyrotropic suppression. Such tumors often become ideal neoplasms for treatment with radioiodine. In some of the older patients who once showed signs of considerable iodine uptake in the metastases, radioiodine often is most beneficial and it can be administered while suppressive doses of thyroxine are also administered.

THYROID CANCER IN CHILDREN. If we were to define a child as someone under the age of 16, it would appear that less than 800 examples of this lesion have been reported in the world literature. Although this disease may be thought of as uncommon, it can no longer be regarded as unusually rare. Winship has made a study of this condition and has developed a registry for these patients. His data indicate that the sites of residence of the patients were widely scattered and that there is no relationship to known goiterous areas. It would appear that thyroid carcinoma in children is more frequently found in areas in which interest in the disease is high. Three-fourths of the patients gave a history of previous irradiation to the head and neck region for treatment of the so-called enlarged thymus, hypertrophied tonsils and adenoids, hemangiomas, cervical adenitis and various skin conditions.

Pathologically, 70 per cent of these cancers are pure or mixed papillary carcinomas and approximately 20 per cent are follicular in type. The remaining are designated as undifferentiated. In only one-fourth of the children was the carcinoma localized to the thyroid gland at the time of the initial examination. Although three-fourths of the patients presented cervical lymph node involvement, there was considerable variation in the therapeutic approach. As one might imagine, in only about one-third of the patients was an operation alone the treatment applied; half of the patients received a combination of operation and external radiation. Twenty per cent of the patients received radioactive iodine and 10 per cent underwent biopsy which was followed only by external radiation.

Very few publications have tabulated patients followed more than ten years. In this regard, children should be ideal subjects for a long follow-up project. Winship has followed 264 of these patients for more than ten years and he reports that their general course seems to resemble that of the disease as found in the adult. Of his entire group, 18 per cent already have died from thyroid cancer. Half of these died during the first ten years, 20 per cent in the second ten-year period and 8 per cent after having had the cancer for 20 years or more. The distribution of cell type among those who died was similar to that for the entire group except for a slightly higher proportion of undifferentiated tumors. Fifty-eight per cent of the patients died of papillary cancer, 13 per cent of follicular and 29 per cent of undifferentiated cancer.

THYROIDITIS

ACUTE AND SUBACUTE THYROIDITIS. The common form of active thyroiditis presents an irregular clinical inflammatory course and usually is nonsuppurative. Some clinicians believe this to be on a viral basis and commonly associated with an antecedent upper respiratory infection. The onset can be sudden, accompanied by a mild fever and tenderness localized to the anatomical extent of the gland. Although the process may begin in one lobe, it usually involves both lobes. The thyroid gland becomes enlarged, tender and painful and occasionally can become so severe as to produce dysphagia and hoarseness. This process is self-limited and usually extends over periods of weeks or even months. In the past, small doses of superficial x-ray therapy were advised, but more recently cortisone has produced dramatic relief of symptoms because of its nonspecific anti-inflammatory action. The patients must be continued on this treatment for a considerable time in order to prevent an immediate recurrence of symptoms whenever the drug is stopped too soon.

In a few instances, acute thyroiditis has been known to go on to suppuration. When this takes place, a localized intraglandular abscess will form which must be drained. Uneventful recovery can be expected following this procedure, although drainage can be expected to continue for three to four weeks in some patients.

CHRONIC THYROIDITIS. In recent years, there seems to be an increased incidence of the various forms of chronic thyroiditis. The most common of these is known as Hashimoto's thyroiditis, or struma lymphomatosa. The second form is known as granulomatous or giant cell thyroiditis and the least common is known as Riedel's struma.

There have been numerous controversial reports on these three forms of thyroiditis relative to etiology, classification, pathogenesis and therapy. In addition, recent statistical studies have indicated that there may be a significant association between the presence of thyroid carcinoma and chronic thyroiditis. These figures have varied between 9 and 22 per cent.

Hashimoto's disease is characteristically found in women in middle life, and it is conjectured that this may be due to some type of reaction in the thyroid gland owing to the presence of circulating antibodies as yet unidentified. If the recent statistics are correct, it is conceivable that antigens from some thyroid neoplasms may be implicated in the development of chronic thyroiditis. Although the present data suggest that thyroiditis may occur secondarily to the presence of thyroid carcinoma, this does not necessarily mean that it should be regarded as a premalignant lesion nor should it be treated by radical operative procedures.

Clinically, the gland is moderately enlarged and quite firm, with definite nodules evident to palpation. The history is that of a very slowly enlarging mass in the area of the thyroid. Microscopically, considerable lymphoid tissue is to be found with varying amounts of fibrous tissue intermixed. The follicular structure of the thyroid is destroyed and the usual clinical hypothyroid state is easily understood.

Diagnosis can sometimes be verified by needle biopsy, but whenever in doubt, biopsy must be performed. This is particularly true as more of these patients are found to harbor simultaneously thyroid carcinoma. After the diagnosis is established, administration of desiccated thyroid over a long period of time will correct the hypothyroidism and in some instances also produce some degree of shrinkage of the gland.

Granulomatous or giant cell thyroiditis represents another form of chronic change within the thyroid gland that appears to be of unknown etiology. On occasion, it has been associated with antecedent upper respiratory infection and in such instances, the onset seemingly has been rather sudden with involvement beginning in one lobe. This may gradually extend to involve the entire gland. It usually does not originate in a gland that has been previously involved by other evident degenerative change. These patients manifest varying degrees of local pressure symptoms, dysphagia, voice changes and varying degrees of the anxiety state which such a symptom complex can understandably produce. Operation is ordinarily not necessary unless the symptoms reach such magnitude as to cause considerable difficulty. In those patients with unilateral involvement, a simple hemithyroidectomy will suffice. In others, subtotal thyroidectomy may be necessary in order to eradicate more completely the mechanical complications this disease produces.

The most infrequent of all of these changes is referred to as Riedel's struma. This rare entity has also been known as ligneous thyroiditis because it presents as a rather invasive fibrous type of change in the thyroid, frequently involving only one lobe. This may involve both lobes and when this occurs, there is a resulting mass of dense fibrous tissue which produces extreme pressure problems in the area of the trachea. As this develops, one can easily imagine how it may grossly simulate a slowly developing carcinoma from its physical signs. The stony hardness and minor irregularity along the surface and considerable fixation to the surrounding tissues all suggest the possibility of carcinoma. On the other hand, the involved lobe or lobes are usually not appreciably enlarged. The situation may be further confused by the fact that the fibroblastic process may invade the adjacent tissues, producing pressure on the esophagus or trachea that appears to be out of proportion to the size of the pathologic change. Although unilateral involvement may displace the trachea, bilateral involvement produces a striking dyspnea because of the significant compression that results. Some of these patients also show some evidence of mild hypothyroidism.

At the time of operation, the attachment of the thyroid lobe to the surrounding fascia, strap muscles and trachea may produce a striking degree of fixation. These attachments to adjacent vital structures make any attempt at thorough removal most hazardous. Frequently, it is almost impossible to find a natural line of cleavage between the tissues, especially in patients in whom the disease has been present for some period of time. These glands are grayish-white, very hard and avascular. The microscopic appearance is that of extreme fibrosis, with destruction of the thyroid epithelium. Although hemithyroidectomy might be the ideal procedure, the surgeon may very often limit the operation to simple removal of the isthmus. This technique itself may be sufficient to free the trachea, allowing the contracted lobes to fall away to either side, and thus alleviating the symptoms secondary to the obvious fibrotic tracheal compression.

THE PARATHYROID GLANDS

The parathyroid glands were discovered only as recently as 1880, and it was not until 1909 that low serum blood calcium levels were associated with hypoparathyroidism. In 1916, Biedl produced excellent experimental evidence to indicate that the parathyroids have an internal secretion, but it was not until 1925 that Mandl successfully applied this information and removed a parathyroid adenoma for the correction of a classic example of advanced osteitis fibrosa cystica. Following this operation, there was definite clinical improvement and recalcification of the bones.

In the years immediately following this dramatic clinical experience, attention was directed solely toward the skeletal system as regards clinical manifestation of primary hyperparathyroidism. In the last 20 years, the work of Cope and others has directed our attention to the urogenital system. It has been found that the urogenital system was involved secondarily by stone formation, or diffuse calcinosis, more often than was the skeletal system involved by either osteitis fibrosis cystica or diffuse osteoporosis. It is now realized that the small parathyroid glands, by controlling the level of serum calcium, have a widespread effect. The metabolic aspect of these glands represents an interesting facet in medicine.

ANATOMY

The parathyroid glands are usually four in number and are oval, yellowish-brown bodies approximately 5 mm. long and 2 mm. thick. Although the glands are usually in close proximity to the thyroid itself, the anatomical location may be variable owing to certain factors of embryogenesis. The inferior parathyroids arise in a symmetrical fashion from the third pharyngeal pouch in close relationship to the origins of the thymus gland. The inferior parathyroid glands migrate caudally with the thymic tissue and tend to show some variation in eventual position in the adult. Thus, it has been shown that parathyroid bodies have been found anywhere between the angle of the jaw to the anterior mediastinum, but not lower than the lowest portion of the thymus gland.

The superior parathyroids arise from the same basic structure in the fourth pouch in close proximity to the ultimobranchial bodies. As a result, the superior parathyroids are generally found located on the posterior aspect of the thyroid at approximately the junction of the upper and middle thirds. The upper pair receive their blood supply from the superior thyroid artery, whereas the lower parathyroids are usually supplied by the inferior thyroid artery. A supernumerary gland, if present, will be found usually associated with the lower pair of parathyroids. The parathyroid glands may lie completely within the thyroid or within a deep crevice.

Histologically, the parathyroids are made up of sheets of epithelial cells separated by sinusoids. The major cell is called the chief cell, which shows a rather scanty cytoplasm and a deeply staining nucleus. The waterclear cells are distinguished by their vacuolated cytoplasm and small nuclei. In addition, there are a group of oxyphil cells which have granules in their cytoplasm that stain red with acid dyes. These do not usually appear until after puberty.

PHYSIOLOGY

The early work done by Hanson in 1923 and Collip in 1925, and the later work of Rasmussen reported in 1961, clearly define the activities of the parathyroid hormone. The parathyroid glands secrete the hormone if serum calcium is low, and a rise in serum calcium lessens the activity of the glands. The hormone increases tubular reabsorption of calcium and increases the tubular excretion of the phosphate ion. Because of the reciprocal relationship between serum calcium and serum phosphate concentrations, loss of phosphate through the kidney results in a rise in serum calcium. Although the parathyroid hormone releases both calcium and phosphate from bone, the kidney excretes the phosphate in much larger amounts, with the result that there is a definite decrease in the level of serum phosphate under such circumstances. In addition, experimentation has proved that parathyroid hormone increases the absorption of calcium in the gastrointestinal tract, thus tending to increase serum calcium and reduce serum phosphate, at the same time maintaining a balance between the levels of the two ions. A recently discovered hormone, named both calcitonin and thyrocalcitonin, has not been sufficiently established by human studies to warrant further description.

PATHOLOGICAL VARIANTS

FUNCTIONAL ADENOMA. Parathyroid adenomas constitute the single largest group of lesions which account for primary hyperparathyroidism. These adenomas are composed of the chief cell type and characteristically are surrounded by a thin collar of compressed normal tissue. Approximately 75 per cent of these adenomas develop in the lower glands and 10 to 15 per cent may be aberrant in location. They can be found in the mediastinum, within the substance of the thyroid gland or behind the esophagus. On rare occasions, two adenomas have been found in the same patient, but never more. In addition, carcinoma of a parathyroid gland can occur and has been known to be able to produce hyperparathyroidism. In these instances, the involved glands become atrophic, a finding which contributes to the diagnosis. Adenomas have been reported in each decade of life from the second to the eighth with a preponderance among females in a ratio of 3:1. No apparent geographical influence has been noted, but at least 14 families have been reported in which the incidence is sufficiently high to suggest the existence of true familial hyperparathyroidism.

Grossly, an adenoma is usually ellipsoidal in shape with three unequal axes. These tumors are smooth, soft and of variable texture, but they are always characteristically encapsulated. This is important in differentiating an adenoma from a malignant lesion.

PRIMARY PARATHYROID HYPERPLASIA. Primary parathyroid hyperplasia involves all the glands in the process of hyperplasia and hypertrophy. All the glands are encapsulated and irregular in shape, and may even have pseudopod projections. Both the chief cell and the water-clear cell are capable of participating in this process of hyperplasia. The work of Cope and his co-workers has done a great deal to clarify the microscopic aspects of this disease. The clinical symptoms produced by the hyperplastic glands are similar to those produced by both adenoma and functioning carcinoma. A large number of patients have shown urinary tract calcifications.

SECONDARY HYPERPARATHYROIDISM. Secondary parathyroid hyperplasia and hyperparathyroidism should be recognized as an entity because the differential diagnosis between the primary and secondary forms may often be of practical importance. Secondary parathyroid hyperplasia is found in connection with renal disease. Retention of phosphate by the damaged kidney leads to elevated serum phosphates and reduction in serum calcium. The parathyroid gland, therefore, responds by producing hyperplasia and serum calcium may either remain low or return to normal. In children with severe renal disease, the secondary parathyroid hyperplasia can produce considerable decalcification of the bony skeleton and the resulting clinical situation is referred to as renal rickets.

PARATHYROID CYSTS. Parathyroid cysts are an uncommon cause of masses in the neck which require surgical intervention. On occasions, these have been reported as functional entities but many have actually been incidental findings at the time of thyroid surgery. If associated with hyperfunction, they may represent cystic degeneration of a previous adenoma. When discovered, they are usually removed for the sake of thoroughness and identification.

Diagnosis of Hyperparathyroidism

Although this diagnosis cannot be established without the aid of exacting laboratory determinations, it should be apparent that a high index of clinical suspicion is necessary for proper screening of these patients. The increased calcium excretion in the urine can lead to renal calculi or to progressive kidney damage with diffuse calcinosis within the renal parenchyma. Even patients with a single renal calculus should be screened for hyperparathyroidism. Polydipsia, polyuria and hypertension are also fairly common findings in advanced phases of this condition. Unfortunately, the renal pathology often persists after correction of the primary hyperparathyroidism is accomplished.

In another group of patients, appreciation of generalized osteoporosis may be quite helpful in reaching the eventual diagnosis. Diagnostic changes in the phalanges and in the lamina dura about the teeth as well as cyst formation within the mandible are classic findings. This process may go on to fracture of the long bones, as well as collapse of vertebral bodies. Only in occasional persons can a diet high in calcium conceal some of these bone changes.

Patients with active peptic ulceration and pancreatitis are infrequently seen with concomitant hyperparathyroidism. For this reason, it has been suggested that all patients with active gastric or duodenal ulceration as well as patients with pancreatitis should be evaluated for this likelihood. In the past, some long-term ulcer patients have demonstrated a high serum calcium level with a normal or high phosphate level along with poor renal function. More recent studies would suggest that this milk-alkali syndrome might very well be on the basis of hyperparathyroidism rather than a complication of prolonged ulcer therapy.

A high level of blood calcium can lead to hypotonicity in skeletal muscle and a generalized diminution in neuromuscular irritability. The simple symptoms of backache and fatigue can often result from this phenomenon. In addition, diminished mental acuity and loss of memory have been found associated with elevated blood calcium levels. In a few patients, severe exacerbations have led to acute parathyroid crises with uncontrollable tachycardia and vomiting, superimposed upon the more common features of generalized weakness, mental deterioration and headaches. Eventual renal failure can contribute to the death of these patients as the unrecognized syndrome progresses.

Once the suspicion of hyperparathyroidism has been entertained, laboratory confirmation by examination of blood and urine becomes a necessity. Of greatest clinical importance is a reliable laboratory with considerable concern over the accuracy of reproducible serum calcium levels. Although there are admitted vagaries in the studies of calcium metabolism, the diagnosis can often be substantiated when a patient exhibits two or three consistently elevated serum calcium values.

The next most reliable indication, serum phosphorus, is helpful in only about 70 per cent of the patients. Calcium and phosphorus levels should be checked and repeated against known normals, followed by calcium excretion studies. If the urinary excretion of calcium is greater than basic calcium intake, this is further confirmatory evidence of the diagnosis of hyperparathyroidism. Chamberlain and his associates have used diffusable serum calcium levels in the diagnosis of primary hyperparathyroidism and this laboratory determination seems to be of considerable importance in eliminating negative exploratory operations.

A radioisotope scanning technique for the identification of hyperactive parathyroid tissue has recently been developed by Potchen. Preoperative scintiscans with a tagged methionine compound that collects in the parathyroids have shown moderate success in localization of adenomas, parathyroid hyperplasia and also malignant neoplasms of the parathyroids. This external monitoring has been made possible by the synthesis of a gamma-emitting analog of methionine, selenium-75 tagged selenomethionine. Selenium substitutes for sulfur in the methionine molecule under these circumstances. The adjacent thyroid tissue is first suppressed by generous doses of triiodothyronine for four to five days prior to the scintiscan. The intravenously injected isotope then accumulates wherever the parathyroid activity is greatest. Four consecutive scans are taken over a 90-minute period. Although both false positives and false negatives have resulted from this technique, it is possible that further improvements may make this a diagnostically valuable tool.

Before an eventual decision is made in favor of surgical exploration, it is obvious that a host of conditions which resemble hyperparathyroidism in one way or another must be eliminated during the clinical evaluation. It is not enough to have knowledge of the conditions entering into the differential diagnosis; rather, one should be assured that the data on which the differential diagnosis depends have been obtained under conditions of rigid control. In addition, the determinations must be repeated, sometimes frequently over a substantial period of time. Hyperparathyroidism, like many other endocrine conditions, tends to fluctuate in intensity and often the diagnosis can be discarded or accepted merely by clinical observation.

SURGICAL EXPLORATION

The glands are located obviously in approximately three-fourths of the patients, whereas in one-fourth they will be located in obscure sites and are often difficult to find. After each has been searched out in turn, identification is necessary and often this means that a definite biopsy must be made. When discovered, the usual procedure is first to remove the enlarged parathyroid mass and submit it for frozen section. If the pathologist is able to identify a delicate rim of normal parathyroid tissue around a central core of tightly packed chief cells, it is most likely that the diagnosis is that of parathyroid adenoma. Upon receiving this report, the surgeon ordinarily will be content to evaluate the other three parathyroids merely to exclude the rare possibility of a second adenoma.

If only hyperplasia is reported, either of the chief cell type or the water-clear type, confirmatory evidence will be found if at least three of the four glands can be identified as also showing hyperplasia. In principle, of course, all four glands should be involved. The treatment of choice is resection of three of the four, and a subtotal resection of the fourth. The number of parathyroids varies from two to six, but up to ten bits of para-

thyroid tissue have been reported in one patient.

On occasion, a thorough search reveals neither an adenoma nor good evidence of hyperplasia. If three atrophic glands have been found, but the fourth cannot be discovered, a total thyroid lobectomy should be done on the site of the missing parathyroid in the hope that it may be found buried within the thyroid lobe itself. The only other alternative is to search the anterior mediastinum. In rare instances, this may require median splitting of the sternum for adequate exposure.

Under normal circumstances following the removal of a functioning adenoma, the serum calcium levels return to normal within 24 to 48 hours. Recalcification of the bones is fairly rapid and the symptoms caused by hypercalcemia disappear. On the other hand, obvious skeletal deformities and permanent renal damage may persist. Early in the postoperative course one may be confronted with the immediate appearance of clinical hypoparathyroidism. Although this may be proof that the significant hyperfunctioning parathyroid tissue has been removed, it should not be a matter of alarm. Severe tetany can be controlled by intravenous calcium and later calcium can be given by mouth until the remaining parathyroid tissue becomes sufficiently functional. On occasion, vitamin D or dihydrotachysterol may be necessary along with the oral calcium.

READING REFERENCES

Adams, H. A., and Murphy, R.: Management of primary hyperparathyroidism. Surg. Gyn. & Obst. *116*:45, 1963.

Albers, G. D.: Branchial anomalies. J.A.M.A. *183*:399, 1963.

Appaix, A.: Tumors of the Thyroid Gland. New York, American Elsevier Publishing Company, 1966.

Arey, L. B.: Developmental Anatomy. 7th ed. Philadelphia, W. B. Saunders Company, 1965.

Barnes, B. A., and Cope, O.: Carcinoma of parathyroid glands: report of 10 cases with endocrine function. J.A.M.A. *178*:556, 1961.

Batsakis, J. G., and Nishiyama, R. H.: Goiter in childhood and adolescence. Arch. Surg. *86*:378, 1963.

Bill, A. H., Jr.: Cysts and sinuses of the neck of thyroglossal and branchial origin. S. Clin. North America *36*:1599, 1956.

Black, B. M.: Problems in the treatment of hyperparathyroidism. S. Clin. North America *41*:1061, 1961.

Bowers, R. F.: Hyperthyroidism: comparative results of medical and (I[131]) surgical therapy. Ann. Surg. *162*:478, 1965.

Bradshaw, H. H., Boyce, W. H., Holleman, I. L., and Smith, L. C.: Long-term results in patients with parathyroid surgery. Ann. Surg. *160*:1017, 1964.

Brown, P. M., and Judd, E. S.: Thyroglossal duct cysts and

sinuses: results of radical (Sistrunk) operation. Am. J. Surg. 102:494, 1961.

Buckner, F., Lyons, C., and Perkins, R.: Management of lacerations of the great vessels of the upper thorax and base of the neck. Surg. Gyn. & Obst. 107:135, 1958.

Carroll, R. E., Haddon, W., Jr., Handy, V. H., and Wieben, E. E., Sr.: Thyroid cancer: cohort analysis of increasing incidence in New York State, 1941-1962. J. Nat. Cancer Inst. 33:277, 1964.

Caswell, H. T., Robbins, R. R., and Rosemond, G. P.: Definitive treatment of 536 cases of hyperthyroidism with I¹³¹ or surgery. Ann. Surg. 164:593, 1966.

Catlin, D.: Surgery for head and neck lymphomas. Surgery 60:1160, 1966.

Catz, B., Petit, D. W., Schwartz, H., Davis, F., McCammon, C., and Stark, P.: Treatment of cancer of the thyroid postoperatively with suppressive thyroid medication, radioactive iodine and thyroid-stimulating hormone. Cancer 12:371, 1959.

Clark, R. L., Ibanez, M. L., and White, E. C.: What constitutes an adequate operation for carcinoma of the thyroid? Arch. Surg. 92:23, 1966.

Colcock, B. P.: Primary hyperthyroidism: results of surgical treatment. S. Clin. North America 42:673, 1962.

Collip, J. B.: The extraction of a parathyroid hormone which will prevent or control parathyroid tetany and which regulates the level of blood calcium. J. Biol. Chem. 63:395, 1925.

Cope, O., Barnes, B. A., Castleman, B., Mueller, G. C. E., and Roth, S. I.: Vicissitudes of parathyroid surgery: trials of diagnosis and management in 51 patients with a variety of disorders. Ann. Surg. 154:491, 1961.

Cutler, R. E., Reiss, E., and Ackerman, L. V.: Familial hyperparathyroidism. New England J. Med. 40:765, 1964.

DeLawter, D. S., and Winship, T.: Follow-up study of adults treated with roentgen rays for thyroid disease. Cancer 16:1028, 1963.

Dische, S.: Radioisotope scan applied to detection of carcinoma in thyroid swelling. Cancer 17:473, 1964.

Dunn, J. T., and Chapman, E. M.: Rising incidence of hypothyroidism after radioactive-iodine therapy in thyrotoxicosis. New England J. Med. 271:1037, 1964.

Fogelman, M. J., and Stewart, R. O.: Penetrating wounds of the neck. Am. J. Surg. 91:581, 1956.

France, C. J., Kouchy, C., Hergt, K., and Brines, O. A.: Relationship of histology to prognosis in thyroid carcinoma. Arch. Surg. 86:583, 1963.

Gaillard, P. J., Talmage, R. V., and Budy, A. M.: The Parathyroid Glands. Chicago, University of Chicago Press, 1965.

Gibbs, J. C., Jr., Halligan, E. J., and McKeown, J. E.: Scintiscanning the thyroid nodule. Arch. Surg. 90:323, 1965.

Goodman, J., McClintock, J., Denton, G. R., and Stein, A.: Cystic hygromas in adults. Arch. Surg. 86:641, 1963.

Gould, E. A., Hirsch, A., and Brecher, I.: Complications arising in the course of thyroidectomy. Arch. Surg. 90:81, 1965.

Halnan, K. E.: Influence of age and sex on incidence and prognosis of thyroid cancer—three hundred forty-four cases followed for 10 years. Cancer. 19:1534, 1966.

Hawk, W. A., Crile, G., Jr., Hazard, J. B., and Barrett, D.L.: Needle biopsy of the thyroid gland. Surg. Gyn. & Obst. 122:1053, 1966.

Hertz, S., and Roberts, A.: Radioactive iodine in the study of thyroid physiology: VII. The use of radioactive iodine therapy in hyperthyroidism. J.A.M.A. 131:81, 1946.

Hirabayashi, R. W., and Lindsay, S.: Relationship of thyroid carcinoma and chronic thyroiditis. Surg. Gyn. & Obst. 121:243, 1965.

Hora, J. F.: Deep neck infections. Arch. Otol. 77:129, 1963.

Hubay, C. A.: Soft tissue injuries of the cervical regions. Internat. Abstr. Surg. 111:511, 1960.

Krach, L. V., Soule, E. H., and Masson, J. K.: Benign and malignant neurilemmomas of the head and neck. Surg. Gyn. & Obst. 111:211, 1960.

Levinson, M. P., and Cooper, J. F.: Urological findings in 58 surgically verified cases of parathyroid adenoma. J. Urol. 96:1, 1965.

Lichtenstein, M. E.: Acute injuries involving the large blood vessels in the neck. Surg. Gyn. & Obst. 85:165, 1947.

Marchetta, F. C., and Sako, K.: Modified neck dissection for carcinoma of thyroid gland. Surg. Gyn. & Obst. 119:551, 1964.

McGinty, C. P., and Lischer, C. E.: Surgical significance of parathyroid cysts. Surg. Gyn. & Obst. 117:703, 1963.

Metropol, H. J., and Myers, R. T.: Hyperthyroidism: review of 277 surgically treated cases. Arch. Surg. 84:615, 1962.

Morfit, H. M.: Cancer of the thyroid. Surgery 59:894, 1966.

Nelson, W. R.: Carotid body tumors. Surgery 51:326, 1962.

Pate, J. W., and Wilson, H.: Arterial injuries of the base of the neck. Arch. Surg. 89:1106, 1964.

Payne, R. L., Jr., and Fitchett, C. W.: Hyperparathyroid crisis; survey of literature and report of two additional cases. Ann. Surg. 161:737, 1965.

Plested, W. G., III, and Pollock, W. F.: Radioactive iodine, antithyroid drugs and surgery in treatment of hyperthyroidism. Arch. Surg. 94:517, 1967.

Plummer, H. S.: Results of administering iodine to patients having exophthalmic goiter. J.A.M.A. 80:1955, 1923.

Potchen, E. J., Wilson, R. E., and Dealy, J. G., Jr.: External parathyroid scanning with selenomethionine-SE⁷⁵ Ann. Surg. 162:492, 1965.

Quinn, J. L., III, and Behinfar, M.: Radioisotope scanning of the thyroid. J.A.M.A. 199:170, 1967.

Rasmussen, H.: Parathyroid hormone. Nature and mechanism of action. Am. J. Med. 30:112, 1961.

Reeve, T. S., Rundle, F. F., Hales, I. B., Epps, R. G., Thomas, I. D., Indyk, J. S., Myhill, J., and Oddie, T. H.: Investigation and management of intrathoracic goiter. Surg. Gyn. & Obst. 115:22, 1962.

Rose, R. G., and Kelsey, M. P.: Radioactive iodine in diagnosis and treatment of thyroid cancer. Cancer 16:896, 1963.

Rosenberg, J. C., and Cushner, G. B.: Biochemical basis of thyroid crisis. Am. Surgeon 31:354, 1965.

Rosvoll, R. V., and Winship, T.: Thyroid carcinoma and pregnancy. Surg. Gyn. & Obst. 121:1039, 1965.

Roth, S. I.: Pathology of the parathyroids in hyperparathyroidism. Arch. Path. 73:495, 1962.

Silliphant, W. M., Klinck, G. H., and Levitan, M. S.: Thyroid carcinoma and death: clinicopathologic study of 193 autopsies. Cancer 17:513, 1964.

Silverberg, S. G., and Vidone, R. A.: Adenoma and carcinoma of the thyroid. Cancer 19:1053, 1966.

Smedal, M. I., Salzman, F. A., and Meissner, W. A.: The value of 2 mv. roentgen-ray therapy in differentiated thyroid carcinoma. Am. J. Roentgenol. 99:352, 1967.

Snedecor, P. A., and Groshong, L. E.: Carcinoma of the thyroglossal duct. Surgery 58:969, 1965.

Socolow, E. L., Hashizuma, A., Neriishi, S., and Niitani, R.: Thyroid carcinoma in man after exposure to ionizing radiation—a summary of the findings in Hiroshima and Nagasaki. New England J. Med. 268:406, 1963.

Stanbury, J. B., and DeGroot, L. J.: Problems of hypothyroidism after I¹³¹ therapy of hyperthyroidism. New England J. Med. 271:195, 1964.

Starr, P., Jaffe, H. L., and Oettinger, L.: Late results of I¹³¹ treatment of hyperthyroidism in 73 children and adults. J. Nucl. Med. 5:81, 1964.

Stevens, L. E., Bloomer, A., and Castleton, K. B.: Familial hyperparathyroidism. Arch. Surg. 94:524, 1967.

Thompson, N. W., and Fry, W. J.: Thyroid crisis. Arch. Surg. 89:512, 1964.

Tollefsen, H. R., DeCosse, J. J., and Hutter, R. V. P.: Papillary carcinoma of the thyroid—a clinical and pathological study of 70 fatal cases. Cancer 17:1035, 1964.

Weissman, S., and Horwitz, S.: Sinus of the first branchial cleft. Plast. & Reconstruct. Surg. 31:79, 1962.

Wetzel, N.: Carotid angiography in diagnosis and treatment of tumors of the neck. Arch. Surg. 94:954, 1957.

Wilder, W. T., Frame, B., and Haubrich, W. S.: Peptic ulcer

in primary hyperparathyroidism: an analysis of 52 cases. Ann. Int. Med. *55*:885, 1961.

Wilson, H.: Carotid body tumors. Surgery *59*:483, 1966.

Wilson, R. E., Bernhard, W. G., Polet, H., and Moore, F. D.: Hyperparathyroidism: problem of acute parathyroid intoxication. Ann. Surg. *159*:79, 1964.

Winship, T., and Rosvoll, R. V.: Childhood thyroid carcinoma. Cancer *14*:734, 1961.

Woolner, L. B., McConahey, W. M., and Beahrs, O. H.: Surgical aspects of thyroiditis. Am. J. Surg. *104*:666, 1962.

Wychulis, A. R., and Beahrs, O. H.: Bilateral chemodectomas. Arch. Surg. *91*:690, 1965.

Chapter 18

THE BREASTS

by
IAN MACDONALD, M.D.

IAN MACDONALD, a Canadian by birth, was educated at McGill University and had an interest in the pathology of tumors, particularly cancer, throughout his medical career. He had the quality of combining an exacting biostatistical and scientific attitude with the surgeon's desire for utilizing every possible therapeutic approach to the cure of cancer. Before his recent tragic death, he meticulously revised this chapter on a subject to which he had devoted many years of his professional life.

INTRODUCTION

In recent years, the female breast has achieved an unjustifiable peak of social significance in the United States of America, with primary emphasis on its volumetric status and anatomic prominence. Such aesthetic preoccupations have been more than matched by an enhancement of clinical and scientific interest in the complex endocrinologic background of mammary growth and development, function and dysfunction, dysplasia and neoplasia.

This is an organ which has commanded the interest of surgeons since the birth of surgical art and practice, from Celsus to Halsted and Meyer. As this century has reached and passed its midpoint by nearly 20 years, the breast would yet be of dominant surgical interest for a single reason—its unenviable distinction as the leading organ-site of cancer in American and European women. This numerical priority was apparent in the earliest reliable data on the relative frequency of malignant neoplasms by anatomic origin. Even more impelling is the failure to achieve any definitive improvement in rates of mortality from breast cancer. For three decades or more a broadening scientific and educational basis for the education and training of surgeons has made proper the expression "the art and science of surgery." But breast cancer has remained singularly resistant both to improvements in surgical techniques and their more general availability in the United States.

The mammary epithelium is entirely dependent on hormonal factors for normal growth and differentiation. There is now satisfactory knowledge of the complex interplay of hormones of hypophyseal, ovarian and adrenocortical origin responsible for the cyclic, lactational and some of the dysplastic changes in mammary tissues. But investigative efforts toward an elucidation of hormonal influences in neoplasia have been uniformly unproductive. The enigmatic relationship of hormonal factors to breast cancer is most apparent in the phenomenon of responsiveness of some disseminated forms of the disease to hormonal alterations. Although the significance of such responsiveness has been recognized for nearly 20 years, has been the subject of repeated clinical investigations, and has stimulated a variety of interdisciplinary research programs seeking a biochemical basis for its identification, there is yet no knowledge of its nature.

The breast provides a double challenge to the surgeon. It is an organ with one disease which is of dominant importance—cancer. It is an organ in which "cancer" indicates a small constellation of disparate malignant neoplasms. As of the year 1968, two premises are inescapable:

The application of the surgical method, which is to say extirpative efforts in its local (primary) and regional (secondary) sites, has been exploited to a maximal level of curative effectiveness. In the remaining and major fraction of patients, systemic dissemination of the neoplasm has occurred before operative treatment is possible.

Any further reduction of mortality and morbidity must await entirely new approaches to treatment or prophylaxis, yet to be born of research. The highly complex hormonal factors on which both normal and abnormal

400   *Chapter 18*   THE BREASTS

growth of mammary epithelium is dependent offer the most promising, immediate avenue to such future objectives.

Other disorders of the human breast, or those of non-neoplastic nature, are of relatively minor importance. Inflammatory states, specific or nonspecific, occur rarely. Developmental abnormalities are seldom noted in Occidental women. Most traumata nowadays are sustained in motor vehicle accidents.

Differential diagnosis of mammary disease is limited, in practical terms, to dysplastic states; benign neoplasms, most often fibroadenoma, and malignant neoplasms, most often carcinoma.

Both the benign and malignant forms of neoplasm share the same single, clinical sign in most instances: the presence of abnormal, indurative change in consistency of mammary tissue, usually amounting to a space-occupying or three-dimensional tumor. But some of the patients, with dysplastic changes only, may also have hyperplastic foci, more often regressive-involutionary changes which are accompanied by three-dimensional lumps as impressive as many carcinomata. The dysplastic focus may mimic carcinoma to the confusion of the most experienced examiner.

Thus, the most important single problem to be determined on physical examination becomes obvious: Is there discoverable a genuine, space-occupying tumor? If so, the physician must take steps toward securing an exact, which is to say, histologic diagnosis. For this dictum, there is but one reason: only by the histologic method is it possible to determine whether the true lump in the breast is neoplastic and whether benign or malignant in nature.

No other maneuvers ancillary to careful physical examination are entirely reliable. Thus, the responsibility of decision for or against diagnostic action must be based on the physician's ability to develop a *tactus eruditus* in examination of the breasts. Development of skill in palpation of the breasts should be regarded as an absolute requirement for every clinician who undertakes such responsibility. Inability of the clinician properly to evaluate changes in mammary texture and consistency leads to many unnecessary exploratory procedures for biopsy of non-existent lesions.

In any unselected group of women whose presenting complaint is of the breast, a majority will be found to have some phase of

Table 1. *Approximate Frequency of Histologic Diagnoses for 100 Excisions of Three-Dimensional Tumors of the Breast*

Dysplasia		35
Gross cysts*	10	
Other space-occupying variants	25	
Inflammatory states		3
Fat necrosis		
Plasma cell mastitis		
Pyogenic mastitis		
Benign neoplasms		10
Fibroadenoma	8	
Ductal papilloma	1	
Lipoma, adenoma and "esoterica"	1	
Malignant neoplasms		52
Carcinoma	51	
Sarcoma	1	

* Aspiration should provide both diagnosis and treatment for most of the gross cysts.

dysplasia, cancer being next most common, followed by fibroadenoma. The small remainder constitute the unusual and esoteric mammary lesions.

About one-third of patients with dysplastic disease will have developed some phase of the process resulting in a three-dimensional tumor: gross cysts, sclerosing reaction or persistent focal hyperplasia. About four out of ten women with complaints concerning the breast present true, mensurable tumors requiring surgical, diagnostic action.

With reasonable skill in physical examination, patients with three-dimensional tumors should be separable from women presenting only changes in texture or consistency in breast tissue but without space-occupying foci. On this basis, for each 100 women who are advised of the need for excision or biopsy of a suspect area, a histologic diagnosis of neoplastic disease should be made nearly twice as often as states of non-neoplasia, as shown in Table 1. An unreasonable relative increase in dysplastic states is a reflection of the clinician's inability to differentiate between true and false lumps.

Clinical competence in diagnosis and evaluation of mammary disease requires a knowledge of anatomic variations, physiology, methods of examination and the natural history of dysplastic and neoplastic states.

ANATOMY

In the female, each mammary gland rests upon the fascia of the pectoralis major muscle. The peripheral limits of the gland are variable from one patient to another, but ordinarily breast tissue extends almost to the midline over the sternum, to the anterior axillary line laterally, and from the level of the second rib above to about the sixth rib inferiorly in a horizontal line drawn through the nipple. The greatest variation in peripheral extension occurs in the axillary area. Most often, there is a blunted, narrow extension of the gland which may still lie on the fascia over the converging fibers of the pectoralis major. In other instances, this so-called axillary tail of the breast is found below or posterior to the pectoralis major muscle in the lower third of the axilla. In unusual instances, the axillary tail may be a prolongation extending into the middle third of the axilla and lying in contact with the pectoralis minor muscle or the intercostal muscles. In such abnormal axillary extensions, the indurative changes of dysplasia may occur, as well as actual neoplasms, and in such instances their origin in mammary tissue may be unrecognized. Still more unusual are the instances of supernumerary foci of mammary glandular tissue, most often without corresponding nipples, which may occur in the axillary area as well as in the anterior axillary line, and below and medial to the normal breast.

Supernumerary foci of mammary tissue may exhibit the cyclic changes which characterize the physiologic response of the breasts to hormonal stimulation.

The superficial fascia of the breasts is attached to the skin, a fact of extraordinary clinical importance. A layer of fat surrounds the gland, except in the area of the nipple and areola. The thickness of the subcutaneous fat is highly variable. In thin women with underdeveloped breasts, the subcutaneous fat layer may be almost nonexistent, so that the reflection of skin from the breast during radical mastectomy requires a meticulous peripheral dissection of extremely thin skin flaps. With increasing obesity, or with fatty replacement of mammary parenchyma, the thickness of the subcutaneous fatty layer increases. The anterior surface of the gland is irregular, owing to the lobulations formed by the deep attachment of fibrous septa, or Cooper's ligaments, which run between the superficial and deep fascia.

The mammary gland is made up of ten to 20 glandular lobes drained by an equal number of tortuous ducts which dilate close to the nipple to form ampullae, and finally divide into minute ducts ending in small openings in the nipples. Each of the orifices in the nipple corresponds roughly to a truncated segment of breast which it drains, a fact of importance in the investigation of bleeding or other discharge from the nipple.

The parenchyma of the breast is composed of two types of epithelium, acinar or secretory, and ductal. Both have a double fibrous covering, the inner periductal or periacinar layer and an outer layer of perilobular connective tissue. The acinar components of the breast are highly variable in quantity during puberty, the reproductive years and even after the climacteric, conditioned upon response to hormonal stimulation. The ductal components are less variable in quantity after maturation, except in the instance of pregnancy and lactation. The acinar epithelium is cuboidal in shape while the epithelium of the ducts is columnar.

In men and in prepubertal females, the gland is rudimentary, with only a few short ducts and ordinarily without genuinely developed acini.

CUTANEOUS LYMPHATICS. There is a continuous intercommunicating network of lymphatics over the entire surface of the chest, neck and abdomen. By this mechanism, the subcutaneous lymphatics over one breast communicate with those of the opposite gland. There are even some lymphatics originating under the skin which drain into the contralateral axillary nodes. For each breast, there is a collecting network of lymphatics under and adjacent to the areola.

INTRAMAMMARY LYMPHATICS. The lymphatics originating within the breast drain by the following pathways (Fig. 1).

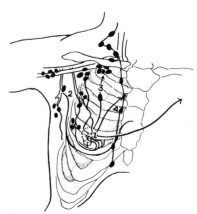

Figure 1. Lymphatics of the breast: 1, subareolar; 2, axillary; 3, transpectoral; 4, internal mammary.

A few follow the ducts and terminate in the subareolar lymphatic network, mainly from the central area.

The principal route is the axillary pathway coming from all parts of the gland and draining directly to the central axillary nodes, the nodes around the axillary vein or the subscapular group. There is also drainage to intercostal nodes in the second and third intercostal spaces.

A transpectoral pathway penetrates the pectoralis major muscle and ends in the supraclavicular nodes. Some may drain into infraclavicular nodes behind the pectoralis minor muscle.

The internal mammary pathway passes through the pectoralis major and intercostal muscles adjacent to the sternum. These lymphatics drain into the nodes of the internal mammary chain. They lie deep to the costal cartilages and surround the internal mammary blood vessels.

PHYSIOLOGY

The hormonal control of the parenchyma of the breast has become well established, both by experimental studies in animals and by biopsies from human mammary glands during various phases of the menstrual cycle, pregnancy and lactation. The development of a normally proliferating ductal epithelium from its anlage requires the conditioning influence of multiple hormones acting in synergism, as provided by the hypophysis, ovary and adrenal cortex. Cellular proliferation by mitosis needs, also, the growth hormone of the pituitary gland. For fulfillment of its expected physiologic function, lactation, the mammary substrate must be conditioned by a constellation of hormonal combinations. The secretory potential begins with acinar differentiation and growth in a pattern which anticipates drainage into the ductal system. With achievement of an anatomically adequate glandular structure, the initiation of lactation depends upon the elaboration of prolactin by the hypophysis, and the maintenance of secretion also is dependent on hypophyseal hormonal support.

In bare outline, the hormonal requirements for growth and function of the mammary parenchyma, from rudimentary state to a fully lactating gland, include hormonal factors from three endocrine sources: gonadotropic, adrenotropic, growth hormone and prolactin from the hypophysis; estrogens and progesterone from the ovaries, and corticosteroid factors from the adrenal glands.

The complexity of the hormonal background of mammary growth and function is of clinical importance in the therapeutic use of hormonal alterations for disseminated carcinoma of the breast. Nearly half of all mammary carcinoma is responsive to such alterations, with longer survival attained than in those patients who are nonresponders. When this clinically determined division first became apparent, more than 20 years ago, the responsive neoplasms were referred to as "estrogen-dependent." Although the fallacy of such specificity is apparent in the perspective provided by the complexity of hormonal growth factors, many clinicians still think in terms of breast cancer activated by estrogens, rather than of neoplasms which are hormonally dependent.

During the years of reproductive potential, there are cyclic changes of ductal and acinar hyperplasia and hypertrophy representing a miniature version of the phenomenon in growth which ends in lactation. These highly variable effects of hormonal origin are of importance in respect to the dysplastic abnormalities of the breasts.

Following the climacteric, the parenchyma of the breasts undergoes a slow, progressive involution in the majority of women. In the first five postmenopausal years, the epithelial structures become atrophic shadows in a process of fatty replacement. Unusual exceptions to such postmenopausal atrophy are found in women in whom the adrenal cortices produce estrogenic steroids in such amount as to prolong the symptoms and objective changes of mammary dysplasia into the postmenopausal years.

EXAMINATION OF THE BREASTS

It is of primary importance that a woman whose complaints are related to the breast should have a general physical examination, unless she has had one performed by a competent physician in the preceding three months. Pelvic examination is essential because of the not infrequent association of gynecologic pathologic states with breast lesions, particularly with dysplastic disease. In functional disturbances of the breast, stigmata of endocrine dysplasia should be searched for, such as hirsutism, abnormal deposits of fat and uterine hypoplasia, as well as indications of hypothyroidism. Should the patient have a three-dimensional tumor which may be carcinoma, methodical examination of such accessible areas as may harbor metastatic foci is essential. If a general physical examination is not to be done, the patient should at least be undressed to the waist and draped with a sheet or a gown.

Preliminary examination should be done with the patient sitting comfortably but erect on the end of the examining table, with the hands resting in the lap and the legs uncrossed. With the patient in this position, the breasts should be inspected for equality of size and similarity of contour, for disparity in the appearance and variation in level of the nipples. It should be obvious that this must be accomplished in a good light.

Approximately one-fourth of all women have some minor degree of inequality of a developmental nature in the size of the breasts. In a very occasional woman, there may be an obvious unilateral hypertrophy, usually unrelated to pregnancy or lactation. It should also be noted that in women who have any degree of scoliosis there will be a distinct lack of symmetry in the breasts, the breast on the side of the convexity of the scoliosis being higher than the opposite breast and the level of the nipples correspondingly altered (Fig. 2).

The color and the consistency of the skin over the breasts should be carefully noted, particularly for areas of erythema or edema. Retraction of the skin due to carcinoma will rarely be noted in this position, except in the instance of an advanced lesion. In fact, distinct retraction of the skin demonstrable with any method of examination is usually an indication of lymphatic permeation and a relatively advanced lesion.

The patient should be asked to bend forward, and the examiner should note whether in a dependent position there is lack of mobility of either breast, alteration in the relative nipple position or evidence of skin retraction in any area.

With the patient again in the sitting position, the patient should be asked to abduct the arms to a 90-degree angle. Inspection is again made for inequalities in the level of the nipples, and for possible areas of skin retraction which may be apparent with the pectoralis fascia under tension, particularly in lesions located in the upper outer quadrant of the breast.

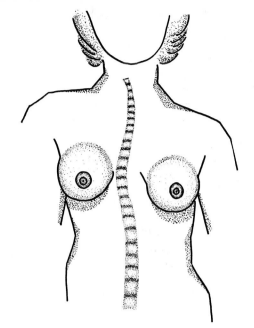

Figure 2. Normal asymmetrical breasts due to scoliosis.

With the patient's arms adducted and without tension on the pectoral fascia, the axillary folds, the supraclavicular and cervical areas and the shoulders should be inspected for any evidence of asymmetry.

By gentle palpation, the neck on both sides and, particularly, the supraclavicular areas should be searched for abnormal nodes. The thyroid should be palpated for abnormal enlargement or displacement. Next, the infraclavicular area should be palpated for possible nodes.

The axillary area on each side should be palpated for lymphadenopathy, the patient's forearm resting on the opposite forearm of the examiner in such a fashion that the patient's upper extremity is entirely relaxed. With the flat of the fingers and beginning at the axillary apex, the axilla is gently palpated. Special attention should be given to the so-called retropectoral area, where nodes lying behind the converging fibers of the pectoralis major muscle may be palpated.

Palpation of the breast, with the patient in the sitting position, yields much less information than that accomplished with the patient supine, except in the central third of the breast. In the latter area, the nipple and areola are carefully examined for indurative changes. With one hand supporting the breast from below, and the other palpating gently from above, abnormality in the ductal system adjacent to the areola may often be detected. The surface of the nipple and areola should be carefully examined for evidences of scaling or erosion, even though of minute degree.

If there seems to be any disparity in the size of the arms, the circumference of each arm should be measured 5 inches from the acromial process on each side.

With the patient in the supine position, each breast is methodically palpated, first with the arm in adduction and then in sharp abduction. In some women, particularly those with bulky breasts, this part of the examination may be facilitated by placing a pillow under the scapular area of the side being examined, particularly to obtain better palpation of the lateral portion and axillary tail of the breast. All of this examination should

be by the flat hand, remembering that the maximum tactile sensitivity is located in the distal two-thirds of the flexor surfaces of the fingers. Finger-point examination has no place in this examination, for it will frequently produce the illusion of a three-dimensional tumor when none is actually present (Fig. 3, *A* and *B*). In order to accomplish systematic palpation of the entire breast, one should begin at some arbitrary axis and, by flat-hand palpation around the circumference of the breast, determine variations in consistency and search for space-occupying lumps. The area of the axillary tail of the breast should be examined separately. Special attention should be given to the inframammary fold, with upward traction on the breast during examination of the latter area.

As experience is gained, one will be able

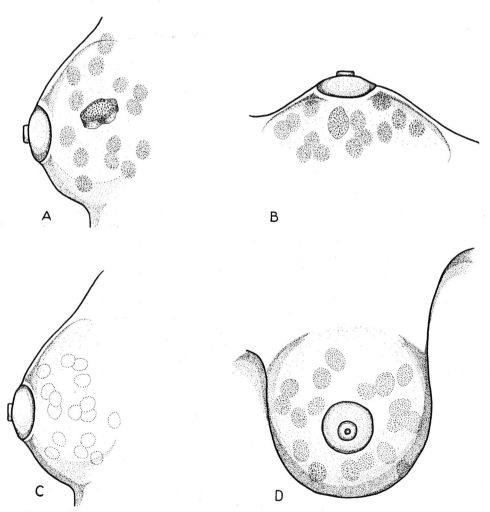

Figure 3. The lesions of both *A* and *B* may resemble lumps by finger palpation with the patient in the sitting position. By flat-hand palpation with the patient in the supine position, the more advanced lesion in *A* is detected as a true lump, that in *B* a pseudolump. *C,* Soft, normal breast lobules not palpable. *D,* Few days' premenstrual breast is fuller, more dense; vague outline of lobules.

to differentiate between varying degrees of consistency in various types of normal breasts. In Figure 3, *C*, is illustrated a soft normal breast in the first half of the menstrual cycle with the lobules not palpable. In *D*, during the few days premenstrual, the breast is fuller and more dense, and careful palpation may suggest the vague outline of lobules throughout the breast. E in Figure 4 is another type of normal breast with considerably different consistency in which, during the early part of the cycle, the lobules are distinctly palpable in the peripheral two-thirds of the breast, while in the central third vaguely outlined radiating areas may suggest the ductal structure. In such a breast, the palpable lobular and ductal architecture will have become considerably exaggerated in the premenstrual phase (F in Fig. 4). The lobules are now palpable to a more distinct degree and the radiating ductal system may also be more apparent in the form of linear, irregular or even slightly beadlike areas. In this type of breast, it is possible by finger-point palpation, and even more by palpation between two sets of opposing fingers, to obtain the sensation of a tumor in one of the well-developed lobular areas. When such an area is gently palpated with the flat of the fingers, the pseudotumor disappears, blending into the adjacent breast tissues.

In these schematic representations, there is implied a uniformity of palpable lobules and ducts along with their premenstrual exaggeration. In fact, the distribution of such palpable normal lobules, either in the resting or hyperplastic stage, usually is extremely irregular.

Represented in Figure 5 are focal areas of persistent abnormal acinar hyperplasia, one represented in the right breast (G), where the lobules are diffusely palpable, and in the left (H), in a soft breast with impalpable lobules. It is possible to interpret these lesions as a lump by fingertip palpation, particularly with the patient in the sitting position. On flat-hand palpation with the patient supine, they should be apparent only as abnormally indurated areas without the circumscription or substance of a space-occupying tumor.

More advanced abnormalities of the hyperplasia-involution cycle are portrayed in the lower part of Figure 5. Represented in the left breast (J) are an area of abnormal hyperplasia large enough in extent to have become a three-dimensional, vaguely cir-

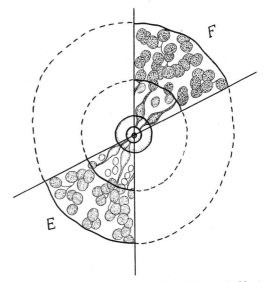

Figure 4. E, Early part of cycle: lobules palpable in peripheral two-thirds, vaguely outlined in central one-third; radiating areas may suggest ductal structure. F, Premenstrual phase: lobules palpable to more distinct degree; radiating ductal structure more apparent.

cumscribed tumor (K), and another area, L, just above the areola, which may also be a three-dimensional lump. The lesser areas indicate indurative changes without the substance of a genuine lump. In the right breast (I) are represented various degrees of the actual cystic phase of dysplastic disease, with two gross cysts, M and N, in the upper hemisphere constituting three-dimensional tumors. In the lower hemisphere are two small cysts which would constitute distinct nodules only if there was sufficient tension of contained fluid within the cyst. The medial nodule, O, represents a combination of the cystic and hyperplastic phases of dysplastic disease.

If a three-dimensional tumor has been satisfactorily outlined, its location should be indicated accurately on a diagrammatic sketch on the patient's record. This may be done either on a free-hand sketch of the breast and adjacent axillary and supraclavicular areas, or a stamped outline. The dimensions of the tumor should be determined as accurately as possible by measurement with a ruler and written on the diagram. Also shown should be the location and approximate size of enlarged regional lymph nodes, if found, or the absence of lymphadenopathy should be indicated. The sketching in of the tumor can also indicate whether it is round, ovoid or irregular in outline.

If possible, one should determine whether

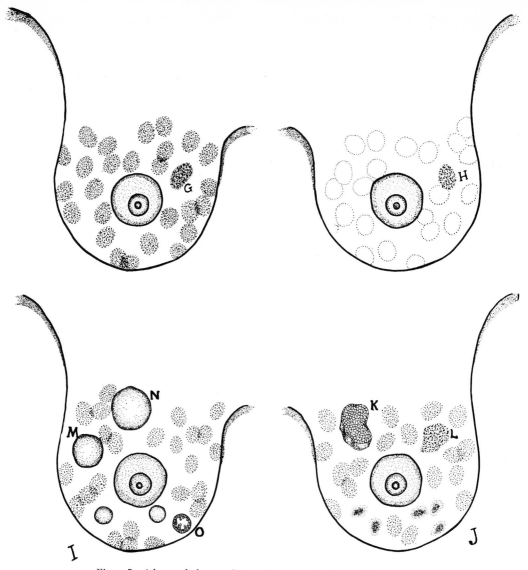

Figure 5.   Advanced abnormalities of the hyperplasia-involution cycle.

Above: The right breast shows diffusely palpable lobules (G). The left breast is soft, with impalpable lobules, except at H.

Below: The right breast, I, shows in its upper hemisphere two gross cysts, M and N, which constitute three-dimensional tumors. In the lower hemisphere are two small cysts which would constitute distinct nodules if only there were sufficient tension of contained fluid. The medial nodule, O, represents a combination of cystic and hyperplastic phases. The left breast, J, has an area of abnormal hyperplasia large enough to be a three-dimensional, vaguely circumscribed tumor (K). Another area above the areola, L, may also be a three-dimensional tumor. Lesser areas indicate indurative changes without the substance of a genuine lump.

the surface of the tumor seems smooth or irregular, usually possible in a patient with small breasts or in tumors superficially located. The degree of mobility, or its impairment in relation to adjacent breast tissue, deserves description. If the tumor is deeply located or bulky in size, the presence or absence of attachment to the pectoral fascia or to the chest wall should be determined and noted. Such a combination of schematic representation and brief description of es-

sential features is informative and accurate, saves time and space, and is of particular importance in those patients requiring subsequent observation of questionable lesions.

In the diagnosis of small carcinomas of the breast, significant changes in the overlying skin usually are so minimal as to be almost subtle. These include an evident impairment of elasticity of the skin overlying the tumor or minor degrees of skin attachment. Such changes may become evident only on changing position of the breast or altering the degree of tension on the pectoral fascia. Skin tension over an area is reduced best when the examiner, with the patient lying supine, gently displaces the breast upward, laterally or medially. Depending on the location of the tumor, the skin may remain taut or slightly depressed over a carcinoma of small size. Decreased mobility of the skin is often best seen with a strong source of illumination lighting the area under investigation tangentially. Occasionally, too, inspection under magnification of two or three diameters may bring out alterations not otherwise seen.

Changes more obvious than these, such as areas of retracted skin, genuine retraction of the nipple, ulceration of the nipple, and distinct erythema or lymphedema, are all signs of advanced disease of the breast, whether inflammatory or neoplastic. The physical signs of early disease of the breast are detected only by exact and meticulous methods of examination and are more suitable for schematic than photographic illustration. Lesions of the breast which are photogenic are so advanced as to be clinically apparent.

Too much emphasis cannot be placed upon development of perceptiveness in the digital, tactile end-organs to the point of performing a type of projected stereognostic function. Such perceptiveness is epicritic, never protopathic. Until such time as more exact methods may be developed, the physician's skill in examination is the most important method for detection of neoplasms of limited, local extent.

Transillumination of the breast is more impressive to the patient than it is informative to the examiner. After having had a considerable vogue some years ago, it is now used by very few clinicians of experience.

Roentgenographic examination of the *breast (mammography)* recently has been the subject of a special study, from which have come indications of its accuracy in general use, and more specific criteria for its application. In 2000 consecutive mammograms interpreted by Egan in a four-year period, 737 had a biopsy performed, thus making possible a control of accuracy by histologic findings. In 418 women, he found radiographic criteria of cancer. In 407 of these (97 per cent), microscopic examination of tissue removed demonstrated its presence. The potential contribution of the technique is emphasized by the fact that, of the 407 women in whom the diagnosis of cancer was made and verified by histopathology, clinical examination had failed to identify the presence of a tumor in 53 (13 per cent). In 313 instances, the radiographic diagnosis of a benign lesion was made and in 284 (90 per cent) microscopy endorsed this conclusion, while the remaining 10 per cent were errors of method, or false-negative reports.

More recently 24 hospitals participated in a study of the reproducibility of the Egan technique. The initial phase consisted of an indoctrination of each contributing radiologist through a five-day period of instruction in technical details and interpretation by Egan, and the opportunity for review of 3000 mammograms. Prebiopsy mammography of 1580 breasts produced 475 radiographic diagnoses of malignant neoplasm, verified by microscopy in 376 patients for a true positive rate of 79 per cent, and a false positive in 21 per cent. A higher degree of accuracy was obtained in the diagnosis of the noncancerous breast, with 90 per cent (999 of 1105) correctly classified.

This study would seem to indicate that other radiologists fell far short of Egan's accuracy, even with preliminary, intensive instruction. Because of differences in the

Figure 6. Mammogram showing a deeply located cyst 2.5 cm. in diameter, with changes of dysplasia in adjacent parenchyma. Note smooth, well demarcated edge of cyst.

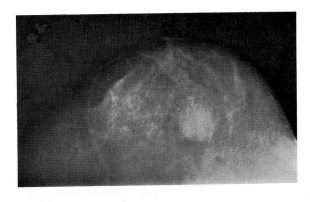

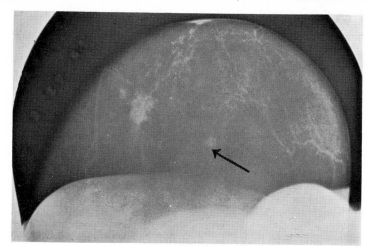

Figure 7. Poorly demarcated, irregular mass about 2.0 cm. in greatest dimensions, with customary spiculated peripheral appearance of carcinoma. More deeply located 0.6 cm. nodule (at arrow) which was missed on sectioning of the specimen, but located after review of films, and was an intramammary metastasis.

two samples of patients, the disparity is not as great as it seems. Egan's studies were done on women admitted to a cancer hospital, many by reference of physicians. The study of reproducibility was much more representative, limited only to women scheduled for biopsy of the breast, and of younger average age than in Egan's sample.

The most important finding in the nationwide survey was the relationship of age to the accuracy of mammographic diagnosis. In women predominantly premenopausal, under age 30, and 30 to 44 years, the "true positive rate" of radiographic diagnosis of cancer was no better than calling heads or tails on a coin (50.0 per cent and 55.6 per cent). In women aged 45 to 59 years, cancer was identified with a percentile accuracy of 77.0, which increased to a 90.3 per cent level in patients 60 or more years of age. The slight luster thus acquired is more than a little tarnished by the inverse relationship of the

"true negative rate," which decreases from a high of 97.2 per cent in women under age 30 years, to a low of 67.9 per cent in the postmenopausal group age 60 or more.

Another finding in the reproducibility survey was an increased accuracy of positive diagnosis of neoplasm in fatty breasts, or in 88.6 per cent versus the overall rate of 79.2 per cent. But in this group also the lowest "true negative rate" occurred—72.9 per cent. In short, both in women over age 60 years, and in patients with fatty breasts, for every ten "negative" reports of mammograms, in three patients cancer actually is present.

These data demand a re-emphasis of the limitations of mammography as a diagnostic aid. The high rate of accuracy in the positive reporting of breast cancer as achieved by Egan was due, in part, to a selected sample studied under ideal conditions. When tested in a more representative patient-population limited only by admission to 24 hospitals for biopsy of the breast, when a majority of selected institutions are teaching hospitals and when instruction in the technique for the radiologists involved has been provided by its originator, the limitations become apparent. Only eight of each ten cancers are identified; in patients less than 45 years of age, the method is only slightly more informative than coin-tossing in its detection of cancers; in women 60 years of age or more, false negative reports occur at a rate of more than three of every ten, and mammography has no present usefulness as a screening technique.

The survey provided sound indications for

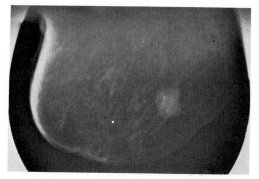

Figure 8. A mass illustrating mammographic features of carcinoma, 1.8 by 1.9 cm., with calcific foci, spiculation of edges of tumor and retraction of overlying skin. (Courtesy of Robert L. Scanlan, M.D.)

the selection of patients in whom mammography is most informative. The most important single criterion is a minimal volume of ductal-acinar parenchyma. Hence the mammogram has maximal accuracy in the postmenopausal years, with 90 per cent true positive reporting after 60 years of age. The method is reliable also in fatty breasts, with 88 per cent identification of cancer. When a dominant area of induration is present but not distinctly space-occupying, mammography may be of value. In the woman who has had a prior carcinoma of the breast, annual mammography of the residual breast may detect a contralateral neoplasm before it is apparent clinically.

Malignant neoplasms are almost always associated with a distinct increase in vascularity of the affected breast. *Infrared photographs* usually demonstrate this circulatory phenomenon rather well.

Malignant epithelial cells in the breast have a somewhat higher *uptake of radioactive phosphorus* than do nonneoplastic cells, but unfortunately the disparity in uptake is not consistently evident until a carcinoma of the breast is of such size as to be clinically obvious.

For the woman who has a *discharge from the nipple,* the first approach should be routine examination in search of a space-occupying tumor. If none is found, the examination is directed toward localization of the duct or ducts from which the discharge originates. In some instances, the patient herself may have discovered a pressure point. If there has been recent bleeding, inspection of the nipple under magnification may reveal an orifice containing dried blood. The most important part of the examination is radial stroking of the breast with a fingertip, with the patient supine, from the periphery toward the areola, repeating the process in clockwise fashion over 12 or more circumferential segments. If this maneuver does not localize the ductal area of origin, it may be repeated with the patient in the sitting position, although the results are not as reliable. If a pressure point is successfully located, it should be marked on the skin with the patient supine, and accurately located on the diagram. The location of the ductal orifice on the nipple through which the discharge exudes should also be indicated. It is advisable to repeat the examination five to seven days later to verify the apparent ductal source of discharge. The only useful cytologic information to be obtained from nipple exudates is the presence or absence of red blood cells; their presence most often is an indication of papillary, ductal lesions which may be malignant. Their absence is a reliable criterion of a simple, exudative phase of dysplasia. Search of exudates for malignant cells has not been productive.

DEVELOPMENTAL ANOMALIES

The least uncommon of the unusual developmental disorders is that of supernumerary nipples or breasts. Practically all such instances of ectopic development occur along the primitive milk line, which extends from the axilla downward across the nipple and thence downward and slightly medially to a point just below the inner third of the inguinal area. The great majority of supernumerary foci occur either in the area above and lateral or below the breast proper.

Racial determinism is a factor of importance in location, frequency and relative incidence by sex. A Japanese study showed 1.5 per cent of males and 5 per cent of females with accessory nipples, while a report from a review of 20,000 school children in England demonstrated an incidence of only 0.4 per cent.

The ectopic focus may be constituted of nipple alone, or of parenchymatous mammary tissue in varying stages of development; more rarely, both may be present. From a standpoint of clinical importance, the most confusing ectopic foci are those of genuinely separate axillary mammary tissue. Many of the so-called supernumerary axillary foci are simply abnormal prolongations of the axillary tail of the breast.

The indicated treatment is surgical excision for cosmetic or diagnostic reasons, or both. The necessity for excision in the axillary area is more urgent, as carcinoma has been known to develop in axillary sites of ectopia.

Complete absence of one or both breasts or segmental failure of development of a breast is so rare that it is unknown to most clinicians. Minor degrees of disparity of size of the breasts is usually of developmental origin, while distinct hypertrophy is more reasonably ascribed to postnatal physiologic disturbances.

The most common malformation of the nipple is that of inversion. Less often, a developmental fissuring of the nipples is seen. Both of these disturbances are, with rare exceptions, bilateral. Their clinical importance is that they be historically established as of developmental origin and not confused with deformities of the nipple secondary to a pathologic process within the breast.

Under the designation of ductal fistula of the breast, Livingston and Arlen have described ten women who presented para-reolar fistulae which were lined with squamous epithelium and occupied by desquamated keratin, usually associated with a congenitally inverted nipple. Adequate treatment required excision of the ductal segment and exteriorization.

There is some academic justification for a belief held by some that two intramammary developmental defects may contribute to some unusual neoplasms in later life. Remnants of the nipple pouch have been noted in the area of the large ducts as late as puberty. This may be the origin of rare epidermoid cysts, with or without squamous carcinoma, and also accounts for at least some instances of Paget's carcinoma of the ducts and nipple. Since the mammary gland represents a modified sweat gland structure, remnants of the mammary buds may be associated with the occasional development of carcinoma of the breast which is of distinct sweat gland structure.

An anomalous muscle which traverses the axilla is a not unusual finding during axillary dissection, and Saitta and Baum have reported one patient in whom the belly of the muscle was so enlarged as to form an axillary mass. It is known by the unsatisfactory name of von Langer's axillary arch, the eponym referring to the author of the first report of the structure in the literature. Usually scanty in amount, the muscle seems to be a slip of the lateral border of the latissimus dorsi extending obliquely across the axilla, over the neurovascular bundle and the coracobrachialis to insert under the insertion of the pectoralis major. It is a regular feature of the axillary anatomy in anthropoid apes, and is said to be present in about 7 per cent of human axillae.

TRAUMA AND FOREIGN BODIES

The breast has a remarkable tolerance for injury and usually will achieve restitution to normal even after extensive extravasation of blood into the parenchyma, fatty and other connective tissue. The most disruptive injury, short of actual laceration, is also the most common of all, that of surgical incision for biopsy or resection. Resection is commonly followed by a period of organization ending in more or less severe fibrosis, which not uncommonly produces a three-dimensional lump more impressive than the tumor which may have originally been present. These postsurgical sclerosing reactions usually regress slowly over a period of months, sometimes completely, sometimes leaving a focus of smooth induration under or adjacent to the scar.

The most common complication of trauma, either accidental or surgical, is the formation of a hematoma. If the blood is in a fluid state and reasonably well localized, it may be aspirated through a 14-gauge needle. Collections of organizing hematoma of more than minor size require incision and evacuation of the blood clot under local anesthesia.

Occasionally, suppurative infection may follow trauma, usually developing in unaspirated or unevacuated areas of hemorrhage. It is of considerable importance that such areas of posttraumatic cellulitis have prompt treatment to forestall ramification of the infection. If evidence of suppuration is lacking, treatment with sulfonamides or antibiotics should be instituted. If an abscess develops, prompt incision and drainage are indicated, preferably with the patient under general anesthesia to permit thorough evacuation of secondary pockets which may be present. This procedure should be followed by use of an antibiotic or antibiotics selected by sensitivity tests, continued for a minimum period of ten days.

A more unusual but frequently confusing complication following trauma is that of *fat necrosis*. This lesion is most apt to develop in obese patients or those with pendulous breasts. Although a history of injury is not obtained in some patients, disruption of fat cells is the mechanism by which the process is initiated. A slow aseptic saponification of fat by blood and tissue lipase develops. The lesion may vary from 1 or 2 cm. to as large as 8 cm. in diameter. The surface is firm and irregular, and frequently the skin becomes attached to the tumor and even retracted, although there is seldom any retraction of the nipple. Fat necrosis can, therefore, simulate carcinoma with such exactness that this is one of the few lesions for which radical mastectomy has been done on the basis of an apparently inescapable clinical diagnosis of carcinoma. Gross examination of the cut section usually differentiates the lesion from carcinoma because of the diffuse yellowish to orange coloration and the greasy consistency. In some of the lesions, cystic degeneration develops with the formation of pools of fat which may be surrounded by foci of hemorrhage. Eventually, in lesions of long duration, calcification occurs in the cystic areas. Treatment is simple excision with a margin of adjacent breast tissue. Diagnosis is readily made by frozen sections.

The most frequent *foreign body* in past years has been paraffin used for cosmetic reasons, resulting in the development of paraffinoma representing a foreign-body granulomatous reaction and producing irregular lumps which may require excision. Some of the nonabsorbable suture materials may produce foreign-body granulomas.

INFLAMMATORY LESIONS

PYOGENIC INFECTIONS. Suppurative infections of the lactating breast, fairly frequent prior to the advent of chemotherapy, have now become unusual, although an occasional patient still progresses to the stage of abscess formation. Very occasionally, a woman with a genuinely cystic phase of dysplasia of the breast will develop a secondary infection in and around gross cysts, an inflammatory process superimposed on the dysplasia. Developing most often in long-standing cystic disease, such infections usually are low grade and slowly progressive. These rare instances represent the one situation in which the old misnomer, chronic cystic mastitis, becomes an apt and accurate designation.

Of even greater rarity are those women who develop pyogenic mastitis by hematogenous dissemination from some distant, primary focus of infection, either apparent or occult.

Abscesses beginning in the subareolar area and involving the central third of the breast have an extraordinary tendency to recur and to be resistant to treatment. Some of these seem to represent an extension of cutaneous adnexal infections. In recurrent abscess of the breast, wide removal of the previous scar or scars, the underlying chronic abscess cavity and the adjacent ductal system should be undertaken during a period of quiescence of the infection. Such wide excisions should be performed only after repeated incision and drainage and use of antibiotics, following which the process may gradually subside over a period of months. Choice of an antibiotic agent by sensitivity tests is of great importance; the strain of *Staphylococcus pyogenes* var. *aureus* most often present is resistant to penicillin.

Irradiation has been of no value except in occasional limited, early foci of cellulitis. In these, a tissue dosage of 300 to 450 r is adequate, divided into two or three treatments.

TUBERCULOSIS. Tuberculosis of the breast is now an exceedingly rare disease. It is invariably either secondary to an active distant focus or results from direct extension of disease in the underlying costal cage. Advanced tuberculosis of the breast is accompanied by multiple sinuses and frequently by involvement of the regional axillary nodes. Thus, the treatment is radical mastectomy.

PLASMA CELL MASTITIS. This rare form of mastitis usually occurs in married women under the age of 40 years. The dominant symptom is pain. There is usually localized erythema overlying a poorly defined bulky mass in the breast, and occasionally there is a milky discharge from the nipple. The skin may become adherent to the mass, is commonly edematous and retraction of the nipple may be present. Thus, the lesion often mimics a carcinoma of the acute or inflammatory type. Enlarged axillary lymph nodes of some size may be present. Clinicians, neglecting the confirmatory evidence of histologic diagnosis, have performed radical mastectomies for this lesion. Some of these purely inflammatory processes, perhaps most, are highly radiosensitive. When confronted by such findings in a married woman under 40 years of age, with no recent history of lactation, information of diagnostic value will probably be obtained from one or more biopsies of the involved skin, including the subcutaneous tissue, and smears from the nipple discharge, if present. This can be done as an office procedure under local anesthesia. If histologic study of the material so obtained fails to show foci of carcinoma cells in the skin or subjacent tissue, or in the smear, one can eliminate the possibility of genuine inflammatory carcinoma with certainty. However, the possibility of carcinoma with erythema of overlying skin cannot be excluded. If the evidence favors the diagnosis of plasma cell mastitis, roentgen therapy in moderate dosage is advised, about 600 rads delivered in two weeks' time. This amount of irradiation over such a period usually induces complete regression of this form of mastitis. If the physical findings are not entirely consistent with this disorder, and in those patients in whom this amount of irradiation does not produce satisfactory regression within three weeks, adequate material for biopsy should be obtained by a surgical approach. Should carcinoma be demonstrated, it is usually biologically inoperable and best treated by intensive radiation therapy.

MAMMARY DUCT ECTASIA (COMEDOMASTITIS). This process may simulate carcinoma in elderly women, to whom it is almost limited. The process is characterized by wide dilatation of the ducts, particularly in the central third of the breast, in which accumulation of fatty debris is accompanied by ductal and periductal inflammation and eventual sclerosis. With severe sclerosis, the ducts may become shortened, thus retracting the nipple so that the physical findings approximate those of subareolar carcinoma of the ducts. In the early stages, the involved ducts can be outlined as individual cirsoid or vermiform structures, with little or no resemblance to a possible neoplasm. In the later stages of sclerosis, induration and nipple retraction, excision and histologic diagnosis become necessary.

It is worthy of note that all three of the inflammatory processes which may simulate cancer—fat necrosis, plasma cell mastitis and duct ectasia—are believed by some to be variants of the same basic disorder of ductal stasis, with trauma playing a determinant part, followed by inflammatory reaction to chemical irritants.

SCLEROSING SUBCUTANEOUS PHLEBITIS (MONDOR'S DISEASE). This relatively rare condition is manifested as a cordlike structure over the breast, extending along the course of the thoracoepigastric vein in the outer quadrants of the breast toward the axilla. The length may be several centimeters to as long as 20 cm. or more. It may turn medially along the inframammary sulcus toward the umbilicus. In some patients, the onset is marked by soreness or even pain, and redness of the overlying skin. It has occasionally followed trauma or respiratory infection. Biopsies taken early in the process show the structure to be venous with inflammatory changes, the end result of which is venous sclerosis. It is not associated with cancer of the breast. No treatment is required; the process is self-limited, although in some it persists for a year or more.

DISORDERS DUE TO ABNORMAL PHYSIOLOGY

PREPUBERTAL HYPERPLASIA. The earliest example of hyperplasia of endocrine origin is that of *neonatal hyperplasia*. Almost one-half of infants, both male and female, exhibit a transient enlargement of the mammary disk as a result of hormonal stimulation through the placental blood. In about one of ten newborn infants, this is accompanied by a scanty secretion of thin fluid from the nipples. This hyperplasia may persist for six months or more, particularly in female nursing infants.

Rare instances of mammary hyperplasia and hypertrophy during the first five years of life, or so-called precocious mammary development, are almost invariably due to hormone-producing neoplasms of the ovary, adrenal cortex or hypophysis, or to hypothalamic lesions.

Later in life, and most often from the ages of eight to 12 years, unilateral hypertrophy unassociated with any recognizable endocrine abnormality is not uncommon. Such female prepubertal hypertrophy may be transient or may persist until puberty, during which period the opposite breast undergoes development equal to that of its fellow.

At the time of puberty, there are rare examples of *hypertrophy* of one breast or even of both. Attempts at control of such hypertrophic abnormalities have been unsuccessful. When they are disfiguring, appropriate plastic surgery is indicated.

GYNECOMASTIA. Enlargement of the breast in the male, either unilateral or bilateral, is most common during the period of puberty and after the age of 40 years. Gynecomastia developing during *puberty* is ordinarily transient and unilateral, with an average duration of 12 to 18 months. It represents an adolescent, mammary dysplasia of functional type, secondary to the profound changes in steroid hormone levels characteristic of adolescence. It is to be found in nearly four of every ten boys between the ages of 14 and 16 years.

The process may be a diffuse, slightly lumpy or even nodular enlargement of the entire gland, in which case the diagnosis is obvious. More often, however, there is a discrete tumefaction, usually subareolar in position, and the area of localized indurative change may be from one to several centimeters in diameter.

The finding of a measurable lump frequently arouses such apprehension in the clinician that he performs an excision for microscopic diagnosis. No such action is necessary because malignant neoplasia in the mammary gland of the adolescent male is unknown. The differential diagnoses of remote chance in boys at this age are dermoid cyst, lipoma, hemangioma and lymphangioma. The only indication is for observation at intervals of several months. It is rare that adolescent gynecomastia persists and is of such a degree as to require treatment, which is subcutaneous mastectomy. Attempts at control of adolescent gynecomastia by hormone treatment are unnecessary, ineffective and not without some hazards.

Gynecomastia developing in the adult male is usually seen in those of middle or late life, is almost invariably unilateral and is also due to functional endocrinologic disturbance. In rare instances, it may be secondary to interstitial cell tumor of the testis, atrophy of the testis, hypophyseal adenoma or adrenocortical lesions. In later life, gynecomastia may be secondary to hepatic cirrhosis, with or without a history of alcoholism, in which instances the lesion presumably is due to the inability of the liver to accomplish intermediate metabolism of steroid hormones.

Examination in the adult should include careful survey of the involved breast for a three-dimensional tumor, palpation of the testes and inquiry as to the possibility of cirrhosis of the liver. If a distinct, circumscribed, three-dimensional tumor is present, it should be excised to rule out carcinoma, although, in the male, fixation of the skin and pectoral fascia is almost invariably present when the diagnosis of carcinoma is first made. Otherwise, no treatment is indicated or useful, unless subcutaneous mastectomy becomes necessary for unsightly enlargement.

DYSPLASIAS OF FEMALE BREAST. The dysplasias of the breast have acquired an unenviable distinction because of an unwarranted complexity of nomenclature. More than 40 separate terms have been used to designate varied phases of mammary dysplasia; some are descriptive of morphologic features, some are eponymic, some are misconceived and not a few disregard the basic pathogenesis of these disorders. All this terminologic overgrowth is readily divisible into four phases of abnormal response to the cyclic hormonal conditioning to which the breast is exposed during a woman's reproductive years.

Normal cyclic changes. An understanding of the abnormalities in response to hormonal influences requires an orientation in normal changes. During the first half of each menstrual cycle the influence of estrone, estradiol and estriol, the classic estrogens, is dominant. Their effect is twofold: ductal hyperplasia and sensitization of the acinar epithelium. The latter effect is necessary for the full effectiveness of progesterone in the latter half of the cycle, the action of which produces acinar hyperplasia and a variable degree of hypertrophy. These responses of ductal and acinar overgrowth are far from uniform throughout the breast each month; individual lobules, or lesser anatomic segments, respond in scattered foci, the extent of which is highly variable and individual. This phase of hyperplasia, ductal and acinar, reaches a peak at the end of each menstrual cycle.

With the onset of menstruation, the foci of hyperplasia in the breast undergo involution which in most women seems to be as complete as the more obvious involutionary shedding of the hyperplastic endometrium. Both mammary and endometrial cyclic hyperplasias are anticipatory, cellular preparations for the nidation of a fertilized ovum; involution in both sites is a recognition of the futility of monthly, hyperplastic preparation.

Even as the hyperplastic mammary foci are involuting, other areas are responding to a new rise in estrogenic secretion with new areas of ductal overgrowth, followed by acinar hyperplasia. These successive phases of epithelial hyperplasia and regression occur with lunar periodicity for 30 years or more in the lives of most women, involving more than 400 times of demand and tissue response, with subsequent quiescence. This is the hyperplasia-involution cycle, the abnormalities of which produce the dysplasias which become manifest in about 30 of every 100 Caucasian women.

The abnormalities of the hyperplasia-involution cycle are divisible into four phases, one of which usually is dominant.

The initial phase most often is a failure of involution, or persistent epithelial hyperplasia, acinar or ductal, or both. In some women hyperplasia may persist as the dominant feature.

Antithetic to the hyperplastic state is an excessive involution, or hyperinvolution. Rather than involuting in normal fashion to a resting phase, the acinar epithelium becomes flattened and blunted. The overinvoluted epithelium begins to shed. The acinar epithelium becomes secretory, usually producing cystic dilatations which, initially, are microcystic. As the process continues by coalescence of contiguous acini under tension of contained fluid, gross cysts of varying size may develop. The obvious designation for this phase is that of its dominant morphology, or cystic disease, a label under which noncystic forms of dysplasia masquerade.

The stromal components of the breast are rarely unaffected by the epithelial changes of dysplasia. In the florid phase of proliferative activity, there is a concomitant though minor degree of fibroplasia, particularly in the periacinar and periductal layers, and this stromal reaction is also subject to either involution or hyperinvolution. When the latter change becomes dominant, progressive hyalinization of the connective tissue occurs, with eventual dense sclerosis. Generally, the sclerosing changes occur in perilobular fashion, but the changes of advancing sclerosis may be extremely irregular. Foci of acinar hyperplasia or microcystic change may become circumscribed and compressed by sclerosing reaction. The same sort of sclerotic reaction may proceed within the walled-off area, isolating contained foci of epithelial elements which may be hyperplastic or cystic, or both. Such circumscribed areas may vary in size from microscopic foci to large areas, representing space-occupying tumors of several centimeters in diameter.

In an advanced area of sclerosing reaction, formerly hyperplastic epithelium becomes compressed and pyknotic. These compressed, distorted, deeply staining cells are the only residual evidence of the florid phase of hyperplasia of former years, now completely overcome by the intensity of the sclerotic stromal reaction. In this phase of dysplasia, as in the others, there may be a histiocytic response, less often some minor foci of lymphocytic infiltrate, probably responsible for the original designation of mastitis. These are the prominent changes in the sclerosing phase.

The least frequent phase of dysplasia is the secretory or exudative response, in which the secretory, acinar function is dominant. Whole lobules of mammary tissue become microcystic, the secretory products drain freely through the ductal system and appear at the nipple in the form of a pseudolactiferous exudate which is rarely profuse. This form of exudative dysplasia constitutes less than 2 per cent of all cases and may be regarded as a variant of the cystic phase.

It should be emphasized that pure examples of hyperplastic, cystic or sclerosing dysplasia are rarely seen. Some degree of all three phases generally will be found in long-standing cases of dysplasia. It is common for one phase to be dominant. It is the variegation of gross and microscopic appearance of acinar, ductal and stromal response which has given rise to the bewildering complexity of nomenclature. For example, dilatation of terminal tubules and acini with the formation of microcysts, usually diffuse, is the hallmark of so-called Schimmelbusch's disease. With this, there is frequently an accompanying epithelial proliferation in the terminal ducts to form intraductal hyperplasia. There is also some degree of proliferative acinar hyperplasia which may spill into the adjacent stroma and resemble, superficially, an infiltrative process. These changes of ductal papillomatosis, adenosis and microcystic formation are to be regarded only as various phases of hyperplasia and involution respectively. In some areas, ductal proliferation produces tubules with a blind ending, referred to as blunt-duct adenosis.

The formation of gross cysts which are clinically palpable occurs in 15 to 20 per cent of women with dysplasia. In some instances a cyst, when exposed surgically, has a bluish color which promptly disappears when the cyst is incised or when the investing layer of tissue is removed. The coloration is simply an optical illusion through the surrounding fat and parenchyma but has acquired a special and unwarranted dignity by the designation of "blue-domed cyst."

In 1 or 2 per cent of women with dysplasia, the sclerosing phase will become so overwhelming as to produce a hard, fixed tumor, occasionally with attachment of the skin, readily mistaken for carcinoma. Even on microscopic examination, especially of frozen sections, the extreme distortion and pyknosis of the formerly hyperplastic cells may mimic carcinoma. This lesion of sclerosing adenosis, or adenomatosis, has probably been the lesion most frequently misdiagnosed as carcinoma. It is most reasonably interpreted as an end phase of a severe sclerosing reaction in dysplasia.

Incidence. Clinically recognizable dysplasia of the breast is probably present in one-fourth to one-third of white women, based on the recognition of abnormal indurative changes. The process is practically always bilateral by objective criteria, although in some instances only one breast may be affected, and occasionally, but one segment of a breast. The process may appear immediately after puberty, but the great majority of dysplasias are seen in women beyond the age of 30 years and up to the climacteric. In the postmenopausal years, the process undergoes gradual resolution, with rare exceptions. Pregnancy has a beneficial effect, particularly in the nulliparous woman. The disorder may improve remarkably after pregnancy or even regress completely.

Symptoms. The most frequent symptoms are soreness, tenderness or even severe pain beginning one to seven days premenstrually, and subsiding rapidly after the onset of menstruation. In some patients, the period of distress is longer, beginning about the time of ovulation each month. Less often, the presenting complaint is a self-discovered lump in the breast with little or no soreness. It is very common for the symptoms to occur in an irregularly periodic pattern, with months or even a year or more between periods of distress. In many women, the severity of symptoms is profoundly influenced by emotional stress, such as domestic difficulties or the death of a relative or friend from cancer of the breast.

Physical findings. When the dysplastic process is in its early phase, most often seen in younger women, the dominant change is most apt to be hyperplastic. The first evidence of such change is the appearance of small foci of abnormally granular or beady thickening, frequently with tenderness sharply localized to the area of altered tissue. In more diffuse forms, larger segments of the breast show granular, or beady, or almost vermiform indurative changes, often linear in arrangement. Not infrequently, these changes vaguely resemble a string of beads of varying size. The hyperplastic phase of the process is that in which pain and soreness are apt to be most distressing.

More advanced changes are those in which some of the proliferative changes have evoked a sclerosing reaction of some degree and the larger lesions may constitute three-dimensional tumors. Such indurative changes, however, can reach several centimeters in diameter and still be distinguishable as diffuse induration without the qualities of a space-occupying tumor.

When it is difficult to differentiate between advanced changes of dysplasia and a three-dimensional tumor in one or more areas, the physical findings may be related to the time of the menstrual cycle. Examination of questionable areas is best done a few days to one week after the onset of menstruation. Not infrequently, what seemed to be a three-dimensional lump during the premenstrual period will have decreased in size, or disappeared entirely on re-examination after the onset of menstruation. For the woman who has the symptomatology and clinical findings of dysplasia, a good working rule is to re-examine "tumors" of 2 cm. diameter or less before proceeding with a surgical biopsy.

When the cystic phase of dysplasia is in the microcystic stage, the physical findings are indistinguishable from those of the hyperplastic or proliferative phase. If the cysts begin to acquire some gross size, even when less than 1 cm. in diameter, they are usually evident as smooth-surfaced moderately movable nodules without attachment to the adjacent breast. Their consistency depends on the amount of contained fluid. When gross cysts reach a size of several centimeters, they may be indistinguishable from solid tumors if the tension of the intracystic fluid is sufficient to distend the wall of the cyst. By this time the surface may seem to be irregular because of overlying indurative change in the surrounding breast, although the largest cysts usually remain mobile and unattached to the skin.

In Figure 9, *A*, is shown the exudative phase with discharge from the nipple. Also indicated is a not infrequent finding in such patients, the presence of a palpable duct or ducts draining the involved segment of the breast from which the pseudolacteal exudate originates. Lacking a space-occupying tumor, the only requirement in this situation is a

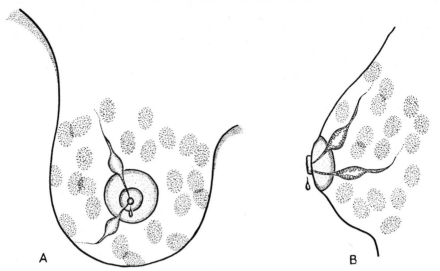

Figure 9.   *A*, Exudative phase with discharge from nipple. Also indicated is the presence of palpable duct or ducts draining involved segment or segments of breast. No space-occupying tumor. *B*, Development of ductal papillomatosis in central third of breast.

smear of the nipple discharge to be examined only for red blood cells. If red blood cells are not found, the only indication is for periodic observation.

Figure 9, *B*, illustrates the development of ductal papillomatosis in the central third of the breast, a ductal hyperplasia producing papillary excrescences of epithelium. Such areas of nodular, epithelial ductal hyperplasia are extraordinarily fragile and a considerable percentage of them give rise to minute amounts of serosanguineous discharge from the nipple. In this situation, one's first effort should be directed toward the search for a space-occupying tumor. If none is found, an effort should be made to locate the ductal area from which the bleeding is originating. If the origin of the bleeding can be consistently demonstrated on two or more examinations, the involved ductal area should be explored. Otherwise, if the patient is premenopausal, continued observation is justifiable. Only once in 20 times will bleeding from the nipple before the menopause indicate the presence of malignant change in ductal epithelium.

Relation of mammary dysplasias to carcinoma. The relation of the dysplasias of the breast to carcinoma is still controversial, but the evidence for dysplasia as a precancerous process is flimsy. If a patient with dysplasia has one breast predominantly affected, she has just as much chance of developing cancer in the less affected breast. Our experience includes over 1500 women

with objective criteria of dysplasia who were followed for periods of two to 15 years. Only five of these patients developed carcinoma of the breast under observation; one had had an excess of mammary carcinoma in her family history. Various degrees of dysplasia are found in surgical specimens showing carcinoma, the frequency depending on the liberality with which the pathologist makes the diagnosis of dysplasia. The only significance of such coexistence is that women with dysplasia may also develop carcinoma.

From our present state of knowledge, the following statements seem permissible in relation to this problem:

The microscopic lesion of blunt-duct adenosis may be a precursor to carcinoma.

The woman with objective changes of dysplasia deserves careful observation for the development of a dominant tumor which may be carcinoma. The development of such a space-occupying tumor, particularly if the dysplastic process is severe, may be masked by the chronic indurative changes. The intervals of observation should be four to six months.

For the woman with well-established dysplasia presenting multiple space-occupying lumps, good management is frequent observation and measurement of the tumors, particularly if the diagnosis has been established by prior excisional biopsy. Many of these lumps will disappear under observation.

Simple mastectomy is rarely, if ever, indicated for mammary dysplasia as a prophylactic procedure. The only reasonable prophylaxis is bilateral mastectomy, a therapeutic absurdity.

Treatment of mammary dysplasias. Three main problems are most pertinent: the patient with symptoms and signs of dysplasia, without a three-dimensional or dominant lump; the patient with a space-occupying solitary tumor; and the patient with nipple discharge.

No DOMINANT LUMP. The patient without a dominant lump usually consults a physician because of soreness, tenderness or pain. For at least half such patients, a careful examination, followed by adequate discussion and explanation of the process, is in itself adequate therapeusis. The reassurance of learning that the symptoms and the process are not related to cancer will satisfactorily diminish the severity of the symptoms. If the indurative changes are more than minimum, examination twice yearly should be recommended. In women with any degree of pendulousness of the breasts, adequate support should be recommended in the form of a fitted brassiere. During the period of greatest discomfort prior to menstruation, the majority of patients obtain great relief from wearing a brassiere at night, for which purpose a "sleeping" brassiere may be obtained if desired. Fitted brassieres should be so designed as to provide adequate uplift to the breasts and relaxation of the suspensory fascia.

These measures of reassurance and proper support of the breasts will produce satisfactory relief of symptoms in at least eight, or possibly nine, of every ten patients. In the remainder, hormonal therapy is usually beneficial, either in the form of small doses of androgenic hormone in the first half of the cycle or progesterone in the latter half. If an androgen is employed, fluoxymesterone (Halotestin) by mouth is as effective as other preparations. It is desirable for the first two months to employ testosterone propionate by intramuscular injection, in dosage of 25 mg. two or three times weekly for two weeks, to measure adequately the response to treatment.

DOMINANT LUMP PRESENT. When a dominant three-dimensional lump is present with physical findings characteristic of dysplasia elsewhere in the breasts, a very useful preliminary diagnostic measure is aspiration of the tumor as an office procedure under local anesthesia. The primary objective of this maneuver is to determine whether the tumor is solid or cystic. If it is cystic and can be evacuated completely, it will fail to refill in at least nine out of ten instances, and thus the patient is spared the distress and expense of a surgical procedure for excision.

In all such instances of successful aspiration of a cyst, the patient should be instructed to return in six weeks for reexamination. If the cyst has refilled, it is preferable to proceed with excision rather than to repeat the aspiration. Reaccumulation of fluid may indicate the presence of papillary changes in the epithelial lining. The development of carcinoma in a gross cyst developing in dysplasia is extremely unusual; not more than 0.5 per cent of all carcinomas of the breast give evidence of intracystic origin.

If the mensurable, three-dimensional tumor in the breast of a woman with dysplasia is solid, it is mandatory that an exact diagnosis be established by histologic study, the only definitive method.

DISCHARGE FROM NIPPLE. If the patient with discharge from the nipple is found to have a space-occupying tumor, the nipple discharge should be disregarded except for cytologic study. Prompt excision of the tumor for diagnosis is recommended. For the patient with nipple discharge but without a three-dimensional lump, the next most important step is to determine whether or not the exudate contains red blood cells. If so, and the segment of the ductal system from which the bleeding originates has been located, the involved area should be exposed through a parareolar incision with the patient under general anesthesia.

Not infrequently, by careful palpation through the wound, nodular involvement of a duct by papillary change can be digitally determined. Prior to incision, it is possible in some instances to pass the blunt end of a straight skin needle into the orifice on the nipple through which the bleeding exudes, and to pass the needle gently into the duct. With or without such localization, a wedge-shaped resection of the involved part of the ductal system should be done, the radial extent of which should be one-third of the distance from the nipple to the periphery of the breast.

If this excised portion of the ductal system fails to show a lesion, and the patient is premenopausal, further action is not indicated, as the ductal papillomatosis coincident with dysplasia of the breast is not known to be a precancerous process. If the patient is postmenopausal, the likelihood of bleeding from the nipple being due to ductal carcinoma increases proportionately with each decade past the menopause. In this instance, if a preliminary, conservative ductal resection fails to demonstrate a benign papilloma, simple mastectomy should be done, particularly if the patient is ten or more years past the menopause. If the excised portion of the ductal system shows an invasive neoplasm, radical mastectomy is indicated.

PSEUDONEOPLASTIC HYPERPLASIA. There are both ductal and acinar states of dysplasia which may resemble closely a genuine neoplastic process. The histologic appearance of some of the more florid of these processes may be so atypical as to make interpretation difficult for the most experienced pathologists. There are occasional situations where the differentiation between hyperplasia with considerable atypism, and neoplasia is difficult.

When there are focal areas of atypical nodular hyperplasia of ductal epithelium, the differentiation from neoplastic ductal papilloma may be extraordinarily difficult. Actually, the differentiation is largely academic, for there is no present evidence that either hyperplastic papillomatosis or the genuine papillomas are precancerous lesions.

Atypical acinar hyperplasia is most often seen where there are areas of long-standing cystic involution with development of papillary excrescences in the epithelial lining of such cysts, a condition referred to by some as papillary cystophorous hyperplasia. As in the ductal lesions, interpretations of such atypical changes are best deferred until permanent sections are available. The distinct criteria of malignant neoplastic change should be agreed upon by several pathologists before radical treatment is undertaken.

Such is the spectrum of the dysplastic disorders of the female breast, with their complexity interpreted in terms of abnormal responses evoked in ductal, acinar and stromal target tissues by an imbalance of endocrinologic factors. Numerically these non-neoplastic states of excessive hyperplasia, involution, sclerosis and secretion constitute the largest fraction of women whose complaint is of the breast. Clinical comprehension of their common genesis as disorders of the hyperplasia-involution cycle has been impaired greatly by the frequency with which

their nomenclatural identification is more of historical than of practical value. Other misconceptions arise from efforts to endow some given phase of dysplasia with the dignity of a separate entity. The most common and persistent misconceptual term is the venerable expression "chronic cystic mastitis" for a process which is never inflammatory and often is noncystic. When this nosologic absurdity is used by pathologists as a histologic diagnosis, it implies a recognition of the limited intellectual capacity of the clinician. There has been a plethora of attempts in the medical literature to create entities from the vagaries of the dysplasias. A symptom was afforded a niche in one classification with the recognition of "mastodynia." Neologistic terms such as "cystophorous hyperplasia" and "mazoplasia" have contributed to conceptual confusion.

There is no satisfactory generic term for all these phases of abnormalities of hyperplasia and involution, but dysplasia seems to provide the best approximation of an all-inclusive label. Originally defined as "abnormalities of development," it indicated gross, regional deformities of development. In recent years, cellular abnormalities of growth short of neoplasia have been designated as "dysplastic" with increasing frequency.

The frequency of symptomatic mammary dysplasia, combined with the continued, unjustifiable emphasis on the early diagnosis of cancer, have produced an increased frequency of unnecessary incisional biopsy procedures. Some of the excisions of nonexistent tumors of the breast are due to the physician's inability to recognize dysplastic abnormalities without a dominant, space-occupying lump. Others are the product of encounters between apprehensively cancer-conscious women and surgeons whose motivation is something less than idealistic.

BENIGN NEOPLASMS

FIBROADENOMA (ADENOFIBROMA). As indicated in Tables 1 and 2, the incidence of this compound neoplasm of fibroblastic and epithelial origin exceeds all other benign neoplasms of the breast by a large margin. It is the only common mammary neoplasm in young women, with a peak of incidence between the ages of 20 and 25. Fibroadenomas occasionally develop during adolescence, a few are seen in women from 30 years of age

Table 2. Mammary Neoplasms

ORIGIN	BENIGN VARIANTS	APPROX. INCIDENCE (PER CENT)	MALIGNANT VARIANTS	APPROX. INCIDENCE (PER CENT)
I. Epithelium				
a. Ductal	Papilloma	18	CARCINOMA	93.0
b. Acinar	Adenoma	2	Lobular Carcinoma	5.0
II. Connective tissue	Lipoma	3	Rare lesions, including lipo-	
	Rare neoplasms, including granu-lar cell myoblastoma, meso-dermal tumors	2	sarcoma, hemangiosarcoma, lymphosarcoma	0.5
III. Compound	FIBROADENOMA	75	Cystosarcoma phyllodes	1.5
		100.0		100.0
Hyperplasia simulating neoplasm	DYSPLASIAS "Cystic" disease; principal phases (a) proliferative (b) cystic (c) sclerosing			

up to the age of menopause, and they are a curiosity in women in the postmenopausal years. Usually, there are no subjective symptoms, although occasionally there may be slight tenderness. This neoplasm has highly characteristic physical criteria in its round or ovoid shape, smooth surface and most of all in its extreme mobility. As indicated in Figure 10, the encapsulation of fibroadenomas is such that gentle pressure over the tumor with a finger will cause displacement of the lump. Multiple fibroadenomas are seen in some 15 per cent of patients with this tumor. Approximately one in ten patients develops one or more additional fibroadenomas after the appearance of an initial tumor.

There is some reasonable evidence to support the thesis that fibroadenomas are related to hyperestrinism. These neoplasms can be induced in animals by administration of estrogenic steroids and it is not uncommon to notice their rapid enlargement during pregnancy. Most of the malignant neoplasms known as cystosarcoma phyllodes have their origin in pre-existing fibroadenomas, which usually have been present for periods of five or more years.

Treatment is that of any undiagnosed three-dimensional tumor of the breast — surgical excision. Because of the characteristic physical findings and their predilection for occurrence in younger women, the accuracy of diagnosis for fibroadenomas is greater than for other space-occupying lesions of the breast.

INTRADUCTAL PAPILLOMA. Genuine benign neoplastic growths in the form of papillomas of the ductal epithelium are a poor second in frequency. They occur in women of almost any age over 20 years. The majority, or about three of four, are located in the ductal system of the central third of the breast, the remainder more peripherally. Minute papillomas several millimeters in diameter may cause significant bleeding from the nipple. Larger papillomas often produce ductal obstruction which, if followed by bleeding into the obstructed portion, will result in severe distention with tenderness, pain and a palpable soft enlargement. Occasionally, there will be periodic, rather profuse bloody discharge from the nipple as a duct alternately is obstructed and drains. Infection may produce retraction of the nipple and secondary axil-

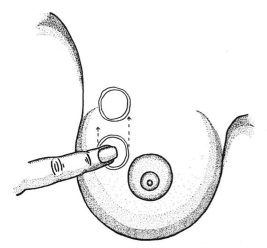

Figure 10. Mobility of an encapsulated fibroadenoma.

lary lymphadenitis, thus imitating a carcinoma of the central third of the breast.

Treatment is the same as for dysplastic ductal papillomatosis. Radical management of this lesion is entirely unjustifiable, for the great majority are localized to a single quadrant and the process does not undergo malignant transition. This latter fact was well documented by a study of 76 patients with intraductal papilloma treated by local excision in whom follow-up for five to ten or more years showed no single instance of subsequent carcinoma.

OTHER BENIGN TUMORS. Other benign neoplasms are so unusual as to occur in a total of not more than 1 per cent of all patients with lesions of the breast. Included are genuine intramammary lipomas, as compared to those developing in the subcutaneous layer of fat, and adenomas.

CARCINOMA OF THE FEMALE BREAST

This epithelial form of mammary cancer is the most common cancer of Caucasian women. As of 1966, it is estimated that this diagnosis was made in over 60,000 patients in the United States. Cancer of the breast will be diagnosed in one of every 18 women over a 72-year lifetime, a probability rate of 5.5 per cent.

The surgical literature provides a reliable indication of the engrossing interest of surgeons in mammary cancer; such reports exceed by a considerable margin their writings on any other single site of cancer. A substantial majority of these contributions are of little significance and, indeed, many are valueless. In recent years, much of the effort, time and reporting by surgeons has been concerned with modifications of the classic operative treatment of carcinoma of the breast. Some advocate anatomic extensions of resection beyond the breast and its regional lymph nodes in the axilla, and others offer evidence supporting their conviction that operations of lesser magnitude are as valuable as the supraradical procedures.

Expanding knowledge of the natural history of mammary carcinoma during the past four years demands that not only treatment, but other features of the disease must be presented in a changed perspective, or with a different emphasis, to achieve a reasonable correlation with the emerging profile of the total life cycle of neoplasia in the epithelial structures of the human breast. Other areas which now require re-evaluation include the concept of early diagnosis, data on survival, the notion of trauma as an etiologic factor and the validity of biologic predeterminism.

The items of evidence which establish the need for a new look at breast cancer are of diverse derivation. Some have been known facts for some years, but acquire a new meaning through illumination provided by more accurate estimates of the perimeters of mammary neoplasia.

MORTALITY RATE. In total numbers, deaths from breast cancer have increased steadily in this century, but only as a function of the increase in female population in the United States. The total toll was 11,000 in 1930, 22,500 in 1958 and nearly 30,000 in 1965. But during these decades, the mortality rate has been almost fixed at 24 to 25 per 100,000.

INCIDENCE. Significant information on rates of incidence is virtually limited to two states, Connecticut and New York. In neither state have any notable trends been apparent in age-adjusted rates of incidence. In upstate New York from 1942 to 1953, incidence rates varied from only 58 to 62 per 100,000 females. In 1941, the incidence rate in Connecticut was about 58, reached a peak of 62 in 1952 and had dropped to 55.5 in 1954 (Fig. 11). Information available for subsequent years does not indicate any significant changes in these rates.

SURVIVAL RATES. When there are stable rates of incidence and of mortality, it must follow with the certainty of a mathematical exercise that rates of survival are stable, assuming that the necessary data are derived from a large, defined population. The information is of value only when the entire sample of patients with breast cancer in the defined population is recorded and followed, without selection or bias. Of all the states, only Connecticut has such total data. In California, the State Tumor Registry has collected information from 40 selected hospitals in the state concerning more than 14,000 women with breast cancer.

The Connecticut experience included a total of over 10,000 patients. In a 15-year interval (1941 to 1956), crude five-year survival—including all causes of death—was 47 to 49 per cent. The relative survival rate, which is obtained by adjustment to exclude causes of death other than from breast cancer, also was fixed with a "range" from 53 to 55 per cent.

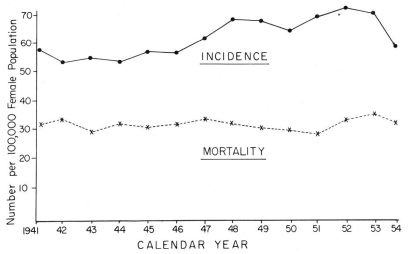

Figure 11. Cancer of the female breast. Connecticut age-adjusted rates of incidence and mortality. (Macdonald, I.: The breast. *In*, Nealon: Management of the Patient with Cancer. W. B. Saunders Company.)

The information from the State Tumor Registry in California provided survival rates for its selected hospital populations from 1942 to 1957. Comparison for the two decades showed no significant improvement (Fig. 12). The proportion of patients diagnosed while still presenting, apparently, local disease in the breast only, increased 2 to 3 per cent. In Connecticut with more reliable data, the proportion of localized neoplasm was fixed at 44 per cent for the two periods. The failure of survival rates to improve in the California sample is the more remarkable because the 40 hospitals in the Tumor Registry include an unrepresentative number of teaching hospitals and institutions with well-organized, departmentalized medical staffs and some degree of special interest in the therapy of cancer, as evident in formal patterns of tumor boards and the like.

RATES OF PREVALENCE. One final epidemiologic measure is the rate of prevalence: the sum of the newly diagnosed cases and those patients surviving still after diagnosis in earlier years, during a given calendar period. With 50 per cent or more of definitively treated patients surviving for five years or more, the total number of women with breast cancer in any calendar year is impressive, or approximately five times the annual incidence of newly diagnosed cases.

This array of epidemiologic data on the ravages of breast cancer in the American female population invalidates a number of long-cherished dogmas, especially those concerning etiology and therapy. To the clinician

Figure 12. Five-year survival rate in carcinoma of the breast for two comparable periods in Connecticut and California. (Macdonald, I.: The breast. *In*, Nealon: Management of the Patient with Cancer. W. B. Saunders Company.)

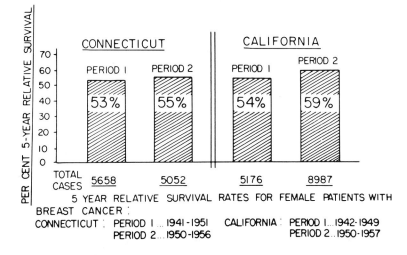

the most important conclusion derived from these dismal facts is that no part of the massive attack which has been mounted against mammary cancer in the past 25 years has produced any alteration in morbidity and mortality from this neoplasm.

For teachers and practitioners of surgery our failure in an improved control of carcinoma of the breast has a twofold meaning. First, the phenomenal increase in centers for sound graduate education and training since World War II has resulted in a highly significant increase in the availability of competent surgical care, of a quality formerly obtained only by those reaching centers of medical education. This achievement has been of no importance to the woman with breast cancer. Second, anatomical extension of operative procedures beyond the limits of the classic radical mastectomy has contributed no apparent improvement in overall survival.

Such a therapeutic stalemate indicates a biologic intransigence, the explanation of which should be discoverable in the natural history of mammary neoplasia.

BIOLOGIC PREDETERMINISM: THE DETERMINANT OF NATURAL HISTORY. A wide variety of malignant neoplasms originate in the epithelial structures of the breast, all of which masquerade as an entity under the generic designation of "carcinoma." The remarkable disparity in behavior, or natural history, of carcinoma of the breast is recognized by any thoughtful clinician with adequate experience. The first indication of the disease may be symptoms evoked by widespread dissemination from a tiny, or even impalpable primary focus in the breast. Occasionally, a woman is seen first with a massive tumor replacing most of the breast, yet which proves to have no extension even to the axillary nodes. Some 5 per cent of all mammary carcinoma is an acute variant which erupts explosively and may be lethal to its host within weeks after its recognized onset. The obverse in relationship of host to neoplasm is provided by patients who survive definitive treatment in good health for many years, only to develop activation of distant metastasis as long as 30 to 40 years after primary treatment. The severe limitations of our nomenclatural vocabulary are obvious in the designation of such a spectrum of neoplastic patterns by a single word—carcinoma.

In a minority of patients the extremes of neoplastic behavior are recognizable by morphologic, usually histologic criteria. In about four out of every five patients no presently available accurate method permits any estimate of neoplastic patterns of activity. Attempts at estimation of the degree of malignancy of an individual breast carcinoma, by histologic observation, is of limited value; the presence and extent of axillary, lymph nodal metastasis provides a predictive gauge of survival for a large sample of patients, but some women with an anaplastic primary focus with involvement of many axillary nodes may survive more than ten years after treatment with no reactivation.

Estimates of chronologic duration, mensurable size of the primary tumor and evidence of extension beyond the breast have provided the basis for separating favorable from unfavorable settings for the clinician and the propagandist alike in this century. Early diagnosis and early treatment are shibboleths which still dominate public education on cancer and, more lamentably, professional education as well. Persistent proponents of such elementary thinking concerning time and size ignore any recognition of valid definitions of earliness. This sort of clinical evangelism has reduced the natural history of cancer to a state of enviable simplicity: the extent of a neoplasm is in direct ratio to the lapse of time since onset of recognizable symptoms or signs.

More than 15 years ago, a correlation of these considerations of time and space-occupation with survival rates in several forms of human cancer led to the following conclusion:

"The behavior of a neoplasm in an individual host is an expression of a biological potential established during the inductive phase of neoplasia. . . . The balance of power between neoplastic and reactive influences in the host has been established in the preclinical phase of the process, and in a clinical sense this concept may be expressed as that of biological predeterminism."

This expression of heterodoxy soon was afforded some support by the growing knowledge of the phase of preinvasive carcinoma in certain sites, notably the uterine cervix, the duration of which was established as from five to as long as 15 years. Chance provided occasional observations of a preinvasive phase in surgically obtained specimens of breast tissue, but without indication of its temporal duration.

LIFE CYCLE OF BREAST CARCINOMA. In more recent years, methods have been developed for estimations of the preclinical phase of human cancers, defined as that interval of time from inception of malignant neoplasia to such size as to permit its clinical recognition. The first requirement was a determination of rates of growth of a given form of neoplasm in a sample of patients. This objective required serial measurements of untreated tumors after the preclinical phase, when the neoplasm had become recognizable, or diagnosable, by some means presently available. The greatest contribution has been made by radiologists, first by serial observations of the growth of lung cancer. Comparable data have been derived by direct observations of the growth of colonic cancer and of experimentally induced neoplasms in animals.

From such observations came the possibility of estimating the time required for an individual cancer to double in its mean diameter, which means an eightfold volumetric increase, and is designated as the "doubling time." The doubling time is an expression of the host-tumor relationship, the kinetic product of neoplastic aggressiveness balanced against hostal factors of resistance.

Estimates of the interval of preclinical growth—from inception to earliest possible clinical recognition—depend upon the retrospective extension of the known doubling time to the origin of the cancer as a single cell, or as is more probable in human cancer, as a focus of neoplastic transition. For this purpose, doubling times are plotted on semi-logarithmic charts against time. Independent applications of this method have produced comparable conclusions for lung cancer. Squamous carcinomas have a mean prediagnostic duration of ten years or more, whereas pulmonary adenocarcinomas average more than 18 years before becoming radiographically detectable at a diameter of 2 cm. For cancers of the colon, to reach a diameter of 1.5 cm., by similar estimates, the total life cycle of the tumor varies from four to more than ten years.

Roentgenographic studies also made possible estimates of the doubling times for mammary carcinoma, in a group of women in whom serial measurements of size were obtained on mammograms prior to a belated recognition of an abnormality, or in whom therapeutic action had been deferred. Some of these tumors were detectable on mammograms before sufficiently large to permit their recognition by palpation, or a maximal diameter of 1 cm. under average conditions. Because of the known, extreme variations in growth rate of breast cancer during its clinical phase, one must assume the total time of growth to be comparably variable; had these estimates indicated any uniformity, the sample studied would have been unrepresentative. In fact, the estimates of doubling time were as disparate as are the established differences of the natural history by clinical observations.

Figure 13 is a schematic representation of

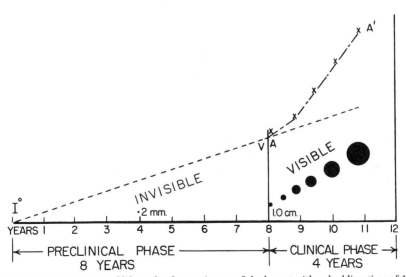

Figure 13.   Schematic representation of life cycle of a carcinoma of the breast with a doubling time of 100 days. I°–V = preclinical phase, assuming a mean diameter of 1.0 cm. as the minimum for palpatory recognition. A–A' = Curve of growth in clinical phase, of which I°–V is the logarithm. (Macdonald, I.: The breast. *In*, Nealon: Management of the Patient with Cancer. W. B. Saunders Company.)

the total life cycle of a cancer of the breast. Clinical orientation requires its division into two phases: the invisible or preclinical period, and the visible or clinical duration. The former is a retrospective, mathematical approximation; the latter is based on serial measurements mainly by mammography, by clinical mensuration in several patients.

Assuming that the size of a neoplastic, epithelial cell of mammary origin is 10μ on average, that breast cancer begins either in a single cell or in a focus of 20 to 30 cells and that the smallest mean diameter at which a cancer becomes palpable is 1 cm., then the initial focus of cancer must undergo 30 doublings in volume before it becomes clinically diagnosable. The doubling time in the clinical phase varied from 23 to 209 days — a difference entirely consistent with the known variations in natural history. Doubling times of short duration indicate an unfavorable, and long duration a favorable host-tumor relationship. In more conventional terms, the doubling time is inversely related to the degree of malignancy.

The schematic outline of the total life cycle of a carcinoma of the breast is based on estimations for a neoplasm of moderate grade of malignancy, in which the preclinical phase occupies a period of eight years. In the most highly malignant of the observed group, with the shortest doubling time, the preclinical duration of the neoplasm was two years, and in the tumors with the most dilatory growth pattern, 17 years. Of even more significance, the relative duration of the preclinical to the clinical phase is such that about two-thirds of the total cycle of the life of a mammary carcinoma has elapsed before it becomes clinically detectable at the earliest moment of time.

No claim is made that these estimates are accurate, and for several reasons. The size of the initial focus of cancerization may be larger than the 20 to 30 cells used in such calculations, especially when the process begins in a multicentric fashion, as seems to be true of many breast cancers. The method also assumes that the volume of occupation of neoplasia is made up entirely of cancer cells, whereas as much as one-half of a tumor mass may be composed of stromal reactive elements, vasculature and other non-neoplastic tissue. But these possible contributions to error would, at most, influence the estimates of intervals of time by considerably less than 50 per cent. Only when the neoplasm approaches the dimensions of clinical recognition do stromal and vascular changes contribute in any degree to volumetric mass. Any error owing to an origin from a single cell or many cells is of less importance; by such time as the occult tumor has reached a diameter of 1 mm., its mass is formed of some 2.5 million cells after 20 doublings.

After the dimensions required for clinical recognition have been reached, fewer doublings produce a greater relative increase in size; for a rapidly growing cancer of 1 cm. in mean diameter, only three more doublings are required to attain a volume which will be apparent in a diameter of 2 cm.

There is no correlation of the doubling time with the microscopic appearance of a breast carcinoma.

There is a positive correlation of doubling time with spread to axillary nodes; in patients whose nodes showed no metastasis after radical mastectomy, the doubling time was 128 days on average, whereas with nodal metastasis doubling time was 85 days.

In breast cancer of moderate grade malignancy, untreated patients survive about three or at most four years; thus the total natural life cycle of such a cancer is 12 years, three-fourths of which has elapsed before any therapeutic interference beomes possible.

These estimations of the life cycle of this neoplasm surely confirm the thesis of biologic predeterminism; when the phase of early clinical detection has been reached, the clinician has to cope with a disease process with a potentiality determined long before he can provide therapeutic interference.

These data, combined with the fixed rates of incidence, mortality and survival, constitute a new perspective in which a number of factors must be re-evaluated.

EPIDEMIOLOGIC (ETIOLOGIC) FACTORS. Inasmuch as we are innocent of any knowledge of the definitive causes of breast cancer, it is preferable to refer to so-called contributory factors, or, in recent language, epidemiologic influences. The failure of the breast to perform its expected physiologic function of lactation has been considered as a predisposing factor in the probability of its becoming the site of cancer. In the past decade, about one-third as many parturient women nursed their infants as did 30 years ago, thus negating their physiologic mammary failure as of any significance. Since the synthetic estrogens became generally available more than 30 years ago, enormous quantities have been prescribed as substitutional therapy for post-menopausal women. For a decade or more many clinicians have ordered estrogens for their patients after treatment for mammary carcinoma, when indicated; no available evidence indicates any harmfulness for such substitutional therapy. Thus, the alarm over such estrogenic therapy in contributing to the incidence of carcinoma of the breast has been effectively dispelled.

Trauma as a causative or augmentative factor is the basis for an ever increasing number of actions at law in recent years. The interval of time elapsing between the allegedly etiologic injury and the diagnosis of breast cancer is usually one year or less; even in those unusual rapidly growing neoplasms with an occult phase of only two or three years, the time relationship is in itself a denial of any causative possibility. Epidemiologic data concerning cases of breast cancer and controls also invalidate any role for trauma in the causation of the disease. Actually, the most frequent and severe injury to the breast occurs when a surgeon does an excisional biopsy for benign disorder; the combined insults of incision, clamping, ligature and closure provide far more injury than is sustained in any but the most severe external trauma. Yet there is no recorded instance of any surgical resection of the breast in which no malignant neoplasm was found but in which a cancer subsequently developed. The claim of injury constituting an augmentative influence is almost equally unsubstantial; careful comparison with the known potential of a given mammary carcinoma, as established by gross and microscopic study, and its course following an alleged injury usually fails to demonstrate any departure from the expected natural history of the neoplasm.

Two factors long recognized and established by careful epidemiologic surveys as increasing the probability of breast cancer are singleness and heredity. Women never married have a 70 per cent higher mortality from the disease than do married females. Though not so dramatic a difference, women who are either the daughters or sisters of patients who have had breast carcinoma are more prone to develop the neoplasm. An increased probability of endometrial carcinoma also is a hazard for women after treatment for tumors of the breast, in whom carcinoma of the uterine corpus is twice as frequent as in other women, although they have a lesser likelihood of developing cancer of the uterine cervix than the female population at large.

EARLY DIAGNOSIS. For more than half of this century physicians and the public alike have been adjured toward greater efforts, in their separate fashions, toward the earlier diagnosis of cancer. For two decades, a crash program has been directed toward breast cancer, although the accumulating evidence indicates that the spectrum of neoplasia which affects the breast is affected little, if any, by an measures of earliness available. The professional propagandists have urged women to undertake monthly self-examination of their breasts with the hope of increasing the detection of small, primary tumors — an objective which many physicians find difficult. An ironic twist of this "do-it-yourself" approach is that the women most concerned over their breasts are those menstruants with dysplastic changes accompanied by symptoms of discomfort or even pain, usually on a cyclic basis. These are the patients in whom the differentiation of a space-occupying tumor from the indurative changes of dysplasia is most difficult even for the experienced examiner. Had the campaign for self-examination been garnished with the reassurance that "cancer of the breast does not hurt," the frenetic concern of many women would have been allayed. By evidence from a number of surgical services, more primary lesions of small dimensions are confirmed as carcinoma of the breast than was the case 20 years ago. In one series of more than 900 patients, the primary focus was 1 cm. or less in nearly one of every four women undergoing mastectomy. Such changes have produced no lessening of mortality, or increase in survival beyond ten years postoperative. It is yet to be proved that any refinements in clinical diagnosis, including mammography, will lessen the toll of breast cancer.

Another and organized pursuit of early diagnosis in cancer is in the shape of "cancer detection clinics." From some of these have come statistical data concerning patients with primary breast cancer of small size, asymptomatic, and discovered only by meticulous physical examination, with or without mammographic techniques. The survival of these fortunate women and the low incidence of axillary nodal involvement by metastasis are said to be proof of the manifest virtues of early detection. Such data are unreliable for the same reason that many surgical reports of the treatment of breast cancer are of a low order of credibility – the factor of selection. The asymptomatic women who patronize the facilities of detection clinics are self-selected; in those who are found to have a small, occult carcinoma of the breast, the biologic balance of tumor and host usually is favorable. The unfavorable lesions are evident by their symptoms and signs, and such women do not go to clinics for well persons.

The educational clamor which has surrounded the discovery of a lump, real or supposed, in the breast has had some undesirable by-products. Chief of these is the sense of urgency created in the public mind which may be so delusional as to engender a belief that the difference between life and death may be measured by the passing of a single day. For the unethical physician such hysteria is an invitation to unnecessary incisional procedures on an emergency basis. Even competent surgeons may be influenced by such fancy phrases as "a high index of suspicion." The interplay of public anxiety and professional zeal is mainly responsible for a furor operandi of such proportion that as many as eight of every ten incisional biopsies produce no semblance of a genuine lump or pathologic evidence of abnormality.

CURABILITY. Happily, the predetermined outcome of the host vs. neoplasm competition for dominance produces a proportion of patients who are curable by treatment presently available. For the greater number, therapy is of distinct value though only in a palliative sense. The process of biologic self-separation into curable and incurable fractions is attended by chronologic intervals which are entirely antithetic to the traditional notions of early diagnosis. In patients in whom the cancer is dominant, the process is notable for a shorter total life cycle; rapid growth and poor hostal response mean a shorter preclinical phase during which regional spread and, usually, distant metastasis occur. When this ominous pattern of growth becomes diagnosable its hyperkinetic qualities commonly produce evidence of its presence in its primary or metastatic sites, recognizable to the patient as symptoms or signs. Thus, she seeks medical advice early in the clinical phase and obtains treatment early, with the probability of an early death. When the host has the upper biologic hand, both the preclinical and clinical phases of growth are long in duration; symptoms usually are absent and the presence of a lump in the breast is the only indication of disease; diagnosis is late and treatment later, and the outcome may be definitive cure.

The most important criterion of curability following surgical treatment is the absence of regional metastasis. Most often, slowly growing primary lesions which lack sufficient biokinetic drive to spread even to axillary nodes are of lesser size than neoplasms of more aggressive behavior. This association of smaller breast cancers with favorable prognosis has served to perpetuate the myth of early diagnosis when, in fact, it is diagnosis late in the long cycle of a favorable pattern of growth which is responsible for the association of little cancers with better end results. The exceptions to such a setting are of great clinical importance: in about two of every ten patients who are eligible for surgical treatment with the intent of cure, a large primary cancer will be without histologic evidence of axillary, nodal metastasis, and the smallest breast cancer, including the clinically occult or impalpable tumor, may have disseminated to a wide variety of organs and tissues.

A new therapeutic perspective should be conditioned upon one hard fact: long before the moment of earliest possible clinical recognition of carcinoma of the breast a determinative relationship between the patient and her neoplasm has been established; the die has been cast for or against her curability by present methods. Faced with such a predetermined status, the clinician should direct his efforts toward an improved recognition of indications of curability and incurability, and toward the most judicious possible selection of curative and palliative treatments. Clinicians in general, and surgeons and radiotherapists especially, face an unpalatable corollary conclusion; the usefulness of treatment is circumscribed by inexorable limitations imposed by the natural history of breast cancer, and these limitations already have been reached. There is no reasonable basis for belief that any further modifications, extensions, higher intensities or combinations of present modalities can improve the current level of end results.

If this be so, the therapeutic future of mammary cancer is expressed best by restatement of a conviction by no means new, or even recent: any real improvement in control of this disease must await entirely new methods in treatment, yet to be born of research.

CLINICAL-PATHOLOGIC CORRELATION. About 95 of each 100 mammary carcinomas are considered by consensus to be of ductal origin. Of this dominant group, nearly 80 are without distinctive morphologic features and may be designated as of no specific type (Table 3). From the standpoint of gross pathologic changes, however, almost all of these common carcinomas provoke a sclerosing stromal reaction of variable intensity which is responsible for the hard, irregular consistency of nearly eight of every ten carcinomas on clinical examination.

When the sclerosing process is advanced, the neoplasm will exhibit a stony-hard consistency. This sclerosing reaction led to their separation in older classifications under the designation of *scirrhous carcinoma*, with the now discredited implication that intense sclerosis implied a more favorable prognosis. The informative value of the scirrhous reaction lies not in prognosis, but in gross diagnosis. It produces on cut section a retracted, gritty surface, with yellowish foci representing minute islands of fat which have become surrounded and isolated. There

are two minor variants of this group, those with mucinous degeneration and those with epidermoid differentiation, representing approximately 2 per cent and 1 per cent respectively of all carcinomas.

There are four recognizable cell types of ductal carcinoma which, when predominant, may permit a favorable prognosis. These, in order of descending importance from a prognostic standpoint, are medullary, papillary, comedo and Paget types of carcinoma.

The *medullary carcinoma* is more apt to occur in women under the age of 50. The tumors are frequently bulky in size, may appear to be encapsulated, and often are mistaken grossly for fibroadenomas. Although they may appear to be highly malignant microscopically, their prognosis is five times more favorable than average because of their inherent tendency to remain localized to the breast and regional nodes for considerable periods.

Papillary cystadenocarcinoma is an unusual neoplasm with a tendency to spread throughout the ductal system and to involve a considerable portion of the breast, often

Table 3. *Mammary Carcinoma: Variants of Clinical Significance for Each 100 Patients*

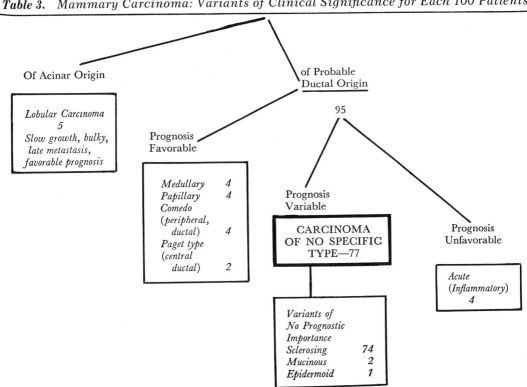

a quadrant or more. Inadequate excision of these neoplasms may be followed some years later by local recurrence without metastasis to regional nodes.

The *comedo carcinoma* is an intraductal process in the beginning and may remain so limited for many months. Necrotic material is extruded into the lumina of the cancerous ducts and, on cut section, compression will cause extrusion of wormlike masses of necrotic tumor, consequently its nomenclatural prefix. Eventually, these neoplasms invariably invade mammary stroma and metastasize to regional nodes.

The term *Paget type* is employed to designate those ductal carcinomas developing in the central third of the breast, in which the first manifestation of the disease may be the development of scaly indurative, erosive or actual ulcerative changes of the nipple and areola, the lesion first described by Paget. Such involvement of the areola is invariably a surface manifestation of an underlying ductal carcinoma, even though no tumor may be palpable. In some instances, the same type of ductal carcinoma may be present without involvement of the areola. This type of mammary carcinoma may remain limited to the central ductal area for varying periods before metastasis occurs.

The most ominous type of mammary carcinoma is that referred to as *acute* or *inflammatory carcinoma*. The lesion is a highly anaplastic variant with a rapid rate of growth and wide lymphatic embolization at an early stage of the process. Obstruction of the subdermal lymphatics by tumor emboli produces congestion with erythema and commonly some degree of lymphedema of the overlying skin. In some instances, no definable three-dimensional tumor is present, as the rapidly advancing neoplasm produces a diffuse, indurative change in the consistency of the affected portion of the breast.

The only excuse for recognizing this as a separate form of mammary carcinoma is the ominous prognostic implication, for this is a surgically incurable form of the disease. Acute carcinoma is more often observed in premenopausal women and is particularly frequent in those carcinomas developing during pregnancy or lactation. It is largely for this reason that carcinoma of the breast in young women is believed by many to be of uniformly bad prognosis. The fact is that, excluding those carcinomas developing during pregnancy or lactation, the prognosis of mammary carcinoma in patients under the age of 30 is somewhat more favorable than for those of all other age groups combined.

CARCINOMA OF ACINAR ORIGIN. Approximately 5 per cent of mammary carcinoma exhibits histologic features consistent with an acinar origin. These lesions are designated as *lobular carcinoma*. Most often, they are slowly growing neoplasms which usually have attained some considerable size when first seen. They have a distinct predilection for long-delayed metastasis to regional nodes. This neoplasm is seen more commonly in young women. It typifies an occasional situation where the clinical setting appears highly unfavorable by reason of a large primary lesion of long duration, yet it has a far better prognosis than the average, indifferent mammary carcinoma of small size. Experience has demonstrated that in situ lobular carcinoma should be treated by simple mastectomy rather than local excision.

GRADING OF MAMMARY CARCINOMA. Apart from recognition of the 20 per cent or more lesions of special types, the pathologist cannot grade carcinoma of the breast with the prognostic accuracy he achieves in most carcinomas of squamous or epidermoid variety. The histologic inconsistencies are well illustrated by the medullary variant in which an anaplastic microscopic appearance is belied by a favorable natural history. The pathologist's recognition of these variants frequently is based on a combination of gross and microscopic features. For the remaining majority of carcinomas, it is possible, by histologic criteria, to label a few as low grade in degree of malignancy, and another small group as having a high grade of malignancy because of striking anaplasia. These relative extremes of histologic architecture account for probably not more than 10 or 12 per cent of the nonspecific carcinomas.

Thus, a major fraction of some 65 per cent are processes which the pathologist can identify only as carcinoma, possibly using the word "ductal" to indicate probable epithelial cell-type. In these instances, information of more prognostic value can be secured from the pathologic extent of the disease and the combined facts of history and physical examination. These factors permit a limited evaluation of the biologic predeterminism inherent in the host-neoplasm relationship for each individual patient. Even in the few mammary carcinomas histologically separable as high or low grade in degree of malignancy, the subsequent course of the disease occasionally belies the histologic assumptions.

DYNAMICS OF GROWTH AND DISSEMINATION. When a patient is seen with a lump in a breast which may be cancer, the clinician must look for evidence of possible extension beyond the breast. Frequently, this search must be made before he is certain that the mammary lesion is, in fact, malignant. But this survey is of great importance to the patient.

The surgeon's first possible opportunity of determining the status of the woman with breast cancer comes when two-thirds or more of its life cycle is completed. At that moment in time he will attempt, with the highly inadequate methods which are available, an orderly clinical expression of the local involvement, of possible regional spread, or distant dissemination. The clinical impression of a predetermined host-tumor relationship is made in terms of anatomic extent and degree of occupation by neoplasm, referred to as "staging." Just as the viewing of a single frame of a motion picture film provides but a hint of the whole, so clinical staging is a static concept of a dynamic biologic complex, as if the restless action in the cellular battle had been frozen for a moment, to give the observer a murky impression of the scene.

The most significant basis for staging in most forms of cancer is that which distinguishes three principal degrees of anatomic extent:

I. Apparently limited to the site of origin
II. Evidence of regional spread, usually in the form of lymphadenopathy
III. Signs of dissemination beyond regional extent, or distant metastasis

In breast cancer, Stage II is divisible usefully into two substages by criteria of anatomic-spatial extent of neoplasm; IIA indicates lesser and IIB greater axillary involvement, with important implications in treatment and prognosis. In some systems of staging these substages of Stage II are given the status of separate stages, by which IIA and IIB become Stages II and III, and distant dissemination becomes Stage IV. The disadvantage of this and even more complex breakdowns is obvious: the basic and most highly significant indications of the stage of disease as local, regional and remote tend to become obscured.

In recent years the International Union Against Cancer has sponsored a movement toward a common language in the staging of cancer; the proposal has gained the endorsement of interested professional organizations in the United States, as well as of several voluntary health agencies, all of which are represented on a Joint Committee on Cancer Staging and End Results Reporting. Functioning under the aegis of this group are separate task forces for the development of clinical stage classifications of major forms or sites of cancer. The systems thus developed have a basis which expresses the desirable concept of staging. Extent of disease is indicated by the use of three capitalized letters; "T" indicates the primary lesion, "N" the lymph nodes and "M" distant metastasis, and hence the plan is designated officially as the "TNM System." Degrees of involvement anatomically are shown by numerals appended to the letter, 0 (zero) indicating no evident involvement, and 1, 2 and 3 progressive extension by neoplasm. Thus, T3, N2, M0 indicates advanced primary disease, unfavorable degree of axillary nodal metastasis but no sign of distant dissemination. From this admirable basis, the architects of the TNM classification became preoccupied with the vagaries of neoplastic activity in breast and axilla, some of which are of little or no prognostic or therapeutic significance. The end result was as complex as any classificatory effort known, with four principal stages, seven substages and a total of 27 descriptive, qualifying conditions. The only stage to escape this confused state was that of distant dissemination as M0 or M1, recognizing any spread beyond homolateral axillary or infraclavicular nodes as distant metastasis. Much of this nomenclatural proliferation arose from an arbitrary designation of tumor size, from artifactual segregation of behavior of the primary lesion and from combining phases of primary and nodal growth to establish substages.

The value of any classification is determined best by its usefulness under working, clinical conditions; experience has demonstrated the failure of the TNM System to meet this crucial test. Under conditions which may prevail with a specially organized clinical service, or in a cancer hospital, the system might be of value in specific investigative projects.

All classifications of breast cancer virtually ignore any criteria of biologic significance, scanty though they may be, stressing only the anatomic extent of and replacement by the neoplasm at that fleeting moment in its life cycle when first subject to clinical evaluation. Though limited, there are features indicating biologic potential which are recognizable readily by the clinician. In some instances such nonanatomic criteria have a significance which far exceeds that of neoplastic space occupation. One is the rate of growth observed by some women; the lump in the breast which has become notably larger in a few weeks up to two or three months, if cancer, is an ominous process. The woman who maintains that her breast lump is unchanged in size for a year or more, if cancer, is more fortunate. Cutaneous erythema or lymphedema apparent to clinician or patient is usually a warning to be heeded before therapeutic decisions are made.

CLINICAL STAGING OUTLINE. In Table 4 is presented an outline for the clinical staging of mammary carcinoma which includes criteria of biologic potential, as well as the more traditional and more important factors of anatomical extent. This outline preserves the basic clinical division of neoplastic extent in the individual patient into primary, regional and distant phases; the variety of factors in Stage II which are pertinent to prognosis, and particularly to treatment, demand its division into two substages. Included also in this outline is a listing of the treatment generally indicated for these several stages, for more timely, subsequent reference.

Patterns of local growth (Stage I clinical). The relative frequency of the sites of intramammary origin of cancer is clinically important. This is most conveniently done by division of the breast into theoretic quadrants and a central or subareolar area, as shown in Figure 14. A distinct excess of carcinoma is found in the upper outer quadrant of the breast, over 40 per cent originating in this quadrant. Next most frequent are the lesions of subareolar origin, accounting for over 20 per cent. In rapidly diminishing sequence of situal frequency are the upper inner, lower outer and lower inner quadrants, with only 5 per cent of lesions originating in the last-named area.

In a few instances, widely separated areas of parenchyma undergo simultaneous cancerization and formation of multiple gross tumors, most often observed in lesions developing during pregnancy or lactation. In

Table 4. Clinical Staging of Mammary Carcinoma by Anatomic and Biologic Criteria

STAGE	AREA	CRITERIA ANATOMIC	BIOLOGIC	TREATMENT
I	T	Disease limited to breast, may include minimal skin changes	Bulky primary tumor without axillary spread usually a favorable setting	Radical mastectomy
	N	No evident lymphadenopathy		
	T	More than minimal changes in skin, up to ulceration		
II A	N	Signs of nodal metastasis Nodes less than 2 cm. in diameter Nodes discrete	History of slow growth	Radical mastectomy
II B	T	Fixed to pectoral fascia Satellite nodules	Rapid growth rate Skin—erythema, edema T small size, N diffuse Acute carcinoma	Test of Radiotherapy: Sensitive: irradiation Resistant: radical mastectomy
	N	Nodes More than 2 cm. diameter Adherent to skin and other nodes Apical Diffuse		
III	T	Fixation to chest wall Contralateral breast		Selective: Irradiation Hormonal alterations—ablative or additive Palliative surgery Chemotherapy
	N	Opposite axillary or supraclavicular		
	M	Evidence of other sites of distant dissemination		

T = Primary tumor of breast.
N = Regional axillary nodes.
M = Distant metastasis.

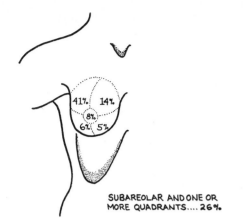

SUBAREOLAR AND ONE OR
MORE QUADRANTS.... 26%.

Figure 14. Distribution of carcinoma in various parts of the breast.

about 1 per cent of all patients, bilateral carcinoma is present on first examination. In patients with only a single lesion demonstrable by gross examination, if scores of microscopic sections are examined from the remainder of the breast, other microscopic foci of carcinoma will occasionally be demonstrated (7 per cent). Further evidence of the biologic abnormality which permits the genesis of mammary carcinoma is the subsequent development of a carcinoma in the remaining breast in 5 per cent of women surviving mastectomy for five or more years. As expressed by Stewart, the most common precancerous condition of the left breast is carcinoma of the right breast, and vice versa.

After reaching three-dimensional size, progressive extension into adjacent mammary tissue usually occurs, most often in irregular, pseudopodic fashion, producing a highly irregular surface and poorly demarcated edge. The rate of growth is not an exponential of time; periods of active local growth alternate with intervals of little or no increase in extent. With advance of the lesion, the skin becomes attached, infiltrated and eventually ulcerated, with subsequent secondary infection, necrosis and hemorrhage. Deep extension becomes attached to the pectoral fascia, which usually acts as a barrier to further direct spread, but extension through fascia and muscle may result in solid fixation to the thoracic cage. In the area of the axilla, the neoplasm may extend directly into and blockade the axillary space.

Notable variations from this average of local growth and extension are seen. In some fortunate patients, a dilatory, progressive ductal process will require several years to produce a palpable mass or to appear clinically as Paget's disease. In such women, dissemination of the disease beyond the breast is long delayed or may never occur. In lobular carcinoma and in the more favorable variants of ductal carcinoma, the tendency is toward a walled-off or even pseudo-encapsulated tumor which may be bulky but is not actively infiltrating. Such neoplasms are expansile rather than infiltrative. Acute, or inflammatory, carcinoma represents a florid, overwhelming variant of infiltrative carcinoma, with multiplicity of origin, rapid extension and the circulatory congestive changes peculiar, in such degree, to this lesion.

A rare variant in local growth is one that may be of great diagnostic difficulty: the primary carcinoma of the breast which remains occult while disseminating widely. In some of these patients, the original lesion can be found only by serial sectioning of the breasts at autopsy. Less striking, but more frequent, are women whose first symptoms are those of either regional or distant metastasis in whom the primary lesion is so small in size as to be detectable only by careful examination.

Secondary changes within mammary carcinoma are most dependent on rapidity of growth and size and are proportional to both. They include areas of hemorrhage, zones of necrosis and secondary infection.

In a few patients, satellite cutaneous nodules develop from subdermal lymphatic tumor emboli, an ominous sign.

Regional metastasis (Stage II clinical). The definition of "regional" is of prime importance. This is the more frequent area of initial spread of cancer beyond its primary site of origin. The usual route of such extension is through lymphatic vessels, those which normally are responsible for lymphatic drainage to regional groups of lymph nodes. This is the route of preference for extension beyond the primary focus manifested by a great majority of malignant neoplasms originating in epithelial structures, or carcinomas. For the sarcomas, lymphatic extension to regional lymph nodes is the exception; most extend beyond their primary site by humoral channels. The breast is no exception to these generalities. In some seven of every ten carcinomas, the first extramammary spread is through lymphatics to the axillary and subscapular groups of nodes. Sarcoma of the breast so rarely takes the lymphatic route that its possibility of so doing is ignored in its therapy.

The proper anatomic definition of "regional" nodes includes the axillary lymph nodal groups and those which are infraclavicular in location. As will be noted in the anatomical representation of lymphatic pathways of drainage from the breast in Figure 1, other and more ominous routes exist, directly to supraclavicular, internal mammary and contralateral axillary groups of lymph nodes. In no anatomic sense are any of these regional, nor should their involvement by neoplastic cells metastatic from the breast be regarded as such. A single nodal focus of metastasis in any of these three areas is as important in prognosis as is spread to viscera or bone.

In a technical, surgical reference the regional nodes are those which should be included in the surgeon's attack on breast cancer. This was the contribution of Halsted and Willy Meyer to the operative treatment of breast cancer—the en bloc resection of breast, pectoral muscles and regional nodes, the first definitive improvement since the pioneering Celsus attempted mastectomy.

The mechanism of intralymphatic spread is usually by embolization, rather than by permeation.

It is probable that some three of every ten breast carcinomas disseminate through hematogenous channels, thus accounting for some of those patients whose axillary nodes are without apparent metastasis, but who develop distant foci of disease.

Distant metastasis (Stage III clinical). The transitional phase from regional to distant metastasis in a few patients seems to occur in an anatomical, orderly sequence through lymphatic pathways. Thus, apical, axillary tumors may next reach supraclavicular nodes, followed by pulmonary or mediastinal nodal metastasis. Or, through the internal mammary pathway, direct spread to the pleura and perhaps lymphangitic pulmonary involvement represent an anatomic sequence.

The vagaries of remote dissemination are such that any orderly, progressive sort of spread is seldom demonstrable. From a practical, clinical standpoint, it is essential to remember that any spread beyond the true, regional nodes is almost invariably an indication of generalized disease.

Of greatest importance to the clinician is a knowledge of the most frequent sites of distant metastasis. From combined information provided by clinical and autopsy studies, distant sites may be listed in order of descending frequency:

Mediastinal nodes, lung and pleura
Bone
Liver and peritoneum
Adrenals
Brain
Ovaries

It is also helpful to have in mind the sites of predilection of skeletal metastases, which in order of diminishing frequency, are:

Ribs
Lumbar spine, pelvis and upper femora
Dorsal and cervical spine
Skull
Upper humeri and scapulae

Skeletal metastasis from carcinoma of the breast is predominantly osteolytic, although some osteoblastic reaction is common at the advancing periphery of bony lesions. Occasionally, osteoblastic metastasis is seen, though rarely is it as sclerosingly eburnated as that common to deposits of prostatic carcinoma.

It is of interest that the only rational explanation for the areas of vertebral involvement is a spread through the paravertebral venous system. The same route probably accounts for cerebral metastasis, as it does for cerebral involvement in bronchogenic carcinoma and pulmonary abscess.

The variegations in patterns and timing of the appearance of metastasis are inexplicable. Activation of skeletal metastasis may occur 30 or more years following radical mastectomy. In some patients, a solitary focus of metastasis will become evident, particularly in bone, several years after primary treatment, and will come under prompt control by palliative management, followed by years of clinical quiescence. At the other extreme of the biologic spectrum, innumerable sites of miliary metastasis may erupt with explosive onset in the first several years after treatment, with a fatal outcome in months or even weeks.

Finally, there are not infrequent instances of spontaneous arrest and regression of metastatic mammary carcinoma, even when widespread. In some instances, the phenomenon is due to a "biologic adrenalectomy," or total replacement of the adrenal glands by metastasis. In menstruants, the same phenomenon may occur due to replacement of the ovaries by metastasis. More often, spontaneous control is of short duration and due to inexplicable changes in host-tumor relationship.

SYMPTOMS. The symptomatology of carcinoma of the breast is influenced by its anatomical extent; the primary lesion most often is asymptomatic, the complaints due to disseminated tumor being limited only by the number of foci and their severity. Nevertheless, it is helpful to correlate symptoms with stages of disease.

In Stage I, or limitation of evident tumor to the breast, the patient is asymptomatic with certain exceptions. In perhaps nine of every ten women the only indication of the presence of a breast cancer is the sign of a symptomless lump usually discovered accidentally. In menstruants, the coincidence of dysplasia with tenderness may lead to an impression that the lump which proves to be cancer was the source of discomfort. To women with symptomatic dysplasia, the information that "cancer of the breast does not produce pain" is of much importance. The rare exception to this generality is provided by a rate of growth which does not permit a gradual adjustment of surrounding breast tissue. Breast carcinoma with a rate of growth more rapid than average produces symptoms which lead to an early diagnosis with a minimal chance of cure.

Symptoms of axillary-nodal metastasis (Stage II clinical) are as unimpressive as in the breast. Even the presence of multiple enlarged nodes 5 or more cm. in diameter may have gone unrecognized by the patient. With a pattern of growth more rapid than ordinary, pressure on the brachial plexus may be the cause of pain in the upper extremity. Only very advanced axillary, untreated disease will produce edema of the arm, or sensory or motor impairment.

In the disseminated (Stage III clinical) phase, symptoms often provide important clues to sites of metastasis. To detail the constellation of symptomatic evidence of metastatic replacement of intrathoracic structures, of osseous and connective tissues, of hepatic, peritoneal, adrenal and cerebral tissues would be redundant. An example will suffice. The skeletal survey by radiography of a woman with a lump in a breast which may be cancer is wasteful of the effort of personnel and money, when used as a routine approach. When such a patient has symptoms of pain or even discomfort of such duration and character as to suggest even the possi-

bility of metastatic cancer, the necessity of special studies becomes mandatory. Similarly, cough, dyspnea or a pleuritic type of pain, headache, visual disturbance and vertigo, if of recent origin, are indications for preoperative investigations.

PHYSICAL SIGNS. The evidence provided by physical examination is objective, and not beset with the subjective uncertainties of symptoms. This is not to imply that clinical objectivity is any guarantee of accuracy; the skillful examiner's ability to determine whether axillary lymphadenopathy is neoplastic is of a low order. For each of the stages of mammary carcinoma, two phases of physical signs will be recognized: the customary evaluation of apparent spatial extent of the neoplasm, and the recognition of physical signs which are not palpable, nor measured volumetrically. These few clues to the biologic potential of a neoplasm are seen in only a minority of patients, but when present they are of more significance than are the anatomic criteria.

The primary carcinoma. Anatomic signs are those of space occupation. In the breast of average size, the cancer must have achieved a volume sufficient to present a diameter in the order of 1 cm. before it becomes palpable by an experienced examiner. When located deeply in a bulky, fatty breast, a three-dimensional tumor several times as large may be missed. Located superficially in a small breast, nodules as small as 0.5 cm. have been palpable. In the instance of larger and obvious primary masses apparent to unskilled or casual observers, no advance in staging is justifiable unless there are concomitant signs of aggressive neoplastic behavior most often evident in alterations in the overlying skin. The earliest of these is a loss of mobility of the skin. When attachment of mammary skin becomes more than minimum, it is a sign of lymphatic spread toward the corium, and is of sufficient prognostic importance to require classification of the neoplastic process as Stage II, even in the absence of apparent axillary metastasis. When such extension occurs centrally, retraction of the nipple is noted, but just as important is an elevation in the level of the areola owing to lesions in a supra-areolar location. Mammary cancer first noted as a plaque-like, indurated replacement of areolar skin, often with ulceration, always is secondary to carcinoma originating in the underlying ducts, and this primary focus may exist without areolar change, often escaping discovery. A minor fraction of patients with cutaneous involvement progress to ulceration of areas of skin over the neoplasm, usually with obvious axillary spread but occasionally, in its absence. A far more serious local extension is toward the chest wall; fixation to pectoral fascia is not a uniformly ominous feature, but infiltrating attachment to the chest wall itself is nearly equivalent to distant metastasis in its significance.

Physical signs of biologic order may be discernible either in apparent growth rate or as mirrored in the skin, in respect to the primary focus. There are occasional women who seek a medical opinion because of their belief that a previously noted breast lump has increased in size in a short interval, usually measured in weeks or several months. The fallacies inherent in such self-observation are obvious, but the credibility which the clinician assigns to such a historical sequence should be related to his evaluation of the woman's capacities. The implication of such a rapid growth pattern is a short doubling time, hence an unfavorable host-tumor relationship. The obverse of this situation is the patient who maintains that her breast lump has been present for long intervals of one year or more, and that she has noted little or no increase in its apparent size. Subject to the same reservations of credibility, such a history may indicate a long doubling time, a dilatory rate of growth and a favorable prognosis.

The cutaneous signs which are biologic indicators are exclusively associated with a poor prognosis and most often are identified with incurability. Both of such skin alterations are the result of vascular abnormalities evoked by an aggressive lesion. Obstruction of superficial lymphatic vessels by neoplastic cells results in varying degrees of edema, so slight as to require magnification for verification, or so severe as to produce the "pig skin" or *peau d'orange* simulation. The gravity of these signs is in proportion to their severity and extent; frequently dependent areas inferior to the level of the primary neoplasm are so involved. More ominous are changes secondary to superficial capillary obstruction or proliferation, with congestion and erythema. The most familiar erythematous manifestation is that of the uniformly lethal and inoperable acute carcinoma. But some other unfavorable breast cancers also are identifiable as much by some degree of erythema in overlying skin as by any other

factor. When present, its significance is greater than any degree of space occupation, for it often is an indicator of inoperability, if not of incurability.

Regional spread. Indications of anatomic axillary metastasis are of much greater importance than those of biologic import. The most important single determinant of prognosis in operable breast carcinoma is the absence or presence of axillary nodal metastasis. If present, its extent of involvement within the axilla is highly important also in estimating probability of survival. Clinical evaluation of regional lymphadenopathy in the woman with carcinoma of the breast is highly inaccurate. For each ten occasions on which a clinical verdict of "no evident metastasis" is recorded, histologic examination will show nodal cancer in four instances. When examination indicates axillary metastasis, it will be disproved in about three of each ten patients. In spite of such inaccuracy in diagnostic evaluation, decisions on therapy must be based upon clinical judgment. Possible metastatic replacement of nodes in the axillary apex is of especial importance. Only when axillary nodal disease becomes so advanced as to be questionably operable does clinical accuracy appear; this is when involved nodes are fixed to each other, or to the skin.

As indicated in Table 4, the size of axillary nodal involvement is one factor which determines IIA or IIB staging, with an arbitrary diameter of 2 cm. usually adopted as the level for separation. Indiscrete nodes, involved apical nodes and very diffuse nodal disease in the axilla are criteria of Stage IIB.

The one regional indication of biologic importance, and equivocally so, is the presence of advanced axillary disease from a small primary lesion. This is analogous to the minute or occult primary focus with wide distant dissemination.

Distant dissemination. The search for evidence of remote spread is simply a meticulous and complete physical examination, remembering that no anatomic area is immune from nidation of tumor emboli in breast cancer. Miliary intracutaneous foci may be found in the extremities. Other sites always to be included in the survey of the woman with a lump in one breast, as yet undiagnosed, are the opposite breast and axilla, cervical nodes, liver, ovary, peritoneum and cerebrum.

Biologic potential is even more evident in the course of distant metastatic disease than in the primary regional complex. The woman who survives in good health for 40 postmastectomy years before a focus of skeletal or other metastasis undergoes activation represents a situation of biologic amity between host and neoplasm so prolonged as to have produced countless assurances of her cure through early diagnosis. The obverse is the woman who succumbs to a fulminating generalized metastatic carcinoma three months after the first recognizable symptom, with the primary site undetermined until, at autopsy, a 4-mm. primary carcinoma of the breast is discovered. If early diagnosis is a function of minimal delay, as is persistently alleged, then this documented history represents an irreducible interval of zero delay.

PATHOLOGIC STAGING. In operable instances of mammary carcinoma, radical mastectomy makes available for microscopic study the contents of the axilla, containing the regional nodes, the clinical evaluation of which has been the surgeon's most difficult preoperative problem. The pathologist has the opportunity of gross and histologic survey of these lymph nodal structures, from which will be derived the most important prognostic information for each patient. From the microscopic examination of these lymph nodes comes a modification of staging; clinical impressionism is replaced by the more accurately objective findings of the microscopist. Thus "clinical staging" is modified to become "pathologic staging," especially in the presence or absence, as well as the anatomic extent, of regional metastasis. Revision of clinical impressions concerning the extent of intramammary disease may also emerge from gross and microscopic study. Rather than the tubular glimpse of neoplastic structure obtained by the pathologist from a biopsy specimen, his thorough study of samplings from the entire neoplasm may require changes of some importance in microdiagnosis.

It is obvious that these conclusions obtained from studies in surgical pathology become the final diagnosis in recording of operable, postoperative patients because of their greater relative accuracy. It is customary to identify staging modified by pathologic criteria by the use of the capitalized letter "P"— but only when the entire product of a radical mastectomy has become available for such study. Clinical staging is signified by a capitalized "C." Thus, following a radical mastectomy, a Stage IIAC may become a Stage IP.

Surgeons and clinicians with any interest in mammary carcinoma tend to overemphasize the importance of pathologic staging. Although it is of somewhat greater accuracy than clinical classification in patients subjected to radical mastectomy, its application is possible only in a selected sample of the total population of women with breast cancer. The principal factor of selection is predeterminism in natural history; for any patient her conformance, or nonconformance to criteria of operability was predetermined in the preclinical phase of neoplastic growth. Among a number of secondary selective factors the most important is the concept of operability as determined by individual surgeons or institutions. The criteria which contribute to decisions on operability determine the relative size of the sample on which definitive operative treatment is employed. The more stringent the criteria, the smaller the operative sample, whereas less exacting criteria may reduce materially the number of women designated as "inoperable." Difference in size of the samples selected for definitive surgical treatment are, inevitably, productive of differences in rates of survival.

Pathologic staging is of only relative accuracy, for two principal reasons—one attributable to the surgeon, and one to inadequacies of techniques in surgical pathology. When the phase of axillary dissection is done meticulously, not less than 15 and up to 30 or more lymph nodes should be found in this portion of the specimen. To the extent that the dissection of the axilla is inadequate, the information from microscopy is unreliable. Histologic discovery of small foci of metastasis in axillary nodes is facilitated by the technique of clearing the gross specimen before nodes are dissected for processing. Such is the added time required that the procedure is inconsistent with the demands of routine work. When clearing has been used after routine processing, in some 20 per cent of axillary tissues reported as free of metastasis, involved nodes have been found. Thus, the number of patients reported as Stage IP should be reduced by some 20 per cent, and the frequency of Stage IIP similarly increased. This represents only an exercise in frustration, but accounts for some Stage IP patients with an unfavorable postoperative course.

It is apparent that the clinical staging of breast carcinoma, in spite of its inaccuracies, is by far the more important of the two systems. Only clinical staging is applicable to the total sample of experience; staging by pathologic information necessarily is limited to a selected, unrepresentative sample of the disease.

A clinical estimate of the extent of the disease is of value for a variety of reasons. It requires of the clinician an orderly evaluation of each patient, accomplished through a comprehensive review of symptoms, signs and physical and laboratory findings; to such extent as is possible with available techniques, a prognostic estimate for each patient is provided; clinical staging provides the only practicable basis for the selection of therapeutic methods.

The first and crucial consideration of treatment demands a decision on one of two alternatives: shall the objective of treatment be the intent of cure, or of palliation?

DIAGNOSTIC PROCEDURE FOR THE PATIENT WITH AN UNDIAGNOSED, THREE-DIMENSIONAL TUMOR IN A BREAST.   As in physical examination of the breasts, an orderly sequence of action toward a diagnosis contributes to orderly thinking, saving of time and effort and may inspire the patient's confidence. A sequence of actions for accurate diagnosis for the woman with a genuine but undiagnosed lump in the breast is outlined in Table 5. This

Table 5.   *Outline for Diagnostic Action for the Woman with an Undiagnosed Three-Dimensional Tumor in a Breast*

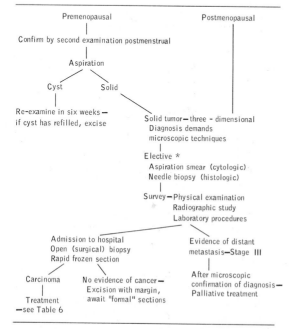

*If employed, of value only if unequivocal diagnosis of cancer is possible; if so, proceed directly to "Treatment."

outline is a replacement of many words used in a narrative account; therefore, certain phases of the outline require comment.

Aspiration of the undiagnosed tumor is a reasonable, initial action in premenopausal patients. At least one-third of the space-occupying tumors due to dysplasia are gross cysts. After aspiration, the area should become impalpable as a definite lump and refilling is uncommon. Re-examination should be done about six weeks following aspiration; in the few patients in whom the cyst has refilled, excision seems preferable to repeated aspirations. Cytologic study of the aspirated fluid or the sediment obtained by centrifuging has been an unproductive gesture.

An 18- or 20-gauge needle is adequate, but the syringe should produce an adequate degree of negative pressure, and this is best obtained by the use of a glass syringe of 20 cc. capacity. Infiltration of the skin with local anesthetic at the site of puncture contributes to the patient's peace of mind.

There is no rational basis for resistance to the advantages of aspiration. A considerable number of women escape the necessity of admission to the hospital and an incisional attack on the breast when aspiration provides a diagnosis and, most of the time, satisfactory treatment as well.

When aspiration has indicated a solid tumor, the surgeon may resort to other nonsurgical methods which may provide a diagnosis. Using the same needle and syringe as for aspiration of fluid from a cyst, with strong suction and gentle movement of the needle-tip within the solid tumor, sufficient tissue may be obtained for a smear to be examined by cytologic technique. More satisfactory, because more often reliably diagnostic, is the use of a needle-like device with which a solid core of tissue may be removed through a small puncture-incision, for examination by histologic method. There is no evidence to indicate any hazard for needle biopsy after more than 20 years of experience. Successful use of needle biopsy requires experience and constant, regular use. Because of the minute volume of the cores obtained, special processing in the laboratory is essential, without which sections of poor quality are obtained.

The surgeon who employs these techniques must remember well two important limitations which attend their diagnostic use: the only report which is of any possible value is that which states unequivocally the presence of cancer; examination either by cytologic or histologic techniques should be done by pathologists experienced in these methods. A positive report under these conditions allows the surgeon to proceed with a definitive operation, thus saving the time involved in a preliminary biopsy.

In the menstruant, re-examination after the onset of the next menstrual flow frequently shows either reduction in size of the lump in the breast or its disappearance. In either event, the possibility of a malignant neoplasm is thus rendered so unlikely that any incisional procedure may be deferred.

Radiographic studies. The absolute preoperative requirement in every patient with an undiagnosed tumor of the breast is roentgenograms of the chest, preferably anterior stereoscopic and lateral views. Some surgeons emphasize routine skeletal surveys, but the yield of positive findings is so low in primary, asymptomatic lesions as to be entirely out of proportion to the burden imposed on the radiologic laboratory and the cost involved. If the tumor is of questionable operability, a simple form of bone survey should be done. This may consist of a large anteroposterior roentgenogram of the lumbosacral spine and pelvis and a similar large film taken laterally. Providing the previously mentioned roentgenograms of the chest have been made with adequate penetration, the ribs and thoracic spine are reasonably visible. If the patient has symptoms which may be due to skeletal metastasis, additional appropriate studies should be ordered.

It should be remembered that the radiographic method is a study in shadows. Considerable destruction of bone may be present without evidence of radiographic abnormality, even with technical work of high quality and expert interpretation. It has been estimated, by study at autopsy, that two-thirds of the diameter of a vertebral body in the exposed plane is usually destroyed before the metastatic focus becomes apparent on the roentgenogram. Clinical evaluation of pain is thus of great importance; persistent, localized pain of increasing intensity, with the added evidence of elevated serum alkaline phosphatase, may be as significant as a questionable area in a roentgenogram.

Clinical laboratory procedures. Unfortunately, there is as yet no specific test for any type of cancer. Nor do any of the current efforts in refinement of nonspecific serologic reactions offer sufficient promise of relative accuracy for routine clinical use.

The *sedimentation rate*, in the absence of concomitant and particularly inflammatory disease, is of some value as it is usually elevated in mammary carcinoma if the primary lesion is bulky or if there is more than minimum axillary nodal spread. Remote metastasis is almost invariably accompanied by highly abnormal rates.

While not as valuable an indication of skeletal metastasis as is acid phosphatase in prostatic carcinoma, the alkaline form of this enzyme is present in concentrations above the average range in some six out of ten women with bony metastasis. When a patient with a known carcinoma of the breast has symptoms consistent with such metastasis, consistently elevated levels of *serum alkaline phosphatase* on two or more determinations are almost confirmatory of skeletal or hepatic metastasis, regardless of roentgenographic findings in respect to bone detail. Pre-existing hepatic disease invalidates these findings.

EVALUATION OF PATIENT. The woman who faces the possibility of an operative procedure for carcinoma of the breast requires both physical and psychologic evaluation.

Physical evaluation. Only severe concomitant disease or extreme senility and deterioration should interfere with the choice of surgical treatment. In women with cardiovascular disease, adequate medical evaluation is indicated, but rarely should it constitute a contraindication to radical mastectomy. Careful medical management before, during and after operation is, of course, mandatory. The same attitude should hold for patients with diabetes or other major medical problems.

Age, as in any other major surgical venture, is more a matter of biology than chronology. Some women of 65 are more senescent than others a decade or two older. The mere fact that a woman has survived past the biblical threescore and ten is usually evidence of a biologic fortitude which will carry her safely through a radical mastectomy, no matter how frail she may appear. We have had an experience of two patients past 90 years of age, both of whom had a smooth convalescence following a hurried but radical mastectomy, one of them surviving four years to die of coronary thrombosis without clinical evidence of recurrence.

Psychologic evaluation. To many women, the prospective mutilating effect of mastectomy seems far more drastic and much more difficult to accept than the most extensive sort of intra-abdominal operation. To such women, the breasts are more closely identified with physical integrity than are any other structures save those of the head and neck. Such an attitude is not peculiar to younger women or to those whose physical attributes command admiration.

In any woman there will be, with rare exceptions, more than a little reluctance to face the situation. Curiously enough, the problem is apt to be less difficult when the patient has had prior, though unrelated, major operations.

For his own protection, the surgeon must inform the woman with an undiagnosed tumor of the breast that a mastectomy may be required, no matter how remote the possibility may seem. Having done so, it seems equally desirable to leave the patient with the impression that a radical procedure will not be required. Sufficient stress is involved for the patient in facing the necessity of excision of an undiagnosed lump. This is a time at which to follow the maxim: Give your patient the benefit of your decisions and keep your doubts to yourself.

When the diagnosis of cancer is established, the frankness with which the situation is discussed, or the evasions which are sometimes almost mandatory, must depend on the clinician's attempt to evaluate the emotional status of each patient, with help from the family when available. The clinician's effort in psychotherapy, amateurish though it may be, is as integral a part of management as the technical details of definitive treatment. Large doses of optimism, warranted or not, are salutary adjuvants to physical therapeusis.

CUTANEOUS BIOPSY IN ACUTE CARCINOMA. When diffuse erythema of the skin overlies a poorly defined, indurative change in mammary texture, with a history of short duration, the possibility of acute carcinoma is confirmed or excluded by obtaining a small wedge of skin and underlying fatty layer for microscopic examination. This can be accomplished easily as an office or outpatient procedure under local, field block anesthesia. A full thickness ellipse of skin and subdermal tissue should be obtained, approximately 1 to 2 cm. in length, and one-half this size in width. In acute carcinoma, emboli of cancer cells in dermal lymphatics are seen; their absence serves to exclude this ominous variant, but does not eliminate the possibility of carcinoma. Some florid variants of mammary carcinoma are accompanied by striking areas of cutaneous erythema, as is plasma cell mastitis.

SURGICAL BIOPSY. The surgical approach to undiagnosed tumors of the breast, whether clinically suspected of cancer or not, should be made with the patient under general anesthesia by a surgeon who is competent in radical mastectomy, with preparations for the latter procedure if it is indicated. The key figure is the pathologist, who must be skilled in the preparation and interpretation of frozen sections. An experienced surgical pathologist can make an exact frozen-section diagnosis in a high percentage of breast lesions, but such accuracy is a product of training, experience and interest in assuming this responsible role. Failing these requirements, either because of disinterest or absence of a full-time pathologist in smaller hospitals, it is best to do excisional biopsies and await the preparation of paraffin sections. If the surgeon has had adequate training in gross pathology, he will be able to make a diagnosis on the physical features of the cut surface of at least seven of every ten carcinomas. Whether he proceeds with a radical mastectomy without histologic confirmation is his own responsibility, for there will be rare instances in which the most typical gross findings are not verified by histologic findings.

Incisions for tumors in different areas of the breast are indicated in Figure 15. Radial incisions should be avoided, for they are more prone to keloidal reaction and stretching than any other and are frequently sensitive, even painful. For exploration of the central third of the breast, including the ductal area, the curved areolar incision permits wide exposure by reflection of skin flaps. The resultant scar is almost invisible after a few months in most patients. An inframammary incision, to expose the undersurface of the gland for a

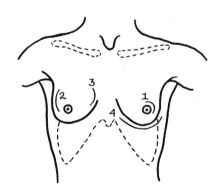

Figure 15. Incisions for exploration and biopsy. 1, Curved areolar for lesions in the central third. 2 and 3, Curved peripheral incisions. 4, Inframammary incision for deeply located tumors.

deeply located tumor, is disadvantageous if a radical mastectomy is indicated.

For tumors with the physical criteria of a benign process, or of small size, excisional biopsy is preferable. In all instances, a margin of adjacent, apparently uninvolved tissue should be removed with the lesion, even though it may seem encapsulated. In tumors clinically suspect of carcinoma, incisional biopsy has theoretical advantages; fewer lymphatic radicles are divided and there is a lesser hazard of cancer cells being spread in the wound or on gloves or instruments.

PRIMARY TREATMENT. The designation "primary" refers to the therapy of previously untreated patients; there is no implication of treatment limited to the primary, or mammary neoplasm.

If one accepts the belief that every woman who presents herself for treatment of a carcinoma of the breast unwittingly has harbored within her body an epic struggle between a malignant neoplasm and such intrinsic defensive reactions as have been possible; that this biologic conflict has already eventuated in a dominance either of the cancer or of the patient early in the life cycle of the neoplasm, and that her survival is mainly dependent on this predetermined balance of power, then it must be obvious that a complete reorientation of our attitudes toward treatment is mandatory.

For more than 30 years the interests of surgeons in cancer of the breast have focused on its therapy to an obsessive degree. Nearly all the surgical literature, the proliferation of modifications in surgical procedures, the views on modalities ancillary to or even replacing surgical therapy, the marshaling of statistical support, with careless disregard of the laws of probability, appear trivial when viewed in the perspective of the natural history of these forms of cancer.

Of first importance is the examination of the most nihilistic of all beliefs: that treatment is valueless.

This dismal interpretation of biologic predeterminism is answerable only by a comparison of significantly sized samples of untreated and treated women, in terms of survival. An adequate sample of untreated patients is obtainable only as a summation of collected series of patients in the earlier years of this century. There is no evidence to suggest that mammary carcinoma has changed in potential since Daland reported one notable group of untreated patients in 1927. The single, speculative difference between treated and untreated concerns the long-term survivors without therapy; it seems certain that these untreated women included a lesser proportion of those with rapidly growing neoplasms. In the sample of patients treated, an obvious necessity is total experience, including those treated with the intent of palliation, as well as those in whom treatment was thought to be curative in intent. A comparison of this sort is shown in Table 6, with estimated relative survival at intervals up to 20 years. Even if it is assumed that the two samples are biologically homogeneous, treatment increases the proportion of ten-year survivors by fourfold (22 per cent versus 5 per cent). If, as speculated, the untreated groups are favored by a lesser relative incidence of neoplasms with rapid growth rate, the superiority of treatment versus no treatment might be in the order of ten times at the tenth year after diagnosis.

With such unequivocal proof of the value of treatment of women with carcinoma of the breast, the next and obvious question is: what type of treatment or combinations of therapy are most effective? A justifiable discontent with the fixed rates of survival, and the minor fraction of patients for whom the end results could be regarded as curative, was responsible for the widely variegated patterns of therapy which began after World War II. None of these therapeutic innovations has improved end results over those obtained around 1930, when examined in terms of total experience, mortality or survival rates for national or state populations. It is a probability that, if data for such a comparison were available, rates of survival have not changed since Halsted modified his cri-

Table 6. *Estimated Survival: Total Clinical Experience Compared to Survival of Untreated Patients*

YEARS OF SURVIVAL	TOTAL EXPERIENCE* (PER CENT SURVIVAL)	UNTREATED PATIENTS (PER CENT SURVIVAL)
1	86	80
2	74	60
3	61	35
5	38	20
10	22	5
15	12	0
20	10	0

* Radical mastectomy and palliative therapy combined.

teria of eligibility for surgical treatment, thus producing a more selective sample in whom his block resection would extend beyond the apparent limits of local-regional disease.

All the extensions of surgical extirpations beyond the classic, radical procedure have been aimed at anatomic areas in which metastasis is not regional, but of distant dissemination. These extraregional sites of extended operation have included the supraclavicular lymph nodal area, the internal mammary nodal groups and the opposite breast and axilla. The combined radical mastectomy and homolateral neck dissection had been employed nearly 50 years before its recent revival; both were admitted to have had no significant effect.

Radiation therapy has a niche of usefulness in the therapy of breast cancer with an ominous potential; its use in general does not approach the effectiveness of surgical treatment in the control of this neoplastic spectrum of disease. No other method is of even slight value in primary treatment, or even as ancillary treatment to definitive surgical therapy.

This forces a single conclusion: the standard, classic or conventional surgical extirpative effort first employed by Halsted is the definitive treatment for the woman with operable breast carcinoma. An outline of therapeutic action based on this belief is presented in Table 7. For operable carcinoma of the breast, which is to say Stages I and IA, radical mastectomy performed immediately after the histological confirmation of its presence is the treatment of greatest effectiveness.

RADICAL MASTECTOMY. This procedure requires a precise knowledge of anatomy and meticulous adherence to operative detail. Competence in the procedure is acquired only by training and experience. Cardinal requirements include:

Wide reflection of thin skin flaps in the area of the primary lesion.

Reflection of skin flaps beyond the midline anteriorly, to the posterior axillary line posteriorly, to the clavicle above and the upper area of the rectus sheath below.

Sacrifice of both pectoral muscles, major and minor.

Meticulous axillary dissection, including the sheath of the axillary vein. If multiple enlarged nodes are found around the axillary vein, its resection will permit a more thorough dissection than is otherwise possible. Resection of the axillary vein entails no increased hazard of postoperative edema of the arm, provided x-ray therapy is not employed.

Various incisions may be employed in radical mastectomy, depending on the location of the primary lesion. When feasible, variants of the transverse or arrowhead incisions are more acceptable from a cosmetic standpoint than the Meyer-Halsted type.

Careful hemostasis is of essential importance in the subsequent healing process. Venous tributaries divided during the axillary dissection are tied with fine ligatures, while chest wall bleeders, including the perforating vessels in the medial portion of the chest wall, are most rapidly controlled by electrocoagulation.

The skin edges should be spared from trauma as much as possible, especially during dissection of the flaps. The use of mosquito hemostats is helpful.

After hemostasis is completed, the wound is irrigated routinely. In recent years, various chemotherapeutic solutions have been employed, but experience with one of the more popular agents, monoxychloresene, has been discouraging. A low local recurrence rate of less than 6 per cent over the past 20 years supports a preference for plain water, although it may well be that the factor of importance is the mechanical effect of liberal washing of the wound, preventing implantation of free neoplastic cells.

Table 7. *Outline of Therapeutic Action for the Patient with Carcinoma of the Breast Confirmed by Microscopy — No Distant Metastasis*

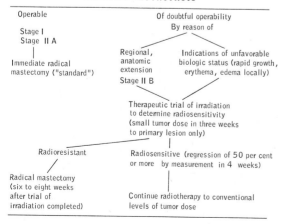

Closure of the wound must be done without undue tension on the thin skin flaps. Split-thickness skin grafts may be required, but in the majority of patients a more satisfactory closure is obtained by using the adjacent skin. This is accomplished by sliding flaps, usually from lateral and lower costal areas.

Postoperative care. Postoperative care is concerned mainly with two important objectives: wound healing and function of the arm. Although the primary contribution to healing is wound closure with minimum tension, a departure from the customary occlusive type of pressure dressing has produced a distinct increase in primary healing. A No. 28 hard rubber catheter, with four or five additional openings cut into the distal 6 cm. of the tube, is inserted through a stab wound below the axilla in the posterior axillary line for dependent drainage. The tube is fixed to the skin with a single suture, which should also make the stab wound airtight. Negative suction through the tube is started in the recovery room or even in the operating room if there has been more than an average amount of generalized bleeding. Negative suction is applied, preferably through a power-operated source such as the Pratt-Chaffin unit, maintaining a constant pressure of about −118 mm. of mercury, although the two-bottle Wangensteen suction can be substituted. This achieves early fixation and revascularization of skin flaps with far greater effectiveness than is accomplished by pressure dressings. Suction is maintained for three to five days or until the amount of exudate recovered in the trap bottle is less than 100 cc. in 24 hours. On the second postoperative day, the patient is taught to disconnect the catheter from the tube to the suction machine so that she can have increasing periods of ambulation and no restriction in bathroom privileges.

Negative suction is employed and no dressing of any sort is used, as it has been demonstrated that complete exposure of the wound provides a combination of drying, cooling and electrolyte and protein environment which is most hostile to bacterial growth. Assuming that there has been meticulous edge-to-edge closure, the wound becomes sealed in less than two hours. During this time, a nonsterile bath towel may be placed over the wound to absorb the early exudate.

With experience in this method of exposure and suction for a period of 12 years in over 400 radical mastectomies, primary healing has occurred in more than 80 per cent of patients. A coincident sharp reduction of the incidence of significant lymphedema of the arm has also been noted.

Antibiotics have not been employed and there is no conclusive evidence of their value as a routine postoperative measure.

Active motion of the arm should begin on the day of operation. The most valuable single exercise in prompt recovery of function of the arm is brushing the hair. The patient should have a hairbrush within reach constantly and be encouraged to spend much of her time using it. She should aim at being able to make the full sweep of the brushing motion on the opposite side of the head in five to seven days after the operation. More varied exercises are of value later.

Ambulation should begin on the evening of operation and increase daily.

OTHER METHODS OF TREATMENT. **Indications.** Any surgeon who has extensive acquaintance with the results of radical mastectomy is aware of the minority of patients in whom the operative procedure seems to exert an unfavorable influence on the course of the disease. Some of these are women in whom the extent of the neoplasm, either locally or in its axillary extension, or both, have marked them as being of borderline operability. In others, the local and regional setting has been well within conventional limits of operability, yet their postoperative course has been highly unfavorable.

These patients usually exhibit one or more of the criteria which suggest biologically unfavorable forms of the neoplasm, and for them an alternative method of treatment is urgently needed. In both groups, it is frequently difficult to assign such patients to the categorically inoperable group. It is for such patients that radiation therapy, used as a therapeutic test, will serve the function of a filter mechanism, dividing the genuinely inoperable patients from those whose best opportunity for effective palliation, if not cure, will be achieved by local and regional ablation of their disease (Table 7).

Radiotherapeutic test for inoperability. A basic consideration in the radiosensitivity of cancer is the general rule that response to irradiation is a function of anaplasia, of rapid and ominous growth patterns. The most radiosensitive neoplasms are generally incurable, such as Ewing's sarcoma and certain of the lymphoblastomas. Mammary carcinoma has a highly variable response to irradiation, consistent with its variegated growth patterns. As might be expected, the most malignant form of the disease, the acute or inflammatory carcinoma, is the most radiosensitive. The current consensus favors an inoperable status for this type, even though irradiation is only palliative. At the other extreme of the biologic scale of growth, the low grade, dilatory forms are almost always radioresistant. Among the remaining major group of infiltrating mammary carcinomas, there is a small group which is distinctly radiosensitive. These tumors are responsive to very modest dosage of irradiation, far less than that ordinarily regarded as being cancericidal.

The radiotherapeutic test is based on the concept that a mammary carcinoma which responds to a relatively low dose of irradiation is radiosensitive and therefore incurable; thus, it must be regarded as inoperable. Evidence indicates that the size of this fraction of breast cancer, including the outright acute carcinomas, is in the order of 15 per cent. Because of their aggressive growth pattern, they are, on the average, more advanced locally and regionally when first diagnosed than are radioresistant neoplasms, and are frequently of borderline operability. In other instances, there are indications of their unfavorable biologic characteristics. The selection of patients for the radiotherapeutic test depends on recognition of one or another of the following situations:

As in Stage IIB, extensive axillary, especially apical nodal involvement
Axillary nodes more than 2.5 cm. in diameter, adherent to each other or to the skin
Satellite nodules in mammary skin
History of rapid growth of primary tumor
Erythema of overlying skin, up to and including acute carcinoma
More than minimum edema of skin over or under the breast tumor
Small primary lesion, diffuse axillary nodal involvement

OUTLINE OF RADIOTHERAPEUTIC TEST. The diagnosis should be established with biopsy, either by a needle biopsy or an open surgical biopsy in the operating room. The primary breast tumor is treated through opposing portals of appropriate size to include several centimeters of margin around the palpable lesion. Delivery of radiation into the chest and lung should be avoided. With a beam of radiation of quality in the order of 1.0 to 2.0 mm. copper, a tumor dose of 1800 to 2000 r is delivered in a period of two weeks.

Within one week after delivery of such a dose, the radiosensitive neoplasms will show a regression, by measurement, of 50 per cent or more. With few exceptions, either this degree of regression, or no significant reduction, will be noted. Such reduction is indication enough of radiosensitivity, and thus of incurability and inoperability. Such patients are then continued on radiotherapy, adding portals to cover axillary and supraclavicular and mediastinal areas. Tumor dose in each of these areas need not exceed 3000 to 3500 r. The customary concept of cancericidal levels of irradiation do not apply in these patients.

In those patients who do not exhibit regression, radiotherapy is discontinued and, other considerations permitting, a radical mastectomy is performed. The amount of irradiation given in the test dose is of no significance in subsequent operative procedures.

TREATMENT IN ELDERLY WOMEN. Using an arbitrary age of 70 or more to define the elderly patient, her ability to undergo a radical mastectomy is remarkably good. Age in itself is no excuse for the performance of simple mastectomies, or of modified radical procedures. In two separate series, followed for more than five years, both 27 in number, survival in women over 70 was 57 per cent and 52 per cent, compared to usual figures of just over 40 per cent in all women treated by standard radical mastectomy. One of these groups included a woman of 95 in whom a radical mastectomy was followed by three years without recurrence before her death from cardiovascular disease.

When the elderly woman, usually through serious concomitant disease, is not thought to be eligible for operation, combined treatment by irradiation in modest dose to the primary tumor, and axilla if involved, and estrogen given orally, has had excellent results. Total tumor dose has been 1200 to 1500 r. Coincident with the irradiation, 15 mg. of diethylstilbestrol is given daily, and this is continued for several months, later lowered to 5 or 10 mg. daily as a maintenance dose. Continuous treatment with the estrogen is essential. Of one series of 21 patients so treated, there was complete regression of the primary and regional disease in 16, major regression in four; after three or more years of such therapy, 15 were still free of evident cancer.

TREATMENT OF PREGNANT OR LACTATING PATIENT. Carcinoma of the breast developing during pregnancy or lactation is usually attended by symptoms and signs indicating an unfavorable biologic pattern, such as rapid growth, bulky primary lesion, cutaneous erythema or extensive axillary nodal involvement. So common is this pattern that the patient with carcinoma of the breast which becomes manifest during pregnancy or lactation came to be regarded as categorically inoperable and incurable. More recently, a number of reports have proved the error of this assumption, with figures as favorable as 30 per cent five-year survival. The same criteria for separation of operable and inoperable cases should be employed as for any carcinoma of the breast, with the expectation that about two-thirds of these patients will present inoperable, incurable disease, best treated by palliative irradiation.

At any stage of pregnancy the carcinoma should be treated as though the patient were not pregnant. Thus, if radical mastectomy is indicated, the procedure is done with little danger of abortion or premature delivery.

There is no satisfactory evidence in favor of advising therapeutic abortion at any stage of pregnancy. In the instance of women who have had definitive treatment for mammary carcinoma, and who are of childbearing age, subsequent pregnancies do not seem to be associated with a greater probability of recurrence or metastasis.

PALLIATIVE TREATMENT

Over 40 per cent of all patients with mammary carcinoma are incurable at the time of initial examination. In some institutions for the indigent, the proportion is considerably higher. The basic reason for incurability of most primary untreated lesions, however, is the unfavorable biologic characteristics of the disease in this fraction of patients. Added to the patients with inoperable primary lesions are those with recurrent or metastatic disease following definitive treatment who also require palliative care. Because at least one-half of operable patients develop recurrence or metastasis within five years after radical mastectomy, it is obvious that palliative management is the clinician's major problem.

At present, palliative treatment depends on control of the disease by irradiation and therapeutic alterations in steroid metabolism, with surgical procedures for removal of local or regional disease occupying a minor but sometimes useful position. Chemotherapy is considerably less effective than hormonal alterations. In general, the best palliation will be secured by conservation of the therapeutic ammunition, reserving the larger-caliber and more drastic bullets until the less spectacular shots have outlived their usefulness. Thus, many women respond well to roentgenotherapy of successive areas of metastatic involvement over a period of years, before the disease becomes so disseminated as to indicate the need for hormonal therapy.

PALLIATIVE RADIOTHERAPY. With one exception, inoperable breast carcinoma, whether primary or recurrent, or a postoperative metastasis, or both, should have preliminary palliative treatment by radiotherapy if the dominant lesions are encompassable by this modality. The exception is that of metastatic lesions of soft tissue in women five years or more postmenopausal. For these patients, primary palliative treatment by estrogens is preferable. The postmenopausal phase is defined as that following the last menstrual period, or what may reasonably be accepted as such.

Even in this situation, however, moderate doses of irradiation will produce more rapid regression than if estrogens alone are employed. It should be noted that "soft tissues" is employed to designate such sites as lymph nodes, contralateral breast, chest wall or subcutaneous areas in any part of the body and does not include visceral metastasis. When employed concurrently with the initiation of hormone therapy, a tumor dose of 1000 to not more than 1500 rads seems to be entirely adequate.

All major areas of skeletal involvement with significant weight-bearing function should have the benefit of x-radiation, regardless of other management. Large tumor doses are not necessary for control of most metastatic lesions in bone. Tumor dosage in the range of 1500 rads will be adequate in most instances and, in some patients, will permit re-treatment of the same area at a later time without concern over skin tolerance.

ALTERATION OF STEROID METABOLISM. Although 20 years have elapsed since the first use of sex hormones for disseminated mam-

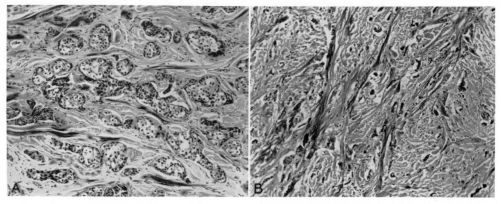

Figure 16. *A*, Photomicrograph of biopsy tissue from a primary inoperable carcinoma of breast before treatment. *B*, Photomicrograph of biopsy tissue from same neoplasm after steroid (estrogenic) hormone therapy, showing major regression. Note diffuse fibrosis and cellular changes.

mary carcinoma, the confusion, disagreement and misunderstanding of clinicians have never been greater than in recent years. One reason for this is the failure of clinical and basic research to discover the mechanism by which hormonal alterations are effective in some patients. Another is the persistence of the early concept that hormonal therapy was a matter of simple antagonist substances. Androgenic hormones were first used with the thought that carcinoma of the breast was an estrogen-dependent neoplasm; later, oophorectomy was performed on the basis that the principal source of endogenous estrogen was removed. Although carcinoma of the breast is in large part hormonally dependent, this dependence is nothing as simple as promotion of growth by a single substance. Both oophorectomy and the additive use of androgens are least effective when ovarian activity is at physiologic flood tide. Removal of the ovaries has a greater incidence of tumor-suppression just before the menopause, and androgens become more effective with each decade beyond the menopause.

The most perplexing evidence against estrogen dependence is the overall superiority of additive estrogens in postmenopausal patients, in the treatment of a neoplasm once thought to be active only in an estrogenic milieu. The complexity of the therapeutic situation deepened with reports of adrenalectomy and hypophysectomy, the major ablations of steroidogenesis, the uncertainties of their effectiveness and the proper time at which to resort to such drastic procedures. Some investigators have claimed that these heavy pieces of ablative artillery should be the initial attack on metastatic disease. There

has been some speculation on using pituitary ablation at an even earlier phase of the disease, as an adjuvant to definitive surgical procedures in Stage II cases.

From large-scale cooperative studies, both on additive and ablative techniques, have come reliable data which permit certain general statements.

The use of any effective method of hormonal alteration divides a treated sample into a smaller group of responsive patients and a larger group of nonresponsive women. Duration of survival in nonresponders is little longer than untreated patients, while the responders live three to four times longer. In general, responders had a longer free interval from definitive treatment to diagnosis of metastasis.

Objective regression is the only exact criterion of response. In brief, objective response requires reduction in size by measurement of the dominant lesion or lesions, with no increased extent of other foci and no new sites of metastasis evident.

Physiologic age, not chronologic, is the main guide to the choice of treatment. The patient with breast cancer reaches the menopause five years later than the usual average age: 52.5 years rather than 47.5.

Any method of hormonal alteration, additive or ablative, deserves continued use with careful observation for a minimum period of three months, providing the disease is not actively progressing. Objective changes are often slow to appear; if the disease appears to be static, treatment should be continued.

The effects of hormonal alterations should not be obscured with other forms of treatment. It is preferable that a patient will have been without any antitumoral treatment for one or more months before the start of hormonal alteration, either initial or secondary. Ablative alterations should not be followed by additive; e.g., oophorectomy should not be "reinforced" with androgens.

Sequential forms of treatment should be the rule, in general reserving the more severe methods, such as major ablations, for patients proved to be responders to prior treatments.

Outline of hormonal treatment. Physiologic age indicates the choice of the first method for hormonal alteration. The dividing line is one year past the menopause, patients who are beyond that level being postmenopausal and those before that physiologic age being regarded, for this purpose, as premenopausal.

PREMENOPAUSAL PATIENTS. By current consensus, the first measure should be induction of the menopause. Bilateral oophorectomy is preferable, but pelvic irradiation is an acceptable substitute if an adequate dose is delivered. In women past 40 years of age, who are still menstruants, 1000 to 1200 r delivered to the midpelvis in a minimum period of ten days is an acceptable dose. In younger women, a proportionately larger dose is required. The effectiveness of radiation-induced menopause may be determined with reasonable accuracy by vaginal smears, which indicate the loss of estrogenic effect.

Objective regression occurs in nearly four of every ten menstruants in whom a menopause is induced, but the effectiveness is greater for women near their menopause than for younger women. Under age 35, responders to oophorectomy are at the 15 per cent level; in older women and up to one year postmenopausal, over 30 per cent achieve regression. The following response rates have been observed, listed by dominant site of metastasis: soft tissue, 40 per cent; skeletal, 38 per cent; and visceral, 18 per cent. In those patients who had not had mastectomy, response was 23 per cent. Survival averaged 31.2 months in the responders, 8.8 months in the nonresponders.

In 28 women who were more than one year beyond the menopause, only one showed objective regression after oophorectomy. In such patients, the ablation of ovaries does not seem indicated unless there is strong evidence of ovarian activity in a highly cornified vaginal smear, and target effect in the breast.

The mean free interval from definitive treatment to diagnosis of metastasis was 32.0 months in the responders to oophorectomy, and 20.9 months in the nonresponders, a highly significant difference.

If a patient has maintained continued objective regression for six months or more after oophorectomy, her probability of obtaining a new regression with either adrenalectomy or hypophysectomy is even better than her chance was of having a remission after the lesser procedure. Similarly, the responders to oophorectomy have an improved chance of remission with the next ablation over those women who had either pituitary or adrenal ablation as their first hormonal alteration. Responders to oophorectomy had a 44.7 per cent (22 out of 49) new regression after one of the major ablations, whereas the overall rate of response to adrenalectomy was 28 per cent (196 out of 690), and to hypophysectomy 32 per cent (111 out of 340). Among the nonresponders to oophorectomy, only 11 per cent (eight out of 71) responded to major ablation.

As for those patients who are nonresponsive to oophorectomy, it is unlikely that additive hormonal therapy will be effective. The use of chemotherapeutic agents is probably preferable for these patients. Similarly, when reactivation of the neoplasm develops after a regression from major ablation, further hormonal measures seldom are helpful, and chemotherapy may then be employed.

POSTMENOPAUSAL PATIENTS. After the first postmenopausal year, the initial treatment should be by additive hormones. In a study of postmenopausal patients treated by androgens (420) and estrogens (357), their effectiveness was similar through the fourth postmenopausal year, less than 20 per cent obtaining regression. Thereafter, the superiority of estrogens was evident at every age level, although both types of hormone became more effective with advancing age. In general, estrogens induced regression in 36 per cent, and androgens in 21 per cent of postmenopausal women. Because of the more distressing side effects of the androgens, estrogens have a clear advantage over androgens.

The standard dosages in additive hormonal therapy are diethylstilbestrol, 15 mg. daily; testosterone propionate, 50 mg. intramuscularly three times weekly. For those unable to tolerate oral estrogen, long-acting preparations such as estradiol valerate (Delestrogen) are available for intramuscular injection. An equivalent dose of this substance is 40 mg. every three to four weeks. Such treatment should be preceded by a two-week trial of a short-acting compound, to eliminate the possibility of hypercalcemia.

In patients who achieve objective regression, continuous therapy should be maintained. After four to six months of treatment in responsive patients, oral stilbestrol may be reduced to 10 mg. daily, and later to 5 mg. daily.

Tolerance of oral preparations is greater if the entire dose is taken at bedtime. The one troublesome side effect of estrogen therapy, uterine bleeding, is usually controlled promptly by increasing the dose of estrogen for several days. Most often, bleeding is a withdrawal effect, caused by failure of the patient to take the drug regularly.

The duration of regression in responsive patients is significantly longer in estrogen-treated than in androgen-treated women; 26 months and 16 months, respectively.

Response to the use of additive hormones is suggestive of a greater probability than average of such patients obtaining regression from adrenalectomy or hypophysectomy. Such responders to hormone therapy should be considered for one of these ablative procedures, assuming their suitability for the major procedure. The chief limiting factor is age. Patients over 60 years of age do not have the same frequency of favorable response as women under this arbitrary level. But the decision should be made more on apparent biologic than chronologic age, for some excellent results have been achieved from major ablation in women well past the 60-year mark.

If the responder with reactivated neoplasm is not suitable for major ablation, it is best to discontinue hormonal therapy for one month, during which some 5 per cent of such women will exhibit a new regression on withdrawal of treatment. Thereafter, the opposite hormone to that which induced the regression may be tried: androgens in lieu of estrogens, and the opposite. When this change in hormonal therapy is ineffective, chemotherapy is the next approach.

Major endocrine ablative procedures. A comparative retrospective study of 801 adrenalectomies and 390 hypophysectomies is available for evaluation of these two methods of hormonal alteration in women with disseminated mammary carcinoma. The two samples, though of unequal size, were biologically comparable as shown by a remarkable uniformity in a number of factors, demonstrating the trend toward homogeneity in populations of breast cancer of adequate size. Evaluation was based on terms of objective evidence only, and response defined as distinct, measurable decrease in one or more dominant foci of metastasis, by clinical and roentgenographic evidence, without appearance of new metastatic lesions or progression of any existing focus. To eliminate the artificial effect of those patients with a favorable natural history, the maintenance of *status quo* postoperatively was designated as failure. Objective regression had to be maintained for a minimum interval of six months; responses for intervals of lesser duration were counted as failures. No credit was assigned to such factors as improved hematopoiesis, anabolic effects, change in calcium balance, gain in weight or resorption of pleural fluid. Of the adrenalectomy series, ovarian influence had been removed by induction of the menopause in all menstruants, either by oophorectomy (468) or irradiation. About one-half of those treated by hypophysectomy had been castrated (oophorectomy in 107, irradiation in 70). A majority had had either prior irradiation of metastasis or additive hormones, or both.

With safeguards established to assure the comparability of the two series of patients and the validity of the evaluations, the results in Table 8 were noted.

By statistical evaluation, none of the differences between hypophysectomy and adrenalectomy were significant. Within the adrenalectomy group, the response of soft tissue and skeletal metastasis was comparable, but of much less effectiveness, in visceral involvement ($P < 0.005$). Within the group treated by hypophysectomy, the only significant difference was in the comparison of response of osseous and visceral lesions ($P < 0.025$). The comparisons relating to the natural history of the disease, or free interval from mastectomy to death, and of the survival of responders and nonresponders were all of a high order of significance. Thus, the outcome of attempts at modification of the hormonal milieu of mammary carcinoma are determined by the biologic characteristics of the neoplasm and its relation with the individual host, the nature of which are not yet apparent.

Table 8. *Comparative Data: Adrenalectomy and Hypophysectomy in Disseminated Mammary Carcinoma*

	ADRENALECTOMY	HYPOPHYSECTOMY
	per cent	*per cent*
Regression (per cent)	28.4	32.6
Average survival (P.O.)	*months*	*months*
Responders	24.2	22.7
Nonresponders	7.7	6.9
Regression	*per cent*	*per cent*
Soft tissue*	34.6	31.1
Bone	37.5	38.8
Viscera	16.4	23.2
Survival by sites	*months*	*months*
Soft tissue and bone		
Responders	25.0	21.8
Nonresponders	9.3	7.6
Viscera		
Responders	22.8	25.2
Nonresponders	6.5	5.4
Mean free interval		
Responders	38.6	42.6†
Nonresponders	30.6	29.4
Mean survival (mastectomy to death)		
Responders	79.2	82.9
Nonresponders	52.4	54.6

* Dominant site of metastasis.
† Responder versus Nonresponder: adrenalectomy, $P < 0.01$; hypophysectomy, $P < 0.005$.

These outlines of sequential management of disseminated carcinoma of the breast in premenopausal and postmenopausal women are summarized in Tables 9 and 10.

Corticosteroid therapy. For women unresponsive to oophorectomy or to additive sex steroidal hormones, there is some evidence that the use of corticosteroids with thyroidal substances will produce some regression of the disease in about one-third of patients, though usually of brief duration. Any of the cortical-adrenal substances of mineralocorticoid nature seem adequate, and in dosage equivalent to cortisone 30 to 50 mg. daily.

For cerebral metastasis, larger doses of corticosteroids produce dramatic results in some patients. The improvement in responsive patients is so immediate as to suggest that some mechanism other than tumor suppression is involved, yet in occasional women the improvement is of such duration that actual regression, on the basis of electroencephalographic evidence, is inescapable.

Chemotherapy. Although distinctly inferior to hormonal alterations, both in incidence of favorable responses and their duration, chemotherapy is of sufficient value to deserve a trial in women who are no longer eligible for hormonal therapy. The alkylating agents are used most often, and experience has indicated the superiority of cyclophosphamide (Cytoxan). This substance has two advantages over earlier versions of alkylating agents: it has a less toxic effect on bone marrow, and is without any deleterious effect on platelets; for continuous therapy, it can be given in oral form.

Table 9. *Sequence of Hormonal Alterations in Premenopausal Patients**

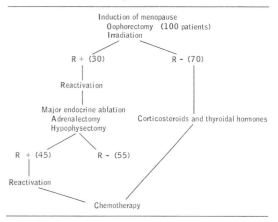

*Including those up to 12 months postmenopausal.
R + indicates an objective response for six months or more.
R − indicates unresponsive by objective criteria.

Table 10. *Sequence of Hormonal Alterations in Postmenopausal Patients*

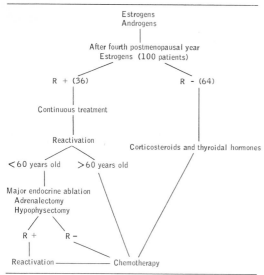

R + indicates an objective response for six months or more.
R - indicates unresponsive by objective criteria.

Initial treatment is given by the intravenous route, and after the first three to four doses the oral preparation is used. As with hormonal therapy, the advantages of continuous therapy have become obvious. The objective should be to maintain a reduction of white blood cells at 3000 per cu. mm. or fewer.

In patients unresponsive, or who have become recalcitrant to Cytoxan, a trial of 5-Fluorouracil or one of its analogues is proper, providing that their hematologic status justifies the use of this highly toxic and potentially lethal agent. Again, continuous rather than intermittent therapy is desirable, and enough patients have been treated, usually at a maintenance dose of 100 mg. weekly, to prove its feasibility in those who have sufficient tolerance of the drug. A practical disadvantage in some patients is the necessity for intravenous administration.

END RESULTS. In clinical language, "end results" constitutes an expression of therapeutic influence on the course of a disease. In itself, such an expression is meaningless unless a yardstick is available with which it can be compared. In a disease of lethal potential, the comparative exercise of basic importance is the survival of treated versus untreated patients. For most sites of cancer, this comparison provides the answer to a crucial question: is the therapy employed of such effectiveness as to alter favorably the natural history of the disease?

When a treatment has demonstrated such improvement in survival beyond peradventure, the availability of untreated patients diminishes rapidly. Soon, the former yardstick of natural history is replaced by the modified profile of survival associated with general use of effective treatment, against which are tested new therapeutic attacks. Often the "new" is a modification of the initial, established modality or, in some diseases, an entirely novel therapy.

In cancer of the breast, no new treatment of any significance has become available since the introduction of the classic radical mastectomy and, later, the advent of the therapeutic use of roentgen rays. Hence, the enormous mass of published data on end results owes most of its bulk to clinical variations in the pattern of surgical and radiotherapeutic management. Many reports are ego-serving essays purportedly demonstrating technologic superiority peculiar to the author, or to the collective acumen of the staff of an institution.

Earlier emphasis on the dominant influence of the natural history of mammary carcinoma has indicated the artificiality of nearly all of such reporting. Although biologic factors established in the preclinical phase predetermine, in a clinical sense, the curability or incurability of each patient, the use of surgical treatment is of great value in this disease, both for cure and for effective palliation. The basic comparison of untreated and treated patients provides emphatic evidence of the value of treatment, with 22 per cent of the treated women surviving for ten years, as against the 5 per cent of the untreated who live for a decade after diagnosis while suffering continuously from the progressive ravages of the disease.

Important as treatment is by these criteria, the ceiling of effectiveness was reached more than 30 years ago; in fact, there is some reasonable basis for supposing that current results are comparable to those obtained by Halsted after he had modified his criteria of operability toward the selection of patients whose gross extent of local-regional disease could be encompassed by his operative procedure.

If this be true, then the variability of end results associated with therapeutic manipulations must be statistically artifactual. The most important and most frequent defect in clinical reports is the failure to express end results in terms of the total sample of experience. Even when this is done the factor of self-selection is not eliminated. For example, if "cancer detection" clinics are limited to examination of asymptomatic women, the discovery of unrecognized breast cancer produces automatically a sample of patients with a more favorable pattern of growth than in the average institution. Self-selection also determines the sample of the disease seen within an institution, sometimes with patient-populations which are highly atypical of breast cancer in general.

A comparison of two specific institutions demonstrates the importance of socioeconomic factors in the production of disparate samples of experience. The Los Angeles County Hospital is the largest teaching hospital in the United States; its patients are almost exclusively indigent in a medical sense and, until very recently, its female patients have been nearly two decades older, on an average, than those in private, voluntary hospitals in the Los Angeles area. Hence, the sample of mammary carcinoma seen in this hospital is atypical; a distinct majority of patients are postmenopausal, their disease is more advanced in anatomical extent than is the case in private patients and more often is associated with physical deterioration due to degenerative disease. The Mayo Clinic is the largest private, group facility in the United States, and provides an antithetic contrast to the experience of a charity hospital, owing to self-selection. Patients must travel to the institution, often from distant areas; their economic resources are superior; women with advanced disease are less apt to seek a distant place for treatment, with or without necessary financial means. These atypical samples of breast cancer are associated with antithetic end results best illustrated by the disparity in operability. With criteria of operability which are roughly comparable, 97.8 per cent of patients were classified as having operable, primary, previously untreated, breast cancer at the Mayo Clinic (9437 of 9649), but less than 50 per cent at the Los Angeles County Hospital. In a recent period at the latter institution, only 52 of 130 women with primary breast cancer were eligible for definitive, surgical treatment with the intent of cure. In the same interval, the number with primary disease was almost equaled by those patients with recurrent or metastatic cancer; hence, on the basis of total experience, only 22 per cent were operable.

Although these are extreme examples of atypical, institutional experience through self-selection, they indicate the probability that the total experience of an institution, and certainly of an individual clinician, may not be representative of the disease. When factors of clinical selection are superimposed on self-selection, the sample becomes still more atypical. The most common method of clinical selection is on the basis of operability; criteria of operability are almost as variable as the natural history of the neoplasm. As such criteria become more restrictive, the "operable" fraction of patients becomes smaller, the sample of the disease thus chosen more favorable and the end results artificially improved. An example of such selectivity is the "triple biopsy," in which lymph nodes from apical axillary, supraclavicular and internal mammary sites are removed. If any of these nodes contain microscopic foci of metastatic neoplasm, the woman is regarded as "inoperable," and is treated by radiotherapy.

This exercise in selective extremism lends a deceptive luster to the end results both by surgical and radiotherapeutic methods. But certain patients are denied the benefits of radical mastectomy of palliative or even curative order; for every 100 women in whom the apical, axillary nodes are involved by metastasis, 20 survive for five or more years without evidence of disease. In the following five years, about one-half of such patients succumb to the neoplasm, but seldom with local-regional disease, whereas those treated by irradiation only are prone to reactivation of cancer in the breast and regional nodes and chest wall.

From all this, it seems apparent that the reporting of end results by individuals and institutions, after treatment by conventional methods, serves no useful purpose. Any future change in the present fixed rates of incidence, mortality and survival will be apparent only in population samples of massive size—national, state or provincial. This is the important function of tumor registries on a state-wide basis, as in Connecticut, California and New York. Smaller samples are most useful in the testing of new treatments yet to be developed, as in recent demonstrations of the relative ineffectiveness of chemotherapy ancillary to radical mastectomy.

Valid reporting of end results requires proper use of the statistical method as applied to a biologic problem. Essentially, statistical testing is numerical estimation of probabilities which permits an expression of the degree of confidence which an observer may have in concluding that observed differences, or similarities, are meaningful. When numerical or percentile differences are apparent in a comparison of two sets of data, the application of statistical testing reflects one of two situations: the disparity is as likely to have been the result of chance as of therapeutic design, and thus is of no significance; or the observed difference is statistically significant, with the probability that it reflects the relative effectiveness of the therapies used. The statistical method measures, also, degrees of probable confidence.

In biologic problems, variable factors of some complexity are often present, the consideration of which distinguishes biometry from statistology. The most precise statistical techniques, unless tempered by sound clinical knowledge of biologic variables, may lead to egregious errors. Biometry is the evaluation of statistical testing as interpreted in terms of established knowledge of biologic variables. Differences which are statistically significant may be of doubtful validity by reason of heterogeneity of the samples under comparison.

Most of the reporting of end results in breast cancer, especially in the surgical literature, is of little or no value. In comparing samples of insignificant size, percentile values are most often the only criteria for expression of differences. Such elementary exercises frequently lead to highly erroneous conclusions, and to the conviction that surgeons often use statistics more for support than for illumination.

If the possible value of a new or modified therapy is to be investigated, it should be mandatory that a protocol be established by conference between clinician and biometrician. The most important objective of such pretrial planning is some assurance that the patient-samples, whether large or small, provide meaningful comparisons of end results; that, if differences do emerge, clinical judgment can be confirmed by statistical measurements. In short, the conclusions which emerge from the comparative study must have validity. In a neoplasm with a wide range of biologic behavior, such as carcinoma of the breast, with our limited resources for evaluation of the biologic potential of primary, untreated patients, the only assurance of obtaining homogeneous samples for comparison is through large size of the samples. Homogeneity in this sense means that each sample would have a predictably comparable pattern of end results without the experimental influence; neither sample is weighted by an unrepresentative proportion of favorable or unfavorable forms of the disease. By current consensus, the minimal size of sample for reasonable assurance of homogeneity is 300 patients. When it is desirable to use smaller samples for preliminary testing, the influence of sample heterogeneity may be measured as in a T test.

For disease which is recurrent or metastatic after definitive, primary treatment, the problem is much less formidable. The meaning of these indications of reactivation of disease, as used here, should be defined. Recurrence refers to active neoplasm appearing in the operative field, most often including the chest wall and axilla. Metastasis indicates active disease in more distant sites, including supraclavicular and contralateral axillary nodes and opposite breast. In these patients, several indications of natural history are available by which relatively small groups may be evaluated to determine their degree of biologic homogeneity. Some of these factors are the result of information obtained by primary treatment, and others of the sequence and timing of events following initial therapy.

Factors related to primary treatment include interval—first recognition of primary tumor to definitive treatment; microscopic grade of neoplasm; extent of axillary nodal metastasis, and evidence of vascular invasion.

Factors related to metastasis in distant sites include mean age at time of diagnosis of metastasis; mean age at mastectomy; if postmenopausal, the mean number of years since menopause, and the number of months from mastectomy to diagnosis of metastasis.

Of all these factors, the "free interval," or the number of months from mastectomy to the diagnosis of metastasis, is the most important indication of neoplastic potential; the longer this interval, the greater the probability of responsiveness to hormonal therapy. If a preliminary analysis of two samples of patients as small as 50 in number shows comparable values for these factors, or most of them, one may be assured of the biologic homogeneity of the two groups.

MEASUREMENT OF END RESULTS. The traditional yardstick of survival at a five-year interval following treatment is of little value in breast cancer; deaths from the disease outnumber those from other causes until ten years after surgical treatment. A far more significant measure is that which has been described by Berkson and Gage as "yearly survivorship function." The logarithm of survivals is plotted as ordinate against time as abscissa, to produce a curve giving the death rate for any given year. If total experience is so recorded, the curve of the death rate, and hence of survival, can be compared to a similarly constructed curve of survivorship for a normal population of comparable age. The uniform use of such reporting would produce significant data on the value of treatment which presently are not available.

When such data are available, biometric evaluation becomes significant. Even small samples of experience thought to be of significance in terms of percentile values can be biometrically tested if yearly survivorship is available. An example of such an exercise might concern a comparison of radical and simple mastectomy in two small samples of patients, as shown in Table 11.

On the basis of simple percentile comparisons, a case could be made for the superiority of the procedure of lesser extent. Seven years postoperative, 55.1 per cent (38 of 69) of patients still survived after simple mastectomy; 48.8 per cent (30 of 62) of those treated by radical mastectomy were survivors. Table 11 shows the yearly decrement of survivors after the two operations, with the differences measured for significance in terms of chi square, only one of which might be of significance, the X^2 of 4.68 after the first year. Expressed in terms of probability of signifi-

Table 12. *Survival of Untreated Patients*

YEARS	PER CENT
1	75
3	40
5	20
10	5

cance, P (probability value) is less than 0.05. Unless nonstatistical considerations of importance are apparent, it is customary to regard as significant only those values which indicate that the probability of a difference being due to chance is less than one in 20, or P = less than 0.05. By a scanning of the other X^2 values for the second to seventh years of follow-up, it is apparent that all the other differences are no more or less than could be expected by chance alone.

This example demonstrates but one of a variety of biostatistical methods used in determining the significance of end results. Different problems require different techniques which the biometrician has at his command.

In summary, the recording of end results should conform to certain desirable requirements so that conclusions of significant value may be derived from their analysis.

Total experience (absolute survival rate) must be reported.

The proportion of patients followed up annually or more often by medical examination should exceed 90 per cent of all patients.

It is preferable to differentiate between survival with and without evidence of disease as determined by clinical examination.

Every neoplasm should be confirmed by histologic examination; exceptions to this rule should be separately tabulated.

End results should be determined by annual survivorship and mortality in preference to the traditional reporting at arbitrary intervals following treatment.

Significant reporting demands samples of experience of adequate size, especially in any comparison of therapies; in carcinoma of the breast, a minimum sample is 300 or more patients, unless biologic homogeneity of the host-tumor relationship has been demonstrated by several criteria.

Reporting of subgroups of patients, as by criteria of eligibility for treatment, must be accompanied always by a statement of total experience.

The end results in mammary carcinoma represent an attempt at estimation of the outcome of the disease "at large," and the influence of treatment upon it by various criteria, as obtained from many sources (Tables 12 to 19). In estimations of survival after definitive

Table 11. *Yearly Decrement of Survivors after Simple and Radical Mastectomy*

YEARS OF SURVIVAL	MASTECTOMY SIMPLE	RADICAL	X^2
1	64/79	58/62	4.68
2	57/69	49/62	0.27
3	53/69	42/62	1.35
4	46/69	38/62	0.41
5	44/69	36/62	0.45
6	42/69	35/62	0.23
7	38/69	30/62	0.58

Table 13.   *Estimated Total Sample—Survival per Each 100 Patients*

YEARS OF SURVIVAL	RADICAL MASTECTOMY (70)	PALLIATIVE THERAPY (30)	SURVIVAL PER 100
1	63	23	86
2	56	18	74
3	49	12	61
5	35	3	38
10	21	1	22
15	12	0	12
20	10	0	10

Table 14.

SURVIVAL (years)	RADICAL MASTECTOMY (per cent)
1	90
2	80
3	70
5	50
10	30
15	18
20	15

Table 15.

SURVIVAL (years)	PALLIATIVE TREATMENT (per cent)
1	75
2	60
3	40
5	10
10	2
15	0

Table 16.   *Average Total Experience in Carcinoma of the Breast (Histologically Confirmed)*

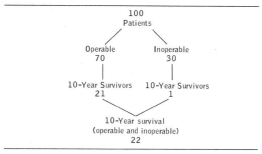

Table 17. *Disseminated Carcinoma of Breast—Response to Sequential Endocrine Ablation in 120 Premenopausal Women*

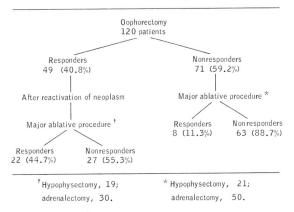

[†]Hypophysectomy, 19; adrenalectomy, 30.

[*]Hypophysectomy, 21; adrenalectomy, 50.

Table 18. Disseminated Carcinoma of Breast—Average Intervals from Mastectomy to Death in Patients Treated by Major Ablative Operations: Responders and Nonresponders

	RESPONDERS		NON-RESPONDERS	
	NO. PATIENTS	MEAN SURVIVAL IN MONTHS	NO. PATIENTS	MEAN SURVIVAL IN MONTHS
Adrenalectomy	147	79.2	427	52.4
Hypophysectomy	77	82.9	194	54.6

"t" Ratio: adrenalectomy vs. hypophysectomy, 0.48.

Table 19. Disseminated Carcinoma of Breast—Survival After Major Endocrine Ablative Operations by Sites of Anatomic Involvement and by Response

	MEAN INTERVAL, ABLATION TO DEATH, IN MONTHS DOMINANT SITES OF METASTASIS			
	SOFT TISSUE AND SKELETAL		VISCERAL	
	R+	R—	R+	R—
Adrenalectomy	25.0	9.3	22.8	6.5
Hypophysectomy	21.8	7.6	25.2	5.4

R+ = Responders.
R— = Nonresponders.

treatment by surgical means, the influence of selection by criteria of operability, both restrictive and liberal, have been eliminated.

CARCINOMA OF THE MALE BREAST

Less than 1 per cent of all mammary carcinoma is of the male breast. The pathologic condition and natural history are the equivalent of the disease in the female. Unfortunately, the lesion is usually relatively advanced and clinically obvious when first seen, probably because of the rudimentary structure of the thin mammary plate with early lymphatic dissemination. Axillary nodal metastasis is usually evident and pulmonary metastasis may also be demonstrated at the initial examination.

If the local and regional evidence of disease fulfill the criteria of operability, radical mastectomy is indicated. More often, even in the absence of distant metastasis, incurability is evident in the form of fixation of primary disease to the chest wall, advanced involvement of axillary nodes including the apical level, or more than minimum involvement of the skin.

The most effective management of inoperable patients is castration, with the use of stilbestrol reserved for the inevitable escape of the disease from the customary interval of postorchiectomy control. Irradiation should not be employed with, or immediately after orchiectomy, so that the responsiveness of the neoplasm to the ablative hormonal alteration may be evaluated, preferably over a period of three months. If the disease is static after three months, or if there is active progression after ablation of the testes, radiotherapy may be used. There are no adequate data permitting an evaluation of the possible usefulness of major endocrine ablations in men who have exhibited responsiveness to orchiectomy.

Survival for five years is less than 10 per cent.

SARCOMA

Sarcomas constitute about 1 per cent of malignant neoplasms. The most frequent connective tissue neoplasm is the *cystosarcoma phyllodes*, generally accepted as arising in a pre-existing fibroadenoma. As is consistent with such an origin, this tumor is actually of compound structure, although the epithelial component is, with rare exceptions, largely overwhelmed by the fibroblastic process.

There is divided opinion on the nature of the neoplasm; some maintain that cystosarcoma phyllodes, in defiance of its ancient nomenclature, occurs in benign and malignant variants, while others state that if a sufficient number of areas are histologically examined genuine sarcoma is invariably found. In rare instances, both epithelial and fibroblastic elements contribute to the structure of a compound, malignant neoplasm.

The tumor is characteristically bulky, nodular and expansile, of slow growth but capable of attaining an impressive size in cases of long duration, giving rise to the term "giant fibroadenoma." Encapsulation is the rule. Metastasis is infrequent and then usually by hematogenous rather than lymphatic routes, with the lungs the most frequent site of deposit. It would seem best to employ the term *adenofibrosarcoma* for this dilatory neoplasm.

For the more bulky variants, simple mastectomy is adequate treatment. When relatively limited in extent, wide resection of the breast is a proper procedure. Axillary dissection is not indicated.

Specific types of sarcoma occur in the breast, but their total number is considerably less than the adenofibrosarcomas. Included are mesenchymoma, even true teratoma, liposarcoma, hemangioendothelioma and sarcoma exhibiting metaplasia to simulate chondrosarcoma and osteosarcoma. The treatment of these rare neoplasms is surgical, of such scope as may be indicated by the extent of the individual lesion. Lymphatic dissemination is so unusual as to preclude concomitant axillary dissection. Prognosis is highly variable but is usually related to the degree of differentiation or anaplasia exhibited by the neoplasm.

READING REFERENCES

Adair, F. E.: Plasma cell mastitis—a lesion simulating carcinoma. Arch. Surg. *26*:735, 1933.

American Joint Committee for Cancer Staging and End Results Reporting: Reporting of cancer survival and end results. 55 East Erie Street, Chicago, Illinois, 1963.

American Joint Committee for Cancer Staging and End Results Reporting: Clinical staging system for cancer of the breast. 55 East Erie Street, Chicago, Illinois, 1962.

Berkson, J., and Gage, R. P.: Calculation of survival rates

for cancer. Proc. Staff Meet. Mayo Clin. 25:270, 1950.

Clark, R. L., and others: Reproducibility of the technic of mammography (Egan) for cancer of the breast. Am. J. Surg. 109:127, 1965.

Collins, V. P., Loeffler, R. K., and Tivey, H.: Observations on growth rates of human tumors. Am. J. Roentgenol. 76:988, 1956.

Daland, E. M.: Untreated cancer of the breast. Surg. Gyn. & Obst. 44:264, 1927.

Editorial: "Early" diagnosis of cancer. New England J. Med. 275:673, 1966.

Egan, R. L.: Mammography, an aid to diagnosis of breast carcinoma. J.A.M.A. 182:839, 1962.

Feinstein, A. R.: Symptoms as an index of biological behaviour and prognosis in human cancer. Nature 209:241, 1966.

Foote, F. W., and Stewart, F. W.: Comparative studies of cancerous versus noncancerous breasts. Ann. Surg. 121:6, 1945.

Garland, L. H., Coulson, W., and Wollin, E.: The rate of growth and apparent duration of untreated primary bronchial carcinoma. Cancer 16:694, 1963.

Gershon-Cohen, J., Berger, S. M., and Klickstein, H. S.: Roentgenography of breast cancer moderating concept of "biologic predeterminism." Cancer 16:961, 1963.

Haagensen, C. D., Stout, A. P., and Phillips, J. S.: The papillary neoplasms of the breast. Ann. Surg. 133:18, 1951.

Hadfield, J.: The effect of hormone deprivation upon breast cancer. Ann. Royal Coll. Surgeons England, 25:1, 1959.

Holleb, A. I., and Farrow, J. H.: The relation of carcinoma of the breast and pregnancy in 283 patients. Surg. Gyn. & Obst. 115:65, 1962.

Lewison, E. F.: Prophylactic versus therapeutic castration in the total treatment of breast cancer. Obst. & Gyn. Survey 17:769, 1962.

Macdonald, I.: Endocrine ablation in disseminated mammary carcinoma. Surg. Gyn. & Obst. 115:215, 1962.

Macdonald, I.: Biological predeterminism in human cancer. Surg. Gyn. & Obst. 92:443, 1951.

Macdonald, I.: Mammary carcinoma: a review of 2,636 cases. Surg. Gyn. & Obst. 74:75, 1942.

Macdonald, I.: The breast. *In*, Nealon, T. F. (Ed.): Management of the Patient with Cancer. Philadelphia, W. B. Saunders Company, 1965.

Macdonald, I.: The natural history of mammary carcinoma. Am. J. Surg. 111:435, 1966.

Moore, O. S., Jr., and Foote, F. W., Jr.: The relatively favorable prognosis of medullary carcinoma of the breast. Cancer 2:635, 1949.

Nathanson, I. T., and Welch, C. E.: Life expectancy and incidence of malignant disease. I. Cancer of the breast. Am. J. Cancer 28:40, 1936.

Paterson, R.: Breast cancer. J. Roy. Coll. Surg. Edinburgh 7:243, 1962.

Rubin, P., Crile, G., Jr., Haagensen, C. D., Miller, E., Urban, J. A., and Moore, G. E.: Current concepts in cancer— No. 13: Carcinoma of the breast. J.A.M.A. 199:732, 1967.

Ryan, J. A., and others: Breast cancer in Connecticut, 1935-53. J.A.M.A. 167:298, 1958.

Shimkin, M. B.: Cancer of the breast. J.A.M.A. 183:146, 1963.

Smithers, D. W., Rigby-Jones, P., Galton, D. A. G., and Payne, P. M.: Cancer of the breast; a review. Brit. J. Radiol. (Suppl. 4), 1952.

Stewart, F. W.: Tumors of the breast. Subcommittee of Oncology, Committee of Pathology, National Research Council, Section IX, Fascicle 34. Washington, D.C., Armed Forces Institute of Pathology, 1950.

Subcommittee on Breast and Genital Cancer, Research Committee, Council on Pharmacy and Chemistry, American Medical Association. Androgens and estrogens in the treatment of disseminated mammary carcinoma (a retrospective study of 945 patients). J.A.M.A. 172:1271, 1960.

Taylor, S. G., III: Endocrine ablation in disseminated mammary carcinoma. Surg. Gyn. & Obst. 115:443, 1962.

Treves, N., and Sunderland, A.: Cystosarcoma of the breast: a malignant and a benign tumor. Cancer 4:1286, 1951.

Urban, J. A., and Adair, F. E.: Sclerosing adenosis. Cancer 2:1286, 1949.

Wynder, E. L., and others. Epidemiology of breast cancer. Cancer 13:559, 1960.

Chapter *19*

THE THORAX, PLEURA AND LUNGS

by
HIRAM T. LANGSTON, M.D.

Hiram Thomas Langston was born to citizens of the United States, Alva and Louise Foe Diuguid Langston, who were engaged in educational missions in Rio de Janeiro for the Southern Baptist Convention. He was educated through the second year of college in Brazil, and subsequently at Georgetown College in Kentucky and the University of Louisville, where he received his degree of Doctor of Medicine. His residency education and training in general and thoracic surgery was received at the University of Michigan, where he earned a Master of Science degree. He is now Professor of Surgery at the University of Illinois College of Medicine. Disciplined instruction and practice upon the violin for eight years in his youth now provides pleasure for him and his wife, who is his pianist accompanist. Attempting to learn the technique of dwarfing plants and keeping contacts with Brazilians, resident in or traveling through the United States, provide avenues which help imbue his son and daughters with principles which make for a full and useful life.

Surgery of the chest is an all-inclusive term which embraces the organ systems within the anatomic thorax, as well as adjacent portions of the neck, abdomen and axilla. A student of surgery can hardly expect to understand the problems presented by the processes of disease within the chest without basic knowledge of anatomy and physiology. The application of these principles to clinical problems constitutes the art of the surgical treatment of diseases of the chest.

TESTS OF CARDIOPULMONARY FUNCTION

An individual's ability to withstand a thoracotomy for mediastinal disease or, more specifically, his ability to survive the loss of part or all of one lung is obviously important. The effect that such an operation may have on breathing during the rest of his life, and the consequences of this physiologic derangement on cardiac reserve are likewise essential prognostic factors.

The search for an answer to these questions begins with clinical evaluation by means of a careful history and physical examination. The gross functional capability of the patient, as brought out by exercise such as walking and climbing stairs, is simple to assess and can be informative. Mobility of the rib cage and diaphragm, as well as the ventilatory capacity, can be objectively estimated by direct inspection or by examination at the fluoroscope. In the majority of instances, these simple observations, when supported by adequate experience, are sufficient in persons with ample reserves.

Limited reserve is indicated by the presence of tachypnea and tachycardia, which disappear but slowly, with rest.

When functional capacity is marginal, or when unusually extensive operations are contemplated so that respiratory crippling or severe cardiac strain might result, more specific methods of estimating function are required. Such have been developed and are constantly being refined.

The tests of pulmonary function hinge upon the patient's ability to inhale and exhale adequate amounts of air, thereby supplying oxygen to the blood and eliminating carbon dioxide from it. The mechanisms involved in supplying air to the alveolar membrane and removing carbon dioxide from the lungs are termed "ventilation," whereas the exchange of carbon dioxide and oxygen across the alveolocapillary membrane is termed "diffusion."

FORCED EXPIRATORY VOLUME (VITAL CAPACITY). Forced expiratory volume is the maximum amount of air in milliliters which can be expelled from the lungs by a single forceful effort following a maximal inspiratory effort. It is most often expressed as percentage of a normal figure which is calculated on the basis of sex, age and height (Fig. 1).

FORCED EXPIRATORY CAPACITY (TIMED VITAL CAPACITY). This determination provides the same figure as vital capacity but measures, in addition, the speed with which the air is expelled. Normal individuals should expel 75 to 80 per cent of the air in the first second.

MAXIMUM VOLUNTARY VENTILATION (MAXIMUM BREATHING CAPACITY). This can be defined as the largest amount of air which an individual can breathe in and out per minute by maximal effort. This air, collected during a 12-second period, is measured and the maximum voluntary ventilation is then expressed in liters per minute. As with the vital capacity, it is most often recorded in percentage of a normal value. The latter is arrived at through a formula which takes into account the individual's body surface area, age and sex.

As the degree of emphysema increases with consequent trapping of air, the patient's ability to move air decreases. The vital capacity, therefore, may at times be relatively normal, but when an attempt is made to move air rapidly through the lungs, as in the forced expiratory capacity, or in determining the maximum voluntary ventilation, a marked fall-off in performance is seen.

BRONCHOSPIROMETRY. By placing a double lumen catheter under topical anesthesia so that each bronchus is individually cannulated, measurements of oxygen consumption and vital capacity from each lung can be made.

Occlusion of the airway to each lung in turn will determine the ability of its opposite member to support life, particularly when it is realized that the occluded lung is being irrigated, but not ventilated, thereby adding the burden of an increased return of unsaturated blood to the left heart.

DIFFUSION. The efficacy of gaseous exchange across the alveolocapillary membrane, as well as the uniformity of gas mixing within the lung can be determined.

Determination of the levels of oxygen and carbon dioxide in blood provide a good measure of how well the lungs are functioning. Serial determinations of these parameters before and after exercise, or before and after occluding the airway to one lung, or in measuring the effect of breathing pure oxygen, will often provide the necessary information. Direct arterial puncture is required for oxygen determinations.

Indirect determinations of oxygen saturation by means of an oximeter may be used if relative or comparative values are acceptable.

PULMONARY CIRCULATION. High P waves and evidence of right axis deviation, which are signs of pulmonary hypertension, can be seen in the electrocardiogram. Sometimes, enlargement of the pulmonary artery is recognized by x-ray. The technique of right heart catheterization, however, permits direct measurement of pressures as well as estimation of blood flow. Certain cardiac lesions, suspected or unsuspected, are also demonstrable by this technique.

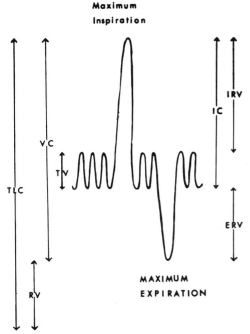

Figure 1. Stylized spirogram tracing, showing its various components. *TLC*, Total lung capacity; *RV*, residual volume; *VC*, vital capacity; *TV*, tidal volume; *IC*, inspiratory capacity; *IRV*, inspiratory reserve volume; and *ERV*, expiratory reserve volume.

Normal Values in Milliliters		
	Males	*Females*
TLC	6000	4200
RV	1200	1000
VC	4800	3200
TV	500	450

In evaluating the patient's suitability for pneumonectomy, for example, the artery to the corresponding lung can be occluded by an inflatable balloon on a special triple lumen catheter. This maneuver effectively eliminates the lung from contributing to respiration and the effect of the occlusion on the level of the pulmonary arterial pressure shows the adaptability of the other lung to receive the increased circulatory load which the resection will impose upon it.

CHEST WALL

The chest wall is made up of extracostal and costal portions. The former comprises the skin, subcutaneous fat, muscle and corresponding fasciae. The latter includes the ribs, intercostal musculature, parietal pleura and associated structures.

The extracostal chest wall is subject to diseases which are common to soft tissues generally.

CONGENITAL ANOMALIES. The anomalies of the chest wall involve principally the bony framework. They occur in approximately 1 per cent of x-rays taken.

Rib anomalies. A common anomaly is the split or bifid rib. Also, fusion of otherwise normal ribs may occur. Neither circumstance is of clinical significance. It is recognized by x-ray but is rarely discovered by other means of examination. Supernumerary ribs can occur in the cervical region. Their clinical significance relates to pressure on the structures in the root of the neck—the subclavian vessels or brachial plexus, or both.

Pectus excavatum (funnel chest). The level of the sternum with respect to the anterior margin of the chest wall on either side of it varies considerably (Fig. 2).

In pectus excavatum, the lower end of the sternum is severely depressed, the rib cage flares outward from this point laterally and little, if any, increase in the anteroposterior diameter of the chest occurs at the level of the xyphoid on inspiration. The lower end of the sternum is relatively fixed.

The pathogenesis of this condition is not well understood. Restriction of ventilation is present in the more severe examples, but may

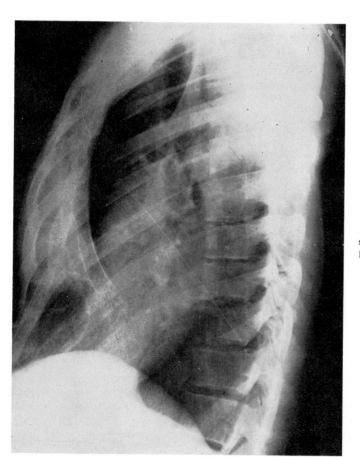

Figure 2. Lateral view of a chest x-ray, showing the marked sternal depression of pectus excavatum in a young adult female.

not be appreciated in the young. Due to the pronounced reduction in the anteroposterior diameter of the chest, the heart may be displaced and rotated. Evaluation of the physiologic derangements encountered in patients with pectus excavatum is difficult and care must be exercised that the deformity is not blamed inappropriately. This is particularly true of cardiac murmurs. In adolescents, the deformity may produce strong emotional conflicts.

In infants, the pliability of the chest wall is such that freeing the xyphoid and the retrosternal attachments has allegedly given a satisfactory result. Older patients, particularly adults, may retain many of the secondary effects on the rib cage even though the sternum is adequately elevated.

The complete repair consists in resecting all of the deformed costal cartilages and the xyphoid process. The sternum is then elevated by freeing all retrosternal attachments. This usually requires an osteotomy of the sternum at its upper end. The new sternal position is then maintained by retrosternal struts of catgut, wire or steel sutures, or bone. Traction from sternum to external supports has largely been discarded. Complete excision of the sternum and its replacement after being turned over has also been advocated.

Pectus carinatum (pigeon breast). Pectus carinatum is a protrusion deformity occurring less often than pectus excavatum and is less likely to produce disability. Its repair is similar in principle to that of pectus excavatum.

Bifid sternum (ectopia cordis). Failure to fuse the embryologic components of the sternum can create a defect which may or may not be further associated with exposure of the heart. Such defects have been successfully repaired.

Hernia of lung. The lung can, on rare occasions, be found to protrude through congenital defects in the chest wall. The commonest site is in the neck through the apical fascia. Bulging of lung through traumatic or surgical defects of the chest wall also occurs. These lesions are usually asymptomatic, are best seen during periods of increased intrathoracic pressure, and generally do not require correction.

INFLAMMATION. Soft tissue abscess. The soft tissues of the chest wall are subject to primary abscesses similar to those elsewhere in the body. One precaution is necessary. In dealing with them, one should consider the possibility that the suppuration lies deeper,

being actually within the pleura, and that the abscess of the chest wall represents a perforation therefrom. A chest x-ray will generally indicate the presence of pleural disease underlying the abscess.

Osteomyelitis of bony framework. Primary osteomyelitis involving a rib occurs infrequently. It is heralded by onset of pain and localized tenderness over the rib. The systemic signs of severe generalized infection are present. As with bony involvement elsewhere, x-ray changes are slow in making their appearance and the diagnosis is established principally on clinical grounds. Drainage of the subperiosteal abscess is indicated.

The ribs or sternum may be involved in suppurative processes secondarily, through surgical incisions which implicate them. If a rib or the sternum is to be resected in the face of suppuration, care should be taken to leave no bone divested of its periosteum. This periosteal envelopment protects against the development of osteomyelitis. Treatment, in the event such infection occurs, is to provide adequate drainage along with the removal of any sequestrated or devitalized portions of bone. The appropriate use of antibiotics expedites healing.

Chondritis. The protective effect of perichondrium is less than that of periosteum. Once a segment of cartilage has become involved in a suppurative process, this will continue until all the cartilage has been eliminated from the wound. Even in the presence of remissions induced by appropriate antibiotic therapy, the outlook for permanent healing is poor. Under these circumstances, it is necessary to resect the entire cartilage back to periosteum-covered bone in order to ensure prompt healing.

It is important to remember that from the sixth costal cartilage downward, the cartilages are fused into an arch, except for ribs 11 and 12.

Because of interference with diaphragmatic function, care should be taken not to excise too much of the costal arch at any one time.

Whereas the ordinary pyogenic organisms are implicated in chondritis, unusual infecting organisms must be kept in mind. This is a common location for the "cold" abscesses of tuberculosis, no doubt originating in the mammary chain of lymph nodes. Osteomyelitis or chondritis due to the Salmonella group of organisms is seen, and fungi must be considered.

NEOPLASMS. Neoplasms of the soft tissues of the chest wall do not differ in any respect from those seen elsewhere. The principles of treatment are also the same.

The bony cage, however, is subject to neoplasia of diverse sorts. The more important members of this group of neoplasms originate in the ribs, but the sternum is not without complicity.

Benign lesions of the chest wall include fibrous dysplasia, eosinophilic granuloma and hemangiomas, as well as some tumors of nerve origin. The osseous neoplasms which may be considered benign are chondromas and osteomas. Caution, however, should be exercised with respect to accepting the benign character of these lesions. Wide excision is justified in all of them because recurrences are to be feared.

The malignant tumors are preponderantly chondrosarcomas, but may include fibrosarcomas as well as Ewing's tumor. Tumors metastatic to rib from a variety of primary sources are also seen.

These lesions are found either by the palpation of a mass, or by the presence of pain or discomfort leading to the demonstration of the neoplasm.

Treatment involves an accurate appraisal of their histologic character and, although preliminary biopsy is frequently attractive, particularly where a mutilating operation such as resection of the sternum is required, the true and full nature of the tumor may not be evident by this maneuver. All such neoplasms believed to be primary probably deserve wide excision of full thickness costal chest wall as well as of any adjacent involved tissues.

The reconstruction of such defects often taxes the ingenuity of the surgeon. The use of tissues from the patient, such as muscle in the form of pedicled grafts or osteoperiosteal flaps, is best if available. Even though a soft spot may be left on the chest wall, this will, in due time, stiffen sufficiently to prevent the adverse physiologic effects of paradoxical motion in most patients.

If autologous tissues cannot be made available, the use of prosthetic material is acceptable.

DISEASES OF THE PLEURA

The pleural cavity is, under usual circumstances, a potential space only, since the lungs remain expanded to fill it.

The various regions of the pleura are conveniently named according to their location as parietal, visceral, diaphragmatic, apical and mediastinal. The subjacent tissues determine the differences that exist between the various portions. For example, the parietal pleura is sensitive to painful stimuli such as cutting and tearing. This is not true of the visceral areas, because the parietal pleura is supplied by the intercostal nerves. In the same manner, the pleura responds to disease processes affecting the subjacent structures. The most dramatic form of such response is the outpouring of fluid—pleural effusion—secondary to lung disease.

PLEURAL EFFUSION. The presence of pleural fluid may be recognized clinically by physical examination or by the characteristic opacification seen in the roentgenogram (Fig. 3).

Physical signs are dullness to percussion, reduced or absent tactile fremitus, decreased or absent breath sounds and reduced transmission of whispered voice. Since even small collections of fluid in the posterior pleural base tend to bulge the thin posterior mediastinal pleura toward the uninvolved side, the presence of a triangle of dullness with the base downward on the uninvolved side (Grocco's triangle) is considered pathognomonic of fluid. Pneumonic consolidation does not displace the mediastinal pleura.

Thoracentesis should be carried out over the area of dullness, generally in the seventh to ninth intercostal spaces along the posterior axillary line. The needle is best inserted at the point where tactile fremitus is least well transmitted.

The skin over the interspace is anesthetized. A needle long enough to reach through the patient's chest wall to the pleura is then introduced and advanced through the successive layers of the chest wall space with further injections of the anesthetic from an attached syringe (Fig. 4). It should pass through the middle of the interspace or immediately above the adjacent rib. Particular care should be taken to anesthetize the pleura. When the needle is advanced through this layer, traction on the plunger of the attached syringe should be rewarded by the aspiration of fluid.

Aspiration of pleural fluid in more than single-syringe amounts should be done using an airtight system to avoid the unwarranted entry of air into the pleura. A stopcock placed between the needle and syringe readily ac-

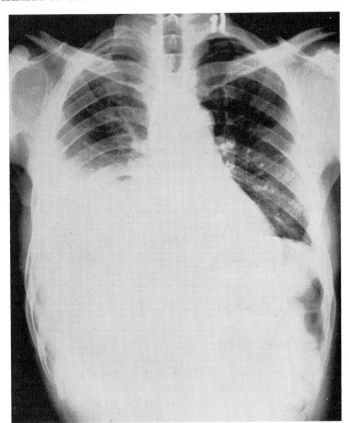

Figure 3. Typical radiographic appearance of a right-sided pleural effusion. The nature of the fluid can be determined only by aspiration.

complishes this. Fluid should be withdrawn slowly and the procedure terminated when cough or pain is incited or discomfort is produced.

The fluid obtained should be subjected to

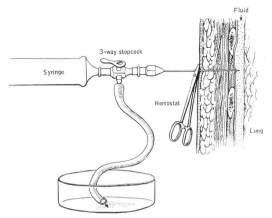

Figure 4. Diagrammatic illustration of technique for thoracentesis. The hemostat locks the needle at appropriate depth. The three-way stopcock is turned to permit withdrawal of fluid from pleura into the syringe and then turned again to evacuate the syringe into the container. This system should be airtight.

complete study of specific gravity, cell count, white blood cell differential, protein determinations, cytology and culture for pyogens, tuberculosis and fungi. This will often permit accurate diagnosis.

Effusions with a specific gravity below 1.016 are generally transudates, whereas values above this figure are usually found in exudates. Various effusions differ in their characteristics.

Cardiac decompensation. Usually the fluid is a transudate and present bilaterally, but right-sided fluid predominates.

Chylothorax. The fluid is turbid and milky, containing fat which can be demonstrated on appropriate staining. It may occur spontaneously, but most often follows trauma or operation. Control may require pleural drainage and interdiction of oral alimentation or, finally, ligation of the thoracic duct.

Neoplasms. Invasion of the pleura by metastatic neoplasm is usually accompanied by effusion. This is characteristically bloody. The finding of neoplastic cells is diagnostic, but caution in establishing this diagnosis is urged since bizarre cell patterns may be seen in nonneoplastic effusions.

The management of these effusions is discouraging. The instillation of anticancerous chemicals or radioactive isotopes, after largely evacuating the pleural content, may be tried along with other appropriate therapy. If the lung is uninvolved by neoplasm so that it can expand to fill the chest cavity, stripping the parietal pleura so that· the reexpanded lung will adhere to this raw surface and create a pleural symphysis may be tried. It may relieve some of the burden of repeated thoracenteses for recurrent dyspnea. This maneuver has the added advantage of supplying histologic instead of merely cytologic proof of the etiology.

The odd association of pleural effusions and ascites with a pelvic neoplasm such as ovarian fibroma may occur.

Hemothorax. This may occur as an accompaniment of spontaneous pneumothorax. Very rarely will hemothorax occur spontaneously without pneumothorax. It is managed as any other hemothorax.

Miscellaneous causes. Pleural fluid occurs also secondary to suppurative processes in adjacent areas, notably below the diaphragm. If unattended, these generally become purulent.

Amebic disease of the liver may extend through the diaphragm. This is best managed by aspiration and emetine and chloroquine. Surgical drainage is required principally for pyogenic complications.

IDIOPATHIC EFFUSION. Pleural effusions for which no etiology can be demonstrated occurring in persons exhibiting skin sensitivity to tuberculin, particularly in the younger age groups, are presumably due to tuberculosis.

EMPYEMA. **Etiology and pathogenesis.** Purulent pleural effusion characteristically follows pneumonia. It may appear during the course of pneumonia, as is commonly the case when streptococci and staphylococci are the responsible organisms, or it may follow pneumonia which is due to pneumococci.

The evolution of the process from effusion to frank empyema basically resembles that of abscesses elsewhere. Invasion of the pleura by the infection results in the outpouring of pleural fluid, which becomes richer in leukocytes and fibrin as the pathologic process advances. The process is initially more or less diffuse even though the greater fluid accumulations occur in the posterior gutter inferiorly because of dependency. As local defenses are mobilized, the pleurae are fused by the fibrinous response around the margins of fluid accumulations, sealing off this portion from the remainder of the space and converting it eventually into a well localized abscess.

At this point, open drainage of the empyema can be carried out without collapsing the lung, a circumstance obviously not possible before such localization occurs. The time of firm pleural symphysis can be postulated when the sediment of the pleural fluid makes up approximately 80 per cent of its total volume after standing overnight.

Premature open drainage, without provision for maintaining lung expansion, accounted for the high mortality seen in the empyemas of World War I. Furthermore, the pneumonia responsible for them was streptococcic, which characteristically produces effusions which are slow to thicken yet invade the pleura during the active pneumonic period. This added the burden of uncontrolled pneumothorax to a patient already ill with pneumonia.

The staphylococcus, as currently encountered, tends to produce pulmonary abscesses. These are prone to perforate into the pleura and produce bronchopleural fistulae. A tension pyopneumothorax may result, particularly in infants, requiring immediate decompression by drainage.

Fungi produce pleural infections occasionally. Surgical drainage is the basis of treatment since chemotherapeutic agents are toxic and offer meager benefits.

Pleural infection may follow surgical operations and be accompanied by a bronchopleural fistula if pulmonary resection has been done. It is managed by the same basic principles applicable to other empyemas.

Diagnosis. The presence of a pleural complication, or extension of disease to the pleura, is suspected on clinical grounds and confirmed by x-ray, physical examination and thoracentesis. The pleural aspirate must be subjected to careful bacteriologic study. Absence of pyogenic organisms on smear or culture speaks strongly in favor of tuberculosis, or more remotely, fungus etiology.

Treatment. If the fluid is recognized when quite thin, intensive treatment by needle aspiration and heavy dosage with a suitable antimicrobial drug may abort the process. Once the exudate is heavy, however, little hope of success can be expected from such a therapeutic program, although use of fibrinolytic enzymes may materially thin the exudate.

In well established empyema, a more continuous form of drainage is required so that the pleura can be kept free of the accumulations which tend to maintain pulmonary collapse. If firm limiting adhesions are not assured by the characteristics of the pleural fluid, insertion of an intercostal catheter connected to a water seal can be considered.

This is accomplished in a manner quite similar to thoracentesis except that a urethral, or other catheter acceptable in size to the selected interspace, is inserted into the pleura. This is most efficiently done through a trocar (Fig. 5). Extra fenestrations in the intrapleural portion of the catheter help maintain its efficacy. The water seal permits egress of pleural fluid or air, yet prevents ingress of outside air with further pulmonary collapse.

Suction added to the water seal further promotes drainage and is often a good adjunctive measure (Fig. 6).

In well established pleural abscesses, open drainage by rib resection provides a bigger outlet for the heavy fibrinous exudate that is often present and is the definitive treatment. Simple catheter drainage suffices in many instances but free and dependent drainage must be assured in order to avoid chronicity.

Rib resection drainage can be done under local infiltration combined with intercostal field block anesthesia. If a bronchopleural fistula is present, the sitting position is generally required.

A vertical incision is made over the empy-

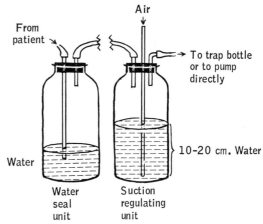

Figure 6. Illustration of a water seal unit on the left. For suction drainage the regulating unit is added. The degree of suction applied is determined by the depth to which the center tube in this unit is introduced below the water surface. As vacuum increases within the system, the water level is progressively lowered within this tube. When it reaches the end of the tube, air is admitted, breaking the suction at this level of negative pressure. A trap bottle in the system, as indicated, affords protection for the source of suction in case fluid from the system spills over.

ema area. This should classically be in the posterior axillary line centering over the eighth or ninth rib. This is deepened to costal level. The field block is carried out over three to five segments through this exposure. Aspiration is carried out from below upward, starting in the ninth intercostal space. If aspiration is required below this starting level, a fresh needle should be used for fear of introducing septic material below the diaphragm. The rib below the lowest interspace yielding pus is selected. A two-inch segment is resected subperiosteally, care being taken to leave no bone denuded of periosteum. The intercostal nerve is best resected back of the posterior rib stump to avoid irritation by the presence of the drainage tube. The vascular bundle is best ligated, both front and back, for security from secondary hemorrhage. The pleura is entered through this bed and emptied of all fibrin clots. A large-caliber tube is placed so as to be dependent in the pleural cavity even if adjustment of the wound is required. Under antibiotic protection, the wound can be loosely closed. The tube is securely anchored by tape and a safety pin.

Healing. Empyema heals by progressive expansion of the lung to obliterate the pleural cavity. In the absence of a bronchial fistula, serial measurements of the volume of the

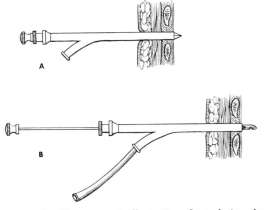

Figure 5. Diagrammatic illustration of a technique by which an intercostal catheter can be inserted in the pleural cavity in order to evacuate air or fluid.

cavity can be carried out. To do this, the patient is placed so that the drain site is uppermost and sterile saline is allowed to run into the cavity filling it. It is emptied by sitting the patient up. Such determinations done serially will clearly show the progress of healing. Visualizing the empyema space on a chest radiograph after the instillation of radiopaque material in it is also helpful.

Drainage tubes should not be removed, except for cleaning and replacement once in seven to ten days, until the pleural space is obliterated. To remove the drainage tube prematurely is to force drainage to take place through whatever sinus may remain, trapping the products of suppuration within the cavity, thereby fostering chronicity.

Complications. CHRONICITY. Persistence of a pleural space and purulent drainage leads to progressive thickening of the empyema wall and continued disability.

Tuberculosis should be suspected, in particular, if the wound is unduly tender. Careful bacteriologic as well as histologic study of the tract may be required to demonstrate this etiologic possibility.

Lack of dependency, or lack of capacity with respect to drainage vent size, will delay healing.

Either by not permitting expansion of the lung or by perpetuating the suppurative process, particularly when accompanied by a bronchopleural fistula, disease of the underlying lung fosters chronicity.

The commonest foreign body is a drainage tube that has slipped into the pleura. A large safety pin through the tube serves admirably for anchoring the tube to the skin with adhesive tape. It also prevents the tube from slipping into the pleural cavity.

The management of chronic empyema, or empyema in which no significant progress in healing can be detected over a period of four to six weeks, depends upon its cause. The various therapeutic maneuvers for most of these are obvious.

Tuberculosis is treated by appropriate chemotherapy; inadequate drainage calls for surgical revision; and a lost drainage tube must be retrieved.

If, however, chronicity is caused by an encasing visceral pleural coat of such nature that lung expansion is mechanically prevented, decortication of the lung should be carried out.

When chronicity occurs secondary to lung disease, particularly if a bronchopleural fistula is an integral part of the disease process, decortication must be combined with some extent of pulmonary resection to ensure obliteration of the pleural cavity by healthy lung.

By decortication is meant the opening of the chest at thoracotomy, preferably by a posterolateral incision, with the objective of freeing the lung from its retaining peel. By incising through the visceral wall of the empyema, a reasonably clear plane can most often be found between it and the lung itself. Along this, the lung is separated and the visceral coat of the empyema is cut away, leaving the lung to expand and fill the chest cavity. Since the parietal peel is an integral part of the empyema, total excision of the empyema sac is advocated as the correct surgical attitude. Healing per primum can be expected with this ideal approach. The parietal peel is separated along the extrapleural plane, which is found immediately deep to the costal level in the thoracotomy incision. The pleural space should be drained to water seal bottles, with or without added suction for three to five days or until the recently freed lung has filled the hemithorax.

When the lung itself is unsalvageable under an empyema because of extensive disease, the only recourse is a pleuropneumonectomy. Complete removal of the empyema sac is then mandatory if any chance of avoiding an empyema postoperatively is to be had.

When attempts to expand the lung have failed, or when it seems ill-advised to attempt this or futile to expect it, obliteration of the remaining pleural space may be accomplished by collapsing the chest wall to meet the lung.

For this purpose, several types of thoracoplasty are recognized.

The Estlander type thoracoplasty calls for the extrapleural resection of ribs subperiosteally over an extent such that the parietal wall of the empyema is decostalized and falls onto the visceral wall, permitting healing.

Even though most empyema spaces are basal, the decostalization must often start well near the apex of the chest in order to secure the degree of collapse desired. It is applied to large spaces rather than small ones. The extent of rib resection is tailored to the needs at hand. If necessary, the procedure may be staged.

The parietal wall of the empyema pocket is excised in toto, removing its full thickness in a Schede type thoracoplasty. The resection of the ribs is carried beyond the margin of the empyema pocket so that no unexposed recesses will remain. The extracostal tissues are allowed to fall against the visceral wall. Healing is by granulation. This is obviously an unattractive procedure, preferably applicable to small residual spaces.

Fowler, Delorme or Ransahoff thoracoplasties utilize the same basic approach as described for the Schede thoracoplasty, but, by adding a maneuver aimed at thinning the parietal "peel," these methods encourage what remaining expansibility exists in the underlying lung. Fowler and Delorme peeled or shaved the visceral coat from the lung, while Ransahoff cross-hatched the visceral coat with incisions down to lung level, expecting the lung to herniate through the defect.

More recently, these classic procedures have been modified, aiming at removing the parietal peel in its entirety, resecting the ribs subperiosteally and allowing the periosteum and intercostal structures to fall in, along with the extracostal tissues.

Under the benefit of antibiotics, more radical procedures, particularly in cases of postpneumonectomy empyema, have been advocated. These are practical and feasible in robust patients and amount to a Schede, or somewhat modified technique thereof, applied to the entire chest wall.

Attempts at sterilizing the empyema space may be considered.

The persistence of a bronchopleural fistula after adequate management of the empyema usually signifies residual pulmonary disease. If the extent of the lung disease is small, it may be the best clinical judgment to accept it as residual pathology rather than resect it in an infected pleural field. The presence of other systemic disease or disability may dictate a similar course. Also, the empyema often has healed to such an extent that only a bronchocutaneous sinus remains. The ingrowth of epithelium from the bronchus along the tract may actually account for the patency of the bronchial stoma, at times, even in the absence of important pulmonary disease. A direct attempt at closing the bronchopleural fistula is, therefore, often clearly indicated. It is the only approach if a pneumonectomy has been performed.

With this objective in mind, one should make sure that all detectable causes for chronicity are eliminated and that the residual pleural space is as small as possible.

The operation then proceeds by opening the residual pleural pocket to divest it completely of any rigid wall. The visceral bed should be thoroughly cleaned and scarified to bring a source of blood for granulation tissue through this coat. The bronchial stoma, or stomata, should be denuded of epithelium and, if possible, actually separated from the surrounding tissues as well, so that it, or they, may be mechanically closed by suturing the freshened edges and burying them beneath adjacent tissues. A pedicled flap of adjacent skeletal muscle, big enough to fill the pleural space completely, is fashioned and sewn snugly into all recesses of the pleural pocket. The remaining extracostal tissues are closed over the area. Pressure dressings are applied to help obliterate, by mechanical means, the air leaks from unclosed or incompletely closed fistulae. Tissue emphysema may occur from these sources, but unless it becomes impressive, is best ignored. Serious infection is an uncommon occurrence under suitable antibiotic protection which supplements the already established local tissue immunity.

Meticulous technique and careful selection of patients will bring success most of the time.

EMPYEMA NECESSITATIS. A neglected pleural abscess may not remain confined. It can break through either the visceral or the parietal wall, and thereby provides for its own drainage. Perforation into the lung and communication with a bronchus may occur with disarming speed and is indicated by the sudden expectoration of large amounts of pus. Prompt evacuation of the pleura and maintenance of proper tracheobronchial toilet is urgent. Proper treatment of the empyema often will permit closure of the bronchopleural fistula, since it is no longer essential to the requirement of drainage.

Perforation of the chest wall occurs less dramatically and is heralded by the appearance of an enlarging local abscess. Suitable treatment of the empyema is urgently called for.

METASTATIC ABSCESS. Under antibiotic control, metastatic abscesses are uncommon. Previously, however, they were annoyingly frequent and the cerebrum was a common site. The prognosis is poor.

AMYLOIDOSIS. Long-standing suppuration may result in deposition of amyloid in various organs, notably liver and kidney, with resultant decrease in their functional capacity.

PRIMARY NEOPLASMS. The pleura can produce neoplasms or be the site of metastatic deposits.

Primary neoplasms of the pleura are uncommon, but occur as two principal types—diffuse and localized fibrous mesotheliomas.

The diffuse type is heralded clinically by effusion. Cytologic studies on the aspirated fluid may permit its recognition. The neoplasm tends to grow along the pleural surface by direct extension, but seeding throughout the pleural cavity undoubtedly speeds its propagation. Large masses of the neoplasm are at times formed and may be recognizable by x-ray. Similar neoplasms occur in the peritoneum and the pericardium.

Surgical excision is usually impossible when the situation is recognized. No other modality of treatment seems to offer appreciable benefit.

Death results from the inexorable growth of the neoplasm, which progressively compromises cardiorespiratory function as well by invasion of the mediastinum, further interfering with fundamental physiologic processes. In the pericardium, progressive tamponade occurs. Regional as well as distant metastases complete the course of malignancy.

The localized, fibrous form is generally seen as a circumscribed intrathoracic mass, which, on direct examination, may lie free in the pleura except for a narrow stalk arising from some pleural margin. Microscopically, the bulk of the tumor is made up of fibrous tissue. Its mesothelial origin is supported by the presence of lacunar spaces within the connective tissue elements which appear to be lined by mesothelium.

That these tumors may have the ability to produce hormones or enzymes is suggested by the occurrence of severe hypertrophic osteoarthropathy in persons harboring them and its often dramatic disappearance on removal of the tumor, which is the proper treatment.

DISEASES OF THE LUNGS AND BRONCHI

Reference to any modern work on pulmonary anatomy confirms the emphasis that is placed on the concept that lungs are divided into lobes, which are in turn made up of segments. The arborization of the bronchus as well as of the pulmonary artery conforms to this pattern.

Not only is this concept valuable to descriptive anatomy, but it is applied constantly by surgeons as they separate these various components along anatomic planes. It should be pointed out, however, that these segments are not isolated from one another, but inosculate through the terminal portions of their vascular beds as well as interalveolar air passages. They are nonetheless separable along planes that can be readily followed without incurring serious leakage of air or blood.

The hilum or "root" of the lung is composed of one pulmonary artery, two pulmonary veins and one bronchus. In similar manner, the hilum of each lobe or segment is rather consistent in its composition.

BRONCHOSCOPY. The bronchoscope is in principle a lighted, rigid, open metal tube, 40 to 45 cm. in length, in diameters of 8 mm. for men, 7 mm. for women and lesser sizes for smaller patients. Under topical anesthesia, the instrument is introduced directly, or with the aid of a laryngoscope, through the larynx into the trachea. The bronchi are then explored. The major divisions of the bronchial tree are available for inspection either directly or by means of a telescopic lens passed through the bronchoscope. Secretions can be collected for cytologic and bacteriologic study, and biopsies may also be obtained.

Various other manipulations can, of course, be carried out through this instrument. Foreign bodies can be recognized and removed, granulation tissue can be cauterized and strictures dilated. Cautery can be effected by silver nitrate or by electrosurgical methods, if appropriate insulation is provided.

BRONCHOGRAPHY. Under topical anesthesia in a manner similar to that utilized for bronchoscopy, contrast material such as Dionosil, Visciodol, Hytrast or Lipiodol is distributed by gravity, guided by posture, to coat the walls of the bronchial tree. Roentgenograms in appropriate projections are made (Fig. 7).

This technique permits the confirmation of bronchial abnormalities of various sorts not only in the major portions inspectable by the bronchoscope, but well beyond these limits. Bronchiectasis is actually not diagnosable unless this technique is employed.

ROENTGENOLOGY. The accuracy and reliability of the chest roentgenogram has made it absolutely indispensable in the evaluation of chest diseases. Not only should it be taken

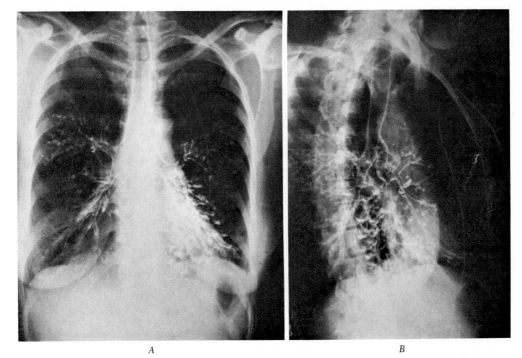

A   *B*

Figure 7. *A*, Posteroanterior view of chest x-ray, following instillation of contrast material. Typical bronchographic appearance of advanced saccular bronchiectasis is seen involving entire left lower lobe and lingular division of left upper lobe. By contrast, the bronchial arborization seen on the right side is essentially normal. All segments are not filled in this film.

B, Oblique projection of bronchogram in same patient as in *A*. This clearly outlines the trachea and main bronchi. The left upper lobe bronchus and its principal subdivisions particularly the inferior division are placed in clear relief. The saccular changes in this latter segment are well seen. The lower lobe bronchus is markedly narrowed. All branches of the lower lobe are crowded together and universally involved by obvious cystic change. The branches of the right lung, although not seen to best advantage in this projection, do show normal arborization where visualized in upper lobe and superior division of the lower lobe, the middle lobe branches being superimposed on those of the left lower lobe.

in posteroanterior projection, but a lateral view should be had, so that the retrocardiac area will be clearly brought to view and lesions accurately localized. Various other projections are indicated on occasion.

Fluoroscopic examination provides the added factor of motion. This is indispensable in determining diaphragmatic paralysis.

Laminagrams, or body section radiographs, are useful in both frontal and lateral views. In tuberculosis, where their use is commonplace, the anteroposterior projections are utilized for the demonstration of residual cavity. The lateral cuts reveal, by showing the fissures, the topographic distribution of disease. This feature can be assessed with amazing accuracy when it is interpreted in combination with a bronchogram.

MALFORMATIONS. The various embryologic elements which go to make up the lung can combine to produce a wide gamut of malformations. The most extensive of these is agenesis of an entire lung.

The organ is represented solely, or principally, by the grosser portions of the bronchial tree in aplasia or hypoplasia, which are less complete anomalies. This frequently produces the bronchographic picture of extensive bronchiectasis. Maldevelopment of the pulmonary vasculature may also occur.

A portion of the lung may become sequestrated from the remainder of the organ. This area of lung is generally characterized by cystic change and the presence of an anomalous artery arising from the aorta as an accessory vessel.

The development of one or more cysts having an epithelial lining, with or without a bronchial communication, is also seen (Fig. 8). Such cysts are to be differentiated from the cystic spaces created by emphysematous changes.

The various degrees of cystic change and similar abnormalities come to attention as a result of infection or hemoptysis. In any event, they most often can be recognized

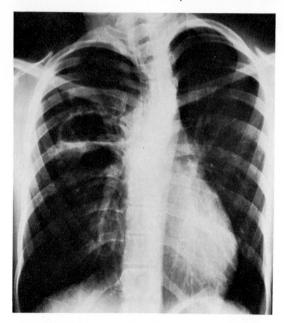

Figure 8. Large epithelium-lined cyst in an adolescent girl who also had a severe pectus excavatum deformity.

for what they are by appropriate clinical investigation. After successful control of the active phase of infection, if present, resection of the involved portion of lung is the treatment of choice. It is to be noted, however, that these lesions may go undetected and be asymptomatic for long periods of time.

Emphysema of obstructive type involving a lobe occurs, possibly on a congenital basis, although its etiology is not clear.

Arteriovenous fistulae of the lung may offer confusion with neoplasms and are of principal interest because of their hemodynamic effects. These include cyanosis and some degree of plethora, but cardiac output is normal, as are the blood pressure, heart size, pulse rate, venous pressure and blood volume. The presence of adventitious sounds over them on auscultation suggests their nature. Demonstration of the fistulous communication by angiocardiography is diagnostic. Resection is the required treatment.

ATELECTASIS. This pathophysiologic state deserves special recognition because it manifests itself in many situations of clinical interest. Atelectasis means airlessness of a portion of lung, resulting in a loss of volume by the area affected due to interference with the airway. In this regard, it is distinguished from the loss of aeration and loss of lung volume secondary to compression of

lung by tumors or other mechanical factors such as pleural effusions. It implies, therefore, a bronchial factor preventing proper aeration of the involved area of lung and the consequent absorption of air distal to the obstruction. In consequence of this obstruction to the airway, the lung parenchyma becomes opaque by virtue of malaeration.

Retention of sputum or bronchial secretions within a lobar or main stem bronchus is the common etiologic factor in atelectasis. Effective plugging of the corresponding airway by this viscid column results. Once sufficient air has been absorbed from the lung parenchyma distal to the point of obstruction, effective expulsion of the column of sputum becomes impossible. The process is progressive and generally requires mechanical aspiration of the offending and obstructing column. The poor respiratory excursions and decreased ventilation incident to postoperative pain and discomfort account for the appearance of this phenomenon as a frequent postoperative complication.

Originally, this process is usually sterile and if not allowed to persist beyond a few hours, no long term residuals need be expected. The clinical symptoms which accompany the usual postoperative atelectasis include dyspnea, cyanosis, tachycardia and fever. Most of these are understandable on the basis of the cardiorespiratory changes present, but the cause of fever is not clearly understood.

Radiographically, the process is characterized by opacification of a lung or some portion thereof with mediastinal shift to the involved side, elevation of the corresponding hemidiaphragm and, at times, recognizable narrowing of the intercostal spaces (Fig. 9).

Other causes for atelectasis are foreign body, neoplasm and stricture of various sorts.

One distinction should be made between the atelectasis of acute obstruction and that produced by the slow growth of a neoplasm or the gradual constriction of an inflammatory stricture. These latter situations are very often accompanied by the superimposition of secondary infection and lead to permanent changes within the lung parenchyma which are not reversible by merely eliminating the obstructing element. Such changes will ultimately be manifested by bronchial distortions consistent with bronchiectasis.

The treatment for acute atelectasis is prompt removal of the obstructing agent. Retained secretions may be expelled in the

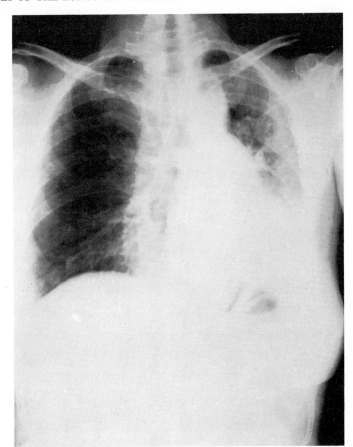

Figure 9. Opacification of the lower left lung field accompanied by shifting of the mediastinal structures to the same side is characteristic of atelectasis. In this patient, it followed an appendectomy.

early phases of the process by insistent cough or, if necessary, by aspiration through a catheter passed via the nose through the glottis into the trachea. This not only aspirates the secretions mechanically, but stimulates strong coughing to help expel them. If gross radiographic changes are present, or if these simpler measures fail, bronchoscopic aspiration is indicated so that the involved areas can be thoroughly emptied. Antibiotics in the acute situation are probably justified to prevent or delay the superimposition of secondary infection. In chronic situations, they can minimize the effects of suppuration.

SPONTANEOUS PNEUMOTHORAX. Realizing that the lung is a rather large and delicately constructed collection of air sacs, it seems remarkable that rupture of this organ and leakage of air into the pleural space does not occur more often. When this does happen it usually occurs with rather dramatic suddenness, but interestingly enough, need not be precipitated by violent exertion. The presence of thoracic discomfort or, at times, acute pain accompanied by dyspnea and varying degrees of weakness or collapse herald the occurrence of this accident. Radiographically, one lung is seen to be collapsed by a varying extent of pneumothorax (Fig. 10). On physical examination, tympany or hyperresonance is noted on percussion and breath sounds are distant on the affected side. Mediastinal displacement, if present, is away from the involved side. If bleeding accompanies the accident, as from a torn adhesion, the presence of even a small amount of intrapleural blood may incite an effusion. In the typical example of spontaneous pneumothorax, however, no such complicating feature is seen.

The etiology of spontaneous pneumothorax has, in the past, been linked to pulmonary tuberculosis, but this connection is not confirmed. There need be no long range implications to a spontaneous pneumothorax.

It occurs typically in the young adult male, probably as the result of some degree of emphysematous change which may be entirely unrecognizable by clinical methods. In spite of the emphysema of advancing years

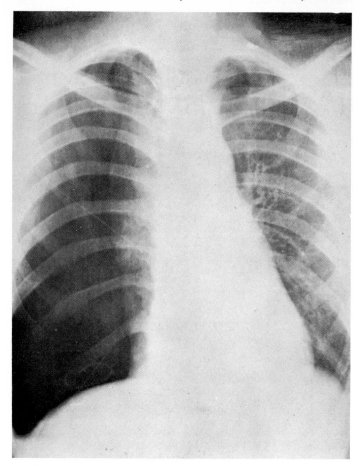

Figure 10. X-ray appearance in a patient with spontaneous pneumothorax. The right lung lies well flattened against the mediastinum. The right hemithorax is otherwise empty, except for a minimal amount of fluid. The mediastinal position is being displaced slightly to the left.

and even the development of large emphysematous blebs or bullae, the incidence in older individuals is not as common as one would expect. When it does occur in the individual with advanced emphysema, moderate degrees of collapse often produce serious cardiorespiratory embarrassment.

Treatment is determined by the extent of the pulmonary collapse. If the degree of collapse is small, amounting merely to a mantle of air surrounding the lung, observation of the patient at bed rest will assure one that no further leakage of air is occurring and should show that slow absorption of the air and ultimate resolution of the process will take place.

If there is more than a mantle of air with a corresponding degree of increased pulmonary collapse, a similar program of observation can be followed, but needle aspiration of air should be practiced to encourage the lung to expand. It should be remembered that the aspiration of air may, of course, re-open a previously sealed pleural leak and bring about additional leakage of air into the pleura, with a resultant return of collapse. Under these circumstances, or when the collapse is 50 per cent or more, the insertion of an intercostal catheter or other decompressive device is in order. This relatively simple procedure permits the decompressing instrument to be connected to water seal drainage, and will often bring about the expansion of the lung in 12 to 24 hours. Radiographic studies are taken to measure the progress.

If the pleural tear remains open or, as sometimes appears to happen, develops a ball-valve effect which permits ingress of air into the pleura but blocks its egress to the bronchial tree, a progressive degree of pulmonary collapse occurs with the appearance of increasing cardiorespiratory embarrassment to an alarming state. This situation is termed "tension pneumothorax." By totally collapsing the involved lung and pushing the mediastinum over so as to compromise the opposite lung, it can be fatal. Immediate decompression of the involved side is required.

Should the insertion of suitable pleural decompression not control the air leak in a reasonable period of time, such as three to five days, it is advisable to carry out a thoracotomy in order to assess the source of the air leak and control it by appropriate measures.

Recurrent pneumothorax occurs, and it has become a generally established policy that after two or more recurrences, or if bilateral pneumothoraces have occurred, a more definitive method of treatment is to be carried out. This generally takes the form of a thoracotomy with the production of a pleural symphysis either by roughening the parietal pleura with gauze, inserting pleural irritants or stripping the parietal pleura so that the expanded lung will be sealed against the chest wall, forestalling the possibility of future collapses.

The introduction of pleural irritants through a needle is advocated by some, but it is tragic indeed if the irritants are placed in the pleura and the lung cannot be immediately expanded, because this collapsed lung will then become covered with a coat of pleural exudate which will subsequently prevent its expansion and may well require decortication to correct an unfortunate iatrogenic condition.

The insertion of an intercostal catheter can be done at the bedside under local anesthesia. A site for introduction of the catheter is selected, either in the axilla above the level of the nipple or more often in the second anterior intercostal space. The skin of the immediate area of the puncture and the tissues of the chest wall are rendered insensitive with local anesthesia. Particular attention should paid to the parietal pleura. A small incision is made in the skin in order to accommodate a trocar of adequate size. The trocar is inserted through this incision and pushed by rotation through the tissues of the chest wall into the pleura. The presence of the pneumothorax is proved by needle at the time of anesthetization, to confirm the clinical and radiographic findings.

Once the trocar is passed into the pleura the stylet is removed and a urethral catheter with additional side openings is threaded through it into the pleura. The trocar is then removed over the intercostal catheter. This is immediately connected to a water seal and the catheter is suitably anchored to the skin, preferably by suture. The area is covered with suitable dressings.

Insertion of a needle is somewhat simpler. The needle should not have a sharp point, since the expanding lung may tear itself on it. In the absence of a trocar, the catheter may be inserted between the jaws of a hemostat and can be passed into the pleura without significant difficulty.

The perforation of pulmonary disease into the pleura may be accompanied by a pneumothorax. The complicating features here have to do with the underlying disease, such as tuberculosis, abscess and so forth.

When the presence of blood produces a pleural effusion, it is suggested that treatment be more insistent since such pleural fluid may well deposit a fibrinous coat over the visceral surface and delay, or possibly prevent, expansion of the lung. Large amounts of blood producing a hemopneumothorax may, of course, require thoracotomy for evacuation of the clotted blood or, on occasion, for control of hemorrhage. In most instances, however, conservative management of spontaneous pneumothorax with hemothorax will ultimately result in recovery.

EMPHYSEMA. Coalescence of alveoli, increased lung volume, as well as loss of inherent contractility are an accompaniment of the aging process. These changes, if kept apace of chronologic age, are entirely within the range of normal. When they occur faster than expected, the clinical problem of emphysema appears.

The physiologic changes which occur in emphysema, as reflected in pulmonary function studies, show the presence of air-trapping due to the loss of inherent contractility, or compliance. Thus, the forced expiratory volume may remain close to normal yet the victim's ability to exhale air is reflected in a lowering of the one-second forced expiratory capacity as well as in a marked lowering of the total amount of air that can be expelled in a given period of time by repeated efforts, maximum voluntary ventilation. Measurements of the residual volume show an increase. These derangements all lead to increased carbon dioxide retention.

It is of importance to realize that in far-advanced stages of emphysema, physiologic derangement may be so marked that the hypercarbia paralyzes the higher respiratory centers in the medulla, leaving the individual to breathe under control of the lower respiratory centers, which are sensitive primarily to oxygen lack. Thus, in the advanced emphysematous patient the administration of oxygen may be hazardous in that it can remove the one remaining respiratory drive—lack of oxygen.

The diagnosis of emphysema is relatively easy once the disease process is fully established. It will be seen that the individual is having obvious respiratory embarrassment. Marked increase in the anteroposterior diameter of the chest, the so-called "barrel chest," will be seen. The costal excursions will be limited by virtue of the marked elevation of the sternum. The accessory respiratory muscles will be utilized. Radiographically, it will be seen that the diaphragms are flattened and the lungs are voluminous (Fig. 11). The excursions of the diaphragms are limited. Pulmonary function studies will corroborate these findings.

Very often in these advanced states the cleansing of the tracheobronchial tree is poor, retention of sputum is common and super-imposed infection results in varying degrees of bronchitis.

Surgically, the basic problem in emphysema cannot be suitably attacked, but one should consider the advisability of resecting localized areas of more advanced disease which take the form of blebs or bullae. These may be encroaching upon lung capable of function adjacent to them. Occasionally, the resection of a segment or lobe of lung is indicated, but most often the simple excision of the air cysts, oversewing the base, will help reduce the mechanical factors which impair pulmonary function. This approach should not be offered indiscriminately to individuals with marginal reserve. After suitable study of pulmonary functions and bronchographic assessment of the amount of lung involved, however, many can be accepted with reasonable prospect of improvement.

BRONCHIECTASIS. The term "bronchiectasis" defies precise definition insofar as a disease process is concerned. Ectasia of the bronchi refers to the bronchographic picture

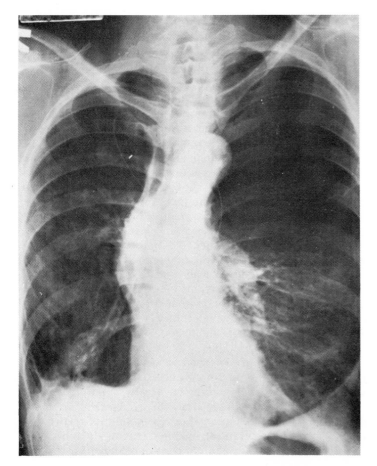

Figure 11. Chest x-ray in advanced pulmonary emphysema. Note the depressed and flattened hemidiaphragms, the loss of lung markings in the upper chest bilaterally. On the left, no evidence of bronchovascular markings is seen in the upper one-half. The increased pressure by trapping of air in this area of emphysematous cystic change is suggested by the compressed and crowded markings evident in the left base. Also, the left hemithorax is seen to be larger than the right. Both bases otherwise show the "stranding" consistent with pulmonary fibrosis. There is marked tortuosity of the aorta.

which depicts the gross anatomic changes that occur. The clinical symptoms are varied. Bronchial dilatation and sacculation in lower lobe bronchi are generally associated with cough and expectoration of heavy purulent sputum, which typically is foul smelling and bad tasting. The clinical disease is the result of chronicity with retention of secretions in the ectatic areas, peribronchial inflammation, interstitial pneumonitis and loss of pulmonary parenchyma by consolidation, fibrosis and contracture. The areas of ectasia are accentuated by the process which originally destroyed the supporting elements of the bronchial wall.

Bronchiectatic changes in upper lobe bronchi are most frequently a sequel of tuberculosis which, in the process of healing, has produced the characteristic distortion. Probably, because of the position of these upper lobe bronchial radicals, drainage is better, retention of secretions less likely and, therefore, symptoms of chronic pulmonary suppuration are less apt to be seen. On the other hand, this "dry" bronchiectasis is prone to ulcerate, leading to hemoptysis. It is true that "wet" bronchiectasis may bleed from the granulation tissue lining the destroyed bronchial tree, but not quite to the same and exclusive degree as in the "dry" type.

The pathogenesis of bronchiectasis is difficult to specify. Two elements appear to be necessary for the production of this process in a previously healthy lung: obstruction and infection. The interplay between the congenital and these acquired factors in the etiology are often not clearly discernible. Furthermore, once ectasia appears, further cicatricial contracture may accentuate the process.

Probably due to the better control of pulmonary infections generally, bronchiectasis is being encountered less often and has presented itself as a clinical problem with decreasing frequency. It is primarily a disease of the younger age groups, developing by adolescence or early maturity.

A sharp distinction, however, should be made between the bronchiectatic patients and individuals who give evidence of chronic pulmonary suppuration due to emphysema and chronic bronchitis.

In the presence of localized bronchiectasis confined to a lobe or a portion thereof, this being the source of symptoms and the cause for the perpetuation of pulmonary suppuration, excision of the area will be curative. In the victim of chronic bronchitis, on the other hand, the process is diffuse, there is no localization and surgical excision of doubtfully ectatic areas in the bronchial tree will be most disappointing insofar as the relief of symptoms is concerned.

Reference is made in the literature to "cylindrical" bronchiectasis as opposed to "saccular" bronchiectasis, but it is doubtful if "cylindrical" bronchiectasis ever becomes a surgical target since it is apt to be part of diffuse bronchial disease.

Areas of bronchial ectasia that are definite and unequivocal, as demonstrated on a bronchogram and confined to a lobe or a portion thereof, is an entirely different disease. The remainder of the lung may be, indeed, quite healthy.

The diagnosis is based on the symptoms as well as the clinical findings. These can be definitive on physical examination in basal bronchiectasis, but are quite apt to be inconclusive in upper lobe disease. Important information can be deduced by bronchoscopy, particularly by localizing the source of sputum. The final and conclusive demonstration of the disease requires a full bronchographic study of the lung fields.

Treatment in the clearly localized unilateral form is excision of the involved segments. The removal of the most extensive areas of bronchiectasis, however, from one lung will often permit gratifying palliation even though small areas of bronchiectasis may be left behind. In selected patients, bilateral excision is justified and rewarding in terms of palliation.

In upper lobe bronchiectasis, an active tuberculous lesion should not be overlooked. If present, appropriate treatment should be instituted before resection is undertaken.

LUNG ABSCESS. The incidence of lung abscesses has dropped considerably since the advent of antibiotics and the better control of pulmonary suppuration. They are, however, still seen as a result of aspiration pneumonitis which may follow vomiting during stuporous states, or may follow any pneumonitis of severe sort, such as that produced by a Friedländer's bacillus. In some instances, it would appear that the abscess is the result of a septic embolus.

In older individuals, the presence of a lung abscess should arouse suspicion that a neoplasm coexists. This neoplasm may be present in the portion of the bronchial tree leading to the area of the abscess, and as a result of this obstruction has produced a suppurative pneumonitis which ultimately excavated with the formation of a true abscess. In this event, the abscess is secondary to a more proximal neoplasm. On the other hand, the abscess cavity recognized on the x-ray film may actually be the neoplasm itself which has excavated and communicated with the bronchial tree.

A lung abscess is characterized clinically by severe illness including a high degree of toxicity, accompanied by a septic course and severe prostration. This varies somewhat with the etiologic agent and the circumstances under which the abscess occurred.

The presence of pneumonitis generally precedes the actual recognition of the abscess either by clinical or radiologic examination.

The radiographic diagnosis of a lung abscess requires the recognition of a cavity. A thick and irregular wall suggests an excavated neoplasm (Fig. 12).

The management of a lung abscess calls for control of the infection by use of the appropriate antibiotics, best chosen on the basis of bacteriologic survey of the sputum. Sup-

porting the use of antibiotics should be all measures designed to promote the expectoration of secretions. These include proper humidification, the use of bronchodilator drugs, the use of expectorants to thin tenacious secretions, insistence upon periodic cough to clear the tracheobronchial tree and the use of postural drainage. General supportive treatment is, obviously, called for. During the course of management, bronchoscopy should invariably be carried out with the view in mind that any obstructing lesion would be recognized and accurately identified. Also, by proper shrinkage of the bronchial mucosa through topical applications to the orifice of the draining bronchus, relief of the edema and consequent promotion of drainage results.

When, by these measures, the disease is brought under clinical control, the radiographic residuals should be assessed. It should be determined whether or not a cavity persists and whether bronchiectasis has resulted from the severe suppuration.

If, after achievement of clinical remission in the course of a lung abscess, the evalua-

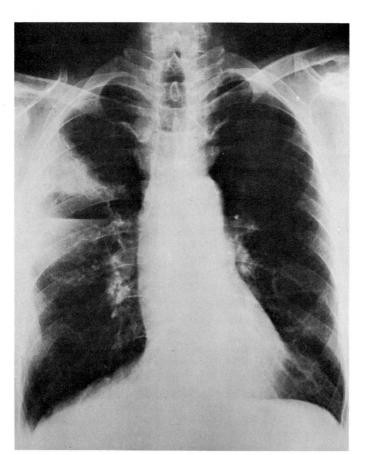

Figure 12. The large area of density in right midlung field contains a cavity and fluid level. This could represent an excavating peripheral carcinoma, but is roentgenographically indistinguishable from a pyogenic lung abscess.

tion by x-ray demonstrates either a persistent cavity or obvious bronchiectasis, serious consideration should be given to resecting the involved areas. The lapse of a suitable time before reaching this decision is justified, however, since small cavities may close through healing of the surrounding lung parenchyma, and minor degrees of bronchiectasis may not be significant as a source of symptoms or recurrences.

However, a cavity which has remained unchanged for six or eight weeks in spite of good clinical control is not apt to close subsequently. Certainly, definite bronchiectatic changes are not reversible. Such residuals, which are indicative of the severity of the original process, can be expected to lead to recurrences.

Drainage of a lung abscess through the chest wall is resorted to infrequently under present-day management. It is required, however, when drainage through the bronchial communications is not adequate, in spite of appropriate management, and the clinical course continues to be active with persistence of significant symptoms.

In this technique, the abscess cavity is localized with respect to the point where it would approach the parietal pleura and be most likely to have a complete pleural symphysis through which drainage might be established. This localization can be done by appropriate x-ray and fluoroscopic studies. The area is often suggested by the presence of tenderness to direct palpation of a rib. This sign is significant of the periostitis which would go with a suppurative process that has approached the parietal pleura.

Preferably under local anesthesia, in order that sputum control may be managed by the patient himself, an incision is made over the area of localization and a segment of one or two ribs is removed subperiosteally for direct inspection of the pleura. If the pleurae appear to be fused, careful incision is made so that the presence of a firm pleural symphysis can be confirmed. Should a free pleural space be recognized underneath the area of rib resection, the incision should not be deepened but a gauze pack should be placed in the area, followed by closure of the wound over it as a foreign body. After a lapse of some two weeks, the wound can be reopened and the pack removed. At this time, a symphysis would be expected to have occurred, in which event the abscess can be entered, preferably by the use of cautery.

The cavity is then carefully emptied and loosely packed with gauze.

Healing of the abscess may be achieved by this maneuver after a somewhat chronic course, but it is to be expected that ultimate resection of the severely diseased portion of lung will be required for final rehabilitation.

FUNGUS INFECTIONS. Pulmonary or pleural infections by fungi are of interest from the standpoint of differential diagnosis because they are easily confused with other chronic granulomatous processes, notably tuberculosis. If they are manifested by solitary nodules, bronchogenic carcinoma must be considered. The fungi which are of interest in the United States are histoplasmosis, coccidioidomycosis, blastomycosis and actinomycosis.

The diagnosis is established by the existence of pulmonary disease and the presence of the organism in sputum or in tissue which may have been made available for study. Positive skin sensitivity test, or a positive complement fixation study, is supporting evidence.

Surgical intervention, usually in the form of pulmonary resection, is required when exclusion of carcinoma is not possible, or for the localized chronic cavitary forms of histoplasmosis and coccidioidomycosis particularly. Drainage is indicated for pleural infections. Amphotericin B is available as a chemotherapeutic agent in blastomycosis particularly, with somewhat more success than in histoplasmosis or coccidioidomycosis. The drug is toxic and treatment is prolonged. A combination of penicillin and sulfa drugs in relatively high dosages is proposed for actinomycosis.

The acute phases of these infections may be highly fatal and are of no surgical interest beyond the possibility of helping to establish a diagnosis.

PULMONARY TUBERCULOSIS. Tuberculosis is the commonest granulomatous disease which involves the lungs and pleura. This diagnosis is justified on clinical grounds if a typical infiltrate is recognized by x-ray in a person with appropriate symptoms who has positive skin sensitivity to tuberculin (Fig. 13).

The recovery of acid-fast bacilli by concentrated smear or culture made from sputum or by culture of fasting gastric content is confirmatory, but indicates the presence of ulceration in the lesion. Careful bacteriologic control is nonetheless important, because

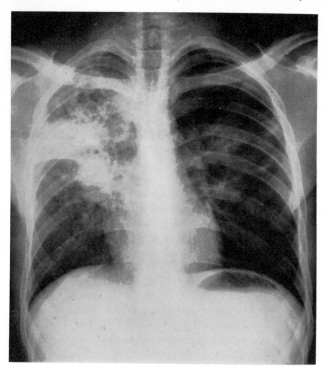

Figure 13. Roentgenogram of a young man, showing extensive bilateral tuberculous disease. Sputum was positive for acid-fast bacilli.

atypical bacilli are assuming clinical significance on the one hand and drug sensitivities offer a logical guide to chemotherapy on the other. Recognition of the atypical mycobacteria as a result of improved and now commonly employed cultural as well as cytochemical methods has become not only possible but necessary.

These atypical mycobacteria differ from *M. tuberculosis* in being more or less resistant to the three standard chemotherapeutic agents and, therefore, require surgical intervention more consistently because of persisting cavitation and failure to convert sputum. Also, transmissibility of the disease associated with these organisms is less clear, and the epidemiologic aspects of the problem are consequently less certain.

Two of the four groups in the Runyon classification of these organisms are consistently associated with pulmonary disease. *M. kansasii* (photochromogen or Group I) and the Battey bacillus (Group III) account for 2 to 8 per cent of the admissions to tuberculosis sanitaria. The other two groups are known as the scotochromogen (Group II) and the rapid growers (Group IV).

Under current concepts of management, pulmonary tuberculosis is treated by antibiotics and chemotherapeutic agents. The principal agents are streptomycin, para-aminosalicylic acid and isoniazid (Fig. 14). Whatever the regimen elected, there is general agreement that isoniazid should be included. Secondary drugs, so called because of their short effective life and high toxicity, include viomycin, pyrazinamide and cycloserine. Ethambutal is under study and has promise.

Surgery is called upon to treat those residuals of lung destruction which cannot or do not respond to these agents, threatening, therefore, the patient's ultimate security.

Timing of surgical intervention. It would seem ideal to observe the course of pulmonary tuberculosis under chemotherapy and resort to surgical intervention only at a time when it could be demonstrated unequivocally that medical management would be inadequate. Because of the fact, however, that these drugs provoke resistance on the part of the tubercle bacillus in due time, and because of the poor results attendant upon resective surgery except when carried out under protection of chemotherapy, this expectant attitude is not advised. Thus it is that, when the disease has been brought under control by chemotherapy so that surgical intervention can be safely carried out, an evaluation of the anatomic residuals is

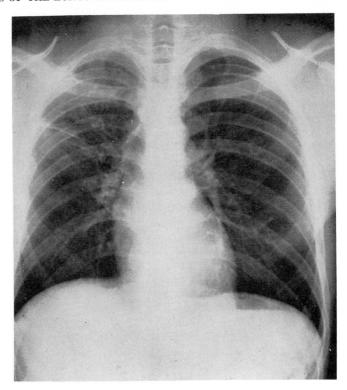

Figure 14. A roentgenogram taken eight months after that in Figure 13. Note the marked improvement brought about by streptomycin, para-aminosalicylic acid and isoniazid.

in order to demonstrate or predict the necessity for surgery.

In general, the disease can be considered to be under control when the process shows radiographic stability and the sputum is negative for tubercle bacilli by ordinary means of examination. The ideal time, therefore, for surgical intervention is that moment when this form of treatment can be seen to be necessary and when chemotherapeutic control is achieved—about six months.

Anatomic residuals. Demonstrable residuals may take several forms. The open cavity is the most obvious surgical target. Whether or not such cavities can actually heal while remaining clearly open is vigorously debated. Until proof of such occurrence is more certain and our ability to recognize this phenomenon more definite, open cavities remain as obvious indications for surgical intervention.

Cavities that are filled, or for that matter areas of focal necrosis that remain and are 1.0 to 1.5 cm. in size, may well be surgical targets. This is particularly true if such lesions tend to conglomerate and present a more impressive volume in their aggregate than they do singly.

Bronchiectasis is another frequently en-

countered lesion, usually following a rather severe tuberculous process. Its importance may be debated, but it had best be considered the sequel of lung disease. It can be regarded as the anatomic expression of lung that has been ravaged by tuberculosis. The changes are irreversible, are not amenable to collapse measures and form a point of insecurity tending to make recurrence or exacerbation likely when chemotherapeutic control is eventually lost.

Carnification due to organization of pneumonic exudates with shrinkage and its counterpart compensating emphysema, all occurring in varying admixtures independent of any consideration of endobronchial disease, represents a final target. These manifestations are likewise an indication of a severe process.

Evaluation of anatomic residuals. The chest x-ray is the basic method of following the course of the disease. Lateral projections are essential in assessing the distribution of lesions by lobes or segments.

Laminagrams taken in anteroposterior projections are reliable in demonstrating residual cavities. In lateral projections, by outlining the fissures, they can clearly give the segmental distribution of lesions. When combined with bronchography, the localization of residual disease of surgical significance can be made with surprising accuracy (Figs. 15 and 16).

Bronchoscopy is important in final evaluation, particularly to recognize any important distortions or significant bronchial inflammation that might predispose to complications in the postoperative period.

Choice of operation. Current philosophy has swung largely to resection of the areas of involved lung and away from collapse measures. The availability and effectiveness of the chemotherapeutic agents has accomplished this. Resection of a tuberculous lung, or portions thereof, could not be performed with any reasonable degree of success prior to the advent of chemotherapy except in cases of quiescent disease, and this only occasionally. Collapse, on the other hand, could be carried out without such protection and was eminently successful. It is obvious that the clean excision of the anatomic residuals of tuberculous disease is a far better approach to management than the "entombment" of these residuals by collapse, such as thoracoplasty.

Since excision cannot always be carried out, for a variety of reasons, a choice of procedures is to be considered. The indication is for resection except when the anticipated amount of lung tissue requiring removal exceeds that which the patient's cardiorespiratory reserve will permit without crippling, or when, because of inadequate control of the tuberculous disease by chemotherapy, the safety of the procedure is doubtful. Under these circumstances, some form of collapse is in order. Patent cavernous disease without significant associated bronchiectasis, located above the fifth rib posteriorly, offers the best prognosis under collapse. Nodular disease, bronchiectasis and carnified lung are relatively unaffected by collapse.

Collapse in the present era means a thoracoplasty (Fig. 17). This must take the form either of a standard seven-rib posterolateral extrapleural costectomy of the Alexander type, usually performed in stages, or a one-stage extraperiosteal separation of a selected area of lung, filling the space so created by a prosthesis (Fig. 18).

These prostheses are foreign bodies and have the detractions generally attributable to them. Paraffin, Lucite spheres and Ivalon

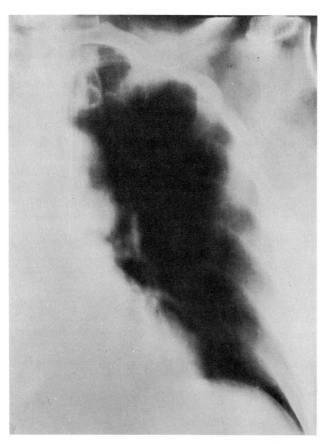

Figure 15.   Anteroposterior laminagram showing left apical tuberculous cavity.

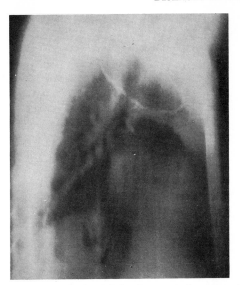

Figure 16. Left lateral laminagram demonstrating large apical anterior cavity in tuberculosis.

are popular materials utilized for this purpose.

The smallest amount of lung which will cleanly extirpate the disease should be resected. Segmental resection is safe and satisfactory but, under conditions of meager or poor chemotherapeutic control, wider resec-

tions to the extent of lobectomy or pneumonectomy are less apt to lead to complications of a tuberculous nature, since they are far more likely to be effected through cleaner planes.

Combinations of resection and thoracoplasty are practicable. When a resection, to be satisfactory in extirpating the disease, leaves behind a piece of lung too small to fill the hemithorax readily, some form of tailoring procedure is necessary. This is done at the time of the resection or better still before the resection, since the concomitant procedure increases morbidity.

An adequate anatomic evaluation preoperatively will permit identification of those portions of lung which will, or probably will, require resection. A tailoring procedure should be done before the definitive operation when an estimate suggests a resection which volumetrically exceeds a lobe. This practice will often forestall a complication which could be expected to follow incomplete or markedly delayed re-expansion of lung, as well as the increased morbidity attendant upon the combined procedure.

Endobronchial tuberculosis. Particularly in women, localized endobronchial lesions resulting in ulceration and healing by cicatrix with stenosis, are seen. This is less

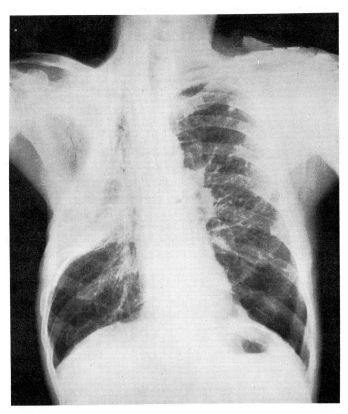

Figure 17. Chest roentgenogram of a middle-aged man illustrating the collapse achieved by a standard posterolateral thoracoplasty on the right.

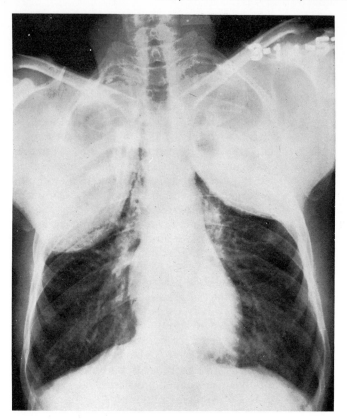

Figure 18. End result of staged bilateral surgical collapse using paraffin as plombage.

common now than formerly, because these lesions respond promptly to chemotherapy. Occasionally, such stenotic lesions can be resected locally, salvaging the distal lung. More often, however, the distal lung is affected irrevocably and must be sacrificed.

Because occasionally and, no doubt, by a happy collusion of several different factors, the complete obliteration of a bronchial lumen has led to negative sputum and clinical remission of disease, interest has been fostered in the concept of surgically closing a bronchus which drains areas containing tuberculous cavitation, when more conventional approaches do not seem practical. The sudden cutting off of an outlet for the products of suppuration seems contrary to accepted principle and cannot be recommended.

Pleural tuberculosis. Tuberculosis may extend to the pleura and produce pleural disease in association with pulmonary disease. It may also occur that pleuritis is the first evidence of clinical tuberculosis, taking the form of a pleural effusion. This is often sterile. The absence of any suitable etiology for the effusion, particularly in young people with positive skin sensitivity to tuberculin, speaks strongly for a tuberculous etiology.

The treatment for the tuberculous effusion is chemotherapy and thoracentesis. Should this regimen not lead to a restoration to normal, decortication may be required. The exact program of management in tuberculous pleuritis becomes complex, depending upon the interplay of the various possible combinations of presence or absence of pyogenic infection and the presence or absence of significant parenchymal tuberculosis. The simplest form which may require no therapy beyond chemotherapy is the clear effusion which rapidly disappears on drugs alone. The most complex is the mixed empyema harboring both tuberculous and pyogenic infection overlying a destroyed lung. This requires pleuropneumonectomy.

Under proper management, tuberculosis can be brought to a point of arrest in approximately 97 per cent of patients with a follow-up of four to five years. The incidence of nontuberculous postoperative complications of significant sort for management by resection should not exceed 4 to 6 per cent and the expected incidence of tuberculous complications should be in the order of 5 or possibly 6 per cent.

MISCELLANEOUS CONDITIONS. Certain miscellaneous conditions are occasionally of surgical interest.

Pneumonia is a medical problem managed by appropriate antibiotics. Pneumonias which fail to resolve promptly should incite curiosity as to possible causes. Studies such as bronchoscopy and bronchography should be performed in an attempt to demonstrate some anatomic change which might account for the slow or delayed resolution.

Pneumonias which undergo organization are not of surgical interest except insofar as they may mimic neoplasms.

Diffuse bilateral pulmonary infiltrates are of surgical interest only as far as diagnosis is concerned (Fig. 19). Excision of the scalene fat pad with its contained lymph nodes may occasionally shed light on the probable etiology. Mediastinoscopy may have a valid place in elucidating this type of clinical problem.

A more direct approach to diagnosis is by lung biopsy, obtaining a specimen for bacteriologic as well as histologic study. This can be carried out by making a submammary incision and resecting a moderate segment of the fourth or fifth rib anterolaterally. The pleura is then entered and the lung is examined within the confines of this exposure. Suitable areas of disease are resected by wedge excision over a clamp with appropriate suturing of the cut edge to control blood and air leak. General anesthesia is recommended and so is pleural drainage. To attempt to obtain pulmonary tissue by needle biopsy through the intact chest wall is not recommended.

Inhalation of oil, notably mineral oil, leads to the formation of lipoid granulomas. These mimic neoplasms.

Amebic disease is rarely, if ever, confined to the lung. The lung may be involved by embolization, but most often the involvement is subdiaphragmatic, secondary to the perforation of an amebic liver abscess into the subdiaphragmatic space. Extension of this through the diaphragm into the pleura produces an empyema. Sputum, when present, is rather characteristic, resembling

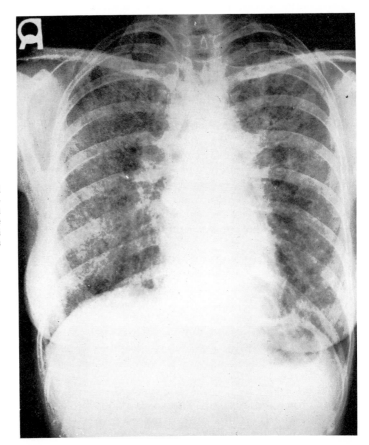

Figure 19. Extensive, diffuse bilateral pulmonary infiltrates accompanied by mediastinal widening, such as are seen in this roentgenogram, can represent any one of many diseases. Biopsy of a skin lesion in this particular patient showed changes typical of sarcoidosis.

tomato catsup or anchovy paste. Suspicion of amebic disease should lead to a clinical trial of antiamebic drugs, particularly emetine. A clear response to emetine is characteristic and diagnostic. The best approach to treatment is the use of emetine or chloroquine with repeated aspirations of any effusion. Surgical drainage is not recommended except under control of emetine or unless pyogenic infection has manifested itself as a superimposed problem.

Echinococcic cysts of the lung are uncommon in the United States.

A common problem presented to anyone interested in pulmonary diseases is the radiograph of an asymptomatic patient showing a solitary nodular density, a "coin" lesion. The important decision is whether or not this shadow represents a neoplasm. Most of these cannot be accurately identified except by direct histologic examination, and thoracotomy is required. The presence of calcium which almost completely fills a lesion in a person who has a demonstrated sensitivity to tuberculin, or to one of the fungi, is fairly conclusive evidence of granulomatous etiology. Absence of calcium would suggest a neoplasm. The bulk of these lesions are either bronchogenic carcinomas or granulomas. The remainder are assorted lesions, such as hamartomas and metastatic carcinomas.

Granulomatous peribronchial lymph nodes which become calcific do occasionally erode into the bronchial lumen, producing hemoptysis or obstruction with its sequels of atelectasis and infection. Although mimicking a bronchogenic carcinoma, the correct diagnosis can often be made by bronchoscopy and possibly bronchography, or thoracotomy. The calcific spicules are sometimes expectorated as lung "stones." Removal of the offending agent by bronchoscopy or at thoracotomy, by an appropriate pulmonary resection, is indicated.

NEOPLASMS. The lung is capable of producing a variety of neoplasms. From a practical standpoint, however, the malignant epithelial tumor (carcinoma) is by far the commonest, making up something like 95 per cent of all pulmonary tumors. This type of pulmonary neoplasm, therefore, deserves first consideration.

Carcinoma. In the early 1900's, the recorded examples of this disease were numbered in the hundreds only. Now some 40,000 to 45,000 yearly deaths are attributed to it in the United States alone.

This sharply increased recognition of carcinoma of the lung has made it outstanding among cancers and has created a sense of near panic among some observers.

Some of this rise in incidence is probably actual and not to be attributed solely to improved methods of diagnosis or to the accurate identification of an otherwise mislabeled disease process.

ETIOLOGY. The sense of panic engendered by this disease has led to a frantic search for etiology. The observation that certain occupational environments such as those of uranium, nickel or cobalt workers, for example, seem to favor the appearance of lung cancer suggested an extrinsic etiologic agent. The consumption of tobacco in the form of cigarettes tending to parallel the rise in recorded deaths from lung cancer soon singled out cigarettes as the chief contender for etiologic supremacy.

Among other and similar pronouncements, the report on Smoking and Health put out by the Surgeon General, U. S. Public Health Service, ultimately led to the placement of a danger label on cigarette packages in the United States by act of Congress.

The evidence incriminating cigarettes in that report came from statistical surveys. Whereas the statistical correlations may show an association between heavy cigarette smoking and the occurrence of lung cancer, clinical facets of the disease strongly dispute the cigarette's role as etiologic agent.

For example, lung cancer is predominantly a disease of males. It exhibits a sharp peak of incidence around 60 years of age and no dosage factor has been demonstrated because those smokers who began smoking at a relatively early age and later do develop lung cancer, do not do so any sooner than the victims who began the habit 15 or 20 years later in life. Cancer is a medical curiosity in the trachea and a rarity on both sides simultaneously. Furthermore, among its victims who have survived the removal of one lung tumor, it is uncommon to see them develop a second and new lung cancer subsequently. Finally, the records of the meticulous German pathologists show the rise in incidence beginning in the early 1900's before cigarettes became popular.

Thus it is not likely, that, if cigarettes ceased to exist, so in large measure would bronchogenic carcinoma.

CLINICAL SYMPTOMS. The clinical symptoms presented by a person bearing a carcinoma of the lung vary, depending upon the location of the neoplasm. There are two areas of the lung which are involved by the neoplasm from a clinical, as well as a topographic standpoint. The first is peripheral, wherein the lesion develops in the lung parenchyma itself; the second is central, when it arises from or involves one of the larger branches of the bronchial tree.

The central location will manifest itself primarily by those symptoms which would be expected from a growth within the bronchial lumen and arising from bronchial mucosa. These will be the signs of obstruction, which include bleeding from the ulcerating tumor and the complications of suppuration distal to a partially or completely obstructed bronchus. They include cough, hemoptysis, production of sputum, varying degrees of dyspnea, chills, fever and the signs of sepsis. The most telltale sign, as well as symptom, in the earlier phases of bronchogenic carcinoma involving a principal portion of the bronchial tree, is a wheeze. This is produced by the distortion of the air column as it rides over the intraluminal lesion. It can be appreciated by the examiner on auscultation but is also very often appreciated by the patient. This wheeze is unilateral.

When the lesion arises from a smaller branch of the bronchial tree in peripheral location, it may not cause symptoms. This is the type of tumor which is discovered on routine roentgenographic surveys. Unfortunately, it may attain relatively large size before discovery.

There are variants in both of these situations. For example, the centrally placed carcinoma may extend into the mediastinum by metastasizing to the lymph nodes or by direct extension to involve adjacent structures. Most dramatically, it may involve the superior vena cava, producing obstruction. It may involve the phrenic nerve along the pericardium and result in diaphragmatic paralysis with further reduction in respiratory reserve. It may extend to involve the recurrent laryngeal nerve, particularly on the left, and produce hoarseness as a sign of its presence. It may invade the pericardium and produce a pericardial effusion; or it is possible for it to invade the esophagus, either directly or through metastatic lymph nodes, and result in dysphagia.

The peripherally placed neoplasm may extend to the pleura where, if it perforates into the free pleura, it will likely evoke an effusion. This effusion then may seed other portions of the pleural space. On the other hand, the pleural space may be obliterated, so that direct invasion of the chest wall occurs. This event is usually accompanied by severe and intractable pain, particularly as ribs are involved. This effect will be recognized on a chest x-ray after the destruction of the bone has made itself manifest (Fig. 21). If this invasion of the chest wall takes place at the thoracic inlet, the consequent invasion of the vertebral bodies and the stellate ganglion, along with the first or second rib and the lower portions of the brachial plexus, results in a typical symptom complex which is called the superior pulmonary sulcus syndrome, the syndrome of Pancoast. Whereas other neoplasms may conceivably produce a similar syndrome, the commonest is a peripheral bronchogenic carcinoma.

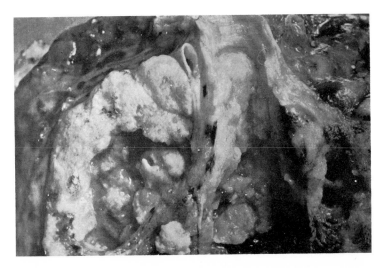

Figure 20. Bronchogenic carcinoma, showing a polypoid tumor projecting into the opened bronchus and its extension as a parabronchial mass.

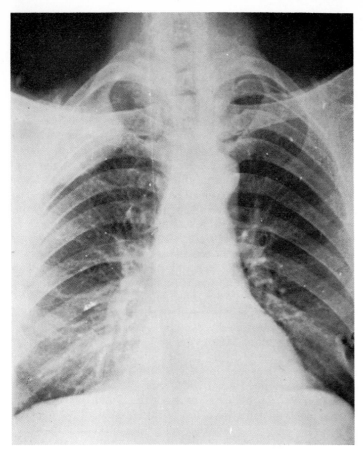

Figure 21.   A peripheral mass is recognized along the lateral upper right chest wall. Its malignant nature is strongly suggested by the erosion of the posterior portion of the third rib, which has been destroyed by the neoplastic process.

Except as a consequence of toxicity from infection or other similar secondary effect of a bronchogenic carcinoma, weight loss or disability is generally indicative of visceral metastases, particularly to the liver. The most striking example of this situation is in the occasional patient who presents with cerebral symptoms when the pulmonary tumor is very small or occasionally still impossible to detect.

DIAGNOSIS.   Once suspected by the clinical symptoms, the first approach to diagnosis is a careful physical examination. This should reveal the parenchymal changes secondary to a centrally placed lesion. In the peripheral carcinoma, however, physical signs, except for those unfortunates with extension to the pleura or the bony portions of the thorax, are absent.

The chest x-ray is the principal means of diagnosis. It is important to point out that in the case of the peripherally located neoplasm appearing as a rounded solitary density in some portion of the lung field, this shadow actually represents the neoplasm itself. In the case of the endobronchial neoplasm centrally placed in the bronchial tree, the x-ray may show extensive changes. These represent atelectasis of one or more lobes with possibly a superimposed pneumonitis. These extensive radiographic changes, however, represent only the effects secondary to the presence of the tumor. The tumor per se may not be visualized at all on a routine or conventional film.

Occasionally, by making laminagraphic cuts through the bronchus supplying the area of atelectasis or pneumonitis, one may recognize the presence of the neoplasm effacing the air column. Extending the same line of reasoning, when one sees that a peripheral neoplasm is cavitated and is, in effect, therefore, an abscess, it is the neoplasm itself which is seen in this peripheral location. In the case of an abscess developing in a lung that has undergone suppurative pneumonitis secondary to obstruction by a centrally placed neoplasm, it is not the neoplasm itself that is visualized, but rather the various secondary manifestations of its presence within the bronchus which are actually recorded on the film.

The bronchoscopic examination of an individual with a rounded solitary density, a peripheral bronchogenic carcinoma, is not apt to be informative insofar as this neoplasm is concerned. Under these circumstances, the examination is done principally to rule out other lesions and possibly for the collection of bronchial secretions for cytologic examination.

Bronchoscopy in the centrally placed lesion is, obviously, mandatory. Direct inspection of the principal portions of the airway can be carried out and biopsies can be obtained. When the lesion involves the depths of an upper lobe, visualization of the tumor may require the use of a telescopic lens.

In all instances, tissue for diagnosis cannot be obtained, but the collection of material for cytologic study may be helpful in indicating the presence of a neoplasm beyond the field of bronchoscopic vision.

Cytologic examination can be carried out on sputum. A fresh specimen immediately fixed is essential for best results.

Any recognized lymphadenopathy should be biopsied in order to obtain tissue for diagnosis, if possible, but more pertinently to find out whether extrathoracic metastases have occurred. When no palpable lymphadenopathy is present, resection of the scalene fat pad or corresponding paratracheal tissue may be warranted. The yield in nodes positive for metastatic carcinoma is low in clinically favorable patients, and does not justify this procedure as a routine.

The technique of scalene node biopsy, which is the approach commonly employed, is simple. Under local anesthesia, an incision parallel to and above the clavicle on the appropriate side, running between the external jugular vein and some portion of the sternocleidomastoid muscle is made. The dissection is deepened to expose the fatty tissue over the anterior scalene muscle and this is dissected off, care being taken not to injure the phrenic nerve or thoracic duct.

Mediastinoscopy is the currently favored approach for examining more succulent lymph nodes deeply situated below the clavicle.

If suspicion of bronchogenic carcinoma exists on clinical or radiologic grounds, the final step in establishing its presence or absence is direct examination of the lung at thoracotomy. Considerable experience and a clear understanding of gross pathology, as well as the limitations and implications of the previously completed diagnostic studies, are required in order to conduct an intelligent exploratory thoracotomy.

Indiscriminate biopsy, or cutting into an excisable tumor in the open surgical field, should not be done. Excision biopsy is far preferable. It may be necessary to remove a lobe or a segment containing the lesion, so that a clean excision of it is accomplished. This is then sent to the pathologist for frozen section and opinion.

It is essential to establish without equivocation the histologic nature of any lesion which is considered to be neoplastic but deemed unresectable.

TYPES OF NEOPLASM. Whereas several classifications for bronchogenic carcinomas have been proposed, the simplest and most commonly utilized considers the following types.

Epidermoid, accounts for something like 50 per cent of the tumors.

Adenocarcinoma, accounts for approximately 15 per cent.

The undifferentiated neoplasm, which may be referred to as an "oat" cell or a small cell carcinoma, accounts for some 30 per cent.

Bronchiolar or alveolar cell carcinoma, accounts for a small percentage of malignant pulmonary neoplasms.

The bronchiolar or alveolar cell carcinoma is a peculiar neoplasm which may even at times be multicentric. It may occur bilaterally; it may extend from one lobe to another and ultimately involve the entire lung or a large portion of both lungs. It is also of interest in that it is histologically reminiscent of a disease recognized in sheep, which is known to be transmissible. Transmissibility of this disease in humans, or the direct parallels of the malignant neoplasm in man to the disease as seen in sheep, and called "jagziekte," has not been clearly established. One feature in common, however, is that there is considerable excess of bronchial secretions present in the disease recognized in sheep and often bronchorrhea is a manifestation of the presence of an alveolar cell tumor in man.

TREATMENT. The best method of treatment for bronchogenic carcinoma is surgical excision. It is becoming increasingly evident that the important prognostic factor has to do with the viability of the metastatic deposits transported through the blood. Whereas these lesions are epithelial tumors and disseminate through the lymphatics, it appears that the ultimate outcome is determined principally by the occurrence of lesions in distant organs, such as the brain, liver and skeleton. Local recurrences or massive mediastinal lymphadenopathy do not account for the bulk of ultimate deaths.

The resection of a bronchogenic carcinoma requires varying degrees of tissue sacrifice. The usual extent of resection calls for the sacrifice of an entire lung, but as experience is gained, smaller resections appear to be adequate. In suitably placed lesions in which an adequate margin can be obtained, a lobectomy is entirely satisfactory. Whereas local resections of sharply limited bronchial carcinomas cannot be recommended as ideal, they may be justified when limited respiratory reserve or other factors demand conservatism.

It has also become evident that excessively radical resections have not improved surgical results commensurate with the magnitude of the operative procedure. On the other hand, there are occasions when invasion by the neoplasm of the chest wall, the pericardium or other adjacent structures which can be sacrificed, calls for courageous extension of the operative procedure. This seems entirely justified and may be crowned with occasional success.

If adequate and secure stumps of the principal vessels and a bronchial stump free of neoplasm can be secured, resection is justified. No one can offer a prognosis for an individual and specific situation.

On the basis of the fundamental concept of cancer surgery, that the adequate operation include the removal of the primary lesion with suitable margin along with the lymphatic bed to which it can be expected to drain, lower lobe lesions peripherally located probably justify pneumonectomy, but should certainly have a complete hilar dissection to include the subcarinal nodes. Upper lobe lesions peripherally located appear to be adequately handled by lobectomy with upper mediastinal dissection. Lesions located endobronchially may require the sacrifice of an adjacent lobe simply because it is impossible to have an adequate margin on the endobronchial portion, while at the same time sparing the bronchus to the adjacent lobe. Thus, the location of the tumor in the bronchial tree will under some circumstances determine the extent of the resection.

Limited excisions of endobronchially located neoplasms call for highly refined techniques and individualized treatment.

Extensions of cancer to the chest wall tend to render more doubtful the ultimate prognosis because the neoplasm has entered a field from which lymphatic extensions cannot be controlled by any added extent of pulmonary resection. Thus the tendency is to remove, by adequate margin, the lesion in the chest wall and in the lung, saving for function in respiration as much lung as is consistent with a relatively wide local excision.

Roentgenotherapy has been the mainstay of treatment, in the hope of palliating those patients who have extensive neoplasms which do not justify surgical excision and those patients who are not resectable.

One of the limitations in roentgenotherapy is the inability of the overlying structures, notably skin, to withstand the amount of x-ray required to deliver a cancerocidal dose to these deeply placed tumors.

Roentgenotherapy from sources such as cobalt[60] provides rays which do less damage to skin and can be focused more directly on the tumor. This has improved the outlook for roentgenotherapy, and it is being pursued with considerable optimism.

The possible combination of preoperative x-ray from a source such as cobalt, followed by resection, is currently being studied in the hope of improving the survival rates from this disease. Some success has been demonstrated, particularly in the superior sulcus tumor.

So far, there has been no encouraging development along the lines of radioactive isotopes.

Likewise, the use of radon seeds or needles placed at the time the neoplasm is found to be unresectable has not brought particularly encouraging results. The use of massive x-ray dosage at the time of thoracotomy has been explored, but no clear results are reported.

A cancerocidal chemical which might be introduced through the intravenous route and, therefore, arrive at the lungs in relatively high concentration would seem to be ideal in lung neoplasms as well as offering control over the viability of distantly implanted metastases. In view of the fact that much of the blood supply to bronchogenic carcinoma is provided by the bronchial circulation, local perfusion also suggests itself. Up to the present time, no agent of serious promise has appeared.

Since this is predominantly a carcinoma of men, the use of hormones has been investigated also, with great disappointment. The use of steroids seems to have benefited no one beyond the nonspecific effect that may come with their use.

INOPERABILITY. Extension of the neoplasm beyond the lung is a relative contraindication to exploration. This is certainly true if the extension can be seen to involve structures that cannot be sacrificed. Involvement of the superior vena cava, for example, generally precludes resection because reconstruction of this channel has not been particularly successful.

Involvement of the phrenic nerve with hemidiaphragmatic paralysis usually means involvement of the pericardium, and most often extension of the neoplasm to the pericardial sac and perhaps to the visceral surface of the heart itself. However, if limited only to the superficial portions of the pericardium, this excision can be carried out along with that of the neoplasm.

The presence of hoarseness produced by paralysis of the left recurrent laryngeal nerve in the presence of a known bronchogenic carcinoma usually means that the neoplasm has involved the nerve where it courses under the aortic arch and, therefore, the likelihood of direct aortic invasion must be considered.

On occasion, resection of the lung can be accomplished with suitable margin when the left recurrent nerve is paralyzed, particularly if the nerve involvement is due to metastatic lymph nodes in this area and not directly due to the primary tumor. Occasionally, only the adventitia of the aorta may be invaded along with the nerve, and separation of the tumor can occur. It should be pointed out, however, that tumors at this level provide a small and often inadequate stump of uninvolved bronchus or artery.

The presence of massive subcarinal lymphadenopathy, as evidenced by widening of the tracheal bifurcation, may preclude a suitable resection.

The presence of a pleural effusion is strongly suggestive of extension of the neoplasm to the pleura, but the fluid may be there from some other cause and need not preclude exploration. If, however, the presence of tumor cells is unquestioned in samples of the aspirated fluid, the likelihood of a successful surgical excision is virtually nil.

The presence of demonstrated metastases at some distant point renders surgical excision futile.

PROGNOSIS AND RESULTS. In round numbers, approximately one-third of the patients suffering from bronchogenic carcinoma are beyond the hope of surgical excision at the time they are first seen. They may be palliated by other avenues of treatment, with prolongation of life in some instances. An additional one-third of the original patients will be found unresectable at the time of surgical exploration. These also require some other modality of therapy in the hope of prolonging life and palliating their remaining days.

The final one-third of these patients will be candidates for resection. Depending upon the extent of the resection and the extension of the surgical maneuvers, as determined by the aggressiveness of the operator, the mortality and morbidity will, of course, vary. For average patients, a mortality rate of around 10 per cent for pneumonectomy and 2 to 3 per cent for lobectomy can be looked upon as acceptable in view of the fact that these individuals will be in the older age groups and may be suffering from other diseases. These figures also express the expected aggressiveness of conscientious operators when dealing with a situation such as bronchogenic carcinoma. Complications in the form of empyema need not be expected in more than 6 per cent of patients.

It is interesting to note that the fatalities from the neoplasm, as it has metastasized to distant organs, is greatest in the first six months following successful pulmonary resection, and the bulk of the patients who succumb to their disease will have done so by the end of 1.5 to two years. A few more will succumb belatedly up to the third or fourth year, after which the chances of recurrence of the neoplasm are materially reduced. Thus, a three-year survival rate is almost as satisfactory as the five-year survival rate. At the end of three to five years, it will be expected that some 20 to 25 per cent of the patients who had the benefit of surgical treatment will be alive and free of their disease.

It is, however, most discouraging to realize that this number represents something like 8 or 10 per cent of the original group of patients.

Adenoma. Into the literature on lung tumors, there has crept the designation of a benign epithelial tumor, namely, the bronchial adenoma. This is a misnomer, in that these lesions are locally invasive and some 10 per cent of them even capable of metastasizing to the regional lymph nodes. An occasional distant metastatic deposit is seen. These lesions can become lethal by obstructing the bronchus and by producing suppuration and abscess formation distal to the obstruction.

They are, therefore, basically malignant. They should not be placed in the broad category of bronchogenic carcinomas, however, because their prognosis for cure is much better.

Adenomas usually occur endobronchially, where they arise deep in the bronchial wall and often are polypoid, being covered by mucosa. They often project extrabronchially through the wall in the manner of an iceberg, which is why bronchoscopic removal usually fails to eradicate the tumor. Also, these neoplasms are prone to bleed and may do so profusely.

There are two general types of adenomas, the carcinoid and the cylindroma. Cylindromas are rare and prone to occur in the trachea, whereas the carcinoid is more common and usually appears in the bronchial tree. Together they account for 3 to 5 per cent of bronchial tumors.

They are recognized by their presenting symptoms, by the radiographic findings and, most importantly, by the bronchoscopic findings. They are rather characteristic in their appearance, and although biopsy is usually definitive, it is important to realize that it may carry some hazard from hemorrhage. Recognizing their presence and their characteristic tan or bluish hue will immediately indicate this possibility and some approach to management, other than endoscopic, is advisable in most instances.

Since they do not respond to any appreciable degree to roentgen therapy, excision remains the only suitable approach. Because of their unusual location in the main stems of the bronchial tree or trachea, their excision must be individualized. The portions of lung which have been diseased secondary to obstruction must be sacrificed. At times, however, they are so located in the bronchial tree that they have not compromised the distal lung, and local excisions with bronchial reconstruction can be done. Local excision is in the majority of instances adequate. The cylindromas have a greater tendency to recurrence, and wider excision seems to be required. This is often embarrassing because their frequent location in the lower trachea may preclude comfortable excisions.

Lymphoblastoma. Lymphoblastomas may appear as isolated lesions in a manner which would suggest primary pulmonary or hilar neoplasms and, therefore, mimic bronchogenic carcinoma. In the absence of any systemic manifestation which might permit the recognition of lymphomatous etiology for a pulmonary or hilar lesion, exploratory thoracotomy is required to establish the diagnosis.

Involvement of the pulmonary parenchyma is, of course, much less common than involvement of the hilar or mediastinal lymph nodes. Bilateral involvement of the hilum along with widening of the superior mediastinum is the characteristic picture. Scalene node biopsy may be diagnostic. Since the lung itself is so often uninvolved, the decision to use roentgenotherapy rather than resection seems wise. The results of roentgenotherapy in such lesions are probably as good as those of surgical excision, and the lung can be spared for use.

Sarcoma. Sarcomas appear in the lung most often as result of metastasis from a distant primary tumor. Primary sarcomas of the lung do occur, however, and are seen as fibrosarcomas and occasionally as leiomyosarcomas. These uncommon neoplasms tend to occur in younger people and cannot be distinguished by clinical methods from other neoplasms. They must be approached directly and are to be treated by resection. The meager experience with them does not permit firm statements with respect to prognosis.

Hamartoma. The hamartoma is a peculiar pulmonary lesion that may occasionally present itself in the bronchus as a chondromatous mass, but more often as a solitary nodule in peripheral location. This is a benign lesion made up of normal elements of the organ involved, but showing an abnormal arrangement. It cannot be accurately identified except by direct examination at thoracotomy. Local excision is adequate. The incidence in infants and children, however, is sufficiently low to raise the question as to when these lesions make their appearance. When they are present endobronchially, management must be individualized.

Metastatic neoplasms. The lung is the obvious depository for a variety of blood-borne neoplasms arising in other organs. Any solitary pulmonary nodule has the potential of being a metastasis from some other source, if a previous neoplasm has been known. If the primary tumor has been successfully treated, the pulmonary deposit may be the only remaining bit of neoplasm, and, therefore, justifies excision for complete rehabilitation of the patient. On the other hand, particularly, in males over 50 years of age, the appearance of a solitary peripheral nodule in a patient who has harbored a successfully treated neoplasm in the past need not lead to the conclusion that it is metastatic in nature. It may represent a second primary neoplasm and must be treated accordingly.

The result of surgical excision of solitary metastatic nodules is directly proportional to the care with which the patients are selected. These metastatic deposits can be managed by limited excision, there being little indication for extended surgical maneuvers to preclude extension from them as sources of daughter metastases.

Other benign tumors. Other tumors do occur in the lung and, particularly, in the bronchus itself. These include fibromas, lipomas and an occasional smooth muscle tumor.

MEDIASTINUM

ANATOMY. The mediastinum is that portion of the interior of the chest between the pleural sacs. It is bounded anteriorly by the sternum and posteriorly by the vertebral column. Within it lie many important structures having diseases peculiar unto themselves.

The most important concept of the mediastinum as a region has to do with its continuity to the neck above and retroperitoneal tissues and abdomen below. The prevertebral, visceral and pretracheal spaces of the neck extend directly into the mediastinum. Infections in the neck can migrate into the mediastinum and, conversely, air from the mediastinum, such as seen in mediastinal emphysema, can and does migrate into the neck. The naturally occurring hiati in the diaphragm to permit the passage of the esophagus, inferior vena cava and aorta provide direct communication with the tissues in the abdomen.

INFLAMMATION. The chronic inflammatory processes, although rare, are attributed generally to such granulomatous diseases as tuberculosis, histoplasmosis and syphilis, to radiation therapy, and possibly to trauma. These agents, no matter how they are carried to the mediastinum, produce a fibrous reaction of the tissues generally. It is presumed that in most instances of tuberculosis and histoplasmosis, the fibrosing mediastinitis is an extension from a similar infection in lymph nodes.

Obstruction of the superior vena cava is the common result of this process. This reduces drastically the return of blood from the upper extremities and head. Because the vena cava is the only direct channel for the return of this large volume of blood, it produces a characteristic appearance of suffusion and edema of the soft tissues with marked bloating and often cyanosis. The appearance is characteristic and can hardly be misinterpreted.

In nonneoplastic obstructions of the superior vena cava, the process may be gradual enough that time is provided for the development of collaterals which will by-pass the superior vena cava. If the obstruction is rapid, as when due to a neoplasm, time is generally not afforded for such collaterals to be established. Efforts at relieving superior vena caval obstruction have not met with great success.

If, however, in benign obstructions the patient can be kept alive until the collaterals have developed, the long term prognosis seems satisfactory. Obviously, if the etiology of the granulomatous process in its early phases can be recognized, appropriately directed treatment may avoid the late cicatrizing effects.

Acute inflammatory processes of the mediastinum can occur as extensions of infections from the neck or the upper abdomen. These sources, however, are much less common than perforations of the esophagus.

The esophagus can be perforated as a result of instrumentation, particularly esophagoscopy or at the time of dilatation of esophageal strictures. The commonest site for instrumental perforation is the upper end of the esophagus at the level of the inferior pharyngeal constrictor with its pinchcock mechanism. Notwithstanding this site of origin, the inflammatory process may find its way promptly into the mediastinum and the findings may even suggest perforation at a lower level.

Spontaneous perforations of the esophagus occur as a result of violent bouts of vomiting, particularly after a full meal. In either situation, the findings are those of a rather painful episode occurring deep in the chest, followed by varying degrees of prostration and shock. Air will generally be palpable in the neck shortly after the accident. Within a matter of hours, a mediastinal phlegmon will be well established. This will be heralded clinically by chills, fever and increasing prostration. Accompanying the air in the mediastinum, there often is a pneumothorax commonly on the left, particularly in the spontaneous perforations. Fluid can be expected to follow the air and an empyema may be well established in 12 to 24 hours.

If a high perforation is known to have occurred, immediate mediastinotomy by an incision along the anterior border of the sternocleidomastoid muscle, exposing the esophagus, locates the defect and permits prompt suture. The cervical mediastinum should be drained.

In the perforations that occur inferiorly, immediately on their recognition, and certainly, before the presence of established infection, a thoracotomy on the side of the pneumothorax or hydrothorax should be carried out, and the esophagus exposed. The mediastinal tissues are to be widely opened and the tear in the esophagus closed. The pleura is drained.

This approach should be insisted upon unless the presence of infection is so obvious that a procedure of this magnitude would be contraindicated. Under these circumstances, drainage of the empyema only is advocated. This may and often does result in an esophagopleural or esophagocutaneous fistula which may take many weeks or months to close. Most esophageal fistulae will ultimately close, but they may, on occasion, require surgical intervention.

The presence of an encapsulated, localized abscess in the mediastinum is probably the only indication for a direct approach through the posterior mediastinum. Under these circumstances, a vertical incision is made, centering over the abscess in the paravertebral area just at the lateral border of the erector spinae muscles. The posterior segments of one or two ribs immediately overlying the abscess are then resected subperiosteally behind the retracted erector spinae musculature. The pleura is then cautiously pushed away and the abscess cavity entered. Tube drainage is generally required.

NEOPLASM. The mediastinum is an area in which many embryologic derivatives are found in the adult organism, and consequently it is subject to a variety of neoplastic processes. Referring to the anatomic divisions of the mediastinum, we can, on the basis of a topographic classification, suggest the possible nature of various tumors.

In the posterior mediastinum, the most common tumor is one of neurogenic origin arising from some of the supporting elements of nerves, most often the intercostals (Fig. 22). In the middle mediastinum, which includes the hilum, tumors of lymphatic origin typically make their appearance (Fig. 23). In the inferior portion of this area, enteric cysts are to be found.

In the anterior mediastinum, tumors of thymic origin or those of teratomatous nature are commonest (Fig. 24). These include dermoid cysts as well as tri-layered teratomas. In the superior mediastinum, the commonest presenting mass is an intrathoracic goiter. In the cardiophrenic angles, pericardial cysts are probably the most common tumor. These, of course, must be differentiated from hernias through the foramen of Morgagni, among other less common possibilities.

Symptoms. Some tumors arising in the mediastinum may be accompanied by suggestive clinical symptoms. Tumors of the thyroid may produce thyrotoxicosis. The association of thymic tumors and myasthenia gravis is frequently alluded to and should be kept in mind when a mediastinal tumor and muscular weakness is encountered. Fibrous tumors of the mediastinum, often of large size, are being related to bouts of hypoglycemia and to chronic disease secondary thereto.

Except for these fairly well-recognized associations, mediastinal tumors generally do not produce symptoms. They are most often found by routine roentgen studies of the chest. They can produce symptoms, however, by their actual enlargement and by encroachment upon vital structures such as the esophagus or the trachea. Also, it is relatively unimportant whether a mediastinal tumor is malignant in the sense of being invasive or not, because it can kill by its bulk alone interfering with vital functions.

Certain misconceptions seem to have crept

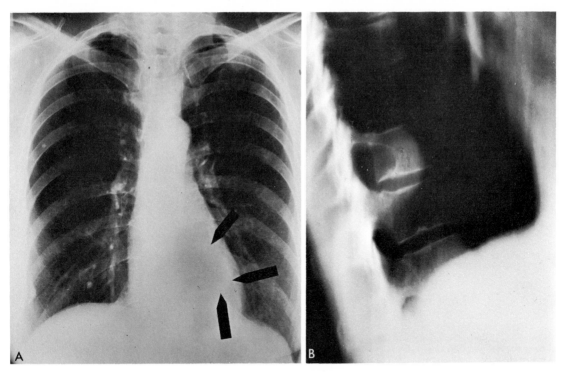

Figure 22. *A*, Posteroanterior chest film which is essentially normal. A posterior mediastinal tumor of neurogenic origin hides behind the heart shadow as indicated by the arrows. *B*, Lateral laminagram showing same posterior mediastinal tumor. The enlarged intervertebral foramen is a common finding in such neoplasms.

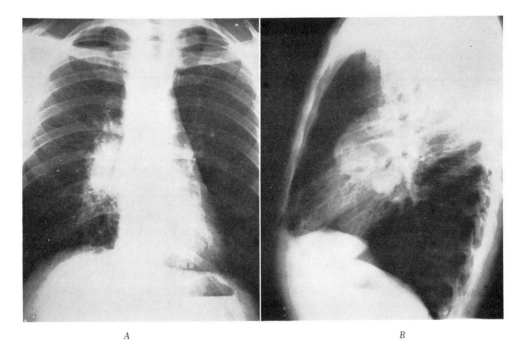

A   *B*

Figure 23. Posteroanterior (*A*) and lateral (*B*) roentgenograms showing a mass in the right hilum. A scalene node removed by a supraclavicular approach showed changes characteristic of Hodgkin's disease. It responded to treatment by nitrogen mustard and irradiation for a time.

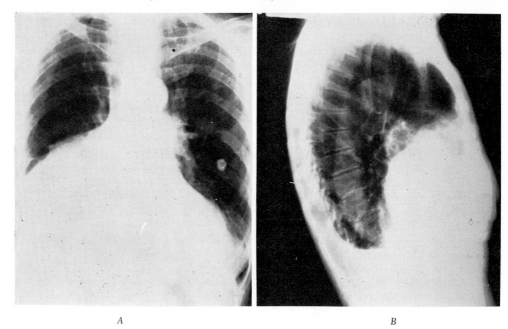

A   *B*

Figure 24. In these roentgenograms (*A*, posteroanterior and *B*, lateral), the large anterior mediastinal tumor is seen to blend with the heart shadow. Although somewhat lower than the typical situation, this lesion was thymic in origin. A calcified solitary "coin" lesion is seen in the left midlung field. It is typical of an ancient granuloma.

into the thinking concerning the mediastinum and the compression of the structures within it. For example, mediastinal emphysema does not kill per se. It is probably impossible to accumulate sufficient air in the mediastinum to obstruct the superior vena cava, or in particular, to compress the trachea or the great arterial trunks in adults. Before any such pressure could be built up in the mediastinum, the pleura should rupture and pneumothorax on one or both sides occur. This mechanism of tension pneumothorax with pulmonary compression is the likely cause of death in mediastinal emphysema. Thus, decompression and evacuation of the pleural air, and the control of the air leak at its source are the important considerations, because the presence of air in the mediastinum itself is of little consequence.

Also, it must be remembered that the mediastinal structures can be displaced greatly, if this displacement occurs relatively slowly, without interfering with their function. This is particularly noticeable in situations such as pulmonary tuberculosis where marked contracture will grossly distort the mediastinum, and its contained structures, yet there may be no evidence of malfunction.

Once a mass in the mediastinum is recognized, some clue as to its intimate nature may be had by its location. It is informative, however, to study the esophagus by radiographic examination. This will indicate any interference with this structure in the way of displacement or invasion. Likewise, a clear visualization of the trachea is in order and many of these lesions should be investigated by bronchoscopy.

Aneurysms must be thought of when considering masses within the mediastinum. This calls for careful fluoroscopy, but may ultimately necessitate the performance of angiocardiography or aortography in order to prove or disprove the presence of a vascular communication. This differential diagnosis may be vexing, but it is relatively important that it be established because if an aneurysm is to be managed at thoracotomy, necessary preparations should be made for support of the patient during this surgical maneuver. On the other hand, no such extended preparations need be made for the mediastinal tumor that is not vascular in origin.

Treatment. The treatment of mediastinal tumors is excisional except for those known to respond promptly and effectively to roentgen therapy, if positively identified. This comprises principally those of the lymphoma group.

More than one approach is available for access to the mediastinum. In lesions that occur in the anterior mediastinum and lie anterior to the great veins, a sternal splitting incision is possible and provides excellent exposure. For neoplasms deeper in the mediastinum that lie behind the great veins, this approach is awkward. For these, the best approach is a right or left lateral thoracotomy through the fourth rib bed or fourth interspace. This will generally provide ready access for the upper portion of the mediastinum. The lower portion of the mediastinum should be approached through a lower level thoracotomy. Most of the neoplasms that are not invasive can be removed by direct enucleation. Those that are invasive require the addition of surgical maneuvers which may compromise the lung, esophagus, pericardium or diaphragm.

Even though the thyroid gland may lie within the thorax, usually it can be removed through the conventional collar-type incision in the neck.

TRAUMA

FRACTURED RIBS. Due to their anatomic relationships, ribs require relatively little treatment when fractured. They usually are well aligned and, in fact, minor degrees of malalignment are of little clinical consequence.

Their principal significance, however, is that pain is repetitiously created at the fracture site by respiratory motion, and function is thereby interfered with. When a single rib is fractured, some degree of immobilization of that side is brought about by voluntary splinting of the chest. This can be enhanced by the use of adhesive strapping. The strapping should not be circumferential to include the opposite side, but some reduction in the motion of the chest by such mechanical means aids voluntary splinting.

If more than one rib is fractured, the degree of discomfort and disability is proportionally increased, and may require an intercostal nerve block in order to interrupt the pain pathways and provide relief. The judicious use of sedatives and narcotics is indicated.

If multiple ribs are fractured in more than one place, there will be a portion of the chest wall which will be flail.

Flail chest is an injury frequently seen in highway accidents. Since the flail area is functionally detached from the rib cage, this portion of the chest wall tends to be displaced inward when the rest of the rib cage is pulled outward in inspiration. The reverse motion occurs when expiration lowers the general level of the rib cage, and the underlying lung forces this flail portion upward. This process is referred to as paradoxical respiration. If the amount of paradoxical respiration and the area involved is small, it can be compensated for by the patient himself. If, however, it is large, a certain degree of rebreathing will occur by exchange of air between the flail segment and adjacent portions of lung, if not to the opposite lung as well.

In any event, this inefficient respiration leads to the production of hypercarbia and hypoxia with increased demand for respiratory effort, which in turn increases the amount of paradoxical motion and the effort of breathing.

Strangely enough, these people often arrive in the emergency department in what appears to be relatively good condition. Thirty to 45 minutes later they may suddenly deteriorate, with marked paradoxical respiration, cyanosis, noisy breathing and a general appearance that is frightening. It would seem that they have been able, in the earlier period immediately following the accident, to splint the side rendered flail, yet still maintain their respiratory requirements. However, this is done on a very marginal basis, and as time goes on, hypercarbia and hypoxia develop to a point such that the respiratory drive will overcome their ability to splint the affected side and they will no longer be able to restrict motion, but must abandon these efforts in favor of increased respiratory excursion. This leads them to the rapid deterioration that is often seen.

The treatment for a flail chest wall is directed at the chest wall itself in an attempt to immobilize it and prevent the repetitive and paradoxical motion. It is further directed at the complications of this situation which involve principally the lung and its ventilatory functions.

The methods by which the chest wall may be immobilized include simple support by sand bags or pressure dressings. If these are inadequate, some form of traction may be applied to the chest wall. This may be obtained by means of inserting towel clips around the ribs or into the margins of the sternum and connecting them to appropriately balanced traction. If the anterolateral portions of the chest wall are affected, Steinmann pins or Kirschner wires can be passed through the mass of the pectoral muscles and these connected to balanced traction.

During the period in which immobilization is being effected, one must not neglect to treat other injuries. A chest film should be obtained as soon after admission as possible in order to determine the presence or absence of pneumothorax, hemothorax or other internal derangements. If pneumothorax is present, and extensive paradoxical motion is anticipated or present, it is imperative that immediate decompression of the pneumothorax by intercostal catheter be carried out. This is particularly important if the degree of paradoxical motion is such that it cannot be satisfactorily controlled, short of placing the patient on a respirator or intubating him under anesthesia, and having his respiratory mechanics taken over by the anesthetist as an emergency procedure. It is obvious that in the presence of a torn lung with pneumothorax, positive endobronchial pressure provided by the anesthetist or a respirator will increase the pneumothorax and compress the lung with the further additional penalty of accentuated hypercarbia and hypoxia.

The performance of a tracheostomy is required in the severely injured, not only as a means through which the bronchial secretions can be aspirated and tracheobronchial toilet maintained, but also because in bypassing the upper portion of the respiratory tract, some reduction in the ventilatory dead space is achieved and some reduction in the amount of paradoxical motion can be expected.

The ultimate approach to controlling the paradoxical respiration is to render the patient apneic and maintain respiration by mechanical means. If this is done with a high flow respirator such as a piston respirator of the Moerch type, an uncuffed tracheostomy is used. If, on the other hand, a tight-fitting circuit is required, as would be the case with a respirator of the Bennett or Bird type, a cuffed tracheostomy should be used. An endotracheal tube can be utilized for 24 to 36 hours in lieu of a tracheostomy.

Pain is a great factor influencing the outcome in these severely injured individuals. This can be controlled by one of several means. Placing the patient in bed in such a fashion that paradoxical motion is reduced

may bring about considerable stability, as well as relief from acute pain. The use of narcotics is in order, but since they tend to depress respiration, reduce the effectiveness of cough and dull the stimulating effect of accumulating bronchial secretions on the cough mechanism, they should be used sparingly and judiciously.

The most important method of controlling pain is intercostal nerve block. This is done in the paravertebral area just lateral to the mass of the paraspinal muscles, where the ribs first become superficial and palpable. Two segments above the area of the involved chest wall and two below is requisite to obtain suitable relief. Two or 3 cc. of an appropriate local anesthetic solution is injected immediately under the rib into the intercostal nerve area of each segment.

Whereas this maneuver will obviously interrupt the nervous pathways mediating pain sensation, it perhaps has an additional function in that, by so doing, it will improve ventilation, mobilize bronchial secretions and aid in effectiveness of cough.

It is also quite likely that the presence of extensive chest wall trauma reflects itself in some degree of bronchorrhea and bronchospasm. Interrupting these reflex pathways may reduce the amount of bronchial secretions present and improve the airway by relieving bronchospasm. Often the result of intercostal nerve block under these circumstances is dramatic.

The process can be repeated as required; usually, the effect will be more lasting after a second or third intercostal block has been carried out.

One must always be mindful of the fact that in these severely injured individuals other lesions may have to be taken into account and treated concomitantly.

PENETRATING WOUNDS. A sucking wound is simply a wound which has involved all layers of the chest wall down to and including the pleura. The soft tissues, therefore, permit the ingress or egress of air between the outside and the pleural space on respiration. It is obvious that this is a serious situation and it is necessary to stop this flow of air to and from the pleura, with its accompanying pneumothorax and consequent lung collapse. To this end, an occlusive dressing is applied over the area of the wound as an emergency measure. This is to be applied at the end of a deep expiratory effort. The wound must be appropriately debrided and ultimately closed.

When the pleura has been injured in such a way that air is allowed to enter it, the amount of pulmonary collapse will be commensurate with and proportionate to the amount of air that has been allowed to enter the pleural space. If the source of this air leak is the lung, and particularly, if air enters the pleural cavity in greater increments than can return through the pulmonary defect, mounting tension occurs. This results in progressive collapse of the lung and displacement of the mediastinum to the opposite side, producing serious embarrassment to respiratory function. This situation must be relieved promptly by adequate decompression.

When such excesses of air occur, the air may well enter the fascial planes of the chest wall and result in extensive subcutaneous emphysema. If the amount of pneumothorax is extensive, particularly if it is bilateral and cannot be controlled by the utilization of one or possibly two large-caliber intercostal catheters supplemented by suction, the presumption is that the tear in the airway is large, possibly even in the trachea or the main stem bronchi, and immediate thoracotomy is indicated. This situation is critical and generally not compatible with life, unless corrected surgically, even though several instances of such survivals are recorded. Even if survival should occur, the rupture in the bronchus, for example, and for that matter, in the trachea, may well stenose and provide a subsequent problem which could have been circumvented by immediate repair of the defect.

Blood which appears in the pleura from a penetrating wound, be it a stab wound or a bullet wound, generally comes from a vessel in the chest wall. It is possible for the lung to bleed seriously, but it is most unlikely unless a hilar vessel has been injured, and under these circumstances, the symptoms are those of gross hemorrhage and not simply moderate hemothorax.

Blood spilled into the pleura is an irritant, and in consequence there is outpouring of pleural fluid. The nature of this effusion varies, depending, probably, upon the amount of bacterial contamination and the degree of lung trauma. If this effusion is serous, it merely dilutes the blood that is present and this will ultimately be absorbed or can be aspirated.

On the other hand, if this effusion is changed in character, it will become exudative in type and richer in fibrin. This deposition of fibrin over the lung will, by subsequent organization, form a coat which will restrain expansion of the lung and entrap it. Aspiration of the more fluid content of such a hemothorax will not change the ultimate situation. Proteolytic enzymes used at this time, when the fibrin has begun its organization, are generally incapable of reversing the process and permitting the lung to expand even though they are entirely capable of lysing unorganized fibrinous masses.

Under these circumstances, and if the process is of sufficient extent and severity, decortication should be carried out in order to free the lung and permit it to fill the chest. Otherwise, serious impairment of ventilation may occur. The appropriate time for the decision for decortication in patients not grossly infected is somewhere between the third and sixth week, at which time the pleural peel is thick enough to be technically handled with accuracy and ease, yet not so dense as to make decortication difficult or incomplete.

Wounds of the lung generally require little or no attention because this organ has remarkable recuperative powers. Lacerations of superficial lung parenchyma will seal themselves off with complete healing. Sealing of air leaks will also occur.

Wounds of the lung which are deep enough to involve the hilum are uncommon and are to be managed according to their particular requirements.

The indications for pulmonary resection as result of trauma are very uncommon if they ever occur.

Foreign bodies retained within the pleural cavity or particularly in the lung, should be removed if they are more than 1.0 to 1.5 cm. in size. These need not be used as an indication for prompt thoracotomy, however. They are, in fact, best treated after the injured lung has had an opportunity to cleanse itself and become fully aerated. The complications of retained foreign bodies in the lung manifest themselves by suppuration or hemoptysis, usually within the first few years following their deposition in the organ. If such has not supervened within this time, the likelihood of delayed trouble is not very great.

GENERAL MANAGEMENT OF TRAUMATIC WOUNDS. The treatment of thoracic trauma is basically conservative. There are, however, certain circumstances which call for immediate action and have been generally agreed upon as the indications for prompt thoracotomy or, at times, laparotomy when penetrating or perforating wounds of the chest have occurred.

Continued intrapleural bleeding that is not controlled by the debridement of the chest wall wound is one indication. The establishment of the diagnosis of continued intrapleural hemorrhage is not based solely upon fluid accumulations within the hemithorax, because a small amount of blood may be followed in 12 to 24 hours by a diluting pleural effusion. Thus, a mere increase in amount of pleural fluid does not necessarily mean further bleeding. The reaccumulating fluid must be whole blood. Determination of hemoglobin and hematocrit on pleural blood may assist in this decision.

On the other hand, if it is suspected that a large vessel may be the cause for the initial blood seen in the pleura, it is best to open the chest and assure oneself that the bleeding vessel is either secured or that it has not, in fact, been injured, because wounds to such structures as the superior vena cava or the innominate or subclavian vessels, particularly the veins, may be quite deceptive. These wounds are quite manageable if promptly treated.

Air leak that cannot be controlled adequately by appropriate decompression is another indication for surgical intervention.

Wounds of the posterior mediastinum which involve or may involve the esophagus are also indications.

Injuries which involve the diaphragm are indications for surgical treatment. If the right side is involved, the abdominal wound is in all likelihood in the dome of the liver. These are prone to bleed severely and recurrently. The leakage of bile is likewise serious. They are best approached by thoracotomy, opening the diaphragm to control the problem in the liver, then re-establishing the identity of the two coelomic cavities by repairing the diaphragmatic wound and providing for wide drainage of the subdiaphragmatic space. The pleura should be drained to get rid of blood and air, and to ensure prompt pulmonary re-expansion. Injury to the lung is usually not very significant.

On the left side, the spleen, stomach or colon may be involved. The approach can be made from above through a thoracolaparot-omy or through separate thoracotomy and laparotomy. In some hands, the preference would be for a laparotomy rather than a thoracotomy. In the presence of an open wound in the diaphragm, once a laparotomy has been performed and the peritoneal cavity entered, a sucking wound of the chest is immediately possible. Also, it is important to realize that in wounds, such as of the stomach, it is possible that gastric content may be present within the pleural cavity, having been sucked there by the negative pressure existing at the time of the perforation. It is also of interest that through a thoracotomy on the left side or a thoraco-laparotomy, excellent access is had not only to the spleen but also the kidney. The stomach can be approached quite satisfactorily.

If injury to small bowel or colon is found, it is preferable to separate the chest from the abdomen and manage the intestinal problems through a separate laparotomy after dealing with the thoracic problem. It is the probability of perforation of a hollow viscus or of injury to the spleen that demands exploration of these individuals, and there is, obviously, a choice as to the method by which this is carried out.

READING REFERENCES

Adams, W. E.: Preoperative evaluation of pulmonary function. *In*, Gibbon, J. H., Jr. (ed.): Surgery of the Chest. Philadelphia, W. B. Saunders Company, 1962.

Avery, E. B., Morch, E. T., and Benson, D. W.: Critically crushed chests. J. Thorac. Surg. 32:291, 1956.

Ballinger, W. F., II: The thoracic wall. *In*, Gibbon, J. H., Jr. (ed.): Surgery of the Chest. Philadelphia, W. B. Saunders Company, 1962.

Barker, W. L., Neuhaus, H., and Langston, H. T.: Ventilatory improvement following decortication in pulmonary tuberculosis. Ann. Thorac. Surg. 1:532, 1965.

Bloedorn, F. G., and Cowley, R. A.: Irradiation and surgery in the treatment of bronchogenic carcinoma. Surg. Gyn. & Obst. 111:141, 1960.

Comroe, J. H., Jr., Forster, R. E., II, Dubois, A. B., Birscoe, W. A., and Carlsen, E.: The Lung—Clinical Physiology and Pulmonary Function Tests. 2nd ed. Chicago, Year Book Publishers, Inc., 1962.

Faber, L. P., Kaiser, G. D., and Langston, H. T.: Preresection radiation for bronchogenic carcinoma. J. Thorac. & Cardiovasc. Surg. 46:227, 1963.

Galofre, M., Payne, W. S., Woolner, L. B., Clagett, O. T., and Gage, R. P.: Pathologic classification and surgical treatment of bronchogenic carcinoma. Surg. Gyn. & Obst. 119:51, 1964.

Gibbon, J. H., Jr., and Nealon, T. F., Jr.: Neoplasms of the lungs and trachea. *In*, Gibbon, J. H., Jr. (Ed.): Surgery of the Chest. Philadelphia, W. B. Saunders Company, 1962.

Godwin, M. C.: Diffuse mesotheliomas with comment on their relation to localized fibrous mesotheliomas. Cancer 10:298, 1957.

Haight, C.: Intratracheal suction in the management of

postoperative pulmonary complications. Ann. Surg. *107*:218, 1938.

Johnson, J., and Kirby, C. K.: Surgery of the Chest. 2nd ed. Chicago, Year Book Publishers, Inc., 1961.

Kent, E. M., and Magovern, G. J.: The mediastinum. *In*, Blades, B. (Ed.): Surgical Diseases of the Chest. 2nd ed. St. Louis, C. V. Mosby Company, 1966.

Kergin, F. G.: An operation for chronic pleural empyema. J. Thorac. Surg. *26*:430, 1953.

Langston, H. T.: Benign endobronchial tumors—a collective review. Surg. Gyn. & Obst. *91*:521, 1950.

Langston, H. T.: Editorial. Etiology by Edict. J. Thorac. & Cardiovasc. Surg. *51*:459, 1966.

Langston, H. T., Barker, W. L., and Pyle, M. M.: Surgery in pulmonary tuberculosis—11 year review of indications and results. Ann. Surg. *164*:567, 1966.

Langston, H. T., and Tuttle, W. M.: Pleuropulmonary tuberculosis. *In*, Blades, B. (ed.): Surgical Diseases of the Chest. 2nd ed. St. Louis, C. V. Mosby Company, 1966.

Maier, H. C.: The pleura. *In*, Gibbon, J. H., Jr. (ed.): Surgery of the Chest. Philadelphia, W. B. Saunders Company, 1962.

Maloney, J. V., Jr., Schmutzer, K. J., and Rashchke, E.: Paradoxical respiration and "pendeluft." J. Thorac. & Cardiovasc. Surg. *41*:291, 1961.

Meade, R. H.: A History of Thoracic Surgery. Springfield, Ill., Charles C Thomas, 1961, Chapters 1 through 8.

Nealon, T. F., Jr.: Trauma to the chest. *In*, Gibbon, J. H., Jr. (ed.): Surgery of the Chest. Philadelphia, W. B. Saunders Company, 1962.

Pascuzzi, C. A., Dahlin, D. C., and Clagett, O. T.: Primary tumors of ribs and sternum. Surg. Gyn. & Obst. *104*: 390, 1957.

Ravitch, M. M.: Operation for correction of pectus excavatum. Surg. Gyn. & Obst. *106*:619, 1958.

Rigdon, R. H., and Kirchoff, H.: Cancer of the lung 1930–1960—a review. Texas Rep. Biol. & Med. *19*:465, 1961.

Sarot, I. A.: Extrapleural pneumonectomy and pleurectomy in pulmonary tuberculosis. Thorax *4*:173, 1949.

Shaw, R. R., Paulson, D. L., and Kee, J. L., Jr.: The Treatment of Bronchial Neoplasms. John Alexander Monograph Series, III. Springfield, Ill., Charles C Thomas, 1959.

Smoking and Health. A Report of the Advisory Committee to the Surgeon General of the Public Health Service. Washington, D.C., U.S. Department of Health, Education and Welfare, Public Health Service Publication 1103, 1964.

Steele, J. D.: The Solitary Pulmonary Nodule. Publication 6, The John Alexander Monograph Series. Springfield, Ill., Charles C Thomas, 1964.

Chapter 20

THE HEART AND GREAT VESSELS

by
NORMAN E. SHUMWAY, M.D.

NORMAN SHUMWAY was born in Kalamazoo, Michigan, but grew up and attended high school in Jackson, Michigan, where his father operated a dairy store. His education at the University of Michigan was interrupted by military service and was resumed at Baylor University. He is a graduate in medicine from Vanderbilt University and was a postdoctoral research fellow of the National Heart Institute at the University of Minnesota. He has pursued his interest in cardiac surgery uninterruptedly. He is Professor of Surgery, Stanford University, and Chief, Division of Cardiovascular Surgery.

Within the last ten years heart surgery has evolved as a separate division of general surgery. In fact today cardiac surgery is as much a speciality as neurological surgery. In addition to important contributions by surgeons, physiologists and biologists have done much to advance the field of cardiac surgery. The impact of successful cardio-pulmonary bypass is evident from the fact that the number of open heart procedures far exceeds those operations which can be done without the artificial heart-lung unit. Extracorporeal circulation was achieved with considerable help from scientists, biologists and engineers who are currently at work on the problems of heart replacement. The specialty of heart surgery has become so intensified that even the close alliance of thoracic and cardiovascular surgery is in danger of abrogation.

CLOSED HEART PROCEDURES

CORRECTIVE OPERATIONS

PATENT DUCTUS ARTERIOSUS. The operation for division and suture of the patent ductus arteriosus is among the half dozen or so really pure surgical procedures. The condition is definitively treated, it can never recur and patients almost always do spectacularly well. Surgical intervention may be urged for every patent ductus arteriosus with a net left-to-right ductus flow regardless of the degree of pulmonary hypertension or vascular resistance. Operation is advised for the small ductus to prevent bacterial endocarditis and to erase the stigmata of any heart disease. Heart failure and pulmonary arteriolar changes are compelling reasons to operate on the large ductus. Serial postoperative heart catheterization studies indicate that changes in pulmonary vascular resistance are reversible, and in certain patients, early operation alone can prevent progression of these changes to the point that ductus flow becomes right-to-left.

Perhaps 90 per cent of the lesions can be diagnosed by the typical machinery murmur with help from the chest x-ray and electrocardiogram. Only patent ductus arteriosus or aortic septal defect produces enlargement of the aorta with biventricular hypertrophy. In infants and children with pulmonary hypertension, the murmur may be detectable only during systole. In adults with pulmonary hypertension and massive dilatation of the pulmonic valvular annulus, the murmur may be confined entirely to diastole, the murmur of pulmonic valvular insufficiency. Heart catheterization is recommended in the atypical patient, and cineangiocardiography may be essential to exclude aortic septal defect which can mimic the atypical ductus in children.

The ductus is a frequent extra anomaly in patients with coarctation of the aorta or ventricular septal defect. This latter combination is so frequently present that every infant with a primary diagnosis of ventricular septal defect and pulmonary hypertension should be carefully studied for a concomitant patent ductus. The use of cardiopulmonary bypass can be lethal in the presence of an unsuspected patent ductus arteriosus. Fortunately, intrapericardial ligation is feasible via midline sternotomy so the staged operative procedure is not obligatory (Fig. 1).

It is our practice to dissect routinely the distal aortic arch before the ductus is clamped. With twill tapes around the aorta above and below the ductus, more ductus length can be made available at the time two Potts clamps are applied for its division. In the case of a huge ductus with essentially balanced pressures, the aorta can be occluded proximal and distal to the ductus with a single Potts coarctation clamp across the ductus. A few degrees of general hypothermia will protect the spinal cord and abdominal viscera for the ten minutes or so needed to suture the aorta at right angles to the pulmonary artery closure. The pericardium is usually widely opened to facilitate dissection of the huge ductus, and the judicious administration of trimethaphan camphorsulfonate (Arfonad) to effect controlled hypotension can be helpful.

COARCTATION OF THE AORTA. For many years coarctation of the aorta was subdivided into adult and infantile types. Because the condition is congenital, such an arbitrary grouping seems unwarranted. In children and adults, the anomaly is readily diagnosed by the combination of upper extremity hypertension and diminished or absent lower extremity pulses. Infants present more of a problem, especially if the ductus is patent. Cine studies are important, and in fact some kind of aortography should be performed before every operative procedure for coarctation. When operations are necessary in in-

fants because of unrelenting heart failure, one may be certain that there is a problem of greater intensity than the coarctation. Endocardial fibroelastosis, ventricular septal defect, aortic valvular or subvalvular stenosis and patent ductus arteriosus are seen commonly in association with coarctation of the aorta in the very sick infant. Excision and repair of the coarctation may be lifesaving, particularly if the anomaly is complicated by the presence of a patent ductus arteriosus. Severe hypertension in the infant constitutes another indication for repair. Several infants have been operated upon because of previous intracerebral bleeding.

Electively, the coarctation should be excised with end-to-end anastomosis around age ten to 12 years. In adults, mobility of the aorta may be so restricted that the use of a Dacron or Teflon graft is required. Only rarely should it be advisable to utilize the left subclavian artery to restore aortic continuity. Similarly, an onlay patch graft is seldom indicated. Wide and careful dissection of the aortic arch and descending aorta is essential to the operation. Abbott's artery must be approached gingerly, but it is almost always present.

Much has been written with respect to interrupted versus continuous anastomotic suture lines. Those without definite prejudices run the posterior row and interrupt the anterior. Time is often at such a premium in infants that the continuous method can be the sine qua non for survival. Mere retraction of the left lung is often poorly tolerated.

VASCULAR RINGS. Vascular rings in general fall into two kinds of malformation: double aortic arch, and aberrant right subclavian artery. In the true double arch, symptoms depend on compression of both trachea and esophagus, whereas in aberrant origin of the subclavian artery esophageal symptoms alone are encountered. The anatomic complex of a right arch and left ligamentum arteriosum also can produce dysphagia.

Surgical treatment is very satisfactory with relief of symptoms occurring almost immediately. Left thoracotomy is routinely used with division of the smaller of the two arches or of the anomalous subclavian artery as it develops from the aorta enroute posterior to the esophagus. The procedure frequently must be done as an emergency during infancy, but the dissection takes little time

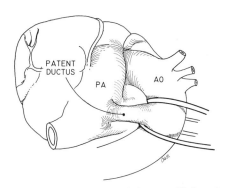

Figure 1. The aorta is looped above and below the patent ductus to achieve control of the high pressure side of the ductus and to facilitate application of the clamps.

and the operation is usually well tolerated. The heart, of course, is normal. In the presence of coarctation, subclavian steal can occur with blood flow from the affected arm to distal aorta.

CONSTRICTIVE PERICARDITIS. At one time in the history of this fascinating disease, most of the world's experience came from tuberculous involvement of the pericardium. Now, the disease is seen most frequently in young adults as the result of viral infection. Concerning its surgical relief long and heated debate once raged between advocates of left ventricular liberation and those who favored freeing the right ventricle, right atrium and venae cavae. Clearly, compromise of left ventricular function is the critical factor, and no one has ever demonstrated a gradient at the atriocaval junctions.

There are few instances when the surgical incision per se can be said to exert paramount importance, but this disease is best treated by a specific approach. The plan of liberation must proceed from left atrium to left ventricle to right ventricle and, finally, right atrium in that order. Anterior approaches are not satisfactory. A long lateral thoracotomy with removal of the fifth rib and costal cartilage gives excellent exposure even for removal of the right ventricular and right atrial peel. Pockets of old hematoma turned to milky liquid are sometimes encountered in the pericardial strata. It must be perfectly clear that the visceral or epicardial pericardial layer is the constricting force, and such simple procedures as pericardial window are to no avail. The operation is somewhat tedious, but results are generally good.

A new cause of constrictive pericarditis has been noted in patients having high voltage irradiation for tumors of the mediastinum. Post-irradiation constrictive pericarditis is a real clinical entity. In constrictive pericarditis, the question always arises concerning the degree of myocardial involvement, but this component can never be satisfactorily evaluated until the heart is divested of its constricting peel. Patients with constrictive pericarditis submitted to operative intervention are given digitalis preoperatively, but varying degrees of cardiac failure and dilatation are often encountered.

PALLIATIVE OPERATIONS

SYSTEMIC–PULMONARY ARTERY SHUNTS. The Blalock-Taussig operation inaugurated the surgical treatment of patients with cyanotic heart disease. Infants with severe grades of tetralogy of Fallot including pulmonic valvular atresia benefit greatly from the subclavian–pulmonary artery anastomosis which is constructed on the side opposite to that of the aortic arch. There is less angulation if the subclavian artery is turned down from the innominate branch rather than directly from the aorta. The anastomosis must be made proximal to the takeoff of the internal mammary and vertebral arteries. Results are good and young patients can be well palliated until age four to eight years when the corrective operation is more easily done. Development of the left ventricle occurs secondary to the increased blood flow from the lungs, and the left heart is perhaps, therefore, better prepared to pump the entire systemic output after total correction.

The first modification of the Blalock operation was suggested by Potts who made a side-to-side anastomosis of the descending thoracic aorta to the left pulmonary artery. Although the procedure was appropriate for the tiny anatomy of the young infant, later takedown prior to full correction of the tetrad often proved catastrophic. When the Potts anastomosis was performed in older patients, the tendency often was to produce a large shunt which later converted the problem into that of too much pulmonary flow resulting in high pulmonary arteriolar resistance. Fallot's anomaly quite literally could be transformed into an Eisenmenger complex through injudicious application of the Potts technique. Today, few indications exist to justify any descending aortic–pulmonary artery anastomosis. Recently, Edwards borrowed a principle used by Blalock and Hanlon in their brilliant method for producing an atrial septal defect in patients with transposition of the great vessels. Edwards applied this idea to the construction of a side-to-side suture union of the ascending aorta and right pulmonary artery within the pericardial cavity. A small right angle noncrushing clamp is used to side-bite the aorta, simultaneously including the right pulmonary artery as it originates from the main pulmonary artery. This ingenious operation has the advantage of application to the smallest infant without prejudicing against a good result with later open correction. Patients with valve atresia and a small main pulmonary artery must be submitted to this procedure as soon as the ductus closes.

In summary, the Blalock-Taussig operation

is preferred in the patient six months to three years old with tetralogy of Fallot who is deeply cyanotic, subject to episodes of loss of consciousness and failing to gain weight. For the symptomatic patient less than six months old, a side-to-side ascending aortic–right pulmonary artery anastomosis is available. The Potts operation should be used only as an alternative procedure. Appropriately in England, some enthusiasm remains for the Brock operation, transventricular pulmonary valvotomy or infundibulectomy. Uneven results from open correction of the tetralogy of Fallot in Europe leave room for the Brock operation, and in the United States some clinics curiously prefer closed operations for pulmonic valvular stenoses. From this latter fact, the inference must be drawn that either bypass techniques are dangerous or it is better not to see the lesions.

BLALOCK-HANLON OPERATION FOR TRANSPOSITION OF THE GREAT VESSELS. The vast majority of patients with transposition of the great vessels die in the first few months of life. Accordingly, a great need was met with the development of the Blalock-Hanlon method for making an atrial septal defect. Nothing can be done for the patient with transposition who already has severe pulmonary vascular changes and a large septal defect of either ventricular or atrial type. Pulmonary banding offers little because the vascular changes seem to progress irrespective of flow diminution. Creation of an atrial septal defect can yield relatively brilliant results in the infant who has two separate circulations and only a patent foramen ovale and perhaps a ductus which is becoming occluded. Occasionally, inflow occlusion with open cardiotomy is necessary to achieve atrial septecomy, but application of a side-biting clamp in such a way as to occlude a sleeve of right atrium and the right pulmonary veins is usually possible and readily accomplished with a lateral thoracotomy through the bed of the fourth rib. In effect, the right pulmonary veins are transplanted above the level of the atrial septum, and a good section of atrial septum is removed. Intra-atrial mixing of arterial and venous blood is thereby promoted, and the patient can be prepared for the corrective procedure at age three to six years. Operative mortality with intensified management such as prolonged tracheal intubation and automatic respiration depends almost entirely on so-called irreversible pulmonary arteriolar changes. Dissection and ligation of the ductus arteriosus can be done from the right thoracotomy and should be routine if plain films of the chest reveal pulmonary overcirculation. Even cineradiography cannot rule out a patent ductus in every patient. Whereas a small patent ductus arteriosus could be beneficial, the large shunt is destructive, and mixing is better located at the atrial level.

PULMONARY ARTERY BANDING. Infants with large left-to-right intracardiac shunts are candidates for pulmonary artery banding. The theory behind this effective palliative operation is that a decreased pulmonary artery cross-sectional area increases right ventricular pressure with a consequent reduction in shunt flow from left-to-right. Whereas some infants with endocardial cushion anomalies and a few infants with transposition of the great vessels may benefit from this procedure, its best application is to tiny infants with ventricular septal defects and low pulmonary vascular resistance. These patients are dying of torrential pulmonary blood flow with secondary heart failure. Banding of the pulmonary artery is easily done with umbilical tape by a small anterolateral incision through the third intercostal space. The pulmonary artery pressure and wave form are monitored as the band is tightened, and a final right ventricular pressure is taken before closing the chest. In addition to gratifying immediate results, pulmonary artery banding is easy to correct at the later definitive operation for ventricular septal defect. Simple longitudinal incision and transverse closure usually suffice, although a pericardial patch may be necessary. Intraventricular bands do not develop in anything like their expected profusion. Little tailoring of the right ventricular corridor is required in the average patient.

MYOCARDIAL REVASCULARIZATION. It is a long jump from the kind of palliation attainable with pulmonary artery banding to that which accrues from the Vineberg–Glover–Beck category of procedures. Despite almost fanatic support for the Vineberg operation, some question must remain concerning its role in the therapy of coronary artery disease. No history of operative surgery is less distinguished than that dealing with myocardial revascularization. The nagging suspicion persists that the Vineberg procedure is akin to internal mammary ligation of ten years ago. Because the clinical condition essentially precludes any control study, it is difficult to assess indirect methods of enhancing myocardial blood flow. Little imagination is needed to visualize any number of aortic-myocardial shunts and tunnels. Some of these are anterior, posterior and even acupuncture into the left ventricle; the approaches are many and obvious. What remains obscure is solid evidence to the effect that the deprived myocardium is truly revascularized. Even the occasional cinearteriogram demonstrating internal mammary coronary artery anastomoses does not provide incontrovertible evidence.

Fortunately, direct coronary artery surgery is becoming more frequent, and some hope exists that this area of cardiac surgery will shed its alchemistic overtones.

SUPERIOR VENA CAVA–PULMONARY ARTERY ANASTOMOSIS; TRICUSPID ATRESIA. Although anastomosis of the superior vena cava to the right pulmonary artery has been performed for a variety of patients with cyanotic heart disease, the so-called Glenn operation is best reserved for patients with tricuspid atresia. The operation is somewhat difficult owing to the tremendous disparity in size between the small pulmonary artery and the large superior vena cava, and during infancy this problem is often insuperable. Moreover, the anastomosis is particularly susceptible to thrombosis because of the low velocity blood flow and the usual elevation in hematocrit. The Glenn operation is particularly ill-advised in patients with tetralogy of Fallot because it adds greatly to the problem of a later corrective operation. When the disparity between superior vena cava and pulmonary artery is too great, a systemic artery–pulmonary artery anastomosis should be made for patients with tricuspid atresia. One possible objection to the Glenn operation in patients with tricuspid atresia lies in the fact that ultimate total correction may depend on homotransplantation of the heart. The Glenn operation would make cardiac transplantation more involved owing to interruption of the superior vena cava and pulmonary artery continuity.

OPEN HEART SURGERY

OPERATIONS PERFORMED WITHOUT ELECTIVE CARDIAC ARREST

ATRIAL SEPTAL DEFECT. The most common form of congenital heart disease appearing for surgical correction is atrial septal defect. Rarely, patients with atrial septal defect uncomplicated by other anomalies come to the attention of physicians early in life. The usual presentation of a patient with atrial septal defect, however, is during school physical examinations, service induction examinations or after the onset of important cardiac arrhythmias, usually in the third to fifth decades of life.

The first successful open heart operation of any kind was repair of an atrial septal defect under hypothermia. Although general hypothermia is still utilized in some clinics, certainly extracorporeal circulation is the modality of access most commonly used.

Defects of the atrial septum may be divided conveniently into two principal types, septum secundum defects and sinus venosus defects. Sinus venosus defects are high in the atrial septum and are almost always accompanied by anomalous pulmonary venous drainage. The pulmonary veins may enter the superior vena cava several centimeters proximal to the atriocaval junction. There is a significant incidence of left superior vena cava with this anatomic complex, and it may be convenient to utilize the right superior vena cava as a conduit for rerouting the anomalous pulmonary venous drainage through the defect into the left atrium. In such a patient, the venous pressure of the upper extremity should be monitored during ligation of the right superior vena cava. It should be ascertained that the left superior vena cava empties into the coronary sinus as it usually does. Anomalous pulmonary veins can be associated with secundum atrial septal defects, and the correction is easily carried out by interposition of the atrial septum. An interesting variant of anomalous pulmonary venous drainage in secundum atrial septal defects is the scimitar deformity, in which the anomalous pulmonary veins enter the inferior vena cava. Correction of this anomaly depends upon partitioning the inferior vena cava, usually with pericardium, in such a way that the anomalous pulmonary veins drain through the atrial septal defect and into the appropriate atrium (Fig. 2).

The mortality involved in the early postoperative period after repair of an atrial septal defect should be negligible. The risk of hepatitis from blood transfusion, approximately 1 per cent in our experience, is greater than the risk of the operative procedure. Some patients will have severe pulmonary hypertension, and in this group tracheostomy is well advised.

ENDOCARDIAL CUSHION ANOMALIES. One

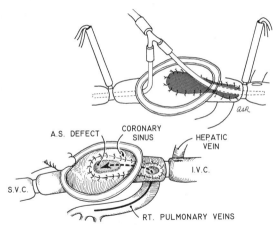

A.S. DEFECT   CORONARY SINUS   HEPATIC VEIN

S.V.C.

I.V.C.

RT. PULMONARY VEINS

Figure 2. The scimitar deformity consists of anomalous right pulmonary veins and a secundum type atrial septal defect. A pericardial patch effectively partitions the inferior vena cava and closes the septal defect.

of the few conditions in infancy in which open correction may be mandatory in the first few months of life is the so-called atrioventricularis communis or complete endocardial cushion anomaly. The atrioventricular valves are extremely primitive in this condition, and their repair is absolutely essential. Closure of the large atrial septal defect and the smaller ventricular defect is possible with careful intracardiac repair. A prosthesis of pericardium or synthetic material is necessary because of the large size of the septal defects. Results of operation are good if particular care is exercised during the postoperative period because these infants have tremendous amounts of tracheobronchial secretions. Most patients have kinetic pulmonary hypertension, and many of them will already have developed significant pulmonary vascular resistances. Left axis deviation of the electrocardiogram and an atrial septal defect in an infant who is in cardiac failure should point directly to the diagnosis of endocardial cushion anomaly.

If the endocardial cushion defect is incomplete, the condition was previously called the ostium primum type atrial septal defect. Important symptomatology may not develop until the second or third decade. Again, the axis deviation is to the left, and the murmur of mitral insufficiency is usually heard in the left axilla. Occasionally, secundum type atrial septal defects are found with left axis deviation, but every patient with endocardial cushion anomaly manifests the typical left axis orientation. Partial atrioventricular canals or endocardial cushion

defects may exist without any lesion of the mitral valve. The most common finding, however, is the large atrial septal defect with a cleft in the aortic leaflet of the mitral valve. It is catastrophic to repair the atrial septal defect and leave the patient with important mitral insufficiency. Owing to regurgitant flow through the cleft in the mitral valve, small fibrotic excrescences are present along each border of the cleft, and their suture union is ordinarily accomplished without difficulty. A prosthesis of pericardium or synthetic cloth should be utilized for closure of the large septal defect. The threat of heart block is always present because sutures must be placed very near the atrioventricular node and along the route of the common bundle of His. This threat is particularly found in patients with total endocardial cushion defects because closure of ventricular septal deficiency can place tension on the septal ridge wherein traverses the common bundle of His. Ordinarily, the aorta is not clamped so the heart will continue beating during the placement of all sutures. Any particular suture which provokes atrioventricular dissociation can be readily detected, removed and repositioned. All sutures should be taken well to the right side of the ventricular septum.

Operative results are good, but some mitral insufficiency is common after repair of the complete or atrioventricular canal variety of endocardial cushion anomaly. Heart block in recent years has essentially disappeared as a complication of open correction.

PULMONIC VALVULAR ATRESIA AND STENOSIS WITH INTACT VENTRICULAR SEPTUM. Pulmonic valvular atresia demands emergency surgical intervention in the newborn. Direct open valvotomy is required under inflow occlusion. If the pulmonary artery segment is also atretic or very poorly developed, the palliative shunt must be constructed. Some general hypothermia protects the nervous system during the three to five minutes of circulatory interruption obligatory to open valvotomy. No deliberate cooling is needed. Body temperature will decrease several degrees merely with the chest open. Midline sternotomy is the best approach; care is taken not to enter either chest cavity. The right heart is so huge that preserving an intact pleura is no real problem. The patent foramen ovale is disregarded. The nasoendotracheal tube remains in place for the next 24 to 48 hours. Usually the tube is so small that it must be removed rather than merely disconnected from the respirator. The infant is closely followed because reintubation is frequently necessary.

Severe pulmonic valvular stenosis in the infant of less than 10 kg. can be operated upon in the same manner. A small pinpoint valvular orifice may only barely separate this kind of patient from one with atresia. This situation is again an emergency, and the valve may be so poorly developed that accurate commissural incision is impossible. Resultant slight pulmonic valvular insufficiency is well tolerated.

Older patients with pressure gradients between 80 and 125 mm. Hg across the pulmonic valve are best operated upon during cardiopulmonary bypass. Precise incision of the commissures can be done in a leisurely fashion, and any septal defect can be detected and repaired. During bypass with the pulmonary artery open, the anesthesiologist continues to ventilate the lungs so that any septal defect can be identified by the issue of arterialized blood from the right ventricle. With right ventricular pressures near systemic levels small ventricular septal defects often pass unnoticed at catheterization. The thunderous murmur of pulmonic valvular stenosis can also obscure the presence of a small patent ductus which becomes quite obvious during cardiopulmonary bypass. Intrapericardial ligation of the surprise ductus should precede the pulmonary artery incision, although suture ligature of the pulmonary arterial ostium of the ductus can be done by extending the arteriotomy to the bifurcation.

With the valvular stenosis abolished, the right ventricular cavity should be inspected for significant muscle bands. Incision of these dense trabeculations does not require a separate ventriculotomy, but absolute identification of the papillary muscles is essential to their preservation.

MITRAL VALVE OPERATIONS. Most operations on the mitral valve can be done with the heart running and the coronary arteries fully perfused. The midline sternal splitting incision is satisfactory with exposure of the mitral valve through a long left atriotomy behind and parallel with the interatrial groove. If retraction of the atrial septum provokes aortic valvular incompetence, the aorta is occluded and the heart cooled. Most patients requiring mitral valve surgery have large to huge left atria, and exposure is good.

The days of closed operations on the mitral valve are gone, but not forgotten are the accidents attendant thereto, such as massive embolism and horrendous insufficiency, particularly with the use of transventricular dilators. An excellent opening snap in a young patient with no history of peripheral embolism constitutes no guarantee that the left atrium will be free of blood clots. Despite many types of mitral valve substitutes now available, the procedure must be carried out with the idea of conserving the patient's own tissue. Valve replacement is done frequently enough because of the high incidence of mitral valvular calcification.

Direct incision of the scarred and difficult-to-recognize commissures saves a certain number of patients from replacement—or, better stated, postpones the hour of replacement. On the other hand, too conservative an approach is even more dangerous than willy-nilly valve replacement because the very sick mitral patient may fail to survive the early postoperative course. The greatest attraction of the ball valve prosthesis is its sound hemodynamic characteristics. Whereas the early postoperative phase of the purple mitral with secondary tricuspid insufficiency is better negotiated with the mechanical valve, a disturbing number of late complications depend entirely on the fact that a prosthesis now fills the mitral annulus. Thus, each patient must be judged on particular features, and no committee can make this decision in advance for the surgeon.

Annuloplasty, or leaflet advancement by means of a free pericardial graft for mitral incompetence, is definitely preferred in young patients with congenital disease. Occasionally, a mitral valve cleft is found as the cause of congenital mitral insufficiency, and operative results are excellent. Children are notoriously difficult to manage with anticoagulant therapy; hence, use of a prosthesis should be done only when all other measures fail. The same philosophy holds for patients with congenital mitral stenosis.

All kinds of artificial heart valves are now available. The most widely used is the ball valve. Low profile lens, flap, and hinge valves are under clinical evaluation. Some deaths with the Starr-Edwards ball valve were surmised to be secondary to the left ventricular space occupying features of that prosthesis. Left ventricular outflow obstruction is assumed to be less when a low profile mechanism is used. The over-all operative or hospital mortality of mitral valve replacement should be 10 per cent, but late deaths and complications detract importantly from the early good results. A few homograft valves have been used for mitral substitutes in patients, and early results are promising. With valve homografts now being used more often for aortic replacement, it would appear that their frequent application as a mitral valve substitute is imminent. It is interesting to note that semilunar homograft valves are more suitable for mitral valve replacement than homograft mitral valves. The day will come almost certainly when tissue valves are used exclusively for the replacement of all diseased heart valves.

TRICUSPID VALVE OPERATIONS. Probably the most important lesson gleaned so far from the management of patients with severe mitral valve disease and secondary tricuspid insufficiency is that the latter requires no specific therapy. With restoration of good mitral function either by repair or replacement, tricuspid annular dilatation almost always regresses without annuloplasty. Organic tricuspid valve disease is another story. Here specific treatment is beneficial. Direct vision commissurotomy is appropriate for patients with tricuspid stenosis who have little or no tricuspid insufficiency. Mixed lesions, however, require valve replacement.

Isolated acquired tricuspid valve disease is rare, but Ebstein's congenital deformity of the tricuspid valve occurs with sufficient frequency to justify consideration of its surgical treatment. Atrialization of the right ventricle and displacement of the tricuspid valve, usually with an atrial septal defect, comprise this anomaly. Plication of the parasitic or defunctionalized right ventricle, with or without valve replacement, has been successful in some patients, and superior vena cava–pulmonary artery bypass of the right heart is available for consideration when the right ventricle is small. Operative results for Ebstein's anomaly are not brilliant.

TOTAL ANOMALOUS PULMONARY VENOUS RETURN. Total anomalous pulmonary venous drainage is a rare congenital anomaly that must be treated in the first few months of life. Cardiopulmonary bypass is justified in the infant of less than 10 kg. for correction of this anatomic complex. Direct cannulation of the aorta, individual catheters in the venae cavae and midline sternotomy permit direct suture of the confluens of anomalous pulmonary veins to the left atrium. The most common variety of total anomalous pulmonary venous drainage shows a characteristic x-ray silhouette termed "the snowman deformity." Pulmonary return reaches the right atrium via a left ascending venous trunk, the innominate vein and the right superior vena cava. The size of the atrial septal defect dictates the severity of the condition. A small patent foramen ovale obviously limits the amount of blood reaching the left heart. The second most common type of total anomalous pulmonary venous return is into the right atrium via a huge coronary sinus, and correction is easily done through a right atriotomy. Drainage below the diaphragm into the portal system is another form of the anomaly.

Very important in the use of cardiopulmonary bypass in the neonate is intrapericardial dissection and ligation of the ductus arteriosus. A good general rule in these tiny infants is to presume its patency and ligate the ductus before placing the patient in conduit with extracorporeal circulation.

CORRECTIVE OPERATION FOR TRANSPOSITION OF THE GREAT VESSELS. In 1954, Albert described an ingenious procedure of intraatrial inflow correction for patients with transposition of the great vessels. The operation achieved little application until Mustard proposed that a large rectangular sheet of autologous pericardium would be the ideal material to effect partitioning of blood flow. At present, any patient with transposition of the great vessels is an eventual candidate for correction if the pulmonary vascular resistance is not prohibitively elevated. The usual sequence of events is to try to identify transposition patients with relatively normal pulmonary vascular resistance, submit them to a Blalock-Hanlon procedure, with or without pulmonary artery banding in the first few months of life, and then to perform the Albert-Mustard operation when the patient is three to six years old. Most patients are carried through infancy with an atrial septal defect or pulmonary artery banding, and the definitive procedure is postponed as long as possible. In a child of 15 kg. or more, the corrective operation goes very well.

CORONARY ENDARTERECTOMY OR ARTERIOPLASTY. With the development of selective coronary cineangiography patients are now being identified with segmental disease, and such patients are candidates for direct coronary artery operation. It is possible to operate on the right coronary artery through a midline sternal splitting incision without cardiopulmonary bypass, but any procedure on the left coronary artery requires enough displacement of the heart that extracorporeal circulation is essential. Medial displacement of the pulmonary artery provides good exposure of the main left coronary artery and its principal divisions. Also with bypass, one can occlude the aorta and examine each coronary ostium for atherosclerotic encroachment.

If the obstructed segment cannot be cleared by endarterectomy, mere incision and implantation of a venous patch graft can yield excellent results. Patient selection is the most important factor in successful coronary artery operations. Whether rapidly improving microsurgical techniques will find application here is unknown.

DESCENDING THORACIC AORTIC ANEURYSM. Traumatic aneurysms of the thoracic aorta develop usually at the site of the ligamentum arteriosum. They are saccular, and restoration of aortic continuity can be accomplished in many patients without use of a graft. The aorta is not diseased, and with adequate mobilization the ends come together surprisingly well.

Arteriosclerotic aneurysms are frequently seen in the thoracic aorta, and a significant number require resection of most of the descending thoracic aorta along with the intercostal arteries. Such a patient should be informed preoperatively of the possibility of at least temporary lower extremity weakness because important contributions are made to the spinal artery by the intercostal vessels. Growth of the aneurysm may occlude many of the intercostals so slowly that adequate collaterals develop to the spinal arteries.

Cardiopulmonary bypass is not complete for the removal of descending thoracic aortic aneurysms, but use of the heart lung machine is helpful because catheters are not needed in the chest and the pericardium remains intact. Both the femoral artery and femoral vein are cannulated, and the pump oxygenator is responsible for perfusion of the body below the occluded aortic segment. The patient's own heart and lungs take care of the perfusion proximal to the isolated segment. Left atrial-femoral artery bypass obviates the need for an oxygenator, but this places a considerable load on the dependent right lung and the retracted left lung. Flow rates of approximately 1 liter per minute suffice to maintain viability of oxygen sensitive organs and spinal cord below the level of the diaphragm.

VENTRICULAR ANEURYSM. Left ventricular aneurysms occasionally develop in the wake of a significant myocardial infarction. Ventricular aneurysms occur most commonly in the area of myocardium served by the left anterior descending coronary artery. The aneurysms are filled with clot and become quite stable, but their presence limits cardiac output, especially during exercise. Longstanding aneurysms become calcified, and removal may eventuate in excision of a considerable portion of the ventricular septum.

Maturation of the aneurysm takes at least two to three months. Earlier surgical intervention may find the edges friable and difficult to suture. The surgical treatment of ventricular aneurysms brings up the feasibility of excising young areas of infarction. The electrical instability of infarcts might be abolished as well as the parasitic area which detracts from effective contraction. Results from excision of ventricular aneurysms are good, but the prognosis depends on the extent of the residual coronary artery disease.

Aneurysms of the right ventricle are almost always postoperative complications of outflow reconstruction for pulmonic annular stenosis. Residual right ventricular hypertension and a weak or prosthetic anterior wall lead to development of the aneurysm. Reoperation with excision is well tolerated because coronary artery disease does not provoke this condition.

ACUTE DISSECTING HEMATOMA OF THE DESCENDING THORACIC AORTA. Previously termed dissecting aneurysms, acute dissecting hematomas of the aorta occur as a result of an intimal and medial tear frequently at a point just below the left subclavian artery. The primary dissection is toward the diaphragm because of the arch branches above. Sudden death from free perforation into the left chest is likely without operation. These patients almost always have a known history of important systemic hypertension, and the acute episode resembles a myocardial infarction, but the electrocardiogram is incompatible with coronary occlusion. A ripping or tearing pain in the chest is the common initial complaint. Shock or near shock follows, and because plain chest films may be relatively normal, aortography is helpful in making the diagnosis. Acute dissection of the aorta should be suspected in any patient with a history of hypertension who appears to have a massive infarct.

Recently, enthusiasm for nonoperative

treatment has come from the work of Wheat and his associates. The patient is heavily sedated, and the method of therapy reminds one of Crile's anoci-association theory in the days of sneak thyroidectomy and thyroid storm. Whatever has been salvaged through the program of intensified medical management in these clinics is better than the 100 per cent operative mortality previously reported by them.

For the acute dissecting hematoma of the descending thoracic aorta, a left posterolateral incision is made through the bed of the fifth rib. Both the femoral artery and femoral vein are cannulated, and the patient is placed on partial cardiopulmonary bypass at flow rates of approximately 1000 to 1500 ml. per minute. The aorta is occluded above and below the affected segment. The aorta is divided, and the area of the intimal tear is resected. A woven prosthetic graft is implanted after obliteration of the false lumen at either end of the aortic resection.

The histopathology usually shows mediocystic necrosis of the aorta. Patients with Marfan's syndrome may manifest the same diathesis without hypertension and at a younger age. Most patients with acute aortic dissection are older than 50 years of age, and men predominate.

TUMORS OF THE HEART. The most common tumor of the heart is myxoma of the left atrium simulating mitral stenosis and frequently connected to the fossa ovalis by a small pedicle. The diagnosis is infrequently made preoperatively, and the tumor is detected in most patients during an operation for mitral stenosis or tricuspid stenosis if formation of the tumor is to the right of the septum.

Histologically, myxomas are benign, but their position makes them malignant. Often, the first evidence of intracavitary myxoma is a nonfatal peripheral embolus. Microscopic examination of the embolus reveals the typical features of myxoma. Cardiotomy should be carried out without delay.

Invasive or truly malignant tumors of the heart do occur but rarely. Their clinical presentation depends on the location. Pulmonic stenosis can be mimicked for example by a rhabdomyosarcoma of the right ventricular outflow tract. Metastatic tumors of the heart and pericardium do occur, but treatment is of little value. The same obtains with the cardiac valvular lesions associated with massive carcinoid disease.

CONGENITAL ANOMALIES OF THE CORONARY ARTERIES. Anomalous origin of the left coronary artery from the pulmonary artery is rare, but the condition is correctable in childhood by simple ligation of the misplaced coronary artery or replantation of the orifice into the aorta. Occasionally, the anomaly is seen during infancy when the persistent anterior infarct pattern of the electrocardiogram is diagnostic. Ligation of the artery before sufficient collaterals have developed can be lethal, and replantation of the coronary artery into the aorta is prohibited by both the tiny patient and the small vessel. In older patients, the anomaly simulates a patent ductus with its continuous murmur. Coronary artery fistulae connect the affected vessel either with a cardiac chamber, usually right ventricle or right atrium, or with a venous network. The former are more readily treated, and the latter can be challenging because of multiple arterial venous fistulae. Care must be taken not to sacrifice distal coronary runoff. Selective cine coronary arteriography is very important in planning the surgical procedure. Cardiac catheterization should be done simultaneously. Endocardial fibroelastosis may complicate the problem of the anomalous origin of the left coronary artery when the anomaly presents itself early in life; however, results of operations during childhood are good.

PULMONARY EMBOLISM. The bubble oxygenator with hemodilution is well suited for the brief periods of cardiopulmonary bypass necessary to carry out pulmonary embolectomy. Most patients with pulmonary emboli do reasonably well on anticoagulant therapy without embolectomy, but the procedure can be lifesaving when applied to the proper situation. Heart catheterization and pulmonary arteriography help to make the diagnosis; however, certain situations are so urgent that elaborate diagnostic studies would take too much time. Radioisotope scanning is another good confirmatory test. Right heart strain on the electrocardiogram provides a simple aid which can be done quickly. Candidates for operation are acutely and critically ill. Pregnancy or a recent abdominal operation frequently precedes the catastrophe.

At operation with emergency cardiopulmonary bypass, the clots erupt from the pulmonary artery incision under pressure. The lungs are carefully massaged to empty the smaller branches. Even counterirrigation of the left atrium can help to dislodge pulmonary arteriolar fragments. The inferior vena cava is ligated at the conclusion of the procedure, and anticoagulants are administered within 24 hours. Plication or special clamps for inferior vena caval obstruction are not necessary. Tracheostomy should be done if the patient has deteriorated to a great degree before operation could be performed. Results are spectacular in selected patients.

ELECTIVE CARDIAC ARREST

Even though operations upon the heart have reached at least daily frequency levels in most centers, resumption of the heart beat after varying periods of elective arrest continues to be one of the wonders of modern medicine (Fig. 3). We have used a particular form of elective cardiac standstill since 1959 with such consistent results that even the smallest ventricular septal defect is repaired in the dry, quiet field afforded by anoxic cold arrest. In fact, the small, difficult-to-locate ventricular septal defect constitutes a prime indication to total control of the heart.

Elective cardiac arrest is induced by cross-clamping the aorta and local cooling with normal saline at 2 to 4° C. A well or sling is made by suturing the pericardium to the wound edges. The level of saline is maintained just below the ventriculotomy or aortotomy. If some of the cold saline enters the cardiac chamber, only slight hemodilution results. Particulate cold or slush is injurious to the thin atrial wall and is not recommended. Experimental work with cardiac homografts has pointed out the difference

between fluid cooling and slush applied to the heart. A higher rate of arrhythmia can be expected from particulate cooling of the heart. Periods of anoxia up to two hours have been well tolerated in the human with topical hypothermia as the only means of myocardial protection. Brief periods of anoxia without hypothermia are not deleterious, but cardiac surgical procedures should not be hurried. With the aorta open, it is possible to see blood continuously emanating from the coronary ostia by way of collaterals from the bronchial circulation, so the use of blood prime is perhaps crucial to this technique of prolonged cardiac arrest. The oxygen carrying capacity of the bronchial circulation is obviously greater with whole blood than with hemodilution methods.

Operations Performed with Elective Cardiac Arrest

VENTRICULAR SEPTAL DEFECTS. Infants with large left-to-right shunts and low pulmonary vascular resistance should undergo pulmonary artery banding. If successive catheterization studies in an infant not previously banded reveal an increasing pulmonary vascular resistance, open correction should be done even in the first two years of life. Any patient with a ventricular septal defect and a left-to-right shunt confirmed by cardiac catheterization and angiocardiogram should be submitted to operation. The incidence of endocarditis over a five-year period in asymptomatic patients with a ventricular septal defect and normal pulmonary artery pressure approached 10 per cent. Any clinic taking the position that every patent ductus arteriosus should be operated upon should likewise urge that every ventricular septal defect with a net left-to-right shunt be closed. The hope of spontaneous closure prevents this apparently sound course of action. Although spontaneous closure of an occasional ventricular septal defect in infancy and childhood has been documented, the lesion basically is an abnormal communication between the ventricles and requires surgical ablation in the vast majority of patients.

Small defects of the membranous septum can be closed by direct suture. Horizontal mattress sutures are advised for their built-in bolster. Simple sutures are likely to pull out. Bites should be kept in the scarred membranous remnants to avoid heart block. Left atrial decompression is used along with local

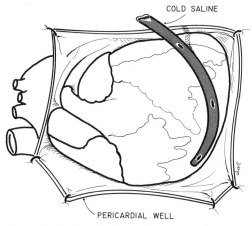

Figure 3. During elective cardiac arrest, the heart is cooled by the constant flow of cold saline into the pericardial well. The level of coolant is maintained just below the aortotomy or cardiotomy. Coronary perfusion of the left ostium protects against calcific emboli during aortic valve removal.

hypothermia. Large ventricular septal defects are repaired with a loosely knitted Teflon or Dacron prosthetic patch sutured circumferentially to the edges of the defect. Mattress sutures are placed first along the perimeter of the defect and then through the slightly oversized patch. The patch is lowered into position, and the sutures are gently tied. With aortic occlusion and local cooling a very small ventriculotomy can be maneuvered anywhere over the septum. The ill effects of temporary cardiac arrest are fleeting, but a long ventriculotomy becomes a permanent scar with varying degrees of functional impairment. Closure of some defects low in the ventricular septal ridge is better done by an atrial incision. A surprise patent ductus is ligated after intrapericardial dissection.

Results of operations for ventricular septal defect are good. An occasional patient with pulmonary hypertension does not respond to closure of the defect, and the pulmonary resistance continues to increase. Such patients cannot be identified preoperatively. Heart block is now a rare complication, but use of a pullout myocardial electrode has erased the significant early mortality of this problem. Gradual closure of the ventricular septal defect associated with a high pulmonary artery pressure has few adherents and probably little place in the surgical approach.

Certain patients with ventricular septal defects also have aortic valvular insufficiency. If operation must be done in early childhood, the ventricular septal defect is closed, and the aortic valve is merely inspected. Any efforts to suture a prolapsed cusp will be only temporarily helpful. The tissue tears easily, and more insufficiency is produced. Homograft cusp replacement or pulmonic cusp autograft substitution should be utilized at a later date when the patient is eight years old or older. Even total aortic valve replacement may be needed, and the fresh valve homograft is preferred to a prosthetic device with its attendant requirement of anticoagulation.

Ventricular septal defects can occur after myocardial infarction. If operation is necessary in the first few weeks following an acute episode, results are poor because of the extreme friability of the septal infarct. Traumatic ventricular septal defects also occur, but their closure is more feasible than repair of postinfarction septal defects.

CORRECTION OF FALLOT'S TETRALOGY. Of all open heart operations, none is more gratifying than complete correction of Fallot's interesting anomaly. There are varying degrees of tetrad depending on the severity of right ventricular outflow obstruction. Acyanotic tetralogy of Fallot does exist, but the shunt reverses itself during exercise. Historical as well as anatomic features distinguish the patient with a large ventricular septal defect and secondary right ventricular corridor obstruction from the patient with so-called acyanotic tetralogy. The patient whose primary disease is ventricular septal defect has a history of heart failure during the neonatal period, with gradual improvement as the left-to-right shunt is diminished by right ventricular hypertrophy. In this patient, the aorta remains small unlike the large aorta of patients with Fallot's tetralogy. Heart failure essentially never occurs in patients with true tetralogy of Fallot. Most patients who undergo surgical correction have cyanosis of some degree with clubbed digits and important activity limitations. If the patient weighs less than 15 kg. and requires operation for tetralogy of Fallot, a systemic-pulmonary artery shunt is recommended. Weight is a better criterion than age for case selection. The right-to-left shunt of patients with tetralogy of Fallot is from the right ventricle to the aorta. The left ventricle is bypassed and remains small, but development of the left ventricle is not impaired, and it readily accepts the full systemic burden after complete correction.

Preoperative evaluation with heart catheterization and cineangiocardiography should be done in each patient with suspected tetralogy. The angiogram shows the right ventricular interior in two planes, and a preliminary surgical plan can be made from it. With infundibular obstruction, which is present in almost every patient with Fallot's complex, the angiogram cannot uniformly delineate the pulmonic valve. Accordingly, such diagnoses as associated valve stenosis rendered by radiology must be confirmed by cardiac catheterization or at operation. Nonetheless, biplane cineangiocardiography has a secure position in the diagnosis of tetralogy of Fallot. Catheter results are interesting in that the femoral oxygen unsaturation is an index to the disease severity. The catheter is a better indicator of separate valvular stenosis if the pulmonary artery can be entered. Ventricular pressures are balanced. Occasionally, an atrial septal defect is present, Fallot's pentalogy, and the diagnosis should be made preoperatively.

Elective cardiac arrest makes the corrective operation relatively easy. The long axis of the huge ventricular septal defect is often in an anteroposterior plane, but with cold cardioplegia the edges of the defect are readily seen even through a small ventriculotomy. Left atrial decompression is essential owing to the tremendous amount of bronchial flow return to the heart. Any previously constructed shunt is dissected and ligated before bypass is instituted. The ventriculotomy is always made with respect for preservation of the coronary artery pattern. The left superior vena cava is sought, especially if the right superior vena cava is small. The ventricular septal defect is closed with a prosthetic patch of loosely knitted Teflon after placement of mattress sutures. The aortic annulus makes excellent footing for the lateral aspect of the suture line. Incision and excision of the dense muscle bands release the right ventricle, and an adequate outflow area is usually provided. If the pulmonic annulus is restrictive, it must be divided. Some patients require a boat-shaped prosthesis to widen the annulus. The crista supraventricularis usually stands as a scarred promontory between the pulmonic valve and the ventricular septal defect. It is not excised, for it makes a good anterior border for sutures to close the ventricular septal defect. Some ventricular septal defects are above the crista, and sutures must be taken in the common annulus of the pulmonary artery and aorta. Again, bites remain well to the right of the defect to avoid heart block. Operative results are dramatic, and the mortality which once stood at 50 per cent is less than 10 per cent now in most clinics. Only in the tetrad with protection of pulmonary vascular bed does one have the opportunity to close the truly huge ventricular defect.

AORTIC VALVE SURGERY. Operations on the aortic valve are readily performed during cold anoxic arrest. No need to perfuse the right coronary artery ever exists, and the cannula in the left coronary artery ostium is helpful principally in keeping calcific particles from embolizing during valvular excision.

Congenital disease of the aortic valve can be either stenosis or insufficiency, and it would now appear that most adults with isolated calcific aortic valve disease have congenitally deformed valves and not rheumatic valvulitis.

Infants with severe aortic valve stenosis must be operated upon early in life with cardiopulmonary bypass if possible, or hypothermia alone, in the neonatal period. Children with left ventricular outflow obstruction can have familial subvalvular muscular hypertrophy. Sudden death of children with aortic stenosis or muscular encroachment is common; hence, pressure gradients should be determined, and operation is advised if the left ventricular aortic pressure differential is greater than 50 mm. Hg. Congenital aortic valve stenosis is not always totally correctable, and one must settle for less than a perfect result lest significant aortic insufficiency be provoked. In the presence of a fibrous subvalvular membrane the valve is usually normal, and operative results are excellent. Poststenotic dilatation of the aorta can be seen in the x-ray in both valvular and subvalvular membrane stenosis, but it is not regularly present with muscular hypertrophy. Supravalvular stenosis occurs rarely, and the huge size of the coronary arteries which lie proximal to the stenosis makes the angiocardiogram very interesting. Incision is made through the annular supravalvular ring, and a prosthetic shield is sutured to its edges. Incision must go deep into the posterior sinus of Valsalva. In the presence of a normal valve the results are excellent.

Acquired or adult aortic valvular disease is best treated usually by excision and replacement. An occasional instance will occur when debridement of the calcified valve can restore good function. Replacement, however, is the rule, and we prefer fresh aortic valve homografts for the procedure (Fig. 4). Prosthetic valves have enjoyed widespread application, but late results are beginning to indicate that the ball valve is not entirely satisfactory. Preserved homograft valves have been used to a great extent in England and New Zealand, but from our laboratory experience, it would appear that the fresh valve homograft taken from a cadaver under sterile precautions comes close to the ideal valve replacement material. In Australia, valve heterografts have been employed, but the incidence of postoperative valvular insufficiency remains significant.

Aneurysms of the ascending aorta in conjunction with aortic valvular disease must be removed with graft implantation. The histopathological diagnosis is almost always

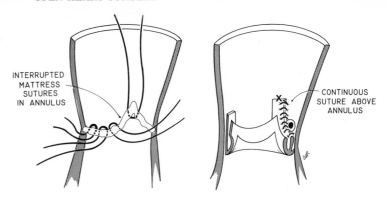

Figure 4.   Suture of the aortic valve homograft is accomplished in two rows, one at the annular level, the other just below each coronary ostium. The deep row is interrupted and of the mattress variety. Tailoring of the annulus is seldom required. Fresh valves are preferred for replacement.

mediocystic necrosis of the aorta. Fortunately, most aneurysms of the ascending aorta narrow at the takeoff of the innominate artery so that conventional perfusion techniques can be used.

MULTIPLE VALVE REPLACEMENT. Local cardiac hypothermia and perfusion of the left coronary artery afford good myocardial protection during open procedures on the aortic and mitral valves. If the tricuspid valve is also diseased, not merely dilated, the aortotomy is closed and the aortic clamp removed before tricuspid valvuloplasty or replacement. The heart is fully perfused while the tricuspid procedure is leisurely completed.

The aortic valve is approached first and excised, and the annulus is measured. With the aortic valve removed, an excellent view of the mitral valve is obtained, and palpation is carefully done through the aortic incision. If the decision is made to replace the mitral valve, its chordae are incised before opening the left atrium behind the interatrial groove. A suction catheter is placed in the left ventricle via the aortotomy while the mitral valve is excised and replaced through the left atrial incision.

After replacement of the mitral valve, the left atriotomy is closed, and attention is then directed to replacement of the aortic valve. All air is expressed from the pulmonary veins, left atrium and left ventricle before suture of the aortotomy. A small needle vent of the ascending aorta above the suture line further protects against air embolism. A #20 needle and syringe suffices without special apparatus. Total bypass time should not exceed two hours for a double valve or 2½ hours when the tricuspid is included. The usual duration of aortic occlusion is less than two hours. If the left coronary artery branches early or fails for some reason to accept a perfusion

cannula easily, local cooling alone protects the heart adequately.

ACUTE DISSECTING HEMATOMA OF THE ASCENDING AORTA. Patients with acute anterior aortic dissection expire for two reasons: heart failure from aortic valvular insufficiency, and cardiac tamponade from intrapericardial perforation of the dissection. Unlike dissections of the descending thoracic aorta, these patients must be operated upon during total cardiopulmonary bypass with occlusion of the aorta at the innominate takeoff. The history of ripping anterior chest pain and intense acute illness plus previously known hypertension should raise the possibility of dissecting hematoma of the aorta. If aortic valvular insufficiency can be diagnosed by the diastolic murmur, there is no need for a confirmatory aortogram, although plain chest films may not be helpful. The patient should be prepared for operation as soon as the diagnosis is made. Acute dissections into the aortic root should not be treated by so-called conservative medical management. The vast majority of such patients are dead within a few days of initial symptomatology.

Peripheral venous cannulation in the neck and groin with femoral artery input from the pump oxygenator can be used on an emergency basis if the patient deteriorates before the chest can be opened. Occlusion of the aorta as far along the arch as possible is the only maneuver needed to attain satisfactory control of the lesion.

The essence of the surgical procedure is to divide and excise the ascending aorta. Continuity is restored by implanting a large tube of woven Dacron or Teflon. Usually, the area of intimal tear is excised with the aorta. The false lumen is oversewn both just above the aortic valve and immediately below the occluding clamp. The hematoma which causes displacement of the aortic valve is removed before closure of the extra lumen. Replacement is not necessary except in the presence of valvular disease. Operative salvage is good if hemorrhage from the friable aortic suture lines does not occur. The blood pressure is kept low with medications during the early recovery period.

With restoration of normal valvular anatomy and excision of the ascending aorta, the two principal causes of sudden death are erased. Long-term survival depends on the prevention of other dissections by weight reduction and medical control of systemic hypertension.

CORRECTED TRANSPOSITION OF THE GREAT VESSELS. This rare anomaly can exist without septal defects or valvular disease and thus provoke no symptoms and only minor cardiac murmurs. Pulmonary blood flow obstruction can be present to the extent that operative intervention is necessary, and all varieties of pulmonary ventricular obstruction with or without ventricular septal defects are seen. Lesions of the atrioventricular valves also may produce symptoms.

Great care must be taken to place the ventriculotomy away from the right coronary artery as it traverses the right ventricle enroute to the atrioventricular groove. The right atrioventricular valve resembles the mitral valve whereas the left atrioventricular valve is tricuspid. The right ventricular interior is smooth rather than heavily trabeculated in the usual manner. The aorta is on the left lateral aspect of the pulmonary artery and forms the left heart border by x-ray. The complex is spoken of as corrected transposition because the aorta does emanate from the left or systemic ventricle even though that chamber is the morphologic right ventricle. Similarly, the pulmonary artery properly derives from the pulmonary ventricle, but it is the morphologic left ventricle. In operations for ventricular septal defect, the danger of heart block is substantially increased owing to the ventricular transposition.

Surgical results have not been brilliant in this condition, but more recent experience is encouraging. Aneurysmal formation of the membranous septum is a frequent cause of obstruction to outflow from the venous ventricle. The cineangiocardiogram may be interpreted to show purely valvular impedance, but the finding of a subvalvular wind sock is not uncommon. Treatment consists of excision and closure of the resultant ventricular

septal defect. Sutures must be taken in the membranous sac away from the muscular septum.

AORTIC SEPTAL DEFECT. The aortic pulmonary window anomaly is readily correctable by operation, and results are excellent if pulmonary vascular resistance is not severe. Inflow occlusion and suture of the defect through an incision in the dilated pulmonary artery will suffice in tiny infants. Cardiopulmonary bypass permits a more leisurely approach in children. The defect usually produces severe symptoms, and diagnostic confusion comes mainly from its similarity to the large ductus in infants and children. Retrograde aortography is essential to separation of the huge patent ductus from aortic septal defect. Occasionally, the defect is distal enough to the heart that it can be ligated after complete dissection of both the pulmonary artery and aorta. Ligation, of course, is not sound and should be done only as a compromise during an emergency operation in a small infant. Accidents were common with persistent efforts to dissect between the window and the heart in the days before successful cardiopulmonary bypass.

MISCELLANEOUS OPERATIONS. Double outlet right ventricle with obstruction of the pulmonary artery can be corrected by direct attack. The ventricular septal defect must be sutured to the base of the aorta by means of a prosthesis, and the pulmonary flow obstruction is then removed or the right ventricle bypassed with a graft from the right ventricle to the distal pulmonary artery. The procedure is best performed in childhood because hopefully entire repair is intraventricular.

The Taussig-Bing anomaly has been definitively treated by Kirklin with a procedure encompassing the Albert-Mustard maneuver after closure of the large ventricular septal defect. The aorta comes off the right ventricle with the pulmonary artery overriding a huge ventricular septal defect. Ordinarily, the pulmonary vascular changes prohibit any consideration of complete repair, but an occasional patient qualifies for ventricular septal defect closure and atrial septal rearrangement.

Correction of a perforated sinus of Valsalva aneurysm is readily carried out by incision into the cardiac chamber with which it communicates. The aorta can be opened to expose the affected sinus, but closure of the fibrous wind sock is quite secure without the additional incision. The right atrium or ventricle is the usual low pressure component of the shunt whereas the right or posterior sinus constitutes the aneurysm. History is generally one of acute onset of cardiac symptoms, and because the aortic valve is normal, operative results are good. Concentric left-to-right shunts can occur if the sinus fistula traverses a membranous ventricular septal defect.

HEART REPLACEMENT AND VENTRICULAR ASSIST DEVICES

Interest is high in the general area of cardiac replacement. There are two primary roads to achievement of this goal, the mechanical heart and the heart transplant. Use of the mechanical heart has not been successful in the laboratory beyond a few hours owing to blood clotting in the device. In fact, survival has been so scarce that the larger problems of power and balance between the systemic and pulmonary circulations have almost escaped identification. Sociological and psychological obstacles lie in the way of the mechanical heart. For example, an implantable power source capable of driving the circulation indefinitely will almost certainly create significant levels of noise. The individual with a mechanical heart will be socially conspicuous and unable to share the anonymity enjoyed by patients with artificial heart valves or pacemakers.

Hopeful of solving the artificial heart problem by increments, many workers are concerning themselves with ventricular assist devices. Vast sums of research money allotted to assist devices can be justified primarily because their development contributes to the major goal of whole heart replacement. Infants and children and even adults with coronary artery disease are not suitable candidates for the use of ventricular assist devices. On the other hand, presently inoperable states in each of these categories are solid indications for heart replacement.

Transplantation of the heart has become a routinely successful laboratory procedure in the dog. Long-term survival up to one year is possible through the administration of presently available immune suppressive chemicals. The current obstacle to orthotopic homotransplantation of the heart revolves around the resuscitation and storage of cadaver hearts. The legal definition of death is under intense study and may be changed so that unpaired organs such as the heart and liver can be taken from patients with irreversible brain damage. It is fair to guess that the proper set of circumstances with respect to cadaver donors and living hosts will permit successful transplantation of the heart long before the problems of the mechanical heart are met and vanquished.

READING REFERENCES

Albert, H. M.: Surgical correction of transposition of the great vessels. Surg. Forum 5:74, 1954.

Barratt-Boyes, B. G., Lowe, J. B., Cole, D. S., and Kelly, D. T.: Homograft valve replacement for aortic valve disease. Thorax 20:495, 1965.

Beck, C. S.: Coronary sclerosis and angina pectoris; treatment by grafting a new blood supply upon myocardium. Surg. Gyn. & Obst. 64:270, 1937.

Blalock, A., and Hanlon, C. R.: Interatrial septal defect—its experimental production under direct vision without interruption of the circulation. Surg. Gyn. & Obst. 87:183, 1948.

Blalock, A., and Taussig, H. B.: The surgical treatment of malformations of the heart in which there is pulmonary stenosis or pulmonary atresia. J.A.M.A. 128:189, 1945.

Bopp, R. K., Larsen, P. B., Caddell, J. L., Patrick, J. R., Hipona, F. A., and Glenn, W. W. L.: Surgical considerations for treatment of congenital tricuspid atresia and stenosis: with particular reference to vena cava–pulmonary artery anastomosis. J. Thorac. & Cardiovasc. Surg. 43:97, 1962.

Brock, R. C.: Pulmonary valvulotomy for the relief of congenital pulmonary stenosis: report of three cases. Brit. Med. J. 1:1121, 1948.

Cross, F. S., and Jones, R. D.: Laboratory and clinical experience with the caged lenticular valve. Dis. Chest 50:307, 1966.

Edwards, W. S., Mohtashemi, M., and Holdefer, W. F., Jr.: Ascending aorta to right pulmonary artery shunt for infants with tetralogy of Fallot. Surgery 59:316, 1966.

Effler, D. B., Jones, F. M., Jr., Groves, L. K., and Suarez, E.: Myocardial revascularization by Vineberg's internal mammary artery implant. J. Thorac. & Cardiovasc. Surg. 50:527, 1965.

El Sayed, H., Cleland, W. P., Bentall, H. H., Melrose, D. G., Bishop, M. B., and Morgan, J.: Corrected transposition of the great arterial trunks: surgical treatment of the associated defects. J. Thorac. & Cardiovasc. Surg. 44:443, 1962.

Gerbode, F., Sanchez, P. A., Arguero, R., Kerth, W. J., Hill, J. D., and deVries, P. A.: Endocardial cushion defects. Presented at the 1967 American Surgical Association meetings, Colorado Springs, Colo., May 11, 12 and 13.

Glover, R. P., Davila, J. C., Kyle, R. H., Beard, J. C., Jr., Trout, R. G., and Kitchell, J. R.: Ligation of the internal mammary arteries as a means of increasing blood supply to the myocardium. J. Thorac. Surg. 34:661, 1957.

Gott, V. L., Daggett, R. L., Botham, R. J., Koepke, D. E., Zarnstorff, W. C., and Young, W. P.: The development of a prosthetic heart valve utilizing a rigid housing and a flexible butterfly-wing leaflet. Tr. Am. Soc. Art. Int. Organs 8:72, 1962.

Hoffman, J. I. E., and Rudolph, A. M.: The natural history of ventricular septal defects in infancy. Am. J. Cardiol. 16:634, 1965.

Kirklin, J. W., and Daicoff, G. R.: Surgery corrects Taussig-Bing heart. J.A.M.A. *199*:41, 1967.

Kirklin, J. W., Harp, R. A., and McGoon, D. C.: Surgical treatment of origin of both vessels from right ventricle, including cases of pulmonary stenosis. J. Thorac. & Cardiovasc. Surg. *48*:1026, 1964.

Kirklin, J. W., Wallace, R. B., McGoon, D. C., and DuShane, J. W.: Early and late results after intracardiac repair of tetralogy of Fallot. Five-year review of 337 patients. Tr. Am. Surg. Assoc. *83*:258, 1965.

Lewis, F. J., and Taufic, J.: Closure of atrial septal defects with the aid of hypothermia; experimental accomplishments and the report of one successful case. Surgery *33*:52, 1953.

Lillehei, C. W., Sellers, R. D., Bonnabeau, R. C., Jr., and Eliot, R. S.: Chronic postsurgical complete heart block with particular reference to prognosis, management, and a new P-wave pacemaker. J. Thorac. & Cardiovasc. Surg. *46*:436, 1963.

Lower, R. R., Dong, E., Jr., and Shumway, N. E.: Long-term survival of cardiac homografts. Surgery *58*:110, 1965.

Malm, J. R.: Discussion of Hallman, G. L., and Cooley, D. A.: Surgical treatment of tetralogy of Fallot: experience with indirect and direct techniques. J. Thorac. & Cardiovasc. Surg. *46*:419, 1963.

Melrose, D. G., Bentall, H. H., McMillan, I. K. R., Flege, J. B., Alvarez Diaz, F. R., Nahas, R. A., Fautley, R., and Carson, J.: The evolution of a mitral-valve prosthesis. Lancet *2*:623, 1964.

Muller, W. H., Jr., and Dammann, J. F., Jr.: The treatment of certain congenital malformations of the heart by the creation of pulmonic stenosis to reduce pulmonary hypertension and excessive pulmonary flow. Surg. Gyn. & Obst. *95*:213, 1952.

Mustard, W. T., Keith, J. D., Trusler, G. A., Fowler, R., and Kidd, L.: The surgical management of transposition of the great vessels. J. Thorac. & Cardiovasc. Surg. *48*:953, 1964.

O'Brien, M. F.: Heterograft aortic valves for human use. J. Thorac. & Cardiovasc. Surg. *53*:392, 1967.

Potts, W. J.: Aortic-pulmonary anastomosis for pulmonary stenosis. J. Thorac. Surg. *17*:223, 1948.

Ross, D.: Homotransplantation of the aortic valve in the subcoronary position. J. Thorac. & Cardiovasc. Surg. *47*:713, 1964.

Shumway, N. E., Lower, R. R., Hurley, E. J., and Pillsbury, R. C.: Results of total surgical correction for Fallot's tetralogy. Cardiovasc. Surg., 1964. American Heart Association, Monograph No. 11, pp. 57-61.

Shumway, N. E., Lower, R. R., and Stofer, R. C.: Selective hypothermia of the heart in anoxic cardiac arrest. Surg. Gyn. & Obst. *109*:750, 1959.

Starr, A., McCord, C. W., Wood, J., Herr, R., and Edwards, M. L.: Surgery for multiple valve disease. Ann. Surg. *160*:596, 1964.

Vineberg, A.: Experimental background of myocardial revascularization by internal mammary artery implantation and supplementary technics, with its clinical application in 125 patients. A review and critical appraisal. Ann. Surg. *159*:185, 1964.

Wheat, M. W., Jr., Palmer, R. F., Bartley, T. D., and Seelman, R. C.: Treatment of dissecting aneurysms of the aorta without surgery. J. Thorac. & Cardiovasc. Surg. *50*:364, 1965.

Chapter 21

THE ABDOMINAL WALL AND PERITONEUM

by
ROBERT A. MACBETH, M.D.
and
WALTER C. MacKENZIE, M.D.

ROBERT ALEXANDER MACBETH, born in Edmonton and the son of a doctor, was educated at the University of Alberta. Trained in surgery at McGill University, he has been a research Fellow of the National Research Council and a teaching Fellow in Anatomy. With the approach of a perfectionist, he has a great interest in medical education, research and history. He is the Professor of Surgery and Director of the Department of Surgery at the University of Alberta.

WALTER CAMPBELL MacKENZIE was born in Nova Scotia, the only son of Canadian-Scottish parents and the grandson of a sea captain. He is the Dean of Medicine and Professor of Surgery at the University of Alberta. His college and medical education were received at Dalhousie University in Halifax. He was a Fellow in Surgery at the Mayo Foundation and Clinic. He served his country as surgical consultant to the Royal Canadian Navy and has played an important role in medical education and research in Canada.

INTRODUCTION

A painstaking examination of the abdomen is one of the most rewarding diagnostic procedures available to the physician. The physician must develop an ability to appreciate even minor variations from normal while conducting this examination. To do this, he must avail himself of every opportunity during his education to examine the abdomens of normal individuals, of patients presenting with abdominal complaints and of postoperative patients.

The physical findings elicited by examination of the abdomen, together with an appreciation of the physiologic mechanisms involved, are the key to the diagnosis of numerous pathologic conditions of the abdominal wall and, more particularly, of the peritoneal cavity. In an acute disease process, physical examination is most rewarding and yields far more information than all laboratory investigations.

Examination of the abdominal wall is of the utmost importance in initially establishing a diagnosis, and repeated examination of the abdomen enables the physician to follow the course of the pathologic process. It should be emphasized that the pathology of disease is a continuing process, and that the clinical findings elicited on abdominal examination vary with the stage of the process present in the abdominal wall or peritoneal cavity.

515

THE ABDOMINAL WALL

EMBRYOLOGY

The Umbilical Region

The essential features in the embryology of the umbilical region are illustrated in Figures 1 to 5.

Figure 1 represents a human embryo 0.7 mm. long. As can be seen, the embryo proper is capped dorsally by its amniotic cavity while it sits ventrally on its relatively large yolk sac. This entire structure is attached to the chorion and thence to the uterine wall by its broad body stalk. The body stalk is seen to contain the fetal vascular pedicle (V) made up of the paired umbilical arteries and umbilical vein and, in addition, the allantois (A) which is a diverticulum of the yolk sac.

By the time the embryo reaches 1.7 mm. long (Fig. 2), its cephalic and caudal extremities have curled ventrally, pinching off the most dorsal portion of the yolk sac, which now takes a form indicative of its future development into the gastrointestinal tract. The allantois (A) arises from that portion of the yolk sac which is taken into the embryo, so that one may now refer to this structure as arising from the primitive hindgut. It is of importance, for understanding future events, to note at this point the depression which is evident at the neck of the yolk sac (X) and which, as a result of further development, is to contribute the coelom.

In the 3.5-mm. embryo (Fig. 3), a stage has been reached at which one may describe an umbilical cord. Enlargement of the amniotic cavity has now compressed the elongated body stalk and the elongated yolk sac stalk into a short compact structure, the anlage of the umbilical cord. The yolk sac stalk may now properly be referred to as the omphalomesenteric (vitelline) duct (M) as it lies free in the extraembryonic coelom, or exocoelom.

The structures in the cord at the 3.5-mm. embryo stage can be best appreciated by reference to Figure 4, which is a cross section of the cord of the embryo in Figure 3 at Y. The patent omphalomesenteric duct, with the accompanying artery and vein on its surface, lies in the exocoelom and occupies the superior portion of the cord. Inferior to it, embedded in mesenchyme, are respectively the umbilical vein, the paired umbilical arteries and the allantois. The umbilical

vein divides, just before entering the embryo, into right and left branches, which pass cephalad to unite with the hepatic circulation.

Figure 5 represents a diagrammatic sagittal view of a 5.2-cm. embryo, approximately ten weeks old. The left umbilical vein is now shown superiorly in the cord as it courses towards the porta hepatis. The right umbilical vein disappears before the embryo is 10 mm. long.

The left vein remains patent until shortly after birth, at which time physiological occlusion occurs. It is subsequently designated the ligamentum teres of the liver. It is, however, capable of cannulation and dilatation even in adult life and, by the technique of umbilical vein catheterization, portal venography, portal pressure studies and portal infusion may be carried out.

The paired umbilical arteries are seen inferiorly, just above and on either side of the allantois. On entering the abdomen, they pass inferiorly on the deep surface of the anterior abdominal wall on either side of the bladder to join their parent trunk, the aorta. After birth, the umbilical arteries become occluded as far proximal as that portion which becomes the internal iliac artery. The fibrous cords representing the remains of the impervious portion are referred to as the lateral umbilical ligaments in the adult.

Normally, the omphalomesenteric duct disappears when the embryo is between 4 and 12 mm. in length, though its vessels persist long after this. At the age indicated, the bowel has already entered the extraembryonic coelom, undergone its rotation and recently re-entered the intraembryonic coelom (peritoneal cavity) and, normally, no vestige of the duct remains. It is depicted in Figure 5 as a patent tube arising from the terminal small bowel, extending to the umbilicus and passing toward the vestigial yolk sac in the extraembryonic coelom. This has been done so that its congenital malformation may be more easily understood.

The allantois, as shown in Figure 5, has differentiated in its most caudal portion into the bladder. In the well-differentiated embryo, its intra-abdominal portion, extending from the apex of the bladder to the umbilicus, is referred to as the urachus. Even in normal embryos, the obliteration of the allantois and the urachus is an irregular phenomenon, and sections at a wide variety of ages may still demonstrate patent segments.

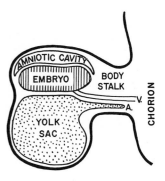

Figure 1. Diagrammatic representation of 0.7-mm. human embryo: A, allantois; V, vascular pedicle.

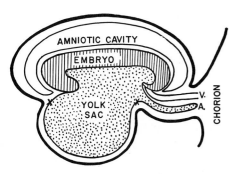

Figure 2. Diagrammatic representation of 1.7-mm. human embryo: A, allantois; V, vascular pedicle.

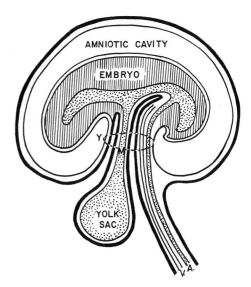

Figure 3. Diagrammatic representation of 3.5-mm. human embryo: A, allantois; M, omphalomesenteric duct; V, vascular pedicle.

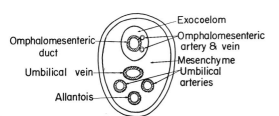

Figure 4. Diagrammatic cross section of umbilical cord of 3.5-mm. human embryo.

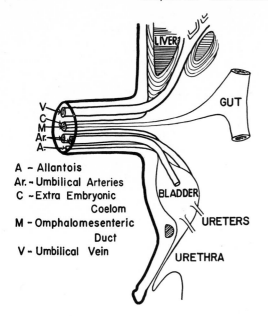

Figure 5. Diagrammatic sagittal section of 5.2-cm. (approximately ten-week) human embryo.

A – Allantois
Ar. – Umbilical Arteries
C – Extra Embryonic
     Coelom
M – Omphalomesenteric
     Duct
V – Umbilical Vein

The Abdominal Wall

Little has been added to our knowledge of the embryology of the abdominal wall since the original researches of Bardeen and Lewis, reported in 1901.

The muscles of the abdominal wall are segmental in origin, arising from the lower thoracic and upper lumbar somites. They arise by differentiation of cells of the myotome which multiply and, in the case of the anterolateral abdominal muscles, migrate into the somatopleure. Here, the muscle fibers take a longitudinal direction, extending between the septa which separate the segments. With further development, muscle fibers of adjacent segments fuse, undergo lamination into layers and, finally, the fibers

of the various laminae modify their direction to conform with the final pattern as seen in the adult. The final step in this process is the fibrous replacement of certain areas of the muscles with formation of their respective aponeuroses. Reference to Figure 6 indicates the source of these muscle fibers.

The basic vasculature of the abdominal wall, too, is derived from the segmental vessels. The arteries arise in pairs from the aorta, contribute a branch to the epaxial muscles, spine and skin of that segment and then course ventrally in the somatopleure to anastomose with the corresponding paired, ventral, longitudinal superior and inferior epigastric vessels. The venous pattern is similar, as is, in essence, the pattern of the

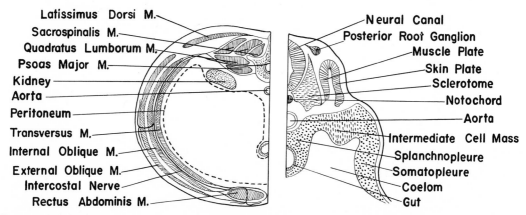

Figure 6. *Left half,* Transverse section showing the structures at the level of the first lumbar segment in the adult. *Right half,* Corresponding section showing diagrammatically the structures of an embryo at three weeks.

peripheral nerves, though no ventral longitudinal nerve completes the analogy.

ANATOMY

The anterior abdominal wall may be looked upon as a laminated structure, of which the middle or myoaponeurotic layer functions as the essential supporting framework. This layer is composed of the anteriorly placed rectus muscles and the laterally situated flat muscles of the abdominal wall, with their aponeuroses. The fibers of the paired recti run longitudinally from the crest of the pubis to their insertion into the cartilages of the fifth, sixth and seventh ribs. Lateral to the recti, and forming what are commonly referred to as the muscles of the anterolateral abdominal wall, are the external oblique, internal oblique and transversus muscles, in that order, from without in. The point at which their muscle fibers become aponeurotic is a feature of some importance. Reference to Figure 7 indicates that the line of transition from muscular to aponeurotic fibers in the case of the external oblique may be represented by a line dropped vertically from the tip of the ninth costal cartilage to join the lateral portion of a line drawn from the anterior superior iliac spine to the umbilicus. In the case of the transversus, the line of transition is indicated by a sigmoid curve, commonly referred to as the linea semilunaris of Spiegel. It is to be noted that in the upper abdomen, muscle fibers of the transversus are found medial to the lateral

border of the rectus, where they contribute to the posterior rectus sheath.

The formation of the rectus sheath superior to the linea semicircularis of Douglas is depicted diagrammatically in the left-hand portion of Figure 6. It may be seen that the aponeurosis of internal oblique splits into two lamellae which enclose, respectively, the anterior and posterior surfaces of the rectus and are joined, in the former instance, by the aponeurosis of external oblique and, in the latter, by the transversus abdominis or its aponeurosis. A feature of some importance surgically is the fact that the aponeurosis of external oblique fuses with the anterior rectus sheath 2 to 3 cm. medial to the lateral margin of the rectus. This fusion allows incision of the deeper of the two leaves of the anterior sheath without disruption of the entire sheath when advancement of portions of the aponeurosis is used in herniorrhaphy. Below the linea semicircularis, which is usually situated about midway between the symphysis pubis and the navel, the aponeuroses of all three anterolateral muscles pass anterior to the rectus muscle, with the result that no posterior sheath exists and the rectus lies on the transversalis fascia. The decussation of the anterior and posterior rectus sheaths in the ventral midline forms the linea alba.

The structures superficial to the myoaponeurotic layer consist of the skin, superficial fascia and deep fascia, from without in. The skin of this area requires little special comment. Cosmetic considerations are seldom of paramount importance in the placement of abdominal incisions, but where they are, the long axis of the incision should parallel the tension lines of Langer.

The superficial fascia of the anterior abdominal wall has a characteristic feature in that the fibrous stroma which supports the fat cells is condensed, in its inferior portion, to form a rather well-defined fibrous layer. This layer replaces the soft fatty tissue in the deepest portion of the superficial fascia and is referred to as Scarpa's fascia. In children, it has occasionally been mistaken by the uninitiated for the aponeurosis of the external oblique muscle during herniorrhaphy. Many surgeons repair it as a separate layer in lower abdominal wound closure.

The deep fascia of the anterior abdominal wall has no peculiar features, save that while it is readily demonstrable over the muscular portion of the external oblique, it becomes

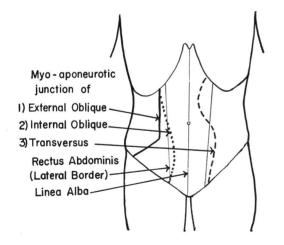

Figure 7. Myoaponeurotic junctions of the anterolateral abdominal muscles.

fused with and inseparable from the apo-neurotic portion of this muscle.

The structures deep to the myoaponeurotic layer consist of the transversalis fascia, the extraperitoneal fat and the peritoneum, from without in. The transversalis fascia is characterized by its firm attachment medially to the posterior rectus sheath, its loose attachment to the transversus abdominis muscle and its uninterrupted continuity posteriorly with the fascia over the quadratus lumborum and psoas muscles. Superiorly, it is continuous with the fascia on the inferior surface of the diaphragm and, inferiorly, with that on the visceral surface of the muscle lining the pelvic cavity.

The distribution of the nerves of the abdominal wall is of importance. The lower five intercostal nerves and subcostal nerve pass downward and medially in the plane between the internal oblique and transversus muscles. They pierce the posterior leaflet of the aponeurosis of the internal oblique muscle at the lateral margin of the rectus sheath, continue their course posterior to the rectus muscle and terminate by supplying branches to this muscle and the overlying skin. The distribution of the iliohypogastric and ilioinguinal nerves from the first lumbar segment is slightly different. They pierce the internal oblique muscle just medial to the anterior superior spine, and thus lie in the plane between the internal oblique muscle and the aponeurosis of the external oblique, in which situation they are displayed at herniorrhaphy.

The segmental arteries, the posterior intercostal and lumbar branches of the aorta, follow the distribution of the corresponding nerves and terminate in anastomoses deep to the rectus muscle with the superior and inferior epigastric arteries. In their course, they anastomose with the ascending branch of the deep circumflex iliac artery deep to the internal oblique muscle. The veins of the abdominal wall course with their corresponding arteries.

The lymphatic drainage of the abdominal wall is of importance with regard to the spread of infections and malignant disease (Fig. 8). On the right-hand side of the figure, the superficial drainage is shown. A line drawn around the body, from just above the umbilicus to the disk between the second and third lumbar vertebrae, separates the superior from the inferior watershed. The medial portion of the superior watershed drains into the pectoral group and the lateral portion

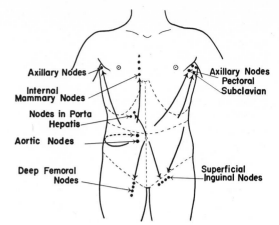

Figure 8. Lymphatic drainage of the abdominal wall. *Right half,* Drainage of superficial structures. *Left half,* Drainage of deep structures.

into the subscapular group of the axillary nodes. The inferior watershed, including the integumentum of the umbilicus, drains into the superficial inguinal nodes. There are no significant anastomoses between the superficial lymphatics of the left and right sides of the abdominal wall except at the umbilicus.

The lymphatic drainage of the deep structures of the abdominal wall is shown on the left half of the figure. The lymphatics are seen to course to the internal mammary, the axillary, the abdominal aortic and the deep femoral nodes from fairly well-defined areas of the wall. Again, the unilaterality of the lymphatic drainage is preserved except for the area immediately around the umbilicus. The umbilical lymphatics communicate freely with channels which pass to all four drainage areas bilaterally and also, by means of lymphatics traveling along the round ligament of the liver, drainage may be to nodes in the porta hepatis.

CONGENITAL ABNORMALITIES

Abnormalities of the Muscles of the Abdominal Wall

Agenesis or absence of the muscles of the abdominal wall is a rare abnormality and extreme deficiency rather than absence would appear to be a more appropriate term. It has been noted that the transversus abdominis, the portion of the rectus abdominis below the navel, the internal oblique, the external oblique and the rectus abdominis above the navel are affected, in decreasing order of frequency. An interesting sex incidence is recorded in that only two of 45 acceptable instances occurred in female children. Associated lesions of the urinary tract are very common and considerable discussion centers around which of the two lesions is the primary one. Congenital malformations of the gastrointestinal tract, mainly in the form of malrotation, occur in at least 20 per cent of patients. Respiratory and urinary infections have been the most common fatal complications. Treatment consists of external support to the abdominal wall, early surgical correction of associated urinary and gastrointestinal abnormalities, and general measures directed toward the maintenance of an optimal nutritional state and the prevention of complicating infections.

Abnormalities in the Region of the Umbilicus

OMPHALOMESENTERIC DUCT ANOMALIES (Fig. 9). Meckel's diverticulum is by far the most common lesion in this class, occurring in some 2 to 4 per cent of persons. Instances of completely patent omphalomesenteric duct are extremely rare. The diagnosis should be suspected in a newborn infant presenting with a reddish, moist, pouting collection of intestinal mucosa at the navel. The intestinal origin of the tissue, as opposed to the more common umbilical granulation, may be suspected by the clinical demonstration of the mucoid nature of its secretion. Intestinal mucosa may, of course, also occur at the navel in association with umbilical polyps and umbilical sinuses, but these three can usually be differentiated by judicious probing and by means of x-ray examination following Lipiodol injection of the sinus, if one exists. The diagnosis is immediately confirmed if, on crying or straining, the infant is observed to pass gas or discharge fecal material from the navel.

Complacency should be avoided in those instances in which normal gastrointestinal tract function appears to exist in the presence of a completely patent omphalomesenteric duct. Ileal prolapse may occur suddenly and rapidly endanger life. The degrees of ileal prolapse are illustrated in Figure 10. The treatment consists of complete excision of the umbilicus and the tract. The ileum is closed transversely following longitudinal excision of the tract from its wall. When the

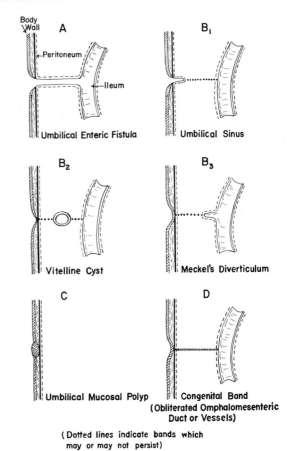

Figure 9. Congenital omphalomesenteric duct anomalies.

operation is carried out before ileal prolapse with vascular embarrassment has occurred, the mortality is minimal.

Umbilical sinuses and polyps are treated by excision. Vitelline cysts are usually asymptomatic unless obstruction occurs around the congenital band which joins them to the ileum or to the navel. Small cysts situated close to the navel or within the abdominal wall, or larger cysts occurring more proximally along the duct, may be palpable. The only satisfactory treatment is excision.

Congenital bands, of either omphalomesenteric duct or vascular origin, are of importance only as an etiologic factor in intestinal obstruction. Bremer makes the interesting observation that a band derived from the obliterated omphalomesenteric artery corresponds in position to that shown for the congenital band in D of Figure 9, while that derived from the corresponding vein runs, not to the antimesenteric border of the bowel, but rather to the base of the mesentery at a more proximal level, or to the porta hepatis.

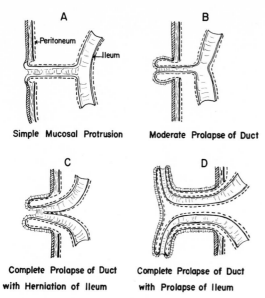

Figure 10. Degrees of prolapse associated with completely patent omphalomesenteric duct.

URACHAL ANOMALIES (Fig. 11). Congenital, completely patent urachus is characterized clinically by the intermittent discharge of urine from the navel, the quantity and the frequency depending on the caliber of the fistula and the presence or absence

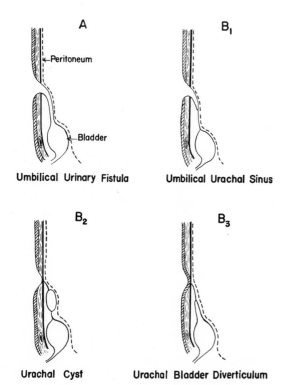

Figure 11. Congenital urachal anomalies.

of some degree of obstruction of the lower urinary tract. A small granular tumor may mark the site of the ostium at the umbilicus, or the navel may appear normal on superficial examination. No symptoms, apart from the discharge, are associated with the anomaly unless infection occurs. Surgical excision is the only satisfactory treatment, but this should be performed only after the patency of the urethra has been confirmed. The entire tract is excised and the site of attachment to the bladder is ligated and inverted with a purse-string suture. In the absence of preexisting infection, the procedure can usually be accomplished extraperitoneally with minimal risk.

In the so-called acquired type of completely patent urachus, no abnormality is apparent at birth and only at some later date does intermittent discharge of urine occur. This condition is almost invariably associated with lower urinary obstruction which forces urine through an incompletely obliterated urachal channel. Treatment is excision following correction of the obstructing lesion. The acquired type of anomaly is more common than the congenital type.

Umbilical urachal sinuses present no additional features except that the discharge is minimal and watery and is not urine. Treatment consists of surgical excision.

Urachal cysts are the most common urachal abnormality. If uninfected they are usually asymptomatic and, when small, are recognized only at surgery or autopsy as an incidental finding. Larger cysts may be apparent to the patient as a subumbilical fullness or swelling, or may be discovered incidentally by the surgeon in the course of abdominal examination. Infection is common and this is the usual method of clinical presentation. The symptoms are those of an acute inflammation deep in the subumbilical abdominal wall. In patients in whom the cyst is not infected, extraperitoneal excision is the treatment of choice and usually presents no difficulties unless the cyst is of large size. It is wise in such instances to demonstrate the cord, which almost invariably runs from the cyst to the bladder, and to deal with it as though it were patent. This precaution is also desirable with umbilical urachal sinus. Excision without peritoneal contamination of infected urchal cysts is virtually impossible; treatment should be restricted to incision, drainage and loose packing of the cavity with gauze. Frequently, as a result of the infection, the transitional epithelium of the wall of the cyst is destroyed and the simple drainage procedure results in permanent cure.

VASCULAR ANOMALIES. Vascular anomalies involving the omphalomesenteric vessels are rare and of little clinical significance. Aberrations in the normal fate of the umbilical vessels are apparently rare if one excludes the possibility that portal vein obstruction may be due to extension into that vessel of the obliterative process that is normally limited to the umbilical vein and ductus venosus. Anomalies of the urachal vessels are apparently of little or no clinical significance.

SOMATIC ANOMALIES. Omphalocele, umbilical hernia and exstrophy of the urinary bladder are somatic anomalies which occur frequently enough to require serious consideration for surgical treatment.

Endometriosis of the umbilicus is rare. It usually presents as a small mass at the umbilicus which enlarges and becomes tender at the time of the menstrual period. External bleeding may also occur. Treatment is by simple excision. Coexistent pelvic endometriosis will require separate treatment.

INFECTIONS OF THE ABDOMINAL WALL

Infections of the abdominal wall proper are essentially similar to superficial infections occurring elsewhere in the body. Progressive bacterial synergistic gangrene and other relatively rare infections of this area may produce serious postoperative complications.

Infections of the Umbilicus

OMPHALITIS IN THE NEWBORN. While this condition is much less common now than 25 or more years ago, it may be a serious lesion and, therefore, demands prompt recognition and treatment. It usually arises as a result of contamination of the cord at the time of section or during subsequent dressing of the umbilicus. The common organisms are the *Staphylococcus aureus* and the hemolytic streptococcus. The widespread lymphatic drainage and the persistence of patent vascular channels in this area account for the rapid dissemination of the infection.

Locally, the condition is manifest by redness, heat, swelling and tenderness which may spread centrifugally from the navel with alarming rapidity. Usually, pus exudes from the folds of the umbilicus. Occasionally, widespread sloughing of skin occurs. Blood stream invasion may occur along the incompletely obliterated umbilical vein or umbilical arteries with signs of septicemia. Spread sometimes occurs to the adjacent peritoneum with signs of fulminating peritonitis.

Treatment of the omphalitis must be initiated promptly with antibiotics, local hot moist compresses and surgical incision of any purulent collections. The localized type of omphalitis usually responds rapidly to treatment, but once septicemia or peritonitis has occurred the outlook is grave.

OMPHALITIS IN THE ADULT. Unlike neonatal omphalitis, umbilical infections in the adult tend to pursue a relatively benign and chronic course. They are commonly seen in office practice but seldom require hospital care. The one common etiologic factor in almost all patients appears to be neglect of personal hygiene in this area. Congenital aberrations in the depth and configuration of the umbilicus may contribute by making cleansing of the area difficult.

The usual complaints are of tenderness in or around the navel and the presence of a seropurulent discharge with an offensive odor. Examination reveals the base of the umbilicus thrown up into a cluster of red, moist, swollen, angry-looking folds which exude the offensive discharge. Extension into periumbilical tissues is uncommon but may occur along with inguinal adenitis.

In the acute phase, omphalitis usually responds rapidly to warm, moist saline compresses. Antibiotics are seldom indicated unless systemic manifestations ensue. Once the acute symptoms have subsided, the patient should be instructed to wash the umbilicus carefully while bathing and dry it with equal care afterward. Gentle cleansing with alcohol-dipped absorbent cotton on the end of an applicator is a useful means of eliminating moisture and excoriation in deep clefts.

TRAUMA TO THE ABDOMINAL WALL

Injuries to the abdominal wall often tax the diagnostic acumen of the examiner. The major problem is to differentiate those lesions limited to the wall from those traumatic intra-abdominal lesions which may rapidly endanger life and for which immediate surgical intervention is mandatory.

Wounds of the abdominal wall, as opposed to blunt trauma where no open wound exists, may be considered under two broad headings. By convention, involvement of the peritoneum is considered the dividing line between these two types of injury.

Nonpenetrating wounds involve only the abdominal wall proper. Like wounds elsewhere, they show all gradations from clean incised wounds to gaping defects with much loss of tissue. In depth, they vary from disruption of skin continuity alone to involvement of all layers including muscle. Apart from those wounds associated with considerable loss of tissue, where some type of plastic procedure may be necessary, the treatment of nonpenetrating abdominal wounds is similar to that of wounds elsewhere in the body and follows the principles laid down for the surgical care of soft tissues.

Penetrating wounds constitute an entirely different problem. Such injuries occur mainly as a result of gunshot and stab wounds, although almost every conceivable foreign body has at some time been recorded as the traumatizing agent. Not all gunshot and stab wounds are, of course, penetrating. Loria, reviewing a series of 4341 such patients encountered at the New Orleans Charity Hospital, reports approximately two-thirds to be penetrating and one-third to be nonpenetrating. There is rather universal agreement, however, that unless such a puncture type of wound is very obviously nonpenetrating, it should receive prompt surgical attention. In penetrating trauma, the injury to the abdominal wall is usually of minor importance and the demonstration and correction of the intra-abdominal component are the prime considerations.

It is usually unwise to attempt to probe the wound tract. If the depth of the wound cannot be determined, it is far better to examine the parietal peritoneum through a planned, initially small incision adjacent to the wound. This incision may be closed, if the peritoneum is intact, or rapidly extended to give wide access to the abdominal cavity, if peritoneal penetration has occurred. When wounds of entrance and exit exist, the incision is selected which will give the best access to the anticipated intraperitoneal damage, and no attempt should be made to incorporate such wounds into the incision. On completion of the intraperi-

toneal procedure and after consideration of the condition of the patient, the puncture wounds may be either simply cleansed and dressed or excised and closed, depending on their character and degree of contamination.

Blunt trauma to the abdomen is linked in the minds of surgeons with the multitude of puzzling intra-abdominal lesions which so frequently accompany this form of injury, and little attention is usually given to isolated abdominal wall lesions which may occur. Contusion and hematomas of the subcutaneous tissue and muscle layers are common but seldom are of serious significance or require more than symptomatic treatment. Their main interest stems from the pain and muscle spasm which they produce and which must be differentiated from similar symptoms and signs produced reflexly by intra-abdominal injury. Occasionally, as a result of blunt trauma, subcutaneous rupture of the muscles of the abdominal wall occurs without disruption of the skin.

Spasm of the Muscles of the Abdominal Wall

Spasm of muscles of the abdominal wall, particularly the rectus abdominis, is a common finding on examination. A relatively simple classification of the causes of abdominal wall spasm includes:

Central or cerebral origin:
Organic, as seen in spastic paraplegia. Psychogenic, as seen in the nervous patient, the patient anticipating some painful experience and in psychopathic drug addiction.

Spinal cord origin, as seen in those diseases characterized by irritation of spinal cord neurons, as for example tabes dorsalis.

Thoracic nerve trunk origin, as seen in pleurisy, infections of the chest wall, chest and spinal column injury, epidemic pleurodynia and severe alcoholic neuritis.

Reflex origin, as seen when the peritoneum is irritated by infection, blood or foreign material or when juxtaperitoneal organs are the origin of extremely painful stimuli, as in renal colic.

Local origin, as seen in local trauma to, or infection of, the abdominal wall.

While peritonitis, in its broadest sense, is by far the most common cause of true abdominal wall rigidity, the interpretation of this finding after abdominal trauma is of extreme importance. It may arise, on the one hand, from a relatively benign injury to the abdominal wall or, on the other, from a grave intraperitoneal insult which will be rapidly fatal if surgical treatment is withheld. It should be possible in every patient to differentiate these two on a basis of complete and careful abdominal examination.

Abdominal wall rigidity, as an early manifestation of purely thoracic wounds, is now well recognized. Frequently the rigidity, which is usually ipsilateral but may be bilateral, is associated with subcostal tenderness of such intensity, in the early hours after injury, that one is tempted to carry out a laparotomy with a diagnosis of ruptured intra-abdominal viscus. The knowledge that this syndrome may exist, along with the absence of signs of peritoneal contamination, should enable one to avoid needless laparotomy. The abdominal findings rarely persist over 48 to 72 hours.

The converse situation is frequently observed, namely, unilateral restriction of movement of the thoracic cage and diminished air entry into the base of the lung on that side, following injury restricted to the abdominal wall. Percussion of the chest along with radiologic examination will quickly clarify the situation.

Hematoma of the Rectus Sheath

In recent years, this uncommon condition has aroused much interest because of the fact that it may mimic acute intra-abdominal disease. It is seldom diagnosed preoperatively because it is not considered. In approximately 90 per cent of instances, the hematoma is situated below the navel; it lies to the right of the midline about twice as often as it does to the left. The frequent occurrence of the hematoma below the semicircular line of Douglas, causing peritoneal irritation, is considered to account for the gastrointestinal manifestations which are often seen. It is seldom possible to demonstrate the exact site of hemorrhage, but the inferior epigastric vein is more commonly the source than the artery.

There is general agreement that the condition is more frequent during pregnancy. Even in this group, it is usually possible to elicit a history of indirect trauma or upper respiratory infection with cough as the immediate cause of the hemorrhage. Apart from pregnancy, the patients may be broadly classified into those associated with:

Trauma, either direct or indirect, of which the latter is far more common.

Infections and *debilitating disease,* in which case a severe paroxysm of coughing is often the immediate cause of the hemorrhage.

Degenerative vascular disease, blood dyscrasias and *abnormalities of coagulation,* including an increasing number of cases ascribed to anticoagulant therapy.

The postoperative patient, in whom the injudicious positioning of rectus muscle retractors or retention sutures is usually the cause.

Idiopathic, which implies a lesion that can occur spontaneously without associated disease or injury. This appears most unlikely and it is probable that one of the above factors is present, though overlooked, in patients so classified.

The symptomatology is classic. Following trauma, which may be mild or severe, there is usually a rather sudden onset of excruciating abdominal pain. When bleeding occurs slowly, the pain will be more gradual in onset and of less severity. It is usually localized to the site of rupture but may be generalized. Nausea and vomiting are relatively common and constipation may occur. Characteristically, after a period of increased pain, there is a gradual improvement which leaves in its wake a persistent dull ache.

Apart from the occasional patient who appears acutely ill and shocked, the significant findings are limited to the abdomen. A hard, exquisitely tender mass may be palpated in one or the other rectus, which may be misinterpreted as localized muscle spasm. If one demonstrates that the mass is restricted to the confines of the rectus sheath and that tenderness and rigidity in the adjacent lateral abdominal muscles are lacking, the diagnosis is supported.

Fothergill has described a sign which assists in differentiating abdominal wall masses from those arising within the peritoneal cavity. When the recti are contracted, as in attempting to sit up, a mass situated in the wall may still be felt and is fixed, while an intra-abdominal mass is no longer easily palpable. An additional late sign is the appearance of ecchymosis about the umbilicus.

The hematoma is usually accompanied by a mild elevation of temperature and pulse and moderate polymorphonuclear leukocytosis is common, further simulating acute intra-abdominal disease.

The natural history of the disease is usually one of spontaneous recovery, with cessation of pain after a few days and gradual disappearance of the mass in the course of three to four weeks. Occasionally, the hematoma becomes infected and forms an abscess or persists and calcifies to give rise to continuing pain.

Some surgeons feel that the safest and surest treatment is to confirm the diagnosis by means of a short paramedian incision, evacuate the clot and ligate the epigastric artery and vein above and below the assumed point of hemorrhage. It is our belief that most of these patients can be successfully managed conservatively. It should be pointed out that some patients will be operated upon in error with a preoperative diagnosis of appendicitis or some other intra-abdominal lesion. In this group, surgical control of the hemorrhage is readily carried out.

TUMORS OF THE ABDOMINAL WALL

Tumors of the abdominal wall frequently present unique problems which warrant their study as an isolated group.

Benign Tumors

Benign tumors constitute 60 per cent of all neoplasms and 80 per cent of the primary neoplasms of the abdominal wall, according to Pack and Ehrlich. In order of frequency, the more common types of benign tumors encountered are lipomas, neuronevi, hemangiomas, epithelial papillomas, fibromas, neurofibromas, keratoses and desmoid tumors. Lipomas, constituting 20 per cent of the benign neoplasms, are the most common.

The treatment of these lesions is similar to that recommended in other situations and presents no special problem. Lipomas, papillomas, fibromas and keratoses are treated by simple excision. Hemangiomas should be excised when the lesion occurs in the abdominal wall, since cure is rapidly achieved and the resulting scar is of little consequence.

Neurofibromas of the solitary type are easily excised surgically, but in over half the patients in whom this lesion presents in the abdominal wall it takes the form of the plexiform von Recklinghausen type. This lesion, with its known predisposition to malignant transformation, is often extensive and invasive and requires wide excision, sometimes in stages.

Nevi of the abdominal wall must be treated with considerable respect. A number of pigmented nevi may be malignant melanomas. A high percentage of melanomas follow chronic irritation of a pre-existing mole. It is obvious that any such lesion should be widely excised surgically, especially if it presents in an area in which irritation from a belt, girdle or other clothing occurs.

Desmoid Tumors

Desmoid tumors are essentially hard, non-encapsulated fibromas arising from the deep fascial and myoaponeurotic layers of the anterior abdominal wall. They are characteristically infiltrative and may attain large size. The etiology is unknown. The preponderance in the female, frequently within a year of parturition, has led to the suggestion that stretching of the abdominal wall during pregnancy, or some gestational endocrine factor, may be important etiologically. However, their occurrence in the male and in the nulliparous female would tend to minimize the etiologic significance of pregnancy. A history of antecedent trauma is also rare, but their occurrence in laparotomy scars is too frequent to be dismissed as incidental.

Clinically, the patient usually presents complaining of the presence of an abdominal mass or a sensation of weight in the abdomen. Less commonly, a vague feeling of pressure on the bladder or bizarre abdominal pains may cause the patient to seek advice. On examination, a mass is usually palpated deep to the skin and unattached to it. Characteristically, it is firm, smooth and discrete. Bouchacourt's sign, which is similar to that of Fothergill but applies to intramural masses situated anywhere in the anterior abdominal wall, is helpful in localizing the mass to the muscular layer of the abdominal wall. The rectus abdominis is the muscle most commonly affected, but the infiltrative nature of the tumor frequently results in multiple muscle involvement.

The gross pathologic features of the tumor are its denseness and hardness, its glistening white or pinkish color and its apparent infiltrative character. Microscopically, it varies from an acellular fibroma to a low-grade cellular fibrosarcoma and the inclusion at its periphery of engulfed and sequestrated degenerating muscle fibers is characteristic.

Desmoid tumors are clinically benign and metastases do not occur. Local recurrence is the rule, unless excision has been complete. Treatment is by wide surgical resection which, because of the large size of some of these tumors, often results in defects which require plastic procedures for closure. The place of radiation therapy in the management of these tumors is controversial and no opinion as to its value is possible at this time.

Malignant Tumors

Malignant tumors constitute about one third of all neoplasms of the abdominal wall, and secondary malignant tumors are as common as primary malignant growths. This is in marked contrast to other soft tissue areas, where secondary deposits are extremely rare. The initial presentation of malignant lymphoma may be an abdominal wall mass.

PRIMARY MALIGNANT TUMORS. Of this group approximately one-half are sarcomas. The more common sarcomas, in order of frequency, are neurogenic sarcoma, spindle cell sarcoma, synovioma and rhabdomyosarcoma. Carcinomas are mainly epidermoid in type, with occasional basal cell lesions and very rarely an adenocarcinoma.

Most sarcomas arise from the deeper layers of the wall and not infrequently give rise to blood-borne metastases, though lymph node involvement does not occur. As a group, these sarcomas tend to be radioresistant and the treatment, if treatment is possible, consists of wide excision of the full thickness of the abdominal wall, including the peritoneum. Synoviomas and rhabdomyosarcomas appear to have a particularly unfavorable prognosis.

Carcinoma of the skin of the abdominal wall is relatively uncommon, as compared with its occurrence elsewhere in the body. It does, however, present some interesting and rather unusual features when it occurs in this situation. Epidermoid carcinoma may arise in an area of pre-existing tissue abnormality, such as an abdominal scar, an abdominal sinus or an area of radiation dermatitis. Epidermoid carcinoma, arising in normal skin, has a relatively good prognosis following total surgical removal. Superficial

lymphatics are scarce in the abdominal wall and lymph node metastases are unusual. Epidermoid carcinoma arising in laparotomy scars and postoperative draining sinuses is a clinical entity with an extremely grave prognosis, for while lymph node metastases are rare, early extensive involvement of the peritoneum is common.

Melanomas appear to be relatively uncommon in the abdominal wall. These lesions appear to have a predilection for the area about the umbilicus, which is a most undesirable situation from the standpoint of facility of lymphatic and venous spread. Melanoma carries with it a grave prognosis and since these lesions are rarely radiosensitive, radical surgical excision is the only available treatment which offers any hope of eradication of the disease. Wide local excision of the lesion is mandatory and this, at the umbilicus, includes ample excision of the full thickness of the abdominal wall and the round ligament of the liver. Block dissection of lymphatic glands in areas of apparent spread should be carried out. If the lesion is situated in a quadrant of the abdomen where its lymphatic drainage can be predicted with assurance, then block dissection of the regional lymphatics should be carried out even in the absence of clinically demonstrable metastases. The principle of excision of the primary lesion with dissection of the regional lymphatic nodes in continuity can frequently be effectively employed in the case of the abdominal wall.

SECONDARY MALIGNANT TUMORS. There is a relatively frequent occurrence of secondary malignant spread to the abdominal wall in contrast to the infrequency of such spread to other soft tissue areas. The source of the metastatic deposit is most commonly a carcinoma. According to Pack and Ehrlich, the common sources in order of frequency are the ovary, stomach, uterus, bronchus, kidney, breast and sigmoid colon. Metastatic carcinoma of the abdominal wall most commonly occurs in the region of the umbilicus.

An interesting story is often told in this connection. Sister Joseph, who was in charge of St. Mary's Hospital in Rochester, and who functioned as the able assistant to Dr. William Mayo in the early days of the Mayo Clinic, is said to have initially drawn to Dr. Mayo's attention her observation that, in the preparation of patients for gastric operations, she occasionally noted a very firm mass at the patient's umbilicus. She further observed that patients so afflicted did particularly poorly following operation. This astute observation is often acknowledged by applying the term "Sister Joseph's sign" to the demonstration of umbilical metastatic deposits in patients with intra-abdominal malignancy.

The presence of secondary malignant deposits in the abdominal wall, with one notable exception, is a sign of advanced disease and inoperability. The one exception is the implantation carcinoma which is occasionally seen in the scars of operations carried out for malignant disease. These lesions, surprisingly, do not tend to invade the peritoneal cavity and while lymph node metastases may occur, wide surgical excision of the implanted lesion, along with block dissection of involved nodes, may be rewarded by long-term survival.

THE PERITONEUM

EMBRYOLOGY

The primitive coelom is partially divided by the septum transversum, or future diaphragm, into a pericardial cavity and a peritoneal cavity in the fourth week of intrauterine life. For a time, the two cavities communicate over the dorsal edge of the thick septum transversum by the paired pleural canals (Fig. 12). By the seventh week, the peritoneal cavity is completely separated from the pleural canals by the pleural-peritoneal membranes.

Initially, the peritoneal cavity is separated into right and left halves by the primitive gut and its mesentery. The mesentery is designated as ventral or dorsal, according to its relationship to the gut (Fig. 13). The ventral mesentery then disappears, except for the lesser omentum and falciform ligament, its contributions to the diaphragm

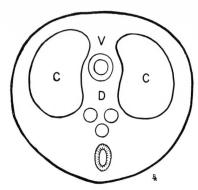

Figure 13. Cross section through the level of the foregut. The peritoneal portion of the coelom (C) is initially divided into two cavities by the gut, the transient ventral mesentery (V) and the dorsal mesentery (D).

and the suspensory ligament of the bladder. With resorption of the greater part of the ventral mesentery, the coelom becomes a single cavity.

That portion of the gut which will become the second part of the duodenum gives rise to two evaginations (Fig. 14). Into the ventral mesentery grows the hepatic diverticulum, from which branches the accessory pancreas. Into the dorsal mesentery grows the diverticulum which is to become the main pancreas. In the dorsal mesogastrium, the spleen develops in relation to blood vessels, not the lymphatics, and then bulges into the left leaf of the mesentery (Fig. 15).

The mesenteries of the foregut shift their attachments as the stomach rotates 90 degrees on a long axis and as overgrowth takes place on the greater curvature side (Fig. 16). The ventral mesentery, bearing the hepatic diverticulum, shifts to the right and cranially to become the lesser omentum.

The rotation of the foregut is accompanied by a modification in the attachment of its dorsal mesentery. In its cranial portion, in which the spleen is developing, the rotation of the stomach carries the dorsal mesogastrium to the left with its contained spleen. Fusion of a portion of the left leaf of the dorsal mesogastrium with the posterior parietal peritoneum results in the apparent origin of the dorsal mesogastrium, gastrolienal and lienorenal ligaments, from a site well to the left of the midline in this situation. Immediately caudal to the spleen containing dorsal mesogastrium, the ballooned-out mesogastrium overlaps the transverse colon and its mesocolon and subsequently fuses with the latter. Its further overgrowth in this situation and the subsequent fusion of its adjacent

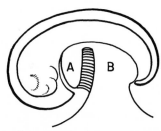

Figure 12. Parasagittal section of an embryo at four weeks. The thick septum transversum divides the coelom into the pericardial cavity (A) and the peritoneal cavity (B). The two cavities communicate over the dorsal aspect of the septum transversum by means of the pleural canals.

Figure 14. Cross section through that level of the gut destined to become the second part of the duodenum. There is no ventral mesentery at this level and the peritoneal cavity is a continuous space. The hepatic diverticulum (H) arises by evagination ventrally and will give rise to the ventral contribution to the pancreas and to the biliary tree and liver. The pancreatic diverticulum (P) arises by dorsal evagination and forms the major portion of the pancreas.

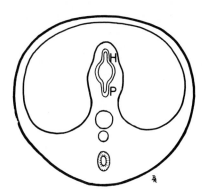

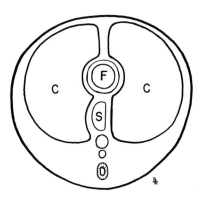

Figure 15. Cross section somewhat cranial to that shown in Figure 14. The peritoneal cavity lies on either side of that portion of the foregut (F) destined to become the stomach. The spleen arises in the dorsal mesogastrium. The hepatic diverticulum, after giving off the ventral pancreas, will grow cranially in the ventral mesogastrium and septum transversum to give rise to the liver. The pancreatic diverticulum will extend cranially in the dorsal mesogastrium and come to lie dorsal to the spleen. Subsequent rotation of the stomach with its mesenteries will cause these structures to lie to the right (liver) and left (spleen and pancreas) of the stomach.

Figure 16. Cross section through a four-month fetus at approximately the level shown in Figure 15. The liver and pancreas have grown cranially from their points of origin shown in Figure 14. Rotation has converted the right half of the peritoneal cavity shown in Figure 15 into the lesser sac. It can be seen that fundamentally the spleen and pancreas lie in the dorsal mesentery of the stomach.

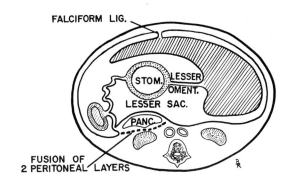

Figure 17. Diagrammatic sagittal section through a fetus, showing the relations of the greater and lesser peritoneal sacs. The two layers of the greater omentum have not yet fused. Basically the greater omentum is the dorsal mesentery of the stomach which has fused with the transverse mesocolon.

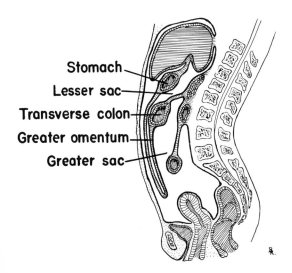

layers forms the greater omentum (Fig. 17) which, therefore, appears to gain attachment to both stomach and transverse colon. More caudal still, the dorsal mesogastrium containing the pancreatic diverticulum is carried to the right as a result of displacement of the duodenum. In this situation, there is more extensive fusion of the right leaf of the dorsal mesogastrium with the parietal peritoneum, as a result of which both pancreas and second portion of duodenum assume a retroperitoneal position.

ANATOMY

GROSS ANATOMY. The peritoneal cavity was mentioned in the *Papyrus Ebers* some 3500 years ago, but it was not thoroughly described until 1730, when James Douglas of Edinburgh published a lucid account which has not been appreciably improved upon to this day.

The peritoneum is a serous membrane which lines the peritoneal cavity and invests a number of abdominal structures. Except for the openings of the fallopian tubes, the peritoneum is a completely closed sac. In a strict sense, the peritoneal cavity does not contain any organs, since the entire gastrointestinal tract and its derivatives are really retroperitoneal in position. It is customary to speak of those structures which are almost completely enfolded by peritoneum, such as stomach, jejunum, ileum, transverse colon, sigmoid colon, appendix, cecum, liver, gallbladder and spleen, as being intraperitoneal.

That portion of the peritoneum which invests the intraperitoneal organs, and which makes up the coverings of the mesenteries, is the visceral peritoneum. That portion which lines the anterior, lateral and posterior abdominal walls, the undersurface of the diaphragm and the floor of the pelvis is the parietal peritoneum. Although these are parts of the same membrane, the distinction is of some importance in regard to differences in sensory innervation. The peritoneum of the anterior and lateral abdominal wall is reinforced by the transversalis fascia.

The peritoneal cavity is divided into the general peritoneal cavity, or greater sac, and the lesser sac (Fig. 17). The latter has, as its only natural opening, the foramen of Winslow. It is bounded anteriorly by gastrohepatic ligament, stomach and gastrocolic ligament and by parietal peritoneum posteriorly.

Hanging from the transverse colon, and covering much of the ventral aspect of the lower abdominal viscera, is the greater omentum. This structure has a rich vascular supply and carries a variable amount of fat.

The surface area of the peritoneum is about 2 square meters and approximates that of the skin. Unlike skin, however, the peritoneum is a highly permeable membrane. This fact has a number of important physiologic implications.

Normally, the peritoneal cavity contains 75 to 100 cc. of clear, straw-colored fluid, which facilitates the normal lubricating function of the membrane.

MICROSCOPIC ANATOMY. The peritoneum consists of a surface layer of mesothelium and a deeper, loose connective-tissue layer containing collagen and elastic fibers, fat cells, reticulum cells and macrophages. The mesothelium is a simple squamous cell layer. As a result of irritation, these cells may become cuboidal and enclose small cystic spaces, a reaction which the pathologist must distinguish from neoplasia.

Normal peritoneal fluid contains 2000 to 2500 cells per cubic millimeter. The majority of these are macrophages with some desquamated mesothelial cells and lymphocytes. There are few polymorphonuclear neutrophils or eosinophils, but the number of granulocytes is greatly increased in the presence of inflammation. Peritoneal aspiration may be of value, not only to obtain fluid for culture and chemical analysis, but also because immediate study of the cells in the fluid may facilitate the diagnosis of tumors, inflammatory conditions and intraperitoneal trauma.

PHYSIOLOGY

RELATION TO EXTRACELLULAR FLUID COMPARTMENT. Since the peritoneum is a highly permeable membrane of considerable surface area, peritoneal fluid is a physiologically active collection constituting part of the extracellular fluid. Deuterium oxide placed in the peritoneal cavity very rapidly becomes equilibrated with the plasma and interstitial fluid of the patient. The intraperitoneal route of fluid administration is used in experimental animals. Not only are water, electrolytes and urea rapidly transported across the peritoneal membrane, but endogenous and exogenous toxic substances are freely absorbed. Rapid absorption of bacterial toxins is one of several reasons for the very high mortality in untreated peritonitis. In bowel obstruction with distention and impairment of circulation, transperitoneal absorption of bacterial toxins, even without peritonitis, is probable. It has been proved by the introduction of antibiotics and iron-dextran into the peritoneal cavity that the peritoneum is an efficient absorbing surface.

In addition to the intimate relation of peritoneum to the circulating blood, there are communications between the peritoneal and pleural cavities which appear to be independent of the blood stream. In patients with Meigs' syndrome, colloidal radioactive gold (Au[198]) instilled into one serous sac rapidly appears in the other, probably as a result of transdiaphragmatic lymphatic transport.

SENSORY INNERVATION. The parietal peritoneum is well supplied with somatic afferent nerves and is sensitive to all forms of stimuli. This is particularly true of the anterior parietal peritoneum, which, along with the rest of the anterior abdominal wall, is supplied by the lower six thoracic nerves. The parietal peritoneum posteriorly and in the pelvis is somewhat less sensitive. The ability of the parietal peritoneum of the anterior abdominal wall to initiate the sensation of sharp pain in response to an adjacent inflammatory process and to permit localization of its origin is of the utmost importance in the diagnosis of acute abdominal conditions. In the case of the parietal peritoneum of the diaphragm, irritation of the peripheral portion is perceived in the vicinity of the adjacent body wall whereas that of the central portion is referred to the shoulder as a result of central misinterpretation. The sharp, well localized pain of parietal peritoneal irritation is in marked contrast to that which arises from the relatively insensitive visceral peritoneum.

In addition to causing sharp and well localized pain, stimulation of the parietal peritoneum may cause involuntary rigidity of the abdominal musculature, tenderness, and rebound tenderness, if the stimulus is sufficiently intense. These characteristics identify the parietal peritoneum as the source of the pain, identify the pain stimuli as being inflammatory and localize the site of the stimuli. Without the pain fibers of the parietal peritoneum, the clinical diagnosis of an acute abdomen would be impossible.

The visceral peritoneum is relatively insensitive, but it does register stimuli if they are sufficiently strong or prolonged, particularly in the presence of pre-existing inflammation. The root of the mesentery is quite sensitive to traction.

Most visceral afferent nerve fibers for pain run in the splanchnic nerves to the same six segments of the cord that receive somatic afferent fibers. The stimulus of visceral sensation is usually tension, whether the result of increased intraluminal pressure or increased tissue pressure from inflammation. Visceral pain is usually dull and vaguely localized to the central portion of the abdomen, although there are some exceptions to this rule, notably visceral pain initiated by the biliary tree.

Healing of Peritoneal Defects

The speed with which intra-abdominal areas denuded of peritoneum rapidly undergo reperitonealization has long been a source of wonder to surgeons. Available evidence suggests that reperitonealization may be accomplished in one of, or a combination of, three ways. Firstly, the denuded area may be seeded by viable mesothelial cells shed from adjacent peritoneal surfaces, which subsequently proliferate to form islands which coalesce. Secondly, the surface may be covered by ingrowth of mesothelium from intact adjacent peritoneum. Finally, there is evidence that blood monocytes and tissue histiocytes may be capable of migrating to the denuded surface from deeper layers and then differentiating to form mesothelial cells.

INFLAMMATION OF THE PERITONEUM

Peritonitis is an inflammation of the peritoneum. The process may be acute or chronic, it may be septic or aseptic and it may be primary or secondary. The most frequently encountered type is an acute bacterial inflammation of the peritoneum, which is almost always secondary to contamination. This particular variety of peritonitis is usually called, simply, "peritonitis" without any qualification.

Peritonitis due to contamination is common because the peritoneum is a serous sac completely surrounded by pathogens. Within it is the gastrointestinal tract teeming with microorganisms. Externally, the environment harbors streptococci and staphylococci. Above and below are the lungs and the pelvic organs, occasionally a source of bacteria which invade the peritoneal cavity.

Historical

Peritonitis has been well known since antiquity, and death from peritonitis has been the terminal event in many disease processes.

Inability to prevent or to treat peritonitis effectively was the chief obstacle to the early development of abdominal surgery. In the pre-Listerian era, laparotomy was almost invariably followed by the development of peritonitis and this infection, once established, progressed in most cases to a fatal outcome. A considerable part of modern surgical ritual in abdominal surgery is directed at the prevention of infection, particularly infection of the peritoneum.

Acute Bacterial Peritonitis Secondary to Contamination

INCIDENCE. In 5 to 7 per cent of all autopsies, peritonitis is the primary, or a contributory, cause of death. Generalized peritonitis, while no longer the overwhelming problem it once was, is still the most common cause of death following abdominal surgery.

ETIOLOGY. Maingot states that the common lesions responsible for acute secondary bacterial peritonitis are appendicitis (40 per cent), perforated peptic ulcer (20 per cent), operative contamination (20 per cent), pelvic inflammation (7 per cent), intestinal obstruction and strangulation (7 per cent), and rupture of the intestine (2 per cent).

A wide variety of organisms may be responsible for peritonitis, and not infrequently more than one species of bacterium may be involved. It may be difficult to determine the relative pathogenicity of each organism, as organisms often act synergistically to produce severe systemic effects.

The organisms frequently found in peritonitis are: *Escherichia coli*, streptococci, both aerobic and anaerobic, staphylococci, pneumococci, Friedländer's organisms, *Pseudomonas aeruginosa*, gonococci, *Proteus vulgaris*, *Clostridium perfringens* and other anaerobes.

The two most common and important pathogens are *E. coli* and *Streptococcus pyogenes*. This may be of some importance, as all streptococci are sensitive to penicillin, whereas the coliforms, which usually exist concomitantly, not only resist penicillin but destroy it by producing penicillinase. In a pure infection, the hemolytic streptococcus produces a highly virulent and rapidly lethal infection, whereas the coliforms tend to produce a relatively low-grade infection.

The degree of contamination is an additional factor in determining whether the infection will be rapidly walled off and controlled, or whether the infection will spread and become generalized in the peritoneal cavity.

The role of bacterial toxins in producing the lethal effects of peritonitis is unsettled, but there is evidence that toxins produced by clostridia and endotoxins from lysis of coliforms play a part in the peripheral circulatory failure which marks the end stage of the disease.

PATHOGENESIS. It is important to appreciate the manner in which infection is disseminated in the peritoneal cavity, and the way in which the peritoneum reacts to combat infection. Insight into this physiologic process enables one to assist the peritoneum and avoid interfering with its beneficial activity by misguided therapeutic efforts.

The outcome of peritonitis depends upon the number, virulence and species of the infecting organisms and the resistance of the host. In addition, the peritoneum exhibits certain peculiar weaknesses and special defensive mechanisms.

The first weakness of the peritoneal cavity is that it constitutes a continuous space through which a contaminant may freely and rapidly spread, aided by respiratory, intestinal and abdominal movements. Dissemination is also aided by the exudation of fluid into the cavity. In addition, mucus and partially digested intestinal contents from a bowel perforation may further promote multiplication and dissemination of bacteria and interfere with phagocytosis. This outpouring of intestinal contents or pus, and the pressure of increasing inflammatory exudates, perhaps aided by gas from bacterial fermentation, all tend to prevent early protective localization of the inflammatory process by fibrinous adhesions. An additional weakness of the peritoneum resides in its extensive absorptive surface which permits rapid absorption of bacterial toxins.

One of the strengths of the peritoneum is

that it is exceptionally well adapted to produce an effective inflammatory reaction and to combat infection providing that the contamination is not massive or prolonged. Inflammation here, as elsewhere in the body, is the basic defense mechanism to an irritant. It consists, in essence, of the vascular response, aided by humoral agents and phagocytic activity. A second and rather specific mechanism by which the peritoneum defends itself is by localization of an irritant. Localization is accomplished by bowel, mesentery and particularly the omentum, adhering to inflamed areas. At the site of inflammation, these structures are arrested by the abundant, sticky, fibrinous exudate which progressively increases the adherence of the localizing structures. Approximately 36 hours is required for the formation of reasonably secure fibrinous adhesions which protect against diffuse peritonitis. Localization of infection is further aided by sympathetic inhibition of peristalsis to produce a paralytic ileus. It is true that prolonged ileus may kill the patient because of the effects of distention and inanition, but it provides temporary protection against continued spread of peritonitis.

These factors determine whether or not the patient will survive. If the organisms are virulent and contamination is sudden and massive, if the infection is rapidly disseminated over the whole of the peritoneal cavity, or if attempts at localization by the peritoneum are thwarted by injudicious surgery or by stimulation of the bowel, the infection may become overwhelming. If the organisms are less virulent, if there is no source of continuing contamination, if drainage is provided for those instances in which increasing pressure in a poorly walled-off area would otherwise soil the remainder of the peritoneum, if the efforts of the peritoneum to localize the infection are respected, if the patient is adequately supported by intravenous therapy and by gastrointestinal decompression, and if the number of pathogens can be kept below the critical level by antibodies and by antibiotics, then the cellular defenses of the peritoneum can be expected to overcome the infection.

PATHOLOGY. Acute bacterial peritonitis secondary to contamination may be either generalized or localized.

In generalized peritonitis, the peritoneal cavity contains several hundred cubic centimeters of fluid, which may be thin, watery and odorless in the case of a hemolytic streptococcal infection, or which may be purulent, contain flakes of fibrin and have a strong fecal odor in the case of coliform infection. The entire bowel is dilated, its serosa is congested, edematous and covered with a purulent or fibrinous exudate which may glue together the loops of small bowel. Between the loops of intestine may be loculated collections of pus. The omentum is usually attracted to the site of the infection, but it may occupy a normal position or be matted into a firm mass. The subperitoneal vessels are dilated and there is edema of the areolar tissue beneath the mesothelium. The process may go on to abscess formation, repair by fibrosis or complete resolution.

In localized peritonitis, the changes are similar but confined to one portion of the peritoneal cavity by adherence of mesentery, bowel and omentum to the source of contamination. After a week or ten days, when the adhesions have become fibrous, the walled-off area may gradually become converted into a shaggy, walled abscess.

The microscopic findings include congestion, edema and leukocytic infiltration, with patchy areas of tissue necrosis.

PATHOPHYSIOLOGY. An understanding of some of the clinical manifestations of peritonitis, as well as a rational approach to therapy, is contingent upon an appreciation of the physiologic aberrations which occur in relation to fluid and electrolyte, and to circulatory, homeostasis. The most important of the former is the translocation of fluid, electrolytes and protein into a third space where they are, for a time, lost to the body economy. There are really three subdivisions of this third space:

The peritoneal cavity, where fluid is lost primarily by "weeping" of the peritoneum. Fluid lost by exudation has an electrolyte and nitrogen content similar to that of extracellular fluid. In addition, fluid may be lost into the peritoneal cavity by outpouring from the alimentary canal, the biliary tree, the pancreas or the urinary tract.

The loose connective tissue beneath the mesothelium of the bowel, mesenteries and parietes, where protein-rich fluid accumulates as edema of the peritoneum.

The atonic, dilated gastrointestinal tract where fluid of varying chemical composition is deposited.

Because of this loss of fluid into the third space, many surgeons have compared the physiologic derangement in peritonitis to that of an extensive burn. The comparison is valid in that there is temporary sequestration of a large amount of fluid having approximately the same composition as plasma. Also, as in the burned patient, fluid sequestered in the third space eventually is reabsorbed and becomes available to the body economy with the production of a diuresis if the patient survives and has been well maintained. However, the interval before resolution of the third space begins is longer and more variable in the patient with peritonitis than in the patient with a burn.

In addition to the creation of a third space, additional fluid deficits occur as a result of cessation of oral fluid intake, vomiting and possibly diarrhea, severely taxing the renal mechanisms by which fluid and electrolyte homeostasis is normally maintained. The fluid and electrolyte abnormalities may be further modified by the metabolic response to the stressful situation, and this reaction may be magnified by surgical measures employed in the treatment of the peritonitis.

The effect of peritonitis on the fluid and electrolyte balance of the body, providing that it is not modified by therapy, is the production of a metabolic hypokalemic alkalosis with marked dehydration.

The shock seen in peritonitis may be due to any one of, or a combination of, several causes. Foremost in this group, and probably the most lethal, is septic shock, which is probably the result of liberation of potent endotoxins from the cell wall of dead bacteria in the circulation. Other causes include reduction of plasma volume, toxic myocardial failure, adrenal cortical insufficiency, fat embolism and hepatorenal insufficiency.

CLINICAL MANIFESTATIONS. The clinical course of acute bacterial peritonitis secondary to contamination is highly variable. In an overwhelming peritonitis, the patient may succumb within a few hours from toxemia and shock. More often, the fatal case terminates after a difficult downhill course. As a result of improved therapy, the natural history of the disease today is localization of the infection with gradual control of the process. Peritonitis sometimes masquerades as prolonged postoperative ileus and may be undiagnosed.

SYMPTOMS AND HISTORY. If the patient is seen early in the course of his disease, the symptoms may do no more than suggest a diagnosis. Even if the diagnosis of peritonitis is obvious, a detailed history is of considerable importance in establishing the nature of the initial lesion, as management may be contingent upon this consideration.

Pain may vary in intensity, but it is the most important and constant symptom. Visceral pain, which may be either steady or crampy, is vague and poorly localized. Pain produced by irritation of the parietal peritoneum is usually sharp, well localized and virtually pathognomonic of an inflammatory process. The fact that it can be localized is of diagnostic importance. Changes in the location and intensity of pain originating in the parietal peritoneum may yield valuable information during a period of observation. Increasing pain, and pain not relieved by drugs, suggest spread of peritonitis. Pain is likely to be most intense over the spreading edge of the inflammatory process. Pain which subsides in intensity and decreases in area suggests a localizing process. The pain experienced by elderly and debilitated patients is minimal and not always in keeping with the underlying pathologic process. It is well to bear in mind that the posterior and pelvic portions of the parietal peritoneum are not very sensitive, and an inflamed organ in these locations may exhibit a more advanced pathologic state than one might suspect from the severity of the pain.

Vomiting is also a common symptom, but its nature and mechanism vary with the stage of the disease. Early in peritonitis, vomiting is reflex in origin and the vomitus consists of gastric contents. Later, it is said to be toxic and the vomitus is brownish or bile stained. In the terminal stages of the disease, vomiting accompanies paralytic ileus and the feculent bowel fluid wells up from the mouth without effort on the part of the patient.

PHYSICAL FINDINGS. The diagnosis of peritonitis can usually be confirmed on the basis of the physical findings, but often examination is not as revealing as interrogation in suggesting the precipitating lesion. When the physical findings are equivocal, there is no substitute for repeated, thorough examination, gently performed, at frequent intervals.

In the early stages of peritonitis, temperature, pulse, respiratory rate and blood pressure, which are indices of the systemic effects of the disease, may be normal or there may be only tachycardia and a low-grade fever.

The physical examination should be complete and not just confined to the abdomen.

A red throat, a dilated fixed pupil, a few rales in a lung base, icterus or a diminished femoral pulse may provide a clue to the cause of abdominal pain. Rectal examination is an important part of the physical examination of the patient with an acute abdomen. Inflammation in the pelvis may not cause significant abdominal findings, but the exquisite tenderness elicited by rectal examination may be diagnostic.

The patient with peritonitis usually lies very still because he has found that all movements aggravate his pain. His thighs and knees may be flexed in order to relax his abdominal muscles. His breathing is shallow so as to avoid movements of the abdominal wall. After inspection is completed, the abdominal wall should be very gently palpated for minor degrees of involuntary guarding, all efforts being made to reassure the patient and eliminate voluntary contraction of abdominal muscles. Only after this maneuver is carried out should one complete the abdominal examination. Guarding is of greater significance than tenderness, but once the patient has been hurt, it is difficult to detect minor degrees of this important physical finding. Point tenderness, referred tenderness and rebound tenderness on palpation, along with involuntary guarding, point to irritation of the parietal peritoneum. Their presence is important and their location corresponds to that of the underlying inflammatory area.

Auscultation of the abdomen must always be part of the abdominal examination. The stethoscope is the key to distinguishing pain due to simple obstruction from that due to peritonitis. The silent abdomen indicates peritonitis.

Percussion has its place in the examination of the abdomen but does not often yield valuable information. Generalized hyperresonance due to the presence of gas-filled bowel may be elicited in ileus. Occasionally, obliteration of the area of liver dullness will be found, suggesting free gas in the peritoneal cavity.

Examination for costovertebral angle and flank tenderness and the use of the psoas and internal obturator tests are also useful.

TERMINAL PHASE. In the end stages of the disease, the previously high fever falls to normal or subnormal and the pulse becomes weak and very rapid, an ominous combination. The pain is severe and steady, the abdomen distended and silent, and the vomiting is effortless. Hippocrates, who must have seen it often, described the dusky pallor, anxious expression, sunken staring eyes, dry, fissured tongue and wet skin that mark the end of the struggle. Death is due to peripheral circulatory and renal failure.

LABORATORY AIDS. The diagnosis of peritonitis is made on clinical grounds, although laboratory aids may confirm the diagnosis. The most important of these is a series of plain x-ray films of the abdomen. Plain films of the abdomen should be taken in three positions: anteroposterior supine, anteroposterior upright and left lateral decubitus. If the peritonitis is localized, there may be a segmental ileus of some part of the bowel in only one region of the abdomen. With general peritonitis, the dilatation of the gastrointestinal tract within the abdomen is widespread (Fig. 18). Jejunum, ileum and colon contain air and can be identified by their typical patterns. The dilatation is usually less than in mechanical obstruction and the distribution of small bowel, while central, forms a mosaic pattern rather than horizontal loops with sharp hairpin turns as seen in mechanical obstruction. There is diffuse haziness, due to accumulation of exudate, with obliteration of the peritoneal fat line and psoas shadows. There is thickness of bowel wall between adjacent gas shadows due to edema of the bowel wall and the exu-

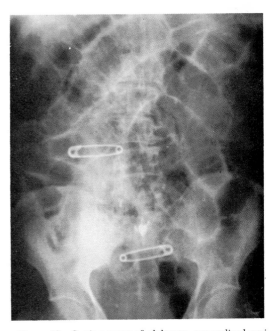

Figure 18. Supine x-ray of abdomen, generalized peritonitis (postoperative). Marked dilatation of large and small bowel is seen and there is thickening between adjacent intestinal loops.

date. Free gas may be seen if peritonitis is due to perforation of bowel. Contrast studies are generally unnecessary and the administration of barium by mouth is contraindicated.

Periodic blood chemistry determinations may be of considerable value as guides to the supportive therapy of the patient. The white blood count is almost always markedly elevated, with a preponderance of polymorphonuclear granulocytes.

DIAGNOSIS. There is no substitute for experience in developing diagnostic acumen in the management of patients with peritonitis. The salient clinical features, stated briefly, are abdominal pain, sharp, steady and localized; the signs of irritation of the parietal peritoneum; and a silent abdomen. As Maingot points out, "It is easier to diagnose the presence than the cause of peritonitis." The differential diagnosis is that of an acute abdomen.

COMPLICATIONS. Paralytic ileus, inanition, dehydration, electrolyte abnormalities, toxemia and shock are usually considered characteristic features of the disease, rather than complications. Septicemia and spread of infection by lymphatics to the retroperitoneum are less common and may be considered complications. The spread of localized peritonitis to become a diffuse infection is, at the same time, a complication of one and the pathogenesis of the other.

When a patient lives beyond a seven- or eight-day period and the infection persists, this may lead to so-called chronic septic peritonitis in which there are numerous pockets of pus walled off by adhesions and coils of bowel. Frequently, these patients die of toxemia or paralytic ileus, or from mechanical bowel obstruction.

A much more common outcome is a localized version of the same process, an intraperitoneal abscess. Most abscesses are confined to their site of origin (e.g., periappendiceal) or are pelvic. Therapy is frequently directed toward obtaining localization of the infection in the pelvis. Less common is the subphrenic abscess, difficult of diagnosis and exacting in management.

Another complication which can occur after peritonitis is mechanical small bowel obstruction due to fibrinous adhesions.

PROGNOSIS. Thirty years ago one-third of patients with peritonitis could be expected to succumb. At the present time, with earlier and more accurate diagnosis, better understanding of the deranged physiology, improved fluid and electrolyte therapy, the use of whole blood where indicated, sulfonamides and antibiotics, gastrointestinal decompression and safer anesthesia, the mortality is between 5 and 10 per cent.

TREATMENT. **Prophylactic treatment.** A number of special procedures, such as preoperative bowel preparation, use of drains when indicated and preservation of blood supply, are particularly concerned with the prevention of postoperative peritonitis.

One question which repeatedly arises in connection with laparotomy for the purpose of preventing peritonitis is whether drainage should be carried out. An old axiom says, "When in doubt, drain." W. J. Mayo turned this about to read, "When in doubt, don't drain." The arguments against prophylactic drainage are that the drain tract is a source of infection from the outside; that it is impossible to drain the peritoneal cavity; and that a Penrose drain is ineffective after six or eight hours because it becomes sealed. All of these statements are true. It is possible and often desirable, however, to drain a localized portion of the peritoneal cavity. The last-named obstacle can be overcome by periodic loosening of the Penrose drain or by use of a sump drain. The decision as to whether to drain is often a matter of judgment and sometimes of personal preference. In general, prophylactic drainage is advised when a localized area of peritonitis exists around which secure adhesions have not yet formed; in operations on the extrahepatic biliary tract; injury to or operations on the liver, where there is a possibility of bile leakage; in the presence of a gastrointestinal suture line which is insecure and not protected by other measures; possible continued leakage of fluid, even though it is sterile at the time of surgery, and involvement of a retroperitoneal area.

A drain can be put down to the vicinity of the source of a fluid or contaminant, or it can be placed to drain a low point to which fluid can be expected to gravitate, or both.

A second group of prophylactic measures, of no less interest to the surgeon, has to do with early diagnosis and treatment of lesions likely to culminate in peritonitis if not adequately treated.

Definitive treatment. The definitive treatment of bacterial peritonitis is based upon an understanding of the etiology, pathogenesis, pathology and physiologic derangements. Treatment can be resolved into five facets.

A decision must be made as to whether there is continuing contamination of the peritoneal cavity and, if there is, operative correction should be undertaken, provided other circumstances do not contraindicate surgical interference.

All possible measures must be carried out to assist the peritoneum in localizing the infection, preferably in a location favorable for future drainage, and in overcoming that infection.

The gastrointestinal tract must be decompressed with a long tube, while the defensive nature of the paralytic ileus is respected.

Supportive treatment should be given to maintain the patient through his illness; this includes relief of pain, treatment of shock, maintenance of fluid and electrolyte balance and correction of hypoproteinemia.

Repeated clinical observations must be made for confirmation of diagnosis, to ascertain effectiveness of therapy and to note the progress of the disease.

Surgical intervention. The decision to operate depends on the presence of continuing peritoneal contamination, and this in turn depends upon the primary lesion more than on any other factor. However, the time interval since onset, the progress of the disease and the general condition of the patient all modify this decision. The peritoneum is well adapted to deal with infection, but it is overwhelmed by continuing contamination.

If the peritonitis is caused by acute diverticulitis with perforation, infection is probably well localized and the perforation is usually small and readily sealed off by natural defenses. If the diagnosis is certain, operation in such a patient is useless or even harmful, unless the peritonitis is spreading.

If a peptic ulcer perforates, one usually operates if the patient presents himself during the first 36 hours. During the first 36 hours, there is usually continuing contamination, whereas after that the perforation has frequently sealed off. Operation, in the patient moribund from his generalized peritonitis, carries a higher risk than active conservative measures alone, if the perforation has sealed off.

In acute appendicitis with generalized peritonitis, continuing contamination can probably be expected for several days and the appendix should be removed, especially in children, if the patient's condition is such that he will tolerate an operation. The mortality rate in generalized peritonitis from acute appendicitis is about twice as high (13 per cent) with conservative treatment as it is with surgical removal of the appendix and intensive supportive measures.

Conservative measures are justified in the treatment of localized peritonitis from acute appendicitis provided that the patient is an adult, is first seen between two and five days after the onset, is very ill and the infection seems to be localizing satisfactorily. This Ochsner-Sherren treatment must be carried out "at the door of the operating room," that is, with continuous observation and readiness to intervene surgically if the peritonitis begins to spread. This plan has no place in the treatment of children and is only occasionally employed for adults.

When surgical intervention is indicated, a few hours of supportive measures may be required to prepare the seriously ill patient for operation.

First, the source of contamination is removed or closed, or, in the case of a gallbladder with impending perforation, it may be simply drained. Second, intraperitoneal fluid or exudate is aspirated to decrease the massiveness of the contamination. Third, if it appears advisable, a drain may be put down to the source of contamination or to the site where fluid is likely to collect. Fourth, one may utilize the opportunity to guide a long tube, which is introduced through the usual nasal route, past the pylorus and into the small bowel. Finally, aseptic decompression of the bowel by means of an enterostomy in the proximal jejunum with passage of a long tube through the dilated bowel, emptying the loops individually, is undoubtedly the most satisfactory method of effecting decompression. These maneuvers should be carried out as quickly as possible and without disseminating infection.

Localizing and combating infection. The great advances in modern drug therapy of infection should not be permitted to overshadow the importance of some basic and simple therapeutic measures. Rest for the patient and for his gastrointestinal tract is essential in order to permit localization of the peritonitis.

The site of localization is important, for should complete resolution of the infection fail and abscess formation result, the abscess will have to be located and drained. The pelvis is a very desirable location; the subphrenic region is a dangerous area for localization of an abscess. It has been shown that when a patient lies flat in bed, the paracolic gutter is 1 inch lower than the pelvis and it is well known that the right paracolic gutter communicates with the subphrenic spaces on the right side. To encourage drainage of fluid from the flank to the pelvis, the head of the bed must be elevated 60 to 70 degrees or, as Fowler advocated, 8 to 14 inches higher than the foot of the bed. The patient's trunk, then, should be oblique, with the patient either flat on a sloping bed or else in a semisitting position. The knees should not be bent and, if the patient tends to slip down in bed, it is good for his venous circulation if he must push his feet against a footboard from time to time to regain his position.

The basic defense against infection is phagocytosis, aided by other natural defense mechanisms. Sulfonamides and antibiotics must play a secondary role in that they only assist these natural processes. Pulaski has shown that any antibiotic which suppresses the total number of microorganisms to below a critical value of about 1×10^5 per milliliter of exudate permits the body's defenses to cope with the remaining bacteria. Thus, it is not necessary to give a specific drug to eliminate completely each of the several bacterial species which may be present; the objective is only to lower the bacterial population below the critical level.

At the present time, it appears that the drugs of choice for the treatment of peritonitis from intestinal contamination are oxytetracycline, chlortetracycline, chloramphenicol, the combination of streptomycin and penicillin, and the sulfonamides. Penicillin is very effective against all streptococci, but it is inactivated by the penicillinase produced by various coliforms. This can be overcome by the use of a penicillin-streptomycin mixture, the only antibiotic combination which appears to have any advantage over the administration of a single drug.

The dose of sulfonamide or antibiotic administered should be large enough so that the partially resistant strains are not just replaced by totally resistant organisms. At the same time, it is well to remember that these drugs are toxic substances and that it is not unusual to encounter complications which necessitate reduction of dose or change of drug. If renal function is inadequate, the blood level of the antibiotics may parallel that of the nonprotein nitrogen. Vitamin K should be given by vein when broad-spectrum antibiotics are given for more than a few days. The patient should be watched for any evidence of agranulocytosis, diarrhea or mycotic overgrowth in the mouth, pharynx and lungs.

The drugs should be given intravenously or intramuscularly in peritonitis. Rarely, the oral route can be used. The question of intraperitoneal administration has not been settled as yet; this route appears to have advantages but is not without danger. Deaths from respiratory arrest have occurred as a result of intraperitoneal administration of neomycin, although there is reason to believe that when this has occurred overdosage has been a factor. Chlortetracycline, tetracycline and streptomycin have been shown to be toxic when given intraperitoneally to experimental animals.

Gastrointestinal decompression. The gastrointestinal tract must be decompressed to prevent the secondary effects of distention upon the circulation in the bowel wall and also upon the patient's respiratory and circulatory systems. Recently, attention has been drawn to a syndrome of high-output respiratory failure as an important cause of death in peritonitis. Respiratory function is considered as the primary defect in this lesion. The factors which lead to insufficient ventilation for the metabolic demands of the patient include the increased minute oxygen utilization due to fever or inflammation, and inability to increase ventilation because of fatigue, pain and an elevated diaphragm due to intraperitoneal fluid or distended intestines. Obesity or previous loss of pulmonary reserve accentuates these factors. When the patient cannot meet the increased oxygen demands, hypoxic acidosis develops and cardiac arrest eventually ensues if specific treatment is not given. Treatment consists of early operative relief of intraperitoneal distention, tracheostomy and artificial ventilation with a mechanical respirator.

Gastric suction is effective to some degree, but the use of a long intestinal tube is preferable for nonoperative gastrointestinal decompression. A rectal tube and application of heat to the abdomen are of value after bowel function begins to return. The use of Prostigmine, Pitressin and all such drugs to stimulate the bowel is definitely contraindicated.

Supportive therapy. The fluid and electrolyte requirements of the patient with peritonitis must be supplied by the intravenous route. The plan of treatment depends on calculation of the static deficit, the dynamic losses and the base line requirements, as outlined by Randall. Estimation of the first of these, and to some extent the second, is nothing more than an educated guess and must be revised by noting the patient's response to therapy. It is helpful to realize that the fluid lost into the third space amounts to several liters and that its composition resembles that of plasma. The use of an indwelling catheter to make certain that a urine flow of 25 to 50 cc. per hour is being maintained, along with other clinical assessment of the state of hydration, will aid in determining the quantity of fluid to be administered.

One can judge the mineral requirements of the patient. Some of the common pitfalls of fluid and electrolyte therapy must be kept in mind in the difficult task of caring for these patients:

A low serum sodium level of 125 to 130 mEq. per liter is to be expected for 48 to 72 hours after severe stress.

Serum potassium is a poor index of the intracellular level. Potassium should be withheld for 48 hours after operation, or in the presence of renal insufficiency or elevated nonprotein nitrogen. Otherwise, it should be given at the rate of about 80 mEq. per day in order to avoid intracellular depletion and prolonged ileus.

Overhydration is a danger in the elderly and after resorption from the third space begins.

Depleted serum proteins must also be replaced by the administration of whole blood, serum albumin or plasma stored at room temperature. Protein hydrolysates can be used to reduce the degree of the negative nitrogen balance, provided that one can simultaneously supply enough calories in the form of glucose to meet the demands of the elevated metabolic rate. For the patient with prolonged ileus, intravenous fat preparations may be used to combat inanition.

As a rule, the use of cortisone and hydrocortisone in the presence of an infection, and particularly if it is due to an ulcerative lesion of the gastrointestinal tract, is contraindicated. Their use is occasionally justified, however, in patients who show signs of adrenocortical insufficiency, i.e., persistent hypotension and vasoconstriction after adequate blood replacement and a high circulating eosinophil count. This state may result from previous adrenal disease, adrenal atrophy due to previous cortisone administration, or from adrenal exhaustion due to the peritonitis.

Relief of pain is part of supportive therapy. Morphine or meperidine (Demerol) should be administered often enough and in adequate dosage to guarantee the patient pain-free periods when he can obtain necessary rest.

Continued observation. Finally, the patient with peritonitis must be frequently reassessed. The diagnosis of the causative lesion, if it has not been confirmed by exploration, is not always clear cut. Response of the patient to the therapy administered should be evaluated several times daily during the acute phase of the illness. Awareness of the complications of the disease and their treatment is essential. Repeated examination of the abdomen for evidence of localization or spread of the peritonitis and careful observation of the course of the disease are as much the responsibility of the physician as are the initial diagnosis and original plan of management.

Less Common Types of Peritonitis

PRIMARY ("IDIOPATHIC") PERITONITIS. Primary peritonitis is an infection which is not secondary to an operation or a wound, to an inflammatory, perforative or other disease process in or near the peritoneal cavity, or to known hematogenous spread of an infection elsewhere. Obviously, the origin of the disease is obscure and the term "idiopathic" seems appropriate.

Primary peritonitis was fairly common prior to the advent of sulfonamides and antibiotics, but it is rare today. The majority of cases occur in girls, usually between the ages of two and ten years, but it has been described at all ages.

About two-thirds of the instances of primary peritonitis are due to hemolytic streptococci and about one-third are due to pneumococci. Only a single organism is involved in any case; hence it differs from the polymicrobiotic character of secondary peritonitis. Occasionally, primary peritonitis is said to be due to coliforms, but such a diagnosis must always be suspect. About half of the pneumococcal cases occur in children with nephrosis.

One concept regarding the pathogenesis of primary peritonitis is that the organisms gain entry through the vagina and fallopian tubes. This is supported by the observation that the disease is one of the underprivileged classes and of unhygienic conditions. The alkaline pH of the vagina in children may account for the age incidence mentioned. Another suggestion has been that most of the infections are really hematogenous. The proponents of this theory point to a high incidence of an associated focus of infection. Neither view completely explains the sex distribution.

Streptococcal infections cause a fulminating infection with a watery, odorless exudate and the pathologic features of streptococcal peritonitis. Pneumococcal infections are less fulminating and cause a characteristic gelatinous, sticky, pale green, odorless exudate with abundant fibrin formation.

The child is most often under five years of age. A pre-existing upper respiratory infection, otitis media or pneumonia may mask for a while the onset of the peritonitis. The main clinical features are rapid onset of diffuse abdominal pain, high fever, often chills, restlessness, irritability, vomiting, diarrhea in half the patients, sometimes hematemesis or melena, and manifestations of extreme toxicity.

The child usually has a temperature of 104° F., appears very ill and may be markedly dehydrated with dry mucous membranes and sunken eyes. The abdomen may be protuberant and diffusely tender. There may be abundant fluid in the abdomen and sometimes shifting dullness can be demonstrated. The consistency of the abdominal wall varies from doughy in infants to boardlike in older children. Peristaltic activity is increased at first and is then followed shortly by paralytic ileus. In pneumococcal peritonitis there may be cyanosis and herpetic lesions on the lips of the patient.

The white blood count usually ranges from 20,000 to 50,000 with polymorphonuclear neutrophils predominating. In cases superimposed on nephrosis, there is a heavy albuminuria. Blood culture is usually positive for streptococci or pneumococci.

Pneumonia should be ruled out. This diagnosis may be difficult in patients in whom there is a paucity of physical and x-ray findings in the chest. A rapid respiratory rate and lack of abdominal tenderness will aid in the differentiation. The two conditions may coexist.

A more difficult problem is the differentiation between primary peritonitis and secondary peritonitis, usually from a perforated appendix. The rapidity of onset and stormy course, particularly if accompanied by a chill, the finding of generalized rather than right-sided tenderness, the degree of fever and leukocytosis during the entire illness, the finding of a primary focus and a history of nephrosis or a finding of heavy albuminuria may favor a diagnosis of primary peritonitis.

The physician rarely accepts a diagnosis of primary peritonitis while acute appendicitis, which is far more common, remains a possibility. In moribund children, and in instances when the diagnosis of primary peritonitis seems almost certain because of known nephrosis or a known coexisting focus of infection and septicemia, the matter may be settled by peritoneal aspiration under local anesthesia. A smear of the exudate showing pure streptococci or pure pneumococci will allow one to proceed with conservative therapy with assurance.

In the majority of instances, the diagnosis will be made at exploration. A right lower quadrant incision can be very limited in extent if one suspects a primary peritonitis. Gross recommends the following procedure: obtain some exudate for a smear to prove the diagnosis—this is done by an assistant immediately, not postoperatively—and culture; confirm that the appendix is not the source of the infection; put a small drain down into the right iliac fossa; do not remove the appendix if it is normal. Postoperatively, an antiperitonitis regimen should be followed. Sulfonamides and penicillin are the specific drugs of choice.

BACTERIAL PERITONITIS DUE TO HEMATOGENOUS SPREAD. This entity is blood borne from a known infection elsewhere in the body, so that it is really a secondary peritonitis. It differs from contamination peritonitis in that it does not arise from a lesion in the vicinity of the peritoneum.

The source of the infection may or may not be apparent. Many surgeons believe that in many patients primary peritonitis is actually due to a hidden focus. Thus, it is really hematogenous and so belongs in this group. The fact that the majority of the organisms are streptococci and pneumococci favors this point of view.

The clinical features are identical to those which have been described for primary peritonitis.

This disease, like primary peritonitis, should be treated conservatively when the diagnosis can be made.

TUBERCULOUS PERITONITIS. Tuberculous peritonitis was at one time fairly common, but fortunately it is now rarely seen. It is almost always associated with tuberculosis elsewhere.

Tuberculous peritonitis is somewhat more common in females. Both children and adults may be affected, the usual age range being between ten and 40 years.

The infecting organism is *Mycobacterium tuberculosis* of either the human or the bovine type. The primary lesion is most often tuberculous ulceration of the bowel, but infection may also arise from tuberculous mesenteric lymph nodes, tuberculosis of the fallopian tubes, lymphatic spread from the lung or pleura or hematogenous spread from distant sites.

Basically, there are two types of tuberculous peritonitis: the moist variety and the dry form. Tubercles are found in both varieties, but they may not be immediately apparent on gross examination because of fibrinous or purulent exudate, caseation or fibrous adhesions. In the dry form, there is usually a dense inflammatory exudate and numerous adhesions matting the coils of bowel together. Fecal fistula formation may occur in either type, particularly in the dry form, and in children the fistula may communicate with the umbilicus. In the moist form, the patient is likely to be a child and the ascites may be massive. The fluid is usually thin and lemon yellow, and it may coagulate spontaneously. Its specific gravity is over 1.018 and its protein content over 4 per cent, thus distinguishing the fluid from a transudate. The encysted variety is a combination of both of these forms, with a localized area of fluid which may be mistaken for some other cystic lesion.

The condition is of fairly acute onset in two-thirds of the patients. The moist form is likely to run a more insidious course than the dry. There are systemic manifestations, consisting of wasting, anorexia and fever, accompanied by abdominal pain, vomiting, diarrhea and enlargement of the abdomen. In the moist form, the abdomen may become very distended and tense with dilatation of the veins of the abdominal wall and, if the tunica vaginalis is patent, a simulated hydrocele. Redness of the umbilicus may precede formation of a fecal fistula.

The diagnosis is usually not difficult, as there is evidence of tuberculous infection elsewhere. In the ascitic variety, peritoneal fluid may be aspirated for culture and guinea-pig inoculation. The differential diagnosis includes pyogenic peritonitis, carcinomatosis, other forms of ascites, abdominal tumor and celiac disease.

The chief complications are cachexia and intestinal obstruction. In the preantibiotic era, the mortality was 40 per cent, death often being due to toxemia, tuberculosis elsewhere or rarely to amyloidosis.

The treatment consists chiefly of general supportive measures for tuberculosis, which should be carried out in a sanatorium. The use of the antituberculous drugs—streptomycin, para-aminosalicylic acid and isonicotinic acid hydrazide—has improved the prognosis markedly. In the ascitic variety, laparotomy and evacuation of the fluid seem to have a beneficial effect. In the dry form, operation should be avoided, except when made mandatory by intestinal obstruction. When laparotomy has been carried out in the presence of tuberculous peritonitis, drainage and exteriorization of bowel should be avoided.

ASEPTIC PERITONITIS. Aseptic peritonitis is important for two reasons. A variety of sterile materials which may gain entrance to the peritoneal cavity are irritants and set up aseptic inflammatory reactions which give rise to sequelae and clinical symptoms. Secondly, the chemical peritonitis produced by any of these substances may be followed by a superimposed bacterial peritonitis.

Foreign bodies may reach the peritoneal cavity from operative procedures, e.g., sponges, suture material and instruments. They may result from penetrating wounds, missiles and bits of clothing. The gastrointestinal and genitourinary tracts may be the source of fish bones, wood splinters, needles, pins and glass. Such foreign bodies usually cause one of three types of reaction: bacterial inflammation in which the foreign body is incidental; aseptic inflammation, which usually results in a localized sterile abscess as the peritoneum walls off the foreign body, and a similar process with formation of a sinus or fistula. The relative amounts of exudation and fibrosis vary greatly with the nature of the foreign body.

The clinical manifestations of a sterile intraperitoneal foreign body are highly variable. A surgical sponge may give rise to an abscess with a mass, fever, chills and toxic manifestations; there are also legal implications. This type of foreign body must be removed. Intraperitoneal shrapnel, if sterile, may be simply walled off by fibrous tissue and give rise to few if any manifestations in the emotionally stable patient. The surgeon must guard against being persuaded by the patient to undertake a search for this type of foreign body, on the basis of vague subjective complaints.

Bile may ooze through the wall of a gallbladder which is distended but intact. More commonly, bile reaches the peritoneal cavity as a result of biliary tract rupture or as a sequel to operations on the biliary system. Sterile bile is a mild irritant in its own right, but should it become secondarily infected, it may give rise to a virulent type of peritonitis. To prevent this unfortunate sequel, the adequate routine drainage of Morison's hepatorenal space is recommended after biliary surgery or liver trauma.

Blood is only a mild irritant and it is slowly absorbed. However, blood in the peritoneal cavity may serve as a nidus for bacterial infection. For this reason, it should always be evacuated at the end of an operation. An oozing surface, capable of producing hematoma, should be drained.

A most interesting entity is meconium or fetal peritonitis, which was first described by Sir James Young Simpson in 1838. The disease results from perforation of the bowel and inflammation of the peritoneal membrane due to sterile meconium. The perforation of the intestine may occur any time from the third fetal month to the neonatal period. It may result from meconium ileus, congenital bands, hernia, volvulus or intussusception. If the opening is still present at birth or if perforation occurs after birth, secondary bacterial infection is a rule and the outlook in such cases is very poor.

Gastric juice is very irritating and the chemical peritonitis which is set up by a perforated ulcer is followed, after several hours, by bacterial infection. Sterile urine from traumatic intraperitoneal rupture of the bladder is also an irritating fluid and this chemical insult is frequently followed by secondary infection. These lesions must be diagnosed early and treated by appropriate operation.

Intraperitoneal pancreatic juice usually becomes infected and, in hemorrhagic pancreatitis, superadded bacterial infection should always be anticipated. Intensive antibiotic therapy deals adequately with this infection in most instances, but occasionally an abscess or collection will have to be drained ten to 14 days after the onset.

Granulomatous Lesions of the Peritoneum

Separation of foreign body granulomas of the peritoneum from aseptic peritonitis due to foreign bodies is somewhat arbitrary. The basic pathologic process is the same – the response of the peritoneum to a noninfected irritant. The varying degrees of exudation and fibrosis distinguish the two reactions.

Some of the substances which are more commonly reported as causes of granulomatous reaction by the peritoneal membrane are talc, starch, lycopodium spores, mineral oil and silica. These etiologic agents are often introduced into the peritoneal cavity by the surgeon.

In the past, granulomatous lesions due to talc were often seen, because this substance was widely used as a glove powder. Talc is composed mainly of hydrated magnesium silicate and incites a very intense fibroblastic reaction which may give rise to dense adhesions within a few weeks, or the process may take years. In an attempt to overcome this problem, powdered starch was introduced as a glove powder. The starch is made from either corn or rice and should be relatively innocuous because it is gradually absorbed by the peritoneum. Unfortunately, it has been found that starch may also give rise to a foreign-body reaction, although less frequently and to a lesser degree than talc.

It appears that soluble starch is the glove powder of choice at the present time. Gloves should be washed or wiped off before hands are put into the peritoneal cavity and care should be taken to avoid spillage of glove powder, should a glove be torn during an operation.

The gross appearance of these granulomatous lesions ranges from a studding of the serous membranes with nodules resembling tubercles or larger masses, to the formation of dense fibrous adhesions.

Microscopically, the reaction is seen to be the formation of a chronic granuloma. There may be monocytes, epithelioid cells, multinucleated giant cells, lymphocytes, plasma cells, fibroblasts and sometimes areas of necrosis. Particles of the particular foreign material responsible can often be identified in the monocytes or giant cells by its characteristic appearance.

Intraperitoneal Abscesses

An intraperitoneal abscess may be regarded as a complication or sequel of either localized or generalized peritonitis. If the peritoneum succeeds in completely walling off the infectious process, but is not able to overcome the infection, an abscess develops. The situation may be looked upon as a stalemate between host and pathogen. However, the patient may be very ill from the infection and the presence of the abscess constitutes a constant threat to the life of the individual.

An intraperitoneal abscess may arise in one of two ways. First, it may result from a slowly advancing inflammatory process within the abdomen, in which case the abscess will develop in the immediate vicinity of the diseased organ, because the defenses of the peritoneum have had sufficient time to localize the infection. An appendiceal abscess is the most common example of this variety, but much the same process may occur from an acutely inflamed gallbladder with perforation, from acute diverticulitis, from hemorrhagic pancreatitis, from acute salpingitis and numerous other conditions which give rise, as a rule, to localized rather than generalized peritonitis. In the second group, there is usually sudden massive contamination of the entire peritoneal cavity, as in a perforated peptic ulcer or a penetrating wound with injury to bowel, in which, if the patient survives, the infection becomes secondarily localized. Such localization generally occurs in dependent parts of the abdominal cavity, to which the infected exudate tends to gravitate. These abscesses usually occur in the pelvis, and this is a favorable location, or in the subphrenic region, which is a very undesirable site.

PERIAPPENDICEAL ABSCESS. Most periappendiceal abscesses lie in the right iliac fossa, but, largely because of the variable position of the appendix, the abscess may be pelvic, may lie in the paracolic gutter, may be in front of or behind the distal ileum, or may be retroperitoneal in position. A postappendectomy abscess is essentially similar to a periappendicular abscess except that the appendix has been previously removed in the former case.

An abscess need not arise from perforation of an organ. Infection may pass through the inflamed but intact wall, as is usually the case with peridiverticular abscess. In the patient with appendicitis, however, perforation usually has occurred by the time an abscess is diagnosed. As a result of inflammation and exudation of fibrin, omentum, mesentery and bowel become adherent about the appendix and localize the infection. There is no sharp demarcation between localized peritonitis and abscess formation. The exudate becomes progressively more purulent, the fibrinous adhesions become organized and within five to ten days an abscess has developed.

The pus of a periappendiceal abscess is never sterile. The organisms are those found in peritonitis. Mixed infections are not uncommon.

The symptoms of a periappendicular abscess follow and cannot be sharply distinguished from those of the preceding appendicitis and localized peritonitis. In the instance of a postappendectomy abscess, there may be an apparently smooth postoperative course with nothing unusual except a low grade fever and slight tachycardia about the time that discharge from hospital is being considered. If antibiotics have been given, the abscess may not be apparent for several weeks or even several months.

In either case, the abscess eventually presents with fever, spiking to 104° or 105° F., and chills are not unusual. There is usually malaise and abdominal pain and there may be associated anorexia, nausea and vomiting. Constipation and some abdominal distention may result from a localized area of paralytic ileus. In a longstanding neglected infection, there may be marked weight loss.

The patient with an abscess usually looks ill. He may be dehydrated and either flushed from fever or pale from associated anemia. Usually, a mass is palpated in the right iliac fossa on abdominal examination and there is associated tenderness and guarding. The mass may be palpable by rectal examination and may be fluctuant. When an abscess is present, leukocytosis is usually marked with a predominance of polymorphonuclear neutrophils.

Periappendiceal abscess may give rise to

other complications, including generalized peritonitis, spontaneous drainage into the bowel, fecal fistula, pylephlebitis, paralytic ileus, mechanical bowel obstruction, septicemia and death.

A periappendicular abscess in occasional patients resolves with conservative treatment alone. The process is probably a localized cellulitis or peritonitis presented with an indurated mass, rather than a true abscess. However, there is no way to distinguish clinically between the abscess which resolves on conservative measures alone and the one which requires surgical drainage because both may present similar symptoms, even to the spiking fever. It is customary to initiate supportive measures and observe the patient for the first 24 to 48 hours. Supportive measures include bed rest, intubation, antibiotics, heat to the abdomen, relief of pain and intravenous fluids often including blood. It is probable that the patient with a true abscess invariably requires surgical intervention to achieve cure. Occasionally, in the very ill patient with a hectic fever, adequate drainage of the abscess is required as soon as dehydration and ketosis have been corrected.

The operation for periappendiceal abscess has three objectives: to drain the abscess, to avoid contamination of the general peritoneal cavity and to remove the appendix. The first two are essential; the third is not. Although the majority of appendices in such circumstances can be removed, it is better to leave the appendix than to disseminate infection. An extraperitoneal approach should be used, a small incision being made either over the most prominent part of the mass or else lateral to the mass. If it becomes apparent that the uninvolved peritoneal cavity will be traversed, the wound should be closed and a more suitable site for incision chosen. Needle aspiration is a blind procedure and is neither safe nor adequate. The pus should be completely evacuated and a Penrose drain placed in the depth of the cavity.

PELVIC ABSCESS. A pelvic abscess may result from disease which is primary in that location or by gravitation of infected exudate from peritonitis elsewhere into the pelvis. The latter development is encouraged by positioning of the patient, because if abscess formation cannot be avoided, the pelvis is a relatively favorable location. A pelvic abscess is preferable to a subphrenic abscess because it does not interfere with respiratory function; it is relatively easy to diagnose

and to drain, or if drainage is spontaneous, it is usually into the large bowel.

The symptomatology of a pelvic abscess resembles that of a periappendiceal abscess in almost every respect. One significant difference, however, is that pelvic abscess is often characterized by diarrhea. Pain, tenderness and guarding are usually less marked and, of course, the mass is not felt as well abdominally as it is by rectal or bimanual examination.

Supportive therapy of a pelvic abscess is similar to that for a periappendiceal abscess, except that if the mass is not fluctuant, it may be encouraged to point toward the rectum by means of warm enemas. The daily rectal examinations, which are carried out to evaluate the abscess, may be enough to encourage spontaneous rupture into the rectum.

If spontaneous rupture does not occur, severe symptoms and finding of fluctuation may serve as criteria for operative intervention. The abscess may be opened through the posterior fornix of the vagina, if the abscess lies in the cul-de-sac in the female, or through the anterior wall of the rectum. These approaches should be used rather cautiously, because a loop of adherent bowel may be mistaken for loculated pus. If the rectal route is chosen, dilatation of the anal sphincter will promote continuous drainage. If the abscess is not pointing toward rectum or vagina, and particularly if the mass can be felt suprapubically, it is better to open it by an abdominal incision and by an extraperitoneal route.

SUBPHRENIC ABSCESS. A subphrenic abscess is an abscess located in the space between the diaphragm and the transverse mesocolon. These abscesses are not common, compared to other intraperitoneal abscesses. They are important because they are difficult to diagnose and treat and because the life of the patient may depend upon adequate management. Untreated, they carry a 90 per cent mortality. Improperly treated, that is drained through the pleural or peritoneal cavity, the mortality rate is 35 per cent to 40 per cent. Early diagnosis and proper treatment reduce the mortality rate to approximately 10 per cent.

Anatomy. The location of a subphrenic abscess influences the clinical symptoms and the surgical approach indicated to provide drainage. The subphrenic region is subdivided into various spaces. A subphrenic abscess, because it is walled off by inflammatory adhesions, may not exactly coincide with the space in which it is situated. As a rule, an abscess is found to occupy only one subphrenic space. When the right posterior superior space is involved, however, the right subhepatic space is frequently involved by an extension of the process.

There are six intraperitoneal subphrenic spaces or potential spaces. The liver conveniently divides the subphrenic compartment into suprahepatic and subhepatic areas, and the falciform ligament and ligamentum venosum demarcate the right and left sides. There are three spaces above the liver and three below; there are three on the right and three on the left:

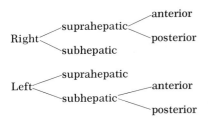

On the right side, there are two suprahepatic spaces and one subhepatic space (Fig. 19). The right anterior-superior space is a large space between the right lobe of the liver and diaphragm which is limited posteriorly by the anterior leaf of the coronary ligament and which communicates with the general peritoneal cavity anteriorly over the free edge of the liver. The right posterior-superior space is a small recess bounded by diaphragm, liver and posterior leaf of coronary ligament. This right posterior-superior space is really an upward extension of the right subhepatic space. The reason for designating the right posterior-superior space as

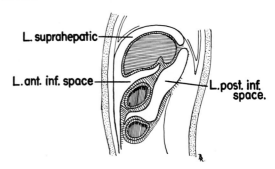

Figure 20. Diagrammatic representation of subphrenic spaces on the left side in parasagittal section. The left posterior-inferior space is the lesser peritoneal sac.

a separate subphrenic space is that it is the site of a subphrenic abscess more often than any other. Exudate from the right paracolic gutter drains to this area in a recumbent patient. The right subhepatic space corresponds to the hepatorenal pouch of Morison.

On the left side, there is only one suprahepatic space but two subhepatic spaces (Fig. 20). The left suprahepatic space lies between the left lobe of the liver and the diaphragm and is bounded posteriorly by the left triangular ligament. Anteriorly, this space communicates over the liver edge with the left anterior-inferior space. The left anterior-inferior space lies below the left lobe of the liver in front of the gastrohepatic ligament, stomach and gastrocolic ligament, and it is sometimes designated the perigastric space. The left posterior-inferior space corresponds to the lesser peritoneal sac. Abscesses in the lesser sac are comparatively rare and are sealed off by adhesions about the foramen of Winslow.

Incidence. Subphrenic abscess is relatively uncommon. It is more often found in males than females, correlating with the higher incidence of primary etiologic lesions in males. In the first quarter of the present century, the disease was more common in the second through the fourth decades, whereas it is now more common in the fifth and sixth decades of life. This may reflect earlier and better treatment of acute appendicitis and other abdominal emergencies, and an increasing number of elective operations on the gastrointestinal tract of older patients.

Etiology. Subphrenic abscess is usually a sequel to abdominal surgery or to suppurative and perforative intra-abdominal lesions. At one time, surgery was not a common cause, but elective operations now precede

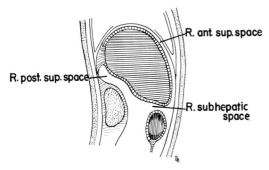

Figure 19. Diagrammatic representation of subphrenic spaces on the right side in parasagittal section. Note that the right posterior-superior space is really a recess arising from the right subhepatic space.

almost half the cases. Over half of the remainder follow appendicitis, perforated peptic ulcer and suppurative disease of the biliary tract. Occasionally, it follows pancreatitis. Only 10 per cent of abscesses arise from a primary focus outside of the abdomen.

The infection either originates in the subphrenic region or it begins elsewhere in the abdomen and reaches the subphrenic region by spread of contamination over the peritoneal surface. Subphrenic abscess occasionally arises by hematogenous or lymphatic dissemination, by rupture of a liver abscess or by spread from a retroperitoneal phlegmon.

The organisms are the pyogenic bacteria which cause peritonitis. Tubercle bacilli are rarely the etiologic agent today. Occasionally in the southern United States, subphrenic abscess is due to *Entamoeba histolytica.*

Pathology. Subphrenic contamination is often overcome by the peritoneum with or without the aid of antibiotics. It has been estimated that only 30 per cent of subphrenic infections go on to suppuration.

Subphrenic abscess is found on the right side far more often than on the left. Gas is present in 25 per cent of subphrenic abscesses. It results from the pneumoperitoneum following perforation of bowel, as a sequel to operation or from gas-forming organisms.

Most complications of subphrenic abscess are thoracic and the most common is pleural effusion. Other complications include pneumonitis, empyema, bronchopleural fistula, lung abscess, perforation of the diaphragm, pericarditis, perforation into a hollow abdominal viscus, spontaneous drainage to the outside, generalized peritonitis and hepatic suppuration. Occasionally, death may supervene without complications. Complications are the result of delayed diagnosis and treatment and markedly influence the prognosis. The mortality is three times as high when thoracic complications have been allowed to develop as when they are absent.

Symptoms and signs. The length of time that may elapse between operation or the onset of the primary disease, on the one hand, and the time the diagnosis is made, on the other, varies from a few days to over a year and the average is five months. A long latent period has always characterized a number of subphrenic abscesses, but has been noted in an increasing proportion of cases since the introduction of antibiotics.

The onset of clinical symptoms may be abrupt, insidious or may blend imperceptibly with the initiating intra-abdominal infection.

Any abscess produces two groups of manifestations: the systemic indications of suppuration and the symptoms and signs which are peculiar to the location of the abscess. The inaccessible and deep-seated location of subphrenic abscess results in the localizing manifestations becoming apparent late in the course of the disease. Typically, subphrenic abscess is characterized early by systemic evidences of an abscess and little to indicate its location. Maingot quotes Barnard in the well-known axiom, "Signs of pus somewhere, signs of pus nowhere, signs of pus there." At the present time, the problem of diagnosis is often made still more difficult by the use of antibiotics.

The administration of antibiotics to treat a fever of undetermined origin is wrong in principle. However, when a patient develops a fever five to ten days following operation, and conscientious investigation reveals no cause, giving antibiotics for a few days is reasonable and justified. No doubt this practice aborts many subphrenic infections, although some progress to suppuration despite the drugs. The physician must appreciate that he is increasing his responsibility to detect lesions which may be masked by the drugs when he elects such a course.

The systemic manifestations of an untreated subphrenic abscess are those of any suppurative process: spiking fever, chills, rapid pulse, dehydration, toxemia and leukocytosis. If the infection has been masked by antibiotics, there may be little or no fever and only such nonspecific symptoms as weakness, malaise, anorexia and, as Blades has expressed it, "a lack of a sense of well-being." It is apparent that if antibiotics are being administered, minimal systemic symptomatology calls for a thorough inquiry and examination for local symptoms and signs.

The most important of the local symptoms is pain, which is usually present but which varies greatly in intensity. The pain is felt in the upper abdomen, along the costal margin, in the flank and renal region, or in the neck or shoulder. The site of pain is of some localizing value. Pain is aggravated by deep inspiration or movements of the trunk. In addition, there may be hiccup, cough or dyspnea.

The most consistent and valuable of the local physical findings is tenderness, the location of which may suggest the site of the abscess. There may be tenderness over the twelfth rib posteriorly with a posterior-superior space abscess, tenderness along the costal margin in an anterior-superior space infection and tenderness with muscle guarding over the upper rectus in a subhepatic space abscess. Tenderness between the two heads of the sternocleidomastoid muscle due to irritation of the phrenic nerve has been described. There may be limitation of respiratory excursion, findings of pleural effusion, elevation and limited movement of a hemidiaphragm or crepitations in a lung base. Occasionally, four distinct levels can be percussed: resonance (normal lung), dullness (pleural effusion), resonance (gas in abscess) and dullness (fluid of abscess and liver). In suprahepatic infections, the liver will be displaced downward.

Minimal clinical suspicion demands preliminary x-ray studies. If fluoroscopy or chest films in full inspiration and full expiration show elevation, limited movement or thickening of a hemidiaphragm or pleural effusion, a full-scale radiologic investigation is necessary (Figs. 21 and 22). This includes planigrams and views in several positions with a horizontal x-ray beam in an attempt to demonstrate an air-fluid level and to try to distinguish elevated diaphragm from pleural fluid. If these studies are unrewarding, they may have to be repeated, because it is absolutely essential to establish the diagnosis and highly desirable to determine

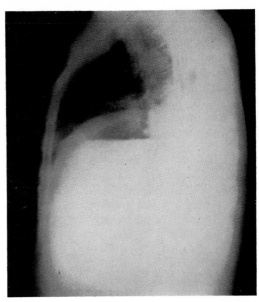

Figure 22. Lateral view of the patient in Figure 21, showing the same three diagnostic features. These two films are unusual in that the typical features are seldom seen so well demonstrated.

the location, should a subphrenic abscess exist.

Diagnosis. The first requisite for early diagnosis is awareness of the disease. The very obvious systemic manifestations without other apparent cause demand a searching investigation for physical signs and radiologic evidences of subphrenic abscess. If antibiotics are being administered, a still higher index of suspicion is necessary. If a patient has recently undergone surgery, or has had an intra-abdominal infection and has only minimal symptoms under antibiotic cover, physical and radiologic examination is warranted. If no evidence of subphrenic abscess is found at this point, antibiotic therapy should be discontinued and the disease allowed to declare itself. A swinging fever and other full-blown systemic manifestations, as well as localizing symptoms and signs, will soon become apparent if the vague symptoms have been due to a suppressed subphrenic infection. It is better to allow the disease to become manifest and then proceed with proper therapy than to allow the masked process to progress.

If, after all other investigative measures have been carried out, there is still doubt about the presence of a subphrenic abscess, surgical exploration may be necessary as an ultimate diagnostic procedure. Aspiration is not a permissible diagnostic or therapeutic procedure.

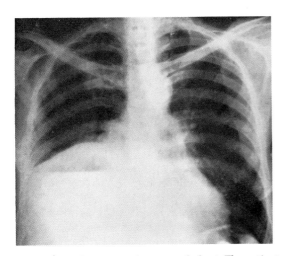

Figure 21. Posteroanterior x-ray of chest. The patient has a subphrenic abscess involving the right anterior-superior space. Note the elevation and thickening of the right hemidiaphragm and the presence of an air-fluid level beneath it.

Prophylaxis. Measures for prevention of subphrenic abscesses are identical with those carried out in the prevention and treatment of peritonitis. Of particular importance is positioning of the patient so that infective exudate drains toward the pelvis and away from the subphrenic area.

Treatment. The treatment consists of both supportive measures and surgical drainage. It is absolutely essential that drainage be carried out by a route that avoids contamination of the unprotected pleural or peritoneal cavities.

For abscess of the posterior-superior and subhepatic spaces on the right side, the "extraserous route" of Ochsner and Nather, through the bed of the twelfth rib, is employed. Although it is true that one actually goes through peritoneum to drain the subhepatic abscess, the suppurative process is walled off anteriorly and there is no general dissemination of infection. For the right anterior-superior and left suprahepatic spaces, the anterior incision of Clairmont and Meyer, along the costal margin, is used. Left anterior-inferior and left posterior-inferior space infections are sufficiently well walled off by omentum and transverse colon that they may be drained by cautious approach through the anterior abdominal wall.

After free drainage has been established, several soft rubber drains are put into the depth of the cavity and are slowly withdrawn over a period of several weeks. If fever does not subside rapidly after drainage, serious consideration of the possibility of a second subphrenic abscess is indicated and appropriate investigation initiated.

Adhesions and Bands

Adhesions are abnormal attachments between peritoneal surfaces; they may be either fibrinous or fibrous. A band is a long, narrow, fibrous adhesion.

ETIOLOGY. Most adhesions are inflammatory in origin and follow either a surgical operation or peritonitis. Some adhesions are thought to be congenital. Others are due to mechanical violence and foreign bodies, but for the most part they may be considered to be inflammatory.

The amount of fibrin produced from the inflamed mesothelial surface of the peritoneum varies according to the chemical irritant or the microorganisms involved. If the action of the irritant is of only a few days' duration, the fibrin is usually absorbed. Intact mesothelium is necessary for resorption of fibrin. If the fibrinous adhesions are not absorbed for any reason, they are invaded by fibroblasts and capillaries and organization begins between five and ten days after the initial insult.

Factors favoring the development of fibrous adhesions following chemical or bacterial peritonitis include continuing action of the irritant, necrosis of the mesothelium due to intense action of the irritant and a predisposition in certain individuals which is not well understood.

A surgical operation promotes fibrinous exudation by mechanical factors; i.e., handling viscera, sponges, instruments, foreign bodies, blood and, in some instances, low-grade and unsuspected infection. Fibrinous adhesions become fibrous in postoperative patients for the same reasons that they do in postperitonitic patients, but in the former there may be an additional factor of denudation of mesothelium — areas which are not adequately reperitonealized at the conclusion of operation. Fortunately, even fibrous adhesions may become attenuated and disappear in time.

Formation of adhesions is a protective process, without which irritants could not be localized and abdominal surgery would be impossible. These beneficial effects should be considered before attempts are made to abolish adhesion formation by means of drugs and chemicals.

PATHOLOGY. The chief complication of adhesions and bands is intestinal obstruction. At the present time, this lesion has displaced external hernia as the most common single cause of mechanical intestinal obstruction. The adhesions and bands may involve intestine, mesentery, parietes, omentum or any other abdominal structure. They are usually fibrous by the time they give rise to obstruction. Small bowel is most often obstructed, usually the distal ileum. This is probably because more inflammations and operations occur in the right lower quadrant than in any other location.

Adhesions and bands obstruct the bowel by several mechanisms. Adhesions, by contracture of the fibrous tissue, may kink, compress or otherwise distort the bowel to cause a nonstrangulating obstruction. A pocket may form into which bowel prolapses, or a narrow aperture may be produced through which a loop of bowel may herniate. A band may also serve as a pivot point for a volvulus.

Before the days of antibiotics a blend of paralytic ileus and mechanical obstruction frequently followed operations for perforated appendicitis with peritonitis. Today, this is a rare complication and when it does occur the extent of the mechanical obstruction can be accurately assessed by the oral administration of sodium diatrizoate solution followed by roentgenographic studies of the small bowel.

SYMPTOMS AND SIGNS. Adhesions may produce symptoms other than those of intestinal obstruction, but this happens rarely and such a diagnosis should be made with reservations. The great majority of patients present with a mechanical small bowel obstruction and an abdominal scar. The obstruction may be strangulating or nonstrangulating, a differentiation which frequently cannot be made with assurance on clinical grounds.

PREVENTION. There is no reliable way by which the formation of adhesions can be prevented, even if it were desirable to do so. The most a surgeon can hope to accomplish is the reduction of adhesion formation to a minimum. Of all the methods that have been tried to minimize adhesions, nothing has been shown to be as worthwhile as careful attention to the details of surgical technique.

All denuded areas should be reperitonealized; attention should be paid to hemostasis, and blood should be evacuated from the peritoneal cavity at the end of the operation; tissues should be handled gently; warm, moist sponges and padded retractors should be used; preoperative bowel preparation by mechanical cleansing and enteric antibiotics and sulfonamides before intestinal surgery is helpful; the area about an open viscus should be packed off and spillage should be avoided, and drains should be used where indicated but should be removed as soon as it is safe to do so. Local use of sulfonamides and antibiotics has no advantage over systemic administration and these chemicals may act as foreign bodies and irritants.

TREATMENT. When a mechanical small bowel obstruction develops within a week or ten days after operation, or after peritonitis without surgical operation, and one believes that the obstruction is due to fibrinous adhesions, the patient may be treated with supportive measures and a long intestinal tube.

The patient must be watched carefully and, if there is no response to this management, operative intervention may be necessary. As a rule, the tube will pass through the small bowel and the obstruction will be relieved.

In cases of mechanical small bowel obstruction due to fibrous adhesions, the patient will require an operation. Supportive measures and the use of the long tube are part of the preoperative preparation and not a substitute for operation.

In patients with a predisposition to form adhesions, ordinary methods of prophylaxis and treatment will prove futile. The most satisfactory solution to this problem is to recognize that a patient of this kind will inevitably re-form adhesions, and to replace haphazard adhesions with an organized pattern of nonobstructing adhesions such as one obtains with the Noble plication procedure.

INTRA-ABDOMINAL TRAUMA

Abdominal injuries, like peritonitis, have afflicted mankind from the remote past to the present day. It is a sad reflection upon our species that an undue proportion of these have been sustained in warfare. Today, a very large number of abdominal injuries result from automobile accidents. Abdominal trauma makes up approximately 10 per cent of incapacitating injuries.

Injuries to the abdomen may be divided into penetrating and nonpenetrating, the latter being more common. These may be subdivided into injuries of solid or hollow viscera.

All types of abdominal trauma, penetrating or nonpenetrating, and regardless of the organ injured, may produce shock and peritonitis, singly or together. At the present time one-half to two-thirds of deaths from abdominal injuries are due to shock. Modern methods of treating peritonitis have greatly reduced the mortality from this complication.

Penetrating Injuries

A penetrating wound is one in which a foreign body has entered or traversed the abdominal cavity.

Penetrating injuries of the abdomen are usually produced by weapons and are important in military surgery. They are by no means rare among civilians.

Wounds of the abdominal wall should be considered penetrating until proved otherwise. An external wound of the chest, back, buttock or perineum, in fact any wound from the shoulders to the knees, may penetrate the abdominal cavity.

If there are wounds of entry and exit, the path of the blade or missile, unless it has been deflected by bone, may be plotted as a straight line; this is of some value in determining the probability of injury to the fixed organs. Any penetrating wound of the abdomen must be assumed to have perforated bowel wall, unless there is very good evidence to the contrary.

The organ most frequently injured is small intestine. Less frequently, there is injury to liver, spleen, large bowel, stomach, mesenteries and major vessels. Several abdominal organs may be injured and there may be associated injuries, often of the thorax or urinary system. Trauma to multiple organs markedly increases the mortality.

The history should include information on the type of weapon and the position of the patient when wounded. The patient's symptoms will be of some value in diagnosing and localizing injuries, but one should not attach too much importance to the patient's denial of symptoms, especially if he is in shock or has multiple injuries. Often by the time a patient complains of symptoms, much valuable time has been lost.

Physical examination yields more information than does the history. The circulatory status, the blood pressure and the pulse, and their response following treatment are of the utmost importance in determining the presence of continued bleeding. Shock is to be expected, but if ordinary resuscitative measures restore pulse and blood pressure to normal and these remain stable, one may assume that there is no continuing hemorrhage.

The appearance of the wound may be deceptive. A small wound may be the only visual evidence of an underlying potentially lethal injury.

The most reliable evidence of injury to a hollow viscus is the absence of bowel sounds. If they remain absent for over an hour, abdominal exploration is mandatory. Abdominal tenderness and guarding may be present with either intraperitoneal blood or injury to a hollow viscus. Rectal examination should be carried out and it should be ascertained that the patient can pass urine normally. Stool and urine should be checked for blood.

If there is any likelihood of a kidney injury, an intravenous pyelogram should be obtained early. The kidneys will usually excrete the dye even in the presence of moderate shock. This is essential not only to establish whether a kidney has been injured, but also whether the opposite kidney is functioning normally. Similarly, if there is any possibility of a bladder injury, there is only one reliable diagnostic procedure: cystography following instillation of 250 cc. of radiopaque dye, 5 per cent sodium iodide.

A chest film and plain supine and upright, or left lateral decubitus, films of the abdomen should be taken to search for free intraperitoneal and retroperitoneal gas, missile fragments, ileus and evidence of fluid.

The supportive treatment will often be initiated even before preliminary assessment of the patient is completed. Blood is drawn for cross-matching, even if there is no immediate intention of giving a transfusion. Intravenous fluids are started through a large needle or cut-down. A Levin tube of generous diameter is placed in the stomach for decompression. In the shocked patient, urinary output as measured by a Foley catheter in the bladder is often a useful guide to the quantity of intravenous fluid required. A penetrating wound of the abdomen is one of the few instances in which prophylactic administration of antibiotics is justified. Narcotics are not administered to the patient with abdominal trauma until the surgeon responsible has had an opportunity to examine the patient and has made a decision regarding operative intervention.

The patient with a penetrating injury to the abdomen will almost always require exploration. In this regard, Sir Gordon Gordon-Taylor stated, "A penetrating wound in the abdomen probably means a penetrating wound of the bowel or other abdominal viscus and demands the earliest surgical intervention, unless a wisdom of prescience born of great experience justifies restraint." The only two instances when laparotomy may be deferred are when a patient is moribund and in the occasional instance in which thorough and repeated examination of the patient reveals no abnormality whatsoever.

Usually, a patient should not be taken to the operating room until he has been resuscitated and his pulse and blood pressure are stabilized. When a patient is actively bleeding as fast as one can pump blood into him, immediate intervention is indicated. If one is able to locate a controllable hemorrhage, the patient's condition will improve almost miraculously on the operating table.

When resuscitation may be carried out at a more leisurely pace, the outlook for the patient is improved, but operation should not be delayed beyond a few hours. Three factors influence the mortality: the severity of the injury, the duration of shock and the duration of peritoneal contamination. The objectives of operation are to control bleeding and to prevent continuing contamination of the peritoneal cavity.

Nonpenetrating Injuries

A more appropriate term for the type of injury to be described would be blunt or closed abdominal trauma because some surgeons limit the use of the term nonpenetrating injury to penetrating wounds restricted to the abdominal wall in which the peritoneum has not been violated. Blunt abdominal trauma is more important than penetrating injury because it is more common in civilian practice, except for certain geographic areas, and because it is more difficult to manage since clear-cut indications for operative intervention may be absent.

Approximately half of the serious blunt injuries to the abdomen which occur in North America are caused by automobile accidents. The steering wheel is a particularly dangerous instrument. Falls, athletic injuries and industrial accidents account for most of the remainder.

The forces which produce the injury to the abdominal contents are of four types: an anterior-posterior or lateral squeezing force which crushes the viscus, usually against unyielding bone; a tangential force which moves a viscus beyond the limits of its mobility, with a tearing of its attachments or capsule; a sudden compressing force which, in effect, bursts a hollow organ as if it were a paper bag, and a blasting force which causes widespread shattering of tissues and petechial hemorrhages.

Fixed organs are more likely to be injured than those which are more mobile. The organs injured, in approximate order of frequency, are spleen, liver, small bowel, large bowel, kidneys, stomach, bladder, diaphragm (left side) and, rarely, a pregnant uterus. The proximal jejunum and distal ileum, near points of fixation, are the parts of the small intestine most frequently injured and bowel is more often injured on its antimesenteric border. The same lesion may spill fecal material and bleed profusely. The vulnerable portion of the duodenum is the third part where it crosses the body of the third lumbar vertebra. A hollow viscus is always more susceptible to injury when distended than when empty.

The injuries frequently involve more than one organ, in which case the mortality rate is increased from less than 10 per cent to more than 30 per cent. The lethal factors—shock and peritoneal contamination—frequently coexist in the same patient.

Delayed hemorrhage may occur. The most frequent type arises from delayed rupture of the spleen. This variety of injury occurs once in six instances of splenic rupture. Delayed intra-abdominal hemorrhage may also result from injury to liver, to duodenum and pancreas and to kidney.

The difficult clinical problem in blunt trauma to the abdomen is to establish the diagnosis of a potentially lethal injury sufficiently early to avoid the high mortality rate which results from prolonged contamination of the peritoneal cavity. A ruptured hollow viscus may produce few symptoms during the most favorable time for closure. The physical findings may be no more than could be explained on the basis of a small amount of blood in the peritoneal cavity, or on the basis of a retroperitoneal hemorrhage. Routine operation is not a solution to this problem because a negative exploration also carries an increased mortality. The only answer is thorough initial investigation and frequent re-evaluation by the same surgeon.

The history may be very misleading. The initial trauma may be remarkably trivial. A history of a severe blow to the abdomen followed by rapid recovery and an interval of several hours without symptoms in no way rules out intra-abdominal injury. The nature and location of the blunt trauma will enable the physician to visualize the possible underlying injuries. The presence and location of pain are of some diagnostic value. A history of persistent vomiting is suggestive of bowel rupture, particularly if the vomitus is bloody. Difficulty in voiding or hematuria will direct attention to the urinary tract.

The history will only suggest the presence of a serious lesion. The diagnosis must be made from the physical findings supported by laboratory aids, chiefly the x-ray films.

The patient with significant nonpenetrating trauma to the abdomen will usually be in shock on admission, although this need not be true, particularly in patients with splenic or gastrointestinal rupture. Resuscitation with whole blood should be carried out concomitantly with the clinical assessment of the patient. Military experience in Korea has indicated that severely injured persons may require quantities of blood far in excess of the amount of blood lost from hemorrhage or the amount of fluid displaced into traumatized tissues. These resuscitative measures are, in a sense, diagnostic as well as therapeutic. Failure of the patient to respond to liberal administration of whole blood, or a temporary response to blood, indicates either very severe trauma or continued hemorrhage.

One should search for an area of contusion on the abdominal wall. Tenderness, guarding and rebound tenderness are usually due to rupture of a hollow viscus but can be caused by blood in the peritoneal cavity. The absence of bowel sounds always suggests severe injury, but it is not by itself an absolute criterion for exploration, as paralytic ileus may be caused by a retroperitoneal hematoma. Obliteration of liver dullness is almost pathognomonic of rupture of some part of the gastrointestinal tract. Shifting dullness in the flanks and fluid in the cul-de-sac on rectal examination are occasionally noted.

Scout films of the abdomen and chest should be taken. Fractured lower ribs should alert one to the possibility of rupture of spleen or liver, but rib fractures are found in only 50 per cent of fatal cases. Finding of free gas on the upright or left lateral decubitus films will make exploration mandatory. A fracture of the pelvis in the vicinity of the pubic rami or which opens up the pelvic ring makes a cystogram absolutely indispensable. If there is any suspicion of kidney trauma, intravenous pyelography should be carried out early.

Four quadrant peritoneal aspiration under local anesthesia is a useful diagnostic adjunct. The finding of blood, bile, fecal material or fluid with a high amylase content may influence the management.

Whether or not operation is indicated, a program of supportive therapy should be instituted.

The objectives of operation are the same for both penetrating and nonpenetrating trauma to the abdomen: control of hemorrhage and prevention of continued contamination of the peritoneal cavity. The treatment of bleeding from a ruptured spleen has high priority and the hemorrhage often becomes profuse when the abdomen is opened. Splenectomy is the only permissible procedure. The essential considerations in the treatment of liver injuries are to stop bleeding, to excise devitalized fragments and to drain. Bleeding may be controlled with mattress sutures and hemostatic sponges; packs should not be used. Hepatic lobectomy has recently been shown to be lifesaving in the treatment of certain patients with massive laceration or fragmentation of the liver. Drainage is essential because bile leakage will occur and may lead to fatal peritonitis. Injuries to the tail of the pancreas are best treated by resection. Elsewhere in the pancreas, drainage alone is often the only procedure possible, although various ingenious pancreaticojejunal anastomoses have been described and have found occasional application. An opening in the stomach may be treated by excision of the wound edges and closure with sutures. The small bowel should be systematically inspected from the ligament of Treitz to the ileocecal valve; wounds are treated either by resection or by a method of suture which does not narrow the lumen. The anterior surface of the duodenum should be inspected for an intraperitoneal rupture, which can usually be closed with sutures. At the same time, one should be alert for bile-stained blood and gas behind the peritoneum, indicating a retroperitoneal rupture of the duodenum; this requires mobilization of the duodenum, suture and drainage. As a general rule, the traumatized colon should be exteriorized in patients with colonic perforation. In the rectum, where this is not possible, closure with proximal colostomy is the treatment of choice. This latter procedure may also find occasional application in left colon lesions, and more particularly in those of the right colon, where protection is afforded by catheter cecostomy. A wound of the gallbladder is treated by cholecystectomy. Injury to the common bile duct is treated by suture and T-tube drainage. Bladder wounds are closed, the usual care being exercised not to put chromic catgut or nonabsorbable sutures through the mucosa. A urethral catheter or suprapubic tube is inserted and the extraperitoneal tissues about the bladder are drained. Nephrectomy is seldom necessary unless the kidney is severely fragmented.

HEMOPERITONEUM

Hemoperitoneum may be either traumatic or spontaneous. The trauma may be trivial, especially if bleeding comes from a previously diseased organ. Delayed hemorrhage from nonpenetrating trauma to the abdomen may also occur.

The lesions which may cause spontaneous hemoperitoneum include ectopic pregnancy, blood dyscrasias, rupture of an artery which is the seat of a degenerative process, torsion of omentum, spleen, fibroid tumor or ovarian cyst, mesenteric vascular occlusion and pancreatitis.

The most probable source of a large amount of blood in the male is rupture of the spleen. In the female of childbearing age, it is ectopic pregnancy.

Hemorrhage should be controlled and the blood evacuated. Blood in the peritoneal cavity is a much greater hazard to the patient than any possible benefit that might accrue from having this blood as a source of iron.

PNEUMOPERITONEUM

Pneumoperitoneum is the presence of gas within the peritoneal cavity. The detection of free intraperitoneal gas is of great value in the diagnosis of a perforated abdominal viscus. There are, however, other important causes of pneumoperitoneum which are included in the following etiologic classification.

Classification of Pneumoperitoneum

From Within the Lumen of the Gastrointestinal Tract
    Perforated peptic ulcer
    Other perforative disease
    Blunt and penetrating trauma to the abdomen
    Endoscopic instrumentation
    Infections
    Postanesthetic
From Outside the Lumen of the Gastrointestinal Tract
    Postoperative
    Diagnostic
      Rubin Test
      Needle
    Therapeutic
    Penetrating trauma
Idiopathic

PERFORATED VISCUS. Perforated peptic ulcer is the commonest disease process producing pneumoperitoneum. The demonstration of free intraperitoneal air in a patient with an acute abdomen usually indicates a perforation of the gastrointestinal tract.

Demonstrable pneumoperitoneum occurs in the majority of patients with perforated peptic ulcers. The detection of air depends upon many factors, including the time elapsed since perforation, the location and size of the perforation, the effectiveness of reaction in walling off the perforation, the amount of air in the stomach at the time of perforation, and the amount swallowed subsequently.

Benign and malignant ulcerating lesions and obstructing lesions in which perforation of the gastrointestinal tract occasionally occurs may produce pneumoperitoneum.

Free gas in the peritoneal cavity seeks the highest level and, in the upright position, tends to accumulate under the diaphragm. Although absence of liver dullness in the midaxillary line is clinically indicative of pneumoperitoneum, accurate detection requires careful radiologic examination (Figs. 23 and 24). A few cubic centimeters of air may be seen on a scout film of the abdomen if sufficient time is allowed for the gas to collect in whatever part of the cavity is up-

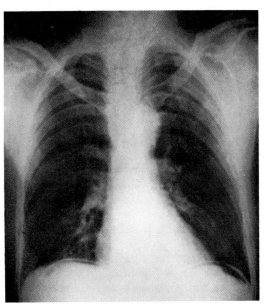

Figure 23. Posteroanterior x-ray of chest, showing a thin rim of free air beneath both leaves of the diaphragm. The patient has a perforated peptic ulcer, the most common cause of pneumoperitoneum other than laparotomy.

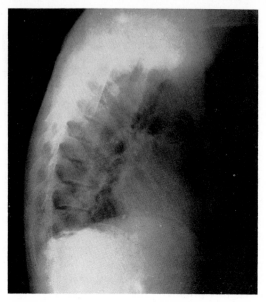

Figure 24. Lateral view of the same patient as in Figure 23. These films were taken in the upright position. If patient is too ill to be upright for a few minutes before films are taken, the left lateral decubitus position should be used, with patient lying on his left side.

permost. Erect and left lateral decubitus views are commonly used.

TRAUMATIC. Pneumoperitoneum following blunt trauma to the abdomen indicates a perforated viscus. Pneumoperitoneum following a penetrating or perforating abdominal wound reveals only peritoneal entrance, since air may enter with the missile. Visceral involvement, however, is common if the peritoneum is entered, and the detection of free intraperitoneal air is a positive indication for laparotomy.

ACCIDENTAL. Instrumental visualization of abdominal organs, often accompanied by air insufflation, may perforate a normal or diseased viscus and produce pneumoperitoneum. Perforation during sigmoidoscopy under direct vision is rare. Pneumoperitoneum occasionally follows gastroscopy, but usually gross perforation is not found at laparotomy. In the absence of clinical peritonitis, these patients have been successfully treated conservatively.

BACTERIAL. Certain gas-forming organisms may cause pneumoperitoneum in an intra-abdominal abscess. *Clostridium welchii* and related bacteria are the commonest infecting organisms that produce gas, but *Escherichia coli*, anaerobic streptococci and *Proteus* have also occasionally been cultured. The formation of gas in an abdominal ab-

scess may be a valuable aid in diagnosis and localization.

POSTANESTHETIC. Pneumoperitoneum following operation is occasionally related to anesthesia. Excessive airway pressure during assisted respiration, or rapid oxygen flow through a nasal catheter, may produce gastric dilatation and, rarely, gastric perforation. Intraperitoneal gas following anesthesia is not always associated with perforation or peritonitis; the gas may diffuse beneath the mucosa along the vessels of the stomach into the peritoneal cavity.

POSTOPERATIVE. The most frequent cause of pneumoperitoneum is abdominal surgery. The peritoneal cavity is normally a potential space in which there is a negative pressure. When the peritoneum is opened at operation, an inrush of air may be noted. The duration of postoperative pneumoperitoneum is variable; small quantities of air are usually absorbed within a few days. In the majority of patients, the air has disappeared by 14 days, but rarely it may persist for as long as six weeks.

There is no apparent correlation between pneumoperitoneum and postoperative pulmonary complications. The presence of intraperitoneal air following operation may confuse the assessment of postoperative abdominal complications.

DIAGNOSTIC. Direct injection of gas into the peritoneal cavity to outline the abdominal and pelvic organs has been used in selected patients as an aid in the radiologic diagnosis.

The potential communication between the peritoneal cavity and the exterior existing in the normal female, via the fallopian tubes and the uterine cavity, is utilized in the Rubin test.

THERAPEUTIC. Artificial pneumoperitoneum has been used in the treatment of pulmonary and abdominal tuberculosis for many years. Five hundred to 1000 cc. of air or oxygen is injected directly into the peritoneal cavity with periodic refills. Elevation of the diaphragms with reduction of pulmonary volume tends to promote collapse of tuberculous cavities, particularly if they are located in the base of the lungs. This treatment often combined with phrenicectomy and chemotherapy is considered of value in some instances. Another use therapeutically is the preparation of the patient with a very large ventral hernia for operation. The air is introduced into the peritoneal cavity while the hernia is under control with strapping. This has been a very useful procedure in selected cases.

IDIOPATHIC OR UNDETERMINED CAUSE. Spontaneous idiopathic pneumoperitoneum occurs rarely with no demonstrable perforation of a viscus, known exogenous cause or underlying disease process. It produces few clinical manifestations and usually subsides without ill effect.

TUMORS OF THE PERITONEUM

The great majority of peritoneal tumors are secondary. Primary tumors of the peritoneum or of any serous membrane are very rare.

Primary Tumors

Neoplasms may arise from any of the fibrous, fatty, vascular or reticular tissues which lie beneath the peritoneal mesothelium, but such are best regarded as tumors of the viscera, parietes or retroperitoneum. Although it is very rare, most pathologists agree that the primary peritoneal mesothelioma is a recognizable entity. Both benign and malignant varieties of mesothelioma exist. The lesions may be localized or diffuse and they occur in plaquelike and nodular forms. The tumor may spread over and encompass the viscera, producing fibrous thickening of the peritoneum and shortening of the mesentery. Intestinal obstruction, viscid ascites and obliteration of the peritoneal cavity have been reported. Even malignant forms do not invade until late and seldom metastasize.

The neoplasm may have the microscopic appearance of a papillary, fibrous, acinar or even squamous cell tumor. It is very difficult for the pathologist to establish the diagnosis on the basis of examination of ascitic fluid or a small amount of biopsy material.

The benign form, if localized, can be effectively treated by surgical excision.

Secondary Tumors

Most secondary tumors of the peritoneum are metastatic carcinomas. The malignant tumor reaches the peritoneal surface by permeation through the wall of a viscus, by hematogenous and lymphatic spread and, occasionally, by inoculation at the time of surgery. Once in the peritoneal cavity, tumor may be disseminated over the serosal surface.

The gross appearance of secondary tumors varies widely, according to the primary lesion and the mode of spread. The main features are ascites and tumor nodules. The ascitic fluid is usually bloody and often contains exfoliated tumor cells. The tumor ranges from minute deposits, a millimeter or less in diameter, studded diffusely over the peritoneal membrane, to large plaques and masses of neoplastic tissue. As a rule, the tumor nodules are less than a centimeter in diameter. The omentum may be so infiltrated with tumor that it is converted into a hard mass. There may be drop metastases to the cul-de-sac, giving rise to a rectal shelf. Sometimes a reticular pattern of white lymphatics, permeated with tumor, is seen beneath serosa. It may be difficult to distinguish grossly the nodular lesions of secondary peritoneal tumor from those of tuberculosis, fat necrosis or foreign body granuloma.

Not all secondary tumors are malignant. One benign secondary lesion is the parasitic fibroid, a leiomyoma that has become detached from the uterus and taken up a new attachment on the peritoneal surface. Similarly, dermoid cysts of the ovary sometimes become secondarily attached to peritoneum.

An interesting form of secondary tumor of the peritoneum is pseudomyxoma peritonaei, which arises from rupture of a pseudomucinous cystadenoma of the ovary or rarely of the appendix. A lesion of similar appearance may be produced by rupture of a mucocele of the appendix, in which case the mucus acts as an irritant and produces chemical peritonitis. The mucus-producing cells become implanted on the peritoneum and continue to produce a gelatinous exudate, causing the so-called jelly belly.

The patient with metastases to the peritoneum usually has advanced symptoms of the primary lesion. He may complain of pain, discomfort or cardiorespiratory symptoms from abdominal distention. Cachexia, pallor and ascites are often present when the patient is seen for the first time. One may palpate tumor tissue in the form of a primary lesion, a Virchow's node, liver nodules, an omental mass or a rectal shelf.

If there is no evidence of metastatic malignancy other than the ascites, abdominal fluid may be examined cytologically. This examination is subject to the limitations inherent in the cytologic method.

Treatment can only be symptomatic. Abdominal tapping may be done for the comfort of the patient. Instillation of colloidal Au[198], or radiomimetic drugs, may reduce ascites when the tumor nodules are only a few millimeters in diameter and there is no block at the porta hepatis.

MESENTERIES AND OMENTUM

ANATOMY AND PHYSIOLOGY

The stomach, jejunoileum, appendix, transverse colon, sigmoid colon, liver and spleen are attached to the posterior wall of the abdominal cavity by mesenteries, which carry their respective blood vessels, lymphatics and lymph nodes. The gastrohepatic ligament is the ventral mesentery of the stomach and first part of the duodenum, but it is also, in a sense, a dorsal mesentery of the liver and gallbladder. The gastrocolic ligament is continuous with the anterior layer of the greater omentum. The mesentery of the jejunoileum is described as fan-shaped, averaging 12 to 25 cm. in height. Its junction with parietal peritoneum is only 15 cm. long, whereas its other border, where it enfolds small bowel, is about 700 cm. in length. This marked disparity in the lengths of its two borders can only be reconciled by numerous folds toward the enteric border. All mesenteries consist of two layers of mesothelium enclosing a variable amount of fatty and loose connective tissue, vessels and lymph nodes.

The mesenteries of the duodenum, pancreas, ascending colon and descending colon have disappeared in fetal life because of fusion with parietal peritoneum. Fortunately for the surgeon, these planes of fusion can usually be converted into planes of cleavage, restoring the primitive state. The mesentery thus created has only one layer of mesothelium, the posterior parietal peritoneum, but it carries in its fatty areolar tissue the blood vessels, lymphatics and lymph nodes of the organ in question.

The greater omentum is a double fold of mesentery embryologically. One might expect it to contain four mesothelial layers, but the central two have fused and vanished. The size and fat content of the greater omentum are highly variable. Its role as the "abdominal policeman" seems well supported by experimental and clinical evidence. The areolar tissue of the omentum is rich in macrophages. Bacteria or carbon particles injected into the peritoneal cavity are rapidly removed by the omentum and are subsequently seen to be situated in phagocytes beneath its mesothelium. The ability of the omentum to adhere to sites of inflammation and perforation has been mentioned in the discussion of peritonitis. Foreign bodies in the peritoneal cavity, such as a bullet or a sponge, are often found completely wrapped in omentum.

The presence of the greater omentum is not always beneficial. Adhesions and bands between the omentum and either parietes or viscera, or openings made in the omentum at surgical operations, may lead to intestinal obstruction. Once a patient has had some such difficulty originating in the omentum, surgical excision of the omentum will circumvent further complications.

MESENTERIC LYMPHADENITIS

Acute Nonspecific Mesenteric Lymphadenitis

Over the past 30 years, this disease has been delineated from tuberculous lymphadenitis and has gradually gained wide acceptance as a clinical entity. Its chief importance lies in the fact that it produces the picture of an acute abdomen and must be considered in the differential diagnosis of appendicitis.

Acute nonspecific mesenteric lymphadenitis is uncommon and, in our experience, the incidence is diminishing. Most patients are between five and 15 years of age and it is somewhat more frequent in boys.

The etiology is unknown and there may be more than one cause. Cultures from the enlarged mesenteric lymph nodes are usually negative. Associated low-grade inflammatory changes in the appendix and distal ileum have been reported in a large proportion of cases and may have a bearing on the etiology.

The appendix is grossly normal. There is discrete enlargement of the mesenteric lymph nodes in the ileocecal angle, particularly those in the juxtaintestinal group. Lymph nodes in this region are prominent in children and normal lymph nodes must be distinguished from those which are pathologic. The nodes vary from soft and pink in the early stage of the disease to firm and white later. Microscopically, the lymph nodes show only hyperplasia, edema and hyperemia.

The child with acute nonspecific mesenteric lymphadenitis usually presents with colicky abdominal pain vaguely situated about the umbilicus, right side or right lower quadrant. The pain is of variable intensity, but in between the cramps the child feels fairly well. There is often a recent upper respiratory infection, which may still be present. There is a history of previous attacks, separated by intervals of several months, in over half the cases. Malaise, anorexia, nausea and vomiting are also frequently present or reported in earlier attacks.

The child does not look or act ill. There is fever, usually under 100° F. The patient is flushed and there may be circumoral pallor. The pharynx is often injected and the cervical lymph nodes may be enlarged. Abdominal tenderness is higher, more medial, less well localized and more variable from one time to another than in appendicitis. A shift in the point of maximum tenderness to the left when the child lies on the left side, due to change in position of the mesentery and nodes, is said to be characteristic but is often absent. The white blood count may be increased to 10,000 to 15,000 per cu. mm.

Indiscriminate appendectomy cannot be condoned. However, if one suspects acute appendicitis the matter should be settled by laparotomy. On the other hand, if one can be reasonably confident of a diagnosis of mesenteric adenitis, a few hours of observation may be confirmatory. The signs and symptoms of this latter disease will subside or improve in less than 24 hours.

If, at laparotomy, one finds a normal appendix and the characteristic lymphadenopathy in the ileocecal angle, appendectomy should be carried out. It is not advisable to remove a lymph node for biopsy, because bowel may become adherent to the site. Postoperative respiratory complications should be anticipated. A small proportion of these patients may have further attacks after appendectomy, but there is an overall tendency toward recovery.

Tuberculous Mesenteric Lymphadenitis

Involvement of mesenteric lymph nodes by tubercle bacilli is now uncommon. The disease may be primary, in which case the organisms, usually bovine, gain entry through intact mucosa to Peyer's patches and then reach the nodes. The disease may be secondary to tuberculosis of lungs or bowel.

Tubercle formation, caseation and eventually calcification are present as in tuberculous lymphadenitis elsewhere. The disease may be complicated by peritoneal adhesions, tuberculous peritonitis or secondary pyogenic infection.

The disease is seen in acute and chronic forms and its manifestations are highly variable. The salient features are fever, general ill health, weight loss, diarrhea and cramping abdominal pain.

X-ray examination of the abdomen in a clinically well person may show calcified lymph nodes in the right iliac fossa—the so-called chalky tombstones of tubercle bacilli, which may or may not be dead.

In general, the treatment should be conservative, with antituberculous drugs and supportive measures.

Mesenteric and Omental Cysts

A variety of unusual cysts may be found in the mesenteries and omentum. These include enterogenous cysts or congenital reduplications; lymphatic cysts, either cavernous lymphangiomas or cystic lymphangiectasis; dermoid cysts; and hydatid cysts.

The cysts may produce no symptoms or only abdominal enlargement and vague discomfort. Occasionally, a patient presents with intestinal hemorrhage or obstruction. Cysts of the omentum may give rise to secondary torsion and the clinical picture of an acute abdomen. The characteristic physical finding is a "floating tumor." Those in the mesentery have greater mobility from side to side than in a vertical direction.

If surgical intervention is necessary, the ideal treatment is to shell out the cyst. Unfortunately, this is seldom possible in the mesentery, as vessels supplying the bowel are adherent to the cyst wall. It may be necessary to resect bowel. A cyst of the omentum is easily treated by excision. Hydatid cyst may be treated by deep x-ray therapy or by excision with care not to spill the fluid, which would reinfect the patient or cause a severe anaphylactic reaction.

INFARCTION OF THE OMENTUM

Infarction of the greater omentum may be due to torsion, thrombosis, polyarteritis nodosa, embolism, trauma or of unknown etiology.

Idiopathic segmental infarction of the omentum is rare. It is most often found in well-nourished men in the third decade. The cause is obscure, but it is thought to be related to venous engorgement and mild trauma, or increase in intra-abdominal pressure leading to thrombosis. Usually, the right, lower, free margin of the omentum is infarcted.

Patients present with steady, severe right lower quadrant pain, the onset of which may be gradual or sudden. Nausea and vomiting are unusual. On examination, the tenderness is usually higher than one would expect for appendicitis and a mass may be palpable. Cutaneous hyperesthesia is said to be characteristic.

The correct diagnosis is never made preoperatively; most cases are diagnosed as acute appendicitis. The finding of a normal appendix and some serosanguineous fluid in the peritoneal cavity should always direct one's attention to disease elsewhere. The infarcted area forms a firm, red to purplish-black mass. Treatment is wide excision of the involved omentum.

Torsion of the Omentum

Torsion of the omentum may be classified as primary and secondary. Secondary torsion is more common and is subdivided into bipolar and unipolar types, depending on whether or not there is a secondary fixation of the omentum. Among the causes are hernias, adhesions, cysts and tumors.

In primary torsion of the omentum there is no apparent cause, although vigorous exercise, movement of the omentum by intestinal peristalsis and hemodynamic forces have been blamed. The torsion is always unipolar and may be either complete or incomplete. In the complete type, there may be up to six full turns. The omentum is usually quite large and fatty with a long pedicle and a narrow attachment. It is often the right, free margin of the omentum that is involved in the torsion.

The clinical symptoms and treatment of torsion of the omentum are similar to those of infarction of the omentum.

Appendices Epiploicae

The appendices epiploicae are fat-laden pouches of peritoneum which are found on the large bowel and, rarely on the appendix. They are usually arranged in two rows, one medial to the taenia libera and one lateral to the taenia omentalis. These are the sites at which some of the vessels enter the bowel wall. One will recall that diverticula also are situated in these positions.

The appendices epiploicae may be the sites of a number of diseases, the most common of which is epiploic appendicitis. This may be due to torsion or thrombosis and so may be regarded as a miniature counterpart of torsion and infarction of the omentum. Epiploic appendicitis is found chiefly in the sigmoid and cecal regions. Other disease processes in which the appendices epiploicae may be involved include acute and chronic inflammation secondary to diverticulitis, degeneration to form an intraperitoneal loose body, initiation of an intussusception and incarceration in a hernia.

The presenting symptom of epiploic appendicitis is lower abdominal pain on either the right or left side. The correct diagnosis is seldom made preoperatively. Treatment is excision with care not to open up a diverticulum.

RETROPERITONEAL SPACE

Anatomy

The retroperitoneal space from the surgeon's viewpoint is a potential space extending from the respiratory diaphragm above to the pelvic diaphragm below. Its posterior boundaries are the vertebral bodies, the psoas and quadratus lumborum muscles and the aponeurotic portions of the transverse abdominis muscles. Below the iliac crests, it is bounded by the sacrum and the psoas and piriformis muscles posteriorly, and by the iliacus and obturatorius internus muscles laterally. The anterior boundary of the retroperitoneal space is chiefly the posterior parietal peritoneum, but in addition the anterior boundary is made up of the posterior surface of the liver, the ascending and descending portions of the large intestine, the retroperitoneal portion of the duodenum and the rectum.

The major organs of the retroperitoneal space are the kidneys and ureters, the adrenals and the pancreas. The space is also occupied by the great systemic vessels and their branches, veins of the portal system, lymphatic vessels and lymph nodes, somatic nerves, sympathetic chains and autonomic plexuses and an abundance of fatty and areolar connective tissue.

RETROPERITONEAL HEMORRHAGE

Bleeding into the retroperitoneal space is a sequel to blunt trauma to the trunk, fractures of the pelvis or lumbar vertebrae, especially of their transverse processes, and lacerations of the kidney. Because the blood is irritating to both somatic and autonomic nerves, the symptoms of peritonitis may be simulated. There may be abdominal pain, nausea, vomiting, abdominal guarding, low-grade fever and leukocytosis. This syndrome may proceed to adynamic ileus characterized by a silent distended abdomen. Except for rupture of an aortic aneurysm and rare instances of severe trauma to the kidney or renal vessels, retroperitoneal bleeding seldom presents as an exsanguinating hemorrhage.

Retroperitoneal bleeding should be recognized early and the ileus and gastric dilatation treated by gastrointestinal decompression. The possibility of a more serious intra-abdominal lesion initially presenting with a similar clinical picture should be considered. The differential diagnosis is difficult and must occasionally be made at laparotomy.

RETROPERITONEAL FIBROSIS

Idiopathic retroperitoneal fibrosis is relatively infrequent, and is reported to be encountered more commonly in the male. The process consists of a fibrous plaque, or mass, which extends into the retroperitoneal tissues above the sacral promontory, extending laterally to involve the ureters, upward to the renal pedicles or even into the mediastinum and downwards to the upper border of the pelvis. The fibrous sheet of tissue is sharply delineated but not encapsulated, obstructing the structures within the retroperitoneal space but not invading them. The clinical symptoms are often fatigue, weight loss, flank and low back pain, occasionally associated with urinary disturbances, including a high urine output as the bilateral hydronephrosis develops. The most dramatic presenting symptom may be anuria. The urographic findings usually include dilatation of the upper ureters and pelves with a narrowing or obliteration and medial deviation of the midureter. Surgical treatment has consisted of temporary nephrostomy and ureterolysis, with the occasional regression of the fibrous tissue under radiation therapy or treatment with cortisone.

RETROPERITONEAL TUMORS

It is customary to exclude tumors of the kidneys, ureters, adrenals, pancreas and bowel as well as metastatic tumors to the retroperitoneal lymph nodes from the group of neoplasms designated as retroperitoneal tumors.

The most common of the primary tumors seen in the retroperitoneal space are lymphosarcoma, Hodgkin's disease and reticulum cell sarcoma. The second most common is the liposarcoma—a noteworthy oddity, since elsewhere in the body benign fatty tumors are quite common and malignant fatty tumors are almost unknown. The remaining tumors are those which arise from the mesodermal tissues in the retroperitoneal space. The majority are malignant, and one-third have metastasized at the time they are diagnosed. Those which are benign tend to recur after removal.

Because the retroperitoneum is a distensible space, these tumors may reach very large size before they are diagnosed. About half the patients present with pain and one-third with an abdominal mass. Gastrointestinal symptoms, backache, pain and swelling in a leg, genitourinary symptoms and fever are occasionally early symptoms.

The most common physical finding is a fixed or movable mass, usually nontender. Varicocele, edema or varicosities of a leg, a forward protrusion of the liver, lumbar dullness on percussion and occasionally a neurologic deficit, especially with dumbbell tumors, may be found.

The chief laboratory aid is the x-ray and the most important investigation is the pyelogram with anteroposterior and lateral views. The ureters, which are adherent to the posterior parietal peritoneum, are seen to be displaced forward or laterally. The function of each kidney should be assessed, as one kidney may need to be sacrificed at operation in order to encompass the lesion. The next most important radiologic procedure is a gastrointestinal series. Presacral oxygen insufflation may be useful to outline the contents of the retroperitoneal area. Aortography and venography may be useful, as the great vessels are often displaced.

At the time of operative intervention, most retroperitoneal tumors will have surrounded or invaded major organs and vessels. Curative operation is possible in about 20 per cent and the operative mortality ranges from 10 to 25 per cent.

Operation is required to assess the tumor and establish a diagnosis. A proportion of the tumors are amenable to surgical treatment, but each case must be individually evaluated. Close cooperation between the surgeon and the pathologist is necessary in order to determine the curability of the lesion and the extent of surgical extirpation which is justified. It may be necessary to sacrifice one kidney or the vena cava below the renal veins. If complete excision is impossible, the residual tumors will be radiosensitive to some degree in about three-quarters of the cases. These remaining patients should be treated with radiation or radiomimetic drugs.

READING REFERENCES

Bardeen, C. R., and Lewis, W. H.: The development of the limbs, body-wall and back in man. Am. J. Anat. *1*:1, 1901-1902.

Berens, J. J., Gray, H. K., and Dockerty, M. B.: Subphrenic abscess. Surg. Gyn. & Obst. *96*:463, 1953.

Blades, B.: Subphrenic abscess. (Editorial.) Surg. Gyn. & Obst. *103*:765, 1956.

Bremer, J. L.: Congenital Anomalies of the Viscera: Their Embryological Basis. Cambridge, Massachusetts, Harvard University Press, 1957.

Brödel, M.: Lesions of the rectus abdominis muscle simulating an acute intra-abdominal condition. I. Anatomy of the rectus muscle. Bull. Johns Hopkins Hosp. *61*:295, 1937.

Burke, J. F., Pontoppiden, H., and Welch, C. E.: High output respiratory failure: an important cause of death following peritonitis or ileus. Trans. Am. Surg. Assoc., 1963.

Cullen, T. S.: Lesions of the rectus abdominis muscle simulating an acute intra-abdominal condition. II. Hemorrhage into or beneath the rectus muscle simulating an acute abdominal condition. Bull. Johns Hopkins Hosp. *61*:317, 1937.

Cullen, T. S.: Embryology, Anatomy and Diseases of the Umbilicus Together with Diseases of the Urachus. Philadelphia, W. B. Saunders Company, 1916.

Donhauser, J. L.: Primary acute mesenteric lymphadenitis. Arch. Surg. *74*:528, 1957.

Fothergill, W. E.: Haematoma in the abdominal wall simulating pelvic new growth. Brit. M.J. *1*:941, 1926.

Gaston, B. H., and Mulholland, J. H.: Treatment of penetrating abdominal wounds. S. Clin. North America *35*:463, 1955.

Jamieson, R. A.: Subcutaneous rupture of the muscles of the abdomen. Brit. J. Surg. *36*:434, 1949.

Johnson, F. R., and Whitting, H. W.: Repair of parietal peritoneum. Brit. J. Surg. *49*:653, 1962.

Kessler, R. E., and Zimmon, D. S.: Umbilical Vein Catheterization in Man. Surg. Gyn. & Obst. *124*:594, 1967.

Lampe, E. W.: Surgical anatomy of the abdominal wall. S. Clin. North America *32*:545, 1952.

Levene, G., and Kaufman, S. A.: Roentgenologic findings in acute diseases in the abdomen. M. Clin. North America *41*:1303, 1957.

Loria, F. L.: Historical aspects of penetrating wounds of the abdomen. Surg. Gyn. & Obst. (Internat. Abstr. Surg.) *87*:521, 1948.

Macbeth, R. A.: Blunt abdominal trauma. Canad. J. Surg. *9*:384, 1966.

Macbeth, R. A., and Harrison, R. C.: Fluid, electrolyte and metabolic problems associated with surgical emergencies. S. Clin. North America *40*:1414, 1960.

MacKenzie, W. C., and Small, J.: Primary idiopathic segmental infarction of the greater omentum. Canadian M.A.J. *55*:144, 1946.

Maingot, R.: Abdominal Operations. 3rd ed. New York, Appleton-Century-Crofts, 1955.

Moore, S. W.: The physiological basis for diagnostic signs of an acute abdomen. S. Clin. North America *38*:371, 1958.

Murray, S. D., and Burger, R. E.: Rupture of the inferior epigastric vessels. Ann. Surg. *139*:90, 1954.

Ochsner, A., and DeBakey, M.: Subphrenic abscess. Internat. Abstr. Surg. *66*:426, 1938.

Ormond, J. K.: Bilateral ureteral obstruction due to envelopment and compression by an inflammatory retroperitoneal process. J. Urol. *59*:1072, 1948.

Pack, G. T., and Ehrlich, H. E.: Neoplasms of the anterior abdominal wall with special consideration of desmoid tumors. Internat. Abstr. Surg. *79*:177, 1944.

Paul, M.: The surgery of the congenital anomalies of the midline ventral abdominal wall. Ann. Roy. Coll. Surgeons England *13*:313, 1953.

Pulaski, E. J., Noyes, H. E., and Brame, R. A.: The influence of antibiotics on experimental endogenous peritonitis. Surg. Gyn. & Obst. *99*:341, 1954.

Randall, H. T.: Water and electrolyte balance in surgery. S. Clin. North America *32*:445, 1952.

Robinson, S. C.: Observations on the peritoneum as an absorbing surface. Am. J. Obst. & Gyn. *83*:446, 1962.

Silverman, F. N., and Huang, N.: Congenital absence of the abdominal muscles. Am. J. Dis. Child. *80*:91, 1950.

Soutar, S. F., Douglas, D. M., and Dennison, W. M.: Patent vitello-intestinal duct: the risk of obstruction due to prolapse. Brit. J. Surg. *45*:617, 1958.

Trimingham, H. L., and McDonald, J. R.: Congenital anomalies in the region of the umbilicus. Surg. Gyn. & Obst. *80*:152, 1945.

Vest, B., and Margulis, A. R.: The roentgen diagnosis of postoperative ileus-obstruction. Surg. Gyn. & Obst. *115*:421, 1962.

Welch, C. E., and Richardson, G. S.: Early operative treatment of generalized peritonitis due to appendicitis. *In*, Current Surgical Management. (Mulholland, J. H., Ellison, F. H., and Friesen, S. R., eds.) Philadelphia, W. B. Saunders Company, 1957.

Chapter 22

THE HERNIAS

by
CHESTER B. McVAY, M.D.

CHESTER BIDWELL McVAY left Yankton, South Dakota, his birthplace, to receive his medical education, do graduate degree work in anatomy at Northwestern University and receive his surgical education and training at the University of Michigan. After military service in World War II, he returned to Yankton to practice and is now Clinical Professor of Surgery and Associate Professor of Anatomy at the University of South Dakota. His union of anatomy and surgery has made him an authoritative and stimulating investigator of the surgical problems of the hernias.

Historically, the development of operations for hernia is one of the most interesting chapters in the field of medicine, since hernias have always been the most common visible affliction of man amenable to surgical treatment. Its common occurrence, the enigma of its etiologic background and the methods of its cure through the ages have made the hernia story an absorbing narrative which has few peers even in the field of fiction. The story in the past 70 years is a monument to the surgeons' ingenuity, but the multiplicity of modern operations for inguinal and femoral hernias is a record of basic misunderstanding of the anatomy involved.

DEFINITION. The classic definition of a hernia is "the protrusion of a viscus from its normal cavity through a congenital or an acquired aperture." While this definition suffices in a general way, it requires some elucidation. For example, a patient may have a hernia consisting entirely of preperitoneal fat, without a peritoneal sac and without the protrusion of a viscus. This is quite common in epigastric and femoral hernias in the early stages. Occasionally, in indirect inguinal hernias, the entire presenting mass is a pedunculated process of preperitoneal fat. These fatty protrusions are attached to the parietal peritoneum, and if the aperture through which the fat protrudes is not repaired at this stage, more and more fat gradually extrudes and eventually pulls a diverticulum of peritoneum with it. Into this peritoneal pouch, then, a viscus may herniate. This is the mechanism of the development of epigastric hernias and is referred to as the lipoma theory of Cloquet.

If one adheres to the classic definition, these fatty protrusions do not represent hernias; nevertheless, they produce a palpable mass which is usually tender and symptoms which bring the patient to the doctor. These fatty protrusions are usually irreducible and in the inguinal canal may not be differentiated from a bowel-containing process of peritoneum. Another aberration of this definition is the reducible hernia, and the majority of hernias are reducible in their early stages of development. A patient who has had a loop of bowel protruding through an aperture in the abdominal wall, and then has this loop of bowel returned to the abdominal cavity, certainly has a hernia from a practical standpoint, although the viscus no longer protrudes.

Many patients live their entire lives with a congenital processus vaginalis in the inguinal canal without bowel or omentum ever entering this pre-formed sac. Therefore, from their standpoint or that of an examining physician, they have never had a hernia. A peritoneal sac is generally considered to be a component of a hernia, but this is not necessarily so. Traumatic hernias of the diaphragm rarely have a peritoneal sac unless they begin as small ruptures of the musculoaponeurotic structure which leave the peritoneum and pleura intact. A wound dehiscence is certainly a protrusion of abdominal viscera without a peritoneal covering.

Thus, it is apparent that the definition of a hernia is not such a simple matter. Furthermore, the mass or size of the hernia, whether it is contained in a peritoneal sac and whether

561

it is reducible or irreducible are not the important considerations. The important point is the defect in musculoaponeurotic and fascial continuity or, more simply, the hole through the parietal abdominal wall, respiratory or pelvic diaphragms. It is the size of this defect which is the crux of the repair problem. The fixation and rigidity of the hernial ring are frequently important factors in reducibility and the incidence of strangulation. The size of the hernial sac is of no particular consequence from the standpoint of repair except in the very large variety where the replacement of viscera long outside the abdominal cavity may present a spatial problem.

Therefore, perhaps a better definition of a hernia would be one directed at the defect. An abdominal hernia is a defect in the normal musculoaponeurotic and fascial continuity of the abdominal wall, respiratory or pelvic diaphragms, either congenital or acquired, which permits the egress of any structures other than those which normally pass through the parietes.

Thus, intermittency of protrusion, peritoneal sac or not, viscus or fat, would not confuse the definition. If one could diagnose a peritoneal sac with relative certainty, as in cryptorchidism or intermittent hydrocele, a diagnosis of hernia could then be made even though there had never been an intra-abdominal viscus in the hernial sac.

CLASSIFICATION. There are many descriptive adjectives used in any discussion of hernias.

Topographic refers to the regional location of the hernia, e.g., inguinal, femoral, umbilical or epigastric.

Congenital or *acquired* hernias would seem to be clear-cut terms and, as the words imply, divide all hernias into those present at birth and those which come in later life, but some hernias are not categorized that easily. While there is not much doubt about absent segments of the respiratory diaphragm and omphalocele being congenital hernias, certain hernias considered to be acquired have a congenital predisposition to development. For example, the indirect inguinal hernia that develops in adulthood has had the peritoneal sac since the descent of the processus vaginalis which preceded the descent of the testis.

Reducible, irreducible or *incarcerated* refers to whether or not the contents of the hernia can be pushed back into the abdomen. Incisional hernias frequently have both reducible and irreducible components.

Strangulated hernia is an irreducible hernia with compression obstruction of the blood supply to the incarcerated loop of bowel. If this is not relieved surgically in a few hours, the strangulated hernia becomes gangrenous.

An *incisional* hernia occurs through a surgical incision or scar, is man-made and in this instance there is no question that the hernia is acquired.

Recurrent hernia is one which recurs following an operation for a similar type of hernia. In the inguinal region, this becomes a moot point. After repair of an indirect inguinal hernia, if the patient develops a direct inguinal hernia or a femoral hernia, does this represent a recurrence; is it a separate, subsequently acquired hernia; was this second hernia present all the time and simply missed at the original operation, or did the surgeon damage the posterior inguinal wall at the original operation and thereby lay the groundwork for the development of the second hernia?

Double usually refers to bilateral inguinal or femoral hernias, but is also used to describe a direct-indirect inguinal hernia on a single side. A direct-indirect inguinal hernia, with the double sac straddling the inferior epigastric blood vessels, is also known as a *pantaloon* hernia.

Very occasionally, one encounters a direct inguinal, an indirect inguinal and a femoral hernia on the same side. In this event, it is known as a *triple* hernia.

An *external* hernia is one that protrudes to the outside where it is visible and palpable. An *internal* hernia is one that remains within the confines of the body cavities. Diaphragmatic hernia is an example of an internal hernia. Occasionally, one sees a hernia through the foramen of Winslow, into a deep peritoneal recess or pouch, or through a traumatic rent in the omentum or mesentery. However, hernias of this type are extremely rare and most so-called internal hernias within the abdominal cavity represent congenital malrotations of the intestinal tract.

A *sliding* hernia is one in which a viscus forms part of the wall on the hernial sac.

Hernia adiposa is one in which the mass consists entirely of preperitoneal fat and is commonly seen in the epigastrium.

Lavater's hernia (Richter's hernia) is a type of incarcerated or strangulated hernia in which only a portion of the circumference of the bowel is caught in the hernial ring. The vermiform appendix, or a Meckel's diverticulum, may be incarcerated or even strangulated in an inguinal or femoral hernia. In the latter instance it is usually referred to as a Littre's hernia. These eponymic hernias may cause a strangulating obstruction without the signs and symptoms of intestinal obstruction.

Spiegel's hernia occurs in the linea semilunaris at or below the linea semicircularis but above the point at which the inferior epigastric vessels cross the lateral border of the rectus abdominis muscle. If it occurs below the inferior epigastric vessels, then it must be termed a direct inguinal hernia. Spiegel's hernia is usually interstitial at the outset and, because it is covered by the intact external oblique aponeurosis, a diagnosis is difficult to establish.

An *interstitial* hernia develops and enlarges between the musculoaponeurotic laminae of the abdominal wall rather than in the subcutaneous fascia.

Complete or *incomplete* usually refers to the indirect inguinal hernia and the extent of the congenital peritoneal sac. A complete indirect inguinal hernia is one in which no portion of the processus vaginalis has become obliterated so that the hernial contents extend into the tunica vaginalis of the testis (inset, Fig. 4, *a*). An incomplete indirect inguinal hernia may also extend into the scrotum, but the sac does not communicate with the tunica vaginalis of the testis because the lower portion of the processus vaginalis has become obliterated (inset, Fig. 2, *a*).

ETIOLOGY. The etiologic basis of a given hernia may be an obvious single defect, but more commonly the cause is a combination of predisposing factors. The *congenital* hernias of infancy may be ascribed to a single etiologic factor which is either a congenital defect, such as omphalocele congenitalis, or failure of segmental development, as in the absence of a portion of the abdominal wall or respiratory diaphragm. An additional type of truly congenital hernia is the indirect inguinal hernia which appears at birth or soon thereafter. This distinction in timing in the development of the most common of all hernias is made to eliminate the contributing factors, such as increased intra-abdominal pressure and muscle relaxation, which are etiologic in the development of the indirect inguinal hernia in adulthood. Rarely, trauma to the abdominal wall is the direct cause of a hernia, but, aside from penetrating wounds, the effect of trauma is usually transmitted

to the weakest point and may be at some distance from the point of the injury. A blunt force to the central portion of the abdominal wall may result in the occurrence of a diaphragmatic hernia, a direct inguinal hernia, an indirect inguinal hernia or a femoral hernia. In the latter two examples, however, congenital predisposition is also an important factor. For example, unless there is a preformed sac in the inguinal canal, no amount of trauma will produce an indirect inguinal hernia. In the case of the femoral hernia, the point is debatable. In an incisional hernia, the cause is the previous operative incision, although here again there are contributing factors such as hemorrhage, infection or increased intra-abdominal pressure in the immediate postoperative period.

Heredity, or a familial tendency to hernia, is an obvious fact when one reviews the patient records of many hernias. Persistence of the processus vaginalis in the inguinal canal, with an abdominal inguinal ring large enough to permit the development of a hernia, is certainly a familial tendency. Likewise, the generalized weakness of connective tissue, as seen in the asthenic individual with visceroptosis and varicose veins, is hereditary and these individuals more commonly develop hernias than does the general population. Any statistical evaluation of the hereditary influence on the incidence of hernia must, however, be plotted against the overall incidence of hernia in the general population, variously estimated at between 1:8 and 1:15. Racial differences are probably more related to habits of nutrition and physical development than to any racial characteristic.

Age as an etiologic factor has two considerations. First, the incidence of all types of hernias as related to age and, second, age as related to a specific type of hernia. For example, direct inguinal hernia is a disease of advancing years and is rarely seen in children. Indirect inguinal hernia is more common in persons in the younger years, having its greatest incidence in the first year of life and a gradually decreasing incidence after that until the mid-teens, when there is a sharp rise which lasts until the mid-twenties. This is undoubtedly due to the fact that this is the period in which the most vigorous physical exercise occurs. The incidence of indirect inguinal hernia then stays rather stationary until the sixth decade, when it again falls off.

Sex as a determining factor in the development of a hernia is concerned with the type of hernia and developmental factors peculiar to the sex. The indirect inguinal hernia is nine times more common in the male than in the female because of the embryologic descent of the testes. Femoral hernia is three times more common in the female than in the male, presumably because of the difference in the inclination of the pelvis and the common occurrence of increased intra-abdominal pressure due to pregnancy. Adult umbilical hernia is two to three times more common in the female because of the element of pregnancy. Direct inguinal hernia is a rarity in the female for reasons unknown, but, from cadaver examination and examination of the posterior inguinal wall during the repair of indirect inguinal and femoral hernias in the female, it would appear that the posterior inguinal wall is a much heavier aponeurotic layer in the female than in the male.

Obesity in the young adult probably has very little effect upon the incidence of the various hernias, but in the older age groups it very definitely increases the incidence of epigastric and umbilical hernias, especially in the pregnant female. Obesity operates in two ways to increase the incidence of these two hernias: first, by increasing intra-abdominal pressure and, second, by forcing fat into tiny apertures, such as the perforating blood vessel foramina in the linea alba above the umbilicus or through a persistent defect at the umbilicus. In the aged obese patient, one can observe fatty infiltration of the aponeurotic laminae with multiple herniae adiposae in the epigastrium. The incidence of incisional hernia is much greater in the obese patient.

Musculoaponeurotic deficiencies of the abdominal wall are an anatomic fact with considerable variation in the strength of the flat muscles of the abdominal wall. This undoubtedly is a primary factor in the development of the direct inguinal hernia. A congenitally narrow insertion of the transversus abdominis aponeurosis into Cooper's ligament may be the principal etiologic factor in the development of a femoral hernia.

Increased intra-abdominal pressure is the major etiologic factor in the development of all acquired hernias and is the precipitating cause in the development of the indirect inguinal hernia, in spite of the existence of a congenital sac. Gradually increasing and steady pressure is not so likely to produce a hernia as are repeated and sudden surges of increased pressure, as in coughing, or an extreme muscular effort, especially when associated with the element of surprise. The shutter action of the abdominal inguinal ring and of the inguinal canal is a fact which largely explains why a physically active man does not develop an indirect inguinal hernia during his active years but suddenly develops the hernia in old age. The congenital sac was always there, but the abdominal inguinal ring was effectively closed by muscular effort until he reached the age of poor muscle tone and developed a chronic cough, or suddenly engaged in a severe muscular effort. Occasionally, one sees the first evidence of a small umbilical defect with the development of ascites, in which event the fluid-containing umbilical bulge becomes a barometer of the degree of ascites. Intra-abdominal neoplasms rarely cause a hernia because they develop so slowly that there is no significant increase in intra-abdominal pressure. This is due to the gradual stretching of the abdominal musculature.

INCIDENCE. The relative frequency of the various common hernias has been tabulated many times. It is interesting that the percentages have remained roughly the same in the past 50 years, with the exception that incisional hernias are increasing in number. This is a natural sequence to the increasing number of operations performed each year.

SYMPTOMS AND DIAGNOSIS. The subjective symptoms caused by a hernia are extremely variable and depend more upon the pressure exerted on the contents than upon the size of the hernia. A large hernia containing several feet of intestine and a large piece of omentum may cause the patient only the vaguest of symptoms, whereas a small hernia tightly constricting a knuckle of bowel or omentum can cause severe local pain, referred pain and nausea. When a hernia becomes strangulated, the symptoms are severe, progressive and, unless corrected promptly, lead to serious consequences and even death.

An indirect inguinal hernia containing incarcerated omentum may cause only slight discomfort locally but by traction on the omentum can cause a more distressing epigastric pain which may be mistaken for that due to a duodenal ulcer or gallbladder disease. The small epigastric or umbilical hernia can have all of the symptoms referred to the epigastrium by traction on the omentum.

A small and unrecognized femoral hernia may contain an incarcerated knuckle of urinary bladder and be attended with frequency, urgency, terminal dysuria, and even hematuria. An esophageal hiatus hernia may cause palpitation and substernal pressure by pressure from the dilated stomach, as it lies in the posterior mediastinum. A traumatic diaphragmatic hernia may be accompanied by shortness of breath due to compression of the lung; pain in the base of the neck due to diaphragmatic irritation; or, if the parietal pleura is irritated, a typical pleuritic pain aggravated by deep breathing.

Whenever there is compression of the bowel lumen, there are the added and usually progressive symptoms of bowel obstruction. Even partial obstruction of the lumen, as in a Littre's hernia, can cause symptoms of bowel obstruction. When the blood supply to a viscus is compressed, there are added signs and symptoms of a strangulating obstruction.

If the hernia is visible or palpable and the mass is painful, there is little doubt on the part of either the patient or the physician as to the diagnosis. Small epigastric hernias, especially in the obese, are difficult to detect. Hernias of the respiratory diaphragm are diagnosed with certainty only by an x-ray examination, usually augmented by a contrast medium. Internal hernias are usually diagnosed only during an operation for intestinal obstruction.

Most hernias have a somatic component of local pain plus a referred element of visceral pain. Pain at the hernial site is directly related to the degree of irritation of the parietal peritoneum and adjacent somatically innervated structures. Pressure and inflammation are the precipitating factors. The pressure upon a contained viscus, or its subsequent vascular injury, is felt by the patient as pain in the epigastrium. Some patients who have had a troublesome hernia for a long time seem to learn to localize visceral pain and, hence, have no referred symptoms.

Certainly, the most common complaint of a patient with a hernia is a painful lump, and it is the pain which usually brings the patient to the doctor. However, concern over the presence of a tumor, even when painless, will usually cause the patient to seek medical advice. The pain is intermittent when the hernia is reducible. It is absent when the hernia is reduced and usually mild when the hernia is "out," if it is of long standing. Especially in hernias with small rings and in hernias that have just made their appearance, the pain is quite sharp when the hernia comes down and again at the moment when it reduces.

The objective characteristics of a hernia are the presence of an abnormal swelling which may be so soft as to feel fluctuant, firm or hard, depending upon the contents of the sac and the pressure exerted. Omentum has a rather characteristic doughy feel, but so does a loop of sigmoid colon containing feces. A loop of gas-filled intestine may be soft and compressible or tense, depending upon the degree of incarceration. If a loop of intestine is strangulated, it is tense and exquisitely tender. Except when incarcerated, the mass of the hernia can be made to disappear with gentle pressure, especially with the patient in the supine position. The patient is frequently more adept at reducing the hernia than is the examining physician, because of long practice and the fact that his muscles are more relaxed when he is not afraid that the physician will hurt him.

Another classic characteristic of a hernia is the reappearance of the tumor with straining or coughing after it has been previously reduced. Associated with the reappearance of the hernia are the sensations imparted to the physician's examining finger. This sensation has been variously described but can most simply be expressed as a push or impulse. An incarcerated hernia or a strangulated hernia is fixed, will not reduce and, of course, has no impulse on palpation. Transillumination with a strong light in a darkened room is a useful aid in differentiating a hydrocele of the cord from an incarcerated indirect inguinal hernia. The hydrocele will transilluminate, whereas the hernia containing bowel or omentum will not because of its greater density.

Percussion of a hernial mass will serve to differentiate a gas-containing viscus from a solid piece of omentum. Auscultation over the hernial mass will occasionally serve to confirm the impression of an incarcerated loop of intestine. Auscultation over the abdomen is more important in determining the degree or status of intestinal obstruction when an incarcerated hernia is present and there are other signs of intestinal obstruction. X-ray examination of the intestinal tract with a contrast medium is rarely necessary for the diagnosis of a hernia of the abdominal wall. Occasionally, however, the barium enema examination of the colon will furnish the only evidence of an incarcerated knuckle of sigmoid colon in an indirect inguinal hernial sac.

TREATMENT. The treatment of a hernia is surgical correction of the defect in normal musculoaponeurotic structure. The operation should have as its principal objective the restoration of the hernial area to as near the normal status as is possible. Except in patients with large incisional hernias and in those with congenital absence of portions of the abdominal wall or respiratory diaphragm, normal anatomy can usually be restored.

The injection treatment of hernias was a popular method in Europe for years and gained its greatest popularity in this country in the 1930's, but experience has shown that it rarely cures a hernia and it has been abandoned. In the first few years of its use, it apparently cured small indirect inguinal hernias but, eventually, most of these hernias reappeared. The scarring incident to the injected sclerosing solution makes the surgical repair extremely difficult.

Some patients refuse operation even though the need is urgent. In other instances, there is a strong contraindication to subjecting the patient to the risk of an operation because of associated serious systemic disease. Such patients whose hernia is amenable to compression reduction should be fitted with an appropriate truss. The only hernia that can be controlled with a truss is the small indirect inguinal hernia. Because this hernia can be repaired under local anesthesia without risk, for all practical purposes there is no recommended treatment other than surgical correction.

Even in infants there is rarely a contraindication to the surgical repair of a hernia. The common indirect inguinal hernia in infancy should be repaired as soon as the diagnosis is established. The umbilical hernia of infancy should not be operated upon when the patient is under one year of age because most of these hernias close spontaneously. The yarn truss for inguinal hernias and the compression treatment of the umbilical hernia are of historical interest only.

The argument continues about contralateral exploration in the infant with a unilateral indirect inguinal hernia. Contralateral exploration is not indicated unless there is a suggestive history of a bulge observed by the parent or the physician. Because the overall incidence of bilaterality of the inguinal hernia can be generously stated as 20 per cent, the routine exploration of the opposite side represents unnecessary surgery. The finding of a small diverticulum of peritoneum on the contralateral side does not necessarily constitute a hernia and one must realize that the obliteration of the processus vaginalis may take up to two years to be complete.

In planning a hernia operation, the surgeon should carefully consider the patient as a whole. This is especially true in persons of the older age groups. The cardiovascular and renal systems should be carefully evaluated. Even though the x-ray film of the chest shows no abnormality, this evidence may be of the most vital importance in evaluating postoperative pulmonary complications. In the older group of patients who suddenly develop a hernia, causes of increased intra-abdominal pressure should be carefully searched for. The patient with an obstructing carcinoma of the colon, or urethral obstruction due to benign prostatic hypertrophy, or carcinoma should not be subjected to a hernia operation unless the hernia is strangulated. If at all possible, the obese patient should be reduced to near normal weight before undergoing an elective hernia operation. The operation is not only more difficult technically, but the incidence of recurrence and postoperative complications is much higher in the obese patient than in one of normal weight.

HERNIAS OF THE INGUINOFEMORAL REGION

It has been customary in the past to discuss the femoral hernia as a separate entity, but the point should be emphasized that a femoral hernia is in reality a type of inguinal hernia. Although the etiologic factors of the indirect inguinal hernia, the direct inguinal hernia and the femoral hernia are different, the effect of these hernias upon the posterior inguinal wall is so interrelated that they must be considered together if one is to understand, first, the altered anatomic structure and, second, the rational repair.

Although the sac of the femoral hernia lies in the fossa ovalis of the femoral region, the defect which allows the hernia to develop is just as truly inguinal in location as is the defect which permits the development of a

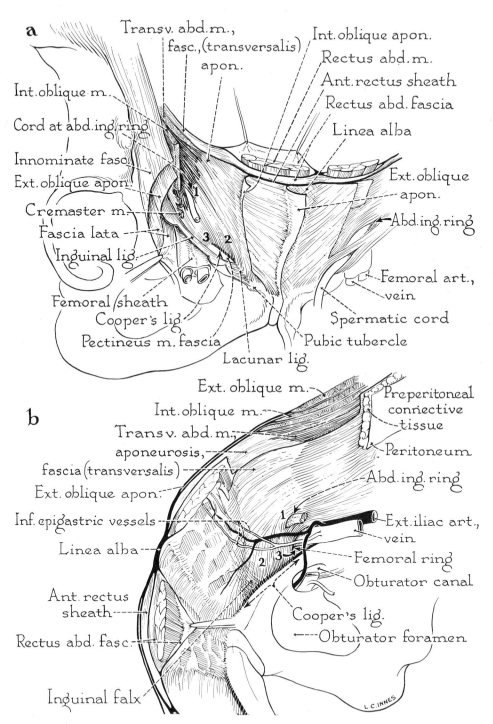

Figure 1. The normal anatomic structure of the inguinofemoral region. *a*, Anterior view. *b*, Posterior view. The numbers 1, 2 and 3 represent the sites of origin respectively of the indirect inguinal, the direct inguinal and the femoral hernia.

direct inguinal hernia, or the enlarged abdominal inguinal ring of an indirect inguinal hernia even though the sac of the latter may extend into the scrotum.

INDIRECT INGUINAL HERNIA

DEFINITION.   An indirect inguinal hernia is one which passes through the abdominal inguinal ring and follows the course of the spermatic cord in the inguinal canal and then emerges through the subcutaneous inguinal ring. A very small sac may be confined to the inguinal canal, whereas the complete congenital peritoneal sac extends into the scrotum to communicate with the tunica vaginalis of the testis (Fig. 4, *a* and inset).

ANATOMY.   The normal anatomic structure of the inguinofemoral region is presented in Figure 1, *a* and *b*. The distortion of the normal anatomic relationship by the presence of an indirect inguinal hernia can best be presented by dividing the indirect inguinal hernias into three categories, depending upon the size of the dilated abdominal inguinal ring. The length of the sac or the quantity of the contents of the hernia is of no particular importance. The crux of the repair problem concerns the size of the abdominal inguinal ring.

Small indirect inguinal hernia. All indirect inguinal hernias are in this category at their outset. Irrespective of the length of the congenital peritoneal sac, there is only slight dilatation of the abdominal inguinal ring (Fig. 2, *a*). Aside from the presence of the congenital peritoneal sac, the only alteration of the normal anatomic state is the minimal stretching of the abdominal ring (Fig. 2, *b* and *c*). The posterior inguinal wall is intact, the femoral ring is small and even the continuity of the transversalis fascia into the anterior femoral sheath medial to the slightly dilated abdominal inguinal ring is normal. Therefore, it should be apparent that the repair of this most common of all hernias should be a simple problem.

Medium indirect inguinal hernia. The small indirect inguinal hernia has only the slightest alteration from normal anatomic relationships (Fig. 3, *a*). The large indirect inguinal hernia may cause complete destruction of the posterior inguinal wall, and its repair involves the same problems as the direct inguinal hernia. In between these two extremes, there is great variation in the dilatation of the abdominal inguinal ring. As the ring is enlarged slowly by the presence of the hernia, it expands medially for the most part. Eventually a point is reached which determines whether the hernia can be repaired by simple closure of the dilated abdominal inguinal ring, or whether the posterior wall must be reconstructed. This point is a line drawn cephalad from the femoral ring. If the dilated abdominal inguinal ring extends medially beyond this line, the hernia must be repaired as for a large indirect inguinal hernia and, conversely, if it remains lateral to this line the hernia may be simply repaired by closing the dilated abdominal inguinal ring.

The term medium indirect inguinal hernia refers to a hernia with an abdominal inguinal ring which has dilated up to this line (Fig. 3, *b* and *c*). In this hernia, in addition to the congenital peritoneal sac, the pathologic anatomy consists of complete destruction of the continuity of the transversalis fascia into the anterior femoral sheath by the enlarged abdominal inguinal ring. However, the posterior inguinal wall and its insertion into Cooper's ligament are undisturbed.

Two other variations of the normal anatomic relationship are common in both this size of indirect inguinal hernia and in the large variety: protrusion of pedunculated processes of preperitoneal fat among the cord structures (Fig. 3, *b*), and the incorporation of a hollow viscus in the wall of the hernial sac, known as a sliding hernia.

Large indirect inguinal hernia. This hernia begins as a small variety and in sequence is a medium indirect inguinal hernia before becoming a large indirect inguinal hernia (Fig. 4, *a*). It takes considerable time for this type of hernia to develop. Any indirect inguinal hernia, with the abdominal inguinal ring dilated medially beyond a line drawn cephalad from the medial margin of the femoral ring, is termed a large indirect inguinal hernia. Just as there is considerable variation between the size of a small and a medium indirect inguinal hernia, there is also a great variety of sizes of dilated abdominal rings between the medium indirect and the largest possible indirect inguinal hernia, which are all designated large indirect inguinal hernias. In the large variety, the medial margin of the dilated abdominal inguinal ring extends to the lateral margin of the rectus abdominis muscle (Fig. 4, *b* and *c*). Anatomically, this means that a posterior inguinal wall is nonexistent.

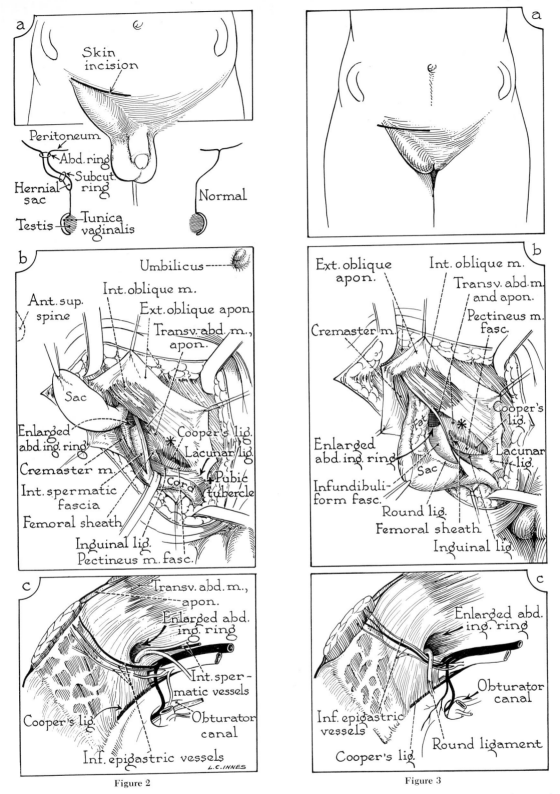

Figure 2

Figure 3

Figure 2. *a,* Appearance of a small indirect inguinal hernia and skin incision used for all groin hernias. *Left inset,* An incomplete hernial sac. *Right inset,* Normal obliteration of processus vaginalis. *b,* Anterior view of the anatomy of a small indirect inguinal hernia. The line of separation of the cremaster muscle from the internal oblique is denoted by an asterisk (*). *c,* Posterior view of the slightly dilated abdominal inguinal ring.

Figure 3. *a,* Appearance of a medium-sized indirect inguinal hernia in the female. *b,* Anterior view of the anatomy of a medium indirect inguinal hernia in the female. The line of separation of the cremaster muscle from the internal oblique is denoted by an asterisk (*). *c,* Posterior view of the moderately dilated abdominal inguinal ring.

569

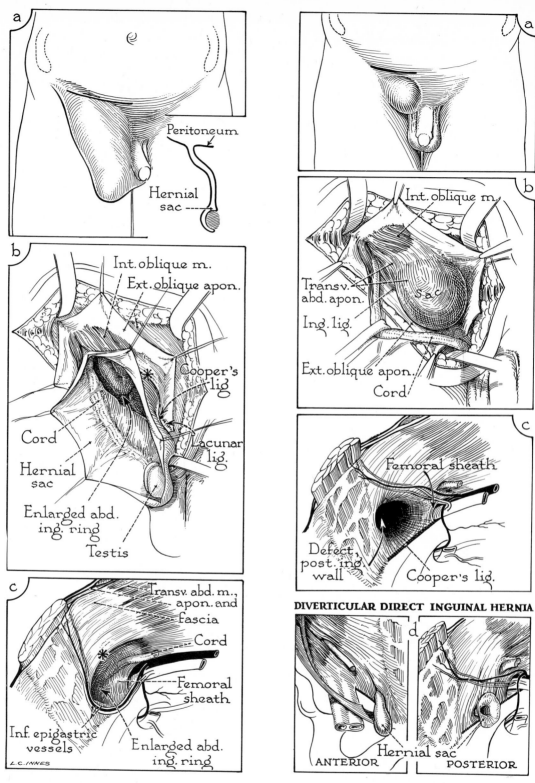

Figure 4.

Figure 5

Figure 4. *a*, Appearance of a large indirect inguinal hernia. *Inset*, Complete, congenital hernial sac. *b*, Anterior view of the anatomy of a large indirect inguinal hernia. The junction of weak and strong posterior inguinal wall is denoted by an asterisk (*). *c*, Posterior view of the greatly dilated abdominal inguinal ring. The edge of remaining strong posterior inguinal wall is denoted by an asterisk (*).

Figure 5. *a*, Appearance of a direct inguinal hernia. *b*, Anterior view of the anatomy of a direct inguinal hernia. *c*, posterior view of the direct hernia defect in the posterior inguinal wall. *d*, Anterior and posterior views of the anatomy of the diverticular type of direct inguinal hernia.

In the slow transition of a small indirect inguinal hernia into the large variety, there are several features which are of importance. In the indirect inguinal hernia, the peritoneal sac is always on the anteromedial aspect of the spermatic cord as it lies in the inguinal canal, except in the recurrent indirect inguinal hernia, where it may bear any relationship to the cord structures. This constant position of the peritoneal sac goes back to the embryologic descent of the testis. Prior to the descent of the testis, the processus vaginalis of the peritoneum descends into the scrotum. The testis, which is a retroperitoneal structure, slides into the scrotum behind and slightly caudad to the peritoneal sac; therefore, when the processus vaginalis fails to obliterate, the indirect inguinal hernial sac is already in position waiting to receive a viscus and become an indirect inguinal hernia.

As the abdominal inguinal ring enlarges in the transition from a small to a medium to a large indirect inguinal hernia, this enlargement takes place predominantly in a medial direction. The origin of the lower fibers of the internal oblique and transversus abdominis muscles from the fascia lata lateral to the abdominal inguinal ring prevents any significant enlargement in this direction. Inferiorly or caudally, the inguinal ligament over the iliac vessels and, more medially, the superior ramus of the pubic bone prevent enlargement in this direction. Superiorly, there is some extension, but the abdominal musculature prevents much enlargement in this direction. Therefore, with rather rigid restrictions superiorly, laterally and inferiorly, the abdominal inguinal ring enlarges medially at the expense of the posterior inguinal wall.

As the posterior inguinal wall is stretched and attenuated, it is pushed outward and becomes part of the internal spermatic fascial investment of the hernial sac. The lateral border of the rectus abdominis muscle and tendon of origin stop the medial enlargement of the abdominal inguinal ring. When a ring of this size is reached, there is never any significant increase in size no matter how long the hernia persists or how many of the abdominal viscera descend into the hernial sac. In the enormous scrotal hernias, there is some stretching of the musculature along the superior margin of the ring, but, for all practical purposes, the rectus muscle is the final delimiting factor in the size of the ring.

TREATMENT. In the *small indirect inguinal hernia*, there is practically no alteration of the normal anatomic structure. The persistent processus vaginalis which is the hernial sac must, of course, be removed and the adequate removal of this sac with high ligation has long been a standard procedure. After dissecting the peritoneal sac free from the cord structures well up through the abdominal inguinal ring, all that needs to be done to return the inguinal region to normal is to tighten the ring to normal size (Fig. 6, *a* and *b*). Any additional approximation or plication of the layers is not only unnecessary but may damage an otherwise normal posterior inguinal wall. After the abdominal inguinal ring is returned to normal size, the spermatic cord is dropped back into its normal position and the external oblique aponeurosis is sutured together making a snug subcutaneous inguinal ring (Fig. 6, *c*).

After the hernial sac is removed, the medial margin of the slightly dilated abdominal inguinal ring is delineated by sharp dissection. This is simply accomplished by cutting the internal spermatic fascia at its point of origin from the transversalis fascia. This clearly demonstrates the margin of the medial half of the slightly dilated abdominal inguinal ring without disturbing the fascial and muscular attachments of the lateral half of the ring, which need not be disturbed. It also demonstrates the fascial continuity of the transversalis fascia into the anterior layer of the femoral sheath. It is upon this anatomic fact that the rationale for the repair of this type of hernia is based. The dilated abdominal inguinal ring is reduced to normal size by suturing the transversalis fascia to the anterior layer of the femoral sheath (Fig. 6, *b*). Frequently, the external spermatic vessels do not pass through the abdominal inguinal ring but through a separate foramen more medially placed. If they cannot be pulled lateralward into the abdominal inguinal ring, they are cut between ligatures to avoid leaving an aperture through which fat might protrude.

The repair of a *medium indirect inguinal hernia* is essentially similar, except that the abdominal inguinal ring is larger and it takes more sutures to return the ring to normal size (Fig. 7, *b*). The principle of repair is identical in that the transversalis fascia is sutured to the anterior layer of the femoral sheath. When an indirect inguinal hernia is repaired in the female, the round ligament is removed with the hernial sac, which per-

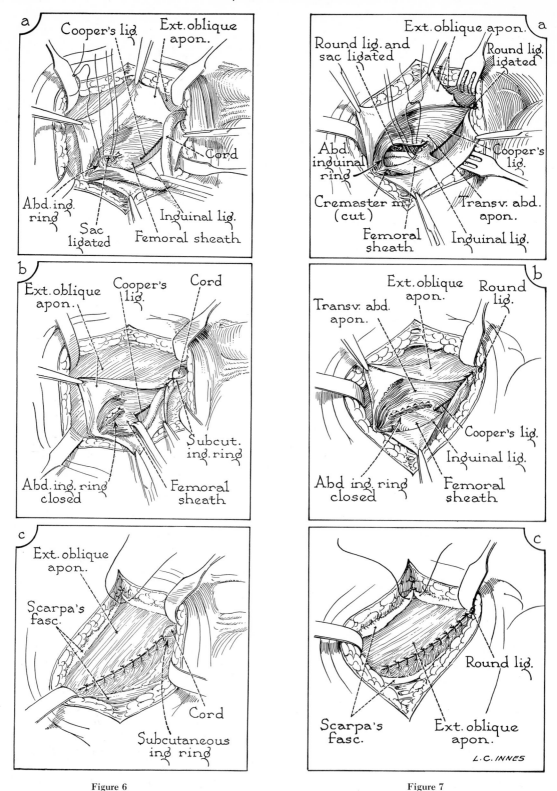

Figure 6

Figure 7

Figure 6. Hernioplasty for small indirect inguinal hernia (viewed from right). *a, b* and *c,* Successive steps in the operation.

Figure 7. Hernioplasty for medium indirect inguinal hernia (viewed from right) in the female. *a, b* and *c,* Successive steps in the operation showing obliteration of the abdominal inguinal ring.

mits complete closure of the abdominal inguinal ring. This is the ideal hernia repair for the beginner to undertake, because the continuity of layers is clear and one is not faced with the complicating feature of structures passing through the inguinal canal.

In addition to the presence of the congenital hernial sac, *a large indirect inguinal hernia*, because of the greatly enlarged abdominal inguinal ring, has destroyed the posterior wall of the inguinal canal. In accomplishing the repair of this type of hernia, one must not only remove the hernial sac and make a snug abdominal inguinal ring, but also reconstruct a new posterior inguinal wall (Fig. 8).

Through the years, innumerable devices have been used to obtain muscular, aponeurotic and fascial material to replace the posterior inguinal wall. Some of them have merit while others are based on false anatomic premises. Any hernioplasty which fastens the new posterior inguinal wall to the inguinal ligament is anatomically unsound. It should be the object of every hernia operation to return the region to the normal anatomic state.

When the posterior inguinal wall is destroyed in part or in toto by a large indirect inguinal hernia, aponeuroticofascial tissue must be borrowed somewhere to close the defect. The simplest device is to use the aponeurosis and fused fasciae of the transversus abdominis immediately above and medial to the defect (Fig. 8). This aponeuroticofascial plate also contains the lowest aponeurotic fibers of the internal oblique muscle. Where it lies over the rectus abdominis muscle, it is known as the rectus sheath. This layer is the ideal material because it is primarily aponeurotic. The fasciae, of which the innermost layer is the transversalis fascia, serve to bind the aponeurotic fibers together into a firm and intact layer. Fascia or muscle does not meet the requirements for a satisfactory layer to close a hernial defect.

Another sound surgical principle is that layers should be approximated without tension. If one sutures the strong edge of the transversus abdominis aponeurosis to Cooper's ligament, there is considerable tension on the suture line. The same difficulty is encountered in the classic herniorrhaphies which use the inguinal ligament as the anchoring structure. To obviate tension, the relaxing incision (Fig. 8) should be used in every instance in which the posterior in-

guinal wall is reconstructed. A modification of the relaxing incision is the turning downward of a triangular flap of the rectus sheath. The slide of the rectus sheath made possible by the relaxing incision seems more physiologic than the flap method because the normal direction of musculoaponeurotic pull is maintained.

Preserved fascia, cutis grafts, osteoperiosteal grafts and flaps of fascia lata have all been used as patches for the posterior inguinal wall. While these methods have been used successfully by their proponents, we have rarely found it necessary to resort to transplanted material. However, should it seem advisable to reinforce the posterior inguinal wall after its reconstruction, it would seem preferable to use a wire mesh or a plastic mesh.

Before the new posterior inguinal wall can be transferred into position, all of the attenuated old posterior inguinal wall and hypertrophied cord fasciae must be excised (Fig. 8). The peritoneal hernial sac must be dissected out and the neck of the sac ligated as for any indirect inguinal hernia. For an accurate repair of this hernia, one must have an evenly cut margin of transversus abdominis aponeurosis above, from abdominal inguinal ring to Cooper's ligament. Below, the glistening margin of Cooper's ligament must be seen medially and the edge of the anterior femoral sheath laterally. When these margins have been carefully dissected and the peritoneal sac excised, one is then ready to repair the hernia (Fig. 8, c).

After making the relaxing incision (Fig. 8, a and b), the strong cut edge of the transversus abdominis aponeurosis is sutured to Cooper's ligament from the pubic tubercle to within a few millimeters of the external iliac vein (Fig. 8, d). This maneuver not only reconstructs the posterior inguinal wall, but it re-establishes a normally broad insertion into Cooper's ligament and thus obviates the possibility of the development of a femoral hernia. It should be noted that the relaxing incision (Fig. 8, d) is now a considerable defect in the rectus sheath, protected behind by the rectus and pyramidalis muscles and their fasciae.

The next suture is the transition suture which approximates the edge of the transversus abdominis aponeurosis to the medial wall of the femoral sheath and pectineus muscle fascia. This suture is necessary to close the angle and permit the line of closure

Large Indirect Inguinal Hernia **Direct Inguinal Hernia**

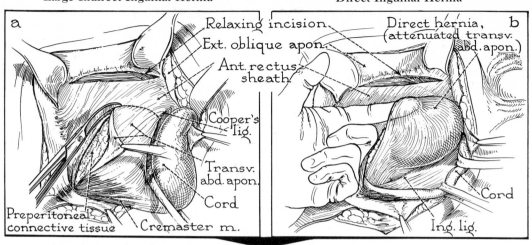

RECONSTRUCTION OF THE POSTERIOR INGUINAL WALL

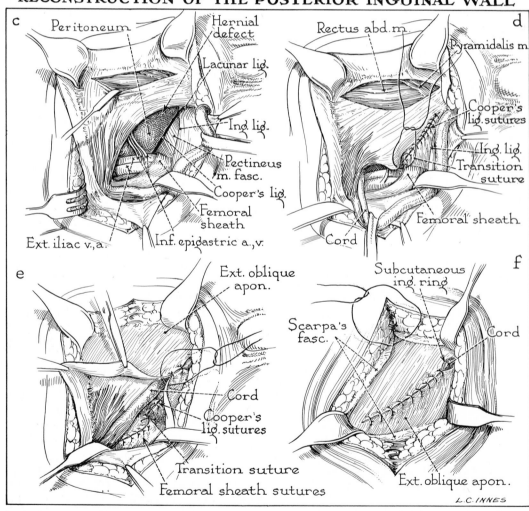

L.C.INNES

Figure 8. Hernioplasty for large indirect and direct inguinal hernias. *a*, Cutting out the attentuated portion of the posterior inguinal wall in a large indirect inguinal hernia. *b*, Attenuated posterior inguinal wall that is to be removed in a direct inguinal hernia. *c*, *d*, *e* and *f*, Successive steps in the reconstruction of the posterior inguinal wall. Hernioplasty for both large indirect and direct inguinal hernias.

to come up from the level of Cooper's ligament to the more superficial level of the anterior femoral sheath. This distance is represented by the diameter of the external iliac vein.

The remaining defect is closed by suturing the transversus abdominis aponeurosis, or in case the layer is muscular at this point, the transversalis fascia, to the anterior layer of the femoral sheath. This re-establishes the normal continuity of transversalis fascia into the anterior femoral sheath. This line of sutures is continued laterally until a snug abdominal inguinal ring is made just as it is done for the repair of the small- to medium-sized indirect inguinal hernia. The spermatic cord is dropped in against the new posterior inguinal wall and the external oblique aponeurosis closed over it (Fig. 8, *e* and *f*), thus re-establishing the obliquity of the inguinal canal. The subcutaneous inguinal ring is snugly closed.

DIRECT INGUINAL HERNIA

DEFINITION. A direct inguinal hernia is one that passes through the posterior inguinal wall medial to the inferior epigastric vessels in the area bounded by Hesselbach's triangle (Fig. 5, *a, b* and *c*).

ANATOMY. The normal anatomy of the inguinofemoral region is presented in Figure 1, in which the number 2 represents the site of direct inguinal hernia. Whatever combination of factors operates to cause a direct inguinal hernia, the immediate cause is a dissolution of the integrity of the posterior inguinal wall.

The most common type of direct inguinal hernia is not an actual hole through the posterior inguinal wall, but a gradual attenuation of an intact but congenitally weak transversus abdominis aponeurosis. It is weak because of a deficient number of aponeurotic fibers. As the bulge of the hernia becomes larger and larger, the aponeurotic fibers are spread farther and farther apart. The fasciae, of which the innermost or transversalis fascia is the heaviest, stretch but maintain the continuity of this layer (Fig. 5, *b*).

As the transversus abdominis layer gives way and bulges forward, the overlying internal oblique muscle is stretched and pushed superiorly. The spermatic cord, with its investing cremaster, usually remains below the bulge of the hernia. This is due to the disrup-

tion of the delicate fascial connection between the lower edge of the internal oblique and the cremaster. A strong musculoaponeurotic internal oblique layer may slow down the development of a direct inguinal hernia, but it cannot prevent it if the underlying transversus abdominis layer gives way. The significance of the so-called inguinal triangle in the causation of a direct inguinal hernia is certainly questionable. However, a deficient internal oblique layer in the inguinal region is frequently associated with a deficient transversus abdominis layer. The important point is that the transversus abdominis aponeurosis, with its investing fasciae, is the key to the development of a direct inguinal hernia. If this layer is strong and intact, a direct inguinal hernia will not develop, even though the internal oblique and external oblique layers are very weak or deficient. On the other hand, if the transversus abdominis layer begins to attenuate and bulge, the patient will develop a direct inguinal hernia in spite of a strong overlying internal oblique muscle.

The strength of the external oblique aponeurosis is of even less importance than the internal oblique muscle, for the developing hernia easily protrudes through this layer between the crura of the subcutaneous inguinal ring. This space between the aponeurotic crura of the external oblique aponeurosis is commonly referred to as a ring. Actually, it is a long triangle with the aponeurotic defect bridged by the innominate fascia. It is variable in strength, depending upon the number of intercrural fibers. When the hernia has passed through the external oblique layer, it enlarges in size in the subcutaneous fascia in the vicinity of the subcutaneous inguinal ring.

Hesselbach's triangle, bounded by the inguinal ligament, the inferior epigastric vessels and the lateral border of the rectus abdominis muscle, is a convenient descriptive area. Direct inguinal hernias must pass through this triangle. If a hernia occurs lateral to the inferior epigastric vessels, it is an indirect inguinal hernia. If a hernia occurs below the inguinal ligament, it is a femoral hernia. If a hernia occurs above the inferior epigastric vessels in the linea semilunaris, it is a Spiegel's hernia.

Rarely, one sees a direct inguinal hernia with a small neck. This is described as a diverticular type of direct inguinal hernia (Fig. 5, *d*). This hernia proceeds through the layers of the abdominal wall in a similar manner and pushes out through the subcutaneous inguinal ring. It may also extend into the scrotum. This type of hernia has been seen following a previous repair of an indirect inguinal hernia, and probably represents a tear in the posterior inguinal wall at the time of surgery. When it develops without a previous operation, it is probably on the basis of the lipoma theory of Cloquet.

TREATMENT.   The rational repair of a direct inguinal hernia must include the replacement of the destroyed posterior inguinal wall. In general, the only difference in the repair of the large indirect and direct hernias is the different management of the peritoneal sac and the fact that the direct inguinal hernia usually destroys more of the posterior inguinal wall. Whereas dissection and high ligation of the peritoneal sac are mandatory in the operation for indirect inguinal hernia, the diffuse bulging of the direct inguinal hernial sac with its broad neck does not necessitate even opening the peritoneum. The sac is simply pushed in and held with a retractor while the posterior wall is reconstructed. In the rare diverticular type of direct inguinal hernia, and when there is any question about adherent viscera to the larger sac, the sac is always opened; but it must be remembered that the urinary bladder forms its medial wall. In the event that there is an associated indirect inguinal or a femoral hernia, the excess of peritoneum in the direct inguinal hernial sac is pulled into the other sac which, of course, must be opened.

Before beginning the reconstruction of the posterior inguinal wall (Fig. 8), it should be emphasized that the abdominal inguinal ring should be carefully explored from within to rule out the possibility of an incipient indirect inguinal hernia. Also, the contents of the femoral canal should be examined to rule out the possibility of a femoral hernia. In the obese patient, there is frequently a large amount of preperitoneal fat down in the femoral canal and this is always removed before beginning the hernia repair.

After disposing of the hernial sac, or sacs, as the case may be, the reconstruction of the posterior inguinal wall is performed exactly as described for the large indirect inguinal hernia (Fig. 8). In repairing the diverticular type of direct inguinal hernia, most of the posterior inguinal wall can be saved, but, even so, the relaxing incision is made to avoid any tension on the suture line.

In the large indirect inguinal hernia, there is frequently a small triangle of posterior inguinal wall which remains in the angle between Cooper's ligament and the lateral border of the rectus muscle. This represents the inguinal falx in many patients and the attachment of the new posterior inguinal wall can begin here. In the large direct inguinal hernia, however, the suturing must begin at the pubic tubercle.

FEMORAL HERNIA

DEFINITION.   A femoral hernia is one which passes through the femoral ring and down the femoral canal to become subcutaneous in the fossa ovalis. It is simply a third variety of inguinal hernia.

ANATOMY.   In Figure 1, the number 3 represents the site of the femoral ring. This is where the femoral hernia begins. The broad attachment of the transversus abdominis aponeurosis and the narrow femoral ring, as shown in posterior view (Fig. 1, *b*), are the normal state and prevent the development of a femoral hernia. The site of origin of a femoral hernia is as truly inguinal as either the indirect inguinal or the direct inguinal hernia.

By comparing the anterior and posterior views (Fig. 1, *a* and *b*), it will be readily apparent that the lacunar ligament is not the medial wall of the femoral ring. The medial wall or margin of the femoral ring is the lateralmost attachment of the posterior inguinal wall into Cooper's ligament. The lacunar ligament lies more medially by at least 1 cm. and in a more superficial plane. The inguinal and lacunar ligaments cannot be seen in a posterior view of the inguinal region. In the presence of a femoral hernia, the medial wall of the neck of the hernia abuts against the lacunar ligament (Fig. 9, *b* and *c*), but this is a pathologic state. The inguinal and lacunar ligaments are not the primary ring of the hernial defect, although they are the final restraining structures. When it is necessary to cut the inguinal ligament to reduce a femoral hernia, it can be plainly seen that the true ring of the femoral hernial defect is the femoral sheath and the aponeuroticofascial fibers of the posterior inguinal wall en route to an insertion into Cooper's ligament (Fig. 9, *b* and *c*).

Irrespective of the number of factors

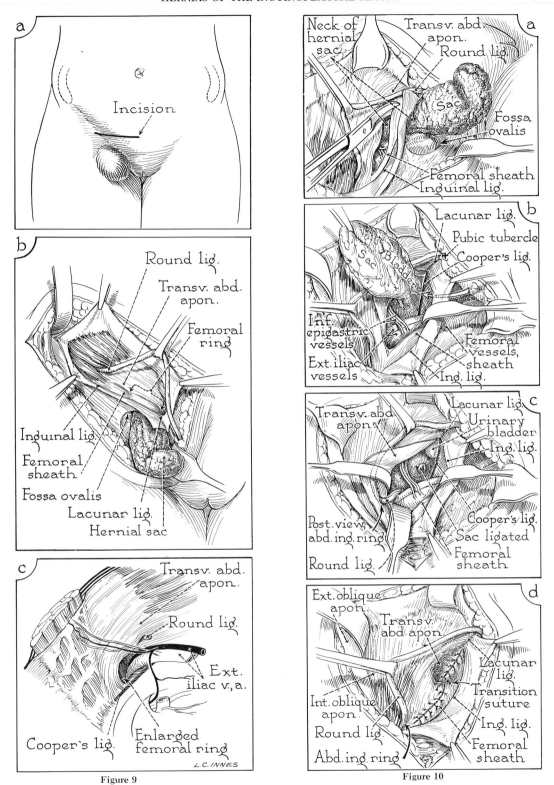

Figure 9

Figure 10

Figure 9. *a*, Appearance of a femoral hernia with location of skin incision. *b*, Anterior view of the anatomy of a femoral hernia. *c*, Posterior view of the dilated femoral ring.

Figure 10. Successive steps in the femoral hernioplasty (viewed from right). *a*, Opening of the lower inguinal region to expose the neck of the femoral hernia. *b*, Conversion of the femoral hernial sac into the position of a direct inguinal hernial sac. *c*, Sac excised and the anatomy of the area prior to the hernioplasty; relaxing incision not necessary. *d*, Femoral hernioplasty; note similarity to Figure 8, *d* and *c*.

which combine to permit the development of a femoral hernia, several progressive changes take place as the hernia enlarges. This hernia begins as a plug of fat in the femoral canal which gradually enlarges and eventually pulls a diverticulum of peritoneum through the femoral ring and down into the femoral canal. As more and more peritoneum pushes out through the femoral ring, the urinary bladder invariably becomes a part of the medial wall of the hernial mass. The hernial sac characteristically has a liberal covering of preperitoneal fat, and the bladder on the medial wall is not immediately apparent (Fig. 10, *a* and *b*). The course of the developing hernia is down the femoral canal where it is forced out of the fossa ovalis by the vessels and the deep fascia. It becomes subcutaneous, pushing the cribriform fascia ahead of it, and at this point the hernia is femoral in location and appears as illustrated in Figure 9, *a*. As the hernia increases further in size, it turns cephalad and may eventually lie in part above the level of the inguinal ligament.

The most important anatomic change takes place at the femoral ring, for as the ring enlarges it pushes the lateral attachment of the transversus abdominis aponeurosis into Cooper's ligament medially, thereby progressively narrowing this tendinous insertion (Fig. 9, *c*) until the more superficially placed lacunar ligament is reached. This is the final and greatest size of the femoral ring. It is a rigid and unyielding ring and accounts for the high incidence of incarceration and strangulation in this type of hernia. The immediate anterior boundary of the femoral ring in both normal anatomy and in the presence of a femoral hernia is the anterior femoral sheath, reinforced more superficially by the inguinal ligament. The direct inguinal hernia and the large indirect inguinal hernia destroy the posterior inguinal wall completely (Figs. 4, *c* and 5, *c*). A femoral hernia destroys the lateral half of the inferior portion of the posterior inguinal wall (Fig. 9, *c*).

TREATMENT. The variety of operations described for the repair of a femoral hernia almost equals the number recorded for the repair of indirect and direct inguinal hernias and, in like measure, reflects basic misunderstanding of the pathologic anatomy.

The femoral approach is anatomically unsound. The many techniques in which an attempt is made to suture the inguinal ligament to Cooper's ligament even by the inguinal approach are likewise an anatomic mistake. The inguinal ligament has mobility in a cephalad direction, but it is a taut cord when attempts are made to displace it posteriorly and approximate it to Cooper's ligament as far laterally as the femoral vein. In any event, suturing the inguinal ligament to Cooper's ligament, by either the femoral or the inguinal approach, is an unanatomic and unsound surgical procedure, for the defect is more deeply placed. The defect in a femoral hernia, irrespective of the causative factors, is a narrowing of the insertion of the transversus abdominis aponeurosis and its fused fasciae into Cooper's ligament. The repair of a femoral hernia, after removal of the hernial sac, is correctly accomplished by broadening this insertion so as to obliterate the femoral ring.

The skin incision for a femoral hernioplasty is the same as that for the other inguinal hernias (Fig. 9, *a*). The external oblique aponeurosis is incised and the inguinal region exposed by elevating the spermatic cord or the round ligament exactly as for an inguinal hernioplasty (Fig. 9, *b*). At this point, the posterior inguinal wall and the abdominal inguinal ring are carefully inspected for associated hernias. The abdominal inguinal ring is inspected again later from within. The hernial sac is shelled out of its subcutaneous femoral position (Fig. 10, *a*) until the neck of the sac is reached. If there is any question of nonviable contents, the sac should be opened at this time for careful inspection before releasing the constriction of the femoral ring. It is a disquieting experience to have a loop of bowel disappear into the abdominal cavity before it is examined. Should this happen, one is then obliged to inspect the adjacent colon and all of the small bowel with a mesentery sufficiently long to permit its entrance into the hernial sac. This precaution, as regards releasing the constriction at the neck of the hernia, applies to all types of hernias with questionably strangulated contents.

An incision is made in the femoral sheath immediately above the inguinal ligament and carried over the bulge of the neck of the hernia and down to Cooper's ligament (Fig. 10, *a*). This allows access to the neck of the hernia and, later, for the repair of the hernia. When this incision is made, the preperitoneal space has been entered and the next step is to separate the neck of the hernia from the external iliac vein. This is easily accomplished, as there is always a nice plane of cleavage due to the areolar tissue surrounding the vein. Tributary blood vessels must be searched for carefully, doubly ligated and cut. This is especially true when an aberrant obturator artery has been pushed forward by the hernia. Aberrant obturator veins are commonly seen. The pubic artery and vein, which course along the edge of Cooper's ligament, are invariably present.

After the external iliac vein is identified, a small retractor is used to elevate the inguinal ligament so that the constricting ring of the femoral sheath may be cut. For most femoral hernias this maneuver suffices for the reduction of the hernia. However, if by a combination of gentle traction above and pressure from below the hernia cannot be reduced, the lacunar portion of the inguinal ligament is cut part way through or, if necessary, completely divided. After the sac has been pulled out of the femoral canal, it is in the position of a diverticular direct inguinal hernia (Fig. 10, b). A femoral hernial sac must always be opened because it frequently contains adherent omentum or viscera. The surgeon should bear in mind that the urinary bladder is part of the medial wall of the fatty envelope which surrounds the peritoneal sac (Fig. 10, b). With the sac opened, one should pass a finger into the abdominal cavity and feel for the opening of an indirect inguinal hernial sac, combining this with direct inspection of the abdominal inguinal ring. The hernial sac is next ligated at its base and the excess excised, again remembering the position of the urinary bladder.

The hernia is then repaired by suturing the cut edge of the posterior inguinal wall to Cooper's ligament up to within a few millimeters of the vein (Fig. 10, d). This not only reconstructs a normally attached posterior inguinal wall but closes the femoral ring and thus corrects the defect which permitted the hernia to develop. The relaxing incision is not necessary. The transition suture (Fig. 10, d) picks up the fragmented end of the anterior femoral sheath and a liberal bite of the pectineus muscle fascia and approximates them to the posterior inguinal wall. This suture not only re-establishes the medial wall of the femoral sheath but is necessary to close the angle between the level of Cooper's ligament and the more superficial anterior layer of the femoral sheath. The operation is completed by approximating the transversalis fascia to the anterior layer of the femoral sheath (Fig. 10, d). The external oblique aponeurosis is closed over the cord or round ligament and the subcutaneous fascia and skin are sutured as for the other groin hernias.

PREPERITONEAL HERNIOPLASTY. The recent studies of Nyhus, Condon and Harkins have re-emphasized the retropubic or preperitoneal approach to the repair of the groin hernias, as originally described by Cheatle. The femoral hernia lends itself ideally to this approach and it is the method of choice in a strangulated femoral hernia when an intestinal resection is likely. However, for the usual femoral hernia and the other inguinal hernias, the conventional anterior approach is preferable. If the preperitoneal approach is used, it is well to remember that the patient is exposed to the incidence of the recurrence of his original hernia plus the incidence of an incisional hernia. It is an unsound method for the large indirect and direct inguinal hernias because a relaxing incision is not used and because the iliopubic tract is used as the anchoring structure instead of the normal insertion which is Cooper's ligament.

SLIDING HERNIA

The sliding hernia is not a special type of hernia but rather represents a complication in the management of the hernial sac in several types of hernias. A sliding hernia occurs most commonly in the indirect inguinal hernia because this is the most common of all hernias, but it should be understood that there is a sliding hernia of the urinary bladder in almost all femoral hernias (Fig. 11, c) and direct inguinal hernias.

In the early stages of an indirect inguinal hernia, the hernial sac consists solely of the congenital diverticulum of peritoneum, and the hernia may enlarge considerably by stretching of the sac. However, when the hernia is of long standing and because of the pressure of its contents, further enlargement of the hernial sac comes from a sliding downward of parietal peritoneum. The peritoneum proximal to the orifice of the hernia is least tightly fixed in the iliac fossa. As this peritoneum is pulled into the hernial sac, the cecum (Fig. 11, a) or sigmoid colon (Fig. 11, b), with a short or absent mesentery, becomes part of the posterolateral wall of the hernial sac. The bowel is outside the lumen of the hernial sac and presents an additional prob-

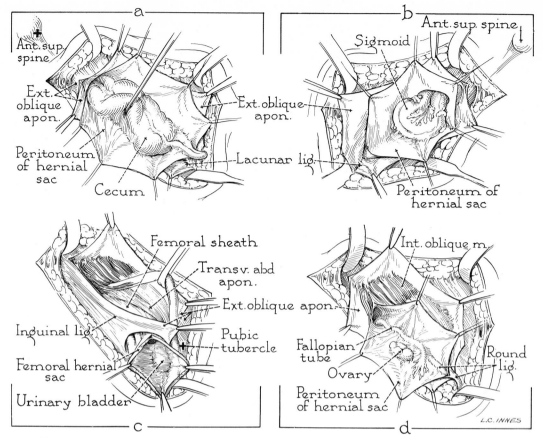

Figure 11.   Varieties of sliding hernia. *a,* Cecum in a right indirect inguinal hernia. *b,* Sigmoid colon in a left indirect inguinal hernia. *c,* Urinary bladder in a femoral hernia. *d,* Fallopian tube and ovary in a right indirect inguinal hernia.

lem in the high ligation of the sac. The peritoneum cannot be dissected off the viscus because it is visceral peritoneum. Therefore, the viscus is simply cut out of the side of the hernial sac which leaves a rent in the wall of the sac. The management of this is a technical problem which is easily handled. Care must be exercised in dissecting the viscus away from the hernial sac because of the mesenteric vessels.

Another mechanism for the development of a sliding type of hernia is seen in incomplete descent of the testis, or in the abnormal descent of an ovary into the inguinal canal (Fig. 11, *d*). In the former, this is simply an arrest in the normal mechanism of the descent of the testis into the scrotum. In the latter, the mechanism is the same although it is an abnormality for the ovary to descend into the inguinal canal. When either of these two abnormalities exists, there is invariably an indirect inguinal hernia associated, al-

though the peritoneal sac may not contain a viscus.

In a diaphragmatic hernia, a variety of retroperitoneal viscera may slide into the thoracic cavity. We have observed the spleen, liver, kidney, adrenal and tail of pancreas in a left-sided diaphragmatic hernia, in addition to the several hollow viscera. On the right side, the liver, adrenal gland and even the superior pole of a kidney have been found in a posterior diaphragmatic hernia through the pleuroperitoneal foramen of Bochdalek.

HERNIAS OF THE LINEA ALBA AND THE LINEA SEMILUNARIS

These hernias are grouped together since they have many features in common and occur along lines of aponeurotic fusion. The principles involved in their surgical repair are also similar. Figure 12 is a posterior view

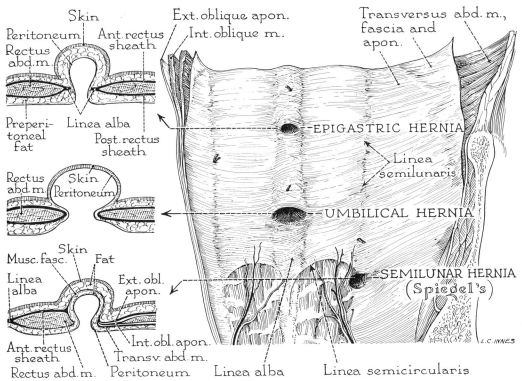

Figure 12. Posterior view of the anterior abdominal wall showing the musculoaponeurotic defects in an epigastric, an umbilical and a semilunar (Spiegel's) hernia. On the left are transverse sections through these hernial defects with the peritoneum and preperitoneal connective tissue added.

of the abdominal wall showing the aponeurotic defect in an epigastric, an adult umbilical and a semilunar (Spiegel's) hernia.

UMBILICAL HERNIA

DEFINITION. An umbilical hernia is one that passes through the umbilical ring and includes three types: omphalocele, or fetal umbilical hernia (Fig. 13, *a*), which is a failure of a portion of the intestinal tract to return to the abdominal cavity during early fetal development; infantile umbilical hernia (Fig. 13, *b*), which is a failure of the umbilical ring to obliterate; adult umbilical hernia (Fig. 13, *c*), which is the acquired dilatation of an imperfectly closed umbilical ring.

ANATOMY. Normally, the umbilical defect is small at birth and just accommodates the umbilical arteries, the umbilical vein, the urachus and a small amount of embryonic connective tissue. After ligation of the umbilical cord, the blood vessels become throm-

bosed back to their nearest collateral and eventually become fibrous cords. The umbilical vein becomes the round ligament of the liver lying in the free margin of the falciform ligament of the liver. The umbilical arteries become the obliterated hypogastric arteries which elevate the peritoneum into the lateral umbilical folds. The urachus obliterates and becomes the middle umbilical ligament over which the peritoneum folds as the middle umbilical fold.

The defunctionalized umbilical vessels and urachus apparently cannot keep the umbilicus open or it is possibly the pressure of the circulating blood in these vessels which prevents the umbilicus from closing prematurely with disastrous results for the fetus. It is also likely that the contraction of the abdominal musculature after birth exerts a shutter-like action at the umbilicus. In any event, irrespective of where the cord is ligated, the slough extends down to the aponeurotic aperture and, in studying the disposition of the aponeurotic fibers about the umbilicus (Fig. 12), it is easy to understand

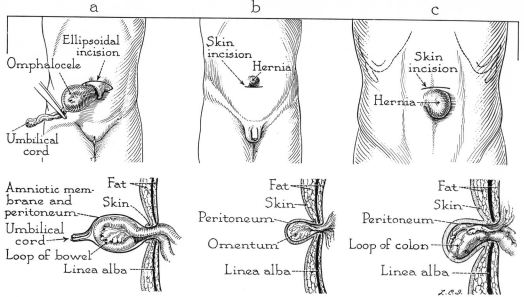

Figure 13.   The appearance of the three types of umbilical hernias in anterior view and sagittal section. *a*, Fetal umbilical hernia or omphalocele. *b*, Infantile umbilical hernia. *c*, Adult umbilical hernia.

how lateral muscle pull tends to close the umbilicus and tightly constrict the structures passing through it. When the cord sloughs, a granulating defect is left which adds scar tissue to the approximated aponeurotic fibers and forms a very dense composite wall that no amount of pressure will disrupt to result in an umbilical hernia. The umbilical skin grows in circumferentially under the umbilical eschar which accounts for the fixation of the umbilical skin to the linea alba.

Aberrations in this pattern of closure result in umbilical herniation. First, is the fetal umbilical hernia (Fig. 13, *a*), or omphalocele, in which the defect cannot close because one or more viscera have been protruding through the umbilicus since the sixth week of intrauterine life and prevent normal development of the aponeurotic elements of the lateral musculature. The size of this defect depends upon the bulk of the protruding viscera. Ordinarily, the viscera which protruded into the umbilical cord have returned by the tenth or eleventh week of intrauterine life, have grown considerably and have completed the rotation that brings the transverse colon over the superior mesenteric vessels. When the viscera fail to return completely into the abdominal cavity, it is because the cavity has not enlarged sufficiently to receive them. When a child is born with an omphalocele, a situation exists which is not present in any other hernia and it demands prompt correction. The viscera lying in the umbilical cord

are not covered with skin but by a thin, translucent membrane which consists of fused peritoneum and amniotic membrane. With exposure to air, it rapidly dries and becomes necrotic so that peritonitis supervenes in a matter of hours.

The second type of umbilical hernia is the infantile umbilical hernia (Fig. 13, *b*) which makes its appearance either shortly after birth or in the first year or two of life, usually following an episode of increased intraabdominal pressure, which can be an almost hourly event attending crying, straining and coughing. This type of hernia is covered with the everted umbilical skin. The skin at the apex of the umbilical dimple is densely adherent to the linea alba at the umbilicus. On the posterior aspect of the umbilicus the peritoneum is equally adherent. Therefore, there is peritoneum, umbilical scar and skin without the interposition of adipose tissue. This accounts for the thin covering of these hernias when a defect persists in the umbilicus. Between the peritoneum of the hernial sac and the everted umbilical skin, there is only the thinnest of areolar tissue layers.

The healing of the umbilicus is essentially the same in all infants with approximately the same amount of scar tissue incident to the healing process. The arrangement that permits this hernia to develop must, therefore, be an abnormality in the disposition of the aponeurotic fibers about the fetal umbilical defect. When muscle fibers contract, the corresponding aponeurotic fibers attempt to make a straight line from their point of insertion. The interdigitation of aponeurotic fibers about the umbilicus in three different planes, corresponding to their origin from the muscle fibers of the two obliques and one transverse anterolateral abdominal muscle, would tend to close effectively an aperture at the umbilicus. The protrusion of extraperitoneal fat is not an etiologic factor, as it is in epigastric and other hernias; neither are there perforating blood vessels other than the fetal ones.

The third type of umbilical hernia is the adult umbilical (Fig. 13, c). It is most commonly seen in persons of middle age, although not uncommonly in the obese multiparous female in her early twenties. Although increased intra-abdominal pressure is the precipitating cause of this hernia, the underlying etiologic condition is the persistence of a small defect from birth. The normally healed umbilicus will not develop a hernia. Small asymptomatic defects in the umbilicus, without a sac and without an impulse, are a fairly common finding in routine physical examinations. Another common finding is a small pea-sized irreducible and nontender lump in the umbilical dimple. This is incarcerated omentum, as can be demonstrated by intra-abdominal exploration at the time of celiotomy performed for some other reason.

With a small defect containing a tag of omentum, it is not difficult to see that this is the entering wedge for the development of a typical umbilical hernia in the adult. Increased intra-abdominal pressure, from whatever cause, gradually pushes more and more omentum into the defect and, eventually, transverse colon enters the hernia as the first viscus. Pregnancy is the most common etiologic factor. Obesity is an important contributing factor and ascitic fluid in an umbilical hernial sac may be the first indication that the patient has a hernia. Once established, the hernia progressively enlarges in size unless the cause of the pressure is relieved. It is not uncommon for an umbilical hernia to decrease in size and become asymptomatic after a woman has delivered. In this event, the woman with a previously painful umbilical hernia may refuse operation only to find that with the next pregnancy the hernia becomes larger and more symptomatic.

TREATMENT. The fetal umbilical hernia, or omphalocele, demands immediate surgical treatment, which means within the first few hours after birth. In the small omphalocele, this presents no special problem because, properly managed, the infant withstands an operation well. The loop of intestine is easily reduced because there is no distention of the intestine with food and air. The repair of the aponeurotic defect is the same as for the infantile umbilical hernia. The only difference is that no attempt is made to fashion an umbilical dimple out of the cuff of periumbilical skin. This cuff of skin is excised as an ellipsoidal segment and removed with the omphalocele sac (Fig. 13, a). For the management of the large omphalocele, or when the abdominal cavity is too small to accommodate comfortably the exteriorized viscera, the two-stage procedure of Gross is certainly the operation of choice.

The infantile umbilical hernia which appears shortly after birth does not need immediate surgical correction unless it becomes incarcerated, but this is a rare occurrence. Many of these hernias gradually disappear without any treatment owing to the gradual constriction of the defect by aponeurotic pull across the midline

In recent years, no attempt has been made to keep a small umbilical hernia in an infant reduced, yet most of them still obliterate by one year of age. If the hernia persists and is symptomatic after one year, it should be repaired. If it persists and is asymptomatic, an elective operation can be performed at any time. A large umbilical hernia in an infant should be repaired without delay.

The infantile umbilical hernia is repaired quite simply through a small transverse incision either just above or just below the umbilicus (Fig. 13, b). The umbilical skin is carefully dissected off the hernial sac and the sac dissected free through the aponeurotic defect. After the sac is opened to be sure that there are no incarcerated contents, the neck of the sac is ligated with a fine silk suture (Fig. 14, a). The defect is then closed in the transverse plane as illustrated in Figure 14, b. Although closure of this defect in the vertical plane has given good results, the transverse closure is under less tension and should have a lower incidence of recurrent herniation. The umbilical skin is then inverted and the apex of the cone is sutured to the linea alba (Fig. 14, b). The subcutaneous fascia is next closed so that dead space is obliterated around the new umbilicus (Fig. 14, c). In applying the dressing, a stent of fine-mesh gauze or silver foil is packed into

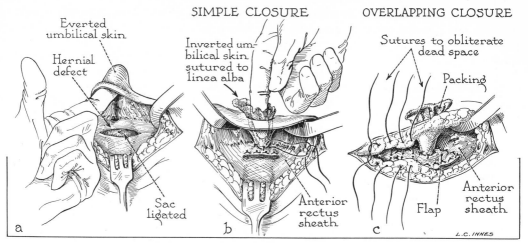

Figure 14. Umbilical hernioplasty. *a*, The sac ligated and the aponeurotic margins of the hernial defect ready to close. *b*, Simple transverse linear closure with the umbilical skin inverted and sutured to the linea alba. *c*, An alternative method in larger umbilical defects. The overlapping, vest-over-pants or Mayo operation.

the umbilical funnel so that a normal-appearing umbilicus is present after the wound has healed.

The only suitable treatment for an adult umbilical hernia is surgical repair. Although an occasional patient can wear a truss with a soft cushion if the hernia is reducible, in general a truss should not be worn: first, because it will not stay in place and, second, because the pressure is painful and dangerous. The small variety of adult umbilical hernia is repaired in exactly the same manner as the infantile umbilical hernia (Fig. 14, *b*). The large umbilical hernia presents some technical problems because, to gain mobility of the rigid aponeurotic flaps, it is necessary to cut into the anterior and posterior rectus sheaths on either side. The Mayo overlapping closure (Fig. 14, *c*) is better than simple linear closure for the large umbilical hernia. An umbilical dimple should also be reconstructed in the adult.

EPIGASTRIC HERNIA

DEFINITION.   Strictly speaking, any hernia which occurs in the topographic designation of the epigastrium would be an epigastric hernia. However, for practical purposes, this is a hernia of the linea alba anywhere between the xiphoid process and the umbilicus. Except for incisional hernias in the epigastrium, hernias other than those in the linea alba are an extreme rarity.

ANATOMY.   These hernias occur almost entirely in the linea alba between the xiphoid process and the umbilicus. Rarely, a hernia is seen in the linea alba just below the umbilicus and, while this hernia occurs in the linea alba, it can hardly be designated an epigastric hernia because of its topographic location. By common usage, however, a hernia in the linea alba just above the umbilicus is called an epigastric hernia even though it lies within the topographic limits of the umbilical region. Hernias through the rectus sheath, or the linea semilunaris in the epigastrium, are rare.

Surgeons frequently fall into the error of referring to the rectus sheaths as fasciae. While it is true that the laminae of the rectus sheaths are invested by fascial layers, the fasciae are very thin and densely adherent to the main structure of the sheaths which is, of course, the aponeurotic or tendon fibers of the anterolateral abdominal musculature. The fasciae by themselves have little intrinsic strength and from a practical surgical standpoint serve only to bind the aponeurotic fibers more closely together. If one dissects the innominate fascia off the external oblique muscle toward the midline, it becomes difficult grossly to differentiate the fasciae from the epitendineum. This is similarly true with the transversalis fascia on the posterior surface of the abdominal wall. With the clear understanding that the rectus sheaths are aponeurotic plates, the next step is to realize that the linea alba is also an aponeurotic structure and not just a fusion of fascial layers. It represents the mutual insertion of six flat muscles and, quite understandably, it is a heavy aponeurotic plate. It is much thicker than either rectus sheath and mathematically should be four times as thick and strong as one layer of the rectus sheath. Because of the different course of the musculoaponeurotic fibers of the external oblique, the internal oblique and the transversus abdominis muscles, there is considerable criss-crossing and actual interdigitation of aponeurotic fibers within the laminae of the rectus sheaths. While there is considerable variation from level to level and between the anterior and the posterior rectus sheath in the degree of this intermingling, it is this woven pattern closely covered by the fasciae which has led surgeons to refer to the sheaths loosely as fasciae and to cut them indiscriminately.

The aponeurotic fibers in the rectus sheaths maintain their various directions as they mingle in their mutual insertion at the midline and form the linea alba. By careful dissection, and sometimes with the use of a magnifying glass, it is possible to trace a given aponeurotic fiber through the linea alba into the opposite rectus sheath. It is undoubtedly this characteristic which led some of the earlier anatomists to consider the six anterolateral abdominal muscles as three digastric muscles. This serves to remind the surgeon that midline hernias are in effect hernias through the tendons of the digastric muscles, and that the repair of the hernia should take into consideration the lines of musculoaponeurotic pull.

If one carefully examines the linea alba in a large number of cadavers, it will be noted that there is considerable variation in the concentration of the aponeurotic fibers from level to level. It is possible that a congenitally weak area is responsible for the development of an epigastric hernia. However, it can also be observed that there are occasional blood vessels which also pass through the linea alba, either in the midline or eccentrically placed next to borders of the rectus muscles. It is the tiny foramina through which these blood vessels pass that provide the opening for the beginning of an epigastric hernia. This opinion is strengthened by the observation that even a small epigastric hernia is accompanied by one or more small blood vessels which will bleed significantly if the neck of the protruding fat is not ligated.

There is rarely any significant amount of preperitoneal fat in the posterior aspect of the upper abdominal wall and the peritoneum is closely adherent to the transversalis fascia. However, even in a slender individual, there is always some adipose tissue between the folds of the falciform ligament of the liver. It is this fat that is the presenting part of an epigastric hernia and, in the small hernia adiposa, represents the entire hernial mass. It is this characteristic of the epigastric hernia which justifies the lipoma theory of Cloquet as the explanation of the cause of this hernia. It is certain that all epigastric hernias begin by the protrusion of a small lobule of fat which, in most instances at least, pushes through a perforating blood vessel foramen. As more fat is pushed out through the defect, the attached peritoneum is eventually pulled through and then a hernia with a peritoneal sac exists. As the hernia enlarges, omentum and the hollow viscera enter the sac. Most of these hernias are repaired when quite small because they are painful and the patient seeks help early in their development. However, they can attain large size with marked displacement of the corresponding rectus muscle.

Most epigastric hernias occur either roughly half the distance between the xiphoid process and the umbilicus or immediately above the umbilicus. It is important to inspect the linea alba just above the umbilicus when repairing an umbilical hernia because, occasionally, one will find an incipient epigastric hernia in this location. It is also important in repairing these hernias to examine carefully the linea alba within the limits of the incision because small defects with hernia adiposa are frequently found adjacent to the main hernial defect. This is especially true in patients in the older age groups in whom fatty infiltration or replacement affects the linea alba as it does many other parts of the body.

TREATMENT. The only treatment for the epigastric hernia is surgical. The pressure of any type of truss is intolerable because most of these hernias are irreducible and tender. A transverse incision is made over the hernial mass and the subcutaneous fascia is dissected off the hernia and the surrounding linea alba. The hernia is usually tightly incarcerated so that the linea alba must be incised on one or both sides to accomplish reduction. A small lobule of fat may be simply pushed in, but larger lobules should be inspected for a peritoneal sac. If a sac is present, it should be opened to rule out the possibility of incarcerated omentum or viscera. Pedunculated processes of fat should be ligated at their base before excision because of the blood vessels. As a rule, a defect that is no broader than the linea alba can be repaired by simple linear closure in the transverse plane. The method of closure or the type of suture material is of less importance than tight closure in preventing fat lobules from pushing out between the sutures in the postoperative period, because this will inevitably manifest itself by recurrent epigastric herniation. Epigastric hernias, with an aponeurotic defect larger than the width of the linea alba, which extend into one or both rectus sheaths, present technical problems in repair. The surgical principle that the subcutaneous fascia should be carefully closed to avoid leaving a dead space applies to any incision.

Semilunar (Spiegel's) Hernia

The extreme variation in the position and formation of the linea semicircularis, along with variation in the structural strength of the transversus abdominis aponeurosis, is the key to the development of this rare type of hernia. Variations in the internal oblique and external oblique layers, while common, are of lesser importance. In reviewing statistical data obtained from observations upon the structure of the anterior abdominal wall in 250 cadavers, it is amazing that clinical evidence of herniation through or near the linea semilunaris in the lower abdomen is not common. It is possible, since most cadavers are the bodies of aged persons, that these defects in aponeurotic structure represent a degenerative process. It is also likely that protrusions of preperitoneal fat through the aponeurotic fibers of the transversus abdominis layer are slow in their development into discrete hernias.

Although hernias in the linea semilunaris above the level of the linea semicircularis have been described, aponeurotic deficiency at this level has not been observed. On the contrary, this line of aponeurotic fusion is extremely dense and strong. They must represent hernias through blood vessel foramina. The angle where the linea semicircularis joins the linea semilunaris is the point at which the transversus abdominis aponeurotic fibers of the posterior rectus sheath change

over into the anterior rectus sheath. Weakness in this angle, as evidenced by separation of the aponeurotic fibers, was repeatedly observed and especially in those cadavers in which the change-over occurred at several levels so as to give, in effect, two, and sometimes three, margins that could be termed linea semicircularis.

A protrusion of preperitoneal fat between the aponeurotic fibers of the transversus abdominis due to an aponeurotic defect is the etiologic basis of this hernia whatever the contributing causes may be. Perforating blood vessels in this angle have not been observed, although a small vein which runs parallel to the lateral border of the rectus abdominis muscle is a constant finding at this level. Small protrusions of preperitoneal fat through the transversus abdominis aponeurosis are occasionally seen above the area of a direct inguinal hernia, so this region should be carefully inspected whenever a direct inguinal hernia is being repaired. Simple reduction and closure of the aponeurotic defects with fine silk sutures seems to be sufficient. Should the hernial defect occur below the point at which the inferior epigastric vessels cross the linea semilunaris, it must be termed a diverticular direct inguinal hernia. The variation in the position of the linea semilunaris allows considerable variation in the vertical location of this hernia.

The presenting mass is preperitoneal fat and it remains for a long time as a vague and slightly tender lump in the interstitial position beneath the external oblique aponeurosis. Fully developed hernial sacs with incarcerated contents have been reported, but usually the hernial mass consists of preperitoneal fat and a small empty hernial sac. To repair this hernia, the transversus abdominis aponeurotic fibers, along with the overlying and interdigitating internal oblique aponeurotic fibers, are closed transversely. The overlying external oblique aponeurosis is closed in the oblique direction of its fibers.

INCISIONAL HERNIA

Definition. An incisional hernia is one which develops in the scar of a surgical incision.

Etiology. Irrespective of the many contributing causes to the development of an incisional hernia, it is fundamentally a failure of the approximated musculoaponeurotic and fascial layers to remain in apposition.

Wound infection is probably the most important factor in the development of an incisional hernia. Suppurative necrosis destroys the approximated margins of the aponeuroticofascial layers, regardless of the type of suture material used. If catgut suture has been used, it undergoes dissolution and fragmentation at a rapid rate.

Drains through the abdominal wall greatly increase the incidence of incisional hernia, as evidenced by the number of these hernias that develop at drain sites. This is due to incomplete closure of the wound plus the added element of infection. Other causes of incisional hernia may be grouped under several headings.

Faulty wound technique includes a host of errors of both omission and commission. The most important include inadequate hemostasis, avascular necrosis of the layers due to sutures too tightly tied, faulty closure of the posterior rectus sheath or transversus abdominis layer, rough handling of tissue and wound contamination from several sources.

The *preoperative status* of the patient, which includes obesity, malnutrition, hypoproteinemia, vitamin C deficiency and tissue edema, may be a factor.

The *postoperative status* of the patient, which includes abdominal distention, chronic cough and inadequate nutrition, may also play an important role.

The *type of incision* also has some bearing upon the incidence of incisional herniation. All other factors being equal, there is not only a higher incidence of herniation through vertical incisions than there is through transverse muscle-splitting incisions, but hernias through vertical surgical scars are more difficult to repair than those through transverse scars.

INCIDENCE. It is impossible to ascertain the true incidence of incisional herniation because no long-term follow-up studies are available on a large series of patients. However, the percentage of incisional hernioplasties in recent series of consecutive hernioplasties would indicate that the incidence of this hernia is increasing. This percentage, of course, is no index of the incidence of incisional hernia after celiotomy. It is also true that the number of operations performed is increasing year by year. Whatever the true incidence of incisional hernia may

be, as related to the total number of celiotomies, it is distressingly high when one considers the almost insurmountable difficulties encountered in the repair of many of them. The surgeon should thoughtfully consider the fate of his surgical incision as he cures the patient of some intra-abdominal disease.

ANATOMY. The pathologic anatomy of the incisional hernia is a story of surgical failure. Every surgeon has had the disquieting experience of seeing a hernia develop in some surgical wounds, and even though it is due to circumstances beyond his control, it is a tragedy for the patient. The surgeon who has a thorough knowledge of the anatomy of the abdominal wall, who understands the importance of the transversus abdominis layer, and who makes his incisions accordingly and practices sound principles of surgical technique, only occasionally will be confronted with this difficult problem.

We favor the transverse abdominal incision, which preserves the greatest number of musculoaponeurotic fibers, since this incision carries the lowest incidence of incisional herniation. In certain patients, the additional exposure afforded by a long vertical rectus incision makes the increased chances of the development of an incisional hernia a justified risk. In the hands of a competent surgeon and in a slender patient with healthy tissues, the vertical wound heals well with a low incidence of herniation. However, the surgeon is faced with the problem of many seriously ill patients with various degrees of malnutrition whose wounds heal poorly under optimum conditions. In this group, and in the obese with their added problems of wound tension and incidence of infection, the transverse incision that carefully preserves the integrity of the transversus abdominis layer carries a much lower incidence of wound hernia.

The anterior and posterior rectus sheaths represent an intermingling and interdigitation of the aponeurotic fibers of insertion of these three muscles as they approach a mutual insertion in the linea alba. The interdigitation of these aponeurotic fibers within the rectus sheaths becomes so complex at times as to suggest the warp and woof of a carpet. The weave is further strengthened by the epitendinea and the fascial laminae, so that at a casual glance the rectus sheath appears to be a dense, tightly woven structure which can be cut in any direction with impunity. However, incisions in the rectus sheath should take into consideration the lines of force of musculoaponeurotic pull.

Above the level of the linea semicircularis, the aponeurotic fibers of the transversus abdominis and internal oblique muscles in the posterior rectus sheath have a predominantly transverse course toward their insertion in the linea alba. As the costal margin is approached, these fibers course in a slightly oblique direction cephalad as they pass from the lateral edge of the sheath to the linea alba. The number of internal oblique aponeurotic fibers gradually decreases until, in the upper epigastrium, the posterior rectus sheath consists entirely of the transversus abdominis musculoaponeurotic fibers. Therefore, in the posterior rectus sheath there can be no question about the direction that a surgical incision should take. If the linea alba and the posterior rectus sheath or sheaths are carefully approximated in the wound closure, the patient has, in effect, a normal posterior layer for the abdominal wall, since no musculoaponeurotic fibers have been cut. The contraction of the transversus muscle in the postoperative period only tends to approximate more tightly the aponeurotic fibers which have been separated during the operation.

The musculoaponeurotic dynamics in the anterior rectus sheath are not quite so simple. The external oblique aponeurotic fibers course obliquely downward, and the aponeurotic fibers of the internal oblique in the anterior rectus sheath course obliquely upward. As their respective aponeurotic fibers enter into the formation of the anterior rectus sheath, there is an intimate intermingling and interdigitation. Because these aponeurotic fibers are rather firmly united, they act as a unit. The predominant force of their combined pull is still in the transverse plane, although some fibers of the external oblique will tend to pull the superior margin of the incision cephalad and some fibers of the internal oblique will tend to pull the inferior margin of the incision caudad. While a transverse incision in the anterior rectus sheath is not ideal because aponeurotic fibers are cut, it is the best available direction for cutting the anterior rectus sheath.

The ideal abdominal incision is the small muscle- and aponeurosis-splitting right lower quadrant incision used for an appendectomy. The external oblique aponeurosis is divided obliquely in the direction of its fibers and the edges are retracted. At this level, the transversus abdominis and internal oblique

musculoaponeurotic layers have an identical course and so these fibers are separated parallel with their course, which is in the transverse plane. This incision, properly made, does not cut a single musculoaponeurotic fiber. If the transversus abdominis and its fascia are carefully closed so that preperitoneal fat cannot push out between the fibers, this wound is as strong after the operation as a normal abdominal wall. The incision should never result in incisional herniation unless it has been necessary to leave a drain through the abdominal wall. The larger transverse abdominal incision is a compromise to adequate exposure. More accurately, it is a compromise only in regard to the anterior rectus sheath, for the posterior rectus sheath and the transversus abdominis muscle fibers can be separated from one side of the body to the other without cutting tendon fibers. The transversus abdominis musculoaponeurotic layer is the most important bulwark against the development of an incisional hernia. If a defect develops in the transversus layer a hernia is born, irrespective of the integrity of the more superficial musculoaponeurotic layers. On the other hand, if the transversus abdominis layer remains intact, a hernia will not develop even though the more superficial musculoaponeurotic layers are imperfectly approximated or subsequently become separated in the postoperative period. The rectus abdominis muscle can be sectioned within its sheath with impunity. If the epigastric blood vessels which course within the muscle substance are ligated to avoid a hematoma, the severed rectus abdominis muscle heals as an auxiliary tendinous inscription.

The vertical rectus incision cuts all the aponeurotic fibers in the rectus sheaths for the length of the incision. As soon as the patient recovers from the anesthetic, the contraction of the muscle fibers whose aponeurotic fibers have been cut puts tremendous tension upon the line of wound closure. By letting the patient come out of the anesthetic until he can close the glottis and strain, we have found the power of the muscle pull to be as high as 40 pounds in a well-developed male. When a transverse incision is used, the divided fibers of the transversus abdominis snap together and can be sutured without any tension. This, of course, does not apply to the anterior sheath which is composed of internal oblique and external oblique fibers and a pull of up to 12 pounds has been necessary to approximate the anterior sheath with the glottis closed. However, it is the transversus abdominis layer which is of the greatest importance in the prevention of wound hernia.

Incisional hernias frequently present multiple defects with septa separating the apertures. These septa represent portions of the wound closure that have held together. In addition to the aponeurotic defects, which represent separate hernial rings, the omentum that is invariably present and incarcerated within the hernial sac will make additional secondary hernial rings which account for the fact that these hernias are so frequently irreducible. It is also common to find a portion of the hernia regularly reducible while other segments cannot be reduced into the abdominal cavity. Frequent findings at the time of operation are unsuspected interstitial components of the hernia which have dissected between the rectus sheaths. Incisional hernias may attain enormous size and contain all of the viscera with a mesentery plus some of the so-called fixed viscera as components of a sliding hernia. While these patients are usually confined to a sedentary life, they are usually free of symptoms of intestinal obstruction.

The hernial sac of an incisional hernia which is fully developed lies immediately beneath the skin, so that peristaltic movement can be plainly seen. At times the skin is so tightly stretched that it appears about to break. Trophic changes in the skin over a large incisional hernia are common along with ulcers that are due to simple avascular necrosis.

TREATMENT. The repair of an incisional hernia is a complex problem. This hernia is a perfect example of the old aphorism that an ounce of prevention is worth a pound of cure. Once a large incisional hernia has developed in a vertical rectus incision, all methods of surgical repair are at best only makeshift and the incidence of recurrent herniation is appalling. The most important single feature in the prevention of an incisional hernia is the careful preservation of the integrity of the transversus abdominis muscle and its aponeurosis. This is accomplished by separating the musculoaponeurotic fibers in the transverse plane.

In general, a small incisional hernia should be repaired by developing the layers of the three anterolateral abdominal musculoaponeurotic laminae and approximating each in the direction of its fibers, with special attention to the reconstruction of a firm transversus abdominis layer. When this is impossible, the fused layers should be approximated in the transverse plane with an overlapping closure. When tension precludes such a vest-over-pants closure, simple linear closure with less tension is the better procedure.

Unfortunately, long vertical oval defects are commonly seen. For these, there is no good solution. They cannot be approximated in the transverse plane, and to reapproximate the edges forcibly in the vertical plane carries a high incidence of recurrent herniation. It is for this reason that various prosthetic devices have been tried to strengthen the line of closure or to fill in the gap when the edges cannot be approximated. Some of the devices that have been used are broad homologous sutures of fascia lata, aponeuroticofascial flaps either turned with their blood supply preserved or transplanted from another part of the body, patches of ox fascia, patches of plastic cloth, full-thickness or split-thickness patches of skin and sheets of metallic wire mesh. None of these is a complete answer to the problem, and all of them, with the exception of the musculoaponeurotic flap with its blood supply intact, eventually result in a layer of scar tissue as the sole bulwark against recurrent herniation. Scar tissue slowly stretches and the broader the amount of scar tissue in a wound, the greater will be the eventual attenuation of the hernial repair. While it is ideal to turn a musculoaponeurotic flap with its blood supply intact in the repair of a midabdominal defect, the technical problems are insurmountable.

Many prosthetic devices have been tried, but reliance has been placed principally upon stainless steel wire mesh. However, it eventually fragments rather completely, and occasionally, the difficult problem arises of repairing a recurrent hernia through the separated fragments of the wire mesh.

Marlex mesh seems to be more inert than the metallic meshes, and does not fragment. It continues to give strength to the wound. An additional advantage is the ability of Marlex to withstand minor wound infection and not be extruded.

HERNIAS OF THE RESPIRATORY DIAPHRAGM

DEFINITION. A diaphragmatic hernia represents the protrusion of an abdominal viscus or viscera into the thoracic cavity through an aperture in the respiratory diaphragm.

ANATOMY. All but the traumatic hernias have their inception in a developmental fault. A thorough knowledge of the normal anatomy of the diaphragm is essential for proper surgical repair of these hernias. Likewise, the origins of the various segments and their musculoaponeurotic composition and mutual insertion in the central tendon are essential information.

Complete absence of the respiratory diaphragm is a rare autopsy finding in the newborn, but, by careful dissection, fragments of the septum transversum and a cuff of costal attachment can be found. Diaphragmatic hernias due to a developmental anomaly are usually concerned with a segmental failure of development in the posterior pleuroperitoneal component, and are known as pleuroperitoneal hernias or hernias through the pleuroperitoneal foramen of Bochdalek (Fig. 15). This segment may be absent in part or completely absent. Occasionally, the corresponding part of the septum transversum is also deficient, so that the hemidiaphragm is totally wanting. Segmental absence of the diaphragm is six times more common on the left side than on the right, presumably owing to the presence of the large right lobe of the liver. When the pleuroperitoneal segment is missing, there is free communication between the abdominal cavity and the hemithorax, which means that there is no hernial sac of either peritoneum or pleura. In this type of defect, the hemithorax is completely filled with abdominal viscera and not only is the homolateral lung collapsed, but there is shift of the heart and mediastinal structures to the opposite side with partial compression of the opposite lung. This situation is not compatible with life, and unless corrected

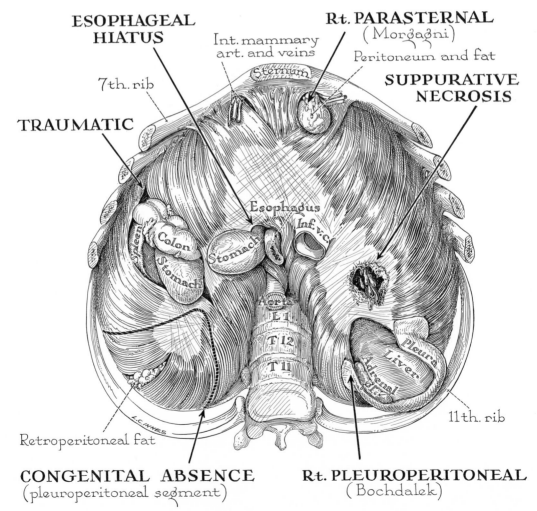

Figure 15. Hernias of the respiratory diaphragm: a view of the superior surface.

shortly after birth results in death of the infant.

A common finding in cadaver dissections is a small cleft over the lateral lumbocostal arch, in which the pleura is in direct contact with the retroperitoneal fat adjacent to the superior pole of the kidney. This may be considered the final line of closure of the pleuroperitoneal segment. In between this small cleft, which may be considered normal, and complete absence of the pleuroperitoneal segment, various quantitative deficiencies exist. The larger ones do not have a pleuroperitoneal sac and are symptomatic immediately after birth. The smaller hernias of this type represent failure of the muscle to develop between the layers of the pleura and the peritoneum and, therefore, they have a combined pleural and peritoneal sac. More commonly, they develop so far posteriorly that the retroperitoneal organs protrude into the thorax with pleura alone forming the hernial sac. The smaller pleuroperitoneal defects prevent immediate herniation and the hernia develops slowly so that symptoms, or diagnostic evidence of herniation, may not appear until adulthood or they may remain so small that they are an incidental autopsy finding.

Of the lesser apertures through the respiratory diaphragm, only one permits the development of a hernia. This is the cleft between the costal and sternal attachments of the diaphragm through which the superior epigastric vessels regularly pass. These vessels are surrounded by a small amount of fat and areolar tissue that is continuous above with the areolar tissue in the anterior mediastinum and below with the preperitoneal connective tissue. A hernia through this cleft is known as a parasternal hernia or hernia of Morgagni. In any statistical analysis, this is a rare hernia; it is due to deficient muscular development about the foramen of Morgagni. When discovered in infancy, it must be due to a developmental defect for it has a peritoneal sac and may contain liver or a loop of a hollow viscus. In the adult, a congenitally large foramen of Morgagni must be the underlying etiologic factor, but the secondary factors of obesity and increased intra-abdominal pressure also play a role, because the presenting mass of the hernia is preperitoneal fat with the peritoneum pulled through secondarily. This hernia is never large, but instances have been reported in which it protruded into the pericardial sac.

The remaining type that is congenital in origin is the esophageal hiatus hernia. In adult statistics, this appears as the most common of all the diaphragmatic hernias. Hernias through the two other major apertures, the aortic and inferior vena caval hiatuses, have not been recorded. The pathologic anatomy of the esophageal hiatus hernia may be very simply described as a hiatus that is too large, so that a pouch of peritoneum and the adjacent fundus of the stomach are forced through the hiatus by the differential pressures within the abdomen and the thorax. The esophagogastric junction may remain fixed at its normal level below the diaphragm, so that the hernia consists of fundus and eventually a portion of the body of the stomach, or the esophagogastric junction may advance through the hiatus as the leading part of the hernia. When this situation prevails, the hernia must be differentiated from an additional variety of esophageal hiatus hernia that is due to a congenitally short esophagus. In most such instances, however, the esophagus has become foreshortened by scar tissue contracture secondary to peptic esophagitis.

Whereas congenital factors exist in both types of hiatus hernias, when there is a congenitally short esophagus, the child is born with the upper portion of the stomach in the posterior mediastinum. When the esophagus is of normal length and the hernia develops because of a large hiatus, the hernia appears gradually after birth and the establishment of negative intrathoracic pressure. The rapidity with which an esophageal hiatus hernia develops is directly related to the size of the hiatus. Although the construction of the esophageal hiatus by the crural fibers of the diaphragm is figured correctly in a general way, there is considerable variation in the size of the hiatus as well as the strength of the muscular margins. There is also considerable variation in the manner in which the crura form the esophageal hiatus. The most common arrangement is to find the margins of the hiatus formed entirely by the right crus. In other instances, varying amounts of the left crus may help to form the esophageal hiatus.

The hiatus is never a fixed or rigid aperture. This can be demonstrated during any upper abdominal celiotomy by the fact that one or two fingers may be passed into the hiatus along the side of the esophagus. If this were not so, a large bolus of food could not pass through the distal esophagus. It is not possible to state just what the measurements of a normal hiatus should be because of the variation in size of cadavers that do not have an associated hernia. The frequency with which small hiatus hernias are found in the obese adult population suggests that there is an acquired element in the development of some of these hernias which is secondary to obesity and increased intraabdominal pressure. A roentgenologically demonstrable and symptomatic hiatus hernia in an obese patient or a pregnant woman will frequently become asymptomatic with weight reduction or after delivery.

Most traumatic diaphragmatic hernias involve the tendinous dome of the left hemidiaphragm because the right lobe of the liver will seal small perforating wounds and dissipate the indirect force so evenly that the right dome is rarely lacerated. A small perforating wound of the left hemidiaphragm, which permits a tag of omentum to enter the left pleural space, is the beginning of a diaphragmatic hernia that may take a long time to develop into a symptomatic hernia. Large rents in the diaphragm due either to direct or indirect violence result in the immediate development of a hernia. The traumatic diaphragmatic hernia does not have a peritoneal sac, although adhesions may prevent open communication between the abdominal and pleural cavities. Aside from the perforating wounds so common in warfare, crushing injuries are the most common cause of this hernia. The force may be due to abdominal trauma and the diaphragm may be torn by the force of the sudden increase in intraabdominal pressure. More commonly, the tear is due to force applied directly to the circumference of the lower thorax. The fracture of a rib along the costal origin may tear the adjacent diaphragm, and the sudden anteroposterior or lateral compression of the thorax, with the diaphragm contracted, may tear the central tendon without rib fracture. After a small rent in either hemidiaphragm, the constant pressure differential after a time may result in bizarre findings at operation. For example, we have seen half of the right lobe of the liver in the right pleural space connected to the infradiaphragmatic portion by a 5-cm. isthmus that represented the diameter of the defect in the diaphragm. On the left, we have observed the spleen as a bilobate organ with the edge of the hernial defect almost bisecting it. This same "oozing" of a solid viscus through an aperture much smaller than the organ itself we have also observed in a right pleuroperitoneal hernia.

Another type of diaphragmatic hernia is that due to suppurative necrosis from a subdiaphragmatic abscess. While this mechanism in the production of a diaphragmatic hernia has been described, suppurative necrosis of the diaphragm more commonly results in a fistulous connection with a lower lobe bronchus. This is because the diaphragmatic surface of the lower pulmonary lobe becomes adherent to the infected diaphragm long before an actual perforation exists.

TREATMENT. The asymptomatic esophageal hiatus hernia does not require treatment. A hernia adiposa of the parasternal foramen of Morgagni and a herniation of the liver through a right-sided pleuroperitoneal foramen of Bochdalek do not need treatment when asymptomatic, if one can be sure of the diagnosis. However, they so closely resemble extrapulmonary but intrathoracic solid neoplasms that an operation is usually indicated.

The obese patient with a symptomatic esophageal hiatus hernia may become completely asymptomatic with the proper weight reduction. Some patients become asymptomatic by observing a few simple precautions such as remaining upright after a meal, avoiding overeating and the drinking of carbonated beverages, eating slowly, reducing their weight and avoiding heavy lifting. When these remedies fail, surgical correction of the hernia is indicated.

The congenital diaphragmatic hernias in the newborn require immediate surgical correction. Increasing difficulties and disaster attend procrastination in infants with congenital, segmental absence of the diaphragm. Properly managed, the newborn withstands an operation well, and the technical problem of restoring the viscera to the abdominal cavity is simplified if operation is performed before the intestinal tract contains food and air.

Because the affected hemithorax communicates freely with the abdominal cavity, positive pressure anesthesia must be instituted before the abdominal cavity is opened. The anesthetic mixture must be high in oxygen content. A special infant anesthetic machine must be used because these patients cannot circulate the gases in an adult type of closed system because of their small respiratory excursion.

Blood loss should be carefully estimated during the operation because the infant's circulating blood volume is small. The amount of blood lost by ordinary standards may be minimal, but for the newborn infant it may prove exsanguinating.

The costal margin of the infant usually flares widely and is very resilient, which makes the diaphragm readily available for the repair. The abdominal approach permits the surgeon to examine the abdominal viscera for associated anomalies of development and the hernia is more easily repaired with the abdominal viscera delivered onto the abdominal wall. The infant tolerates surgical evisceration very well, if the viscera are protected by a warm moist pack.

In older children, or in patients having an esophageal hiatus hernia with an associated short esophagus, the thoracic approach is usually preferable. A congenital diaphragmatic hernia present for some time may develop adhesions between the viscera and the pleura that are more easily severed by the thoracic approach. In any event, time has ruled out associated congenital anomalies of the intestinal tract, and the abdominal cavity is sufficiently large after a few months to accommodate the herniated viscera. If the child has survived for a time, the hernia cannot be massive and the quantitative replacement problem is not so great as in those subjects in whom immediate operation is required. In this group, the technical problems of repairing the diaphragmatic defect are more easily handled from above.

Patients with a congenitally short esophagus and a thoracoabdominal stomach may be repaired from the thoracic approach. However, in recent years it seems that the so-called congenitally short esophagus is more commonly an acquired shortening of the esophagus due to peptic esophagitis. In this group, we have usually added vagotomy and a drainage procedure to the hiatal hernioplasty, and so have returned to the abdominal approach.

Preoperative and postoperative decompression of the gastrointestinal tract is a necessity in most types of diaphragmatic hernia. In recent years, we have routinely done a gastrostomy after intestinal surgery on infants and used the gastrostomy tube for gastric suction, which in turn, can be used for trial feedings. If a long intestinal tube has been passed preoperatively, the upper gastric and esophageal portion is simply pulled out of the gastrotomy wound and used in the same manner. This greatly reduces the problems

in the postoperative period and is followed by a lowered incidence of tracheobronchitis and pneumonia.

In the traumatic type of diaphragmatic hernia, the thoracic approach is always used unless it is advisable to explore all the abdominal viscera for associated injuries. If operation is delayed for some time after the injury, the thoracic approach is mandatory because of the high incidence of very dense adhesions, frequently as high as the apex of the pleural space. Hemorrhage at the time of the injury may firmly encase an atelectatic lobe or lung in a fibrous envelope so that it will not expand without decortication, and this can only be accomplished by the thoracic approach.

The careful anatomic studies of Allison have served to clarify the problem of esophageal hiatus hernia repair. His method, which has been subsequently modified by Effler, is the basis for a sound anatomic hernioplasty. The importance of restoring the esophagogastric angle by including the phrenicoesophageal ligament in the repair is fundamental. The technique of abdominal truncal vagotomy destroys the phrenicoesophageal ligament which is tenuous at best. The drainage procedure which accompanies the vagotomy may prevent reflux, or the intrinsic musculature at the cardioesophageal junction may remain competent in spite of the loss of the fascial attachment of the phrenicoesophageal ligament. It is curious that during the past 20 years thousands of truncal vagotomies have been performed without any significant incidence of postoperative esophageal reflux.

The repair of the traumatic diaphragmatic defect must adhere to sound surgical principles. The strong musculoaponeurotic margins should be approximated in the direction of the fibers of that portion of the diaphragm involved. Most surgeons now agree that the esophageal hiatus should be narrowed to normal size by approximating the crura posterior to the esophagus. In the large hiatal defect, it is usually necessary to make part of the closure anterior to the esophagus. When the margins of a congenital defect cannot be approximated, the costal attachment of the diaphragm can be advanced superiorly to make a flat transverse diaphragm, gaining additional musculoaponeurotic material for closure of the defect. The size of the hemithorax can be decreased at diaphragmatic level by resecting adjacent ribs, or a sheet of Marlex can be sewn into the defect.

READING REFERENCES

Allison, P. R.: Reflux esophagitis, sliding hiatal hernia, and the anatomy of repair. Surg. Gyn. & Obst. *92*:419, 1951.

Andrews, E., and Bissell, A. D.: Direct hernia: a record of surgical failure. Surg. Gyn. & Obst. *58*:753, 1934.

Anson, B. J., and McVay, C. B.: The anatomy of the inguinal and hypogastric regions of the abdominal wall. Anat. Rec. *70*:211, 1938.

Anson, B. J., and McVay, C. B.: The anatomy of the inguinal region. Surg. Gyn. & Obst. *66*:186, 1938.

Anson, B. J., Morgan, E. H., and McVay, C. B.: The anatomy of the hernial regions. I. Inguinal hernia. Surg. Gyn. & Obst. *89*:417, 1949.

Ashley, F. L., and Anson, B. J.: The anatomy of the region of inguinal hernia. II. The parietal coverings and related structures in indirect inguinal hernia in the male. Quart. Bull. Northwestern Univ. M. School *15*:114, 1941.

Bassini, E.: Spora 100 casi di cura radicale dell'ernia inguinale operata col metodo dell'autore. Arch. Atti Soc. Ital. Chir. *5*:315, 1888.

Bloodgood, J. C.: The transplantation of the rectus muscle or its sheath for the cure of inguinal hernia when the conjoined tendon is obliterated. Ann. Surg. *70*:81, 1919.

Cheatle, Sir G. L.: An operation for the radical cure of inguinal and femoral hernia. Brit. M. J. *2*:68, 1920.

Cloquet, J.: Recherches anatomiques sur les hernies de l'abdomen. Paris, These, 1817.

Dickson, A. R.: Femoral hernia. Surg. Gyn. & Obst. *63*:665, 1936.

Effler, D. B.: Allison's repair of hiatal hernia: late complication of diaphragmatic counterincision and technique to avoid it. J. Thorac. and Cardiovasc. Surg. *49*:669, 1965.

Fallis, L. S.: Direct inguinal hernia. Ann. Surg. *107*:572, 1938.

Ferguson, A. M.: Oblique inguinal hernia; typical operation for its radical cure. J.A.M.A. *33*:6, 1899.

Halsted, W. S.: The cure of the more difficult as well as the simpler inguinal ruptures. Bull. Johns Hopkins Hosp. *14*:208, 1903.

Halsted, W. S.: The radical cure of hernia. Bull. Johns Hopkins Hosp. *1*:12, 1889.

Harrington, S. W.: Various types of diaphragmatic hernia treated surgically. Surg. Gyn. & Obst. *86*:735, 1948.

Hoguet, J. P.: Direct inguinal hernia. Surgery *72*:671, 1920.

Koontz, A. R.: Tantalum mesh in the repair of ventral and inguinal hernias. Southern Surgeon *16*:1143, 1950.

Koontz, A. R.: Dead (preserved) fascia grafts for hernia repair. J.A.M.A. *89*:1230, 1927.

Lotheissen, G.: Zur Radikaloperation der Schenkelhernien. Zentralbl. Chir. *25*:548, 1898.

Marcy, H. O.: The cure of hernia. J.A.M.A. *8*:589, 1887.

McVay, C. B.: The anatomy of the relaxing incision in inguinal hernioplasty. Quart. Bull. Northwestern Univ. M. School *36*:245, 1962.

McVay, C. B.: The Pathologic Anatomy of the More Common Hernias and Their Anatomic Repair. Springfield, Illinois, Charles C Thomas, 1954.

McVay, C. B.: Inguinal and femoral hernioplasty: anatomic repair. Arch. Surg. *57*:524, 1948.

McVay, C. B.: A fundamental error in the Bassini operation for direct inguinal hernia. Univ. Hosp. Bull., Ann Arbor *5*:14, 1939.

McVay, C. B.: Preperitoneal hernioplasty. Surg. Gyn. & Obst. *123*:349, 1966.

McVay, C. B.: Inguinal hernioplasty. Common mistakes and pitfalls. S. Clin. North America *46*:1089, 1966.

McVay, C. B.: Inguinal hernioplasty in infancy: The case against exploration of the contralateral side. *In*, Ellison, E. H., Friesen, S. R., and Mulholland, J. H. (eds.): Current Surgical Management III. Philadelphia, W. B. Saunders Company, 1965, p. 482.

McVay, C. B., and Anson, B. J.: Inguinal and femoral hernioplasty. Surg. Gyn. & Obst. *88*:473, 1949.

McVay, C. B., and Anson, B. J.: A fundamental error in current methods of inguinal herniorrhaphy. Surg. Gyn. & Obst. *74*:746, 1942.

McVay, C. B., and Anson, B. J.: Aponeurotic and fascial continuities in the abdomen, pelvis and thigh. Anat. Rec. *76*:213, 1940.

McVay, C. B., and Anson, B. J.: Composition of the rectus sheath. Anat. Rec. *77*:213, 1940.

McVay, C. B., and Chapp, J. D.: Inguinal and femoral hernioplasty—the evaluation of a basic concept. Ann. Surg. *148*:499, 1958.

McVay, C. B., and Savage, L. E.: Etiology of femoral hernia. Ann. Surg. *154* (No. 6):25, 1961.

Nyhus, L. M., Condon, R. E., and Harkins, H. N.: Clinical experiences with preperitoneal hernial repair of all types of hernia of the groin. Am. J. Surg. *100*:234, 1960.

Polya, E.: Die Ursachen der Recidive nach Radikaloperation des Leistenbruches. Arch. Klin. Chir. *99*:816, 1912.

Rienhoff, W. F.: The use of the rectus fascia for closure of the lower or critical angle of the wound in the repair of inguinal hernia. Surgery *8*:326, 1940.

Usher, F. C., and Gannon, J. P.: Marlex mesh: a new plastic mesh for replacing tissue defects. I. Experimental studies. Arch. Surg. *78*:131, 1959.

Veal, J. R., and Baker, D. D.: Repair of direct inguinal hernia by osteoperiosteal graft to the pectineal line of the pubis. Surgery *3*:585, 1938.

Wangensteen, O. H.: Repair of recurrent and difficult hernias. Surg. Gyn. & Obst. *59*:766, 1934.

Zimmerman, L. M.: Recent advances in surgery of the inguinal hernia. S. Clin. North America *32*:135, 1952.

Zimmerman, L. M., and Anson, B. J.: The Anatomy and Surgery of Hernia. Baltimore, The Williams & Wilkins Company, 1953.

Chapter 23

THE ALIMENTARY CANAL

Congenital Malformations

by
ORVAR SWENSON, M.D.

ORVAR SWENSON was born in Hälsingborg, Sweden, but attended elementary and high school in Independence, Missouri, a combination of circumstances which, it might be rightly conjectured, resulted in an individual of pertinacity and with regard for logical and accurate evidence. He received a Bachelor of Arts degree from William Jewell College and a Doctor of Medicine degree from Harvard Medical School. His surgical education and training were obtained at the Peter Bent Brigham Hospital, the Children's Hospital of Boston, and in the research laboratory as an Arthur Tracy Cabot Fellow. Dr. Swenson is Professor of Surgery at Northwestern University, and Surgeon-in-Chief of The Children's Memorial Hospital in Chicago.

Anomalies of the gastrointestinal tract which produce symptoms are limited chiefly to the pediatric age group. Consequently, the surgeon who deals primarily with adults, but who occasionally sees patients in the pediatric group, must keep in mind that he is dealing with conditions almost entirely different from those usually encountered in adults. A basic knowledge of embryology is essential to an understanding of these congenital malformations.

Although many surgeons hesitate to treat the more complicated congenital anomalies in the pediatric age group, and quite wisely so because of limitations in facilities and ancillary professional services, all physicians should be cognizant of the diagnostic features of these conditions so that prompt diagnosis can be made. What a surgeon undertakes to do when faced with a neonate having a complicated lesion is a matter of judgment and appraisal of his own facilities. It is true today that, with fine medical centers scattered throughout the country, many of the more rare and complicated conditions can be cared for best in a large institution where a number of similar problems have been seen. Disposition of the patient is reserved for the surgeon's judgment and is a decision which he alone can determine.

In the neonatal age group, there are certain bits of information in the history which should alert the obstetrician, physician or pediatrician to the possibility of an obstructive congenital malformation of the gastrointestinal tract. First, if there is a history of previous malformations, particularly of the gastrointestinal tract, the physician should be alert for a repetition of the lesion in the newborn sibling. Although quite rare, in certain conditions such as Hirschsprung's disease, it occurs frequently enough that one should be aware that the disease has a familial tendency. Although this tendency is less definite in other conditions, repetition of anomalies in siblings does occur, and the physician should be alert to the possibility whenever there is a history of anomalies of the gastrointestinal tract in older siblings.

The second item of information important in the history is the presence of hydramnios at the time of delivery. If the pediatrician learns that this condition was present, he should immediately be on his guard for some obstruction in the gastrointestinal tract. Careful attention to the history with regard to these points may enable the physician to make an earlier diagnosis than if he had permitted all the clinical symptoms to develop over a period of two or three days. A third sign, which should alert the surgeon, is absence of an umbilical artery which becomes apparent when the cord is cut.

CONGENITAL ATRESIA OF THE ESOPHAGUS AND TRACHEOESOPHAGEAL FISTULA

PATHOLOGY. Malformations of the esophagus occur frequently enough that the physician caring for the newborn should be well versed in the features of this condition. First, it is important to have an understanding of the types of malformations one is likely to encounter. In the most common form of atresia of the esophagus and tracheoesophageal fistula, there is discontinuity of the esophagus; the upper segment ends as a blind pouch at the level of the second or third dorsal vertebra, and the lower esophagus communicates with the trachea either at the carina or somewhere above it (Fig. 1). This form of the anomaly occurs in about 95 per cent of instances. The next most common form of the anomaly also features discontinuity of the esophagus, but the lower segment terminates in a blind end and does not communicate with the trachea. Next most frequent in occurrence is the malformation in which both trachea and esophagus are intact, but in which there is a fistula joining the two structures, producing an H-configuration. A more rare form of the anomaly is that in which the lower segment ends blindly and does not communicate with the respiratory system, and the upper segment communicates with the trachea by means of a fistula. In still another most unusual form, both segments of the esophagus communicate with

the trachea, forming a double tracheoesophageal fistula.

CLINICAL MANIFESTATIONS. The great majority of patients with tracheoesophageal fistula appear fairly normal immediately after birth, except that they seem to need frequent suctioning. They do not necessarily have more saliva than do normal infants, but their inability to dispose of it causes the characteristic bubbling and sputtering. This is such a minor variation from normal that usually this phase of the symptomatology is not sufficient to warn the nurse or attending physician of the serious nature of the anomaly present in the neonate. The first feeding, however, initiates a dramatic train of events; the baby takes a small amount of the feeding and aspirates it, and the aspirated fluid activates a massive spasm of the respiratory system. The patient becomes cyanotic, but in another three or four minutes recovers and becomes pink again. This sequence of events is so clear-cut in patients with tracheoesophageal fistula with atresia of the esophagus that, once seen, it is easily recognized as a feature of the disease. If it is suspected, the attending physician should take a small, fairly stiff, rubber catheter and pass it down through the nostril to see if it enters the stomach. This test may give misinformation if a soft rubber catheter is used, as the catheter may curl up in the dilated upper esophageal segment. As soon as the catheter meets resistance, it should be taped in place.

The patient should then be taken to the x-ray department, where a small amount of Lipiodol should be injected through the catheter under fluoroscopic control so that the roentgenologist can outline the upper segment and detect the rare occurrence of a

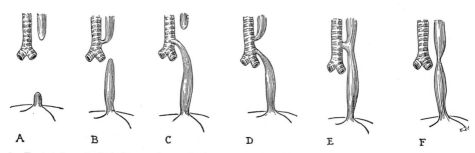

Figure 1. Types of congenital abnormalities of the esophagus. *A,* Esophageal atresia, no esophageal communication with the trachea. Under such circumstances, the lower esophageal end is very apt to be quite short. *B,* Esophageal atresia, the upper segment communicating with the trachea. *C,* Esophageal atresia, the lower segment communicating with the back of the trachea; over 95 per cent of all esophageal malformations fall into this group. *D,* Esophageal atresia, both segments communicating with the trachea. *E,* Esophagus has no disruption of its continuity, but has a tracheoesophageal fistula. *F,* Esophageal stenosis. (From Gross, R. E.: Surgery of Infancy and Childhood.)

fistula between the upper segment and the trachea (Fig. 2). An x-ray film of the abdomen is essential. If this reveals an air pattern in association with the esophageal atresia, it is positive evidence that there is a communication between the esophagus and the trachea. In those patients with isolated atresia of the esophagus with no fistulous communication to the respiratory system, there will be no gas in the gastrointestinal system.

The most difficult lesions to diagnose are those with the H-type of fistula. These patients may do rather well except for considerable coughing associated with feedings. If there is a constant association of coughing and sputtering with feeding, and if the baby fails to do well, the H-type fistula should be suspected. This lesion may be missed by the usual roentgenologic techniques, and the most reliable diagnostic procedure is to make a motion-picture film of the patient taking contrast material by mouth. If the fistulous connection to the trachea is not noted at the fluoroscopic screen, it may be seen when the film is projected. Another method of diagnosis is bronchoscopy, bringing the posterior aspect of the trachea under direct vision so that the end of the fistula may be seen. This is not possible with straight, simple bronchoscopes; it is necessary to have a magnification system such as is found in a cystoscope. One may use a small cystoscope with a foroblique lens to secure a good view of the posterior tracheal wall, thus verifying the diagnosis. If the fistula is high, it may be difficult to see; however, a low fistula can be visualized without difficulty by this technique.

TREATMENT. Once the diagnosis has been made, it is well to keep the patient in a semi-upright position with a small plastic catheter placed in the upper segment and connected to intermittent suction. This keeps the upper esophageal segment empty and prevents further aspiration, to a large extent. The management of these patients depends not only on the type of anomaly, but also on their general condition and weight. Premature infants are the most difficult to treat; the mortality has been quite high. In babies weighing less than 4 pounds, it may be advisable to do a series of operations rather than an immediate primary repair.

One such program, which holds some promise, is to perform a gastrostomy and divide the fistula, closing both ends. Nasogastric suction is then depended upon to keep the upper pouch empty and prevent aspiration. This program permits the babies to gain weight. There have been reports of small series of patients in which this procedure yielded a good percentage of survival in premature infants. When a weight of 6 to 8 pounds has been achieved, it is possible to do a primary anastomosis of the esophagus, thus restoring continuity. Some premature infants cannot be managed with suction on the upper esophageal segment, and it may be necessary to exteriorize the upper esophageal segment to the skin to prevent repeated aspirations. This can be taken down and put back in the mediastinum and an end-to-end anastomosis performed, although this is a more difficult procedure than when the upper segment is left in place.

In the full-term baby without any other complicating lesion, primary repair with an end-to-end anastomosis of the esophagus is the procedure of choice. It is best to let the infant rest for 24 hours or so in the hospital before undertaking surgical therapy. There are indications that performing a gastrostomy shortly after admission may have some advantage. The open gastrostomy decompresses the stomach and reduces the risk of gastric regurgitation into the lungs. This is particularly useful in patients with severe pneumonia. The definitive operation may be de-

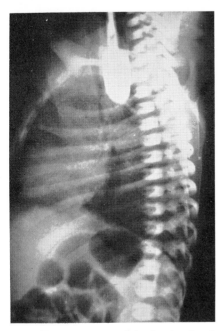

Figure 2. Roentgenogram of the fistula after instillation of contrast material into the upper esophageal pouch. This demonstrates atresia of the esophagus. Air in the intestinal tract proves the presence of a tracheoesophageal fistula.

layed until the child's pulmonary condition has improved. The operation is performed with endotracheal anesthesia. The extrapleural approach seems to have the advantage of retrieving probably 10 to 15 per cent more patients than the transpleural approach. The transpleural approach may reduce the length of the procedure by 15 to 30 minutes, but the results are often fatal if a leak develops at the anastomosis and one is confronted with an esophagopleural fistula. It is unusual, in fact, to have such a patient recover, simply because oral feedings tend to be regurgitated into the esophagus and leak into the pleural cavity. On the other hand, if an extrapleural approach has been used and the anastomosis breaks down, the patient develops an esophagocutaneous fistula, which is not a serious complication because spontaneous closure is the rule and the infant's condition is not affected.

To secure the best result in the treatment of patients with tracheoesophageal fistula, which at best carries a 25 per cent mortality, the most excellent facilities are required. The services of a pediatric anesthesiologist are of great help. The surgeon should have pediatric surgical education and training, so that he can handle the delicate tissues through the small exposure without inflicting undue trauma.

A simple end-to-end anastomosis which joins the mucosa and muscularis of the two segments in two separate layers is most effective. Postoperatively, these patients should not be given large amounts of fluid; about 1200 ml. per square meter of body surface area per day will suffice. High humidity and oxygen are helpful in maintaining these patients in optimum condition. In 24 hours, if the patient is in good condition, he is returned to the operating room and a Stamm gastrostomy is performed under local anesthesia. This is the routine when a preoperative gastrostomy has not been done. On the tenth postoperative day, an esophagram is made. If the esophagus is healed, oral feedings are started and the gastrostomy tube removed. In patients who exhibit some narrowing of the esophagus, it is well to leave the gastrostomy tube in place, but to clamp it off so that the gastrostomy can be utilized if subsequent dilatations are required.

In patients with an H-type fistula which is above the thoracic cavity, an approach can be made through the neck. This is important for operations on a high fistula, because it is much more simple than approaching such lesions through the chest. On the other hand, if the fistula is in the thoracic cavity, it can be exposed extrapleurally and both ends sewn over. This procedure yields excellent results.

In defense of the extrapleural approach, it has now been possible to publish data on a series of patients with 80 per cent survival, although no patients were eliminated from the series on the basis of prematurity or other severe malformations. The best figures available for the transpleural approach are about 15 per cent less. The difference in the survival rate in the two groups undoubtedly may be attributed to the fact that, with the transpleural approach, a leak at the anastomosis is often a lethal complication; on the other hand, this complication carried almost no mortality with the extrapleural approach.

HIATUS HERNIA

True hiatus hernia is rarely encountered in the neonate and the small child. It does occur, however, and it should be considered in the differential diagnosis when an infant vomits persistently. The pathology is not clearly understood. It has been postulated that patients with achalasia, that is, relaxation of the esophagocardiac junction with reflux of gastric contents into the esophagus, have a small hiatus hernia. Achalasia is common in the neonatal age group and should be considered when there is vomiting with no apparent cause. In some infants, the condition persists despite treatment with thickened feedings and sitting the patient upright for 20 minutes to half an hour after feedings. In such situations, a hiatus hernia may develop. In most patients, however, a hiatus hernia is detectable from birth if the infant is examined for it, and it is probably a separate congenital malformation of the diaphragm itself.

Vomiting is the first symptom, and often there is blood in the vomitus. Patients may fail to gain weight, or may lose weight, during acute episodes of prolonged vomiting. The diagnosis can be made readily by an experienced roentgenologist, particularly if he places the patient in the Trendelenburg position and is alert to the possibility of a hiatus hernia. The lesion is usually paraesophageal and may be associated with a shortened esophagus. Whether this latter feature is due to a congenital malformation or to an inflammatory process is difficult to determine. Both situations probably exist. Shortness of the esophagus is present in some neonates and, therefore, probably is a separate congenital malformation. In older children with short esophagus, one cannot rule out the possibility that an inflammatory condition is the cause of the deformity.

Repair of the hiatus hernia is performed most readily by the transthoracic route. It is essential to free the esophagus at the cardia. If at all possible, it is advisable to spare the fibers of the vagi. The esophageal opening should be made appropriate in size. Then, with fine interrupted sutures, the esophago-gastric junction should be attached to the periphery of the defect in the diaphragm. When this is not done, there is a high incidence of recurrence.

Infants who have undergone repair of a hiatus hernia may have a little difficulty in swallowing postoperatively. However, as the swelling subsides, they usually have no difficulty, despite the fact that the opening in the diaphragm appears rather small at the time of the operation.

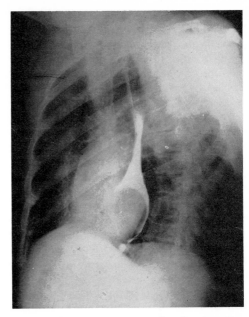

Figure 3. A roentgenogram made after ingestion of barium, showing a large, rounded filling defect in the lower portion of the esophagus produced by a duplication of the esophagus.

DUPLICATION OF THE ESOPHAGUS

Occasionally, in small infants or children, a roentgenogram of the chest reveals a filling defect, particularly in the left side of the chest. Roentgenographic examinations are prompted by repeated bouts of pulmonary infection. The possibility of a duplication of the esophagus must be considered seriously in such situations. At times, it may be necessary to have a barium contrast study of the esophagus to outline the lesion (Fig. 3). These structures are adjacent to the esophagus and usually do not communicate with it. Pathologically, they have a common muscular wall with the esophagus. The cavity itself is lined with mucosa which, in part, may be gastric in type, and consequently the secretions found in the cyst usually are acid. On rare occasions, duplication of the esophagus may ulcerate and perforate, forming a communication with the tracheobronchial tree. When this occurs, the patient has a chronic productive cough which brings up a great deal of thin, blood-tinged material.

When such a lesion is diagnosed, surgical removal is wise because of the possible complications. In the past, some surgeons thought it wise to marsupialize this type of lesion through the thoracic cage to the skin, and then destroy gradually the gastric mucosa by curettage or application of a sclerosing agent. This has the disadvantage of being a long, drawn-out procedure. Also, at times the destruction of the gastric mucosa is extremely difficult. A far wiser course to follow is surgical excision of the duplication. It is well to excise the mass, and in the area adjacent to the esophagus to remove only the mucosa of the duplication, thus leaving a muscular wall intact on the esophagus. Although it is not extremely dangerous to enter the esophagus, it is possible to accomplish the repair without doing so. If one does enter the esophagus, it is wise to close it with fine, interrupted silk sutures and place the patient on catheter drainage of the chest. On the other hand, when a duplication is excised without entering the esophagus, the lung can be expanded and the chest closed without any type of drainage.

STRICTURE OF THE ESOPHAGUS

Strictures of the esophagus are divided into those above the cardia and those at the cardia. Strictures above the cardia probably are congenital in origin, and make themselves known early in life because of vomiting or inability to gain weight. Patients with this condition also have a great deal of difficulty with saliva and may have bouts of pneumonia which can only be understood fully when the lesion in the esophagus is detected. Usually, the stricture is fairly severe, and very early in life the infant has so much trouble that it becomes necessary to resort to roentgenographic study of the esophagus, which clearly demonstrates the lesion. On occasion, there may be tracheoesophageal fistula associated with the stricture; in such patients, the symptomatology is far more drastic than when a simple stricture is present. In patients with an associated tracheoesophageal fistula, taking liquids produces a great deal of coughing even after the stricture has been dilated to the point where it is not the cause of any particular trouble on its own account.

Most esophageal strictures can be dealt with by dilatation. This can be achieved by esophagoscopy, threading a filiform through the stricture and then attaching graduated dilators to the filiforms, so that the dilators will be guided through the stricture without any danger of perforation of the esophagus. In most instances, particularly when the stricture is of the diaphragmatic type, one or two dilatations will suffice to cure the patient. On occasion, however, the stricture may be longer and more resistant to dilatation. Rarely, it may be necessary to resect the stricture and make an end-to-end anastomosis of the esophagus.

The second type of esophageal stricture is that which is at the cardia. This is a lesion quite similar to cardiospasm in the adult, and occurs in older children. The symptomatology may be quite obscure. In some situations, the child may develop a chronic cough from the overflow of material from the massively dilated esophagus into the tracheobronchial tree. At night, particles of food may be found on the child's pillow. It is not unusual for such a lesion to be overlooked for some time, because most of the symptomatology may be referred to the pulmonary tree and, consequently, the appropriate studies may not be carried out promptly to detect the true nature of the lesion. In some patients, a plain chest x-ray may show a rounded convex shadow projecting into the right thoracic lung field. When such a curved line is noted next to the mediastinum, the possibility of megaesophagus must be considered. The diagnosis is readily made by esophagogram.

The treatment of such patients is difficult.

In a few instances, vigorous dilatation of the cardia may be all that is required. In more than half the patients, the lesion probably will yield to vigorous dilatation. This is best performed by an inflatable bag technique, and the dilatation must be vigorous to achieve results. If a reasonable series of four to six dilatations does not relieve the situation, one must resort to operative treatment. There are a number of procedures designed to relieve this apparent obstruction of the lower end of the esophagus, which is probably neurogenic in origin. The best procedure in the hands of most surgeons is an operation which is performed with a vertical incision through the muscular coats of the esophagus and then through the mucosa, with suturing in the opposite plane. In some patients, one can achieve excellent results by cutting only the muscular coat and sewing it in the opposite direction, and not opening the mucosa.

ATRESIA OF THE INTESTINE

ETIOLOGY. A defect producing complete obliteration of the lumen may occur at any point along the small or large intestine. Statistics indicate that these lesions are far more rare in the colon than in the small intestine. The etiology of this condition has been explained on the basis of a congenital malformation. This is based on the embryologic changes which the intestine, particularly the duodenum, undergoes during its formation. Initially, it is a solid cord which forms vacuoles, and these coalesce to produce a lumen. It may well be that the process fails at some point in the development of the intestinal tract, thereby producing a defect in the continuity of the intestine. More recently, it has been pointed out that this may not be the only explanation, for there is a certain amount of clinical evidence to support the thesis that some of the atresias may be related to an intrauterine vascular accident with segmental necrosis of the intestine and production of an atretic lesion.

Some experimental work has been performed which demonstrates that this type of lesion can be produced in animals by a special technique which produces vascular occlusion to a limited segment of intestine. It has also been postulated that intrauterine intussusception may lead to vascular necrosis and an atretic lesion. In examining resected specimens of atresia under the microscope, it has been possible to identify material which indicates that meconium was in the area at an earlier stage. This is taken as further evidence that a break in continuity has healed and produced the atretic lesion.

CLINICAL MANIFESTATIONS. Intestinal atresia is not a common lesion. However, when a newborn begins to vomit bile-stained material, the indications are that some type of mechanical or neurogenic obstruction exists. In the newborn infant who vomits bile-stained material, becomes distended and is obstipated, the diagnosis of small bowel obstruction must be given serious consideration. One of the leading causes of small bowel obstruction, particularly in the neonate, is atresia of the intestine. The diagnosis of small bowel obstruction can definitely be established, but the exact nature of the obstruction is difficult to ascertain preoperatively. In an infant who has bile-stained vomitus, abdominal distention and obstipation, a history of hydramnios in the maternity record should cause one to consider seriously the diagnosis of mechanical obstruction of the intestinal tract.

When the diagnosis of mechanical obstruction of the intestine is under serious consideration, it is prudent for the attending physician to order plain roentgenograms of the abdomen. These should be made in the prone and the upright positions. The presence of dilated loops of intestine with fluid levels supports the clinical diagnosis of intestinal obstruction; however, precautions must be taken in the neonate because it is impossible to differentiate small bowel from large bowel in the plain film. This distinction can be made readily in adults because of the peculiar configuration of the large intestinal gas pattern compared to that of the small intestine, but this is not true of the neonate. The identification of the precise portion of the intestinal tract which has undergone dilatation can only be made by performing a barium enema examination. Should this examination reveal a colon which is small, and obviously an organ of disuse, the diagnosis of small bowel obstruction can be made with certainty. On the other hand, should the barium enema study reveal a dilated colon, the diagnosis of small bowel obstruction must be discarded and such diagnoses as congenital megacolon and meconium plug syndrome should be given serious consideration.

The Farber test is of some value in determining whether one is dealing with mechanical obstruction. This test depends upon the presence of large desquamated epithelial cells in the meconium. Providing that a specimen is obtained well up in the anal canal, away from the skin of the perineum, the material can be spread on a slide and stained with methylene blue and the large cells readily identified. In the patient with a congenital obstruction which has permitted no meconium to pass, the epithelial cells will not be present. Actually, this is an interesting test but in a practical situation it is not of great value. This test is difficult to perform because contamination from the skin of the anal canal may make the results unreliable. If care is taken to avoid this pitfall, the test is valid.

TREATMENT. Once the diagnosis has been made, the treatment is that for intestinal obstruction. If the diagnosis is made in the first 24 to 48 hours of life, abdominal distention is not excessive and electrolyte changes are minimal, although the patient may be somewhat dehydrated from vomiting. In patients in whom diagnosis is made later than 48 hours, one can anticipate a fairly marked degree of dehydration and considerable derangement of the electrolyte pattern. Preoperative preparation is directly related to the age of the neonate. As soon as the infant is hydrated and a beginning has been made to correct any electrolyte deficiency, the child is ready for operation. During the period of preparation, it is well to keep these infants on nasogastric suction so that vomiting is reduced to a minimum and the danger of aspiration is minimized.

General anesthesia is to be preferred except in the most debilitated infants. In such instances, local anesthesia with 0.25 to 0.50 per cent Novocain is useful. The extent to which local anesthesia is used in these patients is related to a considerable degree to the availability of a pediatric anesthesiologist competent to give a general anesthetic to debilitated small infants.

The exploration is performed through a right rectus muscle-retracting incision. This type of incision is not time-consuming to make, gives adequate exposure and can be closed in a manner which practically eliminates postoperative dehiscence. It is well to eviscerate the child and search for multiple lesions. A serious mistake can be made by discovering and correcting one atretic lesion, only to find postoperatively that a second or third lesion actually was present. For this reason, it is imperative to go through the entire length of the gastrointestinal tract during the course of the operation, to make sure of its continuity.

A variety of procedures have been used to treat this condition. In atretic lesions low in the small intestine, exteriorization operations have been favored, but these require second- and third-stage procedures. It would seem that a direct attack on the lesion with an end-to-end anastomosis provides the best overall result. Side-to-side anastomoses are to be condemned because of the fact that blind loop syndrome develops in such patients and can be quite troublesome, not only early in the postoperative course, but later if the infant survives. It is well to resect a segment 8 to 12 cm. in length to remove the bulbous dilatation in the small intestine just proximal to the atretic lesion. There is some evidence that these vastly overdistended hypertrophied segments do not have normal peristaltic activity and may serve as a form of physiologic obstruction when left in place. Therefore, whenever it is possible, it is well to resect back to bowel which is not greatly dilated. It is also well to decompress the intestine proximal to the proposed resection with a catheter, small trocar or large needle. The device used is inconsequential; the important point is that decompression be accomplished. Various techniques have been used to make the anastomosis. The two-layer anastomosis is common. Although this serves well in the hands of many surgeons, it would seem that the preferred anastomosis is that with a single layer of interrupted Halsted sutures. This latter provides an adequate lumen and is a clean operation which minimizes contamination.

By closing the abdominal wound in layers using interrupted silk sutures to the peritoneum, fascia, subcutaneous tissue and skin, one can virtually eliminate dehiscence. Dehiscence in the neonatal group is not an uncommon complication in many reported series, and it has an associated high mortality. For this reason, it is worthwhile to take the time to make a careful closure of the abdominal wall.

Postoperatively, fluids should be administered in reasonable amounts. It is best to give maintenance fluids on the basis of 1200 ml. per square meter of body surface area. One must supplement this with a sufficient volume to cover any loss through a nasogastric suction system.

As soon as peristaltic activity returns, nasogastric suction can be discontinued and oral feedings started. It is well to build up to a food formula as rapidly as tolerated, usually 24 to 48 hours after oral feedings are begun.

STENOSIS OF THE INTESTINE

Stenosis is a more rare lesion than atresia of the intestine, and it may be of such mild character that the diagnosis is not made until

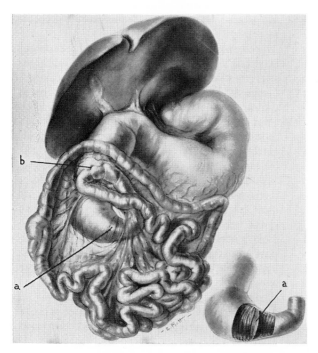

Figure 4. The septum across the duodenum: *a*, the result of the arrest of development at the solid stage; *b*, duodenojejunostomy for relief of the duodenum obstruction caused by *a*.

the patient is several months or even years of age. Infants with this lesion tend simply not to do well. Vomiting may not be a prominent part of the picture. The baby fails to gain weight at a normal rate. The diagnosis can be made by a small bowel roentgenographic examination. Barium is followed through the small bowel with a series of films and the dilated loops are detected by this technique. The treatment of this condition is resection of the stenotic area with end-to-end anastomosis. A common site for the stenosis is the duodenum, and a duodenojejunostomy will relieve the obstruction. (Fig. 4).

CONGENITAL PYLORIC STENOSIS

ETIOLOGY AND PATHOLOGY. The incidence of congenital pyloric stenosis is quite frequent, and all surgeons and physicians should be aware of its diagnosis and treatment. The etiology has been discussed in the medical literature for many years, but no well-documented explanation has been brought forth. Apparently, this condition is a congenital lesion which becomes manifest in the first few weeks of life. Grossly, it is a hypertrophy of the musculature of the pylorus which reaches such a degree that mechanical obstruction is produced at the gastric outlet. This lesion commonly occurs in the first-born male of a family. It is far more rare in females; consequently, one should be cautious in making the diagnosis in a female neonate.

CLINICAL MANIFESTATIONS. The clinical syndrome is quite characteristic. These infants are perfectly well at birth, and may go for a period of a week or ten days to two or three weeks doing perfectly well. Then vomiting begins mildly, and rapidly progresses to a projectile type. The vomiting is extremely forceful as the obstruction becomes more complete. Infants who vomit for other causes are apt to be uninterested in eating owing to their illness, but infants with pyloric stenosis are eager to eat and, therefore, take feedings eagerly even immediately after vomiting. The vomitus is never bile-stained, although it may be light yellow owing to the type of formula or vitamins being offered the baby. Characteristically, these babies have scanty stools and a dark, concentrated urine. Soon after the onset of vigorous vomiting, the baby fails to gain weight and may actually lose weight. The diagnosis can only be suspected from the clinical history. There are a number of conditions which produce or simulate the type of vomiting seen in pyloric stenosis; therefore, one must rely on other factors for establishment of the diagnosis.

The simplest way to make the diagnosis is to palpate the pyloric enlargement. This is detected as an olive-sized oblong mass 1.5 cm. in length and 1 cm. in width. The manner in which one attempts to find this tumor mass in the abdomen determines how successful the examining physician is in detecting it. It is well to palpate directly through the rectus muscle, pressing the tumor against the posterior abdominal wall and rolling it under the fingers. It is possible to palpate the tumor in about 85 to 90 per cent of the patients, providing that the examiner is persistent and has had some experience in detecting this lesion. The optimal time to palpate the tumor is immediately after the baby has vomited, which empties the enlarged stomach and facilitates examination. It may be necessary in some of these babies to use a nasogastric tube to empty the stomach and then palpate for the tumor.

In a small number, the tumor may not be detected on abdominal examination and one must resort to roentgenographic examination. This is a difficult diagnosis to make roentgenographically. Delay of passage of material through the pylorus is not conclusive. Only by depicting the elongated narrow canal can the roentgenologist be sure that he is dealing with pyloric stenosis. Visible gastric peristaltic waves are invariably present in pyloric stenosis. They also may be present in conditions such as subdural hematomas and other lesions of the central nervous system, and they have been observed in patients with impending uremia. Consequently, one should be reluctant to regard this physical finding as pathognomonic of pyloric stenosis.

TREATMENT. Treatment of this condition is simpler today than it was two decades ago. In the past, these babies usually were brought for surgical attention after the disease had been present for several weeks. Marked dehydration and loss of weight contributed to postoperative complications. In such patients, the postoperative fluid and electrolyte treatment was an important feature in their survival. Today, the diagnosis usually is made early and dehydration is minimal. As a matter of fact, a proportion of the patients may be operated on without any preoperative parenteral fluids; however, in half of them, dehydration is present and replacement of fluid and correction of electrolyte imbalance are extremely important before operation is undertaken. It is well to remember that some of these neonates are deficient in potassium, and this must be corrected.

The surgical management of these babies is fairly simple. General anesthesia should be used. It is well to have a nasogastric tube in place before the anesthetic is initiated in order to decompress the stomach. This improves respiratory ventilation and facilitates the induction of anesthesia. It is also of value during the operative procedure, in allowing more room for the surgeon and preventing regurgitation of material into the nasopharynx during the operative procedure.

In determining which type of incision to use, it is important to recall that dehiscence is a serious complication for these infants, particularly if the disease is advanced. When a right rectus muscle-splitting incision is used, there is a likelihood of dehiscence occurring. This complication has led many surgeons to utilize a gridiron type of incision in the right upper quadrant. The procedure is somewhat more difficult to perform with this type of incision, but on the other hand, the complication of dehiscence is eliminated. It is important in making this type of incision to place it well laterally away from the broad rectus muscle in the infant. On opening the peritoneal cavity, one should not seek out the tumor initially. Rather, a portion of the dilated stomach is delivered through the incision and gentle traction on this brings the pyloric tumor through the incision. With the operator's left index finger in the duodenal end of the tumor, an incision is made through the peritoneum and slightly into the muscle with the scalpel along the anterior superior border of the pyloric tumor. This area can readily be seen as the most avascular portion of the structure. Once the incision has been made through the superficial structures, blunt dissection is used to separate the tumor. The hypertrophied musculature can be split readily by blunt dissection and by pushing laterally on the two segments with a forceps. The mucosa is freed in this manner to the extent that it is even with the surface of the tumor at the end of the procedure. One must use care to divide completely the muscular ring at the duodenal end. This carries some hazard, because the mucosa is folded back at this point and may readily be perforated; however, with care, this complication can be avoided. When it does occur, closure of the small opening with a fine chromic suture is all that is required. No attempt should be made to stop the bleeding. This occurs owing to the venous

congestion from having delivered the pylorus through the incision, and no serious bleeding will occur after the structures are returned to the peritoneal cavity.

When duodenal perforation has taken place, the infant must be kept on nasogastric suction for about 72 hours after the operation. Following an uncomplicated operation, the infant should be started on feedings of sweetened water four to six hours after operation. A weak formula can then be begun, and usually within 48 hours of operation the baby can be advanced to a fairly normal formula.

About 50 per cent of these infants vomit postoperatively. This should cease by the fifth or sixth postoperative day and should not recur.

MALROTATION OR INCOMPLETE ROTATION OF THE INTESTINE

ETIOLOGY AND PATHOLOGY.   Malrotation is a fairly common condition encountered in the pediatric age group, particularly in the neonate, as a form of high intestinal obstruction. In order to understand the variety of mechanical factors which can produce duodenal obstruction, one must recall the embryologic development of the intestine, particularly during the early phase from the fifth to the twelfth week. Just prior to this period, the intestine grows voluminously, reaching such a mass that the abdominal cavity cannot accommodate it. Consequently, there develops at the base of the yolk-stalk a virtual omphalocele which houses the intestine during this period of rapid growth. The midgut, or that portion of the small intestine supplied by the superior mesenteric artery, is the principal component of this temporary omphalocele. As the abdominal cavity accommodates to the mass, there is a return of the intestine to the abdominal cavity. The proximal portion of the midgut returns first and literally folds from right to left to form the distal portion of the duodenum. The rest of the intestine then enters the cavity and the colon rotates from left to right. Failure of this process of normal rotation produces the clinical entity referred to as malrotation. Perhaps a more accurate descriptive term would be "incomplete rotation of the colon."

In many patients, incomplete rotation may be present without producing any symptoms. It is only when some portion of the intestinal tract is impinged upon and obstruction produced that the patient exhibits symptoms. There are two essential features which produce duodenal obstruction. First, the cecum may have become attached in the right upper quadrant laterally over the duodenum, or there may be bands crossing the duodenum. Second, in most patients with malrotation, the mesenteric attachment of the small intestine does not follow along the normal broad line from the left upper to the right lower quadrant, but rather is limited to the pedicle of the vascular supply to the small intestine. Thus, the whole of the midgut is free to twist or volvulate. When this occurs, tension is placed on the duodenum; and, as it wraps around the vascular stalk, duodenal obstruction is produced. Vascular obstruction occurs, particularly venous, and becomes an important part of the pathology. This type of duodenal obstruction is intermittent in character and is directly related to the twisting of the midgut and the spontaneous correction of this twisting. It should be borne in mind that there are many forms of malrotation, as the developmental process can be arrested at any point. This is disturbing to the young surgeon who expects to find a set anatomic pattern in all patients with malrotation.

Patients can be divided into two groups. The first consists of those who, as newborns, present symptoms of intestinal obstruction. They vomit bile-stained material. Distention is present only in the upper abdomen. There may be some associated obstipation. Usually, the diagnosis can be made on the basis of plain roentgenograms of the abdomen which demonstrate a large gas bubble contained in the stomach and a second smaller gas bubble to the right of the gastric structure, representing air in the dilated duodenum (Fig. 5). One cannot be positive as to the exact cause of the duodenal obstruction when such a roentgen appearance is noted; but in a good percentage of patients the cause of the obstruction is malrotation. In these patients, the duodenum usually is attached quite firmly in the right upper quadrant and there are bands holding the cecum in place, thus producing constant duodenal obstruction. This may be augmented by volvulus, which pulls the duodenum toward the midline and produces a taut band across the duodenum. The other patients have intermittent duodenal obstruction; they are usually in the younger age group, although the condition may be present in older children. In such situations, there is no duodenal obstruction except when volvulus of the mid-

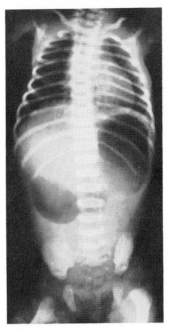

Figure 5. Roentgenogram of a patient with atresia of the duodenum, which shows clearly the point of obstruction without the administration of barium.

gut takes place, producing tension on the duodenum. Many times, the obstruction is in the intestine adjacent to the vascular pedicle of the midgut.

Patients who are examined during the first 24 to 48 hours of life usually are in excellent general condition despite some vomiting. As a rule, there is neither disturbance of the electrolyte pattern nor marked dehydration. In patients beyond 48 hours of age, the degree of electrolyte imbalance and dehydration depends on the duration of the symptoms. The correction of such defects is mandatory before surgical intervention is undertaken.

The operation is performed through a right rectus muscle-retracting incision. The important finding in patients with malrotation is that one does not encounter the colon; all the intestine present on first inspection is small intestine. The first step is to eviscerate the patient completely in order to gain a clear view of the mesentery of the small intestine. Only by this means can one be sure to detect the presence of volvulus.

Usually, volvulus is associated with malrotation, although this is not invariably true. The second step is to free the cecum from its attachment in the right upper quadrant, if this is present, and then to free the duodenum so that it takes a straight course down the right gutter (Fig. 6). This may be quite time-con-

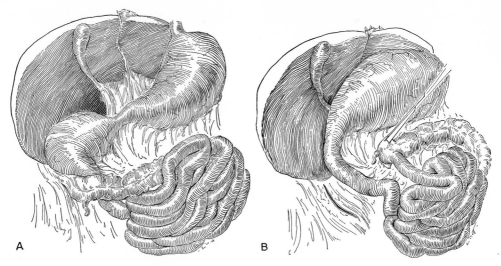

Figure 6. *A*, Drawing showing the obstruction and dilatation of the duodenum caused by the mesenteric attachment of an unrotated and undescended cecum. *B*, After completion of the operation for malrotation and nondescent of the cecum with volvulus of the midgut. The duodenum is exposed throughout its entire length, and the cecum and appendix now lie in the left upper quadrant.

suming, as the duodenum may be pulled toward the midline in the area of the vascular pedicle, and careful dissection in this region must be performed in order to avoid damage to large vessels. The cecum is then returned to the abdominal cavity and placed in the left upper quadrant, after which all the intestine is returned to the abdominal cavity. The incidence of recurrence after this operation is quite small. Undoubtedly, the procedure is so extensive that usually enough adhesion develops to fix the cecum in the left upper quadrant and thus prevent future trouble. It is well during the course of the procedure to perform an appendectomy so that later in life the patient will not have the problem of an atypical appendicitis due to the location of the appendix in the left upper quadrant. If appendectomy is not deemed advisable during the operation, it is well to warn the parents of the possibility of atypical appendicitis at some future time.

MECONIUM ILEUS

Originally, meconium ileus was thought to be an entity which involved the gastrointestinal tract primarily. It is recognized now to be part of a generalized disease resulting from a primary deficiency in pancreatic function, and in abnormalities of other glands, particularly those of the tracheobronchial mucosa. Fibrosis of the pancreas is associated with pancreatic juices deficient in elements essential in digestion. The result is that the meconium is thick and putty-like and causes intestinal obstruction. The pulmonary lesion results in a thick mucus, and those patients who undergo successful treatment of the intestinal manifestations of the disease often succumb to the pulmonary complication.

The intestinal symptoms produced by fibrocystic disease of the pancreas are quite similar to those of mechanical obstruction of the small intestine. The neonate develops abdominal distention, vomiting of bile-stained material and obstipation. Examination of the patient often enables one to suspect the correct diagnosis, owing to the readily palpable dilated loops of intestine which can be determined to be filled with putty-like material rather than to be distended by gas. The diagnosis is supported by plain roentgenograms of the abdomen, which outline the dilated loops without fluid levels in the upright film. Also, the inspissated meconium may produce a fairly characteristic granular appearance in the roentgenogram. Although this may be seen in other conditions, it is unusual except in meconium ileus. This appearance is due to the nature of the meconium, and perhaps to the small bubbles of gas interspersed in it, which produce the particular granularity noted in the roentgenogram.

In mild forms of the disease, it may be sufficient to relieve the obstruction by the use of cleansing enemas. Addition of pancreatic enzymes to the enema fluid probably has some advantage. Some surgeons recommend oral administration of pancreatic material; however, this carries the risk of aspiration of the pancreatic material which may produce quite a severe inflammatory reaction in the lungs. In most patients, the intestinal obstruction can be relieved only by an operative procedure. The type of procedure used varies; one group advocates the use of a double-barreled ileostomy with instillation of pancreatic material to clean out the colon distal to the obstruction. Another form of treatment calls for opening of the intestine and removal of as much of the inspissated material as possible, and in such situations it may be necessary to resect some of the intestine. To clean out the meconium, hydrogen peroxide has been most effective. It is well to remember, however, that one can encounter complications arising from a too vigorous use of hydrogen peroxide, because the material is absorbed with a subsequent release of oxygen into the blood. This may be of such proportion that a cushion of bubbles forms in the right side of the heart, affecting its efficiency. Providing that the intestinal tract can be cleared by the use of hydrogen peroxide, it is possible to make an end-to-end anastomosis if resection has been done, or to close the opening in the intestine if only irrigation has been performed. The advantage of this type of treatment is that it can be accomplished in one operative procedure, whereas treatment calling for an ileostomy requires a second operation for closure.

In the few patients who survive and have a return of intestinal function, long-term therapy is extremely important. The use of Nutramigen as a feeding material is advocated by many. It is well to add pancreatic granules to the feedings to compensate for the patient's deficiency of this substance.

An equally important phase of postoperative treatment concerns the almost inevitable pulmonary complications. The use of antibiotics and various forms of inhalation therapy may be lifesaving in these patients. In the patients who survive over a long period of time, the pulmonary complications become less severe. The number of such survivals, however, is not large.

MECKEL'S DIVERTICULUM

In the first few weeks of life, there is a communication between the midgut and the yolk sac. This omphalomesenteric duct normally is obliterated in the first few weeks of life; however, in about 3 per cent of the population some remnant of this duct persists. In most instances, this consists of a diverticulum projecting from the antemesenteric border of the small intestine in the distal part of the ileum. This was first described by Meckel in 1815, and the anomaly has become known as Meckel's diverticulum.

There are three anatomic features of a persistent omphalomesenteric duct which result in clinical symptomatology. The most important is that, in a certain percentage of patients with Meckel's diverticulum, there is gastric mucosa lining a part of the diverticulum (Fig. 7). As the acidic juice drains onto the normal intestinal mucosa, it may produce ulceration, bleeding and possibly perforation. The second feature of this anomaly is that, in some instances, the diverticulum remains attached to the anterior abdominal wall by means of a fibrous cord. This cord may be the cause of a band-like obstruction across the small intestine, thus constituting a potential cause of intestinal obstruction. The third anatomic feature, which is perhaps the most rare cause of clinical symptomatology in relation to this anomaly, is the persistence of a communication with the umbilicus. Thus, one may have a persistent and patent omphalomesenteric duct between the small intestine and the umbilicus. There are also situations in which the duct has become obliterated in the intra-abdominal portion, and there remains a cyst-like structure in the depths of the umbilicus which may present as a mass or a chronic draining sinus.

Bearing in mind the details of the anatomic arrangement of the anomaly, one can anticipate the type of clinical symptomatology that one might encounter in the patient with some form of Meckel's diverticulum. The most common clinical symptom is that of rectal bleeding. The patient with bleeding from an ulcerated Meckel's diverticulum is usually a young child who has been perfectly well prior to the onset of bleeding, which is sudden and copious. The patient passes a currant-jelly stool; this may be repeated once or twice, after which the stool becomes quite normal. During this time, the patient has no other associated symptomatology. Rarely is the bleeding sufficient to produce shock, although this has been reported in older children. With these bouts of bleeding, there is a drop in hemoglobin.

The diagnosis of this lesion is one of exclusion. The type of bleeding is quite characteristic, and this is the strongest clinical

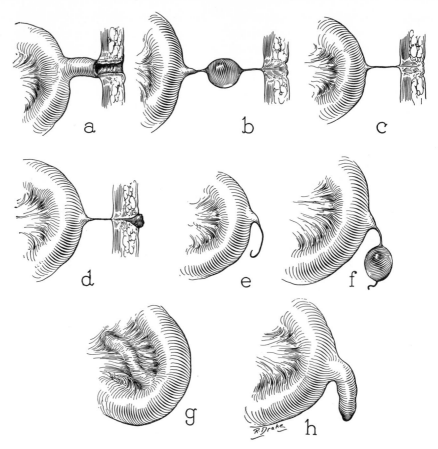

Figure 7.   *a*, Persistent omphalomesenteric duct with umbilical fistula. *b*, Incomplete closure of duct, with midportion presenting a cyst. *c*, Closure of duct with persistent fibrous remnant. *d*, Closure of duct, with umbilical cyst persisting. *e*, Same as *c* without attachment to umbilical region. *f*, Same as *b* without attachment to umbilical region. *g*, Atypical Meckel's diverticulum almost covered by mesentery. *h*, Typical appearance of Meckel's diverticulum. (Dixon, C. F., and Steward, J. A.: S. Clin. North America, Vol. 12, 1932.)

evidence that one has to substantiate the diagnosis of Meckel's diverticulum. One must proceed first to rule out esophageal varices by way of esophagograms. To be sure, most patients with esophageal varices have vomiting of blood as well as blood in the stool. Furthermore, in these latter patients, the blood in the stool tends to be black; there is not the brick-red or currant-jelly type of stool commonly seen in bleeding from a Meckel's diverticulum. There should be proctoscopy to exclude the possibility of polyps in the rectosigmoid and distal sigmoid. Rectal examination may reveal the presence of a polyp within reach of the examining finger. Barium enema examination is important to rule out polyps in the colon. It is impossible, in the vast majority of instances, to outline a Meckel's diverticulum by roentgenologic technique. There have been instances in which there was a fortuitous filling of a Meckel's diverticulum dur-

ing the course of a barium study of the small intestine, but this is so extremely rare that it cannot be relied upon as a routine measure in the diagnosis. Thus, one must establish the diagnosis on the basis of the clinical history and the exclusion of other lesions.

Treatment of this condition is excision of the Meckel's diverticulum. This can be accomplished in one of several ways. It is well to recall that the gastric mucosa occupies the wall of the Meckel's diverticulum and the ulceration usually is beyond this in the rim of the diverticulum. It is well to remove the ulcer. This is not absolutely essential, but if it is not done, there may be some postoperative bleeding. One must be sure that the lumen of the intestine is not narrowed at the point of excision. One can accomplish removal of the diverticulum, avoid narrowing of the lumen, and also be assured of removal of the ulcer by performing a V-shaped excision.

Occasionally, there will be perforation of the Meckel's diverticulum as well as bleeding from the ulceration. The perforation usually occurs slowly, so that a mass develops rather than an acute perforation with generalized peritonitis. The possibility of a perforated Meckel's diverticulum should be considered in a patient who has developed a mass and has had rectal bleeding. Patients with this combination of symptoms are quite sick and face a greater danger than those with bleeding. When perforation has taken place alone, removal of the Meckel's diverticulum necessitates dissection in acutely and chronically inflamed tissues, rendering the procedure difficult and increasing the likelihood of postoperative complications. Patients with a band between the Meckel's diverticulum and the anterior abdominal wall may develop intestinal obstruction. Plain x-ray films reveal the dilated loops of small intestine with fluid levels on the upright projection. The treatment in this case is that for acute intestinal obstruction.

In the third group of patients, there is a discharge from the umbilicus. In determining the cause of chronic umbilical discharge, one should first consider the possibility of a granuloma; this can be seen readily on close inspection and treated by cauterization. When one fails to find a granuloma, one should resort to gentle probing. If a tract is found, the patient in all likelihood has either a cystic remnant of the omphalomesenteric duct, or a tract leading to Meckel's diverticulum. Such patients should be subjected to exploration to rule out the possibility of a band underneath the umbilicus leading to a Meckel's diverticulum.

One other possible clinical situation may be related to Meckel's diverticulum, and this occurs when the diverticulum becomes the leading point of an intussusception. In such patients, the classic symptoms of intussusception with abdominal pain, vomiting and distention are present. When this is encountered, resection is often necessary. Some use a Mikulicz type of resection, leaving the patient with an ileostomy which later must be closed. Gradually, it is becoming evident that resection with a primary end-to-end anastomosis has many advantages in this type of situation.

DUPLICATION OF THE INTESTINE

Various forms of duplication may occur in the intestine, and their presence can best be explained on the basis of a defect in the embryologic development of the intestine. Early in the development of the intestine, there is formation of vacuoles and subsequent breakdown and coalescence of these vacuoles to form the intestinal lumen. It is postulated that duplication occurs where the breakdown of vacuoles has been incomplete. Thus, a portion of intestine could exist completely separate from the rest of the gastrointestinal tract, and this is a common type of duplication which presents as a cystic structure in the mesentery of the intestine adjacent to the lumen. Various other forms of the anomaly occur in which the duplication communicates with the intestinal lumen. Duplications vary in length, and instances have been reported in which virtually the entire colon was duplicated.

The opening into the intestinal lumen may occur at the proximal or the distal end of the duplication, or both, and the site of the communication is of considerable clinical significance. When it is proximal, the duplicated segment forms a blind pouch into which material is forced by peristaltic action. In such situations, the duplicated segment is dilated and pain may be associated with this distention. When the communication is distal, the duplicated segment empties and dilatation of the segment does not occur (Fig. 8).

Some details of anatomy and histology of duplication are important to the clinician. The lining of the duplicated segment often contains gastric mucosa, and consequently the secretion of acid leads, not unusually, to ulceration and bleeding. This is particularly true of the communicating type of duplication. Duplications are situated invariably in the mesentery adjacent to the intestine and have a common muscular wall. The clinical manifestations of duplication depend on the form the duplication takes. The most common site for duplication of the gastrointestinal tract is the ileocecal region. When the duplication is at the ileocecal valve, even a small cystic dilatation will produce a leading point for chronic or recurrent intussusception; such patients have bouts of abdominal pain, vomiting and distention. If a barium enema examination is performed during one of these attacks, the intussusception may be seen. In other patients, a routine form of intussusception occurs, usually in older children. There is an acute onset of abdominal cramping pain with vomiting and progressive abdominal distention. At operation, the intussusception

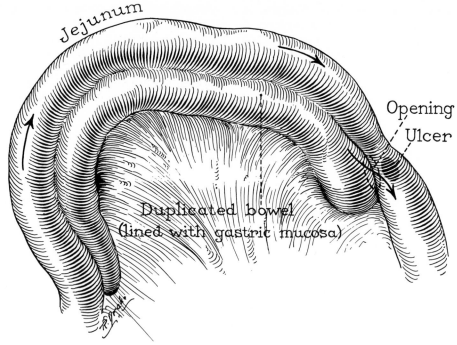

Figure 8. Duplication of small intestine. (Johnston, J. B., Hallenbeck, G. A., Ochsner, A., and DuShane, J. W.: Arch. Surg. Vol. 68, 1954.)

may have a leading point which on rare occasions is found to be a duplication of the terminal ileum.

In an occasional patient, routine physical examination may reveal an abdominal mass which is movable, and which has the interesting feature of change of position in the abdominal cavity from time to time. This set of circumstances suggests the finding of a large duplication of the small intestine which does not communicate with the intestinal tract. In some patients, the duplication may serve as a focal point for torsion of a segment of intestine, and obstruction may occur. In others, the mass is asymptomatic and is detected by the parents or the physician on palpation of the abdomen. A third manifestation of the duplication is chronic rectal bleeding. The diagnosis of duplication should be considered as a possible explanation of bleeding into the gastrointestinal tract. If the duplication communicates proximally, it can be detected by a contrast study of the intestinal tract with the use of barium. In such situations, the barium enters the duplication through the proximal communication, remains there for some time, and can be detected on a roentgen film. When the duplication communicates distally rather than proximally, there may be bleeding. Of course, this type of lesion cannot be detected

by contrast studies; only abdominal exploration can reveal the presence of the lesion. Even then, it may be quite elusive because the duplicated intestine may not be greatly different from normal intestine, and only careful palpation and observation bring to light the fact that the intestine is somewhat more bulky in one section than in another, thus revealing the presence of the duplication.

Duplication of the gastrointestinal tract should be treated by resection wherever possible. This is the treatment of choice in patients with a small duplication which has produced an intussusception, and also with an isolated duplication which does not communicate with the intestinal tract. End-to-end anastomosis of the intestine after resection is the treatment of choice. Whether a one-layer anastomosis or a two-layer anastomosis is used depends upon the surgeon's experience. The advantage of a closed one-layer anastomosis is that there is no contamination of the peritoneal cavity. This is of some importance and some surgeons prefer this type of anastomosis.

If the duplication occurs over a long segment and communicates with the lumen of the intestine, the treatment may be more complicated. In such situations, if the duplication is not too long, resection of the segment of intestine with end-to-end anastomosis is to be preferred. In some patients with a long duplication, this form of treatment may not be feasible. When the duplication communicates proximally, it may be desirable to open the septum between the two segments so that the duplicated segment drains and does not become dilated. However, this procedure does not permit removal of the gastric mucosa, which may be the primary cause of bleeding. The treatment of patients with extensive duplication may be quite difficult.

HIRSCHSPRUNG'S DISEASE

The clinical entity of Hirschsprung's disease has long been known. The explanation of the precise congenital lesion responsible for the clinical syndrome has evolved over the last few decades. Early in this century, pathologists described patients with an absence of ganglion cells in the colon; however, clinicians failed to relate this important finding to the therapy of this group of patients. In 1947, it was demonstrated that a colostomy in the dilated portion of the colon in Hirschsprung's disease would relieve the symptomatology. Peristaltic studies were then performed and these indicated that there was an absence of progressive peristaltic waves in the aganglionic segment and that there were normal or hyperactive peristaltic waves in the dilated or hypertrophied part of the colon. This led to a new concept of the therapy of patients with Hirschsprung's disease, namely, the removal of the aganglionic segment rather than the dilated segment, as had been the practice prior to 1947.

The classic state of a patient with Hirschsprung's disease is that of a malnourished older child with massive abdominal distention, obstipation and bouts of vomiting. These clinical symptoms are rarely encountered because the diagnosis is usually made when the child is in the neonatal period. Newborn patients with Hirschsprung's disease present clear-cut clinical symptoms. At birth, these patients are perfectly normal-looking infants; however, during the first day or two of life they become distended, and there may be vomiting and obstipation. In many respects, these patients have the clinical appearance of intestinal obstruction, and it is not unusual for a mistaken diagnosis of small bowel obstruction to be made and an unnecessary operation performed.

For this reason, all neonates who present symptoms of intestinal obstruction should be subjected to a barium enema examination. It is impossible in this age group to determine from plain roentgenograms of the abdomen whether the dilated loops of intestine are small or large bowel. It is only by performing a barium enema that one can identify the colon. When a barium enema examination is done on a patient with the clinical syndrome of intestinal obstruction, and the barium outlines a small colon, the diagnosis of small bowel mechanical obstruction can be made with assurance. On the other hand, in patients with a similar clinical appearance in whom the barium enema examination reveals a dilated colon, the diagnosis of small bowel obstruction must be abandoned. Unfortunately, in this early age group, the barium enema examination is not diagnostic of Hirschsprung's disease. There are other situations which mimic it and, therefore, therapy cannot be instituted on the basis of the barium enema study itself. It is perfectly true that after the patient is several months of age and has had a chance to develop some chronic dilatation of the colon, the barium enema examination then becomes pathognomonic when it outlines a dilated colon ending in the terminal portion in a funnel-like configuration with a narrow segment distal to the lesion and extending to the rectum.

In the newborn group, the diagnosis can be established with certainty by rectal biopsy. When this procedure is performed, the surgeon must be aware of the fact that he must secure a specimen which includes the full thickness of the bowel, that is, both the mucosa and the muscular coats, in order to supply the pathologist with material on which to base a diagnosis. It is true that the ganglion cells of both the myenteric plexus and the plexus of Auerbach are absent in this disease; however, they do not have an absolutely parallel relationship of absence. It is far more difficult for the average pathologist to make a diagnosis on the basis of absence of ganglion cells in the myenteric plexus. Therefore, it is wise to secure a biopsy through the entire thickness of the bowel wall. A second point to remember is that this biopsy must be taken high – above the internal sphincter which is at least 2 cm. above the mucocutaneous margin.

In the older patient with Hirschsprung's disease, the symptoms are quite classic. There is marked abdominal distention and chronic constipation. One can make a distinction between habitual constipation and Hirschsprung's disease in such patients on the basis of several clinical points: a history of symptoms of intestinal obstruction in the first day or two of life; a history of constipation dating back to birth; the finding of considerable abdominal distention of the gaseous type; and the finding, on rectal examination, of an empty rectum or a rectum with a small amount of fecal material. Impactions, if present, are above the rectosigmoid. In chronic constipation, the impactions are at the sphincter, and when this is found one can virtually eliminate the diagnosis of Hirschsprung's disease. A history of soiling will also enable one to discard the diagnosis of Hirschsprung's disease. In older children, the diagnosis can be made with absolute certainty by having an experienced roentgenologist examine the patient by barium enema (Fig. 9). The examination must be performed carefully so that the colon is not overdistended and a clear outline of the sigmoid, rectosigmoid and rectum is obtained.

It is well to remember that some patients with Hirschsprung's disease have a neurogenic defect of the urinary bladder. Intravenous urograms, cystograms and, particularly, the determination of residual urine are of value in detecting the patients with associated lesions of the urinary system.

Once the diagnosis has been established, the treatment is fairly standard. In the neonatal age group, the safest procedure probably is a colostomy performed at the level of the aganglionic lesion. This level can be established by biopsy of the colon. The surgeon must be warned that a colostomy made in the aganglionic segment will not function well. We have seen a number of patients in whom this has been done, and they have had considerable difficulty. Some have had to undergo revision of the colostomy so that it is placed above the aganglionic lesion in order for the patient to thrive. When patients are about one year of age or have attained a weight of 20 to 25 pounds, they can be subjected to resection of the aganglionic segment. This includes resection of the colostomy, thus limiting operative treatment of these patients to a two-stage operation.

In older patients with Hirschsprung's disease, primary resection can be accomplished in about 75 per cent. In those who are extremely ill, debilitated or acutely obstructed, a colostomy must be resorted to as a preliminary step before resection is performed.

The long-term results are extremely good. We have now followed patients up to 20 years after operation, and these adults are essentially normal. On the other hand, we have seen a number of patients in whom the resection has not been carried down to within 2 cm. of the mucocutaneous margin, and these patients have not done well. For this reason, the suggested procedure of leaving the rectum in place is open to question so far as long-term results are concerned. Leaving a considerable portion of the lesion behind opens the way for recurrence. This may take several years, but when recurrence does take place the eventual treatment of such patients is extremely difficult. It is well to caution the surgeon that resection of the aganglionic segment is an extremely tedious and difficult procedure. We have seen a number of complications arise, usually in patients who have been treated by surgeons with little experience in the surgical treatment of Hirschsprung's disease. The operation should not be attempted unless one has had prior experience with it and unless one has access to the facilities which are so essential to good results in this group of patients.

MALFORMATION OF THE ANUS AND RECTUM

Anomalies of the perineum which affect the intestinal tract are quite common. Recogni-

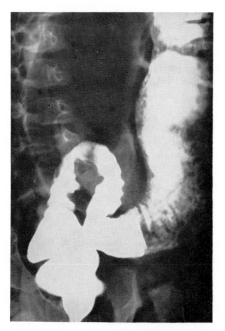

Figure 9.   Roentgenogram with barium in distal colon. Note the dilated descending colon with narrowing beyond. This is diagnostic of Hirschsprung's disease.

tion of these anomalies is not difficult, providing that the attending physician is thorough in his examination of the newborn baby. The treatment of these lesions is of considerable importance, because a great deal can be accomplished for such patients when a good result is obtained from surgical therapy. Congenital malformation of the anus and rectum assumes several different forms. The simple imperforate anus without a fistula to an adjacent structure may occur in both males and females. Here, the lesion may be adjacent to the skin or it may be some distance from the perineum. In extremely rare instances, one may encounter a true atresia of the rectum; such patients have a normal anal canal with an atresia proximal to it.

Over half the instances of perineal anomalies are complicated by fistulas to adjacent structures (Figs. 10 and 11). In the male, it is common for the colon to end in a fistulous tract which communicates with the bladder or posterior urethra. Occasionally, there may be fistulous communication with the skin that extends for a considerable distance in the midline of the perineum, opening onto the skin at the base of the scrotum or even on the scrotum itself. In the female, the majority of patients with anomalies of the perineum have associated fistulas communicating with the vagina. Most of these are low, at the posterior fourchette, but occasionally the fistula may be high in the vagina, at the level of the cervix. In extremely unusual situations, there may be a double fistula, one to the vagina and a second to the urinary bladder.

The diagnosis of these conditions can be readily made if the attending physician makes a careful inspection of the perineum. Probably, the most difficult to diagnose of all these anomalies is the unusual situation in which the rectum actually terminates in a fairly large perineal fistula. In such patients, there is stricture of the anal canal which can be detected on examination. The neonate should have an anal opening which admits the examiner's fifth finger fairly readily; if it is smaller than this, the possibility of what appears to be the rectum and anal canal actually being a fistula must be given serious consideration. Before embarking on surgical therapy, the exact nature of the anomaly must be established in order to assure selection of the proper procedure.

The first question which needs to be answered is whether there is a communication to the urinary bladder in the male patient. This can readily be determined by microscopic examination of sediment from a centrifuged urine specimen. If the sediment contains debris and large epithelial cells, one can make the diagnosis of a fistula between the colon and the urinary system with certainty.

In patients with no fistulous communication, it is important to ascertain the distance of the colon from the perineum. This can be accomplished by having roentgenograms made with the patient held in the upside-down position. When doing this, it is well to remember that it takes 12 to 18 hours for air to distend the distal colon fully, and roentgenograms made prior to 12 hours of age may not be entirely reliable. The second point to remember is that the patient must be held upside down for a few minutes before the film is taken. It is well to have a lead marker on the perineum so that the distance between the colon and the perineum can be determined accurately. When this distance is more than 1 or 1.5 cm., the approach should be abdominoperineal; when the distance is less, the operation can be performed from the perineum and an abdominal operation is unnecessary. In males with a fistulous communication to the

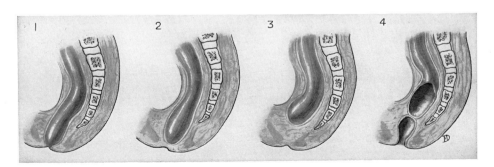

Figure 10.   Types of anal and rectal abnormalities. *1* and *2*, The colonic segment is adjacent to the perineum. These anomalies can be repaired by a perineal operation. *3*, The colon ends above the levator and an abdominoperineal operation is required to correct the defect. *4*, Rare type of anal atresia.

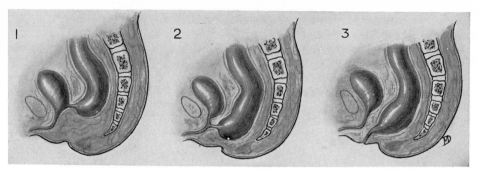

Figure 11.   Types of fistula encountered in male patients. *1*, Fistulous communication between the colon and bladder. *2*, Fistulous communication between the colon and urethra. *3*, Perineal fistula.

urinary system, an abdominoperineal operation is mandatory in order to make an adequate closure of the rectovesical or rectourethral fistula. In females in whom the fistula is in the distal part of the vagina, particularly at the posterior fourchette, a perineal operation will suffice. When the communication to the vagina is high in the region of the cervix, it is necessary to perform an abdominoperineal operation in order to achieve good results.

There is considerable debate regarding the wisdom of performing preliminary colostomies in these patients. This depends upon several factors, first of which is the condition of the infant. If the patient is massively distended and quite ill, or has an associated anomaly, particularly a cardiac malformation, it may be advisable to perform a preliminary colostomy. It is well to place these colostomies high in the sigmoid so that there is sufficient length of the colon beyond the colostomy for the abdominoperineal operation to be performed at a later date. In full term infants in good condition without any associated serious anomalies, it is possible to perform an abdominoperineal operation with satisfactory results. In patients with perineal fistulas, or rectovaginal fistulas which are low, one can perform a primary anoplasty without a preliminary colostomy, providing that the surgeon has had some experience with this type of operation. If he has not, it is best to perform a preliminary colostomy.

When a preliminary colostomy is made, the question arises as to the optimal time for performance of the definitive anoplasty. When the patient has made a good recovery and is gaining weight six to eight weeks after birth, the definitive operation can be performed.

The postoperative care and long term follow-up of patients with imperforate anus are extremely important. Parents and physicians alike are worried about fecal continence, and it is perfectly true that these patients are not normal so far as absolute rectal control is concerned. However, with proper care they can be managed perfectly well. It is not often understood that the underlying problem in this condition is one of severe colonic inertia. It is difficult to explain this phenomenon. It may be that such patients lack the normal urge to evacuate the colon and, therefore, tend to accumulate large fecal impactions. When this occurs, they tend to have diarrhea around the impaction which they cannot control; this excoriates the perineum and creates a very troublesome situation.

Daily stimulation to empty the colon completely is the program that one must institute. This can best be accomplished by the use of suppositories or small irritating enemas. Suppositories are the more common convenient means of stimulating colonic evacuation, and these should be tried first. If these prove ineffective, one must resort to various types of irritating or large-volume enemas. These should be done at regular intervals, preferably each day at a particular time, so that a habit pattern will be established. When dealing with patients with anomalies of the perineum, it is well to remember that the incidence of associated malformations of the genitourinary system is probably as high as 10 to 15 per cent and, therefore, it is mandatory that all have at least an excretory urogram to determine the status of the urinary system.

READING REFERENCES

Abrami, G., and Dennison, W. M.: Duplication of the stomach. Surgery 49:794, 1961.

Benson, C. D., Lloyd, J. R., and Smith, J. D.: Resection and primary anastomosis in the management of stenosis and atresia of the jejunum and ileum. Pediatrics 26: 265, 1960.

Berenberg, W., and Neuhauser, E. B.: Cardioesophageal relaxation (chalasia) as a cause of vomiting in infants. Pediatrics 5:44, 1950.

Bremer, J. L.: Diverticula and duplications of the intestinal tract. Arch. Path. 38:132, 1944.

Cohn, B. D.: Congenital atresia of the colon. Am. J. Surg. 104:861, 1962.

Donovan, E. J.: Congenital hypertrophic pyloric stenosis. Ann. Surg. 124:708, 1946.

Dott, N. M.: Anomalies of intestinal rotation: their embryological and surgical aspects with report of five cases. Brit. J. Surg. 11:251, 1923.

Forbes, G. B., and Erganian, J. A.: Parenteral administration of ammonium chloride for alkalosis of congenital hypertrophic pyloric stenosis. Am. J. Dis. Childh. 72:649, 1946.

Hurwitt, E. S., and Arnheim, E. E.: Meconium ileus associated with stenosis of pancreatic ducts: clinical, pathologic and embryologic study. Am. J. Dis. Childh. 64:443, 1942.

Ladd, W. E.: Congenital duodenal obstruction. Surgery 1:878, 1937.

Louw, J. H.: Congenital intestinal atresia and stenosis in the newborn. Ann. Roy. Coll. Surg. 25:209, 1959.

Mall, F. P.: Development of the human intestine and its position in the adult. Bull. Johns Hopkins Hosp. 9:197, 1898.

Mellish, R. W. P., and Koop, C. E.: Clinical manifestations of duplication of the bowel. Pediatrics 27:397, 1961.

Neville, W. E., and Clowes, G. H. A.: Colon replacement of the esophagus in children for congenital and acquired disease. J. Thorac. Cardiovasc. Surg. 40:507, 1960.

Oeconomopoulos, C. T.: Congenital anomalies of the anus and rectum. The technique of perineal proctoplasty. Am. J. Proctol. 12:363, 1961.

Rhea, W. G., Headrick, J. R., and Stephenson, S. E.: Hypertrophic pyloric stenosis with jaundice. Surgery 51:687, 1962.

Rheinlander, H. R., and Swenson, O.: The diagnosis and management of congenital hypertrophic pyloric stenosis. J. Pediat. 41:314, 1952.

Rhodes, M. P., Geller, M. J., and Becker, J. M.: Meconium peritonitis secondary to intestinal atresia. Surgery 48:812, 1960.

Santulli, T. V., and Blanc, W. A.: Congenital atresia of the intestine. Ann. Surg. 154:939, 1961.

Stephens, F. D.: Congenital malformations of the rectum and anus in female children. Australian & New Zealand J. Surg. 31:90, 1961.

Swenson, O., and Bill, A. H., Jr.: Resection of rectum and rectosigmoid with preservation of the sphincter for benign spastic lesions producing megacolon. An experimental study. Surgery 24:212, 1948.

Swenson, O., Fisher, J. H. and MacMahon, H. E.: Rectal biopsy as an aid in the diagnosis of Hirschsprung's disease. New England J. Med. 253:632, 1955.

Swenson, O., Lipman, R., Fisher, J. H., and DeLuca, F. G.: Repair and complications of esophageal atresia and tracheoesophageal fistula. New England J. Med. 267:960, 1962.

Swenson, O., Neuhauser, E. B. D., and Pickett, L. K.: New concepts of the etiology, diagnosis, and treatment of congenital megacolon (Hirschsprung's disease). Pediatrics 4:201, 1949.

Swenson, O., and Oeconomopoulos, C. T.: Achalasia of the esophagus in children. J. Thorac. Cardiovasc. Surg. 41:49, 1961.

The Esophagus

by
F. HENRY ELLIS, JR., M.D.

FRANKLIN HENRY ELLIS, JR., was born in the nation's capital and educated at St. Mark's School. From there he logically and traditionally entered and was graduated from Yale University. He received his Doctor of Medicine degree from Columbia University College of Physicians and Surgeons, was an intern at Bellevue Hospital, and was educated and trained as a surgeon at the Mayo Clinic. He developed an interest in thoracic surgery and received a Doctor of Philosophy degree from the University of Minnesota. Dr. Ellis' curiosity about the physiology of the esophagus and intracardiac surgical problems has continued to influence his investigative projects. He is Professor of Surgery in the Mayo Graduate School of Medicine, University of Minnesota, and Consultant, Section of Surgery, Mayo Clinic. His writings, presentations, scientific exhibits and motion picture films are characterized by the attributes of an excellent teacher.

INTRODUCTION AND HISTORICAL COMMENTS

Surgical treatment for esophageal disease has shared in the recent rapid developments of all aspects of thoracic surgery. Until intrathoracic operations became possible, only the cervical esophagus could be treated surgically; hence, so far as we know, the earlier operations on this organ were limited to cervical esophagotomy for removal of foreign bodies. By the latter part of the nineteenth century, malignant lesions of the cervical esophagus had been added to the surgeon's domain, largely through the efforts of Billroth and of Czerny. In 1886, Wheeler first successfully resected a pharyngoesophageal diverticulum. Achalasia of the esophagus, though known to physicians for many years, was not treated surgically until von Mikulicz, in 1900, dilated the esophagogastric junction in a retrograde manner through a gastric opening. Heller's double cardiomyotomy, modifications of which are now widely employed, was first performed in 1913.

Operations on the intrathoracic portion of the esophagus continued to resist the surgeon's efforts, although reconstructive procedures using skin-lined tubes and portions of the bowel were proposed and used during the early 1900's in the treatment of corrosive stricture of the esophagus. The first successful resection for carcinoma of the thoracic esophagus was performed by Torek in 1913, employing an antethoracic skin tube for reconstruction. Successful one-stage transpleural esophageal resection and esophagogastrostomy for carcinoma remained an unattainable goal until Ohsawa's report in 1933. In 1937, the first successful esophagogastrectomy in the United States was performed by Marshall.

After that, esophageal operations became commonplace; and advances in anesthesia, blood replacement and surgical technique lowered the mortality and morbidity to acceptable levels. Unfortunately, these remarkable advances were not matched by similar advances in the basic understanding of the function of the esophagus. Only in very recent years has such information become available, largely through studies of esophageal motility. The laboratories of Ingelfinger and Code have made major contributions to current knowledge of esophageal function in health and disease. As a result, it is now possible for the surgeon to emphasize function as well as surgical technique; proper patient selection has been facilitated, and the surgeon can base his operative efforts on sound physiologic grounds.

ANATOMY

The esophagus is a long muscular tube extending from the pharynx at the level of the sixth cervical vertebra to the stomach (Fig. 12). In the neck, it has a midline position immediately behind the trachea. After entering the thorax, the esophagus inclines posteriorly with the trachea behind the great vessels and curves slightly to the left to pass behind the left main bronchus, then slightly to the right as it continues in the posterior mediastinum. Behind the pericardial sac, it curves more strongly to the left, running anterior to the thoracic aorta and crossing it to the left of the midline. It reaches the abdomen through the esophageal hiatus, a diaphragmatic noose composed chiefly of the right crus but reinforced on the left by fibers of the left crus.

The exact site of junction between esophagus and stomach has been a subject of confusion, as is manifested by the variety of terms which have been applied to the region. The term "cardia," for example, has become so ingrained in the medical literature that one doubts it will ever be replaced; yet its anatomic boundaries are vague, including as they do the lower esophagus, esophagogastric junction and upper portion of the stomach. Similarly, such terms as "phrenic ampulla," "vestibule" and "constrictor cardiae," while perhaps useful to anatomists and radiologists, are of little value to the surgeon.

Practically, one can view the esophagogastric junction as that point where esophageal tube meets gastric pouch. This is an intra-abdominal point; and accordingly, an esophageal segment of variable length usually has an intra-abdominal location. Another important anatomic structure related to this zone is the diaphragmatic esophageal membrane, or phrenoesophageal ligament. This structure, described by Laimer in 1883, is composed largely of mature collagenous fibers. Arising primarily from the endoabdominal (transversalis) fascia, it separates at the esophageal hiatus into an upper and a lower leaf. The upper leaf inserts into the esophagus for a distance of 2 to 3 cm. above the hiatus, whereas the lower leaf descends to insert into the esophagus at or below the gastroesophageal epithelial junction.

The muscular wall of the esophagus is composed of an inner circular layer and an outer longitudinal layer without a surrounding serosal covering. Although individual variations exist, the muscular layers of the upper portion of the esophagus are striated. Rarely is striated muscle seen in the lower third of the esophagus, where smooth muscle predominates. It is difficult to identify a true anatomic sphincter in the lower esophagus, but thickening of the circular muscle can often be demonstrated in this region. There is a prominent submucosa containing mucous glands, blood vessels, Meissner's plexus of nerves and a rich network of lymphatics.

Although islands of ectopic gastric mucosa

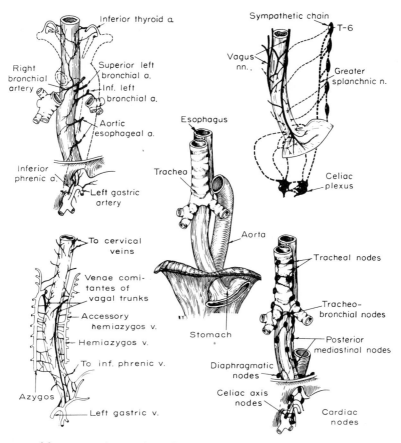

Figure 12. Anatomy of human esophagus. Arterial supply (*upper left*), venous drainage (*lower left*), innervation (*upper right*) and lymph nodes (*lower right*).

have been identified in the mucosal lining of the esophagus, usually in its proximal portions, the mucosal tube characteristically is lined by squamous epithelium. Columnar epithelium, however, makes up the lining of the distal centimeter or so; consequently, the esophagogastric junction cannot be identified accurately by the inner squamocolumnar junction (Fig. 13).

The cervical esophagus is supplied by the inferior thyroid arteries, while the thoracic portion is supplied by branches from the aorta itself and by esophageal branches of the bronchial arteries. These esophageal vessels are supplemented by others descending from vessels at the base of the neck, by ascending branches from arteries on the abdominal side of the diaphragm, and sometimes also by branches from the intercostal arteries.

Subepithelial and submucous venous channels course longitudinally to empty above and below into hypopharyngeal and gastric veins. They also penetrate the esophageal muscle, from which they receive branches, and leave the esophagus to form a periesophageal plexus, the longest trunks of which accompany the vagus nerves. The drainage from the cervical esophagus empties ultimately into the inferior thyroid and vertebral veins, that from the thoracic portion into the azygos and hemiazygos veins, and that from the abdominal portion mostly into the left gastric vein.

The lymphatic vessels, in a pattern completely independent from that of the blood vessels, tend to run longitudinally in the wall of the esophagus before penetrating the muscle layers to reach regional nodes. Hence, malignant lesions of the mid- or upper esophagus may metastasize first to cervical nodes, and lesions of the lower esophagus to gastric and celiac nodes. Once the lymphatic channels leave the esophagus, however, they go to the nearest group of nodes, which within the thorax are usually identified by their location as tracheal, tracheobronchial, posterior mediastinal and diaphragmatic.

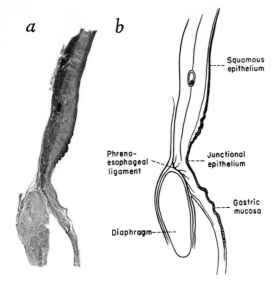

Figure 13. Microscopic anatomy of the esophagogastric junctional region. *a*, Photomicrograph. (Hematoxylin and eosin; ×1.) *b*, Schematic representation, showing origin and insertion of the phrenoesophageal ligament, diaphragm and mucosal lining.

The nerve supply of the esophagus is both from the vagi and from the sympathetic chains. The recurrent nerves supply the upper portion of the esophagus, which also receives branches from the ninth, tenth, cranial root of the eleventh and sympathetic nerves. The vagal trunks send branches to the remaining voluntary muscle and parasympathetic preganglionic fibers to the smooth muscle. Along most of the esophagus, the vagus nerves lie on either side, forming a plexus about it. As the hiatus is approached, two major trunks emerge, the left one coming to lie anteriorly and the right one posteriorly. The vagal plexuses are joined by mediastinal branches from the thoracic sympathetic chain and the splanchnic nerves. The lower end of the esophagus and esophagogastric junctional region also receive branches from the periarterial plexuses along the left gastric, hepatic and left inferior phrenic arteries.

PHYSIOLOGY

The primary function of the esophagus is to convey ingested material from the pharynx to the stomach. A regulatory mechanism exists at either end of the esophageal tube to assist in implementing this function and to

prevent, under ordinary circumstances, free reflux of stomach contents into the esophagus. In 1883, Kronecker and Meltzer first accurately described the peristaltic action of the esophagus, and current knowledge of the physiology of this organ has become possible through refinements of investigative and recording techniques initiated by them.

By means of these techniques, intraesophageal pressures may be detected and recorded. In routine tests, three or four pressure-detecting units are swallowed and positioned at various points in the esophagus, and recordings are made of the pressures at rest and after swallowing. In healthy persons, a pharyngoesophageal sphincter can be identified by a rise in pressure as detecting units are withdrawn from the esophagus into the pharynx. The act of swallowing causes a rise of pressure in the pharynx and a decrease in pressure in the sphincter (Fig. 14), permitting ingested material to be propelled into the esophagus. The sphincter then contracts in peristaltic sequence, with the pharynx above and esophagus below, to initiate the primary peristaltic wave of the esophagus. The resting pressure

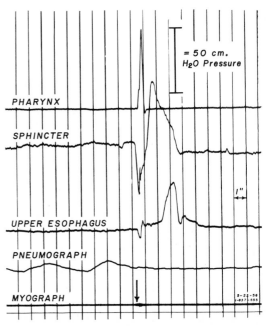

Figure 14. Swallowing pressures at pharyngoesophageal junction. Note relaxation of pressure in sphincter as pressure in pharynx increases. Pressure passes as wave through sphincter into upper part of esophagus. (Reproduced with permission from Code, C. F., and others: An Atlas of Esophageal Motility in Health and Disease. Springfield, Illinois, Charles C Thomas, 1958.)

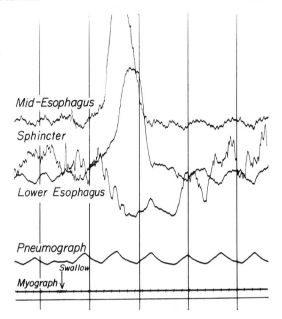

Figure 15. Esophageal and lower sphincteric response to swallowing. Note peristaltic sequence of pressure elevations in mid- and lower esophagus accompanied by relaxation of sphincter.

in the esophagus is subatmospheric, reflecting the negative intrathoracic pressure; but after swallowing, a wave of positive pressure sweeps down it in an orderly peristaltic fashion (Fig. 15). A zone of increased resting pressure 3 to 5 cm. long in the region of the esophagogastric junction identifies the inferior esophageal sphincter (Fig. 16). This sphincter relaxes promptly when a healthy person swallows, the relaxation preceding the arrival of the esophageal peristaltic wave (Fig. 15).

A variety of mechanisms for the prevention of gastroesophageal reflux have been suggested, including the diaphragm, the gastric sling fibers and the oblique angle of entry of esophagus into stomach, the mucosal rosette, and the intrinsic sphincter. Studies of esophageal motility have demonstrated clearly a physiologic sphincter at the lower end of the esophagus. Experimental studies have shown

that even if the influence of the diaphragm, the gastric sling and oblique angle of entry, and the mucosal rosette are removed, the sphincter remains intact and reflux esophagitis does not occur. Gastroesophageal reflux is inevitable when the sphincter is damaged or destroyed by disease or surgery. Accordingly, every effort should be made to preserve this mechanism wholly, or in part, when operations in this region are required.

Details of the esophageal innervation are still under investigation; but it seems evident that the vagi control esophageal peristalsis, for division of these nerves is followed by low simultaneous pressures throughout the body of the esophagus after deglutition. The inferior esophageal sphincter continues to relax on swallowing even in the absence of vagal and sympathetic innervation. Therefore, it must possess a high degree of autonomy.

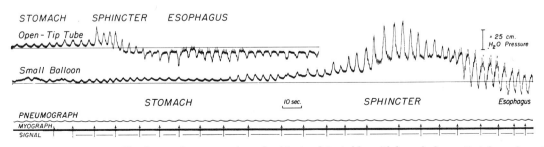

Figure 16. Pressure profile of normal gastroesophageal sphincter detected by withdrawal of open-tip tube and small balloon.

DISORDERS OF ESOPHAGEAL MOTILITY

Although disturbances of esophageal motility vary in detail, from a surgical standpoint they are best classified into two main categories: those characterized by hypomotility and those characterized by hypermotility. The former is typified by the condition known as achalasia of the esophagus, or cardiospasm, the latter by diffuse spasm of the esophagus and hypertensive gastroesophageal sphincter.

HYPOMOTILITY. Esophageal achalasia, or as it is more commonly but inaccurately known, cardiospasm, is a disease of unknown etiology characterized by absence of peristalsis in the body of the esophagus and failure of the inferior esophageal sphincter to relax in response to swallowing. It was first described in 1674 by Willis, who employed dilation in treating his patient. Meltzer and Einhorn, both in 1888, suggested that lack of relaxation of the lower esophagus was the cause of the disease. In 1926, Rake first demonstrated degeneration and decrease in number of the ganglion cells of Auerbach's plexus. These findings have been confirmed by others, and it is generally agreed that neuromuscular incoordination is the basic abnormality in the disease. The cause of this incoordination, however, has not yet been established; nor is it known whether the ganglion-cell abnormalities mentioned are a primary or secondary manifestation of the disease. That the primary site of the disorder may be in the extraesophageal nerve supply, either the vagus nerve itself or its central nuclei, has been suggested by recent pathologic studies of biopsy and autopsy material and by experiments involving selective destruction of the motor nuclei of the vagus nerve in the cat.

In Brazil and other countries where the leishmanial forms of *Trypanosoma cruzi* exist, changes in Auerbach's plexus have been demonstrated in patients with Chagas' disease, who appear to have an esophageal condition indistinguishable from achalasia.

Achalasia of the esophagus occurs with equal frequency in the two sexes. It may occur at any age, but is seen most often between 30 and 50 years. The earliest and most constant symptom is obstruction to swallowing, or dysphagia, which at first may be intermittent but becomes more constant as the disease progresses. As a rule, the patient experiences more difficulty with cold than with warm

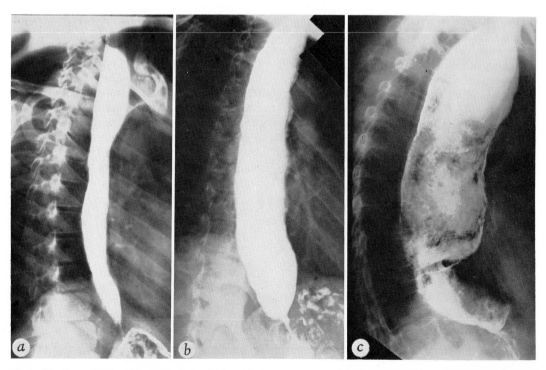

Figure 17. Roentgenographic appearance of (*a*) mild, (*b*) moderate and (*c*) severe achalasia of the esophagus. (Reproduced with permission from Olsen, A. M., and others: The treatment of cardiospasm: analysis of a twelve-year experience. J. Thoracic Surg. 22:164, 1951.)

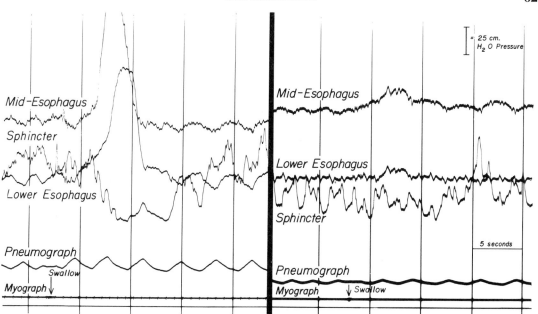

Figure 18. Deglutitive responses in body and lower sphincter of esophagus in health (*left*) and in achalasia (*right*). Note normal peristalsis and sphincteric relaxation in health, and absence of both peristalsis and sphincteric relaxation in achalasia. (Reproduced with permission from Ellis, F. H., Jr., and others: Long esophagomyotomy for diffuse spasm of the esophagus and hypertensive gastroesophageal sphincter. Surgery 48:155, 1960.)

food, and often solid foods are said to pass more easily at first than do liquids. Pain is a relatively infrequent symptom, occurring in a little more than one-fourth of the patients. It is more likely to occur in the early stage of the disease, and becomes less noticeable as the esophagus dilates. Regurgitation is a common symptom, particularly noticeable at night when the patient is reclining. In 10 per cent of patients with achalasia of the esophagus, pulmonary complications in the form of aspiration pneumonitis may develop as a direct result of regurgitation.

The earliest roentgenologic evidences of esophageal achalasia are those of obstruction at the cardia with slight esophageal dilatation proximally. As the disease progresses, the classic roentgenologic signs develop (Fig. 17). The esophagus is dilated and the lower portion of the lumen appears conical and narrowed for a short distance with a beak-like extension directed into the spastic segment. Although esophageal achalasia in its more advanced forms has roentgenographic characteristics which distinguish it from carcinoma, it may not be differentiated thus in its early stages. Therefore, to distinguish carcinoma from early achalasia, esophagoscopy is advisable.

The diagnosis of achalasia can be confirmed by esophageal motility studies which show a slightly elevated pressure in the esophagus, a reflection of esophageal dilatation, and a lack of peristalsis in the body of the esophagus

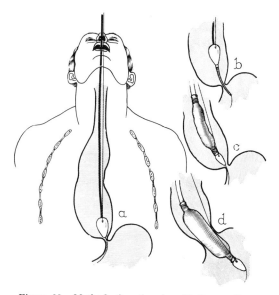

Figure 19. Method of performing dilation. *a*, Passage of 41-F olive-tipped bougie into stomach. *b*, Passage of 50- or 60-F sound into stomach, guided by flexible wire spiral. *c*, Passage of hydrostatic dilator into cardia, and *d*, distention of hydrostatic dilator across cardia. (Reproduced with permission from Olsen, A. M., and others: The treatment of cardiospasm: analysis of a twelve-year experience. J. Thoracic Surg. 22:164, 1951.)

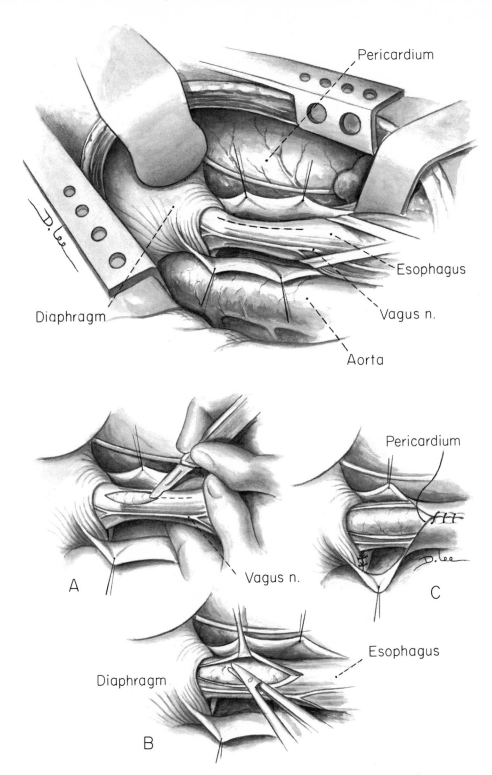

Figure 20.   Technique of esophagomyotomy. *Upper panel:* Operative exposure. Dotted line indicates intended line of incision. *Lower panel: A,* Beginning the incision. *B,* Dissection of mucosa from muscularis. *C,* Restoration of esophagogastric junction to intra-abdominal position with suture narrowing of esophageal hiatus if necessary. (Reproduced with permission from Ellis, F. H., Jr., and others: Esophagomyotomy for esophageal achalasia: experimental, clinical, and manometric aspects. Ann. Surg. *166:*640, 1967.)

following deglutition, the swallowing effort being accompanied rather by feeble elevations in pressure that are simultaneous throughout the body of the esophagus. In contrast to its normal behavior, the inferior esophageal sphincter fails to relax in response to swallowing efforts (Fig. 18).

Treatment by drugs and diet is ineffective. Forcible dilation of the cardia, preferably by hydrostatic pressure, has been employed for a number of years. Though subjecting the patient to a slight but definite risk of rupture, it has proved successful in a high percentage of patients when used by those trained in the technique (Fig. 19). Relatively permanent relief of dysphagia can be obtained by a single course of treatment in approximately 60 per cent of patients. In an additional 20 per cent, the symptoms may be controlled by a second and third course; but there remain approximately 20 per cent of patients who require treatment of some other kind.

Several types of plastic operations have been proposed for destroying or by-passing the esophagogastric junction; but by sacrificing the inferior esophageal sphincter, these procedures invariably lead to gastroesophageal reflux and its debilitating complications.

Such operations no longer have a place in the treatment of achalasia of the esophagus. Esophagomyotomy, first introduced by Heller as a double cardiomyotomy, but since modified to a single incision through the distal esophageal musculature, does not possess these disadvantages. In the present technique, a thoracic approach is preferred because it permits adequate exposure of the distal esophagus, which is the site of the obstruction. A linear incision is made in the distal esophageal musculature. The mucosa is exposed in such a fashion as to free completely the narrowed distal esophageal segment of its circular musculature (Fig. 20). The incision should be carried onto the stomach only far enough to ensure complete division of the distal esophageal musculature. To obviate postoperative development of a diaphragmatic hernia, damage to the esophageal hiatus and its supporting structures should be avoided carefully.

Postoperative studies of esophageal motility in patients treated by this technique demonstrate a lowering of pressure in the region of the inferior esophageal sphincter. A modest pressure barrier, sufficient to prevent gastroesophageal reflux, remains in its subhiatal portion. Symptomatic improvement can be

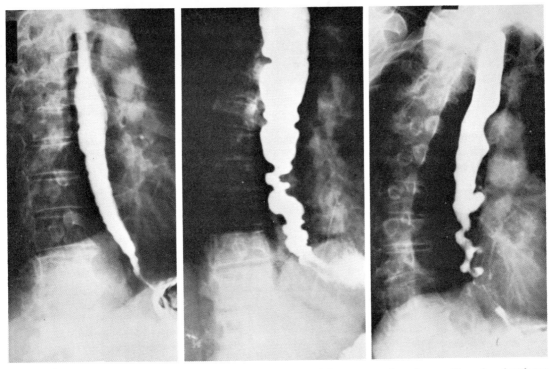

Figure 21. Esophageal roentgenograms from three patients with diffuse spasm of esophagus. (Reproduced with permission from Olsen, A. M., and others: The treatment of cardiospasm: analysis of a twelve-year experience. J. Thoracic Surg. 22:164, 1951.)

expected in more than 90 per cent of patients so treated, and reflux esophagitis rarely occurs.

HYPERMOTILITY. What is generally referred to now as diffuse spasm of the esophagus has been designated in the past by a variety of terms, including "curling or corkscrew esophagus," "idiopathic muscular hypertrophy of the esophagus," and "diffuse nodular myomatosis of the esophagus," which serve to indicate the confusion surrounding the condition. Basically, diffuse esophageal spasm and hypertensive gastroesophageal sphincter are disorders of esophageal motility characterized by elevated intraluminal pressures.

The clinical description of diffuse spasm of the esophagus by Moersch and Camp in 1934 is a classic, as applicable today as it was originally. Pain and dysphagia are the predominant symptoms, the former being more pronounced and dysphagia occurring less commonly, or not at all. The pain varies from a sensation of discomfort beneath the lower half of the sternum to severe, colicky substernal pain extending through to the back. It may mimic cardiac pain. Eating may provoke an attack of pain, or the sensation may come on spontaneously, even awakening the patient at night. Patients with this disease tend to be high-strung and nervous, and a diagnosis of psychoneurosis may be entertained. The symptoms are more likely to be troublesome than incapacitating.

Diffuse spasm may coexist with hypertensive gastroesophageal sphincter, or the two may occur independently. They cannot be distinguished by symptoms; roentgenography usually fails to give positive findings, although minor degrees of hiatal herniation may be present in each. The textbook radiographic picture of diffuse esophageal spasm (Fig. 21) is seen in less than half the patients.

For diagnosis, therefore, special reliance must be placed on studies of esophageal mo-

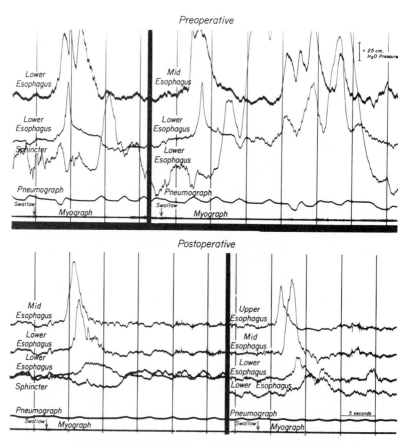

Figure 22. Deglutitive responses in body and sphincter of esophagus before (*upper panels*) and after (*lower panels*) esophagomyotomy. Amplitude, duration and repetitiveness of contractions have been reduced by operation. (Reproduced with permission from Ellis, F. H., Jr., and others: Long esophagomyotomy for diffuse spasm of the esophagus and hypertensive gastroesophageal sphincter. Surgery 48:155, 1960.

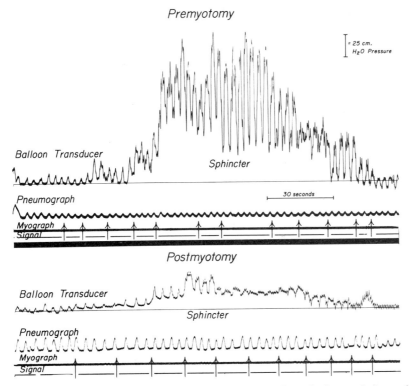

Figure 23. Preoperative and postoperative resting pressures at gastroesophageal sphincter before and after esophago-myotomy in patient with hypertensive gastroesophageal sphincter. Each upright arrow indicates 0.5-cm. withdrawal of recording catheter. Note decrease in length and pressure of sphincter. (Reproduced with permission from Ellis, F. H., Jr., and others: Long esophagomyotomy for diffuse spasm of the esophagus and hypertensive gastroesophageal sphincter. Surgery 48:155, 1960.)

tility. Put briefly, in diffuse spasm powerful, simultaneous, sometimes repetitive and prolonged contractions occur in the lower half or third of the esophagus after swallowing, though usually the sphincter is normal (Fig. 22). In hypertensive gastroesophageal sphincter, the resting sphincteric pressure is excessive, being 140 cm. of water or more as detected by balloon transducers (Fig. 23). There may also be poor relaxation of the sphincter after swallowing.

The hyperactive character of these motility disturbances, and their relatively localized nature, led naturally to the use of an extended modified Heller myotomy procedure in patients with severe symptoms, since other forms of treatment were unsuccessful. The technique resembles in most respects that employed for achalasia of the esophagus. The myotomy is more extensive, however; its limits, defined by the extent of the disease as determined by esophageal motility studies, occasionally reach the aortic arch. Frequently, a small diaphragmatic hernia coexists and must be repaired. Thickening of the distal esophageal musculature will be found at operation in approximately half of the patients.

Although the majority of patients are benefited by this operation and usually maintain an initially good result over the years, the results are not so good as those following esophagomyotomy for achalasia of the esophagus. The reason for the higher incidence of poor results in these patients is not clear, although good results are more likely to follow operation in patients whose preoperative motility studies have shown extreme abnormalities. Currently, operation is advised for these conditions only in the emotionally stable patient with severe disability and a markedly abnormal pattern of esophageal motility.

DIVERTICULA

Esophageal diverticula can be classified by location and mode of development and by their status as true or false diverticula. By location, they are commonly separated into three categories: pharyngoesophageal, thoracic and epiphrenic. Those at the upper and lower ends of the esophagus have been referred to as pulsion diverticula, and frequently may be related to some neuromuscular abnormality. The sac consists primarily of esophageal mucosa and submucosa, and hence these are false diverticula. Thoracic diverticula have been called traction diverticula and usually occur in the midesophagus in the region of the tracheal carina. In contrast to the other two groups, they are more likely to include all layers of the esophageal wall; they are known as true diverticula.

PHARYNGOESOPHAGEAL DIVERTICULA. The pharyngoesophageal diverticulum was first described in 1764 by Ludlow; but Zenker's name has become associated with this condition, for in 1878 he and von Ziemssen collected 22 patient reports from the literature and added five of their own. They recognized the nature and mode of formation of these diverticula, pointing out that they always form between the cricopharyngeus fibers of the inferior esophageal constrictor muscle. Usually, they occur in elderly people; and although a congenital weakness has been postu-

lated as a cause of this lesion, it seems more likely that weakening of the tissues in this region with advancing age may be significant. The suggestion has been made that such diverticula may be the result of achalasia of the cricopharyngeus muscle. Though motility studies have not confirmed this, a number of patients have been treated successfully by cricopharyngeal myotomy.

The chief symptoms are dysphagia, regurgitation and noisy deglutition. Pulmonary manifestations may result from aspiration of diverticular contents during nocturnal regurgitation. The diverticulum inevitably enlarges; and ultimately, if it is untreated, total esophageal obstruction occurs. The diagnosis is made roentgenographically (Fig. 24).

Single-stage resection (Fig. 25) is still the preferred method of treatment for pharyngoesophageal diverticulum. The procedure is readily accomplished through a left vertical or curved transverse cervical incision. The diverticulum itself is exposed by retracting the thyroid gland medially and the carotid sheath laterally. After dissection of the sac up to its neck, which ordinarily is rather narrow, it

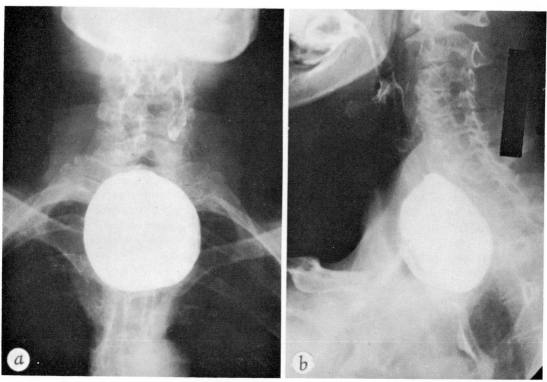

Figure 24.   Classic (*a*) posteroanterior and (*b*) lateral roentgenologic appearance of pharyngoesophageal diverticulum in same patient.

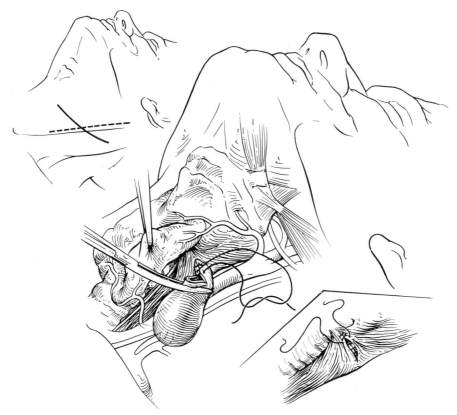

Figure 25. Procedure for removal of pharyngoesophageal diverticulum.

may be divided and removed. The pharyngeal mucosa is closed with interrupted sutures, their knots within the esophageal lumen; the edges of the muscle layer are approximated carefully. The operation carries minimal risk, even in the debilitated and elderly patient. Recurrence is rare.

THORACIC DIVERTICULA. Diverticula seldom develop in the thoracic part of the esophagus, and symptoms are uncommon. The condition has been related to inflammatory carinal nodes secondarily involving the wall of the esophagus with resulting traction on it. The neck of the sac usually is broad, and the diverticulum does not tend to enlarge greatly, for it empties readily and food does not tend to collect within the sac. If esophageal symptoms are present in a patient with a diverticulum of this type, their cause should be looked for elsewhere.

EPIPHRENIC DIVERTICULA. Located just above the diaphragm are epiphrenic diverticula, sometimes called supradiaphragmatic diverticula. They occur less commonly than pharyngoesophageal diverticula and are less likely to produce symptoms. Their primary symptoms are dysphagia and regurgitation, and the radiographic appearance is quite characteristic (Fig. 26). The cause of this condition is not clear; but certainly a neuromuscular disturbance is present in some patients, for conditions such as achalasia of the esophagus and diffuse esophageal spasm have coexisted in a high percentage of instances. To prevent recurrence of symptoms, it is important that the associated conditions be corrected at the time of diverticulectomy. The high incidence of associated diffuse spasm or esophageal achalasia makes it advisable to consider the use of long esophagomyotomy in addition to diverticulectomy. Preoperative studies of esophageal motility help to indicate which patients require an associated procedure.

The technique of diverticulectomy is straightforward, the lesion being approached transthoracically from right or left and dissected up to its narrow neck in preparation for excision and esophageal reconstruction (Fig. 27).

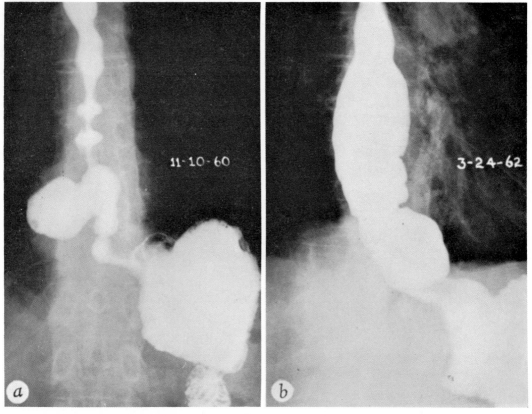

Figure 26.   Esophageal roentgenograms (*a*) before and (*b*) after excision of epiphrenic diverticulum and long esophago-myotomy. Diffuse spasm of esophagus was present also.

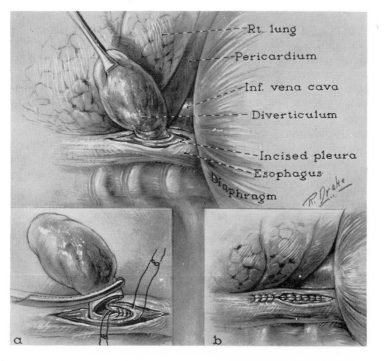

Figure 27.   Technique of epiphrenic diverticulectomy. (Reproduced with permission from Habein, H. C., Jr., and others: Surgical treatment of lower esophageal pulsion diverticula. A.M.A. Arch. Surg. 72:1018, 1956.)

FOREIGN BODIES AND PERFORATION

Children under the age of three years are the patients who most often present with esophageal foreign bodies. Unless a foreign body is unusually large, or has unusual characteristics such as sharp edges or hooks, it will pass readily into the stomach. The most frequent site of arrest of a foreign body is at or just below the cricopharyngeal sphincter. The remainder will be found in the mid- or lower esophagus. Obstruction and perforation are the two main complications of foreign-body ingestion.

The diagnosis should be suspected from the history, obtained either from the family or the patient, and confirmed by roentgenologic visualization of the foreign body in the esophagus. When a nonopaque foreign body is present, roentgenograms made after ingestion of iodized oil (Lipiodol), or methylglucamine diatrizoate (Gastrografin), may demonstrate its nature and location. Endoscopic removal is the procedure of choice and usually can be accomplished by the skilled endoscopist. If not, operative removal by esophagotomy should be undertaken promptly. In any case of esophageal foreign body, care should be taken to exclude an underlying intrinsic lesion of the esophagus.

Perforation of the esophagus can be brought about by ingestion of a foreign body, and also by instrumentation, as during esophagoscopy or bougienage. Perforation accompanying esophagoscopy occurs most frequently at the level of the cricopharyngeus muscle, but occasionally at the gastroesophageal junction. Lower esophageal perforations may follow instrumental dilation for achalasia or malignancy. Other kinds of direct or indirect trauma rarely cause perforation of the esophagus.

Subcutaneous emphysema of the neck follows immediately, or soon after, perforation in the region of the cricopharyngeal muscle during esophagoscopy. The patient experiences pain in the cervical region, aggravated by movement of the head or neck. Lateral roentgenograms reveal air in the prevertebral space with anterior displacement of the trachea. Systemic reaction, characterized by fever and tachycardia, usually develops rapidly. Operative intervention should be undertaken promptly. The cervical esophagus is exposed and the perforation closed, if possible. If operation is delayed, the esophageal tissues become edematous and friable and a retroesophageal abscess may be encountered.

Drainage of the area is the preferred treatment and suffices to relieve the symptoms and permit healing of the perforation.

Perforation of the lower esophagus is characterized usually by pain in the chest, more often on the left than the right. There may also be evidence of peritoneal irritation in the upper part of the abdomen. Thoracic roentgenograms may demonstrate pleural effusion, pneumothorax and occasionally mediastinal emphysema. Surgical intervention should be undertaken without delay and, ordinarily, transthoracic closure of the perforation can be accomplished.

In all instances of esophageal perforation, once the diagnosis has been made, oral feedings should be discontinued, antibiotics administered and nasogastric suction instituted. In some patients, these conservative measures alone may lead to a favorable outcome but operative intervention is the treatment of choice for it usually prevents serious sequelae.

ESOPHAGITIS AND STRICTURE

Esophageal mucosa is highly sensitive to many agents, and particularly to strong acid and alkaline solutions. Such agents may reach the esophagus either by the ingestion of a caustic chemical, or by reflux of acid peptic gastric juices or alkaline intestinal juices. The esophageal lining responds to such insults by an acute inflammatory reaction. Destruction of part or all of the esophageal mucosa and its covering coats may occur, with subsequent formation of stricture.

CORROSIVE ESOPHAGITIS. The condition that develops after the ingestion of a caustic solution, such as a strong alkali or acid, has been termed corrosive esophagitis. Except in attempted suicide, such ingestion usually is accidental and occurs most frequently in young children. Lye, a strong cleansing agent containing sodium hydroxide and sodium carbonate, is the most common offending agent, although a variety of other substances including mineral acids, strong bases, phenol and organic solvents can produce identical injuries. The degree of injury depends upon the nature and concentration of the agent ingested, and whether the ingested material reaches the stomach. In the case of severe burns, the entire mucous membrane of the upper portion of the alimentary tract may slough, with ultimate development of extensive stricture (Fig. 28).

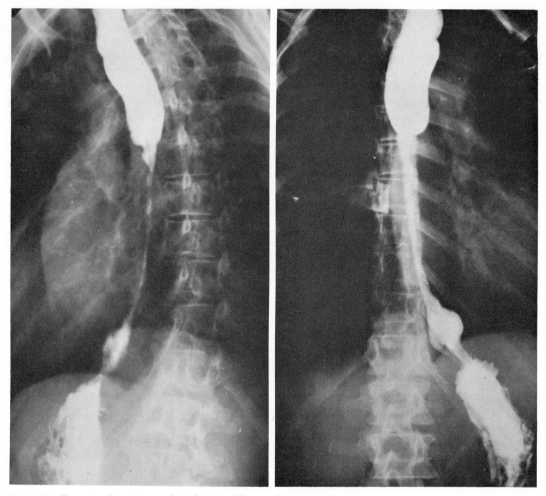

Figure 28. Extensive lye stricture of esophagus: oblique and posteroanterior roentgenograms made in the same patient.

During the acute phase of the reaction, burns of the lips, mouth, tongue and pharynx are evident. The patient complains of pain in the involved region, sometimes associated with vomiting. Painful dysphagia is prominent. The acute phase lasts for several days to several weeks, until the chronic phase is entered and dysphagia becomes predominant as stricture develops.

Neutralizing agents, such as dilute acid or alkaline solutions, should be administered in the acute phase of the process to minimize the effect of the ingested material. Use of cortisone during the acute phase of the burn has been advocated to reduce the incidence and severity of stricture. After the acute phase has subsided, roentgenologic examination of the esophagus helps to delineate the extent of the damage.

Dilation of the strictured zone by bou-

gienage over a swallowed thread may be begun when indicated within a few weeks of the burn. In some patients, such treatment may not be necessary, but others require repeated dilations at intervals for a year or more. Gastrostomy may be necessary, not only for feeding purposes but to permit retrograde dilation.

If it becomes evident that a satisfactory esophageal lumen cannot be maintained, surgical reconstruction of the esophagus becomes essential. Over the years, a variety of operative procedures have been devised which employ skin-lined tubes and segments of intestine, or stomach, for by-passing the obstructed esophagus. For total by-pass, a segment of right or left colon interposed substernally between pharynx and stomach is currently preferred. For lesser degrees of stricture, the site of disease may be approached transthoracically, and either resected or by-passed with a segment of jejunum or colon.

REFLUX ESOPHAGITIS. Sometimes referred to as acid peptic esophagitis, reflux esophagitis results from incompetence of the esophagogastric sphincter mechanism, which permits free reflux of acid gastric juice into the esophagus. This may occur under a variety of circumstances, but in the majority of patients, it is secondary to a sliding esophageal hiatal hernia. Operative procedures which by-pass or destroy the esophagogastric junction lead invariably to gastroesophageal reflux and esophagitis. Prolonged vomiting, as may occur in pregnancy, postoperatively or with obstructing duodenal ulcer, may lead to the same condition. Reflux has been described also in idiopathic incompetency of the cardia or chalasia. After certain operative procedures, such as total gastrectomy with esophagoduodenostomy, reflux esophagitis may ensue because of alkaline regurgitation.

In reflux esophagitis, there is a sequential pattern of tissue destruction and healing. The process may subside at any stage to heal completely, or may progress finally to marked stricture. When secondary to a hiatal hernia, reflux esophagitis usually is limited to a short segment of the esophagus in the region of the esophagogastric junction. Ulceration may occur, but often is superficial and rarely involves the muscularis propria. Nonetheless, stenosis and stricture may develop; and marked degrees of periesophageal reaction are common (Fig. 29). Extended linear esophagitis, a more superficial form of the disease, is more commonly associated with repeated episodes of vomiting.

Recently, Hayward has postulated that the condition known as "lower esophagus lined by columnar epithelium," originally described by Barrett as a congenital lesion, is really a result of reflux esophagitis. In the healing process following mucosal destruction, the columnar epithelium is regenerated more rapidly than the squamous epithelium; so the lower part of the esophagus ultimately may be lined by columnar epithelium for some distance. A stricture may be present at the squamocolumnar junction, and an ulcer frequently occurs in the columnar-lined portion of the tube (Barrett's ulcer).

Dysphagia, regurgitation, substernal and epigastric pain, and heartburn are the common symptoms of esophagitis. Later in the course of the disease, when fibrosis and stricture have occurred, dysphagia may become the predominant symptom and, occasionally, hematemesis or melena may be encountered,

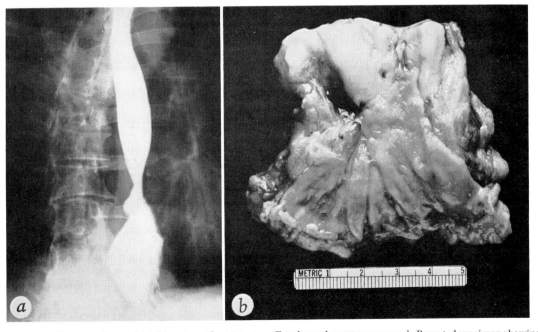

Figure 29. Short-esophagus hiatal hernia with stricture. *a*, Esophageal roentgenogram. *b*, Resected specimen showing ulceration and stricture. (Reproduced with permission from Ellis, F. H., Jr., and others: Treatment of short esophagus with stricture by esophagogastrectomy and antral excision. Ann. Surg. *148*:526, 1958.)

although massive gastrointestinal bleeding is rare. Roentgenography is of little value in diagnosing esophagitis; esophagoscopy is necessary for confirmation, for the disease may be present without the typical symptoms and many patients with regurgitation and heartburn have normal esophageal mucosa.

Nonsurgical treatment similar in most respects to that advocated for duodenal ulcer is indicated in the early stage of the disease. Appropriate diet and supplementary antacids are prescribed. In addition, the patient is advised to sleep with the head of his bed elevated, to lose weight and to avoid wearing constricting garments, for they tend to accentuate gastroesophageal reflux. When reflux esophagitis is associated with a sliding esophageal hiatal hernia, surgical reduction of the hernia is clearly indicated if other conditions permit.

If reflux esophagitis is treated inadequately in its early stages, complications develop. Scarring and fibrosis about the esophagogastric junction may lead to shortening of the esophagus, so that surgical reduction of the

junction to its normal intra-abdominal position becomes impossible. So-called short esophagus is usually, but not always, accompanied by a stricture at the esophagogastric junction, which can be readily demonstrated radiographically (Fig. 29). Other complications of the disease include intractable pain, bleeding and, rarely, perforation.

Often, nonsurgical management of the complications of reflux esophagitis is ineffective in controlling symptoms and preventing progression of the disease. Sometimes, in the absence of severe hemorrhage or stricture, the symptoms of an incompetent cardia and shortened esophagus can be controlled by a gastric drainage procedure such as a Finney or Heineke-Mikulicz pyloroplasty. Esophageal strictures should be dealt with first by dilations. Some patients can be managed for long periods by intermittent dilations; but when this form of treatment fails or the intervals between become too brief, operative intervention is indicated, as it is when hemorrhage has occurred repeatedly.

The diseased tissue must be removed and

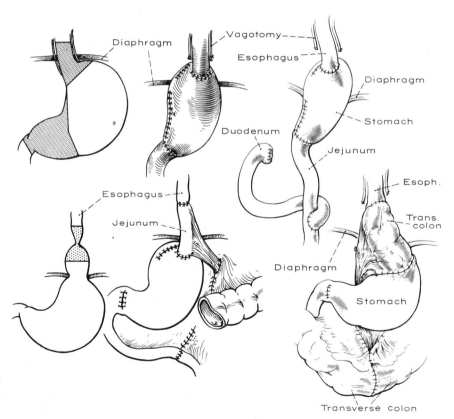

Figure 30.   Operations for esophageal stricture. *Upper,* Esophagogastrectomy and antral excision. *Lower,* Jejunal and colonic interposition procedures. (Reproduced with permission from Ellis, F. H., Jr., and Payne, W. S.: Motility disturbances of the esophagus and its inferior sphincter: recent surgical advances. *In,* Welch, C. E.: Advances in Surgery. Vol. 1. Chicago Year Book Medical Publishers, Inc., 1965, pp. 179-246.)

reflux of acid gastric contents into the esophagus, which would cause the disease to recur, prevented. Several different operative procedures have been employed over the years, but currently two are preferred. A limited esophagogastrectomy with antral excision followed by esophagogastric and gastroduodenal, or Roux-Y gastrojejunal, anastomoses has been used with success as a means of removing the stricture and inducing achlorhydria, thus preventing recurrence of esophagitis (Fig. 30, *upper*). Merendino and Dillard relieved the symptoms of esophageal stricture secondary to reflux esophagitis by interposing a segment of jejunum between the esophagus and stomach after resection of the strictured portion. Some would prefer to interpose a segment of colon (Fig. 30, *lower*). These are extensive operative procedures which carry some risk and accordingly should not be employed unless other methods fail.

NEOPLASMS

Esophageal obstruction in the adult is usually secondary to neoplasia. Both benign and malignant tumors occur in the esophagus, but the vast majority are malignant. Dysphagia is the commonest symptom, regardless of the nature of the neoplasm. Accordingly, the differential diagnosis is based on other features of the disease.

BENIGN TUMORS. Benign tumors of the esophagus, though rare, include leiomyoma, fibrolipoma, papilloma, adenoma, hemangioma, and others. Leiomyomas are by far the most commonly encountered benign esophageal tumors, and together with fibrolipomas, constitute the majority of benign esophageal tumors requiring excision.

Smooth-muscle neoplasms may arise at any level in the wall of the esophagus. Leiomyomas possess an intact mucosal covering and are truly intramural tumors. Microscopically, a pattern of interlacing bundles of spindle-shaped cells is typical. The growths occur more frequently in men than in women. Often, they produce no symptoms and are detected on routine thoracic roentgenography or gastrointestinal radiographic study for unrelated reasons. When present, the symptoms typically are those of slowly progressive dysphagia caused by the size or location of the tumor. In contrast to gastric leiomyomas, they rarely bleed.

Esophageal roentgenograms demonstrate a smooth-bordered filling defect with intact overlying mucosa (Fig. 31). The appearance on esophagoscopic examination is characteristic: a mucosa-covered, freely movable, nonconstricting tumor bulging into the esophageal lumen. Endoscopic biopsy should not be done, for it would add difficulty to the surgical treatment, which involves transthoracic enucleation of the tumor. Excision may be complicated when the leiomyoma straddles the esophagogastric junction to involve both stomach and esophagus. In such patients, esophagogastrectomy may be required for complete removal. Excision is the preferred treatment, not only for symptomatic relief but also to ensure removal of the occasionally present leiomyosarcoma.

Fibrolipomas are polypoid intraluminal esophageal tumors and occur far less frequently than do leiomyomas. They are of considerable interest because of the sensational manner in which they may appear, and because of their fatal potentiality if untreated. Usually, they arise by a long pedicle from either the cervical or upper thoracic esophagus. Multiple tumors have been reported. The mucosa over the surface of the tumor is intact ordinarily, although ulceration may develop. Microscopically, these tumors are a mixture of loose fibrous tissue associated with myxomatous and fatty changes.

Obstruction leads to dysphagia, and the tumor may be regurgitated through the mouth. Thoracic roentgenograms usually reveal mediastinal widening, while roentgenograms of the esophagus after ingestion of barium show esophageal dilatation which may lead to an incorrect diagnosis of esophageal achalasia (Fig. 32.). Esophagoscopy may permit a more accurate diagnosis. Excision is the treatment of choice, and the site of attachment of the pedicle should be determined accurately so that the proper surgical approach will be selected. An occasional tumor may be removed transorally, but most require cervical or thoracic esophagotomy.

MALIGNANT TUMORS. Malignant lesions of the esophagus, while not the most commonly encountered visceral malignant neoplasms, are certainly among the most discouraging to treat. The majority are carcinomas, which predominate especially among men between the ages of 50 and 70 years. The basic cause of the disease is unknown, but a particularly high incidence has been reported in patients with Paterson-Kelly syndrome, achalasia,

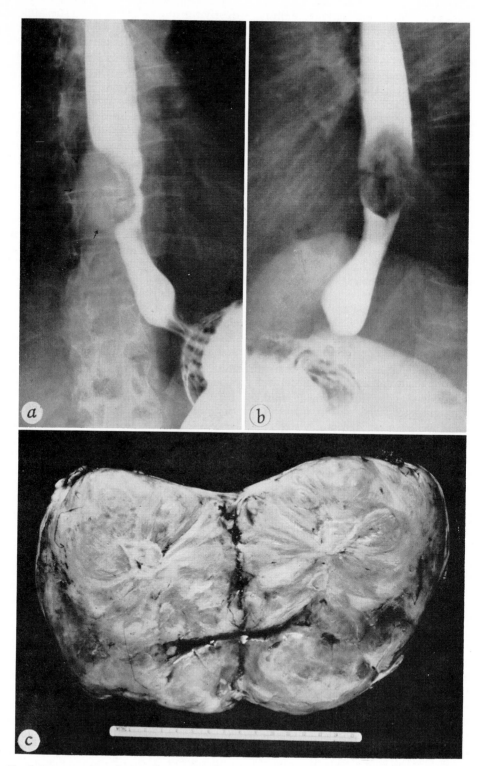

Figure 31.   Leiomyoma of esophagus. *a* and *b*, Esophagograms. *c*, Gross specimen. (Reproduced with permission from Ellis, F. H., Jr.: Surgical management of benign esophageal obstruction. Journal-Lancet *80*:347, 1960.)

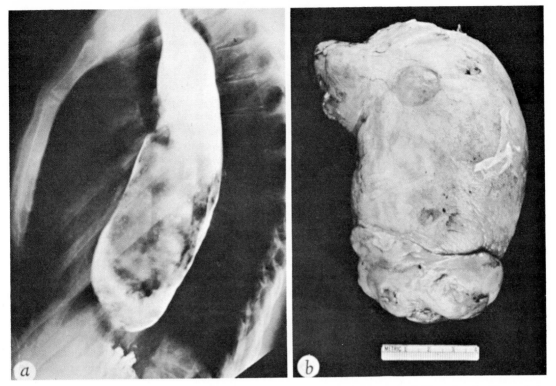

Figure 32. Fibrolipoma of esophagus. *a*, Esophagogram. *b*, Gross specimen (same patient). (Reproduced with permission from Bernatz, P. E., and others: Benign, pedunculated, intraluminal tumors of the esophagus. J. Thoracic Surg. 35:503, 1958.)

corrosive esophagitis and the so-called short-esophagus type of hiatal hernia. There is an unusually high incidence among the Japanese and the South African Bantu, which has been related to the dietary and alcoholic habits of these peoples. Carcinomas involving the esophagogastric junction or cardia, though often of gastric origin, are usually included in any discussion of neoplasms of the esophagus. While malignant lesions can occur at any level of the esophagus, 48.7 per cent arise at the cardia (Fig. 33).

About 90 per cent of all esophageal malignant lesions are squamous cell carcinomas. Most of the remainder are adenocarcinomas, which are usually of gastric origin though occasionally one arises in the esophagus. These lesions are likely to ulcerate and encircle the esophagus. They have a marked tendency to submucosal lymphatic spread and direct involvement of adjacent structures.

Sarcomas, mostly leiomyosarcomas, are distinctly rare. These tumors are predominantly submucosal but in contrast to leiomyomas tend to ulcerate. Carcinosarcoma is another uncommon malignant lesion of the esophagus. It is characteristically a polypoid

tumor and appears to afford a better prognosis than the other malignant neoplasms. Although melanoblasts never have been dem-

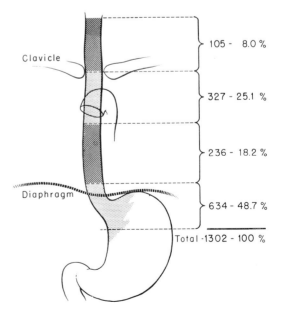

Figure 33. Anatomic location of 1302 malignant lesions of esophagus and cardia encountered at Mayo Clinic from January 1946 through December 1960.

onstrated in the human esophagus, there are a number of well-documented reports of melanomas of this organ.

Dysphagia is by far the most common symptom of carcinoma of the esophagus. Initially, it is noted with ingestion of solid foods, but ultimately, with the relentless progression of the disease, swallowing of liquids becomes difficult. Pain, regurgitation and loss of weight are other common symptoms of the disease. The diagnosis usually is easy to make by esophageal roentgenography, which shows an irregular, ragged mucosal pattern and luminal narrowing, proximal dilatation being rare (Fig. 34). Esophagoscopy should be performed in all patients to obtain a tissue diagnosis, and to determine accurately the upper limits of the lesion. Although findings from endoscopic biopsy usually are positive, cytologic study of smears made from the lesion at the time of endoscopy is a valuable diagnostic adjunct. At the time of esophagoscopic examination of lesions involving the upper esophagus, bronchoscopy should be performed to exclude malignant involvement of the tracheobronchial tree.

Excision of the lesion is the treatment of choice. Not only does it provide the best hope for cure, but it affords excellent palliation. Patients with obvious metastatic disease, or serious associated illnesses, are usually considered unsuitable for surgical treatment. The surgical procedure varies with the site of the lesion. For malignant lesions restricted to the cervical esophagus, the technique perfected and advocated by Wookey, which involves local resection with staged reconstruction employing a cervical flap, is most commonly employed. Concomitant laryngectomy usually is required.

Upper thoracic esophageal lesions are resected through a right thoracotomy or thoracoabdominal incision, continuity being restored either by intrathoracic esophagogastrostomy (Fig. 35) or substernal interposition of a segment of colon (Fig. 36).

Lower esophageal lesions, and those involving the esophagogastric junction, are best approached through either a left thoracotomy or a thoracoabdominal incision followed by esophagogastrectomy, splenectomy and wide resection of the intra-abdominal node-bearing tissues, including a major portion of the acid-secreting portion of the

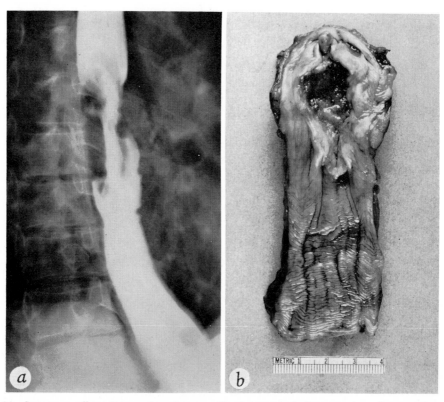

Figure 34.   Squamous cell carcinoma of esophagus. *a,* Esophagogram. *b,* Gross specimen from another patient.

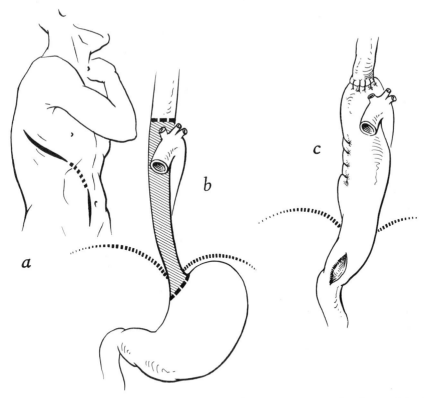

Figure 35. Esophagogastrectomy for lesion of upper thoracic esophagus. *a*, Incision: either thoracoabdominal incision or separate thoracic and abdominal incisions may be used. *b*, Shading indicates portion of esophagus to be resected. *c*, Completed operation with high intrathoracic anastomosis. (Reproduced with permission from Ellis, F. H., Jr.: Treatment of carcinoma of the esophagus and cardia. Proc. Staff Meet., Mayo Clin. 35:653, 1960.)

Figure 36. Esophagectomy with interposition of left colon. *a*, Incisions. *b*, Shading indicates portion to be resected. *c*, Mobilization of colon. *d*, Completed operation. Procedure may be done in one or two stages.

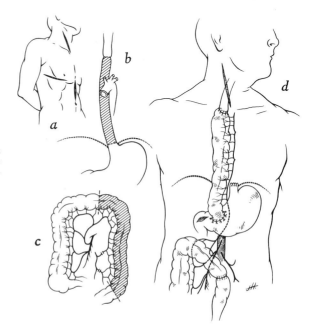

stomach to minimize reflux esophagitis (Fig. 37). Whenever possible, pyloromyotomy should be done at the time of esophageal resection to offset the vagotomy effect.

If exploration discloses that the lesion is inoperable, use of a plastic tube may be of considerable palliative benefit. Even if the impossibility of resection is known prior to exploration, a Celestin tube can be inserted by means of a small abdominal incision and a gastrotomy. Radiation therapy for inoperable lesions may be of considerable symptomatic benefit, particularly for squamous cell carcinomas involving the upper thoracic and cervical esophagus. Some surgeons have advocated preoperative irradiation to increase the resectability rate for middle and upper thoracic esophageal malignant lesions, while others have combined surgical resection with postoperative supervoltage radiation therapy. The ultimate value of such combined therapy has yet to be established.

Over the years, reported hospital mortality for esophageal resection has varied from 5 to 50 per cent. To keep the rate within reasonable limits, considerable care should be devoted to proper preparation of the patient for operation. Restoration of blood volume and proper regulation of the fluid-electrolyte balance, plus administration of supplementary vitamins, including adequate amounts of B complex, C and K, are of obvious benefit. Because of the relatively high incidence of complicating pulmonary problems, the preoperative use of expectorants, antibiotics and bronchodilators may simplify many a postoperative course.

Today, the hospital mortality for esophageal resection should not exceed 10 to 15 per cent. Considerable palliation is afforded, which increases the mean survival period beyond that of untreated patients. Survival varies with the location of the lesion, its cell type and the presence or absence of nodal metastasis. An overall five-year survival rate of 17 per cent for patients surviving resection has been reported. The prognosis for squamous cell lesions of the upper thoracic esoph-

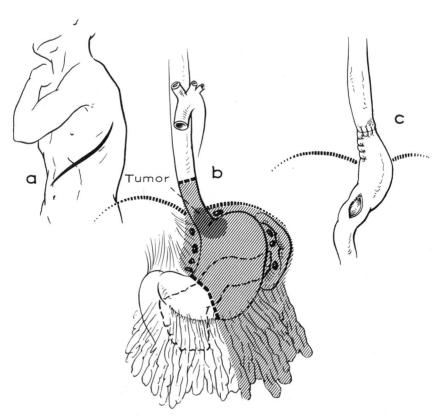

Figure 37.   Esophagogastrectomy for lesions of distal esophagus and esophagogastric junction. *a,* Incision. *b,* Shading indicates tissue to be resected. *c,* Completed operation. (Reproduced with permission from Ellis, F. H., Jr.: Treatment of carcinoma of the esophagus and cardia. Proc. Staff Meet., Mayo Clin. 35:653, 1960.)

agus and for adenocarcinoma of the cardia is the worst, while that for squamous cell carcinoma of the lower esophagus is the best.

ESOPHAGEAL VARICES

The esophageal veins are one of the major collateral pathways between the portal and the systemic venous systems. They respond to elevations of pressure in the portal system by the development of submucosal varicosities, which usually are most prominent at the lower end of the esophagus. Clinically, esophageal varices are associated ordinarily with splenomegaly and often with hepatomegaly and ascites. In some patients, the splenomegaly may lead to secondary hypersplenism. There is a marked tendency for esophageal varices to rupture and bleed massively.

Whipple classified portal hypertension into two main types according to the site of obstruction. Cirrhosis of the liver, which obstructs the portal vein intrahepatically, is by far the commonest cause of portal hypertension. In about 20 per cent of patients, however, portal hypertension results from extrahepatic obstruction affecting either the portal or the splenic vein before it enters the liver. The obstruction may be the result of trauma, infection or congenital abnormalities. Rarely, obstruction to the venous outflow leads to portal hypertension, the so-called Budd-Chiari syndrome.

Whatever the underlying cause of portal hypertension, massive gastrointestinal bleeding is by all odds the commonest symptom of esophageal varices. It has been said that 54 per cent of cirrhotic patients die within a year of the first hemorrhage, 65 per cent within two years, and 70 per cent within four years. The risk among patients with extrahepatic forms of portal hypertension is approximately one-fifth as great as in patients with cirrhosis of the liver.

Disagreement exists concerning the cause of hemorrhage from esophageal varices. Multiple factors probably are involved, for in this region pressure increased by any cause may ultimately result in thinning of the overlying mucosa, making it more susceptible to trauma by ingestion of food or by gastroesophageal reflux, with consequent reflux esophagitis. In some instances thrombocytopenia, which is a reflection of co-existing hypersplenism, must also have an influence.

A diagnosis of hemorrhage from ruptured esophageal varices should be considered seriously in instances of massive hemorrhage from the upper gastrointestinal tract with splenomegaly. Clinical evidence suggesting hepatic disease such as jaundice, enlargement of the liver, vascular spider angiomata and gynecomastia should add support to a correct clinical diagnosis. Hematologic studies may reveal evidence of hypersplenism. Assessment of hepatic function by commonly employed laboratory tests should aid importantly in establishing a diagnosis of hepatic cirrhosis.

Frequently, esophageal roentgenography demonstrates the presence of esophageal varices. Esophagoscopy is another valuable diagnostic aid when performed by a competent endoscopist. Liver biopsy, splenic pulp manometry, and portal venography are three additional diagnostic measures. The latter two procedures are valuable not only in confirming the diagnosis, but more importantly in demonstrating the site of portal vein obstruction and the patency and availability of veins for possible operative shunting procedures (Fig. 38). It is uncommon for bleeding from varices to occur if the splenic pulp pressure is lower than 280 mm. of water. Portal venography is most often performed by transcutaneous splenic puncture, but if the spleen has been resected, direct portal portography may be required. Occasionally, the umbilical vein may be used to permit radiographic visualization of the portal vein and its branches.

During the acute stage of massive hemorrhage from esophageal varices, treatment is directed primarily toward blood replacement and control of bleeding. Balloon tamponade of the bleeding esophageal varices by means of the Sengstaken-Blakemore tube may be a lifesaving measure. Cathartics are employed to remove nitrogenous products from the alimentary tract, for absorption of them would increase the amount of ammonia in the blood. Vitamins, especially B complex and K, should be administered parenterally. If bleeding persists despite proper use of balloon tamponade, or if it recurs immediately after removal of the tube, transesophageal ligation of the varices should be considered. The benefit from this procedure usually is only temporary, however; and if the patient's condition permits, a shunting procedure can be performed, even

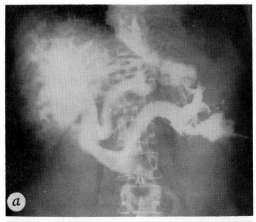
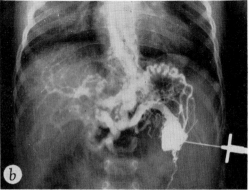

Figure 38. Percutaneous splenic portograms from two patients: (*a*) intrahepatic portal obstruction and (*b*) extrahepatic portal obstruction. Extensive collateral flow with esophageal varices is demonstrated in each, and a sizable splenic vein suitable for shunting is present.

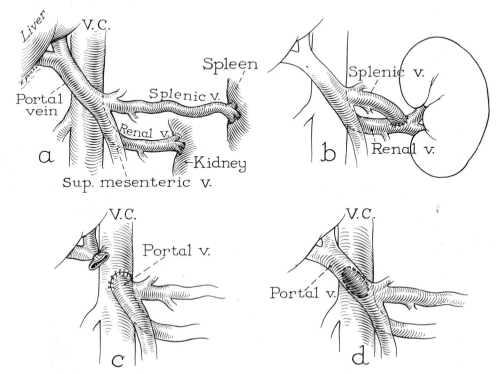

Figure 39. Types of portacaval shunts. *a*, Principal structures involved. *b*, Splenectomy with end-to-side splenorenal anastomosis. *c*, End-to-side portacaval anastomosis. *d*, Side-to-side portacaval anastomosis. (Reproduced with permission from Hallenbeck, G. A.: Portacaval anastomosis: rationale, indications and technique. S. Clin. North America 35:1099, 1955.)

during the acute episode of bleeding. Because the use of supportive measures and balloon tamponade alone has great limitations and because the operative risks of varix ligation and emergency shunting are comparable, the latter procedure is considered by some to be the preferable one during an acute episode of bleeding, providing that hepatic function is adequate.

Elective surgical treatment of the patient with esophageal varices is designed primarily to prevent recurrent hemorrhage. The construction of a shunt between portal and systemic venous systems, first performed experimentally by Eck in 1877, is the best method yet devised to decompress the portal system. Such a procedure may take the form of a splenorenal shunt, an end-to-side portacaval shunt or a side-to-side portacaval shunt (Fig. 39).

In the patient with extrahepatic portal-vein obstruction and bleeding esophageal varices, a splenorenal shunt is the procedure of choice. If splenectomy has been done already, some form of esophagogastrectomy may have to be employed or, if circumstances permit, a mesocaval shunt should be considered. In infants and small children, the size of the vessels may preclude a satisfactory anastomosis, so operation should be delayed if possible.

In selecting cirrhotic patients with esophageal varices for operation, care is necessary to minimize the mortality. Because some patients with cirrhosis of the liver and esophageal varices do not bleed, prophylactic shunting procedures are not routinely employed. The ideal surgical candidate is one who gives a history of serious hemorrhage from esophageal varices, who does not have persistent ascites resistant to medical treatment, and who has adequate hepatic function as evidenced by no more than 25 per cent retention of sulfobromophthalein sodium at the end of one hour, an albumin concentration of 3 gm. or more and total bilirubin of 2 gm. or less per 100 ml. of serum, and a prothrombin time of 24 seconds or less after treatment with vitamin K.

Either splenectomy with splenorenal anastomosis, or a direct portacaval shunt is possible technically in most patients with intrahepatic portal-vein obstruction. The end-to-side portacaval anastomosis is easier technically and decompresses the portal system more effectively than does a splenorenal shunt. The overall mortality of elective shunting procedures of all types is in the neighborhood of 8 per cent, but the rate for splenorenal anastomosis is approximately half of that for portacaval anastomosis. Splenorenal shunts are followed by recurrent bleeding approximately as often as are portacaval shunts, but the long-term survival rate is slightly higher. Most important, however, is the fact that only 5 per cent of splenorenal shunts are followed by disabling portal systemic encephalopathy, as opposed to a 25 per cent incidence among patients who have undergone end-to-side portacaval anastomosis. Side-to-side portacaval shunts have some theoretical advantages which have not been borne out in practice.

MISCELLANEOUS LESIONS

EMETOGENIC INJURY. A common cause is believed to be responsible for both esophagogastric mucosal lacerations (Mallory-Weiss syndrome) and spontaneous rupture of the esophagus (Boerhaave's syndrome). This consists of a sudden increase in intra-abdominal pressure, usually associated with emesis. A history of prolonged retching or vomiting often but not always associated with alcoholism is characteristic.

When such a mechanism leads to gastro-esophageal mucosal lacerations, painless gastrointestinal bleeding may ensue. Although the bleeding may be self-limited, surgical exploration may be required if it persists. Early diagnosis can be facilitated by roentgenographic studies to exclude the possibility of other lesions and by endoscopy to identify the site of the bleeding.

When the lower esophagus ruptures following a sudden increase in intraluminal pressure, the clinical findings are quite different. The patient immediately experiences excruciating pain in the thorax or upper abdomen, symptoms of circulatory collapse develop rapidly, and often subcutaneous emphysema is noted in the neck. Thoracic roentgenograms confirm the presence of air in the mediastinum and of air and fluid in the thorax. Prompt surgical intervention is required. Ordinarily, the rent in the lower esophagus can be closed accurately in layers; if not, the stomach can be pulled up and the fundic wall applied to the defect as a patch.

PATERSON-KELLY SYNDROME. In 1919, Paterson and Kelly independently described a clinical state with which the names of Plummer and Vinson later became associated in the United States. The condition remains of unknown etiology and occurs much less frequently now than heretofore, but most often in women past middle age. A high incidence has been reported from Sweden. Characteristics are atrophic esophagitis and spasm or esophageal web in the cervical portion of the esophagus associated with iron-deficiency anemia. Nutritional deficiency, congenital web, localized esophagitis and hysteria have been suggested as possible mechanisms of the condition. Dysphagia is the most common symptom, and treatment by dilation combined with iron therapy for the hypochromic anemia has often been successful. It should be emphasized that not all patients with Paterson-Kelly syndrome have esophageal webs, nor are esophageal webs seen only in patients with this syndrome. A congenital origin must be postulated in some patients. The condition is said to predispose to carcinoma.

LOWER ESOPHAGEAL RING. Schatzki and Gary first described the radiographic appearance of a ring-like constriction of the lower esophagus in patients with hiatal hernia. This is not an uncommon radiographic finding in such patients and ordinarily has no significance. Dysphagia may occur, however, if the ring is less than 2 cm. in diameter. Esophagoscopy is usually not diagnostic, but pathologic study in the occasional patient in whom part or all of the ring has been excised has revealed submucosal fibrosis at the esophagogastric mucosal junction. In the majority of patients, surgical reduction of the hernia not only provides relief of symptoms but removes the radiographic evidence of a lower esophageal ring. Sometimes, however, a true anatomic obstruction requiring surgical relief is present. Either incision or excision of the constricting ring is then necessary. The etiology of these rings remains obscure. A congenital origin is favored by some, whereas others are of the opinion that they represent sequelae of reflux esophagitis.

SCLERODERMA. Scleroderma is a generalized disease affecting the connective tissues of the body. When the esophagus becomes involved, the characteristic changes are fragmentation and homogenization of the submucosal connective tissue elements. The muscular layers usually are not involved. Dysphagia, regurgitation and heartburn are the typical symptoms. Radiographic studies show lack of motility of the esophagus and narrowing of its lower segment associated with a hiatal hernia and free gastroesophag-

eal reflux. Reflux esophagitis is common, and stricture may occur in the later stages of the disease. Studies show an absence of motility throughout most of the esophagus with marked diminution of tone at the inferior sphincter. Treatment is similar to that for patients with hiatal hernia and gastroesophageal reflux. When stricture develops, dilation may be required. Only rarely should surgical efforts be undertaken, for there is added risk in such procedures and the results leave much to be desired.

NEUROMUSCULAR DISTURBANCES. Swallowing dysfunction is common in patients with neuromuscular disorders, and the details of these abnormalities can be demonstrated by esophageal motility studies. The most striking abnormalities can be seen in patients whose disorders are primarily myotonic in origin such as myasthenia gravis and myotonia dystrophica. Motor failure of the esophagus occurs in both conditions. A variety of nonspecific abnormalities may be seen in patients with central and peripheral neurologic disorders, usually involving changes in peristalsis. Such conditions include Parkinson's disease, amyotrophic lateral sclerosis, and multiple sclerosis.

READING REFERENCES

Allison, P. R.: Reflux esophagitis, sliding hiatal hernia, and the anatomy of repair. Surg. Gyn. & Obst. 92:419, 1951.

Anderson, R. L.: Spontaneous rupture of the esophagus. Am. J. Surg. 93:282, 1957.

Azzopardi, J. G., and Menzies, T.: Primary oesophageal adenocarcinoma: confirmation of its existence by the finding of mucous gland tumours. Brit. J. Surg. 49:497, 1962.

Barrett, N. R.: The lower esophagus lined by columnar epithelium. Surgery 41:881, 1957.

Barrett, N. R.: Chronic peptic ulcer of the oesophagus and "oesophagitis." Brit. J. Surg. 38:175, 1950.

Belsey, R.: Reconstruction of the esophagus with left colon. J. Thoracic & Cardiovasc. Surg. 49:33, 1965.

Belsey, R.: Functional disease of the esophagus. J. Thoracic & Cardiovasc. Surg. 52:164, 1966.

Bernatz, P. E., Smith, J. L., Ellis, F. H., Jr., and Andersen, H. A.: Benign, pedunculated, intraluminal tumors of the esophagus. J. Thoracic Surg. 35:503, 1958.

Billroth, T.: Ueber die Resection des Oesophagus. Arch. klin. Chir. 13:65, 1871.

Bombeck, C. T., Dillard, D. H., and Nyhus, L. M.: Muscular anatomy of the gastroesophageal junction and role of phrenoesophageal ligament: autopsy study of sphincter mechanism. Ann. Surg. 164:643, 1966.

Botha, G. S. M.: Mucosal folds at the cardia as a component of the gastro-oesophageal closing mechanism. Brit. J. Surg. 45:569, 1958.

Boyd, D. P., Adams, H. D., and Salzman, F. A.: Carcinoma of the esophagus. New England J. Med. 258:271, 1958.

Butin, J. W., Olsen, A. M., Moersch, H. J., and Code, C. F.: A study of esophageal pressures in normal persons and patients with cardiospasm. Gastroenterology 23:278, 1953.

Butler, H.: The veins of the oesophagus. Thorax 6:276, 1951.

Byrne, J. J., and Moran, J. M.: The Mallory-Weiss syndrome. New England J. Med. 272:398, 1965.

Carey, J. M., and Hollinshead, W. H.: An anatomic study of the esophageal hiatus. Surg. Gyn. & Obst. 100:196, 1955.

Carveth, S. W., Schlegel, J. F., Code, C. F., and Ellis, F. H., Jr.: Esophageal motility after vagotomy, phrenicotomy, myotomy, and myomectomy in dogs. Surg. Gyn. & Obst. 114:31, 1962.

Cassella, R. R., Brown, A. L., Jr., Sayre, G. P., and Ellis, F. H., Jr.: Achalasia of the esophagus: pathologic and etiologic considerations. Ann. Surg. 160:474, 1964.

Celestin, L. R.: Permanent intubation in inoperable cancer of the oesophagus and cardia: a new tube. Proc. Roy. Coll. Surg. 25:165, 1959.

Clagett, O. T., and Payne W. S.: Surgical treatment of pulsion diverticula of the hypopharynx: one-stage resection in 478 cases. Dis. Chest 37:257, 1960.

Code, C. F., Creamer, B., Schlegel, J. F., Olsen, A. M., Donoghue, F. E., and Andersen, H. A.: An Atlas of Esophageal Motility in Health and Disease. Springfield, Illinois, Charles C Thomas, 1958.

Code, C. F., Schlegel, J. F., Kelley, M. L., Jr., Olsen, A. M., and Ellis, F. H., Jr.: Hypertensive gastroesophageal sphincter. Proc. Staff Meet., Mayo Clin. 35:391, 1960.

Creamer, B., Donoghue, F. E., and Code, C. F.: Pattern of esophageal motility in diffuse spasm. Gastroenterology 34:782, 1958.

Creamer, B., Olsen, A. M., and Code, C. F.: The esophageal sphincters in achalasia of the cardia (cardiospasm). Gastroenterology 33:293, 1957.

Czerny: Neue Operationen: Vorläufige Mittheilung. Zentralbl. Chir. 4:433, 1877.

Dickson, R. J.: Radiation therapy in carcinoma of the esophagus: a review. Am. J. M. Sci. 241:662, 1961.

Effler, D. B., Barr, D., and Groves, L. K.: Epiphrenic diverticulum of the esophagus: surgical treatment. A.M.A. Arch. Surg. 79:459, 1959.

Einhorn, M.: A case of dysphagia with dilatation of the oesophagus. M. Rec. 34:751, 1888.

Ellis, F. H., Jr., Andersen, H. A., and Clagett, O. T.: Treatment of short esophagus with stricture by esophagogastrectomy and antral excision. Ann. Surg. 148:526, 1958.

Ellis, F. H., Jr., Andersen, H. A., and Clagett, O. T.: Surgical management of the complications of reflux esophagitis. A.M.A. Arch. Surg. 73:578, 1956.

Ellis, F. H., Jr., Kiser, J. C., Schlegel, J. F., Earlam, R. J., McVey, J. L., and Olsen, A. M: Esophagomyotomy for esophageal achalasia; experimental, clinical and manometric aspects. Ann. Surg. 166:640, 1967.

Ellis, F. H., Jr., Jackson, R. C., Krueger, J. T., Jr., Moersch, H. J., Clagett, O. T., and Gage, R. P.: Carcinoma of the esophagus and cardia: results of treatment, 1946 to 1956. New England J. Med. 260:351, 1959.

Fischer, R. A., Ellison, G. W., Thayer, W. R., Spiro, H. M., and Glaser, G. H.: Esophageal motility in neuromuscular disorders. Ann. Int. Med. 63:229, 1965.

Fyke, F. E., Jr., and Code, C. F.: Resting and deglutition pressures in pharyngo-esophageal region. Gastroenterology 29:24, 1955.

Fyke, F. E., Jr., Code, C. F., and Schlegel, J. F.: The gastroesophageal sphincter in healthy human beings. Gastroenterologia 86:135, 1956.

Greenwood, R. K., Schlegel, J. F., Code, C. F., and Ellis, F. H., Jr.: The effect of sympathectomy, vagotomy, and oesophageal interruption on the canine gastro-oesophageal sphincter. Thorax 17:310, 1962.

Groves, L. K.: Carcinoma of the esophagus — 1965: evaluation of treatment. Ann. Thoracic Surg. 1:416, 1965.

Habein, H. C., Jr., Kirklin, J. W., Clagett, O. T., and Moersch, H. J.: Surgical treatment of lower esophageal pulsion diverticula. A.M.A. Arch. Surg. 72:1018, 1956.

Hallenbeck, G. A., Wollaeger, E. E., Adson, M. A., and Gage, R. P.: Results after portal-systemic shunts in 120 pa-

tients with cirrhosis of the liver. Surg. Gyn. & Obst. 116:435, 1963.

Hayward, J.: The lower end of the oesophagus. Thorax 16:36, 1961.

Heller, E.: Extramuköse Cardiaplastik beim chronischen Cardiospasmus mit Dilatation des Oesophagus. Mitt. Grenzgeb. Med. Chir. 27:141, 1913.

Hiebert, C. A., and Belsey, R.: Incompetency of the gastric cardia without radiologic evidence of hiatal hernia: the diagnosis and management of 71 cases. J. Thoracic & Cardiovasc. Surg. 42:352, 1961.

Higgs, B., Kerr, F. W. L., and Ellis, F. H., Jr.: The experimental production of esophageal achalasia by electrolytic lesions in the medulla. J. Thoracic & Cardiovasc. Surg. 50:613, 1965.

Ingelfinger, F. J.: Esophageal motility. Physiol. Rev. 38:533, 1958.

Johnston, J. B., Clagett, O. T., and McDonald, J. R.: Smooth-muscle tumours of the esophagus. Thorax 8:251, 1953.

Johnstone, A. S.: Diffuse spasm and diffuse muscle hypertrophy of lower oesophagus. Brit. J. Radiol. 33:723, 1960.

Kegaries, D. L.: The venous plexus of the oesophagus: its clinical significance. Surg. Gyn. & Obst. 58:46, 1934.

Kelly, A. B.: Spasm at the entrance to the oesophagus. J. Laryng. & Otol. 34:285, 1919.

Laimer, E.: Beitrag zur Anatomie des Oesophagus. Med. Jahrb. 1883, pp. 333-388.

Le Roux, B. T.: An analysis of 700 cases of carcinoma of the hypopharynx, the oesophagus, and the proximal stomach. Thorax 16:226, 1961.

Mallory, G. K., and Weiss, S.: Hemorrhages from lacerations of the cardiac orifice of the stomach due to vomiting. Am. J. M. Sci. 178:506, 1929.

Mann, C. V., Schlegel, J. F., Ellis, F. H., Jr., and Code, C. F.: Studies of the isolated gastroesophageal sphincter. Surg. Forum 13:248, 1962.

Meiss, J. H., Grindlay, J. H., and Ellis, F. H., Jr.: The gastroesophageal sphincter mechanism. II. Further experimental studies in the dog. J. Thoracic Surg. 36:156, 1958.

Meltzer, S. G.: Ein Fall von Dysphagie nebst Bemerkungen. Berl. Klin. Wchnschr. 25:140; 173, 1888.

Merendino, K. A., and Dillard, D. H.: The concept of sphincter substitution by an interposed jejunal segment for anatomic and physiologic abnormalities at the esophagogastric junction: with special reference to reflux esophagitis, cardiospasm and esophageal varices. Ann. Surg. 142:486, 1955.

von Mikulicz, J.: Zur Pathologie und Therapie des Cardiospasmus. Deutsche med. Wchnschr. 30:17; 50, 1904.

Moersch, R. N., Ellis, F. H., Jr., and McDonald, J. R.: Pathologic changes occurring in severe reflux esophagitis. Surg. Gyn. & Obst. 108:476, 1959.

Mulder, D. G., Plested, W. G., III, Hanafee, W. N., and Murray, J. F.: Hepatic circulatory and functional alterations following side-to-side portacaval shunt. Surgery 59:923, 1966.

Nakayama, K., Yanagisawa, F., Nabeya, K., Tamiya, T., Kobayashi, S., and Makino, K.: Concentrated preoperative irradiation therapy. Arch. Surg. 87:1003, 1963.

Nardi, G. L.: Surgical treatment of lye strictures of the esophagus by mediastinal colon transplant without resection. New England J. Med. 256:777, 1957.

Neville, W. E., and Clowes, G. H. A., Jr.: Surgical treatment of reflux esophagitis. Arch. Surg. 83:534, 1961.

Orloff, M. J.: Emergency treatment of bleeding esophageal varices in cirrhosis. Curr. Probl. Surg. July, 1966, pp. 13-28.

Panke, W. F., Rousselot, L. M., and Moreno, A. H.: Splenic pulp manometry as an emergency test in the differential diagnosis of acute upper gastrointestinal bleeding. Surg. Gyn. & Obst. 109:270, 1959.

Paterson, D. R.: A clinical type of dysphagia. J. Laryng. & Otol. 34:289, 1919.

Payne, W. S., Ellis, F. H., Jr., and Olsen, A. M.: Achalasia of the esophagus: a follow-up study of patients undergoing esophagomyotomy. Arch. Surg. *81*:411, 1960.

Postlethwait, R. W., and Sealy, W. C.: Surgery of the Esophagus. Springfield, Illinois, Charles C Thomas, 1961.

Sengstaken, R. W., and Blakemore, A. H.: Balloon tamponage for the control of hemorrhage from esophageal varices. Ann. Surg. *131*:781, 1950.

Steichen, F. M., Heller, E., and Ravitch, M. M.: Achalasia of the esophagus. Surgery 47:846, 1960.

Stemmer, E. A., and Adams, W. E.: The incidence of carcinoma at the esophagogastric junction in short esophagus. Arch. Surg. *81*:771, 1960.

Sutherland, H. D.: Cricopharyngeal achalasia. J. Thoracic & Cardiovasc. Surg. 43:114, 1962.

Swigart, L. L., Siekert, R. G., Hambley, W. C., and Anson, B. J.: The esophageal arteries: an anatomic study of 150 specimens. Surg. Gyn. & Obst. *90*:234, 1950.

Thal, A. P., and Hatafuku, T.: Improved operation for esophageal rupture. J.A.M.A. *188*:826, 1964.

Torek, F.: The first successful resection of the thoracic portion of the esophagus for carcinoma: preliminary report. J.A.M.A. *60*:1533, 1913.

Wangensteen, O. H., Sanchez, H., and Sako, Y.: Sensitivity of the esophagus to the acid-pepsin action. Am. J. Physiol. *155*:476, 1948.

Wheeler, W. I.: Pharyngocele and dilatation of pharynx, with existing diverticulum at lower portion of pharynx lying posterior to the oesophagus, cured by pharyngotomy, being the first case of the kind recorded. Dublin J. M. Sci. 82:349, 1886.

Wookey, H.: The surgical treatment of carcinoma of the hypopharynx and the oesophagus. Brit. J. Surg. 35:249, 1948.

Wynder, E. L., and Bross, I. J.: A study of etiological factors in cancer of the esophagus. Cancer *14*:389, 1961.

Yudin, S. S.: The surgical construction of 80 cases of artificial esophagus. Surg. Gyn. & Obst. *78*:561, 1944.

Zenker, F. A., and von Ziemssen, H.: Diseases of the oesophagus. *In*, von Ziemssen, H.: Cyclopaedia of the Practice of Medicine. Vol. 8. New York, Wm. Wood & Co., 1878, pp. 1-214.

The Stomach

by
JOEL W. BAKER, M.D.
and
R. CAMERON HARRISON, M.D.

JOEL W. BAKER is a Virginian who received his education at The University, as he and his fellow statesmen would say. He received his later surgical education and training in Washington, where he is now Chairman of the Department of Surgery at the Virginia Mason Hospital and The Mason Clinic in Seattle. He is an outstanding exponent of the teaching principle that surgery is the art of applying knowledge in the basic sciences to the patient.

ROBERT CAMERON HARRISON is a Canadian by birth. He received his Doctor of Medicine degree from the University of Alberta and, after serving in World War II, pursued graduate training in the Banting Institute, Hospital for Sick Children, and the Toronto General Hospital. He is Professor and Head of Surgery at the University of British Columbia. His interests in surgical research continue to be in gastrointestinal disease, especially the physiology of the upper gastrointestinal tract. His clinical interests are centered in the area of gastroenterology and malignancy, particularly as it concerns the breast.

Indigestion is among the commonest of complaints; diseases of the stomach and duodenum account for a high percentage of all illness. As well as producing symptoms in literally millions of people, this portion of the gastrointestinal tract contributes more than its share to mortality figures. There are approximately 40,000 deaths annually in the United States and Canada from peptic ulceration and carcinoma of the stomach.

ANATOMY

The stomach is a J-shaped mucosa-lined, smooth-muscled organ whose size and shape varies remarkably from person to person and from hour to hour in each individual. It begins with a functional, or cardiac, sphincter at the gastroesophageal junction and ends in an anatomic, or pyloric, sphincter at the junction of the pyloric antrum and duodenum

(Fig. 40). The proximal portion of the stomach is divided into the body, or corpus, and the fundus, which is that portion superior to the gastroesophageal junction. The region immediately distal to the cardiac sphincter is often referred to as the cardiac portion of the stomach. The distal one-quarter is the antrum or pyloric antrum. The medial boundaries of the stomach and duodenum are the lesser curvatures, and the lateral boundaries the greater curvatures. In both instances, the major blood supply is to the lesser curvature. The arterial blood supply of the stomach is of significance in operations; the venous supply is important in the interpretation of alternate venous pathways in portal hypertension, the lymphatic supply in the surgery of malignancy, and the innervation in the treatment of acid-linked diseases.

The arteries of the stomach all take their origin from the celiac axis; the blood supply to the duodenum is supplemented by branches from the superior mesenteric artery. In common with the small bowel, and in contrast to the esophagus and colon, the blood supply to the stomach and duodenum is plentiful. This facilitates healing, but when bleeding occurs it can be life-threatening.

The venous return from the stomach and duodenum is through the portal vein to the liver. In the esophageal area are important anastomoses between the systemic esophageal and azygos veins and the portal gastric veins. In portal hypertension, these become ectatic and may rupture as the result of acid-peptic digestion or trauma.

The parasympathetic innervation of the stomach is by means of gastric branches from the left and right vagal trunks. Because of fetal gastric rotation, these come to occupy an anterior and posterior gastric position near the lesser curvature. The vagal trunks at the gastroesophageal level are often multiple, and the posterior trunk may lie behind the esophagus in the mediastinal tissues. For this reason, it is easily missed by the surgeon not

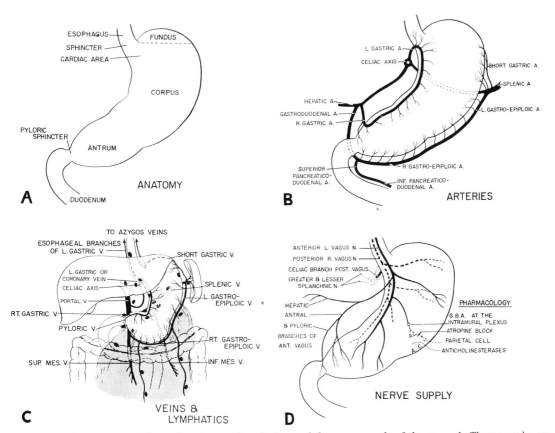

Figure 40. Anatomy, arterial supply, veins and lymphatics, and the nerve supply of the stomach. There may be considerable variation in the venous return, particularly with respect to the left gastric (coronary) vein. This may empty into the splenic rather than the portal vein and may be obstructed in cases of splenic vein thrombosis. The lymphatics are frequently referred to as the inferior gastric, the pyloric, the superior gastric and the pancreaticolienal groups. (G.B.A. = ganglionic blocking agents.)

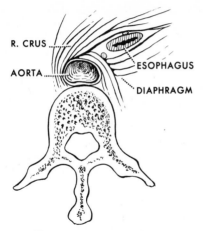

Figure 41. The posterior vagus in this anatomical cross section is not applied closely to the esophagus but is posteromedial. It is easily missed when the esophagus is mobilized, leading to incomplete vagotomy.

completely familiar with the operation of vagotomy (Fig. 41). The posterior vagus sends a large branch to the celiac plexus, a small branch to the liver and several to the stomach. The anterior nerve sends branches to the liver, gallbladder, pancreas and first portion of the duodenum, in addition to its gastric branches. The gastric branches synapse with nerve cells in the submucosal and myenteric plexuses within the stomach wall. Some fibers from the greater and lesser splanchnic nerves synapse with cells in the celiac ganglion, whereas the vagal fibers do not synapse at this level. The sympathetic postganglionic fibers and the vagal, or parasympathetic preganglionic, fibers accompany the blood vessels to the abdominal viscera. In this manner, the celiac portion of the right vagus nerve supplies the duodenum, pancreas, small bowel and possibly the ascending colon. In general, sympathetic stimuli decrease peristalsis and inhibit secretion, while parasympathetic stimuli have the opposite effect. Afferent nerves accompany the parasympathetic and sympathetic fibers to the higher centers. Receptors in the gastric mucosa which are sensitive to temperature, pressure, pH and isotonicity initiate local motor and secretory responses.

HISTOLOGY

The stomach and the first portion of the duodenum are intraperitoneal, whereas the remainder of the duodenum is retroperitoneal. Deep to the serosa are the longitudinal, cir-

cular and oblique sheets of muscle, between which lies the myenteric plexus. Continuing toward the lumen of the stomach is the connective tissue submucosa, in which is situated the submucosal autonomic plexus. The muscularis mucosa, lamina propria and mucosa together constitute the most superficial layer. The stratified squamous epithelium of the esophagus changes at the cardia to a simple columnar epithelium which is mucus-producing. The lamina propria, which is generally occupied by areolar and lymphatic tissue, is almost completely occupied in the stomach by specialized tubular glands which secrete a complex product.

Three types of cells have been identified: the zymogen or chief cells which produce pepsinogen, the parietal or oxyntic cells which produce hydrochloric acid and the goblet cells which produce mucus. The last are specialized mucus-producing cells whose product stains differently from that produced by the columnar epithelium of the gastric mucosa. Pepsinogen is secreted into the lumen of the gland, is converted to pepsin by hydrochloric acid and flows out into the lumen of the stomach as an extremely potent protein digestant. It is difficult to avoid the conclusion that the mucus layer is vitally important in the prevention of epithelial damage. In the antral area, and also in the cardiac portion, the highly specialized acid and pepsin-producing tubular glands are replaced by short

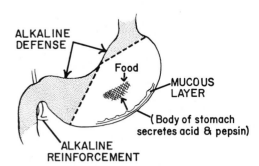

LOCAL DEFENSE MECHANISM
1. Alkaline secretion neutralizes acid
2. Mucous layer protects surface
3. Food buffers the acid

Figure 42. The body and fundus of the stomach are lined by parietal and chief cells secreting hydrochloric acid and pepsin. A narrow rim of cardiac glands above and a three-inch sleeve of antralpyloric glands below this acid-secreting area secrete a highly alkaline neutralizing and mucinous fluid, presumably as a protection to the vulnerable esophagus on the one hand and to the intestine on the other. This alkaline protection is reinforced in the second portion of the duodenum by the alkaline biliary and pancreatic secretions.

tubular glands which secrete an alkaline protective mucus. In the antrum, there must also be specialized cells which produce one or more humoral substances, but these have not yet been identified.

In the duodenum, there are similar glands, which in this location lie deep to the muscularis mucosa rather than in the lamina propria. These submucosal glands (Brunner's), which also secrete an alkaline secretion rich in mucus, are found in large numbers as far as the entrance of the pancreatic and biliary ducts, beyond which they decrease rapidly (Fig. 42).

PHYSIOLOGY

Gastric physiology was born in the 1820's when Prout identified the acid in gastric juice as hydrochloric acid, and an American army surgeon named Beaumont studied the interior of a human stomach. In 1822, Beaumont was stationed on the island of Mackinac when a young French Canadian voyageur, Alexis St. Martin, was brought in with an abdominal shotgun wound. He nursed him back to health but was unable to close the large gastric fistula, which remained open until the voyageur's death some 60 years later. This was not the first patient with a permanent gastric fistula, but until Beaumont no one had perceived that much could be learned from such a preparation. He carried out a series of simple but basic experiments over a period of years and published his findings in 1833. He confirmed that gastric juice contained hydrochloric acid, but demonstrated that it had additional properties which enabled it to digest protein. He determined the gastric emptying time, learned much about the function of the pylorus, demonstrated that finely ground food was digested more rapidly than larger particles and recognized that gastric secretion was increased when food was placed in the stomach. He also observed the effect of emotion on the production of gastric juice. His patient was not always willing, and when St. Martin was in a foul mood his gastric juice was scanty.

In patients, the gastric content can be recovered by a peroral gastric tube or through a surgical gastrostomy. Secretion may be stimulated by hypoglycemia, food or alcohol, histamine and parasympathomimetic drugs.

The mechanism of action of anticholinergic drugs is illustrated in Figure 40. The anticholinesterases prevent the normal breakdown of acetylcholine at both ganglia. The ganglionic blocking agents act at the intramural plexuses, and the atropine-like drugs prevent the action of acetylcholine on the parietal cells, as well as blocking all of the parasympathomimetic agents.

The concentration of acid is measured by an intragastric pH electrode, or by pH or titration methods following its aspiration. Knowing volume and concentration it can be expressed quantitatively. Pepsin is measured as pepsinogen in the blood, uropepsin in the urine or pepsin in the gastric juice.

Animal experiments have contributed essential information in this area. It has become increasingly apparent that the correlation between the results in animals and humans is substantial. Procedures which result in an experimental ulcer will, if applied to man, result in peptic ulceration, and the reverse is also true. Factors which stimulate or suppress acid secretion in the experimental animal have a similar effect in the human.

Prior to the introduction of gastric pouches, animal experiments on gastric secretion had to be limited to the fasting state to avoid admixture with food. In 1878, Heidenhain devised his "little stomach," which was sensitive to all blood-borne stimuli, and made possible for the first time the recovery of pure gastric juice from the nonfasting animal (Fig. 43). His pupil Pavlov preserved some vagal innervation by dividing only the mucosa, and also fashioned a pharyngotomy which permitted sham feeding. This was an extremely useful preparation for studying the effect of the central nervous system on gastric secretion. Pouches with a richer vagal innervation have been prepared since Pavlov by other investigators such as Hollander. Total gastric pouches can also be prepared, either vagally denervated or vagally innervated. The antrum can be separated from the corpus and the duodenum, or both, with or without its vagal supply, and also transplanted to other sites. Similarly, the duodenum and small bowel can be studied as isolated preparations. In both animals and humans, gastric secretion can be collected over a short or a long period, depending on the nature of the subject under investigation. In all research, however, it is difficult to study a physiologic process without grossly altering the normal mechanisms.

As well as measuring acid output quantitatively and qualitatively, many methods have been designed to facilitate the development

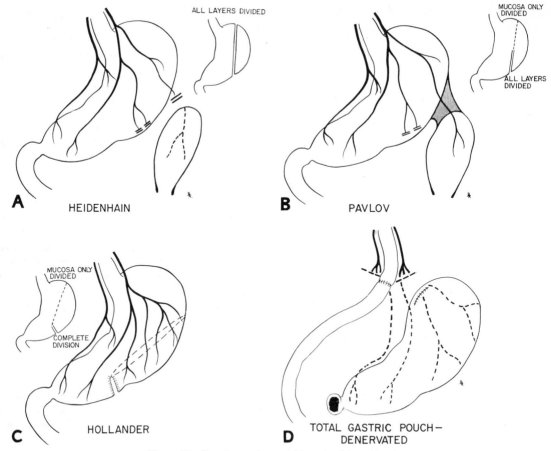

Figure 43. Gastric pouches used in animal investigation.

of an experimental peptic ulcer which can then be used as a control to evaluate known or suspected ulcerogenic factors. The earliest was the Exalto-Mann-Williamson procedure,

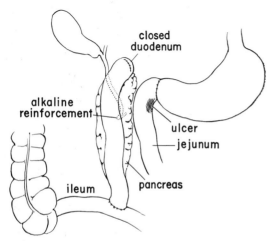

Figure 44. Experimentally produced ulcer resulting from deflection of alkaline defense (Mann-Williamson, dog, 1923).

in which the biliary and pancreatic secretions were diverted to the lower small bowel (Fig. 44). A simpler method is the interposition of a short length of ileum between the first and second portions of the duodenum. This moves the duodenal, pancreatic and biliary secretions spatially down the gastrointestinal tract so that their normal neutralizing and buffering effects are no longer available to protect the ileum (Fig. 45). Unfortunately, most methods of experimental ulcer production increase gastric secretion and many have a specific effect on either the secreting cells, the vagal mechanism or the antral mechanism. Drugs, such as histamine, are frequently employed but they, also, disproportionately affect one of the stimulating or suppressing mechanisms.

The stomach always contains a small quantity of swallowed air, which in the erect position collects in the fundus and may help to prevent reflux into the esophagus. Otherwise, the lumen is only a potential space and the gastric walls are normally closely applied

$$H_2O + CO_2 + NaCl \xrightarrow[\text{Anhydrase}]{\text{Carbonic}} HCl + NaHCO_3.$$

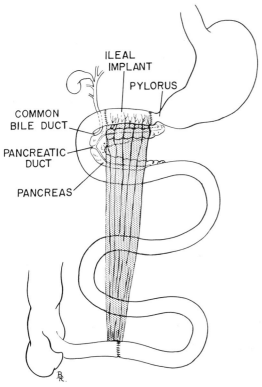

It should be appreciated that the stomach not only secretes hydrochloric acid, pepsin and mucus, but also water and salts such as NaCl and KCl. It is thought that the hydrochloric acid elaborated by the parietal cells is of the same acidity in everyone, but the quantity produced and the extent to which it is diluted by other secretions varies widely. As produced by the parietal cells, it contains 100 mEq. of hydrogen per liter, is 0.16N, 0.5 per cent, and has a pH of 1.0. The number of clinical units are the number of milliliters of 0.1N NaOH required to neutralize 100 ml. of gastric juice, using Topfer's indicator. The concentration of hydrochloric acid may be expressed as pH, mEq. per liter (clinical units), or in terms of its normality (Fig. 46). Quantitatively, the amount of acid is best expressed as mEq., which is obtained by multiplying the concentration in milliequivalents per liter times the volume in liters.

The precursor of pepsinogen is stored as zymogen granules in the chief cells. On stimulation, pepsinogen is secreted and converted to pepsin in the lumen of the tubular glands. Pepsin is an extremely powerful proteolytic enzyme whose optimal

Figure 45. A short length of ileum with its mesentery is interposed after dividing the first portion of the duodenum. Large peptic ulcers develop in the interposed ileum in 80 per cent of the dogs.

to the gastric contents to speed digestion. The stomach is able to adapt to extremely wide variations in content, without any significant change in pressure, in contrast to most smooth-muscled, hollow viscera.

The process of protein digestion begins in earnest through the elaboration of pepsin brought to an optimal pH by the secretion of hydrochloric acid. In addition to being stored, the food is thoroughly mixed and brought to the correct degree of acidity, particle size and isotonicity before being carried by the antropyloric pump to the duodenum. Absorption is limited to water, alcohol and small amounts of carbohydrate. An average meal is evacuated in three to four hours, but this varies widely depending on the bulk of the meal as well as the nature of its contents. Fluid moves along quickly, while fat delays gastric emptying.

Hydrochloric acid is formed in the canaliculi of the parietal cells by a process which is not yet clear. Using water, carbon dioxide and sodium chloride from the blood, the H ion concentration is increased many-fold by these amazing cells:

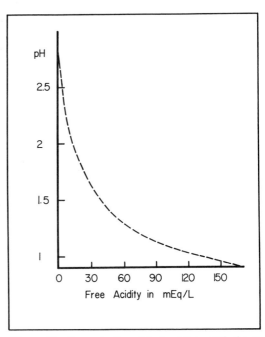

Figure 46. Concentration of hydrochloric acid: the relationship between mEq./L. and pH. (James, A. H., and Pickering, G. W.: The role of gastric acidity in the pathogenesis of peptic ulcer. Clin. Sci., 1949.)

pH for the proteins ingested by man is about 2.0.

It is difficult to study the various mucus substances produced by the cardia, corpus, antrum and duodenum. Deficiencies in mucus production may well be responsible for the development of some types of peptic ulcer, but they are difficult to study qualitatively and quantitatively without markedly altering gastric physiology. The body of the stomach also secretes a factor which combines with vitamin B_{12} to produce a substance essential for hematopiesis.

STIMULATION OF ACID SECRETION

A small amount of gastric acid is produced continuously. This interdigestive phase may be greatly increased in duodenal ulcer.

CEPHALIC, NERVOUS OR VAGAL PHASE. Pavlov fashioned his vagally innervated gastric pouches in a series of dogs and also performed pharyngotomies on them, with the result that their ingested food failed to reach the stomach. In these sham-fed animals, he demonstrated that gastric secretion was stimulated although no food reached the stomach. This also occurred if the animals

thought they were going to be fed, or if they saw or smelled food. In 1910, he demonstrated that division of the vagi abolished this response. Dragstedt and Ellis showed 20 years later that division of the vagi profoundly reduced the subsequent production of gastric acid from a total gastric pouch. This and other experiments by Dragstedt led him to develop the operation of vagotomy for duodenal ulcer in 1943.

Hypoglycemia also stimulates acid secretion by the vagal route, which is now known to be via the anterior hypothalamus to the vagal nuclei (Fig. 47). In 1953, Porter, Movius and French demonstrated that the vagal mechanism could be evoked by electrical stimulation of the anterior hypothalamus, and that this response was abolished by vagotomy.

The gastric branches of the anterior and posterior vagi terminate in the submucosal and myenteric plexuses of the corpus and antrum. Vagal stimulation results in an outpouring of acid by the parietal cells and pepsin by the chief cells in the body of the stomach. For many years, this was thought to be the only aspect of the cephalic phase, until Uvnas found in 1942 that vagal stimulation also stimulated the antrum to produce

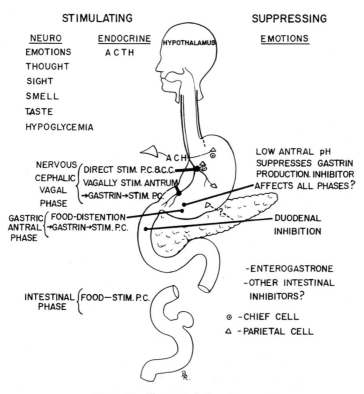

Figure 47. The control of gastric secretion.

gastrin. Direct stimulation of the parietal and chief cells is now called "the direct vagal phase," and the antral aspect of the vagal phase "the vagal-antral phase." Uvnas' findings were doubted for a considerable period but have now been confirmed by other workers. Both aspects of this phase are abolished by vagotomy and are affected by cholinergic drugs.

GASTRIC OR ANTRAL PHASE. After early investigators found that food placed in the stomach excited gastric secretion, this mechanism was intensively studied. The gastric phase was shown to be independent of the cephalic phase, because stimulation of secretion resulted even if the patient or the experimental animal was unaware that food had been introduced directly into the stomach. In 1906, Edkins concluded that the site of stimulation was the gastric antrum, and that it produced a hormone which he called gastrin. He postulated that gastrin was produced by the antrum, and was carried by the blood stream via the portal and systemic circulation to the parietal cells. In succeeding years, it has been demonstrated that the antrum is stimulated to produce gastrin, not only on contact with food, but also if it is distended, and following vagal stimulation. Gastrin-rich extracts have been prepared by numerous investigators. A number of physiologically potent polypeptides structurally related to gastrin have been synthesized and tested clinically.

INTESTINAL PHASE. The double pronged cephalic or vagal phase, and the gastric or antral phase are undoubtedly the major mechanisms of stimulation of gastric secretion. The presence of food, other than fat, in the intestine, or distention of the small bowel, also stimulates the production of acid through a blood-borne mechanism. It was once thought that the blood-borne stimulants were the end products of digestion, but it has been shown by Sircus that a hormone is produced in the intestine, possibly gastrin.

It will be noted that the vagal phase is neuroendocrine, and the other two phases entirely endocrine. There is considerable evidence that these phases potentiate one another in the stimulation of acid secretion. As well as the cholinergic drugs, histamine, alcohol, caffeine and the adrenal steroids stimulate acid secretion.

SUPPRESSION OF ACID SECRETION

CEPHALIC SUPPRESSION. It was noted particularly by Wolf and Wolff that emotional states often result in a suppression of acid secretion. Stimulation of the sympathetic nervous system has a weak but recognizable inhibiting effect.

GASTRIC SUPPRESSION. In 1904, Sokolov in Pavlov's laboratory noted that the introduction of acid into the duodenum suppressed endogenous acid production by the fundus, and in 1955 Day and Webster confirmed this observation.

In 1895, von Eiselsberg developed an operation for duodenal ulcer which was designed to circumvent the danger of transecting the duodenum in the presence of an acute ulcer (Fig. 48). He transected the stomach proximal to the pylorus, closed the distal segment, resected a portion of the stomach and re-established gastrointestinal continuity with an anastomosis between the jejunum and the remainder of the stomach. While this operation was initially safer for the patient, it led to a distressingly high incidence of ulcers at the new stoma; in fact, it proved to be the most ulcerogenic operation ever devised. The resulting ulcer usually healed if the portion of the antrum left behind in contact with the

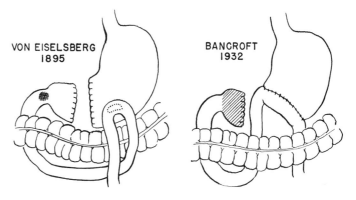

Figure 48. The operative procedure developed by von Eiselsberg: antral exclusion. In 1932, Bancroft modified this by coring out the antral mucosa, reducing its ulcerogenic effect.

VON EISELSBERG 1895

BANCROFT 1932

alkaline duodenal secretion was subsequently excised.

This and other observations persuaded Dragstedt and his associates to study the effect of antral pH on the antrum. They made the fundamental observation in 1950 that stimulation of the parietal cells by the antral mechanism was markedly influenced by the pH of the antral mucosa. If the antral contents were markedly acidic, the introduction of food into the antrum, or its distention, did not result in gastric secretion. Conversely, if the antral pH was raised, the production of acid in response to antral stimulation was greatly augmented. It has subsequently been demonstrated that non-antral mechanisms, direct vagal and intestinal, are also reduced by acidification of the antrum.

The precise mechanism whereby antral pH modifies gastric secretion has been a source of lively controversy. In 1956, experimental evidence was reported that the antrum produces an inhibitor substance which affects all phases of secretion, whereas other investigators have concluded that the antral pH effect is entirely due to a modification of gastrin production. Whatever the mechanism, it is apparent that it is a most important autoregulatory device to prevent an excessive secretion of acid by the parietal cells.

DUODENAL SUPPRESSION. In 1955, Brackney, Thal and Wangensteen showed that a pH-dependent autoregulatory mechanism might also exist in the duodenum.

INTESTINAL SUPPRESSION. Subsequent to the emulsification of ingested fat in the intestine, a humoral agent is produced which is carried by the blood stream to the stomach, where it has an inhibitory effect on gastric acid production. It was termed "enterogastrone" by Ivy. There is considerable evidence that other important inhibitory mechanisms as yet undefined may exist in the pancreas, biliary tree and small intestine.

PEPSIN

Pepsinogen is produced in the chief cells by the breakdown of zymogen granules, small amounts being produced continuously. Some pepsinogen finds its way to the gastric veins and may be measured there, or in the peripheral blood, as blood pepsinogen and in the urine as uropepsin. These levels may not reflect gastric pepsin secretion accurately, but because of their technical facility they have been widely utilized. The prime stimulus for pepsin production is direct vagal stimulation.

The antral and intestinal phases have little effect, but parasympathetic stimulation by cholinergic drugs results in a secretion which is rich in pepsin. Since only a small amount of pepsin is needed to digest ingested protein, an excess is probably not as significant as is an excess of acid which brings the pH down to the optimal range for pepsin activity. This varies with the protein being digested, but appears to be about 2.0 for the type of protein man ingests.

MUCUS

Mucus is produced by the columnar cells lining the body of the stomach, by the goblet cells in the tubular glands of the gastric corpus, and by the mucus-producing glands in the pyloric antrum and duodenum. Although mucus production is stimulated to a slight extent by the vagal mechanism, the most effective stimulant appears to be irritation of the mucous membrane itself. Undoubtedly, mucus production is of prime importance both quantitatively and qualitatively, but its study has proved to be extremely difficult. Adrenal steroids not only interfere with the repair of tissue, but also appear to reduce the viscosity and protective effect of mucus. When steroids are exhibited, the volume of mucus secreted is reduced, and its sialic acid content sharply reduced.

PITUITARY-ADRENAL FACTORS

Porter, Movius and French found that stimulation of the anterior hypothalamus led to an increase in gastric secretion by the vagal route with a prompt increase in acid production. They also found that stimulation of the posterior hypothalamus resulted in a delayed response in acid secretion, which was unaffected by vagotomy but prevented by previous adrenalectomy. The administration of adrenocorticotropic hormone or cortisone in very large doses results in an increase in acid secretion and a rise in uropepsin. These studies suggest that the pituitary-adrenal mechanism may be significant in the control of gastric secretion, but whether this is a major or minor mechanism is debatable.

THE PANCREAS

It has been noted that hypoglycemia results in the stimulation of acid by the vagal mechanism. Insulin-secreting adenomas of the pancreas result in hypoglycemia, but strangely enough are rarely associated with duodenal ulcer. Even stranger is the observation of a high peptic ulcer rate following excision of insulinomas. As first noted by Zollinger and Ellison, non-insulin-secreting tumors of the pancreas can and do result in duodenal and jejunal ulcers which remain intractable until the tumors are completely removed, or until all of the acid-secreting mucosa has been surgically excised. It should be noted that they may be associated with coexisting adenomas in the pituitary, parathyroids or adrenals, and there is a familial history in some of these polyglandular patients. This suggests the importance of the "endocrine orchestra," but these tumors are relatively rare in patients with duodenal ulcer.

As well as the endocrine effects of the pancreas, the alkaline exocrine secretions clearly play a major role in the neutralization of acid chyme in the duodenum. However, ligation of the pancreatic ducts results not only in a loss of this neutralizing secretion, but also results in an increase in the production of acid by the stomach through mechanisms which are as yet undefined.

Suppressing mechanisms for pepsin and mucus have not been investigated. Gastric acid secretion is the end result of an interplay between stimulating and suppressing mechanisms, most of the latter being pH-dependent. Probably the vagal and antral mechanisms are equal importance and together constitute the major stimulating pathways. Vagal stimulation of the antrum appears to be more significant than direct stimulation of the parietal cells and the vagal-antral mechanism appears to be roughly equal to the local antral phase. With respect to the antrum, stimulating mechanisms appear to be more powerful than inhibitory mechanisms. The autoregulation of gastric secretion is obviously an extremely important but as yet imperfectly understood physiologic process.

GASTRIC TRAUMA

Blunt or penetrating trauma to the upper abdomen may result in perforation or laceration of the stomach. The single most important aspect of duodenal injury is the mistake of overlooking it. The majority of duodenal injuries result from penetrating trauma, but because of the fixed position of the duodenum it may be torn or actually divided in its retroperitoneal portion by compression and steering-wheel, blunt-type injuries. To overlook such injury, or to delay in its repair, can be fatal. Discovery requires early laparotomy, on suspicion, with mobilization of the duodenum by the Kocher method, when extravasation or hemorrhage is found in this area. As pointed out by Rosemond, the routine uncovering of a nonexpansile retroperitoneal hematoma can lead to problems of hemostasis. However, free bile staining or emphysema indicates a leak. In his experience with 15 duodenal injuries, Rosemond was able to close primarily all without complication. A small percentage may require a bypass procedure such as gastrojejunostomy. When a larger defect is found than can be safely closed, Kobald and Thal recommend that a loop of jejunum be brought up and sutured over the defect. Coincident injury to the pancreas must be searched for, and suction drainage instituted in the retroperitoneal area.

ACUTE DILATATION

Although the stomach is able to adapt easily to an increase in content without a significant increase in intragastric pressure, this useful adaptive mechanism sometimes exceeds its physiologic limits. Following trauma, operation, or the administration of an inhalation anesthetic with a face mask, the stomach may become enormously distended with fluid and air. The experienced surgeon searches for overdistention of the stomach resulting from the administration of a closed-system anesthetic before closing the abdomen. It is characterized by evidence of shock, by repeated regurgitation or vomiting of small quantities of fluid in the absence of significant pain, and by hiccoughs.

Treatment is simple, but unless the condition is suspected and treated promptly, it may end fatally. The passage of an indwelling tube will substantiate the diagnosis, as large quantities of material are inevitably found and the patient's condition improves remarkably as the stomach is decompressed. Suction is maintained until the stomach has regained its tone, as evidenced by satisfactory gastric emptying when the tube is clamped for increasing periods.

VOLVULUS

Volvulus is usually secondary to other lesions in the immediate vicinity of the stomach, particularly diaphragmatic hernia, but it may be idiopathic. Rotation can occur in three planes. The commonest is a rotation along the axis of the lesser curvature, so that the greater curvature comes to occupy a superior position. If there is marked ptosis of the stomach, the axis of rotation may be through a line passing from the lesser to greater curvatures in a perpendicular direction, the distal portion of the stomach rotating toward the esophageal opening. The third type may occur through the same axis in the absence of ptosis.

It is most frequently seen as an asymptomatic chronic form in elderly patients, in which case treatment is not necessary. It may also present as an acute volvulus characterized by repeated unproductive retching, epigastric pain and sometimes hematemesis. Attempts to pass an indwelling gastric tube may be unsuccessful due to the acute angle at the esophagocardiac junction. If not relieved by aspiration, these patients require early operation because there is danger of strangulation, hemorrhage or perforation.

FOREIGN BODIES

Foreign bodies are frequently swallowed accidentally by children, and occasionally are deliberately swallowed by irresponsible adults. Most articles which will traverse the esophagus will also pass the pyloric and ileocecal valves, and only need to be observed lest they fail to do so. If sharp objects fail to move along on daily fluoroscopic examination, or if signs of peritoneal irritation develop, laparotomy is necessary.

Certain organic material, if repeatedly swallowed, tends to form a round concretion which may then be unable to pass the pylorus. These are termed bezoars, and are usually identified by the radiologist during his investigation of the patient's indigestion.

PROLAPSE OF GASTRIC MUCOUS MEMBRANE

During radiologic examination of the pyloric area, the temporary prolapse of antral mucous membrane through the pylorus is frequently observed. If it is massive and does not return to its normal position with the next peristaltic wave, it can be seriously considered as a cause of obstructive symptoms, but such a sequence of events is rare. A pedunculated gastric polyp in the pyloric area may produce similar symptoms. In the vast majority of patients, the explanation for the symptoms will be found elsewhere. If surgical treatment is employed, resection of the antrum should be done, rather than merely excision of the redundant mucous membrane.

GASTRITIS

ACUTE GASTRITIS. An acute inflammatory reaction can be seen following the ingestion of large quantities of undiluted alcohol, drugs such as salicylates which are irritating to the mucous membrane, and highly spiced foods. Gastritis can also be associated with several infectious diseases such as diphtheria, and can occur as a suppurative, or phlegmonous, gastritis due to streptococci, gas-forming organisms or other bacteria.

Suppurative gastritis is extremely rare. It presents as an acute abdomen with high fever, and should be treated primarily with antibiotics. Corrosive gastritis follows the ingestion of caustic solutions such as lye or strong acid. It is not surprising that caustics do most of their damage in the esophagus, whereas strong acids are more likely to be damaging to the stomach. The emergency treatment consists of copious lavage, and if a stomach tube is not available, the administration of substances which induce vomiting.

CHRONIC GRANULOMATOUS GASTRITIS. Granulomatous gastritis may be associated with Crohn's disease, tuberculosis, syphilis, sarcoidosis, eosinophilic granuloma and nonspecific granulomas. Tuberculosis may produce multiple shallow ulcers in patients with evidence of tuberculosis elsewhere; the treatment is entirely medical. A gastric deformity in a patient with signs of tertiary syphilis raises the question of a gastric gumma in the differential diagnosis. It is tempting to observe these lesions under antiluetic therapy, but the great majority of them prove to be carcinoma and such a plan of treatment results in an undesirable delay.

CHRONIC GASTRITIS. The terms superficial, hypertrophic and atrophic have been coined by gastroscopists to describe what they see through their instruments. The pathologist sees numerous round cells in the lamina propria, which led to the descriptive term "gastritis." The literature on this subject is confusing with respect to classification, clinical significance and correlation, and malignant potential. Palmer believes that these changes are degenerative rather than inflammatory. Superficial gastritis is what the gastroscopist refers to as an edematous, hyperemic mucous membrane which bleeds easily and in which erosions are frequently seen. The microscopic appearance, on the other hand, is frequently normal.

When the gastroscopist visualizes a heaped-up, pebbly mucosa he describes it as hypertrophic gastritis. As this aspect disappears following resection, it is probably due to an increased tone of the underlying muscularis mucosa. Since there are no significant microscopic changes, the term should probably be abandoned.

Atrophic gastritis is seen by the gastroscopist as a thin, translucent mucous membrane which on microscopic examination frequently looks normal or may show hypoplasia of the tubular glands, areas of metaplasia to an intestinal type of epithelium, and replacement of the lamina propria by round cells. Conversely, the mucous membrane may look normal to the gastroscopist and may show the typical microscopic appearances of atrophic gastritis. Gastric atrophy is one area in which there is good correlation; it is uniformly associated with pernicious anemia.

In general, it can be said that superficial gastritis tends to progress to atrophic gastritis; that atrophic gastritis becomes increasingly common with advancing age, and that with it there is a progressive fall in acid production. Some have concluded that the development of superficial and atrophic gastritis is simply an aging process, like wrinkles and gray hair. Others, pointing to a higher incidence of atrophic gastritis in both gastric ulcer and carcinoma, feel strongly that both gastric ulcer and carcinoma are causally related to these changes in the gastric epithelium. Flexible gastroscopes with photographic and direct biopsy attachments have recently been developed which will help to answer the problem of whether gastritis is the cause of symptoms and whether it sets the stage for gastric ulcer and cancer of the stomach.

PEPTIC ULCER

A peptic ulcer is a defect in the epithelium of the gastrointestinal tract which results from the combined action of hydrochloric acid and pepsin. By definition, it penetrates to at least the submucosa; more superficial lesions are erosions. They may occur in the stomach, duodenum or esophagus, in a Meckel's diverticulum, at the site of a surgically created anastomosis and, rarely, in the upper jejunum (Fig. 49). Grossly, the margins of the defect are smooth, the base may be clean or covered by a gray exudate, and both margins and base are firm due to the presence of associated scar tissue. If it penetrates deeply, it can be recognized on the serosal surface by the presence of punctate hemorrhages, by a stellate scar, or by inflammatory adhesions between the involved organ and neighboring viscera.

Marginal, anastomotic, stomal, jejunal and surgical ulcer are synonymous terms. They refer to ulceration developing at the site of a surgically created gastric outlet, usually jejunal. The condition occurs almost exclusively subsequent to operations for duodenal ulcer, being rare after procedures for gastric ulcer.

Ectopic gastric mucosa is frequently found in a Meckel's diverticulum, and when this occurs peptic ulceration frequently develops in the neighboring mucosa. The usual complication is hemorrhage, with perforation less common. It usually presents in childhood as rectal bleeding and is easily solved by excision of the diverticulum.

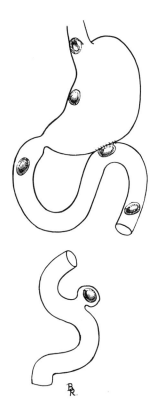

Figure 49. Common sites of peptic ulceration.

GASTRIC AND DUODENAL ULCER

While gastric and duodenal ulcer have much in common, they do have important distinguishing features.

EPIDEMIOLOGY.   Acid peptic digestion of a portion of the gastrointestinal tract is one of the commonest of diseases, affecting 10 per cent or more of the male population during their lifetime. This is more than double the incidence for women, probably because men secrete 50 per cent more acid and pepsin than women after puberty. It has been stated that, of those presenting with the symptoms of indigestion, 20 per cent will be found to have an ulcer. There is some familial tendency, with peptic ulcer commoner in those of blood group O, whereas carcinoma of the stomach is commoner in those of group A. Pregnancy tends to alleviate and lactation to exacerbate ulcer symptoms, again reflecting changes in acid and pepsin secretion during these intervals.

There are about 10,000 deaths annually in the United States and Canada from peptic ulcer, 6500 from gastric ulcer and 3500 from duodenal ulcer. It is said that 30,000 people die of carcinoma of the stomach annually, but it is probable that there is considerable error in the mortality statistics in the gastric ulcer and carcinoma cases. Although the incidence of duodenal ulcer is several times higher, there are more deaths from gastric ulcer. Wangensteen states that half the deaths from peptic ulcer are due to hemorrhage.

The ratio between gastric and duodenal ulcer varies, depending on geography, age, sex, method of diagnosis and material being studied. The ratio is different in the outpatient department, in the hospital, in the operating room and in the morgue. While the incidence of gastric ulcer may exceed duodenal ulcer at postmortem, many of these gastric ulcers are probably terminal in their development. Duodenal ulcer is commoner than gastric ulcer in both sexes, and duodenal ulcer is commoner in males than females.

In women, the ratio of duodenal to gastric ulcer approaches 1 : 1, with duodenal ulcer commoner than gastric ulcer in premenopausal women and the reverse being true in the postmenopausal. In both sexes, the relative incidence of gastric ulcer increases steadily with age. The incidence of gastric ulcer is higher in those of impoverished means, and there is a very slightly increased incidence in duodenal ulcer among the higher income groups.

PATHOGENESIS.   Knowing the properties of gastric juice, it is surprising that peptic ulcer only affects 10 per cent of the population. John Hunter thought that living tissues were immune to digestion by the stomach, but it is now known that even the presence of the vital processes does not protect them against digestion. Any tissue in contact with acid and pepsin may develop a peptic ulcer, but in the absence of acid and pepsin ulcer does not develop. The old dictum "no acid, no ulcer" has stood the test of time.

The literature prior to ten years ago contains several reports of gastric ulcer in patients with achlorhydria. At that time, only a mild gastric stimulant such as a gruel meal or a small dose of histamine was employed, and this occasionally failed to stimulate a measurable amount of free acid. When the antihistamines were introduced, it was disappointing to find that they did not prevent the marked stimulation of gastric acid, for it was thought then that endogenous histamine was an important mechanism in the increased production of acid seen in duodenal ulcer. The fact that the antihistamines prevented the severe side effects of a large dose of histamine, but did not prevent the secretion of acid, was utilized by Conard, Kowalewski and van Geertruyden, and independently by Kay, to investigate further patients found achlorhydric by the previously employed small dose of histamine. Using simultaneously administered histamine and antihistamine, they demonstrated that patients with gastric ulcer did secrete significant quantities of free hydrochloric acid.

Because 90 per cent of the population who do secrete acid and pepsin do not develop peptic ulceration, it must be concluded that a second factor of equal or greater importance is local tissue resistance. The available evidence suggests that duodenal ulcer is largely the result of increased secretion, whereas gastric ulcer is largely the result of decreased local tissue resistance.

When the secretion of hydrochloric acid is compared in patients with duodenal ulcer, those free of ulcer, those with gastric ulcer and those with gastric carcinoma, a decreasing degree of acid secretion is found. This is true whether the determinations are made under fasting conditions, by overnight gastric secretion or following stimulation with a test meal, hypoglycemia or drugs such as alcohol and histamine. While there is some overlap, the average duodenal ulcer patient secretes two to four times the normal amount of acid, whereas the patients with gastric ulcer and carcinoma of the stomach secrete less than normal. Anastomotic ulcer rarely occurs following operations for gastric ulcer, but is not uncommon following operation for duodenal ulcer. If a duodenal ulcer is simply excised, it recurs promptly, whereas simple excision of a gastric ulcer may not be followed by recurrence. There are differences in geographic distribution, social and economic status, sex and age. This is evidence favoring the concept that gastric and duodenal ulcer are different diseases. Both, however, require the presence of acid and pepsin.

Duodenal and gastric ulcers frequently coexist, and this relationship will be more often discerned if all patients with duodenal ulcer are routinely gastroscoped. These patients have the hypersecretory pattern of duodenal ulcer, their duodenal ulcer almost always precedes the gastric ulcer, and the gastric ulcer is usually shallow and in the antrum. There is frequently pyloric stenosis, supporting Dragstedt's concept that stasis in the region of the antrum with resulting antrum hyperfunction plays a role in the pathogenesis of gastric ulcer. There is little danger of malignancy, it usually heals more easily than the duodenal ulcer, and their management should be that of duodenal ulcer.

It is important to distinguish between acute and chronic peptic ulcers. Particularly in the stomach, an erosion may progress to an acute ulcer which heals within days or weeks. Surgeons are particularly concerned with the chronic ulcer, although the acute ulcer may perforate or bleed and be of surgical significance.

HYPERACIDITY IN DUODENAL ULCER. Patients do not have an increased amount of gastric acidity because their parietal cells secrete acid of increased concentration. They do secrete excessive quantities of acid, but it is quantitative rather than qualitative. The increase in acid could be due to increased stimulation along any of the normal pathways, or due to the presence of abnormal stimuli. There is some evidence that more gastrin can be recovered from the resected antrum of patients with duodenal ulcer than from patients operated on for gastric ulcer or carcinoma. Another possibility is that the normal autoregulatory mechanisms are not functioning properly. Antral gastritis is almost invariably found in duodenal ulcer, but there is no good evidence that the autoregulatory mechanisms are deficient. Patients with duodenal ulcer do have an increased number of parietal cells in their stomachs, and a constitutional increase in parietal cells has been advanced as the cause of duodenal ulcer. It has been shown experimentally that stimulation of an experimental animal with a powerful secretagogue, such as histamine, quickly results in a hyperplasia of the parietal cells, so the increased parietal cell count seen in patients with duodenal ulcer could be secondary rather than primary.

The increased duodenal acidity leading to duodenal ulcer could be due to the rapid gastric emptying of acid chyme. There may be a deficiency in duodenal mucin, or in the neutralizing and buffering duodenal, pancreatic and biliary secretions. Again, the suspected deficiencies have not been found. We are left then with the simple fact that patients with duodenal ulcer secrete excessive quantities of acid, and from the therapeutic viewpoint these ulcers can be healed and controlled if this acid secretion can be reduced to one-half or one-third, or effectively neutralized by medication.

NATURE AND CAUSE OF GASTRIC ULCER. A quantitative or qualitative deficiency in mucus production may play a role, but this is only speculative. It has been shown that the gastric and duodenal epithelium is normally replaced at an astonishing rate. The gastroduodenal "patio" must be repaved every three days. Degeneration of the gastric epithelium is probably a normal aging process, but atrophic gastritis is seen with a statistically higher incidence in patients with gastric ulcer, and particularly in patients with carcinoma of the stomach. Most students of this thorny subject have concluded that the gastritis was secondary to the lesion rather than a precursor. Possibly, people who develop a gastric ulcer do so in an area of gastric wall where a premature reduction in epithelial replacement or mucus production has occurred. Certainly, the incidence of gastric ulcer increases progressively with age, and there is considerable evidence that the patient who develops gastric ulcer is predisposed to the subsequent development of carcinoma of the stomach.

Dragstedt believes, on the basis of his experience with the physiologically obstructed stomach following vagotomy, that antral hyperperfusion secondary to stasis is an important ulcerogenic factor in gastric ulcer. There is no question that gastric stasis predisposes to gastric ulcer, even following antrectomy, for it can occur after resection for duodenal ulcer if the gastroduodenal stoma is stenotic.

However, in most patients with gastric ulcer, evidence of antral stasis is lacking, and Dragstedt's suggestion remains an interesting but unproved hypothesis. Healing is promoted in gastric ulcer if gastric drainage is improved, or if acidity is reduced. Moreover, if the ulcer is simply excised, it may not recur.

STRESS ULCER. It is frequently noted in patients with ulcer disease that exacerbations occur subsequent to personal stress and fatigue. The incidence of duodenal ulcer increased during the war, particularly in areas where the conflict had its greatest impact, and the incidence of duodenal ulcer is increasing steadily as our society becomes more complex. Subjecting experimental animals to stress may produce gastric or duodenal ulceration, and in these animals there may be adrenal hypertrophy. At the present time, it is difficult to know the significance of day-to-day stress in the clinical symptoms of the usual patient with peptic ulcer. The influence of the adrenal steroids is also poorly understood. Adrenocorticotropic hormone or cortisone in large doses stimulates acid secretion and uropepsin levels are increased. Pre-existing peptic ulcers in patients with rheumatoid arthritis may perforate or bleed if cortisone is administered. Patients with Addison's disease have a very low incidence of peptic ulcer. The usual dosage of cortisone does not stimulate acid secretion, but steroids do interfere with healing and may interfere with the protective effect of mucin. There is no evidence of increased adrenal activity in the usual case of peptic ulcer, and ulcers can be produced in the adrenalectomized experimental animal. Stress does not stimulate gastric secretion. While constitutional and psychophysiologic factors may prove to be of great importance in the pathogenesis of peptic ulcer, the term "stress ulcer" should be applied strictly to those gastroduodenal ulcers which develop following experimental stress.

CURLING'S ULCER. In 1842, Curling described acute duodenal ulcers associated with burns, and they have been noted following other types of trauma as well as in postoperative patients. Experimentally, there is no increase in gastric secretion, and they can be prevented if hemoconcentration is avoided.

CUSHING'S ULCER. In 1932, Cushing reported acute peptic ulcers associated with intracranial lesions and postulated a relationship. Acute ulcers are frequently seen in patients dying of intracranial lesions as well as other causes, and it is exceedingly difficult to be certain whether the relationship is other than fortuitous. As a terminal event in all illnesses, large duodenal, gastric or esophageal lesions may develop, and perforation is common. Evidence is lacking that intracranial lesions play a significant role in the usual chronic peptic ulcer.

SYMPTOMS AND SIGNS OF PEPTIC ULCER

Pain is the prominent feature of peptic ulcer, although it may be absent, particularly in gastric ulcer. It appears to be secondary to hyperperistalsis, which in turn is stimulated by the action of unbuffered acid, for it can be relieved by neutralization and is aggravated by the artificial introduction of acid. It is generally diffusely localized in the epigastric area and, if there is posterior penetration, it may be felt in the region of the upper lumbar spine. It has a gnawing or burning character, sometimes described as similar to hunger pain, usually only moderate in degree. It is generally relieved temporarily by water, milk, antacids and, in the case of duodenal ulcer, by food. Gastric ulcer pain may be aggravated by meals; much has been made of this differential diagnostic point. The difference in the pain-food sequence is, however, by no means reliable, because the pain of gastric ulcer is often relieved by food and that of duodenal ulcer, in its acute stages, may be aggravated. Ulcer pain often comes on at night, wakens the patient, and is relieved by the taking of food. While it is generally unaffected by posture, repetitive bending as in shoveling, or vibration from driving a heavy vehicle, may be aggravating. It is almost always aggravated by alcohol, particularly beer.

One of the characteristic features of peptic ulcer pain is its periodicity. In the early years of "ulcer trouble," the patient has symptoms for only a few days with long intervals of remission, the symptomatic period often being the Spring and the Fall, even in nonseasonal workers. With the passage of time, the symptomatic periods lengthen and become more frequent until the patient is having ulcer pain much of the time. Anorexia or vomiting is not common unless there is gastric obstruction. Weight loss may occur as the patient becomes a dietary invalid, or the weight may increase because of frequent feedings in an attempt to control the pain. Bleeding, as manifested by hematemesis or tarry stools, occurs at some time in about 20 per cent of patients. In the absence of complications, the physical findings are minimal and are usually limited to tenderness immediately over the ulcer.

LABORATORY FINDINGS. In the diagnosis of duodenal ulcer, x-ray and fluoroscopy have no peer. In duodenal and anastomotic ulcer, they are not too reliable in gauging the progress of healing, amelioration of symptoms being more dependable. In contrast, the radiologic and gastroscopic examination of gastric ulcer are useful in both diagnosis and in assessing the effect of treatment. This is particularly true since image amplification has been added to roentgenologic examination. Neither is completely reliable in making a differential diagnosis between benign and malignant gastric ulcer. The presence of occult blood in the stools indicates continuing activity, and also indicates something other than functional disease, if that diagnosis has been entertained.

Fractional gastric analysis following stimulation by a small quantity of food, alcohol or a small dose of histamine permits a rough measure of the level of gastric secretion. Stimulating the parietal cells with large doses of histamine is particularly useful in determining whether true achlorhydria is present, and is used by some clinicians in an attempt to evaluate the severity of the ulcer diathesis. This procedure takes advantage of the fact that the antihistamines will protect the patient against the systemic reaction of histamine, but do not block the histamine stimulation of the parietal cells. The test was developed by Kowalewski and independently by Kay, and several modifications have been employed. The acid-secreting capacity of the patient can also be evaluated by aspirating the nocturnal secretion of gastric juice continuously from 8 p.m. to 8 a.m. This is actually a measure of the interdigestive phase of secretion, and it is usually expressed in milliequivalents. While the average ulcer-free patient secretes about 18 mEq. of HCl, the average gastric ulcer patient secretes 12 mEq., and the average duodenal ulcer patient about 65 mEq. Patients harboring a functioning pancreatic tumor almost always secrete more than 100 mEq., and levels as high as 300 mEq. of acid have been obtained. Vagal mechanisms can be investigated after stimulation with insulin-induced hypoglycemia, acid secretion being measured during the period when the blood sugar falls below 50 mg. per 100 ml. This method of stimulation can also be used to evaluate pepsin secretion.

DIFFERENTIAL DIAGNOSIS. Upper gastrointestinal symptoms such as fullness, eructation of gas, and poorly defined food intolerances frequently exist in the absence of organic disease. It is not known whether these complaints are psychogenic in origin, or whether they are due to some disturbance in the highly complex smooth muscle coordination of the gastric, duodenal, pancreatic and biliary area. Functional dyspepsia and gastritis are popular diagnoses, but some of these patients undoubtedly have a peptic ulcer which has not been visualized radiologically. Whatever the cause of these vague symptoms, a high percentage are relieved by regular and unhurried meals with or without small doses of sedation and anticholinergic drugs.

Recurrent episodes of biliary colic or cholecystitis are extremely common but can usually be differentiated without difficulty from peptic ulcer disease. Pain usually comes on after a heavy meal, is inclined to be more severe than peptic ulcer pain, and may last from a few hours to several days, during which time the patient is never completely free of pain, in contrast to peptic ulcer. Nausea is more pronounced and there may be vomiting. Except in the occasional patient with an extremely thick abdominal wall, tenderness over the gallbladder can usually be demonstrated.

Esophagitis is an often overlooked cause of high epigastric symptoms. It is characterized by a burning pain behind the xiphoid or lower sternum, often with eructation of sour-tasting fluid brought on by straining or a change in posture. There is generally an associated hiatus hernia, which, in the absence of reflux acid esophagitis, is nearly always asymptomatic.

Recurrent or chronic pancreatitis can be a difficult diagnosis in the differentiation of upper abdominal pain. Like gallbladder disease and gastric ulcer, it is frequently aggravated by food, but there is usually a significant component of back pain similar to that seen in the penetrating duodenal ulcer. The back pain associated with penetrating duodenal ulcer is probably due to a local area of pancreatitis.

Early carcinoma of the body or tail of the pancreas is difficult to diagnose in its early stages as it simply presents as a deep, boring, unrelenting pain which gradually becomes more severe as the weeks pass, and is soon associated with weight loss.

Recurrent pyelonephritis is a not infrequent cause of poorly defined upper abdominal pain. Renal colic is seldom confused with the uncomplicated peptic ulcer but enters into the differential diagnosis in patients with minor leakage from a perforated peptic ulcer.

If there is pyloric stenosis, other causes of high small bowel obstruction must be excluded. The absence of bile in the vomitus in obstruction due to ulcer disease is of great value in the differential diagnosis. If there is hematemesis or blood in the stomach, other sources of bleeding proximal to the ligament of Treitz enter into the diagnosis.

DUODENAL ULCER

CONSERVATIVE MANAGEMENT. In the absence of perforation or uncontrolled hemorrhage, all patients with duodenal ulcer should have a trial of conservative management, which in the majority will be at least temporarily successful. Most physicians believe that medical therapy is of undoubted benefit, that the acute bout can almost always be relieved, and that the incidence of recurrent pain can be reduced if an adequate regimen is followed.

Avery Jones is dubious: "the evidence is regrettably slender that real benefit is derived from the traditional dietary regimen, and over-treatment can undoubtedly be positively harmful. There is, fortunately, a strong natural tendency to recovery for which the patient tends to give credit to his treatment."

Controlled trials have failed to demonstrate that the natural history of duodenal ulcer is affected by medical treatment, but the exacerbations certainly subside, and one has the impression that treatment during the exacerbations speeds recovery. During exacerbations, rest, frequent feedings and anticholinergic drugs are prescribed, and feedings or alkali are taken frequently. Coffee, tobacco and particularly alcohol are prohibited and an attempt is made to encourage the patient to view his environment with equanimity.

INTRACTABILITY. Between 10 and 20 per cent of patients with duodenal ulcer will eventually require operation because of intractability, or one of the complications of duodenal ulcer. This figure varies widely, because intractability is a relative term whose definition varies from doctor to doctor. As in all diseases, the indications for operation have to be compared with the natural history of the disease, the results that can be achieved

with nonsurgical treatment, and the mortality and morbidity associated with surgical treatment. At the Mason Clinic, about 15 per cent of patients with duodenal ulcer are treated surgically. Elective surgical treatment should be considered for the patient who has intractable symptoms unrelieved by an adequate medical regimen, unrelieved or recurring obstruction, and repeated minor hemorrhage.

The indications for surgical intervention, on the basis of intractability, are found in the patient who, in spite of an ideal medical regimen during exacerbations and a sensible regimen during remissions, is seriously affected economically in his day-to-day living; and in the patient who will not or cannot, because of his circumstances, follow an acceptable medical regimen. Examples are the alcoholic, the sailor and the seasonal bush-worker. Obviously, the personality of the patient, his family and home situation, his attitude toward his disease and the facilities available to him for nonmedical treatment influence this often difficult decision. In selecting patients, the surgeon should deny acceptance for operation as long as possible to the asthenic, migrainous patient who is a finicky eater and who is underweight. This introvert finally exhausts his physician's patience and surgical assistance is sought. With any treatment, there will be a high percentage of unsatisfactory results in these patients and an increased percentage of untoward sequelae after operation. Such patients should not have a surgical procedure of any kind without prolonged observation on the part of the surgeon as well as the internist.

Before recommending operation, it is wise to discuss with the patient the possible untoward sequelae in a manner that does not necessarily plant the seed for introspective complaints, but rather provides a protective understanding should they occur. Such sequelae will then be accepted, not as the result of a mistake on the part of the surgeon, but rather as an irreducible premium for control of the more crippling ulcer symptoms.

By the same token, the internist or general physician should not be guilty of procrastination in advising operation in the severe forms of the disease. It is certainly possible to carry on with conservative treatment too long. In defining intractability, the physician should place less reliance on the response of the patient in hospital and more significance on the early relapse after hospital discharge, when the patient resumes his occupation in the habitual environment in which he must continue to work. Too often, the surgeon is asked to treat a grossly obese patient who has been trying to feed his ulcer for years and who faces a higher risk of complications because of his obesity. Again, the surgeon may be asked to take over a patient who is having his fourth bout of pyloric stenosis. The penetration and fibrosis makes management of the duodenum more difficult and earlier recognition of this surgical candidate would result in a lower mortality rate.

Surgical Procedures for Duodenal Ulcer

Procedures for duodenal ulcer must be evaluated in terms of surgical mortality, postoperative morbidity and the incidence of recurrent or anastomotic ulcer after a long interval following operation.

PHYSIOLOGIC PRINCIPLES. Assuming that the greater half of the equation in duodenal ulcer is an increased production of hydrochloric acid, there are four ways in which this secretion can be surgically reduced: by vagal denervation of the corpus, by vagal denervation of the antrum, by excision of the antrum and by excision of a varying percentage of the acid-secreting corpus.

In the experimental animal, the relative importance of these methods has been evaluated, using experimental ulcer as the yardstick. Vagal denervation of the parietal cells is least effective, while vagal denervation of the antrum reduces the ulcer incidence by one-half. If the antrum is removed, the incidence of ulcer is reduced to about one-third. Excision of the acid-secreting mucosa is not effective, unless it exceeds 50 per cent, which is what one would anticipate in a target organ (Fig. 50).

VAGOTOMY. Vagotomy results in a loss of

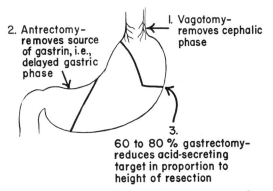

2. Antrectomy—removes source of gastrin, i.e., delayed gastric phase

1. Vagotomy—removes cephalic phase

3. 60 to 80 % gastrectomy—reduces acid-secreting target in proportion to height of resection

Figure 50. Varieties of surgical attack for peptic ulcer. Vagotomy denervates the antrum as well as the acid and pepsin cells in the corpus. As the antrum constitutes about 20 per cent of the stomach, a 60 per cent resection removes the antrum and half the corpus.

gastric tone and must be supplemented by a procedure which facilitates gastric emptying. If deformity and scarring in the pyloric area do not contraindicate it, this can be done by a pyloroplasty to enlarge the pyloric opening and to eliminate its sphincteric action (Fig. 51).

An alternative drainage procedure is gastroenterostomy, which should provide effective gastric drainage. Vagotomy and pyloroplasty, or gastroenterostomy, can be performed with a mortality of less than 1 per cent because the involved duodenum is not divided. Even in experienced hands the recurrence rate is 5 to 10 per cent on a five-year follow-up, and if either of the major vagal trunks is missed at operation, the recurrence rate is higher. Explosive diarrhea is a significant problem in a small percentage of patients when vagotomy is employed to reduce acid secretion. Prolonged symptoms from disruption of the cardioesophageal mechanism may also occur if surgical steps to prevent this have not been taken at the time of vagotomy.

Occasionally, a severe protracted gastric stasis and inanition can seem insurmountable. The referral center inherits this complication, and the problem is appreciated as a real one. The best answer in our experience is to avoid further surgical procedures for at least three weeks, during which time intravenous feedings are handled carefully to support the patient, yet to avoid overload and loss by hypersecretion into the paralyzed stomach, the so-called "gastric kidney." If these measures are unavailing, then gastrostomy to reduce the discomfort and complications of prolonged nasogastric intubation, and a feeding jejunostomy are indicated, and generally preferable to secondary partial gastrectomy.

PARTIAL RESECTION. Partial gastric resection results in excision of the antrum and a portion of the acid secreting mucosa. The amount of stomach removed, including the antrum, varies from 60 to 80 per cent (Fig. 52). One of the major causes of death following gastrectomy is peritonitis caused by subsequent leakage from the duodenal stump. Much of this danger can be eliminated by using vagotomy and pyloroplasty, or gastroenterostomy, when a difficult duodenum is encountered at operation. If this is done, the mortality can be kept in the neighborhood of 1 per cent. Welch and Rodkey employ suction catheter drainage through a duodenostomy, when closure of the duodenal stump seems insecure, and in their recently reported series only had a 1 per cent mortality rate.

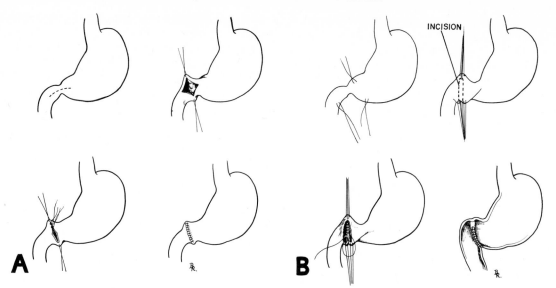

Figure 51.   *A,* Heineke-Mikulicz pyloroplasty. *B,* Finney pyloroplasty. Care must be taken in closure of the Heineke-Mikulicz pyloroplasty, or obstruction will result. Weinberg advocates a one-layer closure without inversion, reinforced if necessary with omentum. The Finney pyloroplasty also provides efficient gastric drainage, and may prove easier and safer in the deformed duodenum.

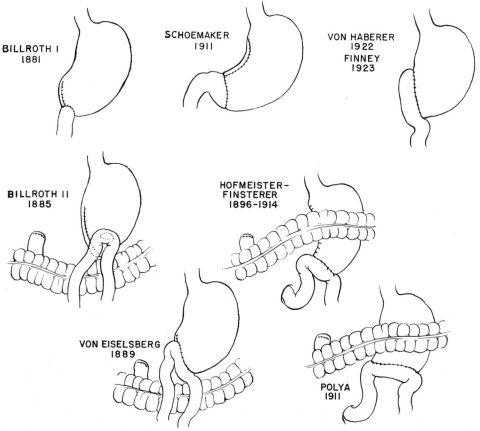

Figure 52.   Methods of anastomosis after partial or subtotal gastrectomy. The upper diagrams illustrate three methods of gastroduodenal reconstruction, and the lower four illustrate alternative methods of gastrojejunal reconstruction. Two of these are antecolic and two are retrocolic. Although not strictly accurate, the terms Billroth I and Billroth II are generally used to describe, respectively, gastroduodenal and gastrojejunal reconstruction following gastric resection. Similar modifications are employed in fashioning a gastroenterostomy (gastrojejunostomy), although of course a resection is not done.

The morbidity following partial resection varies directly with the extent of resection, whereas the recurrent ulcer rate falls progressively as the extent of resection is increased. The incidence of recurrent ulcer varies from 3 to 8 per cent after five years, a two-thirds resection having a recurrence rate of about 4 per cent.

Following resection, gastrointestinal continuity can be established by gastroduodenostomy (Billroth I) or gastrojejunostomy (Billroth II). Gastrojejunostomy is employed most frequently, because the duodenum is often not suitable for anastomosis and gastrojejunostomy can always be accomplished without tension on the suture line. A gastroduodenal reconstruction has been followed by a higher incidence of recurrent ulcer, possibly because the extent of the resection is compromised in order to facilitate reconstruction and avoid tension on the suture line. Theoretically, a gastroduodenal reconstruction should be more physiologic and be followed by fewer nutritional disturbances, but these differences are not impressive.

There are alternative methods of gastroduodenal and gastrojejunal reconstruction. If the afferent jejunal loop is closer to the lesser curvature, it is referred to as an isoperistaltic anastomosis, the reverse being antiperistaltic. There is no evidence that this is of any significance, providing the jejunum drains both the duodenum and the stomach effectively. The decision whether the anastomosis is made in an iso- or antiperistaltic manner should be based on what appears to be the best "fit." The jejunum may be brought through the transverse mesocolon to the left of the midcolic artery as a retrocolic anastomosis, or in front of the colon. While it is unlikely that the jejunum is appreciably more susceptible to ulceration if the proximal loop is slightly longer, as it must be in antecolic reconstructions, the danger of torsion of the afferent and efferent jejunal loops is increased. If stomal ulcer should develop, the danger of penetration into the colon is less after an antecolic reconstruction, and subsequent operation for the stomal ulcer is technically easier. In either event, one should ensure that the anastomosis lies transversely without tension, and that the aperture of the afferent loop is not lower than the efferent loop. Another technical variable is the size of the anastomosis. To discourage rapid gastric emptying, some surgeons advocate restricting the size of the stoma. Others do not consider this significant. Actually, the functional size of the anastomosis is limited by the diameter of the efferent loop.

These principles also apply to the fashioning of a gastroenterostomy after vagotomy, but the prime consideration is free drainage without either afferent or efferent loop obstruction.

VAGOTOMY AND ANTRECTOMY. In 1951, Farmer and Smithwick reported on their experience with vagotomy and excision of the antrum, also called vagotomy and hemigastrectomy, or vagotomy and 50 per cent gastrectomy. In order to be certain that all of the antrum is removed, it is necessary to excise slightly more than half of the lesser curvature and slightly less than half of the greater curvature. This procedure, like partial gastrectomy, requires division and a safe closure of the duodenum. The mortality rate is similar to that for partial gastrectomy, from 1.5 to 5 per cent. If vagotomy were combined instead with pyloroplasty or gastroenterostomy as a substitute for antrectomy in those patients in whom the duodenum is technically unsuitable, the mortality rate could be sharply reduced, and in these precarious patients the greater incidence of recurrent ulcer would be justified. Edwards and his associates report a recurrence rate of less than 1 per cent with a ten-year follow-up record of a large number of patients after vagotomy and antrectomy.

Following excision of the distal portion of the stomach, the specimen can be opened and the junction between antrum and corpus easily identified. In contradistinction to the loose, redundant rugal folds of the fundus, the mucosa of the antrum is smooth and adherent to the submucosa (Fig. 53).

One of the three procedures enumerated here is generally employed for the surgical treatment of duodenal ulcer. The clinical trial initiated by Goligher, Pulvertaft and Franz in 1959 is thus of real significance. If at operation the situation was found favorable for any of the three surgical procedures, the operation done was randomized. They now have a minimum three-year follow-up on over 300 patients, with only eight patients untraced. As can be seen from Table 1, there was no mortality and the difference in the morbidity following the three procedures is not startling. Although the poor results are least in the vagotomy and antrectomy group, the best results are in the partial gastrectomy group. In neither event were these differences statistically significant. Since their trial was closed they have done over 200 operations by vagotomy and pyloroplasty. In their hands the re-

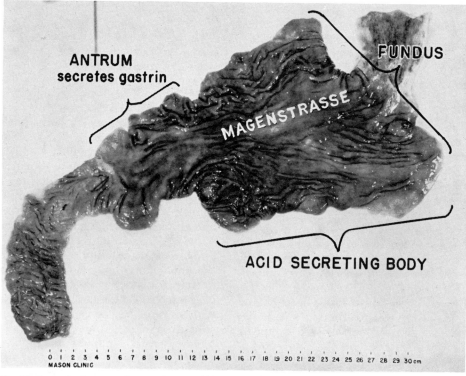

Figure 53.   Photograph of a normal stomach opened longitudinally, showing the terminal end of the esophagus and the first and second portions of the duodenum. The magenstrasse is the lesser curvature. The smooth, fixed mucosa of the the antrum is grossly distinguishable from the rugal folds of the mucosa of the body of the stomach.

sults do not appear to be superior to those obtained by vagotomy and gastroenterostomy.

OTHER PROCEDURES. **Selective vagotomy.** Diarrhea may be one of the complications of any gastric operation, but the incidence appears to be significantly higher following those procedures in which vagotomy is per-

formed. It is much commoner following vagotomy and gastroenterostomy than after simple gastroenterostomy. It has been suggested that the prime cause is vagal denervation of not only the stomach, but also the biliary tree, pancreas and the greater portion of the intestine. We are inclined to think of the vagi as

Table 1.   *Percentage of Problems Encountered in Three Surgical Procedures for Treatment of Duodenal Ulcer*

	VAGOTOMY AND GASTROENTEROSTOMY	VAGOTOMY AND ANTRECTOMY	PARTIAL GASTRECTOMY
Number of cases	126	132	117
Mortality	0	0	0
Early dumping*	15	9	21
Diarrhea*	26	21	12
Less than optimal weight*	2.5	5.6	5.3
Recurrence	4	0	2
Poor result	8	5	8
Severe dumping	0	1	1
Mechanical	2	3	5
Recurrence	4	0	2
Severe diarrhea	2	1	0

* The differences are statistically significant (p = 0.05).

Results from the Leeds-York clinical trial. Early dumping refers to nonhypoglycemic symptoms coming on soon after meals. Mechanical refers to food or bile vomiting, generally blamed on mechanical factors in the gastrointestinal reconstruction. Optimal weight is taken from standard life tables.

efferent nerves. They are 90 per cent afferent, and only a fraction of the 30,000 fibers in each vagus nerve are motor and secretory to the stomach. A limited number of surgeons have recently advocated preserving the hepatic branch of the anterior vagus and the celiac branch of the posterior vagus, a procedure that has been termed "selective gastric vagotomy." It is said that the incidence of gastrointestinal dysfunction following selective vagotomy is less than that in which division of the vagal trunks is employed. The procedure is more time-consuming and until a clinical trial is done we will not know the relative advantages and disadvantages of selective gastric vagotomy.

Vagotomy has been employed following distal partial resection to reduce acid peptic secretion in the residual one-quarter to one-third of the stomach, but this has not afforded any additional protection in terms of recurrent ulceration. It is not advocated, therefore, as a primary ancillary procedure, but should be reserved for the approximately 4 per cent of patients who develop recurrent ulcer after partial gastrectomy.

Duodenal exclusion. The exclusion operation developed by von Eiselsberg resulted in a very high incidence of stomal ulcer because the antrum was left in an alkaline environment. This procedure was modified by Bancroft, who advocated coring out the prepyloric mucosa, following which the muscular layers of the antrum were sutured. This is occasionally employed to avoid transecting a technically unsuitable duodenum, but in this situation it is probably not the best procedure. The antral mucosa may extend as much as a centimeter beyond the pylorus, and one can never be sure that excision of the antral mucosa has been complete. A further technical disadvantage is that the antrum may be devascularized before it is recognized that the duodenum should not be transected, and necrosis of the antral suture line may result.

Segmental resection. Appreciating the importance of the autoregulatory mechanisms, Wangensteen aimed his attack at the acid-secreting corpus. A sleeve of the corpus is resected and gastrointestinal continuity restored by suturing the residual proximal stomach to the antrum. Because the pylorus is vagally denervated by this procedure, a supplementary pyloroplasty is necessary (Fig. 54). A 70 per cent resection of the corpus was successful in preventing ulcer recurrence, but the patient's gastric capacity was seriously compromised and the nutritional

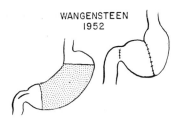

Figure 54. Segmental resection with supplementary pyloroplasty.

problems were as severe as those following a 75 per cent distal partial resection. The excision of the corpus was reduced to 40 per cent, but this was followed by a significant recurrence of ulcer. Wangensteen increased this to 50 per cent of the corpus in the hope that a proper balance could be struck between ulcer recurrence and postoperative morbidity. This procedure has been employed by only a few surgeons up to the present time.

Gastrostomy. A temporary gastrostomy is employed following gastric operations, particularly after vagotomy and pyloroplasty, by many surgeons. This avoids the use of the nasogastric tube, which is annoying to the patient and after prolonged use may give rise to respiratory complications or nasal and pharyngeal ulceration. Farris and Smith insert a Foley catheter into the anterior wall of the stomach, which is inverted at that point by a purse string suture. The catheter is brought through a portion of omentum, which serves as a washer, and the catheter is brought through the abdominal wall at the point where the stomach lies in normal apposition with it. It prevents overdistention of the stomach following vagotomy and avoids the use of a nasogastric tube. However, it is not free of complications and should probably be reserved for the patient in whom it is anticipated that more than one or two days of gastric suction will be required.

Selecting the Procedure for the Patient

There is no ideal operation for duodenal ulcer; all have some mortality and produce some morbidity. Surgeons are frequently asked their opinion as to the best operation; there is no "best" operation. The surgeon's aim is to select the best operative procedure for each patient, and this can be done with considerable assurance. The procedures most commonly employed are vagotomy and pyloroplasty, vagotomy and gastroenterostomy, partial resection, and vagotomy and antrectomy. The choice of procedure is made on the basis of clinical and technical considerations. An attempt is made to assess the ulcerogenic virulence of the patient's disease, ability to withstand operation, emotional status and nutritional needs.

Assessing the virulence of the ulcer disease is by no means exact, but useful information can be obtained by measuring acid and pepsin production.

PREOPERATIVE SECRETORY TESTS. The test most widely employed preoperatively to assess ulcer virulence during the past 15 years has been the augmented or maximum histamine test, or one of its many modifications. It was hoped that by this approach the patient's ulcerogenic potential could be measured and the most suitable operation selected. One of the most thorough clinical studies using this approach was done in the Medical-Surgical Gastro-Intestinal Unit at the Western General Hospital in Edinburgh. Based on the preoperative histamine-stimulated secretion, one of four procedures was selected, the aim being to perform the least possible operation necessary to prevent recurrence in the hope that both recurrence and morbidity would be minimal. The series is impressive in its size, thoroughness and careful follow-up, but the results have disappointed the clinicians in this excellent clinical research unit. The recurrence rate is similar to that generally seen when these procedures are done without the benefit of preoperative histamine-stimulated secretory studies. Many other series of patients now under study may be more encouraging.

A further refinement has been the development of the "medical vagotomy" test described by Kay and his associates. It was designed to evaluate the relative importance of vagal drive in duodenal ulcer patients by measuring the reduction in acid secretion following pharmacological blockade of the vagi. Acid secretion was stimulated by histamine or insulin-induced hypoglycemia, and vagal function depressed by atropine and hexamethonium, or more recently propantheline. Johnston and his associates found the test significant when a large number of patients were assessed, but it was not sufficiently accurate in the preoperative assessment of the individual patient.

The concept of preoperative secretory evaluation is sound, but at the moment the tests are less than ideal. None are specific for the various gastric secretory mechanisms and because of the potentiation of stimuli at the parietal cell level, it is exceedingly difficult to measure any of the mechanisms in its pure form. For example, when the vagal mechanism is stimulated gastrin is produced by vagal stimulation of the antrum, and the two stimuli potentiate each other at the parietal cell level. Histamine is not ideal, for it exerts its major effect on the parietal cell, whereas modern gastric operations are directed at the vagus or the antrum. Because of a reduction in potentiation, the secretory response to histamine is reduced by vagotomy or antrectomy, but histamine tests are not really measuring these mechanisms. Gastrin and the synthetic polypeptides of gastrin are more potent and physiological, but may not prove to be any more practical in assessing ulcer virulence, or dictating the choice of procedure to the surgeon. When it becomes possible to measure gastrin in the peripheral blood, it may be possible to assess the role of the antrum in duodenal ulcer. There is nothing in sight that will accurately assess the relative importance of the vagal stimulating mechanisms in the individual ulcer patient. It is entirely possible that duodenal ulcer patients are homogeneous with respect to the pathogenesis of their hypersecretion, and are not vagal, antral or parietal cell hyperreactors.

The significance of gastric secretory tests may have been overemphasized by clinicians, but there are definite indications for them. All require careful attention to detail, particularly with respect to accurate fluoroscopic positioning of the gastric tube. Unless this is done the tests are not accurate enough to warrant the expenditure of time and money, or the discomfort to the patient. The basal fasting level is high in the Zollinger-Ellison syndrome and may be used as a screening test for this rare condition. Otherwise, as the volume of secretion is small, the error is great. The 12-hour overnight fasting secretion would seem as good as any if the tube is accurately positioned and the suction broken frequently. We do not know if we are measuring the vagi, the antrum or the target cells, but this is also true with respect to the more sophisticated tests. If the overnight secretion is high, the patient probably has a duodenal ulcer; if it exceeds 100 mEq., he probably has a pancreatic adenoma. The old tests of gastric secretion using alcohol or carbohydrate tend to be inaccurate because the secretory volume is small. This is the major advantage of the histamine-antihistamine tests, a large volume and, hence, a smaller error. If in an equivocal situation, the response to histamine is in the duodenal ulcer range, the diagnosis is strengthened. Often in such patients with a classic ulcer history and repeatedly negative x-rays, a channel or pyloric canal ulcer is present. If the basal acid output is high and not significantly increased by histamine, a functioning pancreatic adenoma is suggested. If the diagnosis of stomal ulcer is equivocal, the histamine-stimulated secretion will often be helpful. In testing patients after partial gastrectomy, Holubitsky found those with proved stomal ulcer to have secretory levels of 5 mEq. per hour or more following Histalog stimulation. These tests, however, will not tell what operation should be done, or whether the hypersecretion, if present, is vagal, antral or parietal cell in origin. The search continues on many fronts for reliable measurements to assist the patient and the surgeon.

SURGICAL JUDGMENT. Procedures involving resection of a portion of the stomach are more often followed by gastrointestinal dysfunction and nutritional problems, and the more extensive the resection the greater their severity. Gilbert has shown that postoperative morbidity is much higher in the emotionally labile patient, hence the surgeon is more inclined toward vagotomy and drainage in these patients, although other factors such as a high secretion might tip the scales in favor of distal partial resection or vagotomy and antrectomy. The elderly or poor-risk patient should have the procedure of least magnitude, vagotomy and pyloroplasty, or vagotomy and gastroenterostomy. The female patient, particularly if she is in the childbearing age, does not have as powerful an ulcer diathesis, and vagotomy followed by either of the drainage procedures is the operation of choice. The incidence of stomal ulcer is higher in the menopausal or postmenopausal woman, and many surgeons favor vagotomy and antrectomy, or distal partial resection in these patients.

For the male patient, who constitutes the commonest candidate for the treatment of duodenal ulcer, the surgeon has a logical choice from among three established procedures: partial gastric resection, vagotomy with drainage, and vagotomy with 50 per cent gastric resection, or antrectomy. Resection may be conservative or radical; vagotomy, total or selective. Each leaves something to be desired, and selection should be based on a comparison of effective ulcer control, as balanced against comparative mortality and disagreeable sequelae. Mortality should be a first consideration; this will vary with each procedure in individual hands, depending upon the surgeon's technical experience and good judgment in selectively fitting the procedure to the individual situation.

Conservative resection has a reported mortality varying from 1 to 5 per cent and affords from 96 to 98 per cent protection against recurrent ulcer; antrectomy and vagotomy has the same, or slightly greater mortality, and a comparably greater protection against recurrent ulcer; vagotomy and drainage has the lowest mortality, less than 1 per cent, but gives a protection of only 80 to 95 per cent against recurrent ulcer. Many surgeons have been slow to abandon the conservative 60 to 65 per cent resection as the preferred primary operation in the good risk patient. However, when the ulcer is penetrating and creates an unusual technical hazard to resection, most surgeons leave the ulcer alone, and substitute vagotomy and drainage because of its greater safety. While the large penetrating ulcer may, in expert hands, be excluded or even resected, the increased hazard of resection in handling the duodenal stump makes it unwise to stretch resection to such limits.

By the same reasoning, vagotomy, either total or selective, is more difficult, more hazardous, and apt to be more often incomplete in the overweight patient and in the barrel-chested patient. To accomplish vagotomy, the surgeon is forced to disrupt the hiatal structures and the esophagogastric mechanism by which the esophagus is protected against reflux. The reflux of succus, whether acid or otherwise, is not tolerated well and particularly poorly by the overweight patient. In these patients, therefore, many surgeons find partial resection a technical preference, and at the same time they point out that the patient will obtain a better result, as well as greater ulcer protection, than from vagotomy and drainage. On the other hand, for the occasional thin, underweight patient who is a finicky eater and of introspective temperament, vagotomy and drainage is physiologically preferable and technically easier.

An increasing number of surgeons are employing the third procedure, antrectomy combined with vagotomy. Of the three procedures, it provides the greatest protection against recurrent ulcer. However, if applied primarily it can be argued that it exposes all patients to the hazards of both resection and vagotomy, and to the delayed morbidity of both sacrificing procedures, reduced gastric capacity and total, or near total, achlorhydria. The deciding factor should be the mortality risk. While there are some reports of mortality as low as

1.5 per cent, including perforation and uncontrolled hemorrhage, unpublished experiences in representative hospitals indicate that the mortality following gastric resection for duodenal ulcer can be as high as 5 per cent, compared to 1 per cent mortality for pyloroplasty and vagotomy. This higher mortality rate is not acceptable, and can be reduced by substituting vagotomy and drainage for resection when there is a large, penetrating ulcer. Regarding the disagreeable sequelae following operation, if diarrhea and esophageal reflux disorders, as well as dumping and reduced gastric capacity are considered, they are about the same for conservative gastric resection as for vagotomy and pyloroplasty. Those who prefer resection argue that there is no evidence that the partially gastrectomized state is less desirable than the totally vagotomized state. Those who favor antrectomy and vagotomy claim that the mortality and untoward sequelae are no greater than for simple resection, and that the protection against recurrent ulcer is greater. These differing opinions should serve to emphasize that, while all three procedures are acceptable on a physiologic basis, individual risk and technical hazard should influence the choice in each instance.

A review of any series of resective procedures will demonstrate that most of the postoperative deaths are secondary to duodenal stump leakage. The technically difficult duodenum can be recognized early in the operative procedure and transection of such a duodenum should be strictly avoided. It can be suspected preoperatively, if the patient complains of pain referred to the lower dorsal or upper lumbar region, and can be confirmed at operation, by the presence of an inflammatory mass in the duodenal and pancreatic area, as well as a tendency for the duodenum and pancreas to move as a unit as the surgeon evaluates the local condition of the duodenum.

A deep ulcer penetrating into the pancreas may be felt through the anterior duodenal wall. If such a duodenum is divided, there may be injury to the biliary tree, or the pancreas and its ducts, and it will be difficult to obtain a sound duodenal closure. In such a situation, vagotomy and pyloroplasty, or gastroenterostomy should be performed, even if the surgeon has a strong preference for one of the operations associated with a lower degree of ulcer recurrence. Vagotomy and gastroenterostomy can be performed with safety and, if and when the ulcer recurs, the healed duodenum can usually be safely transected.

If the surgeon embarks on resection and fails to anticipate that the duodenum will be technically difficult, duodenostomy and the use of catheter suction will add a margin of safety, as will duodenal exclusion. With respect to the difficult duodenum, Sir Heneage Ogilvie has sagely remarked, "the best way to keep milk from turning sour is to leave it in the cow."

MANAGEMENT OF PANCREATIC ADENOMA. In 1955, Zollinger and Ellison described a condition in which there is a tremendous stimulation of gastric secretion, associated with the presence of one or more pancreatic adenomas. Over 100 patients with nonbeta, non-insulin-producing islet cell tumors of the pancreas have been reported. Some of these have also had multiple adenomas, or hyperplasia, in other endocrine glands, particularly the pituitary and the parathyroids. These patients secrete large quantities of concentrated acid, are prone to recurrent ulceration, and often suffer from diarrhea. The average overnight secretion is in excess of 100 mEq. and the volume may exceed 1500 ml. At operation, single or multiple tumors may be found in the pancreas, splenic hilum or the duodenal or gastric wall. About one-third of the tumors are multiple and almost half are malignant. When present, only half the metastases are functional, and both the primary lesions and the metastases are slow-growing. As well as being intractable, the peptic ulcers are frequently found in the second or third portion of the duodenum or upper jejunum, because of the massive secretion of gastric juice. The pH in the duodenum remains so high that the pancreatic enzymes function inadequately, which leads to steatorrhea, diarrhea and hypopotassemia. A powerful gastric stimulant similar to gastrin has been recovered from these tumors by Gregory.

The severe ulcer diathesis persists until all of the functioning tumor has been removed and, occasionally, until all of the acid-secreting mucosa has been excised by a total gastrectomy. The decision whether the attack should be directed at the tumor tissue or the stomach is based on the characteristics of the tumor at operation, and whether it can be completely excised.

Postoperative Complications and Management

Vagotomy is followed by a temporary loss of gastric tone, which can become a chronic problem if overdistention occurs in the postoperative period. For this reason, all patients require gastric decompression for several days until tone is partially regained, either by nasogastric or gastrostomy suction. By temporarily discontinuing suction for increasing lengths of time, the period at which it can be permanently discontinued is easily determined. These patients should be advised to avoid large meals for the first postoperative month.

In the past, when a 75 per cent distal partial gastrectomy was generally employed for duodenal ulcer, the incidence of nutritional problems was much higher than it is today. In an attempt to bring the ulcer recurrence rate down to a lower level, the extent of resection was increased, and while this was successful with respect to ulcer recurrence, the larger resections resulted in an increasing incidence of nutritional problems. They are more severe in female patients, and in patients in whom resection is done for duodenal as compared with gastric ulcer. They are encountered to a decreasing degree following distal partial resection, vagotomy and hemigastrectomy, and vagotomy and drainage. It is difficult to compare accurately the frequency and severity of symptoms following gastric operations, because evaluation of the patient is often a matter of opinion. The ability of the patient to carry on with his previous employment and to maintain a satisfactory weight is a reliable, objective standard of evaluation.

It is useful to divide postoperative gastrointestinal dysfunction into two main groups. The first consists of those symptoms which come on shortly after the taking of food and are provoked by food. Included are distention, dumping, bilious vomiting and postprandial hypoglycemia. When present, these symptoms begin shortly after the operation and tend to improve with the passage of time.

The second group consists of those whose symptoms are the result of inadequate ingestion or absorption of food, are not provoked by eating, and may appear immediately or years after the operation. Thus, whereas weight loss may be an immediate problem, the development of megaloblastic anemia often requires a decade or more to reveal itself.

Overeating, or the rapid ingestion of fluid or food, causes a feeling of distention in the majority of patients following partial gastrectomy. This is seldom a serious problem. The patient soon learns to conserve his remaining gastric capacity by eating dry food and taking fluids between rather than with his meals. Capacity tends to improve with time.

Dumping manifests itself toward the end of, or immediately after, a meal. It is characterized by a feeling of weakness, and by perspiration and tachycardia; nausea and abdominal distress may also be present. Such symptoms may be more frequent following a Billroth II operation, compared with a Billroth I gastrointestinal reconstruction. The published incidence of the syndrome varies greatly, but following radical gastric resection it may be as high as 35 per cent; in only 5 to 10 per cent, however, does it cause any significant disability.

The mechanism of the dumping syndrome is not clear, and none of the several theories put forward has been entirely satisfactory. Thus, the concepts of sympathetic shock, a postprandial fall in plasma volume, hypokalemia and excessive serotonin have all been found to be incomplete. There is a functional as well as an organic component in this syndrome. Gilbert has shown what surgeons long suspected, that there is a high degree of correlation between dumping and a neurotic personality. The organic aspect of the problem is secondary to the rapid gastric emptying of hypertonic fluid into the upper jejunum. Sudden jejunal distention results in sympathetic reflexes, and the presence of large quantities of hypertonic fluid leads to the transfer of fluid and electrolytes from the intravascular space to the upper jejunum, with resulting hypotension and hypokalemia.

Treatment is often difficult and consists of reassurance; the avoidance of fluids with meals; six dry, small, high-protein meals daily and, if the symptoms are severe, a period of recumbency following each meal. If the symptoms of dumping are sufficiently troublesome, the patient will reduce his oral intake to the point where weight-failure becomes a problem, and this is the explanation for the inability to gain weight in some patients.

Bile is not tolerated by the stomach. If, due to efferent loop obstruction, it accumulates in significant quantities, vomiting results. It occurs almost exclusively following the Billroth II type of reconstruction, and if severe and persistent the anastomosis may require surgical modification.

Late postprandial hypoglycemia is the result of rapid emptying of the gastric remnant resulting in sudden hyperglycemia, which evokes an excessive secretion of endogenous insulin and secondary hypoglycemia. The effect is aggravated by physical exertion, the symptoms usually coming on between one and two hours after meals. The most effective treatment is the avoidance of easily assimilated carbohydrate and the taking of a high-protein diet. Patients who have been on a conservative ulcer regimen for a long period are inclined to continue their liquid high-carbohydrate, high-sugar diet, and they should be told specifically to avoid such a dietary regimen following operation.

Of the late complications, the most frequent is failure to regain the preoperative weight. This is least marked in those who are obese preoperatively. Although there is an excessive amount of fat in the stool after gastrectomy, the essential problem is an inadequate oral intake, often due to the fear of "dumping." If the patient is underweight preoperatively, and the caloric requirements of his job are high, a radical distal partial gastrectomy may be followed by a severe nutritional problem.

Although steatorrhea and diarrhea may occur after distal partial gastrectomy, they are more common following those procedures in which vagotomy has been done. They may be due to vagal denervation of the extragastric viscera and selective vagotomy may eliminate this problem, although this is not yet established.

A mild normocytic hypochromic anemia is frequent in women who have had a gastric operation during their childbearing period. Macrocytic anemia, presumably from loss of the intrinsic factor secreting mucosa is rare and seldom occurs within five years of operation. Anemia can be corrected appropriately by iron or by vitamin B_{12}.

ANASTOMOTIC OR STOMAL ULCER

The development of stomal ulcer is evidence of the inadequacy for that patient of previous surgical treatment. It is suspected if the patient shows evidence of upper gastrointestinal bleeding, or if ulcer-like pain recurs. The radiologic diagnosis is less exact than it is in duodenal ulcer because the radiologist may mistake a surgically created deformity at the suture line for ulceration, or miss a small ulcer in this area. Occasionally, the gastroscopist can visualize the ulcer, which almost invariably lies beyond or on the suture line. In most instances, it is only a presumptive diagnosis until proved at operation or autopsy. The presence of persistent occult blood, and the demonstration of significant acid secretion after histamine stimulation, reinforces a presumptive diagnosis of stomal ulcer.

Fortunately, stomal ulcer is not as common as it once was, for the incidence was as high as 35 per cent after gastroenterostomy alone. This led eventually to the abandonment of simple gastroenterostomy as a primary operation for ulcer. Following 65 per cent distal gastrectomy, the five-year incidence of recurrent ulcer is 2 to 4 per cent; following vagotomy and gastroenterostomy or pyloroplasty, it is 5 to 10 per cent; and after vagotomy and hemigastrectomy, it is approximately 1 per cent.

In the treatment of recurrent ulcer, medical measures should be tried initially, but they are generally unsuccessful. Stomal ulcer is either the result of failure to accomplish the intent of the original operation, or failure of the operation selected to reduce acidity sufficiently (Fig. 55). If the duodenum was transected, a portion of the antrum may have been left in contact with alkaline duodenal secretion. If resection of the body of the stomach was the primary purpose, it may have been inadequate, and in those patients in whom vagotomy was primarily depended upon, it may have been incomplete. Occasionally, the afferent loop in a gastrojejunal reconstruction is too long, which also favors recurrent ulceration. It is not a simple matter to determine whether vagotomy is complete. The usual test is the measurement of acid secretion after insulin-induced hypoglycemia. Unfortunately, insulin itself tends to inhibit the production of acid by the parietal cells, a direct action which is the opposite of the acid stimulation resulting from hypoglycemia. This may result in bizarre secretory patterns which are difficult to interpret; indeed, there is much confusion as to what constitutes a

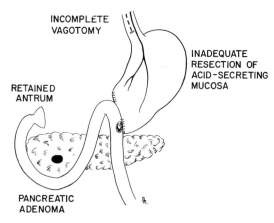

INCOMPLETE VAGOTOMY

INADEQUATE RESECTION OF ACID-SECRETING MUCOSA

RETAINED ANTRUM

PANCREATIC ADENOMA

Figure 55. Factors to consider in the etiology of stomal ulcer.

positive test and with respect to the frequency of incomplete vagotomy. Better tests are needed. 2-Deoxy-D-glucose may be better; it is a glucocytopenic agent in that it interferes with the utilization of sugar by the cell, does not inhibit the parietal cells and is a much more potent stimulator of the vagal mechanism than insulin. It has been employed clinically by Grossman and others.

The diagnosis of an ulcerogenic pancreatic adenoma is best made preoperatively as it may be otherwise difficult at operation to demonstrate the small adenoma in the pancreas, duodenum or splenic hilum. The history of diarrhea and particularly of excessively high levels of gastric acid secretion obligates the surgeon to find the tumor.

At operation, the pancreas and adjoining area are carefully examined for adenoma and if the duodenum was transected, the duodenal stump is inspected for the possibility of retained antrum. A previous incomplete vagotomy is completed and the question of how to reduce acidity further is carefully considered. If the antrum has been completely removed, and an incomplete vagotomy found, completion of the vagotomy should correct the ulcer diathesis. If distal resection was done, the addition of vagotomy is advisable, since Walters found that excellent results were obtained in 70 per cent of the patients previously treated by distal partial resection. If the previous procedure was vagotomy and pyloroplasty, or gastroenterostomy, residual vagus fibers should be searched for, particularly the posterior trunk, and the antrum excised.

The second alternative is a distal resection, which gave good results in 86 per cent of patients managed in this manner by Walters. The mortality following operations for stomal ulcer was 1 per cent following vagotomy, but when resection was necessary, the operative mortality was 15 per cent in Walters' series. There is some difference of opinion as to whether the previous anastomotic area should be excised when it is found to be indurated, even though resection may not be necessary to achieve a further reduction in acid secretion. Most surgeons are loath to disturb this area unless there is associated hemorrhage, obstruction or perforation.

GASTROJEJUNOCOLIC FISTULA. If a stomal ulcer develops following gastrojejunostomy, it may secondarily involve the colon, first by adhesions and later by fistula formation involving all three organs. The incidence of this complication has decreased since the marked decline in the popularity of simple gastro-

enterostomy. This complication of stomal ulcer is suspected if anorexia and diarrhea develop. The colonic contents tend to pass freely into the stomach, which explains the anorexia, and into the jejunum, leading to diarrhea. If left untreated, there is a marked loss of weight. The diagnosis is confirmed roentgenologically with a barium enema. A barium meal less frequently demonstrates the fistula because the pressure gradient is from colon to stomach. If this complication is treated before inanition develops, the jejunum and colon can be disconnected, the defect closed, and a definitive procedure carried out to prevent recurrent ulceration. If the treatment is delayed until the patient's condition becomes critical, the operation will have to be staged, the first stage being either a proximal colostomy, ileostomy or ileocolostomy. In the past 15 years, improvements in diagnosis, preoperative and operative techniques have almost eliminated the need for staged procedures in the treatment of these distressing problems.

OBSTRUCTION IN DUODENAL ULCER

If the peptic ulcer is juxtapyloric, every exacerbation will produce some degree of obstruction, but in the early phases of the disease this is largely due to edema and is only temporary. With each exacerbation and subsequent healing, fibrous tissue is laid down until eventually stenosis results which becomes irreversible. In these patients, vomiting of bile-free fluid is a prominent feature, physical examination will demonstrate the classic signs of a stomach distended with air and fluid, and radiologic examination will confirm that the stomach contains a large residue with markedly delayed emptying.

While an ulcer in the antrum can produce pyloric stenosis, this is much less common than obstruction due to duodenal ulcer. Gastric carcinoma developing in this area will generally have a shorter history, and if the stomach is aspirated prior to the examination, the radiologist can generally make this distinction. Rarely, the obstruction may be due to the adult form of hypertrophic pyloric stenosis, an extrinsic lesion which is usually malignant, or prolapse of a gastric polyp or the gastric mucosa.

Treatment is directed at gastric decompression, either by continuous gastric suction, or by aspiration of the stomach night and morning, combined with a liquid diet. The anticholinergic drugs are contraindicated because they serve to increase the retention. Usually, 48 hours of continuous suction will relieve any superimposed edema, and relief of the obstruction can be evaluated by plotting gastric intake against return. If the obstruction is relieved, an operation should be done, but not until several days of normal alimentation have elapsed. Relief of the obstruction should not lead to further medical procrastination, because these patients are generally overdue for surgical treatment. It is just such a patient who often has a markedly deformed duodenum at operation, and if further delayed, the hazards of operative treatment are thereby increased.

If there is no relief of the obstruction after a few days, operation is indicated. During the period of gastric suction, fluid and electrolyte deficiencies are slowly corrected, and the blood volume is restored if it is found to be reduced. Hypochloremic alkalosis and hypokalemia are frequently present in these patients with pyloric obstruction. In the very elderly or poor-risk patient, it may be necessary to perform a simple gastroenterostomy under local anesthesia. If this is done, the likelihood of subsequent development of stomal ulcer is high, and when their condition improves the addition of vagotomy under a general anesthetic should be seriously considered. When a definitive operation is undertaken in the patient who has suffered prolonged duodenal obstruction, it is wise to consider a concomitant gastrostomy and feeding jejunostomy, as anastomotic lines may be particularly vulnerable to edema and temporary partial obstruction. This is best relieved by administration of whole food via the jejunostomy.

Duodenal and Gastric Perforations

Perforation may complicate duodenal ulcer, gastric ulcer, stomal ulcer or carcinoma of the stomach, in descending order of frequency. Perforation may be minor and close within a short time, but it is generally major and may be associated with some bleeding. The amount of fluid discharged into the peritoneal cavity from perforated gastric and stomal ulcers is generally greater than that from duodenal lesions. The degree of peritoneal soiling is greater when the perforation occurs with a full stomach.

As in other catastrophies of sudden onset, the patient can pinpoint the beginning of symptoms with great accuracy, and the manner in which he relates his story usually makes it unnecessary to ask whether the pain came on suddenly or slowly. The patient is in severe pain and lies very quietly, resenting the slightest movement. Indeed, the peritoneal irritation is so marked that it may even cause distress if the examining table or the patient is jarred during the physical examination. The patient appears shocked and has a fast pulse, but the blood pressure is usually well maintained in the early hours of this catastrophe. The patient may vomit at the outset, but he does not do so repeatedly. Abdominal pain is generalized and may be referred to the acromial areas supplied by the cervical fifth and sixth nerves. Tenderness is generalized, and marked with rebound tenderness and extreme rigidity. The increase in muscle tone is greater than that seen in any other condition and is well named "boardlike." After a few hours, the abdominal rigidity decreases somewhat and signs of hypovolemic shock develop.

If there has been sufficient leakage, a pocket of air will be present which can be percussed in relation to the liver and demonstrated radiologically. For both examinations, the patient must be so positioned that the air which rises can be detected above the solid viscera. With the patient supine, the tympanitic air bubble will be found over the anterior aspect of the liver; with the patient lying on his left side, it will be in the right axillary line area. If the patient is able to stand, a chest film may demonstrate air beneath the left diaphragm, which may be difficult to differentiate from air in the stomach, but there may also be air under the right diaphragm which cannot be misinterpreted. Free air under only the left diaphragm suggests a perforated gastric ulcer. The subdiaphragmatic areas are more adequately demonstrated on a chest than on an abdominal film. If the patient is too ill to stand, he should be positioned lying on his left side with the film at his back in order to demonstrate free air in relation to the liver. If an anteroposterior film is made with the patient on a tilted x-ray table, free air will not be demonstrated unless it is massive. If the proper techniques are employed, free air will be demonstrated in more than three-quarters of these patients.

The differential diagnosis includes all thoracic, cardiac and major blood vessel catastrophies. While in the first six to 12 hours the symptoms may be mistaken for those due to acute pancreatitis, acute cholecystitis or closed-loop intestinal obstruction, after six hours or more, they may be more often mistaken for acute appendicitis. By then, the agonizing pain and rigidity may have been replaced by localized pain and tenderness over the right lower quadrant, and the initial slight leukocytosis will have increased. The changing symptons are due to gravitation of the fluid down the right iliac gutter, with beginning peritonitis in this dependent area.

If free air is not demonstrated, these other possibilities, particularly pancreatitis, should be considered. If the laboratory is equipped to perform a rapid serum amylase determination, it is worth waiting for this result. It is often elevated slightly in perforated ulcer, but not to the marked extent present in acute pancreatitis. The minimal perforation which closes spontaneously within a few hours results in a very confusing picture.

Severe pain presenting in the shoulders or root of the neck suggests a perforation of the lower esophagus, and this possibility should be ruled out before the abdomen is incised. A broadened mediastinum, a pneumothorax or hypdropneumothorax, as demonstrated by chest x-ray films, may be associated with rupture of the esophagus. Supraclavicular surgical emphysema may develop.

Perforation may occur as a complication of acute ulcer, as evidenced by a lack of previous ulcer history, and the lack of induration and scarring characteristic of a chronic ulcer at operation. Of those patients who do not have definitive surgical treatment for their ulcer disease at the time that the perforation is surgically closed, one-third remain symptom-free and will not require subsequent medical or surgical treatment for their ulcer. This group of patients have had a perforation of an acute peptic ulcer, and do not require anything but lifesaving surgery for this catastrophe. Approximately two-thirds of the patients treated by simple closure of the perforation will have significant ulcer symptoms subsequently, and about half this group, or one-third of the total group, have sufficient difficulty that definitive surgery for their chronic ulcer disease becomes necessary in the subsequent months or years.

As in the case of any perforated abdominal viscus, the earlier surgical intervention is accomplished the better. Except for uncontrolled hemorrhage, there is no abdominal surgical emergency in which each of the early hours of delay is more costly. The mortality is negligible in those patients treated within six hours, and increases steadily as the duration between onset and treatment increases. All patients should have a nasogastric tube passed and the stomach emptied, and most require some intravenous fluid. Although cultures from the peritoneal cavity are generally negative when treatment is instituted early, secondary bacterial invasion becomes superimposed upon the chemical peritonitis, and antibiotics are indicated. Those patients coming late for treatment may require preoperative transfusion, and if shock and anemia are present associated bleeding should be suspected.

At operation either simple closure or definitive treatment is employed. In either case, a supportive program is essential.

Simple closure of the perforation is an extremely satisfactory operation for the immediate problem. Through a modest incision, the anterosuperior aspect of the first portion of the duodenum should be inspected. It is here that over 90 per cent of the perforations will be easily located. As suggested by Graham, the most satisfactory method is the tacking of a portion of omentum over the defect. The duodenocolic appendage of the omentum adjacent to the inferior curve of the duodenum, between the duodenum and hepatic flexure of the colon, is easily available (Fig. 56). This is brought over the perforation and tacked with a few fine sutures to the duodenal wall. This seems preferable to a free omental graft, and the sutures do not have to be taken close to the ulcer where the wall is friable. This appendage of omentum has proved so useful in closing perforations and protecting duodenal stump closures after resection that we have termed it the "providential omentum." This does not tend to produce stenosis, as a suture closure of the perforation might do, and there is no danger of the sutures cutting through with secondary leakage. Neither should a purse-string closure of the perforation be attempted.

Definitive treatment, which has as its goal not only the problem of closure of the gastrointestinal tract, but also the correction of the ulcer diathesis, may be used in selected patients. Partial resection has been the standard operation, but in recent years vagotomy and antrectomy, or vagotomy and pyloroplasty, have been advocated. It was feared that mediastinitis would invariably result if the abdominal attic was opened and vagotomy performed in the presence of peritonitis, but this fear has not been realized. In these patients, the duodenum can usually be safely

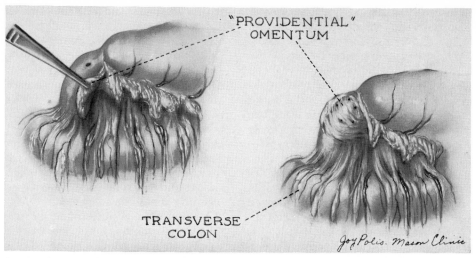

Figure 56.   For closing the perforated duodenal ulcer, the tag of gastrocolic omentum adjacent to the duodenum is tacked in a circumferential manner over the perforation with fine, interrupted nonabsorbable sutures.

transected unless there is an associated posterior duodenal ulcer, and gastrectomy is generally less difficult than when it is performed for obstruction or hemorrhage. Those who advocate pyloroplasty and vagotomy have a technical point in their favor, for the perforation is generally in an area which can be conveniently excised as part of the pyloroplasty procedure. If vagotomy is part of the definitive procedure, the peritoneum in the gastroesophageal area is left open to facilitate drainage from the abdominal attic. It is not clear at this time which of these three definitive procedures is preferable.

There are widely divergent opinions about whether a perforated ulcer should be treated by simple closure or by a definitive operation. Because gastric ulcers are more difficult to close, and because malignancy is always a possibility, resection is favored for the perforated gastric ulcer if the patient's general condition permits, and if frank peritonitis is not present. For duodenal ulcer, some surgeons advocate simple closure for all patients, arguing that the problem at hand is peritonitis and that further treatment is meddlesome. Others advocate definitive treatment almost routinely, restricting simple closure to those with late perforations, the elderly and the poor-risk patients. It is true that, with this selection of patients, a mortality rate for emergency resection comparable to that for elective resection can be achieved, but the overall mortality may be increased.

The majority of surgeons restrict definitive treatment to those patients who, on the basis of a long history and operative findings of a chronic duodenal ulcer, will probably need definitive treatment for their ulcer diathesis; those who are treated within a few hours of perforation but before generalized peritonitis is in evidence; and those who are good surgical risks. The indications for definitive treatment are broadened if the perforation is gastric. Simple closure is employed when the history and operative findings suggest that the ulcer is acute, when the interval since perforation exceeds six to eight hours, and when the patient is not an ideal candidate for operation. This individualization of the problem at hand is the preferable plan of management.

A third alternative, nasogastric suction and supportive treatment as a substitute for operation, has been explored by Seeley and Campbell. It has been adopted by others for the patient encountered late after perforation, and when the clinical symptoms are those of advanced peritonitis rather than perforation. The advocates of this method base their argument on the frequency with which spontaneous closure of the perforation is found at laparotomy. This policy should not be seriously entertained, because perforated ulcers have been found in the operating room, or in the morgue, which have failed to close spontaneously after several days. It is true that this nonoperative treatment may deserve consideration in the desperately ill patient seen late, with severe underlying metabolic, cardiac or respiratory disease.

However, even in the presence of generalized peritonitis and shock, there is an increased risk in diagnostic error; and the delay in treatment of a strangulating obstruction, for example, might deprive the patient of his only hope of survival. Even in the patient encountered late, with generalized peritonitis and advanced distention, the best chance for recovery may be by laparotomy. The thesis for operating upon desperately ill patients with diffuse peritonitis and advanced distention so severe as to create respiratory embarrassment has been expounded by Welch, and is in conformity with our experience.

Laparotomy is for surgical decompression of the intestine and for peritoneal lavage. The small bowel is stripped and aspirated free of gas and intestinal content for its entire length. The Baker long jejunostomy tube provides a facile method to accomplish this with speed and without contaminating spill. This tube, 6 feet in length, has a small, firm balloon at the end to permit traction and thereby easily advance the tube through the length of bowel. Inserted via purse-string suture into the jejunum 1 foot below the ligament of Treitz, it may be left indwelling postoperatively as a protection against distention until peristalsis is regained at about the fifth to seventh postoperative day. At the same time that the long tube is advanced through the intestine, the intra-abdominal fossae and loculated interintestinal pockets of pus are evacuated, the peritoneum being irrigated with copious amounts of saline to which has been added one of the antibiotics. The perforation, which by now may have been sealed over with exudate, is nevertheless securely closed by omentum and a gastrostomy is performed. While the mortality in such desperately late situations may be extremely high, some patients may be saved by these heroic methods: more, it is believed, than by gastric suction alone. This method of treating peritonitis is reserved for the more advanced condition, complicated by distention or obstruction, and the patient who has a septic course. It is admittedly unorthodox and requires more than the presently accumulated experience to prove the superiority that it is believed it should have.

GASTRODUODENAL HEMORRHAGE

Approximately 20 per cent of patients with peptic ulcer bleed at some time, and 5 per cent bleed massively. When the patient presents with gastrointestinal bleeding, the physician faces the problem of determining the site of bleeding and the volume and rate of blood loss. He must promptly pursue a dependable course which will control the emergency. This can be a challenging responsibility. The main difficulty lies in determining which patient will cease bleeding by conservative measures and which will die from lack of surgical control of the hemorrhage. This must be accomplished without permitting the patient to remain hypotensive for more than a very short period. Aird said, "The surgeon's aim is to have the opportunity of treating surgically on the second or third day after bleeding the patient who without surgical treatment would die on the fifth or eighth day."

The surgeon who has seen penetration and erosion into an artery in the base of an ulcer can appreciate that such bleeding can be fatal. Blackford, Smith and Affleck showed that in a six-year period in Seattle, with a population at that time of 350,000, there were 151 deaths from hemorrhaging ulcer. Wangensteen has stated that half the deaths from peptic ulcer disease are due to hemorrhage, and Allen has pointed out that hemorrhage in the older patient is often fatal.

The term "massive hemorrhage" refers to that group of patients in whom the symptoms and signs of hypovolemic shock appear. The blood loss required to produce these symptoms and signs varies with the rapidity of the bleeding and the age and general condition of the patient, but it requires an amount of 1500 ml. or more. After hemodilution, the hematocrit will be below 30 per cent and the erythrocyte count below three million.

Minor degrees of bleeding should be considered in a manner similar to pain as an index of intractability. If the patient is having repeated minor hemorrhages in spite of good ulcer management, operation is indicated. As is true with intractability, procrastination is unwise and, in this instance, much more dangerous, for the next hemorrhage may be massive, with a 5 to 10 per cent mortality. A patient who is subject to gastrointestinal hemorrhage should be operated upon if conservative management does not completely prevent this complication. If the patient's employment takes him far from good surgical treatment, good anesthesia and a plentiful supply of blood, this factor weighs heavily in favor of definitive interval treatment. If there is a specific problem in blood matching, the patient should also have surgical treatment. A follow-up of those patients who had a massive hemorrhage demonstrates that over half subsequently have surgery for their ulcer disease.

ETIOLOGY. The important causes of massive hemorrhage are peptic ulcer, gastric erosions, hemorrhagic gastritis and esophageal varices.

Gastric erosions are superficial epithelial defects which do not penetrate the muscularis as an ulcer does. They are most frequently multiple and often appear as a complication following operation, in association with indwelling gastric tubes and with a severe nonsurgical illness. They have been referred to as "stress" ulcers, although this term should probably be restricted to those ulcers resulting from experimentally induced stress.

The terms "hemorrhagic gastritis" and "gastroduodenal hemorrhagic diathesis" refer to those patients who ooze blood from the gastric mucous membrane in the absence of a frank ulcer or erosion. Hemorrhagic gastritis, usually with erosions, as a cause of minor or massive bleeding, is becoming commoner each year as an increasing number of new drugs are developed. As well as alcohol and the anticoagulants, phenylbutazone (Butazolidin), the Rauwolfia derivatives, cinchophen, steroids and salicylates may cause gastric bleeding. Aspirin is probably the commonest specific cause of hemorrhagic erosions, which are also a frequent complication of steroid therapy. When the bleeding is idiopathic, it is possible that it is the result of pituitaryadrenal mechanisms. Gastroduodenal bleeding may also complicate uremia. In large charity hospitals, esophageal varices may rank second as a cause of massive upper gastrointestinal hemorrhage. Uncommon causes are esophageal ulcer, hiatus hernia, esophageal laceration secondary to vomiting, blood dyscrasias and congenital hemorrhagic telangiectasis. Ulcerating malignancies invade rather than erode vessels and seldom bleed massively. Lymphosarcoma of the stomach is an occasional exception to this.

SYMPTOMS AND SIGNS. Gastrointestinal hemorrhage may manifest itself as hematemesis, melena, or the passage of bright red blood rectally. It is extremely important to bracket the level of bleeding in the gastrointestinal tract. If hematemesis has occurred, the source of the bleeding is proximal to the ligament of Treitz. In the absence of hematemesis, a gastric tube should be passed to determine whether or not the stomach contains blood. If bleeding from the duodenum is rapid, it will enter the stomach, otherwise it will be carried along the gastrointestinal tract. Thus, in massive hemorrhage associated with signs of shock, the presence of blood in the stomach indicates that the bleeding point is proximal to the ligament of Treitz, whereas its absence strongly suggests that it is beyond this point. If the bleeding is not massive, a stomach free of blood does not exclude the duodenum as a possible source. In the presence of massive bleeding, bright red blood per rectum may be coming from a lesion as high as the hypopharynx. The more minor the hemorrhage, the more likely is the source to be in the lower bowel. If the patient passes changed blood, the source of bleeding is proximal to the right hepatic flexure, as the concentration of digestive juices beyond this point is not sufficient to produce the characteristic picture of melena. To improve the accuracy of diagnosis, patients with gastrointestinal bleeding should be investigated while they are bleeding, to the extent that their general condition permits.

Although not completely reliable, the character of the hematemesis or gastric aspirate may provide a clue as to its source. In gastritis, the blood is inclined to be only moderate in amount and bright red; that from varices, darker and massive, whereas blood from an ulcer is flecked with "coffee grounds."

MEDICAL MANAGEMENT. In the medical management of massive upper gastroduodenal hemorrhage, the first 24 hours after admission are utilized for resuscitation and for diagnosis. On admission, blood is taken for determination of the hemoglobin, hematocrit, white blood count, prothrombin index, partial prothrombin time, bleeding time and clotting time, and for matching. If there is a suggestion of esophageal varices, a blood ammonia and serum bilirubin should also be taken; and if uremia is suspected, the blood urea nitrogen level should be determined. Dextran or blood is administered and the patient's clinical record begun.

A history is obtained from the patient, or his relatives, and particular attention is paid to dyspepsia, to any previous radiologic examination, to familial bleeding, and to the use of medication and alcohol. If a history suggestive of ulcer disease is obtained, it is of great value, as is a previous radiologic diagnosis. It is well to remember, however, that this does not necessarily establish the source of the bleeding. Palmer found that gastric erosions were the source of bleeding in many duodenal ulcer patients.

On physical examination, a particular search is carried out for jaundice, melanin spots or telangiectases in the mucous membranes, and for the tell-tale signs of cirrhosis: spider nevi, gynecomastia, liver palms, an enlarged liver or spleen, ascites, testicular atrophy and sparse pubic hair.

During the history and physical examination, the pulse and blood pressure are frequently monitored. At the completion of the physical examination, it will be apparent whether the patient has lost only a few hundred milliliters of blood, or whether he has had a truly massive hemorrhage. When blood becomes available, it should be given quickly until it is apparent that the replacement equals the loss, as manifested by pulse and blood pressure changes. The gastric aspirate may provide some evidence as to whether the bleeding is continuing or has ceased. If the patient's pressure remains low, the blood should be pumped in and a urinary catheter passed. The hourly urinary output should be charted as a measure of the effective renal perfusion. If the history and physical examination strongly suggest portal hypertension, with varices presumed to be the source of the bleeding, a Bromsulphalein determination should be done.

As soon as it is apparent that replacement is having a measurable effect, arrangements should be made for continuing the diagnostic program if the source of the bleeding is not yet known. If a skilled endoscopist is available, the patient's stomach should be washed out with generous quantities of iced water, and esophagoscopy and gastroscopy carried out. In general, the endoscopist is at a disadvantage in such crises, and his examination is less rewarding and more hazardous than a careful barium swallow and examination of the stomach and duodenum done without discontinuing blood replacement. Hemoglobin, hematocrit and, if available, serial blood volume determinations are obtained to supplement the half-hourly pulse and pressure record.

Specific treatment is indicated for those patients bleeding from esophageal or gastric varices. It should be remembered that patients with portal hypertension and varices have a much higher than average incidence of duodenal ulcer, and that 15 per cent of these patients will be bleeding from a duodenal ulcer or from gastric erosions. The radiologist should not terminate his examination when he has demonstrated esophageal varices, but should also examine the stomach and, particularly, the duodenum. A blood ammonia level above 120 is highly suggestive of cirrhosis, as is a Bromsulphalein retention above 30 per cent.

An esophagogastric balloon is not only of therapeutic use, but it is of considerable value in the diagnosis of bleeding varices. The double balloon tube is passed, the gastric balloon well inflated, and the tube pulled back until resistance is met. The tube must be maintained in this position or gastric varices will not be controlled. There are inherent dangers in the careless use of the tube, and if excessive traction is employed it can lead to nasal or pharyngeal ulceration, acute asphyxiation or esophageal rupture. Its position is maintained by taping it to a soft sponge at the nasal opening, following which the esophageal balloon may be inflated. Some surgeons find it unnecessary and hazardous to inflate the esophageal balloon, and depend on traction of the gastric balloon to control bleeding. This is also our experience. Gastroesophageal tamponade and cooling may be combined. If the stomach contains blood, it is washed out through the central lumen of the tube and evidence of further bleeding beyond the gastric balloon is sought. If the patient is being transported by air, particularly in an unpressurized aircraft, the balloon pressure should be reduced. If there is no further bleeding proximal or distal to the balloons, it is presumptive evidence that the bleeding is from varices. After about eight hours, the balloons can be decompressed, but they are left in position lest bleeding recur.

There is a marked difference of opinion among surgeons as to how long tamponade therapy should be continued, and if surgical intervention is carried out, whether it should be simply a ligation of the esophageal and upper gastric veins, or whether an emergency shunt should be done. As an additional diagnostic maneuver and as an aid in the selection of the shunting procedure, a percutaneous transplenic portogram may be done under local anesthesia and the portal pressure measured. If it exceeds 300 mm. of water, the patient almost certainly has portal hypertension and is probably bleeding from varices. Irrespective of whether treatment is conservative or surgical, an attempt is made to hurry the passage of blood out of the gastrointestinal tract, to reduce nitrogenous absorption, and to reduce the bacterial flora with oral antibiotics. It has been reported that nialamide will reduce the level of blood ammonia.

If the administration of as much as 2500 ml. of blood has been necessary during the diagnostic 24-hour period, and the patient shows evidence of continued bleeding from a source other than varices, he should be operated upon at that time. If the patient's condition has not improved significantly after the administration of large quantities of blood, in the absence of evidence of further bleeding, it has been shown that this critical condition may be the result of intractable shock rather than continued bleeding. The hourly output of urine may be reduced out of proportion to the patient's blood pressure, and provide a clue to the evidence of this irreversible state. Prolonged hypotension leads to anemic hypoxia of the brain, heart and kidneys. It is particularly important that prolonged hypotension be avoided in the elderly patient. If such a patient is operated upon, it will often be found that the bleeding has stopped, and that continuing blood loss was not the cause of the patient's critical condition. The mortality in such a situation is prohibitively high and will not be improved by surgery. In this connection, it should be emphasized that all these patients should be seen by a surgeon soon after they are admitted to the hospital, so that he can continue to evaluate their progress and assist in making the decisions regarding conservative and operative treatment.

Even if the patient is bleeding during this diagnostic and resuscitative period, he should be allowed fluid by mouth, which is aspirated by the continuous suction. This helps to keep the tube clear of clots and improves oral hygiene. The majority of patients cease bleeding during this diagnostic and resuscitative 24 hours, particularly those bleeding from hemorrhagic gastritis. If the bleeding has not stopped, operation is indicated. Unfortunately, there is no laboratory test which can be used as a guide to the cessation of hemorrhage. The best rule to follow is constant observation of the patient. If the pulse remains fast, if the blood pressure and hematocrit remain reduced, and if the patient is perspiring, all despite continuous blood replacement, common sense indicates that the bleeding is continuing.

Elderly arteriosclerotic patients tolerate prolonged bleeding badly, and conservative treatment in the face of continued bleeding is particularly hazardous in this group. The mortality over age 50 is six times that under 40 years; the mortality from gastric ulcer is twice that of duodenal ulcer, and the mortality is high in those patients who have hematemesis as well as melena. Operating on all patients as soon as they present with massive upper gastrointestinal hemorrhage has been tried as a plan of management, but a rigid operative program is as unsatisfactory as a rigid conservative program. Neither is a substitute for consultative individualization and careful observation. Those patients who stop bleeding and re-bleed in the hospital should be operated upon promptly, as well as those who continue to bleed.

OPERATIVE MANAGEMENT. Many patients with massive gastrointestinal hemorrhage come to operation after the transfusion of several liters of blood. Citrated blood tends to bind ionized calcium, a deficiency of which may lead to cardiac arrhythmia and interfere with the effectiveness of digitalis in the older patient, particularly in the presence of hyperkalemia. If many transfusions are necessary, 2 ml. of 10 per cent calcium chloride should be added to each unit of blood. If the patient has been on steroid therapy, intravenous preparations should be administered in liberal quantities.

One of the most difficult surgical problems is the operative management of the patient in whom hemorrhage has been so overwhelming that a preoperative investigation could not be done adequately, and in whom the preoperative investigations failed to demonstrate a possible source of the bleeding. Dunphy has outlined the operative management of these patients in a classic manner. An indication of a bleeding tendency is sometimes apparent as the abdominal incision is made. Unfortunately, clotting may be deficient after many transfusions; this will greatly aggravate both the diagnosis and the management.

As the abdomen is opened, evidence of portal hypertension should be looked for in the falciform ligament and omental veins, and as manifested by cirrhosis or ascites. Other intra-abdominal lesions which might explain the gastrointestinal hemorrhage are searched for, following which the esophageal hiatus is palpated, and the stomach carefully inspected and palpated. The duodenum is carefully examined for scarring, thickening or subserosal punctate hemorrhages which may point to an underlying ulcer. The lesser sac is opened so that the stomach can be palpated bimanually, and the duodenum mobilized to facilitate a further examination of the second portion. The surgeon must also consider that the bleeding may have come from the mid- or lower gut, such as a bleeding Meckel's diverticulum.

A 10-cm. incision is made, centered on the pylorus, and the duodenum carefully irrigated until it is free of blood. Rough handling or strong suction may initiate mucosal bleeding, making it impossible to decide whether the source has been found or is iatrogenic. If the examination of the duodenum as far as its curvature is inconclusive, attention should be directed to the stomach. If this cannot be completely examined through the pylorotomy wound with an endoscope, a proximal transverse gastrotomy should be done, and a gastric ulcer, erosions or diffuse bleeding sought. A bilateral truncal vagotomy permits the esophagogastric juncture and gastric fundus to be pulled down to a more accessible position. A gauze pack insinuated between the spleen and diaphragm protects against traction injury to the spleen. The entire inside of the stomach can now be adequately visualized and erosions so common to the upper fundus will be found and can be oversewn. If the source has not by now been found, and if on further examination of the duodenum blood has accumulated in this area, it should be opened at the ligament of Treitz and inspected proximally and distally. If the source of the bleeding still cannot be found, and this should be seldom true if the previously mentioned preoperative and operative methods have been followed, the surgeon must admit defeat and finish with a pyloroplasty, the vagotomy having already been accomplished. This procedure is now favored over blind gastrectomy by an increasing number of experienced surgeons. The source of the bleeding in these instances is usually from hemorrhagic gastritis or undiscovered erosions.

If a gastric ulcer is found, distal gastric resection should be carried out to include the ulcer, and the lesion examined for evidence of malignancy. While malignant gastric ulcers and frank carcinoma of the stomach are a frequent source of blood loss, they are an uncommon cause of massive hemorrhage. Biopsy, suture ligation of the ulcer base, vagotomy and pyloroplasty are being used with increasing frequency to control gastric ulcer bleeding, particularly if the ulcer is proximally situated and if the patient's general condition is poor. It is not yet apparent whether this will prove as satisfactory as resection.

Until recently, the mortality following operations for a massively bleeding duodenal ulcer remained above 5 per cent. In these patients, the ulcer is generally posterior and penetrating, posing a difficult technical problem. Simply excluding the ulcer does not always control the bleeding; when operative treatment is carried out for hemorrhage, the ulcer should be excised if gastrectomy is performed. It is in just this clinical situation that the unsuitable duodenum is frequently encountered, and the surgeon must deal not only with a difficult technical problem but with a desperately ill patient as well. All too frequently, the patient is grossly overweight and has a high-lying stomach.

Over the years, repeated attempts have been made to manage the problem of bleeding ulcer by visualization and ligation of the bleeding point, or ligation of the vessels external to the duodenum. These were unsuccessful in arresting the bleeding, or secondary hemorrhage resulted so frequently that this approach had to be abandoned.

In 1947, Hinton performed vagotomy alone for hemorrhagic gastritis, and in 1952, Dorton reported on pyloroplasty, suture of the ulcer bed and vagotomy. Weinberg and his associates independently reported on a similar approach, and for the first time a significant number of patients were reported upon with no mortality. Because of the previous unhappy experience with a local attack on the bleeding vessel, interest has naturally centered on the incidence of secondary hemorrhage following these more conservative procedures. Secondary hemorrhage in hospital has occurred, but the incidence has been surprisingly low.

In comparing this lesser procedure with gastrectomy, it must be pointed out that, even in this latter group, both in-hospital secondary hemorrhage and recurrent hemorrhage months or years later are by no means unknown. For some reason as yet obscure, there is more to the problem of gastroduodenal hemorrhage than simply the digestive erosion of a vessel wall. There is an increased incidence of postoperative bleeding in these patients both from the remaining gastric stump and from sutures lines remote from the ulcer. Moreover, if these patients develop an ulcer recurrence, they usually manifest it by bleeding rather than by a recurrence of ulcer pain.

Dorton had only one death in over 50 patients; Weinberg's mortality rate was also 2 per cent, and Farris and Smith reported a 4 per cent mortality. The last group had a 2 per cent in-hospital secondary hemorrhage rate, whereas Weinberg had a 4 per cent incidence of secondary in-hospital hemorrhage. Undoubtedly, a higher incidence of recurrent ulceration will follow these procedures than if vagotomy and antrectomy, or distal partial resection, were done; but it is extremely unlikely that these mortality figures can be approached or equaled in these desperately ill patients, if the duodenum is divided.

If the duodenum can be easily transected and the ulcer removed, most surgeons would elect this rather than pyloroplasty, suture of the ulcer bed, and vagotomy, particularly if the patient's general condition is satisfactory, but an increasing number are employing the lesser procedure. The precise role of these operations in the management of massive gastroduodenal hemorrhage awaits a longer evaluation. If the surgical mortality associated with bleeding can be kept below 5 per cent, the indications for surgical arrest of the bleeding can be broadened.

The duodenum is opened as far as necessary distally to expose the ulcer, and the incision extended proximally into the stomach for an equal distance. The ulcer bed is transfixed deeply with two sutures placed at right angles to each other to ensure hemostasis. Both absorbable and nonabsorbable sutures have been recommended, but if catgut is used the swaged needle used for gastrointestinal suturing is inadequate for this purpose. A larger needle such as the Murphy type is satisfactory, and the swaged needle and catgut used for abdominal closure is ideal. The pyloroplasty can be closed in the Finney manner or by Weinberg's modification of the Heineke-Mikulicz procedure.

The operative management of massive hemorrhage from gastric erosions is controversial because the etiology is unknown and no medical center has a large surgical experience. The mortality rate without surgical control is extremely high in those which bleed massively as a postoperative complication. Whether such erosions are from "stress" or drugs, or the bleeding is from activation of previous peptic ulcer, the chance of survival is less with nonintervention than with surgical intervention. In such instances the thoroughness with which the erosion is sought determines the outcome. In these desperately ill patients, it is a temptation to shortcut these steps. Some undiscovered erosions may stop bleeding spontaneously,

some after vagotomy, some after partial resection and some after near total resection. The majority of authorities favor vagotomy and pyloroplasty, reserving the "blind" near total or total resection for the significant number that rebleed. We are convinced that the surgical approach which permits direct inspection of the entire gastroduodenal mucosa seldom fails to disclose the bleeding site, and that, therefore, it is seldom necessary to resort to "blind" measures.

GASTRIC COOLING.   In recent years, gastric cooling has been employed for massive upper gastrointestinal hemorrhage. As developed by Wangensteen, it requires special balloons and a refrigerating apparatus which will pump alcohol at low temperatures through the balloon. It was developed because of the demonstration that acid peptic digestion, like all enzymatic processes, is greatly retarded at lower temperatures, and gastric blood flow is probably also reduced. With the proper equipment, bleeding has been arrested in a promising percentage of patients with duodenal ulcer and varices, more than would be anticipated by the natural history of massive upper gastrointestinal hemorrhage. The vascular supply of the stomach is extremely generous; temperature reduction in the stomach cannot be effected by the mere introduction and withdrawal of cold saline. Outflow temperatures of 10 to 15°C. are optimal. The method is an expedient to control the hemorrhage, it does not protect against recurrent bleeding. Gastric cooling has not been as effective in controlling bleeding from gastric ulcer, and is ineffective in hemorrhagic gastritis and carcinoma.

GASTRIC ULCER

While chronic gastric and duodenal ulcer are both the result of peptic erosion due to either an increase in acid pepsin or a decrease in tissue resistance, they have important differences. Gastric ulcer is less common, occurs in an older average age group, is more evenly divided between the sexes and the symptomatology is less typical than that of duodenal ulcer. Chronic gastric ulcer is more resistant to medical measures, yet is more easily controlled by conservative surgery than duodenal ulcer. Erosions and acute ulcers do not progress to chronic ulcers as frequently as they do in the duodenum. It has been noted that lack of tissue resistance is probably a more important side of the equation in gastric ulcer than hypersecretion, for the average patient with gastric ulcer secretes less than the normal amount of acid and pepsin. Dragstedt's theory of antral hyperfunction, and the question of atrophic gastritis as a precursor of gastric ulcer, have also been noted. In duodenal ulcer, the prime aim of treatment is a reduction in acidity; but in gastric ulcer, the excision of the ulcer, the correction of antral stasis and the reduction of gastric acidity may all be beneficial and favor healing.

MALIGNANT GASTRIC ULCER. The most important difference between duodenal and gastric ulcer is the matter of malignancy. When a patient presents with a gastric ulcer, there is a real possibility that it is malignant. An ulcerated lesion in the stomach whose nature is unknown is well named an "indeterminate" ulcer, because it is possibly benign and possibly malignant. When patients with indeterminate ulcer are first evaluated, it is impossible to rule out malignancy by any or all of the methods available (Table 2). There is a marked overlap in the age groups, and a long ulcer history does not exclude malignancy. In Marshall's series, half the patients had an ulcer-like history of five or more years' duration.

Lesions on the lesser curvative and in the antrum are more likely to be benign, and those on the greater curvature more likely to be malignant. There are, however, many exceptions to this generalization. Extremely small ulcers are generally benign and heal promptly, but some are malignant.

It is the clinician's responsibility to maintain a high index of suspicion when a patient presents himself with indigestion, and ask for a radiologic examination. It is the radiologist's responsibility to find a lesion if one is present, and the newer image amplifiers have increased the accuracy of this examination. Whereas his diagnostic accuracy in cases of frank gastric cancer is high, the radiologist is unable to differentiate accurately between benign and malignant gastric ulcers. There are a number of radiologic signs which are helpful in the differentiation, but the question remains unanswered in a significant percentage of patients.

Gastroscopic examination is also helpful, but even when combined with an experienced radiologic opinion, 10 per cent of the ulcers remain indeterminate. If there is an active duodenal ulcer, the gastric acidity and the secretory pattern will be high, in which case malignancy in the associated gastric lesion is rare. Duodenal deformity in the absence of a duodenal ulcer crater, however, may not be due to present or previous duodenal ulcer disease. Improved methods of cytologic examination and the use of new flexible gastro-

Table 2. *Considerations in Differential Diagnosis of Benign and Malignant Gastric Ulcers**

	BENIGN	MALIGNANT
Age	Younger	Older
Length of history	Long, may be short	Short, may be long
Ulcer-like symptoms	Probably present	Does not exclude if present
Location of ulcer	Low on lesser curve and in antrum: 80% benign	Cardia, body: 50% malignant; greater curve: 85% malignant
Size of ulcer	Very small: usually benign	More common in large ulcers; but some huge ulcers are benign
Radiologic appearance	Ulcer base outside gastric wall	Ulcer base inside gastric wall
Gastroscopic appearance	If well visualized, this and the radiologic examination are 50 to 75% accurate; combined, they reach 90%.	
Gastric acidity	The higher it is, the higher the percentage of benign lesions.	
Duodenal ulcer	If there is an ulcer, the gastric lesion is almost certainly benign; if the duodenum is only deformed, the deformity may not be due to duodenal ulcer disease.	
Gross appearance	Frankly malignant lesions are easy to recognize; even after excision there is a margin of error in the indeterminate ulcer.	
Frozen section		
Cytologic appearance	If any one of these is positive, the diagnosis is established; but if negative, malignancy is not excluded.	
Gastroscopic biopsy		

* Total accuracy: 90 per cent.

scopes with which a biopsy can be taken are establishing the presence of malignancy earlier and in a much higher percentage of cases than was possible a few years ago. False negatives, however, occur frequently and a negative report does not exclude malignancy. Even at operation, some of these ulcers remain indeterminate until a histologic examination is completed. In a large series of patients, these factors show significant differences, but there is always some overlap. When an individual patient is seen for the first time with a gastric ulcer which is not a frank carcinoma obvious to all concerned, the combined intelligence of the internist, the surgeon, the radiologist, the gastroscopist, the cytologist and the director of laboratory services will not reduce the incidence of error below 10 per cent.

MEDICAL MANAGEMENT. Some surgeons have adopted the extreme position of recommending prompt removal of all gastric ulcers. In favor of this policy is the argument that the issue is rapidly and, from the standpoint of cancer, more safely settled. The resection of malignant gastric ulcers, in contrast to gastric cancer, yields a five-year survival rate of approximately 40 per cent. Against this extreme position, however, is the fact that many of these are only acute ulcers which will heal promptly; gastric resection is not without mortality and mobidity, and finally, it is doubtful whether a short period of medical management will significantly affect the survival rate of those lesions which subsequently prove to be malignant. We would not advocate immediate operation except in those ulcers situated on the greater curvature, in which the incidence of malignancy is very high; or when a previous gastric ulcer has recurred; or in those patients in whom medical treatment is almost certain to be unsuccessful. This includes the ulcer that has penetrated deeply beyond the gastric wall, patients in whom there is an associated gastric or pyloric obstruction, and those in whom there is perforation or uncontrolled bleeding.

Some of the acute ulcers may be secondary to drug therapy, particularly salicylates and steroids. Because a decreased local tissue resistance may be an important part of the gastric ulcer equation, anything that will improve the patient's general condition may be beneficial. With the use of anticholinergic drugs, diet and rest, a three-week therapeutic and diagnostic trial is instituted. At the end of this time, the radiologist and gastroscopist should be asked to evaluate the lesion, at which time approximately half these indeterminate ulcers will have healed, or will be measurably reduced in size. The remainder should be operated upon promptly.

Under such a regimen, a significant percentage of these lesions will prove malignant. Marshall reported a series in which 15 per cent were malignant, and Pearson and Jones reported a 9 per cent incidence of malignancy. It should be emphasized that the prognosis in these patients is vastly superior to that for frank carcinoma, and there is no justification for a fatalistic attitude toward this problem.

Of those ulcers which heal, or show evidence of healing under this intensive regimen, a very small percentage will be malignant, because occasionally a malignant ulcer responds to medical management. All these patients should continue their medical treatment, and must have further evaluation of the ulcer over the next three months. If there is any evidence of recurrence or an increase in size, they should be operated upon forthwith.

Patients with ulcers which remain healed should be seen frequently, and the radiologic examination repeated if symptoms recur at any time. They are candidates for the development of recurrent ulcer, a new gastric ulcer or, eventually, of carcinoma. Larson and Hayes have re-emphasized that the long-term results of the medical management of gastric ulcer are poor, and that if these patients are carefully followed, over 10 per cent will eventually develop carcinoma of the stomach. In addition, two-thirds of these patients will have a recurrence of their gastric ulcer within ten years, at which time operation should be advised without a further trial of medical therapy. Malignant ulcers will be found with increasing frequency, and many of these patients will have a frank carcinoma of the stomach. The ulcer may be in a new location, and if gastric cancer has developed, it may arise in an area remote from the previous ulcer. Because of the long time interval, it is doubtful if the late development of malignancy in these patients can be explained on the basis of a slow-growing malignant lesion, and because they may develop malignancy in an area remote from the site of the original ulcer, they are by no means all benign ulcers that have become malignant.

It is extremely difficult to determine

whether benign ulcers become malignant, but it is clear that the stomach which develops a gastric ulcer has a predisposition to the subsequent development of gastric malignancy. Following operation for gastric ulcer, most of the gastric mucous membrane is preserved and this residual gastric mucosa is also susceptible to malignant degeneration. Helsingen followed a series of patients after surgical treatment for duodenal and benign gastric ulcer and found an increased incidence of carcinoma of the residual stomach in those operated upon for benign gastric ulcer.

OPERATIVE MANAGEMENT. As well as recommending surgical treatment for patients whose ulcers fail to heal promptly, and those in whom symptoms continue in spite of good medical management, it must be recognized that there are patients who almost invariably fail to respond to a conservative regimen. In the operative management of gastric ulcer, the question is not whether a gastric ulcer can become malignant, or whether atrophic gastritis predisposes to both gastric ulcer and carcinoma, but whether this indeterminate ulcer is malignant. Evidence of malignancy is sought at operation, an evaluation which is not completely reliable in the absence of metastases. If the lesion is distal and appears to be benign, a conservative distal partial gastrectomy which circumscribes the ulcer is performed. At this time, gross examination of the lesion in the opened stomach and microscopic examination of a frozen section of any suspicious portions of the ulcer margin establish the true nature of the lesion with a high degree of accuracy. If proved to be malignant, a wider resection is performed, including the regional node-bearing structures. Surgical therapy for benign lesions can usually be completed by a gastroduodenal reconstruction, if the duodenum is normal. The mortality rate following distal partial resection for benign gastric ulcer is less than that for duodenal ulcer, and the postoperative morbidity is significantly less.

It has been appreciated for many years that gastric drainage, a reduction in gastric acidity by distal resection, or simple removal of the ulcer may be curative. Kelling and Madlener found that distal resection, leaving an ulcer situated high in the stomach in situ, was frequently followed by healing of the ulcer. Walton treated over 300 patients with gastric ulcer by wedge excision and gastroenter-

ostomy, and reported only a small recurrence rate. On the other hand, Balfour was disappointed with his results in over 500 patients with gastric ulcer, upon whom he did a wedge excision and gastroenterostomy. He personally came to favor distal resection to include the ulcer.

More recently, Movius and Weinberg, and Farris and Smith, have re-explored the role of conservative surgical procedures in the treatment of gastric ulcer. Farris currently recommends leaving the ulcer in situ if multiple biopsies are negative for malignancy, followed by pyloroplasty. If there is an associated duodenal ulcer, he advocates the addition of vagotomy. A long term follow-up of a significant number of patients will be of extreme interest and importance.

Although we advocate distal resection to include the ulcer, a more conservative approach may be indicated for the ulcer situated high on the lesser curvature or in the fundus. At the present time, it is impossible to state the relative importance of vagotomy, antrectomy and pyloroplasty in favoring the healing of a benign gastric ulcer. No ulcer should be left in situ without taking several biopsies from the ulcer margin, and even under these circumstances, an area of malignancy may be missed. In most high ulcers on the lesser curvature the lesion can be safely resected, leaving an adequate amount of the greater curvature of the stomach for anastomosis (Fig. 57). Because in these instances a clamp placed on the lesser curvature above the ulcer might encroach upon the esophageal area, it is placed only part way across the stomach. Under direct vision, a minimal amount of normal tissue is then taken with the ulcer, and the specimen carefully examined for evidence of malignancy. If benign, the lesser curvature can be reconstructed so as not to encroach upon the opening of the esophagus. The "tubed" stomach is then anastomosed, usually to the duodenum. In the absence of malignancy, a total gastrectomy should not be done for these high lesions.

HEMORRHAGE, PERFORATION AND OBSTRUCTION. It has been noted that bleeding from a gastric ulcer carries a higher mortality, and when it is known to be the source of bleeding, it often tips the scales in favor of surgical intervenion. When a gastric perforation is found, the indications for resection rather than simple closure are broadened. Pyloric

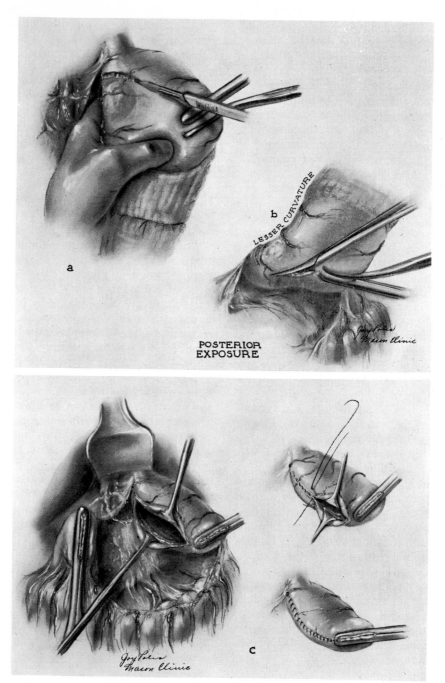

Figure 57.   A method of resecting the ulcer high on the lesser curvature of the stomach. After the stomach is freed and the duodenum transected, the level of resection and anastomosis is marked on the greater curvature by a Payr clamp. Then, without the aid of vertical clamps which might encroach upon the esophagus, the ulcer and lesser curvature are removed by sharp dissection. *a*, Anterior view, and *b*, posterior view. *c*, This vertical lesser curvature incision is then closed under direct vision with two rows of sutures, and the greater curvature stump is anastomosed to either the duodenum or the jejunum.

obstruction from gastric ulcer is often an indication for operation and, less commonly, gastric ulcer may obstruct the body of the stomach.

CARCINOMA

Carcinoma of the stomach is responsible for almost one-quarter of all cancer deaths, killing about 30,000 people in the United States and Canada annually. Relative to population, the actual incidence of carcinoma of the stomach appears to be declining in the United States. Males are affected almost twice as often as females.

Carcinoma of the stomach is approximately three times more common in people with pernicious anemia than in the normal population. Whether this is secondary to the gastric atrophy which is always present is not known. Similarly, there is some question as to whether gastric polyps progress to invasive carcinoma.

PATHOLOGY. Carcinoma of the stomach is grossly polypoid, ulcerating or diffusely infiltrating. Microscopically, it is adenocarcinoma, colloid or undifferentiated carcinoma simplex. The ulcerating form is the commonest gross lesion and the undifferentiated carcinoma is the most malignant. Spread occurs along the tissue planes of the gastric wall, hence pyloric lesions may spread a short distance into the duodenum, and proximal lesions into the lower esophagus.

Lymphatic spread occurs early; even in those patients who appear to be curable, the lymph nodes are involved in 75 per cent, reducing the five-year survival by more than half. Depending on the location of the lesion, the nodes most often involved are those in relation to the greater curvature and pylorus, those along the lesser curvature and celiac axis, and those in relation to the hilus of the spleen and pancreas. The most difficult nodes to remove completely are the celiac nodes and those in relation to the pancreas. Direct extention to the pancreas, colon and other neighboring organs is not uncommon. When the lesion penetrates to the serosa, peritoneal implants flourish, particularly where they are shed onto the greater omentum and into the pelvic cul-de-sac; subsequently, ascitic fluid is formed. Supraclavicular nodes are involved late in the disease. Venous invasion is also common, the organs most often affected being the liver and the lungs.

SYMPTOMS AND SIGNS. These patients may present with indigestion, pyloric obstruction or loss of weight. Frequently, the indigestion is ulcer-like and has a surprisingly long history. Gastrointestinal complaints may be entirely absent, with anemia or fatigue as the prominent symptoms. Anorexia is the most frequent initial symptom.

Those patients with a history of gastric ulcer or pernicious anemia should be followed very carefully, and any patient over 45 years of age who develops anorexia or indigestion for the first time should be considered to have carcinoma of the stomach until proved otherwise. About 15 per cent of patients with gastric cancer present with a change in bowel habit, probably secondary to the anorexia. This may lead to a negative investigation of the colon, allowing the gastric carcinoma to go undiagnosed for several more months. Elderly patients with longstanding complaints, such as a hernia or prostatism, may begin to feel poorly as a result of their developing carcinoma but may attribute this to the obvious condition. Unless the clinician is on his guard, he may easily be misled.

There are no signs in the early stages, but there may be clinical evidence of pyloric obstruction as the lesion advances, or a mass may be palpated in the gastric area. An irregular enlargement of the liver, ascites, a rectal shelf and grossly enlarged supraclavicular nodes are all signs of distant spread.

The clinician's responsibility is to suspect a gastric lesion, and the radiologist's responsibility is to find the lesion, if one is present. The radiologic diagnosis is much more accurate in frank carcinoma of the stomach than in malignant gastric ulcer. Cytologic techniques are quite accurate, but in this situation their use is almost academic, and the same can be said about the high incidence of achlorhydria and hypochlorhydria. Occult blood in the stools should drive the clinician on to find the lesion in the gastrointestinal tract.

DIFFERENTIAL DIAGNOSIS. Ninety-five per cent of gastric tumors seen clinically eventually prove to be carcinoma, the remainder being benign tumors and sarcomas. Because carcinoma of the stomach is so much more common than a gastric gumma, those patients with a positive Wassermann test and a large gastric defect probably have carcinoma of the stomach and should be treated as such, rather than put on a course of antiluetic therapy.

TREATMENT. Having made a presumptive diagnosis of carcinoma of the stomach, the first question to be answered is that of operability. The presence of an epigastric mass is associated with a very poor prognosis, particularly if it is fixed; but it is not an absolute contraindication to laparotomy, because some of these tumors are still resectable. An enlarged, hard and irregular liver generally indicates inoperability, but the presence of tumor in one of these masses should be confirmed by needle biopsy, if no other evidence of inoperability can be found. A high rectal examination should be performed, searching for peritoneal seedings in the pelvic pouch, the well-named "rectal shelf." Ascites also indicates inoperability, which can be proved by aspiration of fluid and a search for malignant cells. A preoperative chest roentgenogram should always be made. Enlargement of the supraclavicular lymph nodes is for some reason the first thing looked for when inoperability is mentioned, even though spread here is generally late. At times, however, this may be the only evidence of inoperability. Suspicious nodes should be biopsied before inoperability is assumed. At operation, a search is made for distant intra-abdominal spread, which denotes incurability in about 25 per cent of patients at the time of laparotomy.

In spite of incurability, a palliative resection can be seriously considered, particularly when obstruction or bleeding has been a prominent feature of the disease. In most instances, however, evidence of incurability at operation terminates the procedure. If these signs are absent, the surgeon must decide whether he can encompass the tissues grossly involved by the malignant process. Involvement of the transverse colon or the body or tail of the pancreas does not preclude resection.

In all curative gastric resections for carcinoma, an attempt is made to remove en bloc the first portion of the duodenum and the subpyloric nodes, all of the greater omentum with the nodes along the greater curvature, the spleen, the gastrohepatic omentum and the nodes in relation to the celiac axis. If the lesion is distal, more duodenum is removed. If the tumor lies in the proximal stomach, a thoracoabdominal approach is usually necessary. It is essential to get at least two inches beyond the gross limits of the tumor. Reconstruction of the gastrointestinal tract is accomplished in the proximal lesions by esophagojejunostomy, and a storage area is created by a long enteroenterostomy (Fig. 58). In selected proximal lesions, the distal portion of the stomach may be preserved and anastomosed to the esophagus after performing a pyloroplasty to facilitate gastric drainage. While anastomosis of the esophagus to the duodenum is technically possible, it is not frequently employed because it leaves the patient with two areas in his reconstructed gastrointestinal tract where local recurrence may produce obstruction. In distal lesions, the tumor is widely encompassed and the gastric remnant sutured to the jejunum.

Total gastrectomy is not employed as a palliative procedure, but when necessary is done to widely encompass the tumor. Its routine employment was unsuccessful in improving the survival rate of patients with prepyloric carcinoma of the stomach.

PROGNOSIS. The reported results vary widely, depending on whether the indeterminate gastric ulcers later proved to be malignant are included with frank carcinoma. The five-year survival rate of 40 per cent for

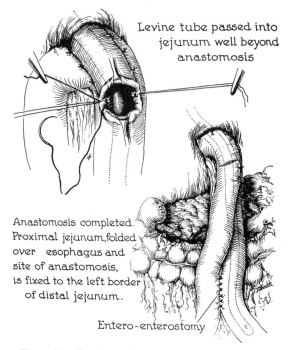

Levine tube passed into jejunum well beyond anastomosis

Anastomosis completed. Proximal jejunum, folded over esophagus and site of anastomosis, is fixed to the left border of distal jejunum.

Entero-enterostomy

Figure 58. Esophagojejunostomy following total gastrectomy, after the technique of Roscoe Graham. The loop of jejunum has been tacked to the diaphragm behind the hiatus, and the infradiaphragmatic portion of the esophagus is laid on the anterior surface of the distal limb of jejunum and fastened there by means of interrupted silk sutures. The anastomosis is then made between the open end of the esophagus and the side or the distal limb of jejunum. (From Graham, R.: A technique for total gastrectomy. Surgery 8:262, 1940.)

malignant gastric ulcer must be compared with the 15 per cent figure for frank carcinoma. If a gastric ulcer previously thought to be benign is treated conservatively, and eventually is recognized to be carcinoma after a long period of medical management, the five-year survival rate approximates that of frank carcinoma rather than the much more favorable figure for malignant gastric ulcer.

If 100 patients present with carcinoma of the stomach, 25 will be clinically inoperable, and at operation the tumor can be resected for cure in only 50. The natural history of carcinoma of the stomach is such that there are no five-year survivors among those patients who could not have a resection for cure. Of the 35 that have positive nodes, only seven will be alive at the end of five years; of those 15 with negative nodes, eight will be alive after five years, for a total of 15 patients. Of those resected for cure, there will be a 25 to 30 per cent five-year survival. The presence of positive nodes reduces the survival rate by more than one-half, a situation which holds generally in surgery for cancer. The operative mortality is approximately 5 per cent, which is scattered among the three groups operated upon. Radiation offers little for these patients and chemotherapy has not been effective in this area to date.

SARCOMAS

About 3 per cent of gastric tumors are either leiomyosarcoma, lymphosarcoma, reticulum cell sarcoma or Hodgkin's disease. Pseudolymphoma of the stomach, a benign condition, may be erroneously diagnosed as lymphosarcoma by the pathologist. Although the last three may represent localized disease in a generalized lymphoblastoma before it has become manifest elsewhere, the results of resection are surprisingly good. The resectability rate and the five-year survival are sufficiently rewarding to justify surgical treatment. In these lesions, in contrast to carcinoma, postoperative radiation is of value and palliation can be achieved in the nonresectable case. A leiomyosarcoma may present as a massive gastric hemorrhage.

BENIGN TUMORS

In order of frequency, benign tumors are polypoid adenomas, leiomyomas, tumors arising from aberrant pancreatic tissue, fibromas, neurogenic tumors, lipomas and vascular tumors. They are usually found on radiologic examination and prove at operation to be other than carcinoma.

Aberrant pancreatic tissue is seen at operation as a submucosal mass in the distal stomach or proximal portion of the duodenum. Adenomatous polyps are generally single but may be multiple, in which case they must be differentiated from inflammatory polyps. Inflammatory polyps do not undergo malignant degeneration, and while histologic evidence of malignancy may be demonstrated in adenomatous polyps, simple removal is almost always curative, as shown by Huppler and Priestley. The management of these at operation is similar to that of large bowel polyps. If single, they can be removed and examined by frozen section, and further treatment is unnecessary unless there is malignant invasion of the stalk. If the stalk is invaded, a more extensive operation should be done. If the polyps are multiple, partial gastrectomy is the method of choice, with fulguration of any polyps left in the remaining portion of the stomach. A polyp with a long pedicle may prolapse through the pylorus and cause symptoms of intermittent pyloric obstruction or gastrointestinal bleeding.

READING REFERENCES

Avery Jones, F.: Modern Trends in Gastroenterology. (Second Series.) London, Butterworth & Co., 1958.

Baker, J. W.: The management of gastric ulcer. Bull. Mason Clinic 15: 101, 1961.

Baker, J. W., Boyd, R. S., and Foster, R. A.: Gastric resection with exclusion of a complicated duodenal ulcer: analysis of 122 cases. Ann. Surg. 142: 519, 1955.

Baker, J. W., and Ritter, K. J.: Complete surgical decompression for late obstruction of the small intestine, with reference to a method. Ann. Surg. 157: 759, 1963.

Beaumont, W.: Experiments and Observations on the Gastric Juice and the Physiology of Digestion. Plattsburg, F. P. Allen, 1833.

Blackford, J. M., Smith, A. L., and Affleck, D. H.: Peptic ulcer emergencies: study of massive hemorrhages and acute perforations treated during diagnosis of 916 private cases suffering from peptic ulcer. Am. J. Digest. Dis. 4:646, 1937.

Brackney, E. L., Thal, A. P., and Wangensteen, O. H.: Role of duodenum in the control of gastric secretion. Proc. Soc. Exper. Biol. Med. 88:302, 1955.

Burke, J. F., Pontoppidan, H., and Welch, C. E.: High output respiratory failure: an important cause of death following peritonitis or ileus. Ann. Surg. 158:581, 1963.

Checketts, R. G., Gillespie, I. E., and Kay, A. W.: Propanthelene as an agent for medical vagotomy. Gut 7:200, 1966.

Dorton, H. E., Webb, J. G., and Royalty, D. M.: Vagotomy and pyloroplasty. A simple safe solution to the bleeding ulcer problem. J. Kentucky State M. Assoc. 50:16, 1952.

Dragstedt, L. R.: The physiology of the gastric antrum. Arch. Surg. 75:552, 1957.

Dragstedt, L. R., and Owens, F. M., Jr.: Supradiaphragmatic section of vagus nerves in treatment of duodenal ulcer. Proc. Soc. Exper. Biol. Med. 53:152, 1943.

Dragstedt, L. R., and others: Quantitative studies on the mechanism of gastric secretion in health and disease. Ann. Surg. 132:626, 1950.

Edwards, L. W., and others: The surgical treatment of duodenal ulcer by vagotomy and antral resection. Am. J. Surg. 105:352, 1963.

Eisenberg, M. M., Emas, G. S., and Grossman, M. J.: Comparison of the effect of 2-deoxy-D-glucose and insulin on gastric acid secretion in dogs. Surgery 60:111, 1966.

Ellison, E. H., and Carey, L.: Diagnosis and management of the Zollinger-Ellison syndrome. Am. J. Surg. 105:383, 1963.

Farmer, D. A., and others: The effect of various surgical procedures upon the acidity of the gastric contents of ulcer patients. Ann. Surg. 134:319, 1951.

Farris, J. M., and Smith, G. K.: Vagotomy and pyloroplasty for bleeding duodenal ulcer. A note on selective vagotomy. Am. J. Surg. 105:388, 1963.

Farris, J. M., and Smith, G. K.: Role of pyloroplasty in the surgical treatment of gastric ulcer. Supplement. Ann. Surg. 154:293, 1961.

Farris, J. M., and Smith, G. K.: An evaluation of temporary gastrostomy—a substitute for nasogastric suction. Ann. Surg. 144:475, 1956.

Gillespie, I. E., and Kay, A. W.: The effect of medical and surgical vagotomy on the augmented histamine test in man. Brit. M.J. 1:1557, 1961.

Goligher, J. C., Pulvertaft, C. N., and Watkinson, G.: Controlled trial of vagotomy and gastroenterostomy, vagotomy and antrectomy and subtotal gastrectomy in elective treatment of duodenal ulcer. Brit. M. J. 1:455, 1964.

Goligher, J. C., Pulvertaft, C. N., and Franz, R. C.: A comparison of surgical methods in the treatment of duodenal ulcer. Personal communication.

Graham, R. R.: Treatment of perforated duodenal ulcers. Surg. Gyn. & Obst. 64:235, 1937.

Gregory, R. A.: Secretory Mechanisms of the Gastrointestinal Tract. London, Edward Arnold, 1962.

Griffith, C. A., Harkins, H. N., and Nyhus, L. M.: Surgery of the Stomach and Duodenum. Boston, Little, Brown & Co., 1962.

Harrison, R. C., Lakey, W. H., and Hyde, H. A.: The production of an acid inhibitor by the gastric antrum. Ann. Surg. 144:441, 1956.

Helsingen, N., and Hillestad, L.: Cancer development in the gastric stump after partial gastrectomy for ulcer. Ann. Surg. 143:173, 1956.

Hollander, F.: The insulin test for the presence of intact nerve fibres after vagal operations for peptic ulcer. Gastroenterology 7:607, 1946.

Huppler, E. G., and others: Diagnosis and results of treatment in gastric polyps. Surg. Gyn. & Obst. 110:309, 1960.

Johnston, D., Goligher, J. C., and Duthie, H. L.: Medical vagotomy: an assessment. Brit. M. J. 2:1481, 1966.

Jordan, G. L., DeBakey, M. E., and Cooley, D. A.: The role of resective therapy in the management of acute gastroduodenal perforation. Am. J. Surg. 105:396, 1963.

Kay, A. W.: Effect of large doses of histamine on gastric secretion of HCl: augmented histamine test. Brit. M. J. 2:77, 1953.

Larson, N. E., Cain, J. C., and Bartholomew, L. G.: Prognosis of the medically treated small gastric ulcer. New England J. Med. 264:119; 330, 1961.

Marshall, S. F.: The relation of gastric ulcer to carcinoma of the stomach. Ann. Surg. 137:891, 1953.

Mixter, G., Jr., and Hinton, J. W.: Massive hemorrhage of the upper gastrointestinal tract: indications for subtotal gastrectomy or vagotomy. Am. J. Gastroenterol. 28:71, 1957.

Moore, F. D.: Surgery in search of a rationale. Eighty years of ulcerogenic surgery. Am. J. Surg. 105:304, 1963.

Movius, J. H., DaGradi, A. E., and Weinberg, J. A.: Conservative resection for gastric ulcer. Am. J. Gastroenterol. 22:136, 1954.

Osborne, M. P., and Dunphy, J. E.: Identification of cause of obscure massive upper gastrointestinal hemorrhage during operation. Arch. Surg. 75:964, 1957.

Palmer, E. D.: Observations on the vigorous diagnostic approach to severe upper gastrointestinal hemorrhage. Ann. Int. Med. 36:1484, 1952.

Porter, R. W., Movius, H. J., and French, J. D.: Hypothalamic influences on hydrochloric acid secretion of the stomach. Surgery 33:875, 1953.

Rosemond, G. P.: Injuries involving hollow viscera both closed and penetrating. *In*, Hawthorne, H. R., Frobese, A. S., and Sterling, J. A.: The Acute Abdomen and Emergent Lesions of the Gastrointestinal Tract. Springfield, Illinois, Charles C Thomas, 1967, p. 354.

Sircus, W.: The intestinal phase of gastric secretion. Quart. J. Exper. Physiol. 38:91, 1953.

Smithwick, R. H., Farmer, D. A., and Harrower, H. W.: Some comments on recurrent ulceration after various operations for duodenal ulcer based upon the acidity and peptic activity of the gastric contents. Am. J. Surg. 105:375, 1963.

Thompson, J. C., and Peskin, G. W.: Collective review. The gastric antrum in the operative treatment of duodenal ulcer. Surg. Gyn. & Obst. 112:1, 1961.

Walters, W., Chance, D. P., and Berkson, J.: A comparison of vagotomy and gastric resection for gastrojejunal ulceration: a follow-up study of 301 cases. Surg. Gyn. & Obst. 100:1, 1955.

Walton, A. J.: *In*, Maingot, R.: Abdominal Operations. New York, D. Appleton-Century Co. Inc., 1940.

Wangensteen, S. L., and others: Intragastric cooling in the management of hemorrhage from the upper gastrointestinal tract. Am. J. Surg. 105:401, 1963.

Weinberg, J. A.: Vagotomy and pyloroplasty in the treatment of duodenal ulcer. Am. J. Surg. 105:347, 1963.

Welch, C. E., and Rodkey, G. V.: A method of management of the duodenal stump after gastrectomy. Surg. Gyn. & Obst. 98:376, 1954.

Westlund, J. C., Movius, H. J., and Weinberg, A. J.: Emergency surgical treatment of the severely bleeding duodenal ulcer. Surgery 43:897, 1958.

Zollinger, R. M., and Ellison, E. H.: Primary peptic ulcerations of the jejunum associated with islet cell tumors of the pancreas. Ann. Surg. 142:709, 1955.

The Small and Large Intestine

by
ROBERT M. ZOLLINGER, M.D.
and
COLIN T. HOWE, B.M., B.Ch.

ROBERT MILTON ZOLLINGER was born in Ohio and educated at Ohio State University and its Medical School. After receiving his education and training in surgery in Boston and Cleveland, he returned to his own medical school as its Professor of Surgery, and Chairman of the Department. The interest of the surgical faculty at Ohio State University in the diseases of the intestinal tract, pancreas and spleen has been long and productive of distinguished contributions. Dr. Zollinger's interest, abilities and energy have been given unsparingly to the area of education and training in surgery. His influence has been important and impressive.

Educated at Winchester College and Magdalen College, Oxford, COLIN HOWE received a Bachelor of Medicine degree and his clinical education in medicine at the Middlesex Hospital, London. After his service in the Royal Army Medical Corps, he was a registrar at Hillingdon Hospital, London. Then followed two years as research clinical assistant in the Department of Surgical Studies, Middlesex Hospital, where his research was devoted to problems in gastroenterology. For one year, he was a Visiting Research Fellow in the Department of Surgery at Ohio State University. He is Senior Lecturer in Surgery at King's College Hospital Medical School and Consultant Surgeon to King's College Hospital, London.

DUODENUM

INTRODUCTION. The duodenum is the first part of the small intestine, and its importance lies in its anatomic and physiologic relationships with the stomach, pancreas and common bile duct. Surgical lesions of the duodenum, apart from benign ulceration, are uncommon; and the relative immunity of this portion of the body to neoplastic disease is one of the most interesting problems of oncology. Because surgical diseases other than ulceration are rare, the duodenum is seldom considered as a possible site of trouble. This fact, combined with the difficulty of radiologic examination and the retroperitoneal position of the duodenum, often leads to delay in diagnosis.

ANATOMY. Except for its first part, the duodenum is retroperitoneal. It consists of four parts, closely applied to the retroperitoneal organs of the area between the bodies of the first and third lumbar vertebrae. Its position varies according to the position of the patient. It is roughly C-shaped, enclosing in its concavity the head of the pancreas, which is adherent to it. The first part, approximately two inches long, ascends from the pylorus to the right and posteriorly. It is anterior to the important structures in the hepatoduodenal ligament and forms the inferior border of the foramen of Winslow. Posterior to it are the inferior vena cava and the upper pole of the right kidney.

The second part of the duodenum is entirely retroperitoneal and lies in the right paravertebral gutter. It is approximately three inches long and is covered by the peritoneum of the infracolic compartment of the peritoneal cavity, which separates it from the coils of small bowel. It is crossed by the transverse colon and its mesentery. The hilum of the right kidney and right renal vessels lie behind it, and the bodies of the lumbar vertebrae and inferior vena cava are medial to it. The head of the pancreas is intimately applied to its inner aspect. The common bile duct and pancreatic duct enter the second part of the duodenum on its posteromedial aspect, their common entry being marked by the papilla on the mucosal aspect of the bowel; but they may enter by separate openings.

The third part of the duodenum arches transversely across the vena cava and aorta at the level of the body of the third lumbar

689

vertebra. It is 3 to 4 inches long and lies behind the peritoneum of the infracolic compartment. The root of the mesentery crosses its terminal portion obliquely, and it is also crossed by the superior mesenteric artery and vein. Superiorly, it is related to the uncinate process of the pancreas.

The fourth part of the duodenum is variable in length and is often difficult to distinguish from the third part. It curves up to the left to the duodenojejunal flexure, to which is attached the suspensory ligament of the duodenum, the ligament of Treitz. This is a band of fibromuscular tissue, which blends above with the right crus of the diaphragm and below with the circular muscle of the bowel wall.

Only the first part of the duodenum is readily accessible to exploration during laparotomy. Kocher's method of mobilization is used to examine the second part. The peritoneum along the lateral border of the second part is incised, and by blunt dissection the duodenum and contained head of the pancreas are lifted anteriorly and medially. This maneuver may be made easier by preliminary mobilization of the overlying hepatic flexure and proximal part of the transverse colon. In some patients, the third and fourth parts may be satisfactorily examined only by mobilizing the entire right side of the colon and transverse colon.

The intimate association of the duodenum with the head of the pancreas and with important structures such as the common bile duct and portal vein means that these are often involved by diseases of the duodenum. Adequate surgical excision of duodenal lesions may involve removal of the head of the pancreas, and reanastomosis of the common bile duct, as well as the pancreatic duct, to the intestinal tract. Its proximity to the right kidney, hepatic flexure and lumbar sympathetic chain accounts for some injuries of the duodenum which have been recorded during operations on these structures.

PHYSIOLOGY. The duodenum receives gastric juice through the pylorus, and biliary and pancreatic secretions through the duodenal papilla. The volume of fluid rich in electrolytes entering the duodenum is approximately 5 to 6 liters per 24 hours. Loss of the duodenal contents, either by vomiting due to obstruction or through an external duodenal fistula, quickly depletes the body of water and electrolytes.

The duodenum plays a role in the control of gastric secretion, the rate of gastric emptying and the motility of the stomach. It is thought that there are "osmoreceptor" cells in the duodenal wall and that when these are stimulated by hyperosmotic fluid discharged from the stomach, they cause contraction of the pyloric musculature. The rate of gastric emptying is reduced, so that only a little at a time is delivered into the duodenum. This mechanism protects the normal individual against the sudden entry of a hypertonic meal into the small bowel soon after its consumption. Such a precipitate emptying of the stomach often occurs after operations which remove or alter the pyloric mechanism, and this causes symptoms.

The release of acid gastric contents into the duodenum depresses the rate of gastric acid secretion. This constitutes a "feed back" mechanism which controls excessive secretion of acid by the stomach. The duodenum also depresses acid production by the elaboration of a specific inhibitor, enterogastrone, when stimulated by a mixture of bile and fat. The duodenal mucosa is also stimulated by contact with acid gastric contents and food to produce secretin and pancreozymin, which stimulates pancreatic exocrine secretion, and enterokinase which activate the pancreatic enzymes. Oral intake is restricted, therefore, in patients with acute pancreatitis in order to reduce stimulation of the pancreas by the secretin and pancreozymin in the duodenum.

The peristaltic movements of the normal duodenum have been studied intensively since cineradiography and image intensification made x-ray studies more precise. The first part is often referred to as the "duodenal pump," since periodically it delivers small quantities of barium into the second part, whence they are carried rapidly through the duodenal loop to the jejunum. The duodenal pump mechanism helps to control the rate of gastric emptying, and the rapid transit of the bolus through the remainder of the duodenum prevents this portion of the bowel from having any major absorptive function.

Brünner's glands, which are characteristic of the duodenal mucosa, start at the pylorus and extend down to the jejunum. They secrete a small amount of viscid, clear mucus. This mucus may protect the duodenal mucosa from digestion by the acid gastric juice. The mechanisms which control the secretion from these glands are unknown, but certainly the entry of acid solutions into the duodenum increases the volume of mucus produced.

CLINICAL SYMPTOMS. The symptoms of all duodenal disease, other than duodenal ulcer, fall into four main groups: pain, obstruction, anemia, and those due to blocking of the adjacent bile and pancreatic ducts (Fig. 59).

The pain is commonly precipitated by meals, and it may be relieved by antacids. However, the characteristic periodicity of ulcer dyspepsia may be lacking and the pain is usually more persistent. The pain is epigastric or right hypochondriac in site, and because of the retroperitoneal situation of the duodenum it often radiates to the back. It may mimic the pain of duodenal ulcer, cholelithiasis or pancreatitis.

Obstruction of the duodenum may occur without pain as a prominent symptom, particularly when the obstructing lesion is in the proximal parts. The cardinal symptom of high duodenal obstruction is a feeling of distention and nausea after meals; it is relieved by vomiting. The character of the vomitus depends on the site of the obstruction. If this is below the entry of the bile and pancreatic duct, the vomitus is bile-stained, but if above that level it is indistinguishable from the vomitus seen in pyloric stenosis.

The metabolic disturbance caused by vomiting from complete duodenal obstruction is particularly severe and rapidly progressive because large volumes of fluid and electrolytes are involved. The exact electrolyte disturbance depends on the site of obstruction. If it is above the duodenal papilla, more chloride is lost than the sodium and potassium combined, and a severe extracellular alkalosis is produced, as in pyloric stenosis. If the obstruction is below the duodenal papilla, the vomitus contains pancreatic juice and bile; therefore, more sodium and potassium than chloride are lost, together with considerable quantities of bicarbonate. Replacement therapy is different in the two conditions; relatively larger amounts of anion are necessary to correct the first condition, and larger amounts of cation to correct the second condition.

A characteristic symptom of a surgical disease of the duodenum is chronic anemia from slow and persistent bleeding. The anemia is of the hypochromic, microcytic, iron deficiency type caused by chronic blood loss. The symptoms are those of the overlying anemia: listlessness, lethargy, poor exercise tolerance, dyspnea and palpitations, and the fecal occult blood test is usually positive. A few patients have severe gastrointestinal hemorrhage and melena.

The common bile duct is often obstructed by lesions in the second part of the duodenum, particularly neoplasms, and the symptoms are indistinguishable from those caused by carcinoma of the bile duct or head of the pancreas. Even pathologic examination may fail to show whether a neoplasm originates in the duodenum or pancreas. Slowly progressive jaundice is the main complaint, with its usual associated symptoms of diarrhea and the passage of pale, offensive and bulky stools. Occult blood in these stools may give them a diagnostic silvery or aluminum appearance. The urine passed is dark, and there may be generalized pruritus.

Investigations specifically directed at duodenal function are few and diagnosis is usually made by an upper gastrointestinal roentgenographic examination. With conventional methods, repeated examinations of duodenum are often necessary before early lesions can be seen, because the barium passes rapidly through the duodenum and the overlying coils of the small bowel often obscure the third and fourth parts.

A recently developed fluoroscopic technique, hypotonic duodenography, gives much clearer pictures of the duodenum. A small nasogastric tube is passed and guided under fluoroscopic control into the first part of the duodenum. The duodenum is then made inert by the instillation of a local anesthetic and the parenteral administration of an atropine-like substance. The immobile duodenum is then outlined by injected radiopaque material. Air or oxygen is then insufflated. This technique gives a very exact outline of the whole of the mucosa of the

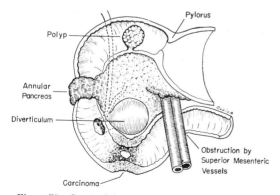

Figure 59. Surgical diseases of the duodenun. All these conditions, except diverticula, are uncommon in comparison with duodenal ulcer.

duodenum and reveals small deviations from normality.

Aspiration of the duodenal contents through a nasogastric tube is used to determine whether there is bleeding and to study pancreatic exocrine function, but it gives no specific information about the function of the duodenum. Cytologic examination of this duodenal aspirate may show the presence of malignant cells, if a carcinoma is present. To exclude anemia, jaundice or body fluid disturbance, the appropriate examination of the blood, liver function and electrolyte levels should be carried out.

Endoscopic examination of the duodenum beyond the first part is not yet possible, despite the recent development of more flexible endoscopes. Blind biopsy through the various appliances for small bowel biopsy rarely obtains representative sections of the suspected lesion, unless the lesion is widespread and affects considerable portions of the bowel mucosa.

An exploratory laparotomy may be the only certain method of determining the existence or exact nature of duodenal disease. Adequate exposure is necessary, and if doubt still exists after thorough palpation of the suspect part, the duodenum should be opened and biopsy performed. Careful closure of duodenal incisions without tension is essential to avoid the dangerous complication of a duodenal fistula.

ANOMALIES. Most congenital lesions of the duodenum present their problem in neonatal or early infant life and demand immediate treatment. Occasionally, however, no symptoms are produced until adult life. This is particularly true when obstruction is caused by an annular pancreas, or by a partial mucosal diaphragm in the duodenum itself. The latter may occur anywhere in the duodenum, and it is due to failure in recanalization of this portion of the gut during development. The degree of obstruction varies, but even when symptoms do not start until adult life, only a small orifice may be present in the diaphragm.

In annular pancreas, a ring of pancreatic tissue surrounds the second part of the duodenum; this is due to persistence and malrotation of the ventral outgrowth of the foregut which forms part of the pancreas. The symptoms are precipitated by an attack of pancreatitis affecting the ectopic pancreatic tissue. This explains the onset of duodenal obstruction rather late in life.

The obstructing mucosal diaphragm is simply excised. Duodenal obstruction due to annular pancreas should be treated by some form of by-pass operation, preferably a duodenojejunostomy. Simple division of the constricting ring of pancreatic tissue may result in a pancreatic fistula.

DUODENAL DIVERTICULUM. Diverticula of varying size are a common incidental finding during radiography of the upper gastrointestinal tract; estimates of their incidence vary from 0.85 to 33 per cent of the population. Diverticula are found more often in women than men, and 90 per cent are solitary. They are usually classified as primary or secondary, the latter group being caused by deformity due to duodenal ulceration or traction by an inflamed gallbladder. Of the primary diverticula, 70 per cent occur in the second part of the duodenum, mostly on its concavity, and the mouth of the diverticulum is immediately adjacent to the site of entry of the common bile duct. Often, this duct and the major pancreatic duct may open into the diverticulum itself. Patients with duodenal diverticula commonly have diverticulosis of the colon as well.

It is difficult to assess the significance of a diverticulum found during routine radiologic examination, particularly when it is the only abnormality found in a patient with vague upper abdominal unhappiness and a tendency to complain.

If a diverticulum produces definite complications, such as obstruction of the bowel or ampulla of Vater, if it becomes inflamed and causes cholangitis or pancreatitis, or if it develops a large enterolith in its cavity, the need for surgical treatment is obvious. When the symptoms are less definite and mimic those of gallbladder disease, ulcer dyspepsia or hiatus hernia, the decision whether to operate is more difficult. Surgical excision of an uncomplicated duodenal diverticulum is rarely advocated unless it is quite large and retains barium for over 24 hours. All other possible sources of the patient's complaints must first be excluded. Surgical treatment may be difficult, owing to the close relationship of many of the diverticula to the biliary and pancreatic ducts. Operation for a duodenal diverticulum should not be lightly advised because it carries a mortality of 5 to 10 per cent.

TRAUMA. The duodenum is protected by the overlying organs and is injured in only 9 per cent of patients with blunt abdominal injury. The retroperitoneal parts are particularly affected, due to their relative fixity and their relationship to the rigid vertebral bodies.

The degree of injury varies from a complete tear of the wall of the duodenum, or transection, to a mere bruising of the wall of the viscus. Sometimes, a large hematoma may form in the wall of the duodenum. This injury presents fairly constant clinical symptoms.

The patient is often a child, and gives a story of mild trauma to the upper abdomen, although this is often concealed to prevent parental punishment. After a period during which they complain little, the patients notice upper abdominal and right hypochondriac pain which may radiate to the back or right shoulder tip. Coincidentally, they start vomiting, the vomit often being copious and bilestained. These various symptoms slowly worsen. A mass may be present in the right upper abdomen with epigastric tenderness and a succussion splash. Such a history and physical findings should suggest the diagnosis and plain roentgenography may confirm it. This may show a dilated stomach and a dilated proximal duodenum, with a gas-fluid level and haziness of the right psoas shadow. If the patient's condition permits, an upper gastrointestinal series should be done. This confirms the duodenal obstruction. A marked leukocytosis is also a constant feature.

The treatment is usually operative, although some patients have improved on a conservative regimen. Laparotomy discloses a large tense hematoma, most often surrounding the second or third parts of the duodenum. The mucosa and serosa are usually intact, although occasionally blood may have leaked out causing a hemoperitoneum. This tense hematoma compresses the lumen of the bowel, thus causing obstruction. It has been suggested that such a hematoma expands slowly by osmotic attraction of fluid into it, like a subdural hematoma. This would explain the slow progression of the symptoms. At operation, the hematoma should be evacuated, but if the mucosa is lacerated as well, a more formal repair is necessary.

Because a small retroperitoneal tear of the duodenum can be missed, diagnosis is often difficult even at laparotomy. Preliminary x-ray examination may show the right kidney outlined by air which has leaked from the duodenum. The mortality from such duodenal injury remains high owing to difficulties in diagnosis and to the associated injuries, particularly of the pancreas. The abdominal cavity should be explored if duodenal injury is suspected, and the torn bowel should be repaired or excised.

DUODENAL ILEUS. In the early part of this century, subacute duodenal obstruction due to compression of the duodenum by the superior mesenteric vessels was commonly described. The patients were characteristically "asthenic" and suffered from "visceroptosis." Later, little was heard of this syndrome and its validity was often questioned. The superior mesenteric vessels cross the third part of the duodenum and are believed to compress the duodenum against the abdominal aorta. Radiologic and manometric evidence of such obstruction has been found in some patients. Typically, the obstruction can be temporarily relieved by having the patient lie face down. Some believe that the obstruction is caused by kinking of the bowel at the attachment of the suspensory ligament.

If a patient with symptoms of partial duodenal obstruction and loss of weight is shown by roentgenographic examination to have a dilated duodenum, and if there is narrowing of the third part which disappears when the patient is prone, operative relief of the obstruction may relieve the symptoms.

TUMORS OF DUODENUM. A primary tumor of the duodenum is rare, and carcinoma at this site comprises only 0.3 per cent of all bowel carcinomas. Duodenal carcinomas may be found anywhere in the duodenum, but approximately two-thirds occur near the papilla, the others being distributed evenly above and below this site. They are adenocarcinomas, and they spread into the pancreas and to the lymph nodes of the porta hepatis, celiac axis and pancreas.

Symptoms of anemia due to occult bleeding, obstructive jaundice, or pain like that of a duodenal ulcer may be present. Pain is a common symptom and is particularly persistent, radiating to the back when the growth invades the pancreas. Fluoroscopically, a carcinoma of the duodenum may be visible as an abnormality of the normal mucosal pattern of the bowel, as a filling defect, as an ulcer or as a fixed narrowing of the lumen of the bowel. The only hope of cure lies in radical excision of the growth and of the lymph nodes likely to be involved, since local excision of a malignant growth of the duodenum is followed rapidly by recurrence. This means that the head of the pancreas must often be excised with the duodenum. Even with radical surgical excision, long-term results are poor. The five-year survival rate after pancreaticoduodenectomy for this condition is less than 30 per cent. Due to delay in diagnosis, many duodenal carcinomas are inoperable when first diagnosed, and only palliation can be offered by some form of by-pass operation.

All types of benign tumors have been described as occurring in the duodenum, such as adenoma, lipoma, leiomyoma and fibroma, but they are all rare. They cause the same symptoms as malignant neoplasms, and their differentiation is often impossible without exploration and biopsy. If the tumor is benign, local excision of the lesion should be adequate, although for technical reasons the head of the pancreas may have to be excised if the growth is in the second part of the duodenum. Malignant forms of all these benign tumors also occur in the duodenum, and they should be treated in the same way as a carcinoma.

Ulcerogenic pancreatic tumors may occur in ectopic pancreatic islet tissue in the wall of the duodenum. When a tumor of the pancreas cannot be found in a patient with intractable peptic ulceration, the duodenum should be explored. Ulcerogenic tumors are usually found on the concavity of the second part of the duodenum, and approximately one-half of them are malignant. The treatment depends on the histology of the growth. A benign tumor may be locally excised, but if it is malignant, radical excision should be attempted. Total gastrectomy to remove the source of acid may be the only way to prevent further ulceration, since the incidence of multifocal sources for this potent hormone has been estimated to occur in at least 50 per cent of patients.

Regional enteritis, scleroderma and carcinoid tumor may affect the duodenum, but these are really surgical curiosities at this site. The symptoms they produce are often indistinguishable from those of other obstructive duodenal disease.

DUODENAL FISTULA. Fistulae between the lumen of the duodenum and adjacent organs or the skin are usually caused by operation, but they may be due to disease. Internal fistulae may connect the duodenum with the biliary apparatus or other organs, such as the colon. A gallstone ulcerating its way into the duodenum may form a fistula between the gallbladder and duodenum. Sometimes, the symptoms of cholelithiasis will be relieved by this discharge of gallstones into the bowel through an internal fistula. Unfortunately, the gallstones may impact in the small intestine and cause an intestinal obstruction or "gallstone ileus." An ulcer or a carcinoma of the duodenum may erode into the gallbladder or bile duct and form a fistula.

The development of a choledochoduodenal fistula due to peptic ulceration is usually marked by an exacerbation of the ulcer symptoms and periodic episodes of jaundice. An internal biliary fistula due to any cause makes the patient liable to attacks of ascending infection of the biliary tree, but this is more common when the fistula is caused by an ulcer or carcinoma of the duodenum. Roentgenography can help in the diagnosis of a fistula. A plain film of the abdomen may show air in the biliary tree, or barium may enter the gallbladder or bile duct during a barium meal examination.

Operation is not always necessary, as for example, when the passage of a gallstone through a fistula has relieved the patient's symptoms and no further stones remain in the gallbladder; but operation should always be recommended if cholangitis has occurred. The treatment for cholecystoduodenal fistula should be cholecystectomy with closure of the defect in the wall of the duodenum. If the fistula is caused by a duodenal ulcer, the ulcer must be excised, the defect in the bile duct closed and a partial gastrectomy performed.

An external duodenal fistula usually results from operation and is commonly caused by complications affecting the duodenal stump after gastrectomy of the Polya—Billroth II type. If the afferent loop becomes obstructed, or if the duodenum is insecurely closed, leakage from the duodenal stump may occur. Duodenal fistulae may also follow inadequate closure of a perforated duodenal ulcer, or damage to the duodenum during right colectomy, nephrectomy, adrenalectomy or even appendectomy. These fistulae cause digestion of the skin at their external opening, and rapid loss of the electrolyte-rich fluid derived from the pancreas and the stomach.

The four aims of treatment are to protect the skin, to replace and reduce the losses of fluid and electrolytes, to maintain adequate nutrition and to induce the fistula to close. The skin must be protected by applying protective aluminum or silicone paste, or by placing the patient so that the fistulous opening is in a dependent position. Continuous suction on a "sump" drain placed well into the fistulous tract is the most efficient way of collecting the secretions and keeping them off the skin. A plastic ileostomy bag which adheres to the skin around the fistulous opening will also give some protection and allow accurate measurement of the fluid loss. The volume of secretions can be reduced by large doses of anticholinergic drugs. The loss of fluid from the fistula should be measured and replaced volume-for-volume by parenteral fluids. A feeding jejunostomy may be needed to maintain nutrition. Some external duodenal fistulae close slowly with such a conservative regimen, but many require operation. Prevention during the time of primary operation is the "best cure" of a duodenal fistula.

AORTODUODENAL FISTULA. After resection of an abdominal aortic aneurysm, with graft replacement, the upper anastomosis is immediately related to the third and fourth parts of the duodenum which lie anteriorly. An increasingly common complication of such operations is the slow erosion of the duodenal wall near the anastomosis, either by direct pressure or by sepsis. Although there may be small warning hemorrhages, the usual end result is a catastrophic bleed through an aortoduodenal fistula, and few patients have survived such an episode.

THE JEJUNUM AND ILEUM

The jejunum and ileum show the same apparent immunity to the development of new growths as the duodenum, despite the evidence that, in this region of the bowel, the normal rate of formation and shedding of the epithelial cells is very high. Since the small intestine is the main area for absorption of digested food, many of its diseases present symptoms of some disorder of absorption. The various malabsorption syndromes usually come under the care of the gastroenterologist, but some can be dealt with by surgical treatment.

ANATOMY. The small intestine measures approximately 20 feet from the duodenojejunal flexure to the ileocecal valve. The mesentery supporting it fans out from an origin only 6 to 8 inches long. This runs on an oblique line crossing the posterior abdominal wall from the left to right, from the duodenojejunal flexure to the right iliac fossa.

There is no sharp distinguishing line between the jejunum and ileum, but there are certain differences between the upper and lower small intestine which can be seen by the naked eye or felt during laparotomy. The lumen of the jejunum is wider than that of the ileum, and its wall is thicker due to the prominent circular folds in its mucous membrane, known as valvulae conniventes. Since the mesentery of the jejunum is not so laden with fat, the lymphatics or "lacteals" are more easily seen. The arterial arcades in the mesentery of the jejunum are short, and the vasa recta are large and long. In contrast, the ileum is narrower, and its wall feels thinner because the valvulae conniventes are less prominent and farther apart. The mesentery is more laden with fat, and its vascular pattern is different from the pattern in the jejunal mesentery. There are more arterial arcades, and the vasa recta are shorter. The differences in the distribution and size of the valvulae conniventes in the two parts of the small bowel are important in distinguishing between distention of the high or low small intestine on x-ray examination.

PHYSIOLOGY. The convolutions, villi and mucosal folds of the small intestine provide an area of approximately nine square meters for the absorption of digested food. Besides absorbing the bulk of the food and fluid ingested each day, the small intestine reabsorbs about 5 liters of the digestive juices produced by the salivary, gastric and pancreatic glands, and the 2.5 liters of digestive juice produced by the jejunum itself. As a result, only 300 ml. of fluid per day enters the cecum. Interference with this absorptive function, whether due to obstruction or to mucosal disease, causes severe changes in the fluid and nutritional economy of the body.

The digestive juice of the jejunum is called succus entericus. It is secreted partly by cells in the crypts of Lieberkühn and partly by the disintegration of mucosal cells containing enzymes. The factors which control the rate of formation of succus entericus are not known, except that the entrance of a meal into the small intestine increases the secretion.

The small intestine can be considered an endocrine organ since it manufactures certain chemical transmitters which influence other organs. Fat and bile salts inhibit both gastric secretion and gastric contractions. The inhibitor may be a hormone, produced by the small intestine and known as entero-gastrone, or it may be a substance produced during the breakdown and assimilation of fat. There is also evidence that, when the small intestine is distended, it manufactures a substance which can stimulate gastric secretion. It is also responsible for the elaboration and absorption of histamine, another stimulant of gastric secretion.

Distributed throughout the small intestine are cells known as argentaffin cells because of their affinity for silver salts. These cells elaborate serotonin (5-hydroxytryptamine). The function of serotonin is unknown, but it may play a part in normal intestinal peristalsis.

The terminal ileum is the principal site for the absorption of vitamin B_{12}, so that disease or excision of this part of the intestine may cause a macrocytic anemia. The ileum is also an important site for the manufacture of vitamins, particularly those of the B complex and vitamin K. These vitamins are synthesized by the bacteria normally present in the bowel lumen. Interference with the normal bacterial flora by the use of broad-spectrum antibiotics or by surgery may prevent their formation.

The assessment of the absorptive function of the small intestine is usually carried out by the physician, using biochemical balance studies. In addition to these biochemical tests, biopsy of the mucosa can be obtained by an ingenious suction device fitted to a tube which is passed through the mouth into the intestine. The material obtained is examined initially under the dissecting microscope or hand lens. The mucosal villi can be clearly seen, and any deformation of shape or atrophy can be assessed. Sections are stained and studied and special stains may be used to detect the presence or absence of specific enzymes.

Roentgenographic examination of the small intestine is of crucial importance in diagnosis, but it is a very time-consuming procedure for both the patient and the roentgenologist; it should not be ordered indiscriminately. Visualization of the small intestine is not easy since the coils of bowel continually change their position in the peritoneal cavity. Repeated fluoroscopy and many photographs during the time when the barium is traveling down the small bowel are necessary to get satisfactory views of suspicious areas. When no lesion can be found in the stomach, duodenum or colon, and the occult blood test is persistently positive, the small bowel should be re-examined repeatedly. When there is a history suggestive of partial occlusion of the superior mesenteric artery, an aortogram should be made. The narrowing at the origin of the artery can be demonstrated by taking lateral films of the abdomen after the injection of dye.

TRAUMATIC INJURIES. The small intestine may be injured either by penetrating wounds or by blunt trauma. Acceleration and deceleration forces may produce injury to the fixed points of the gastrointestinal tract, particularily the duodenojejunal and ileocecal areas. Most of the knowledge of treatment of these conditions comes from experience with battle casualties. As a result of the increase in automobile accidents, abdominal trauma now forms an important part of civilian surgical practice.

Blunt trauma can damage the intestine in several ways. Direct compression may burst it against a rigid structure such as the vertebral bodies, a blow may cause a large hematoma either in the wall or in its mesentery, endangering the blood supply, or a portion of the intestine may be detached from the mesentery. It should be remembered that an external hernia, whether it contains bowel or not, makes a patient more liable to rupture of the intestine.

Perforating injuries are obvious in their effects and easy to diagnose. Any patient with a wound of the abdominal wall should not be subjected to timid probing in the emergency room. This will not help in deciding the extent of intraperitoneal injuries and will only further contaminate an infected wound. After resuscitation, laparotomy is essential for the assessment and the repair of the intraperitoneal damage.

The effects of blunt trauma are more difficult to diagnose since there may be no symptoms or signs of intraperitoneal damage for some time after the injury. A history of a significant blow to the abdomen should, therefore, be sufficient reason to admit the patient to the hospital for detailed observation. Since hemorrhage almost invariably accompanies trauma of the small intestine, the vital signs of pulse rate, blood pressure, respiration rate and temperature should be recorded frequently, and any sudden change reported immediately.

Examination on admission may show general signs of hemorrhage, such as pallor, vasoconstriction, sweating, tachycardia and hypotension. The local evidence of intraperitoneal soiling or hemorrhage may be very slight at first, and only moderate guarding or tenderness may be found. Shifting dullness and the absence of bowel sounds may be the earliest signs of serious intraperitoneal injury. Irritation of the undersurface of the diaphragm by blood or free air may cause referred pain to the tip of the shoulder via the phrenic nerve. Since clotted blood appears to be less irritating to the peritoneal cavity than fresh blood, the physical signs following intraperitoneal trauma frequently alter as clotting occurs. Evidence of gross intraperitoneal soiling or hemorrhage should be obvious, but doubtful cases will remain doubtful, despite scrupulous care in the first examination and meticulous reassessment of the patient while under observation. The common association of other serious injuries, whether cranial, thoracic or to the extremities, makes this assessment difficult.

Roentgenography can help in some patients if it shows the presence of free gas in the peritoneal cavity or under the diaphragm, thus confirming the diagnosis of a perforated intestine.

The simplest way to detect intra-abdominal hemorrhage is by abdominal paracentesis. When properly performed, peritoneal tap is accurate in more than 85 per cent of patients. The abdomen is tapped with a small needle in all four quadrants and the appearance of the material aspirated is noted. Blood or bile in the aspirate confirms the presence of intraperitoneal injury, but negative findings do not rule out the possibility of contamination or hemorrhage in the peritoneal cavity. Peritoneal lavage with saline at the time of needle aspiration may increase the accuracy of this procedure.

Death following abdominal trauma is most often due to massive hemorrhage and shock, or their after-effects. The circulating blood volume must be replaced rapidly by whole blood, plasma substitutes or plasma. It is difficult to assess the amount of colloid needed by a patient even with the aid of present-day laboratory facilities. The amount given and the rate of administration must be based on the patient's response to treatment and by monitoring central venous pressure. A nasogastric tube should be passed to empty the stomach. As soon as transfusion has produced an improvement in the vital signs, the patient is taken to the operating room, if a perforation or continued bleeding is suspected.

A laparotomy incision is made which is large enough to permit examination of all the abdominal contents. All bleeding points are secured as a first step. Replacement therapy is then continued until the blood pressure returns to a normal level. When the bleeding has been controlled and the blood pressure restored to normal, the intestine should be re-examined. Sometimes, on first inspection a portion of the intestine may appear nonviable, but after resuscitation the blood supply will improve; the color becomes normal and the bowel again shows contractility. Any portion of the intestine which still appears doubtful after adequate resuscitation should be resected. Simple perforating wounds are sutured as far as possible in the transverse axis of the bowel, to prevent narrowing. Multiple perforations, areas of extensive bleeding into the mesentery with questionable viability of the intestine, large ragged lacerations and portions detached from their mesentery should be resected.

The abdomen should not be closed until careful examination throughout the peritoneal cavity has shown that no bleeding point has been overlooked. After such an extensive laparotomy, particularly if intestine has been resected, paralytic ileus is common. Decompression, by either a temporary gastrostomy or an inlying nasogastric tube, and intravenous therapy should be continued until normal peristalsis returns. Modern treatment has reduced the mortality to less than 10 per cent, and most deaths now result from the effects of associated injuries or severe hemorrhagic shock, rather than from local complications.

INFECTIONS OF SMALL INTESTINE. Minor attacks of acute gastroenteritis are common, but they seldom engage surgical interest except in children, when they may be difficult to differentiate from acute appendicitis. The sudden and simultaneous onset of vomiting, diarrhea and cramping abdominal pain in gastroenteritis is characteristic. The patient may remember eating unfamiliar or suspect food, and a history of similar trouble in the family, neighborhood or school can often be obtained.

Pseudomembranous staphylococcal enterocolitis is becoming a common and troublesome complicating disease in surgery. It is an acute, fulminating infection of both the large and small intestine. The lumen of the bowel is filled by a protein coagulum, the pseudomembrane. This enterocolitis is caused by replacement of the normal bacterial flora of the intestine by *Staphylococcus pyogenes*, which is resistant to most antibiotics. The overgrowth of resistant bacteria follows the use of broad-spectrum antibiotics. These have either been given to prepare the bowel for resection, or to combat an established infection during the postoperative stages. It is a serious condition, with a mortality of approximately 60 per cent. Since its incidence appears to be increasing, many surgeons have decreased the use of broad-spectrum antibiotics in preparing patients for operation.

Staphylococcal enterocolitis produces a profuse, liquid, green diarrhea. There is a remarkable absence of abdominal pain, but there is severe toxemia and circulatory collapse. The onset is insidious, and the nursing staff must be watchful for the first symptoms, since early and energetic treatment is essential if the patient is to be saved. Any patient who starts passing liquid stools following operation, or after a course of antibiotics, should be isolated immediately.

Examination should exclude any obvious cause of diarrhea, such as fecal impaction or a pelvic or intraperitoneal abscess. A specimen of stool should be immediately stained and examined microscopically; this usually shows multitudes of gram-positive cocci. The feces should be cultured and the sensitivity of the predominant organism to a variety of antibiotics determined, but treatment should not be delayed until the results of this culture are available. Death is due to two causes: a profound toxemia caused by an enterotoxin formed by the organisms in the bowel, and rapid loss of fluid rich in protein and electrolytes. The volume of diarrhea fluid passed may exceed 6 liters a day, and it must be replaced by intravenous therapy.

The management of these patients is much easier if accurate accounts are kept of the volume and chemical make-up of the fluid lost per rectum. The diarrheal fluid has a high protein content, so that the volume lost in each 12-hour period should be replaced with an equivalent volume of plasma. Large losses of potassium also occur, and supplements should be given. Hypovolemic shock occurs rapidly and intravenous replacement of the lost fluid, electrolytes, plasma and whole blood must keep pace with the losses. During the acute stage, in addition to the 3 liters required for maintenance, up to 6 or 8 liters may be required to replace the abnormal rectal losses.

Judicious antibiotic therapy will correct the toxemia caused by large numbers of staphylococci in the bowel. It is safe to assume that these organisms are resistant to standard broad-spectrum antibiotics, and the patient should be given the potent current specific chemotherapy available for the control of staphylococcal infections. Sensitivity of the organism to the various agents should be determined and the appropriate drug reaffirmed. Adrenocorticotropic hormone and intravenous hydrocortisone are also useful supportive measures during the acute stage of staphylococcal enterocolitis. Attempts have been made to displace the staphylococci by administering retention enemas of normal fecal suspensions in the hope that the normal bacterial population will re-establish itself.

Tuberculosis of the small intestine is now rare; it may be primary or secondary. The primary type of intestinal tuberculous infection is unusual owing to the universal pasteurization of milk, but it still occurs, particularly in immigrant groups. This hyperplastic form of the disease usually affects the ileocecal region, because the submucous lymphoid follicles through which the infection enters are prominent and numerous in that area. It causes a localized lesion in the terminal ileum, with ulceration of the mucosa and thickening and fibrosis of the wall. The mesentery of the affected bowel is also thickened and fibrosed, and the adjacent lymph nodes show caseation. There may be small tubercles on the serosal surface, together with redness and loss of its normal lustre. Ileocecal tuberculosis causes diarrhea, intermittent attacks of intestinal obstructive pain, or localized abdominal pain in the right lower quadrant, if there is much serosal involvement. There is usually a history of weight loss, malaise, anorexia and intermittent fever.

Regional enteritis is often suspected, since barium studies show ulceration and deformity of the terminal ileum. Occasionally, tubercle bacilli may be found in or cultured from the feces. This primary type of tuberculosis is usually treated surgically, either because of the onset of intestinal obstruction or because it has been diagnosed as regional enteritis or appendicitis. Resection of the affected intestine, followed by a long course of antituberculous therapy, gives good results. The secondary type of intestinal tuberculosis is often terminal and occurs in patients with pulmonary tuberculosis. It causes acute symptoms and widespread ulceration of the mucosa of the bowel. This is due to continuous swallowing of the infected sputum which the patient coughs up. Treatment is directed at controlling the pulmonary infection.

Regional enteritis, or Crohn's disease, which was first described in 1933, is included among the infectious diseases of the small intestine, although its cause is unknown. This is an inflammatory granulomatous condition which usually affects the terminal ileum, but it is by no means confined to that site. It was originally described as a terminal ileitis, but the disease has since been found in all parts of the gastrointestinal tract, from duodenum to rectum. Therefore, regional enteritis seems a better term.

The pathologic appearances of regional enteritis have been extensively described and investigated in the hope that they would offer some clue to its cause. The diseased bowel presents different appearances, depending upon the duration and severity of the disease. The acute form tends to attack the terminal ileum, the proximal cecum and the appendix. The bowel is red; its serosal surface is dull and covered with a gray fibrinous exudate which sticks the loops of bowel together and to the adjacent parietes. Edema makes the bowel wall boggy and swollen to the touch. The transition to normal intestine at the upper and lower margins is abrupt and easily seen, but other distant segments of the intestine may also be involved. These areas of diseased bowel separated by lengths of normal intestine are often called "skip lesions."

The chronic lesion presents a classic ap-

pearance: fibrosis replaces edema in the bowel wall and mesentery, so that there is thickening and rigidity of both (Fig. 60). The mesenteric fat is thickened and pulled up onto the wall of the bowel, which is hyperemic, and the mesenteric nodes are enlarged and fleshy. Perforation of the intestine may be seen with adjacent abscess cavities, and the loop of bowel may adhere to other parts of the intestine, the abdominal wall or the urinary bladder. Fistulous connections may be found between the affected intestine and the skin or any nearby organs. Upon opening the bowel, the thickening and fibrosis of the walls and the narrowed, constricted lumen are obvious. There is ulceration of the mucosal surface, with underlying edema and vascularity of the submucosal and muscular layers.

Upon microscopic examination, the inflammatory process is seen to affect the whole thickness of the wall. The mucosa is ulcerated, and this is usually more obvious on the mesenteric border. The submucosa is infiltrated by a wide variety of inflammatory cells and shows vascular dilatation. Similar changes are seen in the mesentery and local lymph nodes. Multinuclear giant cells of the epithelioid type are commonly found in regional enteritis. These may occur in the intestinal wall, the mesentery, and the affected lymph nodes. They are large, and contain up to 30 or 40 nuclei. Despite their resemblance to the giant cells seen in tuberculous infection, caseation or breaking down of the lesion is never seen. The resemblance to tuberculosis formerly caused regional enteritis to be labeled frequently as tuberculous. The previous confusion of the two diseases probably explains the increase in the reported incidence of regional enteritis in the 30 years since Crohn's first description.

Despite increased knowledge of the incidence and natural course of the disease, the etiology of regional enteritis remains unknown. Many possibilities have been canvassed. The idea that it was some form of atypical tuberculous infection, or "paratuberculosis," was popular for a long time, but the consistent failure to detect this organism by culture or staining makes this explanation unlikely. The lesions are very similar to those seen in sarcoidosis, but the cause of the latter disease is also unknown. Viral infection, lymphedema due to lymphstasis, a foreign-body reaction to ingested silica or talc in toothpaste, a localized sen-

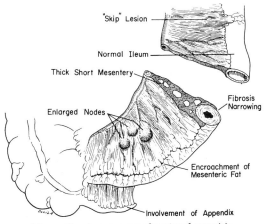

"Skip" Lesion

Normal Ileum

Thick Short Mesentery

Fibrosis Narrowing

Enlarged Nodes

Encroachment of Mesenteric Fat

Involvement of Appendix

Figure 60. Appearance of regional enteritis.

sitivity reaction to foreign proteins, and destruction of the mucosa by an autoimmune process have all been suggested as possible causes of this perplexing disease.

Regional enteritis is mainly a disease of young adults, but it also occurs in childhood and old age. Men are more often affected than women, in the ratio of 5 to 4. There may be a familial tendency to develop the disease.

Regional enteritis may manifest its presence in a variety of ways, and certain general types of the disease can be recognized. One of the common types is as an acute inflammatory intra-abdominal condition. There is usually severe, right-sided abdominal pain which may come on suddenly and is associated with nausea, anorexia and vomiting. Examination shows the patient to have a fever, a coated tongue and signs of peritoneal irritation in the right iliac fossa. A leukocytosis is common. With all these features, it is easy to understand why an inaccurate diagnosis of appendicitis is often made. Prodromal symptoms of general ill health, loss of weight or diarrhea may give a clue to the real nature of the patient's disease. On occasion, the best clinical acumen fails to differentiate between acute appendicitis and regional enteritis, and the diagnosis may be made only at laparotomy.

A second way of presentation is as a chronic relapsing enteritis or enterocolitis with recurrent bouts of cramplike lower abdominal pain and diarrhea. There may be periodic attacks of vomiting with loss of appetite, nausea, weight loss and fever. The diarrhea is difficult to control by medical means, although it may remit temporarily.

The obstructive type of the disease presents with attacks of small bowel colic and vomiting, following a period of intermittent diarrhea. With each attack of colicky pain, the patient may notice abdominal distention, audible bowel sounds and even peristalsis visible through the thin abdominal wall. He may also notice a palpable mass.

The fourth group of patients have fistulae. These frequently form after an appendectomy, laparotomy or drainage of an abdominal abscess, although fistulae between the small intestine and colon or bladder may form spontaneously. It is important to remember that regional enteritis may affect the large bowel and may present as perirectal suppuration or a fistula-in-ano. If a fistula-in-ano is excised, or a perirectal abscess drained, the tissue should always be examined microscopically, so that the diagnosis of regional enteritis is not overlooked. Patients with regional enteritis may also have obvious melena, an iron deficiency anemia due to occult intestinal bleeding, a malabsorption syndrome or a pyrexia of unknown origin.

The classic patient with regional enteritis is, therefore, a young person who has complained for some time of intermittent diarrhea and lower abdominal cramps. There may be a recent history of localized right-sided abdominal pain. His weight has declined and he complains of symptoms due to anemia and intermittent fever. He may also complain of a persistent discharging sinus following an appendectomy early in the course of the disease.

Examination shows the patient to be anemic, and he has signs of recent weight loss. An abdominal mass may be present and there may be signs of subacute intestinal obstruction.

The diagnosis can usually be made on the history and physical examination, but confirmation depends upon radiography. Either a barium meal or a barium enema examination may show the typical strictured appearance of the terminal ileum known as the "string" sign. Careful search should be made for "skip lesions" elsewhere in the gastrointestinal tract. Hematologic study may show an iron deficiency anemia and a leukocytosis. The stools should be cultured to exclude a pathogenic organism causing an enteritis, and other enteropathies should be excluded by appropriate investigation.

Since the cause of regional enteritis is unknown, the treatment, whether medical or surgical, is empirical. As a result, there is still considerable argument concerning treatment. As far as possible, medical measures should be tried first. Iron to correct the anemia, paregorics intermittently to control the diarrhea, a low-residue, high-protein diet, and periods of complete bed rest will give the patient some symptomatic relief. Adrenocorticotropic hormone and corticosteroids have been tried; apart from their general tonic effects, however, they do not appear to influence the course of the illness.

A surgical procedure is necessary to treat the complications of regional enteritis. There are certain absolute indications for operative treatment, such as the onset of intestinal obstruction or the formation of a fistula or an intra-abdominal abscess. In other patients, a continued downhill course on conservative treatment, or progressive anemia, or severe abdominal pain may constitute relative indications for operation.

Two types of operations are possible in regional enteritis. The involved intestine and mesentery can be removed completely, or they can be by-passed by anastomosing healthy bowel above and below the lesion. At present, resection of the diseased segment of intestine is more common, but with either type of operation the chance of recurrence is approximately 35 per cent, and this increases as time goes by. When abdominal exploration shows multiple "skip" areas of diseased bowel, excision is not feasible.

One of the most difficult surgical problems is to decide what to do when regional enteritis is discovered on opening the abdomen for suspected appendicitis. Appendectomy alone should be avoided, because this commonly causes fistula formation. If possible, the affected segment of intestine should be by-passed or resected.

DIVERTICULOSIS. Diverticula of the small intestine may be congenital or acquired. Those of congenital origin, apart from Meckel's type, are rare, and they are usually situated on the antimesenteric border of the bowel. Acquired diverticula are also uncommon. They are usually multiple, and they are more numerous in the upper jejunum than elsewhere in the small intestine. They are pulsion type diverticula and consist of pouches of mucosa only, without a muscular covering. They are usually on the mesenteric border of the bowel at the points of entry of the blood vessels into the wall.

Jejunal diverticulosis is often symptomless and found incidentally during a barium meal examination. The commonest symptoms are flatulent dyspepsia with a bloated feeling after eating, and occasional embarrassing borborygmi. Complications of jejunal diverticulosis are unusual, but among those described are severe intestinal hemorrhage, perforation, intussusception, intestinal obstruction and inflammation of the diverticula. Some patients develop diarrhea and a macrocytic anemia due to bacterial infection of the diverticula. The organisms continually infect the small intestine and they compete with the body for the available vitamin B_{12}, a condition analogous to the "blind loop syndrome." The macrocytic anemia may improve

if antibiotics are given to control the infection. Should any of these complications arise, the portion of the small intestine affected by diverticulosis should be resected.

VASCULAR DISEASE OF SMALL INTESTINE. Occlusion of the superior mesenteric artery due to atheroma is usually an acute catastrophe, but it sometimes occurs as a gradual process. As the vascular supply of the intestine is reduced, it becomes inadequate to provide oxygen for the muscular work of the intestine, or to carry away the waste products. The patient complains of cramplike abdominal pain of varying severity within an hour of each meal. It is analogous to the pain of intermittent claudication or angina pectoris. The pain is less if only a small meal is eaten, so that the patient learns to restrict his diet and begins to lose weight. There may also be evidence of malabsorption as a result of the vascular insufficiency. Morphologic changes similar to villous atrophy have been shown experimentally in chronic intestinal ischemia. This may also contribute to the associated malabsorption.

The diagnosis of mesenteric angina should be suspected in any elderly person who has signs of severe atheroma, and who complains of abdominal pain occurring regularly after meals. Examination of the abdomen may not help unless a bruit is heard over the area of the aorta, and the diagnosis can be confirmed only by aortography. A lateral roentgenogram of the aorta after the injection of dye will show narrowing at the origin of the superior mesenteric artery. It is important to make the diagnosis at this stage of relative vascular insufficiency before complete arterial obstruction causes infarction of the intestine. The atheromatous plaque in the superior mesenteric artery can be removed by endarterectomy, or the obstruction can be by-passed. using an arterial graft.

Similar symptoms of postprandial pain sometimes occur in a much younger group of patients who have no signs of generalized atherosclerosis. Lateral aortography in these patients shows an obstruction of the celiac axis. Subsequent laparotomy has shown the vessel to be compressed by a fibrous band near the median arcuate ligament of the diaphragm. Simple division of this band relieves the symptoms.

More commonly, the obstruction of the superior mesenteric artery is acute. It causes infarction of most of the small bowel and, unless the collateral supply from the inferior mesenteric artery is good, it can cause infarction of part of the large intestine on the right side. Mesenteric thrombosis causes severe and continuous abdominal pain with vomiting and circulatory collapse. The symptoms closely resemble a small bowel strangulation obstruction. The pain increases in intensity, and is accompanied by a rising pulse rate, progression of the abdominal signs and an increase in the white cell count. Some patients may pass bloodstained stools soon after the pain begins.

Examination shows a patient in considerable pain with signs of peritonitis and with absent bowel sounds. Shock and severe peripheral vasoconstriction are common. There is usually extensive infarction of the intestine. Although patients occasionally survive resection, more than 80 per cent die. A similar syndrome is caused when an embolus occludes the superior mesenteric artery. The embolus is usually caused by atrial fibrillation secondary to mitral stenosis. If the diagnosis is made promptly enough, embolectomy may prevent infarction of the intestine.

Extensive gangrene of the intestine has been found in patients in whom there is no gross obstruction of the mesenteric artery. instead, there is widespread thrombosis of the venous tributaries and of the main superior mesenteric vein. This venous type of gangrene appears to be secondary to other conditions such as congestive heart failure, hypertensive disease or a prolonged period of hypotensive shock.

TUMORS OF THE SMALL INTESTINE. Tumors of the small intestine are uncommon, but most types of malignant and benign lesions have been described. The symptoms produced are similar whatever the type of tumor, although progression may be more rapid in the malignant lesions. In two types of tumors, the signs and symptoms have such characteristic features that two syndromes, the carcinoid syndrome and the Peutz-Jeghers syndrome, have been described.

Benign tumors of the jejunum and ileum affect the sexes equally. They usually present between the ages of 30 and 40 years, although no age is immune. The malignant tumors, except for lymphosarcoma, occur later in life. There seems to be an association between adult celiac disease, steatorrhea and the development of malignant neoplasms of the small bowel. The number of instances so far reported is small, but the incidence of neoplasms, particularly of the lymphoma group, is much higher in such patients than in a normal group. All types of growth are seen more frequently in the proximal third of the jejunum, or the distal third of the ileum. Anemia due to chronic and unsuspected blood loss and episodes of obstruction are particularly common.

The symptoms in the early stages are usually dyspeptic in type. Attacks of abdominal pain are precipitated by food, and lead to a limitation of intake or an alteration of the type of food eaten. When the pain is severe, the patient may vomit, which gives partial relief of the symptoms. The patient may notice an abdominal mass which frequently alters its site, or he may complain of symptoms due to an associated anemia from occult intestinal hemorrhage. A hemangioma, for example, may cause no local abdominal symptoms, but only those of anemia. Since these tumors are difficult to visualize on x-ray examination or at laparotomy, they may be extremely difficult to diagnose. The bowel is suggested as the site of hemorrhage only if severe melena occurs.

The symptoms of a small bowel tumor change when obstruction occurs. Abdominal pain is severe and colicky, and causes the patient to double up or writhe around. The patient complains of vomiting and absolute constipation. Obstruction may be due to the intussusception of a submucosal tumor within the lumen. The particular importance of intussusception in an adult is that it rarely occurs spontaneously, and when this condition is found at laparotomy every effort should be made to find a primary cause. This may be either a submucous or a polypoid tumor being propelled along the intestine, a Meckel's diverticulum, or an obstruction situated distally. Obstruction of the bowel is often due to compression of the lumen by a growth and it is precipitated by the impaction of some solid piece of food at the site of narrowing. The symptoms are those of simple intestinal obstruction.

The diagnosis of small bowel tumor is difficult; it usually depends upon barium studies extending over many hours. A persistent stricture or filling defect, an intussusception or abnormal distention of the proximal loops of bowel may be seen. Frequently, however, the diagnosis is first made at operation for acute intestinal obstruction.

The definitive treatment of small bowel neoplasms is surgical. Operation should be postponed, however, until the blood volume has been restored, the fluid and electrolyte deficiencies corrected, and the hourly urinary output determined to be adequate. A nasogastric tube should be passed to decompress the distended intestine before operation.

For benign lesions, local excision is enough. The treatment of malignant tumors of the small intestine is much less satisfactory. Adenocarcinomas of this region tend to be high-grade malignancy and show early metastasis, both to regional nodes and distant sites. Only about 20 per cent of patients survive five years after resection for carcinoma of the ileum. The treatment of the lymphoma group is equally disappointing. These tumors arise in the submucous layers of the intestine and often spread widely to the mesentery and the posterior abdominal wall before operation is undertaken. For this reason, about one-third of these tumors are unresectable. Some palliation can often be given by deep x-ray therapy or cytotoxic drugs. The expected five-year survival rate with this group of tumors is less than 10 per cent.

Carcinoid tumors and the carcinoid syndrome. Throughout the gastrointestinal tract in the submucosa there are cells which have a special affinity for silver stains. They are known as argentaffin, or Kultschitzky cells. They are particularly numerous in the appendix, the crypts of Lieberkühn and the terminal ileum. These cells were known many years ago and tumors arising from them were described, but little was known of their function until it was shown that they secreted a physiologically potent substance called serotonin, or 5-hydroxytryptamine. Serotonin appears to stimulate intestinal peristalsis and it also causes vasoconstriction.

Shortly after the discovery of serotonin, the symptoms of a patient were described, in whom a tumor of argentaffin cell origin produced excessive amounts of serotonin. This caused a combination of symptoms and signs which was termed the "carcinoid syndrome."

The features of this syndrome are characteristic (Fig. 61). First, a malignant carcinoid tumor is present in the abdominal cavity or in the lung. Second, the patient complains of hyperperistalsis and abdominal pain. Third, he suffers from periodic flushing of the face due to capillary dilatation and telangiectasia. Fourth, pulmonary valve stenosis or tricuspid incompetence may develop. Fifth, attacks of dyspnea coincide with the facial flushes. These symptoms are associated with a high

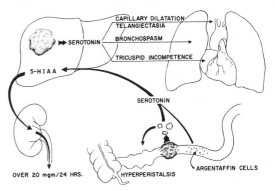

Figure 61. The carcinoid syndrome. Serotonin is produced by the primary tumor and its metastases. It causes a characteristic syndrome and is accompanied by an increased excretion of 5-hydroxyindoleacetic acid.

level of serotonin in the peripheral blood and an increased output, over 20 mg. per 24 hours, of its main breakdown product, 5-hydroxyindoleacetic acid (5-HIAA), in the urine.

Carcinoid tumors are found wherever there are argentaffin cells, but only a small number cause the characteristic syndrome. Approximately 55 per cent occur in the appendix. These affect a young age group, they rarely metastasize, and they are usually found on routine pathologic examination of the appendix. Between 25 and 30 per cent of carcinoids develop in the terminal ileum and, in contrast, more than three-quarters of this group have lymphatic and liver metastases. Ileal carcinoids tend to occur in an older age group, the average age being 52 years. The next most common site is the rectum, where these tumors are small. They are usually found on routine examination and are excised for biopsy. The remaining few carcinoid tumors are widely distributed throughout the alimentary tract and bronchi.

The ileal carcinoid, although it is malignant, is slow-growing, and survival for 25 years after first diagnosis has been reported. Symptoms of the carcinoid syndrome develop only when metastases are present in the liver, so that serotonin is released directly into the systemic circulation. Treatment consists of excising the primary lesion if possible. This will relieve the local symptoms due to the growth. Some palliation can be achieved by excising as much of the metastatic tumor as possible to reduce the bulk of active, secreting tumor tissue. The drugs which antagonize serotonin have so far given only limited symptomatic relief.

Peutz-Jeghers syndrome. This is a rare disease in which multiple adenomatous polyps of the gastrointestinal tract, particularly the small bowel, are associated with spotty melanin pigmentation of the buccal mucous membrane, lips, tongue, face, fingers and toes. It is a familial condition. It affects both sexes equally and commonly presents between the ages of 10 and 30 years. The polyps are found in the small bowel in 50 per cent of the patients and in the large bowel in 40 per cent, but they may occur anywhere in the gastrointestinal tract. The symptoms may be those of bowel obstruction, recurrent intussusception, hematemesis or melena, or iron deficiency anemia. A family history of similar episodes may also be obtained.

Treatment is not influenced by the prospect of malignant changes in the polyps, which is very rare. For this reason, and because of the diffuse distribution of the polyps, treatment should be conservative. However, if intestinal obstruction or severe bleeding occurs, laparotomy is necessary. If the disease is localized, the affected intestine should be resected. The life story of these unfortunate patients is usually punctuated by various surgical operations for intestinal hemorrhage or recurrent intussusception.

THE APPENDIX

Acute appendicitis is the commonest cause of an "acute surgical abdomen," and should always be thought of in any patient who presents symptoms of peritonitis. Although appendectomy is regarded by the layman as a minor operation, appendicitis and its complications cause considerable mortality in this country. It is strange, looking back on the history of appendicitis and the development of appendectomy, that such a common condition should have been unrecognized for so long. Isolated instances of suppuration around the cecum, or "perityphlitis," were reported in the eighteenth and early nineteenth centuries. Both Addison and Bright reported upon such patients, but the recognition of the appendix, and not the cecum, as the primary site of the infection was really due to Reginald Fitz. He described the pathologic findings in 1888, and in 1889 McBurney described the typical clinical findings and the incision which now carries his name. The treatment of the complicated case of appendicitis was described by A. J. Ochsner in the early part of the twentieth century. His regimen of conservative management for patients with peritonitis reduced the mortality rate from 70 to 25 per cent. This was an astonishing achievement for the days before antibiotics and intravenous therapy.

ANATOMY.   The appendix in man is a vestigial organ which develops as part of the midgut. Its size varies, but it is usually 3 to 4 inches long. It arises at the tip of the cecum where the three taenia coli coalesce. The position of the appendix is variable. It may be in the peritoneal cavity, in its characteristic position in the right iliac fossa. It may be buried under the terminal ileum, or it may lie behind the cecum. If the cecum is low, the appendix may be entirely in the true pelvis, or it may hang over the brim of the pelvis, crossing the iliac vessels. If the cecum is high, due to failure to descend during development, the appendix may lie behind it and ascend into the right hypochondrium. The only constant feature of its position is that its base at the cecum is always at the point where the three taeniae coli coalesce. If it proves difficult to find the appendix at operation, the base can always be found by tracing the taeniae downward to the tip of the cecum.

It is supplied by the superior mesenteric artery, through the appendicular branch of the ileocolic artery. Its nerve supply originates at the celiac plexus and accompanies these vessels. The appendix has a small mesentery arising from the mesentery of the terminal ileum, and there are often other small folds of peritoneum running from the appendix to ileum or cecum, which may form a variety of para-appendiceal fossae.

The lumen of the appendix is narrow and lined by epithelium of the large intestinal type. Its walls are muscular with an outer longitudinal and inner circular layer. In the submucosa are lymphoid follicles. These are particularly prominent in children or young adults and may project into and partially occlude the lumen of the appendix.

Acute appendicitis is the commonest surgical emergency, affecting between one in 500 and one in 700 persons. In 60 per cent of the patients, the acute attack is caused by obstruction of the appendix. In the remainder, the cause is unknown. A high proportion of meat in the diet predisposes to appendicitis, and the condition is less common where the staple diet is largely carbohydrate, as in India. It is particularly common in the first three decades of life because of the prominence of the submucosal lymphoid follicles in the appendix. These slowly regress after the age of 30 years. In childhood, measles, glandular fever and other diseases which cause lymphoid hyperplasia may precipitate an attack of appendicitis. Recently, there have been indications that the incidence of appendicitis in this country is slowly falling.

PATHOLOGY. The most common cause of acute inflammation is obstruction of the appendix, and the pathology of acute appendicitis resembles that of intestinl obstruction. The obstructing agent may occur naturally in the lumen, as a fecolith does, or it may be a solid foreign body such as a cherry stone. The obstruction may be caused by disease in the wall of the appendix such as hyperplasia of the lymphoid follicles, a fibrous stricture due to previous inflammation, or a tumor. Obstructions outside the wall are uncommon, although an adhesion may constrict the base of the appendix and obstruct it.

Obstructive appendicitis is a "closed loop" type of intestinal obstruction which progresses to strangulation or perforation. The pressure inside the appendix rises because of the obstruction. As this intraluminal pressure increases, it is transmitted to the wall of the appendix and interferes with the blood supply. At first, the venous return is slowed, causing venous thrombosis and eventual arterial thrombosis. Gangrene and perforation of the appendix follow. Perforation may also be caused by ulceration of the contained fecolith or foreign body through the wall of the appendix.

The effects of perforation depend on its suddenness. If the omentum and adjacent loops of bowel have become adherent to the inflamed appendix, perforation will cause a local mass or abscess. In young children and in old people, perforation occurs rapidly before the infected appendix is walled off. The omentum in children is short and fragile. In old people, arteriosclerosis of the artery leads to its early occlusion. The contents of the necrotic appendix are discharged into the peritoneal cavity, causing a general peritonitis. Paralytic obstruction of the intestine is a common sequel of appendicitis, due to localized or generalized peritonitis.

In 40 per cent of resected appendices, no evidence of obstruction can be found. These are often called cases of catarrhal appendicitis. The infection may be taken to the appendix in the blood stream and is common in children after attacks of tonsillitis or measles. If appendicitis follows measles, typical measles giant cells may be seen on microscopic examination.

CLINICAL SYMPTOMS. The differential diagnosis of a patient with abdominal pain is one of the fascinating exercises of surgery. Minor differences in symptoms and signs may entail major differences in the management or operative approach. In most patients, when a diagnosis has been made, only a short time passes until operation shows the true state of affairs. This is particularly true of the patient with suspected appendicitis, since it must be differentiated from nearly every other intra-abdominal emergency.

The major symptom of acute appendicitis is abdominal pain. Any pain that persists for more than six hours should be regarded seriously. This pain is caused by obstruction of the appendix and is similar in character to the pain caused by any bowel obstruction. It is intermittent and colicky at first and makes the patient feel that passing wind or feces could relieve it. It is this plain "bellyache," in the early stages, which so often makes the patient take a laxative. This is a dangerous practice because it may precipitate perforation of the appendix. The pain returns in waves and makes the patient restless. He tries to obtain relief by wriggling around, doubling up or walking about the room. Because the appendix and the small bowel have the same nerve supply, the pain is at first referred to the epigastrium or periumbilical area.

As the inflammation in the appendix progresses through its wall to involve the serosal covering, the character of the pain changes. Wherever the inflamed serosa of the appendix is in contact with the parietal peritoneum, localized pain is produced. The patient notices that the pain shifts from the epigastrium to the right iliac fossa and its character alters. Whereas at the beginning of the attack, the patient could get some relief by moving around, he now finds that movement makes the pain considerably worse, since the two inflamed serosal surfaces grate against each other. The pain is no longer intermittent, cramplike, and colicky, but continuous and sharp. When the inflamed appendix perforates, the severe pain of intestinal colic abruptly disappears. For a short time, the patient may believe that he is improving, but the onset of severe generalized pain due to peritonitis soon disillusions him. In an explosive attack of appendicitis with the rapid onset of perforation, the pain may start in the right iliac fossa and then spread over the abdomen.

The site of the local pain produced by appendicitis depends on the position of the appendix (Fig. 62). If it is retrocecal, it will lie on the muscles of the posterior abdominal wall and on the kidney, or ureter. The pain of retrocecal appendicitis may then be localized to the loin and flank; it mimics the pain caused by renal disease. In pelvic appendicitis, local abdominal pain may be mild and confined to the hypogastrium. The inflamed appendix may touch the peritoneum over the bladder, rectum or the pelvic organs in the female, and movement of any of these makes the pain worse. The patient also complains that defecation or urination makes the pain worse. It is important to be sure what the patient means when he says, "It hurts to pass water," because the pain of an inflamed pelvic appendix might be attributed to a simple cystitis.

Loss of appetite is nearly invariable in appendicitis, and vomiting is characteristic. This typically starts a short time after the pain. If a patient gives a history of vomiting before the pain starts, appendicitis is unlikely. There is nothing specific about the character of the vomitus, which is reflexly produced in the early stages. Late in the disease, when peritonitis has caused a paralytic ileus, the vomitus may be large in volume and feculent in type.

The effects of appendicitis on the bowel habit are variable. Characteristically, it causes constipation, but this is by no means universal. Diarrhea may occur, particularly in children, and in patients in whom the appendix lies near the rectum and irritates it. If an abscess has formed in the pelvis, it produces a continual urge to defecate, and the patient will pass small quantities of mucus repeatedly.

Appendicitis commonly causes a rise in temperature, but the fever is usually not very high unless serious complications have occurred. A coated tongue, fetor oris, sweating and other generalized symptoms of an abdominal infection may be seen.

PHYSICAL SIGNS. Just as the symptoms of appendicitis depend partly on the position of the appendix, so do the signs of this disease. The examination of the patient must be complete and thorough, as many conditions have to be considered in the differential diagnosis of acute appendicitis, and these may involve any system in the body.

The temperature and pulse are noted for evidence of fever or tachycardia. The tongue may be coated.

The posture and behavior of the patient are also important. He usually avoids movement, and if asked to turn or sit up does so gingerly and gradually, to avoid any jolt which will make the pain worse. He may lie with the right hip slightly flexed. This position relaxes the muscles of the abdominal wall, or the psoas muscle, and gives him some relief from pain. Movement of the abdomen, particularly on the right side, may be less than normal. There is tenderness, muscular guarding, or even rigidity of the muscles over the right iliac fossa.

These signs are maximal at the point described by McBurney: "a point 1.5 to 2 inches medial to the anterior superior spine on a line joining the anterior superior iliac spine to the umbilicus." Release or rebound tenderness may be elicited by suddenly withdrawing the hand from the abdominal wall. Gentle palpation may outline a mass in the right iliac fossa.

If the appendix lies in an unusual position, the local signs of peritoneal irritation are most obvious at points other than the one described by McBurney. Tenderness may be most marked in the flank in retrocecal appendicitis, or in the suprapubic region if the appendix

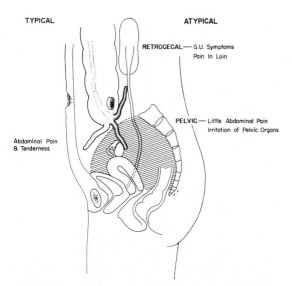

TYPICAL

ATYPICAL

RETROCECAL— G.U. Symptoms
Pain In Loin

PELVIC— Little Abdominal Pain
Irritation of Pelvic Organs

Abdominal Pain
& Tenderness

Figure 62.   The symptoms of acute appendicitis. The position of the appendix governs the symptoms produced. The pelvic appendix is particularly dangerous, as abdominal pain may be minor and imitate other pelvic conditions.

lies in the pelvis. Signs of localized muscle irritation may be elicited by special tests. If the appendix is near the psoas muscle, pain can be produced by stretching the muscle by slight hyperextension of the hip. An appendix hanging down the side wall of the pelvis is adjacent to the obturator internus muscle, and pain can be caused by rotation of the hip joint. Rectal examination and pelvic examination are essential in making the diagnosis of appendicitis, first to exclude definite pelvic pathology such as an ovarian cyst, and second to elicit tenderness in cases of pelvic appendicitis. As the finger is pressed gently against the peritoneum of the pouch of Douglas, the patient will complain of pain in the hypogastrium. True tenderness of the pelvic peritoneum must be distinguished from the mild discomfort which patients commonly feel during rectal examination.

Three investigations are necessary in assessing a patient with suspected appendicitis. These are a differential white blood cell count, roentgenograms of the abdomen and chest, and microscopic examination of the urine deposit. A moderate polymorphonuclear leukocytosis is common in acute appendicitis, but the absence of a raised white cell count should not rule out the diagnosis if the history and signs are at all suggestive.

X-ray examination of the abdomen does not show any appearances diagnostic of appendicitis, although sometimes a few small fluid levels in the small intestine may be seen localized in the right iliac fossa, and sometimes free air may be seen under the diaphragm if the appendix has perforated. On very rare occasions, an appendiceal fecalith may be identified. A plain x-ray film of the abdomen does help to exclude other diseases, such as small bowel obstruction or ureteric calculi. An intravenous pyelogram may be necessary to differentiate a right ureteral calculus from acute appendicitis. A chest x-ray examination should always be done to exclude a right basal pneumonia which may closely mimic appendicitis, particularly in a child.

The urine deposit must be examined in every patient with suspected appendicitis. Red blood cells in the urine can only be due to renal or ureteral disease. Pus cells in the deposit suggest pyelitis or urinary infection, although on occasion an inflamed appendix lying near the ureter or bladder can produce pyuria and microscopic hematuria. The pus cells are usually less numerous if this is the cause. A significant number of organisms in the deposit confirm an infection of the urinary tract.

DIFFERENTIAL DIAGNOSIS. The differential diagnosis of acute appendicitis depends upon three major factors: the age and sex of the patient, the stage of the local pathologic process in the appendix and the anatomic situation of the appendix.

In three groups of patients, the diagnosis is particularly difficult since the presentation is often atypical. In children, particularly of preschool age, the rate of perforation is over 30 per cent, due not only to the anatomic differences but also to the habit of giving a purgative to any small patient with abdominal pain and fever. In pregnant women, the appendix is displaced by the enlarged uterus and the local signs of inflammation may be in different places from usual. In old age, appendicitis is often "silent" and does not cause typical symptoms or signs. Diagnosis is consequently delayed. It is in these three groups of patients that appendicitis still causes morbidity and mortality.

The child with suspected appendicitis presents a particular problem. A coherent and definite history may be difficult to obtain, and this may be due not so much to an inarticulate child as to interruptions from an overarticulate parent. Proper and unhurried examination may also be difficult in a small, frightened patient with severe abdominal pain. The diagnosis is especially difficult before the age of three; appendicitis is uncommon before that age, and the abdominal signs are bizarre and hard to elicit. Simple acute gastroenteritis mimics appendicitis closely in children, but usually the mistake in diagnosis is made the other way around: the patient with appendicitis is treated initially for gastroenteritis. If antibiotics are administered, the symptoms and signs of acute appendicitis may be altered considerably. This makes the differentiation from acute gastroenteritis even more difficult.

Primary mesenteric adenitis is a common cause of abdominal pain in childhood, and it may be impossible to distinguish from appendicitis. The pain sometimes remains more in the center of the abdomen and the local signs on the right side may not be so severe. A lymphocytosis may be found on blood count, and indicate the correct diagnosis. An intussusception may also cause difficulty, as central abdominal colic occurs and the pain may later settle on the right side. When necrotic changes in the intussuscepted bowel cause local peritoneal irritation, it may be impossible to distinguish the two conditions. Usually, the absence of a fever and the presence of blood on rectal examination will help in making the distinction.

Other common causes of a fever or abdominal pain in children are urinary infections, particularly in young girls, or a right basal pneumonia. Inflammation or perforation of a Meckel's diverticulum must also be considered. If a normal appendix is found at operation, the terminal part of the small bowel should always be inspected to exclude the presence of a Meckel's diverticulum. Among the rarer conditions which may cause difficulty in childhood are purpura and primary peritonitis.

In the young man, one expects to obtain a typical history of appendicitis and the list of alternative diagnoses is smaller. A right renal or ureteral calculus, or a hydronephrosis, may cause symptoms similar to appendicitis, particularly a retrocecal one, but appropriate investigation should exclude these other conditions. The most difficult condition to differentiate in this age group is an acute onset of regional enteritis. The only hint is a history of previous attacks of abdominal colic and of sporadic diarrhea for some time before the present acute attack started. Torsion and strangulation of the testicle, or a right-sided epididymitis may sometimes be overlooked when the referred pain in the epigastrium is particularly severe and the local signs in the scrotum are mild.

In young women, diseases of the ovary and the fallopian tubes must be differentiated. Salpingitis may cause the greatest difficulty, but usually the pain is bilateral and low down in the abdomen. It often occurs at the end of a menstrual period, and a previous history of venereal disease, vaginal discharge or deep dyspareunia may be obtained. "Mittelschmerz," the pain produced by ovarian bleeding as the graafian follicle ruptures, may be distinguished by its characteristic onset in mid-cycle. An ectopic pregnancy, or endometriosis of the pelvis, may also resemble appendicitis, and a careful inquiry must always be made into the previous menstrual history. Right-sided pyelitis, particularly when it occurs during pregnancy, can be very difficult to distinguish from appendicitis. The pain of pyelitis characteristically starts in the loin and may later shift to the abdomen. The patient may complain of attacks of shivering, sweating and severe headache, and the temperature is usually much higher than in appendicitis. The signs of acute appendicitis in pregnancy may be altered considerably by the gravid uterus pushing the appendix upward and outward. The greatest tenderness is, therefore, in the right flank and loin, increasing the confusion with pyelitis. Red degeneration of a fibroid during pregnancy may also cause acute abdominal pain; it is usually possible to feel the tender lump attached to the gravid uterus.

In later life, other problems in differential diagnosis arise. A perforated duodenal ulcer may closely resemble appendicitis, particularly if the leak of gastric contents is small and the fluid travels down the right paracolic gutter to pool in the right iliac fossa. The absence of fever and a previous history of ulcer dyspepsia may suggest the correct diagnosis. Acute cholecystitis may also be difficult to identify if the gallbladder is unusually low or the appendix is abnormally high. A carcinoma of the cecum may mimic appendicitis or an abscess of the appendix. A carcinoma on the left side of the colon may also give rise to pain in the right iliac fossa by causing distention of the cecum through back-pressure. This localized pain may be preceded by a history of abdominal colic and constipation, thus closely simulating the onset of appendicitis. Torsion of an ovarian cyst may also produce a typical history of severe upper abdominal cramp followed by localized pain in the lower abdomen; but proper pelvic examination, and on occasion x-ray films, should distinguish this condition. Other conditions to be considered in the elderly are myocardial infarction, rupture of an aneurysm of the abdominal aorta and mesenteric thrombosis.

At all stages of life, acute intestinal obstruction may be very difficult to differentiate from appendicitis. When the appendix lies in the retroileal position, it can easily cause mechanical or paralytic obstruction of the overlying ileum. The possibility that appendicitis may cause an intestinal obstruction in this way should always be remembered.

TREATMENT. The treatment of appendicitis depends on the duration and the stage of the disease. Four stages are usually described: first, acute appendicitis; second, acute appendicitis with local peritonitis; third, acute appendicitis with abscess formation; and fourth, acute appendicitis with general peritonitis. Appendectomy should be carried out in all patients in the first two stages. The mortality from operation in these two types is negligible, and convalescence is usually uncomplicated and rapid. There is no such unanimous agreement about the most effective treatment when a lump can be felt in the right iliac fossa.

The inflamed appendix is at first surrounded by omentum and adjacent loops of bowel, forming a mass or appendix "phlegmon." If this progresses, a true abscess cavity is later formed. Some surgeons feel that the presence of a mass is an indication for conservative or nonoperative treatment, since operation will break down the natural adhesions which are present. These adhesions contain and localize the infection, and prevent its spread to the general peritoneal cavity.

In contrast to this view, others feel that if the situation is dealt with by conservative means, the disease may take a long time to resolve. The phlegmon may progress to an abscess despite the use of an antibiotic, and an abscess may cause severe complications such as bacteriemia, or it may rupture into the peritoneal cavity.

It is probably best to be guided by the duration and severity of the symptoms and the local signs in choosing the correct treatment for a patient with a mass. In certain types of patients, operation should always be advised. In children, in pregnant women, in elderly patients and in patients in whom the diagnosis of abscess formation is in doubt, operation is the best treatment. An arbitrary time limit cannot be set beyond which operation should be forbidden. If a patient is first seen more than two or three days after the start of an attack and the symptoms are subsiding, conservative treatment could be used. Operation may also be delayed if there is reason to believe that regional enteritis or an underlying carcinoma of the cecum is present. If a patient is examined within 24 to 48 hours of onset, appendectomy is the best treatment.

If an abscess of the appendix is treated conservatively, the patient requires the closest supervision, and he should be mentally and physically prepared for operation at any time it may be indicated. The vital signs should be recorded and any change reported immediately. The size of the mass should be recorded accurately, or outlined on the patient's skin, so that the changes in size can be easily noticed. Sedation should be minimal, so that any alteration in the intensity of the pain is not masked. Periodic leukocyte counts should be made to assess progress. Some appendiceal masses will resolve if the patient is restricted to a fluid intake by mouth, but it is safer and wiser to use gastrointestinal suction coupled with intravenous fluids, since resolution will be quicker. Since the sensitivity of the organisms is unknown, a broad-spectrum antibiotic should be given.

With these measures, the majority of appendiceal abscesses treated conservatively will resolve satisfactorily. If, while under treatment, the pain persists for more than 24 hours or becomes more severe, or if there are significant changes in the vital signs, operation should be performed. The appendix should be removed, unless technical difficulties make this too difficult and would prolong the operation unnecessarily. Drainage alone will then have to suffice. If conservative treatment only has been employed, gastrointestinal x-ray studies should be performed to exclude any underlying pathology, such as a carcinoma of the cecum or regional enteritis, before the patient leaves the hospital. The patient should be advised to have an elective appendectomy after an interval of six to eight weeks.

Similarly, there are two alternative treatments for the patient with general peritonitis, but in this instance the emphasis on surgical attack is greater. The perforated, gangrenous appendix may be unguarded by omentum or adhesions, and it forms a reservoir to discharge further infected material into the peritoneal cavity. It should, therefore, be removed, but time must be spent getting the patient into as good condition as possible before operation.

The effects of generalized peritonitis following appendicitis are due to a variety of causes. The inflamed surface of the peritoneum weeps fluid of the same composition as plasma. The intestines are paralyzed and distended with large volumes of secretions. Vomiting causes considerable loss of upper gastrointestinal juices. The bacteria present in the peritoneal cavity cause severe toxemia and hyperpyrexia, particularly in children. These patients require careful clinical and biochemical assessment when they are first seen. The physical signs of electrolyte depletion and dehydration should be sought. A plasma volume deficit may be shown by a tachycardia, hypotension and peripheral vasoconstriction.

Biochemical assessment should start by recording the specific gravity, chloride content, and pH of the urine, and it should also include the plasma electrolyte and blood urea levels, and the hematocrit. When all these figures are available, the approximate size of fluid and electrolyte deficit should be computed and the patient replenished with intravenous fluids. Due to the peritoneal inflammation, a large volume of colloid will have to be given in the form of plasma or blood. The amounts that have to be given are extremely variable and should be determined by the patient's response to treatment. The losses incurred by vomiting must be replaced by normal saline, and the rate of administration checked by periodic determinations of the biochemistry. A catheter may be placed in the bladder so that the hourly urine output can be accurately measured. The intestinal dilatation and paralysis is treated by a nasogastric tube with continuous aspiration, and the infection combated by broad-spectrum antibiotics. An effective analgesic should also be given. If the body temperature is high, it should be reduced by tepid sponging, exposure, and the use of a fan. There is a danger that serious cardiac arrhythmias may develop if such a hyperpyrexic patient is given an anesthetic.

With these measures, the patient's condition should improve sufficiently to allow administration of an anesthetic and removal of the appendix. In the postoperative period, paralytic ileus should be treated by the same methods and the antibiotics continued. These patients with generalized peritonitis are the cause of the continuing small mortality following appendectomy, and they require careful and energetic treatment.

COMPLICATIONS. The most common complication after appendectomy is an infection in the wound. This is particularly likely to happen when the appendix is perforated at the time of the operation, but the infection can be reduced, either by draining the superficial tissues of the wound, or by leaving the skin and subcutaneous tissues open initially and suturing them a few days later by delayed primary suture.

When peritonitis is present at the time of operation, paralytic ileus is common. Postoperative adhesions may cause mechanical obstruction of the bowel, and particular care is needed to distinguish this from simple paralytic obstruction in the early postoperative days. Intraperitoneal abscesses may result, either in the subphrenic space or in the pelvis; they should be looked for specifically

in any patient who runs a fever after operation. Fistula formation is occasionally seen after appendectomy. This may be due to a retained foreign body such as a surgical pack, to distal obstruction of the colon by a neoplasm, to a missed diagnosis of regional enteritis or to infection with Actinomyces. It may sometimes be caused by unsatisfactory closure of the appendix stump due to edema of the cecum, or by erosion of the walls of the bowel caused by a stiff rubber drain left in situ too long. If a fistula does occur, the primary causes listed above should be excluded by x-ray films and pathologic tests. A final complication, rare since the development of antibiotics, is portal pylephlebitis. This is caused by bacterial invasion of the portal venous system, and leads to multiple liver abscesses.

Mortality from acute appendicitis is about 1 per cent. Death occurs most frequently in young children with generalized peritonitis and in older people in whom the diagnosis is delayed by the atypical presenting features of the disease.

OTHER DISEASES OF THE APPENDIX. Chronic appendicitis is a doubtful clinical entity. At one time, chronic infection of the appendix was thought to cause flatulence, dyspepsia, irregularity of the bowels, persistent abdominal pain and other abdominal complaints. These symptoms are not caused by a chronic, perpetual infection of the appendix, and other causes should always be sought.

There is, however, a small group of patients in whom attacks of appendiceal obstruction occur and subside spontaneously. Characteristically, these patients suffer from recurrent bouts of abdominal pain with little localization, and are symptom-free between attacks. Physical examination is usually normal, unless the patient is examined during an attack. An upper gastrointestinal series of x-ray studies should be made, which may show nonfilling of an obstructed appendix, the presence of a fecalith, or immobility and tenderness of the appendix during fluoroscopy. Before appendectomy is advised in such a patient, the entire gastrointestinal tract and genitourinary tract must be thoroughly investigated to exclude any other pathology. The appendix may show fibrosis, partial obliteration of the lumen and infiltration by chronic inflammatory cells. Occasionally, the lumen may be filled with parasitic pinworms, or oxyuria.

If the lumen of the appendix is obstructed and there is no infection, the appendix may slowly distend with the mucus secreted by its mucosal cells to form a "mucocele." Symptoms are few, and the mucocele is often found incidentally at operation for another condition. There may be attacks of low-grade abdominal pain, and occasionally the patient may notice a mass in the right iliac fossa. X-ray examination is inconclusive, but a mucocele may indent the shadow of the cecum. If a mucocele should rupture naturally or be broken during removal, mucosal cells may be implanted in the peritoneal cavity and continue to secrete mucus. A ruptured appendix mucocele is, therefore, one of the causes of pseudomyxoma peritonaei. In this condition, the entire peritoneal cavity is filled by masses of gelatinous mucus.

Infection of the appendix by the fungus *Actinomyces israeli* is now uncommon, and is usually confined to rural districts. It causes a granuloma of the ileocecal region with the formation of a mass and multiple sinuses draining through the skin overlying it. The pus from these sinuses usually contains the characteristic "sulfur granules" of the ray fungus, which may be seen with the naked eye. The diagnosis should always be suspected if a fecal fistula forms after appendectomy. It can be confirmed by histologic examination of the removed appendix. Actinomycosis is treated by a six weeks' course of penicillin, or a long course of treatment with one of the tetracycline group. A course of iodine treatment may also help in resolution of the disease.

Tumors of the appendix are uncommon, and primary carcinoma at this site is extremely rare. A tumor may obtruct the lumen of the appendix and precipitate an attack of acute appendicitis. An unsuspected tumor may be found only on microscopy of the removed appendix. If a carcinoma is found, a standard right hemicolectomy should be performed. This can be done either at the time of operation or later, if the pathologic report is the first indication that cancer is present.

Carcinoid tumors of the appendix are formed from the argentaffin cells, which are more numerous in the walls of the appendix than in any other part of the intestine. More than 50 per cent of carcinoid tumors arise in the appendix, but invasion or spread to the lymphatic system is uncommon. They usually occur at the tip of the appendix, and in view of their benign nature, appendectomy is adequate treatment. If the tumor occurs at the base of the appendix, and if it involves the

wall of the cecum, it is more likely to be invasive and to metastasize; a right hemicolectomy should be performed in such patients.

Mesenteric adenitis is a common condition, and is often the main problem in differential diagnosis when appendicitis is suspected. Enlargement and hyperplasia of the lymph nodes in the mesentery of the terminal ileum and appendix are present. The bowel itself appears normal. Usually, no specific organism can be identified in the bowel or in the nodes. This idiopathic type of mesenteric adenitis is seen in childhood or early adult life, and is characterized by intermittent attacks of abdominal pain with fever and upset bowels. It is probably infectious, since small outbreaks may occur in communities such as schools, and it sometimes follows a sore throat. On microscopic examination, the mesenteric nodes show nonspecific hyperplasia. The disease may be caused by infection with an adenovirus, which sometimes can be recovered from the stools.

Mesenteric adenitis is a benign and self-limiting disease, with the attacks of abdominal pain passing off in early adult life. It has been suggested that it may be the primary cause of regional enteritis by producing lymphatic stasis in the mesentery. It may also be the primary cause for intussusception in children by producing hyperplasia of the submucosal lymphoid follicles of the small bowel. The enlarged follicle may then form the apex of the intussusception.

The symptoms of mesenteric adenitis are very similar, if not identical, to those of acute appendicitis; often, the two conditions cannot be distinguished. Occasionally, a lymphocytosis may be found, or mobile, enlarged nodes may be felt in the right lower quadrant in the well-relaxed abdomen. Enlargement of nodes elsewhere, as in the cervical region and axilla, may also be found. Most commonly, the diagnosis is made at operation for suspected appendicitis. Appendectomy should be performed, and one of the nodes removed to confirm the diagnosis and exclude the presence of lymphoma.

THE COLON

ANATOMY AND PHYSIOLOGY. For most of its path, the colon lies against the posterior abdominal wall, forming a frame around the loops of small intestine. The longitudinal muscle layer is concentrated into three bands, the taeniae coli, which travel the length of the bowel. These appear to be shorter than the colon itself, so that the bowel is drawn into loose folds, or sacculations, which give it its characteristic appearance both in the abdomen and on x-ray examinations.

The large bowel is derived embryologically from the midgut and the hindgut, the boundary between these portions being toward the left of the middle of the transverse colon. The cecum, ascending colon and right part of the transverse colon are, therefore, supplied by the superior mesenteric artery via the ileocolic, right colic and middle colic arteries (Fig. 63). The nerve supply to these parts of the colon is derived from the vagus nerve and the sympathetic fibers from the celiac plexus. The left half of the transverse colon, the descending and sigmoid colon, and most of the rectum get their blood supply from the inferior mesenteric artery through the left colic, sigmoid and superior rectal arteries. Their autonomic nerve supply comes from the nervi erigentes and the presacral plexus. The distribution of referred pain is, therefore, different in lesions of the two parts of the large bowel; pain from the right half is felt in the epigastrium, and pain from the left half is felt in the hypogastrium.

In the normal individual, the transverse and sigmoid colon are the only parts provided with a mesentery; the remainder of the bowel lies retroperitoneally. Due to abnormalities in development, some patients may have a complete mesentery to the right half of the colon and cecum, so that a twisting or volvulus of this part of the bowel can occur. Similarly, an unusually long mesentery of the sigmoid colon with a narrow base predisposes to volvulus of this portion.

The termination of the colon at its junction with the rectum is not a precise anatomic point, and it is loosely described as the "rectosigmoid." Over this portion, the three taeniae coli fan out, so that the bowel once again has a complete covering of longitudinal muscle. This junction of sigmoid colon and rectum lies just below the sacral promontory, approximately 15 cm. from the anal verge on sigmoidoscopic examination.

The functions of the large bowel are absorption and storage. The proximal part, which receives the fluid chyme from the terminal ileum, reabsorbs water so that the feces become more solid as they move through the colon. The left half of the colon is mainly a reservoir for the formed feces; but it still has considerable absorptive power, as has been shown by the effects when this part of the colon is used as a urinary conduit.

The peristaltic activity of the colon is well

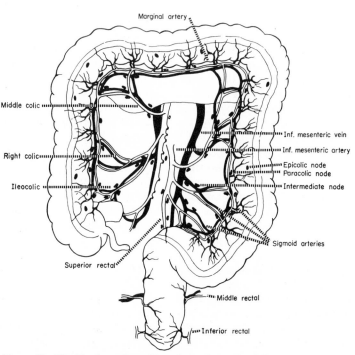

Figure 63. The blood supply and lymphatic drainage of the large bowel.

adapted to these functions. Peristalsis is infrequent and has a mass action, the whole content of stored feces being propelled into the rectum and initiating the reflexes necessary for defecation. This colic peristalsis may be stimulated by eating, resulting in the "gastrocolic reflex," particularly in small babies. More frequent small amplitude waves of contraction do occur, but these are not propulsive. However, they may be of importance if their duration and intensity increase, causing a persistent rise in the intracolonic pressure. This may lead to the formation of diverticula.

The investigation of suspected disease of the colon depends particularly on the hand and eye. In all patients, a great deal of information is to be found in the rectum and the part of the sigmoid colon visible through a sigmoidoscope. The fact that 75 per cent of all neoplasms of the large bowel occur in this area emphasizes the importance of careful digital examination and sigmoidoscopy. Inspection and biopsy of the rectal or sigmoid mucosa may confirm a diagnosis of amebiasis or ulcerative colitis and make further investigation unnecessary. Culture of the stools and the usual laboratory investigation of the blood for anemia or evidence of malnutrition should also be routine.

The final step in investigation should be the barium enema examination. This is an accurate diagnostic procedure, except for showing early lesions of the hepatic or splenic flexures. At the end of the examination, the barium is evacuated and air may be insufflated so that the mucosal pattern of the bowel can be examined more closely; the bowel being distended with air and the mucosa coated with barium. This examination is most important when polyps of the colon are suspected.

TRAUMA. Traumatic lesions of the colon, like those of the small bowel, have become more common with the rising automobile accident rate. Again, knowledge of their treatment stems largely from experience in war. Rupture of the colon may follow blunt trauma, or a penetrating wound by gunshot or knife. The cecum, which is often distended so as to lie immediately under the anterior abdominal wall, is particularly liable to traumatic rupture; but any other part of the colon may be involved. The two flexures lying deep are protected by the rib cage and are less liable to injury except by penetrating wounds. Rupture of the colon following blunt injury is often an insidious process, as the immediate effect of the blow is only a partial splitting of the thin circular muscle coat, or a hematoma of the bowel wall. Complete rupture and peritoneal soiling may occur later, when the patient is no longer under observation.

Rupture of the colon has followed the playful use of compressed air equipment as a makeshift enema during industrial horseplay. The colon and rectum may also be injured by accidental or deliberate impalement of the rectum. The variety of objects which have been described as causing this type of injury makes the imagination boggle; they range from a Japanese paper sunshade to a tin of domestic drain cleanser. Injury of the colon by a sigmoidoscope is uncommon as long as the examination is done gently and no unusual angulations or other difficulties are encountered.

The diagnosis of large bowel injury depends on a careful history as to the severity and site of the blow and complete examination. The physical and x-ray signs of intraperitoneal bleeding or perforation should be looked for, and after suitable resuscitative measures, the patient should be operated on. The safest way of managing ragged lacerations of the colon is to exteriorize the involved loop as a colostomy. Clean, regular holes in the colon may be sutured, and a proximal colostomy added to isolate the injured bowel. This technique is particularly useful in wounds or trauma to the rectum or lower sigmoid when exteriorization of the injured area would be technically impossible.

INFECTIONS. Bacterial infections of the colon, such as cholera and the various types of dysentery, are seldom of surgical importance, except as a diagnostic exercise in distinguishing them from other causes of diarrhea. In contrast, infection with the protozoan parasite *Entamoeba histolytica* is of some importance. Infestation of the bowel by this parasite is endemic in many tropical areas and in certain parts of the United States. Figures for the incidence of symptomless carriers vary, but there was a marked increase after the Second World War, with the return of servicemen from tropical areas. Infection occurs through eating foodstuffs, or water infected with *E. histolytica* in its encysted form. Once in the habitat of the large bowel, the parasite enters the mucous glands. By proliferation in the submucosal layer and the secretion of a proteolytic enzyme, it undermines the mucosa and forms multiple flask-shaped ulcers. The protozoa may enter the portal venous system and thus reach the liver. Secondary infection of the ulcers by bacteria is common, and if the disease persists in a chronic form the identification of the causative protozoon may be very difficult, owing to the overgrowth of enteric bacteria.

Amebiasis may present in three ways: as a localized bowel infection with the typical symptoms of dysentery, including rectal bleeding; as a localized granulomatous lesion which commonly affects the cecum and closely mimics a carcinoma, and by involvement of the liver, causing an amebic hepatitis or amebic liver abscess. The last two groups cause particular difficulty in diagnosis, as the symptoms are remarkably nonspecific.

Amebic infection causes a progressive pyrexial illness, with marked systemic upset, loss of weight, anorexia and diarrhea. If liver involvement has occurred, the disease may resemble infective hepatitis; liver abscesses may present with symptoms due to a sympathetic pleural effusion.

Investigation shows a neutrophil leukocytosis and the presence of *E. histolytica* in a fresh specimen of stool. Sigmoidoscopy will often show a vascular proctocolitis with ulceration of the mucosa, and the parasite may be seen either in scrapings from the ulcers or in a biopsy specimen. The treatment consists of antibiotics to control the secondary infection, with emetine and chloroquine which specifically act against the parasite. If a liver abscess is present with secondary infection, surgical drainage may be needed. In parts of the world where amebiasis is endemic, a course of emetine treatment is routinely given as a therapeutic trial to patients who present with symptoms and signs suggestive of carcinoma of the colon.

ULCERATIVE COLITIS. Idiopathic ulcerative proctocolitis is considered with infections of the colon, although the true etiology remains obscure. The facts known about ulcerative colitis are few and these are confined to its pathology, incidence and prognosis; but the theories as to its cause are legion.

This disease is characterized by widespread superficial ulceration of the mucosa of the colon, with superimposed secondary inflammatory changes of the bowel wall. The primary mucosal nature of the disease distinguishes it from regional enteritis, which affects the submucosal layers as much as the mucosa. The disease has a slight predilection for the Jewish race, but is worldwide in distribution. It may occur at any age, although the peak incidence is between the ages of 20 and 40 years. Women are affected more often than men, in the ratio of 2.5 to 1.

A chronic dysentery due to infection has been suggested as a possible cause of ulcerative colitis, since it often follows an attack of acute amebic or bacillary dysentery. However, repeated investigation of patients with ulcerative colitis has failed to demonstrate a consistent bacterial pathogen. The association of the disease, or its relapses, with periods of emotional stress suggests a psychologic cause. Many of the patients have unstable emotional backgrounds and a family history of insecurity and instability. Psychiatric treatment has helped some patients. Sensitivity to cow's milk, induced in infant life by the early cessation of breast feeding, has been suggested as a contributory cause. Excessive amounts of lysozyme have been found in the feces of patients with ulcerative colitis, and this has also been alleged as a cause. It is probable, though, that the excessive lysozyme is produced by the large numbers of pus cells in the bowel as a result of the acute inflammation. More recently, it has been suggested that an autoimmune reaction is involved. This causes sensitization and destruction of the colonic mucosa, and these superficial lesions of the mucosa are then enlarged and perpetuated by secondary bacterial invasion.

Characteristically, ulcerative colitis is a chronic disease liable to remit spontaneously for a variable time. There are three clinical types. In the first of these, acute fulminating colitis, the whole colon and rectum are affected and the ulceration is extensive and deep. This type affects approximately 20 per cent of the patients. In the second type, continuous colitis, the symptoms persist from the onset and vary in severity. Usually, only the left side of the colon is affected. The third type is often called recurrent colitis, in which the attacks are limited and separated by varying periods of remission.

The symptoms may vary from those of a mild rectal irritation to those of an acute severe infective enteritis. Diarrhea and urgency of defecation, bleeding at stool, attacks of cramplike abdominal pain and perianal soreness are common in the early stages. In other patients, the disease may be explosive, with the sudden onset of acute diarrhea and frequent bloody stools, continuous abdominal pain, rapid loss of weight and a persistent pyrexia. Some patients first seek advice only because of the occurrence of complications such as arthritis or perianal suppuration.

The diagnosis of ulcerative colitis is not usually difficult, although regional enteritis affecting the colon may be very similar in presentation. In the early stages of the disease, the radiologic appearance of the colon is normal, but examination of the rectal mucosa shows the typical hemorrhagic vascular appearance, with ulceration. The stools should be examined and cultured to exclude amebiasis and simple bacterial infection. Sigmoidoscopy and barium enema examination should exclude other conditions such as carcinoma of the colon or familial polyposis. A biopsy of rectal mucosa may exclude other causes of chronic diarrhea. Later, barium enema examination shows loss of the normal haustral pattern, rigidity and shortening, the so-called "hosepipe colon," due to fibrosis and contraction. As ulceration continues, pseudopolyposis may occur. The islets of mucosa between the ulcerated areas become hydropic and edematous, and show on roentgenograms as apparent polyps throughout the colon. These polyps are not formed by epithelial hyperplasia, but by inflammation and edema. In the acute variety, the right half of the colon may be grossly dilated. Spontaneous perforation of the colon may result from deep ulceration or acute dilatation.

There are many complications of ulcerative colitis, some of which are due to the local condition and some to the systemic effects and the toxemia caused by the inflammation of the colon (Fig. 64). There is rapid loss of fluid, electrolytes and protein due to the frequent passage of liquid, hemorrhagic stools. Malnutrition, electrolyte deficiencies and hypoproteinemia are common, and the loss of blood causes a progressive iron deficiency anemia.

The local complications affecting the colon are particularly important since they often require surgical intervention. Malignant change in the chronically inflamed colon occurs in approximately 12 per cent of the patients who have had ulcerative colitis for more than ten years. Because carcinomata which develop are often anaplastic and multiple, the prognosis is poor. Also, the symptoms of a developing cancer are masked by those of the pre-existing colitis and this

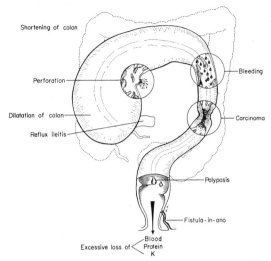

Figure 64.   The complications of ulcerative proctocolitis.

causes delay in investigation, diagnosis and treatment. Acute dilatation of the colon or perforation, particularly after steroid therapy, may occur. Perianal abscesses and fistulae-in-ano commonly occur, and are especially distressing to women. If fibrosis of the colon develops, it may cause a rectal stricture. Among the general complications seen in ulcerative colitis are polyarthritis, uveitis, liver damage, venous thrombosis and skin lesions such as pyoderma gangrenosum.

Treatment. There are no set rules for the treatment of ulcerative colitis and the advice given to any patient must be based on an exact knowledge of the prognosis of this disease, and of the indications for medical or surgical treatment.

The prognosis depends on three main factors; the severity of the symptoms, the length of bowel affected and the age of the patient (Fig. 65). If the symptoms are mild, the disease is localized to a small part of the bowel, usually the rectum and sigmoid, and if the patient is a young adult, he has a 90 per cent chance of remission with medical treatment alone. By contrast, if he is over 60 with severe symptoms and involvement of the whole colon, he has slightly less than a 50 per cent chance of remission on medical management. One would, therefore, recommend surgical intervention much earlier in such a patient. The majority of patients get over their first attack of colitis, but nearly 90 per cent have recurrent attacks during a subsequent ten-year period.

Patients should be admitted for investigation and diagnostic study. Surprising symp-

PROGNOSIS OF ULCERATIVE COLITIS

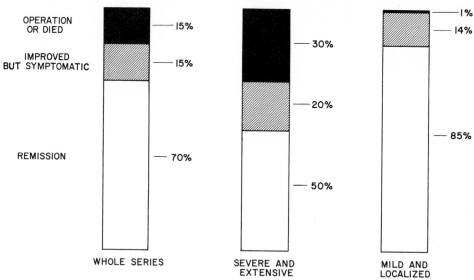

Figure 65.   The prognosis of ulcerative colitis to both surgical and medical therapy is related to its severity.

tomatic improvement results from placing these patients in the disciplined atmosphere of a hospital regimen under moderate sedation. Careful inquiry should be made into their emotional state and psychologic background to see if any factor in home or business life has triggered the attack. Nutrition should be maintained or improved by a high protein diet, if this can be taken, and anemia should be corrected by systemic iron therapy or by blood transfusion. Dramatic improvement may follow a short course of corticosteroid or adrenocorticotropic hormone therapy, the local administration of hydrocortisone enemas, or the use of nonabsorbable sulfonamide preparations. The latter also appear useful in preventing recurrences. There is, however, a wide difference of opinion regarding the advisability of steroid therapy.

In the acute fulminating stage, the symptoms are much more dramatic. There is severe toxemia, shown by persistent high fever and tachycardia, bowel actions are frequent, and blood loss may be severe. Despite the severity of symptoms, approximately two-thirds of these patients remit under careful medical management. This should include antibiotics to control secondary infection, adequate doses of steroids and repeated infusions of blood and plasma to compensate for the continuing losses. In addition, intravenous replacement of elec-

trolytes, particularly potassium, is often necessary.

There are certain definite indications for operation in this disease, the most important being the definite or suspected presence of a carcinoma in the inflamed bowel. Operation is also necessary in the fulminating disease when medical therapy has failed, when acute dilatation or perforation of the colon has recurred, or when blood loss is so severe that excision of the colon is the only way to stop it. In chronic or recurrent colitis, operation may be necessary for local complications, such as a fibrous stricture of the colon, persistent perirectal suppuration or fistula formation, or for the more distant complications such as uveitis or arthritis. Probably, the most important indication in this type of patient is the persistence of bowel symptoms with only short and infrequent remissions.

The first successful surgical treatment in ulcerative colitis was simple ileostomy, the creation of an artificial anus in the abdominal wall, through which ileal contents are discharged into some form of bag appliance. In the early days of surgical treatment for this condition, the diseased colon was left in situ, and it was hoped that this diversion of the fecal stream alone would cause a remission of symptoms.

However, the preservation of the diseased colon caused almost as much trouble as the primary disease, particularly in the continuance of such distant complications as uveitis or arthritis. At present surgical treatment offers three alternatives: first, ileostomy and colectomy, leaving a rectal stump disconnected temporarily, with the possibility that it might be used to re-establish bowel continuity later (Fig. 66, A); second, complete excision of the colon and rectum, leaving the patient with a permanent ileostomy (Fig. 66, B); third, excision of the colon, but re-establishment of continuity immediately by an ileorectal anastomosis (Fig. 66, C).

The arguments in favor of these alternative surgical procedures are finely balanced and they are not yet resolved. The general preference is for panproctocolectomy with permanent ileostomy, but the results are not always reassuring. In emergency for fulminating colitis, the mortality of this operation is ap-

proximately 30 per cent and the morbidity a further 30 per cent. By contrast, in elective circumstances, that is, for a patient with chronic recurrent disease during a remission, the mortality of this major operation is approximately 4 per cent. Unfortunately, the postoperative morbidity remains high.

The main causes of morbidity are complications associated with the ileostomy, difficulties in healing of the perineal wound or subsequent episodes of torsion or adhesive small intestinal obstruction. Stenosis, prolapse or retraction of the ileostomy stoma affects approximately one-fourth of the patients, even using present techniques to fashion the ileostomy exactly. In any series, follow-up records show that a quarter of the patients require further surgical procedures to correct such deformities of the ileostomy stoma. A persistent sinus in the perineal

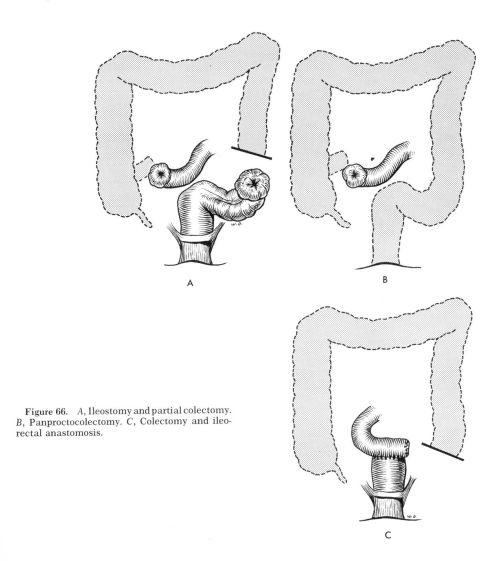

Figure 66. A, Ileostomy and partial colectomy. B, Panproctocolectomy. C, Colectomy and ileorectal anastomosis.

A

B

C

wound is also a common sequel and is particularly likely in patients who have had prolonged steroid therapy before operation.

Episodes of adhesive small bowel obstruction afflict about 15 per cent of postcolectomy patients, but these episodes usually die out after the first three postoperative years. There is, therefore, a continuing morbidity after colectomy and also some further mortality owing to the need for subsequent operations. This combined mortality and morbidity figure probably compares favorably with comparable figures for patients looked after by long-term medical therapy, but it should always be remembered in assessing the necessity or probity of operating on a patient with ulcerative colitis.

Other sequelae of the operation may also cause some distress, such as loss of sexual potency in the male, or loss of control of micturition in either sex.

The main alternative operation, total colectomy with continuity preserved by ileo-rectal anastomosis, has obvious attractions. Any alternative to a permanent ileostomy is particularly attractive in the age group affected by ulcerative colitis, both to the patients and to their medical advisers. Unfortunately, this operation also has its drawbacks.

It should not be used if the patient has any of the rectal complications of ulcerative colitis, such as perianal fistula, ischiorectal abscess or fibrous stricture of the rectum. Preoperative sigmoidoscopic examination should show that the rectum is still supple and distends normally when insufflated with air. There must be absolutely no suspicion of malignancy in the rectal mucosa.

Even with these restrictions of its use, this operation has drawbacks. Continuing frequency of bowel action is common. Systemic complications such as arthritis may persist. The subsequent, or previously unrecognized, development of malignancy in the remaining rectum is a frequent enough occurence to cause concern. The advantage of this particular procedure for colitis is often in the eye of the performer, and there is still wide disagreement as to the eventual symptomatic relief which this operation gives to the patient.

The general preference, therefore, is for panproctocolectomy as the best operative treatment for ulcerative colitis, and the patients should not be misled about the fact that their ileostomy is likely to be a permanent feature of their future life. However,

with modern light, disposable ileostomy bags, this is now much easier to manage. Ileostomy clubs, or associations of patients with this disability, hold regular meetings and have helped many to adjust satisfactorily to this condition.

DIVERTICULOSIS AND DIVERTICULITIS. Diverticulosis of the colon is an acquired disease, the diverticula being of the pulsion type and consisting of pouches of mucosa not covered by muscular tissue. These pouches tend to occur on the circumference of the large bowel, where the blood vessels penetrate the muscular wall to form a point of potential weakness. The diverticula result from a persistently increased intracolonic pressure, which is raised to abnormal heights during peristalsis. The causes of this increased pressure are not known, but it is associated with chronic constipation or bowel irregularity, and is probably a result of uncoordinated muscular activity in the colon. Diverticulosis is a disease of adult life, and the incidence increases with age. Most autopsy studies report an incidence of 30 per cent; and at the age of 80 years, more than two-thirds of the population have diverticula. In 50 per cent of patients, the diverticula are in the sigmoid colon; they occur in the descending colon, transverse colon and cecum in descending order of frequency. The patients are often obese, and hiatus hernia, cholecystitis and duodenal diverticula frequently accompany diverticulosis.

Diverticulosis often produces no symptoms at all, or only a vague, querulous bowel consciousness. Symptoms occur only when pathologic changes in the diverticula cause diverticulitis. The incidence of diverticulitis is increasing, and it appears to have two fairly distinct clinical types. In the elderly patient it runs a benign course, producing moderate bowel symptoms with left-sided abdominal pain, but few complications. When it occurs in the 40-to-60 age group, it is often more virulent. Its onset appears more acute and the complication rate is higher.

Diverticulitis is caused by inflammation of the diverticulum, resulting from inadequate drainage through its narrow neck and from impaction in the sac of a small pellet of feces which becomes inspissated and forms a fecalith. This may ulcerate or erode the wall of the diverticulum. Since the sac contains little muscular tissue, it is difficult for its contents to empty into the lumen of the colon, particularly when the neck of the sac is narrow to start with and is made narrower by inflammatory edema. Stasis occurs, and a perfect site for bacterial proliferation is created in the diverticulum. The colon shows evidence of inflammation surrounding the diverticula, and of gross hypertrophy of the muscular layers, which are thickened and encroach on the lumen of the bowel to give it a ragged appearance.

The patient with diverticulitis usually seeks advice because of symptoms of low-grade bowel obstruction from muscular hypertrophy, and pain in the left iliac fossa due to inflammation of the diverticula on the sigmoid colon, or spasm and segmental dilatation of the sigmoid colon. An alteration in normal bowel habit, with episodes of mucous diarrhea and constipation, is common. Colicky lower abdominal pain occurs with the episodes of constipation and may shift to the left iliac fossa for periods of a few days. When this happens, the pain changes to a sharp persistent ache made worse by movement or coughing. During the acute bouts of pain, the patient may notice a fever, with anorexia and nausea. Rectal bleeding may also occur.

Diverticulitis causes various complications which considerably alter the symptoms it produces (Fig. 67). As a result of pent-up infection in the thin-walled sac, it may rupture. If this happens suddenly before many adhesions have formed, the contents of the infected sac are discharged abruptly into the peritoneal cavity, causing a bacterial peritonitis with severe, sudden abdominal pain.

Sometimes a diverticulum bursts without much previous inflammation and leaves a hole in the wall of the colon through which feces enter the peritoneal cavity, causing a fecal peritonitis. This catastrophe is sometimes precipitated by giving an enema with excessive pressure. More commonly, the diverticulum has been walled off by the omentum and adjacent loops of the bowel before it perforates, and it then causes abscess formation with local pain ad tenderness. This abscess is adherent to adjacent structures, and particularly to the bladder. If it ruptures into the bladder, it causes a vesicocolic fistula, an abnormal communication between the colon and bladder. The patient will then have symptoms of a persistent urinary infection and may complain of pneumaturia, the passage of bubbles of gas in the urine. Lastly, erosion of the wall of the diverticulum by its contained fecalith may expose the blood vessels coursing over the sac and cause severe rectal hemorrhage.

When no acute complication of diverticulitis is present, there is time to assess and investigate the patient fully. A carcinoma of the colon produces practically identical symptoms. Other conditions, such as amebiasis, regional enteritis and ulcerative colitis, should be excluded by appropriate investigation. A barium enema examination must be performed, showing certain features in the affected colon. The diverticula are outlined by the barium, and although there may be marked narrowing of the colon due to the muscular hypertrophy, the normal mucosal pattern can usually be traced through the narrowed area. If there is still doubt as to whether the narrowing is caused by a neoplasm or spasm associated with diverticulitis, an anticholinergic drug should be given. This will relax spasm but will not alter the narrowing due to an organic stricture. The barium may be seen to leave the colon and enter an abscess cavity, or to outline a fistulous track into the bladder.

Unfortunately, both diverticulitis and carcinoma of the colon are common; and since they are frequently present in the same patient, differentiation between the two is often impossible. If there is any doubt in the surgeon's mind, operation should be advised so that tissue can be obtained for histologic examination. Even at laparotomy, it is difficult to distinguish an area of diverticulitis with fibrosis from a carcinoma, and the pathologist must be the final judge.

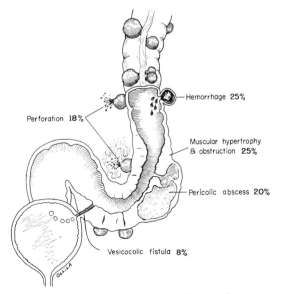

Figure 67. The complications of diverticulitis.

Diverticulitis may present, therefore, as a chronic bowel complaint with sporadic diarrhea and constipation, as an acute abdominal emergency with signs of peritonitis, as an undiagnosed lump in the abdomen due to abscess formation, as rectal hemorrhage, as a large bowel obstruction of low-grade type, or as a urinary infection with pneumaturia. Examination may show nothing at all between attacks. Localized tenderness in the left iliac fossa is usually found, with mild signs of peritoneal irritation or a palpable thickened tender loop of colon. If complications have occurred, there may be signs of a generalized peritonitis, of a pericolic abscess or of a large bowel obstruction.

The treatment of diverticulitis depends on the severity of the symptoms and the presence of complications. With periodic mild upsets in bowel action and left-sided abdominal pain, medical measures may be sufficient, particularly when the patient is elderly. A low-residue diet, reduction in weight, mild analgesics, a bulk laxative of the agar group and antispasmodics may be sufficient to control the attacks. To these one may add periodic short courses of a nonabsorbable antibacterial drug such as phthalylsulfathiazole, which will at least reduce the pathogenic population of the colon.

If the diagnosis is doubtful, if complications have occurred, or if the symptoms are intractable, treatment must be more aggressive. Most of the patients who require operation for diverticulitis have persistent symptoms due to low-grade inflammation and obstruction, but without dramatic complications. The diseased segment of colon should be resected after adequate preparation. A pericolic abscess due to diverticulitis should be drained, and the feces diverted by a proximal colostomy to prevent further fecal contamination of the diseased portion. Peritonitis from a ruptured diverticulum may require drainage and suture of the perforation, combined with a colostomy proximal to the site of perforation. If this program of drainage and a colostomy are carried out, the patient will need two further operations: resection of the diseased colon and closure of the colostomy. As an alternative to this traditional method of treating perforated diverticulitis, primary resection of the diseased segment of bowel may be performed with immediate restoration of continuity. With modern supportive treatment and antibiotics, primary resection produces better results than the older measures do, and it saves the patient considerable expense and hardship. A vesicocolic fistula will not heal without surgical treatment; the diseased segment of colon, the fistula tract and the affected part of the bladder wall are excised completely. The bladder is then repaired and the colon reanastomosed.

ISCHEMIC COLITIS. Like the small bowel, the large bowel may also be damaged by arterial insufficiency. Ischemic colitis has only recently been recognized and has previously masqueraded under a variety of names, such as "necrotizing colitis," "ischemic enterocolitis," or "acute segmental colitis." The portion of colon affected is usually the splenic flexure where the territories supplied by the superior mesenteric and inferior mesenteric arteries meet. Ischemic colitis causes an acute inflammation of a variable length of bowel in this area. This may progress to gangrene, it may partially resolve leaving a fibrous stricture, or it may resolve completely.

This is a disease of the middle-aged or elderly and causes acute lower abdominal pain with vomiting, fever and brisk rectal hemorrhage. The clinical signs closely resemble those of acute diverticulitis of the colon and this is the usual preoperative diagnosis.

At laparotomy, the affected segment of bowel may appear gangrenous or just reddened and swollen. Most patients have been treated by resection of the diseased bowel or some type of exteriorization procedure. Microscopically, the bowel shows the changes of a hemorrhagic infarct, the mucosa being particularly affected. If tissue destruction is severe, virulent organisms of the clostridial group invade the bowel wall. This may alter the microscopic picture so as to give the impression that this disease is primarily bacterial in origin.

NEOPLASMS OF COLON AND RECTUM. The most important and the most numerous benign growths of the large bowel are the polyps (Fig. 68). The word "polyp" applies to any lesion seen projecting into the lumen of the bowel. A polyp with a stalk is pedunculated, and one with no stalk is sessile. True polyps are tumors of epithelial origin. Tumors originating in other tissues such as carcinoid, lipoma, fibroma, angioma or hyperplasia of a lymphoid follicle may all be called polyps. "Polyp" is, therefore, not a histologic description.

Until recently, all epithelial polyps were

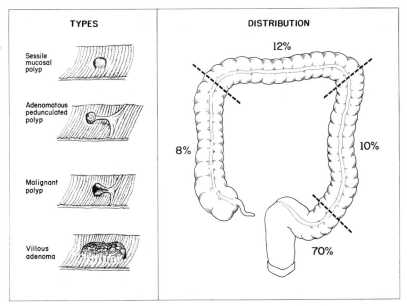

Figure 68. The epithelial polyps and their distribution.

regarded as premalignant conditions, and the treatment was excision of the polyp, either through the sigmoidoscope or by laparotomy. The polyps were regarded as showing a general instability of the colonic mucosa, predisposing to cancerous change. This reasonable conclusion was based on the presence of malignant pathology in many polyps and the common finding of polyps of the colon adjacent to a carcinoma. Areas of abnormal epithelial proliferation are also found in the mucosa near polyps. This simple picture is shrouded in doubt, however, and there is increasing belief that the treatment of polyps of the colon in the past may have been too radical.

Polyps of the colon are of five main types. The most common is the polypoid adenoma, a true adenomatous polyp of the mucosal epithelium. These polyps are found throughout the colon, though approximately 70 per cent are concentrated in the rectum and sigmoid. Since carcinomatous changes may be found in some, polyps should be removed. These changes vary from carcinoma in situ at the apex of the tumor to true invasive carcinoma spreading to the stalk and thence to the bowel wall, although this is an uncommon finding. These polyps have a narrow pedicle or stalk and are, therefore, easily removed with a wire snare or biopsy forceps if visible through a sigmoidoscope. If the polyp lies high up, laparotomy and incision of the colon will be needed to remove it.

Histologic examination of the polyp is essential so that the further management of the patient can be planned. A benign adenoma, or one in which carcinoma in situ is demonstrated, requires no more than local removal. It is wise, however, to keep the patient under supervision with periodic sigmoidoscopic and air contrast examinations to check for recurrences. If the polyp shows frank carcinomatous invasion of the stalk or adjacent mucosa, the standard operation for cancer at that site should be carried out. If it is in the rectum, local excision followed by fulguration may occasionally be sufficient.

The second type of polyp is the villous adenoma. This is a diffuse hyperplastic change in the mucosa over a wide area of the colon or rectum. It may involve the circumference of the bowel and extend for 6 to 10 cm. along its length. Villous adenomas are less common than the polypoid adenoma, and occur in an older age group, but the vast majority affect the rectum and sigmoid colon. Malignant change occurs in a higher proportion, up to 40 per cent, than with the other types. This may be confined to a small portion of the growth in its early stages, and multiple biopsies from various sites should be obtained, since a small piece taken from one site may not truly represent the nature of the tumor. These growths characteristically produce large quantities of mucus and the patient's main complaint is of frequent mucous diarrhea. This mucus is rich in protein and electrolytes, particularly potassium, and the tumor may cause severe electrolyte or protein deficiency and acid-base imbalance. A paralytic ileus mimicking intestinal obstruction may occur as a result of the potassium deficiency. Because the incidence of carcinoma is higher, and because these are more extensive tumors, local treatment through a sigmoidoscope is often not possible. Treatment should be local removal of the affected part of the colon. If pathologic examination shows that carcinoma is present, a more radical operation is needed.

The third type of polyp is the mucous polyp. These may be multiple and scattered throughout the length of the large bowel. They are formed by mucus retention and are not neoplastic or malignant. They can cause severe rectal bleeding, or a polyp may form the apex for an intussusception of the colon. Since these polyps often regress spontaneously, their treatment should not be aggressive. Biopsy of one or two of the polyps should be performed to establish the diagnosis and the patient thereafter kept under periodic observation.

Pseudopolyposis of the colon, the fourth type, is a complication of both the acute and chronic types of ulcerative colitis. These polyps are not true tumors of the mucosal epithelium, but are formed by islands of edematous inflamed mucosa between the ulcerated areas. They are not areas of mucosal overgrowth or hyperplasia, and not premalignant. Their presence, however, indicates a severe or long-lasting type of ulcerative colitis, which is often complicated by the eventual occurrence of carcinoma. The development of pseudopolyposis in a patient with ulcerative colitis may, therefore, be an indication for surgical treatment.

The fifth type of polypoid disease of the colon is familial polyposis (Fig. 69). This is a rare condition which affects both men and women, and is transmitted to half the offspring of an affected patient. Adenomas arise throughout the large bowel, forming a diffuse carpet of polyps over the whole mucosa. For some reason, that part of the cecum bathed in the ileal juices coming through the ileocecal valve is often free of polyps, suggesting that these juices have an antineoplastic, or protective, action on the colon.

These polyps have a definite tendency to become carcinomatous; in fact, if untreated, 60 per cent of the patients eventually develop cancer of the bowel. There is also a high inci-

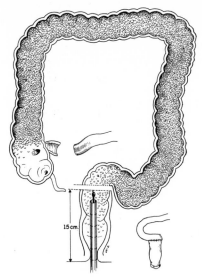

Figure 69.   Familial polyposis of the colon. The polyps are less numerous in the cecum. Most of the colon is excised, leaving a rectal stump in which the polyps are destroyed by electrocoagulation.

dence of carcinoma of the colon among the relatives of these patients, even though they themselves may not have polyposis.

The typical symptoms of polyposis are diarrhea and rectal bleeding, which start when the patient is in the late teens or the early twenties. The diagnosis is made by sigmoidoscopy, which shows multiple polyps in the rectum and sigmoid, and by barium enema examination.

Familial polyposis is treated by total colectomy, leaving a stump of rectum, to which the ileum is anastomosed. The amount of rectum left should be of such a size that the whole stump can be easily seen through a sigmoidoscope. The polyps in the rectum are initially destroyed by electrocoagulation and the patient returns at regular intervals so that any further polyps which develop can be dealt with in the same way. The polyps in the rectum may regress spontaneously after the ileum has been anastomosed to the rectum, further evidence of the antineoplastic effect of the ileal contents. If polyposis of the colon is diagnosed, the patient's family should be called for similar examination and all members should be advised to have regular, routine investigation because of the increased risk of carcinoma of the colon.

The colon may be the site of many other types of benign tumors, such as lipoma, fibroma, leiomyoma or hemangioma; but these are uncommon and they are often difficult or impossible to distinguish from a carcinoma without exploratory operation. Endometriosis also may involve the colon, forming a localized endometrioma of the wall of the bowel. This sometimes causes complete obstruction of the bowel, or may cause intermittent bouts of subacute obstructive symptoms coinciding with menstruation. The involved portion of colon should be excised.

CARCINOMA OF COLON AND RECTUM. Carcinoma of the large bowel is an important and common condition and is responsible for more of the deaths from malignant disease in this country than either cancer of the lung or cancer of the breast. Both sexes are liable to develop it and its incidence reaches a peak between the ages of 50 to 70 years, although it may occur at any age. In general, these tumors are more malignant when they affect young people. They may occur anywhere in the large bowel but are distinctly more frequent in the rectum and sigmoid, where 75 per cent are found (Fig. 70). The diagnosis in three-quarters of the patients can be made by relatively simple digital or visual examination of the lower bowel. It is a sad reflection of both patient and professional neglect that so many patients are first examined late in the

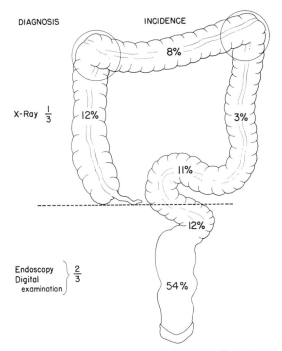

Figure 70. The distribution and diagnosis of carcinoma of the large bowel. Approximately two-thirds of these tumors are within reach of the finger or sigmoidoscope. The remaining third should be visualized by x-ray, but special care is needed to examine the flexures.

disease when curative treatment is impossible. The cause of carcinoma of the large bowel is unknown, but two conditions, familial polyposis and ulcerative colitis, predispose to the formation of cancer.

Carcinoma of the colon forms three main pathologic types when the gross specimen is examined. It may be polypoid, projecting into the lumen of the bowel like a cauliflower; it may be stenotic, forming a constricting ring distorting and narrowing the bowel, or it may be ulcerating, part of the growth at its center having undergone necrosis, which causes a typical malignant ulcer with rolled, everted edges and a floor covered with slough. The histologic appearance ranges from a tumor of low grade malignancy, with well-formed acini which secrete mucus, to a tumor of high grade malignancy which is composed of masses of primitive cells which give little indication of their origin in the bowel mucosa.

Cancer of the colon spreads by invasion of the bowel wall and contiguous tissues, of the lymphatics and the regional lymph nodes, and of the veins which then carry emboli of tumor cells to distant sites. It also spreads by shedding viable tumor cells into the lumen of the bowel and through the bowel wall into the peritoneal cavity. Most attention has been given to the spread of these tumors through the lymphatic system, and to the influence that lymphatic metastasis has on the prognosis after operation. The resected colon is examined microscopically and the lymph nodes in the mesentery are dissected out and similarly examined. The stage of the growth is then worked out according to Duke's classification. Stage A means that the tumor is confined within the bowel wall. Stage B means that it has spread through the bowel wall. In Stage C_1, there is invasion of lymph nodes adjacent to the tumor and bowel wall. Stage C_2 means that the node nearest the point of ligature on the main vessel is invaded. Stage D is reached when distant metastases are present. If the grade, or histologic type, and stage, or degree of lymphatic spread, of the growth are known, the patient's chances of eventual survival can be accurately predicted.

Carcinoma of the left side of the colon or rectum commonly presents as a simple alteration in bowel habit, or with rectal bleeding. A patient who previously has passed normal, formed stools at regular intervals notices either increasing constipation or attacks of diarrhea, or the two conditions alternating with each other. The feces may be narrower than normal, or more liquid, and streaked with mucus and blood. The patient may have a continuous urge to defecate, and a feeling after passing a stool that evacuation has been incomplete. Spasms of lower abdominal colic may occur, which are relieved by the passage of excessive amounts of flatus or liquid feces. Sometimes, the presenting symptom is acute rectal hemorrhage, which can be severe. This is often attributed by the patient to the presence of hemorrhoids and leads to neglect and delay in seeking treatment. Since hemorrhoids may be due to the presence of a growth higher up in the colon, they should never be treated until investigation has excluded the presence of a tumor.

When a carcinoma develops in the cecum or ascending colon, the symptoms are different and more insidious (Fig. 71). Pain is referred to the upper rather than the lower abdomen. Alteration of bowel habit is not so prominent, although diarrhea is common, and the passage of blood from the rectum is not noticed by the patient. The bleeding is occult and commonly causes an iron deficiency anemia. Since the symptoms are less obvious, a carcinoma of the cecum may reach a large size and form an obvious mass in the right iliac fossa before the patient seeks advice. Loss of weight is also a common symptom. Investigation of any patient who has dys-

peptic symptoms and an iron deficiency anemia must include a lower gastrointestinal x-ray examination.

The onset of complications may cause the first symptoms of carcinoma of the colon, such as obstruction of the large bowel, perforation of the tumor to cause a peritonitis or abscess formation, or involvement of other structures by the growth, causing fistulae. The two most common fistulae are gastrocolic and vesicocolic. Pyrexia of unknown origin, due to necrosis and secondary infection of the growth, may occasionally be the presenting symptom.

The conditions which must be distinguished from carcinoma of the colon are obviously varied. In lesions of the right colon, other causes of upper abdominal pain or iron deficiency anemia must be excluded, such as peptic ulceration, cholecystitis or neoplasms of the stomach and small bowel. Appendicitis, appendiceal abscess and ameboma formation must also be considered. In left-sided lesions, diverticulitis, ulcerative colitis and regional enteritis must be excluded. Granulomatous conditions of the rectum such as lymphogranuloma inguinale, syphilis or radiation proctitis may mimic a carcinoma. When peritonitis or abscesses occur, other causes for these conditions such as diverticulitis, appendicitis, or salpingitis may be confused.

The diagnosis of carcinoma of the colon or rectum is made by a proper digital and sig-

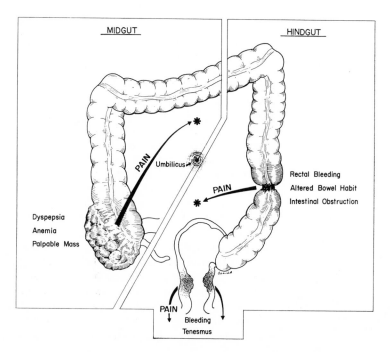

Figure 71. The symptoms of carcinoma of the colon. The symptoms of a tumor of the right colon are different from those of a tumor of the left colon, due to the different embryologic derivation.

moidoscopic examination, by barium enema examination and, occasionally, by finding malignant cells in colonic washings. The abdominal signs may be negligible unless the tumor is so large that it can be felt, or unless complications such as perforation or obstruction have occurred. The diagnostic accuracy of rectal examination combined with barium enema examination is high and when the tumor can be seen through a sigmoidoscope, tissue can be obtained for histologic examination. Barium enema examination shows either a typical shouldered "napkin ring" type of filling defect with loss of the normal mucosal pattern, an ulcer with prominent fixed edges, or a polypoid defect in the normal shadow of the bowel. Lesions of the hepatic and splenic flexure may be difficult to see, and particular care is necessary when examining these two parts. Repeat barium x-ray studies should be carried out, if suspicious symptoms persist, to avoid overlooking a neoplasm.

The only curative treatment for carcinoma of the colon and rectum is operation. The methods of spread of a carcinoma, through the lymphatic channels or the blood stream, and by the shedding of cells into the lumen of the bowel, are of particular importance during operations to remove cancer of the large bowel and certain steps are taken to prevent them (Fig. 72).

Malignant cells are shed into the lumen of the bowel when the primary tumor is handled. Early in the operation, therefore, tapes are placed around the bowel on either side of the tumor to prevent tumor cells in the lumen from escaping into those parts of the bowel which are to be left in place. The bowel is irrigated with a cytotoxic solution to prevent implantation of these cells in the raw area of the anastomosis, which is often a cause of recurrence. Since the number of malignant cells in the venous blood increases during manipulation of the tumor, the main vein is ligated early in the operation to prevent tumor emboli during manipulation. The length of colon resected is largely governed by technical reasons concerned with the blood supply. The aim is to remove the lymphatic field to as high a point as possible. Since the lymph channels accompany the arteries, the main artery is ligated at its point of origin. The whole length of bowel supplied by that artery must be removed, and final anastomosis performed using two ends of intestine with a good vascular supply.

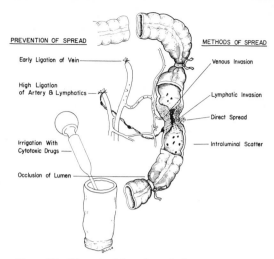

Figure 72. The principles of surgical treatment of cancer of the colon.

In the presence of perforation or abscess formation due to a growth, the operative treatment may be modified. Primary resection and anastomosis may be possible with good antibiotic cover. An alternative is to drain the abscess and perform a colostomy as a preliminary maneuver. The growth is later resected and the colostomy closed. Similarly, in obstruction of the large bowel, a preliminary drainage operation, such as cecostomy or colostomy, followed by resection after an interval, is often safer than primary resection with the immediate suture of distended, unprepared bowel.

Carcinoma of the rectum poses a particular problem, as alternative procedures are possible. The entire rectum can be removed and the patient left with a terminal colostomy, or the rectum can be excised, leaving the anal sphincter mechanism behind so that normal bowel action is preserved. The type of operation performed depends on three factors: the histologic grade of the growth, its situation and the presence of metastases. In general, abdominoperineal resection is used if the growth is in the lower half of the rectum or if it is of high grade malignancy, and also when there are no distant metastases. A sphincter-preserving operation, such as anterior resection is performed if the tumor is in the upper rectum and is of no more than average grade malignancy. This operation is also used as palliation if distant metastases are present, or, exceptionally, if the patient is completely averse to a colostomy, even after a full explanation of the facts. Any tumor which can be felt on digital examination is usually considered too low for a sphincter preserving operation, although there are exceptions.

Colostomy. The prospect of a colostomy, that is, an artificial anus through which bowel contents are discharged onto the abdominal wall, is distasteful and frightening to most patients. It may overshadow all other features of the proposed operation in their minds, and create problems in their postoperative care. The patient and family must be informed of the nature of the procedure. It is helpful if the patient is visited by one who has effectively managed his own colostomy for several years.

The colostomies employed in surgery are either temporary or permanent. Temporary colostomies either of the loop, or "double barreled" type are used to get the patient over some major complication, such as perforation or obstruction of the colon, and they are later closed. The transverse colon is used most commonly for this purpose. A terminal or permanent colostomy is made when the rectum is removed, and the descending colon is used.

A temporary colostomy is readily tolerated by the patient who realizes that it will eventually be closed. A permanent colostomy poses a different problem. Stenosis, prolapse or retraction of the colostomy stoma may occur and require surgical correction. Judicious use of paregoric and bulk laxatives helps achieve a formed stool. Gentle finger dilatation of the colostomy stoma each day also helps to prevent stenosis. The patient should avoid items of diet which disturb the colostomy, items which can only be found out by trial and error. Daily irrigation of the colon through a soft rubber catheter is probably the best way to ensure that the colon is emptied at the beginning of each day. A belt and a light pad over the colostomy opening is then worn. By these means, the patient's life can be made more comfortable and his initial dislike of a colostomy and his fear of social ostracism as a result of it can be surmounted.

Mortality is low, unless complications have risen, and this is due to four factors: improvement in anesthesia, better postoperative management of abdominal and pulmonary complications, better understanding of fluid and electrolyte problems, and preparation of the bowel for operation by the use of nonabsorbable antibiotics. Too much credit has probably been given to the use of antibiotics in preparing the bowel, and reliance on this particular factor may have led to less careful techniques when operating on the colon. No regimen of preoperative antibiotics completely sterilizes the intestine, but it does reduce the bacterial population temporarily, to cover the period of operation, and some tend to assist in emptying the colon as a result of a mild cathartic action.

The prognosis in tumors of the colon varies with the site, type and stage of the carcinoma. For example, an 80 per cent survival to five years can be anticipated in patients with a Stage A growth of the rectum. This figure falls to 40 per cent if the growth is at Stage C. Representative overall figures suggest that a 65 per cent five-year survival rate can be anticipated in all patients without lymph node involvement, but that this figure falls to 35 per cent if the nodes are involved.

VOLVULUS OF THE COLON. The cecum or the sigmoid colon may twist or undergo volvulus, forming two unusual and uncommon causes of intestinal obstruction. Volvulus of the cecum depends on a congenital abnormality of the right half of the colon, which is not retroperitoneal as in normal patients, but suspended on a mesentery continuous with that of the small bowel. It probably constitutes less than 2 per cent of all instances of intestinal obstruction in the Western world, but is more common in Eastern Europe. The axis of rotation is around the superior mesenteric vessels. It produces a characteristic roentgenographic appearance of small bowel obstruction, enormous distention of the right half of the colon, and displacement of the cecum into the upper abdomen. Operation is required for its correction and the best treatment is a right hemicolectomy. If the patient's condition is too poor, then untwisting the volvulus and fixing the cecum to the wall of the right iliac fossa may be sufficient.

Sigmoid volvulus similarly depends on pre-existing anatomic abnormalities. The sigmoid loop is large and redundant; its mesentery is unusually long, but its base is narrow. For some reason, sigmoid volvulus particularly affects psychiatric patients and senile people. The symptoms are those of lower large bowel obstruction with colicky pain, gross distention of the abdomen and constipation. The attacks may be recurrent if the volvulus spontaneously untwists. During an attack, the roentgenograms are typical. On a plain film, the abdomen is filled by huge distended loops of large bowel. When a barium enema examination is made, barium flowing through the narrowed portion of the colon into the volvulus is compressed, causing a typical "bird's beak" or "ace of spades" appearance. A barium enema examination is particularly useful in this condition, since it is not only diagnostic, but may also relieve the volvulus. If this does not happen, a large tube should be passed into the colon through a sigmoidoscope with great care taken not to perforate an edematous or necrotic colon wall. This decompresses the obstructed loop, and in most patients the volvulus untwists as a result. If these measures fail, or if the patient has had recurrent attacks of obstruction, the redundant colon should be excised.

RADIATION INJURY TO THE BOWEL. The increased use of roentgen ray and radiation therapy for a variety of pelvic and intra-abdominal malignant conditions has caused more frequent instances of intestinal damage from radiation. Any part of the intestine may be affected, but injury to the rectum and lower sigmoid colon is particularly common. The use of local sources of radiation, such as cobalt or radium, to treat carcinoma of the cervix is usually the cause. Roentgen ray therapy for a carcinoma of the bladder also may cause injury. The dose necessary to destroy the cancer is enough to cause a considerable reaction in nearby organs, such as the rectum, the colon or the loops of small bowel lying in the pelvis. Similarly, when roentgen ray therapy is given to the aortic nodes after removal of a malignant testicular tumor, the overlying coils of small intestine may be damaged. In view of the number of patients who receive radiation therapy, however, the incidence of bowel complications is relatively small. The early stages of radiation injury to the bowel are similar to a burn, with a considerable acute inflammatory reaction, increased vascularity and sloughing of part of the mucosa. The symptoms depend on the part of the intestine affected, and range from those of acute enteritis to those of a severe proctitis. The acute reaction usually subsides without complications unless a heavy dose of radiation has been given.

The late effects of roentgen ray therapy develop after an interval varying from a few months to many years. The underlying pathology is an obliterative endarteritis, a slow and progressive obliteration of the arterioles with resulting fibrosis or necrosis of the bowel tissue. In the small bowel, these changes may cause intestinal obstruction, a sprue-like syndrome, an enterocutaneous fistula, or even perforation and peritonitis. In the rectum, they may cause a severe fibrous stricture or fistulae between the rectum and adjacent structures, such as the vagina or bladder.

Radiation damage to the bowel is difficult to diagnose, since recurrence of the cancer previously treated causes many of the same symptoms. Satisfactory biopsy specimens to settle the question of recurrence are difficult to get. Surgical attack may cause the formation of more fistulae due to poor healing of the irradiated tissue, including the abdominal wall. Affected parts of the small bowel should be resected. If the rectum is involved, a proximal colostomy or excision of the rectum may be necessary.

THE RECTUM AND ANUS

The rectum and anus form the termination of the alimentary tract. A large number of common surgical lesions occur in this comparatively small part of the intestine, and this explains its particular importance to the surgeon. Nearly half of all large bowel cancers arise in the rectum, and hemorrhoids afflict a large percentage of the population. Surgical and anatomic interest in the rectum and anus has always been great, and there are more eponymous designations per square centimeter for this part of the body than for any other.

ANATOMY. Some knowledge of the anatomy of this region is necessary in order to understand the methods of examination, and the principles employed in treatment (Fig. 73). The rectum starts at its junction with the sigmoid colon just below the sacral promontory. This is an indefinite point, referred to surgically as the rectosigmoid region. It can be identified on the outside of the bowel by the expansion of the three taeniae coli to cover the whole circumference, and is some 15 to 20 cm. from the anus on sigmoidoscopic examination. The upper part of the rectum is in the peritoneal cavity and is covered by peritoneum. The peritoneum continues down over its anterior surface to a lower level than it does posteriorly. The rectum is closely applied to the hollow of the sacrum as it passes downward, and then curves gently forward to its junction with the anal canal at the anorectal ring. When looked at from in front, the rectum is S-

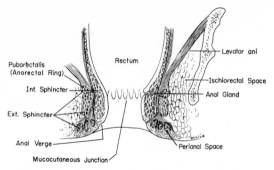

Figure 73. Coronal section of the anorectal region.

shaped, which can be seen when examining the lumen through a sigmoidoscope by three prominent mucosal folds, the valves of Houston. There are usually two of these on the left side and one on the right, but their disposition is variable.

The rectum receives its blood supply from the inferior mesenteric artery through the superior rectal hemorrhoidal artery, and from the internal iliac artery through the middle rectal vessels. Most of the lymphatics accompany the superior rectal artery to the para-aortic nodes, but some go with the middle rectal vessels, above the levator ani, to the side wall of the pelvis.

The anal canal starts at the anorectal ring; this is the point at which the puborectalis, a part of the levator ani muscle, forms a sling around the bowel and angulates it forward. This level also marks the start of the anal sphincter mechanism, which surrounds and compresses the bowel from this point downward.

The upper part of the anal canal is lined by intestinal type of mucosa. Mucosal folds in this area, called the anal columns, run vertically down to an irregular ring of anal valves which mark the junction of the mucosa with the skin. Above each valve is a small recess, the anal crypt, into which open the mouths of ten to 20 small anal mucous glands. The anal canal below the mucocutaneous junction is lined by smooth skin, which becomes cornified at the external opening of the anus. The portion of the anal canal below the mucocutaneous junction is supplied by branches from the pudendal arteries and its lymph drains to the inguinal group of nodes.

The circular muscles of the sphincter surround the anal canal. The internal sphincter is an expansion of the circular muscle of the rectum, and is involuntary in type. Surrounding it are the voluntary muscles of the

external sphincter, grouped into three main parts: the subcutaneous, the superficial and the deep or external sphincters. Between them run strands of muscle derived from the longitudinal muscle layer of the rectum. The puborectalis muscle loops behind the bowel at the level of the anorectal ring and merges with the upper margin of the sphincter.

The mucocutaneous junction forms a watershed between two fields of drainage. Above this level, drainage is into the portal venous system and to the para-aortic nodes. Below this level, venous drainage is to the pudendal veins and lymph drains to the inguinal nodes.

EXAMINATION. Thorough examination of the anus and rectum is an important part of every complete physical examination, particularly if the patient is over 40 years of age. The skin surrounding the anus is examined for evidence of infection, factitious changes due to scratching, and for the presence of fistulous openings, abscesses and condylomata. The anal orifice may show sentinel piles, skin tags, prolapse of piles or prolapse of the rectum itself. After careful inspection, the patient is asked to strain down and the presence of prolapse again noted. A well lubricated finger is next introduced gently into the anal canal, after explaining to the patient what is going to be done. The tone of the anal sphincter muscles is assessed and any induration or spasm of the muscles is noted. The finger then enters the ampulla of the rectum, and the walls are palpated with care. Through the walls can be felt the anterior surface of the lower part of the sacrum, the prostate and seminal vesicles in the male, and the lower part of the rectovesical pouch of the peritoneal cavity. The uterus and other pelvic organs can be similarly palpated in the female.

After digital examination, the rectum is inspected through a sigmoidoscope, provided that there is no local painful lesion in the anal canal which would prevent passage of the instrument. The sigmoidoscope can be passed with the patient in the left lateral position or in the knee-chest position. The latter often gives a better view, as it straightens out the slight kink where the rectum and sigmoid join. Mild preparation of the bowel should be sufficient to empty the rectum if it is full on the first attempt at examination.

The sigmoidoscope is passed pointing forward at first, to follow the direction of the anal canal. The anal canal is approximately

3 to 5 cm. long, so that when the sigmoidoscope has been passed for just over that distance, the obturator is removed and the eyepiece and source of light fitted to it. Since the rectum now passes backward, the instrument should be pointed in that direction and the interior of the rectal ampulla inspected as the instrument is passed up, with gentle inflation to distend the bowel. The only difficult point to negotiate is the junction of rectum and sigmoid; it requires some practice to be able to do this and to reach the lower part of the sigmoid colon.

A quiet, murmuring commentary on the progress of the examination should be given to reassure the patient and prepare him for the rather strange sensations he will have, particularly when the lower sigmoid is entered. Neoplasms or polyps should be obvious, unless they are hidden behind the valves of Houston, and they are biopsied. The color and appearance of the rectal mucosa are also important, because it may be characteristically altered in such conditions as ulcerative colitis, amebiasis, proctitis or melanosis, and again a biopsy should be taken. As the sigmoidoscope is withdrawn, the interior of the bowel is again examined, particularly the areas partially concealed by the rectal valves. As the instrument is withdrawn through the anal canal, internal hemorrhoids may be seen prolapsing into the end of the sigmoidoscope. For the examination and treatment of lesions of the anal canal and the lower part of the rectum, the proctoscope is usually used. It is shorter than the sigmoidoscope and has a larger diameter.

HEMORRHOIDS. Hemorrhoids, or piles (from the Latin *pila*, a ball), are one of the commonest afflictions of the human race and cause a great amount of misery. The term "piles" is nonspecific when used by patients and may describe any local anal condition, particularly if it is painful. The term may, therefore, cover a large number of symptoms, from bleeding due to a rectal neoplasm to the irritation caused by a fungus infection.

Internal hemorrhoids are varicose dilatations of the plexus of veins lying under the mucosa of the upper anal canal. They produce localized bulging of the mucosa over the plexus. The venous plexus lies above the mucocutaneous junction and drains into the three main branches of the superior rectal vein. This vein has one branch on the left and two on the right, a posterior and anterior. The hemorrhoids are situated in these positions in the anal canal, and when seen with the patient in the lithotomy position they are at 4, 7 and 11 o'clock. These are the three primary hemorrhoids. If further dilatation of the hemorrhoidal plexus occurs, then secondary piles may be formed between these primary sites. As the veins dilate, the overlying mucosa is stretched until it eventually protrudes into and down the anal canal, causing prolapse of the hemorrhoid.

The cause of hemorrhoids is not known, but certain factors causing a sustained rise in the pressure in the superior rectal vein will produce back-pressure on the hemorrhoidal plexus and lead to its dilatation. Portal hypertension, for example, can cause varix formation in the anus, just as it does at the gastroesophageal junction. Straining due to an enlarged prostate or a pelvic tumor may also compress the rectal vein. A carcinoma of the upper rectum or sigmoid commonly presents as hemorrhoids, and should be specifically excluded by appropriate examination before treatment is started.

Hemorrhoids are particularly common during pregnancy, and several factors may be responsible for their occurrence during this time. The increased production of progesterone, the increased circulating blood volume in pregnancy, and the pressure of an enlarged uterus have been suggested as causes of hemorrhoids. In addition, the placenta forms a type of arteriovenous fistula in the pelvis, and the dilatation of the hemorrhoidal venous plexus may be the result.

In most patients, no primary cause for the formation of hemorrhoids can be found. They tend to occur in families and to be associated with varicose veins in the legs, which suggests that there may be some underlying abnormality of the veins. Chronic constipation, due to simple causes such as an inadequate fluid intake or a faulty diet, is probably the most common cause, and much improvement can be produced in the early, mild case by restoring sensible bowel habits.

Uncomplicated hemorrhoids are painless, and the principal symptom is bleeding on defecation. The blood is bright red and it may be noticed on the surface of the stool or the toilet paper, or it may actually spurt out during defecation. The bleeding is often unnoticed by the patient, and piles are a relatively common cause of iron deficiency anemia. Examination in any patient with anemia must include a satisfactory proctoscopic examination to exclude hemorrhoidal disease, or a malignant tumor in the rectum. As the hemorrhoids enlarge, the patient may notice, in addition to bleeding, that the piles prolapse through the anus during defecation and then return spontaneously. This is known as a first-degree hemorrhoid. In second-degree hemorrhoids, the prolapsed pile has to be replaced by the patient himself, and in third-degree cases the hemorrhoids are prolapsed all the time. These may be associated with troublesome mucous discharge and pruritus ani.

In addition to prolapse, which is the commonest complication of hemorrhoids apart from bleeding, strangulation or thrombosis may occur. This extremely painful condition is caused by spreading thrombosis in the venous channels in the hemorrhoid. It may be precipitated by prolapse of the pile through the anal sphincter, which then grasps the base tightly. As edema develops, the sphincter muscles contract more powerfully, preventing the return of the hemorrhoid and causing increasing pain. If the strangulation is due to gripping of the base of the pile by the contracted anal sphincter, the patient should be anesthetized and the pile replaced. If strangulation is due to spontaneous thrombosis in a prolapsed pile, replacement is not possible and should not be attempted. A thrombosed or strangulated internal hemorrhoid is best treated by local applications of lead lotion, and the administration of analgesics. It is difficult to carry out any satisfactory operation because of the severe surrounding edema and inflammation. When the acute symptoms have subsided, hemorrhoidectomy should be performed. On very rare occasions, septic thrombosis of a hemorrhoid may be followed by a portal pyemia.

Hemorrhoids may be treated in two ways, by injection and by operation (Fig. 74). The general condition of the patient, the severity of the local disease, and the wishes of the patient govern the choice between the two types of treatment. Injection can be performed in the office and is painless, but like all injection therapy for venous disease, it is only temporarily effective. A sclerosing solution, such as 5 per cent phenol in almond oil, is injected not into the pile itself, but under the mucosa at its base at the anorectal ring, which is insensitive. As long as the injection is given into the right site, the complication rate is negligible. The most common mistake is to place the sclerosant too superficially so that a mucosal ulcer results. This

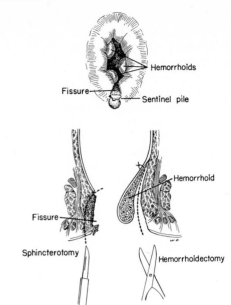

Figure 74.   Common anorectal diseases and their treatment. The usual positions of the primary hemorrhoids and an anal fissure are shown viewed with the patient in the lithotomy position. The basic steps in their operative treatment are shown.

is tiresome but seldom gives more than local trouble before healing. Injections should not be used if there is any perianal infection, thrombosis of the hemorrhoids or a severe degree of prolapse.

The alternative treatment is surgical excision of the piles, and for this purpose a wide variety of operations have been devised. The classic operation consists of excision of the three primary piles with ligation of each pedicle. This leaves three raw areas on the anal canal, which are allowed to heal by secondary intention. This operation has a negligible recurrence rate and a very low incidence of complications, but it has the reputation of being particularly painful.

The alternative types of operation are designed to produce wounds in the anus which can be sutured and which will heal by first intention. These latter operations are less painful than the classic type, as long as primary healing of the wounds occurs, but sutured wounds in the anal region have a bad reputation for becoming infected and causing subsequent fibrosis.

Hemorrhoidectomy is not free from complications. The most urgent is hemorrhage, which may occur shortly after the operation if the ligature on the base of the hemorrhoid slips, or between the seventh and tenth days, due to sloughing and separation of the ligature from the pedicle. As the blood is lost into the cavity of the rectum, which is capacious, no overt signs of bleeding may be present unless a tube has been placed in the rectum at the end of the operation and allows blood to escape. A close watch should be kept for systemic signs of hemorrhage after hemorrhoidectomy. This complication is best treated by passing a Foley catheter into the rectum, inflating the balloon and then pulling it down so that the bleeding point is compressed against the anal sphincter by the balloon.

Retention of urine, especially in the male, is common after hemorrhoidectomy and may require catheterization for a few days. Fecal impaction may also be troublesome, and is caused initially by the patient's fear of pain on defecation. If a proper bowel action has not occurred within 72 hours of operation, suitable laxatives should be given, as well as the usual regimen of enemas, otherwise the feces in the rectum will become scybalous and hard. They irritate the rectum and produce a liquid, spurious diarrhea with continual tenesmus, or painful desire to defecate. Manual removal of the fecal mass under anesthetic may be required to relieve this impaction.

The most troublesome long-term complication of hemorrhoidectomy is an anal stricture. This is more likely to occur after total excision of the pile-bearing area than after the other types of operation. The anus should be gently dilated at regular intervals until the anal wound is well healed. Bulk laxatives to ensure the regular passage of a formed stool help to prevent the formation of a stricture.

THROMBOSED EXTERNAL HEMORRHOID. Thrombosed external hemorrhoid is a misnomer, as it is not a varicose dilatation of a vein, but a hematoma under the perianal skin caused by spontaneous rupture of a vein in the external hemorrhoidal plexus. It is a painful condition, often referred to by the layman as "an acute attack of piles." It is self-limiting and resolves spontaneously with eventual fibrosis of the hematoma. However, it is a simple matter to incise and evacuate the hematoma under local anesthetic, and the patient will be extremely gratified with the complete and dramatic relief of the pain. Any redundant skin should be excised to ensure adequate drainage and to prevent the subsequent formation of irritating skin tags.

FISSURE-IN-ANO. Fissure-in-ano is a linear ulcer of the skin of the anal canal. It is usually caused by the passage of a particularly hard or large fecal mass which overstretches the anal canal. It may be caused by scybala catching on an anal valve and tearing the skin downward. Its symptoms are diagnostic. The patient experiences a severe burning pain in the anal region on defecation, which continues for some hours. Because of this pain, the patient avoids defecation as much as possible, with the result that when he does evacuate, the feces are hard and excoriate the anus. The fissure also causes severe spasm of the anal sphincter, so that the condition constitutes a vicious cycle, with the fissure causing muscular spasm which in turn causes fecal retention.

When the anal region is examined, the site of the fissure may be marked by a small tag of edematous skin at its base, the so-called "sentinel pile." The fissure is usually in the midline posteriorly, but it may be anterior in women. Spasm of the sphincter may be so severe that an examining finger cannot be passed into the anal canal. If the fissure has been present for some time, considerable fibrosis of the perianal tissue may be felt.

The factors which make a fissure persist are anal spasm in the acute case, and inadequate drainage of the fissure in the chronic case. Treatment is directed at stopping the anal spasm, thus breaking the cycle which makes the condition persist. In the more chronic type, operation may be necessary to improve drainage.

In the acute case, the patient is given a local anesthetic jelly to apply to the anus to relieve local pain. An anal dilator should be coated with the jelly and passed twice a day to overcome the anal spasm, and a bulk laxative given to ensure the daily passage of a formed solid stool. With these relatively simple measures, many acute fissures will resolve and heal in about two weeks.

If the fissure persists despite this treatment, or if it presents as a chronic type, more energetic treatment is needed. Forceful dilatation of the anal sphincter under anesthesia causes a temporary paralysis of the muscle, overcomes the spasm, and may allow time for the fissure to heal. This rather crude treatment is often ineffective, however, and the paralysis of the sphincter may be more permanent than was desired. The operation of sphincterotomy is more effective. The lower part of the internal sphincter is pulled down by the fibrosis due to the fissure, and the lower fibers of this muscle can be seen in the floor of the fissure.

This is incised until the fibrous constriction is relieved. The sentinel pile is then excised and the skin trimmed back so that a flat pear-shaped wound is left, which will granulate and epithelize.

PERIANAL SUPPURATION. Abscesses and their sequelae, fistulae, are common in the perianal and perirectal area, and cause disagreeable symptoms, particularly to the fastidious patient.

Abscesses may occur in any of the potential spaces near the anus or rectum, and their etiology varies. In the perianal space, infection usually enters through the skin and forms an acutely painful, tender subcutaneous swelling. The patient soon becomes aware of it because of the pain produced, and it ruptures or is incised before it can reach any great size.

Infections of the ischiorectal fossa are more of a problem. The ischiorectal fossa forms a large potential space on either side of the rectum, communicating posteriorly behind it, and it has extensions forward above the perineal membrane to either side of the prostate. The space is normally filled by large lobules of fat with loose strands of fibrous tissue. Infection in the ischiorectal fossa is insidious, and by the time an abscess is drained, it may have burrowed around the rectum to infect the opposite side.

These abscesses are caused by infection of the anal glands. These small glands lie in the substance of the internal sphincter, and they drain into the anal canal just above the mucocutaneous junction. If the duct of the gland becomes blocked, infection forms an abscess. This may rupture through the sphincter muscle into the ischiorectal fossa, causing an ischiorectal abscess.

The symptoms of this condition are not dramatic at first. The patient notices a dull, aching pain in and around the rectum. The pain may become more severe just before defecation, when the rectum fills with feces. Eventually, as the abscess spreads and comes nearer the surface, the pain becomes more intense and throbbing, and there is local tenderness which keeps the patient from walking or sitting in comfort.

On examination, the patient is often febrile, and there is obvious tenderness, induration and redness lateral to the anus. Rectal examination confirms the presence of a tender mass. A leukocytosis is usually present. Once an ischiorectal abscess is diagnosed, it should be drained, since it may otherwise rupture into the bowel at a high level and make the eventual surgical treatment much more difficult. With adequate drainage, the abscess soon subsides, and most patients heal without further trouble. In a definite percentage, however, the abscess forms a fistula-in-ano, and the patient should be warned of this complication. Meticulous care in dressing the wound after operation will prevent this if the cavity is allowed to heal from the bottom.

Abscesses in the pelvirectal space occur above the levator ani and are usually secondary to intra-abdominal inflammatory conditions or due to blood-borne infection. They are difficult to distinguish from an intraperitoneal pelvic abscess, and their treatment usually depends on treatment of the primary intra-abdominal disease.

FISTULA-IN-ANO. Fistula-in-ano is an abnormal track lined by granulation tissue connecting the lumen of the anal canal with the skin. A fistula usually follows an abscess in the perianal or ischiorectal spaces. It may also be associated with organic disease of the intestine, such as ulcerative colitis, regional enteritis or tuberculosis. For this reason, a portion of the fistulous track should always be examined microscopically after excision to make sure that such conditions are not overlooked. A chest radiograph should also be obtained before treatment is started.

A fistula causes a persistent discharge, often blood-stained. When the track becomes blocked, there are recurrent bouts of inflammation, which usually subside as the discharge starts again. Pruritus ani, anal discomfort and recurrent furunculosis around the anus may also occur. Examination should show the typical puckered orifice or orifices of the fistula near the anus, with underlying induration around the fistulous track. Fistulae with openings in front tend to be simple, but those with the openings posteriorly are complicated and may have extensive ramifications. Goodsall's law of fistulae states that when the external opening of a fistula is situated posteriorly to an imaginary transverse line drawn across the center of the anus, the internal opening is usually in the midline posteriorly and the track of the fistula is curved (Fig. 75). When the external opening is situated anterior to this imaginary line, the track usually travels straight to the internal opening in the anal canal.

Fistulae-in-ano are classified according to their relationship to the muscles of the anal sphincter. The most superficial type runs

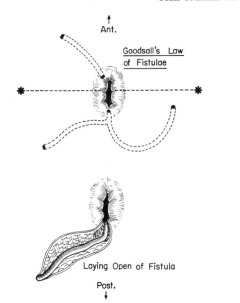

Figure 75. The disposition and treatment of fistula-in-ano.

below the subcutaneous external sphincter, the intermuscular types run through the superficial and deep external sphincters, and an anorectal fistula runs above the puborectalis muscle, or the anorectal ring.

The treatment of fistula-in-ano must be surgical. A probe is placed in the outside opening and manipulated until it emerges through the internal opening. The skin is then incised along this line and the incision carried down to the probe. The skin edges are excised until a wide wound is made which provides adequate drainage. The aftercare of these wounds is as important as the operation itself. They must heal by granulation from the bottom upward, and they must be carefully watched to ensure that the skin is not allowed to heal over too soon, forming a bridge across the cavity and thus leading to a recurrence of the fistula. The "horseshoe" type of fistula may require the excision of a large amount of skin, nearly surrounding the anus, and may take many months to heal completely and satisfactorily.

In any operation for fistula, the puborectalis muscle must not be divided, as continence depends on this muscle. When exteriorization of the fistula requires extensive and deep dissection in the sphincter muscles, it may be difficult to decide how much of the sphincter needs to be divided. A seton may then be inserted. This is a length of braided silk or wire which is threaded through the fistula track. It is then loosely tied around the remaining intact sphincter muscle. After a period to allow fixation of the muscle by the resulting fibrosis, it can be divided with less risk of causing incontinence. Most of the muscles in the sphincter may have to be divided, depending on the level of the internal opening, but the puborectalis must be left intact.

PRURITUS ANI. Pruritus ani is a common and distressing complaint. The patient complains of incessant and intractable irritation around the anus, which is particularly bothersome at night. Some of these patients have an obvious local anal condition causing the pruritus, such as prolapsed hemorrhoids or a fistula-in-ano. Skin tags around the anus may prevent proper toilet of the area. The leakage of mineral oil due to excessive dosage may also cause pruritus. In other patients, worm infestation, local dermatologic diseases such as fungus infections, psoriasis or kraurosis vulvae explain the pruritus. These patients are the most satisfactory to treat, since correction of the primary lesion stops the itching. General diseases, such as diabetes mellitus or Hodgkin's disease, may occasionally have pruritus ani as an initial symptom. For this reason, the urine must always be tested for sugar, a blood count performed, and an x-ray of the chest obtained in any patient with pruritus ani.

There remain a large number of patients with intractable pruritus in whom no primary cause can be found, and they form a very unsatisfactory group. The anus usually appears normal, but it may be surrounded by factitious changes in the skin due to the patient's incessant habit of scratching. The skin is smooth and atrophic, with many superficial abrasions. The scratching perpetuates the pruritus, and the first step in treatment is to try and break this habit. The patient should be scrupulously clean in his habits, washing the perianal area after every bowel action. Local treatment of the anal skin with hydrocortisone ointment often gives dramatic relief. Sedation and the wearing of gloves at night may stop the patient from scratching while asleep. If these measures fail, the cycle may be broken by the injection of long-acting anesthetic to the perianal area. In many patients, however, some deep-seated psychologic abnormality is responsible for the condition, and they do not respond to any physical treatment.

PROLAPSE OF RECTUM. There are three

types of rectal prolapse. In the first group, the rectal mucosa alone prolapses through the anus because of the loose attachment of the mucosa to the submucosal tissues and the weakness of the anal sphincter. In the second group, all layers of the rectum prolapse due to laxity of the pelvic muscles and fascia. In the third group, the upper rectum intussuscepts into the lower bowel and the apex of the intussusception protrudes through the anus.

Patients with rectal prolapse complain of a feeling of weakness in the perineum and of the presence of something protruding after defecation or when they stand up or walk about. The prolapsed bowel produces a profuse mucous discharge, which soils the underclothes, and it occasionally bleeds as well. Because there is associated weakness of the anal sphincter, due to overstretching, incontinence of feces and flatus is common. These unpleasant symptoms and the fear of public disgrace cause many patients with rectal prolapse to live the lives of social hermits.

In the first group, the rectal mucosa is able to slide down, since it is not fixed to the submucosal tissue as in normal people. This type is particularly likely to occur as a result of hemorrhoids stretching the mucosa above them and eventually pulling it down. If the prolapse is caused by hemorrhoids, these should be corrected by operation. Mucosal prolapse can be corrected in its early stages by injecting a sclerosant into the submucous layer, to fix the mucosa to the underlying tissues. An alternative method of accomplishing this is to scarify the mucosa with a cautery at multiple points in a circle around the bowel. In more severe degrees of mucosal prolapse, the protruding length of mucosa is amputated and reanastomosed at its base.

Complete rectal prolapse, or descent of all layers of the rectum, occurs at the extremes of life. In young children, it may follow any illness causing loss of weight or diarrhea. It is particularly common after gastroenteritis, when frequent defecation is combined with the loss of the supporting fat from the ischiorectal and pararectal spaces. In old people, it is much more common in women and often accompanies vaginal and uterine prolapse. It is due to weakness of the pelvic muscular diaphragm, and stretching of the pelvic fascia which normally support the rectum and uterus. In severe cases, the sagging pelvic floor allows the rectum to drag down the pouch of Douglas with it, so that the anterior part of the prolapse may contain a peritoneal sac with coils of small bowel in it. The muscles of the anal sphincter are also very lax and allow the rectum to protrude.

In young children, the prolapse should be replaced. As soon as the precipitating illness has been treated and the infant regains weight, the prolapse should correct itself. During this time, strapping the buttocks together and persuading the child to defecate lying down also helps to prevent recurrence. In old patients, treatment is unsatisfactory, and recurrence may follow any type of operation. In a mild case, when the prolapse is minimal, exercises to strengthen the pelvic muscular diaphragm, and stimulation of the anal sphincter muscles by faradism may produce an improvement.

The simplest operation to cure prolapse is to insert a ring of wire or nylon in the subcutaneous tissue surrounding the anus. This has to be adjusted with nicety so that it prevents descent of the rectum but still allows the passage of feces. This operation is simple, it can easily be repeated if the wire or nylon breaks, and it can be quite successful. Its disadvantages are that it may cause fecal impaction, and that fracture of the wire is common after about a year. Fecal impaction, with its attendant spurious diarrhea, can usually be prevented by intelligent care and the proper use of laxatives.

Many other operations have been described for the treatment of prolapse of the rectum. The redundant bowel can be pulled down, then amputated and reanastomosed outside the anus. In advanced cases, a more radical procedure is used. The redundant sigmoid colon and rectum are excised and the bowel rejoined by end-to-end anastomosis. The "hernial sac" of pelvic peritoneum, which accompanies the prolapse, is excised to obliterate the pouch of Douglas, and the pelvic fascia and the muscular diaphragm plicated. Finally, the rectum is fixed to the sacrum and pararectal tissues. The recurrence rate following such an extensive operation is approximately 10 per cent, but it is a severe procedure for an elderly patient. Its other disadvantage is that it does not correct the laxity of the anal sphincter, so that although the prolapse is corrected, the patient may still complain of incontinence. An alternative is to mobilize the rectum off the sacrum and pull it upward. It can then be fixed in its correct position by wrapping it in a synthetic sponge material which is sutured to the fascia on the front of the sacrum. The mortality and recurrence rates are less than with other operations.

INFLAMMATION OF THE RECTUM. Inflammation of the rectum, or proctitis, may be due to gonorrhea, syphilis or infestation by parasites such as *Schistosoma mansoni*, but these are all very uncommon. Other specific infections, such as dysentery and amebiasis, affect the entire colon.

Idiopathic or granular proctitis is seen frequently. Its cause is unknown, but it may be produced by excessive purgation or may be related to ulcerative colitis. A small percentage of patients who are first seen with granular proctitis later develop full-blown ulcerative colitis. The symptoms are those of any inflammatory condition of the rectum. The bowel habit is altered and diarrhea is common. Rectal bleeding, urgency of defecation and a continuous desire to defecate may occur. There may be continuous, deep-seated discomfort and perianal soreness.

Digital examination is often normal, but the appearances through a sigmoidoscope are characteristic. The lower rectum appears hemorrhagic and granular, and it bleeds easily when touched with a swab or the end of the instrument. As the sigmoidoscope passes upward, one sees an abrupt transition to normal, pale, rectal mucosa. The abnormal mucosa should be biopsied and the feces cultured to exclude any specific infection. Idiopathic proctitis responds well to the intermittent use of hydrocortisone suppositories. Since hydrocortisone has been shown to be absorbed into the body from the rectum, these suppositories should only be given intermittently and for short periods. Because of the good response they produce, this is often all that is necessary.

TUMORS OF THE ANUS. Squamous cell carcinoma and melanoma of the anus are both uncommon tumors. They arise in the anal canal below the mucocutaneous junction. They spread by local invasion into the perirectal spaces, into adjoining structures such as the vagina, or upward into the rectum itself. They usually metastasize to the inguinal group of nodes, unless the tumor invades the rectum. Then, it may metastasize to the para-aortic nodes. These tumors should be treated by abdominoperineal resection of the rectum and anus. Block dissection of the inguinal nodes should be performed if they are involved at the time, or if they become enlarged during the follow-up period.

PILONIDAL SINUS. A pilonidal, or hairbearing, sinus or abscess is a common condition, particularly in young male adults, and is a frequent cause of loss of time from work. The sinus occurs in the upper part of the natal cleft overlying the sacrum. The patient usually complains of a persistent discharge at the base of the spine, and of recurrent episodes of acute pain and tenderness when the sinus becomes blocked and forms an abscess. The patient may not notice the sinus until an abscess forms, and he is then admitted with a tense, fluctuant, painful and tender swelling in the sacral region. A single small puckered orifice with a few hairs protruding is the most common finding, but there may be a complicated network of sinus tracks with multiple openings extending out over the buttocks.

Pilonidal sinus was long regarded as a congenital condition, because it occurs at the same site as the small sacrococcygeal pit commonly seen in children. The evidence, however, is overwhelmingly in favor of the view that a pilonidal sinus is an acquired condition due to implantation of hairs into and under the skin. Similar sinuses are seen in other parts of the body which are hairy, such as the axilla or mons veneris. Pilonidal sinus is a common occupational hazard of barbers, occurring in the clefts between the fingers. Sacral pilonidal sinuses are not found in children, and they are much more common in the hirsute male than in the female.

A pilonidal sinus is formed by the penetration of the skin by short stout hairs, and is caused by movement of the buttocks. The sinus is perpetuated by the hairs and by recurrent bouts of infection. Pilonidal sinus occurred so commonly in the army that the condition was christened "jeep disease." It was thought to be due to continual minor trauma to the sacral region by bumping up and down on the hard seats of a military vehicle.

An abscess due to acute infection of a pilonidal sinus should be incised and adequate drainage provided by excising part of its roof. The treatment of the uncomplicated sinus is not so easy. It may be excised, marsupialized, or exteriorized. When it is excised, an ellipse of skin with the underlying block of subcutaneous tissue containing the sinus is removed. The underlying cavity is obliterated by deep sutures and the skin is then sutured. If the wound heals without complication and by first intention, the patient is able to leave the hospital within ten days, but the recurrence rate after this type of operation is approximately 20 to 30 per cent. Alternatively, after the block of tissue containing the sinus has been excised, the wound may be packed open instead of sutured.

Marsupialization involves laying open the sinus track and all its ramifications. The skin edges are then sutured to the edges of the sinus tracks. The wound is carefully dressed until it has healed by granulation and epithelialization. This process may take four to six weeks, depending on the size of the sinus, but the recurrence rate is negligible. Each of the methods has its advantages and disadvantages, and the alternatives should be discussed with the patient. He would be well advised, after any type of operation, to keep the area free of hair by using a depilatory cream.

INTESTINAL OBSTRUCTION

Obstruction of the small intestine is one of the most common surgical emergencies and comprises approximately 20 per cent of all acute surgical admissions. The mortality rate is still disturbingly high, although it has fallen from the 60 per cent of four decades ago to approximately 10 per cent, if all types of obstruction are considered. Three factors are responsible for the lower mortality rate: intestinal decompression, increased understanding of the fluid and electrolyte problems involved, and the use of antibiotics. The continuing mortality is due to delay in diagnosis, the difficulty in deciding if strangulation has occurred, uncertainty in management, and faults in surgical technique.

ETIOLOGY. Intestinal obstruction may be caused by mechanical factors or by reflex paralysis of the bowel (Table 1). Mechanical obstruction is due to a variety of causes in the lumen, in the wall and outside the wall of the bowel. There are three types of mechanical obstruction. If there is no disturbance of the blood supply to the bowel, the obstruction is called "simple." If there is interference with the blood supply, the obstruction is called a "strangulation obstruction." The third type is the "closed loop obstruction"; in this, both ends of an obstructed loop are occluded. This may be due to an adhesion, a volvulus, or an external or internal hernia. The most common example of a closed loop obstruction is acute obstructive appendicitis.

PATHOLOGY. Mechanical obstruction of the intestine usually starts as a simple obstruction. The bowel proximal to the site of the obstruction becomes distended, and that part beyond the obstruction is collapsed. The distention of the proximal intestine is due to the accumulation of gastrointestinal secretions and gas. It has been estimated that 70 per cent of the gas is swallowed air, the other 30 per cent having diffused through the intestinal wall from the blood. The pressure in the intestine and the mesentery increases, and it interferes with the venous blood flow. This causes edema of the bowel wall and the transudation of plasma into the peritoneal cavity and the bowel lumen. The edema and the increasing pressure eventually obstruct the arterial supply and cause strangulation of the intestine.

Strangulation is, therefore, a gradual process unless it is due to sudden obstruction of the artery itself by thrombosis or embolism. When the blood supply to the intestine is reduced, necrosis of the wall occurs and a perforation results. Necrosis of the bowel wall may be caused by the direct pressure of a constricting band, or of a foreign body tightly impacted in the lumen of the intestine. The highly infected contents of the intestine are then discharged into the peritoneal cavity, causing a peritonitis. Bacteria may also invade the peritoneal cavity before perforation occurs, due to the migration of the organisms through the edematous intestinal wall.

PHYSIOLOGY. The general effects of intestinal obstruction are the same whatever the primary cause, although minor modifications in these effects may be due to the level at which the bowel is obstructed (Fig. 76). Between 7 and 8 liters of electrolyte-rich fluid enter the bowel in each 24 hours, and in normal health the greater part is reabsorbed. When the small intestine is obstructed, a large proportion of this fluid is lost from the body by vomiting or by sequestration in the lumen of the distended intestine and its edematous wall. A loss of 7 or 8 liters of fluid means a deficiency in the average person of half the extracellular fluid volume, and such a deficit may arise in 24 hours or less after the onset of intestinal obstruction. A severe and acute reduction in the extracellular fluid volume due to the loss of salt and water may markedly reduce the circulating blood volume. The same effect may be produced by the loss of plasma and blood into the obstructed segments of intestine or into the peritoneal cavity. It is not unusual to find the equivalent

Table 1. *Clinical and Pathologic Classification of Types of Intestinal Obstruction**

CLINICAL CLASSIFICATION	PATHOLOGIC CLASSIFICATION
I. *Mechanical obstruction*	
A. Narrowing of lumen	
1. Strictures of intestinal wall	Simple
a. Congenital:	(except in complete colon obstruction,
atresia, stenosis, imperforate anus	when distention may have necrotizing
b. Acquired:	effect on wall of bowel)
inflammatory	
traumatic	
vascular	
neoplastic	
2. Obturation	
3. Compression from without (especially in pelvis and	
at retroperitoneal duodenum)	
B. Adhesions and bands:	Either simple or strangulating
congenital	
inflammatory	
traumatic	
neoplastic	
C. Hernia, external or internal	
D. Volvulus	Strangulating
E. Intussusception	
F. Developmental errors giving rise to obstruction (in ad-	
dition to congenital atresia and stenosis)	
II. *Obstruction due to nervous imbalance*	
A. Inhibition ileus (paralytic or adynamic)	Simple
B. Spastic ileus (dynamic)	
III. *Vascular obstruction*	
A. Mesenteric thrombosis or embolism	Strangulating
IV. *Iatrogenic*	
A. Hypokalemia (diuretics)	
B. Potassium chloride strictures	
C. Spasmolytic drugs	
D. Anticoagulants	
E. Antihypertensive drugs	

*Modified from Wangensteen in Christopher: A Textbook of Surgery, 5th ed.

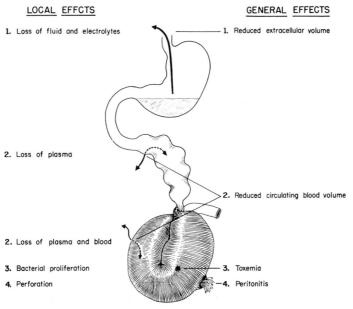

LOCAL EFFCTS	GENERAL EFFECTS
1. Loss of fluid and electrolytes	1. Reduced extracellular volume
2. Loss of plasma	2. Reduced circulating blood volume
2. Loss of plasma and blood	
3. Bacterial proliferation	3. Toxemia
4. Perforation	4. Peritonitis

Figure 76. The pathophysiology of small intestinal obstruction.

of 1.5 to 2 liters of plasma in the peritoneal cavity, and an equivalent amount may be trapped in the lumen and wall of the intestine. The amount of blood lost is difficult to estimate, but the volume of blood sequestrated in an infarcted segment of bowel may be approximately 10 per cent of the total blood volume for every 24 hours of the obstruction, and may be enough to be lethal. The loss of plasma and blood rapidly reduces the circulating blood volume, a much more dangerous situation than simple reduction of the extracellular fluid volume. A reduced circulating blood volume causes hypotension, lowered renal plasma flow, and lowered coronary and cerebral artery flow. Oliguria, anuria, coronary thrombosis and cerebral thrombosis are, therefore, common complications of intestinal obstruction, particularly in the elderly, who have a poor circulatory reserve.

Added to the effects of the reduced extracellular fluid and circulating plasma volumes are the effects of bacterial proliferation in a strangulated portion of intestine. The organisms are usually of the coliform or clostridial groups. Anaerobic organisms of this type grow rapidly in a medium rich in altered blood, as found in a strangulated loop, and form a lethal endotoxin. This toxic material may enter the peritoneal cavity, making the patient gravely ill. It may be suddenly released into the circulation when the strangulation obstruction is relieved by operation. This causes extreme hypotension and circulatory collapse which is very resistant to the usual methods of resuscitation. Endotoxin shock, which may occur before, during or after operation, is one of the causes of the high mortality of strangulation obstruction. Antibiotics should, therefore, be given in adequate doses to prevent the proliferation of organisms in the strangulated bowel and the consequent formation of endotoxin.

CLINICAL SYMPTOMS. The symptoms of intestinal obstruction are characteristic but quite variable in severity. Abdominal pain is always present. This pain is colicky, severe and usually localized around the umbilicus. The spasms make the patient double up or roll about. Vomiting is common, and at first it is reflex. Later, vomiting is caused by the reflux of intestinal contents into the stomach, and the vomitus may be feculent, depending upon the level of obstruction. Absolute constipation for feces and flatus is the rule, but sometimes the patient passes a small amount

of flatus once or twice after the onset of pain, before constipation becomes absolute. The patients may notice abdominal distention due to dilatation of the obstructed bowel. They may also notice the loud borborygmi synchronous with the colicky pain, due to increased intestinal peristalsis.

Certain symptoms are said to be characteristic of strangulation obstruction, but they are an unreliable guide unless they are very obvious. The character of the pain changes from the intermittent colicky type seen in simple obstruction to a severe, continuous pain made worse by any movement. This change is due to the localized peritoneal irritation over the strangulated loop. The patient may get some relief from the earlier colic by changing positions, or doubling himself up. Once strangulation occurs, he finds it better to lie still. If there is much contamination of the peritoneum, the pain may radiate to the shoulder tips, due to irritation of the domes of the diaphragm.

The physical examination of the patient with intestinal obstruction should answer four questions: whether the patient has an intestinal obstruction; whether there is any interference with the blood supply to the bowel; the extent of the fluid, plasma and electrolyte deficit; and the cause and level of the obstruction. No narcotics or analgesics should be given until a definite diagnosis and decision as to treatment have been made.

The diagnosis of obstruction depends on certain local signs in the abdomen. Abdominal distention is usual, unless the obstruction is sited high in the small bowel. The distention may at first be seen in the lower abdomen, since the small bowel normally lies in the pelvis. Visible peristalsis may course along the distended intestinal loops, or this can sometimes be provoked by flicking the abdominal wall with the finger. The loops themselves may form a "ladder pattern," visible through the abdominal wall. Hyperperistalsis of the obstructed bowel causes an increase in the frequency and the intensity of the bowel sounds, which can be appreciated with a stethoscope. The noise may be so obvious that it can be heard while standing at the patient's side. An area of local tenderness and pain may be found over the point where an adhesion is attached to the abdominal wall, particularly when it is attached to the scar of a previous operation. Tenderness may also be found over a distended loop of intestine, but muscular guarding is unusual in simple obstruction. The rectum is empty and not ballooned on rectal examination.

The hernial orifices must be carefully examined when intestinal obstruction is suspected. A strangulated external hernia is the most obvious cause of obstruction; and it should never be missed, especially in the femoral region of elderly females. A small Richter's hernia in the femoral canal may produce intestinal obstruction with minimal external signs of a hernia.

If strangulation has occurred, the physical signs change and there should be evidence of peritoneal irritation. Abdominal tenderness, muscular guarding and rigidity may be more obvious, and rebound tenderness may be present. Bowel sounds are now sparse or absent, rather than increased. Circulatory collapse is more marked. All these signs are relative, and it is often impossible to distinguish a simple from a strangulated obstruction with any certainty by physical examination alone, unless perforation has occurred. There will then be signs of a severe peritonitis and of free air in the peritoneal cavity.

The circulatory state and the state of hydration of the patient should be judged by the pulse rate, blood pressure, degree of venous filling and the absence of normal skin elasticity.

DIFFERENTIAL DIAGNOSIS. Mechanical obstruction of the small intestine may be mistaken for a wide variety of intra-abdominal conditions, and any of these which cause colicky pain must be considered. Since appendicitis is the most common acute abdominal disease, it should always be considered first in the differential diagnosis of intestinal obstruction. The two conditions may be extremely difficult to distinguish, particularly in the early stages of acute obstructive appendicitis before localizing signs appear. The situation is further complicated when the appendix lies in the retroileal position. It may then cause an obstruction, either a paralytic type due to a localized peritonitis or a mechanical type due to surrounding inflammatory adhesions.

One of the most difficult questions to answer when a patient is seen with pain, progressive abdominal distention and constipation is whether the symptoms are due to a paralytic or a mechanical obstruction. Many conditions may present as a paralytic ileus, such as pneumonia, septicemia, pancreatitis, retroperitoneal hemorrhage and a ureteric calculus. The patient should always be asked if he is taking any drugs. Iatrogenic lesions of the small intestine are increasingly common. Enteric-coated potassium chloride capsules, used with diuretics, cause ulceration and a fibrous stricture of the bowel. This causes an organic obstruction. Anticoagulants are also dangerous and may cause obstruction in two ways. A hematoma may form in the layers of the wall of the intestine, thus occluding the lumen, or a spontaneous retroperitoneal hematoma may cause adynamic ileus. This may also be caused by the various ganglion-blocking drugs used to treat hypertension. Knowledge of the patient's current therapy is, therefore, essential to prevent mistakes being made. Although the clinical signs and investigations will usually reveal the primary cause of the paralytic obstruction, failure to recognize its true nature and confusion between mechanical and paralytic obstruction remain two of the common causes of morbidity in the management of intestinal obstruction.

Other causes of spasmodic abdominal pain must be considered in diagnosing intestinal obstruction. Acute cholecystitis may cause severe abdominal colic, and is commonly associated with marked constipation. Acute gastroenteritis may cause difficulty, particularly when vomiting is severe and diarrhea is not. Regional enteritis, inflammation of a Meckel's diverticulum, tuberculous enteritis, and severe and obstinate constipation may all have to be considered.

In the diagnosis of intestinal obstruction, good erect and supine x-ray films of the abdomen, with a metal marker placed on the umbilicus, are probably the most important single investigation. Distention of the bowel with air-fluid levels may be seen on the erect film, and the pattern of distended loops may resemble the ladder pattern seen on physical examination. Occasionally, an obvious cause of obstruction may be seen, such as a radiopaque foreign body or a gallstone. Roentgenograms may suggest the probable site of the obstruction, since the valvulae conniventes of the obstructed jejunum give an entirely different appearance from that of the saclike haustrations of the distended colon. If the obstruction is proximal to the cecum, the normal colonic gas shadows may be absent.

A plain roentgenogram may sometimes distinguish a mechanical obstruction from a paralytic ileus. The films may show an obvious precipitating factor for paralytic obstruction, such as a ureteric calculus, a pneumonia or calcification in the pancreas. Paralytic ileus should also be suspected if both the small and large bowel are distended, if peritoneal fluid is present, if the walls of the distended intestine appear thickened, or if multiple small and scattered air-fluid levels are seen.

Roentgenograms may be deceptive in closed loop obstruction. The loop contains no gas since swallowed air cannot enter it, and it is filled with fluid only. It may not be seen on a plain roentgenogram unless it produces an alteration in the position of nearby normal structures, although films of high quality sometimes outline the loop as a soft tissue shadow.

Plain roentgenograms do not help in the early differentiation of strangulation from a simple obstruction, but an upper gastrointestinal series, using a small amount of barium, may help in a difficult case. Normally, the stomach will start to empty within 60 minutes. If strangulation is present, emptying of the stomach is delayed beyond that time. The dangers of using barium by mouth to study a patient with intestinal obstruction have probably been exaggerated. So long as small amounts are used, the procedure is safe and it may show the site, cause, and degree of the obstruction. In doubtful cases, this examination clinches the diagnosis of obstruction and reduces the delay, due to indecision, before effective treatment is started. In obese patients, it is often impossible to obtain useful plain films. A barium enema and a series of upper gastrointestinal roentgenograms may be the only satisfactory way of visualizing the gastrointestinal tract to see if obstruction is present, as well as to determine the probable location.

A blood count should always be done. An increased hemoglobin concentration, or a raised hematocrit reading, gives a quantitative indication of the fluid loss and the resulting hemoconcentration. A raised white cell count may be the only evidence of strangulation, although it is not invariably elevated in this condition. The sodium, potassium, chloride, bicarbonate and blood urea levels should be measured. It is important to determine the prothrombin concentration, particularly in the elderly or in patients with a history of cardiac disease, who may be taking anticoagulants. The serum amylase should be measured to help differentiate an obstruction from pancreatitis, although it may be elevated in the presence of gangrenous intestine. The specific gravity, the chloride content, and the pH of the urine should be measured.

Abdominal paracentesis is often useful in intestinal obstruction. If the peritoneal fluid is heavily bloodstained, strangulation should be suspected. The amylase content of the fluid aspirated should be measured as it is high in acute pancreatitis. This is not absolutely diagnositic since the amylase may also be raised in a strangulation obstruction, particularly when perforation has occurred. The patient should be weighed, since the changes in weight may be helpful in the management of the fluid and electrolyte therapy.

With the physical signs and the biochemical measurements, the size and type of fluid and electrolyte deficit can be assessed. Two components must be considered: loss of plasma and blood, and loss of water and electrolytes. If the patient is in peripheral circulatory failure due to the loss of water and electrolytes only, there is probably an extracellular deficit equivalent to 6 liters of normal saline. The deficit is approximately 4 liters if there are clinical signs of fluid depletion, and chlorides are absent from the urine. If there are signs of dehydration but chlorides are present in the urine, the deficit is between 1 and 2 liters.

Some guide to the amount of plasma and blood which will be needed can be gained from the length of time the pain has been present. Approximately 500 ml. of colloid will be necessary for each 24-hour period that pain has been present, although more may be needed if a long length of intestine is strangulated.

After deciding that the patient has intestinal obstruction and after assessing the fluid requirements, the only question to be considered is whether strangulation is present. If there is any evidence, either from the examination or the investigations, that there is interference with the blood supply to the bowel, operation must be performed as soon as possible.

TREATMENT. In all patients, sufficient blood is obtained for all the foregoing investigations and for grouping and cross-matching. The needle may be left in place, and through it an infusion of saline and dextrose is started. In all patients, a nasogastric tube is inserted and the stomach aspirated. The volume and chemical make-up of the aspirate will give an indication of the losses of fluid and electrolytes. In early simple obstruction, gastric aspiration, rehydration with glucose and replenishment with physiologic saline may be all that is needed before operation is performed.

A significant number of patients, however, are examined late due to neglect of their symptoms and to delay in diagnosis. When first examined, they may be in peripheral circulatory failure, particularly if strangulation has occurred. The reduced circulating blood volume must be replenished rapidly to prevent complications of prolonged hypotension, such as anuria. Normal saline is given first to replace the losses caused by vomiting. If there is evidence of strangulation, plasma and blood will certainly be needed. The treatment of each patient is an individual physiologic experiment, and the success of the therapy must be judged by frequent observation of its effects on the pulse rate, blood pressure and urine output. The patient should be catheterized to allow accurate measurement of the hourly output of urine. A broad-spectrum antibiotic should also be given from the start of the treatment, since its routine use significantly lowers mortality.

Operation should be delayed until replenishment has stabilized or improved the vital signs, and until the urine volume secreted exceeds 40 to 60 ml. per hour. A patient in shock from intestinal obstruction should not be subjected to the added insult of an anesthetic and an operation. Adequate preparation is essential, although it should not postpone the operation more than six hours.

Certain principles are important in any operation for intestinal obstruction. Particular care is necessary during the induction of anesthesia to prevent the regurgitation of gastric contents and their aspiration into the trachea and bronchi. This may happen to any patient who is given a narcotic and particularly in elderly people in whom an unsuspected hiatus hernia may make regurgitation easy. Although preoperative gastric aspiration will help to empty the stomach, a "cuffed" endotracheal tube should be inserted, after anesthetizing the larynx and trachea, to prevent aspiration of vomitus. Moderate pressure on the cricoid cartilage, while the endotracheal tube is being inserted, also helps to prevent regurgitation. Sometimes, it may be safer to operate with local or regional anesthesia. At the end of the operation, the endotracheal tube should be left in place until the patient is awake and has an adequate cough reflex.

If a local point of tenderness is found or if previous surgical scars are present, the incision should be planned to ensure early vision of the underlying areas. The laparotomy incision should be large enough for rapid and thorough examination of the bowel. The site of obstruction should be found by following a collapsed loop of intestine. This saves exposing masses of distended bowel in an effort to localize the obstruction. Any devitalized intestine must be resected. The signs of nonviability are usually fairly obvious. An unpleasant odor on opening the peritoneal cavity is a sure index of necrotic bowel. The intestine may be black, gray or deeply congested, and there is loss of the normal serosal sheen. Peristalsis is absent in the dead segment and no pulsation of the mesenteric arteries can be felt or seen. Since needless resection and anastomosis of distended, edematous bowel should be avoided, the viability of the intestine should definitely be settled after relief of the obstruction. Intestine which at first appears of doubtful viability will often improve in color if it is wrapped for a short time in warm moist towels, and if the patient's general condition is improved by transfusion and the administration of oxygen. The local circulation can also be improved by the injection of 1 per cent Novocaine into the mesentery. In some instances after these maneuvers, the bowel will appear viable. However, the ischemia may have been severe enough so that healing produces fibrosis and stricture formation, resulting in subsequent repeated bowel obstruction. Resection of a segment of bowel which had been subject to severe ischemia but grossly viable would then be indicated. Unnecessary massive small bowel resection should be avoided to prevent postoperative diarrhea and malabsorption. The ultimate outcome will depend upon whether or not fibrosis and stricture formation occur. Distended bowel should be aspirated until it is as empty as possible, to prevent postoperative paralytic ileus and to allow easier closure of the incision. Lastly, a gastrostomy tube should be inserted to allow postoperative aspiration.

Postoperative care is important. Aspiration of the stomach and intravenous therapy should be continued until normal bowel peristalsis returns. Antibiotics should be continued, since their routine use significantly lowers mortality. Certain complications are particularly likely to occur after any operation for intestinal obstruction; among them are fluid and electrolyte imbalance, paralytic ileus, dehiscence of the wound, peritonitis, abscess formation, aspiration pneumonitis due to inhalation of vomitus, and pulmonary insufficiency due to abdominal distention. Watchful care is needed to note the early signs of all these conditions.

Although some prefer a long intestinal tube of the Miller-Abbott type, it has a limited use in the treatment of intestinal obstruction. This tube has a double lumen and a small bag at its tip, which is inflated when the tip of the tube has passed through the pylorus. Intestinal peristalsis will then carry the tube down through the intestine to the site of the obstruction. The intestinal contents are aspirated as the tube progresses along the bowel; and if all goes well, it produces rapid decompression of the intestine.

The Miller-Abbott tube has several disadvantages in practice. The bulk of the bag and the tube makes it difficult and painful to pass through the nose. Its passage through the pylorus is simple in theory but often difficult in practice, and it involves repeated visits to the x-ray department for fluoroscopy. Even when the tube does pass through into the intestine, its use often causes further delay before definitive treatment is started and gives a false sense of security. For all these reasons, a short gastric tube is now preferred. It is easily inserted and does not lead to procrastination.

The long tube may still be useful in the type of obstruction which occurs postoperatively due to peritonitis, or a localized paralytic ileus. It may also be valuable in the treatment of a patient who has had multiple operations for bowel obstruction due to adhesive peritonitis. It should never be used if strangulation is suspected, and its use should not be continued unless it produces prompt evidence of clinical and roentgenologic improvement in the degree of obstruction.

Common errors in the evaluation of patients with intestinal obstruction are to ignore or underestimate the abdominal pain; to administer a narcotic before the diagnosis has been definitely made, thus masking the pertinent signs; to overlook a tender surgical scar or femoral hernia; and not to distinguish a paralytic obstruction due to retroperitoneal disorders. The management of any patient with acute intestinal obstruction is a test of overall skill as a surgeon, and any operation performed is only an incident in a prolonged application of physiologic knowledge to the patient's problems. With better understanding of the fluid and electrolyte problems involved, mortality figures have improved; they will not improve further until the diagnosis of intestinal obstruction and of strangulation is made earlier and with greater certainty.

SPECIAL TYPES OF OBSTRUCTION. Paralytic ileus, or adynamic obstruction, is a reflex paralysis of the intestine. It is caused by infections in the abdomen, such as a peritonitis or acute pancreatitis and, particularly, infection or hemorrhage in the retroperitoneal tissues. It may complicate an attack of lobar pneumonia, causing the meteorism often seen in that condition. More remote stimuli, such as the application of a plaster cast or even a head injury, may also precipitate paralytic ileus. Any electrolyte imbalance, but particularly a low plasma potassium concentration, predisposes to paralytic intestinal obstruction. Some of the drugs used to treat hypertension may also cause ileus. It may follow any operation, but it is particularly likely after any major resection, or extensive dissection in the retroperitoneal tissues, such as that involved in the resection of an aortic aneurysm.

The treatment of postoperative paralytic ileus starts in the operating room. Careful handling of the bowel and reasonable speed and skill in manipulation will help. Careful technique and scrupulous hemostasis prevent soiling of the peritoneal cavity.

Since a short period of inactivity in the intestine appears to be the normal reaction to any operation, a patient should not be hurried during the immediate postoperative days. A nasogastric tube or gastrostomy tube should be in place after most major operations; aspiration of the gastric contents and the restriction of oral fluids usually prevent the unpleasant complications of paralytic ileus. If intestinal paralysis arises unexpectedly, or continues for an abnormally long time, aspiration of the stomach through a nasogastric tube should be started and intravenous fluids given. The patient's fluid and electrolyte requirements are given intravenously until normal peristalsis is resumed. No specific drug treatment will restore normal mobility to the bowel, but antibiotics should be given to combat any peritoneal infection and appropriate treatment should be started for any primary cause for ileus, such as pancreatitis.

Strangulated external hernia is a common cause of intestinal obstruction, and a tender, irreducible hernia should never be overlooked. Early operation is essential, after preparation of the patient, since it must always be assumed in such cases that strangulation of the bowel is present. When the hernia has been exposed and opened, the viability of the bowel is assessed; and if gangrenous, it is resected. Obstruction may sometimes be caused by a hernia when only a part of the circumference of the bowel is trapped by the neck of the hernial sac. This is called a Richter's hernia, and it is particularly common in a strangulated femoral hernia in women.

An *internal hernia usually* causes a closed loop obstruction. The bowel may herniate into normal peritoneal compartments, for example, into the lesser sac through the epiploic foramen. The intestine may also herniate into abnormal peritoneal fossae, such as those occasionally found near the duodenojejunal flexure or the appendix. The loop of intestine may also be trapped by a postoperative or congenital adhesion. Internal herniation often occurs after partial gastrectomy, when the small bowel becomes trapped behind the limbs of the jejunum going to the gastrojejunal stoma. Internal hernias often present great difficulty in diagnosis, which is usually made only at operation.

Gallstone ileus is obstruction of the bowel by a gallstone in the lumen. This is an uncommon cause of intestinal obstruction, but the incidence is increasing. It occurs predominantly in elderly women, who often give a long history of gallbladder dyspepsia before the onset of cramplike abdominal pain due to intestinal obstruction. The gallstone ulcerates its way from the gallbladder into the intestine and then usually impacts in the terminal ileum or at the ileocecal valve. X-ray examination sometimes shows the stone, if it is radiopaque, as well as evidence of intestinal obstruction. In addition, air is sometimes seen outlining the biliary tree and this confirms the existence of a fistula between the gallbladder and the intestine.

The patient should be operated on and the gallstone removed. It should be milked upward into a healthy piece of intestine before incising the bowel to remove the stone. Gallstone ileus is a dangerous condition; the diagnosis is often delayed, and since it mainly affects the elderly, cardiovascular and pulmonary disease are commonly present.

A *swallowed foreign body* may also cause intestinal obstruction. Children frequently swallow all sorts of objects, but luckily, however irregular in shape, most of the foreign bodies pass through the alimentary tract without causing obstruction. Periodic roentgenograms should be taken to see that the foreign body is progressing, and that it does not cause any significant dilatation of the intestine. In adults, this type of obstruction is most common in patients who have had a partial gastrectomy or a gastroenterostomy. The foreign body usually responsible is a citrus fruit, persimmon or desiccated coconut. Faulty chewing habits, a low gastric acidity, and a large stoma between the stomach and the jejunum allow a poorly masticated bolus to enter the small intestine and obstruct it. The episodes of obstruction are often mild, and preoperative diagnosis is rare. If such an obstruction is found at laparotomy, the mass of fruit fiber can often be milked down into the cecum. If this is not possible, it should be removed through a small incision in the bowel wall.

Multiple intraperitoneal adhesions may cause recurrent attacks of small bowel obstruction. As each episode of obstruction is treated by operation, more adhesions form and cause further episodes. Why some patients have a tendency to form multiple adhesions is unknown, although in a few it may be due to talc, which was once used to powder surgical gloves. Talc in the peritoneal cavity produces multiple foreign body granulomas and adhesions, or so-called talc peritonitis. Further episodes of obstruction can sometimes be prevented in these patients by laying the small bowel in orderly rows and plicating the loops together.

Intussusception is the invagination of a proximal (intussusceptum) part of the intestine into an adjacent distal (intussuscipiens) segment. The most common anatomic type is the ileocolic, in which the terminal ileum enters the cecum and is then propelled along the lumen of the large bowel by peristalsis. This type of intussusception is the most common cause of intestinal obstruction in infants; it usually occurs between the ages of three and 12 months, and affects males more frequently than females, in the ratio of 2 to 1. The cause of infantile intussusception is unknown, but sometimes there is hypertrophy of the submucosal lymphoid follicles of the terminal ileum. A hypertrophic follicle may project sufficiently into the lumen to form the apex of the intussusception. In a few patients, a Meckel's diverticulum may form the starting point of the intussusception.

The history usually obtained is that the infant gets spasms of abdominal pain, shown by attacks of screaming and drawing up the legs. Vomiting may occur, and the child may pass a bloodstained, or a typical "red currant jelly" stool. On examination, a mass may be felt anywhere along the course of the colon, depending on how far the intussusception has progressed. Sometimes, the apex may actually be felt on rectal examination. Characteristically, the right iliac fossa feels empty due to the migration of the cecum. The diagnosis can be confirmed by barium enema examination; sometimes this examination may reduce the intussusception, and the progress of reduction can be watched fluoroscopically. Although this appears to be a simple method of treatment, it is difficult to be certain on roentgenographic evidence alone that the reduction has been complete, or to exclude some primary cause for intussusception, such as a Meckel's diverticulum or an intestinal polyp.

Because of these uncertainties about enema reduction, operation is usually carried out for intussusception. The intussusception is manually reduced if possible, or it is excised if gangrenous changes have occurred in the bowel. The chances of a recurrent intussusception are low, probably under 5 per cent.

In adults, intussusception is an uncommon cause of intestinal obstruction, and it is nearly always due to some primary lesion of the intestine. The primary cause may be a diverticulum invaginated into the bowel, a benign or malignant tumor projecting into the intestinal lumen, or a distal obstruction. Rarely, it is possible to diagnose an intussusception as the cause of an obstruction preoperatively, unless it is shown on a barium enema examination. If the condition is found at laparotomy, a careful search must be made to ensure that a primary cause, particularly a distal obstruction, is not overlooked. The intussuscepted segment of bowel is reduced, if possible, and resection carried out; the amount of intestine resected depends on the nature of the primary lesion.

LARGE BOWEL OBSTRUCTION. The most common cause of obstruction of the large bowel is a carcinoma in the left half of the colon or the rectum, but diverticulitis, rectal stricture, anal stenosis or a sigmoid volvulus may also be responsible. The obstruction is commonly caused by the impaction of a small piece of feces in a part of the bowel narrowed by an annular growth. Therefore, lesions in the descending colon are usually the cause of an obstruction because the feces in this part of the colon are more solid than those in the right colon. There is little risk of

strangulation unless a volvulus occurs, so that the problem is different from that presented by obstruction of the small intestine.

Altered bowel habits and periodic attacks of lower abdominal colic usually precede the onset of large bowel obstruction. The patient complains of severe colicky abdominal pains situated in the hypogastrium, and of absolute constipation with a persistent desire to defecate or pass flatus. He notices distention of the abdomen and loud borborygmi. On examination, the abdomen is distended, resonant and noisy. The distention may be localized to one particular segment of the colon, but usually the cecum and proximal transverse colon are particularly dilated, whatever the site of the obstruction, because they are the most distensible parts of the colon.

The effects of the large bowel obstruction depend on the ileocecal valve (Fig. 77). If this is competent, it prevents reflux of the contents of the cecum into the ileum; and obstruction of the large bowel is, therefore, a closed loop obstruction. The loop is closed at one end by the valve and at the other by the obstructing lesion. Since the cecum bears the brunt of the colonic distention, the chief danger is that the cecum may rupture. Urgent treatment is necessary to prevent this catastrophe. If the ileocecal valve is incompetent, the contents of the cecum reflux into the terminal ileum. This causes distention of the small intestine, and the effects of a small bowel obstruction are added to those of an obstruction of the large bowel.

The managment of large intestinal obstruction is, in some ways, simpler than that of small bowel obstruction. If the diagnosis is suggested by the symptoms and signs, it can readily be confirmed by investigation. Plain roentgenograms of the abdomen show the typical appearance of a distended large bowel. If the ileocecal valve is competent, the cecum is grossly distended; if the valve is incompetent, the small bowel will also be distended and fluid levels will be seen.

The exact site and nature of the obstructive lesion can be discovered by barium enema examination, and if a sigmoid volvulus or intussusception is responsible, the examination may actually relieve the condition. Finally, sigmoidoscopy will show if any lesion in the accessible portion of the bowel is responsible for the obstruction. The degree of electrolyte depletion should be estimated, and treatment begun.

Surgical treatment is essential for obstruc-

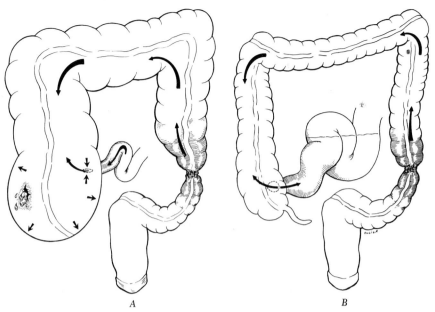

Figure 77.   The effects of large bowel obstruction depend on the competence of the ileocecal valve. *A*, Competent ileocecal valve, showing closed loop type of perforation of cecum. *B*, Incompetent ileocecal valve, showing ileal reflux and small bowel distention.

tion of the large bowel, unless it has been relieved by the barium enema. Spontaneous perforation of the cecum is the main danger, and the colon must be decompressed as soon as the patient's general condition permits.

The patient is prepared for operation, as in small bowel obstruction, and a short gastric tube is inserted to aspirate the stomach.

Various methods can be employed to decompress the distended colon (Fig. 78). A tube

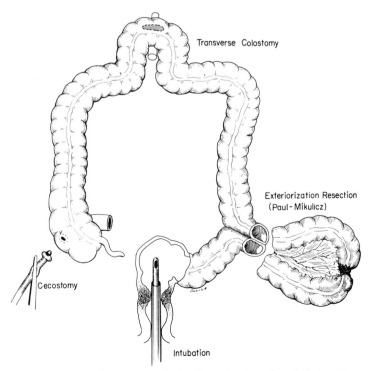

Transverse Colostomy

Exteriorization Resection
(Paul-Mikulicz)

Cecostomy

Intubation

Figure 78.   The alternative methods of treating large bowel obstruction.

can be placed into the cecum; the proximal colon, usually the transverse colon, can be exteriorized as a loop colostomy; or a tube can be manipulated through the obstructing lesion if it is in the lower part of the bowel. Alternatively, the obstructing lesion is resected, and the two ends of the bowel are brought to the surface as a colostomy. This operation is known as "exteriorization resection," or the "Paul-Mikulicz" procedure.

Cecostomy is the simplest of all the methods described. It requires only a small incision and can be performed rapidly and with local anesthesia if necessary. As long as proper care is taken of it after operation, it provides drainage of the distended colon, and it will often close spontaneously without further operation after definitive treatment of the obstructing lesion.

Transverse colostomy is a more efficient drainage operation and does not require as much aftercare as a cecostomy; however, a further operation is necessary to close the colostomy after the original obstructing lesion has been resected. The Paul-Mikulicz procedure, or exteriorization resection, is now not commonly performed for obstruction due to cancer of the colon, since the excision of the lymphatic drainage field is not extensive enough to satisfy the requirements of proper cancer surgery. However, it is still a useful procedure in certain benign conditions, such as diverticulitis of the colon.

Once the emergency situation in large bowel obstruction has been dealt with by decompression of the colon, the patient can be prepared in the usual way for definitive operation on the obstructing lesion. Obstruction of the large bowel is a dangerous complication of carcinoma of the colon particularly in the older age groups. The mortality rate of large bowel obstruction remains at about 12 to 15 per cent.

READING REFERENCES

Abrams, J. S., and Holden, W. D.: Tuberculosis of gastrointestinal tract. Arch. Surg. 89:282, 1964.

Adrwitz, A., Smith, D. F., and Rosensweig, J.: The acutely obstructed colon. Am. J. Surg. 104:474, 1962.

Altemeier, W. A., Bryant, L. R., and Wulsin, J. H.: The surgical significance of jejunal diverticulosis. Arch. Surg. 86:732, 1963.

Asman, H. B.: Radical hemorrhoidectomy. Am. Surg. 28:324, 1962.

Astler, V. B., Miller, E. B., Snyder, R. S., McIntyre, C. H., and Lillie, R. H.: Benign surgical lesions of the cecum. Arch. Surg. 86:435, 1963.

Aylett, S. O.: Three hundred cases of diffuse ulcerative colitis treated by total colectomy and ileo-rectal anastomosis. Brit. Med. J.: 1:1001, 1966.

Bacon, H. E., and McGregor, R. A.: Diverticulitis and its surgical management. Surgery 49:676, 1961.

Bagley, E. C., Crabtree, H., Fish, J. C., and Miller, E. B.: Volvulus of the right colon. Ann. Surg. 154:268, 1961.

Bailey, W. C., and Akers, D. R.: Traumatic intramural hematoma of the duodenum in children. Am. J. Surg. 110:695, 1965.

Barber, K. W., Waugh, J. M., Beahrs, O. H., and Sauer, W. G.: The indications for and the results of the surgical treatment of regional enteritis. Ann. Surg. 156:472, 1962.

Barber, K. W., Waugh, J. M., and Sauer, W. G.: Surgical treatment of complications of regional enteritis. Arch. Surg. 86:442, 1963.

Bargen, J. A.: The nature of the carcinoma associated with ulcerative colitis. Dis. Colon & Rect. 5:536, 1962.

Barnett, W. O.: Experimental strangulated intestinal obstruction—a review. Gastroenterology 39:34, 1960.

Beahrs, O. H., Richards, J. C., and Woolner, L. B.: Carcinoma of the anus. Surg. Gyn. & Obst. 114:475, 1962.

Beahrs, O. H., Vandertoll, D. J., and Baker, N. H.: Complete rectal prolapse: evaluation of surgical treatment. Ann. Surg. 161:221, 1965.

Bennett, R. C.: A review of the results of orthodox treatment for anal fistula. Proc. Roy. Soc. Med. 55:756, 1962.

Benson, C. D., Lloyd, J. R., and Fischer, H.: Intussusception in children. Arch. Surg. 86:745, 1963.

Bierman, H. J., Tocker, A. M., and Tocker, L. R.: Statistical survey of problems in patients with colostomy or ileostomy. Am. J. Surg. 112:647, 1966.

Bockhus, H. L., Tachbjian, V., Ferguson, L. K., Mouhran, Y., and Chamberlain, C.: Adenomatous polyps of colon and rectum, their incidence and relationship to carcinoma. Gastroenterology 43:125, 1961.

Boles, E. T., Ireton, R. J., and Clatworthy, H. W.: Acute appendicitis in children. Surg. 79:447, 1959.

Bolt, D. E., and Hughes, L. E.: Diverticulitis: A follow up of 100 cases. Brit. Med. J. 1:1205, 1966.

Bonilla, K., Hughes, C., and Bowers, W.: Experiences with management of the ruptured appendix. Am. J. Surg. 102:439, 1961.

Brzechwa-Agdukiewicz, A., McCarthy, C. F., Austad, W., Cornes, J., Harrison, W. J., and Read, A. E. A.: Carcinoma, villous atrophy and steatorrhoea. Gut 7:572, 1966.

Brown, D. B., and Toomey, W. F.: Diverticular disease of colon. Brit. J. Surg. 47:485, 1960.

Bruce, D., and Cole, W. H.: Complications of ulcerative colitis. Ann. Surg. 155:768, 1962.

Buetow, G. W., and Crampton, R. S.: Gallstone ileus. Arch. Surg. 86:504, 1963.

Burns, F. J.: Bleeding after hemorrhoidectomy. Dis. Colon & Rect. 5:281, 1962.

Burrus, G. R., Howell, J. F., and Jordan, G. L.: Traumatic duodenal injuries. Trauma 1:96, 1961.

Byrne, J. J.: Unusual aspects of large bowel obstruction. Am. J. Surg. 103:62, 1962.

Chang, W. Y. M., and Burnett, W. E.: Complete colonic obstruction due to carcinoma. Surg. Gyn. & Obst. 114:353, 1962.

Chapman, I.: Adenomatous polyps of large intestine. Incidence and distribution. Ann. Surg. 157:223, 1963.

Cole, J. W., Kalen, A. M., and Powell, J.: The role of ileal contents in the spontaneous regression of rectal adenomas. Dis. Colon & Rect. 4:413, 1961.

Cooke, D. C., and Lewis, E. C.: A thirty year survey of acute intussusception in childhood. Lancet 2:1359, 1960.

Davis, C., and Trueheart, R.: Surgical management of endometrioma of the colon. Am. J. Obst. & Gyn. 89:453, 1964.

Davis, W. D.: Medical aspects of chronic ulcerative colitis. Dis. Colon & Rect. 5:446, 1962.

Devroede, G. T., Tirol, F. T., Lo Russo, V. A., and Narducci, A. E.: Intramural hematoma of the duodenum and jejunum. Am. J. Surg. 112:947, 1966.

Drapanas, T., and Stewart, J. D.: Acute sigmoid volvulus. Am. J. Surg. *101*:70, 1961.

Eisenhammer, S.: The ano-rectal and anovulval fistulous abscesses. Surg. Gyn. & Obst. *113*:519, 1961.

Ewart, W. B., and Lennard-Jones, J. E.: Corticosteroids in preoperative medical management of ulcerative colitis. Lancet 2:60, 1960.

Ferguson, L. K., Boland, J. P., and Thomen, F. J.: Anterior segmental resection for carcinoma of upper rectum, rectosigmoid and sigmoid. Surgery 52:741, 1962.

Fogarty, T. J., and Fletcher, W. S.: Genesis of nonocclusive mesenteric ischemia. Am. J. Surg. *111*:130, 1966.

Garlock, J. H., Lerman, B., Klein, S. H., Lyons, A. S., and Kirschner, P. A.: Twenty-five years' experience with surgical therapy of cancer of the colon and rectum. Dis. Colon & Rect. 5:247, 1962.

Gerber, A., Thompson, R. J., Reiswig, O. M., and Vannix, R. S.: Experiences with primary resection for acute obstruction of the large intestine. Surg. Gyn. & Obst. *115*:593, 1962.

Goldfarb, W. B.: Coumarin-induced intestinal obstruction. Ann. Surg. *161*:27, 1965.

Goldman, M.: Appendicitis – historical survey. Hosp. Med. *1*:42, 1966.

Gooding, R. A., and Couch, R. D.: Mesenteric ischemia without vascular occlusion. Arch. Surg. 85:186, 1962.

Gouistis, M. C.: Hemorrhoidectomy. S. Clin. North America 41:143, 1961.

Hickey, R. C., Tidrick, R. T., and Layton, J. M.: Fulminating ulcerative colitis with colonic wall necrosis. Arch. Surg. 86:764, 1963.

Hubbell, D., Barton, W., and Solomon, D. O.: Appendicitis in older people. Surg. Gyn. & Obst. 110:289, 1960.

Huebner, G. D., and Reed, P. A.: Annular pancreas. Am. J. Surg. *104*:869, 1962.

Hummel, R, P., Altemeier, W. A., and Hill, E. O.: Iatrogenic staphylococcic enteritis. Ann. Surg. *160*:551, 1964.

Irvine, V. M., and Tsangaris, N.: Primary carcinoma of duodenum. Am. Surg. 27:744, 1961.

Jones, S. A., Carter, R., Smith, L. L., and Joergenson, E. J.: Arteriomesenteric duodenal compression. Am. J. Surg. 100:262, 1960.

Jones, T. W., and Merendino, K. A.: The perplexing duodenal diverticulum. Surgery *48*:1068, 1960.

Kelley, D. J., Falk, S., and Olson, K. C.: Hemorrhage from a solitary jejunal diverticulum. Am. J. Surg. 100:597, 1960.

Kerry, R. L., and Glas, W. W.: Traumatic injuries of the pancreas and duodenum. Arch. Surg. 85:813, 1962.

King, R. D., Kaiser, G. C., Lempke, R. E., and Schumacker, H. B.: An evaluation of catheter cecostomy. Surg. Gyn. & Obst. *123*:779, 1966.

Kirk, G. D.: Diverticula of duodenum. Am. J. Surg. 99:233, 1960.

Kirsner, J. B.: Immunologic considerations in ulcerative colitis. S. Clin. North America 42:115, 1962.

Kirsner, J. B., Rider, J. A., Moeller, H. C., Palmer, W. L., and Gold, S. S.: Polyps of the colon and rectum. Gastroenterology 39:178, 1960.

Koffler, D., Minkowitz, S., Rothman, W., and Garlock, J.: Immunocytochemical studies in ulcerative colitis and regional ileitis. Am. J. Path. *41*:733, 1962.

Latham, W. D., Arnold, H. S., and Ede, S.: Kultschitzky cell carcinoma (carcinoid) of the appendix with metastasis. Am. J. Surg. *102*:607, 1961.

Lawrason, F. D., Alpert, E., Mohr, F. L., and McMahon, F. G.: Ulcerative obstructive lesions of small intestine. J.A.M.A. *191*:641, 1965.

Lo, A. M., Evans, W. E., and Carey, L. C.: Review of small bowel obstruction at Milwaukee County General Hospital. Am. J. Surg. *111*:884, 1966.

Lockhart-Mummery, H. E.: Intestinal polyposis; the present position. Proc. Roy. Soc. Med. *60*:381, 1967.

Madden, J. L., and Tan, Y. T.: Primary resection and anastomosis in the treatment of perforated lesions in the colon with abscess or diffusing peritonitis. Surg. Gyn. & Obst. *113*:646, 1961.

Marable, S. A., Molnar, W., and Beman, F. M.: Abdominal pain secondary to celiac axis compression. Am. J. Surg. *111*:493, 1966.

Marston, A., Pheils, M. T., Thomas, M. L., and Morson, B. C.: Ischaemic colitis. Gut 7:1, 1966.

Marx, F. W., and Barker, W. F.: Surgical results in patients with ulcerative colitis treated with and without corticosteroids. Am. J. Surg. *113*:157, 1967.

Mathewson, C., and Morgan, R.: Intramural hematoma of the duodenum. Am. J. Surg. *112*:299, 1966.

Matts, S. G. F.: Combined steroid therapy of fulminating ulcerative colitis. Brit. Med. J. *1*:1045, 1962.

Mavor, G. E., Lyall, A. D., Chrystal, K. M. R., and Tsapogas, M.: Mesenteric infarction as a vascular emergency. Brit. J. Surg. *50*:219, 1962.

McDonald, J. C.: Nonspecific mesenteric adenitis. Surg. Gyn. & Obst. *116*:409, 1963.

McGregor, J. K., and Bacon, H. E.: The surgical management of carcinoma of the mid- and upper rectum. Arch. Surg. 85:807, 1962.

McInerney, G. T., Sauer, W. G., Baggenstoss, A. H., and Hodgson, J. R.: Fulminant ulcerative colitis with marked colonic dilation. Gastroenterology 42:244, 1962.

McLauthlin, C. H., and Packard, G. B.: Acute appendicitis in children. Am. J. Surg. *101*:619, 1961.

McSherry, C. K., and Beal, J. M.: Sigmoidovesical fistulae complicating diverticulitis. Arch. Surg. 85:1024, 1962.

Moertel, C. G., Sauer, W. G., Dockerty, M. B., and Baggenstoss, A. H.: Life history of the carcinoid of the small intestine. Cancer *14*:901, 1961.

Morson, B. C.: Precancerous lesions of colon and rectum. J.A.M.A. *179*:316, 1962.

Morton, D. L., and Goldman, L.: Differential diagnosis of diverticulitis and carcinoma of sigmoid colon. Am. J. Surg. *103*:55, 1962.

Neely, J. C. S.: A ten year analysis of primary disease of the small bowel causing acute small bowel obstruction in adults. Am. J. Surg. *103*:119, 1962.

Palmer, J. A.: Treatment of massive rectal prolapse. Surg. Gyn. & Obst. *112*:502, 1961.

Parks, A. G.: The pathogenesis of fistula-in-ano. Proc. Roy. Soc. Med. 55:751, 1962.

Parks, A. G.: The surgical treatment of haemorrhoids. Brit. J. Surg. 43:23, 1956.

Passi, R. B., and Lansing, A. M.: Experimental intestinal malabsorption produced by vascular insufficiency. Canad. J. Surg. 7:332, 1964.

Prather, J. R., and Bowers, R. F.: Surgical management of volvulus of the sigmoid. Arch. Surg. 85:869, 1962.

Prohaska, J. V., Greer, D., and Ryan, J. F.: Acute dilatation of colon in ulcerative colitis. Arch. Surg. 89:24, 1964.

Prohaska, J. V., Houttuin, E., and Kocandrie, V.: Pathogenesis of fistulization in inflammatory disease of the bowel. Am. J. Surg. *111*:126, 1966.

Prohaska, J., Mock, F., Baker, W., and Collins, R.: Pseudomembranous (staphylococcal) enterocolitis. Surg. Gyn. & Obst. *112*:103, 1961.

Raia, S., and Kreel, L.: Gas-distention double-contrast duodenography using the Scott-Harden gastroduodenal tube. Gut 7:420, 1966.

Ranger, I., and Spence, M. P.: Superior mesenteric artery occlusion treated by ileo-colic aortic anastomosis. Brit. J. Med. 2:95, 1962.

Ridstein, C. B., and Lanter, B.: Etiology and surgical therapy of massive prolapse of the rectum. Ann. Surg. *157*:259, 1963.

River, L. P., Tope, J. W., and Ashley, W. F.: Tumors of the small intestine and intestinal obstruction. Am. J. Surg. *104*:395, 1962.

Romsdahl, M. M., and Cole, W. H.: Diverticulitis of the colon. Arch. Surg. 86:751, 1963.

Rosi, P. A., Cahill, W., and Carey, J.: A ten year study of hemicolectomy in the treatment of carcinoma of the left half of the colon. Surg. Gyn. & Obst. *114*:15, 1962.

Rousselot, L. M., and Cole, D. R.: Intraluminal injection of nitrogen mustard as adjuvant chemotherapy in treatment of carcinoma of colon and rectum. Surg. Gyn. & Obst. *114*:409, 1962.

Saitzstein, E. C., Marshall, W. J., and Freemark, R. J.: Gangrenous intestinal obstruction. Surg. Gyn. & Obst. *114*:695, 1962.

Sanders, R. J.: The management of colon injuries. S. Clin. North America *43*:457, 1963.

Sawyer, R. B., Sawyer, K. C., Jr., and Sawyer, K. C.: Volvulus of the colon. Am. J. Surg. *104*:468, 1962.

Schier, J., Symmonds, R. E., and Dahlin, D. C.: Clinicopathologic aspects of actinic enteritis. Surg. Gyn. & Obst. *119*:1019, 1964.

Sherman, D., and May, A. G.: The ileum, site of vitamin B_{12} absorption. Arch. Surg. *86*:187, 1963.

Shnitka, T. K., Friedman, M. H. W., Kidd, E. G., and Mackenzie, W. C.: Villous tumors of rectum and colon, characterized by severe fluid and electrolyte loss. Surg. Gyn. & Obst. *112*:609, 1961.

Silen, W. M., Hein, M. F., and Goldman, L.: Strangulation obstruction of the small intestine. Arch. Surg. *85*:121, 1962.

Slack, W. W.: Anatomy, pathology and some clinical features of diverticulitis of the colon. Brit. J. Surg. *50*:185, 1962.

Smiley, D. F.: Perforated sigmoid diverticulitis with spreading peritonitis. Am. J. Surg. *111*:431, 1966.

Smith, F. W., Law, D. H., Nickel, W. F., and Sleisenger, M. H.: Fulminant ulcerative colitis with total dilation of the colon. Gastroenterology *42*:233, 1962.

Smith, J. W., and Mathewson, C.: Appendicitis in the aged. Western J. Surg. *70*:225, 1962.

Smithwick, R. H.: Surgical treatment of diverticulitis of the sigmoid. Am. J. Surg. *99*:192, 1960.

Snyder, E. N., and McCranie, D.: Closed loop obstruction of the small bowel. Am. J. Surg. *111*:398, 1966.

Southwick, H. W., Harridge, W. H., and Cole, W. H.: Recurrence at suture line following resection for carcinoma of the colon. Am. J. Surg. *103*:86, 1962.

Speer, C. S., and Bacon, H. E.: Co-existing diverticular and neoplastic disease of the colon. Surgery *52*:733, 1962.

Spratt, J. S., Ackerman, L. V., and Moyer, C. A.: Relationship of polyps of colon to colonic cancer. Ann. Surg. *148*:682, 1958.

Sterns, E. E., Palmer, J. A., and Kergin, F. G.: Surgical significance of radiation injuries to the bowel. Canad. J. Surg. *7*:407, 1964.

Stewart, J. O. R.: Lesser sac hernia. Brit. J. Surg. *50*:321, 1962.

Stewart, W., Bartlett, R., Bishop, H., Campbell, D., Goldsmith, N., Maclean, K., Middleton, E., Musselman, M., Ronnick, G., and Tappan, W.: Carcinoid tumors presenting with acute abdominal signs. Ann. Surg. *154*:112, 1961.

Stoney, R. J., and Wylie, E. J.: Recognition and surgical management of visceral ischemic syndromes. Ann. Surg. *164*:714, 1966.

Vest, B.: Roentgenographic diagnosis of strangulating closed-loop obstruction of the small intestine. Surg. Gyn. & Obst. *115*:561, 1962.

Watne, A. L., and Trevino, E.: Diagnostic features of mucocele of the appendix. Arch. Surg. *84*:517, 1962.

Watts, J. McK., De Dombal, F. T., and Goligher, J. C.: Early results of surgery for ulcerative colitis. Brit. J. Surg. *53*:1005, 1966.

Watts, J. McK., De Dombal, F. T., and Goligher, J. C.: Long term complications and prognosis following major surgery for ulcerative colitis. Brit. J. Surg. *53*:1014, 1966.

Watts, J. McK., De Dombal, F. T., Watkinson, G., and Goligher, J. C.: Early course of ulcerative colitis. Gut *7*:16, 1966.

Weckesser, E. C., and Putnam, T. C.: Perforating injuries of the rectum and sigmoid. Trauma *2*:474, 1962.

Wierman, W. H., Strahan, R. W., and Spencer, J. R.: Small bowel erosion by synthetic aortic grafts. Am. J. Surg. *112*:791, 1966.

Williams, E. D., and Sandler, M.: The classification of carcinoid tumours. Lancet *1*:238, 1963.

Williams, L. F., Hughes, C. W., and Bowens, W. F.: Obstruction of the small bowel. Am. J. Surg. *104*:376, 1962.

Williams, R. D., and Elliott, D. W.: Surgery for ulcerative colitis. Arch. Surg. *86*:761, 1963.

Williams, R. D., Yurko, A. A., Kerr, G., and Zollinger, R. M.: Comparison of anterior and abdomino-perineal resections for low pelvic colon and rectal carcinoma. Am. J. Surg. *111*:114, 1966.

Wilson, H., Storer, E. H., and Star, F. T.: Carcinoid tumors. Am. J. Surg. *105*:35, 1963.

Wilson, R.: Primary carcinoma of the appendix. Am. J. Surg. *104*:238, 1962.

Winsey, H. S., and Jones, P. F.: Acute abdominal pain in childhood: analysis of a years' admissions. Brit. Med. J. *1*:653, 1967.

Wray, C. H., Stark, C. E., Brackney, E. L., and Moretz, W. H.: Surgical problems in amebiasis. Am. Surg. *30*:780, 1964.

Zollinger, R. M., Kinsey, D. L., and Grant, G. N.: Intestinal obstruction. Postgrad. Med. *33*:165, 1963.

Zuidema, G. D.: Surgical management of superior mesenteric arterial emboli. Arch. Surg. *82*:267, 1961.

Chapter 24

THE LIVER AND BILIARY SYSTEM

by
MARSHALL J. ORLOFF, M.D.

A Chicagoan, MARSHALL ORLOFF graduated from the University of Illinois and its medical school. He received a master's degree in pharmacology and completed his surgical residency education at the University of Pennsylvania. He worked on a doctor of philosophy degree in pharmacology at the University of Colorado where he was a member of the faculty of the Department of Surgery. He went to the University of California, Los Angeles, as a Markle Scholar in medical sciences. During these years of study, he made contributions in the fields of neuropharmacology, liver physiology and disease, pediatric surgery, adrenal gland physiology and shock. He is the first Professor and Chairman of the Department of Surgery, University of California, San Diego, School of Medicine.

The Liver

EMBRYOLOGY

The liver arises from the entoderm of the foregut and the mesoderm of the septum transversum. In the 2.5 mm. embryo, approximately four weeks old, a diverticulum develops from the ventral floor of the foregut at the level of the future duodenum and extends into the septum transversum in close association with a capillary plexus that connects to the vitelline veins. The caudal portion of the diverticulum develops into the cystic duct and gallbladder, and the cranial portion becomes the liver. In the early embryo, the two vitelline veins pass through the hepatic anlage to enter the sinus venosus of the heart in conjunction with the paired umbilical veins from the placenta. At a later stage, the vitelline veins form the portal vein and the hepatic veins, whereas the left umbilical vein becomes the ductus venosus which largely bypasses the liver and shunts oxygenated placental blood directly into the inferior vena cava. At birth, the ductus venosus closes and along with the remainder of the obliterated left umbilical vein becomes the ligamentum teres hepatis in the caudal free border of the falciform ligament. The ligamentous attach-ments of the liver are derived from the two layers of the ventral mesentery between which the hepatic anlage develops. The embryonic structures are represented in the adult as follows:

Embryo
Right and left vitelline veins
Left umbilical vein – ductus venosus
Anterior portion of ventral mesentery
Posterior portion of ventral mesentery

Adult
Portal vein, hepatic veins
Ligamentum teres hepatis
Falciform ligament, right and left anterior coronary ligaments, right and left triangular ligaments
Gastrohepatic ligament, hepatoduodenal ligament, right and left posterior coronary ligaments, right and left triangular ligaments

ANATOMY

MICROSCOPIC ANATOMY. The liver is covered by a thick capsule of collagen and elastic

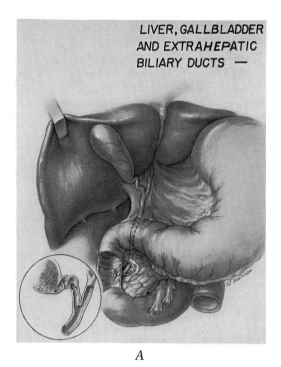

A

B

Figure 1. *A*, Gallbladder and extrahepatic ducts. *Inset*, Schematic detail of junction of cystic with common duct. *B*, Schematic diagram after Hans Elias, portraying the liver as a spongelike structure of cells penetrated by communicating system of cavities or lacunae through which courses the blood from the portal tract to the central vein. These sinusoids are lined with the all-important Kupffer cells.

tissue, called Glisson's capsule, which extends into the parenchyma along the blood vessels and bile ducts. The capsule encases a sponge-like mass of cells arranged in plates through which passes an intricate system of capillaries called sinusoids. The sinusoids differ from ordinary capillaries in that their endothelial lining is made up of specialized phagocytic cells, the Kupffer cells, and they are more permeable to macromolecules than systemic capillaries. The liver cell plates are one cell thick and have an intimate association with the sinusoids. On microscopic examination the hepatic parenchyma appears to be distributed in poorly defined lobules. At the center of each lobule is a central vein, a tributary of the hepatic venous outflow system. At the periphery, between several lobules, is a collection of connective tissue called a portal tract or triad which contains branches of the portal vein, the hepatic artery and the bile duct. The branches of both the portal vein and hepatic artery empty directly into the sinusoids after a series of divisions and ramifications. In addition, branches of the hepatic artery nourish the structures in the portal tracts. The central veins drain into progressively enlarging sublobular veins until connections are made with the major hepatic veins which enter the inferior vena cava. The bile duct system originates as fine bile canaliculi located between the hepatic cells and forming a part of the cell membrane. These bile capillaries drain into intralobular ductules and then into large ducts in the portal tracts.

GROSS ANATOMY. The liver is the largest organ in the body with a weight of from 1200 to 1600 gm. Its superior surface conforms to the undersurface of the diaphragm and its inferior surface rests on the viscera in the upper abdomen. It is held in position mainly by intra-abdominal pressure. The liver is covered by peritoneum except for an area on the posterior superior surface adjacent to the inferior vena cava which is in direct contact

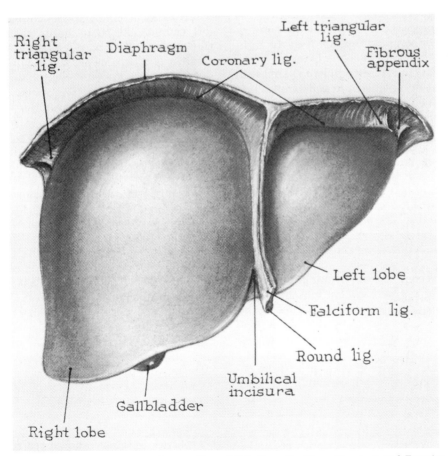

Figure 2. Ligaments of the liver. (From Popper, H., and Schaffner, F.: Liver: Structure and Function. New York, McGraw-Hill Book Co., 1957.)

with the diaphragm and is called the bare area. The peritoneal reflections from the anterior abdominal wall, diaphragm and abdominal viscera to the liver form a number of distinct ligaments (Fig. 2). These are:

The falciform ligament which attaches the liver to the anterior abdominal wall between the diaphragm and umbilicus.

The ligamentum teres hepatis which occupies the lower free border of the falciform ligament and represents the obliterated left umbilical vein.

The gastrohepatic ligament and hepatoduodenal ligament which are the portions of the lesser omentum extending to the liver from the lesser curvature of the stomach and the proximal duodenum. These ligaments contain the hepatic artery, portal vein and common bile duct. The hepatoduodenal ligament forms the anterior boundary of the epiploic foramen of Winslow.

The right and left anterior coronary ligaments and the right and left posterior coronary ligaments which represent the peritoneal reflections from the diaphragm onto the liver.

The right and left triangular ligaments which are produced by fusion of the anterior and posterior coronary ligaments at the right and left lateral borders of the liver.

The liver occupies the right hypochondrium and much of the epigastrium and extends into the left hypochondrium. Except in the epigastrium, the organ is largely surrounded by the thoracic cage and in normal subjects usually cannot be palpated on physical examination. The superior surface of the right lobe extends as high as the right fourth intercostal space or right fifth rib, just below the nipple.

The falciform ligament divides the liver topographically, but not anatomically or functionally, into a large right lobe and a smaller left lobe. In addition, on the visceral surface several fissures and fossae arranged in the shape of an H demarcate two additional lobes, the quadrate and caudate. The crossbar of the H is the porta hepatis in which are found the hepatic artery, portal vein, bile duct branches, lymphatics, nerves and attachment of the lesser omentum (Fig. 3).

Recent interest in and success with resection of portions of the liver have served to re-emphasize the fact that the classic topographic division of the liver into right and left lobes is not anatomically or functionally correct. The liver is similar to the lung in that it can be divided into anatomic segments on the basis of the pattern of branching of the

hepatic artery, portal vein and bile duct. Accordingly, the true anatomic left lobe consists of a medial segment which lies to the right of the falciform ligament and a lateral segment made up of the classic topographic left lobe. The true anatomic right lobe consists of anterior and posterior segments. The line of division between the anatomic right and left lobes is not marked on the surface but follows a line from the gallbladder fossa below to the inferior vena cava fossa above. The topographic caudate lobe is divided, according to its blood supply and bile duct drainage, between the anatomic right and left lobes. The hepatic veins have an interlobar distribution between the liver segments.

The liver is unique among the abdominal viscera in having a dual blood supply. The common hepatic artery arises from the celiac axis along with the left gastric artery and splenic artery, and courses to the liver in the lesser omentum to the left of the common bile duct and anterior to the portal vein. It gives off three major branches, the gastroduodenal artery, supraduodenal artery and right gastric artery, after which it divides into a right and left ramus. The right ramus passes behind the common hepatic duct and gives off the cystic artery before entering the liver. In over 40 per cent of subjects, variations from the classic pattern occur. The surgeon must be aware of these variations if he is to avoid serious operative accidents.

The valveless portal vein carries blood to the liver from the stomach, small intestine, large intestine, pancreas and spleen. It is formed from the junction of the superior mesenteric vein and splenic vein behind the head of the pancreas, and passes posterior to the first part of the duodenum through the hepatoduodenal ligament to the porta hepatis where it divides into right and left branches. The hepatic artery and common bile duct lie anterior to it. The inferior mesenteric vein usually drains into the splenic vein. The tributaries of the portal vein connect with the systemic venous system in several areas. In normal subjects, these communications are of little importance but in patients with portal hypertension they may assume great clinical significance. Portal-systemic anastomoses occur at the following sites:

The left gastric (coronary) vein, a tributary of the portal vein, connects with the esophageal plexus of veins and, in turn, with the azygos vein, hemiazygos vein and other tributaries of the superior vena cava. Esophageal

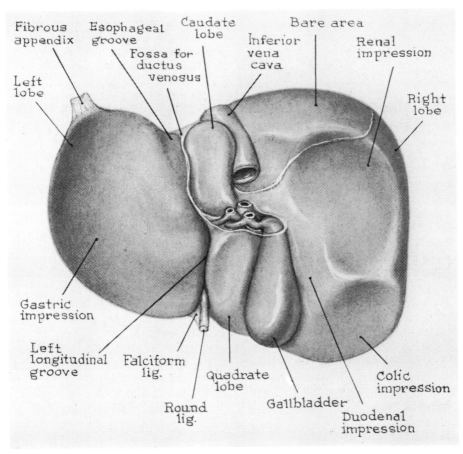

Figure 3. Topographic lobes and impressions of the liver. (From Popper, H., and Schaffner, F.: Liver: Structure and Function. New York, McGraw-Hill Book Co., 1957.)

varices develop in the esophageal plexus as a result of portal hypertension.

The short gastric veins and left gastro-epiploic vein, tributaries of the splenic vein, connect with the esophageal plexus.

The paraumbilical veins, tributaries of the portal vein, and occasionally a persistent umbilical vein anastomose with the inferior and superior epigastric veins of the systemic system. These connections are the site of the caput medusae and the Cruveilhier-Baumgarten syndrome in patients with portal hypertension.

The superior hemorrhoidal vein, a tributary of the inferior mesenteric vein, communicates with the middle and inferior hemorrhoidal veins of the systemic circulation and may form large hemorrhoids in the presence of portal hypertension.

Retroperitoneal veins form communications between the portal vein, superior mesenteric vein, inferior mesenteric vein, pan-

creatic veins and the tributaries of the inferior vena cava.

The venous outflow from the liver is carried by the valveless hepatic veins which enter the inferior vena cava just below the diaphragm (Fig. 4). Beginning with the central veins in the liver lobules, the venous effluent passes through progressively larger sublobular veins and collecting veins into the major right, middle, and left hepatic veins. The middle and left hepatic veins usually join and enter the vena cava as one vessel. Several smaller hepatic veins from the caudate lobe and other parts of the liver are consistently found.

Recent interest in the role of the hepatic lymph in cirrhosis has focused attention on the lymphatic drainage of the liver. Between the liver cell plates and the sinusoids tissue spaces called the perisinusoidal spaces of Disse are found, through which fluid exchange between the blood and the hepatocyte takes

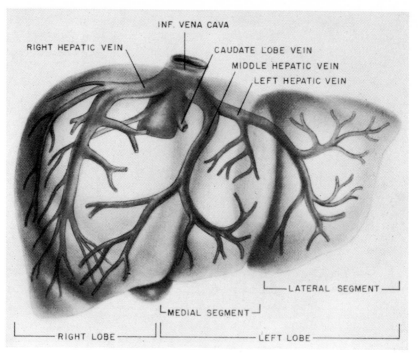

Figure 4. The hepatic venous outflow system. (From Schwartz, S. I.: Surgical Diseases of the Liver. New York, McGraw-Hill Book Co., 1964.)

place. Fluid from these spaces drains into small lymphatic vessels in the portal tracts and then into major lymphatics which leave the liver in the porta hepatis and empty into the cisterna chyli. In addition, lymphatic vessels are found around the hepatic veins, in Glisson's capsule and around the bile ducts. Many of these pass through the diaphragm and empty into the thoracic duct in the thorax. The lymph nodes to which the hepatic lymphatics connect are located in the porta hepatis, which, in turn, connect with the celiac nodes, around the termination of the inferior vena cava, along the left gastric artery, and near the pylorus.

The nerve supply to the liver consists of sympathetic fibers from the seventh to the tenth thoracic segments of the spinal cord and parasympathetic fibers carried in the right and left vagus nerves. The sympathetic nerves pass through the celiac ganglia. The nerves form an anterior and posterior hepatic plexus in the porta hepatis and are distributed throughout the liver along the blood vessels and bile ducts. The afferent innervation is carried in the sympathetic splanchnic nerves and in the right phrenic nerve. Hepatic pain is dull and is distributed over the area occupied by the liver, with occasional radiation to the right shoulder.

PHYSIOLOGY

FUNCTIONS OF THE LIVER. Just as the heart is the focal organ in the circulatory system, and the brain is the hub of integrative activity, the liver is the center of metabolism in the body. The synthesis, modification, storage, breakdown and excretion of many of the substances upon which life depends occur in the liver. The functions of the liver exceed those of all other organs in number and complexity.

Bile formation and excretion. Bile is composed of bilirubin, the salts of bile acids, cholesterol, phospholipids, inorganic salts, mucin, water and a host of metabolites. It is excreted at the rate of 600 to 1000 ml. per day. The liver synthesizes bile acids from cholesterol, and bile represents the main route by which cholesterol is eliminated from the body.

Bilirubin is formed from the breakdown of hemoglobin in the reticuloendothelial system at various sites in the body, but particularly in the bone marrow and spleen. The first step in the process involves the opening of the tetrapyrrole ring in the heme radical to form biliverdin-iron-globin. Next, the iron and globin components are separated to form biliverdin. Reduction of the biliverdin produces unconjugated bilirubin. This compound is largely insoluble in water and does not give the van den Bergh reaction unless it is first treated with agents to make it water soluble. The unconjugated bilirubin is carried to the liver cell in the blood, loosely bound to albumin and alpha globulin. In the liver, bilirubin is conjugated with glucuronic acid and to a much lesser extent with sulfate to form bilirubin diglucuronide and bilirubin sulfate. These compounds are water soluble and give the van den Bergh reaction without pretreatment. In actuality, direct-reacting bilirubin consists of two pigments, I and II, the major of which is bilirubin diglucuronide and the other of which is believed to be the monoglucuronide or unconjugated bilirubin. Conjugated bilirubin is secreted into the bile canaliculi and is excreted via the bile ducts into the intestine where it is reduced by bacteria to colorless compounds, mesobilirubinogen and stercobilinogen, collectively called urobilinogen. Much of the urobilinogen is excreted in the stool where part of it is oxidized to the colored pigment urobilin. However, about one-third to one-half of the urobilinogen is reabsorbed from the intestine in what is called the enterohepatic circulation, and is carried to the liver where it is again excreted or is transformed back to bilirubin. A small amount of the reabsorbed urobilinogen escapes processing by the liver and is excreted in the urine. Figure 5 summarizes the steps in the breakdown of hemoglobin.

Carbohydrate metabolism. Hepatic synthesis, transformation and breakdown of carbohydrates, fats, and proteins are so intimately related that the liver has been referred to as a metabolic pool. The liver is capable of forming these major substances from each other so that separation of the metabolic processes is done mainly for discussion purposes. The liver converts pentoses and hexoses absorbed from the intestine to glycogen, the major form of carbohydrate storage in the body, by enzymatic mechanisms called glycogenesis. In reverse, the liver breaks down glycogen by glycogenolysis, and, thereby, serves as a primary source of glucose for the body. The liver converts glucose, via the hexose monophosphate shunt, to pentoses which have several uses. They are metabolized to provide energy. They are used in the biosynthesis of nucleotides, nucleic acids, and adenosine triphosphate. They are used to produce 3 carbon compounds, such as pyruvic acid, which serve as precursors for

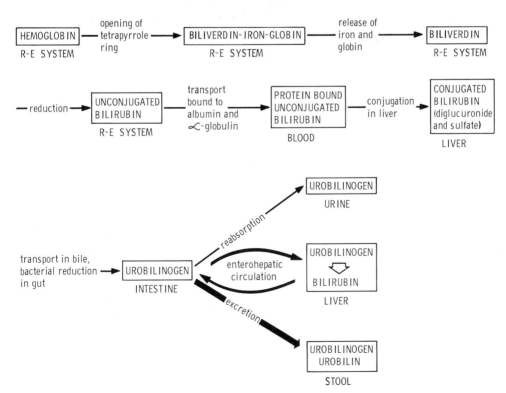

Figure 5.   Hemoglobin breakdown and bile pigment formation.

active acetate, a compound that forms a link between carbohydrate, fat and protein metabolism and plays a central role in the tricarboxylic acid cycle.

Fat metabolism. The liver both synthesizes and catabolizes fatty acids and neutral fats. Fatty acids are transformed into four carbon compounds, the ketone bodies, and into 2 carbon compounds such as active acetate. Similarly, glycerol is broken down into active acetate. The liver is the predominant site of cholesterol synthesis and esterification, and it plays a major role in the synthesis and breakdown of phospholipids and lipoproteins.

Protein metabolism. The liver synthesizes a large variety of proteins from amino acids. By deamination, the liver forms sugars and fatty acids from amino acids, and by transamination it produces amino acids from nonnitrogenous compounds. The liver is the only organ which produces plasma albumin and alpha globulin, and it is the major site for the production of urea, the end product of protein metabolism. Beta-globulin is also formed in the liver.

Blood coagulation. The liver is the primary center for the synthesis of most of the proteins involved in blood coagulation. It manufactures fibrinogen, prothrombin and factors V, VII, IX and X. Vitamin K is required for the formation of prothrombin and several of the other coagulation factors.

Vitamin metabolism. All the vitamins are stored in and utilized by the liver. It is the primary site for the storage of vitamins A, D, E and K.

Detoxification. The liver is the detoxification center of the body. By oxidation, reduction, methylation, acetylation, esterification, and conjugation the liver degrades or modifies a great variety of endogenous substances, such as the steroid hormones, drugs and chemicals.

Phagocytosis and immunity. Through the Kupffer cells of its reticuloendothelial system, the liver serves as a large filter where bacteria, pigments and other debris are removed from the blood by phagocytosis. Furthermore, the Kupffer cells are an important source of gamma-globulin which is involved in immune defense mechanisms.

EFFECTS OF HEPATECTOMY. Studies in hepatectomized dogs have provided important information about liver function and have raised a number of questions not yet answered. Immediately following complete removal of the liver the animals awake from anesthesia and appear normal. After several hours, however, muscular weakness and depressed reflexes develop, followed in a short time by convulsions and death. These abnormalities are due to hypoglycemia and can be prevented by the administration of glucose. The animal treated with glucose survives in good health for up to 48 hours. However, despite the continued provision of sugar, the dog ultimately develops restlessness, vomiting and tachypnea followed by ataxia, spasticity, coma and death. The cause of death is unknown. A number of biochemical abnormalities have been observed, but none has been proved to be responsible for the terminal events. These include a mild increase in blood ammonia, a rise in the amino acid content of blood, cerebrospinal fluid and brain, an elevation of blood uric acid, an increase in serum bilirubin and the appearance of bilirubin in the urine, a decrease in the proteins involved in blood coagulation, and a fall in blood urea.

LIVER REGENERATION. The liver has a striking capacity to regenerate following partial removal or injury. After excision of 75 per cent of the liver, complete restitution of the organ occurs within eight weeks in the dog and three weeks in the rat. A marked increase in mitoses in the liver cells and of hepatic deoxyribonucleic acid formation are important features of the regeneration process. The factors responsible for liver regeneration are incompletely understood. Some studies indicate that the amount of blood flowing to the liver is an important factor, whereas other work suggests that there is a specific hepatotrophic substance in portal venous blood. Although it was believed for many years that diversion of blood from the liver through an Eck fistula prevented regeneration, conclusive recent evidence has shown that liver regeneration is normal in the animal with an Eck fistula.

THE ECK FISTULA DOG. Performance of a portacaval shunt in animals with a normal liver results in a number of serious disturbances which suggest that sudden diversion of portal blood is incompatible with good hepatic function. Such animals develop a syndrome of central nervous system symptoms following the ingestion of meat which has come to be known as meat intoxication. In addition, animals with an Eck fistula have a decreased capacity to synthesize proteins, impaired bile formation, decreased hepatic

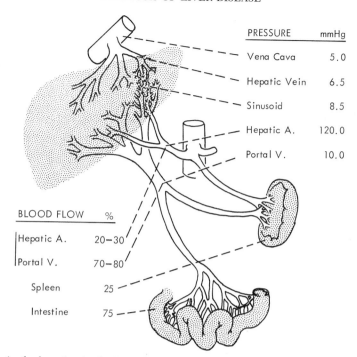

PRESSURE	mmHg
Vena Cava	5.0
Hepatic Vein	6.5
Sinusoid	8.5
Hepatic A.	120.0
Portal V.	10.0

BLOOD FLOW	%
Hepatic A.	20–30
Portal V.	70–80
Spleen	25
Intestine	75

Figure 6. Pressures in the hepatic circulation and the percentage of contribution to hepatic blood flow made by the various components.

storage of glycogen, a fall in serum cholesterol and fatty acids, a progressive rise in blood and urine uric acid and a hypochromic anemia. The liver undergoes atrophy and accumulates fat, and the animal develops polydypsia, polyuria, anorexia, weight loss and lassitude. Unless care is meticulous, the animals do not survive for more than a few months. In dogs with experimental cirrhosis, construction of an Eck fistula does not produce the abnormalities observed in animals with an initially normal liver.

HEPATIC HEMODYNAMICS. Measurements of hepatic blood flow by indirect and direct methods have shown that the liver receives about one-fourth of the cardiac output. Liver blood flow in normal subjects averages 1500 ml. per minute, with a range of from 1000 to 1800 ml. per minute. The hepatic artery contributes about one-fourth of the blood flowing to the liver and the portal vein contributes about three-fourths (Fig. 6). The pressure in the portal vein averages approximately 10 mm. Hg (140 mm. saline), whereas the pressure in the hepatic artery is the same as the systemic arterial pressure. In the hepatic sinusoids, where the two systems join, the pressure is reduced to a mean 8.5 mm. Hg. The pressure in the hepatic veins averages 6.5 mm. Hg and in the inferior vena cava at the level of the diaphragm it is about 5 mm.

Hg. The consecutive pressure gradients assure movement of blood toward the heart. The oxygen content of portal vein blood is higher than that of systemic venous blood, averaging approximately 80 per cent saturation. The flow of blood to the liver is controlled by mechanical, neural, and humoral mechanisms. Rapid and striking changes in hepatic blood flow occur under various conditions such as exercise, fever, and shock. Thus, the liver is important in maintaining circulatory homeostasis.

DIAGNOSIS OF LIVER DISEASE

HISTORY. Diseases of the liver produce a variety of symptoms depending on the etiology and nature of the underlying disturbance, and upon the rapidity with which liver damage occurs. Many of the symptoms are nonspecific. Nevertheless, certain symptoms occur with sufficient frequency in various hepatic diseases to alert the physician to the possibility that a liver disorder is the cause of the patient's illness (Table 1).

Jaundice is a common symptom of many liver diseases and, perhaps, is the complaint which most frequently leads the patient to seek medical attention. Jaundice is often accompanied by dark urine and sometimes by

Table 1. *Common Symptoms and Signs of Liver Disease*

SYMPTOMS

Jaundice, dark urine, pruritus
Fatigue, malaise, myalgia, headache
Anorexia and nausea
Pain in right upper quadrant of abdomen
Fever
Hematemesis and melena
Pedal edema and abdominal enlargement (ascites)
Mental changes, forgetfulness, confusion
Weight loss
Purpura and epistaxis

SIGNS

Jaundice
Hepatomegaly and liver tenderness
Splenomegaly
Fever
Ascites (with shifting dullness) and edema
Spider angiomas
Palmar erythema
Collateral veins in abdominal wall
Tremor, asterixis, mental confusion
Muscle wasting (shoulder girdles, extremities)
Xanthomas
Gynecomastia, testicular atrophy, loss of axillary and pubic hair
Hematemesis, melena, hematochezia
Purpura

light stools. The investigation of a patient with jaundice should include a search for a history of transfusions of blood or blood products, injections, contact with jaundiced individuals, occurrence of jaundice in the family, exposure to chemicals at work or in the home, and a record of travel. The possibility that jaundice is due to biliary obstruction requires questioning about fatty food intolerance, attacks of colic, bloating and belching. Pruritus sometimes accompanies jaundice and may be the patient's predominant complaint.

Fatigue, malaise, headache, myalgia, arthralgia, and fever are frequent symptoms associated with acute hepatic inflammation and necrosis. Anorexia and nausea are striking manifestations of hepatitis, but are also found in chronic liver disease. Pain in the right hypochondrium may occur in most liver diseases as well as in disturbances of the biliary system. The distinction between continuous dull pain and colic is of diagnostic importance.

Hematemesis and melena are complications of chronic liver disturbances, and particularly of cirrhosis. Liver disease must be considered, at least initially, in every patient with upper gastrointestinal bleeding. Similarly, ascites, dependent edema, weight loss, and a bleeding tendency are manifestations of severe and usually longstanding liver damage. Mental abnormalities such as forgetfulness, confusion, inability to concentrate, and personality changes are common symptoms of advanced cirrhosis. A history of alcohol intake and a dietary history are of great importance.

PHYSICAL EXAMINATION. The findings on physical examination again depend on the type of liver disease and its chronicity. Jaundice, seen best in the sclerae, is an important sign. Hepatomegaly and liver tenderness are found frequently in both acute and chronic liver disease, whereas splenomegaly is a common finding in longstanding hepatic disorders. Fever occurs most often in acute inflammation and necrosis of the liver. Circulatory disturbances, such as spider angiomas seen usually on the face, neck, upper trunk and arms, telangiectases over the nose and cheeks, palmar erythema, and collateral veins beneath the skin of the abdomen are characteristic signs of chronic hepatic dysfunction. Similarly, ascites with shifting dullness, dependent edema, gynecomastia, testicular atrophy, loss of axillary and pubic hair, and muscle wasting are classic manifestations of cirrhosis. Neurologic disturbances such as tremor, asterixis, peripheral neuritis, and disorders of consciousness varying from confusion to coma are associated with severe destruction of the hepatic parenchyma. Xanthomas, which occur most often in the skin of the eyelids, extremities, and upper trunk, are found in liver diseases associated with chronic biliary obstruction. An interesting but uncommon sign of advanced liver disease is a sweet, musty odor of the breath called fetor hepaticus.

LIVER FUNCTION TESTS. A large number of laboratory procedures are used to detect the presence of liver disease. Some of these measure functions of the liver, some measure activities which the liver shares with other organs and systems, and many measure biochemical changes which are associated with hepatic injury but have nothing to do with the known functions of the liver. Collectively, these studies are called liver function tests.

Bilirubin metabolism. SERUM BILIRUBIN. The liver conjugates and excretes bilirubin carried to it in the unconjugated form by the blood. Conjugated bilirubin is water-soluble and gives the prompt, direct red diazo reaction of van den Bergh. Unconjugated bilirubin is largely water insoluble and must be pretreated chemically to give the van den Bergh reaction. The total concentration of bilirubin in normal serum is less than 1.2 mg. per 100 ml. and almost all of it is in the unconjugated form. A rise in unconjugated bilirubin in the blood occurs when there is an increased breakdown of hemoglobin and in certain liver disorders in which there is a deficiency of the enzymes involved in bilirubin conjugation. Jaundice due mainly to an increase in conjugated bilirubin in the blood is found in intra- and extrahepatic bile duct obstruction, in hepatocellular damage, and in certain rare diseases in which the transport of bilirubin after conjugation is disturbed.

URINE BILIRUBIN. Normally, bilirubin is not present in the urine because the kidney is capable of excreting only the conjugated form of the pigment. Bilirubin appears in the urine in diseases in which there is an elevated level of conjugated bilirubin in the blood.

URINE UROBILINOGEN. The bilirubin excreted into the intestines is transformed into urobilinogen by intestinal bacteria. A substantial amount of the urobilinogen is reabsorbed, and a small portion of that which is reabsorbed is excreted in the urine (0.2 to 0.3 mg. per day). Absence of urobilinogen in the urine occurs in obstruction to bile flow and when the intestines are sterilized with antibiotics. Increased urine urobilinogen is found in hepatocellular disease and in conditions which produce an increase in hemoglobin breakdown.

FECAL UROBILINOGEN. Normally, fecal urobilinogen excretion ranges from 40 to 280 mg. per day. The excretion rate decreases markedly in biliary obstruction and increases in association with increased bilirubin production. Excretion rates in hepatocellular disease are variable.

Serum enzymes. ALKALINE PHOSPHATASE. This enzyme hydrolyzes phosphate esters in an alkaline medium. It occurs in a number of tissues, including bone, liver, kidney, intestine and placenta. It is excreted from the body in bile. Elevations of serum alkaline phosphatase levels are most striking in conditions which produce bile duct obstruction, but substantial increases occur also in association with liver neoplasms, liver abscesses, bile duct inflammation and diffuse liver damage. For many years, elevation of alkaline phosphatase was attributed solely to mechanical obstruction of the excretory pathway. Recent evidence, however, suggests that overproduction of the enzyme by the liver occurs in response to a variety of stimuli, in the absence of impairment of bile flow.

GLUTAMIC OXALOACETIC TRANSAMINASE (SGOT). This enzyme facilitates the transfer of an amino group from glutamic acid to oxaloacetic acid. It is found in skeletal muscle, kidney, brain, and pancreas but the highest levels occur in liver and heart. Normal serum contains 60 units or less. Elevations of glutamic oxaloacetic transaminase occur following injuries to various tissues, and are found in a variety of hepatic disorders. Marked elevations in excess of 300 units suggest the presence of acute hepatic inflammation or necrosis.

GLUTAMIC PYRUVIC TRANSAMINASE (SGPT). This enzyme promotes the transfer of an amino group from glutamic acid to pyruvic acid. Its concentration in liver greatly exceeds that in other tissues or organs. Normal serum contains 45 units or less. Although it has been suggested that a rise in glutamic pyruvic transaminase is a more specific indicator of liver damage than an elevation of glutamic oxaloacetic transaminase, both enzymes increase in various liver diseases.

CHOLINESTERASE, LEUCINE AMINOPEPTIDASE (LAP), LACTIC DEHYDROGENASE (LDH), ISOCITRIC DEHYDROGENASE (ICD). Abnormal serum levels of these enzymes, and a number of others, have been observed in various hepatic disorders as well as in diseases of other organs. Their determination adds little to the diagnosis of liver disease.

Blood coagulation factors. The liver is the primary site for synthesis of most of the proteins involved in blood coagulation. Methods have been devised for measuring individual factors, such as fibrinogen, factor V, factor VII and prothrombin but they are seldom used. Rather, a composite test is employed which depends on the presence of all the factors in the prothrombin complex and is a sensitive measure of liver disease. This test is called the prothrombin time, and the one-stage clotting method of Quick is most commonly used. Normally, the prothrombin time is at least 80 per cent of the time obtained with control plasma. The prothrombin time is prolonged or, in other terms, the percentage of normal is decreased, in hepatocellular disease due to depressed protein synthesis, and in obstructive jaundice due to impaired absorption of vitamin K which is required for synthesis of the prothrombin complex. Normalization of the prothrombin time following parenteral administration of vitamin K occurs in biliary obstruction and is an important method of distinguishing between hepatocellular and biliary disease.

Dye excretion. BROMSULPHALEIN EXCRETION (BSP). Bromsulphalein is a synthetic dye which is removed from the blood mainly by the liver. Following intravenous injection, the dye is carried to the liver bound to albumin, is taken up by the hepatic cells, is conjugated mainly with glutathione, and is excreted in the bile in both the free and conjugated forms. The dye is not reabsorbed from the intestines. In normal subjects, less than 5 per cent of the injected dose, (5 mg. per kg. body weight), is present in the blood 45 minutes after administration. The Bromsulphalein test is an excellent measure of hepatic functional reserve and retention of the dye is found consistently in patients with significant liver damage. The test is difficult to interpret in the presence of a serum elevation of conjugated bilirubin greater than 5 mg. per 100 ml. because the dye competes with conjugated bilirubin for the excretion pathway, and in obstruction of the bile ducts because the dye is removed from the liver via the biliary system. In shock, Bromsulphalein may be retained because of impaired hepatic blood flow.

INDOCYANINE GREEN EXCRETION (ICG). Indocyanine green is a synthetic dye which is removed from the blood almost exclusively by the liver. It is excreted in the bile in an unconjugated form. Retention of the dye occurs in the presence of hepatocellular disease. Experience with this test is limited, but results thus far suggest that it is a good test of hepatic function.

I[131] ROSE BENGAL EXCRETION. Rose bengal is a synthetic phthalein dye which is removed from the blood almost entirely by the liver parenchymal cells and excreted in the bile. The dye can be labeled with I[131], and by positioning detectors over the head, liver and abdomen its disappearance from the blood, its hepatic uptake and its excretion into the intestines can be determined. It has been suggested that the radioactive rose bengal test makes possible a differentiation between hepatocellular and obstructive jaundice, but the results have not been consistent. Rose bengal and Bromsulphalein are retained under similar circumstances.

Protein metabolism. SERUM ALBUMIN.

The liver is the sole source of serum albumin. In normal subjects, the serum albumin concentration exceeds 4.0 gm. per 100 ml. Serum albumin levels decline in hepatocellular damage and, particularly, when albumin is lost into the peritoneal cavity in ascites. Normal levels are not infrequently found in advanced liver disease, so that measurements of serum albumin do not serve as a sensitive test of liver function.

SERUM GLOBULINS. Hyperglobulinemia occurs in acute and chronic liver disease, as well as in a number of nonhepatic illnesses. The elevations are due mainly to augmented gamma globulin production, although increases in alpha and beta globulins are sometimes found. Because gamma globulin is produced by the hepatic and extrahepatic reticuloendothelial system, it is not certain that the liver is completely responsible for the rise in gamma globulin. Changes in various serum protein fractions are detected by serum electrophoresis.

TURBIDITY AND FLOCCULATION TESTS. There are a number of tests which do not measure liver function, but reflect qualitative and quantitative changes in serum proteins and are frequently positive in the presence of hepatocellular damage. The most frequently used studies in this category are the cephalin-cholesterol flocculation, the thymol turbidity and the zinc sulfate turbidity. Flocculation of a cephalin-cholesterol suspension occurs upon the addition of serum containing decreased or altered albumin, increased or altered gamma globulin, altered alpha and beta globulins, or reduced alpha lipoproteins. Turbidity of a thymol-barbital buffer solution occurs upon exposure to serum containing increased gamma globulin, increased beta globulin, an increase of certain lipoproteins, or decreased or altered albumin. Turbidity of a zinc sulfate solution develops upon addition of serum containing an increase in gamma globulin. In all these tests, the degree of turbidity or flocculation is quantitated in terms of arbitrary units. None of the tests are abnormal in uncomplicated obstructive jaundice in the absence of liver injury. Unfortunately, the tests are often negative in the presence of advanced chronic hepatic disease, and are sometimes positive in disorders unrelated to the liver.

Carbohydrate metabolism. Although the liver plays a central role in carbohydrate metabolism, tests of this hepatic function are of limited value. The standard glucose tolerance test often produces a diabetic curve and gly-cosuria in patients with severe hepatocellular damage. The intravenous galactose tolerance test measures the specific capacity of the liver to convert galactose to glucose. Impaired clearance of galactose from the blood and its appearance in increased quantities in the urine indicate liver dysfunction.

Lipid metabolism. The liver is the major site of cholesterol synthesis and esterifica-tion, and the bile is the primary avenue of cholesterol elimination from the body. Serum cholesterol levels decrease as does the esteri-fied fraction in severe liver damage. Intra- or extrahepatic biliary obstruction, in the ab-sence of severe hepatocellular injury, causes an increase in serum cholesterol. Cholesterol and cholesterol ester determinations are of limited value in the diagnosis of liver disease.

Ammonia metabolism. Ammonia is formed from nitrogenous substances in the intestines by the action of bacteria. Ammonia absorbed into portal blood is largely converted to urea by a highly efficient enzyme system in the liver. In the presence of severe hepatic damage or portal-systemic venous connec-tions, ammonia levels in peripheral arterial blood may rise above the normal concentra-tion of less than 100 micrograms per 100 ml. Although theoretically attractive, determina-tions of blood ammonia show no consistent correlation with the type or extent of hepatic damage and are of limited diagnostic value.

Liver biopsy. Biopsy of the liver is valu-able in the diagnosis of liver disease as well as in the assessment of therapy. It is not a routine procedure, but is indicated in a variety of situations when there is doubt about the diagnosis or uncertainty about the activity of a pathologic process. If necessary, biopsy can be performed under direct vision through an abdominal incision. Usually, however, a per-cutaneous liver biopsy is possible using a cutting or aspirating needle which is inserted through the right eighth or ninth intercostal space between the anterior axillary and mid-axillary lines. When the liver is large, a sub-costal approach may be used. Serious compli-cations of the procedure are infrequent and consist mainly of bleeding and bile peritonitis. In patients with a prothrombin time less than 50 per cent, platelet count below 100,000, or with obstructive jaundice, the risk of needle biopsy is increased. Liver biopsy provides accurate information in patients with diffuse hepatic disease. Focal lesions in the liver may be missed.

Roentgenographic studies. **Barium con-trast upper gastrointestinal series.** In our experience, the upper gastrointestinal series is the simplest and most accurate method of making the diagnosis of esophageal varices (Fig. 7). In a large series, this procedure provided accurate information in over 90 per cent of the patients. Barium contrast x-rays of the esophagus, stomach and duodenum have proved particularly helpful in the differ-ential diagnosis of upper gastrointestinal hemorrhage because they demonstrate the presence or absence of lesions other than varices which may be responsible for bleed-ing, such as duodenal and gastric ulcers.

Portal venography. Visualization of the portal venous system by the injection of con-trast media is most valuable in the diagnosis and evaluation of portal hypertension and occasionally may be helpful in the diagnosis of space-occupying lesions within the liver. Portal venography provides important infor-mation about the site of venous obstruction, the type and extent of portal-systemic col-laterals, the size of the major components of the portal system and, with appropriate timing, the rate of portal venous blood flow. Several methods are available for demon-strating the portal vasculature. The most frequently used technique is that of percu-taneous splenoportography which involves injection of a radiopaque dye into the spleen through a needle inserted through the left ninth or tenth intercostal space between the mid- and posterior axillary lines (Fig. 8).

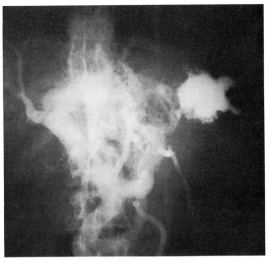

Figure 7.   Barium contrast upper gastrointestinal x-rays showing large esophageal varices.

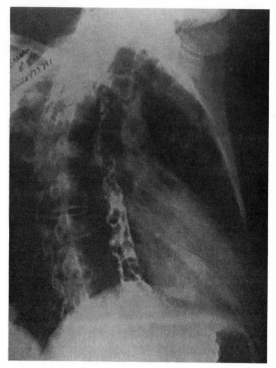

Figure 8. Splenoportogram in a patient with cirrhosis showing enlarged coronary vein connecting with gastro-esophageal varices.

Bleeding from laceration of the spleen is an occasional serious complication of this procedure. Another technique is that of operative portal venography in which a tributary of the portal vein is catheterized under direct vision at laparotomy. Catheterization of the umbilical vein through a small incision in the abdominal wall permits transumbilical portal venography, a technique which is useful in splenectomized patients. Direct percutaneous needle puncture of the portal vein has been used to perform transhepatic portal venography. Finally, splenic arteriography performed by catheterization of the splenic artery via the femoral artery permits visualization of the portal venous system by appropriately timed x-rays. None of these techniques are routine procedures which are required in all patients. All of them are associated with risks which must be weighed against the information to be obtained.

Hepatic arteriography. Percutaneous catheterization of the hepatic artery via the femoral or brachial artery has made possible the visualization of the arterial tree of the liver. This technique may be of value in the diagnosis of space-occupying lesions within the liver.

Cholecystography and cholangiography. These valuable diagnostic techniques are important in the diagnosis of diseases of the biliary system, and may be of help in the differential diagnosis of jaundice.

PORTAL PRESSURE MEASUREMENTS. Measurements of portal venous pressure are helpful in the diagnosis of portal hypertension and in the selection of appropriate surgical therapy. Direct pressure measurements are always made at operations for portal hypertension before a portacaval shunt is undertaken, and include determinations of the inferior vena cava pressure, the pressure in the unoccluded portal vein, and the portal pressure on the hepatic side of a clamp temporarily occluding the portal vein. The later measurement is helpful in determining the severity of hepatic outflow obstruction and in detecting reversal of portal flow.

Nonoperative measurement of portal pressure may be made by percutaneous splenic puncture according to the technique described for splenoportography. This procedure may be performed at the bedside. The splenic pulp pressure is similar to the portal pressure. Another nonoperative method of measuring portal pressure involves umbilical vein catheterization. Finally, catheterization of the hepatic veins via an arm vein permits measurement of the occluded hepatic vein pressure, which approximates portal pressure under most circumstances. In portal hypertension due to an extrahepatic block, the occluded hepatic vein pressure is normal.

ESOPHAGOSCOPY. Many surgeons are of the opinion that esophagoscopy is the best means of determining the presence of esophageal varices and of demonstrating varix hemorrhage. In the face of massive bleeding, endoscopy may be difficult and occasionally hazardous.

RADIOISOTOPE STUDIES. **Hepatic blood flow.** Estimation of hepatic blood flow may be helpful in the assessment of portal hypertension and in the selection of appropriate therapy. Indirect methods for measuring liver blood flow involve the infusion of a tracer substance which is removed mainly, and preferably completely, by the liver. Bromsulphalein was the first tracer used for this purpose and the technique consisted of simultaneous measurements of concentrations in arterial and hepatic venous blood during a continuous intravenous infusion of the dye. Subsequently, simple methods have been developed for measuring the blood disap-

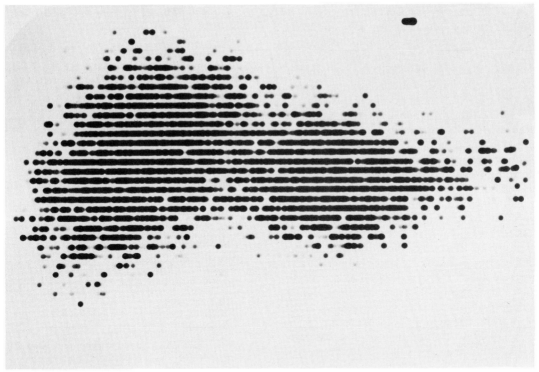

Figure 9. Scintillation scan of normal liver following administration of colloidal human serum albumin I^{131}.

pearance rate of a radioactive tracer which is removed mainly by the liver. Radioactive colloidal chromic phosphate (P^{32}), colloidal gold (Au^{198}), and colloidal human serum albumin (I^{131}) are used for this purpose.

Liver scanning. Scintillation scanning following the administration of a radioisotope which selectively localizes in the liver is helpful in determining liver size and shape and in detecting lesions which occupy space within the hepatic parenchyma or compress the liver from without. Isotopically labeled colloidal gold (Au^{198}), colloidal human serum albumin (I^{131}), rose bengal (I^{131}), ammonium molybdate (Mo^{99}), and pertechnetate (Tc^{99m}) are employed. Figure 9 shows a typical liver scan.

BALLOON TAMPONADE CONTROL OF BLEEDING. Control of upper gastrointestinal hemorrhage by esophageal or gastric balloon tamponade has been interpreted as evidence that the bleeding is coming from esophageal varices. This diagnostic procedure has been accurate in approximately 75 per cent of patients.

HEMATALOGIC STUDIES. Hematologic abnormalities are common in chronic liver disease. Gastrointestinal bleeding, of course, is a major complication of cirrhosis. In addition, chronic anemia is frequently found as a result of a decreased red blood cell survival time and poor nutrition. Hypersplenism, with a depression of any or all of the formed elements of the blood is often associated with portal hypertension. Appropriate hematologic studies, including the usual complete blood count, platelet count, determinations of red cell indices, measurements of serum iron, and determinations of red blood cell survival time and splenic trapping of red cells may be important components of the diagnostic workup.

JAUNDICE

Jaundice or icterus is a yellow discoloration of the tissues that results from staining with bilirubin. It is best observed in sites containing elastic tissue such as the sclerae and skin of the face and neck. Jaundice appears when the conjugated bilirubin concentration in the serum reaches 2 to 3 mg. per 100 ml., or the unconjugated bilirubin level is 3 to 4 mg. per 100 ml. Jaundice occurs in a substantial number of diseases and determination of the precise cause can be one of the more difficult problems in clinical medicine.

There is no satisfactory classification of jaundice which accounts for all conditions. The classic separation of jaundice into hemolytic, hepatocellular, and obstructive types is useful but does not explain all the pathophysiologic mechanisms which recent studies have clarified. Classification on the basis of the type of bilirubin, conjugated or unconjugated, which predominates in the blood is of limited clinical validity because of the frequent occurrence of mixed forms of hyperbilirubinemia. An understanding of bilirubin metabolism and of the stages at which it may be disturbed by disease provides the soundest approach to the differential diagnosis of icterus.

The metabolism and excretion of bilirubin involve the formation of free bilirubin from the breakdown of hemoglobin in the reticuloendothelial system; transport of the unconjugated bilirubin to the liver; conjugation of the bilirubin by the hepatic cell; excretion of the conjugated bilirubin in the bile, and excretion of the bile along the biliary ducts into the intestines, where conjugated bilirubin is converted to urobilinogen. A classification of jaundice according to the stage at which bilirubin metabolism is disturbed is presented in Table 2.

Increased production of bilirubin from hemolysis of red blood cells, impaired transport of bilirubin to the liver, and impaired conjugation of bilirubin by the liver cell result in icterus due to unconjugated hyperbilirubinemia. The term "retention jaundice" has been used to describe this type, and it is not accompanied by impairment of bile flow. The jaundice in most of these disorders is mild, there is no bile in the urine, urine urobilinogen is not increased, and the liver function tests are usually normal.

Impaired transport and excretion of conjugated bilirubin by the hepatic cell produces jaundice with a substantial amount of conjugated bilirubin in the blood. The term "regurgitation jaundice" has been applied to this type. Most of the common liver diseases fall into this category. Because the damaged hepatic cells are unable to conjugate all the bilirubin resulting from normal hemoglobin breakdown, an increase in unconjugated bilirubin develops along with the regurgitated conjugated pigment in the blood. Bile appears in the urine, urine urobilinogen levels rise, and liver function tests are usually abnormal. One group of disorders which produce impaired cellular excretion of conjugated bili-

Table 2. *Classification of Jaundice*

I. *Excessive bilirubin production due to hemolysis ("hemolytic jaundice")*
   A. Inherited hemolytic anemias
   B. Acquired hemolytic disorders
      1. Hemolytic anemias
      2. Sepsis
      3. Hemolysins (snake venom, mushrooms)
      4. Absorption of sequestered blood (hematomas, hemothorax, hemoperitoneum, infarcts)
      5. Burns
      6. Mismatched blood transfusions
      7. Massive blood transfusions
II. *Impaired transport of bilirubin to liver* (Some types of Gilbert's syndrome)
III. *Impaired hepatic conjugation of bilirubin*
   A. Inborn errors
      1. Crigler-Najjar syndrome
      2. Some types of Gilbert's syndrome
   B. Immaturity of enzyme systems
      1. Physiologic jaundice of newborn
      2. Jaundice of prematurity
IV. *Impaired hepatic transport and excretion of bilirubin after conjugation ("hepatocellular jaundice")*
   A. Acquired liver diseases (e.g., hepatitis, cirrhosis, neoplasms)
   B. Dubin-Johnson syndrome and Rotor syndrome
   C. Intrahepatic cholestasis (drug-induced, disease-related, and idiopathic)
V. *Mechanical bile duct obstruction ("obstructive jaundice")*
   A. Extrahepatic (stone, neoplasm, stricture, atresia, etc.)
   B. Intrahepatic

rubin does not conform to the usual pattern of liver disease and presents problems in the differential diagnosis of obstructive jaundice. The term intrahepatic cholestasis has been used to describe these conditions. They are characterized by a clinical and biochemical picture similar to that of bile duct obstruction, normal or mildly abnormal liver function tests, and a histologic picture of bile stasis without mechanical obstruction. A number of drugs, including phenothiazine compounds, certain diuretics, testosterone derivatives, and arsenicals are known to injure the cellular excretion mechanism and cause intrahepatic cholestasis. A similar picture has been observed during pregnancy and, as a transient phenomenon, during viral hepatitis. In some instances, no etiologic agent can be identified.

Mechanical bile duct obstruction results in conjugated hyperbilirubinemia, along with an increase in unconjugated pigment in the blood. The mechanism is similar to that which occurs in primary liver disease, and the jaundice is of the regurgitation type. Bile appears in the urine but, if the obstruction is complete, urobilinogen is absent from the urine and stool and the stools are light or clay colored.

The serum alkaline phosphatase levels are significantly elevated, but the other liver function tests are usually normal early in the course of obstruction. However, repeated or longstanding obstruction or infection results in substantial liver damage and makes it difficult to distinguish the symptoms from those of primary hepatic disease. Prolonged absence of bile from the intestine impairs the absorption of fat-soluble vitamin K and produces a decrease in prothrombin activity which can be corrected by parenteral administration of the vitamin. The prothrombin response to vitamin K is helpful in differentiating liver disease from biliary obstruction.

The first steps in the diagnostic approach to the patient with jaundice, after a thorough history and physical examination are performed, involve determinations of the levels of direct reacting and indirect reacting bilirubin in the blood, and the amounts of bile and urobilinogen in the urine. Hyperbilirubinemia which is mainly of the unconjugated type, combined with the absence of bile in the urine, indicates that the icterus is the retention type. In an adult patient, the odds are overwhelming that the cause is hemolysis of red blood cells. The liver function tests under these circumstances will be normal and appropriate hematologic studies and other tests should be performed to identify the underlying disease.

If a substantial portion of the bilirubin in the blood is the direct reacting variety, as is commonly the case, and there is bile in the urine, the jaundice is the regurgitation type and the problem is usually one of distinguishing between liver disease and bile duct obstruction. Liver function tests, stool color examination, and urine urobilinogen measurements should be performed. Normal liver function tests except for a depressed prothrombin activity and an elevated serum alkaline phosphatase, light or clay colored stools, absence of urobilinogen in the urine, a good prothrombin response to parenteral vitamin K, and a history and physical examination which are compatible indicate clearly that the jaundice is due to biliary obstruction which requires surgical relief. On the other hand, abnormal liver function tests, a normal colored stool, increased urobilinogen in the urine, a negative or incomplete prothrombin response to parenteral vitamin K, an enlarged liver, and the absence of symptoms of biliary tract disease such as abdominal colic and fatty food intolerance indicate that the jaundice is a result of hepatocellular damage and should be treated by nonsurgical measures. Needless to say, the history and physical findings are of great importance in arriving at the correct diagnosis.

In a number of patients, a diagnosis will not be possible on the basis of the initial workup. Additional studies, repeated tests, and a period of observation will be required to determine the etiology of the jaundice. In some patients liver scan, upper gastrointestinal x-rays, cholangiography, and duodenal drainage must be performed. Occasionally, laparotomy must be done for diagnostic as well as therapeutic purposes.

PORTAL HYPERTENSION

Portal hypertension is a manifestation of various diseases of the liver and its circulation. It is the complication of hepatic disease which most frequently requires surgical treatment. Although the portal pressure in normal subjects varies considerably with activity, at rest it ranges from about 40 to 180 mm. saline (3 to 13 mm. Hg). In terms of pressure measurements, portal hypertension may be defined as a portal vein pressure of 250 mm. saline (18 mm. Hg) or greater in the presence of a normal pressure in the inferior vena cava. More important, portal hypertension may be defined in terms of the pathologic disturbances that it produces which compromise health and threaten life. Some of these disorders, such as bleeding esophageal varices and hypersplenism, are a direct reflection of the high pressure in the portal circulation and its collateral communications. Others, such as ascites, hepatic coma, and peptic ulcers, are complicated manifestations of a number of factors including the portal hypertension, the underlying liver disease, and the required treatment.

ETIOLOGY. Table 3 lists the causes of portal hypertension. From both clinical and pathologic standpoints these may be divided into diseases within the liver and diseases of the blood vessels outside of the liver. With the exception of the rare arteriovenous fistulae, all the conditions cause portal hypertension by producing obstruction to portal blood flow.

Intrahepatic obstructive diseases account for over 90 per cent of the patients with portal hypertension. Of these, portal cirrhosis associated with chronic alcoholism is by far the most common etiology in the United States.

Table 3. *Etiology of Portal Hypertension*

I. *Intrahepatic obstructive disease*
   A. Portal cirrhosis (alcoholic, nutritional, Laennec's)
   B. Postnecrotic cirrhosis (posthepatitic)
   C. Biliary cirrhosis
   D. Uncommon forms of cirrhosis and fibrosis (hemochromatosis, Wilson's disease)
   E. Neoplasms and granulomas
   F. Schistosomiasis
II. *Extrahepatic disease*
   A. Portal vein obstruction
      1. Congenital atresia or stenosis
      2. Thrombosis due to infection or trauma
      3. Cavernomatous transformation
      4. Extrinsic compression
   B. Hepatic vein (outflow) obstruction
      1. Budd-Chiari syndrome
      2. Constrictive pericarditis
   C. Excessive portal blood flow
      1. Arteriovenous fistula between hepatic artery and portal vein
      2. Arteriovenous fistula between splenic artery and vein

Postnecrotic cirrhosis due to viral hepatitis is a fairly common cause of portal hypertension, whereas the incidence of biliary cirrhosis due to extrahepatic bile duct obstruction or primary intrahepatic disease is low. The other forms of intrahepatic obstruction are uncommon. Because cirrhosis is largely a disease of adulthood and, particularly in alcoholic cirrhosis, develops slowly over many years, patients with portal hypertension of the intrahepatic type are most often in the fifth or sixth decades of life. Moreover, they are usually in poor health because of the underlying liver disease, and the risk of operative treatment is significant.

Extrahepatic obstruction of the portal vein is most often due to thrombosis. Neonatal omphalitis is a relatively frequent cause but often the etiology of the thrombosis cannot be determined. Cavernomatous transformation is most likely the end result of thrombosis and recanalization of the portal vein. Congenital atresia of the portal vein and extrinsic compression are rare causes of portal hypertension. Extrahepatic portal hypertension usually develops in childhood or early adult life. Furthermore, the patients do not have liver damage, are otherwise in good health, and usually tolerate both the complications of their circulatory disorder and the required surgical therapy quite well.

Extrahepatic obstruction of the hepatic venous outflow system occurs in a group of rare conditions called the Budd-Chiari syndrome. The obstruction is usually due to inflammatory or neoplastic thrombosis of the hepatic veins and, sometimes, of the adjacent inferior vena cava. The etiology of the process is often obscure, although some are associated with polycythemia vera and with neoplasms. Marked hepatomegaly and massive ascites are the most striking clinical findings. The condition has been relieved by performance of a side-to-side portacaval shunt.

PORTAL HYPERTENSION DUE TO CIRRHOSIS

PATHOPHYSIOLOGY. The widespread destruction of the hepatic parenchyma in cirrhosis leads to overgrowth of fibrous tissue and the formation of regenerative nodules in a pathologic rearrangement of liver architecture. As a result, the hepatic blood vessels are compressed and distorted. The branches of the hepatic vein, because of their low pressure and thin protective coat of connective tissue, are affected more than the other components of the vasculature and hepatic venous outflow obstruction develops. This postsinusoidal obstruction is the fundamental hemodynamic lesion in the common forms of cirrhosis. Outflow obstruction leads to an increase in sinusoidal pressure which, in turn, is reflected in an elevation of portal pressure and a decrease in portal blood flow to the liver. In extreme stages of postsinusoidal obstruction, the valveless portal vein may become an outflow tract and conduct blood in a retrograde manner away from the liver. An additional consequence of the disruption of hepatic integrity is the development of communications between the intrahepatic branches of the hepatic artery and portal vein, and between the tributaries of the portal vein and hepatic vein. The arteriovenous shunts contribute to the portal hypertension. Moreover, both types of shunts divert blood away from the hepatic parenchyma and compromise the nutrition of the liver cells. In an unsuccessful attempt to compensate for the reduction in portal flow to the liver, hepatic artery flow increases and the liver becomes dependent upon the hepatic artery for a major portion of its blood supply.

The elevated pressure in the portal vein leads to an enlargement of all the collateral venous connections between the portal and systemic circulations, and development of varicosities. In addition, splenomegaly develops. Blood flow through the collaterals is away from the liver, which further impairs hepatic nutrition. Despite their large size, the portal-systemic anastomoses are insufficient to accommodate the volume flow of

Table 4. *Natural History of Cirrhosis*

AUTHORS	CASES	COMPLICATION	SURVIVAL IN %		
			1 YEAR	2 YEARS	5 YEARS
Ratnoff and Patek (Five New York Hospitals, 1916–1938)	296	Ascites	32	17	7
	245	Jaundice	26	23	5
	106	Hematemesis	28	25	20
Boston Inter-Hospital Liver Group (Seven Boston Hospitals, 1959–1961)	467	Varices	34	21	5½
	288	Varices without bleeding	43	25	8
	179	Varices with bleeding	21	14	1½

portal blood and to overcome portal hypertension. Most prominent among the collaterals are those in the submucosa of the lower esophagus and upper stomach, and those around the umbilicus and anterior abdominal wall. Rupture of the esophageal varices often causes massive hemorrhage and is associated with a high mortality rate.

NATURAL HISTORY OF CIRRHOSIS. Cirrhosis of the liver is a common and highly lethal disease. Table 4 shows the survival rates of patients admitted to general hospitals because of cirrhosis. In the classic study of Ratnoff and Patek, who examined in retrospect the histories of 386 patients admitted to five New York hospitals between 1916 and 1938, only one-third of the patients with ascites were alive after one year and little over a handful survived for five years. Survival rates for patients with jaundice and hematemesis were similar. In the current prospective study of the Boston Inter-Hospital Liver Group, 79 per cent of the patients who bled from esophageal varices were dead within one year of bleeding, and in the entire group of 467 patients, with and without bleeding, only 26 lived for five years. The results of these studies indicate that once a patient entered the hospital for treatment of cirrhosis, his chances of living for one year were similar to those of a patient with acute lym-

phocytic leukemia, and his chances of surviving five years were about the same as those observed in most untreated cancers.

The causes of death in patients with cirrhosis and varices were tabulated by the Boston Group (Table 5). Hemorrhage was responsible for one-third of the deaths, hepatic failure accounted for one-third, renal shutdown for 11 per cent, infection for 9 per cent and miscellaneous causes for the remainder. These figures, which are similar to those obtained in other studies, clearly show that varix bleeding is a major cause of death in cirrhosis. This complication in particular has occupied the attention of surgeons and serves as the major indication for surgical therapy.

BLEEDING ESOPHAGEAL VARICES. The most frequent cause of death from upper gastrointestinal bleeding is rupture of an esophageal varix. Until recently, approximately three out of four cirrhotic patients who entered the hospital with their first episode of bleeding varices failed to leave the hospital alive. Table 6, which shows the results of a number of studies conducted during the past 40 years, indicates that as of 1962 the immediate mortality rate of the first variceal hemorrhage averaged 73 per cent. From these statistics, it is apparent that the emergency treatment of bleeding esophageal varices is the single most important aspect of the therapy of portal hypertension.

The precipitating cause of rupture of esophageal varices is uncertain. It has been proposed that erosion of the mucosa by reflux acid-peptic esophagitis is involved. However, in a gross and microscopic study of the distal esophagus in 20 patients at the time of bleeding, esophagitis was found in only one patient. The evidence strongly suggests that increased hydrostatic pressure is responsible for varix rupture.

DIAGNOSIS. In most patients who enter

Table 5. *Causes of Death in 235 Patients with Cirrhosis and Varices (Boston Inter-Hospital Liver Group, 1959–1961)*

	% OF DEATHS
Hemorrhage	34
Hepatic failure	32
Renal shutdown	11
Infection	9
Indeterminate and other	14

Table 6. *Mortality of First Variceal Hemorrhage in Cirrhosis*

AUTHORS	YEAR REPORTED	TYPE OF HOSPITAL	NUMBER OF PATIENTS	MORTALITY %
Ratnoff and Patek	1942	Five private-teaching	106	40
Higgins	1947	City indigent	45	76
Atik and Simeone	1954	City indigent	59	83
Nachlas, O'Neil and Campbell	1955	City indigent	102	59
Cohn and Blaisdell	1958	City indigent	456	74
Taylor and Jontz	1959	Veterans	102	45
Merigan, Hollister, Gryska, Starkey and Davidson	1960	City indigent	74	76
Orloff	1962	City indigent	87	84
			Total 1031	Mean 73

the hospital with upper gastrointestinal hemorrhage, the diagnosis of bleeding esophageal varices depends on affirmative answers to three questions. Does the patient have cirrhosis? Does the patient have portal hypertension and esophageal varices? Are the varices the site of the bleeding, rather than some other lesion such as a duodenal or gastric ulcer, gastritis or hiatus hernia? Information sufficient to answer these questions usually can be obtained within a few hours of the patient's admission to the hospital by means of an organized diagnostic plan which includes some, and if necessary all, of the following steps:

History and physical examination. A history of chronic alcoholism, hepatitis, jaundice, previous bleeding episodes, melena, abdominal swelling, edema, and mental abnormalities, and the absence of symptoms of peptic ulcer suggest the diagnosis of cirrhosis. The most important physical findings are hepatosplenomegaly, spider angiomas, palmar erythema, collateral abdominal veins, muscle wasting, jaundice, ascites, edema and neurologic signs such as tremor and asterixis. In many patients, all these classic signs are not present.

Blood studies. Blood samples for typing and cross-matching and for studies are drawn immediately on admission. The initial studies include a complete blood count, liver function tests (Bromsulphalein excretion, prothrombin, bilirubin, alkaline phosphatase, albumin, globulin, thymol turbidity, cephalin flocculation, glutamic oxaloacetic transaminase, glutamic pyruvic transaminase, urea nitrogen, electrolytes, pH and blood gases). The liver function tests which are most consistently abnormal and of greatest value are the prothrombin, bilirubin, and Bromsulphalein

excretion, if performed in the absence of marked jaundice and after hypovolemic shock has been corrected.

Upper gastrointestinal x-rays. As soon as shock has been corrected and the patient's condition stabilized, a barium contrast upper gastrointestinal series is obtained. It is to be emphasized that roentgenographic studies are directed at determining the presence or absence not only of esophageal varices but also of other lesions such as a duodenal ulcer, gastric ulcer or hiatus hernia. X-ray studies can be performed safely in almost all patients and have accurately demonstrated esophageal varices at the time of bleeding in 95 per cent of patients.

The emergency diagnosis of bleeding esophageal varices can be made accurately from information obtained in these first steps in over 90 per cent of patients.

Splenic manometry. The splenic pulp pressure can be determined readily at the bedside by percutaneous puncture of the spleen under local anesthesia. Although this procedure does not determine the site of bleeding, it indicates the presence or absence of portal hypertension. Bleeding from esophageal varices infrequently occurs with a splenic pulp pressure below 300 mm. saline and rarely occurs with a pressure below 250 mm. Splenic manometry should be performed only when conventional roentgenography has failed to demonstrate varices, and in the majority of instances it provides confirmation that the patient was not bleeding from varices.

Esophagoscopy. If these measures have failed to provide the diagnosis, esophagoscopy is performed. Although many clinicians rely heavily on esophagoscopy, the results of this procedure are sometimes difficult to interpret in the face of massive bleeding. Esophagoscopy has been required in less than 10 per cent of our patients.

Balloon tamponade control of bleeding. Control of bleeding by esophageal balloon tamponade is presumptive evidence that an esophageal varix is the site of bleeding. This diagnostic test is accurate in approximately three-fourths of patients and may be attempted if the other diagnostic measures are not successful.

Splenoportography. Visualization of the portal venous system is not regularly required for emergency diagnosis of varix hemorrhage in patients with cirrhosis. However, in patients with normal liver function who are suspected of having extrahepatic portal obstruction, this procedure is diagnostic and invaluable. Recently, it has been suggested that splenoportography, by demonstrating the pattern of collateral circulation and the volume of blood perfusing the liver, may be of value in selecting patients with cirrhosis for portacaval shunt. Should further studies establish the validity of this suggestion, the time, effort and risk involved in performing splenoportography as a routine emergency procedure may prove to be worthwhile.

This diagnostic plan was applied to 89 consecutive adult patients in whom cirrhosis and varix hemorrhage were suspected on admission. Table 7 summarizes the results of this diagnostic approach. Upper gastrointestinal x-rays were obtained in all patients and correctly demonstrated the presence or absence of varices in 96 per cent. Roentgenography gave false negative results in 4 per cent of the patients. Splenic manometry was performed in 11 patients in whom x-rays failed to show varices; in two patients, portal hypertension was found and bleeding varices were

demonstrated subsequently at operation, whereas in nine patients the finding of a normal portal pressure corresponded to the absence of varices on x-ray. Esophagoscopy was performed in six patients in whom no varices were demonstrated by roentgenography; in two patients bleeding varices were observed and subsequently proved at operation, whereas in the other four patients the absence of varices was confirmed by endoscopy. In 97 per cent of the patients, the diagnostic workup was completed within six hours of admission to the hospital. Fifty-nine of the 89 patients were subjected to emergency operations with the preoperative diagnosis of cirrhosis and bleeding esophageal varices, and in each instance this diagnosis proved to be correct.

EMERGENCY TREATMENT. Cirrhosis of the liver is a severe, debilitating disease with remote manifestations, only one of which is bleeding from esophageal varices. Death after varix rupture is frequently due to hepatic decompensation, renal failure or infection, rather than to exsanguination. Although control of bleeding is of primary importance, the effectiveness of therapy of the underlying liver disease often determines the outcome. Therefore, there are certain general principles of treatment which apply to all patients, regardless of the specific therapeutic measures used to stop the hemorrhage.

Prompt restoration of the blood volume. Vigorous replacement of blood loss with whole blood transfusions is essential. Every effort is made to obtain fresh blood less than 12 hours old for administration because of the serious defects in coagulation associated with liver disease plus those superimposed by multiple transfusions.

Prevention of hepatic coma. Although the

Table 7. Diagnostic Findings in 89 Consecutive Cirrhotic Patients Suspected of Bleeding from Esophageal Varices*

FINAL DIAGNOSIS	NUMBER OF CASES	HISTORY COMPATIBLE WITH CIRRHOSIS	PHYSICAL EXAM COMPATIBLE WITH CIRRHOSIS	LIVER FUNCTION TESTS COMPATIBLE WITH CIRRHOSIS	VARICES ON UPPER GI X-RAY	OTHER LESION ON UPPER GI X-RAY	PORTAL HYPERTENSION ON SPLENIC MANOMETRY	VARICES ON ESOPHAGOSCOPY
Bleeding varices	74	74	74	74	70/74	4/74	2/2	2/2
Peptic ulcer	6	6	6	6	0/6	6/6	–	0/2
Gastritis	9	9	9	9	0/9	0/9	0/9	0/2

*From Orloff, M. J.: Current Problems in Surgery. Chicago, Year Book Medical Publishers, July, 1966.

nervous disorders associated with liver disease are diverse and poorly understood, the encephalopathy observed in patients with bleeding esophageal varices sometimes appears to be due to the absorption of large quantities of ammonia directly into the systemic circulation via portal-systemic collaterals. For this reason, measures directed at destroying ammonia-forming bacteria and eliminating all nitrogen from the gastrointestinal tract are initiated promptly. These include removal of blood from the stomach by lavage with iced saline, instillation of cathartics and neomycin into the stomach, and thorough and repeated cleansing of the colon with enemas containing neomycin. Although ammonia-binding agents, such as sodium glutamate and arginine, and ion-exchange resins have been used, we have obtained no evidence that agents of this sort have been of value.

Support of the failing liver. Parenterally administered hypertonic glucose solutions containing therapeutic doses of vitamins K, B and C are included in the initial treatment regimen. Appropriate amounts of electrolytes are added to the parenteral fluids to correct any acid-base abnormalities. Severe hypokalemia and metabolic alkalosis are not uncommon and require the administration of sizable quantities of potassium and an acidifying agent.

Frequent monitoring of vital functions. The usual techniques are used to determine the magnitude of bleeding and adequacy of blood volume replacement. These include measurements of vital signs, urine output by way of an indwelling catheter, central venous pressure via a polyethylene catheter threaded through an arm cutdown into the superior vena cava, hematocrit and rate of blood loss by continuous suction through a nasogastric tube.

Emergency measures used specifically to stop varix bleeding may be divided into medical and surgical procedures. Emergency medical therapy includes esophageal balloon tamponade, intravenous posterior pituitary extract and gastroesophageal hypothermia. Although each of these measures is capable of temporarily controlling bleeding esophageal varices, it has been our experience, as well as that reported by many other workers, that they have not significantly influenced the mortality rate of varix hemorrhage in cirrhotic patients.

The most widely used nonoperative method of treatment has been esophageal balloon tamponade (Fig. 10). Since its introduction in 1930 by Westphal, and its popularization in 1950 by Sengstaken and Blakemore, balloon tamponade has been adopted by almost every hospital in the country as standard treatment for bleeding esophageal varices. As shown in Table 8, there is no doubt that this popular mode of therapy has initially stopped varix bleeding in many patients. The disheartening aspect of this form of management has been that many of the patients have resumed bleeding when the balloons were deflated. Moreover, we and others have observed frequent and sometimes lethal complications of balloon tamponade, which include perforation of the esophagus, asphyxiation from regurgitation of the balloon into the pharynx, and aspiration pneumonia. Most important, data from a number of institutions clearly indicate that balloon tamponade has failed to influence measurably the mortality rate of bleeding esophageal varices during a trial of 15 years. For these reasons, we have abandoned the use of balloon tamponade as a definitive form of treatment and use it only on infrequent occasions as a temporary measure to prepare patients for operation when massive bleeding cannot be initially controlled by other means.

It has been shown in both experimental animals and man that posterior pituitary extract reduces portal pressure and blood flow by constricting the splanchnic arterioles. The response is directly related to the dose and rapidity of injection, and in the usual clinical dosage range has a duration of one hour or less. However, as shown in Table 9, the transient reduction of portal pressure has been sufficient to stop varix hemorrhage temporarily in a large percentage of patients. Unfortunately, most of the patients have re-bled unless operation was performed within eight hours of treatment, and subsequent administration of the drug has been much less effective in stopping bleeding. It is apparent, therefore, that posterior pituitary extract alone is not a definitive form of treatment but may be of considerable immediate value while other measures are being readied or the patient is being prepared for operation. Every patient with bleeding esophageal varices is given posterior pituitary extract soon after admission. The agent is administered intravenously over a 15 to 20 minute period in a dose of 20 units diluted in 200 ml. of solution. This measure of therapy has largely replaced esophageal balloon tamponade as a means of obtaining immediate control of hemorrhage.

Use of gastroesophageal hypothermia to

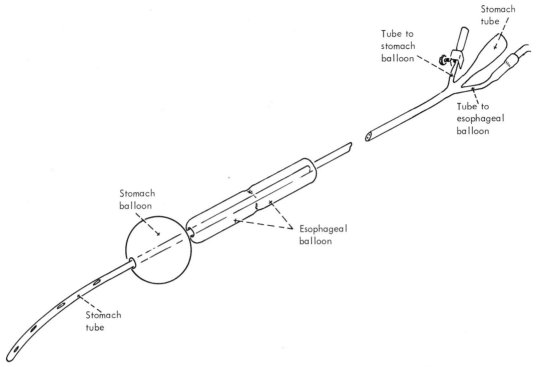

Figure 10. The Sengstaken-Blakemore triple lumen, double balloon tube used to tamponade esophageal varices. The gastric balloon is inflated first and pulled up against the cardia by continuous mild traction. The esophageal balloon directly compresses the varices in the lower esophagus. The third lumen is used for irrigation of the stomach and removal of blood and gastric contents.

Table 8. *Results of Esophageal Balloon Tamponade in Cirrhotic Patients with Bleeding Varices*

AUTHORS	YEAR REPORTED	NUMBER OF PATIENTS	INITIAL CONTROL %	ULTIMATE CONTROL %	MORTALITY %
Reynolds, Freedman, and Winsor	1952	32	66	50	47
Hamilton	1955	20	45	–	75
Ludington	1958	58	75	43	–
Conn	1958	50	70	–	82
Read, Dawson, Kerr, Turner and Sherlock	1960	38	84	24	74
Merigan, Hollister, Gryska, Starkey and Davidson	1960	68	–	–	80
Orloff	1962	45	56	20	82
	Total	311		Mean	74

Table 9. *Results of Intravenous Posterior Pituitary Extract in Cirrhotic Patients with Bleeding Varices*

AUTHORS	NUMBER OF PATIENTS	NUMBER OF TRIALS	INITIAL SUCCESS %	REBLED %	MORTALITY %
Schwartz, Bales, Emerson and Mahoney	11	27	89	Frequent	–
Merigan, Plotkin and Davidson	15	22	73	Frequent	93
Shaldon and Sherlock	8	> 25	100	63	75
Orloff	45	45	88	Immediate operation	–
	18	18	88	83	–

stop varix bleeding is based on the demonstration that lowering the temperature of the stomach to 10 to 14° C. abolishes the digestive activity of gastric juice and produces a significant reduction of blood flow in the stomach. Cooling is accomplished with balloons in the stomach and esophagus through which a cold alcohol-water solution is circulated. The rationale of gastroesophageal cooling in part hinges on the theory that rupture of esophageal varices is the result of reflux acid-peptic esophagitis. However, recently, considerable doubt has been cast on the acid-peptic hypothesis. Experience with gastroesophageal hypothermia has been small but preliminary reports indicate that this technique, although effective in temporarily stopping bleeding, has failed to lower the mortality rate of varix hemorrhage.

Because of the high mortality rate associated with medical treatment of bleeding esophageal varices and the failure to achieve improvement of results during two decades of intensive effort, there has been considerable recent interest in emergency operative management. Results obtained during the past seven years have been encouraging and suggest that immediate operation is the treatment of choice. Experience is insufficient as yet to establish definite criteria for selection of patients for operation; although it is clear that the risk of operation is great in patients with decompensated cirrhosis, it is also certain that such patients have little chance of surviving with nonoperative therapy. Currently, emergency operative treatment is largely confined to the use of two operations, transesophageal varix ligation and the emergency portacaval shunt. Both procedures stop varix bleeding in almost all patients, and the problem associated with them is mainly that of hepatic decompensation which results when a critically ill patient with a severely damaged liver is subjected to anesthesia and major trauma.

Several years ago we undertook a prospective study aimed at evaluating the effectiveness of medical treatment, transesophageal varix ligation and emergency portacaval shunt in the emergency therapy of bleeding varices. Every cirrhotic patient admitted to the hospital with varix bleeding was included in the study with no attempt at selection. The diagnosis was completed within six hours of admission to the hospital and, in the surgical groups, operation was performed within eight hours. The study was conducted in

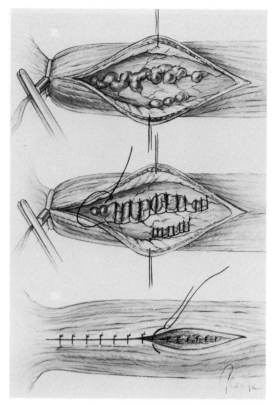

Figure 11. Technique of transesophageal varix ligation. (From Orloff, M. J.: Surgery 52:103, 1962.)

comparable groups of chronic alcoholics with moderate to advanced cirrhosis and massive varix hemorrhage. Approximately half the patients in each group had jaundice and ascites, and one-fourth had hepatic encephalopathy. A total of 82 patients were involved in the program and an additional 45 patients treated just prior to the start of the study were added to the comparison. The results are summarized in Table 10.

The early survival rates following transesophageal varix ligation and emergency portacaval shunt were similar (54 and 53 per cent) and were about three times greater than the survival rate resulting from medical treatment. Long-term survival was strikingly more frequent following operative treatment than after medical management. Of the two forms of surgical therapy, the emergency portacaval shunt resulted in a long-term survival rate (43 per cent) which was twice as high as that produced by varix ligation (21 per cent). Figure 12 shows the cumulative survival rates up to four years after therapy in the three treatment groups.

On the basis of our studies and those of

Table 10. *Comparison of Results of Emergency Portacaval Shunt, Transesophageal Varix Ligation, and Medical Treatment in Patients with Cirrhosis and Bleeding Varices*

	MEDICAL TREATMENT	VARIX LIGATION	EMERGENCY SHUNT
Number of patients	59	28	40
Jaundice	25 (42%)	16 (57%)	23 (58%)
Ascites	24 (41%)	14 (50%)	17 (43%)
Encephalopathy on admission	15 (25%)	7 (25%)	8 (20%)
Mean liver index	2.8	2.8	2.9
Admission hemoglobin 11 gm./100 ml. or less	41 (70%)	20 (71%)	28 (70%)
Varices demonstrated	56 (95%)	28 (100%)	40 (100%)
Volume of blood transfused (mean) – L.	7.2	4.2	4.2
Early survival (30 days and left hospital)	10 (17%)	15 (54%)	21 (53%)
Four-year survival	2 (3%)	6 (21%)	17 (43%) (predicted)

others, it appears that emergency operative management has significantly improved the survival of cirrhotic patients with varix hemorrhage. As with medical treatment, transesophageal varix ligation is not a definitive procedure for the prolonged control of varix bleeding and must be followed by an elective portacaval shunt. This disadvantage, plus the

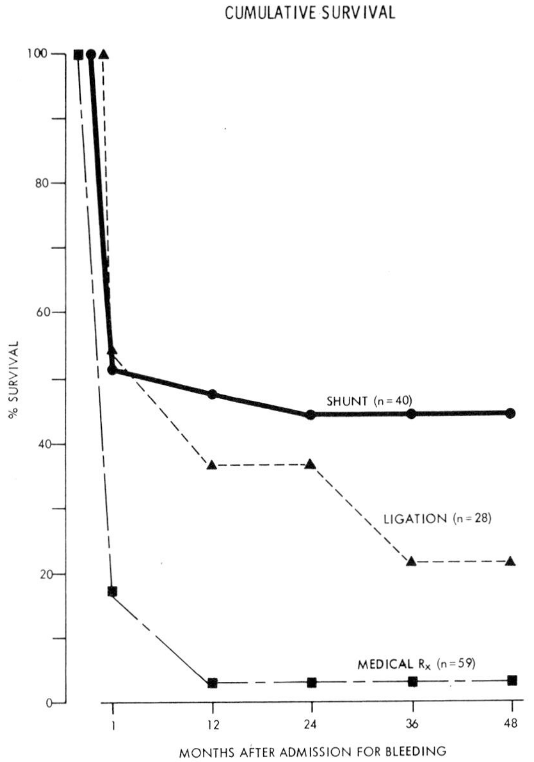

Figure 12. Cumulative survival rates of patients with cirrhosis and varix hemorrhage following emergency portacaval shunt, transesophageal varix ligation and medical treatment; calculated by the life table method. (From Orloff, M. J.: Ann. Surg. *166*:456, 1967.)

lower survival rate following varix ligation, has led to the conclusion that emergency portacaval shunt is the therapy of choice for most cirrhotic patients who bleed from esophageal varices.

ELECTIVE TREATMENT. There is general agreement that patients who have recovered from an episode of bleeding esophageal varices should receive elective surgical treatment directed at overcoming portal hypertension. Our studies of 27 patients who survived their first bleeding episode and qualified for surgical therapy but were not operated upon showed that 93 per cent bled again, 74 per cent died from the subsequent hemorrhage, and all were dead within five years. The portal-systemic shunt is the only definitive treatment for portal hypertension which is consistently effective. Abundant data indicate that the portacaval anastomosis will protect over 90 per cent of patients against subsequent varix bleeding. Therefore, one episode of varix hemorrhage is an indication for elective shunt therapy, provided there is reasonable likelihood that the patient will survive the operation.

The answer to what criteria can be used to predict the likelihood of a patient surviving the shunt procedure is still uncertain, because the criteria for selection of patients for operation have been undergoing progressive change as knowledge regarding the underlying liver disease and its management has accumulated. The decision concerning operation is based on a composite of many features of a patient's disease, determined during a period of intensive medical treatment in the hospital. Certain features are ominous; thus, the presence of substantial jaundice of ascites which cannot be stabilized, of repeated bouts of encephalopathy, of frank muscle wasting and of a poor appetite indicate that operation will carry a high risk and probably should not be undertaken. Studies of hepatic blood flow may prove to be of additional help in selecting patients for operation. If these general criteria have been followed, the operative mortality rate has been in the acceptable range of 10 per cent. It should be emphasized that, whenever possible, patients are prepared for an elective operation during a three- to six-week period in the hospital with a regimen directed at improving nutrition, slowly restoring blood volume and red cell mass, correcting electrolyte and acid-base abnormalities, and unloading excess fluid.

There are several untoward sequelae of the portal-systemic anastomosis. The most important of these is post-shunt encephalopathy which presumably is due to shunting of ammonia, or some nitrogenous substance absorbed from the intestine directly into the systemic circulation. The reported incidence of this disturbing complication has varied considerably, but has been in the range of 10 per cent of patients. Because ammonia is formed by the action of bacteria on nitrogenous substances in the terminal ileum and colon, encephalopathy often can be controlled by limiting the protein content of the diet and by the use of intestinal antibiotics such as neomycin. If these measures fail, operative exclusion of the colon by ileostomy or ileosigmoidostomy may be effective.

The development of peptic ulcer is another potential complication of portal-systemic shunt. In experimental animals, portacaval shunt produces a profound increase in gastric acid secretion and ulcer formation. Evidence indicates that the gastric hypersecretion is due to hepatic bypass of a potent gastric secretogogue or hormone released from the intestines. In man, the effects of portacaval shunt on gastric secretion and ulcer incidence are uncertain. It would seem prudent to institute antacid therapy and a dietary ulcer regimen following shunt operations.

Venous shunt therapy, of course, represents treatment of the complications of cirrhosis and has no direct beneficial effect on the liver disease itself. In contrast to the effects of portacaval shunt in experimental animals with normal livers, the influence of the operation on liver function in humans with cirrhosis and portal hypertension is variable. In our studies, hepatic function did not change or improved moderately in the majority of patients following operation. Deterioration of hepatic function has been more closely related to whether or not the patient resumed the ingestion of alcohol than to any other factor.

Several types of portal-systemic anastomoses are available for relief of portal hypertension (Fig. 13). The end-to-side portacaval shunt accomplishes splanchnic decompression by shunting all splanchnic venous blood into the inferior vena cava, and at the same time decompresses the liver sinusoid by eliminating the contribution of portal venous blood to hepatic inflow and pressure. The side-to-side portacaval shunt produces similar splanchnic decompression and greater hepatic decompression by allowing egress of blood in a retrograde manner through the portal vein into the low pressure vena cava. Portal blood seldom continues to perfuse the liver in the presence of a side-to-side anastomosis, despite the intact portal vein. The splenorenal shunt is a variant of the side-to-side shunt which utilizes tributaries of the portal vein and vena cava; removal of the spleen is usually part of the operation. The mesocaval shunt is an anastomosis between one end of the divided inferior vena cava and the side of the superior mesenteric vein; in principle, it is similar to the side-to-side portacaval shunt.

In patients with cirrhosis, a portacaval shunt is preferable to the smaller splenorenal shunt because it provides greater portal decompression and has a much lower incidence of thrombosis. In rare instances of severe and intractable hypersplenism, a splenectomy, and splenorenal anastomosis are indicated. There is no proven advantage of one type of direct portacaval shunt over the other except in patients with spontaneous reversal of portal flow, in which case the side-to-side anastomosis is clearly the procedure of choice.

Beyond any doubt, the portal-systemic shunt prevents subsequent varix bleeding in the vast majority of patients. Moreover, one-half to three-fourths of the patients subjected to elective treatment have survived five years (Table 11). The crucial question of whether a comparable, selected group of patients who were treated medically rather than surgically would survive as long cannot be answered with certainty. On the basis of our current knowledge, and until adequate information to the contrary is available, the elective

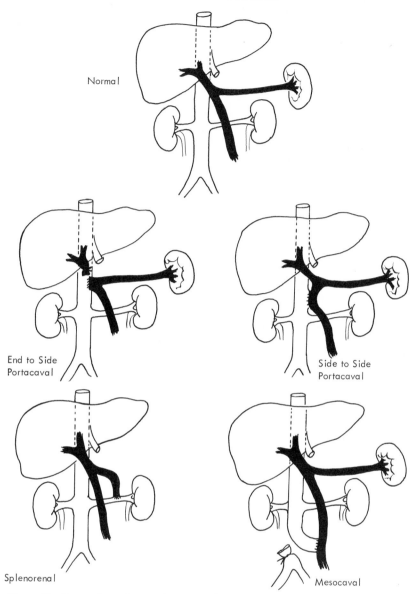

Figure 13. Types of portal-systemic venous shunts used to relieve portal hypertension.

Table 11. *Results of Elective Portal-Systemic Shunt in Patients with Cirrhosis*

AUTHORS	NUMBER OF PATIENTS	TYPE OF SHUNT	OPERATIVE MORTALITY %	VARIX REBLEEDING %	FIVE-YEAR SURVIVAL %
McDermott, Palazzi, Nardi and Mondet	237	166 splenorenal 71 portacaval	23	15	54
Mikkelsen, Turrill and Pattison	173	All portacaval	12	7	44
Linton, Ellis and Geary	169	129 splenorenal 47 portacaval	12	19	50
Wantz and Payne	97	All portacaval	11	5	68 (four-year)
Walker	50	All portacaval	6	12	70
Child	56	All portacaval	12	0	—
Orloff	54	All portacaval	4	2	—

portacaval shunt is indicated in patients who have bled one or more times from esophageal varices.

PROPHYLACTIC SHUNT. Because of the very high mortality rate associated with varix bleeding, some workers have advocated prophylactic performance of portacaval shunts in patients with demonstrable varices who have never bled. This, of course, raises the question of the predictability of bleeding and the answer to this question is not known. Recent reports indicate that prophylactic shunt does not influence the survival of cirrhotic patients. Accordingly, at present there is little to recommend the prophylactic operation.

ASCITES. Ascites is a serious complication of cirrhosis. In many patients, it develops suddenly in association with severe hepatocellular damage and is a manifestation of hepatic decompensation. In others, it develops gradually and persists as a chronic disturbance which leads to progressive discomfort, nutritional depletion and debilitation.

The pathogenesis of ascites is best explained by Starling's hypothesis which states that the exchange of fluid across capillary membranes is a result of the hydrostatic pressure and osmotic pressure on each side of the membrane. Although several factors may be involved in the pathogenesis of ascites, including the serum albumin concentration, the sodium ion and hormones such as aldosterone, results of recent studies indicate that increased pressure within the liver plays a major role in ascites formation and is the primary mechanism responsible for transudation of ascitic fluid. Moreover, substantial evidence suggests that the intrahepatic hypertension in cirrhosis is a result of hepatic venous outflow obstruction.

Experimentally, ascites is produced by any procedure which obstructs hepatic venous outflow but does not result from obstruction of portal venous or hepatic arterial inflow. Furthermore, in experimental ascites the fluid leaks into the peritoneal cavity from the surface and hilum of the liver, a finding which suggests that it originates from some intrahepatic disturbance. Under experimental circumstances, therefore, hepatic outflow obstruction is the sine qua non for ascites formation. In man, a similar striking difference is seen in the ascites-producing effects of outflow and inflow obstruction. In the Budd-Chiari syndrome, a condition resulting from occlusion of the hepatic veins, massive ascites is an invariable complication. In contrast, ascites rarely accompanies extrahepatic obstruction of the portal vein. Comparative observations such as these, both experimental and clinical, plus substantial supporting evidence obtained from hemodynamic and histopathologic studies in man, have led to the conclusion that hepatic outflow block is involved in the pathogenesis of ascites in cirrhosis.

A number of studies have demonstrated a marked increase in the flow of lymph in the hepatic hilar lymphatics and thoracic duct in association with experimental ascites, hepatic outflow obstruction or experimental cirrhosis. A similar increase in lymph flow in the thoracic duct has been observed in humans with cirrhosis and with congestive heart failure, and the marked enlargement of the lymphatics in the hilum of the cirrhotic liver, so familiar to surgeons who have performed operations for portal hypertension, has been documented by careful histopathologic studies. The bulk of evidence indicates that the augmented production of hepatic lymph is in large part a mechanical phenomenon resulting from obstruction to the outflow of blood from the liver sinusoids and the consequent spillover of the plasma portion of the blood into the perisinusoidal spaces and lymphatics. Ascites, in turn, has been attributed to the inability of the lymphatic system to accommodate the excessive formation of lymph, with resultant leakage of fluid into the peritoneal cavity from the overburdened hepatic lymphatics. This chain of events in ascites formation is depicted in Figure 14.

Humans with cirrhosis and ascites present a characteristic picture of marked salt and water retention, secondary hyperaldosteronism, hypervolemia, and dilutional hypona-

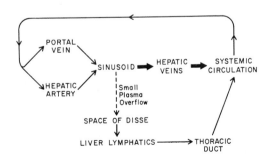

Figure 14. The chain of events in ascites formation. Hepatic venous outflow obstruction and the resultant intrahepatic hypertension play a primary role in causing transudation of ascitic fluid. (From Orloff, M. J., et al.: Arch. Surg. 93:119, 1966.)

tremia. In the majority of such patients, ascites disappears in response to a regimen consisting of abstinence from alcohol, a nourishing diet, salt restriction and one or more of a variety of diuretic and antialdosterone drugs. Nevertheless, in a small but disturbing group of patients, ascites is refractory to these measures. It is for this group that the surgeon has attempted to devise operative measures of relief. If it is assumed, on the basis of substantial evidence, that increased hydrostatic pressure within the liver is important in the pathogenesis of ascites, it should be possible to relieve ascites by reducing the intrahepatic pressure. Theoretically, decompression of the obstructed hepatic vascular bed may be accomplished, to a greater or lesser degree, by reducing the inflow of blood to the liver or by improving the outflow of blood from the liver. Inflow-reducing procedures include ligation of the hepatic artery and the end-to-side portacaval shunt, both of which have been used in the treatment of cirrhotic ascites. Hepatic artery

ligation no longer merits serious consideration, because it is an unpredictable operation which is associated with a high mortality rate. Improving the outflow of blood from the liver by a direct attack on the hepatic veins is not possible. However, numerous studies have demonstrated that the valveless portal vein is capable of serving as an outflow tract and that the objective of hepatic decompression is realized by a side-to-side portacaval shunt.

In a series of experiments, the effects of portacaval shunts on ascites were evaluated. These studies showed that the side-to-side portacaval shunt was effective in relieving ascites, overcoming intrahepatic hypertension, eliminating the hypersecretion of aldosterone which follows hepatic outflow occlusion, and reducing the markedly augmented thoracic duct lymph flow to normal. The end-to-side portacaval anastomosis was much less effective than the lateral anastomosis in relieving the sequelae of increased pressure in the liver.

On the basis of these experimental obser-

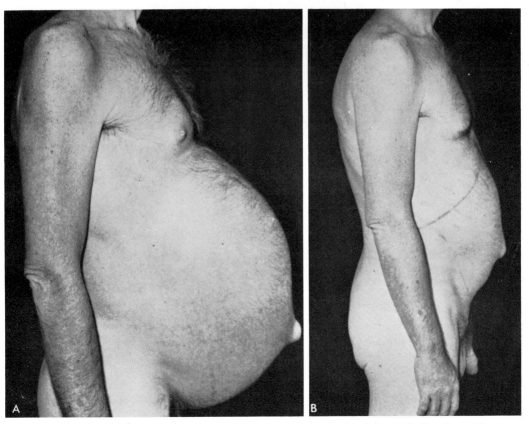

Figure 15. Photographs of a patient with cirrhosis and intractable ascites taken before and after side-to-side portacaval shunt. A, Preoperatively, when ascites was massive. B, Six weeks after side-to-side portacaval shunt. (From Orloff, M. J.: Am. J. Surg. *112*:287, 1966.)

vations, the side-to-side portacaval shunt has been used in a small number of selected patients with cirrhosis and truly intractable ascites. All of our patients failed to respond to prolonged and intensive medical treatment for ascites before operation was considered. Eighty-nine per cent of the patients survived the operation, and all the survivors were relieved of ascites, salt retention and hyperaldosteronism (Fig. 15). Figure 16 shows the effects of the shunt on water and electrolyte balance and on aldosterone excretion in one of these patients. This small but consistent and encouraging clinical experience suggests that further trial of the side-to-side portacaval shunt in carefully selected patients with truly intractable ascites is warranted.

HEPATIC COMA. The central nervous system disorders associated with hepatic cell failure and portal-systemic shunting are included under the umbrella of the term "hepatic coma" and represent the most common terminal event in cirrhosis. The etiology and pathogenesis of most of these disturbances are unknown. In a small percentage of patients, hepatic coma appears to be due to ammonia intoxication resulting from hepatic bypass through spontaneous or surgical portacaval shunts of ammonia absorbed from the intestines or to the inability of the damaged liver to transform ammonia to urea. The symptoms are related to the amount of nitrogen in the intestine and to the level of blood ammonia, and are described by the terms

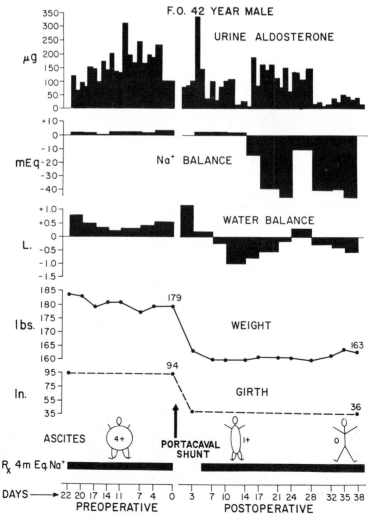

Figure 16.   Results of a metabolic balance study of the patient shown in Figure 23, conducted before and after treatment of intractable ascites by side-to-side shunt. (From Orloff, M. J.: Am. J. Surg. *112*:287, 1966.)

"portal-systemic encephalopathy" and "exogenous hepatic coma." Ammonia is believed to produce central nervous system depression by interfering with aerobic glycolysis in the brain. In most patients with hepatic coma, the neurologic abnormalities are unrelated to intestinal ammonia absorption but appear to be a mysterious manifestation of hepatic failure.

Hepatic coma occurs under a variety of circumstances in patients with advanced liver damage. Often, it is an aspect of progressive clinical deterioration. Not infrequently it occurs following an episode of varix bleeding or after major operations of any type in cirrhotic patients. It may be precipitated by infection, disorders of fluid and electrolyte balance, certain diuretics such as chlorothiazide, sedatives and analgesics, a bout of alcohol ingestion, or paracentesis.

The symptoms and signs are nonspecific and run the gamut of alterations of consciousness. In the early stage, called "hepatic precoma," a variety of personality changes occur, including euphoria, untidiness, inability to concentrate, insomnia and mild confusion. Later, depression and disorientation progressing to stupor and unconsciousness develop. Occasionally, convulsions occur. Asterixis or "liver flap" is a characteristic sign which consists of a flapping, rough tremor best demonstrated by having the patient dorsiflex the hands and spread the fingers. The electroencephalogram shows paroxysms of bilaterally synchronous, high voltage, slow waves. Fluctuations of the symptoms and level of consciousness are usual.

The treatment of hepatic coma is generally supportive and nonspecific. In patients with portal-systemic encephalopathy related to intestinal ammonia absorption, elimination of protein from the diet, removal of nitrogen from the gastrointestinal tract by cathartics and enemas, and administration of intestinal antibiotics such as neomycin may be helpful. In chronic intractable encephalopathy, bypass of the colon by ileostomy or ileosigmoidostomy may be indicated. The use of ammonia-binding agents such as glutamic acid and arginine, and ion exchange resins has met with little success. Treatment of abnormalities known to precipitate hepatic coma and support of liver failure with parenteral glucose and vitamins are of value. Spontaneous recovery from hepatic coma occurs with sufficient frequency to make evaluation of the efficacy of therapy difficult.

PORTAL HYPERTENSION DUE TO EXTRAHEPATIC PORTAL OBSTRUCTION

Portal hypertension due to extrahepatic portal obstruction is a strikingly different condition from intrahepatic portal hypertension. The patients are usually much younger and most often are children. They do not have liver disease and, consequently, have a much greater tolerance for bleeding and for operations. Except in infancy, they rarely have ascites and they do not develop hepatic coma due to liver cell failure. Because the portal vein is usually obliterated, a direct portal vein to vena cava anastomosis cannot be performed for portal decompression. Finally, age and the related technical matter of adequate vessel size influence treatment.

Patients with extrahepatic portal obstruction come to the attention of the surgeon usually because of bleeding from esophageal varices or splenomegaly. Although hematemesis is the most common symptom, the bleeding sometimes presents as melena. Exsanguinating hemorrhage does not occur nearly as often as in cirrhosis. On physical examination, splenomegaly is almost always found but the liver is not palpable. Dilated collateral veins in the abdominal wall may be striking. The liver function tests are normal, but hematologic studies often reveal peripheral cytopenia that reflects hypersplenism. The hypersplenism is usually not severe. Upper gastrointestinal x-rays and, if necessary, esophagoscopy demonstrate esophageal varices. Splenic manometry and splenoportography are crucial diagnostic procedures and regularly demonstrate the presence of portal hypertension, the site of the portal obstruction, and the size of the vessels available for portal decompression.

The definitive treatment of extrahepatic portal obstruction is the portal-systemic venous shunt. However, for technical reasons related to the size of the vessels required for the shunt, temporizing hemostatic measures may have to be used in infants and young children until they have grown to the point where an adequate anastomosis is feasible. The mesocaval shunt usually should not be performed before the age of four, and splenorenal shunt is often not feasible before the age of seven or eight. Consequently, the emergency treatment of varix bleeding in infants and young children consists of blood transfusions and, when necessary, medical measures such as esophageal balloon tamponade and intravenous pituitrin. Failure to control bleeding is an indication for transesophageal varix ligation. Re-bleeding following these temporizing measures is the rule, but it is usually well-tolerated and controllable until the child reaches a suitable age.

The types of portal-systemic anastomoses used in patients with an obliterated portal vein are the superior mesenteric vein–inferior vena cava shunt and the splenorenal shunt. The mesocaval shunt has been followed by a lower incidence of re-bleeding and will probably become the procedure of choice. Both operations have been associated with operative mortality rates below 5 per cent. Other operative procedures, such as esophagogastrectomy with intestinal interposition are associated with a high mortality rate and incidence of failure, and are indicated only when a portal-systemic shunt is impossible.

LIVER TRAUMA

Because of its size, the liver is the most frequent solid viscus injured by perforating wounds of the abdomen; it is involved in approximately 25 per cent of patients who have received perforating trauma. In blunt injuries to the abdomen, liver damage occurs in 5 to 10 per cent of the patients. Because of the marked increase in automobile accidents, blunt liver trauma has become a common clinical entity. Of all the abdominal injuries, those to the liver present the most difficult problems. Moreover, liver wounds are often associated with injuries to other organs which complicate treatment and significantly increase the mortality rate.

As a result of its rich blood supply, hemorrhage and shock dominate the clinical symptoms of liver trauma. In addition, the patient with a liver injury usually complains of pain in the right upper quadrant of the abdomen and on physical examination there are distinct signs of peritoneal irritation such as tenderness and rigidity in the right hypochondrium and hypoactive or absent bowel sounds. Laboratory studies reveal an elevated white blood cell count and a fall in the hematocrit, although early in the course hematocrit determinations may be of no value. Abdominal x-rays are of limited value, but may demonstrate signs of blood in the peritoneal cavity, an elevated right hemidiaphragm, and telltale fractures of the right lower ribs. The most helpful diagnostic procedure is the four-quadrant abdominal tap, which usually shows blood in the peritoneal cavity.

Liver injuries require emergency surgical therapy. The treatment of shock, which includes restoration of the blood volume, and assurance of adequate ventilation are of first priority and precede or accompany operation. Operative treatment hinges on three important principles. The first involves securing hemostasis, a task that is frequently formidable. If possible, hemostasis is obtained by direct suture but resection of the liver and the use of hemostatic agents may be required. The second principle involves the excision of all devitalized hepatic tissue to prevent delayed necrosis, infection and late hemorrhage. The third principle is drainage of the peritoneal cavity to remove the bile that invariably leaks from the hepatic wound and may cause bile peritonitis or localized collections.

The most frequent postoperative complication of liver trauma is infection. Subphrenic abscess, peritonitis and wound infections occur with disturbing frequency. Secondary hemorrhage from necrosis and infection of hepatic tissue is the major cause of delayed death. Bile peritonitis occurs occasionally when adequate drainage has not been provided.

An unusual but interesting complication of liver injury is hemobilia. This disorder follows central rupture of the liver as well as suture of liver lacerations without obliteration of the dead space. The communication between the vasculature and the biliary tract develops as a result of necrosis of a portion of hepatic parenchyma within a closed space. Symptoms commonly appear three to four weeks after injury and consist of episodes of biliary colic due to blood clots in the bile ducts, mild jaundice and gastrointestinal bleeding. Elevations of the serum alkaline phosphatase and bilirubin usually accompany the attacks. Treatment consists of resection of the lesion or ligation of the ends of the contributing blood vessels.

The mortality rate of perforating liver injuries has been reduced to 10 to 15 per cent. In contrast, liver damage from blunt trauma presently carries a mortality rate of 38 to 50 per cent. Associated injuries to other organs are partly responsible for the seriousness of blunt hepatic trauma.

PYOGENIC LIVER ABSCESS

Although pyogenic liver abscess was fairly common prior to the antibiotic era, it now is found infrequently. Invasion of the liver by bacteria occurs along several routes. Ascending biliary infection, cholangitis due to calculi in the common bile duct, or an obstructing cancer is the most frequent cause of hepatic abscess. Hematogenous invasion of the liver via the portal vein from intraperitoneal infections such as suppurative appendicitis, diverticulitis or omphalitis is another relatively common route. Occasionally, such conditions are associated with a suppurative thrombophlebitis of the portal vein, called pyelophlebitis, which gives rise to multiple liver abscesses. Hematogenous spread by way of the hepatic artery occurs in systemic infections such as bacterial endocarditis. Direct extension of infection into the liver from peritonitis or a diseased gallbladder is an unusual mechanism for hepatic abscess formation. Finally, implantation of microorganisms during liver trauma is responsible for some cases of abscess.

The clinical symptoms of pyogenic liver abscess consist of fever often accompanied by chills, pain in the right upper abdomen, anorexia and weight loss. In one-half to two-thirds of the patients, the liver is enlarged and tender. Jaundice and a right-sided pleural effusion occur in one-fourth of patients. Leukocytosis is almost invariable and anemia is common. The liver function tests often show abnormalities similar to those found in viral hepatitis. These include enzyme elevations, Bromsulphalein retention, positive turbidity and flocculation tests, hyperbilirubinemia and, particularly, an elevation of serum alkaline phosphatase. X-rays of the abdomen and chest, and fluoroscopy, show elevation and fixation of the right hemidiaphragm. Occasionally, a diagnostic air-fluid level below the right diaphragm and a pleural effusion above are seen. The liver scan is an important diagnostic procedure, and hepatic arteriography may be helpful. A serious complication of pyogenic liver abscess is rupture into the pleural cavity.

The treatment of pyogenic liver abscess consists of antibiotics and surgical drainage. Selection of the appropriate antibiotics depends on the causative organism; *Escherichia coli* and *Staphylococcus aureus* are the bacteria most frequently found. Surgical drainage may be performed by an extraserous transthoracic approach or by a transabdominal approach, depending upon the location of the lesion. Abscesses most often occur in the right lobe of the liver. Multiple liver abscesses are not uncommon and in such cases effective drainage may be difficult.

AMEBIC LIVER ABSCESS

Infection with *Entamoeba histolytica* involves 10 to 20 per cent of the population of the United States. The reported incidence of amebic liver abscess in patients with intestinal amebiasis has varied from 1 to 25 per cent. Hepatic complications of amebic infection are usually found in middle-aged males. Liver abscess is always due to spread of intestinal amebiasis via the portal vein. However, cysts or trophozoites are found in the stool in less than one-fourth of the patients with hepatic infection. The liver abscess is most often solitary and in the right lobe, and its contents have a characteristic appearance of anchovy paste.

The clinical symptoms of amebic liver abscess consist of pain in the right hypochondrium or lower chest sometimes with radiation to the right shoulder, fever, chills, sweating, anorexia, and weight loss. Diarrhea is an inconstant feature of the present or past history. Hepatomegaly and liver tenderness are the most important physical findings. Pulmonary abnormalities occur in one-fourth of the patients. Jaundice is unusual.

Laboratory studies show a leukocytosis and often an anemia. Elevation of the serum alkaline phosphatase and Bromsulphalein retention are inconsistently found, and the other liver function tests are usually normal. The radiographic and liver scan findings are similar to those observed in pyogenic liver abscess, and are of significance in making the diagnosis. The findings of anchovy sauce material on needle aspiration of the liver is diagnostic. Parasites are found in the aspirate in less than one-third of the patients.

The complications of amebic liver abscess consist of secondary pyogenic infection, which is usually accompanied by a sudden increase in toxic signs and symptoms, and of rupture of the abscess into the lung, pleural cavity or peritoneal cavity. The development of pulmonary signs and symptoms should suggest the possibility of rupture.

The treatment of amebic liver abscess involves chemotherapy and drainage. Patients should receive a course of therapy with an extraintestinal amebicide, such as emetine or chloroquine, followed by therapy with an intestinal amebicide such as diodoquin or chiniofon. Persistence of the abscess after drug therapy is an indication for needle aspiration. If needle aspiration fails to cure the patient, open drainage by an extraserous transthoracic or subcostal approach should be performed.

ECHINOCOCCUS CYST

Hydatid disease is common in many parts of the world, but it is a rare condition in the United States and is found mainly in immigrants who bring the disease to this country. Two forms of the echinococcus tapeworm produce disease in man, *Echinococcus granulosus* and *Echinococcus multilocularis*. The adult tapeworm lives in the intestine of the dog, from which ova are passed in the stool. The ova are ingested by an intermediate host, usually sheep, cattle and pigs but occasionally man, and hatch into embryos in the duodenum. The embryos pass into the portal venous system and are filtered out by the liver, although occasionally they escape to the lung or other organs. In the liver, the embryos reproduce asexually and form multiloculated cysts. The cyst in the liver usually has a well-defined wall with an inner germinative layer and a thick outer laminated layer which often calcifies. The cyst fluid contains numerous embryonal scolices called "hydatid sand." The cycle is completed when a dog feeds on the infected tissues of an intermediate host, and the scolices develop into mature tapeworms in the dog's intestines.

Hydatid cysts frequently are present for many years without producing symptoms. Often, the discovery of a liver mass on physical examination or the pathognomonic finding of a calcified, round mass in the liver on x-ray leads to the diagnosis. Eosinophilia occurs in one-fourth of the cases. A complement fixation test and the response to intradermal injection of cyst fluid are positive in the vast majority of patients.

The major cause of morbidity and mortality associated with echinococcus cyst of the liver is rupture of the cyst. Rupture into the bile ducts produces a syndrome of biliary colic, jaundice, urticaria and fever. Rupture into the peritoneal cavity results in abdominal pain, urticaria, anaphylactic shock and the development of multiple intra-abdominal cysts. Rupture into the pleural cavity causes pain, cough, fever and the development of empyema. Rarely, hydatid cysts rupture into the gastrointestinal tract. Secondary infection of liver cysts with pyogenic bacteria occurs sometimes and produces the signs and symptoms of pyogenic liver abscess.

The treatment of hydatid cyst is surgical removal. Usually the cyst can be removed by shelling out, but occasionally hepatic resection is required. In order to prevent seeding of the cyst contents, preliminary aspiration and instillation of hydrogen peroxide or formalin is done. Care must be taken to avoid spilling viable scolices into the peritoneal cavity. The mortality rate for treatment of uncomplicated cysts is less than 5 per cent.

BENIGN NEOPLASMS AND CYSTS

Usually, benign neoplasms of the liver are of clinical significance only in that they pose problems in differential diagnosis from more serious lesions. The most common benign tumor is the hemangioma, a lesion of blood vessels which presents the microscopic appearance of endothelial-lined cystic spaces filled with blood. The liver is the parenchymatous organ in which hemangiomas are most frequently found. The tumors vary greatly in size. They are usually asymptomatic, although they may grow so large as to compress adjacent viscera. When clinically significant, they present as an abdominal mass and produce x-ray and liver scan abnormalities. The most serious complication of the hepatic hemangioma is rupture with massive intraperitoneal hemorrhage, an event which has been reported with some frequency. Treatment is required when the tumors become clinically significant and consists of excision or hepatic lobectomy. Radiation therapy may be effective and is indicated in inoperable lesions.

Hepatic adenomas are rare tumors of liver cells or bile duct epithelium. They are usually asymptomatic and when discovered at laparotomy may be mistaken for primary or metastatic cancers. They require excision only when large.

Hamartomas are congenital collections of normal hepatic cell plates, bile ducts, blood vessels, and fibrous tissue in an abnormal arrangement. They are developmental disturbances and are not true neoplasms. They may be single or multiple and vary greatly in size. Some are quite large and are palpable on physical examination. Usually, they are asymptomatic. No treatment is necessary unless they are very large. Hamartomas are of clinical significance mainly because of the difficulty in distinguishing them from malignant tumors on gross examination.

Cysts of the liver are uncommon. Most of the solitary cysts are congenital lesions caused by arrest in the development of the bile ducts. Some single cysts originate from trauma, and in rare instances true neoplastic cystadenomas are found. Multiple cysts of the liver, or polycystic disease, represent congenital bile duct anomalies; associated polycystic disease of the kidneys is found in half of the patients and accompanying cystic disease of other organs has been reported. Other congenital anomalies are often found in patients with polycystic disease. Both solitary cysts and polycystic disease are usually not discovered until adulthood.

Cysts of the liver are usually asymptomatic and come to the attention of a physician because of the finding of an enlarged liver or a mass in the abdomen. Liver function is normal. X-rays of the abdomen and liver scan are helpful in demonstrating the presence of a liver mass. Treatment consists of excision of the cyst, hepatic resection, or external drainage with packing. Polycystic disease requires no treatment and is compatible with long life if serious associated anomalies are absent.

MALIGNANT NEOPLASMS

PRIMARY CANCER. Primary cancer of the liver is uncommon in the United States but in Africa and Asia it is one of the most frequent malignant neoplasms. Only the Caucasian race is relatively free of liver cancer. The disease occurs in infants, but predominates in adults in their 40's and 50's. Two-thirds to three-fourths of hepatic cancers develop in patients with cirrhosis.

There are two major forms of liver cancer. These are liver cell carcinoma and bile duct carcinoma. Hepatomas outnumber cholangiocarcinomas five to one. Other primary liver cancers are rare. Carcinoma of the liver metastasizes widely, but the most frequent sites are the lungs and regional lymph nodes.

The clinical features of liver carcinoma most often consist of a rapid increase of signs and symptoms in a patient with cirrhosis and include the appearance of ascites, edema, jaundice, anemia, weakness and weight loss. Occasionally, hepatic carcinoma is responsible for the first episode of bleeding varices. In non-cirrhotic patients, the common symptoms are weakness, weight loss, dull pain in the hypochondrium, abdominal swelling, edema and fever. The usual signs are nodular hepatomegaly and ascites. Hemorrhage into the peritoneal cavity is an occasional terminal event.

All the liver function tests may be abnormal, but elevation of the alkaline phosphatase and glutamic oxaloacetic transaminase, and Bromsulphalein retention are the most consistent biochemical abnormalities. Liver scan, hepatic arteriography, splenoportography, and needle liver biopsy may provide the diagnosis.

The treatment of primary carcinoma of the liver is hepatic resection when the lesion is solitary and there are no regional or distant metastases. Unfortunately, these circumstances rarely occur and cure of the disease is unusual. Duration of life after discovery of hepatic cancer averages only three to four months. Radiation therapy is of no value. Infusion of chemotherapeutic agents, such as methotrexate and 5-fluorouracil, into the hepatic artery has provided brief palliation in occasional patients.

METASTATIC CANCER. Because of its rich and unique blood supply, the liver is the most common organ to be involved by metastatic cancer. One-half to two-thirds of the patients who die from cancer of the gastrointestinal tract, pancreas, breast and ovary, and one-third of the patients who die from lung and kidney cancers develop liver metastases. Neoplasms spread to the liver by way of the portal vein, hepatic artery, lymphatics and by direct extension. Right upper quadrant abdominal pain, nodular hepatomegaly and ascites are common clinical features. Bromsulphalein retention and elevation of serum alkaline phosphatase and glutamic oxaloacetic transaminase are consistent findings. Liver scan, arteriography, portography and needle liver biopsy help to make the diagnosis. Although rare cases of metastatic carcinoma have been cured by hepatic resections, the lesions are essentially incurable.

The Biliary System

ANATOMY

The biliary system and liver develop together from a diverticulum which arises in the embryo from the ventral floor of the foregut and extends into the septum transversum. The caudal portion of this diverticulum becomes the gallbladder, cystic duct and common bile duct, whereas the cranial portion develops into the liver and hepatic bile ducts.

The gallbladder is a thin-walled, pear-shaped organ covered by peritoneum and attached to the inferior surfaces of the right and quadrate lobes of the liver. Normally, it is about 10 cm. long, 3 to 5 cm. in diameter and has a capacity of 30 to 60 ml. Anatomically, it is divided into a fundus or tip which protrudes from the anterior edge of the liver, a corpus or body, an infundibulum called Hartmann's pouch and a narrow neck that leads into the cystic duct.

The cystic duct is about 3 cm. long and contains mucosal duplications called the spiral fold or valve of Heister which regulate the passage of bile to and from the gallbladder. The cystic duct joins the right lateral aspect of the common hepatic duct to form the common bile duct. The common hepatic duct is 2 to 3 cm. long and is formed from the right and left hepatic ducts. The common bile duct, formed from the union of the cystic duct and common hepatic duct is 10 to 15 cm. long. It descends in the hepatoduodenal ligament to the right of the hepatic artery and anterior to the portal vein, passes behind the first part of the duodenum and through the pancreas, and enters the descending duodenum on its medial aspect at the papilla of Vater. The choledochoduodenal junction is an oblique passageway through the duodenal wall occupied by the common bile duct and the main pancreatic duct of Wirsung. These two ducts usually join in a common channel, the ampulla of Vater which opens into the duodenum at the papilla of Vater; however, the two ducts may join before entering the duodenal wall or may empty into the duodenum through separate openings. The muscle of the choledochoduodenal junction, called the sphincter of Oddi, regulates the flow of bile and consists of several components. The two major components are the sphincter choledochus which surrounds the common bile duct within the duodenal wall proximal to its junction with the pancreatic duct, and the sphincter ampullae which surrounds the common ampulla of Vater.

The arterial blood supply to the common bile duct comes mainly from the retroduodenal artery, a branch of the gastroduodenal artery. The gallbladder is nourished by the cystic artery which originates from the right hepatic artery, to the right of the common hepatic duct, and divides into anterior and posterior branches. Venous drainage from the extrahepatic biliary system is into the portal vein. Lymphatic vessels from the gallbladder join those from the liver to empty into the cisterna chyli and thoracic duct. Lymph nodes at the neck of the gallbladder, at the junction of the cystic duct and hepatic ducts, and at the end of the common duct play a prominent role in the lymphatic drainage and are regularly enlarged in cholecystitis. The innervation of the biliary system is similar to that of the liver. Vagal stimulation causes contraction of the gallbladder and relaxation of the sphincter of Oddi, whereas sympathetic stimulation produces the reverse actions.

Histologically, the gallbladder consists of a mucosa of columnar epithelium, a muscularis, a subserosa, and a serosa. Mucous glands are found only in the neck. Gallbladder inflammation characteristically produces invaginations of the mucosa into the muscularis called Rokitansky-Aschoff sinuses. The bile ducts are lined by columnar epithelium and contain mucous glands.

A most striking and, for the surgeon, dangerous feature of the anatomy of the extrahepatic biliary system is its variability. Variations in the bile ducts, cystic artery and hepatic artery are very common. For this reason, biliary operations require extremely careful technique.

PHYSIOLOGY

Bile has a number of important functions. It plays a role in the absorption of lipids through a complex mechanism of emulsification. It is involved in the absorption of minerals such as calcium, iron and copper. It activates and stimulates secretion of certain digestive enzymes, such as pancreatic lipase. It provides alkali for the neutralization of gastric acid in the duodenum. Finally, bile serves as a vehicle for the excretion of numerous compounds metabolized by the liver.

The functions of the extrahepatic biliary system consist of the transport of bile secreted by the liver to the intestines, the regulation of bile flow, and the storage and concentration of bile. The liver secretes 600 to 1000 ml. of bile per day. Liver bile has a specific gravity of 1.011 and 97 per cent of its content is water. The gallbladder concentrates the bile at least five to ten times by absorbing water and electrolytes, and excretes a product with a specific gravity of 1.040.

In the absence of food in the intestine, bile secreted continuously by the liver is retained within the bile ducts as a result of steady contraction of the sphincter of Oddi. As the biliary pressure rises, the bile refluxes into the gallbladder where it is concentrated and stored. Entrance of food into the duodenum causes the release of an intestinal hormone called cholecystokinin. This humoral agent plus nervous stimuli produce contraction of the gallbladder, relaxation of the sphincter of Oddi, and free flow of the bile into the intestine. Fats and proteins are strong stimuli to gallbladder contraction, whereas carbohydrates have little effect on motor activity. Following cholecystectomy, regulation of bile flow is dependent entirely on the sphincter of Oddi.

The bile secretory pressure of the liver varies throughout the day, but averages 300 mm. saline. At rest, the pressure within the gallbladder averages 100 mm., but during contraction it rises to as high as 375 mm. The sphincter of Oddi relaxes when the pressure in the common bile duct reaches 200 to 250 mm. saline. Pressures in the bile ducts greater than 350 mm. cause suppression of hepatic bile secretion.

Pain from the gallbladder and bile ducts is produced by distention and is often accompanied by nausea and vomiting. Such pain is carried by visceral sensory fibers in the sympathetic splanchnic nerves, connected to the seventh to tenth thoracic segments, and is perceived in the epigastrium. As a result of the motor activity in the biliary system and the related changes in pressure, biliary pain often has an intermittent component. Inflammation of the gallbladder causes referral of the visceral sensory impulses to somatic segments, giving rise to pain in the right hypochondrium, infrascapular area, substernal area and occasionally, as a result of connections with the phrenic nerve, right shoulder tip pain. Inflammation of the parietal peritoneum adjacent to the gallbladder causes localized somatic sensory pain. Distention of the gallbladder or bile ducts may cause a reflex decrease in coronary blood flow and cardiac arrhythmias, and is believed to explain the association of biliary tract disease and cardiac abnormalities.

DIAGNOSTIC STUDIES

ROENTGENOGRAPHIC STUDIES. The diagnosis of biliary tract disease is in large part dependent on roentgenographic studies.

Survey x-rays of the abdomen. Plain x-rays of the abdomen may be helpful in directing attention to or making the diagnosis of biliary disease. Between 10 and 15 per cent of gallstones contain sufficient calcium to be seen on survey x-rays. An uncommon condition called milk of calcium bile, which consists of a collection of calcified debris, may opacify the dependent portion of the gallbladder or occupy the entire organ. This sediment of calcium carbonate is associated with obstruction of the cystic duct and chronic gallbladder inflammation. Gas in the bile ducts is a diagnostic sign of an abnormal communication between the biliary system and gastrointestinal tract. Emphysematous cholecystitis is an unusual inflammation of the gallbladder due to gas-producing bacteria which results in gas in the wall and lumen of the gallbladder. Intestinal obstruction due to a gallstone which has eroded through the biliary tree and into the intestine, called gallstone ileus, is a well-known complication of cholecystitis and produces the characteristic roentgenographic signs of dilatation of the bowel. Finally, a dilated loop of small intestine adjacent to an inflamed gallbladder, the so-called sentinel loop, represents a localized ileus and may be of diagnostic significance.

Oral cholecystography. In 1924, Graham and Cole produced radiographic opacification of the gallbladder by the oral administration of an organic iodide-containing dye and initiated a new era in x-ray diagnosis. A wide variety of iodinated organic agents that are absorbed from the intestine, excreted by the liver in the bile, and concentrated in the gallbladder are now available for visualization of the biliary system. Failure of the gallbladder to visualize usually indicates obstruction of the bile ducts or inability of the gallbladder to concentrate the dye. However, other causes of failure must be ruled out and include inadequate dose of dye; failure of intestinal absorption; inadequate hepatic excretion due to liver disease and, rarely, a full gallbladder or improper radiographic technique. Administration of a double dose of dye or administration of dye daily for four days sometimes demonstrates a gallbladder which does not visualize with the standard technique. Visualization of the gallbladder does not usually occur when the serum bilirubin is above 4 mg. per 100 ml.

The two most important diagnostic findings of oral cholecystography are radiolucent shadows in the opaque dye and failure of the gallbladder to visualize. The radiolucent shadows are almost always due to gallstones and are diagnostic of disease (Fig. 17). Failure to visualize, on the other hand, should be cautiously interpreted and requires a careful consideration of the patient's history, physical findings and results of other studies.

Intravenous cholangiography. The development of dyes such as sodium ionapamide which do not require concentration in the gallbladder to visualize the biliary system is the basis of intravenous cholangiography. Although this procedure was originally aimed at demonstrating the extrahepatic bile ducts,

it can be employed to visualize the gallbladder. Intravenous cholangiography is used in patients who cannot take the dye orally, in patients who have had a cholecystectomy, and when demonstration of the extrahepatic bile ducts is desired. If the gallbladder is present, failure to demonstrate it has the same implications as in oral cholecystography. Dilatation or stricture of the bile ducts, choledocholithiasis, choledochal cysts, and cystic duct remnants may be demonstrated by intravenous cholangiography (Fig. 18). A successful study is unusual in the presence of a serum bilirubin greater than 4 mg. per 100 ml. Intravenous cholangiography should not be performed without clear indications, because rare hypersensitivity reactions to the dye resulting in circulatory collapse and death have been reported.

Percutaneous transhepatic cholangiography. Instillation of opaque media into the biliary system by percutaneous needle puncture of a bile duct has been used primarily in jaundiced patients to determine whether biliary obstruction is extrahepatic or intrahepatic. Bleeding and leakage of bile are significant hazards of this technique, and it is generally performed when determination of the site of obstruction may make possible a life-saving operation. When surgical ther-

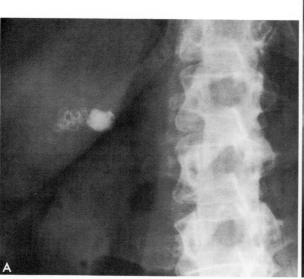
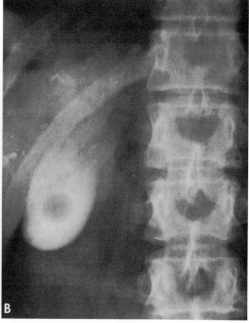

Figure 17.   Calculi in the gallbladder. *A*, Radiopaque stones were discovered on a plain film of the abdomen in a patient who had a gastrointestinal x-ray examination for another disease. *B*, Radiolucent calculi demonstrated by oral cholecystography in a patient with symptoms of chronic cholecystitis.

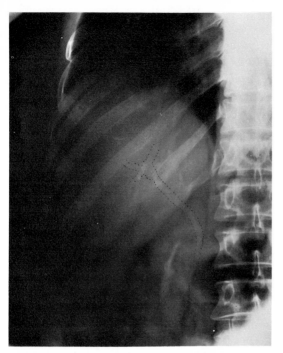

Figure 18. Visualization of normal common bile duct following intravenous administration of iodide-containing dye (intravenous cholangiogram).

apy is indicated, operation is usually undertaken immediately after the cholangiographic study.

Operative and postoperative direct cholangiography. Visualization of the extrahepatic bile ducts by instillation of dye via a catheter in the cystic duct, or common bile duct, during operations on the biliary system has become an important method for identifying stones and other abnormalities. During cholecystectomy, many surgeons perform operative cholangiography routinely to help decide whether or not to explore the common bile duct for stones. Following exploration of the common bile duct, almost all surgeons obtain a tube cholangiogram before terminating the operation to be certain that stones or strictures have not been overlooked. For similar reasons, tube cholangiograms are regularly obtained postoperatively before biliary drainage is discontinued.

Barium contrast upper gastrointestinal x-rays. The upper gastrointestinal series is an important study in the investigation of patients suspected of having biliary disease. Because the symptoms of gastrointestinal diseases, such as peptic ulcer and hiatus hernia, often mimic those of biliary disorders, it is important to establish the presence or absence of extrabiliary disturbances, which may account for symptoms.

The upper gastrointestinal x-rays may be helpful in the differential diagnosis of obstructive jaundice, and particularly in distinguishing between neoplastic and calculus obstruction. Widening of the duodenal sweep, the "reverse 3" sign of Frostberg, distortion of the duodenal mucosa and displacement of the stomach are important radiographic signs of carcinoma of the head of the pancreas.

Duodenal drainage. Aspiration of bile from a tube inserted via the nose or mouth into the duodenum may provide valuable information in the diagnosis of biliary disease, and in the differential diagnosis of jaundice. Instillation of magnesium sulfate or olive oil into the duodenum causes contraction of the gallbladder and permits collection of bile emanating from the gallbladder. By proper timing of specimens, bile from the extrahepatic ducts and fresh liver bile may be obtained. The finding of cholesterol and calcium bilirubinate crystals on microscopic examination of the duodenal aspirate strongly suggests the presence of gallstones. Cytologic studies for cancer cells may provide evidence of carcinoma of the biliary ducts or duodenum. Duodenal drainage is indicated when other diagnostic studies fail to yield positive results in patients with symptoms suggestive of biliary disease.

Biochemical studies. Liver function tests in the differential diagnosis of jaundice are important. Because of the intimate association of diseases of the biliary system and pancreas, determinations of serum amylase and lipase and of urinary diastase are frequently indicated. Elevations of these enzymes are often found in patients with acute biliary inflammations in the absence of gross disease of the pancreas. The frequent occurrence of biliary disorders in patients with diabetes requires determinations of blood and urine sugar.

CHRONIC CHOLECYSTITIS AND CHOLELITHIASIS

GALLSTONES. Except for congenital anomalies, the vast majority of diseases of the extrahepatic biliary system are associated with gallstones. These disorders are among the most common diseases of adult life. Gallstones occur in approximately 10 per cent of the adult population in the United States, and in about 20 per cent of people over the age of 40. The incidence of cholelithiasis increases progressively with age so that approximately one-third of the individuals in the eighth decade of life have calculi. At the same time, the occurrence of gallstones in children associated with hemolytic anemias is by no means rare, and the finding of cholelithiasis in young adults, particularly pregnant women, is not unusual. Women develop biliary calculi about four times more frequently than men.

The pathogenesis of gallstones is not completely understood and, undoubtedly, several mechanisms are involved. The three major organic constituents of bile are the salts of bile acids, bilirubin and cholesterol. Bilirubin is poorly soluble in water and cholesterol is insoluble, yet these substances are normally maintained in a supersaturated aqueous solution, because water makes up 97 per cent of bile. The mechanism whereby this is accomplished depends on the emulsifying action of the bile acids and fatty acids which form micelles with bilirubin and cholesterol. Any chronic disturbance which produces increased concentration of the relatively insoluble components of bile causes them to precipitate and might lead to stone formation. Thus, excessive bilirubin formation such as occurs in hemolytic anemias is associated with a high incidence of pigment stones, and the hypercholesterolemia that occurs in pregnancy, obesity and diabetes may be responsible for the increased frequency of cholesterol-containing stones in these conditions.

Stasis has been proposed as a factor in gallstone formation, in part on the basis of experimental studies regarding the production of calculi. Chronic spasm of the sphincter of Oddi is believed to be a cause of stasis. It is postulated that stasis leads to excessive reabsorption of water by the gallbladder and an increased concentration of bilirubin and cholesterol in bile. The resultant physiochemical imbalance may cause precipitation of the organic constituents and the development of calculi.

The role of infection in the pathogenesis of cholelithiasis is uncertain. Although bacteria are commonly found in inflamed gallbladders and in stones, substantial evidence indicates that normal bile is usually sterile. The inflamed gallbladder mucosa has a markedly altered permeability which permits the absorption of bile acids and the movement of inorganic salts into the gallbladder lumen. It is possible that these changes alter the distribution of the constituents of bile and cause precipitation of cholesterol. Equally important may be the role of excessive cellular debris and increased protein secretion which occur in response to inflammation and may form a nidus for gallstones.

The most common type of biliary calculus is the mixed stone composed of cholesterol, bilirubin, calcium and varying amounts of cellular debris. Other types are the pure cholesterol stones and the bilirubin-calcium stones. The latter are formed only in disorders causing increased bilirubin production.

Symptomatic chronic cholecystitis is almost always associated with cholelithiasis. At the same time, a substantial number of patients with calculi have silent stones that do not produce symptoms. The percentage of calculi which are asymptomatic has been estimated as from 10 per cent to as high as 50 per cent.

PATHOGENESIS OF CHRONIC CHOLECYSTITIS. Chronic cholecystitis is a disease distinguished by the pathologic findings of chronic inflammation, and by a clinical course in which the systemic manifestations of inflammation are not prominent. The pathogenesis of this condition is not clear despite the attention which it has received. It is not a usual bacterial inflammation, although bacteria may play a primary or secondary role. The theories regarding etiology are several. Prominent among these is the proposal that chronic cholecystitis is caused by mechanical or chemical irritation. According to this proposal, gallstones form before inflammation occurs. The calculi then cause inflammation by pressure on the mucosa and lead to the formation of mucosal ulcers. The inflammation is promoted by the irritating effect of constituents of bile, particularly when there is bile stasis. These chemicals may cause inflammation in the absence of stones. Bacterial invasion may occur as a secondary event.

A second theory proposes that bacterial infection is the primary cause of chronic cholecystitis. Bacteria are believed to gain access to the gallbladder along the bile ducts, via the lymphatics, and by way of the arterial and venous circulations. Undoubtedly, some cases of cholecystitis, particularly those associated with systemic infections, have a bacterial etiology. However, the absence of bacteria in normal bile, and the frequent failure to culture organisms in diseased gallbladders casts some doubt on the suggestion that bacteria commonly cause cholecystitis.

DIAGNOSIS. The diagnosis of chronic cholecystitis is based mainly on the history, physical examination and x-ray studies. The symptoms fall into two categories, vague digestive complaints sometimes called dyspepsia, and attacks of biliary colic. The digestive disturbances include postprandial belching, nausea, bloating, flatulence and constipation and are often related to the ingestion of fried or fatty foods or such items as cabbage and onions. These symptoms are due to reflex disorders of gastrointestinal motility and by themselves are nonspecific.

The attacks of biliary colic are quite distinctive. They are due to distention of the biliary tree as a result of a calculus transiently obstructing the cystic duct or common bile duct, or of spasm of the sphincter of Oddi. They often begin after a heavy meal or at night and last for from several hours to several days. The pain is severe and, unlike other forms of colic, is continuous with waves of increasing intensity. The pain begins in the epigastrium and, as it progresses, radiates to the right costal margin, to the back below the tip of the scapula, and sometimes to the right shoulder. Radiation to the substernal area and left hypochondrium is occasionally observed. Deep respiration intensifies the pain, but movement does not. At the height of the pain, nausea and vomiting frequently occur. As the pain subsides, the patient is left with residual soreness.

The physical findings are not striking. Mild to moderate tenderness and guarding in the epigastrium and right hypochondrium are the only significant signs. The gallbladder is usually not palpable except in hydrops of the gallbladder, a condition in which the cystic duct is obliterated and the gallbladder becomes distended with mucus. Fever is usually absent or low grade. Transient bilirubinemia is not uncommon.

Roentgenographic studies represent the best means of confirming the suspicion that a patient has chronic cholecystitis. The demonstration of gallstones by cholecystography or, occasionally, by plain abdominal x-rays provides the only certain evidence of the disease. Failure of the gallbladder to visualize, particularly on repeated studies, strongly suggests chronic cholecystitis if added to a history of typical symptoms. Duodenal drainage may provide important information, and is indicated if the diagnosis is in doubt.

Severe attacks of biliary colic may be confused with a large number of diseases, including peptic ulcer, pancreatitis, hiatus hernia, diverticulitis, mesenteric thrombosis, myocardial infarction, and pleurisy. The importance of ruling out these conditions by appropriate studies, particularly when gallstones are not demonstrable, should be apparent.

TREATMENT. The treatment of symptomatic chronic cholecystitis is surgical removal of the gallbladder. The operative mortality of this procedure is less than 1 per cent. The treatment of a patient with clear-cut symptoms by any means other than cholecystectomy is almost always associated with recurrence of symptoms and often with the development of serious complications.

The treatment of a patient whose gallbladder fails to visualize by cholecystography is a matter of judgment. Under such circumstances, operation should be performed only in the presence of strongly suggestive symptoms and after repeated x-ray studies. Moreover, the absence of other diseases which might account for the symptoms should be demonstrated.

The treatment of patients with silent stones discovered incidentally is controversial. The probability that such calculi will become symptomatic is considerable, and the possibility exists that serious complications such as acute cholecystitis, obstructive jaundice, cholangitis and biliary fistula will develop. The low mortality rate and morbidity of elective cholecystectomy add support to the argument for surgical treatment. Nevertheless, the decision regarding therapy must take into account the health of the patient, risk of operation, and the life expectancy. In general, operation is advisable in patients less than 60 years of age who are in good health.

Symptomatic gallstones have been shown to play a potentiating role in pancreatitis and in coronary insufficiency. Removal of the gallbladder often has a beneficial effect on these diseases and is recommended.

GALLSTONE ILEUS. Intestinal obstruction caused by a gallstone which has eroded into the intestine is an uncommon condition. The site of obstruction is usually the ileum in the region of the ileocecal valve. A biliary-enteric fistula is consistently present, most often between the gallbladder and the duodenum, and gives rise to the diagnostic radiographic sign of gas in the biliary tree. The symptoms and signs are those of acute small intestinal obstruction and prompt surgical treatment is required. Therapy of the biliary disorder is indicated at a later time, provided the patient is in satisfactory condition. Gallstone ileus is a manifestation of advanced biliary disease and is most often seen in elderly patients.

SYMPTOMS AFTER CHOLECYSTECTOMY. Ninety to 95 per cent of patients subjected to cholecystectomy for chronic cholecystitis are relieved of symptoms. However, a small number of patients continue to have symptoms or develop new complaints following operation. The causes of these disturbances are several, and they have been lumped together under the term "postcholecystectomy syndrome." The conditions responsible for symptoms after cholecystectomy may be categorized as follows:

Diseases of other systems. Included in this category are functional disorders and conditions such as peptic ulcer, pancreatitis, hiatus hernia and coronary insufficiency. The discovery of these diseases does not necessarily indicate an initial error in diagnosis, although this is often the case. This group represents the most frequent cause of the postcholecystectomy syndrome.

Organic biliary tract disease. This category includes overlooked cholelithiasis, a large cystic duct stump in which calculi may develop, stenosis of the sphincter of Oddi, and injuries to the biliary ducts. These disorders require surgical correction.

Biliary dyskinesia. This is presumed to be a functional disorder of the bile ducts which causes abnormal elevations of pressure and disturbances of bile flow in the biliary system. The existence of this condition as a demonstrable clinical entity has been questioned.

A significant reduction in the incidence of symptoms after cholecystectomy will occur if every patient is evaluated thoroughly before biliary surgery is undertaken.

ACUTE CHOLECYSTITIS

ETIOLOGY AND PATHOLOGY. Acute cholecystitis is characterized clinically by the presence of systemic and local signs of inflammation, and pathologically by the presence of an acute inflammatory process in the gallbladder. In over 90 per cent of the patients it is associated with gallstones. The failure to find bacteria in over half of the cases suggests that it is not usually caused by a bacterial infection. It is currently believed that acute cholecystitis is a chemical inflammation sometimes with secondary bacterial enhancement.

Acute cholecystitis is initiated by calculus obstruction of the cystic duct. The subsequent overconcentration of the bile trapped in the gallbladder is believed to produce inflammation of the mucosa and an outpouring of fluid which causes marked distention of the gallbladder and the development of a high intraluminal pressure. If the obstruction is not relieved spontaneously or surgically, the blood supply to the gallbladder may be compromised and result in necrosis and perforation. Bacterial invasion produces an empyema of the gallbladder and facilitates necrosis. Gangrene and perforation occur in 10 to 15 per cent of the patients with acute cholecystitis. The perforation is usually walled off by omentum and surrounding organs, producing a pericholecystic abscess, subphrenic abscess or biliary-enteric fistula. Free perforation with bile peritonitis occurs in only 1 per cent of the cases.

DIAGNOSIS. The most prominent symptom of acute cholecystitis is severe abdominal pain. Initially, it may be characteristic of biliary colic, but soon it becomes a continuous pain in the right hypochondrium intensified by movement and respiration. One or two episodes of vomiting accompany the pain. Fever up to 101° or 102° F. regularly occurs and may be accompanied by chills. A history of previous symptoms of chronic cholecystitis is often obtained.

The physical findings consist of marked tenderness and rigidity in the right upper quadrant and epigastrium. A mass representing the gallbladder and adherent omentum is palpable in about one-fourth of the cases. Mild jaundice is common and is usually due to associated inflammation of the bile ducts and liver rather than to biliary obstruction.

Laboratory studies show a polymorphonuclear leukocytosis and often a mild elevation of serum bilirubin and alkaline phosphatase. The serum amylase level is commonly increased. Plain x-rays of the abdomen infrequently show a calculus. If cholecystography or cholangiography is attempted, the gallbladder does not visualize.

The differential diagnosis of acute cholecystitis involves a consideration of most acute abdominal diseases and some extra-abdominal disorders. These include pancreatitis, perforated peptic ulcer, appendicitis, strangulation obstruction of the intestines, mesenteric occlusion, pyelonephritis, salpingitis, acute hepatitis, myocardial infarction, acute congestive heart failure, and right lower lobe pneumonia. In elderly patients, symptoms and signs may not be well developed and diagnosis may be difficult.

TREATMENT. In the past, medical treatment of acute cholecystitis was commonly practiced. Approximately 60 to 75 per cent of patients respond to a medical regimen consisting of nasogastric suction, parenteral fluids and antibiotics, and are well within two to 14 days of the onset of the acute attack. Such patients are subjected to an elective cholecystectomy two to three months later. Failure to respond to medical treatment is an indication for an emergency operation and, because the patient is often seriously ill, simple drainage of the gallbladder may be the only safe procedure possible. A second operation for removal of the gallbladder must be done at a later time.

Because of the failure of medical therapy in a significant number of patients, the frequent necessity to perform a compromise operation in patients who do not respond, the requirement for two periods of hospitalization, the danger of perforation, and the fact that all patients must eventually undergo cholecystectomy, there has been a progressive shift toward early surgical treatment. Moreover, the mortality rate associated with early operation has been only slightly greater than that of elective cholecystectomy. For these reasons, early cholecystectomy has become the treatment of choice for acute cholecystitis in most patients. In elderly patients and diabetics, difficulty in judging the progress of the disease makes early surgical treatment imperative.

CHOLEDOCHOLITHIASIS

Calculi in the extrahepatic bile ducts almost always originate in the gallbladder, although infrequently, particularly after cholecystectomy, they may form in the biliary ducts. Between 10 and 20 per cent of patients with gallbladder stones develop choledocholithiasis. Although stones in the bile ducts may be silent, they usually produce biliary obstruction which is often incomplete and intermittent. In addition, they may be associated with bile duct infection and, if present for long periods, may be responsible for significant liver damage and occasionally for secondary biliary cirrhosis.

DIAGNOSIS. Choledocholithiasis in its classic form produces a syndrome of jaundice, biliary colic, and fever. However, in a substantial number of patients one or more symptoms of this triad are absent. Jaundice occurs in about 80 per cent of the patients and is characteristically fluctuating in nature. Progressive, relentless jaundice is unusual and suggests the presence of neoplastic obstruction rather than stones. The jaundice is accompanied by dark urine and light stools, but clay-colored stools lasting for a significant length of time do not usually occur. Biliary colic due to distention of the bile ducts is a common early symptom of choledocholithiasis. The pain is similar in nature and location to gallbladder colic and is often accompanied by restlessness, nausea and vomiting. Fever and chills occur in only one-third of the patients with bile duct stones. A past history of the dyspeptic symptoms of chronic cholecystitis is common.

Physical findings include tenderness and rigidity in the epigastrium and right hypochondrium in proportion to the existence and severity of infection. The liver is often palpable and tender if cholangitis is present. The gallbladder is usually not palpable, even in the presence of severe biliary obstruction. According to the autopsy studies of Courvoisier in the late nineteenth century, the gallbladder was normal and usually distended in obstructive jaundice due to neoplasm, but was seldom distended in obstructive jaundice due to calculi because of pre-existing cholecystitis and fibrosis. These observations have become known as Courvoisier's law.

The diagnosis of choledocholithiasis usually, although by no means invariably, involves the differential diagnosis of jaundice. The hyperbilirubinemia shows a predominance of conjugated bilirubin, there is bile in the urine, and if the obstruction is complete, urine and stool urobilinogen are decreased. Serum alkaline phosphatase is consistently elevated, even in the absence of jaundice. The enzyme, turbidity, and flocculation liver function tests are usually normal except in longstanding obstruction or if cholangitis is present. Intravenous cholangiography may show calculi, or dilatation of the common bile duct greater than 15 mm. if performed in the absence of marked jaundice.

The finding of crystals in the duodenal aspirate is suggestive of biliary stones.

In patients with jaundice, the most important diagnostic considerations include obstructive jaundice due to neoplasm, intrahepatic cholestasis, and regurgitation jaundice due to primary liver disease. Neoplastic obstruction of the bile ducts is usually complete and relentless, and occurs in a patient with debilitating manifestations of cancer and no history of dyspeptic symptoms; stone obstruction is usually incomplete and fluctuating. Intrahepatic cholestasis usually does not produce pain, a history of ingestion of one of the causative agents may be obtained, and a history of dyspeptic symptoms is usually absent. Jaundice due to hepatic cell damage is regularly associated with typical liver function test abnormalities and the absence of colicky pain. Infrequently, percutaneous transhepatic cholangiography may be required to differentiate these three forms of jaundice.

Other diagnostic possibilities, particularly in patients without jaundice, include renal or intestinal colic, acute porphyria, pancreatitis, myocardial infarct, acute congestive heart failure, acute hepatitis, and the numerous diseases which may produce acute abdominal pain.

TREATMENT. The treatment of choledocholithiasis involves surgical exploration of the common bile duct and removal of the calculi after preparation of the patient for operation, which may require parenteral vitamin K therapy. Usually, this is combined with treatment of the associated gallbladder disease by cholecystectomy. Occasionally, choledochotomy is required for newly formed or overlooked calculi in patients who have previously undergone a cholecystectomy.

In every operation on the gallbladder, the surgeon must decide whether or not to explore the common bile duct. Such explorations are not performed routinely because of the increased morbidity and slightly increased mortality associated with them. The indications for exploring the common bile duct as a supplement to cholecystectomy are palpable stone or mass in the common bile duct; dilatation of the common bile duct greater than 12 mm.; jaundice at the time of operation or in the patient's recent history; evidence of stones on operative cholangiogram; small stones in the gallbladder which are smaller in diameter than the diameter of the cystic duct, and a single faceted stone in the gallbladder.

In some instances, duodenotomy and division or partial resection of the sphincter of Oddi must be added to choledochotomy in order to remove stones impacted in the ampulla of Vater and relieve biliary obstruction. Following choledochotomy, most surgeons drain the common bile duct with a T-tube and perform direct cholangiography before terminating the operation and again seven to ten days postoperatively, prior to removing the T-tube, in order to be certain that biliary calculi have not been overlooked.

ACUTE SUPPURATIVE CHOLANGITIS. An acute and often fulminating suppurative inflammation of the bile ducts sometimes results from the combination of duct obstruction and infection, usually with gram-negative organisms. The obstruction is almost always due to cholelithiasis, although noninflammatory strictures and, rarely, neoplastic obstruction may be responsible. The clinical symptoms are characterized by jaundice, high fever, chills, right upper quadrant pain, hepatomegaly, liver tenderness, and marked leukocytosis. Marked systemic toxicity culminating in shock and prostration may develop. In addition to conjugated hyperbilirubinemia and increased serum alkaline phosphatase, elevations of the glutamic oxaloacetic transaminase and glutamic pyruvic transaminase may be pronounced. Positive blood cultures are often obtained. If surgical treatment is not prompt, multiple liver abscesses complicate the course.

ACQUIRED STRICTURES OF THE BILE DUCTS

Although strictures of the extrahepatic biliary ducts may be due to inflammation, the vast majority are caused by accidental injury during the course of operations on the biliary system, duodenum and stomach. The many and frequent variations in the anatomy of the bile ducts and blood supply to the liver and gallbladder are responsible for operative difficulties which occasionally lead to technical errors.

Biliary strictures are characterized by the clinical manifestations of obstructive jaundice, cholangitis, and liver damage. The jaundice almost always appears within six months of a biliary or gastroduodenal operation and usually fluctuates in severity according to the presence or absence of infection. The cholangitis is usually intermittent and produces attacks of fever, chills, continuous, dull pain in the right hypochondrium, tender hepatomegaly, and leukocytosis. In time, liver damage develops and if the stricture is not corrected the hepatic disorder progresses to biliary cirrhosis and portal hypertension. Hepatic failure, bleeding from esophageal varices and systemic infection are the usual causes of death.

Biliary strictures must be corrected surgically. If injury to the common bile duct is recognized during operation, as is seldom the case, a plastic reconstruction of the duct is usually not difficult. Once a stricture is established, operative correction of the obstruction can be a most demanding technical undertaking. End-to-end anastomosis of the common bile duct is done whenever possible. Other procedures include anastomosis of the proximal end of the bile duct to the duodenum or jejunum and, as a last resort, resection of part of the liver to locate an intrahepatic bile duct which is anastomosed to the jejunum. Approximately 70 per cent of bile duct strictures can be cured. Control of infection, support of the liver, and correction of prothrombin deficiency with parenteral vitamin K are integral aspects of therapy.

PRIMARY SCLEROSING CHOLANGITIS. This is a rare, diffuse, chronic inflammation of unknown etiology that involves the extrahepatic bile ducts. It is known also as stenosing cholangitis and fibrosing cholangitis. Some evidence suggests that it is a hypersensitivity disease. The condition is characterized by marked inflammatory thickening of the bile ducts with severe narrowing of the lumen. The clinical manifestations consist of obstructive jaundice, sometimes with associated chills and fever. The diagnosis has been made only by examination at operation. Treatment consists of prolonged T-tube drainage of the bile ducts or, if necessary, connection of the gallbladder to the intestine to bypass the obstructed common bile duct. Steroid therapy has been reported to have a beneficial influence on the disease. In several of the reported patients, sclerosing carcinoma of the bile ducts was discovered some time after the diagnosis of primary sclerosing cholangitis was made.

BILIARY NEOPLASMS

BENIGN NEOPLASMS. Benign neoplasms of the gallbladder and bile ducts are of little clinical significance and most of them are rare. The only relatively common benign tumors are the papilloma and adenomatous polyps of the gallbladder. These lesions are sometimes seen as radiolucent shadows in cholecystograms and may be confused with calculi. They produce no symptoms and are not of clinical importance.

CARCINOMA OF THE GALLBLADDER. Cancer of the gallbladder makes up about 5 per cent of all cancers and, therefore, is not a common neoplasm. It occurs in females three or four times more commonly than in males and its peak incidence is in the sixth decade of life. From 80 to 90 per cent of the patients have associated cholelithiasis. Adenocarcinoma is by far the most common histologic form; squamous cell carcinoma occurs rarely. The neoplasms spread most often by direct extension to the liver and by the lymphatics to the regional lymph nodes.

The early symptoms are those of the associated calculous cholecystitis. During this stage, the cancer may be discovered incidentally in a gallbladder removed because of inflammation and may be cured. Later, the symptoms include persistent right upper quadrant pain, weight loss, anorexia, nausea, and vomiting. Obstructive jaundice due to invasion of the bile ducts occurs in three-fourths of the patients. In about half the patients, a mass is palpable in the right subcostal area.

The prognosis of carcinoma of the gallbladder is very poor and the overall five-year survival rate is less than 5 per cent. Once the tumor produces symptoms there is almost no chance of cure. Treatment of localized lesions consists of cholecystectomy and resection of the adjacent liver. The mean survival time after discovery of gallbladder cancer is less than six months.

The incidence of cancer in patients with gallstones has been reported to range from 0.7 to 5 per cent. Although not high, this frequency, when combined with the incidence of other complications of cholelithiasis, provides support for the argument that patients with silent stones should have the gallbladder removed.

CARCINOMA OF THE BILE DUCTS. Cancers of the extrahepatic bile ducts are uncommon lesions. Although carcinoma of the ampulla of Vater, more accurately the papilla of Vater, may arise from biliary epithelium, most surgeons believe that it more commonly arises from the duodenal mucosa. Bile duct carcinoma is associated with cholelithiasis in about one-third of the cases and occurs in males more frequently than in females. The neoplasm spreads mainly by extension along the bile ducts, by direct extension into the liver, and by lymphatic invasion to the regional lymph nodes. It produces clinical symptoms characterized by progressive, relentless obstructive jaundice with bile in the urine, clay-colored stools and pruritus. Pain of a continuous, dull nature in the right hypochondrium occurs in two-thirds of the patients. Weight loss and cachexia are frequent. Cholangitis with fever and chills is found in one-fourth of the patients. Hepatomegaly is found in most patients and a distended gallbladder is palpable in about one-half.

The cure rate of bile duct carcinoma, excluding cancer of the ampulla of Vater, is less than 1 per cent. The lesion can be resected only rarely.

CONGENITAL ANOMALIES

Numerous congenital anomalies of the extrahepatic biliary system have been recorded, but only two types are of clinical significance. These are the choledochal cyst and atresia of the bile ducts.

CHOLEDOCHAL CYST. This unusual lesion is a localized cystic dilatation of the common bile duct which usually produces symptoms at some time during the first two decades of life (Fig. 19). The manifestations are often intermittent and are due to filling of the cyst with fluid and resultant compression of the remaining common bile duct. The characteristic clinical symptoms consist of episodes of upper abdominal colicky pain, obstructive jaundice and the development of a palpable mass in the right hypochondrium. The mass can become quite large and often can be shown by barium contrast upper gastrointestinal x-rays to displace the duodenum. Occasionally, persistent jaundice early in life occurs and makes differentiation from biliary atresia difficult. The treatment is surgical and consists of connecting the cyst to the duodenum or jejunum. The results of operative therapy are good.

ATRESIA OF THE BILE DUCTS. During early embryonic life the gallbladder and bile ducts are represented by solid cords. Failure of the cords to canalize leads to atresia of part or all of the biliary system. In the majority of instances the atresia involves the extrahepatic ducts or the intrahepatic ducts and is not amenable to surgical therapy. However, in 10 to 20 per cent of the patients only the distal common bile duct is atretic and correction may be accomplished by connecting the gallbladder or proximal common bile duct to the duodenum or jejunum. The types of biliary atresia are shown in Figure 20.

Biliary atresia causes progressive relentless jaundice beginning a few days after birth. The stools are acholic. In time, the liver

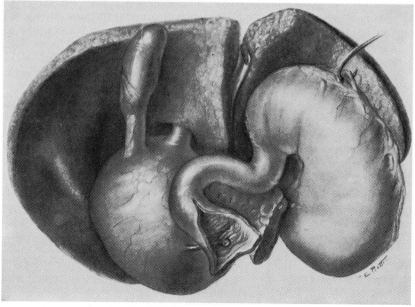

Figure 19. Choledochal cyst. (From Gross, R. E.: The Surgery of Infancy and Childhood. Philadelphia, W. B. Saunders Company, 1953.)

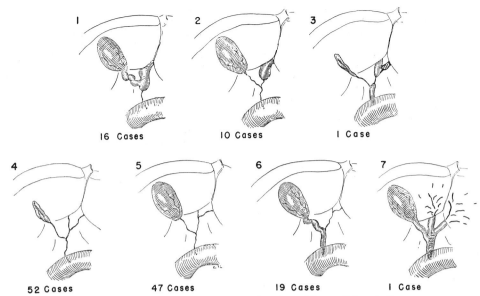

16 Cases   IO Cases   I Case

52 Cases   47 Cases   19 Cases   I Case

Figure 20. Types of biliary atresia encountered by Gross in 146 patients. The conditions in the upper row are surgically correctable; those in the lower row are inoperable. (From Gross, R. E.: The Surgery of Infancy and Childhood. Philadelphia, W. B. Saunders Company, 1953.)

enlarges and develops biliary cirrhosis. The condition is infrequently compatible with more than a year or two of life. Death often is due to hepatic failure, varix hemorrhage, or malnutrition.

The differential diagnosis is usually not difficult because of the progressive, obstructive nature of the jaundice. Physiologic jaundice of the newborn, neonatal hepatitis, and erythroblastosis fetalis must be ruled out early in the course.

All patients with biliary atresia should undergo laparotomy in the hope of finding a correctable lesion. Exploratory operation should be performed before the third month of life to avoid irreversible liver damage.

READING REFERENCES

Alonso-Lej, F., Rever, W. B., Jr., and Pessagno, D. J.: Congenital choledochal cyst, with a report of 2, and an analysis of 94 cases. Surg. Gyn. & Obst. *108*:1, 1959.

Atik, M., and Simeone, F.: Massive gastrointestinal bleeding: a study of 296 patients at City Hospital of Cleveland. A.M.A. Arch. Surg. *69*:355, 1954.

Baker, L. A., Smith, C., and Lieberman, G.: The natural history of esophageal varices. Am. J. Med. *26*:228, 1959.

Bartlett, M. K., and Waddell, W. R.: Indications for common duct exploration. New England J. Med. *258*:164, 1958.

Cattell, R. B., and Braasch, J. W.: Primary repair of benign strictures of the bile duct. Surg. Gyn. & Obst. *109*:531, 1959.

Child, C. G., III.: The Liver and Portal Hypertension. Philadelphia, W. B. Saunders Company, 1964.

Child, C. G., III.: The Shattuck Lecture: The portal circulation. New England J. Med. *252*:837, 1955.

Clarke, J. S., Ozeran, P. S., Hart, J. C., Cruze, K., and Crevling, V.: Peptic ulcer following portacaval shunt. Ann. Surg. *148*:551, 1958.

Clatworthy, H. W., Jr., and Boles, E. T., Jr.: Extrahepatic portal bed block in children: pathogenesis and treatment. Ann. Surg. *150*:371, 1959.

Colcock, B. P., and Liddle, H. V.: Common-bile-duct stones. New England J. Med. *258*:264, 1958.

Colcock, B. P., and Perez, B.: The treatment of cholelithiasis. Surg. Gyn. & Obst. *117*:529, 1963.

Conn, H. O.: Hazards attending the use of esophageal tamponade. New England J. Med. *259*:701, 1958.

Conn, H. O., and Lindenmuth, W. W.: Prophylactic portacaval anastomosis in cirrhotic patients with esophageal varices. New England J. Med. *266*:743, 1962.

Conn, H. O., Mitchell, J. R., and Brodoff, M. G.: A comparison of the radiologic and esophagoscopic diagnosis of esophageal varices. New England J. Med. *265*:160, 1961.

Cronin, K.: Pyogenic abscess of the liver. Gut *2*:53, 1961.

Crosthwait, R. W., Allen, J. E., Murga, F., Beall, A. C., Jr., and DeBakey, M. E.: The surgical management of 640 consecutive liver injuries in civilian practice. Surg. Gyn. & Obst. *114*:650, 1962.

DeBakey, M. E., and Ochsner, A.: Hepatic amebiasis; a twenty year experience and analysis of 263 cases. Surg. Gyn. & Obst. *92*:209, 1951.

Ekman, C. A.: Portal hypertension. Acta Chir. Scandinav. *113*:1, 1957.

Ekman, C. A., and Sandblom, P.: Shunt operation in acute bleeding from esophageal varices. Ann. Surg. *160*:531, 1964.

Fenster, L. F., and Klatskin, G.: Manifestations of metastatic tumors of the liver; a study of 81 patients subjected to needle biopsy. Am. J. Med. *31*:238, 1961.

Garceau, A. J., and the Boston Inter-Hospital Liver Group: The natural history of cirrhosis. I. Survival with esophageal varices. New England J. Med. *268*:469, 1963.

Garceau, A. J., and the Boston Inter-Hospital Liver Group: Controlled trial of prophylactic portacaval shunt surgery. New England J. Med. *270*:496, 1964.

Gerst, P. H.: Primary carcinoma of the gallbladder. A thirty year summary. Ann. Surg. *153*:369, 1961.

Glenn, F., and Mannix, H., Jr.: Biliary enteric fistula. Surg. Gyn. & Obst. *105*:693, 1957.

Glenn, F., and Moody, F. G.: Acute obstructive suppurative cholangitis. Surg. Gyn. & Obst. *113*:265, 1961.

Glenn, F., and Thorbjarnarson, B.: The surgical treatment of acute cholecystitis. Surg. Gyn. & Obst. *116*:61, 1963.

Glenn, F., and Whitsell, J. C., II: Primary sclerosing cholangitis. Surg. Gyn. & Obst. *123*:1037, 1966.

Hunt, A. H.: A Contribution to the Study of Portal Hypertension. London, E. & S. Livingstone, Ltd., 1958.

Hyatt, R. E., and Smith, J. R.: The mechanism of ascites. Am. J. Med. *16*:434, 1954.

Juniper, K. L., Jr.: Physicochemical characteristics of bile and their relation to gallstone formation. Am. J. Med. *39*:98, 1965.

Katz, A. M., and Pan, C.: Echinococcus disease in the United States. Am. J. Med. *25*:759, 1958.

Krovetz, L. J.: Congenital biliary atresia. Surgery *47*:453, 1960.

Kuwayti, K., Baggenstoss, A. H., Stauffer, M. H., and Priestly, J. T.: Carcinoma of the major intrahepatic and the extrahepatic bile ducts exclusive of the papilla of Vater. Surg. Gyn. & Obst. *104*:357, 1957.

Lamont, N. McE., and Pooler, N. R.: Hepatic amebiasis: a study of 250 cases. Quart. J. Med. *27*:389, 1958.

Lester, R., and Schmid, R.: Bilirubin metabolism. New England J. Med. *270*:779, 1964.

Liebowitz, H. R.: Bleeding Esophageal Varices: Portal Hypertension. Springfield, Illinois, Charles C Thomas, 1959.

Longmire, W. P., Jr.: Congenital biliary hypoplasia. Ann. Surg. *159*:335, 1964.

Lund, J.: Surgical indications in cholelithiasis: prophylactic cholecystectomy elucidated on the basis of longterm follow up on 526 nonoperated cases. Ann. Surg. *151*:153, 1960.

MacDonald, R. A.: Primary carcinoma of the liver: a clinicopathologic study of 108 cases. Arch. Int. Med. *99*:266, 1957.

Madden, J. L., Lore, J. M., Jr., Gerold, F. P., and Ravid, J. M.: The pathogenesis of ascites and a consideration of its treatment. Surg. Gyn. & Obst. *99*:385, 1954.

McDermott, W. V., Jr.: Metabolism and toxicity of ammonia. New England J. Med. *257*:1076, 1957.

McDermott, W. V., Palozzi, H., Nardi, G. L., and Mondet, A.: Elective portal systemic shunt. New England J. Med. *264*:419, 1961.

Merigan, T. C., Plotkin, G. R., and Davidson, C. S.: Effect of intravenously administered posterior pituitary extract on hemorrhage from bleeding varices. New England J. Med. *266*:134, 1962.

Mikkelsen, W. P.: Emergency portacaval shunt. Rev. Surg. *19*:141, 1962.

Mikkelsen, W. P., Turrill, F. R., and Pattison, A. C.: Portacaval shunt in cirrhosis of the liver. Clinical and hemodynamic aspects. Am. J. Surg. *104*:204, 1962.

Nachlas, M. M., O'Neil, J. E., and Campbell, A. J. A.: The life history of patients with cirrhosis of the liver and bleeding esophageal varices. Ann. Surg. *141*:10, 1955.

Nagler, W., Bender, M. A., and Blau, M.: Radioisotope photoscanning of the liver. Gastroenterology *44*:36, 1963.

Orloff, M. J.: A comparative study of emergency transesophageal ligation and nonsurgical treatment of bleeding esophageal varices in unselected patients with cirrhosis. Surgery *52*:103, 1962.

Orloff, M. J.: Effect of side-to-side portacaval shunt on intractable ascites, sodium excretion, and aldosterone metabolism in man. Am. J. Surg. *112*:287, 1966.

Orloff, M. J.: Emergency portacaval shunt: a comparative study of shunt, varix ligation and nonsurgical treatment of bleeding esophageal varices in unselected patients with cirrhosis. Ann. Surg. *166*:456, 1967.

Orloff, M. J.: Emergency treatment of bleeding esophageal varices in cirrhosis. *In*, Longmire, W. P., Jr. (ed.): Portal Hypertension. Current Problems in Surgery. Chicago, Year Book Medical Publishers, Inc., July, 1966.

Orloff, M. J.: Surgical treatment of intractable cirrhotic ascites. *In*, Longmire, W. P., Jr. (ed): Portal hypertension. Current Problems in Surgery. Chicago, Year Book Medical Publishers, Inc., July, 1966.

Orloff, M. J., Halasz, N. A., Lipman, C., Schwabe, A. D., Thompson, J. C., and Weidner, W. A.: The complications of cirrhosis of the liver. Ann. Int. Med. *66*:165, 1967.

Orloff, M. J., and Thomas, H. S.: Pathogenesis of esophageal varix rupture: a study based on gross and microscopic examination of the esophagus at the time of bleeding. Arch. Surg. *87*:301, 1963.

Orloff, M. J., and Windsor, C. W. O.: Effect of portacaval shunt on gastric acid secretion in dogs with liver disease, portal hypertension and massive ascites. Ann. Surg. *164*:69, 1966.

Pack, G. T., and Islami, A. H.: Surgical treatment of tumors of the liver. *In*, Treatment of Cancer and Allied Diseases. New York, Paul B. Hoeber, Inc., 1962.

Panke, W. F., Bradley, E. G., Moreno, A. H., Ruzicka, F. F., and Rousselot, L. M.: Technique, hazards and usefulness of percutaneous splenic portography. J.A.M.A. *169*:1032, 1959.

Panke, W. F., Rousselot, L. M., and Moreno, A. H.: Splenic pulp manometry in the differential diagnosis of acute upper gastrointestinal bleeding. Surg. Gyn. & Obst. *109*:270, 1959.

Parker, R. G. F.: Occlusion of the hepatic veins in man. Medicine *38*:369, 1959.

Pines, B., and Rabinovitch, J.: Perforation of the gallbladder in acute cholecystitis. Ann. Surg. *140*:170, 1959.

Popper, H., and Schaffner, F.: Progress in Liver Disease. New York, Grune and Stratton, Inc., Volume I, 1963, Volume II, 1965.

Popper, H., and Schaffner, F.: Liver: Structure and Function, New York, McGraw-Hill Book Company, 1957.

Rains, A. J. H.: Researches concerning the formation of gallstones. Brit. Med. J. *2*:685, 1962.

Ratnoff, O. D., and Patek, A. J., Jr.: Natural history of Laennec's cirrhosis of the liver: analysis of 386 cases. Medicine *21*:207, 1942.

Ravdin, I. S., Fitz-Hugh, T., Jr., Wolferth, C. C., Barbieri, E. A., and Ravdin, R. G.: Relation of gallstone disease to angina pectoris. Arch. Surg. *70*:333, 1955.

Reynolds, T. B., Redeker, A. G., and Geller, H. M.: Wedged hepatic venous pressure; a clinical evaluation. Am. J. Med. *22*:341, 1957.

Rousselot, L. M., Gilbertson, F. E., and Panke, W. F.: Severe hemorrhage from esophagogastric varices. Its emergency management with particular reference to portacaval anastomosis. New England J. Med. *262*:269, 1960.

Sherlock, S.: Diseases of the Liver, 3rd ed. Philadelphia, F. A. Davis Company, 1963.

Sherlock, S.: Jaundice. Brit. Med. J. *1*:1359, 1962.

Sherlock, S.: Needle biopsy of the liver; a review. J. Clin. Path. *15*:291, 1962.

Sherlock, S., and Shaldon, S.: The aetiology and management of ascites in patients with hepatic cirrhosis. A review. Gut *4*:95, 1963.

Smith, R. B., III, Conklin, E. F., and Porter, M. R.: A five year study of choledocholithiasis. Surg. Gyn. & Obst. *116*:731, 1965.

Snell, A. M.: Liver function tests and their interpretation. Gastroenterology *34*:675, 1958.

Sparkman, R. S., and Fogelman, M. J.: Wounds of the liver. Review of 100 cases. Ann. Surg. *139*:690, 1954.

Strohl, E. R., Diffenbaugh, W. G., Baker, J. H., and Cheema, M. H.: Gangrene and perforation of the gallbladder. Surg. Gyn. & Obst. *114*:1, 1962.

Thorbjarnarson, B., Mujahed, Z., and Glenn, F.: Percutaneous transhepatic cholangiography. Ann. Surg. *165*:33, 1967.

Vorhees, A. B., Jr., Harris, R. C., Britton, R. C., Price, J. B., and Santulli, T. V.: Portal hypertension in children: 98 cases. Surgery *58*:540, 1965.

Walters, W., Nixon, J. W., Jr., Hodgins, T. E., and Ramsdell, J. A.: Strictures of the common and hepatic bile ducts. Arch. Surg. *78*:908, 1959.

Wantz, G. E., and Payne, M. A.: Experience with portacaval

shunt for portal hypertension. New England J. Med. 265:721, 1961.

Warren, W. D., and Muller, W. H.: Clarification of some hemodynamic changes in cirrhosis and their surgical significance. Ann. Surg. 150:413, 1959.

Warren, K. W., Athanassiades, S., and Monge, J. I.: Primary sclerosing cholangitis. Am. J. Surg. 111:23, 1966.

Warren, K. W., and McDonald, W. M.: Facts and fiction regarding strictures of the extrahepatic bile ducts. Ann. Surg. 159:996, 1964.

Welch, C. E.: Cholecystectomy for acute cholecystitis. Surgery 49:284, 1961.

Welch, C. S., Welch, H. F., and Carter, J. H.: The treatment of ascites by side-to-side portacaval shunt. Ann. Surg. 150:428, 1959.

Werther, J. L., and Korelitz, B. I.: Chlorpromazine jaundice: analysis of twenty-two cases. Am. J. Med. 22: 351, 1957.

West, J. T., Hillman, F. J., and Rausch, R. L.: Alveolar hydatid disease of the liver: rationale and techniques of surgical treatment. Ann. Surg. 157:548, 1963.

Wright, P. W., and Orloff, M. J.: Traumatic hemobilia. Ann. Surg. 160:42, 1964.

Chapter 25

THE PANCREAS

by
EDWIN H. ELLISON, M.D.
and
LARRY C. CAREY, M.D.

EDWIN HOMER ELLISON is an Ohioan by birth and education through elementary school, high school, college, medical school and surgical education and training. When he left Ohio to become Professor and Chairman of the Department of Surgery at Marquette School of Medicine, he did not break his long established ties with the Midwest. He completed nearly all of the requirements for his doctorate in biochemistry before his interest turned to medicine. He also held faculty rank in the Department of Anatomy. He completed his surgical education and training following service in the Army in World War II. His early leanings toward biochemistry and anatomy have been reflected in his investigations of the problems of malnutrition, electrolyte imbalance and blood volume in surgical patients. His studies of the etiology and treatment of pancreatitis with relation to the endocrine glands and recurrent intractable gastric ulceration continue to add important contributions to the surgical literature.

LARRY CAMPBELL CAREY was born in Coal Grove, Ohio, a town of 2000 inhabitants in the southern tip of Ohio on the Ohio River. He went north to Columbus for his high school, college and medical education. He took an active part in surgical research as a medical student and continued this interest in the residency education and training surgical program at Marquette School of Medicine, where he is an Assistant Professor of Surgery.

ANATOMY

The pancreas lies retroperitoneally in a transverse position across the upper abdomen. It is approximately 25 cm. long, weighs approximately 120 gm. and is arbitrarily divided into head, neck, body, tail and uncinate process. The latter is an inferior projection from the head. The head of the pancreas overlies the vena cava at the level of the second lumbar vertebra and, in addition, its posterior surface is related to the right kidney, renal vein and adrenal gland. The lateral aspect of the head of the pancreas is closely applied to the medial aspect of the duodenal loop.

The common bile duct enters the superior aspect and traverses the head of the pancreas near its posterior surface to enter the second portion of the duodenum. It has long been thought that the intrapancreatic portion of the common duct was surgically unapproachable. Autopsy studies, however, indicate that this portion of the common duct

is easily exposed by a posterolateral approach in 85 per cent of the specimens studied.

At the junction between the head and body of the pancreas, the uncinate process extends inferiorly and its lateral tip lies posterior to the superior mesenteric artery and vein. As these structures course cephalad, they go posterior to the neck of the gland. It is in this area that the portal vein originates from the confluence of the superior mesenteric and splenic veins. The splenic vein courses along the posterior aspect of the body and tail of the gland, a relationship which has occasionally resulted in splenic vein thrombosis as a sequel to pancreatitis.

The arterial blood supply to the pancreas arises from the celiac and superior mesenteric arteries (Fig. 1). The anterior and posterior pancreaticoduodenal arteries provide the blood supply to the head of the gland. The dorsal pancreatic artery has an inconstant origin and supplies the cephalad posterior portion of the neck and body. Branches from the splenic artery identified as caudal

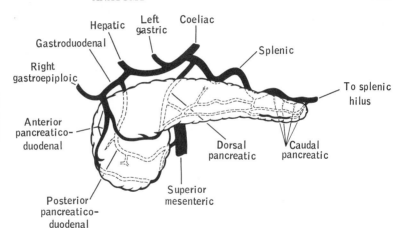

Figure 1. Diagrammatic representation of the extensive arterial blood supply to the pancreas, which arises primarily from branches of the gastroduodenal, splenic and superior mesenteric arteries.

pancreatic arteries are numerous. The venous drainage corresponds to the arterial supply and ultimately empties into the portal circulation.

Thoracic duct pressure and the enzyme content of the thoracic duct lymph are elevated in inflammatory disease of the pancreas. It has been theorized that lymphatic obstruction may be an etiologic factor in chronic pancreatitis, and suggested that direct lymphatic connections between the pancreas and the thoracic duct may be the transport route for insulin, rather than direct vascular absorption. In experimental pancreatitis, red blood cells greatly increase in thoracic duct lymph. As the red cell concentration increases, lymph flow slows and then stops. It has been postulated that the congestion of the lymphatic drainage contributes to the fluid loss in pancreatitis.

The regional lymphatic drainage of the superior pancreas is to the subpyloric nodes, to the nodes of the hepatic artery, the splenic hilum and to the phrenicolienal ligament. Inferiorly, the lymph drains into the superior mesenteric and periaortic nodes.

No portion of pancreatic anatomy has received more attention than the ductal system, which drains the exocrine secretions into the intestinal tract. In 1903, Opie suggested that a common channel shared by the pancreatic and common bile duct might allow bile to reflux into the pancreatic duct and cause pancreatitis. Many studies have been performed in an attempt to establish the incidence of this common channel. A common channel has been reported present in 70 to 80 per cent of all patients at postmortem examination, and in 7 to 30 per cent it exceeded 0.5 cm. in length.

Numerous variations occur in the size and connections of the accessory duct of Santorini, and the major duct of Wirsung. In the majority of reported dissections, Santorini's duct was smaller than the duct of Wirsung and drained the superior portion of the head of the pancreas both into the major duct and into the duodenum (Fig. 2). A recent study indicates that Santorini's duct is obliterated and absent in the majority of instances. This is important, since it is injury to the accessory duct that leads to pancreatic fistula formation following dissection of a posterior penetrating duodenal ulcer. There are two areas of narrowing in the ductal system: one is at the junction of the ducts of Wirsung and Santorini, and the other is found where the pancreas crosses the superior mesenteric vessels.

The mechanism of sphincter action controlling the pancreatic ductal orifice is unknown. Dissection of the sphincter of the pancreatic duct in primates has suggested that the pancreatic and biliary duct sphincters must work in unison.

The pancreas receives both sympathetic and parasympathetic innervation, the former from the greater and lesser splanchnic nerves, principally the greater. The parasympathetic fibers from the vagus are dispersed between the acini and supply both exocrine and endocrine components of the gland. Galvanic stimulation of the pancreas of patients through electrodes implanted at the time of laparotomy has provided information about the localization of pancreatic pain (Fig. 3). Pain arising from the head of the pancreas alone was always referred to the right of the midline; stimulation of the body of the pancreas resulted in epigastric pain and stimulation of the tail of the pancreas

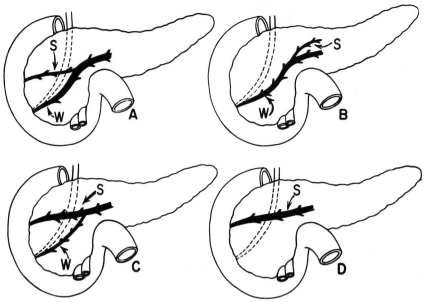

Figure 2. Diagrammatic illustration of several variations in the size and connections of the main duct of Wirsung (W) and the accessory duct of Santorini (S). *A*, The arrangement reported in the majority of dissections. *B*, Santorini's duct draining the midportion of the gland and connecting directly into the duct of Wirsung. *C* and *D*, The duct of Santorini as the major pancreatic duct. *D*, Although relatively rare, obliteration of the duct of Wirsung gives the surgeon great difficulty when attempting to catheterize the pancreatic duct preliminary to a pancreatogram following sphincterotomy.

produced pain in the entire left abdomen. Diffuse pancreatic stimulation resulted in the classic bandlike pain of acute pancreatitis across the upper abdomen, which often radiated to the upper lumbar region. Clinical experience in this study indicated that right splanchnic block alone often relieved the pain of acute pancreatitis. This suggested that the right splanchnic nerve be blocked first in attempts at pain relief, and supports previous experimental studies on animals, which indicated that visceral pain impulses are carried in the right splanchnic trunk.

MICROSCOPIC ANATOMY. The pancreas has exocrine and endocrine functional components. The exocrine portion is a racemose gland similar to the salivary glands. It is made up of oval acini grouped into lobules

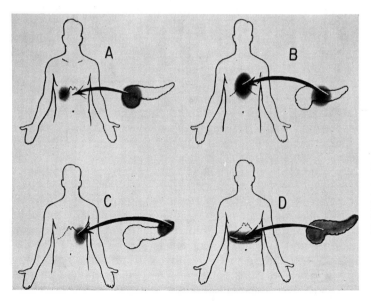

Figure 3. Sites of pain referral on galvanic stimulation of the various portions of the pancreas. *A*, Stimulation of the head of the pancreas resulted in pain to the right of the midline. *B*, Epigastric pain followed stimulation of the body of the pancreas. *C*, Pain was noted left of the midline when the tail of the pancreas was stimulated. *D*, Diffuse stimulation led to the classic bandlike pain across the upper abdomen, frequently seen in acute pancreatitis.

which are separated by connective tissue septa. The acini are composed of blunted pyramidal cells with the blunt end toward the lumen and the broad end resting on a well-defined basement membrane. The nuclei are oval and basally located. The luminal portion of the cytoplasm contains secretory granules, while the basilar aspect of the cytoplasm is granule-free. The larger ducts are lined with columnar epithelium which becomes progressively flattened to a single layer of low cuboidal epithelium toward the acini. The larger ducts contain elastic and fibrous connective tissue but no muscle.

The endocrine portion of the pancreas is composed of at least three separate cell

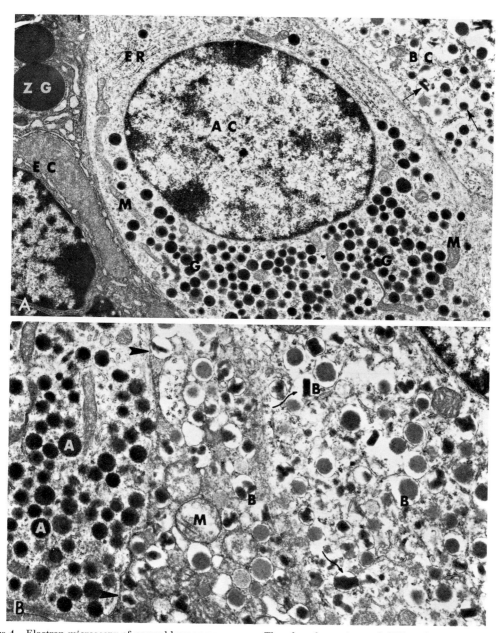

Figure 4. Electron microscopy of normal human pancreas. *a*, The edge of an acinar cell (EC) with zymogen granules (ZG). An alpha cell (AC) with characteristic cytoplasmic granules (G), endoplasmic reticulum (ER), and mitochondria (M). A segment of a beta cell (BC) shows cytoplasmic granules (arrow) with irregular contours. × 12,000. *B*, Higher magnification of adjacent alpha and beta cells demonstrating differences in cytoplasmic granules. Alpha granules (A) consist of a round, electron-dense core separated from a limiting membrane by a less opaque zone. Beta granules (B) have one to several less dense cores which may be angular or round. A clear area (arrow) is present between the limiting membrane and central core. Cell border (arrow head). × 18,000.

types: alpha cells which produce glucagon, a hyperglycemic factor; beta cells which produce insulin; and delta cells to which a function has not been ascribed. These cells are clumped between the acini into the islets of Langerhans, of which there are between 200,000 and 2,000,000. The tail and distal body of the pancreas contain more islets than the head. This fact is of value when searching for an occult islet cell tumor, and makes biopsy or amputation of the distal pancreas likely to be more fruitful in establishing a diagnosis.

Electron microscopy of the normal human pancreas has been performed. Characteristics of exocrine as well as endocrine cells have been established. The pancreatic islet cells can be identified and separated into alpha and beta cells. The cells are characterized by specific kinds of cytoplasmic granules. Those of the alpha cells are round with thin membranes. Beta cells have irregular, angular granules (Fig. 4).

Benign ulcerogenic tumors have granules typical of alpha cells. The malignant tumors are less characteristic but are most like alpha cells. In the malignant tumors, lipoidal bodies and nuclear inclusions have been observed in the acinar cells. The significance of this observation is not clear.

EMBRYOLOGY. The pancreas begins as two separate structures which appear as a dorsal and ventral entodermal pouch from the primitive foregut. They are first discernible between the third and fourth week of intrauterine life. The dorsal portion grows more rapidly and soon develops a longitudinal duct, which becomes the duct of Santorini. The ventral pancreas also has a duct, that of Wirsung. As growth progresses, the ventral pancreas rotates posteriorly, and the movement of the duodenum to the right brings the two primordia into juxtaposition. At about the seventh week, these primordia and their ducts fuse, resulting in the several ductal arrangements.

CONGENITAL ANOMALIES. There are a number of anomalies of the pancreas which are of clinical importance. These include annular and ectopic pancreas and, possibly, cystic fibrosis. The fundamental etiology of these anomalies is not known. It is generally believed that incomplete rotation of the ventral pancreas results in an annular pancreas, which is a band of pancreatic tissue surrounding the duodenum. This anomaly may manifest itself in the newborn by obstruction

of the duodenum and may result in polyhydramnios. The duodenal lumen is quite small and has been thought by some to be atretic. However, if incomplete rotation is the etiologic factor, then the duodenal lumen would not exceed the size of the six- to eight-week embryo and would certainly appear atretic. These infants vomit bile-stained material during the first days of life. A diagnosis of duodenal obstruction is made by the finding of a "double bubble" on roentgenograms of the abdomen, which results from a greatly dilated duodenum and stomach (Fig. 5).

Transection of an annular pancreas in the child is to be avoided since obstruction will not be relieved if the duodenal lumen is atretic. Pancreatitis, cyst formation or fistulization may result if drainage from a segment of still functioning pancreatic tis-

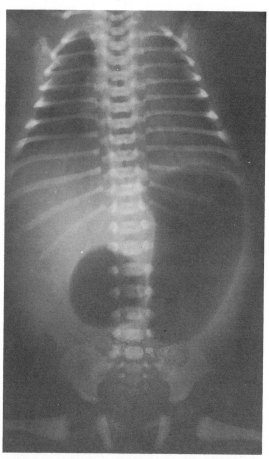

Figure 5. X-ray of a newborn infant with duodenal atresia demonstrating a collection of air in distended stomach and first portion of duodenum forming a "double bubble." Note complete absence of air in bowel distal to atresia.

sue is disturbed. Reported experiences indicate that the symptomatology in the adult occurs frequently from an associated duodenal or gastric ulcer resulting from the partial long-term duodenal obstruction and antral stasis with excessive production of gastrin. The roentgenographic findings are characteristic, and antral drainage by means of a gastroenterostomy is usually sufficient. However, complementary vagotomy should be considered if the patient is known to secrete excessive amounts of hydrochloric acid.

Pancreatic heterotopia is another anomaly which is rather common. While ectopic pancreas may be found in many locations, it is most frequently seen in the wall of the stomach, duodenum or small bowel, and rarely in a Meckel's diverticulum. It is subject to the same disease processes as the normal pancreas. Symptomatology is frequently related to obstruction dependent upon location.

In seven patients, ectopic pancreas was present in the stomach in two. In another, the cystic duct was narrowed; in two others, an ulcerogenic tumor developed in heterotopic pancreas found in the wall of the duodenum. In three patients, aberrant pancreas was located in the upper jejunum. Pancreatitis was present in one of these patients and resection led to relief of unexplained abdominal pain (Fig. 6).

Although perhaps not a true anomaly, cystic fibrosis of the pancreas may result in meconium ileus, a situation necessitating surgical intervention in the newborn. Because of the deficiency of proteolytic enzymes from the pancreas, the meconium fails to liquefy, resulting in a thick, tenacious, ropy

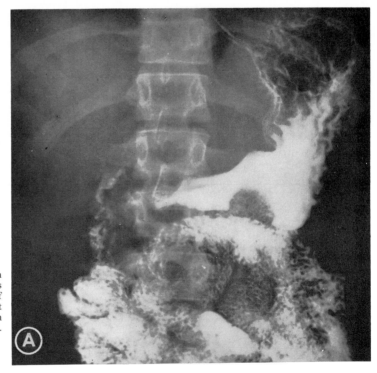

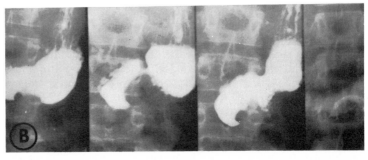

Figure 6. *A*, Typical round, smooth filling defect of an aberrant pancreas occurring on the greater curvature of the stomach. *B*, Fluoroscopy and spot films of the antrum demonstrate an umbilication at the site of a central duct.

material which cannot be propelled through the gastrointestinal tract. The afflicted newborn presents a distended abdomen, fails to pass meconium and may have bile-stained vomitus. It is reported that 7 per cent of all patients with cystic fibrosis have this syndrome, which accounts for 7 to 15 per cent of all intestinal obstruction in the newborn. Roentgenograms of the abdomen are characteristic in one-half the patients, showing a variety of dilated loops containing a homogeneous substance giving a "ground glass" appearance. In the remaining 50 per cent, only small bowel obstruction is found by x-ray examination. If intraperitoneal flecks of calcium are visible, intrauterine meconium peritonitis should be considered. A barium enema should be done on all these infants to eliminate the possibility of congenital megacolon. The surgical management includes construction of a double-barreled ileostomy, permitting irrigations with 1 per cent hydrogen peroxide and pancreatic enzymes to liquefy the meconium.

PHYSIOLOGY

The inaccessible location of the pancreas has made study of pancreatic physiology very difficult. The pancreatic ducts cannot be cannulated as readily as the stomach or intestine. Studies of pancreatic cellular function are not as easily obtained as those of the liver. Fear of precipitating pancreatitis has greatly inhibited more vigorous efforts at exploration. Most of the knowledge of pancreatic function is from research in the canine, whose pancreatic function may be greatly different from man. A few very patient and thoughtful investigators, using tedious and time-consuming methods, have provided information regarding human pancreatic function. These studies have been performed with tubes passed into the duodenum. They are gross at best, but at the moment they provide all the known data about human pancreatic function, the exception being the few studies on patients with pancreatic fistulae.

The pancreas performs both endocrine and exocrine functions. Its endocrine function is primarily the production of insulin by the beta cells of the islets of Langerhans. Other cells in the islets, such as the alpha cells which are thought to produce glucagon, have also been incriminated as the cell type in ulcerogenic tumors of the pancreas.

The exocrine function of the pancreas is very critical. As studies proceed, it is appreciated that the exocrine function is exceedingly complex. At least nine different enzymes are produced in the pancreas. The gland has a great capacity to synthesize protein. Through this protein synthesis, pancreatic enzymes are produced. Care must be taken in patients with pancreatic fistulae to replace the large protein losses. The enzymes of the pancreas have been shown to have the same characteristics as the zymogen granules in acinar cells.

In addition to protein, pancreatic juice is rich in electrolytes. The sodium and potassium contents are equal to plasma, but the bicarbonate content is much higher. It is tempting to give teleological significance to the high bicarbonate content of pancreatic juice, first, to provide the alkaline milieu where enzymes are most active and second, to provide protection of the duodenum by neutralizing the acid chyme from the stomach.

There are both neural and humoral stimuli to pancreatic secretion. The neural stimulation comes from the vagus. Section of the vagus nerves does not appear to have a lasting effect on pancreatic secretion and it is likely that local parasympathetic nerves become effective after vagotomy.

There are now three hormones known to stimulate pancreatic secretion. Secretin, the first substance to be recognized as a hormone, is produced by the duodenal mucosa. The stimulus to its production is a pH in the duodenum of 4.5 or lower. Secretin acts on the pancreas, probably on the ductal epithelium primarily, to cause the outpouring of voluminous thin, watery fluid rich in bicarbonate and poor in enzyme content. Pancreozymin, also produced by the duodenal mucosa and possibly the jejunum and antrum, acts differently. Pancreozymin production is stimulated by the presence of food and affects the acinar cells. From the stimulus, they empty their zymogen granules and the resulting pancreatic juice is rich in enzymes, low in volume, and quite viscous.

Gastrin, the potent stimulus to gastric acid production, has been found to stimulate pancreatic secretion. The hormone can be separated into two fractions: gastrin I and gastrin II. They both have an effect on the pancreas, causing the production of a protein-rich fluid. This observation is relatively recent and not clarified in great detail.

The mechanism of pancreatic ductal

sphincter function is unclear. In dissections in primates, the sphincters of the pancreatic and common bile ducts are intimately related. Cholecystokinin has been found to relax both sphincters. All narcotics tend to increase ductal sphincter tone. Meperidine is the narcotic of choice, because its effect is less than that of morphine. Right splanchnic block successfully relieves pain in pancreatitis and has no tendency to increase ductal pressure. This procedure has been found helpful in controlling pain in acute pancreatitis.

Kanamycin, oleandomycin, sulfonamides, and streptomycin are secreted in pancreatic juice. One or more of these drugs should be given prior to closure of a pancreatic fistula. In acute pancreatitis, blood levels, not pancreatic levels, of antibiotics are important. In most instances, broad-spectrum drugs are preferable because the origin of the infection is the intestinal tract.

TRAUMA

Although located in a relatively protected position, injuries to the pancreas are more common than is generally recognized, and are of considerable significance because of the high mortality and morbidity. In World War II, 56 per cent of the 62 reported injuries to the pancreas proved to be fatal.

PENETRATING TRAUMA. Injury occurs most frequently from penetrating or open abdominal trauma, usually resulting from a high-speed bullet or stabbing with a long knife. Since the acute symptomatology following an isolated wound of the pancreas is delayed for several hours, and depends upon the development of acute pancreatitis, a confirmed diagnosis is rarely made prior to surgical exploration. The occurrence of associated injuries, particularly in gunshot wounds, including trauma to large vessels, hemorrhage, penetration of a hollow viscus and peritoneal contamination, influences the outcome considerably and is of prime importance in deciding upon early operation. The principles of management, therefore, are the same as those advocated for any penetrating abdominal wound.

This in no way lessens the importance of making as accurate a diagnosis as possible, since wounds to the pancreas continue to be overlooked in patients who have severe or multiple abdominal injuries, with disastrous results. For this reason, the surgeon should concern himself with knowledge of the pa-

tient's position at the time of injury. This information, together with an accurate identification of the points of entrance and exit, and roentgenographic localization of any radiopaque foreign body, may lead one to suspect pancreatic involvement. If examination has been delayed, the finding of an elevated serum amylase will be helpful.

BLUNT TRAUMA. Protected as it is by the vertebral column and the lower rib cage, the majority of closed injuries to the pancreas occur from a direct blow to the epigastrium. Physical violence, including participation in active sports, a direct fall on a blunt object or compression of the organ against the spine by the steering column in an automobile collision, are among the most common mechanisms of injury in the adult. Experience at several children's hospitals indicates that the continued forward motion of a youngster falling from a fast-moving bicycle or tricycle may lead to epigastric impalement upon the uppermost and fixed handle bar, resulting in injury to the pancreatic substance and accounting for the majority of pancreatic cysts seen in children.

Even though blunt abdominal trauma involves the pancreas less often than penetrating trauma, it is of considerable clinical importance since intra-abdominal injury may be limited to the pancreas, and the clinical manifestations, dependent upon activation of released pancreatic enzymes or the development of acute pancreatitis, are delayed in onset. In the absence of associated injuries, therefore, the indications for early operation are much less dramatic than in the patient suffering from a penetrating abdominal wound, even if complete transection of the pancreas has occurred.

Often these patients do not seek medical attention for several hours, while others may be examined and discharged soon after injury, only to return a short time later with severe abdominal complaints. A diagnosis of isolated pancreatic trauma, which is sufficiently early to allow for successful operation with minimal complications and late sequelae, requires immediate hospitalization and frequent observation for at least 48 hours of all patients suspected of having sustained blunt trauma to the upper abdomen. Tenderness of the upper abdomen is usually present but often of slight degree. The cessation of bowel sounds and the onset of abdominal distention is an ominous sign and should alert the examiner to a retroperitoneal injury. As time passes, abdominal pain increases and usually is constant and dull, and radiates to the upper lumbar region. The white blood count is elevated, but often not greatly. Admission baseline serum amylase values usually are normal, but will rise significantly within 24 to 36 hours. Scout films of the abdomen usually are nonspecific and show only paralytic ileus. The four-quadrant diagnostic abdominal paracentesis is of great benefit and may be used without fear of complications. The peritoneal fluid obtained in these patients is often clear or slightly sanguineous, and contains large quantities of amylase. It is free of food particles and bacteria, unless the integrity of the gastro-intestinal tract has been disrupted. Once the diagnosis of blunt pancreatic trauma has become highly suspect, immediate operation is indicated.

SURGICAL TREATMENT FOR PANCREATIC INJURY. The principles of operation within 24 hours after injury depend more on the site and extent of damage than on the mechanism of injury. They include control of hemorrhage; external drainage, either alone or combined with repair of the major pancreatic duct; and extirpation of devitalized gland, or provision for some type of internal drainage for the exocrine secretions of a viable distal segment separated from the main gland.

Knife wounds of the pancreas are generally superficial and only rarely result in a complete division of the major pancreatic duct. These and other minor injuries to the pancreatic substance are best treated by simple drainage. A sump drain is preferred since it provides the advantage of suction, thus preventing any further intra-abdominal dissemination of pancreatic juice. Most of the resulting fistulae will be minor and will close spontaneously within a few weeks.

If the major pancreatic duct has been interrupted, it is reconstructed over a small T-tube with fine silk sutures. The T-tube is removed some three weeks later, but only after a postoperative pancreatogram has demonstrated a patent ductal system.

Extensive injury to the tail of the pancreas calls for distal pancreatectomy, including splenectomy with ligation of the major ducts and drainage of the stump of the pancreas. With complete destruction or devitalization of the body of the pancreas, but with the blood supply to the tail still intact, the distal pancreas can be preserved by implantation of the severed end of the pancreas into a defunctionalized segment of jejunum.

Preservation of functioning pancreatic tissue prevents the development of pancreatic diabetes and avoids a deficiency of pancreatic enzymes. Once adequate drainage for the pancreatic secretions from the distal pancreas is provided, fistulization and formation of pseudocysts are minimized.

Bleeding from the surface of the pancreas must be viewed with great concern and handled with meticulous technique, using fine clamps and delicate ligatures. Blind grasping of bleeding points invites catastrophic injury to pancreatic ducts, with ensuing complications. Prior to closing the abdomen, irrigation of the area surrounding the pancreas tends to lessen the enzymatic peritonitis.

Postoperatively, these patients should have nasogastric suction until gastrointestinal motility is re-established. Antibiotics are helpful since the traumatized pancreas and inflamed peritoneum are easily infected. Constant bladder drainage permits accurate measurement of urine output and serves as an aid in the regulation of fluid intake. Drains should not be removed for at least seven to ten days, and then only if there is no drainage.

INFLAMMATORY DISEASES

ACUTE PANCREATITIS. Acute pancreatitis, first clearly described by Fitz in 1889, is by definition a graded inflammatory process of the pancreatic parenchyma which is thought to result from an activation of trypsinogen to trypsin, leading to varying degrees of self-digestion. The seemingly increased incidence of this important and somewhat baffling disease entity has most likely followed a greater awareness of the process and improved methods of diagnosis. Since the symptomatology may be quite varied and even bizarre, acute pancreatitis deserves prominent consideration whenever the diagnosis of acute abdominal disease is necessary.

Acute pancreatitis presents one of the most difficult and challenging problems in clinical medicine. The etiology of the disease remains unknown. A variety of conditions are known to be associated with pancreatitis, but the exact role that these associations play in precipitating the disease remains a mystery (Fig. 7). Acute pancreatitis occurs most commonly in patients with either biliary tract disease or alcoholism, or both. About three of four patients have one of these two problems. The remaining 25 per cent have familial hyperlipemia, hyperparathyroidism, or

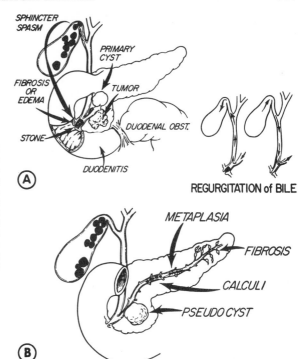

Figure 7. *A*, Conditions associated with and thought to contribute to acute pancreatitis: occlusion of the sphincter of Oddi results in obstruction of the pancreatic duct and permits regurgitation of bile through a common channel; it can result from reflex spasm, stone, fibrosis or edema. Duodenal obstruction distal to the sphincter may cause reflux of duodenal contents. An enlarging tumor or cyst may result in intrapancreatic obstruction. *B*, Recurrent pancreatitis with fibrosis and metaplasia of the ductal epithelium, calculus formation or the development of a pancreatic pseudocyst may lead to secondary obstruction of the pancreatic ducts, thus fostering further attacks.

mumps, or fall into the semantic panacea, idiopathic pancreatitis.

In 1903, Opie suggested that gallstones might obstruct the pancreatic ductal opening as it entered the common duct and cause pancreatitis. There is a vast amount of experimental evidence that pancreatic ductal obstruction, coupled with stimulation, will indeed result in fulminating pancreatitis. Unfortunately, only 8 to 10 per cent of people with pancreatitis and gallstones have common duct stones. To increase the mystery, 90 per cent of those with gallstones will be cured of their pancreatitis by cholecystectomy. The assumption that those without common duct stones may have passed them prior to operation has appeal, but logic does not support it. The excellent results associated with cholecystectomy cannot be denied, however, and so the relationship remains both undeniable and undefined. Recent findings of inflammatory changes in the papilla of Vater suggest that inflammation of the distal common duct may result in cicatrix and partial obstruction.

It is of interest to note the difference in incidence of biliary disease and alcoholism associated with pancreatitis from different areas. In England, the incidence of alcoholism is very low, but in this country, especially in indigent hospitals, it may be as great as 75 per cent. The mechanism by which alco-

hol causes pancreatitis is not clear. Attempts at producing pancreatitis with alcohol alone in animals have been unsuccessful. It is known that parenteral alcohol has little or no effect on pancreatic secretion. Alcohol by mouth affects the pancreas by increasing gastric acid production and, perhaps, by increased gastrin production. Alcohol also causes inflammatory changes in the duodenal mucosa. The combination of duodenitis with swelling and irritation of the sphincter of Oddi and pancreatic stimulation may produce the ductal obstruction and simultaneous stimulation known to be capable of causing pancreatitis.

In the less commonly associated processes, such as hyperparathyroidism and familial hyperlipemia, very little information is available to suggest an etiological relationship, but the incidence seems high enough to be more than coincidental.

A wide variety of drugs have been implicated as inciting agents in pancreatitis. The more common are the thiazide diuretic and steroids. There is little experimental evidence to support the relationship, and the frequency of occurrence is not outside the realm of coincidence.

Pathophysiology. The present state of knowledge of the pathophysiology of pancreatitis is limited. The most appealing theory is a combination of ductal obstruction and pancreatic stimulation. The stagnant enzymes become activated within the ducts and then through back pressure, or through a break in ductal epithelium, attack the parenchyma of the gland. Experimental evidence suggests that a small amount of blood may greatly enhance the speed and intensity of the reaction. There is also good evidence that obstruction of small arteries or veins may accelerate the process. Such vascular obstruction could result from transmitted ductal pressure or edema. The earliest stage of the process seems to be primarily edema. It may stop, or it may progress to a hemorrhagic state, and then to a necrotizing state with complete glandular destruction.

The major disturbance associated with pancreatitis seems to be the loss of large volumes of fluid into the retroperitoneal, peripancreatic tissue, and the free abdominal cavity. This loss of fluid may be extensive and constitute as much as 30 per cent of the total plasma volume. The reason for its loss is unclear. Lymphatic obstruction by plugging with red cells has been shown in experimental pancreatitis.

There has been some suggestion that vasoactive substances and bradykinin, in particular, are released from the inflamed and necrotic pancreas. If these substances are released, their effect is probably local because attempts to show systemic effects have been unsuccessful. Their local effect may increase fluid loss by altering local vascular permeability.

In addition to pancreatic inflammation and fluid loss, other changes occur. Shock is frequently seen with pancreatitis and when present is often associated with death. The shock is certainly related to fluid loss, but other factors are important. Large volumes of electrolyte and colloid solutions as well as whole blood do not always succeed in resuscitating the patient with pancreatitis. The edematous and inflamed gland is very susceptible to infection. The inoculum may be hematogenous or may come from the lymphatics of the gastrointestinal tract and specifically the transverse colon.

Parenchymal digestion is associated with the severe forms of necrotizing pancreatitis. Attempts at proving increase in active proteolytic enzymes in the parenchyma have had varied results. It seems reasonable to relate active proteolysis from enzyme activity and, specifically, trypsin to the necrosis of acute pancreatitis. An additional enzyme incriminated in pancreatitis is elastase, which attacks the elastic substance of blood vessels and may result in the hemorrhage observed in the more severe forms of the disease. Metabolic alterations may be serious complicating factors in pancreatitis. Extensive destruction of the gland and islets of Langerhans may result in acute diabetes mellitus. Metabolic acidosis may result from diabetes or simply from anaerobic metabolism secondary to poor peripheral perfusion. Lipase released into the peritoneal cavity digests fat tissue to fatty acids saponified with calcium ions. This binding of calcium may produce hypocalcemia and tetany. When serum calcium levels fall below 9 mg. per cent, mortality is greatly increased. Fat necrosis, presumably from circulating lipase, has been seen in the subcutaneous tissue as well as in the central nervous system.

The presence of large amounts of proteolytic enzyme inhibitor in the normal circulation has greatly hampered attempts at measuring circulating enzymes. If trypsin plays a role in pancreatitis, and it seems most likely that it does, the mechanism of action remains undefined.

Symptomatology and diagnosis. For approximately 30 years after the turn of the century, pancreatitis was usually diagnosed either at autopsy or at the operating table. The preoperative diagnosis was rarely correct. In 1934, Somogyi described the blood diastase test. For some time, any patient with abdominal symptoms and an amylase elevation was assumed to have pancreatitis. More recent work has shown that the serum amylase may be elevated in a variety of diseases, and is not always elevated in pancreatitis. These findings have served to reemphasize the importance of clinical evaluation used in conjunction with a combination of laboratory and radiographic procedures.

The patient's history and a thorough physical examination are still of prime importance in the diagnosis. The disease process occurs more commonly in females than males, and the age of occurrence usually is from 20 to 50 years. The patients typically have severe upper abdominal pain which is boring and unrelenting, and often radiates into the back. As the process continues, a copious exudate of a plasma-like fluid with a high content of activated pancreatic enzymes collects in the lesser sac. The resultant chemical peritonitis frequently leads to obstruction of the foramen of Winslow (Fig. 8). Continued collection of

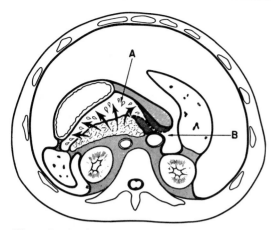

Figure 8. As the inflammatory process continues, a copious exudate of plasma-like fluid with a high content of activated pancreatic enzymes collects in the lesser sac (A). Edema may close off the foramen of Winslow (B).

this fluid in the lesser sac leads to involvement of the diaphragmatic peritoneum, and pain is referred from the central portion of the diaphragm to the shoulder and from the peripheral portion of the diaphragm to the groin (Fig. 9).

Usually, there is associated vomiting. Epigastric tenderness is common and the abdomen may have a rigid, boardlike character with absent bowel sounds. In severe cases, prostration, hypotension and cyanosis may be evident along with hyperpyrexia.

Hypocalcemia, when present, is manifest by a positive Chevostek and Trousseau sign or overt tetany, depending on its severity. A serum calcium below 9 mg. per 100 ml. is considered to indicate a poor prognosis. A bluish discoloration of the umbilicus secondary to an accumulation of bloody abdominal fluid may be found occasionally. Other skin manifestations include ecchymosis and dis-

coloration in one or both flanks at the level of the umbilicus, as a result of hemorrhage into and out of the gland with dissection from the retroperitoneal space into the subcutaneous extraperitoneal fat (Fig. 10). Livedo reticularis, a patchy, slightly gray discolaration of the skin, results from metastatic fat necrosis. A left-sided pleural effusion is commonly present and rupture of the spleen may occur.

Although the laboratory approach to the diagnosis of pancreatitis has undergone some changes in recent years, the amylase test is still of prime importance and should be used as a screening test in all patients presenting abdominal pain. It should be remembered, however, that elevations to more than twice the normal occur in 20 per cent of patients with a perforated ulcer, in one out of ten suffering from acute cholecystitis, and in the majority with strangulating intestinal obstruction. Although some believe that the disease should be suspect in any patient whose serum amylase is elevated above the normal, most authorities agree that an elevation to more than 1000 Somogyi units per 100 cc. of serum is diagnostic of acute pancreatitis. The increase, however, is transitory and persists only a few days. For this reason, it is important to realize that the urinary amylase is usually elevated longer than that in the serum and may be a useful measurement when the patient is seen late in the course of an acute attack (Fig. 11).

The degree of elevation of serum amylase bears little relationship to the severity of the disease, and there is some evidence that the amylase value is more a function of pancreatic duct obstruction than parenchymal

Figure 9. Continued collection of an enzyme-rich fluid leads to irritation and inflammation of the left diaphragm, with pain referred to the shoulder from the central diaphragm and to the groin from the peripheral diaphragm.

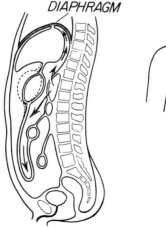

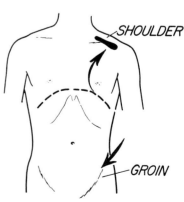

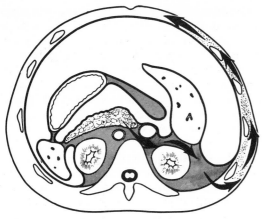

Figure 10. Hemorrhage through the retroperitoneal space into the subcutaneous fat leads to ecchymosis and discoloration in one or both flanks (Gray-Turner sign). A deposit of iron salts may lead to permanent discoloration.

whom the laboratory and roentgenographic studies are inconclusive, a diagnostic peritoneal tap may be profitable. The amylase values in the peritoneal fluid of patients with acute pancreatitis rise to several times the corresponding values of the serum, and tend to remain significantly elevated for two to four days after serum values have fallen to normal. The procedure, therefore, is useful if pancreatitis is suspected when the patient is seen relatively late in the course of the disease.

Because of the high concentration of amylase in acute pancreatitis, only a small amount of peritoneal fluid is required. As little as 0.2 cc. may be diluted ten times and a satisfactory determination obtained by the Somogyi method. Analysis of this fluid for bile and titration of total acidity may be of value in the differential diagnosis of perforated peptic ulcer. In acute nonhemorrhagic pancreatitis, one can expect turbid fluid with an alkaline pH, no bile, no food particles or bacteria, and a very high amylase. In hemorrhagic pancreatitis, the fluid is blood-red and has high amylase levels. A smear and culture should always be included. Measurement of the serum antithrombin, although not commonly performed, may be of value. Reportedly, it has a low incidence of false positives, but a fairly high incidence of false negatives. Loewi's test consists of a mydriasis following adrenalin in the conjunctival sac, which has not proved to be of great help; but coupled with present laboratory aids, it may be of some assistance. Increased total serum fat content is another suggestive finding. A

necrosis. There may be an inverse relationship when the majority of pancreatic tissue has been destroyed by the acute process. It is now known that the serum amylases migrate with different electrophoretic mobility, and that the amylase from the pancreas migrates with the gamma globulin. These studies may lead to the development of a pancreatic amylase test which will measure the specific fraction arising from the pancreas and thus increase the value of this laboratory observation. Recent observations on lipase determinations suggest a higher diagnostic accuracy and closer correlation to the clinical course.

In unusual patients with abdominal pain, signs of peritonitis and paralytic ileus, in

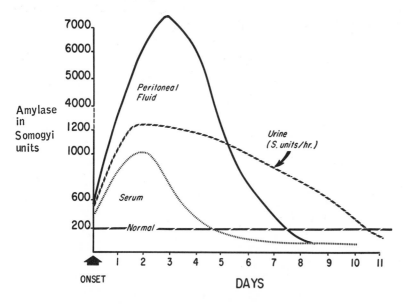

Figure 11. Knowledge of the relative amylase values in the serum, urine and peritoneal fluid is helpful when subsiding pancreatitis is suspected.

transient glycosuria, a moderate to marked leukocytosis, a low serum prothrombin and a rising hematocrit also are seen. The increasing hematocrit is of especial importance, since it usually is a reflection of lowered plasma volume and may be very misleading if used as a guide to blood administration.

Emergency roentgenograms are useful in excluding several conditions which simulate acute pancreatitis, and may include findings which support the clinical diagnosis. A flat and upright film of the abdomen and an upright chest film are recommended on all suspect patients. The demonstration of clear lung fields excludes a pneumonic process which might simulate an acute abdominal condition, and the finding of pleural fluid, usually on the left side, gives added support to the diagnosis of acute pancreatitis (Fig. 12, A). If needle thoracentesis is believed advisable, the amylase content of the fluid collected should be determined and will be markedly elevated in acute pancreatitis. The visualization of calcified shadows in the gallbladder area suggests gallstones. It may aid in establishing the diagnosis, but may also indicate acute cholecystitis, which can be ruled out through visualization of the gallbladder by intravenous cholangiography.

The finding of calcified shadows in the area occupied by any portion of the pancreas is strongly suggestive of an acute inflammatory process superimposed on, or resulting from a chronic calcific pancreatitis. The presence of a single dilated loop of small intestine with a fluid level also is helpful when located in the vicinity of the pancreas (Fig. 12, B). If the patient's condition permits, a barium swallow may demonstrate an enlarged C-loop with an irregular duodenal wall and anterior displacement of the stomach, resulting from edema and enlargement of the pancreas or a beginning collection of fluid in the lesser sac.

Treatment. The treatment of acute pancreatitis in its initial stages is nonsurgical and directed toward the relief of pain, the lowering of intraductal pressure, the control of pancreatic secretion, the neutralization of proteolytic enzymes, the restoration of lost plasma volume and the prevention of secondary infection.

The choice of an agent to relieve pain is difficult, since many narcotics have been shown to increase intraductal pressure. The drug of choice probably is meperidine because of its lesser effect on the sphincter of Oddi.

When the pain is severe and protracted, splanchnic blocks are effective and should be considered. The right splanchnic nerves are blocked first because this procedure alone may prove effective. If pain continues, however, the left side also is blocked.

Continuous gastric aspiration is necessary, since the passage of gastric acid into the duodenum is a major stimulus for pancreatic secretion. In addition, it is useful in controlling nausea, vomiting and distention. To be of value, the tube must be properly positioned in the antrum of the stomach and inspected frequently to insure proper func-

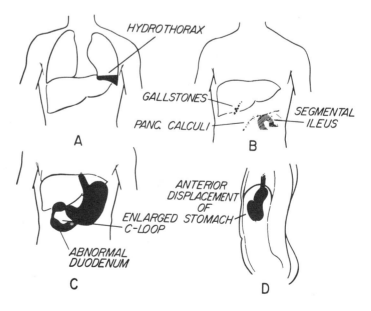

Figure 12. Some of the more common roentgenographic findings in acute pancreatitis.

tion. Vagal stimulation is partially controlled by anticholinergic drugs, which to be effective must be given in sufficient dosage to manifest a systemic response including blurred vision and a dry mouth. Carbonic anhydrase inhibitors are thought to depress pancreatic secretions at the cellular area and may be of value. The use of antiproteolytic substances to neutralize the action of trypsin is of theoretical value, but recent clinical and experimental studies have been encouraging.

The most important factor in decreasing mortality of pancreatitis is the adequate replacement of fluid and electrolytes, especially colloid, which is lost in large amounts into the retroperitoneal and intraperitoneal spaces and by vomiting, diarrhea and gastric suction. It is not unusual for these patients to need the equivalent of 1500 cc. of plasma or whole blood and 4500 cc. of noncolloid fluid in the first 24 hours of therapy. Although plasma is known to contain a naturally occurring antitryptic factor, its major value results from its colloid osmotic effect following restoration of the depleted blood volume. For similar reasons, human serum albumin is especially beneficial since each 50 cc. unit is equivalent to the albumin present in 1500 cc. of whole blood. One or two units daily for three to four days is particularly helpful. The loss of potassium is especially severe and may be manifested as acute psychosis. Intravenous calcium is necessary also, especially when fat necrosis is extensive, and many advocate the routine administration of three ampules of calcium gluconate daily during the acute phase. One should avoid alkalosis, which increases the symptoms of hypocalcemia.

Antibiotics have a definite role in the treatment of pancreatitis because of the possibility of secondary infection. One of the broad-spectrum drugs such as tetracycline should be used. Hyperpyrexia is common and requires intravenous salicylate plus a cooling blanket. Other therapeutic measures which appear beneficial, but lack final evaluation, include the administration of corticosteroids and the induction of hypothermia.

Other details of management include bed rest, nothing by mouth, frequent abdominal examination and checks on the vital signs. Recording of an accurate intake and output, including initially the hourly urinary excretion by means of an indwelling catheter, are important in monitoring the effectiveness of fluid therapy. Repeated determinations of the white blood cell count, hematocrit, amylase, calcium and electrolytes are particularly important if the patient's progress is unsatisfactory. A persistently elevated amylase and a subsiding symptomatology suggest the formation of a pancreatic pseudocyst.

The duration of therapy depends upon the course of the disease and may require ten days or more. The majority of patients, however, will improve considerably within three to four days. Gastric suction had best be continued several days after subsidence of symptoms. Stimulation of the pancreas too early by food frequently leads to a recurrence of the acute process. The initial diet should be bland, fat-free and above all should include no stimulants such as coffee, tea or cocoa.

Surgical treatment in acute pancreatitis is to be avoided. It may be necessary if the disease process is accompanied by acute cholecystitis or occurs in the presence of rapidly increasing jaundice which is presumably the result of a common duct stone impacted in the ampulla of Vater. Depending on the patient's condition, cholecystostomy alone may be indicated, and more definitive surgery postponed until the patient is completely recovered. On the other hand, removal of the common duct stone blocking the pancreatic duct may be a life saving procedure. Jaundice during the recovery phase usually is transient and does not alter the therapy.

Hemorrhage during the attack, either from eroded pancreatic vessels, severe gastritis or duodenitis, or from a duodenal or gastric ulceration is best treated by replacement alone.

When suppuration occurs, drainage of any resultant abscesses may be indicated. In rare instances, a persistent, progressive process may be aborted by adequate drainage of the necrotic pancreas. The prognosis in this instance is extremely poor.

Cholecystostomy may be of value when unexpected acute pancreatitis is found at laparotomy. If necrotizing pancreatitis is discovered, drainage of the lesser sac and the area occupied by the pancreas may prevent the formation of a lesser sac abscess or pseudocyst.

Notwithstanding the many advances in understanding and treating pancreatitis, the overall mortality in acute cases is 10 to 20 per cent; the majority of these deaths occur in the necrotizing and hemorrhagic form of the disease.

After subsidence of the acute attack, roentgenographic studies including a cholecystogram and upper gastrointestinal series are performed. The cholecystogram should be delayed for at least a week following recovery so as to assure reliability of the findings. If biliary tract disease is demonstrated, it should be corrected so as to avoid further attacks. The best results are obtained by delaying operation for several months so as to allow complete resolution of the inflammatory process within the pancreas.

POSTOPERATIVE ACUTE PANCREATITIS. Acute pancreatitis occurring as a postoperative complication is of such grave significance that the surgeon must be ever mindful of its dire consequences. Direct surgical trauma may be partly responsible, as the disease process occurs most often following operation upon the stomach, duodenum, biliary tract, spleen and pancreas proper. On the other hand, many times it has followed an operation on organs and areas quite remote from the pancreas. Concurrent biliary tract disease may play some role in these patients.

Fortunately, the complication is uncommon and occurs in less than 1 per cent of gastrectomies. The reported mortality, however, approximates 50 per cent. The incidence of postoperative pancreatitis following subtotal gastrectomy and gastroduodenostomy is reportedly less than after reconstruction by means of a gastroenterostomy. This may be related to the practice of buttressing the duodenal stump against the pancreas with interrupted sutures when duodenal closure is thought to be insecure.

The symptoms of postoperative pancreatitis may be overlooked in the early postoperative period because they are masked by changes and complaints directly related to the surgical procedure. Perhaps, lack of early recognition and treatment account for the high mortality. Abdominal pain out of proportion to that anticipated for the procedure is the heralding symptom, followed quickly by tachycardia, elevated serum amylase, prostration, tachypnea, hyperpyrexia and often cyanosis, shock and death. Treatment is the same as for acute pancreatitis and must be prompt and vigorous.

RECURRENT AND CHRONIC PANCREATITIS. It is generally agreed that once an attack of acute pancreatitis has occurred the likelihood of recurrence is around 50 per cent. The decision as to what constitutes recurrent, chronic, or chronic recurrent pancreatitis is somewhat arbitrary and requires definition. Any patient who has had more than one attack of acute inflammation of the pancreas with recovery, and no loss of pancreatic function, is said to have *recurrent pancreatitis*. In contrast, *chronic pancreatitis* refers to the clinical entity resulting from one or more attacks of acute inflammation with sufficient destruction of the pancreatic parenchyma to cause some loss in pancreatic function. The severity of the process ranges from at least one documented attack of pancreatitis, with minimal metabolic changes, to the complete stage of exocrine and endocrine insufficiency resulting from nearly total destruction of the organ.

On rare occasions, this occurs with no knowledge of previous acute attacks. In some patients, secondary obstruction of the pancreatic ducts results from fibrosis and scarrings, the development of a pancreatic pseudocyst or the formation of pancreatic calculi, and predisposes to further attacks of acute inflammation. The latter is referred to as *chronic recurrent pancreatitis*. The continued destruction of acinar tissue leads to a "burned out" pancreas, and acute pancreatitis is then no longer possible.

If after one attack of acute pancreatitis, biliary tract disease is demonstrable, operative intervention is indicated. Care must be taken not to institute roentgenographic investigation too soon, or false-positive findings may occur. Operation on the biliary tract is generally delayed 6 to 8 weeks in order to allow inflammatory reaction to subside. In those patients in whom biliary disease is not demonstrable, and in the absence of an alcoholic history or hyperparathyroidism, operation is indicated after two well-documented attacks of acute pancreatitis.

Symptoms and findings. The symptoms of pancreatitis in its chronic form are pain, weight loss and jaundice, in order of incidence. Associated conditions, in addition to biliary tract disease and alcoholism, include addiction to narcotics, peptic ulcer, hepatic cirrhosis, diabetes, malabsorption and steatorrhea. In time, intraductal obstruction occurs from stricture or pancreatic calculi, and pancreatic pseudocyst is frequently noted. Experience indicates that any patient with adult diabetes, steatorrhea and a heavy alcohol consumption should be suspected of harboring chronic pancreatitis and should be studied.

The patients first seen with far advanced pancreatic disease are difficult diagnostic problems, especially if coexisting biliary disease is absent. It has been said that chronic pancreatitis may be the most frequently mis-diagnosed organic disease in the abdomen. In most instances, however, a systematic approach will result in establishing the correct diagnosis. Roentgenograms are helpful when pancreatic calcification is present, and it is said to occur in 40 to 60 per cent of patients (Fig. 13). Other positive findings may include a heavy alcoholic intake, objective and subjective evidence of weight loss and a history of abdominal pain, which is common but not universal. Drug addiction is present in about one-third of the patients. Most often, the differential diagnosis is easily narrowed to an evaluation of the type of malabsorption present. An examination of the stool in all patients with unexplained recurrent abdominal pain will usually lead to further pursuit of the correct diagnosis. The presence of steatorrhea with bulky, foul and fatty stools is classic. On the other hand, the finding of undigested meat fibers and increased fat content in grossly normal stools warrants more extensive studies. A battery of three tests for chronic pancreatitis has been suggested: provocative serum enzyme test with pancreozymin and secretin, the starch tolerance test and I^{131} triolein uptake test. In addition, the presence of normal d-xylose absorption is helpful in ruling out other types of the malabsorption syndrome. Once the diagnosis of chronic pancreatitis has been established, the choice of

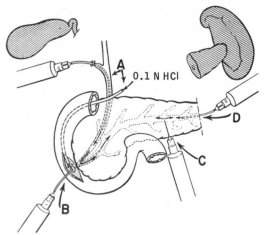

Figure 14. Techniques of obtaining operative pancreato-grams. *A*, Hydrochloric acid is dripped into the second portion of the duodenum, causing spasm of the sphincter of Oddi. Radiopaque dye is then injected into the common duct by means of a catheter threaded into the cystic duct; if a common channel is present, the dye refluxes into the pancreatic ducts. *B*, Following sphincterectomy, the pancreatic duct is identified and cannulated. *C*, The radiopaque dye is injected directly into a dilated pancreatic duct presenting on the surface of the gland. *D*, Amputation of the distal pancreas including splenectomy permits retrograde injection of the dye.

treatment is best made on the basis of etiology and the presence or absence of an obstruction of the pancreatic duct.

In those patients with correctable biliary tract disease, good results may be anticipated in 80 to 90 per cent. Surgical treatment consists of correction of the biliary tract disease and, in some patients, sphincterotomy permitting roentgenographic study of the pancreaticobiliary system (Figs. 14 and 15). The removal of a noncalculous gallbladder is of no value unless chronic cholecystitis is present, nor is hemigastrectomy unless ulcer disease is coexistent. The latter casts some doubt on the role of gastric acid in pancreatitis.

In alcoholic pancreatitis, the results are much less gratifying and these patients constitute the majority of surgical failures. If obstruction of the pancreatic ducts has not occurred, total abstinence from alcohol will lead to complete recovery, including pancreatic regeneration after two or three years of good dietary management. In turn, the inability of these patients to control their alcohol intake is tantamount to recurrent disease.

In 1954, several surgeons first described amputation of the distal pancreas and retrograde drainage into the jejunum, with good results in the absence of multiple points of

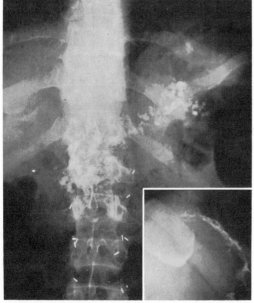

Figure 13. Roentgenogram in severe chronic calcific pancreatitis. *Inset*, Calcified pancreatic cyst which is very unusual and may indicate the presence of Echinococcus.

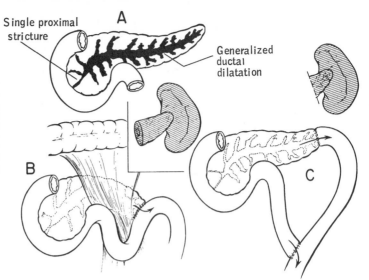

Figure 15. *A*, Diagrammatic representation of an operative pancreatogram, showing single proximal stricture. In this instance, distal pancreatectomy and splenectomy permit retrograde drainage of the ductal system by one of two methods: *B*, End-to-side pancreaticojejunostomy, and *C*, Roux-en-y procedure, which minimizes reflux of intestinal contents in the pancreas.

ductal obstruction. The pancreatic duct has been split in its long axis, and after removing the intraductal calculi, the filleted gland has been anastomosed to a defunctionalized segment of jejunum (Fig. 16). The results of this operation and the several modifications which preserve all pancreatic tissue are reportedly good in 50 to 70 per cent of patients. If, however, the patient continues to consume alcohol, pancreatic function continues to deteriorate.

Prior to the advent of the several drainage operations, total or extensive subtotal pancreatectomy had been proposed as a possible justified operative approach for patients with alcoholic or idiopathic chronic pancreatitis. There has been recent renewal of enthusiasm for this approach. Ninety-five per cent distal pancreatectomy has been performed in a group of patients with far advanced pancreatic destruction and no dilated ducts. The results in terms of pain relief have been good.

Several operations on the sympathetic nervous system have been utilized to improve pancreatic drainage, to alter exocrine secretions or to control the pain of chronic pancreatitis. Anterior and posterior truncal vagotomy, both of which supply parasympathetic fibers to the pancreas through the celiac ganglion, combined with a gastric drainage procedure or antrectomy, has been utilized in the hope of relaxing the sphincter of Oddi and diminishing pancreatic secretion with varied success (Fig. 17, *A*). A right bilateral splanchnic resection controls pain, but contributes nothing to the prevention of

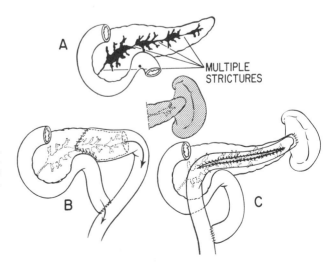

Figure 16. Diagrammatic representation of an operative pancreatogram, showing multiple strictures of the pancreatic ductal system and the "chain of lakes" effect. *B*, Splitting of pancreatic duct on its long axis and anastomosis to defunctionalized segment of jejunum. *C*, Modification procedure permitting preservation of all pancreatic tissue, which can be accomplished without mobilizing the pancreas or disturbing the spleen.

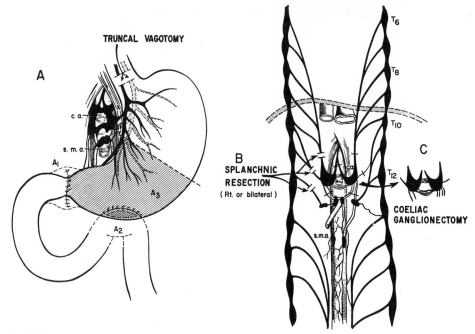

Figure 17. *A*, Parasympathetic innervation, and *B*, sympathetic innervation of the pancreas, demonstrating the several procedures employed to interrupt the innervation.

further painless attacks of pancreatitis (Fig. 17, *B*). Celiac ganglionectomy, if complete, should offer the advantages of control of pain and pancreatic secretion without the necessity of draining the stomach, since the gastric branches of the vagus are left intact (Fig. 17, *C*).

In those patients with hyperparathyroidism and chronic recurrent pancreatitis, surgical relief of the parathyroid problem frequently prevents further attacks. Priority, therefore, should be given to the control of the hyperparathyroidism.

Replacement therapy. In case of extensive pancreatic resection, or in far advanced disease, both the exocrine and the endocrine function of the pancreas may be greatly diminished. While an occasional patient will require no treatment, the majority need permanent replacement therapy.

The diabetes following pancreatectomy can be very labile and may be due to the absence of glucagon, an insulin antagonist. Some surgeons, therefore, have advocated preserving a small portion of the pancreas to avoid this problem. Initially, following total pancreatectomy, 10 units of NPH insulin is given daily and the dose is gradually increased until the diabetes is controlled; 25 to 40 units may be required daily. Satisfactory replacement of the exocrine function is more difficult.

There may be associated liver disease in these patients, which is not surprising since both seem related to low protein intake. It has been suggested that treatment of both organs, when one was known to be involved, results in a greater degree of response. This relationship may not be direct, since some find little correlation between pancreatic function and the degree of hepatic cirrhosis using the secretin test.

PANCREATIC PSEUDOCYST

Pancreatic pseudocyst is a term used to describe a collection of liquefying necrotic tissue which includes pancreas and pancreatic secretory products either within or without the organ. It is surrounded by a fibrous sac without an epithelial lining. Pseudocyst formation depends initially upon disruption of a major pancreatic duct, either by trauma or as a consequence of acute pancreatitis, with necrosis and spillage of activated enzymes into the soft tissues surrounding the pancreas or into the lesser sac. It is of clinical significance primarily as a result of a persistent communication with the ductal system.

A pseudocyst may develop as early as 72 hours after the initial insult or may require several weeks. In the case of trauma, this complication may be prevented if early and adequate drainage of the injured pancreas is accomplished.

DIAGNOSIS. The symptomatology associated with a developing pseudocyst may be somewhat vague and nonspecific. One must be vigilant during an attack of acute pancreatitis if an early diagnosis is to be made. Persistent or increased pain and continued weight loss commonly occur, and nausea and vomiting may become prominent as pressure on adjacent organs increases. Jaundice may appear if the cyst is developing in the head of the pancreas. The finding of an upper abdominal mass is often the first clue to the development of a pseudocyst. The mass is usually globular, slightly tender, fixed, seems cystic or tense to palpation and may grow to be quite large. In this instance, fluid loss may be important. Once diagnosed, care should be taken to avoid accidental rupture, which greatly increases the mortality. Diabetes is found in about 10 per cent of patients who develop a pancreatic pseudocyst.

Roentgenographic findings associated with pseudocyst formation are dependent upon displacement or distortion of the stomach, duodenum or colon. A pseudocyst developing in the head of the pancreas widens the duodenal C-loop and smooths the mucosal pattern of its medial wall (Fig. 18). If arising from the tail of the pancreas, the stomach is displaced anteriorly and medially, and medial displacement may simulate an enlarged spleen (Fig. 19). When developing within the transverse mesocolon, distortion or even obstruction of the colon results and may simulate colon malignancy. If the cyst presents through the hepatogastric ligament, the stomach is displaced anteriorly and inferiorly; if through the gastrocolic ligament, the stomach is displaced anteriorly, superiorly and to the right. A persistent hydrothorax is also suggestive and indicates the need for further x-ray evaluation.

MANAGEMENT. The management of pseudocyst includes a period of close observation, as the cyst may resolve spontaneously. This allows for development of a well-defined wall which aids surgical treatment when required.

External drainage of the pseudocyst has been the classic method of treatment until recent years, and catheter drainage remains the procedure of choice for isolated cysts of the head of the pancreas (Fig. 20, A_1). Marsupialization is now used only for large cysts arising from the body of the pancreas. This involves suturing an opening in the cyst to the parietal peritoneum surrounding an incision in the anterior abdominal wall (Fig. 20, A_2). This procedure is particularly useful in pseudocysts with thin friable walls, and in patients in whom expedient surgery is necessary. The major deterrents to external drainage include persistence of the resultant pancreatic fistula, requiring further operation, and recurrence of

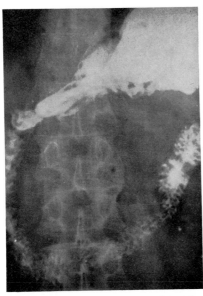
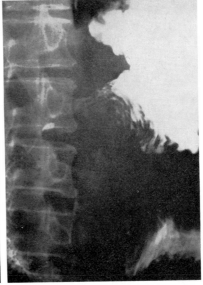

Figure 18. Roentgenographic findings of a pseudocyst in the head of the pancreas, demonstrating the widened duodenal C-loop and the smooth mucosal pattern of the medial wall of the duodenum.

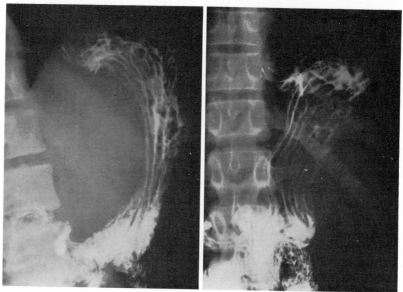

Figure 19.   Roentgenographic findings of a pseudocyst arising in the tail of the pancreas, displacing the stomach anteriorly and to the right.

the cyst when the drainage tract is allowed to close in the presence of a proximal obstruction.

Excision is the most desirable method of treatment but, unfortunately, is not often possible (Fig. 20, *B*). The inflammatory nature of the lesion results in extensive adhesions and tenacious adherence to surrounding tissue, making dissection difficult. Internal drainage procedures, therefore, have now come to be the preferred method of management. The several methods of internal drainage which are shown in Figure 20, C_1, include

a transgastric cystogastrostomy, a cystoduodenostomy and a cystojejunostomy, which may be accomplished in a direct fashion or on the principle of a Roux-en-y procedure.

Cystadenoma and cystadenocarcinoma are rare pancreatic lesions which are much more common in females than in males. They occur most frequently in the body and tail of the gland. The principal symptom is epigastric pain with radiation to the back, along with dyspepsia. These lesions have papillary excrescences on their inner surfaces and, when encountered, should be totally excised.

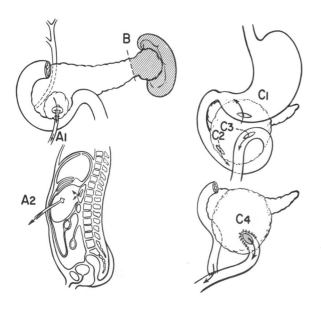

Figure 20. Surgical treatment of pancreatic pseudocysts. A_1, Simple catheter drainage; A_2, marsupialization; B, excision; C_1, transvisceral cystogastrostomy; C_2 cystoduodenostomy; C_3, cystojejunostomy; and C_4, Roux-en-y cystojejunostomy.

PANCREATIC FISTULA

There are few problems which are more disconcerting than the development of a pancreatic fistula. The diagnosis, once suspected, is simple and depends upon the finding of a high amylase content in the drainage fluid.

ETIOLOGY. Since the pancreas presents a ductal system with a physiologic intermittent distal obstruction, the sphincter of Oddi, the tendency for fistulization is great whenever the duct system is interrupted by trauma, inflammatory disease or a surgical procedure.

Surgical trauma is most likely to occur with operations about the stomach and duodenum, biliary tract, spleen or the pancreas proper. The duct of Santorini may be divided while dissecting an edematous and inflamed duodenum away from the pancreas when operating for ulcer. Ducts in the tail of the pancreas may be injured while dividing the vessels in the splenic hilus during a difficult splenectomy. A pancreatic fistula occurs in nearly all patients surviving an emergency drainage of the lesser sac for either hemorrhagic or traumatic pancreatitis, and is obligatory following external drainage or marsupialization of a pancreatic pseudocyst. The persistence of an internal fistula following internal drainage of a pseudocyst prevents recurrence of the cyst even though proximal duct obstruction is present (Fig. 21). The remaining external fistulae are usually a result of pancreatic biopsy, or occur as a complication following anastomosis of a surgically divided pancreas to the gastrointestinal tract.

TREATMENT. Although most pancreatic fistulae close spontaneously, the time varies from a few weeks to many months or occasionally years. In the latter instance, distal obstruction, continued infection and epithelialization of the tract, either with or without an associated tumor or foreign body, must be excluded.

Once diagnosed, steps must be taken to maintain a maximum state of well-being in the patient while awaiting closure. Adequate drainage by means of a catheter or sump drain with suction must be provided to avoid skin changes and to assure obliteration of the tract at the pancreatic level first, thus minimizing the possibility of pseudocyst formation, chemical peritonitis or recurrence.

As soon as gastrointestinal activity resumes, the patient may be re-fed his pancreatic drainage either by nasogastric tube or by ingestion with fruit juice. If this is unacceptable

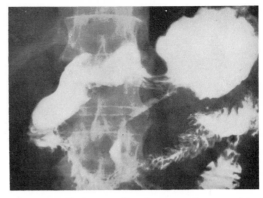

Figure 21. Barium swallow demonstrating a persistent internal pancreatic fistula following a cystogastrostomy for a large pseudocyst of the body of the pancreas.

to the patient, there are balanced electrolyte formulas available which can be taken in fruit juice or soft drinks.

Attempts to decrease the drainage from the pancreas have been almost uniformly unsuccessful. However, the carbonic anhydrase inhibitor, Diamox, will decrease bicarbonate and water secretion as much as 35 per cent and may be useful in total fistulae. Cessation of oral alimentation greatly diminishes pancreatic secretion but is not a practical approach to the problem.

Although the drainage from pancreatic fistulae, which are uncontaminated by other gastrointestinal secretions, contains only inactivated enzymes, skin maceration will occur if collection of the drainage is incomplete. In this instance, frequent dressing changes, the use of aluminum paste or skim milk powder on the surrounding skin, and intermittent use of a heat lamp two or three times a day may be required.

Water, protein and electrolyte losses must be replaced. Pancreatic juice is rich in bicarbonate and protein, as well as sodium, chloride and potassium. This is of particular importance in the first few days when electrolyte imbalance is at a maximum. The provision of pancreatic enzymes for continued digestion of foodstuffs is important only if the fistula is complete.

Once the fistulous tract is well established in five to seven days, a roentgenographic study of the fistula should be done. This can be safely accomplished with the instillation of 30 to 50 cc. of water soluble contrast material into the drainage catheter. This should be done very gently, since injection into the pancreatic ducts under pressure is a well

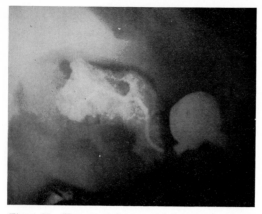

Figure 22. Hypaque injection of fistulous tract demonstrates that the tail of the pancreas is the site of origin and that a complete obstruction is present in the neck of the pancreas. In this instance, a retrograde pancreatico-jejunostomy is indicated. Note opacification of entire pancreas by the radiopaque dye.

recognized method for producing pancreatitis. If the roentgenograms show any degree of obstruction of the pancreatic ductal system between the fistula and the papilla of Vater, there is little hope for spontaneous closure, and surgical intervention should be planned as soon as the patient's general condition will allow (Fig. 22). On the other hand, if there is no obstruction in the ductal system, one is justified in waiting a considerable number of months for spontaneous closure.

Surgical intervention, when necessary, is aimed toward correction of the ductal obstruction per se, or the provision of other suitable internal drainage of that portion of the pancreas in continuity with the fistula.

TUMORS OF THE PANCREAS

Tumors of the pancreas may arise from any of the various cellular elements present in the gland. The most common tumors originate from the ductal and acinar cells. These lesions are nearly always malignant. Next in frequency are tumors of islet cell origin which are often functional and make a variety of hormones. Much more rare are the tumors of stromal cell origin.

ADENOCARCINOMA. Adenocarcinoma of the pancreas as a cause of death increased in frequency between 1953 and 1963 at a greater rate than any cancer afflicting man except cancer of the lung. If the present trend continues, it is estimated that pancreatic carcinoma will cause more deaths than any tumor of the digestive tract except cancer of

the colon. Cancer of the pancreas is a very discouraging disease because it is usually diagnosed at a stage too far advanced to permit cure. The resectability rate reported by various authors varies from 5 to 25 per cent, but 10 per cent may be taken as a mean figure. This low rate of resectable tumors is caused by the silence of the tumor until metastasis has occurred, or until local invasion into vital structures has made resection technically impossible.

Symptoms. Cancer of the head of the pancreas is a painful disease. This point cannot be emphasized too strongly. Although exceptions do occur, between 70 and 90 per cent of patients with pancreatic cancer have pain as an initial symptom. The pain characteristically is dull, vague, and epigastric in location, with radiation to the back. Patients often volunteer that relief can be gained by lying on the side with knees flexed.

Jaundice is nearly always present with cancer of the head of the pancreas before the diagnosis is suspected. The jaundice is unrelenting, whereas in ampullary cancer it may wax and wane. Associated pruritus may be severe.

Weight loss is the third of the major three symptoms and may be the most dramatic. The patient may complain of losing a pound a day, and losses of 30 to 50 pounds are frequent.

The rapidity of loss has been suggested as a differential diagnostic point because it is less severe with other periampullary malignancies and much less severe with nonmalignant causes of jaundice.

The triad of pain, jaundice, and weight loss are the cardinal manifestations of cancer of the head of the pancreas. Other less frequent symptoms are nausea, vomiting, and steatorrhea.

Carcinoma of the body and tail of the pancreas is diagnosed even later than cancer of the head of the gland, and frequently by serendipity. Fortunately, it is less common than cancer of the head of the gland. The only early symptom may be a deep-boring epigastric pain radiating to the back. Suspicion of herniated nucleus pulposus is not uncommon, and many patients undergo myelography. A poorly understood phenomenon with carcinoma of the body of the pancreas is mental disturbance. It is not unusual to have the patients admitted to the hospital psychiatric ward. Peritoneal metastasis and ascites are often present before the diagnosis is made, and five-year survivals are rare.

Physical findings. Jaundice is the most prominent physical finding of cancer of the head of the pancreas. Between one-quarter and one-third of the patients have a palpable gallbladder. A palpable gallbladder in a jaundiced patient in the absence of acute cholecystitis suggests ductal obstruction from tumor. The gallbladder, chronically inflamed, thickened, and containing stones, cannot distend in response to common duct obstruction (Fig. 23).

Laboratory findings. The laboratory findings of cancer of the pancreas do not differ greatly from those of any cause of obstructive jaundice. The bilirubin is elevated and serial determinations show a relentless increase. Elevation of the alkaline phosphatase parallels that of the bilirubin. Tests of hepatic cellular function are usually not abnormal unless the obstruction has been present for four weeks or longer.

Various enzyme determinations have been evaluated in search of a specific diagnostic tool, but none have proved beneficial. Serum leucine aminopeptidase showed early promise, but lack of specificity has made it valueless. Abnormal glucose tolerance tests are found in about half the patients, but do not help in making the diagnosis. Clinical diabetes is much less common and probably only slightly higher than in the general populace.

Although not widely performed, cytology of duodenal aspirate following secretin stimulation has been quite accurate in a few centers. Undoubtedly, the technical difficulties of collecting the specimens and the uncertainties of the cytology have hindered wider acceptance of this test.

Roentgenography. Routine upper gastrointestinal examinations are of assistance in less than one-third of the patients. Widening of the duodenal **C**-loop and the "inverted 3" sign and evidence of external pressure on the duodenum are helpful when present (Fig. 24). Positive findings are too often associated with nonresectable lesions. Percutaneous transhepatic cholangiography has been of benefit. It is wise to be prepared to perform a laparotomy immediately after the examination. More recent attempts at diagnosis with selective arteriography of the celiac axis have received attention. The reports to date are of varying accuracy, and further clinical trial is warranted. To date, all attempts at radiographic visualization of the pancreas have proved fruitless, and the various isotope scanning techniques have been of little value.

Treatment. After an era of pessimism, there has been a recrudescence of enthusiasm for pancreaticoduodenectomy for carcinoma of the pancreas. The last ten years have shown an increase in five-year survivals, so that now figures of 10 per cent are becoming more common. Of further consequence is the observation that those patients undergoing resection for cure rather than palliative surgery survive two to three times as long. In 1935, Whipple described the operation of pancreaticoduodenectomy. Some recent experiences suggest that operative mortality may be lowered considerably by reverting to the older method of performing the operation in two stages, the first stage being directed at biliary decompression prior to the resection.

In a patient with clinical signs of carcinoma of the pancreas, laparotomy should be performed. Many times a remedial nonmalignant process is found, such as a common duct stone. Even if a nonresectable tumor is present, significant palliation can be attained by

Figure 23. Courvoisier's law. *A*, Hydrops. *B*, Thick-walled and chronically infected gallbladder with stones, which cannot distend in response to the common duct obstruction from stone. *C*, Normal gallbladder which has distended in response to the malignant obstruction of the common duct; it should be palpable.

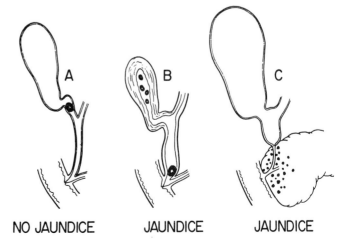

NO JAUNDICE   JAUNDICE   JAUNDICE

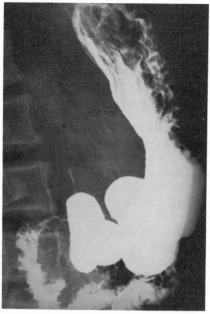

Figure 24. The "inverted 3" sign in a patient with an advanced adenocarcinoma of the head of the pancreas. Note the associated smoothing of the duodenal mucosal pattern.

biliary decompression. There is some evidence that pain relief may be achieved by vagotomy and celiac ganglionectomy.

At the time of exploration, every attempt to establish a tissue diagnosis should be made. There has been considerable reluctance to biopsy the pancreas because of the high incidence of complication and the frequency of nondiagnostic biopsy. Various operative findings have been described to suggest cancer as the diagnosis and encourage resection without tissue diagnosis. Positive lymph node biopsy should not prevent resection of an otherwise removable tumor because as many as 50 per cent of the five-year survivals have had positive nodes. The low resectability rate of this disease is most often related to local invasion into the portal vein or the superior mesenteric vessels.

If resection is not possible, the biliary bypass to relieve jaundice becomes important. A variety of procedures is available to decompress the biliary tract into the intestinal tract (Fig. 25). Cholecystenterostomy is probably the best. Decompression of the duct of Wirsung via pancreatic jejunostomy may be worthwhile. It provides some pain relief as well as improving nutrition by restoring pancreatic enzymes to the digestive tract. Gastrojejunostomy is indicated if vagotomy has been done or if duodenal obstruction is present or impending.

In nonresectable tumors, chemotherapy has

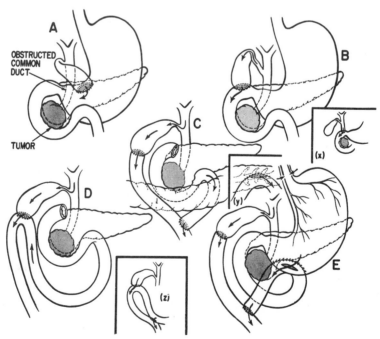

Figure 25. Palliative procedures for nonresectable tumors of the head of the pancreas. *A*, Cholecystogastrostomy. *B*, Cholecystoduodenostomy and (x), choledochoduodenostomy. *C, D* and (z), Several modifications of a cholecystojejunostomy. (y), Drainage of an obstructed pancreatic duct into the jejunum. *E*, Gastroenterostomy included to prevent duodenal obstruction. Vagotomy is added as a precaution against peptic ulceration, since the alkaline juices of the biliary tract have been routed away from the gastrojejunostomy.

given significant palliation in some patients. It is best used in combination with biliary decompression. The drug of choice is 5-fluorouracil in doses of 8 to 10 mg. per kg. per day. The drug is given intravenously in an infusion of 1000 cc. of dextrose and water to lessen its toxicity. Once good results have been obtained, maintenance therapy can be achieved on an outpatient basis with weekly injections.

ISLET CELL TUMORS. **Insulinoma.** Hyperfunction of the beta cells of the pancreatic islets results in excess production of insulin. This situation may prevail with hyperplasia but is much more often the result of an islet cell tumor.

Hyperinsulinism, with its attendant hypoglycemia, causes a clinical syndrome which may be a diagnostic travail for the doctor. The medical literature is replete with patients tragically admitted with psychiatric diagnosis who are subsequently discovered to have hypoglycemia. The first symptoms of hypoglycemia are from an excess epinephrine secretion which may result in nervousness, sweating, tremulousness, and excitability. As the blood sugar falls further, central nervous system symptoms of bizarre behavior, combativeness, and eventually coma occur. Less severe symptoms may be associated with functional hypoglycemia. Functional hypoglycemia is an abnormal hypoglycemic response to a normal stimulus and may be difficult to distinguish from insulinoma. In general, the patients with a functional disorder do not show fasting hypoglycemia or progression of their symptoms, and coma is uncommon. The physician should remember that hypoglycemia may also result from excess insulin administration. Insulin-like substances originating in large retroperitoneal or intrathoracic mesenchymal tumors may produce a syndrome which is very difficult to differentiate from insulinoma. In addition, pituitary or adrenal insufficiency, advanced liver disease, or sensitivity to certain amino acids such as leucine, may cause hypoglycemia.

DIAGNOSIS. The prime diagnostic test for insulin-producing tumors was first described by Whipple. It consists of fasting the patient until symptoms of hypoglycemia occur, substantiating the hypoglycemia with blood sugar determinations, and then eliminating the symptoms by the administration of sugar. If fasting alone does not produce symptoms, exercise may be added. Less than 48 hours of fasting is usually sufficient, but as long as 72 hours may be necessary. The tolbutamide infusion test is also helpful. Intravenous tolbutamide is infused and the blood sugar monitored. If an insulinoma is present, the blood sugar will fall precipitously within 30 minutes and fail to return to 75 or 80 per cent of control levels in three hours. Additional information concerning liver, pituitary, and adrenal function is helpful, as false positives may occur with pathological changes in these organs. Insulin assays are the most reliable when available and will indicate blood levels well above normal, especially in response to tolbutamide or a glucose load.

TREATMENT. Islet cell tumors are often small and very difficult to palpate. Complete examination of the pancreas is mandatory (Fig. 26). If a small single adenoma is found, its removal is adequate treatment. Multiple tumors exist in 12 to 14 per cent, and ectopic tumors occur occasionally. For large tumors in the head of the gland, a Whipple operation is indicated. In cases of hyperplasia, total pancreatectomy may be necessary. In one case in ten, the tumors are malignant. If metastases have occurred, the tumors should be removed if possible. Distal pancreatectomy should be performed when no tumor can be found. Although this procedure may not always result in removing a small tumor or detecting hyperplasia, it may be successful and is preferable to doing nothing.

The cure rate from operation for insulinoma is about 80 per cent. If the patient is not cured, it is usually because metastases have occurred. Functioning insulin-producing metastases present an exceedingly difficult clinical problem. The patients seldom succumb from metastatic disease, but from the sequelae of hypoglycemia, which is virtually uncontrollable. A diuretic, diazoxide, has recently been found effective in controlling hypoglycemia from insulinoma as well as leucine sensitivity. The drug is given orally in doses of 400 to 600 mg. per day. Its only side effect to date has been elevated blood uric acid. Experience is not great, but the drug shows promise and may solve what has traditionally been a perplexing clinical problem.

Glucagon-producing tumors. One islet cell tumor of the pancreas which produced glucagon has been reported. Electron microscopy of the tumor demonstrated cells similar to the alpha cell of the pancreatic islets. The patient was diabetic and had an unusual skin rash. The tumor had the same slow growth characteristic of islet cell tumors. There is

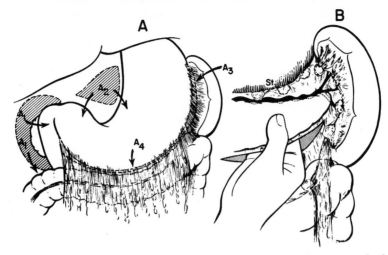

Figure 26. *A,* Diagrammatic illustration of the techniques employed in exploring the pancreas for functioning islet cell tumors. A₁, Kocher maneuver. A₂, Opening of lesser sac through gastrohepatic ligament. A₃ and A₄, Division of gastrosplenic ligament and detachment of greater omentum from colon permits exposure shown in *B.* In *B,* the distal pancreas has been mobilized through an incision in the peritoneum inferior to the pancreas, permitting direct palpation between the thumb and fingers. (St.), Greater curvature of stomach.

not enough known at present to make definite statements regarding the clinical syndrome of excess glucagon. The patient reported did have a decreased response to exogenous glucagon, and this test may be the diagnostic tool of importance.

Ulcerogenic tumors. In 1955, Zollinger and Ellison, based on experience with two patients, suggested that certain non-beta islet cell tumors of the pancreas were related to severe atypical peptic ulcer disease. It was postulated in their initial report that "an ulcerogenic humoral factor of pancreatic islet cell origin" was responsible for the ulcer diathesis. In the ensuing 12 years, over 600 patients were studied and documented and the hormonal hypothesis substantiated.

The presenting complaints are those of severe peptic ulcer resistive to the usual medications. The disease may develop in a patient who has not previously had ulcer symptoms. Often a patient who has had mild symptoms for several years may have rapid acceleration and become completely resistive to all treatment. Unless the physician suspects an ulcerogenic tumor, a standard operation for peptic ulcer may be done. Patients so treated frequently perforate or hemorrhage from recurrent ulcer within days of the operation. Such was the case with the original two patients. Suspicion of an ulcerogenic tumor is often aroused because of unusually large amounts of gastric secretion or ulcer recurrence after a gastric operation. In nearly 40

per cent of the patients, diarrhea is associated with ulcer symptoms. The diarrhea may antedate the ulcer complaints and in a few patients diarrhea may be the only complaint. The cause of the diarrhea is not known but it has been produced experimentally by the infusion of large volumes of acid into the gastrointestinal tract. Complete tumor removal or total gastrectomy has also resulted in cessation of the diarrhea. Rare instances of diarrhea associated with islet cell tumor but without excess gastric acid production have been reported. A different hormone capable of producing diarrhea has been postulated in these patients. The pathophysiology of the diarrhea in the patients without gastric hypersecretion remains obscure. Associated endocrine tumors of the pituitary, adrenals, parathyroids, and beta cells of the pancreatic islets occur in 5 to 10 per cent of the patients. Proper investigations to diagnose associated endocrine conditions should be performed.

The pathophysiology of ulcer diathesis associated with pancreatic non-beta islet cell tumors has been greatly elucidated by evidence that gastrin is present in the tumors (Fig. 27). A gastric secretagogue has also been shown to be present in the circulation of patients with the Zollinger-Ellison syndrome. Tedious counting of the parietal cells in the stomach mucosa of patients with ulcerogenic tumors has usually demonstrated a much greater parietal cell mass in all areas of the gastric mucosa. Whether the increase in the

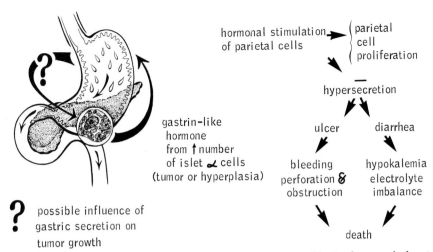

Figure 27. The elaboration of a gastrin-like hormone from the islet cell tumor(s) stimulates marked gastric hypersecretion and may result in a variety of symptoms. The effect of total gastrectomy on tumor growth is still unknown. (Modified from Ellison, E. H., and Wilson, S. D.: Ulcerogenic tumors of the pancreas. *In* Ariel, I. M. [ed.]: Progress in Clinical Cancer, Vol. III. New York, Grune and Stratton 1966.)

number of parietal cells precedes or follows the excess stimulation from the tumor hormone is not known.

DIAGNOSIS. Progress has been made in the laboratory diagnosis of the ulcerogenic tumor. The augmented histamine test has proved most useful. This test involves the administration of a dose of histamine which stimulates the parietal cell mass to its maximal capacity for acid production. In normal or routine ulcer patients, a great increase in acid production is observed after histamine injection. In the majority of ulcerogenic tumor patients, very high gastric secretory rates are present under basal conditions and little or no increase in acid production over baseline values is observed after histamine stimulation (Fig. 28). The implication is that the parietal cell mass in the stomach of the patient with an ulcerogenic tumor is under maximal stimulation from the circulating gastrin and cannot respond further from histamine stimulation. Twelve-hour overnight secretory rates in patients with ulcerogenic tumors are alarming. Volumes in excess of 1000 cc. with an acid content of more than 100 mEq. are common. It is interesting to note that in patients who have associated diarrhea and gastric hypersecretion, the diarrhea may be relieved during aspiration of the gastric acid.

Radiographic studies in this disease may be quite helpful. A typical location of the ulcers in the distal duodenum or proximal jejunum is almost pathognomonic; however, most patients still present with ulcer disease in the more usual locations. Duodenal ileus is common. Changes in the mucosal pattern of the small bowel with a thickened edematous appearance are characteristic, along with increased transit time. Large hypertrophied mucosal folds in a large hypomotile stomach are often seen.

A bioassay technique for evaluating the activity of the tumor has been utilized. It consists of the infusion of the patient's serum into a rat while monitoring the animal's gas-

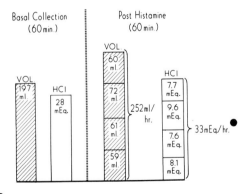

Figure 28. The augmented histamine study in this patient with an ulcerogenic tumor demonstrates little increase in the amount of acid secretion after histamine stimulation. The post histamine columns show four contiguous 15-minute collections.

tric secretion. If an increase in acid production occurs, an ulcerogenic tumor is suspected.

At present, a definitive diagnosis still cannot be made preoperatively. The operating surgeon must prove the diagnosis with biopsy and frozen section techniques (Fig. 29). Small tumors are often located outside the pancreas proper. Common sites are in the wall of the duodenum, peripancreatic and mesenteric lymph nodes. A thorough search for tumor, often with multiple lymph node biopsies, may be necessary. Resection of the tail of the pancreas in search of microadenomas or hyperplasia is warranted if the index of suspicion is high and tumor has not been found.

Successful production of antibodies to human gastrin may soon provide a serologic method for detecting elevated gastrin levels in patients suspected of harboring ulcerogenic tumors. A preoperative diagnosis would then be possible.

TREATMENT. A sufficient number of patients have now been reported in the literature to permit more specific criteria regarding the treatment of ulcerogenic tumors. As with insulinoma, the ulcerogenic tumors of the pancreatic islets are rather slow-growing and the lethality of these lesions is more often related to their endocrine activity than their malignancy. Best results have been obtained with total gastrectomy (Fig. 30). Although removal of all the tumor without gastric resection would be desirable, it is the exception when complete excision of the gastrin-producing

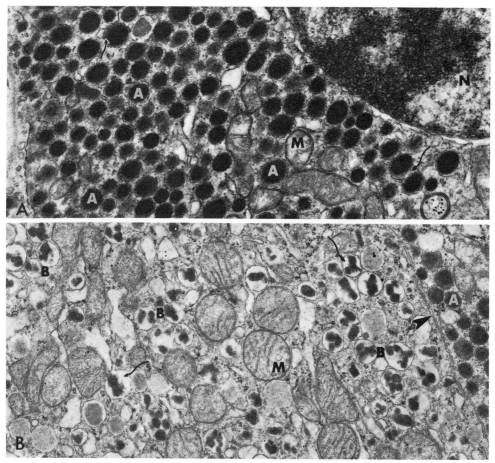

Figure 29. *A,* Electron micrograph from an ulcerogenic tumor of the pancreas composed exclusively of alpha cells. Numerous alpha granules (A) are present in the cytoplasm of the tumor cell. The granules consist of a dense central core separated from the limiting membrane by a less opaque zone (arrows). Mitochondria (M), nucleus (N). × 30,000. *B,* An electron micrograph from an infant with severe hypoglycemia and associated islet cell hyperplasia. Predominantly beta cells were present in the islets of Langerhans. The cytoplasmic granules (B) in a beta cell consist of one to several angular central cores. A clear area (arrows) is between the limiting membrane and central core. Alpha granules (A) are seen in an adjacent alpha cell. Mitochondria (M), cell membrane (arrow head). × 18,000.

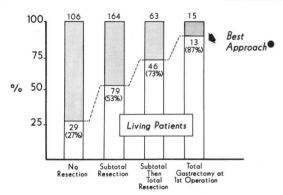

Figure 30. Total gastrectomy at the initial surgical procedure has resulted in the greatest survival. Death in those patients undergoing total gastric resection after previous gastric surgery has been related to the need for emergency operations in poor risk patients. (From Wilson, S. D., and Ellison, E. H.: Am. J. Surg. *111*:787, 1966.)

tion of the gland to the groin of dogs with direct vascular anastomoses. Without protection by immunosuppression, homotransplanted glands have been rejected in seven to 21 days. It has been a consistent observation that the exocrine pancreas ceases function before the endocrine pancreas. Some investigators have observed that the endocrine parenchyma seems more resistant histologically to rejection than the exocrine portion of the gland.

Pancreatectomized animals are able to maintain normal blood sugar levels with a pancreatic homograph long after exocrine function has ceased. Preliminary studies of the exocrine function of pancreatic homographs have shown high basal secretion but impaired response to food and hormonal stimulus.

lesion(s) is possible. More than 60 per cent of the tumors are malignant and most have metastasis at the time of discovery. The benign lesions are often multiple. Diffuse islet cell hyperplasia with or without other tumors may also result in the ulcerogenic syndrome. Any of the preceding varieties of tumor growth would make complete removal of the gastrin-producing lesion(s) most difficult. Lack of success with attempted tumor removal alone, or when combined with subtotal gastrectomy, is evident by the fact that more than half the recorded deaths in patients with this syndrome have occurred shortly following a surgical attempt to control the sequelae of gastric hypersecretion in which some gastric mucosa and residual tumor remain.

Surgeons have been very reluctant to perform total gastrectomies on children, fearing the effect on growth and development. Experience with several patients under 15 with the Zollinger-Ellison syndrome who have undergone total gastrectomy has shown that these children have tolerated total gastrectomy remarkably well with little effect on growth.

Unlike the patients with the gastrin-producing pancreatic lesions, the group of patients with diarrhea, islet cell tumors, and low or no gastric secretory capability are not benefited by gastric resection. The diarrhea in these patients is not the result of gastric hypersecretion and thus gastrectomy is not indicated. Management of these patients should be directed toward tumor removal.

TRANSPLANTATION. Methods have been perfected to transplant the canine pancreas. Most experiments have involved transplanta-

READING REFERENCES

Altemeier, W. A., and Alexander, J. W.: Pancreatic abscess. Arch. Surg. 87:80, 1963.

Anderson, M. C.: Pancreatic hemorrhage: relationship to necrotizing pancreatitis. Arch. Surg. 83:467, 1961.

Anderson, M., and Bergan, J.: Significance of vascular injuries as a factor in the pathogenesis of pancreatitis. Ann. Surg. 154:58, 1961.

Anderson, M., Mehn, W., and Method, H.: An evaluation of the common channel theory as a factor in pancreatic or biliary disease. Ann. Surg. 151:379, 1960.

Anderson, M., Mueller, J., and Snyder, D.: Depression of pancreatic exocrine secretion with a carbonic anhydrase inhibitor. Am. J. Dig. Dis. 5:714, 1960.

Barnett, W. O., Hardy, J. D., and Yelverton, R. L.: Pancreatic trauma, a review of 23 cases. Ann. Surg. 163:892, 1966.

Berkowitz, D., Greenberg, L., and Glassman, S.: The intravenous tolbutamide test as an aid to diagnosis in carcinoma of the pancreas. Am. J. Med. Sci. 243:228, 1962.

Berman, L. G., Prior, J. T., Abramow, S. M., and Ziegler, D. D.: A study of the pancreatic duct system in man by the use of vinyl acetate cast of postmortem preparations. Surg. Gyn. & Obst. 110:391, 1960.

Bernhard, H., Criscone, J., and Moyer, C.: Pathologic significance of serum amylase concentration. Arch. Surg. 79:311, 1959.

Berryman, D., and George, W.: The evaluation of serum amylase levels in non-pancreatic disease. Arch. Surg. 80:482, 1960.

Blandy, J. P., Hamblen, D. L., and Kerr, W. F.: Isolated injury of the pancreas from non-penetrating abdominal trauma. Brit. J. Surg. 47:150, 1959.

Bliss, R., Burch, B., Martin, M., and Zollinger, R. M.: Localization of referred pancreatic pain induced by electric stimulation. Gastroenterology 16:317, 1950.

Boyden, E. H.: The pancreatic sphincters of the baboon as revealed by serial sections of the choledochoduodenal junction. Surgery 60:487, 1966.

Buffkin, W. J., Smith, P. E., and Krementz, E. T.: Evaluation of palliative operations for carcinoma of the pancreas. Arch. Surg. 94:240, 1967.

Carey, L. C., and Rodgers, R. E.: Pathophysiologic alterations in experimental pancreatitis. Surgery 60:171, 1966.

Childs, G., and Kahn, D.: Current status of therapy of pancreatitis: report to the council. J.A.M.A. 179:363, 1962.

Coltar, A., Shelby, J., Massari, F., Hudson, T., Kaplan, M., and Cohn, J., Jr.: Adrenocortical hormones in experimental acute hemorrhagic pancreatitis. Am. J. Dig. Dis. 7:127, 1962.

Cooperative Study: A ten-year experience with carcinoma of the pancreas. Arch. Surg. 94:322, 1967.

Crocker, D. W., and Veith, F. J.: Mesodermal tumors associated with hypoglycemia. Ann. Surg. 161:418, 1965.

Doubilet, H., and Mulholland, J. H.: Surgical treatment of chronic pancreatitis. J.A.M.A. 175:177, 1961.

Doubilet, H., and Mulholland, J. H.: Surgical management of injury to the pancreas. Ann. Surg. 150:854, 1959.

Dowdy, G. S., Jr., Waldron, G. W., and Brown, W. G.: Surgical anatomy of the pancreaticobiliary system: observations. Arch. Surg. 84:229, 1962.

Drash, A., and Wolff, F.: Drug therapy in leucine-sensitive hypoglycemia. Metabolism 13:487, 1964.

Dreiling, D., and Ashikari, H.: Physiologic studies of the heterotopic autotransplanted pancreas. Surg. Forum 12:203, 1966.

Dreiling, D., Nieburgs, H., and Janowitz, H.: The combined secretion and cytologic tests in diagnosis of pancreatic and biliary tract cancer. M. Clin. North America 44:801, 1960.

Dumont, A. E., Doubilet, H., and Mulholland, J. H.: Lymphatic pathways of pancreatic secretions in man. Ann. Surg. 152:403, 1960.

Dumont, A. E., and Mulholland, J. H.: Changes in thoracic duct chyle affected by the pancreas. Surg. Forum 10:243, 1960.

Duval, M. K., Jr., and Enquist, I. F.: The surgical treatment of chronic pancreatitis by pancreaticojejunostomy: an 8-year reappraisal. Surgery 50:965, 1961.

Edlundy, Y., and Ekhom, R.: Microstructure and ultrastructure of human pancreas. Acta Chir. Scandinav. 113:469, 1957.

Edmondson, H., and Berne, C.: Calcium changes in acute pancreatic necrosis. Surg. Gyn. & Obst. 79:240, 1944.

Eklof, O.: Accessory pancreas in the stomach and duodenum: clinical features, diagnosis and therapy. Acta Chir. Scandinav. 121:19, 1961.

Elliott, D., Zollinger, R., Moore, R., and Ellison, E.: The use of serum albumin in the management of acute pancreatitis. Gastroenterology 28:563, 1955.

Elliott, D. W., Zollinger, R. M., and Williams, R. D.: Alterations in the pancreatic resistance to bile in the pathogenesis of acute pancreatitis. Ann. Surg. 146:669, 1957.

Ellison, E. H.: The islet delta cell "ulcerogenic" tumor of the pancreas. *In*, Treatment of Cancer and Allied Diseases. (Pack, G. T., and Ariel, I. M., eds.) Volume 5. New York, Hoeber Medical Division, Harper & Row, 1962.

Ellison, E. H., and Carey, L.: Diagnosis and management of the Zollinger-Ellison syndrome. Am. J. Surg. 105:383, 1963.

Ellison, E. H., and Wilson, S. D.: The Zollinger-Ellison syndrome: re-appraisal and evaluation of 260 registered cases. Ann. Surg. 160:512, 1964.

Elmslie, R. G., White, T. T., and Magee, D. F.: Observations on pancreatic function in eight patients with controlled pancreatic fistulas. Ann. Surg. 160:937, 1964.

Enquist, I., Rosen, R., Allello, R., and Ikezono, E.: Effect of hypothermia on experimental pancreatitis. Arch. Surg. 82:281, 1961.

Ernesdi, M., Mitchell, M. L., Raben, M. S., and Gilboa, Y.: Control of hypoglycemia with diazoxide and human growth hormone. Lancet 1:628, 1965.

Fajans, S., Schnieder, J., Schteingart, T., and Conn, J.: The diagnostic value of sodium tolbutamide in hypoglycemic states. J. Clin. Endo. Metab. 21:371, 1961.

Farringer, J. L., Robbins, L. B., II, and Pickens, J. R.: Abscess of the pancreas: diagnosis and treatment. Ann. Surg. 33:139, 1967.

Fitz, R.: Acute pancreatitis: a consideration of pancreatic hemorrhage, hemorrhagic, suppurative and gangrenous pancreatitis, and of disseminated fat necrosis. M. Rec. 35:197, 1889.

Fitzgerald, J. B., Crawford, E. S., and DeBakey, M. E.:

Surgical considerations of non-penetrating abdominal injuries. Am. J. Surg. 100:22, 1960.

Fogelman, M. J., and Robison, L. J.: Wounds of the pancreas. Am. J. Surg. 101:698, 1961.

Friedlander, E.: Hyperinsulinism secondary to disease of the pancreas and organs adjacent to the pancreas; a review of the world literature. Ann. Int. Med. 52:838, 1960.

Gillesby, W. J., and Puestow, C. B.: Surgery for chronic recurrent pancreatitis. S. Clin. North America 47:83, 1961.

Ginsberg, D. M.: Hypoglycemia associated with extrapancreatic neoplasms. Adv. Int. Med. 12:33, 1964.

Glenn, F., and Frey, C.: Re-evaluation of the treatment of pancreatitis associated with biliary tract disease. Ann. Surg. 160:723, 1964.

Gregory, R. A., Grossman, M. I., Tracy, H. J., and Bentley, P. H.: Nature of the gastric secretagogue in Zollinger-Ellison tumours. Lancet 2:543, 1967.

Gregory, R. A., and Tracy, H. J.: The constitution and properties of two gastrins extracted from hog antral mucosa. Gut 5:103, 1964.

Gregory, R. A., Tracy, H. J., French, J. M., and Sircus, W.: Extraction of a gastrin-like substance from a pancreatic tumour in a case of Zollinger-Ellison syndrome. Lancet 1:1045, 1960.

Greider, M. H., and Elliott, D. W.: Electron microscopy of human pancreatic tumors of islet cell origin. Am. J. Path. 44:663, 1964.

Greider, M. H., and Elliott, D. W.: An electron microscope study of islet cell adenomas. J.A.M.A. 184:217, 1963.

Grozinger, K. H.: Pancreatitis: progress in management. Surgery 59:319, 1966.

Grozinger, K. H., Hollis, A., and Artz, P.: Experimental studies on the prevention of fatal pancreatitis. J.A.M.A. 184:213, 1963.

Hays, D. M., Greaney, E. M., Jr., and Hill, J. T.: The annular pancreas as a cause of acute neonatal duodenal obstruction. Ann. Surg. 153:103, 1961.

Hermann, R., and Davis, J.: The role of incomplete pancreatic duct obstruction in the etiology of pancreatitis. Surgery 48:349, 1960.

Hoerr, S. O.: Value of two-stage pancreatic duodenectomy. Ann. J. Surg. 112:419, 1966.

Howard, J., and Ehrlich, E.: The etiology of pancreatitis: a review of clinical experience. Ann. Surg. 152:135, 1960.

Janowitz, H. D.: Laboratory aspects of pancreatic evaluation. Am. J. Dig. Dis. 6:441, 1961.

Kowlessar, O. D.: The diagnostic value of serum enzyme determinations in pancreatic disease. M. Clin. North America 44:817, 1960.

Lacy, P. E.: Electron microscopic and fluorescent anti-body studies in islets of Langerhans. Exp. Cell Res. 7:296, 1959.

Lacy, P. E., and Hartroft, W. S.: Electron microscopy of the islets of Langerhans. Ann. New York Acad. Sci. 82:287, 1959.

Lafler, C. J., and Hinerman, D. L.: A morphologic study of pancreatic carcinoma with reference to multiple thrombi. Cancer 14:944, 1961.

MacDonald, J. A., and Trusler, G. A.: Meconium ileus: an eleven-year review at the Hospital for Sick Children, Toronto. Canadian M.A.J. 83:881, 1960.

Mange, J. J., Judd, E. S., and Gage, R. P.: Radical pancreaticoduodenectomy: a 22 year experience with the complications, mortality rate, and survival rate. Ann. Surg. 160:711, 1964.

Marks, V., Rose, C. F., and Sarnols, E.: Hyperinsulinism due to metastasizing insulinoma. Treatment with diazoxide. Proc. Roy. Soc. Med. 58:77, 1965.

McCutcheon, A., and Race, D.: Experimental pancreatitis: a possible etiology of post-operative pancreatitis. Ann. Surg. 155:523, 1962.

McDermott, W.: Portal hypertension secondary to pancreatic disease. Ann. Surg. 152:147, 1960.

McGavran, M. H., Unger, R. H., Recant, L., Polk, H. C., Kilo,

C., and Levin, M. E.: Glucagon-secreting alpha-cell carcinoma of the pancreas. New England J. Med. 274:1408, 1966.

McGeachin, R., and Lewis, J.: Electrophoretic behavior of serum amylase. J. Biol. Chem. 234:795, 1959.

McHardy, G., Craighead, C., Balart, Z., Cardic, H., and LaGrange, C.: Pancreatitis: intrapancreatic proteolytic trypsin activity. J.A.M.A. 183:527, 1962.

Menguy, R. B., Hallenbeck, G. H., Bollman, J. L., and Grandley, J. H.: Intraductal pressures and sphincter resistance in canine pancreatic and biliary ducts after various stimuli. Surg. Gyn. & Obst. 106:306, 1958.

Mikal, S.: Operative criteria for diagnosis of cancer in a mass of the head of the pancreas. Ann. Surg. 161:395, 1965.

Miller, D. R.: Functioning adenomas of the pancreas with hyperinsulinism. Arch. Surg. 90:509, 1965.

Mosley, P., Bonanns, C., and Grace, W.: Diabetes and steatorrhea in primary carcinoma of the pancreas. Ann. Int. Med. 52:1147, 1960.

Murphy, R. F., and Hinkamp, J. F.: Pancreatic pseudocysts: report of 35 cases. Arch. Surg. 81:564, 1960.

Nardi, G. L.: Pancreaticoduodenal cancer. Ann. Surg. 33:105, 1967.

Nardi, G. L., and Acosta, J. M.: Papillitis as a cause of pancreatitis and abdominal pain. Ann. Surg. 164:611, 1966.

Opie, E. L.: The etiology of acute hemorrhagic pancreatitis. Bull. Johns Hopkins Hosp. 12:182, 1901.

Opie, E. L., and Meakins, J. C.: The etiology of acute hemorrhagic pancreatitis. J. Exp. Med. 11:561, 1909.

Patt, H. H., Kramer, S. P., Wall, G., and Seligman, A. M.: Serum lipase determination in acute pancreatitis. Arch. Surg. 92:718, 1966.

Paulino-Metto, A., Dreiling, D., and Baronotsky, I.: The relationship between pancreatic calcification and cancer of the pancreas. Ann. Surg. 151:530, 1960.

Preshaw, R. M., Cooke, A. R., and Grossman, M. J.: Stimulation of pancreatic secretion by a hormonal agent from the pyloric area of the stomach. Gastroenterology 49:617, 1965.

Preston, F. W., and Kukral, J. C.: Surgical physiology of the pancreas. S. Clin. North America 48:203, 1962.

Probstein, J., and Blumenthal, H.: Twenty-five years' experience with pancreatitis. Am. J. Gastroenterol. 35:602, 1961.

Randall, R. V.: Hypoglycemia. Mayo Clinic Proc. 41:390, 1966.

Reemtsma, K., Lucas, J. F., Jr., Rogers, R. E., Schmidt, F. E., and Davis, F. N.: Islet cell function of the transplanted canine pancreas. Ann. Surg. 158:645, 1963.

Reinhoff, W. F.: An evaluation of pancreatic cysts treated at The Johns Hopkins Hospital. Surgery 47:188, 1960.

Rittenburg, M.: Pancreatitis in the elderly patient. Am. Surg. 27:475, 1961.

Salmon, P. A.: Carcinoma of the pancreas and extrahepatic biliary system. Surgery 60:554, 1966.

Seddon, J. A., and Howard, J. M.: The endocrine function of the homotransplanted pancreas. Surgery 59:235, 1966.

Seddon, J. A., and Howard, J. M.: The exocrine behavior of the homotransplanted pancreas. Surgery 59:226, 1966.

Shader, A. E., and Paxton, J. R.: Fatal pancreatitis. Am. J. Surg. 111:369, 1966.

Shapiro, H., Wruble, L. D., and Britt, L. G.: The possible mechanism of alcohol in the production of acute pancreatitis. Surgery 60:1108, 1966.

Silen, W., and Goldman, L.: A clinical analysis of acute pancreatitis. Arch. Surg. 86:1032, 1963.

Sim, D. N., Duprez, A., and Anderson, M. C.: Alterations of the lymphatic circulation during acute experimental pancreatitis. Surgery 60:1175, 1966.

Singleton, A., and Cunningham, P.: Islet cell tumors of the pancreas. Ann. Surg. 155:663, 1962.

Somogyi, M.: Blood diastase as an indicator of liver function. Proc. Soc. Exper. Biol. Med. 32:538, 1934.

Stiegmann, F.: The ominous reciprocity between liver disease and pancreatitis. Am. J. Gastroenterol. 33:459, 1960.

Sturin, H. S.: Surgical management of traumatic transection of the pancreas. Ann. Surg. 163:399, 1966.

Swerdlow, A., Berman, M., Gibbel, M., and Valatais, J.: Subcutaneous fat necrosis associated with acute pancreatitis. J.A.M.A. 173:765, 1960.

Taylor, D. H.: Angiographic visualization of the secretin stimulated pancreas. Radiology 87:525, 1966.

Teixeira, E., Sharkey, E., Colwell, J., and Bergan, J. J.: Insulin and glucose levels following pancreas allografting. Surg. Forum 12:205, 1966.

Trapnell, J. E., and Anderson, M. C.: Role of early laparotomy in acute pancreatitis. Ann. Surg. 165:49, 1967.

von Kalsrud, W., and Longmire, W., Jr.: Occurrence of pancreatic antibodies and experimental production of pancreatitis with pancreatic antiserum. Surgery 50:134, 1961.

Warren, K. W.: Islet cell tumors and hyperinsulinism. S. Clin. North America 47:709, 1962.

Warren, K. W.: Surgical aspects of pancreatic disease. Am. J. Dig. Dis. 6:402, 1961.

Warren, K. W., Athanassiades, S., Frederick, P., and Rune, G. A.: Surgical treatment of pancreatic cysts. Ann. Surg. 163:886, 1966.

Warren, K. W., Cahill, R., Blackburn, T., and Nora, P.: A long term appraisal of pancreatic duodenal resection for periampullary carcinoma. Ann. Surg. 155:652, 1962.

Welbourn, R. B.: Surgical aspects of hypoglycemia. J. Roy. Coll. Surg. Edin. 10:196, 1965.

Whipple, A., and Frantz, V.: Adenoma of islet cells with hyperinsulinism. Ann. Surg. 101:1299, 1935.

Whipple, A., Parsons, W., and Mullins, C.: Treatment of carcinoma of the ampulla of Vater. Ann. Surg. 102:763, 1935.

White, T. T., Elmslie, R. G., and Magee, D. F.: Observations on human intraductal pancreatic pressure. Surg. Gyn. & Obst. 118:1043, 1964.

White, T. T., Lawinski, M., Stacher, G., Tea, J. P. T., Michoulier, J., Murat, J., and Mallet-Guy, P.: Treatment of pancreatitis by left splanchnic and celiac ganglionectomy. Am. J. Surg. 112:195, 1966.

White, T. T., Lenninger, S. G., Elmslie, R. G., and Magee, D. F.: Effect of truncal and selective vagotomy on duodenal aspirates in man. Ann. Surg. 164:257, 1966.

Wilson, S. D., and Ellison, E. H.: Total gastric resection in children with the Zollinger-Ellison syndrome. Arch. Surg. 91:165, 1965.

Wilson, S. D., and Ellison, E. H.: Survival in patients with the Zollinger-Ellison syndrome treated by total gastrectomy. Am. J. Surg. 111:787, 1966.

Wilson, S. D., Hurley, J. D., and Ellison, E. H.: Heterologous transplantation and growth in tissue culture of ulcerogenic tumour cells from patients with the Zollinger-Ellison syndrome. Lancet 2:1307, 1962.

Zollinger, R., and Ellison, E.: Primary peptic ulceration of the jejunum associated with islet cell tumors of the pancreas Ann. Surg. 142:709, 1955.

Chapter 26

THE ADRENAL GLANDS

by

H. WILLIAM SCOTT, JR., M.D.
and
ROBERT K. RHAMY, M.D.

In answer to a comment about the new beautiful buildings on the Duke University campus, a graduate of the University of North Carolina qualified his agreement by calling attention to the lack of ivy. H. WILLIAM SCOTT, JR., has pursued his medical education in ivy-covered institutions beginning in Chapel Hill, North Carolina, and progressing to Boston and Baltimore. He began his surgical education at the Peter Bent Brigham Hospital and The Children's Hospital in Boston where he became the Harvey Cushing Fellow in Neurosurgery. He continued his education in surgery at The Johns Hopkins Hospital and advanced to the rank of Associate Professor of Surgery at The Johns Hopkins University School of Medicine. He was appointed Professor and Chairman of the Department of Surgery at Vanderbilt University School of Medicine in 1952. His scholarly attainments were rewarded throughout his education. His teaching talents are attested to by the numerous visiting professorships he has held. His professional abilities and personality have been recognized by numerous society memberships.

ROBERT K. RHAMY received his undergraduate medical schooling and postgraduate education in urology at the Indiana University Medical Center. He is Professor and Chairman of the Division of Urology at Vanderbilt University School of Medicine.

More than a century has passed since Thomas Addison described the syndrome of adrenal insufficiency which bears his name. He described the clinical syndrome with such clarity in the 11 patients whom he reported upon and elaborated the etiologic conditions so pointedly that little can be added even today. Efforts to provide substitutive therapy in adrenal cortical insufficiency were attempted as early as 1856. However, it remained for Kendall and Reichstein, in the late 1930's, to elaborate the biochemical studies which led to the many important discoveries concerning the synthesis and pathophysiology of the adrenal cortical steroids.

Although epinephrine has been recognized as an important hormonal product of the adrenal medulla since the nineteenth century, the isolation of norepinephrine in tissues by Von Euler and his associates in 1946, and in the adrenal gland by Holtz et al. in 1947, and the subsequent elucidation of its role and that of the other catecholamines in physiologic and pathophysiologic states, form an equally important contribution to knowledge of adrenal function. As a consequence, the clinician of today can approach the diagnosis of adrenal disease with a great deal more accuracy and sophistication than was available even a few short years ago. This, coupled with the ability to provide adequate replacement for total absence of the adrenal glands, has affected the field of adrenal surgery to a most remarkable degree.

SURGICAL ANATOMY AND EMBRYOLOGY

The two adrenal glands in man sit as caps over the upper poles of the kidneys. The convex surface of the kidney produces a concave impression on the inferior surface of each gland. The right suprarenal gland is roughly triangular in outline and its anterior surface touches the inferior vena cava posteriorly and medially, the liver laterally and the upper pole of the right kidney inferiorly. The left adrenal is crescentic in its outline and lies between the anteromedial border of the left kidney and the left lateral edge of the aorta. The glands are a darker yellow and firmer than the perirenal fat in which they lie. They are situated in the upper extension of a compartment enclosed by Gerota's fascia and are held in position by numerous fibrous bands as well as vascular attachments. Their relationship to the kidney has been overemphasized. When the kidney is depressed inferiorly the suprarenal glands remain in a relatively fixed position.

The weight of the normal adrenal gland may vary considerably but usually is in the range of 3 to 5 gm. The adrenal gland in the male is usually 30 per cent heavier than its female counterpart. The glands vary from 40 to 60 mm. in length, 20 to 30 mm. in width and 2 to 8 mm. in thickness, except at the bases where they are considerably thicker. The sectioned gland is seen grossly to consist of an outer cortical layer and an inner medullary portion which constitutes approximately 10 per cent of its weight. The outer cortex is yellowish and has a firmer consistency than the reddish-brown medullary portion.

The adrenal glands have an abundant arterial supply by branches of the inferior phrenic artery superiorly, the aorta medially and the renal artery inferiorly. In addition, branches from the ovarian and internal spermatic artery on the left side and from the intercostals bilaterally are found in many patients. As many as 50 or 60 small adrenal vessels have been observed in some individuals. These vessels break up into large sinusoids and blood flows of 6 to 7 ml. per gram of tissue per minute have been measured. After traversing the gland, the blood drains into large venous lacunae in the medulla, from which it is collected into a large venous trunk as well as a number of smaller veins. On the right, the short adrenal veins drain directly into the inferior vena cava, whereas the left adrenal vein drains into either the left renal vein or the vena cava. A small vein on each side courses along with the inferior phrenic vessels. On the left, small venous channels leave the cortex to join the vena cava and the splenic and pancreatic veins. In this way, a small part of the venous return reaches the portal system.

The lymphatic channels of the adrenals form two plexuses, one directly under the capsule and another one in the medulla. The lymphatics of the right adrenal drain into lymph nodes near the aorta and near the crus of the diaphragm. On the left side, they connect with lymph nodes at the origin of the left renal artery and with the lymph nodes along the aorta. The nerve supply is derived primarily from the splanchnic nerves. These nerves then form the suprarenal plexuses and connect with the renal and celiac plexuses and celiac ganglia. Stimulation of the adrenal nerves brings about a prompt release of medullary hormones without influencing cortical activity.

Histologic examination of the cortex reveals three distinct areas as viewed from the periphery medially. The zona glomerulosa, a thin outer layer of short loops of glomeruloid clusters of irregularly arranged cells lying just beneath the capsule of the adrenal, apparently secretes materials having to do with electrolyte exchange. The zona fasciculata, which is the widest cortical zone, consists of radially oriented strands of cells which elaborate hormones having to do with organic metabolism. Most centrally located is the zona reticularis, with its net-like cords of cells, which borders on the edge of the medulla and which elaborates hormones with androgenic and estrogenic effects. In contrast to the cortex, the medulla is structurally uniform, consisting of networks of anastomosing cords of polyhedral cells which secrete the hormonally active catecholamines, epinephrine, norepinephrine, dopamine and other precursors which currently seem to be biologically inert. Epinephrine comprises approximately 75 to 80 per cent of the medullary secretion and its inotropic effect on the myocardium causes an increase in cardiac output, whereas norepinephrine exerts a pressor effect by increasing peripheral resistance by vasoconstriction.

Embryologically, development of the adrenal gland represents the union of certain cells from the neural crest which form the adrenal medulla and cells from the splanchnic mesoderm which comprise the cortex. These two elements in lower vertebrates such as the fish are permanently separated. In embryos at the 5- to 6-mm. stage, the mesothelium at the upper level of the mesonephros proliferates and sends cords of cells laterally into the mesenchyme of the dorsal mesentery. Crowder states that there are three different types of cells comprising the adrenal cortex, two of which derive from the celomic epithelium and one which arises from the Bowman's capsule cells of the mesonephron. The fetal cortex is composed of the same cell types as the adult cortex but proportions and arrangements differ. Crowder maintains that both in the fetus and the adult all three types of cells of the cortex are renewed from the glomerulosa and migrate inwardly. Somewhat later than is the case with the adrenal cortex, the chromaphil cells of the medulla begin to develop. The medullary cells are ectodermal in origin and derive from sympathetic ganglia. The cells are of two types, sympathoblasts which eventually give rise to mature sympathetic ganglion cells, and pheochromoblasts which subsequently develop into the characteristic chromaffin cells of the adrenal medulla. By the 20-mm. stage in the human embryo, these chromaffin cells migrate along the lateral dorsal mesentery and penetrate the cortical analge. At the 100-mm. stage the chromaffin cells have reached the central vein and have formed a true medulla.

During the third and fourth months of fetal life the adrenals are enormous in size and actually exceed the kidneys in total mass. Most of this enlargement is caused by the growth of the fetal cortex. Subsequently, the adrenals grow less rapidly than the developing adjacent structures and at the sixth month of fetal life they are only half as large as the kidneys. At birth, the adrenals are approximately one-third as large as the kidneys.

The cells of the fetal cortex are most closely related to the zona reticularis. The normal human fetal adrenal cortex comprises approximately 80 per cent of the total adrenal mass throughout most of fetal life. At birth and occasionally immediately preceding birth, the fetal zone undergoes rather marked changes. These changes are characterized by necrosis, hemorrhage, vascular engorgement, loss of cellular detail and fragmentation of cells. This degeneration is compensated for in part by proliferation of the zona fasciculata and by the fifth to sixth postnatal week the adrenal cortex has obtained a more adult type of appearance. By the end of the first year of life, there is total disappearance of the fetal adrenal cortex. The rate of disappearance is the same for prematures and full term infants and seems to be related to the changes induced by birth and not by the actual age of the adrenal cortex.

PHYSIOLOGY

More than 50 different steroids have been isolated from the adrenal cortex. Of these only a few are secreted normally into the blood, whereas the rest are intracellular intermediates. Seven of these which are endowed with the capacity to support adrenalectomized animals have been identified: hydrocortisone, cortisone, corticosterone, dehydrocorticosterone, desoxycorticosterone, aldosterone and progesterone.

Recent studies, based on the isolation and characterization of circulating adrenal corticosteroids in the adrenal vein blood of animals and man, and on the identification of specific steroids secreted by perfused, mammalian adrenal glands, have demonstrated that the predominant hormones actually produced by the adrenal cortex are hydrocortisone, corticosterone, aldosterone, 11-hydroxyandrostenedione, androstenedione, and in all likelihood dehydroepiandrosterone. Smaller quantities of other steroids such as cortisone, 11-dehydrocorticosterone and 11-deoxyhydrocortisone are also apparently produced (Fig. 1).

No secretory nerves to the adrenal cortex in man have been demonstrated in contrast to the rich supply to the medulla. Growth of the adrenal cortex, as well as secretory activity of all its hormones except aldosterone, is regulated by the pituitary hormone, adrenocorticotropin. Pure corticotropin has been isolated in sheep and hogs by Li, who has shown it to be a polypeptide with 39 amino acids and a molecular weight of about 4540. Human corticotropin has been purified but has not yet been accurately chemically delineated. Certain of the basophils of the anterior pituitary gland as well as some of the large chromophobe cells are apparently the source of corticotropin. The basophilic cells increase in number after adrenalectomy and thus are presumably a source of corticotropin. The anterior pituitary may show sheaths of basophils in patients who have died of Addison's disease and their excess has been associated with elevated blood levels of corticotropin. Figure 2 demonstrates the stress mechanism of secretion of adrenocorticotropin from the anterior pituitary gland.

The corticotropin releasing factor seems to be the stimulatory factor to the anterior pituitary to release corticotropin. As can be seen there is a feedback mechanism which delicately controls the amount of corticotropin released from the anterior hypophysis. Adrenocorticotropin apparently initiates a biochemical reaction in the cortex of the adrenal glands which leads to enhancement of corti-

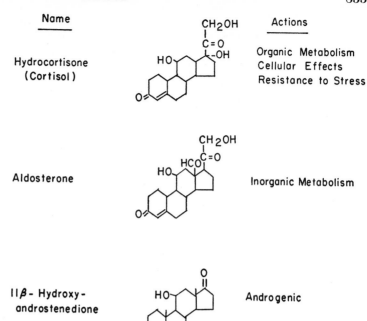

Name		Actions
Hydrocortisone (Cortisol)		Organic Metabolism Cellular Effects Resistance to Stress
Aldosterone		Inorganic Metabolism
11β-Hydroxy-androstenedione		Androgenic

Figure 1. Formulas of major adrenal cortical steroid hormones. (From Campbell, M. F.: Urology, 2nd ed. Philadelphia, W. B. Saunders Company, 1963.)

coid production. Cholesterol, which constitutes 5 per cent of the wet weight of the adrenal cortex, diminishes after adrenocorticotropin stimulation and shortly after this corticosteroids may be found to be increasing in the venous effluent from the adrenal gland.

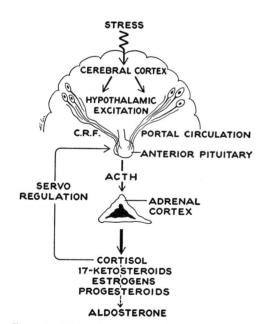

Figure 2. Schematic representation of mechanisms involved in the release of corticotropin from the anterior pituitary gland. (From Williams, R. H. [ed.]: Textbook of Endocrinology, 3rd ed. Philadelphia, W. B. Saunders Company, 1962.)

Among the various adrenal steroids, apparently only hydrocortisone has a physiologically significant role in regulating the rate of adrenocorticotropin secretion. The reciprocal relationship between these two hormones maintains the constancy of plasma cortisol within rather narrow limits in the absence of stress.

Both organic and inorganic metabolism are affected by the adrenal cortical steroid hormones. The organic functions are controlled by the glucocorticoids, especially the catabolic cortisol and corticosterone; the 17-ketosteroids, such as dehydroepiandrosterone, which are anabolic and androgenic; estrogens in small amounts, and various precursors of active corticoids. The inorganic functions include sodium retention and potassium excretion and are principally influenced by the mineralocorticoids aldosterone and desoxycorticosterone. The adrenal corticoids have both specific actions and permissive functions in affecting metabolic processes.

According to Williams, there is considerable functional overlap between glucocorticoids and mineralocorticoids. For instance, aldosterone has 500 times the activity of cortisol in sodium retention, yet only one-third its gluconeogenetic potency. Cortisol, however, has a significant effect on electrolyte metabolism because it is secreted in a quantity of about 20 mg. per day as contrasted to 150 μg. per day of aldosterone.

Cortisol and cortisone are the most important glucocorticoids. They enhance gluconeogenesis and in excess produce protein depletion and diabetes. They also induce a centripetal distribution of fat, hyperlipemia and hypercholesterolemia. They enhance water diuresis and assist in maintenance of the homeostasis of extracellular fluid volume by preventing the shift of water into the cell. Their hematologic effects are to increase the number of circulating erythrocytes, platelets and neutrophils while reducing the number of eosinophils, basophils and lymphocytes.

Physiologically, cortisol maintains the homeostasis of muscle protein and function. In its absence, striated muscles become weak and with excess cortisol, muscle protein is depleted. In the central nervous system cortisol lowers the threshold for electrical excitation. Psychiatric disturbances are common both with lack of cortisol and with its excess. In the gastrointestinal tract, gastric acidity is increased by cortisol and peptic ulcer formation is enhanced, possibly also by gastric mucus suppression, in the presence of excess cortisol. Cortisol blocks new bone formation at the level of the protein matrix, antagonizes the action of vitamin D, impedes the absorption of calcium from the gut, and increases the urinary clearance of calcium. Thus, in excess it enhances every phase of osteoporosis.

A most important physiologic effect of cortisol on the cardiovascular system is its permissive effect in sensitizing the arterioles to the pressor effects of norepinephrine and related compounds. Prolonged excess of cortisol enhances atherosclerosis. The glucocorticoids reduce the inflammatory process and the cellular response to injury, and cortisol inhibits hypersensitivity responses to antigen-antibody complexes. In excess, it reduces the production of antibodies, lyses plasma cells and lymphocytes and depresses immunologic responses.

The half-life of free cortisol in plasma is normally about 90 minutes. Its principal site of metabolic degradation is the liver where it undergoes enzymatic reduction and conjugation. The Porter-Silber chromogens or 17-hydroxycorticosteroids are easily measured urinary metabolites of cortisol and related glucocorticoids.

The anabolic, androgenic 17-ketosteroids enhance the synthesis of proteins from amino acids and antagonize the catabolic effects of the glucocorticoids. In excess, increases in muscle mass, virilization, hirsutism, acne, deepening of the voice and other masculinizing features result. The 17-ketosteroids are metabolized in the liver and are excreted in the urine chiefly as sulfate conjugates.

The mineralocorticoids, aldosterone and desoxycorticosterone, effect sodium retention and potassium loss. Sodium is exchanged for potassium and hydrogen ion in the renal tubule and similar exchanges which take place in sweat glands, salivary glands, intestinal mucosa and in general between intracellular and extracellular fluid are controlled by these corticoids. Aldosterone, which has 30 times the sodium retaining potency of desoxycorticosterone, is secreted by the zona glomerulosa of the adrenal cortex. This part of the cortex maintains its integrity after hypophysectomy and is apparently not controlled by adrenocorticotropin. Rather, aldosterone secretion is closely related to the renin-angiotensin system of the renal juxtaglomerular apparatus and responds to and delicately controls intra- and extravascular fluid volumes.

The adrenal medullary secretory activity is dependent on stimulation or excitation of its sympathetic nerves. Unlike the cortex, there is no known direct hormonal control over the medullary secretion. Epinephrine, norepinephrine and dopamine are secreted by at least two types of chromaffin cells in the medulla. These catecholamines are synthe-

Table 1. *Comparison of Pharmacologic Effects of Norepinephrine and Epinephrine*[*]

NOREPINEPHRINE		EPINEPHRINE
++++	Pressor effect	+
+++	Lipolysis	++
±	Increased cardiac output	++
+	Hyperglycemia	++++
++	Increased basal metabolic rate	++++
+	Eosinopenia	++++
0	Central nervous system excitation	++++

*From Williams, R. H. (ed.): Textbook of Endocrinology. 3rd ed. Philadelphia, W. B. Saunders Co., 1962.

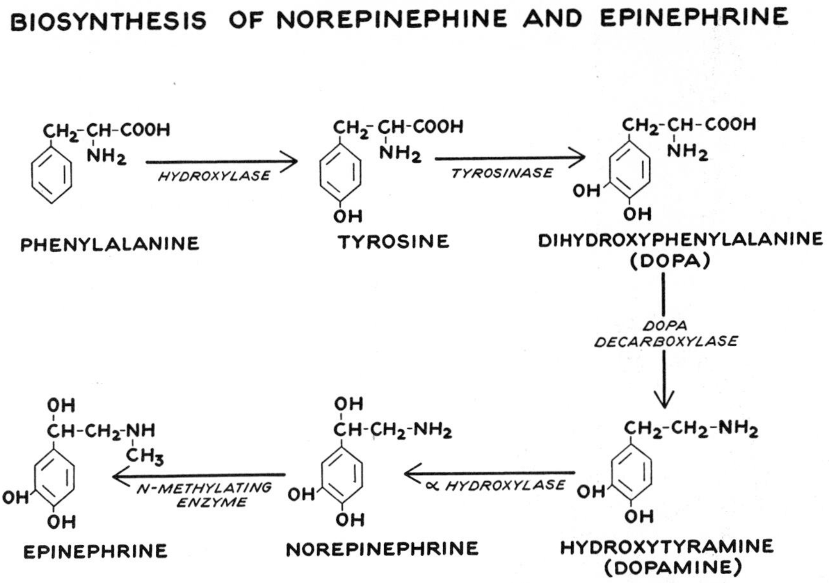

BIOSYNTHESIS OF NOREPINEPHINE AND EPINEPHRINE

Figure 3.   Principal pathways in the synthesis of catecholamines. (From Williams, R. H. (ed.): Textbook of Endocrinology, 3rd ed. Philadelphia, W. B. Saunders Company, 1962.)

sized from tyrosine by pathways indicated in Figure 3.

The physiologically more significant compounds are norepinephrine and epinephrine. Apparently the cells which store norepinephrine are incapable of methylating this catecholamine. Most of the extra-adrenal chromaffin tissues, including sympathetic ganglia and nerve endings, also largely lack the methylating mechanism. Accordingly, these extra-adrenal tissues produce chiefly norepinephrine and dopamine.

The catecholamines differ in their pharmacophysiologic effects, although a good deal of overlap exists. Table 1 summarizes their effects and differences.

Epinephrine has greater excitatory, hyperglycemic and metabolic effects and induces fright. Both compounds enhance the liberation of free fatty acids from fat depots and raise the circulating plasma levels. The catecholamines are normally metabolized rapidly by orthomethylation and oxidative deamination. About 40 per cent of the catecholamine secretion appears in the urine as conjugated 3-methoxy,4-hydroxymandelic acid.

RADIOGRAPHIC DIAGNOSIS

Except in unusually large tumors of the adrenal gland, adrenal tissue is not well seen on plain roentgenograms of the abdomen. Although the kidney and suprarenal gland are surrounded by a relatively radiolucent fat pad, the radiodensity of the suprarenal gland in relationship to the upper pole of the kidney and to the medial structures does not make its outline immediately and easily apparent. With enlargement of the adrenal gland the most usual roentgenographic sign seen on the plain abdominal or K. U. B. film is displacement of the renal mass inferiorly and laterally with the kidney on the same side of the tumor shifting its upper pole to a more lateral position. Sometimes even in bilateral adrenal hyperplasia when no tumor is present, the upper pole of the kidney may be subtly changed in its position and can be visualized in the plain roentgenogram.

The upright film with the presence of contrast media in the kidney will in most instances delineate the separation of the kidney and the adrenal, if the adrenal is enlarged. Laminography will greatly improve the delineation of the contours of the adrenals, particularly when combined with the presence of contrast media in the kidney. However, additional procedures are often required to demonstrate adrenal enlargement.

Retroperitoneal pneumography has long been a valuable procedure for delineation of the outlines of the adrenal gland. Refinements in technique and the utilization of more highly soluble gases have eliminated many of the previous complications of this type of study. The use of carbon dioxide or nitrous

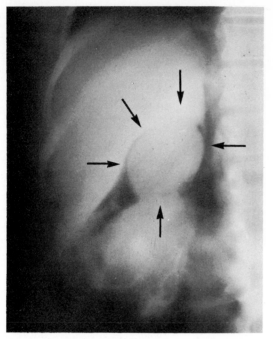

Figure 4. Radiographic visualization of adrenal tumor using retroperitoneal CO_2 insufflation. (From Scott, H. W., Jr., et al.: Ann. Surg. *162*:505, 1965.)

oxide has reduced the hazards of gas embolism. The availablity of image intensification has also greatly increased the diagnostic accuracy of this technique. A direct needle injection into the perirenal or presacral fat of nitrous oxide with control of the volume of gas by image intensification to delineate the adrenals is preferred (Fig. 4). With this technique not only adrenal tumors but adrenal hyperplasia can be recognized.

Adrenal angiography at times is clearly desirable but owing to the difficulties of filling of overlying vessels and the technical problems of selective adrenal angiography, this procedure is infrequently used. Occasionally, it may be helpful in the differentiation between benign and malignant adrenal tumors.

SURGICAL APPROACHES

Four different surgical approaches to the adrenals have been advocated. The approach chosen must be individualized on the basis of the diagnostic findings and the physical characteristics of the patient. Cahill has advocated the transabdominal approach because of the advantage of simultaneous bilateral exploration through a single incision. However, this approach is more time consuming,

difficult and associated with greater morbidity in the obese patient than some of the other approaches. It is most useful in thin patients, especially those with pheochromocytoma in whom opportunities for exploration of sites of aberrant adrenal tissue would be contemplated and in patients of normal habitus with adrenal tumor who have intercurrent abdominal disease which needs correction.

The thoracoabdominal approach affords the optimal exposure of a single adrenal and the contents of the ipsilateral renal fossa. It is indicated when large tumors are encountered, especially pheochromocytomas and adrenal carcinomas. This approach, however, does have the drawback of providing less than optimal exposure of the contralateral adrenal.

The most commonly used approach is that originally described by Young and is a bilateral posterior approach. In Young's approach to the adrenal gland, the patient is placed on the operating table in the prone position and the trunk is flexed. Usually a subperiosteal resection of the eleventh or twelfth rib is done. This approach has the advantage of being extraperitoneal, extrapleural and subdiaphragmatic. It is particularly advantageous where bilateral adrenalectomy is to be carried out when there may be an adrenal cortical adenoma or aldosteronoma in which exposure of both adrenal glands is a necessity. The main disadvantage is the limited operative exposure afforded. The postoperative morbidity is usually impressively reduced.

The posterolateral approach affords a wide field of operation with direct access to the suprarenal region on one side at a time, and is extremely useful when an adrenal tumor has been accurately localized prior to operation or when the patient is too large or obese to consider an approach by either the anterior or the posterior route.

CLINICAL CONDITIONS

Adrenal cortical insufficiency may be primary as in Addison's disease, or secondary as a result of pituitary corticotropic insufficiency. It may be overt or latent, organic or functional. Whether primary or secondary, the clinical syndromes manifest deficiencies in adrenal steroids. In 1855, Thomas Addison wrote: "The leading and characteristic features of the morbid state to which I would direct attention are anemia, general languor, and debility, remarkable feebleness of the heart's action, irritability of the stomach and a peculiar change of color in the skin occurring in connection with a diseased condition of the 'suprarenal capsules.'" His brilliant descriptions of the clinical manifestations of this disease require essentially no alterations even today. However, our understanding of the metabolic aspects and effects of this syndrome is considerably more complete. A classification of the etiologic agents is presented in Table 2.

ACUTE ADRENAL INSUFFICIENCY (ADDISONIAN CRISIS). Acute loss of adrenal function is attended by profound changes in blood pressure, electrolytes and carbohydrate metabolism. This dramatic condition often demands heroic methods of emergency treatment. The syndrome is classically manifested by anorexia, nausea, vomiting, headache, diarrhea, abdominal pain, dehydration, hypotension, hypoglycemia, marked weakness and extreme lethargy. Hyperpyrexia normally is present with coma and vascular collapse rapidly following. Acute adrenal cortical failure may follow hemorrhage into the adrenals as a result of trauma, infection, tumor or adrenal vascular thrombosis. Hemorrhage into the adrenal glands of the newborn is responsible for about 1 per cent of neonatal deaths, occurring most commonly after a difficult labor and fetal anoxia. The fulminating form of meningococcal meningitis, other severe infections with organisms such as pneumococcus, staphylococcus, hemolytic streptococcus, and other bacteremic and viremic states including smallpox and diphtheria may show hyponatremia, hyperkalemia, hypoglycemia and azotemia.

The treatment of the adrenal crisis is aimed at provision of adequate cortical hormone, the control of infection, and support of the cardiovascular system. In babies and young children, and immediate intravenous injection of 50 mg. of hydrocortisone is followed by a maintenance infusion of 100 to 200 mg. of hydrocortisone dissolved in 5 per cent dextrose and normal saline of appropriate volume and administered by intravenous drip over a period of 24 to 48 hours. Infection, which so commonly accompanies this syndrome, should be treated with appropriate antibiotics. If hypotension persists after the initiation of the hydrocortisone, a Neo-Synephrine drip, 5 to 10 mg. per liter, may be added to maintain blood pressure. Because these patients are usually hypovolemic, blood transfusions may be necessary if the shock persists. After the emergency period of treatment, hydrocortisone dosage is reduced by daily decrements until oral therapy with hydrocortisone in the range of 0.3 mg. per kilogram can be initiated. The addition of 0.05 to 0.1 mg. of fluorohydrocortisone daily is adjusted to maintain normal blood pressure. The need for maintenance dosage on a long-term basis must be determined by careful endocrine studies.

CHRONIC ADRENAL INSUFFICIENCY (ADDISON'S DISEASE). Addison's disease is relatively rare. The death rate from this disorder

Table 2. *Adrenal Insufficiency Syndromes—Classification of Adrenal Cortical Hypofunction**

I. Primary—deficiency of corticosteroids, aldosterone, and adrenal androgen
    A. *Acute*—Addisonian crisis
        1. Impaired adrenal secretory capacity—the demand for hormone exceeds the amount that can be produced
        2. Adrenal "apoplexy"—trauma, overwhelming infection, hemorrhage
        3. Adrenalectomy
        4. Atrophy due to prolonged steroid therapy
    B. *Chronic*—Addison's disease
        1. Complete
            a. Primary atrophy of the adrenal
            b. Destruction or replacement of cortical tissue by various diseases, e.g., tuberculosis, amyloidosis, etc.
            c. Adrenalectomy
        2. Incomplete
            a. Partial replacement of the gland, e.g., tumor, infection, hemorrhage
            b. Reduced adrenal cortical function—inanition (?), cachexia
II. Secondary—reduced cortisol secretion as a result of ACTH deficiency
    A. Hypopituitarism—complete, fractional, or unitropic deficiency of ACTH production
    B. Inhibition of ACTH synthesis and/or release due to glucocorticoid administration or hypothalamic-portal system defect
III. Altered adrenal cortisol metabolism
    A. Spontaneous and induced defects of cortisol synthesis—reduced or absent capacity to secrete cortisol as seen in the adrenogenital syndrome or after specific drugs
    B. Accelerated cortisol catabolism—thyroid storm; insulin-induced hypoglycemia

*From Frawley, T. F.: Adrenal cortical insufficiency. *In*, Eisenstein, A. B. (ed.): The Adrenal Cortex, Boston, Little, Brown and Company, 1967.

in the United States is approximately 0.3 per 100,000. It is predominantly a disease of adult life. The majority of patients are in the second and the fifth decades and males and females are affected with equal distribution. Basic to the physiopathology of the disease is a loss of adrenal cortical substance. Prior to 1950, 70 to 88 per cent of instances of Addison's disease were ascribed to adrenal tuberculosis, whereas the remainder were believed to be due to primary atrophy of the gland.

Currently, tuberculosis probably accounts for about 50 per cent of instances of Addison's disease. In the remainder, various other lesions may be encountered, including bilateral tumor metastases, leukemic infiltration, amyloidosis, hemochromatosis, histoplasmosis, coccidioidomycosis, cryptococcosis, blastomycosis, reticuloendotheliosis, giant cell granuloma, diphtheria, measles, scarlet fever and smallpox, typhoid fever, influenza, syphilis, malaria, amebiasis, and pyogenic infections. In addition, in rare instances familial Addison's disease has been described.

In Addison's disease due to tuberculosis of the adrenals, the lesions are always found bilaterally because the disease does not become symptomatic until 90 per cent or more of the glandular tissue has been destroyed. Although fibrosis is usually present, calcification of the caseous material occurs on rare occasions and may be demonstrated on x-ray examination. Tuberculosis of the adrenal glands is always secondary to an extra-adrenal focus and, therefore, pulmonary or renal tuberculosis should be looked for.

Addison's disease is usually insidious in its onset. Mild to severe weight loss is invariably present. Easy fatigability and muscular weakness occur in almost every patient. The muscular weakness which is commonly improved by sleep and rest also improves markedly when glucocorticoid administration restores carbohydrate metabolism to normal. Hyperpigmentation has been commonly observed in this disease. It is present in approximately 90 per cent of patients with Addison's disease. It is most marked in exposed areas of the skin, particularly in scars and on mucosal surfaces. The hyperpigmentation in patients with primary adrenal cortical insufficiency results from increased release in the pituitary gland of peptide hormones that cause the melanocytes to darken. Hyperpigmentation improves with treatment. Vitiligo is said to occur in 10 to 20 per cent of patients with Addison's disease. Hypotension, which is seen in ap-

proximately 90 per cent of patients with the disease, results from a combination of dehydration, decreased plasma volume and diminished peripheral vascular tone. Symptomatically, it is reflected by syncope, vertigo, weakness and postural hypotension. The symptoms most commonly presented by the patient are those associated with the gastrointestinal tract; anorexia, nausea and vomiting are present in the majority of patients. Abdominal pain may be seen in a few instances along with constipation or diarrhea. Hypoglycemic symptoms are described in approximately 60 per cent of patients with Addison's disease. The mental and nervous symptoms in Addison's disease are undoubtedly due in a large measure to hypoglycemic episodes. Loss of libido, impotence and reduced virility reflect the decreased androgenic function. Amenorrhea is noticed frequently in the female. The common laboratory findings in Addison's disease are increased urinary sodium and chloride excretion; increased serum sodium concentration; increased serum potassium concentration; decreased plasma 17-hydroxy corticosteroids; decreased urinary 17-ketosteroid and 17-hydroxy corticosteroid excretion; hypoglycemia; abnormal electroencephalogram; low voltage electrocardiogram with prolonged PR and QT intervals, with nonspecific T wave changes; decreased basal metabolism, and anemia.

Radiographically, skull films may aid in the differential diagnosis between primary and secondary adrenal cortical insufficiency. Enlargements of the sella turcica and erosion of the clinoids often occur with pituitary tumors and adrenal insufficiency may be secondary to destruction or failure of the anterior pituitary. Calcification of the pinna of the ear has been described in Addison's disease but also is seen in other conditions. Calcification of costal cartilages has been reported by Jarvis in 93 of 104 patients with Addison's disease. The chest film may reveal the source of the tuberculous infection, and the cardiac silhouette is ordinarily decreased in size in this condition. Abdominal films reveal calcification of the adrenal in about 12 per cent of patients.

The definitive diagnosis of adrenal insufficiency is largely, if not entirely, dependent upon the results of laboratory tests which measure adrenal function. The test procedures generally used can be divided into indirect and direct categories. The indirect tests of adrenal function are impaired water diuresis; salt deprivation; serum Na:K ratio; salivary Na:K ratio; absolute level of circulating eosinophils, and insulin-glucose tolerance test. Direct tests of adrenal function are basal levels of urinary steroid excretion; plasma level of cortisol, and response to adrenocorticotropin stimulation.

The diagnosis of Addison's disease can be best confirmed by the poor response to adrenal stimulation using an intravenous infusion of adrenocorticotropin over a period of eight hours with simultaneous measurement of urinary corticosteroid excretion.

The treatment of chronic adrenal insufficiency is dependent upon the relative deficiencies of the various corticosteroid compounds. The addisonian patient normally does not require special dietary measures; however, with extreme physical activity compensation in total caloric requirement should be made. During periods of stress or infection, foods which are high in carbohydrates and contain considerable sodium are to be preferred. If the addisonian patient works in a hot environment or travels to a region of high ambient temperatures, the need for salt and fluids must be recognized and the losses compensated. In adults, the usual maintenance dose of steroid necessary in complete adrenal insufficiency is approximately 20 to 40 mg. of hydrocortisone daily. Usually two-thirds of the dosage is given in the morning and the remainder in the late afternoon or evening. If weakness, hypoglycemia or other symptoms of adrenal insufficiency appear, the steroid dosage must be increased. The predominance of gastrointestinal symptoms in adrenal insufficiency makes these an excellent clinical indicator of insufficient maintenance dosage. Therefore, when nausea and vomiting occur the patient should take additional steroid medication. As far as other corticosteroids are concerned, symptoms as listed in Table 3 give an adequate guideline for replacement therapy.

HYPERADRENOCORTICISM. Clinical syndromes of hyperadrenocorticism are much more common than adrenal cortical insufficiency. Because the adrenal gland is capable of secreting glucocorticoids, mineralocorticoids, androgens and estrogens the spectrum of manifestations of disease in hyperadrenocorticism is wide. The clinical patterns of hyperadrenocorticism are listed in Table 4.

CUSHING'S SYNDROME. During the past decade, a number of developments have combined to increase the ease and accuracy with which Cushing's syndrome can be diagnosed

Table 3. *Selection Basis for Specific Steroid Therapy**

1. Glucocorticoids:
   Weakness
   Hypoglycemia
   Anorexia and gastrointestinal disturbances
   Central nervous system disturbances
   Hyperpigmentation
   Impaired water tolerance
   Drugs:
   a. Hydrocortisone, 10–40 mg. by mouth daily in divided doses
   b. Cortisone, 25–50 mg. by mouth daily in divided doses
2. Mineralocorticoids:
   Dehydration and weight loss
   Hypotension and small heart size
   Weakness
   Low serum sodium, high serum potassium
   Elevated urinary, salivary, sweat sodium
   Drugs:
   a. Desoxycorticosterone acetate in oil, 3–5 mg. intramuscularly daily
   b. Desoxycorticosterone trimethylacetate, 50–100 mg. intramuscularly every 4–6 weeks
   c. Fluorohydrocortisone acetate, 0.1–2 mg. by mouth daily
   d. Sodium chloride, 3–6 gm. daily
3. Androgenic-anabolic hormones:
   Anemia
   Impotence
   Diminished axillary and pubic hair
   Weakness and decreased muscle mass
   Drugs:
   a. Fluoxymestrone, 2 mg. by mouth daily 5 days per week
   b. Testosterone cyclopentylproprionate, 50 mg. intramuscularly every 4–6 weeks

*From Frawley, T. F.: Adrenal cortical insufficiency. *In*, Eisenstein, A. B. (ed.): The Adrenal Cortex. Boston, Little, Brown and Company, 1967.

Table 4. Clinical Patterns of Hyperadrenocorticism

ADRENAL SECRETION	PRINCIPAL HORMONE	RESULTS OF EXCESSIVE SECRETION
Glucocorticoid	Hydrocortisone	Cushing's syndrome
Mineralocorticoid	Aldosterone	Hyperaldosteronism (Conn's syndrome)
Androgen	Androstenedione	Virilism in females
	Dehydroepiandrosterone	Precocious puberty in males
Estrogen	Estradiol-17B	Feminization in males

and treated. In his classic description of the syndrome in 1932, Harvey Cushing emphasized the clinical features of central obesity, osteoporosis, amenorrhea, hirsutism, striae, hypertension and weakness. At that time, he attributed these changes to pituitary basophilism. Anderson and her co-workers were among the first to present evidence that the probable common denominator in all patients with Cushing's syndrome was hyperactivity of the adrenal cortex. We may now define Cushing's syndrome as a group of clinical and metabolic disorders which result from an excess of cortisol (hydrocortisone).

Apart from the medicinal use of hormones, an excess of cortisol results most commonly from bilateral adrenal cortical hyperplasia under the stimulatory effect of increased secretion of adrenocorticotropin by the pituitary. The latter may or may not contain an adenoma. In what is probably the next most common situation, Cushing's syndrome results from a nonendocrine tumor which secretes adrenocorticotropin or an adrenocorticotropin-like polypeptide. The next most common cause of the syndrome is adrenocortical tumor. In the past 30 years, it has become established that unrecognized and untreated Cushing's syndrome is a highly incapacitating and lethal disorder. With accurate recognition and treatment, the results are now very good.

In recent years, it has been the impression of some physicians that Cushing's syndrome is on the increase. However, it appears more likely that this represents better implementation of diagnostic methods which promote wider recognition of the disease rather than an absolute increase. In spite of the increased number of reported patients, Cushing's syndrome still remains comparatively rare. The incidence of spontaneous Cushing's syndrome is probably about six per million population. It occurs most frequently in young adults and is three to five times more common in females than in males. In 69 patients studied in the past decade, the age range was from nine months to 57 years of age and two-thirds of the patients were females. In Heeg's recent series 67 per cent had hyperplasia, 23 per cent had adrenal cortical carcinoma and 10 per cent had benign adrenal cortical adenoma. In children aged 13 years or less, however, adrenal cortical carcinoma as a cause of Cushing's syndrome accounts for approximately 60 per cent of the recorded patients and an additional 15 per cent are due to benign cortical adenoma. Thus, it appears that about 75 per cent of cases of Cushing's syndrome in children are due to adrenal cortical tumor. The most common cause of naturally occurring Cushing's syndrome is bilateral adrenal hyperplasia, infrequently with accompanying pituitary tumor; second is adrenal cortical adenoma; third is ectopic adrenocorticotropin producing extraendocrine malignant tumor, and fourth is adrenal cortical carcinoma.

Excessive production of corticoids results in a catabolic effect which leads to protein depletion and diminution in the mass of connective tissue and muscle of the individual. The thin, delicate skin and increased capillary fragility which are manifested by easy bruisability as well as abdominal striae are characteristic of the severe protein depletion. Children usually show growth retardation, muscular weakness and osteoporosis with loss of strength of bones; pathological fractures are common. Cutaneous striae result where the protein-depleted corium of the skin is stretched and split by underlying accumulations of adipose tissue. The accelerated protein breakdown results in increased gluconeogenesis and diminished carbohydrate tolerance. Overt diabetes may result from these processes. Another common result of altered protein and carbohydrate metabolism is impairment of wound healing. The integument is sometimes so friable that it may be denuded merely by removal of adhesive tape.

The serum gamma globulin tends to be decreased and this coupled with altered metabolism of protein and carbohydrate makes these patients particularly subject to infections. Accompanying the excessive protein breakdown is an abnormal accumulation of fat with deposition especially in the face, neck, back and trunk. The cervicodorsal fat pad has been characterized as a "buffalo hump."

The anterior pituitary gland may show cytologic abnormalities characterized by basophilic cytoplasmic hyalinization, vacuolization and degranulation. Cushing described these changes originally as "pituitary basophilism." True basophilic adenomas, if they occur, are incredibly rare, but mixed basophilic and chromophobe tumors and pure chromophobe adenomas of the pituitary do occur in Cushing's disease.

Among a large group of patients with suspected Cushing's syndrome studied by Liddle and his associates between 1956 and 1964, 46 patients proved to have Cushing's disease or pituitary dependent hyperadrenocorticism. Six of this group showed erosion of the sella turcica at the time the diagnosis of hyperadrenocorticism was made. A few patients subsequently developed pituitary tumors after excision of the adrenals. In 14 other patients with Cushing's syndrome verified during this period, adrenal cortical tumors were present and in approximately one-third of these the tumor was adrenal carcinoma. Summaries of many patients reported in the literature have demonstrated that approximately 55 per cent of adrenal tumors occur on the left, 35 per cent on the right and 10 per cent bilaterally. In nine patients with Cushing's syndrome hyperadrenocorticism resulted from the effects of a malignant extraendocrine tumor, most commonly carcinoma of lung, which secreted adrenocorticotropin or adrenocorticotropin-like polypeptides.

Histologically, bilateral hyperplasia of the zona fasciculata of the adrenal cortex is most apt to be present when the clinical diagnosis is pituitary-dependent Cushing's syndrome or so-called "Cushing's disease." Unilateral adrenocortical hyperplasia has been reported on rare occasions. A small percentage of patients with Cushing's syndrome exhibit no structural abnormality of the adrenal glands, grossly or histologically.

Measurement of the daily urinary excretion of 17-hydroxycorticosteroids, the metabolites of hydrocortisone, has proved to be a practical index of cortisol secretion. Normal adults usually excrete 3 to 10 mg. of 17-hydroxycorticosteroids in 24 hours and patients with Cushing's syndrome usually excrete in excess of 12 mg. per day.

The relations between the adrenocorticotropic hormone of the pituitary and cortisol in normal individuals and in patients with Cushing's syndrome have been studied extensively by many investigators and form the basis for precise diagnostic studies. Liddle and his associates have previously described a standardized adrenocorticotropin suppression test of great practical use in the diagnosis of Cushing's syndrome. In the normal individual adrenocorticotropin secretion by the pituitary governs the secretion of cortisol by the adrenal cortex. Cortisol in turn has a suppressive effect on the secretion of adrenocorticotropin. This relationship can be depicted as a servo-mechanism in which cortisol levels tend to be self-regulating. In Cushing's syndrome, the fact that cortisol levels are elevated indicates that the normal restraint on pituitary or adrenal function is not operating properly. Two possibilities are apparent: either the adrenocorticotropin-secreting mechanism is not restrained by normal levels of cortisol or else the adrenal cortex is no longer dependent on the stimulatory effect of adrenocorticotropin and secretes excessive cortisol autonomously.

Liddle's suppression test is based on the urinary 17-hydroxycorticosteroid response to small doses of potent synthetic steroids, $\Delta9\alpha$-fluorocortisol (ΔFF) or dexamethasone, which have 30 times the potency of cortisol and which like cortisol can suppress adrenocorticotropin secretion by the pituitary. In normals 0.5 mg. of ΔFF or dexamethasone every six hours causes a drop in urinary excretion of 17-hydroxycorticosteroids to less than 2.5 mg. per day in 48 hours. In a study of 30 patients with Cushing's syndrome, 29 individuals showed resistance to the normally suppressive effect of this small dose of ΔFF. In 23 of 24 patients with adrenocortical hyperplasia a larger dose of ΔFF or dexamethasone caused a suppression of the daily urinary output of 17-hydroxycorticosteroids. This response indicates adrenocorticotropin-dependent Cushing's syndrome. In patients with Cushing's syndrome due to an adrenocortical tumor, ΔFF and dexamethasone in both small and large doses as a rule failed to show suppression. This absolute resistance to suppression is characteristic of nonadrenocorticotropin-dependent Cushing's syndrome and suggests the autonomous secretion of cortisol by an adrenocortical tumor which is not under the control of the pituitary. A practical schema for the use of the suppression test in suspected Cushing's syndrome as used by Liddle is seen in Figure 5.

The standard adrenocorticotropin stimulation test offers further diagnostic information. In normals the urinary 17-hydroxycorticosteroid response to eight-hour infusion of 50 units of adrenocorticotropic hormone is in the range of 20 to 40 mg. per 24 hours. In Cushing's syndrome due to adrenal hyperplasia in our series the basal levels were elevated and the response was in the 30- to 80-mg. range. In the majority of instances the patients with adrenal hyperplasia responded by excreting over 50 mg. of 17-hydroxycorticosteroids. In Cushing's syndrome due to adrenal tumor most patients are resistant to adrenocorticotropin stimulation and show no change in urinary 17-hydroxycorticosteroid excretion in response to the standard infusion. Patients with adrenal carcinoma are uniformly resistant to adrenocorticotropin stimulation. However, about half the patients with adrenal adenoma show an increase in urinary 17-hydroxycorticosteroid excretion following infusion of adrenocorticotropic hormone.

Other endocrine studies which are helpful in the diagnosis of Cushing's syndrome and the differentiation between tumor and hyperplasia include the measurement of plasma adrenocorticotropin levels, the Metyrapone (SU 4885) test and measurement of urinary 17-ketosteroid levels. The drug Metyrapone blocks the conversion of compound S to cortisol in the adrenal cortex. When patients with Cushing's syndrome are tested with the drug, those with hyperplasia usually show pituitary responsiveness with an increase in urinary 17-hydroxycorticosteroid excretion and those with adrenocortical tumor do not respond. In general the measurement of daily urinary 17-hydroxycorticosteroid output, the adrenocorticotropin suppression, and stimulation tests will establish the diagnosis of Cushing's syndrome and delineate the underlying cause with a high degree of accuracy.

A correct diagnosis of tumor can be made before operation using these diagnostic concepts. Removal of the tumor is followed by regression of symptoms and prompt relief of hypertension. In our experience, there has been no evidence of recurrence of either the benign or malignant tumors during a follow-up period of three to 11 years.

In the management of Cushing's syndrome associated with bilateral adrenal cortical hyperplasia, there has been much less uniformity in both method and result. Our own experience reflects the evolutionary aspects

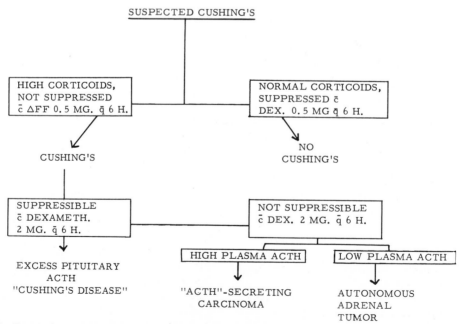

Figure 5.   Practical use of the synthetic steroid (ΔFF or dexamethasone) test (Liddle) for evaluation of the patient with suspected Cushing's syndrome. (From Scott, H. W., Jr., and Foster, J. H.: Surgical considerations in hypertension. *In*, Current Problems in Surgery. Chicago, Year Book Medical Publishers, 1964.)

of clinical treatment in adrenocorticotropin-dependent hyperadrenocorticism.

Inappropriately high secretion of adrenocorticotropin in these patients was found to be of pituitary origin. In contrast to the excessive secretion in the functioning extra-endocrine carcinomas suppression of adrenocorticotropic hormone activity can be demonstrated by the use of dexamethasone in patients with "Cushing's disease."

Bilateral total adrenalectomy was used in treatment of most instances of pituitary-dependent hypercortisolism. Elimination of the target organ, the adrenal cortex, is the most dependably accurate means of effecting prompt regression of symptoms in these patients. The addisonian state which is produced as a substitute can be managed currently with considerable ease and accuracy. More recently, pituitary irradiation with radioactive cobalt (CO^{60}) has been found to be increasingly satisfactory in controlling Cushing's disease and bilateral adrenalectomy has been reserved for patients with severe symptoms and for those who fail to respond satisfactorily to pituitary irradiation.

A careful regimen of adrenal substitution therapy has been required by the patients treated by total adrenalectomy. In most of the patients with unilateral adrenalectomy for tumor, supportive adrenal substitution therapy has been needed only in the early postoperative period. In a few exceptions, several weeks or months of steroid support have been required. The patients treated by pituitary irradiation alone who have obtained a good result have not required adrenal substitution therapy.

The management of the patients with the Cushing syndrome due to an extraendocrine tumor which produces adrenocorticotropic hormone or an adrenocorticotropic hormone-like polypeptide is apt to be most unsatisfactory. In the majority of such patients the source of the ectopic hormone is a highly malignant tumor which has most often reached an incurable stage by the time the manifestations of Cushing's syndrome are recognized. The ectopic adrenocorticotropic hormone which stimulates the adrenal cortex to produce hypercortisolism is not responsive to dexamethasone suppression. The incidence of extremely high corticosteroid levels is greater in this syndrome than with the other varieties of the disease.

Liddle has pointed out that many patients with this syndrome lack the characteristic cushingesque central obesity. The only explanation offered for this is that these patients eat poorly and fail to gain weight as a result of the advanced primary malignant tumor.

The logical treatment of the ectopic adrenocorticotropic hormone syndrome is removal of the primary tumor. Unfortunately, this is rarely possible because of the invasive and metastatic state of the tumor. Palliation of the syndrome can be provided by bilateral total adrenalectomy. The prognosis in most patients is very poor.

The present program of treatment of Cushing's syndrome can be summarized as follows. In patients with Cushing's syndrome due to adrenal cortical tumor, unilateral adrenalectomy with removal of the tumor is clearly indicated. The posterior retroperitoneal operative approach is preferable unless a massive tumor is present, in which case a thoracoabdominal exposure is desirable. In most patients with Cushing's disease due to pituitary tumor, and in those with bilateral adrenal cortical hyperplasia due to excess pituitary adrenocorticotropin with manifestations of moderate degree, pituitary irradiation should be given a trial. If radiation is unsuccessful in producing a satisfactory and lasting remission in these patients, removal of the pituitary tumor, if present, or bilateral total adrenalectomy should be performed. In patients with florid manifestations of Cushing's syndrome due to adrenal cortical hyperplasia, especially with severe progressive hypertension and morbidly symptomatic osteoporosis, and for palliation of the ectopic adrenocorticotropic hormone syndrome, bilateral total adrenalectomy should be done. The bilateral posterior retroperitoneal approach to each gland is preferred.

ALDOSTERONISM. In 1955, Conn reported a clinical syndrome which he designated "primary aldosteronism." He described this as a syndrome of mineralocorticoid excess induced by the adrenal cortical elaboration of excessive amounts of aldosterone and characterized by abnormally large amounts of urinary aldosterone and normal amounts of urinary 17-hydroxycorticoids and 17-ketosteroids. The symptomatology of Conn's syndrome in its full-blown state includes intermittent or recurrent bouts of muscular weakness, occasionally progressing to flaccid paralysis of the lower extremities; headache, usually severe; polydipsia and polyuria with nocturia, and paresthesias consisting of prickling and tingling of hands and feet and bouts of carpopedal spasm. The most prominent physical finding in the syndrome is hypertension which may vary from a mild, benign form to malignant hypertension with papilledema and hemorrhagic retinopathy. Chvostek's and Trousseau's signs may be present. Zimmerman has described a dramatic clinical sign which should alert the physician to the possibility of the presence of aldosteronism. This is the production of carpal spasm at the time the blood pressure cuff is inflated, coupled with the recording of hypertension.

Women are afflicted more commonly than men in a ratio of 2.5:1. Although children and young adults occasionally have primary aldosteronism, the majority of patients fall into the age range of 30 to 50 years.

The clinical syndrome of primary aldosteronism is most commonly produced by functioning, benign, adrenal cortical adenoma, usually single but occasionally multiple. These adenomas are usually small and well encapsulated, although large lesions up to 90 gm. in weight have been reported. Less frequently, bilateral adrenal hyperfunction, with or without gross or microscopic evidence of hyperplasia, has been found. This has been more common in young adults and in children. The least common cause of primary aldosteronism has been an adrenal cortical carcinoma.

The small cortical adenomas which commonly are found to be the cause of the syndrome are usually soft, orange to yellow, spherical lesions. On microscopic examination, the adenomas are composed of uniform, clear cells of the type seen in the zona glomerulosa of the adrenal cortex from which they are believed to arise.

The characteristic laboratory findings in primary aldosteronism are hypokalemia, hypernatremia and alkalosis accompanied by large urine volumes with low specific gravity and a neutral or alkaline reaction. Proteinuria is commonly observed. The typical changes of hypokalemia are usually present in the electrocardiogram. On a normal salt intake, urinary potassium levels are usually elevated to 30 mEq. per liter or more. Urinary aldosterone excretion of the free hormone is increased in most instances from the normal 2 to 12 μg. per 24 hours to the range of 12 to 40 μg. per 24 hours.

Measurement of the rate of aldosterone secretion using radioisotopic techniques has become accepted as the most accurate laboratory method for establishing the diagnosis of hyperaldosteronism. Coppage and his associates found the rate of secretion of aldosterone in 15 normal subjects on unrestricted diets with liberal sodium intakes to range from 95 to 249 μg. per day. Normal persons on low-sodium diets and patients with either primary or secondary hyperaldosteronism are found to have secretory rates greatly in excess, up to 2000+ μg. per day, of this normal range.

In making a diagnosis of primary aldosteronism, the syndrome must be differentiated from the various secondary states of excess aldosterone secretion which may occur in decompensated cirrhosis of the liver, the nephrotic syndrome, congestive heart failure and various hypertensive diseases. The common use of the chlorothiazide diuretics in the management of hypertension results in symptoms which may obscure or be confused with Conn's syndrome. The recognition of the significant combination of hypertension and hypokalemia associated with metabolic alkalosis in the absence of the stigmata of Cushing's syndrome, or the states which produce secondary aldosteronism, becomes the initial basis for the diagnosis of the primary disorder. It has been repeatedly stressed that the diagnosis of this disease largely depends on precise laboratory studies. Hypokalemic alkalosis is usually present and is accompanied by excessive urinary potassium losses. In the presence of normal salt intake, hypernatremia is commonly observed. Conn has demonstrated that secondary hyperaldosteronism may occur in patients with advanced essential hypertension, renovascular hypertension and unilateral renal disease with malignant hypertension. In secondary aldosteronism, potassuric hypokalemic alkalosis may be present but hypernatremia is absent and hyponatremia is common.

The double isotope derivative assay for aldosterone secretion described by Kliman and Peterson makes the investigation of aldosterone secretion rate more reliable and, therefore, in evaluation of patients fewer aldosterone secretion rate determinations are necessary. Although making the spadework of evaluation easier and more uniform, this new method does not add to the differentiation between primary and secondary aldosteronism.

The role of angiotensin in circulatory homeostasis has recently been clarified. In addition to its role in constriction of the arterioles, angiotensin stimulates the adrenal glands and causes the production of aldosterone. Renin produced by the renal juxtaglomerular cells acts on a liver substrate α-2 globulin to form angiotensin I, which is then converted by a plasma enzyme into the active peptide, angiotensin II. The relationships of renin, angiotensin and aldosterone in primary and secondary aldosteronism are shown in Figure 6.

With the development of a bioassay for the measurement of human plasma renin activity levels, the diagnostic criteria for primary aldosteronism have been sharpened. Only those hypertensive patients with an elevated aldosterone secretion rate on high sodium intake and a low plasma renin activity on a low sodium diet can be considered to fulfill the present criteria for the diagnosis of primary aldosteronism. The relationships between aldosterone secretion rate and plasma renin activity in primary and secondary aldosteronism under different conditions of salt balance are shown in Table 5.

The major differentiating finding is a low plasma renin activity on a low sodium diet in patients with primary aldosteronism. The value of plasma renin activity in differentiating primary from secondary aldosteronism has led to a practical approach to the diagnosis of primary aldosteronism. Definitive diagnosis can only be made by demonstrating inappropriately and autonomously elevated aldosterone secretion rate, but this determination in every hypertensive patient is not practical at present. Priority for evaluation should be given to patients who manifest hypokalemia and the classic clinical findings. Suspected patients should have plasma renin activity response to low sodium diet tested first. This determination yields diagnostically crucial information and is less expensive and more efficient as a screening procedure than determination of the aldosterone secretion

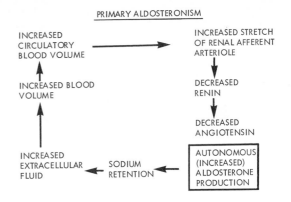

PRIMARY ALDOSTERONISM

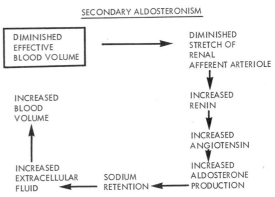

SECONDARY ALDOSTERONISM

Figure 6. Pathogenesis of hyperaldosteronism—primary and secondary types.

rate. Patients unable to increase plasma renin activity in response to a low sodium diet and upright posture should have the aldosterone secretion rate determined while on a high sodium diet.

Conn attributes the renal defect in tubular reabsorption of water in hyperaldosteronism, as well as the kidney's inability to acidify the urine normally, to the effect of chronic de-

Table 5. *Effects of Variation in Sodium Intake on Aldosterone Secretion Rate and Plasma Renin Activity in the Normal Subject and in States of Hyperaldosteronism*

CLINICAL STATE	NA INTAKE	ALDOSTERONE SECRETION RATE	PLASMA RENIN ACTIVITY
Normal	High sodium	↓	↓
	Low sodium	↑	↑
Secondary aldosteronism	High sodium	↑	↑
	Low sodium	↑ ↑	↑ ↑
Primary aldosteronism	High sodium	↑	↓
	Low sodium	↑	↓

pletion of body potassium on renal function and structure. The histopathologic lesions have been designated "kaliopenic nephropathy." These are concentrated in the proximal tubules and consist mainly of vascular degeneration progressing in severe cases to tubular necrosis and calcification. Much of the tubular lesion is thought to be reversible with potassium repletion.

Because of the small size of the adenomas which cause primary aldosteronism, preoperative efforts to localize or lateralize the tumor are not likely to be successful, although the less common larger tumors may be identified by the use of retroperitoneal pneumography, aortography or pyelography, alone or in combination. After the diagnosis is established, efforts to eliminate severe hypokalemic alkalosis are in order and usually require large amounts of supplemental potassium, up to 300 mEq. per day, for many days. Failure to correct the severe electrolyte imbalance prior to operation may increase the likelihood of arrhythmias, respiratory paralysis and irreversible shock with the stress of anesthesia and operation. Zimmerman attributes these complications to inadequate repletion of severe potassium deficits. He also warns against the use of the curare-like compounds during anesthesia in these patients because of the synergistic effects of such drugs and potassium deficiency.

In the surgical treatment of primary aldosteronism, careful bilateral exploration of the adrenal glands seems to be clearly indicated. This can readily be accomplished by a transperitoneal approach using an upper abdominal transverse or "bucket-handle" incision.

Careful search for adenoma in each adrenal gland is required and removal of a localized adenoma with preservation of residual normal adrenal tissue is the aim of the operation. This can be accomplished in the majority of patients. If no adenoma can be found and the clinical and laboratory diagnosis of primary aldosteronism is unequivocal, bilateral total or near total adrenalectomy is indicated. Postoperatively, adrenal substitution therapy is usually required only if total adrenalectomy has been necessary. Potassium supplements to diet may be required, however, for several weeks to restore the total body deficits.

In general, the results of operative removal of the source of excessive aldosterone secretion have been dramatically good. In most instances, the entire syndrome is relieved with prompt disappearance of symptoms, the initiation of a sodium diuresis, cessation of excessive potassium losses and restoration of acid-base balance. In addition, hypertension disappeared completely in two-thirds of Conn's patients within three months and did not recur during follow-up. In about one-fourth of his patients, there was marked reduction but not total elimination of hypertension, and in only a small percentage did hypertension persist and in these, severe renal damage is suspected.

In 12 patients with primary aldosteronism, the average age was 40 years, with a range from 21 to 26 years; three-fourths of the patients were female. Preoperative blood pressures ranged from 160 to 240 systolic and 90 to 140 diastolic. Serum potassium concentrations averaged 2.7 mEq. per liter, with a range of 1.8 to 3.9 mEq. per liter. Ninety-six per cent of the patients were hypokalemic and 90 per cent showed changes in the electrocardiogram indicative of electrolyte imbalance.

Aldosterone excretion was measured in two patients in this group whereas in the remaining patients, aldosterone secretion rates were determined by a double isotope derivative method. The normal aldosterone secretion rate in our laboratory is less than 150 μg. per day in a patient equilibrated on a 100 mEq. sodium diet. The range in these 10 patients was 169 to 10,000 μg. per day with an average of 397 μg. per day, excluding the 10,000 μg. per day value. This latter value was measured in a young woman in the sixth month or pregnancy.

Plasma renin activity was also measured in eight patients by modification of the bioassay of Boucher. After four days of a 10 mEq. sodium diet and after having been upright for at least four hours, normal subjects have a plasma renin activity greater than 600 nanograms per 100 ml. The range of values in these patients with primary aldosteronism was 0 to 401 nanograms per 100 ml. with an average of 127 nanograms per 100 ml.

Adrenal adenomas were present in 11 of these 12 patients. One patient had no demonstrable abnormality of the adrenal gland and no ectopic adrenal tissue with adenoma could be found at operation. In two-thirds of the patients, the adenoma was in the right adrenal and one patient had bilateral tumors. All the tumors were benign and varied in size from 1 to 22 gm. In each instance, bilateral adrenal exploration was carried out and in the last ten patients the bilateral posterior retroperitoneal approach was used. In the 11 patients in whom adrenal adenomas were found and removed, hypertension and other manifestations of hyperaldosteronism regressed rapidly, although in a few patients mild hypertension persisted for six to 12 months.

Conn has recently suggested that 10 to 20 per cent of patients with so-called essential hypertension probably harbor a small aldosterone-secreting cortical tumor. Evaluation of a large series of relatively unselected hypertensive patients has led us to believe that probably no more than 3 per cent of such patients actually fulfill the present criteria for the diagnosis of primary aldosteronism. However, until the currently accurate diagnostic methods are applied on a wide scale, the true incidence of aldosteronism in essential hypertension must remain unknown.

CONGENITAL ADRENAL HYPERPLASIA (ADRENOGENITAL SYNDROME). This syndrome is an inherited, inborn error of metabolism and is related to specific enzymatic defects in biosynthesis of steroids by the adrenal cortex. Congenital adrenal hyperplasia occurs frequently in siblings but the parents show no evidence of endocrine dysfunction, and consanguinity is rare. Childs has deduced that this syndrome is due to a nonsex-linked recessive mutant gene, which can only express itself clinically in homozygous offspring. The detection of the disease in twins, first cousins and half-sisters is in accordance with this mode of inheritance. The greater frequency of the disease in females is an artifact caused by the difficulty in diagnosis in males. Childs has found there is at least one affected child per 62,500 persons in the state of Maryland. Discovery of the efficacy of cortisone therapy by Wilkins, and the more recent elucidation of the enzymatic defects concerned with this syndrome, have greatly improved our understanding of the diagnosis, pathophysiology and treatment of the disease.

Congenital bilateral adrenal cortical hyperplasia produces pseudohermaphroditism in females and macrogenitosomia praecox in males. This may manifest itself in the prenatal period or in the postnatal years.

The exact set of symptoms rising in each individual depends upon the enzymatic block which is present in the biosynthesis of cortisone. The four major types of congenital adrenal hyperplasia are the simple virilizing form; the sodium-losing form; the hypertensive form, and the $3,\alpha$-hydroxysteroid dehydrogenase defect.

Because of the impaired cortisol synthesis there is a hypersecretion of adrenocorticotropin by the pituitary gland which in turn leads to adrenal hyperplasia. The excess secretion of the adrenal androgens and the virilism that is characteristic of this syndrome are responses to hypersecretion of the pituitary hormone. In the male infant, the internal and external genitalia are quite normal, although the penis may be slightly enlarged. Female infants present as pseudohermaphrodites in that they have a small phallus but otherwise normal external and internal genitalia. The phallus may be represented by any extreme from a simple hypertrophied clitoris to a penile-appearing organ with scrotum-like labia without testes and a urogenital sinus opening at the end of the phallus. The genital abnormality may be so extreme as to present the appearance of a cryptorchid male, but the chromosome structure is that of the female with congenital adrenal hyperplasia. In such patients, the müllerian tubercle fails to descend normally and the vagina and the urogenital sinus can be at a considerable distance from each other. Sometimes, the müllerian tubercle fails to canalize so that no communication with the vagina can be demonstrated. The degree of masculinization depends both upon the time in fetal life in which the androgens begin to exert their influence and upon the degree of androgen secretion. The postnatal development of children with this disorder is one of progressive virilization. In boys, the penis continues to grow rapidly and its large size is certainly obvious by the second year. The scrotum expands also but the testes remain infantile. In girls, the gonads remain infantile also and the external genitalia virilize. The clitoris enlarges and may reach a length of 2 to 3 inches and may have erections. The labia majora grow and project forward and appear like a split scrotum. Pubic hair usually appears in both sexes at about three years of age and acquires a more masculine distribution. Axillary hair usually appears a few years later and a mustache may appear between nine and 12 years of age.

Other characteristics include the skin changes of acne, light brown coloration generally and deep pigmentation in the anogenital regions. The skeletal changes include premature epiphyseal closure with complete absence of the female contour. These individuals usually have a short, stocky build with wide thorax and shoulders and narrow pelvis. The limbs are short in relationship to the trunk which is usually of normal length. Muscular development is extremely good and they are usually stronger than other children their own age and most have a rather athletic build when they get older. In adult life, their appearance remains essentially a progression of the childhood traits; their physiques remain masculine and the female is, of course, bothered by considerable increase in facial and body hair. The infertility in these patients is attributed to hypogonadism and the males have obviously hypoplastic testes. Primary amenorrhea is always a feature in the females, although, infrequently, scanty menses have been reported. In the simple virilizing form, the usual clinical appearance is that of a female child with ambiguous external genitalia. The establishment of the correct sex assignment of this group is essential early in life.

The salt-losing form of congenital adrenal hyperplasia is also more frequent in females than in males. In addition to the virilization seen in the simple type, these children also have symptoms of acute adrenal insufficiency. Because of equilibrium with the maternal circulation, the symptoms usually do not appear until approximately five to ten days of age. A lack of appetite, apathy, vomiting, diarrhea, hypoglycemia, dusky color of the skin, convulsions and sudden circulatory collapse are common features. Many of the deaths have been due to a combination of hypovolemia and hyperkalemia. Laboratory studies in these children show low serum sodium and bicarbonate and high serum potassium. They also exhibit increased excretion of 17-ketosteroids and pregnenetriol. The salt-losing type is associated with a defect of 21-hydroxylase enzyme.

In the hypertensive form, there is a defect of the 11-β-hydroxylase enzyme. This leads to a deficient cortisol synthesis and to hypersecretion of adrenocorticotropin. The patients exhibit virilization as well as a mildly elevated blood pressure, although in a few the blood pressure has been quite high. It has been suggested that the hypertension is due to excessive secretion of desoxycorticosterone.

A rare type of adrenogenital syndrome is associated with 3-β-hydroxysteroid dehydrogenase defect. This causes a block in the synthesis of cortisol at a much earlier stage and is manifested by virilization but to a smaller degree in females than in the other types of perineal hypospadias in males. The presence of perineal hypospadias in males suggests a role of this enzyme in androgen synthesis by the testes as well as by the adrenals.

Diagnosis of this condition can be expedited by determination of nuclear sex chromatin, which is extremely helpful when combined with endocrine studies to establish the sex in this type of ambiguous external genitalia and to differentiate this from other forms of pseudohermaphroditism; radiologic and cystoscopic examination of the lower genitourinary tract; increased excretion of 17-ketosteroids and pregnenetriol, along with normal or diminished excretion of corticosteroids, and suppression of abnormal urinary excretion of steroids with cortisol or dexamethasone stimulation. When uncertainty still exists, exploratory operation must be undertaken in order to determine the true nature of the gonads. Wilkins has demonstrated in recent years the efficacy of cortisone or hydrocortisone in treatment of patients with bilateral adrenal hyperplasia. With this therapy, there is a striking reduction in the secretion of adrenal adrogens, presumably on the basis of inhibition of adrenocorticotropic hormone production by the anterior pituitary.

Using the level of urinary 17-ketosteroid excretion as a guide, dosage must be individualized throughout the period of treatment. The dosage level employed should be the least amount of cortisone necessary to suppress the 17-ketosteroid excretion to a normal level for the age and sex of the individual. This usually is in the neighborhood of 50 mg. per day in older children and 25 mg. in infants and younger children. Maximum suppression of 17-ketosteroid excretion should occur approximately five to ten days after initiation of treatment and maintenance doses are usually half of initial dosage. Oral cortisol is usually less effective in maintenance therapy than that given intramuscularly and the dosage needed accordingly is two to three times greater. The length of therapy is presumably for a lifetime. It is essential in this syndrome that diagnosis and accurate therapy be initiated as soon as possible so that the child can be raised in his respective genetic sex orientation.

FEMINIZING TUMORS OF THE ADRENAL CORTEX. In rare instances, tumors of the adrenal cortex may produce feminizing effects. Most of these tumors are highly malignant. Of the 52 patients with feminizing tumors reported in males, 41 were carcinomas, seven were adenomas and in four it could not be determined whether the tumor was malignant or benign. These tumors almost always occur in males and only two are reported in young females. Most feminizing tumors occur in patients between 25 and 45 years of age, although several patients as old as 50 to 66 years of age have been reported. Gynecomastia is the most common symptom and is usually rather prominent with tender bilateral fullness of the breasts, although on occasion it may be unilateral. In addition to this, patients exhibit impotence and loss of libido but very few other hypoandrogenic features. A palpable tumor is present in many individuals and local pain due to neoplastic growth is frequent. Calcification in the tumor has occurred in four patients. Urinary estrogen levels are usually markedly elevated and are higher in the patient with carcinoma than with adenoma. In several patients, estrogen excretion was increased 100-fold. Although these are feminizing tumors, the levels of urinary 17-ketosteroid excretion are also elevated in most patients. Urinary gonadotropin excretion has showed no significant variation from the normal in the patients in whom it has been measured.

In the malignant tumors there are two cell types. The predominant type closely resembles the cells of the zona reticularis. The cells are variable in size and shape; sometimes fusiform or spindle shapes are most common but usually the cells are eosinophilic, rounded and polygonal. They contain an abundance of finely granular cytoplasm and small hyperchromatic nuclei, located generally in a central position. Upon differential staining the tumor cells show characteristics of the cells of the zona reticularis. The second cell type is much larger and more polygonal in shape, containing large amounts of homogeneous, clear or slightly foamy cytoplasm. The nuclei are large, bizarre and hyperchromatic. These elements closely resemble the cells of the zona fasciculata, although they are lacking in the characteristic cord or columnar arrangement. The diagnosis of malignancy is based upon capsular invasion, venous invasion and distant metastasis. The testes show profound changes with total absence of spermatogenesis and no recognizable spermatogonia. Sertoli cells are not significantly altered and Leydig cells have not been found. The hypophysis appears normal but slightly enlarged.

The feminizing tumor should obviously be removed as soon as the diagnosis is established and postsurgical radiotherapy is usually advisable. Because some of these tumors also produce increased amounts of cortisol, substitution therapy postoperatively is usually indicated. After operation, gynecomastia regresses and libido usually returns to normal as does spermatogenesis. Unfortunately in most patients, metastases appear in a short time with or without return of urinary steroids to the preoperative levels. Recurrence and spread of tumor often occur within one year of the primary operation. In the rare instances in which the tumor was an adenoma, cures have been obtained.

PHEOCHROMOCYTOMA. Considerable progress has been made in the last ten years in the recognition and management of pheochromocytoma, undoubtedly the most dramatic and treacherous of the various surgically correctable causes of hypertension. Although the tumor was described as early as 1886 by Frankel and given its name pheochromocytoma or "black celled tumor" by Pick in 1912, it was not until 1922 that the clear demonstration of the association of the tumor with hypertension of a paroxysmal nature was made by Labbé and his associates. Although Roux and Charles Mayo are credited with early successful surgical removal of pheochromocytomas during the 1920's, the first correct preoperative diagnosis of the tumor was apparently made in 1929 by Pincoffs with subsequent successful removal of the lesion. In 1929, Rabin demonstrated an epinephrine-like substance in a pheochromocytoma and for a time the syndrome of paroxysmal hypertension was thought to be the only manifestation of the "epinephrine-producing" tumor of the adrenal medulla. However, in 1938, both Binger and Craig and Palmer and Castleman described instances of pheochromocytoma with sustained hypertension. In 1946, the studies of von Euler and his associates demonstrated the presence of norepinephrine at the terminals of adrenergic nerve fibers and in the adrenal medulla. Holton in 1949 and Goldenberg in 1950 demonstrated the presence of norepinephrine in pheochromocytomas. It thus became apparent that the clinical manifestations of these neoplasms were related at times to their secretion of norepinephrine as well as epinephrine.

The cells of the chromaffin type which give rise to pheochromocytoma are located in the adrenal medulla, in the sympathetic nervous system, and in the aberrant chromaffin tissue distributed along the sympathetic chain extending from the base of the brain to the pelvis. In the adult, these cells are concentrated in the adrenal medulla and most tumors originate in this site. Extra-adrenal tumors, however, may develop in chromaffin tissue scattered along the sympathetic system from the bladder to the brain. Apparently about 10 per cent of pheochromocytomas are extra-adrenal in location.

From the work of von Euler and others it has become clear that the clinical manifestations of pheochromocytoma are related to the secretory output of catecholamines by the tumor. In normal man, there are three naturally occurring catecholamines: dopamine, norepinephrine and epinephrine. Each of these can be identified in adrenal medullary tissue but at postganglionic sympathetic nerve endings apparently only dopamine and norepinephrine can be identified in other than the most minute concentrations. It has been suggested that efficient methylation of norepinephrine to form epinephrine occurs only in the well-organized tissue of the adrenal medulla. In normal man at rest, the adrenal medulla is said to secrete 0.07 μg. per kg. per minute of epinephrine and 0.2 μg per kg. per minute of norepinephrine. In tumors amounts of these catecholamines greatly in excess of normal levels occur and ratios vary widely. For a time it was thought that pheochromocytomas which occur in the periphery could produce only norepinephrine whereas tumors of the adrenal medulla could produce both epinephrine and norepinephrine. Recently, however, two epinephrine-producing pheochromocytomas of the organ of Zuckerkandl at the aortic bifurcation have been described. Goodall has cited two instances of pure epinephrine-producing tumors of the medulla which have been studied by von Euler. In general, it would appear despite these rare exceptions that the majority of extra-adrenal pheochromocytomas are pure norepinephrine producers, whereas the tumors which arise in the adrenal medulla for the most part produce both epinephrine and norepinephrine; very rarely pure epinephrine-producing tumors of the adrenal medulla and the periphery are encountered.

Pheochromocytomas are relatively uncommon tumors but are by no means rarities. The incidence has been variously determined as 0.4 to 2 per cent of all hypertensives but some investigators believe the actual incidence to be higher. The majority of pheochromocy-

tomas occur in adults but about one-fifth of the reported tumors have occurred in children. In the latter, 39 per cent are either bilateral or multiple. The tumor occurs in women with greater frequency than in men and many are first recognized during pregnancy. The tumor has a very definite association with von Recklinghausen's neurofibromatosis and has an increased incidence in this disorder. A familial tendency has been recorded.

Most pheochromocytomas are grossly well encapsulated tumors of yellow-brown or reddish-brown color. Often an attenuated adrenal gland can be seen overlying a portion or all of the tumor. Microscopically, the structure is somewhat variable. The cells are usually large, polyhedral or irregularly shaped with granular, slightly acidophilic cytoplasm and a large eccentric vesicular nucleus. For the most part, the cells are arranged in an alveolar pattern, but this is by no means constant. Pleomorphism, lymphatic, blood vessel and capsular invasion frequently occur and cannot be considered signs of malignancy. The majority of these tumors are benign and only the finding of direct invasion of surrounding structures and distant metastases provides the justification for the diagnosis of malignancy. From the literature it would appear that the incidence of malignant tumors in both children and adult age groups ranges around 2 to 3 per cent.

The tumors vary greatly in size and weight. The largest on record weighed 2000 gm. with its contained cystic fluid. Usual weight range is from 1 to 75 gm. For reasons that are unknown, right-sided tumors are more common than those on the left and the incidence of bilaterality or of multiplicity of pheochromocytoma ranges from 7 to 11 per cent of reported cases.

The symptoms and signs of pheochromocytoma are those which result from the release of excessive amounts of epinephrine or norepinephrine. Although epinephrine and norepinephrine are similar in metabolic action, epinephrine is 30 to 100 times more potent than norepinephrine in this regard (Table 6). Norepinephrine is thought to be the more potent general vasoconstrictor. Paroxysms of hypertension occur in 30 to 50 per cent of patients with pheochromocytoma. These apparently represent episodes of massive release of hormone, either epinephrine or norepinephrine or both, and are precipitated by a variety of stimuli, including various

Table 6. *Comparison of the Effects of Epinephrine and Norepinephrine**

EFFECTOR	NOREPINEPHRINE	EPINEPHRINE
Heart		
Isolated	Positive inotropic	Positive inotropic
	Positive chronotropic	Positive chronotropic
In vivo	Positive inotropic	Positive inotropic
	Negative chronotropic	Positive chronotropic
Blood pressure		
Systolic	Increase	Increase
Diastolic	Increase	Slight increase
Peripheral resistance	Increase	Slight increase or decrease
Cardiac output	Slight increase or unchanged	Increase
Liver	Vasoconstriction	Vasodilation
Skeletal muscle	Vasoconstriction	Vasodilation
Skin	Vasoconstriction	Vasoconstriction
Kidneys	Vasoconstriction	Vasoconstriction
Intestinal smooth muscle	Relaxation	Relaxation
Sweat glands	Slight activation	Activation
Pupils	Slight dilatation	Dilatation
Central nervous system,		
nervousness and apprehension	No effect	Marked effect
Basal metabolic rate	Slight increase	Increase
Blood sugar	Slight increase	Increase
Plasma nonesterified		
fatty acid level	Increase	Increase

*From Scott, H. W., Jr., et al.: Surgical management of pheochromocytoma. Surg. Gyn. & Obst. *120*:707, 1965.

forms of stress such as trauma, exercise, massage of tumor, sexual intercourse and emptying of the bladder. Paroxysms are characterized by extreme levels of hypertension, blanching, occasionally flushing, tachycardia, syncope, sweating, angina and headache.

Three clinical patterns of hypertension occur with pheochromocytomas. First, there is the classic situation in which blood pressure is normal between hypertensive paroxysms. This was long thought to be the only manifestation of the tumor. Second, blood pressure may be elevated in a sustained fashion without paroxysms and may resemble essential hypertension. Third, blood pressure may be elevated constantly and in addition extreme paroxysmal hypertensive crises may be superimposed.

The signs and symptoms of hypermetabolism are evident in many patients with pheochromocytomas and reflect the intensive metabolic activity of the catecholamines secreted by the tumor. Symptoms simulating hyperthyroidism with tremor, tachycardia and elevated basal metabolic rate may be present. The manifestations of diabetes, including glycosuria and a diabetic type of glucose tolerance curve may occur. Weight loss is quite common in these individuals

and the majority of patients with pheochromocytoma are thin. Fever, vasomotor phenomena, headache, angina, nausea and anxiety attacks are quite common. Death is apt to occur during a paroxysmal episode. The causes of death from pheochromocytoma include cerebrovascular accidents, congestive heart failure with pulmonary edema and ventricular fibrillation. Rarely, a malignant pheochromocytoma has recurred after its operative removal and widely distributed metastases have caused the patient's death.

Since the introduction of the histamine provocative test by Roth and Kvale, a variety of pharmacologic tests have been devised as aids in diagnosis of pheochromocytoma. The histamine test is based on the direct stimulating effect of the drug on chromaffin cells with release of catecholamines; a prompt rise in blood pressure usually occurs in a patient who has a pheochromocytoma. Phentolamine (Regitine), introduced by Longino, Grimson et al., causes a fall in blood pressure in patients with pheochromocytoma by blocking the effector cell for catecholamines. Other pharmacologic tests based on the patient's blood pressure responses to such drugs as Mecholyl, benzodioxane, Dibenamine and tetraethylammonium bromide have been developed but have not proved to be of much additional value in diagnosis of these tumors. In the last decade, the indirect pharmacologic tests have been used more as screening procedures and have been supplanted to a great extent by direct chemical methods of estimating the levels of the catecholamines in plasma and the excretion of both free and conjugated hormones and their metabolites in urine. Fluorometric estimates of urinary catecholamine excretion in resting normal individuals usually range below 200 μg. per 24-hour urine volume, whereas patients with pheochromocytoma usually excrete in excess of 300 μg. per 24 hours. An alternative or confirmatory direct chemical diagnostic procedure is to measure the excretion of the catecholamine metabolite 3-methoxy,4-hydroxymandolic acid, which is usually excreted in amounts in excess of 12 mg. per 24 hours in patients with the tumor.

Once the diagnosis of pheochromocytoma has been established, the next clinical problem is that of localization of the tumor. By far the great majority develop in the adrenal medulla and even those which originate in extra-adrenal chromaffin tissue have a predilection for the renal fossae. Cervical, mediastinal and pelvic sites of origin, however, occur with rarity but there are several reports of pheochromocytoma originating in such bizarre sites as the jugular foramen and the wall of the urinary bladder.

In attempting to localize a pheochromocytoma, intravenous pyelography should always be used but cannot be counted on to locate the tumor unless the latter is quite large. Abdominal laminagrams occasionally indicate the tumor's density or identify flecks of calcification in the lesion. Retroperitoneal pneumography with carbon dioxide can contribute valuable localizing information, either alone or combined with aortography. Mahoney and his associates have described an ingenious localizing technique based on vena caval catheterization with plasma catecholamine determinations on blood samples drawn at intervals as the catheter is passed along the cava.

The favorable results of prompt and aggressive surgical treatment of pheochromocytoma are well documented. Prompt regression of the blood pressure to the range of normal is the rule and recurrence of the tumor is rare. Experience emphasizes the treacherous nature of pheochromocytoma, the hazards of failure by clinicians to recognize the presence of the tumor, and the importance of proceeding to remove pheochromocytoma once it is recognized by well-planned surgical operation without delay.

It is important in successful management of pheochromocytoma to realize that the small lesions frequently cannot be lateralized or localized by currently available preoperative diagnostic techniques. Overzealous and prolonged diagnostic efforts to localize the tumor may lead to catastrophic delay in treatment. Because well over 90 per cent of these tumors originate in the adrenals and their immediate environs, well-planned surgical exploration of the adrenal fossae can quickly and efficiently localize the tumor and permit its safe removal. Even when the larger tumors can be accurately lateralized, it is desirable to use an operative approach which permits examination of both adrenal fossae and the entire abdominal cavity. For this purpose in patients of average habitus with suspected pheochromocytoma, it is preferable to use a transverse upper abdominal incision for transperitoneal bilateral adrenal exploration. After lateralizing an adrenal pheochromocytoma, the incision can be extended across the costal margin into a lower intercostal space and wide thoracoabdominal exposure of the tumor obtained.

This permits gentle, atraumatic, nonmanipulative dissection of the tumor with early ligation of the major adrenal vein, which is highly desirable to minimize hypertensive crises during the operation. Anesthesia for these operations should be undertaken only by an expert. There is a paramount need for the anesthesiologist to employ a smooth, nonstressful induction and atraumatic intubation and to avoid anesthetics which stimulate catecholamine release or enhance responsiveness to the hormones. Both phentolamine (Regitine) and norepinephrine should be readily available. Small (2.5 to 5 mg.) repeated doses of phentolamine are used to control hypertensive crises during induction, intubation and maintenance of anesthesia in these patients. In most instances as soon as the adrenal vein is interrupted or the tumor removed, hypotension ensues which requires a norepinephrine infusion for several hours to several days. Intravenous pentothal induction with anectine and gas–oxygen–ether maintenance was formerly used quite satisfactorily. More recently, induction with Pentothal and Anectine and maintenance with Fluothane have been favored by most anesthesiologists.

NEUROBLASTOMA. Excepting leukemia and tumors of the central nervous system collectively, neuroblastoma is the most common malignant tumor that occurs in infancy and early childhood. Although it most commonly arises in the adrenal medulla, neuroblastoma can develop from sympathetic tissue anywhere in the body. Although it may occur in the brain, it is much more common in structures outside the central nervous system. Although neuroblastomas are highly malignant, metastasize early and have an exceedingly serious prognosis, they are not uniformly fatal. Spontaneous regression of the tumor may rarely occur, and therapeutic efforts have resulted in a number of cures.

In the development of the sympathetic nervous system and the adrenal medulla, the precursor cell is known as the sympathogon which forms the ganglionic anlage. The sympathoblast derives from the ganglion crest and migrates into the visceral areas to form the anlage of the sympathetic nervous system and adrenal medulla, finally differentiating into unipolar and multipolar neuroblasts. Further differentiation produces mature ganglion cells. Neoplasia in this cellular system may produce an extremely primitive tumor which can be designated a sympathogonioma or a sympathoblastoma. Collectively, these malignant tumors are called neuroblastomas. Neoplastic changes in the ganglion cell may produce a benign tumor, the ganglioneuroma, and rarely, an intermediate type of tumor which contains both immature and mature ganglion cells and which has been called ganglioneuroblastoma. The highly malignant neuroblastoma is much more common than the benign ganglioneuroma.

Grossly, neuroblastoma, whether originating in the adrenal medulla or in the areas of the sympathetic nervous system, usually has a nodular or lobulated surface with a rubbery firm consistency. The tumors are often grayish red, with a fine vascular network over the surface. Areas of hemorrhagic necrosis are frequent. The neuroblastoma of the adrenal medulla may arise on either side of the vertebral column but has a strong tendency to invade across the midline. The tumor may extend upward and downward in the retroperitoneal plane and up through the diaphragmatic hiatuses in the retropleural plane. It usually grows rapidly to large size. Often the growth will infiltrate adjacent viscera such as the kidney, the body of pancreas and root of the mesentery. At times, the tumor may remain relatively well localized and seemingly encapsulated but in most instances extensive retroperitoneal invasion occurs early.

Metastases take place by lymphatic and blood invasion. In addition to regional nodes, there is a predilection for metastasis to the skeletal system and often extensive replacement of bone marrow occurs. Metastases to the skull and orbits by this tumor were described by Hutchinson in 1907 and came to be known as the Hutchinson syndrome, whereas diffuse invasion of the liver by the tumor was described by Pepper a few years earlier and has in the past been referred to as the Pepper syndrome. These eponymous terms no longer have any real value except for historic interest. Gross points out that the tumor had metastasized in 60 per cent of neuroblastomas by the time the patient was hospitalized. Pulmonary metastases tend to occur later in the course of the disease than do those to bone, marrow, liver, orbit and skin.

Microscopically, neuroblastomas are highly cellular tumors consisting of broad sheets of small cells with dark, round nuclei between wide areas of pale fibrillar stroma. Rosette formation is characteristic of many neuroblastomas with clusters of cells in ring-like formation in the center of which neurofibrils may be demonstrated with phosphotungstic acid–hematoxylin stain. In the less differentiated and more malignant forms of neuroblastoma, the cells are usually a little smaller and often no rosettes or fibrils can be identified. Conversely, in the less malignant and more favorable varieties of the tumor there may be areas in which ganglion cells are present, suggesting that the tumor is a neuroblastoma which is differentiating into a ganglioneuroma.

Although neuroblastomas may occur at any age in children, they are most commonly found in infants and very young children; 80 per cent have been observed in the first five years of life. The tumor occurs with equal frequency in boys and girls. Children with adrenal neuroblastomas usually present with a complaint of painless abdominal swelling accompanied by pallor, fatigue, loss of appetite and often weight loss of several months' duration. All too often, the manifestations of distant metastases present with the development of headache and vomiting from cerebral metastases, the pain and deformity of a pathologic fracture or the proptosis of an orbital site of spread.

The principal finding on abdominal examination with adrenal neuroblastoma is the presence of a firm nodular mass occupying one side of the abdomen. Unlike Wilms' tumor from which adrenal neuroblastoma must always be differentiated, the neuroblastoma is not reniform in shape or smooth in outline. Rather, the neuroblastoma usually presents as a nondescript, nodular, vaguely rounded mass which often does not permit clear delineation of contour on physical examination. Often, the tumors are fixed in the flank and do not move with inspiration. There may be a palpable extension of the mass across the midline. Other significant physical findings are apt to be those associated with the metastases of the tumor.

Laboratory studies often show a mild degree of anemia. It is very rare for urinalysis to show any abnormalities. In a very small percentage of patients with invasion of the renal pelvis, hematuria may present. If a profound anemia is present, bone marrow invasion should be suspected and marrow aspiration may reveal metastatic neuroblastoma. Chemical analysis of 24-hour collections of urine for the metabolites of norepinephrine and its precursors, dopamine and dopa, may show abnormally high levels of homovanillic acid and vanilmandelic acid.

Plain films of the abdomen may show a nonspecific radiopaque mass above a kidney. Calcification can be detected as fine, stippled or flocculent densities in about half of these tumors, being more common in older children than in infants. Intravenous or retrograde pyelography commonly shows displacement of the kidney and deformity of the pelvis but Gross states that such studies may fail to differentiate with certainty between neuroblastoma, Wilms' tumor and retroperitoneal teratoma. Angiography may be helpful in this differentiation.

A skeletal survey and films of the chest are mandatory parts of the evaluation of the patient with suspected neuroblastoma. Skeletal metastases are found at the time of initial examination in about 35 per cent of patients. The preferential sites of bony metastases are the skull, femur, humerus, vertebrae, pelvis and ribs in descending order of frequency. The moth-eaten, spotty rarefactions of neuroblastoma's bony metastases have a characteristic roentgenographic appearance (Fig. 7). The more extensive lesions tend to be symmetrically distributed. Proliferative bone lesions may occur and at times may produce

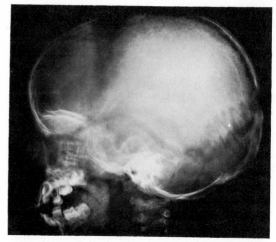

Figure 7. Roentgenogram of child's skull with moth-eaten, spotty rarefactions of bone, characteristic of neuroblastoma metastases to the skull and facial bones.

sclerosing changes in the skull, spine or pelvis which resemble Paget's disease.

Unless contraindicated by extensive metastases, primary treatment of adrenal neuroblastoma in infants and children is always surgical resection of the tumor. If a total removal of the tumor cannot be safely done, Gross advises that as much of the bulk of the tumor as possible be resected. In either case, whether total or subtotal resection has been possible, postoperative radiation therapy should be used.

The surgical approach most commonly used is a long, transverse, supraumbilical abdominal incision which is extended into the loin on the side of the lesion; occasionally, an extension of the incision across the coastal margins into a lower interspace is needed to provide optimal exposure. In assessing the resectability of the tumor, the surgeon should look for metastases in liver and other abdominal viscera and should inspect and palpate the posterior and medial attachments of the lesion. Because of the close proximity and early invasion of the renal capsule and kidney, the resection usually involves removal of the kidney with the tumor. Accordingly, assurance of the functional integrity of the contralateral kidney is always requisite. As with the operation for Wilms' tumor of kidney, early ligation of the hilar vessels is desirable before extensive operative manipulation of the tumor. Unless the lesion has metastasized or invaded diffusely, radical surgical removal of the contents of the renal fossa is indicated. On the left side large tumors may compromise the splenic vessels and the tail of the pancreas, often necessitating resection of the tail of the pancreas and spleen with the kidney and tumor (Fig. 8). On the right side invasion in and around the vena cava may prevent complete removal of the lesion. Unless the tumor is so friable, necrotic and vascular that it cannot be resected with safety, subtotal removal of a diffusely invasive tumor can be accomplished by dividing the tumor tissue lateral to the great vessels between clamps. The residual tumor should be outlined by clips to aid the roentgenologist in postoperative radiotherapy.

Most neuroblastomas are radiosensitive and to date the best results have occurred when the combination of surgical resection and radiotherapy has been used. Radiotherapy of individual metastatic sites in skin or bone may provide transitory palliative relief of pain and parental anxiety but, unfortunately, in most instances not much more. Widespread metastases to skin or skeleton cannot be safely treated with "spray" x-ray therapy because of the depressant effect of extensive radiation on the hematopoietic system. Complications of radiation therapy in these tumors must be equated with the theoretically curative potential of such postoperative therapy. In general with widespread skeletal metastases, radiotherapy has very little to offer and the prognosis after radiation in widespread osseous lesions is uniformly bad.

Chemotherapy has proved to be increasingly valuable in treatment of disseminated neuroblastoma as well as an adjunct to surgical resection. Farber and his associates initiated the use of treatment with nitrogen mustard and folic acid antagonists as early as 1951 and have subsequently observed remission or objective regression of extensive tumor in sporadic instances with a variety of other chemotherapeutic agents. Bodian has had enthusiasm for vitamin B_{12} in large doses. However, none of the many agents used has proved to be consistently effective.

Two of the more promising newer drugs which have been tried in treatment of neuroblastoma are the alkylating agent, cyclophosphamide, and the alkaloid, vincristine sulfate. Transitory objective tumor regression has been reported in less than half of children with neuroblastoma who have received these drugs individually. However, the combination of the two drugs was recently reported by James and his associates to provide objective tumor regression in each of nine children with unresectable neuroblastomas and "complete remission" for periods as long as 12 to 26 months in seven of the group. In two of the youngsters given this treatment subsequent complete surgical excision of the primary tumor was accomplished.

Despite the lethal potential and continued high fatality rate of neuroblastoma, patients with this malignant neoplasm have shown an increased number of favorable responses to treatment in the last two decades. Prior to 1930, neuroblastoma was considered a hopeless condition; with no effort to treat it there were no cures. As surgeons and radiologists mounted a combined attack on the problem in the period of 1930 to 1950, a few cures began to appear. In the period since 1950 with an aggressive approach to the tumor, combining surgery, radiotherapy and chemotherapy, the cure rate has definitely increased. Judgment of response to therapy, however, must take cognizance of spontaneous regression of the tumor.

Other factors which apparently influence response to treatment include age of patient, location of tumor and its metastases as well as the type of treatment used. Gross reports that in those patients in whom there are no demonstrable metastases and the treatment has consisted of total excision of the tumor followed by local x-ray therapy, a cure rate

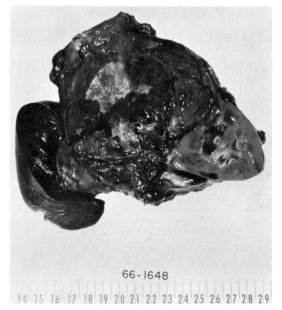

66-1648

Figure 8. Photograph of gross specimen removed at operation from two-year old child with left adrenal neuroblastoma involving kidney, spleen and tail of pancreas.

of 88 per cent has been obtained. Babies under a year of age have had the best response to treatment. When total removal of the tumor has not been possible, partial surgical removal followed by radiation and tumor chemotherapy has provided a cure rate as high as 64 per cent. Unfortunately if skeletal metastases are present, few cures have been observed with the most aggressive therapy. However, recent reports on the remarkable responses to the combination of cyclophosphamide and vincristine both with and without surgery and radiation bring a further note of optimism.

READING REFERENCES

Addison, T.: Disease of suprarenal capsules. London Med. Gaz. 43:517, 1849.

Anderson, E., Haymaker, W., and Joseph, M.: Hormonal and electrolyte studies of patients with hyperadrenocortical syndrome (Cushing's syndrome). Endocrinology 23:398, 1938.

Baulieu, E. E., Peillon, F., and Migeon, C. J.: Adrenogenital syndrome. In, Eisenstein, A. B. (ed.): The Adrenal Cortex. Boston, Little, Brown and Company, 1967.

Binger, M. W., and Craig, W. M.: Atypical case of hypertension with tumor of adrenal gland. Proc. Staff Meet. Mayo Clinic 13:17, 1938.

Bodian, M.: Neuroblastoma. Pediat. Clin. North America 6:449, 1959.

Boucher, R., et. al.: New procedures for measurement of human plasma angiotensin and renin activity levels. Canad. Med. A. J. 90:194, 1964.

Cahill, G. F.: Hormonal tumors of the adrenal. Surgery 16:233, 1944.

Carelli, M. D.: Sur le pneumoperitoine et sur une methode personelle pour voir le rein sans pneumoperitoine. J. Bull. Soc. Med. Hop., Paris 45:1409, 1921.

Childs, B., Grumbach, M. M., and Van Wyk, J. J.: Virilizing adrenal hyperplasia: a genetic and hormonal study. J. Clin. Invest. 35:213, 1956.

Conn, J. W.: Aldosteronism and hypertension: primary aldosteronism versus hypertensive disease with secondary aldosteronism. Arch. Int. Med. 107:813, 1961.

Conn, J. W.: Evolution of primary aldosteronism as a highly specific clinical entity. J.A.M.A. 172:1650, 1960.

Conn, J. W.: Presidential address. II. Primary aldosteronism: a new clinical syndrome. J. Lab. & Clin. Med. 45:6, 1955.

Conn, J. W., Cohen, E. L., Rovner, D. R., and Nesbit, R. M.: Normokalemic primary aldosteronism. J.A.M.A. 193: 101, 1965.

Conn, J. W., Knopf, R. F., and Nesbit, R. M.: Clinical characteristics of primary aldosteronism from an analysis of 145 cases. Am. J. Surg. 107:159, 1964.

Coppage, W. S., Island, D. P., Conner, A. E., and Liddle, G. W.: The metabolism of aldosterone in normal subjects and in patients with hepatic cirrhosis. J. Clin. Invest. 41:1672, 1962.

Crowder, R. E.: Developments of the adrenal gland in man with special reference to origin and all of the locations, cell types, and evidence in favor of cell migration (theory). Contrib. Embryol. 36:193, 1957.

Cushing, H.: The basophil adenomas of the pituitary body and their clinical manifestations. Bull. Johns Hopkins Hosp. 50:137, 1932.

Cushing, H., and Wolbach, S. B.: The transformation of a malignant paravertebral sympathicoblastoma into a benign ganglioneuroma. Am. J. Path. 3:203, 1927.

Davis, J. O.: The regulation of aldosterone secretion. In, Eisenstein, A. B. (ed.): The Adrenal Cortex. Boston, Little, Brown and Company, 1967.

Forsham, P. H.: The adrenals. In, Williams, R. H. (ed.): Textbook of Endocrinology. 3rd ed. Philadelphia, W. B. Saunders Company, 1962.

Frankel, F.: Ein Fall von doppelseitigen, vollig latent verlaufenen Nebennieren-tumor und gleich zeitiger Nephritis mit Veranderungen am Circulations-apparat und Retinitis. Arch. Path. Anat. 103:224, 1886.

Frawley, T. F.: Adrenal cortical insufficiency. In, Eisenstein, A. B. (ed.): The Adrenal Cortex. Boston, Little, Brown and Company, 1967.

Goldenberg, M., et al.: Pheochromocytoma and essential hypertensive vascular disease. Arch Int. Med. 86:823, 1950.

Goodall, M. C., and Stone, C.: Adrenaline and noradrenaline producing tumors of the adrenal medulla and sympathetic nerves. Ann. Surg. 151:391, 1960.

Gross, R. E., Farber, S., and Martin, L. W.: Neuroblastoma sympatheticum. Pediatrics 23:1179, 1959.

Heeg, M. M.: Urological spectrum of adrenal surgery. J. Urol. 96:427, 1966.

Holton, P.: Noradrenaline in adrenal medullary tumors. Nature, London 163:217, 1949.

Holtz, P., Credner, K., and Kroneberg, G.: Ueber das sympathicomimetische pressorische Prinzip des Harns ("Urosympathin"). Arch. Exp. Path., Opz 204:228, 1947.

Hume, D. M.: Pheochromocytoma in the adult and in the child. Am. J. Surg. 99:458, 1960.

James, D. H., Hustu, O., Wrenn, E. L., Jr., and Pinkel, D.: Combination chemotherapy of childhood neuroblastoma. J.A.M.A. 194:123, 1965.

Jarvis, L., Jenkins, D., Sosman, M., and Thorn, G.: Roentgenologic observations in Addison's disease. Radiology 62:16, 1954.

Kendall, E. C.: The chemistry and partial synthesis of adrenal steroids. Ann. New York Acad. Sc. 50:540, 1949.

Kliman, B., and Peterson, R. E.: Double isotope derivative assay of aldosterone in biological extracts. J. Biol. Chem. 235:1639, 1960.

Kvale, W. F., et al.: Present-day diagnosis and treatment of pheochromocytoma. J.A.M.A. 164:854, 1957.

Labbe, M., Tinel, J., and Doumer, A.: Crises solaires et hypertension paroxystique en rapport avec une tumeur surrenale. Bull. et Mém. Soc. Méd. Hôp. Paris 46:982, 1922.

Lance, E. M., et al.: Clinical experiences with pheochromocytoma. Surg. Gyn. & Obst. 106:25, 1958.

Li, C. H., Simpson, M. E., and Evans, H. M.: Isolation of adrenocorticotropic hormone from sheep pituitaries. Science 96:450, 1942.

Li, C. H., Evans, H. M., and Simpson, M. E.: Adrenocorticotropic hormone. J. Biol. Chem. 149:413, 1943.

Liddle, G. W.: Cushing's syndrome. In, Eisenstein, A. B. (ed.): The Adrenal Cortex. Boston, Little, Brown and Company, 1967.

Liddle, G. W.: Tests of pituitary-adrenal suppressibility in the diagnosis of Cushing's syndrome. J. Clin. Endocr. 20:1539, 1960.

Liddle, G. W., Givens, J. R., Nicholson, W. E., and Island, D. P.: The ectopic ACTH syndrome. Cancer Res. 25: 1057, 1965.

Longino, F. H., et al.: Effects of a new quaternary amine and a new imidazole derivative on the autonomic nervous system. Surgery 26:421, 1949.

Mahoney, E. M.: Localization of (adrenal and extra-adrenal) pheochromocytomas by vena caval blood sampling. Surg. Forum 14:495, 1963.

Mayo, C. H.: Paroxysmal hypertension with tumor or retroperitoneal nerve. J.A.M.A. 89:1047, 1927.

Palmer, R. S., and Castleman, B.: Paraganglioma of adrenal gland simulating malignant hypertension. Report of a case. New England J. Med. 219:793, 1938.

Pick, L.: Das Ganglioma embryonale sympathicium. Klin. Wchnschr. 19:16, 1912.

Pincoffs, M. C.: A case of paroxysmal hypertension associated with suprarenal tumor. Tr. A. Am. Physicians 44:295, 1929.

Rabin, C. B.: Chromaffin cell tumor of suprarenal medulla. Arch. Path. 7:228, 1929.

Reichstein, T., and Shopper, C. W.: The hormones of the adrenal cortex. Vitamins & Hormones 1:345, 1943.

Roth, G. M., and Kvale, W. F.: Tentative test for pheochromocytoma. Am. J. M. Sc. 210:653, 1945.

Scott, H. W., Jr., Liddle, G. W., Harris, A. P., and Foster, J. H.: Diagnosis and treatment of Cushing's syndrome. Ann. Surg. 155:696, 1962.

Scott, H. W., Jr., and Rhamy, R. K.: Surgical Procedures. Vol. 2, No. 9, October, 1965.

Scott, H. W., Jr., Riddell, D. H., and Brockman, S. K.: Surgical management of pheochromocytoma. Surg. Gyn. & Obst. 120:707, 1965.

von Euler, U. S.: Increased urinary excretion of noradrenaline in cases of pheochromocytoma. Ann. Surg. 134:929, 1951.

von Euler, U. S.: Specific sympathomimetic ergone in adrenergic nerve fibers (sympathin) and its relation to adrenaline and noradrenaline. Acta Physiol. Scandinav. 12:73, 1946.

Wilkins, L.: The diagnosis and treatment of endocrine disorders in childhood and adolescence. 3rd ed. Springfield, Illinois, Charles C Thomas, 1965.

Wilkins, L., Lewis, R. A., Klein, R., and Rosenberg, E.: The suppression of androgen excretion by cortisone in a case of congenital adrenal hyperplasia. Bull. Johns Hopkins Hosp. 86:249, 1950.

Williams, C. M., and Greer, M.: Homovanillic acid and vanilmandelic acid in diagnosis of neuroblastoma. J.A.M.A. 183:836, 1963.

Young, H. H.: Genital abnormalities, hermaphroditism and related adrenal diseases. Baltimore, Williams and Wilkins, Company, 1937.

Zimmerman, B., and Moran, W. H.: Aldosterone. Am. J. Surg. 99:503, 1960.

Chapter 27

THE SPLEEN

by

ROGER D. WILLIAMS, M.D.

ROGER DAVIS WILLIAMS is Professor of Surgery, University of Texas Medical Branch in Galveston. His undergraduate education was at Duke University and his graduate education at Ohio State University where he was on the faculty before moving to Texas.

The spleen continues to be one of the most interesting yet least understood organs within the abdomen. It is often involved in many generalized systemic disease processes, and primary splenic abnormalities may produce widespread effects. Abnormalities of splenic physiology, which have been more clearly delineated in recent years, are not necessarily associated with splenomegaly. The unwary physician may be misled unless he is familiar with the many diseases of this organ.

The changing concepts of splenic function make difficult the classification of splenic diseases under categories wherein there may be indication or contraindication for splenectomy. It may be assumed that trauma usually presents the most common indication for splenectomy in the United States. Whereas some consider surgery of no value in aplastic anemia and leukemia, many reports of the favorable results of splenectomy in certain cases tend to refute earlier impressions. Certainly, no set rules regarding surgery can substitute for competent hematologic evaluation of patients with splenic disease.

SURGICAL ANATOMY

Lying beneath the left ninth, tenth and eleventh ribs, the spleen is rarely palpable unless enlarged. In the adult it averages 11 by 7 by 4 cm. in size and weighs approximately 200 gm. It is usually shaped like a large coffee bean and often has a notch along its antero-medial border. The medial concave surface is bordered by the stomach, to which the upper pole may be closely attached. The lateral con-vex surface lies against the left diaphragm and kidney.

The peritoneal attachments of the spleen are of great surgical importance. Three of these form ligamentous attachments through which course the arteries and veins (Fig. 1). The presplenic fold, coursing from the lower pole and hilum of the spleen to join the gastrocolic ligament, is thin and moderately vascular. The gastrosplenic fold extends as a double peritoneal layer from the splenic hilum to the greater curvature of the stomach. Through these layers course the short gastric arteries and veins, which form large collaterals when there is impairment of flow in the splenic artery or vein. This ligament is greatly shortened as the superior hilum lies in close contact with the stomach. The splenorenal ligament, another double peritoneal fold, stretches from the tail of the pancreas to the splenic hilum and contains the splenic artery and vein. Several smaller peritoneal attachments between the spleen and diaphragm, and between the spleen and colon, may be prominent when the spleen is enlarged or when there is portal venous hypertension.

The splenic artery, the largest branch of the celiac axis, follows an irregular course over the superior border of the pancreas to divide into several branches near the hilum. Of the four branches commonly noted, three supply the spleen and two supply the greater curvature of the stomach. The superior and inferior terminal arteries and the superior polar artery all give branches into the spleen. The latter, in addition, gives off the short gastric vessels to the fundus of the stomach. The gastroepi-ploic artery branches off to the greater curva-

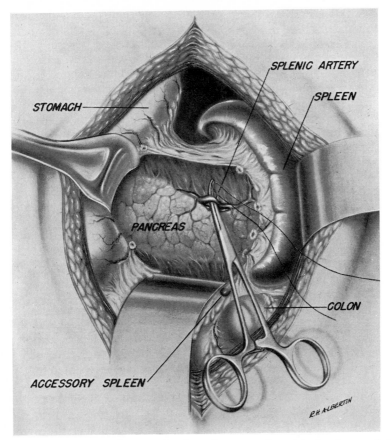

Figure 1. The spleen and its relations to the stomach, colon and pancreas. An opening has been made through the gastro-splenic ligament showing a suture being passed beneath the splenic artery proximal to the splenic pedicle.

ture of the stomach. The splenic vein follows a similar course to the artery, except that its course is usually inferior and straighter. Frequently, it is partially embedded within the pancreas. The lymphatic drainage of the spleen follows the vessels, along which there may be numerous lymph nodes.

INTERNAL ANATOMY

The internal anatomy of the spleen is less readily defined. The larger arteries which enter at the hilum branch into the trabeculae, the fibromuscular tissue framework of the spleen. Several trabeculae may form a small, almost microscopic lobule. The trabecular arteries branch into a zone of lymphoid tissue, the malpighian body. Continuing from this lymph follicle are the penicillate arteries which communicate either directly, through capillaries, or indirectly, through the splenic sinuses, with the venules. Direct communication through multiple pre-formed channels

have been noted. More recently, studies well documented by photographs and movies strongly support a combined open and closed system in which blood flows from the arteries into both pulp spaces and venous channels.

The splenic pulp is composed of sinuses and several types of cellular elements. The pulp contains lymphocytes, granulocytes and erythrocytes. There are numerous branching strands of lymphoid tissue, known as the cords of Billroth. The sinuses occupy most of the pulp and are lined by a reticular network which becomes continuous with pulp partitions. Within this network are phagocytic cells. In the congested spleen, the line between sinus and parenchyma may be poorly defined and changes which occur with certain splenic dysfunctions are somewhat inconstant.

PHYSIOLOGY

Normal physiologic functions of the spleen are of much less importance than splenic hyperfunction. The spleen is important, primarily, as a large part of the reticuloendothelial system and, secondarily, because of its position in the portal venous circulation. Since the spleen is not essential to life, because its functions are readily assumed by the remainder of the reticuloendothelial system, normal function has been difficult to evaluate.

Several functions may be ascribed to the spleen. It may act as a reservoir, yielding increased quantities of blood during stress or exercise. Gradual changes in volume take place under normal situations. In the embryo, the spleen takes part in blood formation. Although this function ceases after birth, it may be taken up again under demand. Lymphocytes continue to be formed throughout life. Blood destruction also occurs in the spleen, as in all reticuloendothelial tissue. Although phagocytosis is probably insignificant, fragmentation of red cells during periods of relative splenic congestion probably occurs. There is some evidence that the spleen has a regulatory action to increase red cell fragility. The spleen plays an active part in defense mechanisms, which include the formation of antibodies.

Several studies suggest that the spleen may have an endocrinologic function. The spleen has been considered a regulator of bone marrow, controlling the emission of its various elements by a humoral mechanism. Some splenic extracts stimulate and others depress the bone marrow. Serum from patients with cytopenias considered due to hypersplenism or dyssplenism has produced similar cytopenias when injected into a normal individual. These functions are probably cytoimmunologic and often can be suppressed by adrenocorticotropin (ACTH) and cortisone. The release of a vasodilator substance, in combination with peripheral cytologic changes resulting from stress, has been considered due to a substance called "splenin" by Ungar. This response to stress is inhibited by splenectomy.

There has been considerable recent interest in the relationship of the spleen and splenic extracts to tissue and organ transplantation. The splenic cells are apparently immunologically competent to produce both sensitization and, perhaps, desensitization. Although there are many varying reports, it appears that pretreatment with adequate numbers of donor spleen cells may significantly increase the survival of a subsequent organ allograft from the same donor.

ANOMALIES

Except for accessory spleens, anomalies of the spleen are rare. Congenital absence has been associated with several other anomalies, including an anomalous relationship of the inferior vena cava and abdominal aorta. Ectopic position of the spleen rarely occurs, and may require splenectomy because of torsion of the pedicle.

ACCESSORY SPLEENS. An accessory spleen consists of a separate encapsulated mass of splenic tissue which was probably pinched off from the main splenic mass during embryologic development. It has been suggested that many occur in the embryo but disappear after birth, unless perpetuated by increased demand in such diseases as congenital hemolytic icterus or thrombocytopenic purpura. They occur most commonly in the splenic hilum, the splenic pedicle or tail of the pancreas, the gastrosplenic ligament and the gastrocolic ligament. Rarely, they are found over the left kidney or even in the scrotum. Accessory spleens are reported in 18 to 30 per cent of patients undergoing splenectomy. They number from one to five or more, and vary in size from a few millimeters to several centimeters. Although they have the same gross appearance as the spleen, they are readily confused with lymph nodes. Often the accessory spleen not only has its own small artery and vein, but also a separate pedicle. When splenectomy is performed for hypersplenism, it is important to remove all accessory spleens since they may be the cause for continuation or recurrence of the disease.

TRAUMA

Splenic injuries are common, and if rupture of the spleen is remembered as a possibility, its diagnosis is not usually difficult. Rupture or contusion of the spleen should be considered in most automobile accidents of severity, particularly when the abdomen or left thorax is involved. Fractured ribs may direct attention to the underlying spleen, yet the association of rib fractures with splenic rupture occurs in only about one out of five patients.

Classification of open or closed wounds serves little purpose. Most open wounds occur with war injuries or stab wounds, and are usually obvious. Contusion or laceration of the spleen is more common, yet less readily diagnosed. Either contusion or rupture may follow a violent blow and rupture may occur without obvious trauma.

Two peculiarities of splenic rupture are often observed. The first of these is spontaneous rupture without a history of trauma, occurring usually in a soft, friable, diseased spleen. It has been reported to occur with malaria, typhoid fever, several of the lymphomas, Boeck's sarcoid and infectious mononucleosis. In addition, spontaneous rupture occurs even in the normal spleen, although this is rare.

The second peculiarity of the spleen is its tendency to secondary rupture at varying intervals following the episode of trauma. This phenomenon occurs in approximately one out of six patients, any time from one to 30 or more days after injury. Nearly 75 per cent take place during the first two weeks following trauma. The recurrence of hemorrhage may be due to continuous increase in a subcapsular hematoma or failure of the omentum or a clot to offer complete tamponade of the spleen.

The symptoms are those of blood loss into the peritoneal cavity. The signs may be minimal or marked. If the blood loss is great, weakness, abdominal pain and muscle spasm, either generalized or localized in the left upper quadrant, and depression of abdominal breathing are noted. Rebound tenderness is common and may be more noticeable than tenderness to palpation. Reference of pain to the left shoulder occurs in nearly three-fourths of the patients and is diagnostically significant. It may be produced by placing the patient in the Trendelenburg position. All symptoms may be overshadowed by shock and other bodily injuries. A palpable tender mass, fixed dullness in the left flank, or shifting dullness due to free blood in the peritoneal cavity is a less common finding.

Leukocytosis, with a white cell count of over 12,000, is of more diagnostic importance than is early anemia. With rapid hemorrhage, hemoconcentration may precede the lowering of hemoglobin or red blood cell count. Abdominal x-ray study is rarely much help until other findings are also diagnostic. Miniature paracentesis, if performed carefully, will give helpful information more often. This peritoneal tap is readily performed utilizing a No. 20 or 18 spinal needle and a 10-cc. syringe. If blood is encountered, the diagnosis of internal bleeding is confirmed and the possibility of splenic rupture strongly considered. A negative tap does not eliminate the diagnosis of splenic rupture.

The only safe treatment for splenic rupture is splenectomy, which should be performed without hesitation. When the diagnosis is in doubt but there is strong evidence of intra-abdominal injury, exploratory laparotomy is justified. Suture of tears is not satisfactory. Whole blood should be made readily available and usually one or more transfusions are required. Following splenectomy, complete exploration of the entire abdomen is an absolute necessity in order that the possibility of other intra-abdominal injuries may be eliminated.

The results of splenectomy largely depend upon the extent of other injuries. Nearly half the patients with ruptured spleen have other injuries to the head, chest or extremities which divert attention from the diagnosis of splenic injury and increase mortality. Approximately one-third of the patients have other intra-abdominal injuries to the kidney, bladder or intestinal tract. Multiple injuries are often found, since the most common cause of splenic rupture is an automobile accident. If a ruptured spleen is the only significant injury, the mortality is low. When multiple injuries occur, mortality will depend upon the time and adequacy of treatment of all injuries.

HYPERSPLENISM

Several clinical entities, in which there is a depression of one or more of the formed elements of the blood, are considered to be due to splenic overactivity. Whether the spleen acts directly to produce an increased breakdown of peripheral blood elements, elaborates a humoral substance which affects the productivity of the bone marrow, or produces antibodies which act on the cellular elements is debated by hematologists. Regardless of the mechanisms of hypersplenism, the resulting decrease in red cells, platelets, white cells or all three of these elements produces well-known clinical diseases. These diseases are classified as primary hypersplenism if congenital, hereditary or of unknown cause, and as secondary hypersplenism if they occur during the course of another chronic disease process.

Four clinical diseases comprise the syndrome of primary hypersplenism (Fig. 2). Depression of circulating blood platelets due to splenic overactivity results in essential, or primary, thrombocytopenic purpura. The destruction of red blood cells produces congenital hemolytic anemia. Because the sphero-

PRIMARY HYPERSPLENISM

1. PLATELETS

2. RED CELLS   **+**

3. WHITE CELLS

4. ALL ELEMENTS

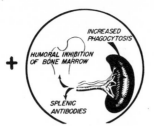

HYPERACTIVE SPLEEN

= **1. ESSENTIAL THROMBOCYTO-**
    PENIC **PURPURA**

2. CONGENITAL HEMOLYTIC
    ANEMIA

3. PRIMARY SPLENIC
    NEUTROPENIA

4. PRIMARY SPLENIC
    PANHEMATOPENIA

Figure 2. Several mechanisms may occur whereby a decrease of blood platelets, red cells, white cells or all three elements by a hyperactive spleen produces four clinical disease entities, depending upon which element or elements is decreased.

cytic red cells in this disease are unchanged by splenectomy and are more rapidly destroyed than normal cells, even by a normal spleen, many authorities do not consider this disorder hypersplenism. Primary splenic neutropenia and panhematopenia are two more recently recognized diseases, in which there is a depression of granulocytes or all three of the formed elements of the blood. In all four of these disease processes, splenectomy effects excellent results.

Secondary hypersplenism produces identical cytopenias, but the splenic dysfunction develops secondary to another chronic disease. The primary chronic diseases include leukemia, Banti's disease, Gaucher's disease, Hodgkin's disease, the other lymphomas, tuberculosis, Boeck's sarcoid and other chronic infections. Secondary hemolytic anemia, thrombocytopenia, neutropenia or panhematopenia may occur as a complication during any phase of one of these chronic disease processes. Although splenectomy may produce dramatic remission of the hypersplenism, and thereby lengthen life, the primary disease continues its course.

Another group of hematologic disorders in which there is bone marrow depression as well as overactivity of the spleen and other reticuloendothelial tissue has recently been treated by splenectomy. This group includes myelofibrosis, polycythemia vera with myelofibrosis, and aplastic anemia. Although there is still debate regarding the benefits of surgery, effect on prognosis, and acceptance of a high surgical risk in these disorders, several recent reports suggest real benefit in a reasonable proportion of carefully evaluated patients.

An accurate diagnosis is the prerequisite to

good results in the management of hypersplenism. Splenomegaly, peripheral blood cytopenia and a hyperplastic bone marrow compose a triad which should cause the diagnosis to be considered. History and physical examination are important; toxic cytopenias are suggested by history. The spleen is usually but not always palpable; the larger spleens occur in patients with secondary hypersplenism. Routine blood studies may suggest hypersplenism, but more specific studies are required to confirm the diagnosis in most instances. These include chest and gastrointestinal roentgenographic studies, blood cultures, skin tests, serum electrophoresis, and liver and lymph node biopsies. Bone marrow studies must be made and interpreted by a competent hematologist.

The concepts of hypersplenism have been variously expressed by several hematologists. It may be seen from a study of several disease entities that the spleen plays a varying role in the production of the pathophysiologic changes comprising them. An understanding of these factors is helpful to an appreciation of both the results of splenectomy and the need for careful hematologic evaluation.

PRIMARY (IDIOPATHIC) THROMBOCYTOPENIC PURPURA. Primary hypersplenism, associated with reduced blood platelets and abnormal bleeding, has been called essential thrombocytopenic purpura, idiopathic thrombocytopenic purpura and Werlhof's disease. Clinical manifestations, due to pathologic bleeding, are the result of a combination of abnormal capillary permeability and a lowered blood platelet level. With an onset early in life, the disease may be continuous or intermittent.

One of three mechanisms responsible for

the reduction of platelets is thought to be primary hypersequestration and lysis in the spleen. A second mechanism may be abnormal platelet production in the bone marrow from a humoral substance liberated from the spleen. The production of thrombocytopenia in the normal individual by injection of serum from a patient with thrombocytopenic purpura, the occurrence of thrombocytopenic purpura in the newborn, and the response of many patients with this disease to adrenocorticotropic hormone and cortisone add weight to the contention of a number of recent investigators that immunologic factors are of great etiologic importance.

Recent reports show that idiopathic thrombocytopenic purpura occurs in two forms. One, an acute, usually self-limiting disease, occurring in infants and children, frequently develops spontaneous remission over a period of several weeks to a year. Evidence for hereditary factors is inconclusive, and there is nearly equal sex distribution. The other is a chronic disease, occasionally with temporary but incomplete remissions in young adults, or usually requiring splenectomy after failure of permanent responses to adrenocorticotropin or cortisone. Females are more commonly affected with this form.

Easy bruising, an otherwise asymptomatic rash, nosebleeds or menorrhagia may be the first symptoms. The signs and symptoms depend upon the severity of the thrombocytopenia. Although frequent ecchymoses may follow trauma in mild cases, spontaneous skin, mucous membrane, gastrointestinal or cerebral hemorrhages are usually associated with platelet levels well below 70,000. Menorrhagia is a common first symptom which probably is treated at its onset without diagnosis of thrombopenia, since there are frequent associated gynecologic abnormalities. Intracranial hemorrhage presents a serious problem in approximately 10 per cent of the patients.

The diagnosis depends upon the symptomatology and the hematologic findings. Splenomegaly is uncommon and, when found, suggests other diagnoses such as secondary hypersplenism due to leukemia, Hodgkin's disease or some chronic systemic infection. Purpura, or spontaneous hemorrhage, is found to be due to markedly lowered blood platelet levels. Bleeding time is prolonged, clotting time is normal and clot retraction delayed or absent. Demonstration of an abnormal coagulation mechanism can be made, however, by the finding of a defective prothrombin consumption. When a tourniquet is applied to the arm for ten minutes at a pressure midway between systolic and diastolic levels, numerous petechiae of the skin occur. This positive test is known as the Rumpel-Leede phenomenon.

Differentiation can be made between purpura haemorrhagica and hemophilia by the history and a prolonged clotting time, normal clot retraction, a negative reaction to the tourniquet test and a normal platelet count in patients with hemophilia. Hyperplasia of the megakaryocytes of the bone marrow must be present. Erythroid hyperplasia is also usually present to a degree consistent with the anemia. This finding of marrow hyperplasia is of utmost value in differentiating essential thrombocytopenic purpura from other purpuras due to the effects of toxins, tumors or infections of the bone marrow.

The dramatic subsidence of bleeding and the low mortality have made splenectomy the treatment of choice in most adult patients with this disease. Spontaneous remissions are common in childhood, however, and the results of splenectomy do not indicate an advantage over medical therapy. Adrenocorticotropin and cortisone decrease bleeding tendency by their effect on capillary permeability plus an elevation of platelet levels. They have been of great value in deferring operation. In patients failing to respond to these drugs, and in those with chronic thrombocytopenia which relapses after drug therapy is stopped, splenectomy is indicated.

Operation should not be delayed in the face of continuously lowered platelet levels because of the danger of intracranial hemorrhage. Preoperative fresh whole blood transfusions have been recommended, not only as a source of platelets but also to raise the lowered blood volume found consistently in these patients. In those patients with inadequate platelet response to splenectomy, adrenocorticotropin or cortisone may be of value following removal of the spleen.

PRIMARY (CONGENITAL) HEMOLYTIC ANEMIA. Of the several forms of hemolytic anemia, the spleen probably plays the most important role in congenital hemolytic anemia. This disease has been described under the terms congenital hemolytic jaundice, acholuric jaundice and spherocytic icterus, all of which point to the clinical features of anemia, jaundice without bile in the urine and the typical spherical characteristic of the red cells. Careful history and hematologic evaluation of several members of the family may be necessary to establish the diagnosis, since mild cases may be entirely asymptomatic. Despite the persistence of spheroidal cells with increased susceptibility to hemolysis, splenectomy is usually curative.

The symptoms vary markedly with the severity of the disease. One member of the family may have severe anemia, splenomegaly and jaundice, while all others have only the characteristic spherocytosis without significant anemia. Latent forms of the disease may become active any time between infancy and the fifth decade of life. Remissions and exacerbations are then common. Mild jaundice, weakness and malaise are the most common symptoms. These patients are not actually sick, except when hemolytic crisis, an acute exacerbation of hemolytic activity, occurs. Dull pain or dragging discomfort in the left upper abdomen is occasionally found and splenic tenderness with splenomegaly increases during exacerbations of hemolysis. Nausea and vomiting, abdominal pain and a rapid increase in jaundice are noted with a hemolytic crisis.

As with all jaundiced patients, the diagnosis depends upon an accurate history plus certain laboratory data. Confirmation of the familial nature of the disease is important. The peripheral blood shows microcytic anemia with 2 to 4 million erythrocytes per cubic millimeter, and 4 to 12 gm. of hemoglobin per 100 cc. Counts below 1 million occur with hemolytic crisis. Spherocytosis and a marked reticulocytosis of 5 to 20 per cent are invariably present. The spheroidal red cells show increased fragility with hemolysis in 0.7 to 0.5 per cent saline, as compared with 0.45 per cent for normal cells. The bone marrow shows an erythroid hyperplasia of a degree dependent upon the degree of anemia. Bone marrow studies are absolutely necessary to rule out other forms of anemia. In the indirect van den Bergh test, the value is elevated. There is an increase of urobilin in the urine and stool, but bile is absent in the urine, while urobilin is increased. Splenomegaly is common, the spleen usually weighing 1000 to 1500 gm., but it may not be palpable in patients having mild or asymptomatic anemia.

The only acceptable treatment is splenectomy. If the diagnosis is correctly established, the results of splenectomy are immediate and dramatic. Preoperative transfusions are contraindicated since the danger of producing hemolytic crisis is greater than splenectomy in a moderately anemic patient. Rarely, with a severe hemolytic crisis and a megaloblastic bone marrow, both folic acid and transfusions may be tried before emergency surgery is planned. Once the splenic artery is ligated, blood replacement should follow. Although spherocytosis and increased red cell fragility are not changed, hemolysis ceases following splenectomy.

PRIMARY SPLENIC NEUTROPENIA. Neutropenia and granulocytopenia due to primary hypersplenism were first described in 1939. The decrease in white cells due to overactivity of the spleen and the response to splenectomy have been confirmed by numerous observers.

The symptoms are usually those of a recurrent or chronic infectious process. Oropharyngeal and skin infections may be associated with weakness, malaise and intermittent fever. Infections respond poorly to the usual methods of therapy. In some patients, markedly severe anemia and mild jaundice have been noted. Splenomegaly is usually present and the large spleen may cause abdominal discomfort. Joint pains may be present in some patients.

The diagnosis depends upon the findings of neutropenia, for which there is compensatory myeloid hyperplasia of the bone marrow. Care must be taken to rule out toxic neutropenias in which the bone marrow is not hyperplastic and shows myeloid maturation arrest. Although splenectomy is the treatment of choice, the neutropenia usually runs a cyclic course and operation may await an optimum peak in peripheral white cell count.

PRIMARY SPLENIC PANHEMATOPENIA. The simultaneous occurrence of thrombopenia, neutropenia and hemolytic anemia due to hyperactivity of the spleen has been delineated as a clinical entity called splenic panhematopenia. Although the degree of the various cytopenias may differ, their mechanism of development is considered similar.

Symptoms of panhematopenia vary, being somewhat dependent upon the severity of the specific cytopenia. Weakness, malaise, scattered recurrent infections, easy bruising, petechiae and jaundice are the most common symptoms. When platelet counts are markedly lowered, spontaneous mucosal hemorrhage ensues. Splenomegaly is a consistent finding. The differential diagnosis may be difficult; hypoplasia of bone marrow and secondary hypersplenism must be considered. A compensatory hyperplasia of all the cellular elements of the bone marrow must be found to confirm the diagnosis. Even then, lymph node biopsy may lead to the discovery of another systemic disease process, changing the diagnosis to secondary hypersplenism.

Splenectomy is indicated. The indications and contraindications to preoperative transfusions, antibiotics, adrenocorticotropin or cortisone, and the decision of optimum time for operation, are problems which try the judgment of a competent hematologist. Surgical results will depend upon the adequacy of preoperative evaluation.

SECONDARY HYPERSPLENISM. During the course of certain chronic disease processes which involve the reticuloendothelial system, associated hypersplenism occasionally develops. This produces cytopenias identical with those which occur in various forms of primary hypersplenism. The typical features are those of the various specific blood cytopenias or panhematopenia with a definite compensatory bone marrow hyperplasia. Secondary thrombocytopenic purpura, hemolytic anemia, neutropenia and pancytopenia have all been recognized. Since complications of the hypersplenic cytopenias can be expected, splenectomy is indicated.

The diagnostic criteria in secondary hypersplenism are similar to those of the primary form of this syndrome. Signs and symptoms vary widely and may be complicated by those of the primary disease. The spleen is almost invariably enlarged to a much greater degree than in patients having primary hypersplenism. Splenomegaly is due in large part to involvement in the primary chronic disease process.

If surgical mortality and morbidity are to be kept low, great attention must be given to preoperative preparation in these patients. Owing to the nature of the diseases with which hypersplenism is associated, most of the patients are poor surgical risks. They are generally of an older age group, often with much deterioration resulting from the original disease. The principles of surgery include attention to details in the preoperative preparation, with the establishment of optimum nitrogen balance, blood volume levels and pulmonary reserve. Close cooperation with a hematologist is mandatory. Although splenectomy cannot be expected to affect the ultimate outcome in the chronic disease with which secondary hypersplenism is associated, the hematologic improvement following splenectomy, after adequate preparation, strongly justifies surgery even in many debilitated patients.

ACQUIRED HEMOLYTIC ANEMIA

While the etiologic basis of primary and secondary hemolytic anemia is ascribed to a defect in the red cell and a selective sequestration in the spleen, the mechanisms of acquired hemolytic anemia include the factors of increased red cell fragility, destructive agents in the blood serum and erythrophagocytosis. The overproduction of serum hemolysins unantagonized by antihemolysins results in red cell destruction. Autoagglutinins, autohemolysins and isohemolysins have all been found in the blood serum.

Hyperactivity of the reticuloendothelial system is probably the cause of hemolytic anemia in some patients. The spleen may, therefore, be only one part of the system causing abnormal red cell destruction. Unless the spleen is of great importance in the individual patient, at times a diagnostic problem even to the most astute hematologist, splenectomy will be of little value.

Recent use of chromium tagging of red cells has helped to indicate those patients most likely to respond to splenectomy. Using the patient's own cells, a half-survival of cells of less than 20 days is considered significant evidence of hemolysis. This is associated with an increased radioactivity over the spleen; the splenic count should be over twice that noted over the liver.

The course of this disease is usually more severe than that of congenital hemolytic anemia. Red cell counts are usually below 2,000,000 and hemolytic crises may cause anemia beyond the regenerative capacity of the bone marrow. Red cell fragility in saline solutions may not be greatly altered. The spleen is usually greatly enlarged. Reticulocytosis is marked and normoblasts may be found in the peripheral blood. Autoagglutinins are often present and the blood serum may contain hemolysins. Reaction to the antihuman globulin test is usually positive.

When the cause of excessive hemolysis cannot be accurately determined, splenectomy is usually considered. At least in part, the anemia in many patients is directly due to splenic hyperactivity. Results of splenectomy cannot always be accurately determined preoperatively. Once the diagnosis is established, adrenocorticotropin or cortisone should be given a trial of therapy. Failure of response to these drugs initially, or failure of response to an exacerbation after good initial response, warrants splenectomy. Response of acquired hemolytic anemia to splenectomy occurs in only about 50 per cent of the patients; however, in those failing to respond, adrenocorticotropin or cortisone may be of benefit after splenectomy.

CYSTS

Cysts of the spleen are classified as nonparasitic or parasitic. All are rare. Nonparasitic cysts may be divided into primary (true) and secondary (pseudocysts), depending upon whether an epithelial or mesothelial lining exists. They may be of various sizes and either multiple or single. The more common type is the single, subcapsular, secondary cyst, usually resulting from degeneration in an infarct or tumor or the breakdown of a hematoma.

The hydatid cyst is the only parasitic cyst. It occurs in less than 2 per cent of patients with the Echinococcus infection.

Symptoms vary with the size and type of cyst. Most of the smaller cysts are asymptomatic, while the larger ones cause abdominal discomfort and are confused with omental, pancreatic and ovarian cysts. Calcification of the cyst wall may simplify the diagnosis. Eosinophilia and a positive reaction to the skin test may differentiate hydatid from nonparasitic cysts.

Treatment consists of splenectomy, if the cyst is centrally located, and marsupialization for drainage, if the cyst is located peripherally and associated with many adhesions. Splenectomy carries a low mortality and is the treatment of choice. Aspiration is dangerous when hydatid cyst is suspected, since spillage of cyst contents causes an anaphylactoid reaction.

TUMORS

Tumors of the spleen, both primary and secondary, are even more rare than cysts. All types have been described and include angioma, lymphoma, endothelioma, reticulum cell sarcoma, dermoid epithelial cyst, mesothelial inclusion cyst, fibrosarcoma, fibroma and leiomyoma. The only important benign tumor is hemangioma, and the only important malignant tumor is sarcoma.

Tumors of the spleen rarely produce symptoms. The spleen is rarely palpated except when there is a malignant inoperable tumor. Splenectomy is the treatment of choice and leads to cure for benign tumors, carrying a mortality of about 2 per cent. Since sarcoma is the most common malignant tumor, the operative mortality is higher and the five-year cure rate practically zero.

ANEURYSM OF THE SPLENIC ARTERY

The rare finding of aneurysm of the splenic artery at autopsy is even less often noted clinically, despite the more recent use of contrast arteriography. This aneurysm is the second most common within the abdomen, occurring more often in women than in men. It may be due to arteriosclerosis, trauma or congenital defect, but the majority are due to arteriosclerosis. Spontaneous rupture may occur and produce a fatal outcome.

The symptoms vary, but pain, nausea, anorexia, weight loss and, occasionally, a palpable mass have been noted. These symptoms usually simulate those of chronic pancreatitis, so that diagnosis has been accurately made in less than 10 per cent of the patients. Calcification in the walls of the aneurysm is the only diagnostic radiographic finding, other than that disclosed by the use of aortography.

Treatment consists of excision of the aneurysm if possible, or proximal and distal ligation when excision is considered unsafe. Splenectomy need not necessarily follow ligation of the splenic artery.

INFECTIONS

During recent years, acute infections involving the spleen have been extremely rare, probably owing to widespread use of antibiotics. Chronic infectious processes, primarily or secondarily involving the spleen, are somewhat more common.

Abscess of the spleen may develop with infection in an area of hemorrhage or devitalized splenic pulp. During its early stage, the abscess remains within the capsule and may cause no symptoms. With enlargement, perisplenitis may cause pain, chills, fever and splenomegaly. If drainage is not instituted or splenectomy performed, the possibility of splenic rupture, with a high mortality, exists. If diagnosis can be made early, splenectomy is the treatment of choice.

Several chronic infections are characterized by splenomegaly. Splenectomy may produce remission of general symptoms, or may be beneficial to the patient in whom secondary hypersplenism is associated. The chronic infections with which the spleen may become involved include malaria, tuberculosis and Boeck's sarcoid.

The involvement of the spleen in patients with malaria is well known. In certain instances of chronic malaria, the disease may not be diagnosed from peripheral blood smears alone, whereas numerous parasites are harbored within the spleen. No significant diagnostic criteria of malarial infection are present, other than splenomegaly, without other known cause in patients who have been known to have malaria. The problem presented by the enlarged spleen is the occasional discomfort which it may cause and the susceptibility to either spontaneous or easy traumatic rupture, both of which are direct indications for splenectomy. In the tropics, splenomegaly may be associated with chronic hemolytic anemia, lymphocytic sinusoidal infiltration of the liver, and increased antibody titers to malaria which may be due to an abnormal immune response to malaria.

As with other portions of the reticuloendothelial system, the spleen may become involved in the chronic systemic disease processes, tuberculosis and Boeck's sarcoid. The importance of this involvement lies in whether the disease is active and whether it produces hematologic complications. Thrombocytopenia is common but may not necessarily be due to hypersplenism. Other forms of hypersplenism secondary to these chronic disease processes, however, have been reported and the results of splenectomy in the relief of various cytopenias have been quite favorable. The only other indication for operation in these patients is the occasional markedly enlarged spleen, causing enough abdominal discomfort to warrant its removal.

MISCELLANEOUS DISEASES

BANTI'S DISEASE. Portal hypertension is the common denominator of the group of hepatosplenopathies loosely termed Banti's disease. Whether intrahepatic (cirrhosis) or extrahepatic (thrombosis) portal obstruction is present, the splenic changes are similar.

The spleen is invariably enlarged. The capsule is thickened and there are usually numerous vascular adhesions. The splenic parenchyma is firm, deep red in color and markedly congested. Fibrosis, with hyperplasia of the reticuloendothelial lining of dilated sinuses, is prominent.

MEDITERRANEAN ANEMIA. This is a familial chronic hemolytic anemia, also called erythroblastic or Cooley's anemia, which occurs usually in children descended from parents of Mediterranean countries. The abnormalities producing anemia consist of a defect in hemoglobin formation and an increased resistance of the red cells to hypotonic saline. Characteristic thickening of the frontal bone, with depression of the nasal bridge, and a mongoloid slant to the eyes help to differentiate this disease. The microcytic anemia may be associated with leukocytosis and is invariably associated with marked hyperplasia of the bone marrow. Splenectomy has been advocated when marked hemolytic activity is present. Most patients will at least maintain a higher red cell count and hemoglobin level and require fewer transfusions following splenectomy.

Felty's syndrome. Felty's syndrome is a clinical entity consisting of splenomegaly, anemia and neutropenia, and occurring most often in association with chronic rheumatoid arthritis in women between the ages of 40 and 60 years. The pathologic findings in the spleen are not characteristic and the etiologic basis is controversial. The leukopenia may be the result of multiple chronic infections or a splenic hyperfunction of unknown origin. Leukopenia occurs in variable degrees and the arthritis is of several years' duration prior to the onset of the syndrome. The symptoms consist of weakness, frequent episodes of fever, weight loss, swollen and painful joints and multiple skin or oral infections.

Splenectomy has given variable success, but in a number of patients has produced relief not only of the neutropenia and anemia, but also marked improvement in the joint symptoms. Adrenocorticotropin and cortisone may also give temporary and, at times, longstanding symptomatic relief.

STORAGE DISEASES. Several diseases due to abnormal lipid metabolism may produce splenomegaly of surgical importance. These include Gaucher's disease, Niemann-Pick disease and Hand-Schüller-Christian disease, in which there is abnormal reticuloendothelial storage respectively of cerebrosides, sphingomyelin and cholesterols. Only in Gaucher's disease is splenectomy frequently indicated.

Idiopathic splenomegaly is a term formerly used to denote Gaucher's disease. Patchy pigmentation of the face, conjunctival thickening, hepatomegaly, splenomegaly, flaring of the distal end of the femur, thrombocytopenia and neutropenia may suggest the diagnosis; this can be confirmed by findings of foam cells in the bone marrow. The thrombocytopenia and neutropenia are often due to hypersplenism. The diagnosis of Gaucher's disease as the cause of secondary hypersplenism is often not made, however, until the time of splenectomy. Thrombocytopenia and neutropenia may be greatly relieved by splenectomy, but improvement in anemia is only temporary.

INFECTIONS AFTER SPLENECTOMY

Since 1952, there has been considerable concern that splenectomy in children may be followed by an increased susceptibility to infection. Fatal infections, most often owing to pneumococcus or meningococcus, have been rather frequently reported. A review of the literature suggests that splenectomy for idiopathic thrombocytopenic purpura, congenital hemolytic anemia, traumatic rupture and portal hypertension is not associated with an increased post-splenectomy infection rate. On the other hand, patients with a serious primary disease, such as Cooley's anemia, lipidosis, or histiocytosis, carry a high risk of subsequent fatal infection.

READING REFERENCES

Collier, R. L., and Brush, B. E.: Hematologic disorder in Felty's syndrome: prolonged benefits of splenectomy. Am. J. Surg. *112*:869, 1966.

Curtis, G. M., and Movitz, D.: Surgical significance of accessory spleens. Ann. Surg. *123*:276, 1946.

Daire, J. V.: Acquired hemolytic anemia; with special reference to the antiglobulin (Coombs') reaction. Blood 8:813, 1953.

Dameshek, W., and Welch, C. S.: Hypersplenism and Surgery of the Spleen. New York, Grune & Stratton, 1952.

Doan, C. A., Wiseman, B. K., and Bouroncle, B. A.: Hypersplenic cytopenic syndromes: a twenty-five year experience with special reference to splenectomy. Proc. Internat. Soc. Hematol. *1*:429, 1956.

Doan, C. A., and Wright, C. S.: Primary congenital and secondary acquired splenic panhematopenia. Blood *1*:10, 1946.

Dunphy, J. E.: Splenectomy for trauma. Am. J. Surg. *71*: 450, 1946.

Elliott, L. D., Cramer, G. G., and Amplatz, K.: The anomalous relationship of the inferior vena cava and abdominal aorta as a specific angiocardiographic sign in asplenia. Radiology 87:859, 1966.

Ellison, E. H.: Spontaneous rupture of the diseased spleen. Arch. Surg. 59:299, 1949.

Eraklis, A. J., Kevy, S. V., Diamond, L. K., and Gross, R. E.: Hazard of overwhelming infection after splenectomy in childhood. New England J. Med. 276:1225, 1967.

Fowler, R. H.: Non-parasitic benign cystic tumors of the spleen. Internat. Abstr. Surg. 96:209, 1953.

Harrington, W. J., and others: Immunologic mechanisms in idiopathic and neonatal thrombocytopenic purpura. Ann. Int. Med. 38:433, 1953.

Heaton, L. D., Crosby, W. H., and Cohen, A.: Splenectomy in the treatment of hypoplasia on the bone marrow. Ann. Surg. 146:637, 1957.

Macpherson, A. I. S.: Late results of splenectomy; review of 240 cases. J. Roy. Coll. Surg. Edinburgh 4:305, 1959.

McSherry, C. K., and Dineen, P.: Significance of splenic abscess. Am. J. Surg. *103*:618, 1962.

Medoff, A. S., and Bayrd, E. D.: Gaucher's disease in 29 cases; hematologic complications and effect of splenectomy. Ann. Int. Med. 40:481, 1953.

Owens, J. C., and Coffey, R. J.: Aneurysm of the splenic artery, including report of six additional cases. Internat. Abstr. Surg. 97:313, 1953.

Robb-Smith, A. H. T.: The reticuloses. Lancet 2:619, 1953.

Rousselot, L. M., and Stein, C.: Malignant neoplasms of the spleen, primary and secondary. S. Clin. North America 33:493, 1953.

Sandusky, W. R., Leavell, B. S., and Benjamin, B. I.: Splenectomy: Indications and results in hematologic disorders. Ann. Surg. *159*:695, 1964.

Shirkey, A. L., Wukasch, D. C., Beall, A. C., Jr., Gordon, W. B., Jr., and DeBakey, M. E.: Surgical management of splenic injuries. Am. J. Surg. *108*:630, 1964.

Trusler, G. A., and Bartlett, G. S.: The role of splenectomy and the treatment of thalassemia major. J. Pediat. Surg. 2:55, 1967.

Ungar, G.: Endocrine function of the spleen and its participation in the pituitary-adrenal responses to stress. Endocrinology 37:329, 1945.

Wagner, H. N., Jr., and Bardfeld, P. A.: Evaluation of structure and function of the spleen with radioactive tracers. J.A.M.A. *199*:202, 1967.

Weed, R. I., and Weiss, L.: The relationship of red cell fragmentation occurring within the spleen to cell destruction. Tr. A. Am. Physicians 79:426, 1966.

Whipple, A. O., Parpart, A. J., and Chang, J. J.: A study of the circulation of the blood in the spleen of the living mouse. Ann. Surg. *140*:266, 1954.

Williams, R. D., and Zollinger, R. M.: Diagnostic and prognostic factors in abdominal trauma. Am. J. Surg. 97:575, 1959.

Williams, R. D., and Ellison, E. H.: Complications following splenectomy. *In*, Artz, C. P., and Hardy, J. D.: Complications in Surgery and Their Management. Philadelphia, W. B. Saunders Company. 1967.

Wiseman, B. K., and Doan, C. A.: Primary splenic neutropenia. Ann. Int. Med. 16:1097, 1942.

Zollinger, R. M., and Williams, R. D.: Surgery of the spleen. Minnesota Med. 42:881, 1959.

Chapter 28

THE URINARY SYSTEM

by

JOHN T. GRAYHACK, M.D.

JOHN THOMAS GRAYHACK was born in Kankakee, Illinois, and received his undergraduate and medical education at the University of Chicago. He was an intern in general surgery at The Johns Hopkins Hospital and there pursued his education in urology. He is the Professor and Chairman of the Department of Urology at Northwestern University where he directs an active investigative and teaching program in urology utilizing the facilities of the Herman Kretschmer Laboratory.

INTRODUCTION

Historically, operative procedures for removal of bladder calculi were undoubtedly carried out by the ancients. In the middle ages, itinerant lithotomists who retained the secrets of their art for their family carried out this procedure. However, the development of urology as a recognized, respected surgical specialty depended primarily on the introduction of specialized roentgenographic and endoscopic diagnostic techniques. Specialized therapeutic procedures were conceived and improved once diagnoses could be established with regularity. Similarly, proper treatment today demands accurate diagnosis. This in turn requires a painstaking history, a complete physical examination, a careful examination of the urine with employment of special tests as indicated, and utilization of appropriate x-ray, isotope, and endoscopic studies. All are essential to establish a diagnosis.

A patient may have a life-threatening disease of the genitourinary tract with few if any symptoms. However, the following symptoms are suggestive of urinary tract disease.

Nocturia, awakening at night to void, is unnecessary for the normal individual. Nocturia may be caused by lower urinary tract disease, such as bladder neck obstruction, neurogenic dysfunction, infection and calculus; metabolic disorder, such as diabetes mellitus or diabetes insipidus; congestive heart failure; renal failure, and habitual excessive fluid or drug intake.

The normal person voids three to five times a day. Increased *frequency* may be due to organic or psychogenic causes. Diurnal frequency in the absence of nocturia suggests a functional disorder.

Polyuria means larger than normal total urine volume and is characteristic of metabolic disorders, renal disease, and excessive fluid intake.

Oliguria is utilized to describe diminished urine volume; usually 400 ml. is considered the minimum obligatory urine output.

Anuria is complete suppression of urine formation.

Urgency is a precipitous desire to void, making control difficult or impossible.

Dysuria means pain or discomfort on urination. When it is severe, it is called strangury. Bladder spasm or tenesmus often follows voiding in the presence of an irritated or infected bladder.

Hesitancy denotes undue delay and difficulty in initiating voiding.

Intermittency is the term used to describe the interrupted urinary stream thought to be due to detrusor fatigue in the presence of bladder neck obstruction. Usually there is an associated decrease in size and force of the urinary stream.

Incontinence is involuntary loss of urine. It is further characterized as true when caused by abnormalities such as sphincter injury or fistula; as paradoxical or overflow when resulting from urinary leakage from an overdistended bladder; as stress when associated with coughing or straining, or as

869

urgency when it is preceded by a desire to void as may occur with neurogenic dysfunction or inflammatory lesions.

Pyuria is used to denote the presence of pus in the urine. It is due to inflammation and may be associated with an undesirable odor.

Crystalluria due to precipitated urinary solutes is similar in gross appearance to pyuria.

Hematuria may be gross or microscopic, painless or painful. Hemoglobinuria, beeturia, red bladder dyes, and the brickdust color of uric acid crystals may be confused grossly with hematuria. Hematuria may be further characterized by its relationship to the act of micturition. Initial hematuria is noted only at the beginning of urination and usually is secondary to pathology distal to the neck or the bladder. Terminal hematuria is noted at the end of urination and is secondary to pathology in the region of the trigone, bladder neck, and posterior urethra such as a calculus, bladder neoplasm, or prostatitis. When blood is passed throughout urination, the descriptive term total is utilized. The common causes for hematuria vary with age and sex. (Table 1). Although there are over 100 causes for hematuria, consideration of tumor of the bladder, tumor of the kidney, stone, tuberculosis, acute hemorrhagic cystitis, trauma, and blood dyscrasia as causes of gross hematuria in the adult is a useful diagnostic framework. Benign prostatic hypertrophy is probably the commonest cause of bleeding in males over the age of 55. Blood dyscrasias have assumed greater importance with the increased use of anticoagulants.

Lithuria is used to describe the passage of urinary calculi.

Pneumaturia, passing gas in the urine, may be due to an enterovesical fistula, gasforming organisms, or urologic instrumentation.

Pain from a renal lesion may vary from a dull, aching flank discomfort to a severe, sharp flank pain radiating into the lower abdomen or the gluteal region. The pain may be episodic or persistent. Often, it is associated with anorexia, nausea, and vomiting. No relationship is evident to the intake of food or to movement. Occasionally, as in the presence of ureteral reflux, the pain may be precipitated by voiding, or as in the occasional rare instance in which renal ptosis is obstructing, by the assumption of an erect position. In general, pain is as likely to awaken a patient as to occur during waking hours. Usually, with severe discomfort the patient tends to move about restlessly and to indicate the site of discomfort by grasping the flank between his thumb and forefingers. Renal pathology may be responsible for bizarre abdominal complaints. Pain from ureteral colic often causes flank discomfort associated with severe abdominal discomfort, nausea, and vomiting. As the site of the calculus or clot responsible for the discomfort progresses inferiorly, the pain tends to radiate into the lower abdomen, genitalia, and occasionally the thigh. If a calculus lodges at the ureterovesical junction it may also cause associated frequency, urgency, and dysuria.

Pain from bladder pathology is often dull and aching and confined to the suprapubic area. It may, as in the case of an acute infection, be severe and associated primarily with voiding or a desire to void. Discomfort of the glans penis, particularly at the end of voiding, often results from pathology in the region of the neck of the bladder.

All patients with urologic complaints deserve a complete physical examination, including a neurological evaluation. Inspection of the abdomen in the presence of a distended bladder may disclose a lower midline mass tending to flatten rather than accentuate the lower abdominal crease. Neither the dis-

Table 1.   *Common Causes of Hematuria in Various Age Groups Listed in Order of Frequency*

MALE AND FEMALE			MALE			FEMALE		
1–5	5–10	11–30	31–40	41–50	51–60	31–40	41–50	51–60
Inf. Gl.Neph.	Gl.Neph. Inf.	Inf. Cal. Bl.Neo.	Inf. Bl.Neo. Cal.	Bl.Neo. Cal. Inf.	Bl.Neo. B.P.H. Cal. Inf.	Inf. Cal. Bl.Neo.	Inf. Cal. Bl.Neo.	Bl.Neo. Inf. Cal.

Inf.—Inflammatory lesion; Gl.Neph.—glomerulonephritis; Cal.—calculus; Bl.Neo.—bladder neoplasm; B.P.H.—benign prostatic hypertrophy.

tended bladder nor the hydronephrotic kidney is easy to delineate on palpation. Palpation of the kidney should usually be initiated with the patient supine and with one examining hand on the flank and the other hand anteriorly on the abdomen. Utilization of both the lateral margin and tips of the fingers of the anterior examining hand is an aid in the examination. Observation of the changes in position of a palpable mass with respiration and change to a lateral or erect position of the patient is of value in identifying the mass, as is recognition of a landmark such as the renal hilum. In a child, a hydronephrotic kidney will occasionally transilluminate. Sudden pressure in the costovertebral angle may elicit pain in the diseased kidney; this does not require delivery of a blow to the flank. On many occasions, the site of maximal abdominal tenderness is best localized by examination with a single finger or by having the patient cough or strain and identify the site of discomfort. Pressure over a full bladder often precipitates a desire to void.

Accurate diagnosis is usually dependent on judicious utilization of the many laboratory studies now available. This in turn requires an understanding of the test and its limitation.

Urinalysis should be preceded by cleansing of the genitalia, particularly in the female. In the male a two- or three-glass urine specimen assists in localizing the abnormality found in the urinary sediment. The first glass should contain the initial 30 to 60 ml. and the third glass, if employed, the final 30 ml. of voided urine. In the female, midstream urine should be utilized; if properly collected, the sample is likely to reflect the findings in the urinary tract, particularly if negative. Under some circumstances, catheterization is required in the female to obtain a representative specimen. Assessment of findings on urinalysis and urine culture is discussed in the section on infection.

Evaluation of total and often individual renal function is of importance in patients with suspected or proved pathology of the urinary tract. Clinically, evaluation of total renal function is achieved by measurement of the degree of retention in the blood of endogenous wastes such as *urea* or *creatinine* and excretion of these substances or of exogenous chemicals such as *inulin, paraminohippurate,* or *phenolsulfonphthalein.* The blood urea nitrogen is a less accurate indicator of renal function than the serum creatinine level. Although both are excreted primarily by glomerular filtration, the amount of the former available for excretion is variable. For example, excessive protein breakdown following hemorrhage may result in a marked increase in total urea production. Creatinine is produced in essentially constant amounts. The blood urea level often seems more indicative of the clinical status of the patient, although urea itself is a nontoxic substance. In clinical practice, the creatinine clearance and phenolsulfonphthalein excretion tests are popular. The latter apparently reflects primarily renal blood flow. It correlates well with the creatinine clearance and has the advantage that it can be performed rapidly by the physician with little specialized equipment. The creatinine clearance test is a satisfactory measure of glomerular filtration rate and may be performed in most hospital laboratories. Inulin clearance, an extremely accurate measure of glomerular filtration, is utilized as an investigative tool. Paraminohippurate is secreted by the proximal tubule and is a measure of renal plasma flow. All excretory tests are dependent on total urine collection for accuracy and may yield inaccurate results in patients with significant residual urine unless this is corrected. Knowledge of the concentrating ability of the kidney is of value in assessing renal functional status and in studying patients with possible diabetes insipidus. Individual renal function may be assessed crudely by cystoscopic observation of concentration of a chromogen such as indigo carmine excreted by each ureter or more accurately by the insertion of ureteral catheters bilaterally and collection of individual urine for clearance studies — split function studies.

In addition, the *radioisotope renogram* may be utilized to indicate the functional status of the individual kidney in a qualitative fashion (Fig. 1). This test is carried out by placing a scintillation counter over each renal area and measuring the accumulation of radioactivity following the intravenous injection of an organic iodide labeled with isotopic iodine, either I^{131} or I^{125}. Efforts to permit quantitation of this test are continuing.

Development of special instruments, useful both in diagnosis and treatment, has greatly benefited the patient with genitourinary disorders. *Catheters* of varying construction have been utilized since ancient times. They are employed to bypass and relieve obstruction, to measure residual urine, to introduce and remove solutions or other substances, or

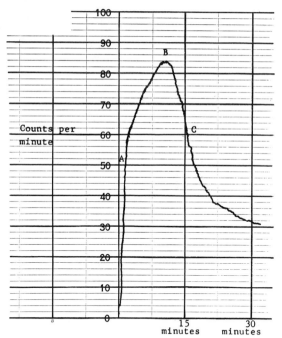

Figure 1. Normal renogram. The initial vascular spike (A) is the result of blood-borne radioactivity supplemented by tubular function. The accumulation or tubular phase (B) represents the excess of tubular secretion over excretion. The excretory phase (C) is dependent on the ability of the pelvis and ureter to transport the radioactive substance from the renal area.

to collect specimens. These hollow tubes come in varying sizes and are made of a variety of materials (Fig. 2). Properly utilized for a reasonable indication, they can provide important information and may be

lifesaving; employed indiscriminately in an unskilled fashion, they can cause serious complications.

Cystometry (Fig. 3), a method of assessing the pressure response of the bladder to distention, may be performed by infusing fluid through a urethral or suprapubic catheter and recording the pressure response. Bladder capacity and voiding pressure may be noted. This method is of value in evaluating neurogenic dysfunction.

A *bougie* (Fig. 4) is an acorn-tipped instrument usually utilized for calibration of the urethra.

Sounds are metal instruments of various shapes primarily employed to dilate the urethra. A *filiform* is a thin threaded guide used to bypass a difficult stricture or tortuous area of the urethra and act as a guide for larger, less flexible sounds or catheters.

Direct visualization of the bladder and urethra has been achieved by development of an excellent group of endoscopic instruments (Fig. 5). In general, the *cystoscope* combines a hollow tube or sheath with a light source and a lens system. Employment of water as an irrigating fluid distends the portion of the lower urinary tract being studied and permits visualization. Proper combinations of instruments permit complete inspection of the lower urinary tract. In addition the instruments may be utilized to pass other diagnostic aids such as ureteral catheters and may be employed for a number of therapeutic purposes such as ureteral stone extraction

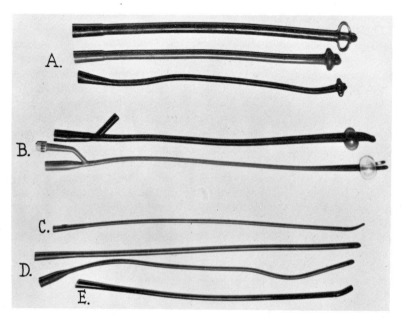

Figure 2. Types of catheters. *A* and *B* represent self-retaining catheters made of rubber. *A* shows a Malecot and two de Pezzer catheters. *B* shows a coudé and conical tip Foley catheter. *C* is a red rubber coudé catheter. *D* shows a polyvinyl and red rubber Nélaton catheter. *E* is a woven silk coudé catheter. Many other materials and shapes are utilized in the manufacture of catheters for special purposes.

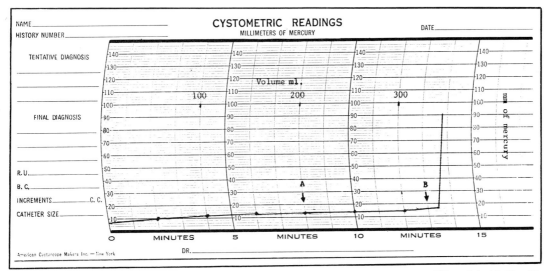

CYSTOMETRIC READINGS
MILLIMETERS OF MERCURY

Figure 3. Normal cystometrogram. Pressure response is recorded to gradual or intermittent filling of the bladder. First desire to void (A) is usually at 150 to 250 ml. Sensation of discomfort (B) precedes voiding. Voiding pressure is usually 40 mm. of mercury or more. Residual urine determination and testing of sensation of bladder to heat and cold are carried out as part of the test. The initial pressures may be set at 0 or utilized as a zero point as in this drawing.

and fulguration of bleeding areas or bladder neoplasms.

The *resectoscope* is an endoscopic instrument which permits excision of prostatic and bladder tissue through the urethra. The tissue is excised with a movable wire loop by employing a high frequency current; bleeding is controlled by fulguration.

Roentgenographic study of the urinary tract has been a great asset in increasing accurate diagnosis of genitourinary pathology. A scout film of the abdomen taken with a soft tissue technique (KUB – Kidneys, Ureter, Bladder) may demonstrate normal structure – e.g., the size, shape, and position of the kidney, the psoas shadow, and the bony structures of the pelvis and lumbar spine (Fig. 6). In addition, significant abnormalities such as soft tissue masses or radiopacities representing possible calculi may be seen. Visualization of the various portions of the urinary tract by employing contrast media has added to the value of x-ray as a diagnostic tool. These studies should always be preceded

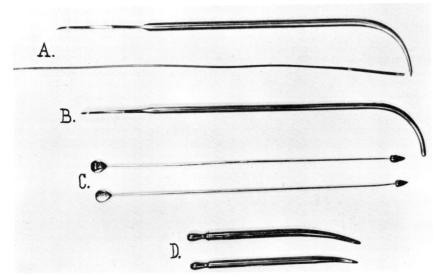

Figure 4. Urethral instruments. *A*, Filiform and LeForte (following) urethral sounds. *B*, Van Buren urethral sound. *C*, Otis bougie à boule. *D*, Walther female dilator-catheter. Many other specialized instruments exist for diagnostic and therapeutic manipulation of the urethra.

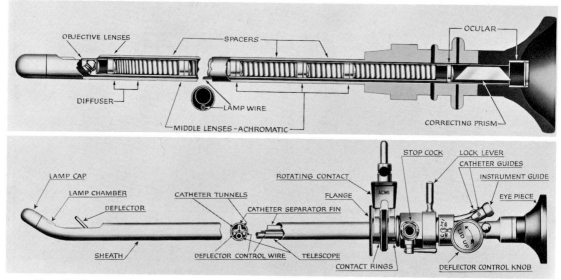

Figure 5. Diagram of typical cystoscope. (Reproduced with permission of American Cystoscope Makers, Inc.)

by a plain film to permit accurate interpretation.

The *intravenous pyelogram* (Fig. 7) is a technique for achieving visualization of the urinary tract that employs the intravenous injection of an organic iodide and is dependent on renal function. The contrast medium is excreted, primarily by glomerular filtration, and concentrated because of re-

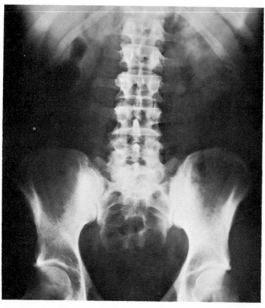

Figure 6. The renal and psoas shadows are visible as well as the bony structures. An estimate of renal size as well as evaluation of renal shape and position is possible. Small radiodensities in the left side of the pelvis represent phleboliths.

absorption of water. The collecting system of the kidney is visualized as an opacity because of the absorbed x-rays. Visualization can usually be improved by increasing water reabsorption as occurs in a dehydrated patient. Administration of large amounts of contrast media increases the amount filtered and may achieve visualization even in patients with some degree of impaired renal function.

The *nephrotomogram* (Fig. 8) is an x-ray study in which opacification of the renal parenchyma is achieved by prolonged intravenous infusion of a high concentration of an organic iodide. Functioning tissue concentrates the media homogeneously; nonfunctioning vascular tissue such as a neoplasm shows irregular pooling of the media; in avascular tissue such a cyst lacks opacification. Tomography is a body sectioning x-ray technique that allows reduction of interfering shadows overlying an organ.

Aortography (Fig. 9) is an x-ray technique utilized to visualize the renal arteries. It is dependent on delivery of a sizable concentrated bolus of contrast media to the renal arterial system and is independent of function. The contrast medium is commonly introduced through a needle placed in the lumbar aorta from the back, through a catheter threaded into the lumbar aorta from the femoral artery, or through a needle inserted in the brachial artery. The retrograde catheter technique is currently favored by many and has the advantage of allowing selective catheterization of individual renal arteries.

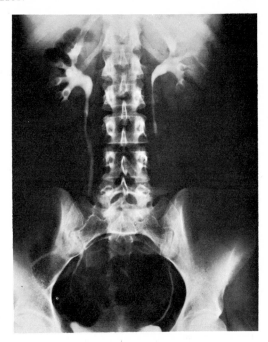

Figure 7. Intravenous pyelogram. Excellent visualization of the renal collecting system is achieved bilaterally. The distal collecting tubules are faintly visualized near the tip of the papilla, causing a fan-like effect within some of the minor calyces. The calyces do not lie in one plane so that they may be seen in an "end-on" view at times. The patchy visualization of the ureter is the result of normal peristaltic activity.

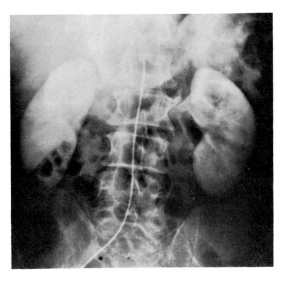

Figure 8. Nephrogram. Opacification of the renal parenchyma resulting from functional accumulation of contrast media by kidney. Tomogram technique is unnecessary in this postaortogram study because of absence of interfering shadows.

Figure 9. Brachial angiogram performed by retrograde pressure injection of contrast media through a needle inserted in the brachial artery. Both main renal arteries and major branches are visualized. Visualization of other abdominal vessels decreases clarity of renal vessels to some degree.

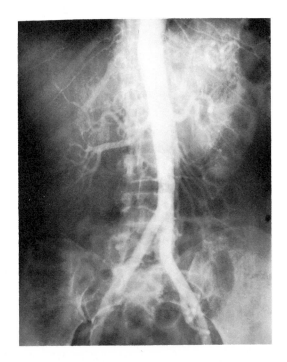

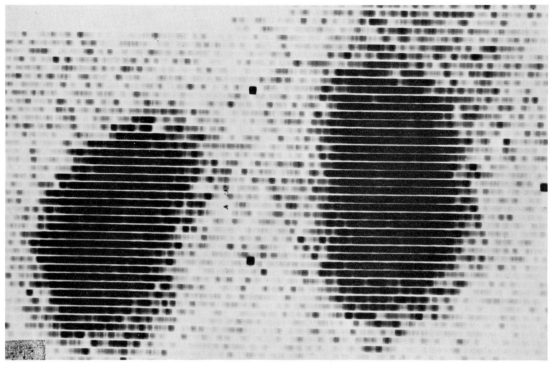

Figure 10.   Mercury[203] renal scan. Functioning renal tissue concentrates the radioisotope.

X-ray studies utilizing intravascular injection of contrast media introduce the risk of various allergic reactions, including anaphylactic shock. Damage to the arterial system or the kidney may also occur after intra-arterial injection. The possibility of these infrequent complications must be recognized.

A *radioactive renal scintiscan* (Fig. 10) may be carried out by injecting a radioisotope-labeled compound such as chlormerodrin Hg^{203} or Hg^{197} which is concentrated throughout the functioning renal tissue. Areas composed of nonfunctioning tissue, such as cyst or tumor, fail to concentrate the isotope. The routine renal scan provides information similar to that obtained with a nephrotomogram. Modifications of the method to increase its value are being studied.

Combinations of instrumentation and instillation of contrast media have the advantage of permitting complete visualization of the portion of the urinary tract being studied passively and do not rely on function. They are disadvantageous in that instrumentation must be possible and that it introduces risk, although minimal, of infection, bleeding, or perforation.

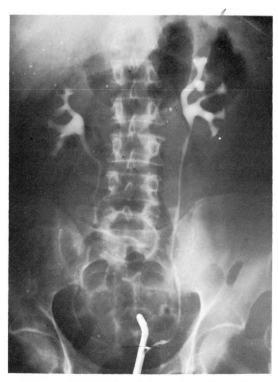

Figure 11.   Retrograde pyeloureterogram obtained by instillation of an organic iodide through an acorn tip ureteral catheter.

The *retrograde pyelogram* (Fig. 11) is accomplished by the instillation of contrast media through a small catheter inserted in the ureter or wedged into the ureteral orifice.

The *retrograde cystogram* (Fig. 12) is made by gravity instillation of contrast media through a catheter into the bladder. This study has considerable value in demonstrating ureteral reflux and in delineating abnormalities such as bladder diverticula and urinary extravasation. X-rays taken as the patient voids the contrast media may disclose ureteral reflux, or bladder neck or urethral pathology.

A *retrograde urethrogram* (Fig. 13) ac-

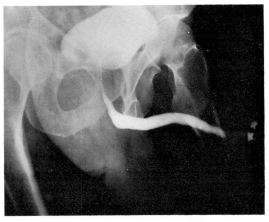

Figure 13. Retrograde urethrogram. Oblique view of the urethra of a male with a bladder neck contracture as it is being filled with a viscous radiopaque medium.

complished by instilling a thick contrast medium in the urethra may also be of assistance in demonstrating urethral pathology such as strictures and diverticula.

CALCULOUS DISEASE OF THE URINARY TRACT

Calculous disease of the urinary tract has been the object of diagnostic and therapeutic effort since ancient times. A urinary calculus is usually composed of a crystalline component and an organic matrix. Table 2 lists the common crystalline composition of calculi received from patients and the frequency with which they are found. The organic matrix is a mixture of mucoprotein and mucopolysaccharide. The factors initiating calculus formation are controversial. However, a typical calculus can be made to form artificially without an organic matrix. On the other hand, so-called matrix calculi with crystalloids present in minute traces form clinically. Currently, the crystalloid component is thought to be critical under ordinary circumstances.

Areas of high incidence of stone formation are recognized throughout the world. The etiological factors in this phenomenon are unknown. In general, stone formation is facilitated by factors which increase solute concentration in the urine, alter urinary pH, and provide a nidus for precipitation. Recognized abnormalities contributing to stone formation are stasis; infection with alteration in pH and nidus formation; immobilization

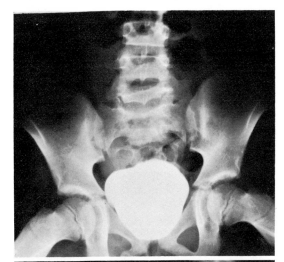

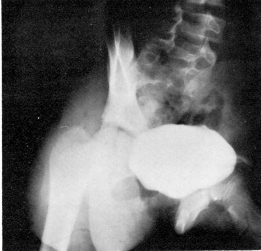

Figure 12. Retrograde cystogram. Anteroposterior and oblique views of bladder filled with opaque media instilled in a retrograde manner. Note that the bladder wall is smooth, filling defects are absent, and the contour is nearly symmetrical.

Table 2. *Composition of Urinary Calculi**

Urinary pH usually acid; urine usually sterile:	
Calcium oxalate	33%
Calcium oxalate + apatite	34%
Uric acid	6%
Cystine	3%
Urinary pH usually alkaline; urine usually infected:	
Mg NH$_4$PO$_4$ ·6 H$_2$O – apatite calculi	22%
Calcium hydrogen phosphate	2%

* Percentages are those reported in 1000 calculi by Prien (J. Urol. *61*:821, 1949).

impairing transport of urine and altering calcium metabolism; dehydration; metabolic disorders, e.g., hyperparathyroidism, hyperuricemia, cystinuria, and oxalosis; hypercalciuria secondary to neoplasm or sarcoidosis, or occurring without apparent cause; vitamin D intoxication; prolonged ingestion of excessive quantities of milk and absorbable alkali, the so-called milk alkali syndrome; abnormal renal function altering urine composition, e.g., renal tubular acidosis or Fanconi syndrome, and a foreign body, e.g., catheter.

The patient with urinary tract calculi may present with any one or a combination of symptom complexes: pain, severity and site being dependent on the site and effect of the calculus; systemic or local symptoms of infection—fever, chills, frequency, dysuria, urgency, pain; hematuria; anuria, if complete obstruction of only functioning or both kidneys; uremia-nausea, vomiting, diarrhea, mental confusion and somnolence, muscular irritability, and weight loss.

Physical findings in the presence of an uncomplicated urinary calculus are minimal. There may be slight abdominal or costovertebral angle tenderness and muscle spasm with guarding over the site of a ureteral calculus. If infection or obstruction is present, characteristic physical findings may be evident.

Urinalysis usually discloses the presence of erythrocytes but not always. Leukocytes may be present in the presence or absence of bacteria. The pH of the urine may assist in reasonable speculation regarding the composition of the calculus once its presence is established. Calcium oxalate, uric acid, or cystine calculi usually are found in acid urine. Crystals such as the hexagonal crystal of cystine may be present. Culture of the urine and determination of calcium or cystine excretion may aid in evaluation of cause or complications of calculous disease.

The diagnosis depends primarily on in-direct methods of evaluating the urinary tract, namely, roentgenography. The plain film of the abdomen usually discloses a radiopacity due to the calculus (Fig. 14), providing that the size and composition of the stone permit sufficient absorption of the x-rays to cause this, and that surrounding or overlying structures permit its recognition. The radiopaque stones are primarily those containing a heavy metal, such as calcium or magnesium; cystine calculi are radiopaque presumably because of their sulfur content. Uric acid calculi are radiolucent and therefore not seen on a plain film. Not all radiopacities seen on x-ray of the abdomen are urinary calculi. It is necessary to establish a constant relationship of the opacity to the urinary tract to justify the presumptive diagnosis of urinary calculus. To achieve this, visualization of the urinary tract by intravenous or retrograde pyelography is necessary. Radiolucent calculi cause a filling defect on pyelography (Fig. 15). Calculi may be diagnosed by other indirect methods such as the clank resulting when a urethral sound strikes a bladder stone or the scratch resulting on a waxed ureteral catheter when it bypasses a ureteral calculus, but these methods are primarily of historical interest. On the other hand, direct visualization of bladder calculi by cystoscopy is commonly employed and is extremely useful. Extension of endoscopic techniques for visualization of calculi in other areas is being investigated.

The therapy of urinary calculi may consist mainly of observation to prevent serious complications from occurring. Medical therapy utilizing such rational measures as forcing fluid, and alteration of urinary pH in uric acid and cystine calculi may be initiated. Drugs may be given to reduce production or excretion of components of the calculus, such as allopurinol in patients with uric acid calculi, penicillamine in patients with cystine calculi, and for the treatment of urinary infection. Similarly, surgical removal of calculi by various techniques, both endoscopic and open surgery, may be required and surgical procedures may be urgently necessary to correct the complication resulting from the presence of urinary calculus. Obstruction, infection, and recurrent or persistent pain are the usual indications for surgical intervention.

Between 10 and 20 per cent of patients with urinary calculi develop so-called "malignant stone disease," a life-threatening process.

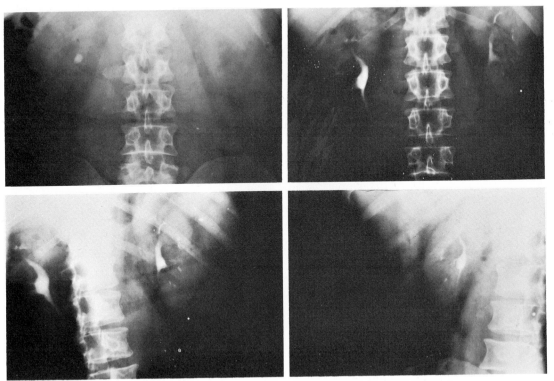

Figure 14. Renal calculus. Radiopacity in renal area on KUB; the opacity maintains a constant relationship to the renal collecting system in all views of the intravenous pyelogram, supporting the diagnosis of renal calculus.

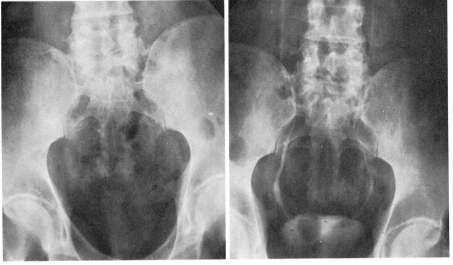

Figure 15. Radiolucent bladder calculus not evident on scout film (KUB) but appearing as a filling defect in the cystogram of the intravenous pyelogram.

URINARY TRACT INFECTION

Bacteriuria may be defined as significant presence of pathogenic bacteria in the urine. Bacteriuria is usually thought to be indicative of a urinary tract infection. However, if an infection in the urinary tract is defined as a tissue reaction resulting from the presence of a foreign organism, bacteriuria and urinary tract infection need not always be synonymous.

In any consideration of urinary tract infection, the resistance of the normal urinary tract to infection must be emphasized. Consequently, persistence or recurrence of urinary tract infection must be assumed to be associated with a local or systemic abnormality. Any systemic abnormality decreasing the host's ability to resist infection may contribute significantly to the development and persistence of infection, such as malnutrition, diseases causing severe liver dysfunction, or diabetes mellitus. The local factors usually considered are urinary stasis and the presence of a calculus, essentially a foreign body (Fig. 16). Urinary stasis may result from obstruction, neuromuscular dysfunction, or a congenital or acquired abnormality such as ureteral reflux. The presence of any foreign body such as an indwelling catheter or a calculus acts as a nidus for continued infection and makes eradication of infection extremely difficult if not impossible. Trauma is a third local factor which is employed experimentally to permit development of infection and which has probable clinical significance in the urinary tract infections developing after instrumentation and in the common occurrence of so-called "honeymoon cystitis."

Bacteria do not enter the urinary tract by normal filtration. The mechanisms by which they do enter the urinary tract are hematogenous, as in the coccal infections of the kidney; ascending, as in the presumed entrance of bacteria into the bladder via the female urethra or into the kidney from the bladder; direct extension, as in the bladder infection at times associated with a diverticulitis of the colon, and lymphatic. The organisms infecting the urinary tract are commonly gram-negative bacilli. However, infections of the urinary and adjacent genital organs may be caused by parasites such as Echinococcus, primarily in the kidney, and *Schistosoma haematobium* and *mansoni*, primarily in the bladder; by Protozoa, such as Trichomonas, primarily in the prostate and the female urethra, and by *Entamoeba histolytica;* by yeast, usually occurring in debilitated patients treated repeatedly with antibiotics; by the tubercle bacillus, and by other specific organisms such as the Gonococcus which causes an anterior urethritis in the male. The common bacterial organisms causing urinary tract infection are *E. coli, Pseudomonas aeruginosa, Aerobacter aerogenes, Proteus vulgaris,* Staphylococcus, Streptococcus, *Alcaligenes faecalis,* and Paracolon organisms. Among these, Proteus is recognized for its ability to split urea with liberation of ammonia. The resulting alkalinization may be important, not only in stone formation, but also in permitting persistence of infection. Subcellular forms of bacteria such as protoplasts may play a role in the persistence of urinary tract infections and their presence and importance are currently the focus of investigative activity.

The patient presenting with an acute urinary tract infection has symptoms related to the site and severity of the infection. Acute pyelonephritis is usually associated with flank pain, chills, fever, and often nausea and vomiting. Acute cystitis is associated with frequency, dysuria, urgency, suprapubic pain, and hematuria. The patient with a chronic urinary tract infection may experience the symptoms associated with acute urinary tract infection chronically or periodically or may be virtually asymptomatic until renal failure develops.

The physical findings in urinary tract infection vary with the site and severity of the infection. Marked flank tenderness and muscle spasm are characteristic of acute pyelonephritis. Equivocal flank tenderness may be the only physical finding in chronic pyelonephritis or there may be none. Occasionally, a physical finding makes a diagnosis highly probable, as in the beading of the vas deferens or the scrotal fistula seen with tuberculosis of the vas deferens and epididymis.

Examination of the urine is the most important tool employed in establishing a diagnosis of urinary tract infection. Gross inspection of the urine may yield valuable clues. As an

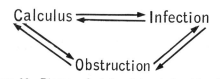

Figure 16. Diagram depicting interrelationship of obstruction, stone formation, and urinary tract infection.

example, the first portion of the voided urine of the patient with prostatitis usually contains shreds.

The number of white blood cells which must be present on microscopic examination of the urine to cause suspicion of a urinary tract infection is not clearly established. If the uncentrifuged urine is employed, ten white cells per 20 high power fields must be regarded with suspicion. If a 10-ml. random midstream urine sample is centrifuged at 2500 r.p.m. for five minutes, one or two white blood cells per high power field require further evaluation. One or more red blood cells per high power field must be regarded as abnormal. White cell casts in the urinary sediment are a significant abnormality and and indicative of renal infection, past or present, until this presumption has been disproved. Visualization of bacteria on a wet smear or on Gram stain of the urine is an excellent indicator of bacteriuria. Occasionally, as in the gonococcal infections, the stained smear remains the practical method of establishing a diagnosis.

A persistently alkaline urinary pH or the finding of abnormal amounts of protein may be the result of urinary tract infection, although other causes warrant equal consideration.

The urine culture is the definitive laboratory test for establishing the presence of bacteria in the urine and the diagnosis of urinary tract infection. Identification of the bacteria is of value in directing therapy and sensitivity testing is of even greater assistance. Normal urine is sterile. The sterility is maintained in the bladder but because the urethra frequently contains a few bacteria, the urine collected after passage through the urethra often contains bacteria. Passage of a catheter through the urethra also occasionally yields a contaminated urine and is not entirely free of risk. The problem, then, is to obtain a urine sample which satisfactorily reflects the status of the bladder urine and to obtain this with a minimum of risk. Urine may be obtained by voiding, catheterization, or suprapubic aspiration. A voided urine sample should be obtained after satisfactory cleansing of the genitalia by utilizing a two- or three-glass collection technique for urine to be examined microscopically and by employing a midstream specimen for culture. The voided urine reflects the bacteriologic status of the urinary tract more accurately in the male than in the female. In either sex

it has a great significance if it is sterile and free of abnormality on examination of the sediment. In an attempt to assess the significance of finding bacteria in the urine, quantitative techniques have been employed to count numbers of bacteria present. Because urine is an excellent culture medium and because the bladder is a reservoir usually emptying at three- to four-hour intervals, one can predict that bacteria present in the bladder will multiply and be present in great numbers in the urine. Observations have confirmed this postulation. Further, on studying urine samples obtained by both catheter and voided techniques there seem to be two groups, one with little or no bacterial growth, and a second with over 100,000 colonies per ml. The finding of a colony count exceeding 100,000 organisms per ml. is employed clinically to increase the possibility to over 90 per cent that bacteria found in the urine are representative of the state of the bladder urine. However, with a voided urine, particularly in the female, this may represent contamination or mishandling of the specimen. Furthermore, a urinary tract infection may be present with a colony count of less than 1000 colonies per ml. Routine use of the catheter increases the reliability of the urine sample, particularly in the female. However, catheterization of a patient with a sterile urinary tract may introduce a urinary tract infection. Therefore, as much reliable information as possible should be obtained from the voided specimen. Catheterization is a valuable tool and should be employed when indicated.

Urinary enzymes and other constituents of urine may eventually prove invaluable in establishing the diagnosis of urinary tract infection.

Biopsy may yield isolated evidence of infection of a genitourinary organ in rare instances. The x-ray studies of the upper urinary tract may be characteristic of a urinary tract infection such as tuberculosis and occasionally chronic pyelonephritis. The presence of characteristic anatomical changes makes a diagnosis highly probable even in the absence of bacteriological confirmation on examination of the urine.

Although infection of any portion of the urinary tract constitutes a risk to other organs and both ascending and descending infection occur, isolated infection of an organ such as the bladder or prostate does occur and is relatively common. Although the possible effect on renal function is of primary concern, not all or even the majority of urinary tract infections are pyelonephritis. In addition to local effects of a urinary tract infection, the systemic effects of a chronic infection, such as weight loss, weakness, and easy fatigability, may be evident. Furthermore, the bacteria in the urinary tract are a potential cause of bacteremia, septicemia, and occasionally bacteremic shock.

Once the diagnosis of infection is established, the fact that a single urinary tract infection in the male, or a recurrent infection in the female, is likely to be related to an underlying systemic or local cause must be emphasized. Stasis, stone, diabetes, and other abnormalities must be sought by repeated examination.

Treatment should be directed at elimination or control of the underlying causes for the infection, elimination of the bacterial agent by employment of antibiotic or chemotherapeutic agents indicated by culture, and re-examination at intervals following treatment to be certain that the infection has been eliminated.

OBSTRUCTION OF THE URINARY TRACT

Obstruction to the free egress of urine in response to normal contracture of the musculature of any portion of the urinary tract results in a series of events which may eventually result in destruction of the portions of the urinary tract above the obstructive site. The sequence of events following an obstruction may usually be divided into the following stages:

Trauma. The site of the obstruction and the areas above it may show hemorrhagic areas and the urine above the site may increase both in volume and hemoglobin content.

Muscular hypertrophy. It is presumed that muscular hypertrophy is related to development of increased pressure required to overcome the obstruction. The portion of the urinary tract just above the obstruction shows these changes first. In the urinary bladder, the hypertrophied muscle associated with a distal obstruction is evident on gross inspection as prominent ridges called trabeculae.

Dilatation and destruction. Dilatation resulting in the anatomic changes, hydroureter, hydronephrosis, caliectasis, recognized as a consequence of obstruction, may be marked. Accompanying the progression of this change,

there is usually a replacement of functioning tissue, muscle, or nephrons by fibrous tissue.

ETIOLOGY. The causes of an obstructive lesion in the urinary tract may be *congenital* or *acquired, intrinsic* or *extrinsic* (Fig. 17). The obstruction may be partial or complete. The effects of an obstructive lesion depend on the site, degree, and duration of the obstruction. Any obstructive lesion below the site of the ureteral orifices is likely to affect the functional status of both kidneys as well as making both kidneys subject to any complications that may occur.

With regard to the development of hydronephrosis, the kidney is unique in that even following total obstruction urine formation continues (Fig. 18). Following the develop-

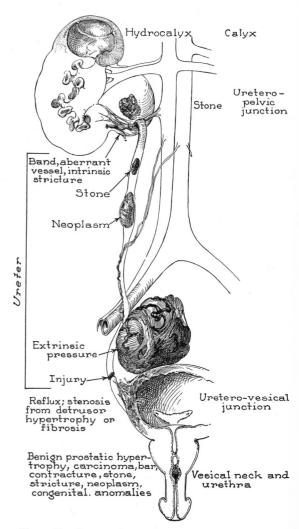

Figure 17. Causes of urinary tract obstruction. (From Hinman, F., Jr.: The pathophysiology of urinary obstruction. *In* Campbell: Urology, 2nd ed., W. B. Saunders Company.)

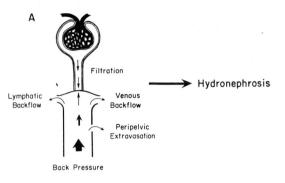

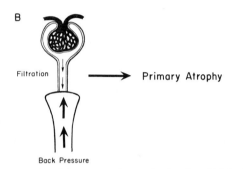

Figure 18. *A* represents the mechanism by which hydronephrosis is thought to develop; if reabsorption failed, as shown in *B*, it is postulated that a small contracted kidney would result from primary atrophy.

ment of an obstructive lesion, the intraluminal pressure above the site of obstruction rises rapidly. One would suspect that as this pressure reached filtration pressure glomerular filtration would cease and tubular secretion would be minimal. However, active reabsorption of urine occurs by pyelovenous, pyelolymphatic, tubulovenous, and tubulolymphatic routes and by peripelvic extravasation. This permits continued urine formation by filtration. Although there is an immediate increase in blood flow from the renal vein, with an acute obstruction this rapidly diminishes to levels well below normal. The resulting anoxia adds to the tissue destruction resulting from the back pressure. This sequence of events, continued secretion of urine with gradual destruction of tissue, probably accounts for the dilatation of the kidney usually found as the result of ureteral obstruction. Otherwise, primary atrophy would be expected. Experimentally, respiration of cortical tissue falls markedly within 48 hours after obstruction but the respiration of medullary tissue is unaltered. Anaerobic glycolytic ability of the cortical tissue increases markedly in the same period after occlusion.

CLINICAL SYMPTOMS. The patient with urinary tract obstruction may present with one of the following symptom complexes: obvious symptoms related to obstruction, as in the patient with bladder neck obstruction presenting with hesitancy, intermittency, decrease in size and force of the urinary stream, frequency, and nocturia; symptoms related to the primary pathology causing the obstruction, as in the patient presenting with hematuria from stone or bladder tumor; symptoms related to the presence of abdominal mass, such as the epigastric distress that may accompany a hydronephrosis, and symptoms resulting from the complication of the obstruction, as in the patient presenting with nausea, vomiting, diarrhea, muscular irritability, mental confusion, and somnolence as the result of renal failure, or in the patient presenting with chills, fever, and flank pain as the result of infection of an obstructed kidney.

The significant physical findings in a patient with obstruction may be those associated with the pathology causing the obstruction, such as the enlarged prostate causing bladder neck obstruction. They may be due to the enlarged distended organ, such as the palpable midline abdominal mass associated with dullness on percussion characteristic of a distended bladder. They may be the result of the development of a complication of an obstruction, such as the flank tenderness and muscle spasm associated with infection of the obstructed kidney.

Unfortunately, there are no characteristic findings of obstruction on urinalysis or blood chemistry studies. The findings on urinalysis may be due to the primary pathology, such as red blood cells seen with a calculus, or to a complication such as bacteria or pyuria seen with a urinary tract infection. Similarly, findings of elevated serum creatinine, blood urea nitrogen, serum phosphorous, and serum potassium associated with decreased serum calcium, characteristic of renal failure, raise the question of the presence of an obstructive lesion but do not assist in establishing this diagnosis.

The diagnosis of an obstruction in the urinary tract is dependent on one of the following: demonstration of abnormal retention of urine by recovery by catheter, by visualization of dilatation and delayed drainage by intravenous pyelography, or by showing abnormal retention of contrast media instilled in a retrograde fashion; demonstration of the obstructing pathology by cystoscopic visuali-

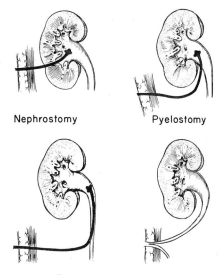

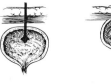

Figure 19. Representative methods of achieving temporary diversion of urine at various sites in the urinary tract.

zation of the obstructing prostatic tissue or x-ray visualization of the calculus, or demonstration of secondary pathology usually due to obstruction, trabeculation and diverticulum of the bladder, by cystoscopy or cystogram.

Treatment is directed toward relieving the obstruction (Fig. 19). This is often easily accomplished by as simple a maneuver as passage of a catheter. The effects of even longstanding obstruction including renal failure are potentially reversible with this relief. Correction of the cause of the obstruction is a secondary consideration to the relief of the obstruction.

DISEASES OF THE KIDNEY AND URETER

ANOMALIES OF THE KIDNEY

Anomalous development of the upper urinary tract can be life-threatening in the patient with renal hypoplasia or polycystic renal disease, or may predispose to acquired disease, as in partial ureteral duplication. Urogenital malformations comprise 35 to 40 per cent of all congenital abnormalities and are frequently one of multiple abnormalities. In some patients, an association of particular defects exists, such as aneurysm of cerebral vessels with polycystic kidney and nerve deafness with congenital renal parenchymal failure. Anomalies of the genital organs and kidney frequently coexist. The complex embryologic development of the kidney with serial maturation of the pronephros, mesonephros, and metanephros, the independent development of the collecting system prior to joining the renal parenchyma, and the ascent and rotation from a pelvic to a flank position provide multiple opportunities for maldevelopment of the upper urinary tract. The renal anomalies are usually classified as anomalies of number, including bilateral agenesis, unilateral agenesis, and supernumerary kidney; anomalies of position, including simple ectopia such as pelvic kidney, crossed ectopia with or without fusion, and nephroptosis or movable kidney; anomalies of form, including horseshoe, disk, L-shaped, lump, hour-glass, lobulated, and round kidney; anomalies of rotation; anomalies of volume and structure, such as hypoplasia, congenital hypertrophy, solitary cystic, multicystic, parapelvic cyst, sponge kidney, and polycystic disease, and anomalies of the renal pelvis, including duplication or so-called double kidney and congenital hydronephrosis.

All these lesions have clinical importance. Knowledge that a patient without an abdominal scar may have been born with only one kidney can be critical even if the incidence of this abnormality is one in 1200. Recognition that a palpable mass may be a functioning renal mass can prevent serious errors in diagnosis and treatment. The relative frequency of urogenital abnormalities requires consideration of this possibility in patients with abdominal complaints or physical findings of an obscure nature. These lesions may become manifest at any age. Employment of modern diagnostic techniques should permit uniformly accurate assessment of the anatomical status of the upper urinary tract.

CYSTIC DISEASE

Solitary cysts of the kidney are probably the most common renal mass recognized clinically. They are thought to result from a malunion or obstruction of the tubules when the etiology is congenital, and from tubular obstruction associated with localized vascular insufficiency when the lesion is acquired. Solitary renal cysts are bluish, thin-walled, smooth masses characteristically containing a clear serous fluid with small quantities of albumin, chlorides, globulin, urea, cholesterol, epithelial cells, and leukocytes. They are rarely seen before adulthood and are most common in the fourth, fifth, and sixth decades. Renal cysts are often asymptomatic. They may be associated with slight flank discomfort, mild gastrointestinal complaints, or infrequently with hematuria. Even less commonly, the cyst may be associated with excessive production of erythropoietin and consequent polycythemia. Infection of the cyst is a possibility. The definite diagnosis of solitary cyst is dependent on the diagnostic studies employed to demonstrate a renal mass and on the characteristic gross and histologic appearance in the absence of neoplasm. The treatment of solitary renal cyst is partial excision of the cyst wall with oversewing of the remaining edge. If nonoperative differentiation of solitary cyst and renal neoplasm were certain, many would not require operative therapy.

Peripelvic cyst is essentially a simple serous cyst located in the hilum of the kidney. It characteristically exerts lateral pressure on the collecting system and shows no evidence of renal parenchymal distortion on aortography or nephrotomography.

Medullary sponge kidney is a term applied to describe a dilatation of the distal collecting tubules of the kidney. This anatomical deformity probably results either from a developmental defect or an acquired abnormality. The characteristic dilated tubules seen at the renal papilla on intravenous pyelography suggest the diagnosis. Tuberculous lesions of the kidney may mimic the changes seen in medullary sponge kidney. Rarely the lesion may be localized to one segment of the kidney and partial resection may be employed because of complications such as persistent infection or calculous disease.

Medullary cystic disease of the kidney is an infrequent lesion often associated with renal failure and salt losing. At present this disease has no surgical significance.

Multicystic renal disease usually presents as an abdominal mass in infancy. Older patients may complain of dull abdominal pain. The lesion consists of multiple thin-walled cysts resembling a bunch of grapes. There is no associated renal parenchyma. The ureter is characteristically rudimentary and not connected with the cystic mass. Unfortunately, an abnormality of the opposite kidney may be associated with this lesion.

Although a developmental similarity seems to exist between the various types of renal cystic disease, congenital polycystic disease is an inherited renal abnormality. The adult variety is probably transmitted as a mendelian dominant, the infant variety as a recessive. The disease must be considered bilateral unless proved otherwise.

Oasthanondh and Potter have described four types of polycystic disease: Type I, due to hyperplasia of interstitial portions of the collecting tubules; Type II, due to inhibition of ampullary activity resulting in marked reduction of the number of generations of tubules derived from the ureteral bud; Type III, consisting of multiple developmental renal defects, and Type IV, due to urethral obstruction. In polycystic disease the kidneys are usually several times larger than normal and studded with cysts of varying sizes. Cysts of the liver and pancreas and aneurysms of the circle of Willis are recognized as associated lesions infrequently.

Clinically, the disease becomes manifest either in infancy or in early adulthood. Some patients with polycystic disease have a normal longevity. The symptoms calling attention to polycystic disease are pain, hematuria, abdominal mass, or the symptoms of renal

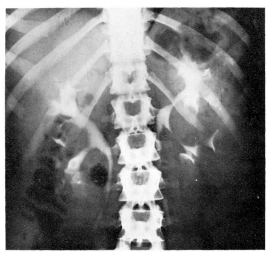

Figure 20. Intravenous pyelogram demonstrating typical configuration of polycystic renal disease. Note enlarged renal shadow, flat minor calyces, and deformity and elongation of infundibulum.

failure or hypertension. The physical examination characteristically discloses palpable, irregular, enlarged renal masses bilaterally. Hypertension is common. Urinalysis characteristically shows proteinuria; pyuria and hematuria may be present. Evidence of renal failure may become apparent on testing as the disease progresses. The diagnosis is made from the history, the physical findings, and the demonstration on intravenous or retrograde pyelography of bilateral renal enlargement with flattening of the minor calyces, elongation of the infundibula, and other evidences of multiple space-occupying lesions (Fig. 20). Progressive renal failure is the rule in recognized disease in the adult.

Hematuria, infection, obstruction, and calculous disease occasionally require surgical intervention in these patients. All attempts to preserve renal function permanently have been unsuccessful to date. These patients constitute a group in whom renal transplantation has been attempted. The disease presents a continuing challenge because many of the patients have satisfactory renal function when first seen.

CONGENITAL OBSTRUCTION OF THE UPPER URINARY TRACT

Although obstruction at such other sites as the ureterovesical junction may be on a congenital basis, congenital obstruction of the upper urinary tract occurs most frequently at the ureteropelvic junction. The obstruction at this site may be due to an aberrant renal vessel, adhesions, intrinsic stenosis, and perhaps a functional abnormality of this segment, either alone or in combination. The lesions may be bilateral. The patient with a congenital ureteral pelvic junction obstruction usually presents with intermittent flank pain, often associated with nausea and vomiting, hematuria, or evidence of a urinary tract infection. In children, an abdominal mass is commonly palpable. The lesion may not become symptomatic until early adulthood or late in life. The diagnosis is usually established by x-ray studies demonstrating the dilatation of the pelvis or calyces characteristic of a hydronephrotic kidney and the site of obstruction at the ureteropelvic junction (Fig. 21). Functional impairment may be sufficiently great to prevent visualization by intravenous pyelography.

Decisions to operate on the patient with a

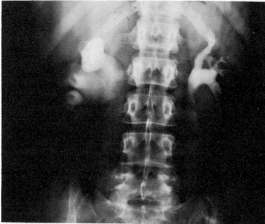
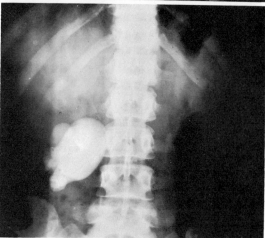

Figure 21. Intravenous pyelogram demonstrating typical deformity of hydronephrosis resulting from ureteropelvic junction obstruction. Note abrupt absence of contrast media below this site.

congenital obstruction are guided by the presence of functional impairment, complications such as infection or stone, and symptomatic complaints related to the obstruction. Whether removal of the hydronephrotic kidney or repair of the obstruction is the preferable course depends on assessment of the probable degree of function retained in the diseased kidney, as well as the status of the opposite kidney. A number of ingenious techniques have been devised to permit repair of a stenotic ureteropelvic junction with a high degree of success.

ANOMALIES OF THE URETER

Anomalies of the ureter and kidney are often associated. However, the ureteral anomalies are usually considered separately to facilitate presentation. The following is a commonly employed classification: anomalies of number – agenesis, duplication, triplication; anomalies of form, caliber, and structure – aplasia, congenital stricture, congenital valves, megaloureter, congenital diverticula; anomalies of origin and termination – ectopia, ureterocele, blind ending, ureteropelvic defect, postcaval ureter.

From a clinical standpoint, the anomalies of origin and termination are of primary importance. Ureteral ectopia in the female may be the cause of a disturbing clinical symptom complex which requires knowledge of its existence to permit its recognition and treatment. The patient presents with a history of constant dribbling incontinence with intermittent normal voiding. Usually, the offending ectopic ureter is in the upper segment of a duplicated collecting system. The extravesical source of the urinary leak can be demonstrated by instilling a colored fluid in the bladder and observing the persistent loss of clear urine. The site of the extravesical orifice can often be demonstrated. Removal of the portion of the kidney supplying the aberrant ureter is the common method of treatment.

Ureterocele is a cystic dilatation of the lower end of the ureter. The ureteral orifice is narrowed. The intravesical dilatation of the ureter is covered externally by bladder mucosa and lined internally by ureteral mucosa. The lesion is of importance because it may be a cause of significant obstruction to the ipsilateral ureter and also because it may give rise to mechanical obstruction to the bladder neck with its attendant complications, particularly renal failure. The lesion can often be recognized by a characteristic cobra head deformity of the lower ureter on intravenous pyelography. Cystoscopic examination yields the definite diagnosis.

Neoplasms

Renal neoplasms may be benign or malignant, primary or secondary. A satisfactory classification is presented in Table 3. Clinically, carcinoma of the kidney, the so-called hypernephroma, is the common (80 to 85 per cent) primary adult malignancy. Nephroblastoma, Wilms' tumor, is the common primary renal tumor of infancy and childhood. Metastatic involvement of the kidney by lesions such as lymphosarcoma, leukemia, and carcinoma of the breast occur with greater frequency than their clinical recognition would indicate.

Table 3. *Abbreviated Classification of Renal Tumors*

Tumors of mature renal parenchyma – adenoma, adenocarcinoma

Tumors of immature renal parenchyma – nephroblastoma (Wilms' tumor)

Tumors of renal pelvis – transitional cell, squamous cell

Other primary renal tumors – hemangioma, hamartoma, fibroma, leiomyoma, sarcoma

Secondary renal tumors – carcinoma of breast, sarcoma

RENAL CELL CARCINOMA. Carcinoma of the kidney occurs predominantly in the 50 to 70 year age group and very infrequently below 30 years of age. Males are affected about twice as frequently as females. Each kidney is involved with about equal frequency. Histologically two cell types are recognized, clear and granular. In addition, a variable degree of differentiation of the tumor cells can be recognized which permits histologic grading of the tumor. The ultimate prognosis is better with the more differentiated (Grade I) tumor than with the undifferentiated (Grade IV). Metastases from renal cell carcinoma are both hematogenous to the lungs, liver, and bone in addition to the renal vein, and lymphatic to the regional lymph nodes. Although a renal cell carcinoma can be induced in the male hamster with estrogen and in the rat with dimethylnitrosamine, no etiologic relationship has been established for the human renal cell carcinoma.

The common symptoms associated with primary renal tumor are the triad of hematuria, mass, and flank pain. Any of these may be present alone. When all three are present the lesion is usually far advanced. In addition, fever is commonly associated with renal carcinoma. Erythrocythemia and anemia may also be associated with this lesion. The primary renal lesion is often silent and found only when systemic symptoms such as weakness, fatigue, anorexia, and weight loss signal the presence of a neoplasm.

Physical examination may reveal a flank mass which is firm and nodular. The lesion may be so sizable that it is fixed and definite identification of its association with the kidney is impossible.

Clinical recognition of the possibility of a renal mass is primarily dependent upon x-ray studies. The plain film of the abdomen may show evidence of a distortion of the renal outline (Fig. 22A). Retroperitoneal carbon dioxide injection or tomograms may serve to demonstrate this more clearly. The intravenous pyelogram may reveal nonfunction, usually due to obstruction of the renal vein, or may show distortion of the collecting system compatible with the presence of a space-occupying lesion in the renal parenchyma (Fig. 22*B*). The nephrotomogram is of considerable assistance in further identifying the renal mass and in indicating the vascularity of the lesion (Fig. 23). The aortogram identifies the abnormal arterial and venous pattern frequently seen with a renal carcinoma (Fig. 24).

Those x-ray studies which simply indicate the presence of a mass do not establish the presence of a renal carcinoma. Any lesion which occupies space in the kidney, such as a carbuncle, a tuberculous granuloma, or a simple cyst, may cause similar distortion. Of these, the simple serous cyst is seen with five to eight times the frequency of a renal neoplasm. The renal cyst is avascular so that demonstration of blood supply to the mass on nephrotomography or aortography makes the diagnosis of renal neoplasm highly probable. Unfortunately, the demonstration of an avascular lesion does not eliminate the possibility of the presence of a tumor which

has undergone necrosis, a well-recognized phenomenon.

The presence of symptoms such as hematuria or pain increases the possibility that a renal mass is a neoplasm. Current attempts to utilize urinary enzymes to assist in establishing the diagnosis have been inconclusive. Histologic study of the lesion is required to establish its nature. Although needle biopsy and examination of aspirated material have been utilized for this purpose, the presumed danger of spread by these techniques has made them unpopular. At present, open exploration and biopsy, if necessary, are utilized in most instances to establish the diagnosis.

The established method of treatment for carcinoma of the kidney is excision of the kidney with its surrounding fat, Gerota's fascia, and adherent peritoneum. The regional nodes are removed systematically by some. The desirability of occlusion of the renal vessels prior to manipulation of the renal neoplasm has been repeatedly emphasized on theoretical grounds. Prior to nephrectomy, the presence of a contralateral kidney with life-sustaining functional ability is essential. Knowledge of the absence of demonstrable metastases at common sites is important. X-ray therapy prior to or following

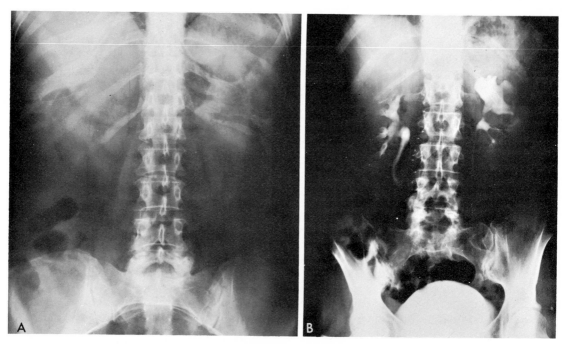

Figure 22. *A,* KUB demonstrating a mass at the lower pole of the right kidney. *B,* Intravenous pyelogram demonstrating deformity of collecting system by a mass occupying the midportion of the left kidney.

nephrectomy may be therapeutically useful. The chemotherapeutic agents and hormones such as progesterone must be regarded as having no established role in the treatment of this disease.

The five-year survival rates for patients with renal carcinoma subjected to nephrectomy have approached 50 per cent in recent communications. The ten-year rate approximates 30 per cent in these studies. Renal neoplasm is one of the tumors known to undergo spontaneous remission of metastatic lesions. This regression has occurred following nephrectomy in a few patients. The lesion is also known occasionally to follow an indolent course with metastases developing as late as 20 years after removal of the primary growth.

CARCINOMA OF THE RENAL PELVIS AND URETER. Carcinoma of the renal pelvis is most common in the fifth, sixth, and seventh decades. Males are affected four times as often as females. Each kidney is affected with equal frequency. Bilateral tumors occur in under 5 per cent of the patients. The common pelvic neoplasm is a transitional cell one, although adenocarcinoma and squamous cell

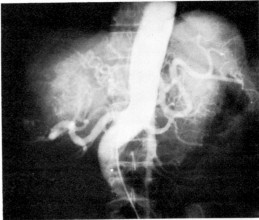

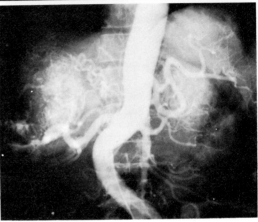

Figure 24. Aortogram demonstrating extreme vascularity with pooling of contrast media typical of renal cell carcinoma. Rapid visualization of veins is characteristic of arteriovenous fistula.

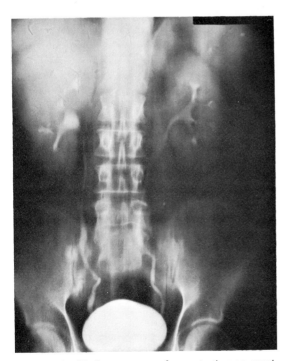

Figure 23. Nephrotomogram demonstrating an opacified mass at the upper pole of the right kidney. Opacification following injection of contrast media indicates vascularity of a mass and is typical of a neoplasm.

tumors occur. The prognosis with the latter lesion is uniformly bad. Transitional cell carcinoma tends to be associated with development of multiple lesions in the ureter and bladder either because of multicentric origin or because of metastatic spread or implantation. Other sites of metastases are lung, liver, bone, and lymph nodes. As with bladder tumors, the greater the degree of infiltration of the tumor, the poorer the prognosis. All tumors, even the typical papilloma, are to be regarded as potentially malignant.

Hematuria is the common symptom in a patient with a tumor of the renal pelvis. Pain may accompany the passage of a clot or tissue fragment in the ureter. Physical examination commonly reveals no abnormality. The diagnosis is suspected by the demonstration of filling defects on intravenous or retrograde pyelography (Fig. 25). In a pyelogram of good quality these defects may represent tumor,

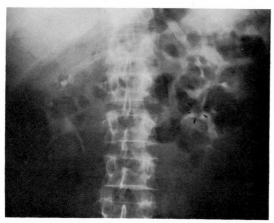

Figure 25. Intravenous pyelogram demonstrating filling defect of renal pelvis compatible with transitional cell tumor. Similar deformity may be caused by blood clot and nonopaque calculus. Retrograde pyelogram confirmed the filling defect. Exploration revealed a transitional cell carcinoma of the renal pelvis.

a nonopaque calculus, blood clot, or air. Urinary cytology and repeat x-ray studies carried out after passage of two to three weeks often help to differentiate these.

The treatment of choice in the presence of a normal contralateral kidney is nephroureterectomy with removal of a cuff of adjacent bladder. If a portion of the ureter remains, neoplasm develops in about 50 per cent of the patients. The five-year survival rate after nephroureterectomy is approximately 50 per cent. Occasionally, local resection, or destruction of a transitional cell neoplasm of the pelvis or ureter, has apparently resulted in long-term survival without recurrence.

NEPHROBLASTOMA OF THE KIDNEY (WILMS' TUMOR). Nephroblastoma of the kidney is a mixed tumor containing epithelial, muscular, and connective tissue elements. In a recent survey, 89 per cent were recognized before or at six years of age, 64 per cent being identified before four years of age. An occasional nephroblastoma is seen in an adult. There is no predilection for sex or side. Metastases occur by direct invasion of organs such as the liver, spleen, and intestine or by bloodborne spread to the lung, bone, and occasionally brain. Bilateral tumors do occur, perhaps as often as 5 per cent of the time.

Discovery of an abdominal mass in an infant by a parent or an examiner is the frequent presenting complaint in the presence of a Wilms' tumor. About 20 per cent of the abdominal masses noted in infancy arise from the genitourinary tract; about one-third of these represent malignant neoplasms. Pain

and vomiting are occasionally associated with a Wilms' tumor. Gross hematuria is an infrequent complaint, being present in about 15 per cent of the patients. Fever of an irregular character and degree may be present.

On physical examination, the characteristic mass noted on palpation is usually spherical, of variable consistency from soft to rubbery, and confined to the flank. The desirability of avoiding repeated palpation of the flank in the presence of Wilms' tumor has been emphasized by many surgeons. Hypertension has been noted in association with Wilms' tumor in from 60 to 95 per cent of the patients.

The diagnosis is established by the diagnostic studies employed to establish the presence of a renal cell carcinoma, although aortography is employed with less regularity in the child. Nonfunction on intravenous pyelography is unusual in Wilms' tumor as is calcification of the mass seen on x-ray. The collecting system is usually distorted from the presence of the mass. Hydronephrosis is usually differentiated from Wilms' tumor by the x-ray studies. Neuroblastoma, another common retroperitoneal tumor of infancy and childhood, is more difficult to identify; these tumors show a much higher incidence of calcification. Tuberculosis, retroperitoneal lymph gland tumors, and pancreatic, splenic, and hepatic enlargement may cause confusion.

The basic treatment of Wilms' tumor is nephrectomy. The tumor is very radiosensitive; x-ray therapy is employed preoperatively infrequently and postoperatively commonly. In addition, the nephroblastoma is apparently responsive to the administration of chemotherapeutic agents, the most widely used at present being actinomycin D.

The prognosis with current therapeutic techniques is difficult to estimate. The usual reported overall control with Wilms' tumor approximates 30 per cent. Current efforts are undoubtedly exceeding this rate. There is no question that a Wilms' tumor treated before one year of age has a better prognosis than one treated after this age. A control rate of as high as 80 per cent has been reported for patients less than one year of age. Survival for a period equal to the time required for the initial tumor to become clinically manifest, age plus gestation period, has been utilized as an indicator of control of the neoplasm by Collins. A two-year survival period seems to be of equal value.

RENAL INFECTIONS

Renal infections are commonly divided on the basis of the infecting organism into *nonspecific*, which includes the common pathogenic organisms, and *specific*, which includes tuberculosis, actinomycosis, and echinococcus. Routes of entry of infection include hematogenous, lymphogenous, ascending, and direct extension.

Pyelonephritis is the term applied to the common diffuse parenchymal infection of the kidney. As the name implies, both the pelvis and parenchyma are involved. The exact incidence of pyelonephritis is difficult to determine. Clinically, it is definitely recognized in less than 1 per cent of hospital admissions. Pathologically, chronic pyelonephritis has been reported to be present in from 2.8 to 9 per cent of autopsies. The incidence of an active lesion is high at death but the significance of this observation is questionable. In younger groups, the lesion is found predominantly in women; in the older age groups, men predominate. The common infecting organisms are *E. coli, Pseudomonas aeruginosa, Aerobacter aerogenes, Proteus vulgaris,* Staphylococcus, Streptococcus, *Alcaligenes fecalis* and Paracolon organisms.

The kidney with acute pyelonephritis is a swollen, tense organ with multiple subcapsular whitish areas. The mucous membrane of the pelvis and calyces may be edematous and erythematous. Microscopically, there are accumulations of leukocytes with some lymphocytes and plasma cells scattered between and within tubules but usually sparing the glomerulus. The patient with acute pyelonephritis may first note the onset of frequency, dysuria, and urgency followed by the onset of chills, high fever, and flank pain, often associated with nausea and vomiting. At other times the chills, fever, and flank pain occur initially, often followed by frequency, urgency, and dysuria. Characteristically, the patient has a tachycardia and appears ill. Flank tenderness is often marked. When the symptoms of chills, high fever, flank pain, and the findings of flank tenderness are accompanied by bacilluria on wet smear, stain, or culture, the urinary tract infection present is presumed to have affected the kidney. A moderate leukocytosis is usually present.

Treatment is administration of a chemotherapeutic or antibiotic agent selected initially on the basis of findings on smear and continued or changed on the basis of culture and sensitivity studies when they become available. General supportive measures such as the maintenance of fluid balance initially by the administration of intravenous fluids, and then by encouraging copious oral intake, use of analgesics, or antipyretic agents are essential. Urinary output and body weight should be observed. As in all patients with a bacteremia due to a urinary tract infection, a few of these patients may develop bacteremic shock. The response to therapy of a patient with an uncomplicated pyelonephritis is usually prompt. Following the subsidence of the acute episode or during it, if it does not respond promptly, a search for local and systemic causes of the infection should be initiated. In addition to looking for evidence of obstruction and calculous disease, the possibility of ureteral reflux should be considered, especially in patients with repeated episodes of acute pyelonephritis. If urinary stasis is present, relief, at least by catheter drainage, may be required to allow control of the infection. Subsequently, correction of the primary cause of the stasis, such as removal of an obstructing stone or relief of an intrinsic ureteral stenosis or bladder neck obstruction, may be accomplished. Evidence that the pathogenic bacteria have been eradicated should be sought by culture rather than relying upon absence of symptoms as evidence of cure of the infection.

Chronic pyelonephritis may be associated with a predisposing cause or may occur without a contributory abnormality which can be recognized with current techniques. Grossly, the kidney with chronic pyelonephritis is a pale, firm, shrunken organ with scarred, irregular surface depressions and adherent capsule. Etiology of an end stage or contracted kidney is difficult to identify with certainty. The pelvis and calyces may be normal or thickened and fibrotic.

Microscopically, lymphocytes, plasma cells, monocytes, and neutrophils may be present. Fibrosis of the medulla and cortex with involvement of the glomeruli may be seen. The tubules may be normal or dilated with their lumen containing colloid-like casts. Varying degrees of sclerosis may occur in the arteries. Fever, chills, flank pain, frequency, dysuria and urgency, symptoms of recurring or persistent urinary tract infection, may be present. Or, the patient may be essentially asymptomatic until nausea, vomiting, diarrhea, gastrointestinal bleeding, muscular irritability, drowsiness, weakness, and fatigue, symptoms of renal failure, develop. Urinalysis may show white cell casts, white blood cells, red blood cells, and protein alone or in combination.

Diagnosis is complicated by the occasional absence or intermittent presence of bacteria from the urine in patients with longstanding disease. Recognition of the infecting organisms by smear or culture is essential to establish the diagnosis of urinary tract infection. Similarly, isolation of the organism from ureteral urine supports the involvement of the upper urinary tract in the infectious process. X-ray changes of reduced renal size, irregular renal contour, calyceal blunting or clubbing, and infundibular narrowing are often sufficiently suggestive to make the diagnosis highly probable. Renal biopsy may be essential to establish the diagnosis of chronic pyelonephritis. In this type of chronic infection, search for a contributory cause such as bladder neck obstruction secondary to benign prostatic hypertrophy or neurogenic bladder dysfunction assumes great importance. If found, these must be corrected.

Treatment is directed to control or elimination of the bacterial infection by prolonged administration of antibiotic or chemotherapeutic agents indicated by culture. Repeated urine cultures are utilized to guide therapy. Careful repeated evaluation of renal function is essential to permit evaluation of the effects of therapy. Occasionally, chronic pyelonephritis may be unilateral; if the infection cannot be eliminated, nephrectomy may be necessary. Similarly, unilateral chronic pyelonephritis may occasionally be a cause of renovascular hypertension which may be alleviated by nephrectomy.

A form of renal damage in which the tip of the papilla is partially or completely destroyed occurs in association with diabetes and obstruction. The necrotic papilla often sloughs. This condition, known as *papillary necrosis*, has recently been recognized in association with other abnormalities, such as sickle cell trait and massive prolonged intake of phenacetin. The sloughing papilla can obstruct and necessitate measures to relieve the obstruction.

Urinary tract infection and pyelonephritis are recognized complications of *pregnancy*. The incidence of recognized pyelonephritis in pregnancy approximates 2 per cent. The hydroureteronephrosis which is commonly present, particularly on the right side, is an important contributory factor. These upper tract changes are thought to be due to mechanical pressure on the ureter and to some degree of ureteral hypotonia. There is an accompanying increase in vascularity and some edema of both upper and lower urinary tracts. Recent observations indicate that ureteral reflux may play a role in the etiology of pyelonephritis. The diagnosis is established as in the nonpregnant female. Treatment is similar to that usually employed but may include use of the knee-chest position or in unusual circumstances insertion of a ureteral catheter to reduce urinary stasis. Postpartum evaluation is essential in these patients. Evidence of persistence of infection or any deviation from expected course demands a search for etiologic factors not related to pregnancy.

Staphylococcic infections of the kidney are generally hematogenous and are usually related to a focus elsewhere in the body. The infection is primarily in the cortex of the kidney. It may subside or progress to multiple abscesses, carbuncle formation, or if rupture into the perinephric space occurs, to a perinephric abscess.

Symptoms vary considerably with the stage of the infection and the patient's status. Generally chills, high fever, lumbar or abdominal pain, and generalized malaise and weakness are present. Tenderness in the renal area and occasionally an enlarged kidney may be evident on physical examination. Leukocytosis is usually marked. The urine may show a few red and white cells on microscopic examination. Isolation of the organism is characteristically difficult. Both urine culture and smear should be utilized.

X-ray studies may show evidence of renal enlargement, obliteration of the psoas shadow, and curvature of the spine away from the infected kidney. The intravenous or retrograde pyelogram may show deformity characteristic of a space-occupying lesion or may show little deviation from normal. With perinephritic involvement, either directly or indirectly, fixation of the kidney develops and it does not show normal movement on respiration or the assumption of an erect position. This finding can be demonstrated by lack of blurring of the renal image on x-ray during respiratory movement.

Treatment is primarily by antibiotic therapy if the lesion is confined to the kidney. Often sensitivity studies are not available and selection of the antibiotic is empirical. If a perinephric abscess is present, or if the response to therapy is poor suggesting a persistent renal abscess, surgical drainage is necessary. Nephrectomy is rarely required.

Perinephric abscess may develop from causes other than staphylococcic infection of the kidney. The infection of the perinephric space may be metastatic or may result from a suppurative process in adjacent organs. It may be secondary to renal infection other than a cortical abscess, such as calculous pyonephrosis. Physical, laboratory, and x-ray findings are similar to those of renal abscess, except that distortion of the renal collecting system is often absent. In general, the patients have symptoms for a prolonged period before a diagnosis is established. Perinephric abscess should be considered in any patient with prolonged sepsis of unknown etiology. Needle aspiration of the perinephric space may assist in establishing the diagnosis. Treatment is by incision and retroperitoneal drainage. If renal disease is present and severe, primary or secondary nephrectomy may be necessary.

Tuberculosis of the urinary tract is a hematogenous disease which, in the United States, usually is secondary to pulmonary tuberculosis. The primary tuberculous lesion may heal, whereas the renal tuberculosis progresses. The initial renal lesions are in the renal cortex and in the glomeruli. The medulla is involved secondarily. Initial bilateral involvement is thought to be the rule. Bilateral or unilateral healing of the disease follows the initial hematogenous dissemination in some patients. Once the medulla is involved, the disease tends to progress and cavitation in the region of the renal papilla occurs. Renal tuberculosis is found in males more often than females. Its highest incidence is in the third decade.

The symptoms associated with renal tuberculosis are those of secondary tuberculous cystitis. Hematuria, dysuria, frequency, urgency, and nocturia draw attention to the presence of this urinary tract infection. Flank pain, usually mild but occasionally of a severe degree, may also be present. Physical examination may disclose evidence of genital tuberculosis, such as a scrotal fistula, beading of the vas deferens, or irregular nodular involvement of the prostate and seminal vesicles. The findings on urinalysis may vary from gross hematuria and pyuria to minimal microscopic hematuria and pyuria or in some instances to a normal urine. Bacteriologic studies of the urine, including smear, culture, and guinea pig inoculation, permit accurate diagnosis. Usually three pooled morning urine samples, or concentrates of 24-hour urine samples, are utilized for study. Repeated bacteriologic studies are often necessary to establish the diagnosis.

Active, diffuse tuberculosis may be present without x-ray evidence. The classic changes noted on intravenous pyelogram are calcification, evidence of a renal mass, ulceration of the papilla, causing a moth-eaten appearance, and stricture formation in the infundibulum. A nonfunctioning mass of putty-like calcium deposits is characteristic of the autonephrectomy seen as a result of a far advanced tuberculous infection. Tuberculosis of the ureter secondary to renal tuberculosis may result in stricture formation or in a dilated fibrotic ureter which becomes almost "lead pipe" in character and which has a gaping "golf hole" type of orifice. Tuberculosis of the bladder is characterized by ulceration and tubercle formation.

Currently, the majority of patients with urinary tuberculosis are treated with antituberculous drug therapy. Usually, this includes streptomycin, isoniazid, and para-aminosalicylic acid. Variations in this drug regimen may be necessitated by the patient's tolerance or by the development of a drug-resistant organism. Nephrectomy for persistent active unilateral tuberculous infection, or because of secondary infection of a poorly functioning kidney, is occasionally necessary. Similarly, surgical correction of a ureteral stricture following therapy is occasionally necessary, as is a procedure to enlarge the small contracted bladder which may sometimes persist following treatment. In general, tuberculosis of the ureter and bladder are secondary to renal tuberculosis and even prior to institution of chemotherapy they would subside once the renal tuberculosis had been eliminated. Genital and urinary tuberculosis are commonly associated.

RENAL AND URETERAL CALCULI

Calculi may occur in the kidney at any age but are more common in the third and fourth decades. They may be single or multiple, impacted or free. The calculi may be confined to the tubules at the tip of the papilla as in nephrocalcinosis (Fig. 26), may be a cast of the collecting system as in a staghorn

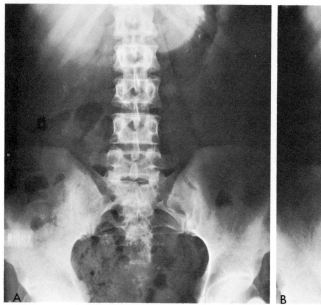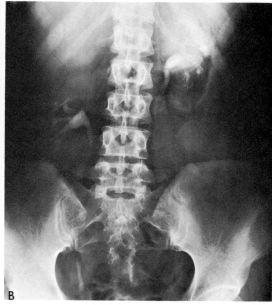

Figure 26. Nephrocalcinosis. *A,* Typical stippled calcification of kidney, demonstrated on intravenous pyelogram (*B*) to be associated with collecting ducts in the tip of the papillae.

calculus (Fig. 27), or may be in any of a variety of shapes. In about 15 per cent of patients the calculi are bilateral. They may result in renal destruction by causing obstruction, infection, or both.

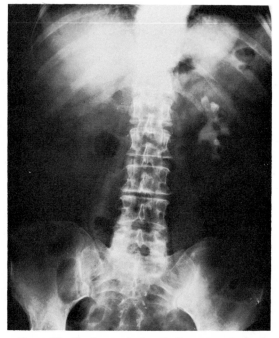

Figure 27. Staghorn calculus. Radiopaque calculus is seen to be a cast of the collecting system of the left kidney.

Renal calculi may cause pain, hematuria, or symptoms of vague abdominal distress. If associated with infection, chills, fever, frequency, urgency, and dysuria are present. They may be entirely asymptomatic even when large and result in serious renal damage. Characteristically, renal calculi cause severe, sharp flank pains which are often acute in onset and present intermittently. The pain may radiate into the lower abdomen or buttocks and is often associated with nausea, vomiting, and gross or microscopic hematuria. The patient usually moves about restlessly seeking relief. At other times, gross hematuria or routinely discovered microscopic hematuria may be the only indication of the presence of the calculus. Not infrequently, the symptoms or urinary findings of a urinary tract infection will lead to evaluation leading to the diagnosis.

Physical findings in patients with renal calculi may be entirely normal or may yield nonspecific evidence of renal pathology, such as tenderness, muscle spasm, or a palpable mass. Tenderness and muscle spasm are usually minimal even when present. On microscopic examination of the urine sediment, hematuria is present in about 75 per cent of patients even in the absence of colic. Pyuria and bacilluria may be present. Occasionally, characteristic crystalluria is noted. Observations of the urinary pH may assist in directing attention to the composition of the calculus. The diagnosis is usually dependent on x-ray demonstration of the calculus. In the presence of a calcium-containing stone, a radiopacity maintaining a constant relationship to the kidney and its collecting system will usually be demonstrated on plain film of the abdomen and intravenous or retrograde pyelogram. If the calculus is composed of uric acid, or another nonopaque substance, its presence will be evident only as a filling defect following visualization of the urinary tract with contrast media.

Treatment of renal calculi is dependent on their size, composition, the presence or absence of symptoms, and complications such as infection or obstruction. A cause for the calculus is always sought and an attempt made to correct it. Observation utilizing analgesics for relief of acute episodes of pain, forcing fluids, and employing such measures as alkalinization and administration of allopurinol in known uric acid calculi, or alkalinization and d-penicillamine in known cystine calculi, may be indicated. If life or renal function is threatened, or if symptoms are severe with little hope of spontaneous passage of the calculus, removal by incising the renal pelvis or the renal parenchymal or both may be indicated. If the kidney is irreparably destroyed, if infection is confined to one stone-bearing kidney, or if the condition of the patient dictates, unilateral nephrectomy may be the desirable course. The recovered stone should always be analyzed to serve as a guide for future therapy.

Ureteral calculi are presumed to arise in the kidney and pass into the ureter. Their composition is essentially the same as renal calculi. They occur primarily in middle age and with equal frequency on each side. Men are affected about twice as frequently as women. Pain, either typical colic or indefinite or indistinct abdominal discomfort, is present in the overwhelming majority of patients. Hematuria, symptoms of infection, or anuria may also cause the patient to seek aid. The local physical findings are usually limited to minimal localized tenderness. Flank tenderness and guarding may be noted when obstruction is present.

Urinalysis shows red blood cells in most patients with ureteral calculi. A ureteral calculus may be present in the absence of abnormality on urinalysis but this finding should increase suspicion that a presumed diagnosis of ureteral calculus is in error. The diagnosis is established by x-ray studies. Demonstration of a constant relationship of a presumed stone to the urinary tract is essential. Most ureteral calculi pass spontaneously. They tend to impact at the ureteropelvic junction, the area over the iliac vessels, or in the lower third of the ureter, particularly in the ureterovesical area. Relief of pain of ureteral colic often requires large amounts of narcotics. Nausea and vomiting may necessitate fluid replacement. If symptoms are prolonged, they may be relieved by bypassing the calculus with a catheter. Similarly, catheter drainage of an obstructed kidney may be necessary to permit control of infection. Persistent obstruction, infection, and severe recurrent pain are the general indications for operative removal of ureteral calculi. Instrumental removal of stones is frequently accomplished with a variety of baskets and catheters; most limit the use of baskets to stones in the lower third of the ureter.

The operative approach employed for ureterolithotomy is dependent on the site of the impaction of the calculus. Every effort should be made to recover all stones and analyze them. A search for an etiological factor, such as hyperparathyroidism in calcium-containing stones, should be made routinely. Measures such as elimination of infection and obstruction and encouraging fluid intake should be undertaken to prevent recurrence.

VASCULAR DISEASE OF THE KIDNEY

Diseases of the renal artery have been recognized with increasing frequency since aortography became a relatively safe, readily available diagnostic tool. These arterial lesions have clinical importance if they are a cause of bleeding, contribute to renal functional impairment, or cause alteration in renal blood supply sufficiently severe to stimulate excessive production of renin and consequent hypertension.

ANEURYSM OF THE RENAL ARTERY. Arteriosclerotic saccular aneurysm of the renal artery is commonly asymptomatic. Occasionally, rupture of the aneurysm causes massive hemorrhage or the aneurysm may be associated with hypertension. Typically, these lesions are recognized as faintly calcified ring-like shadows near the hilum of the kidney. If the lesion is small, asymptomatic, and seemingly completely surrounded by calcification, treatment is not necessary. If bleeding or hypertension secondary to the aneurysm occurs, or if the aneurysm has a significant uncalcified portion, resection of the aneurysm or nephrectomy may be desirable. Bleeding is rarely associated with a calcified aneurysm. In addition to the saccular aneurysm, the renal artery may be the site of a dissecting aneurysm, poststenotic aneurysm, multiple microaneurysms, or a fusiform aneurysm. When present, they are often associated with fibrotic stenosis of the renal artery in hypertensive patients.

ARTERIOVENOUS FISTULA. Arteriovenous fistula, either extra- or intrarenal, is also being recognized with increasing frequency. Surgical trauma, including needle biopsy, accident and neoplasm are the common causes of the acquired fistula. Some are thought to be congenital in origin. Pain and hematuria may be presenting complaints as are complaints related to hypertension and congestive failure. A localized bruit is the outstanding physical finding. The diagnosis is made by rapid visualization of the renal veins on aortography. The treatment has shifted in recent years toward a reconstructive approach rather than nephrectomy.

OCCLUSIVE DISEASE. Occlusive disease of the renal artery has assumed clinical importance with the recognition that it is a cause of hypertension. It has become increasingly apparent that renovascular hypertension may run almost any course. However, a renal cause should be particularly suspected in patients with hypertension of abrupt onset, in patients under 35 years of age, in patients with malignant hypertension of abrupt onset, in patients with symptoms of atherosclerosis preceding the onset of hypertension, and in patients with an epigastric bruit.

Atherosclerosis is the commonest cause of occlusive lesions of the renal artery. These lesions are usually well localized and characteristically occur near the orifice of the renal artery, although other sites are affected. Fibromuscular hyperplasia constitutes the other sizable group of patients with occlusive lesions of the renal artery. Pathologically, fibromuscular hyperplasia includes a variety of lesions resulting in derangement of the media and intima of the artery. This lesion occurs eight to nine times more frequently in women than in men. About one-half of the patients have bilateral lesions, which are characteristically located in the middle and distal thirds of the renal artery.

An abdominal bruit is the only physical finding suggesting the presence of renal artery stenosis. Establishing the diagnosis of a significant renal artery lesion is dependent on laboratory studies. The intravenous pyelogram may show a discrepancy in renal size of 1 cm. or more, a delay in the appearance of contrast media, or nonfunction, or a late hyperconcentration of contrast media on the side of the arterial lesion. The radioactive renogram is almost always abnormal on the affected side but the nature of the abnormality may be variable. The aortogram will show evidence of an anatomical lesion of the artery which may or may not have functional significance. Differential renal function studies must be carried out to determine this. The characteristic physiologic changes associated with significant narrowing of the renal artery are a reduction in glomerular filtration rate, an excessive tubular reabsorption of water, and an even greater reabsorption of sodium. As a consequence, the urine from a kidney with a significant renal artery lesion is reduced in volume, shows a slight decrease in sodium concentration, and marked increase in the concentration of creatinine, inulin, and paraminohippurate which are filtered or secreted high in the tubule and not reabsorbed. The demonstration of these characteristic changes in the urine from the kidney with a renal artery lesion makes an abnormality of this organ a highly probable cause of hypertension. Currently, renin levels in renal venous blood are being determined in an effort to identify a kidney responsible for hypertension with greater certainty. Segmental artery disease and renal infarct may also cause hypertension.

Treatment of renovascular hypertension is dependent on the general condition of the patient, the nature of the renal artery disease, and the bilateral status of the renal parenchyma. Reconstruction of the renal artery, bypass of an arterial lesion, partial nephrectomy, and nephrectomy all are utilized depending on these findings. Relief or marked improvement in the hypertension may be expected in about three-fourths of the patients treated when properly selected.

Renal failure as a consequence of major renal artery disease has been recognized infrequently. This possibility warrants consideration in patients with renal failure of unknown etiology despite its infrequent occurrence because the possibility of reversal of the renal malfunction exists.

RENAL VEIN THROMBOSIS. Renal vein occlusion has been recognized infrequently in the past, and then almost always in infants. The infants usually present with evidence of systemic illness, hematuria, and an abdominal mass. Blood studies often show a diminished platelet count. Adults present with lumbar or abdominal pain, occasionally an enlarged kidney, and occasionally symptoms and findings compatible with the nephrotic syndrome. Cardiac failure is a frequent associated finding. As methods of visualizing the renal veins become more accurate and available, disease of the renal vein will be recognized more frequently. In at least some circumstances, the occluding thrombi may be amenable to surgical removal.

RENAL AND URETERAL TRAUMA

Renal trauma may be secondary to a penetrating injury or to a blunt force. Penetrating injuries of the abdomen usually require exploration and, therefore, constitute less of a problem in diagnosis than does blunt abdominal trauma. Although renal trauma usually follows severe injury and is often associated with injury of other organs, seemingly minor falls or blows may occasionally produce severe renal injury. Aside from the direct effect of force on the kidney, injury may apparently result from the forceful whip-like movement of the kidney on its pedicle. Although spontaneous renal rupture occurs infrequently, the kidney diseased by reason of obstruction or tumor is more easily injured by trauma than is a normal kidney.

The types of renal injury are depicted in Figure 28. Depending on the type and extent of injury, the immediate complications of renal injury are those related to blood loss and urinary extravasation. Rarely, in bilateral injury or injury of a single kidney, acute renal failure may be a primary result of the renal trauma.

Hematuria is the primary finding in trauma to the urinary tract. It is often gross but may be microscopic or absent. Abdominal pain is usually present, located in the flank or upper abdomen, and variable in severity. Physical examination may disclose evidence of shock as well as local tenderness, swelling, and ecchymosis. Usually, muscle spasm is marked in the flank and upper quadrant of the abdomen. A mass is usually not palpable early in injuries other than renal pedicle injuries.

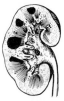 Contusion (Minor)

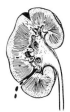 Laceration With & Without Urinary Extravasation (Major)

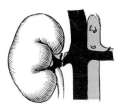 Pedicle Injury (Critical)

Figure 28. Diagram representing the various types of renal injury. Laceration with urinary extravasation usually requires drainage. Pedicle injury demands prompt control of hemorrhage.

An expanding mass with recurrent evidence of severe blood loss is evidence of a type 3 or pedicle injury.

The diagnosis is usually made by the finding of hematuria associated with the physical findings suggesting renal trauma and evidence of renal malfunction or distortion on pyelography. In addition to providing evidence of renal abnormality, the intravenous pyelogram provides invaluable evidence of the presence of a contralateral functioning kidney. Occasionally, other x-ray studies such as aortography, nephrotomography, or mercury scan may be indicated to delineate the extent and nature of the trauma. The possibility that the hematuria noted may be related to lower urinary tract injury must be kept in mind and investigated, usually with a cystogram, in any questionable instance.

If a diagnosis of renal pedicle injury is suspected by the clinical course of the patient, prompt exploration and control of the hemorrhage are indicated. Even in these circumstances demonstration of a contralateral functioning kidney by intravenous pyelography is usually possible by temporary restoration of the blood pressure and a single film taken after injection of contrast media on the way to the operating room. Other renal injuries associated with blunt trauma usually do not require immediate intervention. Bed rest, analgesics for relief of pain, and observation coupled with investigation of renal status as indicated by the patient's course compose the usual treatment. Aside from hemorrhage, the presence of urinary extravasation or development of infection may necessitate surgical intervention. If an operative procedure is performed, it may vary from simple drainage to partial or total nephrectomy. Usually, a delay of two to three days after trauma before exposure of the kidney simplifies the surgical procedure. The majority of patients with renal injury can be treated without operative intervention. Upper urinary tract extravasation is better tolerated than lower urinary tract extravasation and is not subjected to drainage by all urologists. Secondary hemorrhage from renal parenchymal injury may occur and dictates caution in allowing the patient out of bed. In many instances in patients with multiple injuries, the ideal treatment of the renal injury must be compromised.

URETERAL INJURY. Ureteral injury is an uncommon complication of penetrating or blunt trauma. In penetrating trauma, symptoms due to other involved organs often mask symptoms due to ureteral involvement. In blunt trauma, the evidence of urinary tract involvement is so slight that diagnosis of ureteral injury is delayed. Tenderness and muscle spasm due to urinary extravasation and development of signs of infection usually cause x-ray evaluation of the urinary tract. Intravenous or retrograde pyelography discloses the urinary extravasation and often identifies the site of injury. Drainage of extravasated urine and relief of obstruction are essential. Reconstruction of the disrupted ureter may be attempted by a number of techniques. In the past, the resultant damage associated with injury and delay in recognition has made nephrectomy a frequent necessity. The ureter is subject to iatrogenic injury with much greater frequency than it is to injury from external trauma. These injuries result from both open surgical and endoscopic surgical technique. Some of the more common types of injury are seen in Figure 29. These may result in silent destruction of the kidney from unilateral hydronephrosis or in acute renal failure if a single ureter or both are ligated. Between these extremes urinary

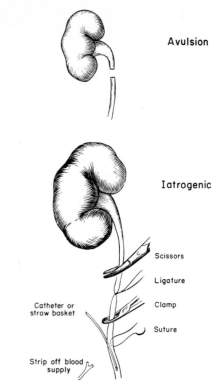

Figure 29. Diagrammatic representation of various types of ureteral injury.

Avulsion

Iatrogenic

Scissors

Ligature

Clamp

Catheter or straw basket

Suture

Strip off blood supply

extravasation with eventual infection and fistula between the ureter and the skin, vagina, and uterus may result. In treating iatrogenic ureteral injuries, both relief of obstruction and drainage of extravasated urine must be achieved promptly. Reconstruction of the defect may then be attempted as indicated by the general and local condition of the patient.

THE BLADDER

ANOMALIES

Agenesis and *duplication* of the bladder occur but are very rare. *Congenital diverticulum* is rare and definite differentiation from acquired diverticulum is difficult. The presence of muscle fibers in the diverticular wall, thought to be characteristic of congenital lesions, is probably not a valid differential feature. The symptoms of a congenital and an acquired diverticulum are similar.

Exstrophy of the bladder is an embryologic catastrophe in which there is an absence of the lower abdominal and anterior vesical walls. The posterior bladder wall is exposed. There is an accompanying epispadiac deformity of the urethra and separation of the pubes. This abnormality occurs in about one in 50,000 births, with males predominating three to one. Recently, Muecke has produced the defect experimentally in the chicken by utilizing a plastic graft to interfere with normal cloacal membrane regression. In addition to the social inconvenience occasioned by total incontinence, upper urinary tract infection is common and often leads to death. Attempts to reconstruct the bladder are frequently unsuccessful and diversion of the urine by placing the ureters in the large bowel, or in an isolated loop of ileum with an external orifice, is necessary (Fig. 30).

Urachal abnormalities vary from persistent fistula due to the failure of closure of the allantoic duct to cyst formation, persistent umbilical sinus, or a diverticulum of the dome of the bladder due to failure of fusion of a portion of the duct.

Ureteral reflux may be congenital in origin. The responsible defect is a maldevelopment of the trigone of the bladder with the trigone

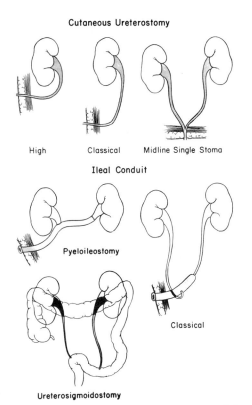

Cutaneous Ureterostomy

High   Classical   Midline Single Stoma

Ileal Conduit

Pyeloileostomy

Classical

Ureterosigmoidostomy

Figure 30. Methods of permanent supravesical diversion.

being large and the ureter being laterally placed with a short intramural tunnel. At times, these defects are accompanied by a thin-walled bladder with a large capacity, so-called *megacystis syndrome.*

TUMORS OF THE URINARY BLADDER

Malignant tumors of the urinary bladder account for about 3 per cent of the deaths from cancer in the United States. Males are affected approximately 2.5 to four times as often as females. Epithelial tumors are rare in children but may occur at any age in adults. The peak incidence is in the sixth and seventh decades in both males and females. The overwhelming majority of bladder neoplasms are epithelial in origin. Grossly, they are commonly exophytic, protruding into the vesical lumen. They may vary from a papillary configuration with a narrow stalk and multiple frond-like projections to a sessile serpiginous growth. Ulceration and encrustation with calcium salts may occur. Approximately 40 per cent of the tumors involve the trigone and an additional 45 per cent the posterior and lateral bladder walls. Multiple tumors are common, being present in approximately 25 per cent of the patients on diagnosis, and becoming evident in as high as 50 per cent of the patients with a so-called benign papilloma, Grade I carcinoma, in a five-year period.

Classification of the epithelial tumors of the bladder has been and is confusing. Histologically, these tumors are primarily transitional cell or squamous in cell type. Undifferentiated carcinoma, adenocarcinoma, and mucus-forming adenocarcinoma are also recognized. Some utilize a designation of benign papilloma for well-differentiated epithelial tumors; others prefer to utilize the term Grade I carcinoma because patients with these tumors show a tendency to reappearance of neoplasm as well as to development of a more advanced neoplasm. Grading of the tumor on the basis of cellular differentiation has clinical significance; the most differentiated tumors are designated Grade I and the undifferentiated or poorly differentiated, Grade IV. Degree of cellular differentiation varies throughout a tumor approximately 50 per cent of the time. The transitional, squamous, or undifferentiated cell type of the tumor is commonly maintained throughout.

The demonstration by Jewett and Strong that depth of infiltration of a bladder tumor is related to the presence of recognizable metastasis at autopsy was an important observation (Fig. 31). They observed no evidence of metastases in patients with invasion confined to the submucosa, metastatic spread in 14 per cent of patients with invasion confined to the muscularis, and in 74 per cent of the patients with invasion of the perivesical tissue. Subsequent clinical experience has tended to confirm the potential survival without evidence of neoplasm in patients with superficially infiltrating lesions and the poor prognosis of patients with deeply infiltrating lesions.

Nonepithelial tumors of the bladder are mesenchymal in origin and may be benign such as fibroma or leiomyoma, or malignant such as sarcoma. Metastases to the bladder are unusual.

Bladder cancer is known to be associated with exposure to two chemicals, beta-naphthylamine and xenylamine. In addition, a higher incidence of bladder tumors is recognized in smokers than in nonsmokers. Bladder infestation with *Schistosoma haematobium* is also recognized as predisposing to the development of a bladder neoplasm.

Gross hematuria is the presenting complaint in about 70 per cent of the patients with bladder neoplasm. The hematuria is usually total but may be initial or terminal. Microscopic hematuria is present in an even greater proportion of patients. Symptoms of vesical irritability, such as urgency, frequency, and dysuria, constitute the other common group of complaints in patients with bladder tumors.

Physical examination is usually normal in the patient with a bladder tumor unless the lesion has spread beyond the bladder. The diagnosis of a bladder neoplasm warrants serious consideration in any patient with gross or microscopic hematuria, or recurrent episodes of vesical irritability. Presence of a filling defect on the cystogram of the intravenous pyelogram or on a retrograde cystogram should increase the suspicion of a bladder tumor. Definitive diagnosis is dependent on cystoscopic visualization of a mucosal abnormality and biopsy with confirmation of the presence of a neoplasm on histologic examination. Studies of urinary cytology may yield evidence of neoplastic change not identified by cystoscopy. Currently, efforts are being made to utilize drug-induced fluorescence with ultraviolet light to aid in cystoscopic identification of bladder tumors not readily identified by routine light cystoscopy. In any patient with a bladder neoplasm, the kidneys and ureters should be visualized to eliminate the possibility that a transitional cell neoplasm of the upper urinary tract is seeding the bladder.

Once the diagnosis of bladder neoplasm is established, clinical staging of the neoplasm is important to permit rational therapy and prognosis. The staging is based on the pathologic observations correlating tumor spread with degree of tumor invasion as confirmed and modified by clinical experience. The gross appearance of the bladder tumor assists in staging, with the more advanced lesions tending to have a broader, flatter base with evidence of fixation of the bladder wall. Similar fixation of the bladder wall may be evident on retrograde cystography. The single most important observation in staging is the depth of infiltration of the bladder tumor. To allow assessment of the infiltration, an adequate biopsy of the tumor and of the muscle at its base, as well as deep biopsy of any other suspicious area in the bladder and prostate, is essential. If biopsy indicates infiltration limited to the superficial portion of the muscle, prognosis is good. Infiltration deep in the muscle is associated with a poor prognosis. Bimanual examination under anesthesia is also of value in clinical staging. Induration of any type indicates a poor prognosis but this is particularly true if the induration extends beyond the bladder. If histologic evidence of invasion of the prostate, or involvement of the iliac lymph nodes, is obtained, the prognosis for cure becomes so poor that vigorous therapeutic attempts are usually avoided in favor of palliative procedures. In general, evidence of lymphatic invasion on biopsy is a poor prog-

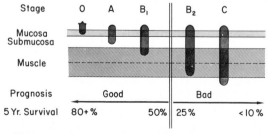

Figure 31. Staging of bladder tumors (after Jewett). Solid vertical bars indicate depth of infiltration. If lymph node or prostatic involvement is demonstrated, "D" classification is utilized by some.

nostic sign as is evidence of ureteral obstruction. Squamous carcinomas often are a higher stage than indicated by biopsy.

Therapy of bladder tumors may be curative or palliative. The results achieved with any type of therapeutic approach seem more related to the stage of the tumor at the initiation of therapy than to the therapy itself. Untreated, the majority of the patients with carcinoma of the bladder die directly or indirectly from their disease. Renal failure from obstruction and infection is a prominent cause of death. Carcinomatosis is also common, with frequent involvement of the regional nodes, liver, lungs, and vertebra in that order. Uncontrolled hemorrhage from the bladder tumor also contributes to mortality.

Attempts to eradicate the neoplasm employ surgery or radiation therapy. Operative procedures utilized in the treatment of bladder tumors are directed to the local destruction or excision of the neoplasm or to removal of the entire bladder. The procedures utilized in local destruction of the neoplasm include:

Transurethral fulguration or transurethral excision and fulguration carried out with an endoscopic instrument per urethram; this is limited by size and location of the lesion.

Suprapubic excision and fulguration approached through a cystotomy incision; the excision is followed by local destruction.

Segmental resection of bladder with or without ureteral reimplantation. Location and extent of the tumor have limited the utilization of partial excision of the bladder, as has the tendency for tumors to be multiple. Current techniques for ureteral reimplantation have permitted more enthusiastic employment of this technique when resection includes the ureteral orifice.

Various techniques for local application of radon packs, radon seeds, and radioactive suture materials.

Instillation of chemotherapeutic agents has been utilized with some success in noninvasive tumors.

Cystectomy is employed in the treatment of higher stage neoplasms, in patients with multiple recurrent tumors, or in treatment failures by locally destructive techniques. It is rarely employed in the presence of metastases to iliac nodes or the prostate unless some local complication, such as bleeding, dictates the palliative removal of the bladder. Cystectomy necessitates diversion of the urine. Utilization of an ileal conduit to divert the ureteral urine to the skin affords the best

long-term results currently. However, the surgical procedure involves moderate risk. For this reason diversion of the ureter to the skin is employed at times. Placement of the ureters into the intact large bowel is also employed. It has the advantage of providing urinary continence. The disadvantages of this technique are its frequent failure to preserve renal function and the development of hyperchloremic acidosis in some patients from the reabsorption of urine by the bowel.

Palliation of the patient with bladder neoplasm may be a very difficult problem. The local complications of hemorrhage, frequency, pain, and ureteral obstruction may necessitate utilization of the procedures employed in an attempt to eradicate the neoplasm. Locally destructive procedures or urinary diversion often provide required relief.

INFLAMMATORY LESIONS OF THE BLADDER

Bacterial cystitis is characterized by urinary frequency, nocturia, urgency, and dysuria. In women, acute hemorrhagic cystitis is probably the commonest cause of hematuria. As in any urinary tract infection, cystitis may be secondary to upper or lower urinary tract disease or to a systemic illness and requires thorough evaluation if recurrent or persistent in the female. Males should be evaluated after a single episode. Classically, the diagnosis is based on the symptoms, the finding of a two-glass pyuria, and the identification of bacteria by smear or culture.

The symptoms of *tuberculous cystitis* are those of bacterial cystitis. Hematuria is often present. The small contracted bladder is rarely seen at present. Tuberculous cystitis is usually secondary to tuberculosis of the upper urinary tract.

Interstitial cystitis is an inflammatory disease of the bladder, the etiology of which is unknown. It occurs predominantly in women. Frequency, nocturia, urgency, dysuria, and lower abdominal pain are prominent symptoms. The physical examination reveals no abnormality. The urinalysis and urine culture are normal. The diagnosis is established by the demonstration on cystoscopy carried out under anesthesia of an extremely small bladder capacity and evidence of ulceration and cracking of the bladder wall with hydraulic distention. Hydraulic distention of the bladder is also therapeutic, temporarily increasing bladder capacity. Other therapy has included instillation of various mild caustic solutions in the bladder. Occasionally, intractable discomfort and frequency necessitate use of a patch of bowel to increase bladder capacity and on occasion diversion of the urine has been necessary.

URETERAL REFLUX

Despite development of high voiding pressures by the detrusor muscle, urine does not normally reflux from the bladder into the ureters on voiding. The oblique submucosal course of the intravesical ureter combined with the normal ureteral peristalsis is thought to prevent backflow of urine from the bladder into the ureter. Ureteral reflux has come to be recognized as an important abnormality of the urinary tract contributing to persistent or recurrent infection and possibly to renal damage in the absence of infection. The recognized causes of ureteral reflux are congenital deformity, bladder outflow obstruction, neurogenic dysfunction, surgical alteration of the intravesical ureter, and infection. In the latter instance, the reflux stops when the infection subsides. Patients with reflux commonly present with symptoms of persistent or recurrent urinary tract infection. Occasional intermittent flank pain with voiding may be the result of ureteral reflux. Although reflux may be identified by cystoscopic techniques employing a chromogen or by isotope studies, the voiding cystourethrogram and the retrograde cystogram have permitted recognition of this phenomenon with ease (Fig. 32). Ureteral reflux has been recognized with greater frequency in children than in adults, and in females than in males. In some patients, reflux may subside with elimination of a contributory cause, such as infection or obstruction. In others, institution of simple techniques, such as double and triple voiding coupled with treatment of infection, eliminates infection and prevents renal damage. When the intravesical ureter is abnormal, restoration of the normal anatomical relationship of the bladder and the tunneled intravesical ureter may be achieved by any of a number of techniques, usually employing reimplantation of the ureter. With elimination of reflux, the control of infection is usually possible.

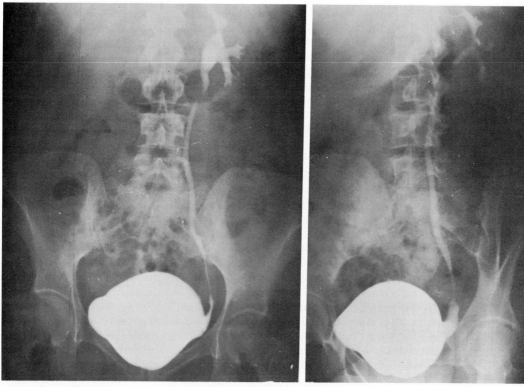

Figure 32.   Ureteral reflux on left demonstrated on cystogram study in adult female with recurrent left pyelonephritis.

BLADDER CALCULI

In the United States, bladder calculi are a disease of the adult male. In other parts of the world, children are primarily affected. Calcium oxalate stones are the commonest type found in the bladder. They may assume a mulberry or jackstone configuration. Dull or sharp pain, aggravated by movement and relieved by rest, and hematuria are the common symptoms. The pain may be referred to the tip of the penis. Occasionally, the patient experiences periodic retention from the ball valve action of the calculus or passes calculi per urethram. The physical examination rarely aids in establishing a diagnosis. The urinalysis characteristically shows red blood cells and may disclose white blood cells. Only about half of the bladder calculi are visible on x-ray, either because of their size, composition, or overlying structures. Characteristically, stones lying free in the bladder lie in the midline. Whenever bladder calculi are present in the adult, the possibility of urinary stasis either on an obstructed or a neurogenic basis becomes paramount. Other causes of calculus formation also warrant consideration. Treatment consists in removal of the stone either by endoscopic or open surgical techniques. Often, smaller calculi may be removed by irrigation through an endoscopic sheath. Occasionally, fracture of the calculus may be carried out by either a blind or a visual technique to facilitate its transurethral removal. If an open surgical technique is utilized, the suprapubic route is usually employed. After removal of the calculi, prevention of recurrence is dependent on correction of the underlying cause for their development.

BLADDER DIVERTICULUM

A bladder diverticulum is an outpouching of the bladder wall. It may be congenital or acquired. Differentiation on the basis of etiology is often difficult; it seems probable that congenital abnormality may play a role in the diverticula developing as the result of obstructive lesions. The majority of bladder diverticula are associated with and probably secondary to obstruction at or distal to the bladder neck. Neurogenic bladder dysfunction may also lead to their formation.

Diverticula of the bladder may be single or multiple, small or large. They form most commonly in the region of the ureteral orifices on the posterior or lateral bladder wall. The diverticular wall usually consists of bladder mucosa with few, if any, investing muscular fibers. The patient with a bladder diverticulum usually presents with symptoms of bladder neck obstruction such as hesitancy, intermittency, weak urinary stream, and nocturia. None of these symptoms suggests that the bladder neck obstruction has been complicated by the development of a diverticulum. Similarly, the presence of a urinary tract infection or bladder calculus may result from the stasis of urine occasioned by a nonemptying diverticulum and cause symptoms leading to its discovery. Occasionally, an asymmetrical lower abdominal cystic mass will be evident on inspection or palpation of the abdomen of a thin patient but the physical examination rarely aids in establishing the diagnosis.

Cystoscopic visualization of the orifice or base of the diverticulum and visualization of a smooth asymmetrical outpouching of the bladder wall on retrograde cystogram are useful in establishing the diagnosis. Indirect visualization of the diverticulum by the cystogram is particularly important, because it allows an assessment of the size, the presence or absence of pathologic change on the wall, and the ability of the diverticulum to empty.

Bladder diverticula are usually secondary to obstruction at or below the bladder neck; therefore, relief of this obstruction is essential to their treatment. If the size or configuration of the diverticulum does not permit it to empty despite relief of obstruction, or if complications of stasis such as stone or persistent infection are present, measures to ensure emptying are required. Under these circumstances the diverticulum is usually excised and the bladder wall reconstructed to eliminate the defect permitting its development. Occasionally, the presence or suspicion of a neoplasm in a diverticulum is an indication for its removal.

BLADDER TRAUMA

Perforation of the urinary bladder is a surgical emergency requiring prompt recognition and treatment. Spontaneous perforation is extremely rare and almost always associated with disease of the bladder, such as infection or neoplasm. Bladder rupture may result from blunt or penetrating wounds of the abdomen. A full bladder predisposes to

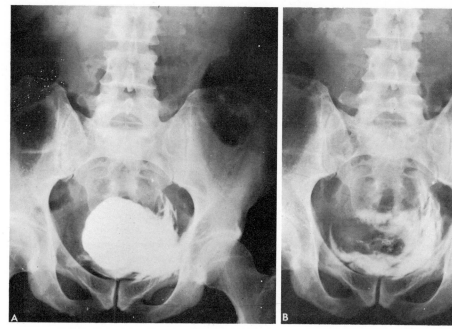

Figure 33.   Retrograde cystogram demonstrating extravasation. *A*, Filling phase; *B*, postevacuation.

rupture. Injuries of the bladder and urethra are associated with fractures of the pelvis with sufficient frequency to warrant consideration in patients with this type of trauma. Instrumentation and endoscopic operative procedures have assumed major importance as a cause of bladder perforation. Because a peritoneal injury may accompany the bladder injury, the extravasation may be intraperitoneal, extraperitoneal, or both. The inferior extension of the extravasated urine is usually limited by the urogenital diaphragm.

Severe abdominal pain and hematuria, or inability to void, are common symptoms. Tenderness, rebound tenderness, and muscular rigidity are commonly seen with perforation of the bladder. Shock is not uncommon. However, the symptoms and signs of bladder rupture may be insignificant and insidious if the possibility is not considered. Although procedures such as measuring return of instilled irrigating fluid and cystoscopy may assist in recognition of perforation of the bladder, they are often misleading. The retrograde cystogram is the most useful and reliable diagnostic tool (Fig. 33). It should always be preceded by a plain film of the abdomen because the extravasated contrast media can be difficult to recognize in an intraperitoneal perforation.

Once the diagnosis of ruptured bladder is made or strongly suspected, treatment should be prompt because mortality increases mark-

edly with delay. The essential therapeutic maneuver is institution of adequate suprapubic drainage. Repair of the bladder defect, although desirable, is unnecessary if adequate drainage is achieved. Repair of the peritoneal rent in patients with intraperitoneal extravasation should be carried out if possible.

NEUROGENIC BLADDER

Two components of the bladder, smooth muscle and nerves, are concerned in the functional anatomy of neurogenic bladder.

The detrusor has the intrinsic quality of all smooth muscle in that it maintains tone even after all motor nerves to the bladder are blocked. An example of this persistence of tone is seen after spinal anesthesia. The characteristics of the bladder, whether innervated or denervated, are such that during filling a constant pressure is maintained. Alterations in this property of accommodation occur after overstretching of the bladder or in instances in which there are too many motor impulses to the bladder, usually as a result of a short circuit of the reflex arc by injury or with excessive sensory stimuli from the bladder. In Figure 34 are illustrated the sources of nerve impulses to and from the bladder. The supply is double: parasympathetic and somatic. The sympathetic nerves are an unimportant portion of the nerve supply. The parasympathetic supply constitutes the main reflex arc and is carried by way of the hypogastric plexus and the pelvic nerve. Stimulation causes contraction of the detrusor. Section first causes complete inability to empty the bladder, but later weak uncoordinated contractions of the detrusor occur.

The somatic supply is carried through the pudendal nerve. Stimulation causes closure of the external sphincter, a striated muscle. Section results in relaxation of the external sphincter. Incontinence occurs only if both the internal sphincter and external sphincter are absent.

PHYSIOLOGY. Normal urination is accomplished in five phases: cerebral release of inhibition, detrusor contraction (parasympathetic), opening of the internal sphincter (detrusor action), relaxation of the external sphincter (somatic via pudendal) and, finally, contraction of the external sphincter, bulb and perineal musculature at the termination of urination (Fig. 35).

The reflex arcs involved in urination are: proprioceptive sensation from the filling of

THE NEUROANATOMY OF VESICAL FUNCTION

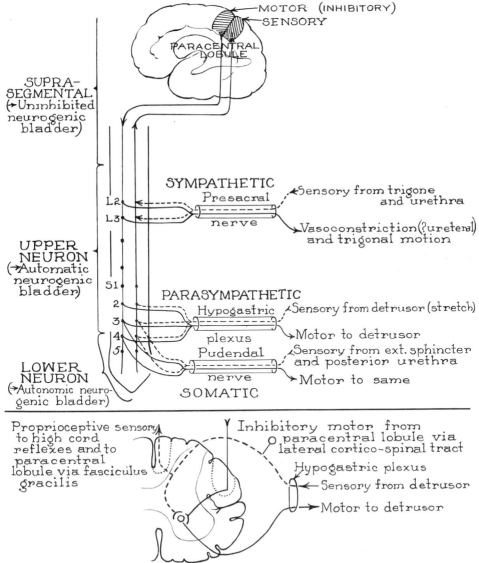

Figure 34. Nerve pathways to and from the bladder.

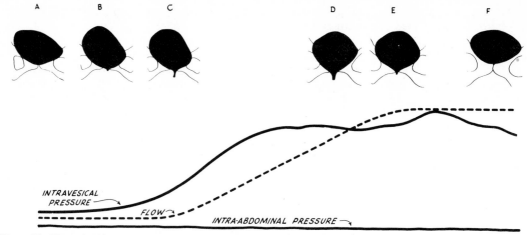

Figure 35.   Normal voiding. *A*, Resting bladder. *B*, Opening of internal sphincter by detrusor contraction and concomitant lowering of base of bladder. *C*, Opening of external sphincter and start of flow. *D*, Flow established. *E*, Closure of external sphincter. *F*, Closure of internal sphincter with relaxation of the detrusor.

the bladder passes over the parasympathetic fibers of the pelvic nerve, by way of the hypogastric plexus, to the spinal cord and ascends by way of the fasciculus gracilis to consciousness in the sensory cortex, resulting in inhibition if necessary, thence to the cerebral motor cortex and down the lateral corticospinal tracts to parasympathetic fibers by way of hypogastric plexus and pelvic nerve to the detrusor.

It is important to recognize that this reflex arc can be deficient in any part. Consequently, disease or trauma can produce an almost infinite variety of functional results. This fact, of course, makes it hard to formulate an exact classification, since the groups are actually continuous with each other.

In classifying the individual patient, the site and degree of the nerve lesion should be determined first. This in turn will suggest the effect on the bladder. It is necessary to utilize all the historical information, neurologic data and urologic findings that can be obtained about the patient. Often the type of neurologic lesion is determined by its effect on bladder function. The examination of the individual patient should include the following procedures:

A neurologic examination should be performed to establish the level and severity of the lesion as it affects the sensory and motor components of the somatic structures. Little can be learned of bladder and rectal function from the usual neurologic examination, but it is needed for correlation and to allow classification of the neurogenic bladder. It also offers a background for application of methods of therapy, particularly those employing blocking or sectioning of nerves.

Cystometry is done by measuring intravesical pressure during filling of the bladder. With each 50 cc. increment of fluid there is accommodation by the bladder so that the pressure remains at a little below 10 cm. of water pressure until bladder capacity is reached, between 400 and 450 cc. At this time the patient is instructed to cease inhibition of his voiding reflex; that is, he is told to void, which he does around the catheter.

Cystoscopy, or better, panendoscopy, with observation of the vesical neck and external sphincter, is helpful in the diagnosis of neurogenic bladder. For instance, long-standing failure to relax the internal sphincter results in a collar of tissue at the vesical neck which is obstructive in itself. Spasm and lack of relaxation of the external sphincter are also observed and, in addition, any actual obstructive hypertrophy of the prostate in older patients may be observed at this time. The condition of the bladder wall, such as the degree and type of detrusor hypertrophy, may also be seen. Concomitant abnormalities are also noted, the principal ones being vesical diverticula, which make restoration of normal bladder function more difficult, and abnormal ureteral orifices associated with reflux.

Intravenous urography permits observation of changes of the upper urinary tract secondary to disorders of the bladder. A cystogram in conjunction with a voiding film will allow detection of dilatation of the bladder neck such as is found with lesions of the cauda equina. In addition, ureteral reflux, which results in renal damage, may be seen. Reflux means that the use of tidal drainage will cause further renal damage.

Determination of sphincteric resistance is important in the diagnosis of imbalance of the bladder since voiding depends on a vesical pressure higher than the opposing urethral resistance. Normal values of urethral resistance are between 20 and 30 mm. of mercury, but often only the strength of the sphincteric contraction is measured since the patient cannot relax the reflexly contracted external sphincter. If the vesical imbalance is found to be due to increased urethral resistance, its location should be determined by urethrography and panendoscopy, to see whether it is from the external sphincter or from the prostate.

The function test is perhaps the most important of all, since normal bladder function depends on a correct balance between the forces of filling and expulsion against the resistance of the sphincters and urethra. The crucial test, therefore, is measurement of the vesical capacity and of the residual urine, since an adequately functioning bladder, normal or neurogenic, should have a capacity greater than 200 cc. and have less than 30 cc. of residual urine. These conditions are desirable if serious chronic infection and renal damage are to be avoided. Anything short of this cannot be called adequate.

TREATMENT OF SPINAL SHOCK. After an injury to the spinal cord, almost regardless of site or degree, a period follows of absence of voluntary function and reflex activity below the site of injury. During this period of spinal shock, the bladder functions as a denervated organ. Since it is unable to empty itself because intrinsic detrusor tone is less than urethral resistance, the bladder distends with urine. If the distention persists, the result is a flaccid, atonic bladder. Consequently, the aim of immediate therapy after a spinal cord injury should be to prevent overdistention, which can be accomplished occasionally by intermittent catheterization, more commonly by retention catheterization, or even by suprapubic cystostomy. The last should be reserved for patients treated under conditions where sterile handling of urethral catheters is impossible. The catheter is connected to a Y-tube closed system with a Kelly bottle filled with 0.25 per cent acetic acid solution, which allows manual filling and evacuation of the bladder at intervals. In addition, it is wise to begin prophylactic sulfonamide chemother-

apy to reduce the chance of invasive infection, since it is too often impossible to keep the bladder sterile no matter what form of indwelling catheter is used or what antibiotic is given. As soon as the bladder regains function, the catheter can be removed.

A neurologic approach to vesical dysfunction recognizes three main areas for interference with nerve pathways from the bladder: the suprasegmental, which mainly concerns inhibition of lower reflexes; the upper motor neuron, which concerns the long extravesical reflexes, release of which results in something like normal voiding; and the lower motor neuron, which means short extravesical and mainly intravesical reflexes which leave the detrusor to its own devices. These sites are usually involved by lesions cutting both sensory and motor pathways. If only sensory pathways are interrupted, or if the motor pathways are cut, dysfunctions with other characteristics result. It is obvious that all degrees and modalities can occur, but if these major groups are kept in mind, any particular group of bladder symptoms can be loosely classified (Table 4).

The *uninhibited neurogenic bladder* results from decreased cerebral inhibition of bladder reflexes. In the normal infant, urination occurs whenever vesical or other regional stimuli reach a sufficient height to act through an upper motor neuron reflex arc. As the child grows older, bladder training allows the cerebral cortex to exercise an inhibitory effect over this simple reflex arc so that reflex emptying can be delayed. Inhibition is obtained first during the waking hours and subsequently becomes so patterned that it is present even during sleep, and enuresis ceases.

In some children, however, the cerebral inhibitory control does not become developed, perhaps as a result of deficient pathways or from psychologic defect, and the child continues to have uninhibited contractions (Fig. 36). There is then urinary frequency during the daytime and enuresis at night. The characteristics of this type of bladder are normal or increased tone and decreased capacity without residual urine.

Two groups are recognized: a congenital group and an acquired one. In the congenital group, administration of atropine in dosage sufficient to atropinize a child, if effective, is diagnostic of the uninhibited neurogenic bladder and, in addition, is therapeutic. The acquired group, composed of individuals with

Table 4.　Characteristics of Neurogenic Bladders

I. UNINHIBITED	II. AUTOMATIC (REFLEX)	III. AUTONOMOUS	IV. SENSORY (ATONIC)	V. MOTOR
SITE OF LESION				
Cerebral or high cord (underdeveloped central control)	A and B: Upper neuron	A and B: Lower neuron	Dorsal columns	Anterior horn cells
CHARACTERISTICS				
Voiding reflexes to filling are not suppressed	A, Spastic (imbalanced): Bladder takes part in general hypertonicity B, "Normal" (balanced): Bladder independent of control but reflex arc functions well	A, Flaccid (imbalanced): No external nervous control, but atonic B, "Normal" (balanced): No external nervous control, but bladder tone adequate for urethral resistance	Loss of sensation allowed excess filling, ending in flaccidity and atony	Sensation normal, but motor paralysis
DISEASE PROCESS				
A, Congenital: Delayed development of inhibitory pathway B, Acquired: Hemiplegia, brain tumors, multiple sclerosis	A and B: Transection of cord	A and B: Transection of conus or cauda equina	Tabes, pernicious anemia, multiple sclerosis, diabetes, syringomyelia	Poliomyelitis
SYMPTOMS				
Enuresis, urgency and frequency; occasional incontinence	A: Reflex, involuntary voiding without sensation B: Same; occasional trigger zones cause voiding	A: Overflow incontinence B: Continence by periodic forceful evacuation	Painless overflow incontinence	Painful overflow incontinence
TONE				
Normal or increased	A: Increased B: Normal or increased	A: Decreased B: Decreased	Decreased (late)	Increased (early)
CAPACITY				
Decreased	A: Decreased B: Normal or increased	A: Increased B: Increased	Increased	Increased (late)
RESIDUAL URINE				
0	A: 20–50 cc. B:　0–50 cc.	A: ± 300 cc. B: ± 30 cc.	500 cc. +	300 cc.+
TREATMENT				
Atropinization (parasympathetic block)	A: 1, Remove irritants (infection, calculi); 2, Sacral neurotomy; 3, alcohol subarachnoid block B: None	A and B: 1, Presacral neurectomy; 2, pudendal block; 3, TUR; 4, Crede; (5, Urecholine)	1, Preserve bladder tone; 2, evacuate with straining; (3, presacral neurotomy if sphincter tight; 4, pudendal block; 5, Urecholine)	Catheter drainage expectantly
RESULTS				
Good in children	A: Fair if treatment prolonged. B: Good	A: Poor B: Fair	Poor	Good

cerebral or high cord damage, is less susceptible to this form of treatment.

The *automatic neurogenic bladder* typically results from a complete transection of the cord at a level above the conus. It may also result from a disturbance of the suprasegmental arc which simulates transection of the cord. The result is a reflex arc running from the bladder to the sacral cord, synapsing and running back down to the bladder. The bladder, then, is an organ controlled by a simple reflex. The lesions which cause this syndrome are usually injuries to the thoracic or lumbar cord which result in paraplegia.

The diagnosis of automatic neurogenic bladder rests upon locating the site and degree of injury and upon determining the type of bladder function which results. The bladder empties by reflex activity arising either from intrinsic stimuli from the bladder wall itself or from extrinsic stimuli which provoke mass movement. These patients have no real sensation of vesical filling, but the increasing size of the bladder as the urine accumulates produces sensations within the abdomen which they may interpret as a full bladder. Urination occurs without warning as soon as the reflex arc is closed, by summation of afferent stimuli.

Two major types of automatic bladders are recognized. The more usual is the spastic type; the other is the so-called normal reflex neurogenic bladder. The former is seen in patients with spasticity of the extremities. It is characterized by small capacity with more or less residual urine. Since urination is of necessity frequent because of the spasticity and small capacity, urination is precipitant and inconvenient (Fig. 37). The goal of therapy is a so-called normal reflex neurogenic bladder. If this is obtained, bladder capacity may be as high as 300 cc. Visceral sensation of bladder filling may be enough to give the patient opportunity to reach a convenient place for voiding. Residual urine is low.

The therapeutic aim is first to remove all irritative foci, since the bladder is a purely reflex organ with the sensory stimuli arising within the bladder wall itself, both from the mucosa and from the muscle, as a stretch reflex. Bladder infection and calculi increase the sensory component of the reflex arc and thereby cause increased stimuli for contraction.

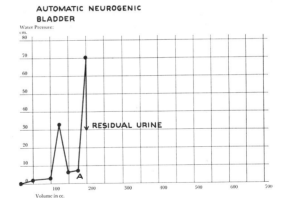

CYSTOMETROGRAM

AUTOMATIC NEUROGENIC BLADDER

A. UNABLE TO RESIST VOIDING.

REFLEX CONTRACTIONS, UNCONTROLLED, DURING FILLING, ENDING IN FORCEFUL, INCOMPLETE EMPTYING.

Figure 37.

A patient is observed over a period of months and then restudied to learn what sort of bladder function will result from these simple measures. If spasticity persists, blocking of the sensory nerve impulses is necessary and may be accomplished either by alcohol block or by sectioning the sacral roots. Intradural alcohol injection of the lower spinal cord blocks all long reflexes and produces an autonomous neurogenic bladder. The result is greater capacity and relative freedom from the inconvenient reflex voiding of the automatic bladder. A more direct approach is to block the sensory roots of the third, fourth and fifth sacral nerves to cut off the sensory components arising from the irritable bladder and so interrupt the reflex arc. The bladder is then free to relax and to attain a normal capacity. In addition, the irritative stimuli arising from the posterior urethra are cut off, releasing the reflex spasm of the sphincter. Thus, sphincteric tone is more nearly normal. These procedures may assist patients with automatic bladders to regain almost normal control.

The *autonomous neurogenic bladder* results from section of the cauda equina and conus, usually by trauma, but occasionally by inflammatory lesions and often from such congenital anomalies as meningocele with spina bifida. In contrast to a lesion across the spinal cord above the conus, a lesion through the cauda equina leaves the bladder autonomous (Fig. 38), possessing little or no outside reflex arc. It acts merely by the intrinsic reflex arc through the detrusor ganglia.

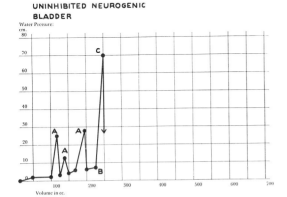

CYSTOMETROGRAM

UNINHIBITED NEUROGENIC BLADDER

A. DESIRE TO VOID.
B. STRONG DESIRE TO VOID.
C. VOIDED AROUND CATHETER.

MANY SMALL CONTRACTIONS, NOT CONTROLLED BY PATIENT, ENDING IN STRONGER CONTRACTION AND VOIDING.

Figure 36.

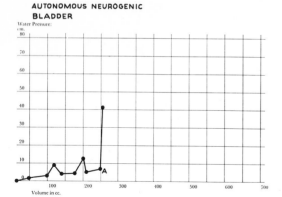

A. STRAIN TO VOID.

NO SENSATION OF FILLING.
VOIDS BY STRAINING AND LITTLE REFLEX ACTIVITY.

Figure 38.

Sensation is diminished and coordinated reflex stimulus to the detrusor is absent. The bladder fills against the intrinsic detrusor tone and urination is irregular and incomplete. Depending on the degree of resistance at the vesical neck, the patient will be able to void more or less of the bladder contents by increasing abdominal pressure or by the use of manual pressure over the bladder. The capacity of the bladder may be as high as 350 cc., but the residual urine is, of course, also quite high.

Treatment of these patients is directed at balancing urethral resistance against intravesical pressure. For emptying to occur, the ineffective detrusor contractions, supplemented by the pressure of the abdomen and the hand, must overcome urethral resistance. If urethral resistance is too high, retention of urine will result. On the other hand, if urethral resistance is too low, incontinence occurs.

Several measures have been proposed to decrease urethral resistance, since the strength of detrusor contraction can seldom be affected directly by therapy, even by such agents as the parasympathomimetic drug Urecholine.

Pudendal nerve block and section, either unilateral or bilateral, will cause partial paralysis of the external sphincter. Transurethral resection of the prostatic urethra, especially when definite obstructive elements are seen with the panendoscope, will quantitatively reduce urethral resistance. Often more than one resection must be done to secure a good result, since initial overenthusiasm can result in total incontinence.

The *sensory neurogenic bladder* occurs after interruption of the sensory side of the reflex arc. Tabes dorsalis, occasionally pernicious anemia and multiple sclerosis, and syringomyelia are followed by this dysfunction. The patient does not know when his bladder is full because the afferent stimuli are cut off, so that, after a time, gross overdistention occurs, which results in atony. This atonic bladder devoid of motor power is the end result of the sensory defect. The bladder has a large capacity and urination occurs by overflow during straining. Incontinence often brings these patients to the doctor. They are able to empty their bladders only by forceful abdominal pressure and manual compression. A cystometrogram would show a low filling pressure with a very large capacity and no contractions of any sort. Cystoscopically, fine trabeculations are seen. The neck of the bladder is open and relaxed, as are the other portions of the detrusor. The external sphincter is not involved by the atony, so that its resistance is the cause of the retention of urine and overflow incontinence.

The object of treatment is primarily preventive. If the patients are seen early, before bladder tone is destroyed, they can be instructed to void at predetermined intervals, perhaps every two or three hours. Their bladders then will not become overdistended. After overdistention and atony have occurred, the object of therapy can only be to reduce the amount of residual urine and hope for return of bladder tone. The patient should be instructed to strain at each voiding and supplement the straining by manual pressure on the bladder. Urecholine may be of some assistance in increasing detrusor activity. In very severe cases, a period of drainage by an indwelling catheter will occasionally reduce capacity to a more normal level and restore some tone. The fundamental disease process should be treated. Transurethral resection of the bladder neck is of little value to these patients since the bladder neck is already widely open. Section of the pudendal nerve, either unilaterally or bilaterally, in certain cases will promote reduced urethral resistance because of partial paralysis of the normally active external sphincter and so will decrease the amount of residual urine.

The *motor neurogenic bladder* is the result

of loss of the motor side of the reflex arc. It is most commonly seen after poliomyelitis in adults. Sensation is normal so that distention is painful, but overdistention occurs because the bladder is unable to contract as a result of loss of efferent stimuli to the detrusor. If catheter drainage is not instituted, overdistention and atony will result.

In the immediate care of the paralyzed bladder, the first aim should be to prevent atrophy resulting from overdistention by catheter drainage; the second, to avoid and repress infection; and the third, to reduce the possibility of stone formation by recommending ambulation, irrigation and a high fluid intake.

In later care, the establishment of the optimum reflex activity must be sought; it often occurs only after six months or longer.

Testing allows differentiation of the automatic bladder, which results from the higher spinal cord lesion, from the autonomous bladder secondary to injury of the cauda equina. But the final goal is balance and the final question is what can the bladder do?

For example, a patient with a high lesion voids small amounts frequently. His residual urine is low, but his capacity is also low and interpretation of the cystometrogram indicates a quick voiding reflex after small increments during filling. This is an automatic neurogenic bladder. To achieve balance, the bladder must be calmed by reducing afferent sensations which set off the premature reflex activity. This can be done either by decreasing infection in the bladder and removing stones, or by blocking the afferent nerves by sacral nerve block or subarachnoid alcohol block. If residual urine persists, a transurethral resection of the bladder neck will reduce urethral resistance and help achieve balance.

For another example, a patient suffers a low lesion in the cauda equina resulting in an autonomous neurogenic bladder. He voids by straining, but empties his bladder only partially. Interpretation of the cystometrogram indicates that the capacity is good, but adequate voiding pressure is reached only by abdominal compression and straining. To achieve balance in this case, urethral resistance must be decreased. Pudendal block, which interrupts the somatic nerves to the external sphincter, may help. More often, transurethral resection of the bladder neck performed in stages so that total incontinence does not result will achieve balance between the reduced vesical pressure and the surgically reduced urethral resistance.

READING REFERENCES

Bors, E.: Neurogenic bladder. Urol. Survey 7:177, 1957.

Butt, J. B.: Treatment of Urinary Lithiasis. Springfield, Illinois, Charles C Thomas, 1960.

Colby, F. H.: Pyelonephritis. Baltimore, Williams and Wilkins Company, 1959.

Creevy, C. D.: Outline of Urology. New York, McGraw-Hill, 1964.

Emmett, J. L.: Clinical Urography, an Atlas and Textbook of Roentgenologic Diagnosis. 2nd ed. Philadelphia, W. B. Saunders Company, 1964.

Farber, S.: Chemotherapy in the treatment of leukemia and Wilms' tumor, J.A.M.A. 198:826, 1966.

Higgins, C. C., and Straffon, R. A.: Urolithiasis. In, Campbell, M. (ed.): Urology, Vol. 1. 2nd ed. Philadelphia, W. B. Saunders Company, 1963.

Hinman, F., Jr: The pathophysiology of urinary obstruction. In, Campbell, M. (ed.): Urology, Vol. 1. 2nd ed. Philadelphia, W. B. Saunders Company, 1963.

Hodges, C. V., Gilbert, D. R., and Scott, W. W.: Renal trauma. J. Urol. 66:627, 1951.

Jewett, H. J.: Tumors of the bladder. In, Campbell, M. (ed.): Urology, Vol. 2. 2nd ed. Philadelphia, W. B. Saunders Company, 1963.

Jewett, H. J., and Strong, G. H.: Infiltrating carcinoma of the bladder; relation of depth of penetration of bladder wall to incidence of local extension and metastases. J. Urol. 55:366, 1946.

Kuru, M.: Nervous control of micturition. Physiol. Rev. 45:425, 1965.

Kunin, C. M.: Epidemiology and natural history of urinary tract infection in school children. Bull. New York Acad. Med. 40:767, 1964.

Lattimer, J. K., and Kohen, R. J.: Renal tuberculosis. Am. J. Med. 17:533, 1954.

Marshall, V. F., et al.: Symposium on Bladder Tumors. Philadelphia, J. B. Lippincott Company, 1956.

Marshall, V. F.: Text Book of Urology. 2nd ed. New York, Harper & Row, 1964.

Mostofi, F.: The Kidney. Baltimore, Williams and Wilkins Company, 1966.

Ney, C., and Friedenberg, R. M.: Radiographic Atlas of the Genitourinary System. Philadelphia, J. B. Lippincott Company, 1966.

Prather, G. C., and Kaiser, T. F.: The bladder in fracture of the bony pelvis. The significance of a "tear drop bladder" as shown by cystogram. J. Urol. 63:1019, 1950.

Poutasse, E. F.: Surgical treatment of renal hypertension. Am. J. Surg. 107:97, 1964.

Reynolds, C. J.: The diagnosis and a new treatment of traumatic rupture of the posterior urethra. South. M. J. 35:825, 1942.

Riches, E.: Tumor of the Kidney and Ureter. Edinburgh and London, E. & S. Livingstone, 1964.

Schirmer, H. K. A., et al.: Renal metabolism with proximal or distal ureteral occlusion. Surg. Gyn. & Obst. 123: 539, 1966.

Scott, R., et al.: Initial managment of non-penetrating renal injuries: clinical review of 111 cases. J. Urol. 90:535, 1963.

Smith, D. R.: General Urology, Los Altos, California, Lange Medical Publications, 1966.

Stamey, T. M.: Localization and treatment of urinary tract infections: role of bactericidal urine levels as opposed to serum levels. Medicine 44:1, 1965.

Stamey, T. M.: Renovascular Hypertension. Baltimore, Williams and Wilkins Company, 1963.

Quinn, E. L., and Koss, E. H.: Biology of Pyelonephritis. Boston, Little, Brown & Company, 1960.

Winter, C. C.: Radioisotope Renography. Baltimore, Williams and Wilkins Company, 1963.

Chapter 29

THE MALE REPRODUCTIVE SYSTEM

by

HENRY M. WEYRAUCH, M.D.

and

ARJAN D. AMAR, M.D.

The late HENRY M. WEYRAUCH was born in a village which nestles in the foothills of the Shawangunk Mountains, one of the small ranges of the Catskills. He became the organist of the First Baptist Church in this village at a salary of fifty cents a week. This first paying job started him off on a career as an organist and choirmaster, which helped pay his tuition through Union College and Johns Hopkins Medical School. His interest in organs was maintained by establishment of a unique store in San Francisco, which featured organs of every description. He received his training in general surgery at the Presbyterian Hospital in New York, and in Urology at the University of Pennsylvania, Duke University and the University of California. Formerly Clinical Professor of Surgery and Chief of the Division of Urology at Stanford University School of Medicine, Doctor Weyrauch was Chief of the Department of Urology, Presbyterian Medical Center, San Francisco. He passed away soon after he and his co-author completed the revision of this chapter.

ARJAN D. AMAR was born in Shorkot, a small town in the Province of Punjab, India, now in West Pakistan. The youngest of seven children, he was assisted through medical school by an older brother physician after his father suffered severe financial losses. He won many honors in the Medical College of the University of Punjab, from which he was graduated in 1951. He left Pakistan under threat of death because of differences with the Moslem religion. He received his post-graduate education in urologic surgery at the University of Michigan. He is Chief, Department of Urology, Kaiser Foundation Hospital, Walnut Creek, California, and a member of the staff of the Presbyterian Medical Center, San Francisco.

The male reproductive organs consist of the *external genitalia*, made up of the penis and scrotal contents, and the *internal genitalia*, comprising the prostate, seminal vesicles and Cowper's glands (Fig. 1). The functions of the male reproductive system are to produce spermatozoa, to perform copulation and to produce and secrete hormones.

The penis, which is primarily composed of erectile bodies, provides a conduit for the urethra and serves the important function of copulation. The testes produce both spermatozoa and hormones. The epididymides, vasa deferentia and ejaculatory ducts form the efferent tract by which spermatozoa are collected and conveyed to the urethra, which serves as a channel for both seminal fluid and urine. The prostate gland, the seminal vesicles and Cowper's glands play an accessory role in providing glandular secretions which serve as a vehicle for spermatozoa and facilitate their passage.

EXTERNAL GENITALIA

Although the organs of the external genitalia are in close association, they constitute three anatomic units: the penis and urethra; the scrotum and scrotal contents; and the inguinal lymphatic system.

PENIS AND URETHRA

The penis is primarily a sexual organ; secondarily, it encompasses a portion of the urethra. The three erectile tissue components

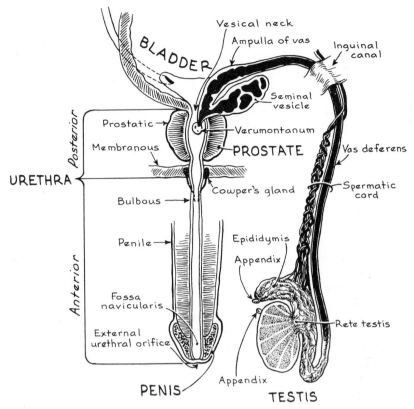

Figure 1. The male reproductive system.

are the two corpora cavernosa situated dorsally and the corpus spongiosum penis on the ventral surface (Fig. 2). The corpus spongiosum contains the urethra and is capped distally by the glans penis. The corpora are enclosed in fascial sheaths. All in turn are surrounded and bound together by a dense fibrous envelope known as Buck's fascia. This serves as a barrier against extravasation of urine and the spread of infectious processes. The corpora cavernosa are anchored to the ischiopubic rami. Passing between and below them, the corpus spongiosum surrounds the urethra in its bulbous extent before the urethra enters the external layer of the urogenital diaphragm. The penis is fixed to the pubis at its root by the suspensory ligament. The lax elastic composition of the penile skin permits

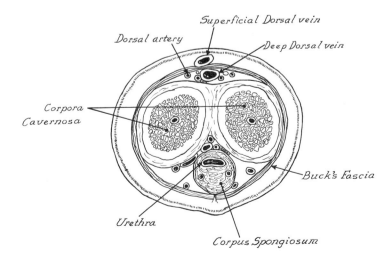

Figure 2. Cross section of penis.

enormous inflammatory edema and extensive burrowing of subcutaneous blood.

The penis derives a rich blood supply from the internal pudendal arteries. Venous drainage is provided by the dorsal veins of the penis which pass through the prostatic plexuses. This unusually rich vascularity is advantageous in controlling infections and in favoring wound healing. The lymphatic drainage from the penis is to the superficial and subinguinal lymph nodes; that from the glans penis is to the subinguinal and external iliac nodes. The lymphatics from the urethra empty into the hypogastric lymph nodes.

Although the mechanism of erection is poorly understood, it is produced by rapid engorgement of the cavernous bodies by blood through psychic and nervous stimuli. When the blood supply to the penis is impaired, or when the nervous supply is damaged, the ability to attain erections may be impaired or lost.

The penile urethra is that extent of the anterior urethra which lies within the pendulous portion of the penis. It extends from the external urethral orifice to the penoscrotal junction, where it becomes the bulbous portion of the urethra. The bulbous portion consists of a dilation of the anterior urethra located in the perineum, distal to the anterior leaf of the urogenital diaphragm. Cowper's glands lie within the urogenital diaphragm and empty through ducts into the floor of the bulbous portion of the urethra.

Anomalies

The common anomalies of the penis are phimosis and those in which the urethra is primarily at fault. Anomalies such as absence of the penis, double penis, micropenis, congenital torsion and transposition of the penis and scrotum are rarely encountered in clinical practice. They are likely to be associated with severe abnormalities in other parts of the body which are incompatible with life. Penile anomalies are caused by maldevelopment of the genital tubercle and of those portions of the urogenital sinus involved in the formation of the external genitalia.

PHIMOSIS. Phimosis designates the condition in which the orifice of the prepuce is too small to permit retraction behind the glans penis. It may be either congenital or acquired. Acquired phimosis usually arises from infection and subsequent edema and scarring. Phimosis predisposes to infection of the glans penis and prepuce.

Calculi sometimes form in the preputial sac. In extreme degree, phimosis causes obstruction to the outflow of urine and the development of obstructive changes in the bladder and upper urinary tract. Chronic infection and irritation associated with phimosis frequently lead to malignant neoplasms of the penis.

During adult life, phimosis impairs the transmission of normal sensation from the nerve endings of the corona of the penis during coitus. Infection may lead to dyspareunia and difficulty in performing coitus.

Treatment of phimosis consists of circumcision. This operation should be performed during infancy to prevent the described complications. When there is marked infection, antibacterial agents and local application of heat should be used to control infection preliminary to operation. Failing in conservative therapy a dorsal slit should be performed to establish drainage and control the inflammatory reaction.

At the time of performing circumcision, it is important to release any adhesions between the prepuce and the glans penis, and to be certain that the external urethral orifice is of adequate size. If the orifice is smaller than normal, it should be enlarged by external urethrotomy at the time of circumcision.

HYPOSPADIAS. This is a common deformity of the penis and urethra, in which the anterior urethra terminates at some point on the undersurface of the penis, proximal to the normal position at the tip of the glans. Embryologically, hypospadias results from imperfect closure of the urethral groove, the margins of which normally fuse in the midline to form the floor of the urethra. It is a hermaphroditic manifestation, in which the urogenital derivatives in the male tend to develop toward the female side.

Depending upon the degree of hypospadias, the types are designated as balanic or glandular, penile, penoscrotal and perineal (Fig. 3). The fundamental defect is in the urethra and the corpus spongiosum which, excepting in the balanic type, produces a shortening of the ventral aspect of the penis. This causes a downward curvature of the penis which is most marked during erection, known as chordee (Fig. 3, *d*). Deficiency of the prepuce on the ventral aspect causes the dorsal portion to be prominent, giving a hooded appearance (Fig. 3, *d*). When the orifice is in the scrotal or perineal area, the scrotum is bifid and may resemble the labia majora of the female. In addition, the penis may be small,

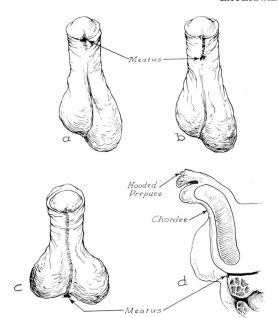

Figure 3. Types of hypospadias: *a*, glandular; *b*, mid-penile; *c*, perineal; *d*, side view, perineal.

simulating a large clitoris. Male infants may thus be mistaken for females.

Although balanic hypospadias is largely asymptomatic, the other types lead to difficulty in urination due to the abnormal location of the external urethral orifice, and to difficulty in coitus caused by chordee. Since the defect is confined to the anterior urethra, there is no deficiency of the urinary sphincters and no urinary incontinence.

Diagnosis of hypospadias and an associated hermaphroditism is established by examination of the external genitalia, cystourethroscopy, buccal smears and testicular biopsy. In most forms of uncomplicated hypospadias examination of the external genitalia suffices. When there is bilateral cryptorchidism or a vaginal tract, other tests may become necessary. Cystourethroscopy shows the presence or absence of a prostatic urethra and verumontanum. Penoscrotal and perineal types of hypospadias are usually associated with an enlarged verumontanum which represents the remnant of the fused ends of the Müllerian ducts. Study of the chromosomes in cells obtained by buccal smear and the cytology of gonadal cells seen in biopsy specimens provide definitive information.

The treatment is surgical, to enable the patient to urinate and to copulate in the normal manner. As a general rule, disability is so slight in the balanic type that treatment is not required, other than enlarging the external

urethral orifice, if it is small. In some cases of balanic hypospadias, the orifice is minute. Meatotomy is performed toward the glans, instead of in the usual ventral direction. A tiny sinus tract, leading toward the tip of the glans, is usually present. Incising into this tract to enlarge the orifice decreases the balanic deformity. Incision in the opposite direction would increase the deformity.

Surgical treatment of the other types consist of correcting the chordee by excision of fibrous tissue and constructing a new urethra by plastic operation. Circumcision should be avoided in hypospadias since the skin of the prepuce often proves useful in surgical correction of the anomaly.

Corrective surgical procedures should be completed before five years of age. This avoids embarrassment when the child enters school.

EPISPADIAS. Epispadias is a congenital absence of the upper wall of the urethra at some point proximal to the glans, which has a "spadelike" appearance. It is an inevitable counterpart of exstrophy of the urinary bladder in the male; when it occurs alone it may be considered as a mild exstrophy. Although epispadias is much less common than hypospadias, it is more disabling. The usual site of the urethral opening is at the abdomino-penile junction. There is commonly an associated defect of the urinary sphincters which causes urinary incontinence.

Treatment is accomplished by plastic repair of the penis and formation of an anterior urethra. The objectives are to provide urinary continence and the ability to copulate. If it is impossible to achieve urinary continence, some type of supravesical diversion of urine is required.

Trauma

With the exception of paraphimosis, injuries of the penis are extremely rare. Self-mutilation, such as contusion from pressing or pinching during masturbation, or strangulation from forcing the organ into the neck of a bottle or other firm constricting ring, accounts for many injuries. Incised or gunshot wounds may lead to profuse hemorrhage. A severely injured penis will usually heal promptly if immediately sutured.

PARAPHIMOSIS. Paraphimosis is a condition in which the prepuce, when once retracted behind the glans penis, cannot be replaced in its normal position. It is frequent in the uncircumcised, particularly during in-

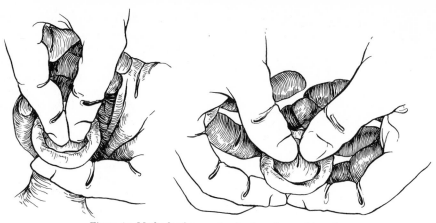

Figure 4.   Methods of manual reduction of paraphimosis.

fancy. Infection of the prepuce predisposes to development of this abnormality. A tight ring of skin, proximal to the corona of the glans penis, produces venous occlusion. This leads to edema of the glans and increases the disproportion between the size of the glans and the preputial opening. If the paraphimosis is not reduced, the arterial supply of the glans may be impaired or entirely cut off, with resulting gangrene.

Paraphimosis can usually be reduced manually, hyaluronidase being first injected into the subcutaneous tissues (Fig. 4). In chronic cases, and particularly when infection is marked, dorsal slit of the prepuce may be required. Circumcision should be carried out when the inflammatory reaction has subsided. Prophylaxis, performing circumcision when the prepuce is tight or redundant, and cautioning mothers in the care of infants to avoid leaving the prepuce in the unretracted position are important.

DISLOCATION.   Dislocation of the penis results from severe trauma in the erectile state. There is usually associated rupture of the urethra. The penis is inverted and disappears into the scrotum or the adjacent tissues of the inguinal or suprapubic region. There may be considerable swelling from subcutaneous hemorrhage and urinary extravasation. Immediate operation is indicated to evacuate blood clots, suture the penis in its normal position and repair urethral damage.

Infections

Aside from the venereal infections, which rarely constitute a surgical problem, the penis is relatively immune to infection. The abundant blood supply is helpful in com-

bating pyogenic infection such as cellulitis, erysipelas and furuncles. Nonvenereal infections of the urethra are usually secondary to obstruction or urethral instrumentation.

POSTHITIS, BALANITIS AND BALANOPOSTHITIS. Balanitis is inflammation of the glans penis, posthitis of the prepuce; the combined inflammatory lesion is known as balanoposthitis. These inflammations are usually caused by retention of secretions and bacteria beneath a redundant prepuce.

Local signs and symptoms vary according to the severity and etiology of the infection. The patient usually complains of local itching, burning and pain, and in the more virulent infections, a purulent discharge is present. The presence of a discharge may cause confusion in making a differential diagnosis between urethritis and balanoposthitis. When the infection is not a complication of gonococcal urethritis or other specific disease, the treatment is routine cleansing and drying of the involved surfaces. In acute infection, the type of bacteria is determined by smear and culture and appropriate antibacterial agents are administered. In infections which resist treatment, a dorsal slit is performed to facilitate drainage. When the acute process has receded, circumcision is usually indicated to prevent recurrence.

HERPES PROGENITALIS.   This common lesion of the penis is caused by a virus. It is manifest by groups of vesicles on the surface of the glans or prepuce along the distribution of the dorsal penile nerve. The lesions appear as small red areas which become vesiculated and rupture, leaving superficial ulceration. Mild itching and burning are the chief symptoms.

Unfortunately there is no specific treatment. Local cleansing with a bland soap, careful drying and application of zinc stearate are helpful. If the prepuce is redundant, circumcision usually eliminates recurrences. In resistant cases, the daily application of Penotrane jelly (phenylmercuric dinaphthylmethane disulfonate) accelerates the healing process.

CONDYLOMATA ACUMINATA. Condylomata acuminata, usually known as venereal warts, are soft, painless, cauliflower-like growths which appear on the prepuce, glans penis and within the adjacent urethra. The lesion is aggravated by secretions and dampness. A redundant prepuce is usually the chief predisposing factor. Despite the common name, it is doubtful that they are contracted by sexual contact. Like herpes, they are caused by a virus. The lesions are usually numerous and vary in size from a few millimeters to a centimeter in diameter. Occasionally, they attain tremendous size.

Cleanliness and dryness are the important factors in prophylaxis and in preventing recurrence. For this reason, circumsion is helpful. Once developed, the lesions can usually be eradicated by local application of 25 per cent podophyllin in tincture of benzoin. Care must be exercised to avoid application of the drug to uninvolved portions of the skin and mucous membrane. In resistant cases, electrofulguration proves effective.

CAVERNOSITIS. Cavernositis is an infection of the erectile bodies of the penis, usually secondary to acute gonorrhea or acute nonspecific urethritis. It may complicate trauma, especially with urinary extravasation, and occurs in some systemic diseases, such as leukemia.

The condition is evident as a tender, indurated area in one of the cavernous bodies. The urethra may be compressed, causing difficult urination. Occasionally, cavernositis leads to priapism. Like periurethral abscess, a cavernous abscess may rupture into the urethra. Treatment consists of specific antimicrobial therapy, and incision and drainage in resistant cases.

Neoplasms

Carcinoma of the penis, the usual malignant lesion, comprises only 1 per cent of all cancers of the urogenital tract in the United States. In China and Southeast Asia, it consitutes 20 per cent of all urogenital malignancies. It is the commonest malignancy in men in Uganda, being exceeded in frequency only by malignant lymphoma and carcinoma of the cervix uteri. In Uganda, it accounts for 12.2 per cent of all male cancers; 90 per cent of the patients are uncircumcised.

In the diagnosis of neoplasms of the penis, such common skin neoplasms as nevi, hemangioma and papilloma offer little clinical difficulty. Local excision provides both the diagnosis and definitive treatment.

CARCINOMA OF PENIS. Carcinoma of the penis usually develops in men over 50 years of age. Circumcision in infancy grants almost complete immunity. Circumcision later in life is valuable, but decreasingly so as the patient becomes older. These considerations suggest that the exciting cause operates over a period of many years, apparently contributed to by preputial secretion or chronic bacterial irritation, or both.

Most of these carcinomas are composed of squamous cells. They may be divided into the verrucous and ulcerated types. The papillomatous may originate from condylomata acuminata and tend to grow quite large, although they are less invasive and are of a lower grade of malignancy than flat, ulcerative types. Metastasis is chiefly by way of the lymphatics, so that the inguinal and femoral lymph nodes must be carefully examined in every suspected instance. However, it must be determined by biopsy whether enlargement of these nodes is caused by secondary infection or carcinomatous invasion. Distant metastasis from carcinoma of the penis occurs late. Since a portion of the lymphatic drainage of the penis extends directly to the pelvic and iliac lymph nodes, these nodes may become involved without invasion of the superficial inguinal lymph nodes.

Symptoms consist of the presence of a painless, slow-growing lesion, most frequent on the glans penis, which may be obscured by a redundant prepuce. Persistent ulceration and the presence of a discharge are common complaints – "a sore which does not heal."

Differential diagnosis must be made with ulcerative lesions of the penis such as chancre and chancroid. Carcinoma is not excluded by a positive serologic test for syphilis. Diagnosis is established by biopsy. With the use of local anesthesia, a small wedge of tissue is removed from non-necrotic tissue at the edge of the ulcer.

In the treatment of carcinoma of the penis, surgical therapy remains the method of choice. There is still disagreement as to the most appropriate type of operation; as to whether amputation of the penis 2 cm. proximal to all visible and palpable evidence of the neoplasm suffices, or whether this should be combined with extirpation of the inguinal, femoral and pelvic lymph nodes. Radiation therapy, previously employed in treatment, has proved ineffectual and has been largely abandoned.

Special Diseases

In addition to conditions of known etiology, there are some penile lesions of idiopathic or protean manifestations.

PLASTIC INDURATION OF PENIS (PEYRONIE'S DISEASE). Plastic induration of the penis is a common lesion of the fibrous coverings of the corpora cavernosa, usually involving the dorsal aspect and intercavernous septum of these bodies. It appears as a painless plaque of fibrotic tissue similar to keloid formation and to Dupuytren's contracture of the palmar fascia of the hand. Although in most instances the etiology is unknown, in some it arises as a sequel of trauma.

The incidental finding of a firm area in the penis may call attention to the lesion. As it progresses, the fibrotic area limits erection. The penis remains bent in the direction of the involved area. This leads to difficult coitus and sometimes precludes penetration; erection may be accompanied by pain. In most instances, the deformity progresses slowly and is subject to long periods of remission regardless of whether or not treatment is instituted. Spontaneous regression occasionally occurs.

Diagnosis is established by palpation of the shaft of the penis. This reveals a well-defined plaque of firm tissue, usually located in the midline of the dorsum and near the base of the organ. Occasionally, it is placed distally, laterally, or deep between the corpora cavernosa. X-ray films sometimes reveal signs of calcification in the area of involvement.

Numerous forms of treatment have been advocated, and their multiplicity bears evidence to the ineffectiveness of them all. Of reputed value are x-ray or radium, vitamin E, ultrasonic wave therapy and administration of fibrolytic agents such as Potaba (potassium para-aminobenzoate).

Surgical extirpation of the plaque has not proved successful. Excision tends to increase rather than to decrease the curvature. With healing, more fibrous tissue forms. This adds still more to the deformity.

PRIAPISM. Priapism is a rare affliction manifest by prolonged painful erection of the penis, unaccompanied by sexual desire. In most instances, the etiology is unknown. Sometimes, there are specific causes such as leukemia, sickle cell anemia, invasion of the base of the penis by carcinoma of the prostate, penis or urethra, trauma to the corpora, or injury to the spinal cord.

Excluding the few patients who are cured by treatment of a neurologic disorder, the forms of attempted therapy have proved notably ineffective. Because blood in the cavernous spaces becomes sludge-like, rather than clotted, temporary relief is afforded by aspiration with a large bore needle, followed by irrigation with an anticoagulant solution. Thickened blood can sometimes be expressed into the venous circulation by manual massage under regional anesthesia. A venous by-pass by anastomosis of the saphenous vein to the corpus cavernosum has been created in a few patients. Incision and drainage have been employed without remarkable improvement. In most instances, prolonged priapism is followed by partial or complete loss of power to attain erections.

URETHRA

The male urethra is divided into anterior and posterior portions. The posterior is made up of the prostatic and membranous urethra. The latter lies within the triangular ligament. Fixed to the arch of the symphysis pubis, it is the frequent site of rupture, owing to straddle injury or fracture of the pelvis. Encircling the urethra at this point is the external urinary sphincter. The anterior urethra lies distal to the triangular ligament.

The latter marks the point where the bacteria-free posterior urethra joins the anterior urethra, which provides normal habitat for bacteria, similar to the nose and throat. Since it is impossible to sterilize the anterior urethra by any innocuous method, the passing of a catheter always creates the danger of introducing infection, no matter how painstaking the technique. For this reason, catheterization and cystoscopic procedures are avoided whenever possible, especially in the presence of obstruction in which the danger of infection is imminent. In addition to employing strict asepsis, precautionary measures to avoid introducing infection consist of giving the patient a broad-spectrum antibacterial drug and irrigating the bladder with a mild antiseptic solution, such as Zephiran, 1:20,000.

The anterior urethra is divided into the bulbous portion, which takes off from the posterior urethra, and the more distal penile or pendulous urethra which lies within the penis. Cowper's glands open by way of their ducts into the floor of the bulbous urethra. Ducts from the testicles, prostate, seminal vesicles and Cowper's gland release their components of spermatic fluid into the urethra during ejaculation. The widest portions of the urethra are the prostatic and the bulbous extents.

Congenital abnormalities of the anterior urethra consist of duplication of the urethra, accessory urethral channels and hypospadias. In the posterior urethra, congenital valves in the region of the verumontanum provide one of the causes of urinary obstruction. Congenital narrowing is most common at either extremity: stenosis of the external urethral orifice and contracture of the vesical neck.

The common forms of urethral stricture are inflammatory, such as postgonococcal stricture of the bulbomembranous portion of the urethra, and posttraumatic. The latter occurs most commonly at the fixed part of the urethra, where it is attached to the arch of the pubis. This is at the level of the urogenital diaphragm. Rupture results from fracture of the pelvis or from shearing injury to the urethra from straddle injuries to the perineum. Posttraumatic stricture also occurs at the vesical neck following operation on the prostate and vesical neck, and at the fossa navicularis following transurethral operative procedures.

Diagnosis of urethral obstruction is made on the basis of the history of a poor urinary stream, dribbling, hesitancy, urgency and frequency of urination. It should be suspected when there is recurrent or persisting urinary infection. Attempts at passage of a urethral catheter, sound or cystoscope disclose the presence of a stricture; valvelike obstructions are recognized on urethroscopy. Cystourethrography is also a valuable diagnostic aid. Prolonged urethral obstruction from any cause leads to changes in the bladder and upper urinary tract.

Treatment of accessory channels consists of surgical excision. Valves are destroyed by transurethral fulguration with high frequency electrosurgical currents. Areas of narrowing are widened by surgical procedures, such as external urethrotomy for stenosis of the external urethral orifice, or wedge excision of a contracted vesical neck.

The usual treatment for urethral stricture is dilation with urethral sounds. If the stricture is not located in close proximity to the external urinary sphincter, it may be widened by cutting a channel dorsally with the electrosurgical knife of the resectoscope. Unfortunately, there is recurrence in approximately one-half the patients following this procedure. A two-stage operation is more satisfactory; at the first stage, the strictured area is excised. After several months, a plastic operation is performed to reconstruct the urethral channel.

Urethral stricture can be largely prevented by prompt treatment of gonococcal urethritis, by careful urethral instrumentation and by immediate repair of rupture.

Carcinoma of the male urethra is a rare form of neoplasm, usually of the epidermoid type. It leads to slowing of the urinary stream, hematuria and a urethral discharge. Differentiation from urethral stricture is established by biopsy. Treatment consists of radical surgical extirpation. Prognosis is poor.

SCROTUM

The scrotal sac encloses the testes, epididymides and structures of the spermatic cords. Under the corrugated skin lie the dartos fibers; within this layer are three fascial layers derived from the abdominal wall during testicular descent. The scrotum is divided into two compartments by a septum of connective tissue.

The function of the scrotum is the regulatory maintenance of temperature of the testes. Normal spermatogenesis in men requires a temperature several degrees lower than that within the abdomen. The scrotal wall adjusts by responding to changes in external temperature. The dartos muscle contracts in cold weather; it relaxes in a warm temperature. Aided by the cremaster the dartos withdraws the testicles and reduces the size of the scrotum to increase the intrascrotal temperature. To lower the temperature, the muscles relax, the scrotal compartment is increased in size and the testicles hang free.

The arteries which supply the scrotum arise from the femoral, internal pudendal and inferior epigastric arteries. The veins are paired with the arteries. The lymphatics drain into the superficial inguinal and sub-inguinal lymph nodes.

The diagnosis of most scrotal masses can be made by careful palpation and identification of each structure, combined with transillumination, and occasionally by radiography. When doubt remains, exploration of the scrotum may be simply and safely performed.

Anomalies

Anomalies of the scrotum are usually associated with anomalies in other parts of the reproductive system. The most common are a bilobate scrotum resulting from arrest of fetal development and failure of union of the lateral halves along the line of the median raphe. This results in the formation of a separate pouch for each testicle, frequently associated with perineal hypospadias. When there is congenital absence of the testicle, or cryptorchism, the affected side of the scrotum fails to develop.

Trauma

Although scrotal injuries are few, trauma is occasionally sustained by kicks, blows or gunshot wounds. In any penetrating injury, the chief concern is whether there has been damage to the scrotal contents and whether any foreign material has been introduced. Such wounds should be promptly debrided and tetanus antitoxin administered. As a general rule, a compression bandage will check mild hemorrhage, but arterial bleeders require ligation. Unless this is promptly executed, a large scrotal hematoma will develop. The scrotal skin has a great capacity for regeneration and its loss does not usually require skin grafting, although in reconstruction of the scrotum, the testicles may be initially left in a bizarre position. The presence of urinary extravasation, as from a coincident rupture of the urethra, demands definitive treatment. Serious infection may ensue unless the urine is diverted, proper drainage of the involved tissues instituted and appropriate antimicrobial agents administered.

Infections

Most infections of the scrotum are secondary to infection of the testicle, urethra or rectum, or to urinary extravasation. Scrotal cellulitis and furunculosis are similar to these infections elsewhere on the skin surface.

Special Diseases

SCROTAL EDEMA. Because of the laxity of the scrotal skin and subcutaneous tissues, edema may progress to startling dimensions. The penis may be similarly involved and so dislocated by invagination as to cause interference with urination. If the urine is discharged over the scrotum, the skin becomes macerated, predisposing to infection and ulceration. Scrotal edema is frequently associated with cardiac or renal disease, blood dyscrasia or abdominal neoplasms which interfere with venous and lymphatic return. On the other hand, it may be secondary to infection of the testicle or other adjacent structures. Treatment of scrotal edema consists of a high scrotal support while definitive treatment is being applied to the primary cause. In the absence of complicating infection, surgical drainage is unnecessary and contraindicated because of the danger of producing cellulitis and bacteremia.

ELEPHANTIASIS. Elephantiasis is a chronic disease caused by interruption of the lymphatic drainage of the scrotum, leading to hypertrophy of the skin and edema of the subcutaneous tissue with tremendous enlargement of the affected areas. There are two forms: the nonfilarial and the filarial, which is limited to tropical and semitropical regions. Nonparasitic elephantiasis may result from excision or postoperative sclerosis of the inguinal lymph nodes into which the scrotal lymphatics drain. Parasitic elephantiasis is common in many Asian countries, especially India. The condition results from infection with the nematode *Wuchereria bancrofti*, an organism which utilizes two hosts, man and certain mosquitoes, to complete its life cycle. Filaria are blood-borne to the lymphatics, where they interrupt drainage of the regional lymph nodes.

In the early stages, scrotal edema may be present. This must be differentiated from that caused by torsion of the spermatic cord or appendices of the testis or epididymis. With filarial infection, the inguinal lymph nodes usually enlarge and become tender.

During the acute phase blood drawn during the night hours, when the nematodes are circulating in greater numbers, provides the best opportunity to establish the diagnosis.

In elephantiasis, the scrotum may enlarge to such an extent as to reach the level of the knees or even touch the ground as the patient walks. The tissues have a brawny hardness attributable to fibrous infiltration and hyperplasia of the cutaneous tissues, which become coarse in texture. Since the cutaneous blood supply is preserved, gangrene seldom develops.

In the differential diagnosis, it is important to recognize that pyogenic inflammation of the scrotum and urinary extravasation may simulate elephantiasis.

Aside from treating the primary disease if it is recognizable, treatment of elephantiasis consists of plastic excision of the scrotum, preserving the testicles, which are unaffected by the lesion.

SCROTAL GANGRENE. Scrotal gangrene is caused by interference with the cutaneous blood supply of the scrotum. It may result from any one of several causes: infected wounds; chemothermal or mechanical trauma without infection; any condition such as cardiorenal disease leading to scrotal edema; systemic diseases such as diabetes, which predispose to infection; and urinary extravasation with secondary infection.

Diagnosis is made by inspection. Gangrenous areas of skin show a purple, dark green or black discoloration. Treatment consists of appropriate antimicrobial therapy when there is complicating infection, together with excision of gangrenous tissues. Incision and drainage prove inadequate. After separation of the slough, skin grafting may be required.

Neoplasms

Neoplasms of the scrotum are extremely rare. Although a few benign tumors such as polyps, fibromas, adenomas, lipomas and hemangiomas have been reported, a malignant skin neoplasm, *chimney-sweeps' cancer*, holds chief clinical interest. It is occupational, being associated with prolonged exposure to bacterial or chemical products which contain carcinogens. Persons working in some metallurgic occupations are also prone to develop scrotal cancer. The exciting cause is prolonged contact with coal tar derivatives which emanate from lubricating oils rich in anthracene. The selective localization of these tumors to the scrotum is attributable to the voluminous number of sebaceous glands in the scrotal skin, coupled with the liposolubility of carcinogens in the lubricants.

Diagnosis is made by biopsy. Treatment consists of wide excision, with removal of one or both testicles and regional lymphadenectomy if indicated in advanced stages of the neoplasm. Radiation therapy has limited applicability.

TESTES

The testes are two ovoid, tunic-covered organs, suspended in the scrotum by the spermatic cord. At the upper pole of each is a· small pedunculated body, the appendix testis. The testes are enclosed in a dense fibrous capsule, the tunica albuginea, which forms into fibrous septa which penetrate the glandular structure, converging at the hilum. Between the septa are the spermatic tubules, which produce and conduct spermatozoa to the vasa efferentia and thence to the epididymis. Within the framework of the septa are the interstitial cells of Leydig. These cells elaborate an androgenic hormone which influences sexual development and activity. Posterolaterally, the testes are attached to the epididymides. Elsewhere, they are firmly covered by the tunica albuginea, which forms the visceral layer of their investment by the tunica vaginalis testis.

The blood supply to the testis is closely associated with that to the kidney because of the common embryonal origin of the two organs. The arteries to the testis, the internal spermatic, arise from the aorta below the renal artery. The venous return is through the pampiniform plexus of the spermatic cord to the spermatic vein. On the right, the spermatic vein enters the vena cava below the right renal vein; on the left, it empties into the renal vein. The longer blood column on the left, with its increased hydrostatic pressure, may be a participating cause of varicocele.

The lymphatic drainage from the testis is to the common iliac and lumbar lymph nodes, which in turn communicate with the mediastinal and supraclavicular chains, an anatomic arrangement intimately concerned with the spread of carcinoma of the testis.

The testicular nerves are from the aortic and renal plexuses by way of the spermatic cord. Because of the intimate connection of the spermatic, aortic and solar plexuses, abdominal pain may be produced by trauma to or acute infection of the testicle. For the same reason, testicular pain may be referred from acute abdominal and retroperitoneal conditions, such as acute appendicitis and rupture of an aortic aneurysm, and in the passage of a calculus through the ureter.

The testes have a twofold function, to produce spermatozoa and secrete male hormone. Derangement or impairment of one function may occur without affecting the other. One normal testis is adequate for this dual purpose.

Anomalies

Of the congenital anomalies of the testicle, anomalous location is the most frequent; cryptorchism much more so than ectopy. Absence of one or both testes or their duplication is a rare anomaly. Hypoplasia is unusual in the normally descended organ. The possible variations are listed in Tables 1 and 2.

CRYPTORCHISM. Cryptorchism, or undescended testicle, is the most common of all anomalies of the male reproductive system. The term connotes the existence of a hidden testicle. The location may be any place along the course of normal descent: intra-abdominal, inguinal or prepubic (Fig. 5). In many animals, the testes do not descend normally until after birth. In some, they descend only during the mating season; in others, they remain in the abdominal cavity at all times. In man, the testes usually descend between the eighth and ninth fetal months. However, an estimated 1 to 10 per cent of male infants

Table 1. *Anomalous Location of Testes*

Cryptorchism	Interrupted during descent	Abdominal Inguinal Prepubic
Ectopic	Vicarious excursion	Superficial inguinal Symphysial Penile Femoral Crural Perineal

are born with undescended testes. In half, the testes migrate into the scrotum spontaneously, most within the first year of life, a small number up to the time of puberty. They may be temporarily retracted from the scrotum by an active cremasteric reflex which is stimulated by cold or emotion.

The cause of cryptorchism is obscure. In less than 15 per cent of patients, it is the result of endocrine dysfunction, such as hypopituitarism. At one time, mechanical factors were considered to be the cause. In recent years, more emphasis has been given to an incapacity of the testis to respond to normal stimuli. The disclosures of testicular biopsy indicate that there is inherent testicular deficiency which may be the cause of arrested descent. Biopsy has shown that in undescended testes there is failure of tubular development which normally takes place after the age of ten years. This failure is observed even after orchiopexy.

The chief diagnostic signs of cryptorchism are absence of the testicle from the scrotum and underdevelopment of the empty scrotal sac. If these findings are complemented by the palpation of a testicle in the inguinal or prepubic region, the diagnosis is established. However, if the testicle is in the abdomen and cannot be palpated, cryptorchism must be differentiated from agenesis. As the testicle is palpated in the inguinal canal or abdomen,

Table 2. *Anomalies of Development of Testes*

In number	Deficient	Complete absence (bilateral anorchism) Lack of one (unilateral anorchism)
	Excess	Polyorchism
In size	Deficient Excess	Hypoplasia Hypertrophy
Abnormal position	Lower pole upward Posterior aspect anterior	Inversion Retroversion
Fusion anomaly	Synorchism	

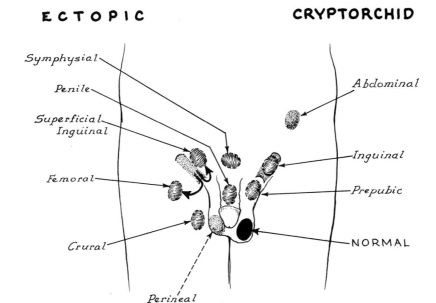

ECTOPIC **CRYPTORCHID**

Symphysial

Penile

Superficial Inguinal

Femoral

Crural

Abdominal

Inguinal

Prepubic

NORMAL

Perineal (behind scrotum)

Figure 5. Anomalous positions of testicle.

the patient may feel the typical sensation of the testicle being compressed. The examiner should have warm hands, make certain that the patient is fully relaxed, and conduct the examination as gently as possible.

It may prove difficult to differentiate the retractile testicle from true cryptorchism. Examination of the genitalia may be required on more than one occasion. It is difficult to palpate retractile testicles in obese sensitive boys. When the patient is relaxed it may be possible to milk the testicle into the scrotum. Having the patient sit in a tub of warm water may induce the retractile testicle to descend, a maneuver which cannot be accomplished with the undescended member. Once the testicle is palpated in the scrotum cryptorchism is ruled out.

In cryptorchism, androgens are secreted, but sperms are not produced. As a result, the adult with bilateral cryptorchism yields an azoospermatic ejaculate, although he has normal libido and potentia. Most adults with unilateral cryptorchism are normally fertile. The normal scrotal testis provides the sperm.

Pain in an undescended testicle usually signals the onset of some complication such as inguinal hernia, torsion of the spermatic cord, inflammation or neoplasm. The inguinal testis is relatively fixed and is more easily injured than the mobile scrotal testis.

In undescended testis, there is a higher rate of malignancy than in the scrotal testis. The abdominal testis is more vulnerable than the inguinal testis. Orchiopexy does not reduce the increased rate.

Since the processus vaginalis precedes the testis in its descent, it may reach the scrotum independently and remain patent, even when the testis remains in the abdominal cavity. The condition must be recognized at operation so that the sac can be obliterated and the danger of development of a hernia allayed.

For the treatment of cryptorchism, chorionic gonadotropin may be used in an attempt to produce descent; 500 to 1000 units given parenterally twice weekly for six weeks constitutes a fair trial. If there is hypothyroidism, thyroid extract should be given in doses commensurate with the degree. In assessing the value of hormonal therapy, it must be recognized that normal descent may take place up to the time of puberty.

If descent fails to occur spontaneously or following hormonal therapy, three alternatives are possible: continued observation, orchiopexy or orchiectomy. The stated objectives of treatment are to produce fertility, to eliminate a potential focus of malignant degeneration, to correct an associated inguinal hernia, and for cosmetic effect. Unfortunately, operation does not reduce the incidence of carcinoma. One advantage is that, after orchiopexy, the testis is in a better location for observation to detect the earliest changes of malignancy.

In attempting to promote spermatogenesis, some advise that orchiopexy be performed before the patient reaches the age of five years; others think that ten years is sufficiently early. Still others maintain that operation never promotes spermatogenesis and cite the presence of an associated inguinal hernia as the only indication for operation.

Most surgeons believe that orchiectomy is indicated at the time of operation when it is found that it is not possible to bring an undescended testis into the scrotum, providing the opposite testis is normal and located in the scrotum.

ECTOPIC TESTIS. In rare instances, the testicle lies outside its line of normal descent. Vicarious excursion usually takes place after the testicle has emerged from the inguinal canal. The most common site is in the superficial inguinal region; less common are the subcutaneous tissues of the perineal and femoral regions. The penile position is extremely rare.

Diagnosis is made by palpating the ectopic testis in its anomalous position. The testis should be placed in the scrotum by a surgical procedure.

Trauma

Because of their mobility and the protection afforded by the pelvic arch, the testes are seldom injured. Occasionally, straddle or perforating injuries lead to contusion, laceration, puncture or dislocation. Extravasation of blood may cause infarction and atrophy of the testis. Trauma to the testicle, even mild, may cause excruciating pain, nausea, vomiting, faintness and shock. On rare occasions, a severe blow to the scrotum dislocates the testicle into the abdomen, the subcutaneous tissues of the penis or the perineum. Diagnosis is made on the basis of the history and local signs of injury. Operation is indicated for evacuation of blood and to replace the dislocated organ. Penetrating wounds require suture of the tunica albuginea and scrotal lacerations. When irreparably damaged, the testicle should be removed. This avoids such complications as gangrene, atrophy and infection.

Torsion of the appendix testis is primarily a prepubertal condition. The cause is unknown. It leads to exquisite testicular pain and tenderness on palpation. In the early stages, the diagnosis can sometimes be established by palpation of the tiny indurated body; later, with edema, diagnosis may not be made until operation. The condition is frequently mistaken for torsion of the spermatic cord or acute epididymitis.

The important aspect of management of torsion of the testis is its distinction from torsion of the spermatic cord which is the outstanding surgical emergency of the scrotal contents. In any doubtful situation, immediate exploratory operation is indicated. The proper treatment for torsion of the appendix testis is excision of the appendage.

Infections

In contrast to the epididymis, which is usually invaded by pyogenic bacteria, the testis is usually invaded by viruses. Bacterial orchitis almost always represents an extension from infection of the epididymides. Only in rare instances, as during bacteremia, do metastatic foci develop in the testis without first infecting the epididymis.

Of the infections, mumps orchitis is most frequent. It rarely develops before puberty, but complicates epidemic parotitis in one-fifth of male patients beyond the age of puberty. It begins four to six days after the onset of parotitis, in most instances is unilateral and causes fever.

Physical examination reveals an enlarged, tender testis. Differentiation is made from acute epididymitis by a lack of induration in the epididymis, and a sharp sulcus dividing the testis from an inflamed epididymis. The testicle is not elevated, as it is in torsion of the spermatic cord. Clinical evidence of parotitis, or of systemic viral infection, aids the diagnosis. Less common than mumps orchitis is that which complicates smallpox, varicella, measles, influenza and dengue fever.

Prophylaxis consists of keeping patients with viral infections in bed during the acute illness. The scrotum should be elevated and either warm or cold applications used to relieve pain. Estrogens and cortisone have been used with some favorable results. Infiltration of the spermatic cord with a local anesthetic agent is said to accelerate the course.

Although the testis retains its hormonal function following viral orchitis, in approximately one-third of the patients, the tubules undergo atrophy and spermatogenesis is terminated.

Tuberculous orchitis is usually secondary to tuberculous epididymitis. Syphilitic orchitis has been rendered a medical curiosity by the modern treatment of syphilis.

Neoplasms

Fortunately, tumors of the testis are uncommon, for they are one of the most dangerous forms of malignancy in the male. The onset is insidious, growth is rapid and early metastasis is frequent. Whereas nearly all tumors of the epididymis are benign, practically all tumors of the testis are malignant. Testicular neoplasms comprise from 1 to 2 per cent of all malignant tumors and account for about 3 per cent of the malignant conditions of the male urogenital tract. Although their age range is from infancy to old age, most are found in patients during the ages of greatest sexual activity, 20 to 40 years.

Indicted by many as a cause, injury has nothing to do with initiating a testicular neoplasm. It may call attention to an existing tumor. The cryptorchid testis is more likely to be the site of a neoplasm than is a normally descended gonad. If the patient has bilateral cryptorchid testes and carcinoma in one, there is such a high incidence of carcinoma in the opposite testis that bilateral orchiectomy is justified.

Testicular neoplasms are best grouped into germinal and nongerminal tumors.

Germinal tumors arise from totipotent sex cells capable of reproducing any of the tissue derived from the three primary germ layers. The following classification is based on the experience of the Armed Forces Institute of Pathology:

Pure seminoma is of relatively low malignancy. Thirty-five to 50 per cent of germinal tumors are pure seminomas. The neoplasm replaces the testis with a firm, uniform mass. On section, it bulges as a homogeneous grayish white structure. Microscopically, it consists of uniform, closely packed round or polyhedral cells with clear cytoplasm and hyperchromatic nuclei. This tumor has a low incidence of metastases; with proper treatment the prognosis is good.

Embryonal carcinoma, pure or with seminoma, comprises 30 to 35 per cent of germinal tumors. Grossly smaller than seminomas, they usually replace only part of the testis. The histologic pattern is myriad. It may be completely undifferentiated, with large pleomorphic anaplastic cells with irregular nuclei and numerous mitotic figures. Areas of hemorrhage and necrosis are frequent.

Teratoma, pure or with seminoma, comprises about 10 per cent of germinal tumors. They vary considerably in size. The cut surface is usually honeycombed. Cartilage and bone are sometimes identified. Microscopically, various tissues, including squamous epithelium, gastrointestinal or respiratory epithelium, thyroid, smooth muscle, cartilage and lymphoid tissue are seen.

Teratoma with embryonal carcinoma or choriocarcinoma with or without seminoma comprises about 32 per cent. These tumors vary considerably in size; the tumor usually replaces a large portion of the testis. Microscopically, a combination of adult teratoma, embryonal carcinoma or choriocarcinoma is seen.

Choriocarcinoma, pure with seminoma or with embryonal carcinoma, comprises about 10 per cent of germinal tumors. They are among the most malignant of all human cancers. Metastases are frequently present at the time of diagnosis. The tumor may be so small that the external surface of testis may appear normal. The microscopic appearance resembles chorioepithelioma seen in the uterus; closely packed trophoblasts with clear cytoplasm and uniform nuclei, and containing typical syncytial trophoblasts with large multinucleated cells with deep eosinophilic vacuolated cytoplasm and many irregular dark-staining nuclei. Despite treatment prognosis is poor.

The nongerminal neoplasms include interstitial cell tumor, also known as Leydig cell tumor, and androblastoma. They comprise 4 to 5 per cent of all testicular tumors, which also include stromal tumors, lymphomas, reticulum sarcomas and plasmacytomas. Interstitial cell tumors produce hormones which cause virilism and precocious puberty in children. In adults, they may produce impotence and gynecomastia. Androblastomas are homologous with ovarian arrhenoblastomas and may produce feminization of the male.

Early diagnosis of testicular neoplasms is difficult because of a lack of symptoms. Despite the relatively exposed position of the testicle, patients may be unaware of the tumor for a long time. The initial symptom is usually a painless swelling in the scrotum. With further growth, a dull, dragging sensation develops. In the later stages, an abdominal mass, representing metastatic lesions in the lymph nodes, may be noted. Gynecomastia has occurred in patients unaware of any testicular swelling, as a result of hormonal secretion by the tumor.

Not infrequently, the first manifestation of a testicular neoplasm arises from a metastatic lesion, such as hemoptysis from pulmonary metastasis. Dissemination is commonly by way of lymph channels, although the blood also may be responsible, especially in the more malignant types (Fig. 6). Metastatic lesions tend to advance rapidly. Sometimes, the cellular pattern of the metastatic lesion differs from that of the primary neoplasm. Since lymphatic drainage from the testicle is periaortic, rather than to the inguinal lymph nodes, extension is to the periiliac and thence to the periaortic lymphatics. The metastasis tends to skip glands and to cross to the opposite side. Involvement of the glands surrounding the renal pedicle causes displacement of the kidney and upper portion of the ureter. Spread may be as high as the mediastinum and supraclavicular lymph chains. The thoracic duct and its surrounding lymphatics are frequently involved. Bloodborne metastasis is commonly to the lungs and the liver.

The size of the primary tumor bears no close correlation with the time of onset or multiplicity of metastatic lesions. Many neoplasms one centimeter or less in diameter may spread to other organs. In some patients, the primary growth is discovered only after metastatic lesions appear; others come to necropsy before the true nature of the metastasis becomes known.

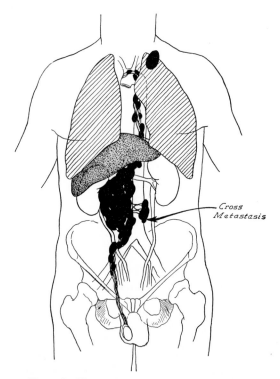

Figure 6.   Metastatic areas, carcinoma of testis.

In examination of the external genitalia, it is important to determine whether any scrotal mass lies in the testis or in the epididymis, since enlargement of the epididymis is usually benign. The typical characteristic of a testicular neoplasm is a stony-hard mass of increased weight confluent with the structure of the testis. Although tumors are rarely painful, the fact that tenderness is present does not rule out a neoplasm. Occasionally, a tumor coexists with epididymitis. Increased vascularity of the scrotum and invasion of the spermatic cord are late signs. With extensive lymphatic involvement, there may be edema of the lower extremities.

Auxiliary diagnostic studies are x-rays of the chest and intravenous urograms. The former discloses pulmonary metastasis; the latter, displacement of the kidney or ureter by enlarged periaortic lymph nodes (Fig. 6). The urine should be examined for chorionic gonadotropin since this hormone is excreted in many testicular tumors. It is most marked in choriocarcinoma, less so in embryonal carcinoma and seminomas; it usually does not occur in the teratoid group. Since hormonal tests may be negative in all types of tumor, their value in this diagnosis is limited.

Lymphangiography and phlebography of the inferior vena cava provide evidence of lymph node involvement and caval obstruction by metastatic nodes.

Testicular neoplasms have been mistaken for hydrocele, spermatocele, hematocele, epididymitis, torsion of the spermatic cord and orchitis. If hydrocele is present, aspiration of the fluid permits better examination of the testis. Whenever the nature of an intrascrotal enlargement is doubtful, operation should be performed.

Exploratory operation is performed through an inguinal incision. After occluding the spermatic cord with a noncrushing clamp at the internal inguinal ring, the testis is gently delivered into the wound and examined. Biopsy and frozen tissue examination are made if the diagnosis cannot be made by gross inspection. If the diagnosis of neoplasm is established, the testicle is removed by amputating the spermatic cord at the level of the internal ring.

Further definitive treatment is predicated upon the microscopic findings. Radical retroperitoneal lymph node dissection or radiation of these areas may be selected. For pure seminomas which are highly radiosensitive, radical retroperitoneal lymph node dissection is not indicated (Fig. 7). Pure choriocarci-

```
* * * *  SEMINOMA
            600 to 800 r
            (1000 r adequate dosage)
   * *   CARCINOMA
            2000 to 3000 r
    *    CHORIOEPITHELIOMA
            5000 to 6000 r
Lethal dose for mature TERATOMA cannot
be reached with safety.
```

Figure 7. Radiosensitivity of testicular neoplasms.

nomas metastasize by way of the blood, and radical lymph node dissection is not advisable.

Radiation therapy is usually directed to the iliac, umbilical, epigastric, lumbar and lower dorsal regions. The umbilical area is of greatest importance because it is the region most commonly involved with metastases. Supervoltage therapy is now used extensively in this country. For pure seminomas 2000 to 3800 r is considered the optimum tumor dose. For relatively radioresistant tumors, including embryonal carcinoma and teratocarcinoma, 4500 to 6000 r is needed. With the use of linear accelerator and cobalt-60 sources, serious complications have not been encountered.

Several studies indicate that radical retroperitoneal lymph node dissection and radiation should be done for all germinal tumors except pure seminomas and choriocarcinomas. A long incision is made from the xiphoid process to the pubis. Lymph nodes, connective tissue and fat are stripped from above the renal veins bilaterally, the renal arteries and veins are cleared to the kidney hila, lymph node–bearing tissues are stripped from the anterior surface of the aorta and vena cava, and dissection is carried out between the aorta and vena cava. A block dissection is then made down either side of the aorta and vena cava, extending laterally for 4 to 5 cm. on each side, down to the branching of the common iliac arteries. The average number of lymph nodes removed by this method is less than 75 per cent of the total lymph nodes present in the area. Mortality and morbidity following radical retroperitoneal lymph node dissection are slight. If no positive lymph nodes have been recovered, many urologists withhold radiation therapy. When positive lymph nodes are found, radiation therapy is given and the mediastinal area is included.

Chemotherapy has been used in palliation of recurrent or advanced tumors. In 5 per cent, complete disappearance of tumors has occurred.

Prognosis depends largely upon the type of neoplasm. Teratomas without malignant elements can be cured by orchiectomy alone. Seminomas respond well to orchiectomy and deep x-ray therapy. Embryonal carcinomas and teratocarcinomas have a higher mortality rate, and chorioepitheliomas are the most malignant. As a general rule, decrease in the chorionic gonadotropic hormone indicates removal or regression of chorionic tumor tissue; increase means spread of the disease. However, after operation, negative hormonal tests are occasionally noted in the presence of widespread metastasis.

EPIDIDYMIDES

The epididymides are a pair of crescentic structures composed of tremendously coiled ducts. They lie posterolateral to the testes, to which the rete testis provides communication. The appendix epididymis is a small, pedunculated body attached to the upper pole. The elongated upper end of each epididymis, termed the globus major, is flattened against the testis; the body comprises the midportion; the lower end, the globus minor, gives rise to the vas deferens. An infection in the globus minor may seal off the spermatic ducts, causing sterility of the involved testis.

In addition to providing conduits, the epididymides contribute to the maturation of spermatozoa. Spermatozoa first become motile after passage through the head of the epididymis. However, the fertilizing capacity of spermatozoa recovered from the head is low; those recovered from the body or tail are more fertile.

The epididymal epithelium is under the control of hormones produced by the Leydig cells of the testis. Deterioration of the Leydig cells causes involution of the epididymal epithelium. Spermatozoa passing through defective epithelium fail to mature in the normal manner. In addition to its stimulative role, the epididymis serves as a way-station for the storing of spermatozoa.

The arterial supply to the epididymis comes from the internal spermatic artery and the artery of the vas deferens. The venous drainage is through the pampiniform plexus into the spermatic vein. The lymphatics drain into the external iliac and hypogastric lymph nodes.

Anomalies

The most usual anomaly is found in the epididymis which lies anterior rather than posterior to the testis. Lack of fusion between the epididymis and testis has been reported. Congenital absence of the epididymis is extremely rare.

Trauma

Injuries of the epididymis accompany trauma to the testis. Differential diagnosis is made at operation. Clinical recognition and treatment are similar to those of injury of the testis.

Infection

Epididymitis is the most common disease of the scrotal contents and is relatively frequent in males of all ages. It may be nonspecific, gonococcal or tuberculous.

NONSPECIFIC EPIDIDYMITIS. Nonspecific epididymitis is commonly a sequel to prostatitis and posterior urethritis. The usual pathway of invasion is retrograde extension through the lumen of the vas deferens. Any bacteria which invade the urinary tract may thus cause epididymitis. Hematogenous spread, from a distant focus of infection, is rare.

Acute epididymitis. Acute epididymitis is a fulminating process manifest by diffuse cellulitis with swelling and edema. The inflammation usually arises in the tail of the epididymis and thereafter involves the entire organ. The chief symptoms are pain and swelling. There is frequently a prodromal ache in the inguinal region or discomfort along the spermatic cord. Chills, fever, headache, nausea and vomiting may occur with more virulent infection.

Diagnosis is established by gently palpating the enlarged, exquisitely tender epididymis. An important physical sign is detection of the sulcus between the enlarged epididymis and the testis. Involvement of the vas deferens by coincident vasitis contributes evidence of epididymitis. The spermatic cord may be thickened by edema. Hydrocele may develop secondary to infection. Specific diagnosis is made by identifying the bacteria present in a urethral discharge or in the urine. Digital rectal examination should be performed to learn whether there is coincident prostatitis or seminal vesiculitis. Palpation must be gentle to avoid producing bacteremia and dissemination of the genital infection.

In making a differential diagnosis, it is important to rule out torsion of the spermatic cord or of the testicular appendages. Elevation of the scrotum usually relieves the pain of epididymitis but not of torsion. In torsion of the spermatic cord, the testicle lies high in the scrotum. When examination is unsatisfactory because of exquisite tenderness, injection of the spermatic cord with 1 per cent Xylocaine will facilitate the procedure. The physical findings in trauma to the testicle may simulate those of acute epididymitis, but the history of injury and the absence of a urethral discharge or pyuria aid in differentiation. Other conditions which may be confused with acute epididymitis are strangulated inguinal hernia, tumor of the testis with thrombosis, virus orchitis and hematocele of the tunica vaginalis testis. When doubt exists, diagnosis is established by operation.

Treatment consists of prompt administration of the appropriate antimicrobial agent, and elevation and immobilization of the scrotum. The patient with acute epididymitis should be kept in bed until fever subsides, in order to help limit spread of the infection.

Epididymitis secondary to operation on the prostate has been largely eliminated by performing bilateral vasectomy before or at the time of prostatectomy.

Abscess formation may follow resolution of acute epididymitis. This is more usual in tuberculous epididymitis. The abscess may extend into the testis. Some drain spontaneously when surgical measures are delayed.

Chronic epididymitis. Chronic epididymitis is usually a sequel of acute epididymitis, but at times arises insidiously as a subacute process giving rise to little pain or discomfort. In chronic infection, the organ is thickened and slightly enlarged. It may or may not be tender. Differential diagnosis must be made from tumor of the testis by carefully palpating the testicle to be certain that any induration is confined to the epididymis. Since the two may occur together, whenever there is a coincident mass in the testis, operation is indicated to learn the true state of affairs.

Nonspecific epididymitis is treated by eliminating the source of the infection, usually a prostatic infection. In such cases, vasectomy usually prevents acute exacerbations. If chronic epididymitis causes persistent pain, epididymectomy is indicated. Administration of antimicrobial agents is usually fruitless. Epididymovasostomy, with anastomosis of the vas to the upper part of the epididymis, may be performed in patients with bilateral occlusion of the globus minor, as from fibrosis. This short-circuiting operation does not always restore patency, however, and sperm from the head of the epididymis is usually immature.

GONOCOCCAL EPIDIDYMITIS. This formerly was a common complication of gonococcal urethritis. With the reduced incidence of gonorrhea, it is now rare. The infection nearly always results from improper treatment of anterior gonococcal urethritis, allowing extension to the posterior urethra and thence down the vas deferens to the epididymis. The lesions and symptoms of both acute and chronic gonococcal epididymitis are similar to those of nonspecific epididymitis, with one significant difference. With resolution of the acute inflammation, the tissues affected by the gonococcal process are more likely to be replaced by scar tissue which occludes the epididymal tubules. If this is bilateral, sterility results. Scar tissue, easily palpable, causes permanent induration in the globus minor of the epididymis.

TUBERCULOUS EPIDIDYMITIS. The epididymis is one of the common sites of urogenital tuberculosis. The incidence of epididymitis is highest in patients from 20 to 45 years old, and is usually secondary to tuberculous prostatitis or seminal vesiculitis. Extension is usually by way of the vas deferens; less commonly, it spreads by means of the blood from a distant focus, for example in the lungs or kidneys. Tuberculous epididymitis usually presents as an indurated enlargement of the organ. Upon palpation, nodularity and thickening are noted, a process which may involve the vas deferens. There is usually little tenderness, despite considerable involvement of the epididymis. In advanced cases, caseation takes place. The process may then involve the subcutaneous tissues and the skin, causing edema, ulceration and fistula formation. The testis is invaded late, being relatively immune to the tubercle bacillus. Secondary infection may take place, giving rise to all the manifestations of acute nonspecific epididymitis.

With respect to diagnosis, the history and presence of tuberculosis elsewhere, particularly in the urogenital tract, should suggest tuberculosis. Proof is obtained by isolating tubercle bacilli in the urine, spermatic fluid, or discharge from a sinus, and, with surgical exploration, by microscopic examination of the tissue. In chronic cases, calcification may be noted on x-ray of the scrotum. Differential diagnosis must be made between nonspecific epididymitis, coccidiodomycosis and tumor of the testis or epididymis.

If the lesion is not far advanced, chemotherapy and general measures directed to tuberculosis elsewhere in the body may suffice. If there is caseation and particularly if there is scrotal fistula, operation is indicated, excising the vas deferens, epididymis and involved tissues of the scrotum.

Neoplasms

Tumors of the epididymis are extremely rare and, in contrast to testicular neoplasms, most are benign. These include angioma, myoma, leiomyoma, adenomatoid tumors and dermoid cysts. Examination demonstrates a firm mass in the epididymis, which does not transilluminate. Tumors may be mistaken for tuberculous epididymitis. The precise diagnosis will seldom be made without microscopic examination of tissue. Malignant neoplasms of the epididymis are chiefly adenocarcinoma, although occasionally a sarcoma is present. Since these tumors grow rapidly, and frequently invade the testis, they may be mistaken for testicular neoplasm. The testicle should be removed, followed by radiation. The prognosis is usually poor.

Miscellaneous Conditions

A spermatocele consists of a diverticulum of the epididymis (Fig. 8, a). It is a single or multilocular cystic structure communicating with the vasa efferentia. It contains a cloudy fluid usually found to be teeming with motile spermatozoa. The typical spermatocele is a small, cystic, nontender, spherical mass which transilluminates, usually attached to the upper pole of the epididymis. Usually, the condition is asymptomatic and discovered as an incidental finding on examination of the scrotal contents. One to 2 per cent of all adult males have spermatoceles. They are most common from ages 30 to 50. Treatment is not indicated unless the spermatocele attains considerable size and causes pain, in which case excision is indicated. The differential diagnosis lies chiefly between various types of hydrocele, or the rare epididymal neoplasm. The cystic consistency of the mass and the

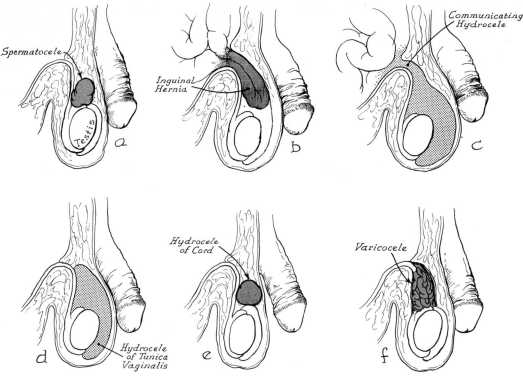

Figure 8.   Common lesions causing a mass in the scrotum.

characteristic of transillumination establish the diagnosis. Aspiration of the spermatocele yields fluid containing spermatozoa. However, this procedure is followed by recurrence and there is the hazard of producing hemorrhage and infection.

Sperm granulomas result from escape of spermatozoa from their normal intratubular habitat into surrounding interstitial tissue. They usually occur at the globus minor of the epididymis or at the site of surgical vasectomy. A foreign body reaction results in a sterile inflammatory process with the development of a granulomatous mass 1 to 2 cm. in diameter. Tenderness may be present. The condition may be confused with tuberculosis of the vas or epididymis. In doubtful cases, excision of the mass provides the correct diagnosis and treatment.

TUNICA VAGINALIS TESTIS

The tunica vaginalis testis is a pouch formed by two layers of connective tissue. It is a remnant of the peritoneal prolongation into the scrotum. The visceral layer covers most of the epididymis and is firmly attached to the tunica albuginea testis. The parietal layer forms the outer covering. A secretion from the cells of the endothelial lining lubricates the space between the two. When excess fluid accumulates, a hydrocele is produced. Although the processus vaginalis is usually open at birth, it closes within the first month in most infants.

Anomalies

When the processus vaginalis fails to close, and remains patent in its course through the inguinal canal and spermatic cord, it predisposes to an indirect hernia and to communicating hydrocele. The diagnosis of an inguinal hernia is made on the basis of physical signs (Fig. 8, *b*). The scrotal mass is soft, compressible, usually reducible and does not transilluminate. Auscultation may disclose peristaltic sounds or gurgling from intestinal contents. The presence of a communicating hydrocele is not usually distinguished from a hydrocele of the tunica vaginalis testis, until at operation a communication with the peritoneal cavity is found (Fig. 8, *c*).

Trauma

Injury of the tunica vaginalis is nearly always caused by a blow to the scrotum. The response of the tunica may be the production of a large serous effusion known as a traumatic hydrocele (Fig. 8, *d*). If the cavity becomes filled with blood, it is known as hematocele. A scrotal hematoma is a collection of blood in tissues outside the tunica. Acute hydrocele is similar to idiopathic hydrocele. Spontaneous hematocele has been observed in arterial disease such as arteriosclerosis and in blood dyscrasias such as purpura. Traumatic lesions may or may not be painful.

Hematocele does not transilluminate. The blood may be under such tension that the surface feels stony hard and heavy, findings similar to those in tumor of the testis. The treatment of hematocele is surgical evacuation of the blood with excision or reflection of the tunica. Usually, the diagnosis of hematocele is evident because of the history of trauma. In addition to tumor of the testis, differential diagnosis must be made from torsion of the spermatic cord and acute epididymitis.

Hydrocele

Hydrocele is the term applied to an abnormal accumulation of serous fluid between the two layers of the tunica vaginalis testis (Fig. 8, *d*). Most hydroceles are idiopathic.

Congenital hydrocele is caused by failure of obliteration of the processus vaginalis testis. It is continuous with the peritoneal cavity and may be referred to as a communicating hydrocele (Fig. 8, *c*). Sometimes, there is an associated inguinal hernia. Spontaneous closure of the processus vaginalis occasionally takes place during infancy, rarely in older children, with disappearance of the hydrocele.

Acquired hydrocele may be secondary to any type of epididymitis or orchitis or to scrotal trauma. It may also be associated with a tumor of the testis.

Hydrocele of the spermatic cord results from a sealing off of the processus vaginalis above and below the accumulation of fluid (Fig. 8, *e*).

Hydrocele is one of the most common causes of scrotal swelling. Small hydroceles are asymptomatic and go unrecognized by the patient. With large accumulations of fluid, the prevailing complaint is of a mass in the scrotum, sometimes with a dragging sensation. Occasionally, hydroceles attain such tremendous size as to interfere with walking and sexual intercourse.

The diagnosis is made on the basis of a symmetrical, cystic mass which is not tender. Hydrocele of the tunica vaginalis testis is confluent with the testis which is observed posterolaterally on transillumination of the scrotum. In hydrocele of the spermatic cord, the testicle is felt apart from the cystic mass and in large hydrocele is displaced to the base of the scrotum.

A hydrocele of long standing may evoke fibrous tissue or calcification in the wall. It may fail to transmit light and thus be mistaken for neoplasm or hematocele. Elephantiasis of the scrotum is easily differentiated, because the scrotal edema is bilateral and unaccompanied by a cystic mass within the scrotum.

Small hydroceles require no treatment. Those observed in infants and secondary to epididymitis may recede spontaneously. Whereas aspiration and injection of a sclerosing material has been attended with some success, this method of treatment may lead to infection and hemorrhage; it is not recommended. The parietal tunica vaginalis testis should be excised, or reflected behind the testicle to prevent the reaccumulation of fluid. In addition to yielding a permanent cure, operation affords accurate examination of the scrotal contents for any associated hernia, tumor or other abnormality.

SPERMATIC CORD

The spermatic cord is composed of the vas deferens, the artery of the testis, the epididymis, the pampiniform plexus, the lymphatics and the autonomic nervous supply. In addition, there may be a patent or partially obliterated processus vaginalis, which may lead to inguinal hernia or hydrocele of the cord.

The vas deferens extends from the epididymis to the inguinal canal and, thence, retroperitoneally to an ampulla before it joins the outlet of the seminal vesicle to form the ejaculatory duct.

It provides a passageway for spermatozoa. Its narrow lumen is surrounded by a layer of longitudinal muscle fibers which contract to convey sperm. The ampulla serves as a receptacle for sperm until it is expelled.

In partial vasectomy for sterilization purposes, or to prevent retrograde infection from the prostate and urethra to the epididymis, a small segment of each vas is excised in the upper part of the scrotal extent. Reanastomosis of the vas may be performed to restore fertility. This operation is successful in a high percentage of patients, even after many years of interruption.

Anomalies

Anomalies of the vas deferens consist either of an absence or aplasia of the structure which, if bilateral, accounts for isolated cases of sterility. These are an occasional accompaniment of renal agenesis or hypoplasia.

Torsion

Torsion of the spermatic cord is an axial rotation, a twisting of the cord upon itself. The rotation may be only a quarter turn, but as many as five complete turns have been reported. Unrelieved, serious interference with the blood supply causes gangrene of the testicle (Fig. 9, *A*).

Atrophy of the testicle depends upon the length of time and degree to which the blood supply is reduced or terminated before operation is performed. In instances of complete strangulation, if the torsion is relieved within four hours, complete return of function may be anticipated. With partial strangulation up to 12 hours is probably the upper limit of safety. Of 500 patients reported up to 1963, 90 per cent of the involved testes were lost, 80 per cent by orchiectomy, and 10 per cent by subsequent atrophy. Delay, for a variety of reasons, including wrong initial diagnosis, was the main reason for this loss. The most frequent misdiagnosis was epididymitis. If the results are to be improved, it is important that parents, emergency room doctors, pediatricians and surgeons realize the urgent need for immediate correction of the abnormality.

The condition is almost limited to boys nearing the age of puberty. It may occur in the cryptorchid testis, as well as in the normally descended gonad. Although torsion is frequently attributed to a laxness of the tunica vaginalis testis, this is not always pres-ent. Torsion may take place within the tunica vaginalis or outside the tunica vaginalis.

Apparently, the lesion is produced by a violent contraction of the cremaster muscle. Sometimes, there is a history of strenuous physical activity, such as running or jumping, but in other instances, torsion develops as the patient lies quietly in bed.

Predisposing factors are low insertion of the fibers of the cremaster muscle; separation of the epididymis from the testis by an abnormally long mesorchium; loose areolar planes of fascia surrounding the testis and spermatic cord, and proximal extension of the tunica vaginalis around the spermatic cord.

Rarely, torsion corrects itself spontaneously. Some patients experience recurrent attacks. Since the condition is likely to be bilateral, when operation is performed to correct torsion on one side, it is advisable to also suture the opposite testicle in place.

The typical onset of torsion is manifest by exquisite testicular pain and swelling. Abdominal pain, nausea and vomiting are common accompaniments. Rotation of the spermatic cord leads to elevation of the testicle, a valuable diagnostic sign. When untreated, the local process continues to cause acute symptoms for two or three days, after which gangrene ensues with lessening of pain and relative anesthesia of the involved structures. Atrophy takes place over a period of several months.

A valuable diagnostic sign is that the testicle under torsion lies at a higher level than the normal organ. In assessing this sign, it is important to allow for the fact that the left testicle is normally at a lower level than the right. The chief error in differential diagnosis is to mistake torsion for acute epididymitis. In the latter condition, the urine usually contains pus cells and bacteria, and physical examination of the scrotum is of considerable help. In torsion, it is impossible to make out a sulcus, as one can between an enlarged, tender epididymis and an uninvolved testis. The entire testicle is exquisitely tender and is palpated as one boggy or indurated mass.

Torsion of the appendix epididymis and appendix testis must also be considered in differential diagnosis. These may twist on their pedicles, producing a similar but more localized and less violent reaction. Soon after it occurs, torsion of an appendage produces a tender, indurated nubbin at the upper pole of the testicle; later, scrotal edema obscures this sign.

Since examination may be extremely pain-

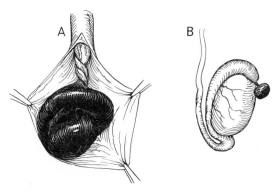

Figure 9.   *A*, Torsion of spermatic cord causing gangrene of testis and epididymis. *B*, Torsion of appendix testis.

ful in acute conditions, it is helpful to infiltrate the spermatic cord at the level of the external inguinal ring with a solution of 1 per cent Xylocaine. This relieves pain and makes it possible to palpate the structures in the scrotum. Aspiration of bloody fluid from the tunica vaginalis testis is a diagnostic sign of torsion. Blood is not present in epididymitis or orchitis. Whenever the diagnosis is in doubt, immediate exploratory operation is indicated. In torsion of the spermatic cord, immediate surgical correction offers the only hope of preserving the testicle.

In many patients, orchiectomy is necessary because of gangrene. After the torsion is relieved, the testis remains black and incision into the parenchyma excites no bleeding.

Whenever torsion is corrected, the testis is stitched in place by an anchor suture to prevent recurrence. The opposite testis is likewise fixed because the tendency to torsion is frequently bilateral.

Infection

Funiculitis, inflammation of the spermatic cord, is usually a complication of epididymitis or of vasitis. Acute funiculitis causes swelling of the cord with tenderness and induration. In chronic funiculitis, the cord may be edematous and increase of connective tissue may suggest a mistaken diagnosis of hernia. Infection of the vas deferens extends upward from concurrent epididymitis below, or downward from prostatic infection above. In the latter instance, if vasectomy has been performed, the process ends abruptly at the operative site, preventing extension to the epididymis. In acute vasitis there may be local tenderness, but this is mild in comparison to that in epididymitis. There is no febrile reaction from vasitis, as is usual in epididymitis. In chronic vasitis, the vas becomes fibrosed, beaded or nodular; the latter is common in tuberculosis.

Neoplasm

Tumors of the spermatic cord are usually secondary to tumors of the testis. Primary tumors of the vas deferens are extremely rare. A few have been observed, similar to those of the epididymis.

Varicocele

Varicocele is characterized by elongation, dilation and tortuosity of the veins of the pampiniform plexus, usually on the left side. Most varicoceles are idiopathic. They usually develop at the time of puberty, being observed in about 8 per cent of otherwise normal men. They usually persist throughout life unless corrected by operation.

Secondary varicocele results from obstruction to the spermatic vein. This may result from the growth of abdominal or retroperitoneal neoplasms, particularly tumors of the kidney.

Small varicoceles rarely cause symptoms. If large, they may give rise to scrotal and inguinal pain. This results from venous congestion or traction on the spermatic cord, produced by the weight of the varicocele.

Diagnosis is suspected on inspection, the wormlike configuration of the dilated veins being seen through the scrotal skin. This observation is confirmed by palpating enlarged, soft, dilated veins within the spermatic cord.

For asymptomatic varicocele, treatment is not indicated. When there is discomfort or pain, a snugly fitting scrotal suspensory may provide relief. Operation is indicated for large varicoceles which cause pain. The dilated segment of veins is excised, and the testicle suspended by suturing the distal stump to the external inguinal ring.

Infertility has been attributed to varicocele, through the mechanism of any interference with spermatogenesis is obscure. Improvement in the quality of semen has been observed in subfertile males who underwent varicocelectomy.

INGUINAL LYMPHATICS

The inguinal lymphatics warrant consideration since they are intimately concerned with many of the lesions of the penis and scrotum. There are three groups of superficial inguinal lymph nodes which lie above and external to the saphenous opening. A deep group is situated around the femoral vein at the level of the saphenous opening. The lymphatics of the shaft of the penis, the penile skin and scrotum drain into the superficial inguinal lymph nodes; those of the urethra into the deep inguinal and hypogastric nodes, and those from the glans penis to the external iliac nodes.

Inguinal Adenitis

Inguinal adenitis may be secondary to infections of the penis or scrotum. In an acute process, the nodes usually become enlarged and tender and the condition may progress to suppuration. In the chronic form, the nodes are discrete and painless. Suitable treatment of the local primary inflammation of the genitalia minimizes the development of secondary adenitis. Treatment of acute lymphadenitis consists of appropriate antimicrobial therapy, rest in bed and cold application to the affected areas. Chronic adenitis rarely requires treatment. Chancroidal bubo represents a lymphatic extension from a chancroid, usually on the penis. This lesion tends to suppurate and requires surgical drainage.

Granuloma Inguinale

Granuloma inguinale is a superficial ulcerative skin lesion with complicating inguinal adenitis. The etiologic agent is an intracellular monocystic Donovan body transmitted by sexual contact. Although the lesion is prevalent in tropical areas, it has a low incidence in the United States. It is seen more frequently in the southern states and in the Negro population. The lesion is essentially an indolent granuloma of the skin. There are usually multiple painless lesions. Advancing borders leave dense scars in their wake. Secondary infection is common. Diagnosis is made by finding the Donovan bodies in the smear of the exudate. Treatment consists of administration of streptomycin and tetracycline or their derivatives.

Lymphogranuloma Venereum

Lymphogranuloma venereum (lymphopathia venereum, lymphogranuloma inguinale) is a rare inguinal adenitis produced by a filtrable virus transmitted by sexual contact. Blockage of the inguinal lymphatics may cause elephantiasis of the penis and scrotum. Diagnosis is suggested by inguinal adenitis and fistulas from involved lymph nodes. Confirmation is made by the intradermal Frei test and complement-fixation test. Although tetracycline is useful in treatment, surgical excision of the involved areas is frequently required when there is secondary infection.

Metastatic Neoplasm

Neoplastic invasion of the inguinal lymph nodes is a common sequela of carcinoma of the penis and of the scrotum. Differential diagnosis between lymphadenitis and carcinomatous invasion can be established only by biopsy, since secondary infection is so frequent in carcinoma of the genitals.

Since the lymphatic drainage of the penis and urethra is not only to the inguinal nodes but also, by a separate route, to the hypogastric and iliac groups of the pelvis, excision of the inguinal nodes is insufficient if radical operation is to be performed for carcinoma of these organs.

INTERNAL GENITALIA

The internal genitalia are the prostate, seminal vesicles and Cowper's glands. Their function is to provide secretions for storage of spermatozoa and to convey them during copulation. It has been suggested that the prostate may produce a hormone, but the evidence is not convincing. Ninety-five per cent of a total volume of 2 to 4 ml. of spermatic fluid is provided by the prostate and seminal vesicles.

The function of the prostate and seminal vesicles is dependent upon stimulation by male hormone. Fructose, which is elaborated by the seminal vesicles, provides nutrient for spermatozoa. The survival of spermatozoa in ejaculated semen is largely dependent upon the amount of free sugar which is present.

PROSTATE

The prostate is a musculoglandular body surrounding the vesical neck (Fig. 10). Through its central portion, it transmits the posterior urethra; posteriorly, it is perforated by the ejaculatory ducts. These open into the verumontanum on the floor of the prostatic urethra. The normal prostate weighs about 20 gm. and is roughly pyramidal. It lies deep within the pelvic cavity below the symphysis pubis, being supported anteriorly by the puboprostatic ligaments and inferiorly by the urogenital diaphragm. In the embryo, the gland is derived from five epithelial evaginations of the posterior urethra, which form into compound alveolar glands and empty into ducts opening into the posterior urethra.

The prostatic glands consist of two groups which have functional differences and a separate embryologic origin. An anterior group is in intimate association with the urethra. These are known as the periurethral glands. In later life, they give rise to benign prostatic hyperplasia. A posterior group constitutes the main portion of the prostate and

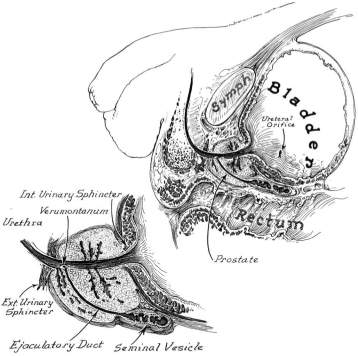

Int. Urinary Sphincter
Verumontanum
Urethra

Ext. Urinary
Sphincter

Ejaculatory Duct Seminal Vesicle

Symph
Bladder
Ureteral Orifice
Rectum
Prostate

Figure 10. Anatomy and relationships of prostate.

in later life provides the origin for carcinoma of the prostate.

The blood supply to the prostate is from the inferior vesical and internal pudendal arteries. The prostatic veins form plexuses about the sides of the gland and drain into the internal iliac veins. The nerves are derived from the pelvic plexus. The lymphatic drainage is into the nodes lying beside the external iliac and hypogastric blood vessels. There are intercommunications with the lymphatics of the bladder, seminal vesicles, vasa deferentia and rectum.

Anomalies

Of chief surgical interest are contracture of the vesical neck, valves of the posterior urethra, hypertrophy of the verumontanum, cysts of the prostate and müllerian duct cyst. The great danger is urinary obstruction, which may cause profound renal damage. The symptoms are similar to those of prostatic obstructions of later life. Treatment consists of surgical excision.

Trauma

Because of its protected position, the prostate is rarely injured. Injury may be caused by puncture or gunshot wounds and by inexpert urethral instrumentation. In severe injury, treatment consists of immediate repair to avoid urethral stricture and permanent damage to the adjacent external urinary sphincter.

Infections

Infections of the prostate comprise a large portion of the problems encountered in the practice of urology. In view of an intimate association with the urethra and the vasa deferentia, the prostate is prone to infection from either of these sources. Less commonly infection is by way of the blood, through the lymphatics or by direct extension.

NONSPECIFIC INFECTION. From a surgical standpoint, the chief importance of the nonspecific infections is their coincidence with obstructive lesions of the prostate. Any obstructive lesion predisposes to infection and, once infection is established, it usually cannot be eradicated without first removing the obstruction. Any of the common pyogenic bacteria may infect the prostate either alone or in combination. *Escherichia coli* and other gram-negative bacilli are the most common invaders.

Acute prostatitis. Acute prostatitis is an

inflammation of the prostatic parenchyma, inevitably complicated by posterior urethritis. Unless there is coincident obstruction, it may resolve without progression to chronic prostatitis or to abscess. In acute prostatitis, frequency and urgency of urination, nocturia and dysuria may be extreme. There may be hematuria and urethral discharge. The patient may complain of perineal aching or rectal or low back pain. Systemic symptoms of fever and, occasionally, chills occur. Inflammatory edema may lead to urinary retention. Digital examination reveals an exquisitely tender, enlarged prostate, usually firm. Examination of an acutely inflamed prostate should be most gentle. Massage may lead to epididymitis, bacteremia and severe systemic reaction.

Of chief importance in differential diagnosis is acute urinary infection, such as cystitis and pyelonephritis. The site of an acute infection is usually revealed by tenderness over the involved organ. Acute congestion of the prostate from retained secretion may lead to symptoms typical of prostatitis.

Treatment of acute prostatitis consists of appropriate antimicrobial agents selected according to the results of microscopic and cultural studies of the urine, urethral discharge and prostatic secretion. Instrumentation other than the passage of a small urethral catheter to relieve urinary retention is contraindicated during the acute phase. Continuous catheter drainage is preferable to repeated catheterization, which is more injurious to the urethra and prostate.

Chronic prostatitis. Chronic prostatitis is usually either a sequela to acute prostatitis, or occurs as a complication of some prostatic obstruction. The condition may be asymptomatic. A few men complain of an aching pain or fullness in the perineum, or of symptoms of mild vesical irritability. There may be a scant urethral discharge. Digital examination of the rectum may reveal a normal, boggy or indurated prostate. Epididymitis, either acute or chronic, may be a complication.

Diagnosis is established by the finding of pus cells, with or without bacteria, in the prostatic secretion. The chief error in differential diagnosis is in mistaking chronic, nonspecific urethritis for chronic prostatitis. The error is avoided by having the patient void prior to massage of the prostate. This removes any secretion from the urethra before prostatic secretion is expressed. Up to 5 per cent pus in the cellular elements of the prostatic

secretion is a normal finding. Cystitis may be confused with prostatitis. Diseases of the anus and rectum may cause urinary symptoms and lead to the mistaken diagnosis of prostatitis.

Treatment of chronic nonspecific prostatitis should be directed to any contributory cause such as an obstructive process. Antimicrobial therapy is usually ineffective. Occasionally, judicious prostatic massage is helpful. This should be carried out no oftener than once a week, or once every two weeks, with the most gentle manipulation. Frequent massage injures the prostate and induces acute infection. Massage is contraindicated in the presence of prostatic calculi. The rationale of prostatic massage is that it dislodges cellular exudates which obstruct the prostatic ducts and impede drainage. Sexual intercourse encourages drainage without injuring the prostate.

Granulomatous prostatitis is a multifocal, abacterial, inflammatory process. Extravasation of prostatic secretion from the glandular acini into the interstitial tissues initiates this histiocytic granulomatous reaction.

The striking clinical feature of the disease is that many times it is initially misdiagnosed as prostatic carcinoma. Digital rectal examination discloses irregular, stony hard induration of the prostate which suggests malignancy. This re-emphasizes the necessity for histologic confirmation before establishing the diagnosis of prostatic carcinoma.

The condition may be asymptomatic or may be ushered in with urgency and frequency of urination, or with a febrile course. The latter suggests that bacterial invasion may sometimes be the cause of escape of prostatic fluid into the parenchymatous tissues. When there are obstructive signs, as in the frequently associated benign prostatic hyperplasia, transurethral resection is the preferable method of treatment.

Trichomonas infestation of the prostate may produce symptoms and signs similar to nonspecific prostatitis. Diagnosis is established by identification of mobile trichomonas in a fresh drop of urine or prostatic secretion. Repeat examinations, culture and isolation of trichomonas of the sexual partner of suspects aid in making the diagnosis. Treatment consists of administration of oral metronidazole of both sexual partners.

Prostatic abscess. Prostatic abscess is an occasional complication of acute prostatitis. Sometimes, it can be recognized as a fluctuant area on rectal examination. Such an abscess may resolve, if small, or it may rupture spontaneously into the urethra. If not, prostatotomy becomes necessary. Symptomatic treatment consists of analgesics, hot sitz baths and bed rest. Fluids should not be forced unless an indwelling urethral catheter is in place, because frequent voiding causes irritation of the bladder and urethra.

Tuberculous prostatitis. Tuberculous prostatitis is usually secondary to tuberculosis of the kidney. The symptoms are generally overshadowed by the symptoms of involvement of the urinary tract: dysuria, frequency of urination and hematuria. On rectal examination, the prostate is found to be markedly indurated. It may be stony hard, suggesting carcinoma. However, in contrast to carcinoma, the condition usually occurs in the young. Differentiation is made by the finding of tubercle bacilli in the urine, and the recognition of tuberculosis elsewhere in the urogenital tract. Tuberculous prostatitis usually responds promptly to chemotherapy.

Prostatic Enlargement

Since the prostate completely surrounds the posterior urethra, any abnormality of this gland is a potential source of urinary obstruction. Some pathologic conditions are more likely to produce obstruction than others. Lesions such as benign hyperplasia progress slowly. Others, such as acute prostatitis, cause only temporary obstruction and still others, such as prostatic calculi, are less prone to cause obstruction. *Prostatism* is a clinical term which refers to the symptomatic and pathologic complex which results from any obstruction at the vesical neck. The symptoms and diagnostic measures are quite similar for the different lesions. The symptoms fall roughly into four groups.

The symptoms of mechanical obstruction are caused by encroachment on the vesical neck and by the reaction of the bladder to obstruction. Nocturia is usually the earliest symptom and, in most instances, serves as a rough index of the stage of a lesion. Less noticeable, but occurring with nocturia, are diurnal frequency of urination and a diminution in the size and force of the urinary stream. Later, there are hesitancy and dribbling on urination, urgency of urination and incontinence. Hematuria may be another symptom of obstruction. The force exercised during difficult urination incites bleeding. With the development of residual urine, the patient may note a mass low in the abdomen and have a feeling of incomplete emptying of the bladder. Complete obstruction may supervene.

When an obstruction is complicated by acute urinary infection, all previous symptoms exacerbate markedly.

In some instances, the symptoms of azotemia, secondary to hydronephrosis, are the first to call attention to a lower urinary obstruction.

Some patients with prostatic enlargement have increased potency; in others, it is diminished. As a general rule, decreased potency is a more frequent accompaniment of carcinoma of the prostate than of a benign lesion.

Obstructions to the vesical neck and posterior urethra impede the outflow of urine from the bladder. This leads to back-pressure changes in the bladder: hypertrophy of the trigone, trabeculation of the detrusor, and the formation of cellules and diverticula. During an initial stage of compensation, the capacity of the bladder becomes decreased to 250 ml. or less. Later, the kidney is destroyed by hydronephrosis caused by compression of the intramural portion of the ureter by the hypertrophied bladder musculature. Later, with decompensation, the bladder becomes widely distended, to 1000 ml. or more, and overflow incontinence results. Infection and the formation of calculi in the bladder are frequent complications.

As a part of the study of the patient with prostatic obstruction, kidney function tests are necessary to reveal whether there has been any impairment of renal function. Intravenous urograms are obtained, if renal function is adequate, to learn the condition of the kidneys, ureter and bladder. The after-voiding film will show residual urine without the danger of introducing infection, which accompanies catheterization.

BENIGN HYPERPLASIA OF PROSTATE. Of all obstructions which arise from the prostate, benign hyperplasia is the most common, occurring in over 50 per cent of men past the age of 50 years, and 75 per cent of those past 80 years of age. Although the cause of benign hyperplasia remains in doubt, some hormonal imbalance seems to be either a predisposing or aggravating factor. In contradistinction to carcinoma of the prostate, which arises from the prostatic cortex, benign hyperplasia arises from the glandular acini in the immediate vicinity of the mucosa of the prostatic urethra (Fig. 11). For this reason, it is more logically

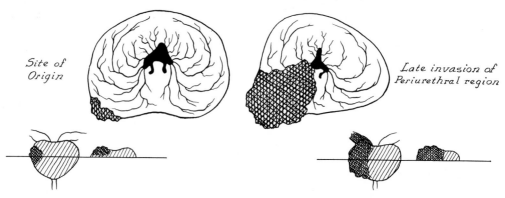

NORMAL PROSTATE

Periurethral Glands

True Prostatic Glands

BENIGN PROSTATIC HYPERPLASIA

False (surgical) Capsule

Anatomic Capsule

True Prostate compressed

CARCINOMA OF PROSTATE

Site of Origin

Late invasion of Periurethral region

Figure 11.   Site of origin of benign prostatic hyperplasia contrasted with that of carcinoma of prostate.

referred to as periurethral adenoma than benign prostatic hyperplasia. It is not a neoplasm, but is an overgrowth of normal glandular and muscular elements. As prostatic hyperplasia progresses, the true glands of the prostate are compressed peripherally. Between the two, a plane of cleavage develops, known as the surgical capsule, a plane which permits the surgeon to shell out a periurethral adenoma from within the prostate at open operation (Fig. 12).

Benign prostatic hyperplasia is referred to according to the location of hyperplastic glands. Median lobe and lateral lobe enlargements are the most common (Fig. 13). On rectal examination in lateral lobe hyperplasia, the gland is symmetrical and elastic throughout. In median lobe hyperplasia, the findings may be confined to the vesical side without detectable enlargement on digital rectal examination. A large median lobe enlargement with normal rectal findings is shown on intravenous urography in Figure 14. Other signs demonstrated by this test are thickening of the bladder wall, a "halo" surrounding the

media in the bladder, irregularity of the interior of the bladder due to trabeculation, and "fish-hooking" of the lower ends of the ureters as they are displaced upward by an enlarged prostate (Fig. 15).

Treatment of benign prostatic hyperplasia is surgical. Large adenomas should be removed by open operation; small adenomas by transurethral prostatectomy. In conservative prostatectomy, only enlargements within the prostate or at the vesical neck are removed (Fig. 16). The true prostate is left in place.

Conservative measures for treatment of benign hyperplasia, such as prostatic massage and passage of urethral sounds, have been abandoned. It was found that by their use there is danger of introducing infection or lighting up a latent infection. Nor has any drug or hormone proved effective in reducing the enlargement. Antibacterial drugs are useful in controlling infection until the obstruction is removed. Antispasmodics provide symptomatic relief.

MEDIAN BAR.   Next in frequency of occurrence of benign hyperplasia is median bar.

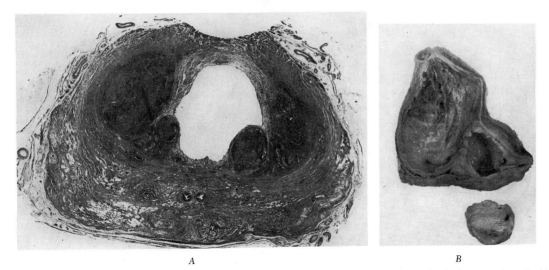

A   B

Figure 12. Surgical capsule between benign prostatic hyperplasia and compressed capsule. *A*, Cross section of mid-prostatic region showing spheroids of hyperplasia around urethra within true prostate. *B*, Hyperplasia enucleated from within rim of true prostatic tissue.

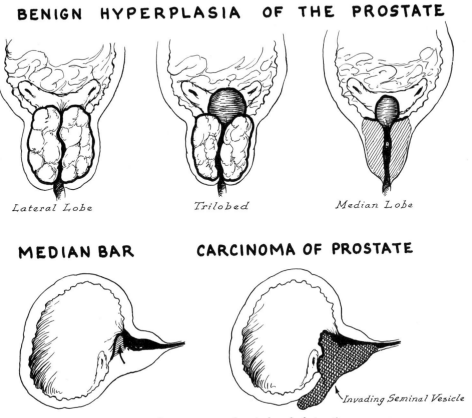

Figure 13. Common types of vesical neck obstruction.

This lesion develops in a younger age group than does benign hyperplasia of the prostate. The lesion is a fibromuscular elevation of the posterior vesical lip which distorts the normally smooth vesicourethral outlet. The bar is separate from the prostate. Although it has been said to be secondary to prostatitis, in most instances of median bar, prostatic tissue is normal. When a rim of fibrous tissue completely encircles the vesical neck, the condition is contracture of the vesical neck. This may be congenital or secondary to infection or to prostatectomy. The diagnosis of both these lesions is established by cystourethroscopy.

CARCINOMA OF PROSTATE.   Of the prostatic neoplasms, adenocarcinoma is the most common. It has been estimated that 15 per cent of all men over 50 years of age develop cancer of the prostate. However, many carcinomas are small and do not come to clinical recognition. Like most neoplasms, prostatic carcinoma has no known cause. It develops in the cortex of the prostate, whereas benign hyperplasia develops immediately around the urethra. Its progress is so slow that by the time it produces symptoms of obstruction to the outflow of urine, metastasis has occurred in many cases. Lesions amenable to surgical cure are

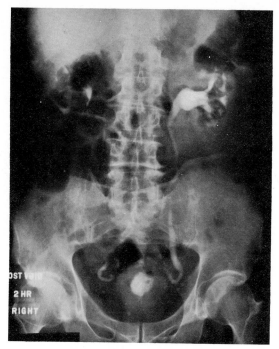

Figure 15. Signs of marked vesical neck obstruction shown on intravenous urography. Thickened bladder wall ("halo") surrounds contrast medium in the bladder; lower ends of ureters curve up ("fish-hooking" of ureters) owing to upward displacement by large benign hyperplasia of prostate. There is also mild left hydroureter and left hydronephrosis owing to early back pressure on the upper urinary tract.

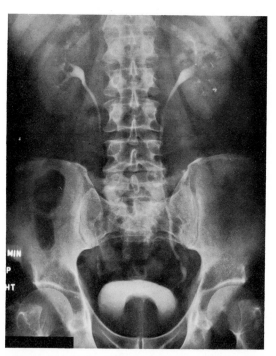

Figure 14. Median lobe prostatic hyperplasia, which projects into bladder shown on cystogram of intravenous urography. Prostate normal on digital rectal examination.

those discovered as incidental findings on routine rectal examination, or those that occur with benign prostatic hyperplasia which leads to their discovery. The earliest sign on rectal examination is a stony-hard area within the prostate. If it lies superficial to the rectal surface, palpation usually reveals irregularity. In advanced carcinoma, the prostate becomes fixed and there is asymmetric involvement of the entire gland. Typical areas of invasion are to the seminal vesicles, the base of the bladder and the membranous urethra.

Carcinoma of the prostate spreads both by way of the lymphatics and the blood, the latter giving rise to osseous metastasis most frequently in the lumbosacral spine, the bony pelvis and upper portions of the femur (Fig. 17).

A peculiar feature of prostatic tissue is the production of a large quantity of enzyme known as acid phosphatase. In the normal prostate, most of this enzyme drains into the urethra and is carried off in the urine, so that the blood level remains low. When enormous quantities are produced, the blood acid phosphatase level becomes elevated, indicating metastatic carcinoma of the prostate. Since the blood acid phosphatase in all metastatic carcinomas is not elevated, a negative finding does not rule out dissemination. A source of error in this test is in obtaining blood for examination within 48 hours of prostatic massage, a manipulation which will carry the enzyme into the blood stream from the normal prostate.

Differential diagnosis must be made from chronic prostatitis, either nonspecific or tuberculous, with fibrous tissue reaction which may similate the stony-hard induration of carcinoma. Also, areas of calcification or calculi may yield rectal findings suggestive of carcinoma. The ultimate diagnosis, particularly in early cases amenable to surgical cure, is made by biopsy. This is usually best accomplished after perineal exposure of the gland when tissue is examined by frozen section. If the diagnosis proves positive, immediate prostatovesiculectomy is carried out at the same time. In advanced cases, the diagnosis usually presents little difficulty. In addition to the typical rectal findings, there is frequent elevation of the blood acid phosphatase and osseous metastasis. However, even in advanced cases, it is important to establish the diagnosis with certainty before starting treatment. This can be done by needle biopsy through the perineum or rectum, or by transurethral resection of tissue. Transurethral resection is frequently indicated in patients with carcinoma because of associated benign prostatic hyperplasia which is not affected by hormonal therapy.

The only proved cure for prostatic carcinoma is total prostatovesiculectomy (Fig. 18). This is applicable to no more than 5 per cent of patients at the time of clinical recognition.

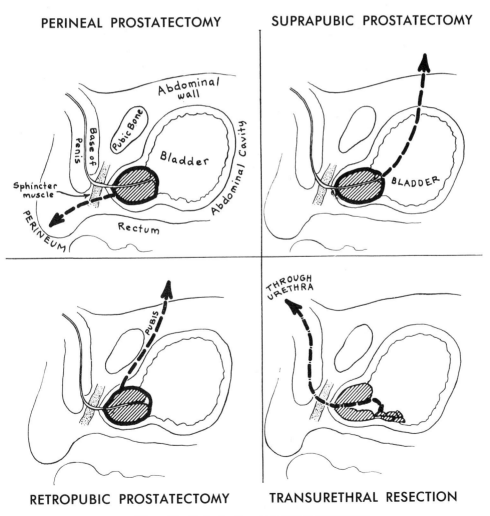

PERINEAL PROSTATECTOMY

SUPRAPUBIC PROSTATECTOMY

RETROPUBIC PROSTATECTOMY

TRANSURETHRAL RESECTION

Figure 16.   Methods of conservative prostatectomy.

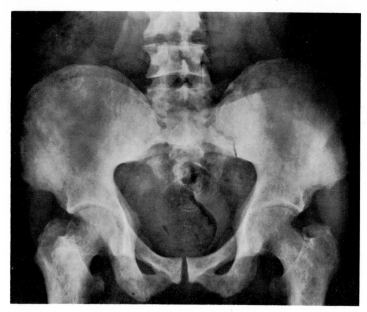

Figure 17. Areas of bone condensation in lower spine, pelvis and upper right femur, typical of osseous metastasis from carcinoma of the prostate.

The disease is so silent in its early development in most patients that it is no longer localized when they seek medical aid. Urinary complaints, or complaints from spread, as in osseous metastasis, usually in the lumbosacral region, occur late. Metastatic foci produce constant pain, whether or not the body is immobile. Pains caused by arthritis usually cease when the patient is quiet.

Early tumors, suitable for radical operation, come to attention when digital rectal examination discloses a stony hard area limited to and within the prostate. Nor do all such pa-

tients have localized carcinoma. Before performing radical operation, all possible evidence must be obtained which would indicate spread: chest x-rays and skeletal survey for metastasis, cystoscopy and intravenous urograms to rule out extension into the bladder and intramural portion of one or both ureters, causing hydroureter or hydronephrosis, and a blood test to detect any elevation of the serum acid phosphatase.

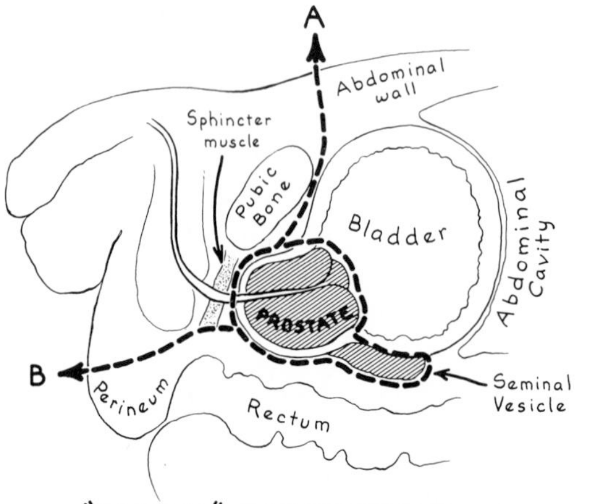

When there is local invasion which eliminates the feasibility of radical operation, evidence of metastasis or when patients are poor surgical risks or elderly, conservative treatment is indicated. The outlook in patients with advanced carcinoma of the prostate has been remarkably brightened by hormonal therapy. In 1940, Huggins reported that, in many patients, castration favorably influences the course of prostatic carcinoma. Shortly thereafter, he stated that the administration of estrogens produces the same effect. Estrogen suppresses the function of androgen-forming cells of the testis, which promote activity of prostatic carcinoma. Although the effect of neoplastic stimulation has been abundantly proved, it has never been demonstrated that androgens initiate carcinoma of the prostate. With removal of androgen stimulation, there is a cessation or regression in many patients, to such an extent that the rectal signs of carcinoma entirely recede. Likewise, the blood acid phosphatase activity is suppressed and osseous metastasis recedes.

"RADICAL" PROSTATECTOMY

Figure 18. Total prostatovesiculectomy for carcinoma of the prostate: removal of prostate, seminal vesicles and surrounding fascia. *A*, Retropubic route. *B*, Perineal route.

Unfortunately, although patients may obtain relief for periods of several months or several years, there is a tendency sooner or later for the carcinoma to escape from hormonal control, either with estrogens alone or castration alone, or with both. Apparently, the use of both methods is the most advisable.

After escape of the carcinoma from hormonal control, other measures may be applied, such as administration of tremendous dosages of estrogens or the use of adrenal steroid hormones. At this stage, androgens occasionally prove beneficial. Neither hypophysectomy nor adrenalectomy has proved its worth in treatment of prostatic carcinoma although both operations have been helpful in isolated instances.

Many supplementary measures prove helpful in conservative management of advanced prostatic carcinoma, such as transurethral resection for hormonally resistant carcinoma. Chemotherapy has limited usefulness. Radiation therapy relieves the pain of osseous metastasis. Intravenous administration of P^{32} localizes this radioactive isotope to the area of metastatic cells within bone.

During the past few years, supervoltage radiation has been used in the attempt to cure early prostatic carcinoma limited to the prostate or with minimal local spread and encouraging results have been shown. Although long-term evaluation is required for accurate assessment, the method has already shown proved value. It bears the advantage of retention of sexual powers, eliminated both by radical operation and hormonal methods of treatment. With supervoltage radiation, there are few untoward complications and a low morbidity rate.

Sarcoma and secondary neoplasms, such as invasion of carcinoma of the rectum, are less common and usually can be treated only by palliative resection and symptomatic treatment.

PROSTATIC CALCULI. Calculi sometimes form in the glandular acini and ducts of the prostate. With growth, they assume the contour of the units in which they lie. They may involve segments on one or both sides, or the entire gland. Large calculi impart a stony hardness to the prostate, observed on rectal examination; occasionally, they yield crepitation. Diagnosis is established by demonstrating their presence on x-ray of the prostatic region (Fig. 19).

From a clinical standpoint, calculi are of threefold significance: they may lead to the mistaken diagnosis of carcinoma; they frequently occur in association with obstructive processes, such as benign hyperplasia and carcinoma of the prostate; and calculi may cause urinary obstruction or contribute to infection, thus providing an indication for operation. If they are asymptomatic and do not produce urinary obstruction or contribute to infection, no treatment is indicated.

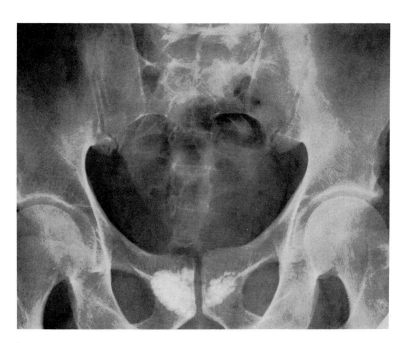

Figure 19. X-ray showing prostatic calculi which have assumed conformation of prostatic ducts.

SEMINAL VESICLES

The seminal vesicles are a pair of mono-tubular structures located just above the prostate between the floor of the bladder and the rectum. Joined medially by the ampullae of the vasa deferentia, they unite to form the ejaculatory ducts. The function of the seminal vesicles is to secrete a tenacious mucus and serve as a reservoir for spermatic fluid. Their muscular wall contracts during ejaculation to expel secretion.

The intimate relationship of the seminal vesicles to the vesical trigone, the prostate, the posterior urethra and the rectum explains why seminal vesiculitis, the condition of most surgical concern, may cause urinary frequency, dysuria and painful defecation.

Anomalies

Congenital anomalies of the seminal vesicles usually accompany ipsilateral maldevelopment of the upper urinary tract. They are extremely rare and of little clinical importance.

Trauma

Injuries of the seminal vesicles are likewise extremely rare. They are usually a complication of fracture of the bony pelvis. Treatment is the same as for trauma to the prostate.

Infection

Inflammation of the seminal vesicles is usually with pyogenic bacteria secondary to infection of the posterior urethra and prostate. Failure to recognize seminal vesiculitis may lead to confusion in explaining obscure symptoms of low backache, perineal discomfort and urinary irritability. Perhaps, one important cause of continued difficulty from seminal vesiculitis is occlusion of the ejaculatory duct which prevents escape of infected products.

Acute seminal vesiculitis is readily diagnosed by the palpation of an enlarged tender seminal vesicle, an oblong-shaped, cystic mass above the prostate. In chronic seminal vesiculitis, the seminal vesicle becomes indurated and fixed. Diagnosis can sometimes be established by stripping the seminal vesicle and recovering vesicle fluid impregnated with pus cells and bacteria.

The treatment is similar to that of pros-tatitis. In chronic infection, gentle stripping of the vesicles may induce resolution of the process. Occasionally, in chronic infection, seminal vesiculectomy becomes indicated. Since this operation may produce sexual impotence, it should not be lightly considered in young men.

Neoplasms

Carcinoma of the seminal vesicles has been described rarely. The growth of the neoplasm is so rapid as to make it difficult to determine the site of origin. Secondary invasion of the seminal vesicles by carcinoma of the prostate by way of the perineural lymphatics is quite common. Extension is revealed by rectal palpation.

COWPER'S GLANDS

The bulbomembranous glands of Cowper are paired glands between the layers of the urogenital diaphragm, which drain by ducts which empty into the floor of the bulbous urethra. They provide a clear, alkaline, mucoid secretion which supplements the spermatic fluid. This secretion apparently alkalinizes the urethral channel to prepare the way for expulsion of semen. In the normal state, Cowper's glands are not palpable. When they become infected, they enlarge and, on rectal examination, can be palpated adjacent to and lateral to the membranous urethra. Sometimes, pressure over an infected gland yields pus from the urethra.

Carcinoma of Cowper's glands is extremely rare; only 12 instances have been reported in the English literature. The disease causes perineal pain and difficult urination. Digital rectal examination reveals a stony hard mass distal to the apex of the prostate. In early stages, cure can be attained by local excision; in advanced tumors, a more radical operation is required.

DIFFUSE ANOMALIES AFFECTING REPRODUCTIVE SYSTEM

SEXUAL IMPOTENCE

Impotence signifies the inability to perform properly the sexual act. This may be manifest by a loss of libido, by the inability to gain or to sustain an erection, or by difficulties related to ejaculation. The mechanism of coitus entails a complex coordination of nervous, vascular, muscular and chemohormonal influences. When any or all of these factors are deficient, impotence may develop. It has been estimated that impotence affects 25 to 35 per cent of all adult males.

In 90 to 95 per cent of men complaining of impotence, the inadequacy is emotional rather than physical. The practice of withdrawal as a means of preventing pregnancy is sometimes the sole cause. Psychogenic influences which lead to impotence are guilt, anxiety or jealousy, or frigidity of the female partner. Common among the neurogenic causes are tabes dorsalis, hemiplegia, multiple sclerosis and other diseases affecting the spinal cord. Extensive pelvic operations for carcinoma of the rectum or prostate may damage the nerves and blood vessels of the penis. Coarctation of the aorta may cause impotence by interference with vascular supply. A chemohormonal cause of impotence is absence of both testes, either congenital or acquired. Atrophic testes usually provide adequate androgen to establish secondary sex characteristics and to perform coitus despite defective spermatogenesis. In Cushing's disease, impotence may result from decreased gonadotropic activity and loss of androgen secretion. Bilateral orchiectomy performed after puberty sometimes, but not universally, produces impotence. The administration of estrogens, as in the treatment of carcinoma of the prostate, almost invariably produces impotence because of the inhibitory effect on the pituitary gland. Patients with pituitary adrenogenital syndrome do not develop secondary sex characteristics and are impotent. Impotence may also develop in profound systemic disorders, febrile and cachectic states.

Congestion and infection of the prostate, prostatic urethra and verumontanum tend to produce premature ejaculation, apparently because of mechanical irritation. Carcinoma of the prostate may produce impotence, particularly in the advanced stages. It is obvious that almost all lesions of the penis may either cause or contribute to impotence.

In the study of a patient with impotence, the examination must be sufficiently complete to differentiate between systemic, local, organic and psychologic causes, for without accurate diagnosis, treatment cannot be intelligently administered. Cystourethroscopy should be a part of the examination to disclose any abnormality of the vesical neck or posterior urethra. Treatment is directed to the cause. In most young males, this is psychiatric. Since sexual problems are among the most difficult to treat, they usually require more skill than the physician without psychiatric training can give.

INFERTILITY

Fertility is the capacity to procreate. Infertility signifies impairment of a normal capacity to produce offspring. With complete and permanent incapacity, the condition is known as sterility. Studies indicate that the male is the sole cause of infertility in 20 to 40 per cent of all barren marriages. The fertility of the male is established through studies of the spermatic fluid, including a count of the number of spermatozoa, the percentage of abnormal forms and their viability. If sperma are absent or defective, biopsy of the testis is indicated to differentiate between the types of intrinsic deficiency of the germ cells, This study will also reveal instances in which there is normal spermatogenesis and azospermia caused by obstruction to the conductive system. A lack of fructose in the semen indicates deficient seminal vesicles. About 20 per cent of patients with azospermia have congenital absence of the seminal vesicles and vasa deferentia. Because the substrate for coagulation of spermatic fluid is manufactured by the seminal vesicles, this fluid remains liquid when the vesicles are absent.

The causes of male infertility are one or more of the following factors:

It has been estimated that 95 per cent of infertile males suffer from intrinsic spermatogenic defects. The germ cells of the seminiferous tubules may be congenitally defective; they may have been damaged by infection, as in mumps orchitis, or by trauma, as in destruction of the blood supply; or the defect may be chemohormonal, as in hypopituitarism. The cryptorchid testis is almost invariably deficient in spermatogenesis. Although this was previously presumed to be due to damage from increased temperature in the undescended position, the inability to restore normal spermatogenesis by orchiopexy, no matter how early in life the operation is performed, suggests that the defect may be congenital.

The usual cause of obstructions to the

conductive system is bilateral stenosis due to epididymitis, usually gonococcal. Occasionally, there is congenital absence of the vas deferens. This includes acquired defects, such as bilateral vasectomy.

Obviously, the impotent male has difficulty in the delivery of spermatozoa, although his capacity to produce normal spermatozoa may not be impaired. Thus, the patient may by impotent yet fertile, or he may be potent yet sterile.

In the clinical study of a patient complaining of inability to reproduce, a careful history should be taken of all possible etiologic factors, such as mumps orchitis, tuberculosis, deficiency diseases, operations such as repair of inguinal hernia or orchiopexy, trauma to the genitalia and genital infections such as epididymitis. The patient should be questioned about the course of any pregnancies he has induced and about his performance of the sexual act.

Physical examination should be painstaking, seeking out any neurologic cause or endocrine dyscrasia. Careful examination should be made of the genitalia with particular attention to the prostate, seminal vesicles, vasa deferentia, epididymides and testes. In obscure cases, cystourethroscopy should be carried out to seek any abnormality of the posterior urethra or verumontanum. The urine and prostatic secretion should be examined for pus cells which would indicate a complicating infection.

The most important step in the study of a patient of suspected infertility is examination of the spermatic fluid. Care should be taken in collection to avoid contamination with chemicals, such as those which might be present on a condom. The best specimen is produced by masturbation following four days of abstinence from intercourse. Examination should be made within a few hours after collection to learn of the motility of the spermatozoa. The normal sperm count ranges from 90 to 100 million per ml., with an average volume of 3.5 ml. after three days of abstinence. The cytology of the sperm is an important factor in fertility; normally, 60 per cent or more are perfectly formed adult cells. The percentage of defective forms should be calculated. Testicular biopsy provides the final information concerning spermatogenesis, giving indication of the degree and type of any impairment.

The results of treatment of infertility in the male are not encouraging. Measures should be instituted to improve the general health. Frequently, when infertility is mild, a vacation supplemented by rest and an adequate diet will produce the desired result. Sexual technique should be discussed with the patient. Frequently, the timing of intercourse to the period of fertility in the female will prove successful. Intercourse at this time should be carried out after three or four days of celibacy, since this helps increase the number and vigor of spermatozoa. In overweight men, a reducing diet should be prescribed.

Of the various forms of hormonal therapy, thyroid has proved most effective, particularly in cases of hypothyroidism. Gonadotropins would theoretically aid the development of the seminiferous tubules, but their use has not proved successful, perhaps because preparations thus far developed are not sufficiently powerful. Androgens are contraindicated since they depress rather than stimulate spermatogenesis. There is one exception to this rule, in that the rebound following administration of testosterone has proved effective in some instances. In this method, testosterone is given for three to six months, providing there is no blockage to the conductive system. Following cessation of treatment, a rebound may result in increased spermatogenesis.

Vasovasostomy in cases of previous vasoligation will result in success in 60 to 80 per cent, when the operation is performed bilaterally. Epididymovasostomy, if azospermia is caused by occlusion of the ducts in the globus minor, has a very low rate of cure. This operation attempts to divert sperm from the globus minor of the epididymis to the vas deferens. Technically, the operation leaves much to be desired and it may be followed by stenosis. There is a possibility of restoring fertility in bilateral cryptorchism by bringing both undescended testes into the scrotum. The operation should be performed before six to eight years of age. There is no possibility of producing spermatogenesis if orchiopexy is delayed until the time of puberty.

INTERSEX STATES

The intersex states produce external manifestations of both sexes to an abnormal degree. Hermaphrodism makes it difficult or impossible to determine on external inspection the sex of the patient. The entire appearance such as the breasts, distribution of hair, shape of the body and tone of the voice may suggest the sex opposite the one represented by the gonads. Deformities of the external genitalia which throw doubt upon the true sex of the individual should be recognized during childhood. Temporizing is not only disastrous to the emotional balance of the child but may contribute to omission of appropriate forms of therapy.

The clinical management of patients with anomalous sexual development presents many difficult therapeutic problems. Of primary concern is the importance of making an early decision regarding the sex in which the child is to be reared. The choice must rest upon multiple factors, such as possibilities presented by surgical procedures and hormonal therapy, and the age and psychologic status of the patient when the diagnosis is reached. Observations indicate that an alteration of sex in rearing is feasible until the age of one and a half years, sometimes until two and a half years. After this age, sexual gender alteration may cause serious psychologic disturbance.

The basic components of the sex of an individual are the aggregate of the chromosomal pattern established at the time of fertilization of the ovum. The somatic cell of the human contains 46 chromosomes, 44 autosomes and two sex chromosomes. The sex-determining genes known as the X and Y chromosomes influence the direction of sexual development through the development of the gonads. By counting the chromosomes of cells grown in tissue culture, it can be determined whether a given individual has a female (XX) or male (XY) pattern of sex chromosomes. Anomalies of sexual development are caused by faulty sex chromosomes, or chromosome patterns.

The nuclear components of the cell can be determined by examination of the polymorphonuclear leukocytes of the blood, or by examination of cells obtained by skin biopsy or scrapings from the buccal mucosa. A peripheral chromatin nuclear mass is noted in 20 per cent of females, rarely in males. Males are, therefore, designated as sex chromatin negative.

Gonadal sex is based on histologic evidence obtained from biopsy of the individual's germinal tissues. Hormonal determination of sex rests upon the excretion of ketosteroids and estrogens in the urine. The

gender role is the legal and sociologic attitude in which the patient is reared. Confusion arises from the fact that there is frequently little correlation between these criteria, the appearance of the external genitalia, and the secondary sexual characteristics of the individual.

MALE PSEUDOHERMAPHRODITISM

Male pseudohermaphroditism results from failure of the fetal testis to stimulate complete male differentiation. Although the testicles develop, they usually descend only as far as the inguinal region. The external genitalia tend toward the female type. Perineal hypospadias with a bifid, rudimentary scrotum, resembling a vulva, is a form of this anomaly. The chromosome pattern is XY. The nuclear sex is male, or chromatin negative.

Diagnostic features are the presence of testicles in the inguinal region, as confirmed by biopsy; the presence of a rudimentary vagina in the perineum; and demonstration of male components by skin biopsy, buccal smear or leukocyte examination.

When there is a preponderance of female characteristics, these children are reared most successfully as girls. Estrogen therapy started at puberty accentuates development in the female direction. Since the testicles may provide a source of embarrassment in later life, orchiectomy is sometimes performed.

FEMALE PSEUDOHERMAPHRODITISM

Congenital adrenal hyperplasia with defective synthesis of steroids in the adrenal cortex accounts for most instances of this anomaly. The patient has normal ovaries, uterus, fallopian tubes and vagina. The vagina, however, usually communicates with the urethra, which, in turn, opens at the base of an enlarged clitoris that resembles a penis. The labia are hypertrophied, simulating a bifid scrotum. The external appearance simulates perineal hypospadias with cryptorchism.

Excess androgenic activity is occasionally so marked as to make a female child appear male to external appearance, except for absence of gonads from the scrotum. There is usually other evidence of abnormal adrenal function, such as salt loss and other electrolyte imbalance. Premature growth of pubic hair and other androgenic manifestations associated with absence of testes from the scrotum may cause inquiry to be made.

In typical instances, 70 per cent or more of the cells show the female (XX) pattern. Final diagnosis depends upon abdominal exploration and biopsy of gonadal tissue.

Female pseudohermaphrodites adjust best as females. Patients treated with cortisone sufficiently early in childhood may achieve normal female development. Surgical measures consist of separating the urethra from the vagina, and amputation of the clitoris to produce the female appearance. The female constitution may be simulated by the administration of large doses of hormones, as in a regimen used to combat habitual abortion.

TRUE HERMAPHRODITISM

True hermaphroditism is extremely rare. It may be manifest as one ovary and one testis on either or both sides, or an ovotestis on either or both sides.

The chromosomal sex is either XX or XY. Surgical correction is directed toward establishing the patient's predominant gender role by removing the opposite gonadal tissue and modifying the appearance of the external genitalia to resemble the appropriate sex.

MALE HYPOGONADISM, GONADAL DYSGENESIS AND THE EUNUCHOID STATE

The pathogenesis of these syndromes is poorly understood and their classification unsatisfactory. They are variously attributed to inadequate, abnormal and absent testicular development. Some are caused wholly, or in part, by concurrent glandular disorders of the pituitary, adrenal and thyroid.

Since androgens derived from the testes exert no influence on the development of secondary sexual characteristics until the time of puberty, the effects of these disorders frequently go unrecognized until this stage of life.

Male hypogenitalism is characterized by inadequate development. It may result from testicular hypoplasia or from lack of, or destructive disease of, the anterior hypophysis.

Inadequate pituitary function is evidenced by reduction or absence of urinary gonadotropins. Pituitary infantilism is known as Frölich's syndrome. In Klinefelter's syndrome, the testes are small and exhibit tubular fibrosis; the secondary sexual characteristics vary from the eunuchoid to complete virilization; gynecomastia is occasionally observed in patients with high gonadotropic excretion.

Eunuchoidism results from congenital absence of hypoplasia of both testes, or from total destruction of the testes before puberty. It is manifest by absence of secondary sexual development.

Turner's syndrome is characterized by testes of normal size, yet histologic examination demonstrates that spermatogenic cells are arrested. The penis and prostate are hypoplastic.

Except the eunuchoid state, which is benefited by androgen therapy, clearly defined indications for hormonal administration in these syndromes have not been established. There is advantage in knowing that no permanent damage has been known to result from hormone medication. Although this is not to be construed as encouragement for indiscriminate hormone therapy, it seems preferable to test the effect in too many rather than in too few of these patients.

SEXUAL PRECOCITY

Adrenocortical hyperplasia is the most common cause of precocious sexual development in the male. The external genitalia may be noticeably enlarged at birth and at times a mild degree of hypospadias is present. Since excess androgens act only upon secondary sex characteristics, there is lack of concurrent spermatogenesis. Cortical tumors of the adrenal gland and tumors involving the hypothalamus, either primary or secondary, especially of the posterior segment, also cause precocious male puberty.

TRANSSEXUALISM

Some males with normal male genitalia harbor an intense desire to become females. The etiology may incorporate genetic and endocrine factors. The principle of therapy should be to adjust the mind to the body.

Sometimes, estrogen therapy is of benefit. In cases of failure, consideration may be given to alter the body to adjust to the mind. Prolonged observation and psychiatric consultation should always precede operation. Thirty-one patients are on record who have undergone penectomy, 23 with castration and 25 with creation of an artificial vagina. Excellent results were obtained in 16; six patients were married as females after operation.

READING REFERENCES

Altman, B. L., and Malament, M.: Carcinoma of testis following orchiopexy. J. Urol. 97:498, 1967.

Amar, A. D.: Probable *Trichomonas vaginalis* epididymitis. J.A.M.A. 200:417, 1967.

Aquino, J. A., Cunningham, R. M., and Filbee, J. F.: Peyronie's disease. J. Urol. 97:492, 1967.

Barr, M. L.: Sex chromatin and phenotype in man. Science 130:679, 1959.

Batson, O. V.: Function of the vertebral veins and their role in the spread of metastases. Ann. Surg. 112:138, 1940.

Bonner, C. D., and others: Prostatic serum acid phosphatase level in cancer of the prostate. J.A.M.A. 164:1070, 1957.

Charny, C. W.: Male infertility as a concern of the gynecologist. J.A.M.A. 186:842, 1963.

Charny, C. W., and Wolgin, W.: Cryptorchism. New York, Paul B. Hoeber, 1957.

Clarke, B. G.: Incidence of varicocele in normal men and among men of different ages. J.A.M.A. 198:1121, 1966.

Colston, J. A. C.: Differential diagnosis and management of the senile prostate showing twenty-five years of progress. Am. Surgeon 21:581, 1955.

Culp, O. S.: Struggles and triumphs with hypospadias and associated anomalies: review of 400 cases. J. Urol. 96:339, 1966.

Dodge, O. G., and Linsell, C. A.: Carcinoma of penis in Uganda and Kenya Africans. Cancer 16:1255, 1963.

Edman, P., and Qvist, O.: Torsion of appendix testis: an analysis of 121 cases. Acta Chir. Scand. 125:370, 1963.

Emmett, J. L., Greene, L. F., and Papantoniou, A.: Endocrine therapy in carcinoma of prostate gland. J. Urol. 83:471, 1960.

Flocks, R. H.: Clinical cancer of the prostate: a study of 4000 cases. J.A.M.A. 193:559, 1965.

Fox, M.: The natural history and significance of stone formation in the prostate gland. J. Urol. 89:716, 1963.

Garrett, R. A., and Rhamy, D. E.: Priapism: management with corpus saphenous shunt. J. Urol. 95:65, 1966.

Gartman, E.: Torsion of the spermatic cord in adult scrotal testes; a review of eighteen cases managed surgically. Am. J. Surg. 94:787, 1957.

Getzoff, P. L.: Clinical evaluation of testicular biopsy and the rebound phenomenon. Fertil. & Steril. 6:465, 1955.

Gibson, T. E.: Tumors of the seminal vesicles. *In*, Urology. (Campbell, M. F., ed.) 2nd ed. Philadelphia, W. B. Saunders Company, 1963, pp. 1284–1290.

Hand, J. R.: Treatment of undescended testis and its complications. J.A.M.A. 164:1185, 1957.

Henry, W. L., and others: True hermaphroditism. J. Nat. M. A. 49:212, 1957.

Hinman, F., Jr.: Intersexuality. Pediat. Clin. North America 4:905, 1957.

Hotchkiss, R. S.: Infertility in the male. *In*, Urology. (Campbell, M. F., ed.) 2nd ed. Philadelphia, W. B. Saunders Company, 1963, pp. 643–679.

Hutfield, D. C.: Herpes genitalis: survey of 30 cases and effect of treatment with penotrane jelly. Brit. J. Ven. Dis. 39:181, 1963.

Johnsen, S. G.: The management of male hypogonadism. Acta Endocrinol. Suppl. 66, Periodica, Cophenhagen, 1962.

Jones, H. W., and Scott, W. W.: Hermaphroditism, Genital Anomalies and Related Endocrine Disorders. Baltimore, Williams and Wilkins Company, 1958.

Leeson, C. R.: Electron microscopic study of cryptorchid and scrotal human testes. Invest. Urol. 3:498, 1966.

Lyon, R. P.: Torsion of testicle in childhood: a painless emergency requiring contralateral orchiopexy. J.A.M.A. 178:702, 1961.

Lyon, R. P., and Bruyn, H. B.: Mumps epididymo-orchitis: treatment by anesthetic block of spermatic cord. J.A.M.A. 196:736, 1966.

Mandler, J. I., and Pool, T. L.: Primary carcinoma of male urethra. J. Urol. 96:67, 1966.

McCormack, J. L., Kretz, A. W. and Tocantins, R.: Traumatic rupture of the testicle. J. Urol. 96:80, 1966.

McIntosh, H. W.: Syndromes of hypogonadism in the male. Postgrad. Med. 22:102, 1957.

Mittemeyer, B. T., Lennox, K. W., and Borski, A. A.: Epididymitis: a review of 610 cases. J. Urol. 95:390, 1966.

Morris, J. M.: Intersexuality. J.A.M.A. 163:538, 1957.

Nelson, W. O., and Boccabella, R. A.: Application of the sex chromatin test. Fertil. & Steril. 8:333, 1957.

Nesbit, R. M., and Baum, W. C.: Endocrine control of prostatic carcinoma: clinical and statistical survey of 1818 cases. J.A.M.A. 143:1317, 1950.

O'Shaughnessy, E. J., Parrino, P. S., and White, J. D.: Chronic prostatitis—fact or fiction? J.A.M.A. 160:540. 1956.

Patton, J. F., and Mallis, N.: Tumors of the testis. J. Urol. 81:457, 1959.

Patton, J. F., Seitzman, D. N., and Zone, R. A.: Diagnosis and treatment of testicular tumors. Am. J. Surg. 99:525, 1960.

Scorer, C. G.: Descent of testicle in the first year of life. Brit. J. Urol. 27:374, 1955.

Scott, W. W., and Toole, W. N.: Carcinoma of the prostate. *In*, Urology. (Campbell, M. F., ed.) 2nd ed. Philadelphia, W. B. Saunders Company, 1963, pp. 1173–1221.

Smith, D. R.: General Urology. 5th ed. Los Altos, California, Lange Medical Publications, 1966.

Staubitz, W. J., and others: Management of testicular tumors. J.A.M.A. 166:751, 1958.

Thomson, I. M., Wear, J., Jr., Almond, C., Schewe, E. J., and Sala, J.: An analytical survey of one hundred and seventy-eight testicular tumors. J. Urol. 85:173, 1961.

Thompson, R. V., and Mostofi, F. K.: Benign hyperplasia of the prostate gland. *In*, Urology. (Campbell, M. F., ed.) 2nd ed. Philadelphia, W. B. Saunders Company, 1963, pp. 1101–1142.

Tyler, E. T., and Singher, H. O.: Male infertility—status of treatment, prevention, and current research. J.A.M.A. 160:91, 1956.

Weyrauch, H. M.: Surgery of the Prostate. Philadelphia, W. B. Saunders Company, 1959.

Whitesel, J. A.: Lymphography: its place in urology. J. Urol. 91:613, 1964.

Whitmore, W. F.: Some experience with retroperitoneal lymph node dissection and chemotherapy in the management of testis neoplasms. Brit. J. Urol. 34:436, 1962.

Williams, D. I., and Eckstein, H. B.: Obstructive valves in posterior urethra. J. Urol. 93:236, 1965.

Chapter 30

THE FEMALE REPRODUCTIVE SYSTEM

by
LANGDON PARSONS, M.D.

Born and reared in Massachusetts, LANGDON PARSONS graduated from Yale University in 1921, "with a brief time out when I protected these shores as Quartermaster, 2nd Class, USNR in World War I. After two years in the financial world, where I found I could sell bonds but didn't know why, I entered Harvard Medical School and graduated in 1927." Langdon Parsons served with U.S. General Hospital No. 6, in World War II in North Africa and Italy, and later with the 52nd Station Hospital, a Maxillo-Facial Center. "My associates did such an excellent job that I received the Legion of .Merit as a Lieutenant Colonel." Dr. Parsons is Emeritus Clinical Professor of Gynecology at Harvard Medical School.

The great majority of the complaints referable to the female reproductive system are functional in nature and fall within the province of internal medicine. The surgeon, therefore, has a broad spectrum of medicine to consider when he attempts to evaluate the three major gynecologic symptoms of bleeding, discharge and pain.

In the physical examination of the patient he must depend upon what he sees in the external genitalia and vagina, and upon what he can feel on vaginal or rectal examination, which revolves largely around the size, position, contour and degree of fixation of the uterus and adnexae. Systemic, local, developmental, endocrinologic, functional or organic causes may be the explanation for the presenting symptoms.

The same facts gathered from the history and physical examination often have varying significance, depending on the time in a woman's life when they occur. In many instances, the underlying pathology, etiology and symptomatology are the same for all ages, but the treatment must of necessity be different. The surgeon must screen the facts and evaluate them properly before he can establish a basis for operative interference. The nature of his surgical attack must then be modified by the desire of both surgeon and patient to preserve menstrual as well as reproductive function.

Problems in Puberty and Adolescence

CONGENITAL ANOMALIES

The chief problems in girls at puberty and adolescence have to do with growth and the establishment of a regular menstrual pattern. Most of the gynecologic problems in adolescence are concerned with the failure of gonadal structure to develop properly or the ovary and uterus to function in a consistent pattern. Many of the congenital anomalies and a few of the functional entities require surgery. Two other problems which may call for surgical operation in this age group are primary dysmenorrhea and neoplastic or physiologic ovarian tumor formation.

IMPERFORATE HYMEN. The young patient may have difficulty in extruding the products of menstruation when they appear at puberty, simply because an imperforate hymen provides an anatomic block. Normally, the hymen is patent, but at times it is represented by a complete partition or a thin veil of tissue which has only a few inadequate perforations in it. Depending on the extent of the obstruction, blood accumulates and distends the vagina and, occasionally, the uterus and tubes to the point where a mass can be felt on both abdominal and rectal examination. On inspection of the external genitalia, the hymen is seen to bulge outward because of the pressure of blood trapped in the vagina.

The symptomatology varies from moderate degrees of discomfort to actual pain localized in the vagina, abdomen and low back. A large amount of blood can accumulate over a period of months following the onset of menstruation without creating anything more than mild discomfort. Conversely, a small collection may produce severe abdominal pain.

At puberty, the hymen should be excised under anesthesia rather than incised. This must be done with care to prevent subsequent bands of scar tissue that may constrict the outlet. It is important that the vagina be completely and thoroughly drained of all accumulated blood. Any retained products tend to serve as a culture medium, and secondary infections are prone to occur. If an adequate vent has been produced, the local and intra-uterine mass will gradually disappear.

If the mass does not disappear, or if it seems to be eccentrically placed when the pelvis is examined at the time of hymenectomy, it is advisable to perform a dilatation and curettage to rule out congenital anomalies of the uterus.

In uterus bicornis unicolis, a rare lesion, one horn of the duplex uterus does not communicate with the cervix or vagina. The endometrial epithelium, however, responds to the same hormonal stimulation and the patient menstruates into the blind cavity. This may undergo progressive enlargement, since its only outlet is by way of the tube. If the diagnosis is confirmed at the time of examination under anesthesia, the rudimentary cornua should be excised.

TRANSVERSE PARTITION OF VAGINA. On rare occasions, the vagina may be obstructed at its midportion. If the partition is imperforate, the patient may have the same problem in extruding menstrual products as she would if the block were at the introitus. This condition is sometimes confused with congenital absence of the vagina. The obstructing partition can be easily excised and the vaginal epithelium reapposed without constricting the vaginal outlet.

LONGITUDINAL PARTITION OF VAGINA. The major factor of importance when a septum runs in the long axis of the vagina is the possible association with other developmental defects in the genitourinary tract. Since they result from failure or improper fusion of the müllerian duct elements, a wide variety of anomalies have been reported. There may be a single uterus and a double vagina, or a double uterus and a double vagina, or any variation thereof.

The problems which require surgical treatment arise after the patient has married and experiences difficulty in becoming pregnant, maintaining a pregnancy or delivering it, due to the presence of anatomic defects in the uterus or vagina.

CONGENITAL ABSENCE OF VAGINA. In the patient who has a true congenital absence of the vagina, the buccal smear shows a feminine sex chromatin body, despite occasional X chromosomes. Generally, however, it is true that such a patient also has other defects in the internal genitalia. The reported instances of a normally functioning uterus vary from 4 to 14 per cent. In some instances, the uterus may be absent or incompletely developed, but the ovaries and tubes are normal.

Because there are so many departures from the normal, a laparotomy should be performed to establish the extent of the defect in development of the internal genitalia, particularly if nothing resembling a uterus can be felt on rectal examination.

If it can be shown that the patient will never menstruate, construction of an artificial vagina should be postponed until a few months before she plans to marry. The best results from plastic reconstruction of a vagina come when the new canal is kept dilated by regular intercourse. If it is not kept open, there is a tendency for the vagina to stenose with loss of length as well as breadth. When the operation is performed too far ahead of the date set for marriage the patient must wear an obturator.

Construction of a vagina is a relatively simple operation. After identifying the course of the urethra, a transverse incision is made in the skin, anterior to the anal opening. With one finger in the rectum as a guide to protect it, the surgeon carries the dissection deeper and soon enters a space which is readily enlarged, in a bloodless field, as the areolar tissues are pushed aside. When the opening is large enough to receive an obturator the dissection is discontinued. A split thickness skin graft is then taken, with an electric dermatome, from the patient's buttock with the patient lying prone. The graft is immediately transferred to the obturator and carefully tailored to cover it with the skin surface in contact with the obturator. It is then inserted in the newly constructed opening and is both sutured in space and held in place by a male type of cotton binder. The graft will take in approximately ten days. The obturator is then removed, the area cleansed and inspected and the obturator replaced and worn intermittently. The patient can function adequately as a female, although she will never menstruate or bear a child.

AMENORRHEA

In the absence of any congenital defect, amenorrhea is most likely due to faulty endocrine function of some portion of the pituitary, ovary, adrenal and uterine axis. Before attributing the cause entirely to endocrine malfunction, such factors as obesity, disturbances in thyroid function, malnutrition and psychic disorders must be considered. Endocrine therapy is ineffective until these factors have been brought into balance.

ADRENAL GLAND FUNCTION. Disturbances in the function of the adrenal gland are not uncommon, and they are occasionally the explanation of amenorrhea. The basic defect is more often hyperplasia than tumor of the adrenal gland. The differentiation between a virilizing tumor of the adrenal gland and congenital hyperplasia can be made by serum testosterone determinations. Dexamethasone suppression, adrenocorticotropic hormone stimulation as well as metipyrone response tests may differentiate the immune response of hyperplasia from the independent secretion rate of a tumor.

Cushing's syndrome is another possibility, since the basic fault lies in the overproduction of the cortisone family. The chief symptoms are hirsutism and diminished ovarian function. Development of the breast, labia, vagina and uterus may be in abeyance. The clitoris is not necessarily enlarged.

The treatment is primarily surgical and is directed toward the adrenal gland. Roentgen ray therapy has been notoriously unsuccessful. Suppression therapy over a long period of time usually fails because of sodium retention and the development of both hypertension and psychosis. Operation has the additional advantage of helping to distinguish between adrenal hyperplasia and adrenal cortical tumor. The results of surgical excision are often dramatic.

POLYCYSTIC OVARY (STEIN-LEVENTHAL) SYNDROME. The Stein-Leventhal syndrome is a more advanced manifestation of the polycystic ovary syndrome. As originally described, the patient has all the symptoms and physical findings ascribed to the polycystic ovary syndrome, as well as most of the physical findings. In the Stein-Leventhal syndrome, however, the cystic enlargement of the ovaries is much more pronounced and is easily the most striking feature found on physical examination.

The two terms, Stein-Leventhal and polycystic ovary syndrome, are interchangeably used. The latter is very common whereas the former is relatively rare.

The patient has either never menstruated or develops amenorrhea over a period of time. In most instances, she begins to have normal and regular cycles, and then the flow becomes excessive. The bleeding always takes place from an anovulatory endometrium. Gradually, the patient begins to skip periods, until finally menstruation either ceases or occurs only once or twice a year. In addition, the adolescent girl or young woman in her early twenties, who has this syndrome, frequently has a mild degree of hirsutism of the male type, hypoplasia of the uterus and bilaterally enlarged polycystic ovaries. She may or may not be obese.

Many endocrine abnormalities produce the same gross and microscopic pathologic picture in the ovary. There is, therefore, nothing pathognomonic about the finding of polycystic ovaries.

Hyperfunction of the adrenal gland is the most likely source of confusion in establishing a diagnosis. Estimation of the 17-ketosteroid excretion is often helpful in distinguishing adrenal hyperplasia from the polycystic ovary syndrome. It is usually elevated in the former, but normal in the latter. On rare occasions, the 17-ketosteroids are elevated in the polycystic ovary syndrome. The use of corticoid drugs can also be given as a test. When prednisone, 5 to 10 mg., hydrocortisone, 25 to 40 mg., or cortisone, 37.5 to 50 mg. per day is given, the periods may resume a normal pattern, despite the fact that the 17-ketosteroid estimations were not elevated.

Although some patients respond to corticoid therapy, it still does not necessarily prove that the adrenal gland is implicated. Recently, experimental evidence suggests that a steroid enzyme block may be present in the ovary which responds in the same fashion as the hyperplastic adrenal.

Chlomophene citrate has now been made available for the treatment of the polycystic ovary syndrome. A dosage schedule of 100 mg. for five days at monthly intervals has proved to be effective in creating ovulatory cycles and on occasion pregnancies have resulted. It is well to keep in mind when chlomophene is used that there is not sufficient evidence available to permit an estimate of what long-term effect this drug will have upon the ovary. It is an excellent drug to use when the primary object is correction of an immediate fertility problem. Whether a permanent ovulatory condition can be created which will persist without the necessity of continuing administration of chlomophene is not yet known.

If the patient does not respond to chlomophene citrate or cortisone therapy, abdominal exploration is indicated, particularly if culdoscopic examination shows bilaterally enlarged ovaries. Characteristically, the ovaries resemble an oyster, with a smooth gray-white surface punctuated with small translucent areas which reflect the presence of small cysts lying beneath. No suggestion of corpora lutea, either new or old, can usually be found.

At the time of operation, curettage will reveal a small, underdeveloped uterus with scanty endometrium which is invariably in the proliferative phase. There are few gynecologic procedures which produce such dramatic results as bilateral simple wedge resection of the ovary. An incision extending down into the hilar portion is made, either longitudinally or transversely, and the multiple small follicular cysts are punctured. On cut section, there is always a thick fibrous capsule with multiple small follicle cysts lying beneath it. The ovarian capsule is then restored with interrupted catgut sutures.

Excellent results may be expected in at least 75 per cent of patients operated on, with a 50 per cent chance of fertility among those who are married and desire children. In addition to the restoration of the ovulatory cycle, there is marked improvement in feminization, particularly in the breast.

ARRHENOBLASTOMA. Functioning tumors of the ovary do, on rare occasions, appear in childhood and early adolescence. Primarily, they are of the feminizing type such as the granulosal cell tumor, secreting estrogens and producing precocious menstruation and secondary sex characteristics. The masculinizing tumors such as arrhenoblastoma, which secrete the male hormone, have amenorrhea as their most prominent symptom as well as masculine manifestations in development.

No patient under the age of 13 years has been reported, but there is a marked tendency

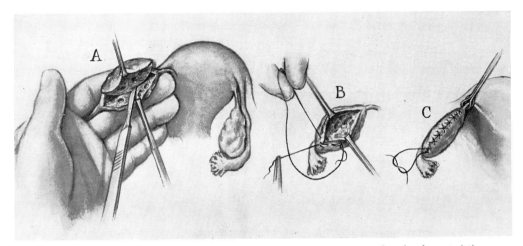

Figure 1.   Wedge resection of the ovary for the Stein-Leventhal syndrome. The ovary has the characteristic appearance of multiple small follicular cysts and a heavy, thick cortical covering. Reduction of the bulk of the ovarian substance may correct the condition. A, The wedge-shaped section is excised. B, A Babcock clamp steadies the ovarian ligament medially, and the edges of the cavity are held apart with Allis forceps while the raw edges of the ovary are approximated by a suture which includes the base of the cavity. C, The running suture is completed by returning to its point of origin. Since the pathologic state is always bilateral, this procedure must be repeated on the opposite side.

for the tumor to concentrate in numbers around the age of puberty. In most instances, they are discovered in the course of investigative studies to determine the cause of the amenorrhea.

Because the girl has reached full maturity before the masculinizing hormones exert their influence, there are no congenital defects. The masculinizing and virilizing elements are obvious and dramatic. The body contour and musculature are those of the male type, the breasts are atrophied, the clitoris is hypertrophied, the voice deep in tone and hair distribution follows the male pattern. After removal of the tumor, all these male characteristics disappear except the deep voice, and pregnancies have been reported.

Although the malignant potential is high among the tumors found in adults, one can afford to be conservative in the adolescent, provided the tumor is small and completely encapsulated. The solitary tumor alone may be removed. If there is any suggestion on gross inspection that the tumor capsule is involved or that the tumor is attached to any other structure, radical removal of the uterus and opposite ovary is indicated. If the operation has been conservative and there is any evidence of recurrence, the patient should be operated upon again to remove the uterus and adnexae.

DYSGERMINOMA. There is a marked tendency for dysgerminoma of the ovary to be discovered at the time of puberty. While this tumor does not secrete any hormone to alter menstrual function, its symptoms suggest endocrine influence.

The patient usually presents evidence of sexual and gonadal underdevelopment. The most striking finding is the gross enlargement of the clitoris which may simulate the appearance of a small penis. One, therefore, suspects an inherent masculinizing factor. The tumor, however, is hormonally inert. The ambiguity of the external genitalia is due to the fact that dysgerminomas are frequently associated with congenital adrenal hyperplasia. The patient is, therefore, a hermaphrodite. Despite the presence of the tumor, she may have ovulating periods and become pregnant.

Although dysgerminomas are usually discovered at puberty, they may be encountered at any time during the menstrual life of women. The degree of malignancy varies, despite the fact that the malignant potential is high. The microscopic appearance is often frightening.

Nevertheless, there is a rightful place for a conservative operation when a unilateral encapsulated tumor is found in an adolescent child. Experience has shown that when this situation exists the surgeon may justifiably remove only the involved ovary and tube. The tumor metastasizes to the nodes along the inferior vena cava or aorta rather early in its course, even though it is seemingly confined to the ovary. It is fortunate that the dysgerminoma is extremely sensitive to radiation. It is essential that external radiation therapy be given to supplement the unilateral adnexal excision. The uterus and opposite ovary are heavily screened while a relatively low tumor dose, in the range of 1500 gamma roentgens, is administered to the entire abdomen. The cure rate reported from this type of therapy for unilateral encapsulated tumors in this adolescent group is in the range of 80 per cent, with few recurrences. Additionally, a number of subsequent pregnancies have been recorded.

Therapy must be much more drastic when the tumor appears bilaterally or gives any indication that it has broken through its capsule. Because dysgerminomas are frequently bilateral, the surgeon will be well advised, before he embarks on a conservative course of management, to split the opposite, normal-appearing ovary and inspect the interior. When the tumor has broken through the capsule, total hysterectomy with bilateral salpingo-oophorectomy, followed by external radiation, is the only acceptable form of therapy. The results are poor.

After a simple removal of the tube and ovary, the appearance of ascites, or any suggestion of recurrence, calls for immediate re-exploration with removal of the uterus and remaining adnexa, providing that the extent of the recurrence is not too great. Postoperative roentgen ray treatments should be given as adjuvant therapy.

ABNORMAL UTERINE BLEEDING

It is common for the adolescent patient to have an irregular bleeding pattern at the beginning of her menstrual life. She may bleed irregularly or not at all. From the surgical point of view, interest is greatest in the patient who bleeds either excessively or persistently.

The adolescent patient bleeds from an anovulatory proliferative type of endometrium, largely because the ovary is not yet mature enough to respond in regular fashion to the stimulating effects of the pituitary gonadotropic hormones. It often takes several years following the menarche for the menstrual periods to acquire an adult pattern, complete with ovulation and a progestational type of endometrium.

There is enough estrin to stimulate the endometrium and cause it to proliferate, but the balancing effect of progestin is absent. The primary defect is a lack of progestin. On rare occasions, the patient may bleed from an inactive or atrophic endometrium. The explanation for this type of bleeding is not quite clear. It is a relatively rare but significant condition, however, for it cannot be reversed by giving hormones. The patient continues to bleed so persistently that curettage is necessary.

In this age group, there is little reason to associate the abnormal bleeding pattern with malignant disease. The child may have too frequent and excessive bleeding from a follicle cyst of the ovary or, less often, a granulosal cell tumor. Both produce anovulatory bleeding, but their presence should be suspected on vaginal or rectal examination.

The great majority of patients at puberty establish a normal menstrual pattern spontaneously after a few periods of anovulatory bleeding. Others have irregular spotting, or too frequent periods for a time, but never lose enough blood to warrant a surgical procedure.

Most of the patients undergo spontaneous cure, and a normal pattern can be created for those who do not by giving progestational hormones. The degree of success depends partially on the patient's nutritional and emotional state, as well as normal thyroid function. It is important to keep in mind that hypofunction of the thyroid may be responsible for excessive menstrual bleeding, and that thrombopenic purpura may manifest itself for the first time at puberty.

Although excessive menstrual bleeding can be controlled with oral or intramuscular progesterone, the best method of controlling hemorrhage is by curettage. Three things are accomplished: pelvic examination under anesthesia will permit better evaluation of the adnexal areas, thereby eliminating any possibility that ovarian tumors may be the cause of the bleeding; the bleeding is immediately controlled; and histologic examination of the endometrium will provide a sound, rational basis for the management of any abnormal bleeding which may reappear in later months. In most instances, curettage stops the immediate hemorrhage and corrects the disturbed bleeding pattern for the future. If it reappears, the surgeon may institute hormone therapy, or repeat curettage.

VAGINAL DISCHARGE

Vaginal discharge is a troublesome symptom in this or any age group, but it does not carry with it the serious implications of malignant disease that it does in adulthood. The most common causes of vaginal discharge, in addition to foreign bodies in the vagina, are protozoan infection by *Trichomonas vaginalis* and *Monilia albicans*. The diagnosis is indicated by the symptoms, which are chiefly a malodorous discharge associated with burning and itching in the vagina, and it is confirmed by the finding of characteristic organisms on wet smear preparations.

Occasionally, Skene's or Bartholin's glands develop abscesses which require incision and drainage, marsupialization, or excision. If the process is thoroughly established in the cervix and does not respond to antibiotic therapy, on rare occasions there may be a reason for cervical cauterization.

A common cause of vaginal discharge in this age group is congenital erosion of the cervix. It is not an erosion in the sense that the normal epithelium has been denuded by chronic infection or other cause, but rather is a prolapse downward of the glandular mucosa of the endocervix. There is no occasion to do anything about it unless the discharge becomes profuse or malodorous. Radial cauterization can then be carried out as an office procedure, provided the vagina will distend sufficiently. If not, anesthesia is required.

PELVIC PAIN

There are many local and extragenital conditions which produce pain, but the three most common causes in adolescence are twisted ovarian cyst, mittelschmerz and primary dysmenorrhea.

OVARIAN CYST. Simple benign cysts and

dermoid cysts of the ovary are common in the adolescent age group, and are a frequent source of pelvic pain. They lie free in the abdominal cavity, unattached to other structures, and grow on a pedicle which contains the blood supply to the ovary. A sudden shift in the position of the tumor may cause the pedicle to twist.

Interference with the blood supply to the ovary containing the cyst produces varying degrees of pelvic pain, depending upon the extent of the obstruction and its permanence. A complete obstruction which does not relieve itself will produce severe colicky pain which comes in waves because of the ischemia created by loss of blood supply, and sudden hemorrhage into the cyst cavity. The latter produces a sudden stretching of the visceral peritoneum covering the cyst. There are very few nerve endings in the peritoneum, so that an ovary which slowly enlarges rarely produces pain. The patient may have a large cyst and never know it. This is why carcinoma of the ovary has such an insidious growth pattern.

A sudden hemorrhage within the cyst cavity stretches the capsule and produces pain. The acute colicky pain is not always persistent, but may either disappear entirely or recur intermittently, depending upon the position of the tumor. If it reverts to its former position, the torsion of the ovarian pedicle is relieved and pain subsides, only to recur again if the twist reappears.

In most instances, the acute colicky abdominal pain suggests that acute disease has developed in the lower pelvic cavity. The symptoms are similar to those produced by appendicitis, intussusception, acute Meckel's diverticulum, renal stone and acute pelvic inflammation. These entities must be ruled out by a careful history and physical examination. The presence of a palpable pelvic mass, which is tender to touch, should suggest the correct diagnosis. Immediate abdominal operation is indicated. Because of the possibility of an error in preoperative estimate of the cause, the incision should be made in the midline.

MITTELSCHMERZ. Patients in this age group are prone to have fairly severe lower abdominal pain, frequently localized in the right lower quadrant at the time of ovulation. The parietal peritoneum is particularly sensitive to the spillage of blood or cystic fluid. When the developing follicle ruptures, it may do so explosively, with leakage of follicular fluid and sometimes blood. All the symptoms and signs of acute appendicitis may develop, including an elevated white blood corpuscle count. At times, the differential diagnosis cannot be made, and exploratory laparotomy through a midline incision is indicated.

PRIMARY DYSMENORRHEA. One of the most common and disturbing complaints in adolescence is primary dysmenorrhea. It is called primary because the patient has no palpable pelvic pathology to explain the cramplike menstrual pain.

Characteristically, the pain comes 24 to 48 hours before the menstrual flow begins and persists for a varying time thereafter. It is most severe in the first six to 12 hours.

The pain is of two types: a sharp gripping cramplike pain similar to that produced by an intestinal colic, and a steady dull ache or bearing down sensation localized to the upper thighs, low back and suprapubic area.

The severity of the pain and the response of the patient to it vary widely in different individuals. There can be no question that there is a large psychogenic component in patients who have dysmenorrhea. In addition to abdominal pain, these patients also complain of abdominal distention, painful breasts, nausea and vomiting, premenstrual tension, depression, irritability and a host of other difficulties. Pain is only one portion of the symptom complex. Since primary dysmenorrhea also appears to be a self-limited process, and disappears as the patient becomes older, the indication for definitive surgical treatment is sharply limited. It should be considered only when all other methods have failed in a patient who is incapacitated and totally unable to carry out her social life, her studies or her work.

Before advocating an intra-abdominal operation, the surgeon should try hormonal therapy. If this fails, dilatation and curettage should be performed. This procedure provides a clean base for the hormones to work upon and disrupts the nerve plexus in the region of the internal os. Approximately 50 per cent of patients can be relieved in this manner.

Presacral nerve resection is a satisfactory operation, provided the patient is properly selected. The chances of success improve if the patient has first responded satisfactorily to hormone suppression of ovulation, but regressed when the hormone support was withdrawn. The rationale for the use of hormones to suppress ovulation is based on the fact that anovulatory bleeding occurs without cramps. The operation can be counted on to relieve only pain which is located in the midline. It will be unsuccessful if the patient has lateral pain or pain in her back.

The success of the operation is based on interruption of the transmission of painful impulses and improvement in the vascular flow to the uterus by releasing vasoconstriction. All the nerve, and not a small segment, must be removed.

Problems in the 20 to 30 Age Group

The gynecologic problems within the 20 to 30 age group have a particular association with pregnancy, since the fertility curve is highest at this time. In evaluating the three major symptoms of bleeding, pain and discharge, accidents to the pregnancy must receive prime consideration. In addition, there are problems amenable to surgical correction which are concerned with the inability of the patient to become pregnant, as well as those which follow the complications of pregnancy. Functional bleeding problems occur and malignant disease appears occasionally, but for the most part pregnancy is implicated in one way or another.

STERILITY

The primary problem in the treatment of female sterility is determination of the cause, which may be endocrinologic, nutritional, psychologic or anatomic. Surgery concerns itself largely with the correction of any defect which prevents the union of the sperm and ovum. Other problems appear when congenital abnormalities are found, which either prevent the patient from becoming pregnant, or interfere with the normal progression of pregnancy.

EROSION OF THE CERVIX AND ENDOCERVICITIS. Chronic infection in the cervix may create a medium unfavorable to the survival of the sperm in the cervical canal, or prevent their passage into the endometrial cavity.

Chronic cervicitis is the most common cause of leukorrhea. The discharge is invariably thick, gelatinous and mucoid, and frequently is mixed with pus. A mucoid plug often fills the cervical canal, and because it is not easily detached, it creates a mechanical block to the transmission of sperm. If the history is suggestive, smears and cultures should be made to rule out gonorrhea.

Chronic cervicitis rarely produces any more serious symptom than annoyance at having a discharge. Because of the exposed position of the cervix, the patient may experience bleeding or spotting after intercourse or following the use of a douche. Because these are the same symptoms one finds in early cancer of the cervix, a Papanicolaou smear and a biopsy should be made to rule out carcinoma.

In evaluating the various factors concerned with the etiology of cervical cancer, greater emphasis is placed on the age when intercourse was first experienced than on the age of marriage, or the initial pregnancy. Because the modern generation has a different attitude toward sex, we may expect to find more cases of pre-, as well as invasive, carcinoma of the cervix than formerly. This is the period of a woman's life when she is most fertile. The problems involved in the management of cancer of the cervix are compounded in the presence of pregnancy. It is essential, then, that Papanicolaou smears be taken routinely in this age group.

The treatment of choice is electrocoagulation carried out in the office, using no anesthesia or possibly a local application of carbocaine, provided that there is no stenosis of the endocervical canal and that the infection seems relatively superficial. Only a moderate degree of heat in the cautery tip should be used, because too much heat creates excessive destruction and often results in severe bleeding later when the slough separates. If a deep endocervical infection is present in a lacerated cervix, cauterization must be made deeper into the substance of the cervix. Hospitalization and cauterization under anesthesia are then indicated.

Cauterization should be carried out about one week after completion of the menstrual flow. The two methods by which the infected glands in the cervix may be destroyed with an electric cautery are radial cauterization and conization. In the former, the cautery tip is inserted to the level of the internal os and linear cauterizations are made at the 12, 2, 4, 6, 8 and 10 o'clock positions. In conization, a special cautery tip is used. The tip is passed to the level of the internal os and the instrument is rotated slowly in clockwise fashion. A figure-of-eight suture placed deep into the cervical musculature at the level of the internal os secures the cervical branches of the uterine artery and minimizes postoperative bleeding. In the convalescent period, some bleeding is to be expected when the slough separates. The patient should return for weekly office visits so that the endocervical canal can be dilated, thereby preventing stenosis. Complete reepithelization can be expected in about six weeks.

THE UTERUS. The initiation of pregnancy may be denied by such factors as stenosis of the cervical canal, intrauterine polyps, submucous leiomyomata, retroversion and congenital anomalies of the uterus.

Stenosis of the cervical canal can be corrected by dilation, and endometrial polyps can be removed by curettage. Because polyps of the endometrium are highly mobile on a stalk base, they may escape the curette. It is advisable, therefore, to explore the cavity after curettage with some type of grasping instrument such as a common duct forceps.

The surgeon should think twice before advising operation for either malpositions of the uterus or fibroid tumors, when the primary consideration is fertility. The normally fertile woman is not denied pregnancy because of the position of the uterus. When all else fails, uterine suspension may be justified in the subfertile patient.

Similarly, the majority of leiomyomata do not interfere with insemination or the conduct of a normal pregnancy. It is the position of the tumor which is of prime importance in the problem of fertility. Normally, an intramural fibroid does not interfere with conception, but if it happens to be placed at either the internal os or the cornual portion of the endometrial cavity, the tumor can cause obstruction to the passage of sperm into the uterus from below, or deny passage to the sperm or ovum at the point where the tube enters the uterus. A large intramural fibroid which encroaches on, or a submucous tumor which arises within the endometrial cavity, may interfere with proper implantation of the fertilized ovum, or complicate the normal progression of pregnancy.

OVARIAN TUMORS. It is possible to have orange-sized physiologic cysts of the ovary, such as the follicle or corpus luteum cysts, in this age group. Unlike neoplasms, the physi-ological cysts may alter the character of the menstrual pattern. The follicle cyst frequently creates an early or foreshortened cycle, whereas a persistent corpus luteum cyst may delay the onset of menstruation. Frequently, they rupture and disappear spontaneously. The palpation of an ovarian cyst which persists for several months calls for surgical intervention. A cyst which is larger than 5 cm. and does not disappear after a few menstrual periods is pathologic, regardless of its etiology.

TUBAL PATHOLOGY. Pelvic infections, whether they are produced by streptococci secondary to abortion, instrumentation of the cervix or endometrium, gonococcal or tuberculous infection, frequently create intrinsic or extrinsic damage to the tube and make conception impossible, more difficult or dangerous.

Primarily, streptococcal infections produce perisalpingitis and interfere with conception through loss of tubal motility. In severe infections, the tube becomes fixed in the pelvic mass. The gonococci, on the other hand, tend to destroy the mucosa of the tube, thereby producing obstruction to the passage of sperm or ovum, at either the uterine or the fimbriated end of the tube. Tuberculous infections are primarily tubal, but the endometrial cavity becomes involved approximately 50 per cent of the time. The patient is usually unaware of its existence and the diagnosis is apparent only when endometrial biopsy is performed to determine the cause of the patient's infertility. It may be missed then unless the biopsy is taken immediately before the onset of the menstrual period. The tubes are usually badly distorted, irregular, stony hard and totally devoid of any mucosa.

In general, whenever thickening, fixation and tenderness of the pelvic floor are noted on pelvic examination, and particularly when pelvic masses can be felt, chronic pelvic inflammatory disease should be suspected. Its treatment should take precedence over the investigation for sterility.

Any surgical operation on the tube for the purpose of improving fecundity should be preceded by an endometrial biopsy to determine the state of the endometrium and whether ovulation is occurring normally. Carbon dioxide insufflation of the tube or stereosalpingography should be employed to establish patency. Hysterosalpingography is also useful to detect any interference with the motility of the tubes which may be caused

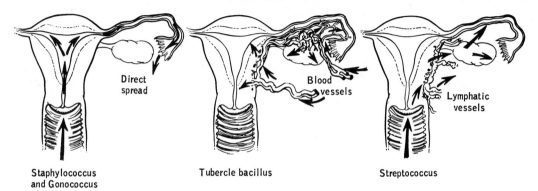

Direct
spread

Blood
vessels

Lymphatic
vessels

Staphylococcus
and Gonococcus

Tubercle bacillus

Streptococcus

Figure 2. Comparison of the modes of invasion of four important bacterial infections of the female genitalia. The gonorrheal and staphylococcal infections spread upward along surfaces to reach the peritoneal cavity. Tuberculosis is blood-borne. Streptococci penetrate through the lymphatics and veins to reach the parametrium.

by peritubal adhesions. The husband's ability to fertilize an ovum should also be tested by postcoital semen analysis.

More precise information concerning the conditions in the lower pelvis and, particularly, the tubes can be obtained by performing a culdoscopy. This requires anesthesia and hospitalization. A further check on tubal patency can be obtained if tubal lavage is performed at the time of culdoscopy.

Surgical procedures to restore the tube to a functional state are usually not rewarding. They are more successful when the obstruction centers on the fimbriated end of the tube. Encouraging successes have been reported in the use of polyethylene tubing to maintain patency, and a plastic cover to prevent adhesions from negating the reconstruction procedure on the fimbriated end of the tubes. The tubing and plastic cover must be removed at a second operation. Operations which call for resection of the cornual end of the tube and reimplantation of the distal portion over an inlying stint which passes through the tubal lumen into the endometrial cavity have been increasingly successful in establishing patency. Unfortunately, the pregnancy rate at present continues to be low. Greater rewards come when there is normal patency, and the primary problem is disturbed motility from peritubal adhesions.

CONGENITAL MALFORMATIONS. Although it is desirable to recognize anatomic variations in the uterus and vagina as early in life as possible, many congenital abnormalities are not discovered until investigations are conducted to determine the reason why the patient cannot become pregnant or cannot maintain a pregnancy. They produce few symptoms and frequently cannot be detected on routine physical examination.

All manner of duplications and partitionings of the uterus occur, ranging from double uterus and vagina, with normal tubes and ovaries, to the most common anomaly, which is a heart-shaped uterus with an indentation on the fundal portion. They are obvious examples of either complete or partial failure of union of the two müllerian ducts. The finding of a single cavity and one tube and ovary is an example of unilateral failure in development. Figure 3 depicts the types of anomaly as classified by Jarcho. Approximately 1 in 1500 obstetric, and 1 in 2000 gynecologic patients show some variation from the normal.

The clinical importance of congenital malformations lies in the fact that they produce so many obstetric complications. Fertility is impaired, and there is also a marked tendency for the pregnant, malformed uterus to abort spontaneously. This is particularly likely to occur in a septate uterus, whether partial or complete. Conversely, twin infants have been delivered from a uterus didelphys. If the pregnancy does go to term, a number of complications tend to appear, such as fetal prematurity, postmaturity, prolonged labor, breech and transverse presentations and retained placentas. Labor is usually prolonged and the rate of cesarean section is high.

One of the most drastic and dangerous complications occurs when pregnancy takes place in a rudimentary horn of a bicornuate uterus. Intra-abdominal rupture will take place if the condition is not recognized. The condition is similar to that existing in an ectopic pregnancy, but occurs near the tenth week of pregnancy.

Uterosalpingography, which provides visible evidence of the congenital defect, is the chief detecting device. The history of repeated miscarriage suggests its presence, as

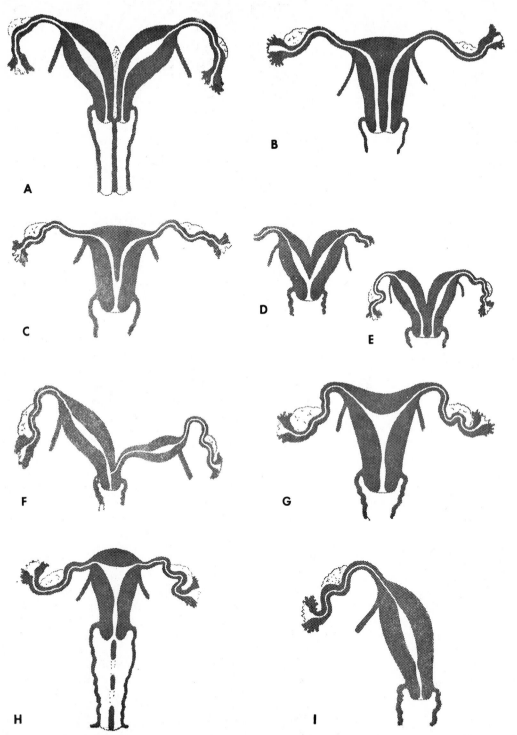

Figure 3.   Diagram of uterine anomalies. *A,* Uterus didelphys with double vagina; *B,* uterus septus duplex with single vagina; *C,* uterus subseptus unicollis; *D,* uterus bicornis unicollis, a variant of so-called bipartite uterus; *E,* uterus duplex; *F,* uterus bicornis unicollis with one connected rudimentary horn: in a related anomaly the smaller horn is unconnected; *G,* uterus arcuatus; *H,* septations of vagina; and *I,* uterus unicornis.

does the palpation of an eccentrically placed uterine mass. If a congenital anomaly is discovered in the uterus, the urinary system should be examined for additional malformations.

Though the fetal mortality rate is nearly ten times higher in the malformed uterus, the maternal mortality rate is in the range of 0 to 1.5 per cent. Unless the patient has a history of repeated abortions, or many complicated and protracted labors, there is no indication to operate simply to correct a known deformity. If, on the other hand, the patient with a septate, subseptate or arcuate uterus has had such a history, there is every reason to resect the septum by longitudinal section of the uterine body, followed by reconstruction of the uterus so that a single endometrial cavity is created. If the patient is found to have a rudimentary horn, it should be removed. There is no valid reason for surgical excision or reconstructive procedures in a patient with a double uterus, as long as there is no vaginal partition to interfere with intercourse. If abnormal bleeding patterns develop in a patient with a double uterus, both cavities should be curetted. Instances of carcinoma of the fundus on one side only have been recorded.

OBSTETRIC COMPLICATIONS. The basic problems in sterility are concerned not only with the initiation of pregnancy but also with the inability to retain it. Among the problems are habitual abortion, threatened abortion, incomplete abortion, missed abortion and ectopic pregnancy.

Approximately 10 per cent of all pregnancies end in spontaneous abortion early in their course. Some of this is due to chance, and the patient who has such an experience in one pregnancy need not repeat it in another. When three or more pregnancies have so terminated, there is undoubtedly a basic defect. The defect may be faulty germ plasm, an unfavorable environment within the uterus which prevents proper implantation of the fertilized ovum, or biochemical alterations within the endometrium which interfere with adequate nourishment to the implanted conceptus.

Habitual abortion. The treatment of habitual abortion is basically a medical problem. In recent years, surgical treatment has been employed to correct the incompetent cervix. The operation takes one of two forms: the endocervical canal and the internal os are constricted by wedge-shaped removal of sections and closure, or the caliber of the os is reduced from without by placing a constricting band of fascia, Mersilene gauze or poly-ethylene-encased O-Surgiloid sutures beneath the vaginal epithelium but around the cervix. This is generally done after the patient has become pregnant, but it may be employed in anticipation of this.

There are two courses available for management of pregnancy at term. The constricting band may be divided to allow normal delivery through the vagina, or it may be left in situ and cesarean section performed.

Threatened and inevitable abortion. A distinction must be made between threatened and inevitable abortion, in order that proper therapy may be instituted early enough to do any good. Bleeding in the first trimester of pregnancy is not uncommon. Unfortunately, the amount of blood loss, whether estimated by patient or doctor, is not helpful in establishing the differential diagnosis. The diagnosis of abortion can be made if the immunological test for pregnancy shifts from positive to negative.

Every effort should be made to save the pregnancy if abortion is threatened. Bed rest, thyroid and progesterone supplements should be given, with mild sedatives to relieve apprehension. Heavy sedation or narcotics must be avoided because the differential diagnosis between threatened abortion and ectopic pregnancy is not always easily established.

If the bleeding is excessive and the cervix is either dilated or effaced, and particularly if recognizable fetal tissue can be seen at the external os, uterine evacuation should be encouraged by an intravenous Syntocinon drip. Curettage is usually advisable to ensure complete emptying of the uterus. The blood loss should be replaced by transfusion when required, and antibiotics should be given to prevent the development of any infection which may have been caused by intrauterine manipulation.

The consensus is that curettage can be performed immediately with minimal morbidity and mortality, based on the fact that the infection is apt to be saprophytic and confined to the retained products of conception. Morbidity is believed to be due to toxic absorption rather than to uterine infection. To be successful, the uterus must be thoroughly cleaned and no products of conception left behind. There is less likelihood that destructive secondary infection will arise when the uterus is emptied early. Transfusions and antibiotic drugs are given as adjuvant therapy.

Missed abortion. At times, the initial episode of bleeding and the accompanying abdominal cramps subside, and the threat of abortion seems to have passed. It is well to remember that some patients may have received progestational hormones which may have delayed uterine evacuation. The patient and surgeon hope that the pregnancy has simply been threatened, but the uterus does not increase in size as it should with a viable fetus. The problem then arises whether to allow the patient to extrude the dead fetus herself, or to empty the uterus by curettage.

Curettage is the best choice. There is less emotional strain on the patient, and there is always some chance of developing afibrinogenemia even in early pregnancy. The symptoms of missed abortion and chorioepithelioma are identical. Measurement of chorionic gonadotropin in these patients is not much help, for it only indicates that viable trophoblasts persist. It does not distinguish pregnancy or missed abortion from a trophoblastic tumor.

Septic abortion. An infected abortion is a common complication in the pregnant patient, despite the widespread use of antibiotics. It is usually the result of introduction of an instrument or solution into the uterine cavity in the hope that pregnancy will be interrupted. Rarely does a missed abortion become infected as long as the cervix is closed. In many instances, a careful history unearths the fact that some foreign body or substance has been inserted in the pregnant uterus in an attempt to produce an abortion, but the great majority of patients deny any such act. Important information can be obtained from the history, however, such as the date of the last normal period, as well as the duration and nature of the present bleeding episode. It is helpful to know the character of any abdominal pain, where it is located and whether the elevated temperature has been accompanied by chills.

In addition to the necessity of ruling out extragenital sources as a cause of elevated temperature in a patient who may be trying to abort, it is also of basic importance to decide whether the infection is confined to the uterus or has spread to involve the parametrium and the tubes. The nature of the treatment depends on the extent of the inflammatory disease.

The decisive factor in differential diagnosis is the degree of pelvic floor tenderness. The history or presence of chills and fever in a septic abortion is indicative of an extensive infection. Uterine infection alone is usually accompanied by temperatures of 100 to 103° F. The leukocyte count varies from normal to 20,000. There is less bleeding but more discharge. The size of the uterus depends on the duration of the pregnancy and how much of its contents have been evacuated. On rectal examination, the pelvic floor is neither tender nor thickened. Abdominal wall tenderness is elicited if the infected uterus is pushed against the sensitive parietal peritoneum, but on moving the uterine cervix alone only uterine tenderness is noted.

Pelvic tenderness usually suggests parametrial extension but the surgeon should always keep in mind that in these patients there may be a large psychic component which makes evaluation of the degree of pelvic tenderness difficult.

The primary site of infection in septic abortion lies in the fetal membranes. It is important that the uterus be emptied at the earliest possible moment to prevent spread of the infection beyond the uterus. There is much to lose by waiting until the cervix is dilated.

Since the bleeding is rarely excessive, time can be taken to assess the patient's condition by obtaining the hematocrit, white blood count and differential, urine output, cervical smear and culture, and an upright x-ray film of the abdomen to rule out foreign body or perforated viscus. Intramuscular penicillin, erythromycin or chloromycetin may be given. It is sometimes a good idea to add intravenous fluid with Syntocinon. After six to 12 hours of observation, the patient is usually afebrile and the uterus can safely be emptied by curettage. The antibiotic regimen should be maintained intramuscularly or orally for at least five days.

The common variety of septic abortion is usually not a dangerous condition, but occasionally the patient will suddenly go into shock while antibiotic therapy is being given in preparation for curettage. There is little evidence of blood loss and the fall in blood pressure cannot be corrected by transfusions alone. The peripheral collapse is due to toxic absorption from an overwhelming infection in the placenta and membranes within the uterus.

The patient must be placed in the best possible condition at the earliest possible time. Massive doses of antibiotics should be given. One of the reasons for the persistence of falling blood pressure may be pooling of the extracellular fluid in the splanchnic bed. The patient's circulating blood volume must be restored to normal. A catheter in the axillary vein, which permits monitoring of the central venous pressure, provides a clinical guide to impending congestive heart failure. The central venous pressure gives more accurate information than can be obtained by observing the arterial pressure. Rarely is it essential to employ pressor drugs such as Metraminol or levarterenol. If a pressor drug is needed, the drug of choice is isoproterenol (Isoprel). The advantage of this agent is that it has a sympathomimetic effect which tends to improve coronary perfusion and cardiac output without cutting down on the blood flow to other vital organs.

With the axillary catheter in place and the central venous pressure maintained, blood can be given under better control and a better estimate can be made of the circulatory volume. With improvement in the patient's clinical condition, the patient should begin to diurese as extracellular fluid returns from the splanchnic bed.

At this point, under the protection of massive doses of antibiotics, the uterus can be emptied by curettage. If the cervix is closed and there is doubt whether the uterus can be completely evacuated, a hysterectomy should be done.

When the infection has spread beyond the uterus the patient has a fulminating case of acute pelvic inflammation and is seriously ill. She may develop pelvic cellulitis, thrombophlebitis, pelvic abscess or pulmonary infarct. The infecting organism is almost always the Streptococcus, and the severity of the infection varies with its virulence.

The symptoms and physical findings are those of acute pelvic inflammation from any cause. The treatment should be conservative and supportive. Little will be gained from a curettage because, in most instances, the abortion is complete. The patient may be expected to have rebound tenderness, spasm and even rigidity of the lower abdominal wall, combined with exquisite pelvic tenderness when abdominorectal examination is done. The pelvic tenderness is often so extreme that it is impossible to determine the size of the uterus or whether pelvic masses are present. Pelvic peritonitis may become generalized. The temperature rarely falls below 103° F., and peaks occur as high as 105°.

Massive doses of penicillin and streptomycin should be given along with intravenous fluids to replace the electrolytes. Blood transfusions should be given to counteract sepsis,

not to combat blood loss. The bowel should be decompressed with a Miller-Abbott tube and the patient should rest in Fowler's position.

The infection frequently disappears in a couple of weeks, leaving either no residual, or else pelvic masses which can be easily felt and may require incision and drainage. Occasionally, the patient may not respond rapidly and may throw off septic emboli to the lung, which can be fatal. At this point, the surgeon may be forced to ligate the inferior vena cava and the ovarian veins.

ECTOPIC PREGNANCY

One of the more common and dramatic forms of abnormal uterine bleeding occurs when the patient has an ectopic pregnancy. When implanted outside the endometrial cavity, a beginning pregnancy may be found in any portion of the fallopian tube, in the ovary or on the peritoneal surface of the abdomen. In most instances, it is found in the outer or ampullary portion of the fallopian tube.

The etiology of an ectopic tubal pregnancy is linked to mechanical interference with the passage of the fertilized ovum. Certain disease entities, such as gonorrhea, attack the tubal epithelium primarily and create an endosalpingitis. If the destruction is not too great, the tube may be sufficiently patent to admit sperm but not dilated enough to allow the escape of the larger fertilized ovum into the endometrial cavity.

A previous streptococcal pelvic infection may have produced a perisalpingitis, which creates kinking and interferes with normal motility of the tube. The fertilized ovum then becomes trapped in the tube. It is possible that abnormal physiology and intrinsic metabolism of the tubal epithelium may be as important as the patency of the tubal lumen. Ectopic pregnancies have been known to occur as the first pregnancy in a patient who has no obstructive element in the tube itself.

The embryo implanted in an ectopic position tries to grow in the same manner it did in the endometrial cavity, but it has far less of a base in which to grow. The tubal epithelium lacks the elements necessary to nourish and sustain the fetus, because it was never designed to do so and cannot readily adapt to the new demand. The voracious trophoblast invades the muscle wall of the tube in search of sustenance. The eroding chorionic villi

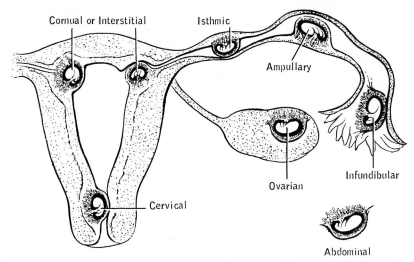

Figure 4.   Implantation sites in ectopic pregnancy: the uterus, tube, ovary and peritoneal cavity.

progressively weaken the tubal wall and infiltrate the underlying vessels, producing hemorrhage both within the embryonic sac and between it and the tubal wall. This usually takes place within the first ten weeks of the pregnancy.

Once the embryo dies, several things may happen. The blood-filled chorionic sac may rupture into the tubal lumen, forming a so-called tubal mole. If the bleeding is not too extensive, it may absorb wholly or in part, with mild lower abdominal pain as the only indication of its presence. If the hemorrhage is sudden and severe, tubal contraction often forces the abortus out through the open end of the tube, either partially or completely. The fallopian tube may rupture abruptly and explosively into the peritoneal cavity, or develop a slow hemorrhagic leak.

The symptoms and physical findings vary according to the nature of the growth pattern. The abdominal symptoms are usually sufficiently pronounced to warrant exploration. The symptoms are extreme when actual rupture of the tube occurs or when extensive bleeding takes place from the open end of the tube in a complete tubal abortion. They are not pathognomonic of tubal rupture, but rather of an intraperitoneal hemorrhage. If the distention of the tube occurs gradually and forceful contractions do not take place, the condition may go unrecognized and may either absorb completely or develop a palpable mass which is undistinguishable from pelvic inflammation. The symptoms then will be minimal and consist chiefly of a delay in the onset of the period followed by slight staining and moderate cramplike pains in the lower

abdomen. The same symptoms arise when the patient bleeds intra-abdominally from a persistent corpus luteum. A biological or immunological test of pregnancy is usually done but it is not particularly helpful. Primarily, the diagnosis of ectopic pregnancy in an unruptured state is made upon suspicion.

At times, there is great difficulty in distinguishing an early ectopic pregnancy from a threatened abortion. Posterior colpotomy, culdoscopy and needle puncture of the cul-de-sac all can contribute to the diagnosis. They do not necessarily rule out an ectopic pregnancy, which is still in the tube, simply because the patient may not be leaking blood into the cul-de-sac, and on culdoscopy, the entire length of both tubes may not be seen.

A curettage should be helpful, but there is a natural reluctance to do it if there is any chance that a viable pregnancy remains in the uterus. If an abnormal amount of vaginal bleeding is of long standing and the diagnosis is still in doubt, curettage may establish the diagnosis. If the curetted material shows decidua without villi, one may then reasonably assume that either an ectopic pregnancy is present or that complete abortion has taken place. Unfortunately, this is not complete proof because regeneration of the endometrium may have taken place and a secretory endometrium may be present with a live trophoblast in the tube.

When ectopic pregnancy is suspected, the patient should be hospitalized. If the patient is admitted with symptoms suggesting early unruptured ectopic pregnancy, and an abdominal mass is felt, immediate abdominal exploration should be done. Too frequently, rupture occurs spontaneously while the patient is under observation on the ward, or following discharge from the hospital.

It has been the custom to remove the involved tube when exploration reveals the presence of an ectopic pregnancy within it. This is probably advisable if there has been a history of pelvic infection, particularly gonorrhea, for the endothelium of the tube has been compromised and the tube is basically defective. One may take a calculated risk and incise the tube overlying the pregnancy, evulse it and close the defect rather than sacrifice the tube in a young patient with normal genital development and no history of tubal infection.

When tubal rupture occurs explosively, the patient usually has abdominal pain so severe that she faints. She may recover temporarily only to collapse and go into shock when further intraperitoneal hemorrhage occurs. The extent to which the classic picture of shock is present depends on how rapidly a large amount of blood is lost. It is the rapidity of the loss which is the important factor. The symptoms and physical findings are those of intra-abdominal hemorrhage; they are not pathognomonic of ruptured ectopic pregnancy.

The most important element in therapy is abdominal exploration performed as soon as possible after shock has been corrected by intravenous solutions and blood replacement. It is a basic surgical principle that the patient's condition be stable before operation is performed. However, the patient may be bleeding massively into the peritoneal cavity, and there may not be enough time to restore her to good condition. Arterial transfusion, followed by abdominal exploration, arrest of the hemorrhage and blood replacement as the operation proceeds, may be the only choice.

With the abdomen open, upward traction on the uterus usually controls the immediate hemorrhage. With the bleeding controlled, the emergency phase passes. If a rupture has occurred in the tubal lumen, the damaged tube should be removed. The ovary should also be removed if it is matted together in one mass with the tube, otherwise the ovary should be spared. If the ectopic pregnancy is being extruded from the fimbriated end, it may be milked out of the open end and the tube spared, provided it can be established that the abortion is complete. All obvious blood clot should be removed if the patient is in reasonably good condition. Under these circumstances, the appendix can also be removed, but if the patient's condition is equivocal, the part of wisdom is to remove the tube as quickly as possible and leave the old blood and appendix undisturbed.

TROPHOBLASTIC DISEASE

In early gestation, the level of human chorionic gonadotropin is normally in the high range. For this reason, the determination of the amount of circulating gonadotropin is not helpful in establishing the diagnosis of a suspected hydatidiform mole. The quantitative measurement of human chorionic gonadotropin, however, is extremely important in following the course of the known presence of trophoblastic disease both during and after treatment.

With the diagnosis of a mole established, the surgeon is concerned with the earliest possible evacuation of the uterus. In the past, this was usually accomplished by either curettage or hysterotomy. The latter is preferred because it gives the pathologist an opportunity of examining the implantation site of the mole. It would be at this point that the mole might be invasive or an element of choriocarcinoma might appear. In most instances, evacuation of the uterine cavity can be accomplished by the intravenous use of Syntocinon, and rarely is hysterotomy necessary. Following extrusion of the mole, curettage should be done to ensure the complete evacuation of the uterine contents. This can produce an excessive amount of bleeding. The surgeon must be prepared to replace several units of blood, with the amount dependent upon the extent of blood loss.

Since approximately 10 per cent of hydatidiform moles undergo malignant change, the surgeon will be well advised to administer chemotherapeutic drugs just before, or immediately following, evacuation of the mole. If the kidney function is normal, the average dose given should be 25 mg. of methotrexate intramuscularly over a five-day period. If the surgeon prefers, he may give actinomycin D rather than methotrexate on a dosage schedule of 400 to 500 gamma per day, for a period of four to five days.

Periodic estimates of the levels of human chorionic gonadotropin should follow the treatment regimen outlined. If the titer has returned to normal nonpregnancy levels of 50 to 200 mouse units, the patient should have monthly tests for total gonadotropin for at least one year before she can be permitted to have another pregnancy. If the total gonadotropin titer has not returned to the normal non-pregnant level of 50 to 200 mouse units, the surgeon should be alert to the possibility that persistent trophoblastic disease is present. It is important to stress the fact that the chorionic gonadotropin levels should not be made by the usual pregnancy test. A negative pregnancy test can be misleading. Total gonadotropin titers should be done and be in the normal range before one can be sure that trophoblastic disease no longer exists.

If, at the end of six weeks following evacuation of the mole, the gonadotropin is still elevated, it is very likely that the mole has a malignant component which must be vigorously treated. This can best be accomplished in various centers that have recently been established. To evaluate properly the extent and localization of the disease, it is essential that the patient have such examinations as electroencephalogram and chest x-ray, intravenous pyelograms, pelvic arteriograms and liver scans as well as liver function studies. Because the effectiveness of the drugs used is closely related to the toxicity created by the drug, the courses of chemotherapy are given as frequently as the effect on the hematopoietic system, particularly the bone marrow, permits. In addition, the toxic reaction of the drug on the gastrointestinal and genitourinary tracts must be carefully observed. Because 70 per cent of the methotrexate is eliminated by the kidney, it is important that kidney function be adequate. The treatment schedules are carried out until the titers of chorionic gonadotropin are reduced to the normal range. The drugs are usually given intramuscularly but in special instances, when the metastases can be identified in a specific area, it may be possible to treat the lesion by arterial infusion. Excellent results have been reported when the chemotherapeutic drugs are used in this fashion and operation is indicated less often than in the past. In special instances, when the metastases are readily accessible, it is still possible and reasonable to excise the metastatic area.

The chemotherapeutic agents presently employed are methotrexate and actinomycin D. Newer drugs such as Velban and Cytoxan have been used when the trophoblastic disease has proved to be resistant to methotrexate and actinomycin D. On the other side of the coin, it is well recognized that spontaneous cures do occur.

We recognize that trophoblastic disease often follows, or is present in association with, a hydatidiform mole. It is well to keep in mind that on rare occasions it may follow a normal pregnancy, a gestation in either tube or ovary, or appear after an abortion.

TUMORS IN ASSOCIATION WITH PREGNANCY

Benign and malignant neoplasms occur in young women who are pregnant. The surgical problems are concerned with whether the tumor is malignant, or if benign, how it will interfere with the normal progress of labor.

CANCER OF THE CERVIX. Approximately 1.5 per cent of all cervical cancers are associated with pregnancy. The lesions have the same appearance and give rise to the same symptoms as those which appear in the nonpregnant state. Cancer of the cervix in pregnancy is commonly said to have a poor prognosis. This is not due to any alteration in the growth pattern, but to the fact that the lesions are more advanced.

Any patient who presents symptoms of abnormal bleeding and discharge, and who has a suspicious lesion on the cervix which is ulcerated or bleeds easily, should have a biopsy and a smear test. If the smear is suggestive, there is no contraindication to performing a cold knife conization. The pregnancy will not be interrupted.

If the histologic review reveals carcinoma in situ, the pregnancy can be allowed to continue provided the patient is examined regularly with smear and biopsy. Whether the uterus should be removed at the termination of the pregnancy depends on the age, parity and the desire to have children.

The choice of therapy for invasive cancer depends on the extent of the invasion and the trimester of pregnancy in which the diagnosis is made. The two modes of therapy are operation and radiation.

In the first trimester, the optimum treatment for a Stage I lesion is a Wertheim hysterectomy with pelvic lymphadenectomy. The technical difficulties presented by an enlarged soft uterus and the increased vascularity are more than balanced by the edema of the tissue spaces. The advantage of the surgical approach lies in the fact that there is less chance of disseminating tumor cells, for it will not be necessary to abort the patient prior to treatment.

Attempts to treat cancer of the cervix and salvage the embryo by radiation therapy have resulted in such a high incidence of congenital malformations that it can no longer be recommended. If radiation is to be used, the uterus must be emptied either by curettage or roentgen ray treatment of the ovaries.

When the cancer has spread beyond the confines of the cervix and the tissues adjacent to it, operation should not be considered. It will then be wise to empty the uterus and proceed with the radiation program.

The basic therapy for cancer of the cervix later in pregnancy is radiation. An abdominal hysterotomy should be done as a preliminary step. The uterus must be emptied because it is unwise to allow the patient to extrude the large fetus through an undilated cervix that contains carcinoma, and because radiation of the ovaries at this phase of pregnancy will not produce a spontaneous abortion.

When the pregnancy approaches term, it is advisable to delay definitive therapy until there is a chance of obtaining a viable infant. A cesarean section should then be performed, followed by radiation therapy, approximately two weeks later.

OVARIAN CYSTS. Ovarian cysts, particularly the larger ones, contribute to the complications of pregnancy and may require operation. The cyst may undergo torsion of the pedicle and require immediate operation; the position of the cyst may interfere with the mechanics of delivery; and the adnexal tumor may be malignant.

The risk of torsion increases markedly after the third or fourth month as the pregnant uterus rises out of the pelvis. In the early months, the pregnancy usually terminates in abortion, while premature labor appears when the pregnancy is more advanced. The risks of torsion of the pedicle are not over when the delivery is finally accomplished, since the incidence rises as the uterus involutes.

A large cyst impacted in the pelvis may be so traumatized that the cyst wall ruptures during delivery, producing peritonitis. This is more apt to occur if the cyst is a dermoid because its contents are very irritating. Cesarean section is indicated, because the maternal mortality rate, as well as that of the infant, is appreciable when the cyst ruptures during a normal delivery.

LEIOMYOMA. The presence of a fibroid in the uterus not only makes it more difficult for the patient to become pregnant and harder for her to maintain a pregnancy, but also it may complicate delivery.

Whether or not complications arise depends on the size of the tumor, its location and the degree of fixation to other structures.

A pedunculated fibroid, like an ovarian cyst, is prone to twist on its pedicle and compromise its blood supply. This is the only type of fibroid tumor which can successfully be removed without disturbing the pregnancy.

Large tumors, or those occupying strategic positions within the uterus, are apt to produce abortion, premature labor, abnormal presentations and dystocia. For example, a submucous myoma either aborts early or has a high incidence of placenta previa, abnormally adherent placenta or abnormal presentations. There is no indication for operation because abortion will surely follow.

The presence of a large fibroid in the lower uterine segment which juts out posteriorly so that the fetal head cannot become properly engaged, is a proper indication for cesarean section. This is particularly true if the tumor is adherent in the cul-de-sac. Usually, the tumor will rise as the uterus enlarges, but it cannot do so if it is impacted. These patients tend to have uterine inertia, difficulty in separating and delivering the placenta, and postpartum hemorrhage. The tumor should be excised, following the delivery of the fetus by cesarean section.

Red degeneration of a myoma produces the most difficulty in management. It results from interference with the blood supply to the tumor located within the wall of the uterus. The degree of necrosis within the tumor varies markedly, and with it, the nature of the symptomatology. Red degeneration often occurs with dramatic effects in the middle stages of pregnancy, when the uterus is undergoing its greatest period of enlargement.

The preferred treatment of red degeneration is supportive and expectant. The thought of operation should be entertained only if the diagnosis is in doubt. In most instances, the process will subside. Surgical intervention commonly results in the loss of the fetus, while the chance of sepsis increases.

PELVIC INFLAMMATION

ACUTE PELVIC INFLAMMATION. In the acute form of pelvic inflammation there is little reason for performing surgical procedures. Supportive measures plus an intensive antibiotic regimen are preferable modes of therapy. This is particularly true when the infection is of gonorrheal origin.

Except for the excision, marsupialization, or incision and drainage of Bartholin's glands, and the incision and destruction of the multiple miliary abscesses which occur in Skene's glands with gonococcal infections, there is no indication for operation in acute infections which occur below the level of the cervix. In those infections which spread to involve the uterus, fallopian tubes, ovaries and lower pelvic cavity, the only indication for surgical intervention appears when pelvic abscesses develop. They may require drainage because of the danger that they may rupture into the peritoneal cavity and produce a generalized peritonitis. The chief problem from a surgical point of view is the uncertainty of the primary diagnosis. The same symptoms, which are actually those of a localized pelvic peritonitis, can be produced by other pathologic entities which may require immediate operation. The differential diagnosis includes appendicitis, ectopic pregnancy, twisted ovarian cyst and acute pyelitis. At times, the differential diagnosis cannot be made and the patient has to be operated upon. If the diagnosis is in error, and the tubes are acutely inflamed, they should be left alone.

The history may provide the clue. The history of a previous abortion, disturbed menstrual cycles or operative treatment of the cervix, suggest a streptococcal infection as the explanation for the pelvic inflammation. If there is a history of coitus immediately preceding menstruation, or an acute vaginal discharge appears following it, then gonorrhea should be suspected.

There are many points of similarity between acute pyelitis and acute pelvic inflammation. Both produce a high temperature, abdominal distention, nausea and vomiting, lower abdominal tenderness, chills and elevated white blood counts. The urinary sediment may show no pus cells, particularly if there is a ureteral block. The history of onset, however, is different. The chills in pyelitis usually precede the onset of pain, whereas in acute pelvic inflammation, the pain is there and the chills are simply evidence of further spread of the local infection.

CHRONIC PELVIC INFLAMMATION. In the recurring and chronic stage of pelvic inflammation, the indications for operation and the type of operation performed are controlled by the disability produced, the desire for and likelihood of maintaining reproductive capability, as well as the psychologic need for continued menstrual function.

An acute pelvic inflammation of gonorrheal origin may become chronic if the original tubal infection was extensive, the patient resistant to therapy, the antibiotic regimen inadequate or the patient refused further treatment. The patient is then apt to develop a pyosalpinx because the fimbriated ends seal over and become adherent to the ovary and adjacent peritoneum. As a result of the pus tubes and localized pelvic abscesses, the patient is apt to have recurring attacks of pelvic inflammation. These patients are usually seriously ill, with much more peritoneal involvement than in the original attack. The abdominal distention is more pronounced and the white blood count is consistently over 20,000. The severity of the infection is not due to the gonococci, but to secondary invaders, chiefly *Escherichia coli.*

Even though it is well recognized that antibiotic therapy will resolve a tubo-ovarian abscess or pyosalpinx, it is wiser to wait for a period of remission rather than attempt a curative operation during an acute flareup. The only exception is the uncertainty of whether the palpable adnexal masses or abscesses are about to rupture into the general peritoneal cavity.

The actual operation is tailored to the patient's need as to the location and extent of the pathology, and the desirability of attempting to preserve the reproductive capacity. In the older patient whose family is complete, or the younger patient whose internal genitalia are hopelessly compromised by the pathology, the best procedure is total hysterectomy and bilateral salpingectomy. The ovaries can be left in the younger woman if they are not involved in a tubo-ovarian abscess. Infections involving the interior of the ovary do not respond to antibiotic therapy, however intense it may be.

The patient may wish to preserve her reproductive function if it is at all possible. Rarely is this possible when the underlying cause is gonorrhea, because infections from this organism usually produce severe damage to the tubal epithelium and it is almost invariably bilateral. Only 5 per cent return to normal function. The surgeon must then decide whether there is enough chance of success to warrant a tuboplasty.

The type of operation on the tube depends on the extent of the damage and the localization of the pathology within the tube. Rarely does the surgeon find simple uncomplicated adhesions which produce kinking of the tube, but if he does, lysis of these adhesions and uterine suspension may suffice. In the majority of instances, the fimbriated ends of the tube are closed and more sophisticated surgical procedures are required to restore normality. If preoperative gas insufflation or hysterosalpingography indicates that the remaining portion of the tube is patent, resection of the involved fimbria and plastic reconstruction can be a rewarding operation. In 75 per cent of the patients, tubal patency is achieved, and 33 per cent become pregnant. If the fimbria are open but the block occurs at the uterine end of the tube, it is possible to resect the damaged cornual portion and insert the fish-mouthed end of the proximal portion of the tube into the endometrial cavity. The results for subsequent conception are poor, although the patency of the tube may be maintained.

Except for the rare opportunity of freeing tubal adhesions following a mild attack of streptococcal infection, total hysterectomy or drainage of localized pelvic abscesses should be performed.

In the absence of any indication of encapsulated pus, the longer any operation is postponed the better. When the following situations arise, it may become necessary to operate on the patient if, under the protection of heavy doses of the antibiotics: the attacks recur too frequently; the pain is persistent and incapacitating; the recurring episodes are accompanied by signs of peritonitis; and signs of intestinal obstruction appear.

Localized abscesses take longer to develop when the patient is subjected to heavy antibiotic therapy. They may not appear for several months. They are suspected by the presence of pitting edema or soft spots within an indurated area. The area where localization takes place varies, but there is a marked tendency for pus pockets to point on the lower abdominal wall close to the symphysis on either side. In this situation, it is possible to drain the abscess extraperitoneally, thereby avoiding the danger of contaminating the peritoneal cavity. Incisions are made in the groin overlying the abscess. The presence of pus is confirmed by needle aspiration. The anatomical relationship of the peritoneum to the wall of the abscess is established and the pus pocket drained.

The basic therapy for tuberculosis of the genital tract is antibiotic therapy. Isonicotinic acid hydrazide, para-aminosalicylic acid and streptomycin are used in various combinations. At times, all three may be given. Modern drug therapy has been very effective, and the surgeon can afford to delay operative procedures to await the response to medical therapy.

However, there is still a place for surgical therapy in tuberculosis, for a variety of reasons: the diagnosis is not made preoperatively, the dense adhesions which frequently follow tuberculous salpingitis do not disappear with medical therapy, the disease may reactivate after years of successful medical treatment, the bleeding pattern may be excessive and depleting, and fistulous tracts may develop which will not heal.

The extent of the operation is tailored to the extent of disease and, within the framework of good judgment, the desires of the patient. Under the protection of antituberculous drugs, one may remove the tubes, the main source of the infection, and leave the uterus and ovaries; sacrifice the uterus and tubes, but save the ovaries; or excise uterus, tubes and ovaries. With drug protection for the patient, the surgeon need no longer fear that a general systemic flareup will follow the surgical procedure.

Problems in the 30 to 40 Age Group

The patient between the ages of 30 and 40 presents a variety of problems of a surgical nature. They become complex because the surgeon is uncertain when he should be conservative and preserve menstrual and reproductive function. The chief entities which create this problem are abnormal bleeding of functional nature, endometriosis, carcinoma in situ of the cervix, leiomyomata and physiologic and neoplastic tumors of the ovary.

ABNORMAL BLEEDING

In contrast to the patient in the 20 to 30 age group, where the predominant cause of the abnormal bleeding lies in some abnormality of pregnancy, either inside or outside the uterus, the most likely explanation in the later reproductive years is a functional one. The patient may still become pregnant and she may have malignant disease in the background, but bleeding of functional nature is the most common finding. In general, abnormal bleeding appears because of derangements in endocrine balance, blood dyscrasias or organic disease within the uterus.

The manifestations of the abnormal bleeding pattern are many and varied. The majority of patients have menorrhagia, which is the term used to describe the profuse period, often prolonged, which occurs at regular monthly intervals. The flow may be either ovulatory or anovulatory. Less often, bleeding may be prolonged for several weeks after a normal period, occur without regard to the normal cycle, or appear as intermenstrual spotting either continuously or at irregular intervals throughout the cycle, but usually just before the period.

In taking the history, which is the most important step in investigating the cause of the abnormal bleeding pattern, particular attention should be paid to the amount of blood loss; the number of pads used in the abnormal period as compared with the normal flow; the timing of the period within the cycle; the duration of menstruation, and the character of the bleeding. The most important factor is the duration of the flow. Any extension of the bleeding beyond a week may be regarded as pathologic.

There are other factors in the history which should be investigated, since it is well known that systemic disease, metabolic disturbances, and emotional strain may influence the menstrual pattern.

Physical examination often provides useful information, but it must be general as well as local. A pelvic and rectal examination can only disclose gross pathology in the uterus and adnexae. It will not reveal blood dyscrasia, anemia, systemic disease or metabolic disturbances. Laboratory studies to determine the degree as well as the character of the anemia, and thyroid function tests such as blood cholesterol, basal metabolic studies, protein bound iodine and radioactive iodine determinations are needed to confirm the suspicions aroused by the history and general physical examination.

Before instituting therapy, it is important to establish as far as possible the underlying cause of the abnormal uterine bleeding. Although disturbances in hormonal imbalance explain most of the abnormal bleeding patterns, the spectrum of causes is so broad that therapy often seems to be empirical and with little physiologic background. The major problem is to differentiate between functional and organic causes.

This is frequently no easy problem because in most instances, the patient with gross palpable organic abnormalities, who bleeds abnormally, does so because she has an endocrine imbalance rather than tumor or pelvic infection. This factor is not well understood. It applies particularly to leiomyomata of the uterus, but equally well to pelvic inflammation, ovarian tumors and endometriosis. A patient may have a large fibroid, extensive pelvic endometriosis or inflammation, and have no menstrual disturbance. The only fibroids which bleed per se are the submucous fibroids, or the intramural fibroid which occupies a submucosal position in the endometrial cavity, neither of which can be detected on physical examination.

The patient who has gross pelvic disease, which can be felt, bleeds from a proliferative endometrium, not a secretory one. The bleeding is anovulatory in character. The estrin stimulation is unbalanced by progestin, as shown by the fact that secretory endometrium is not recovered regardless of the stage of the cycle, and no recent corpora lutea are seen in the ovaries when abdominal exploration is done.

On the other hand, the patient with an endometrial polyp or a submucous fibroid bleeds because she has them. The former may bleed excessively but it is discovered only when curettage is done. The presence of a submucously placed fibroid, though it cannot be felt, may be suspected from the history. Characteristically, the patients have an unpredictable gushing flow of such quantity that they have to put a protective cover on the bed linen at night. Frequently, they are afraid of having an embarrassing accident during the day and will not leave the house during the time of the menstrual period. If flow of these proportions has occurred in successive cycles, the hemoglobin is often in the range of 6 to 7 gm. Rarely is the anemia this profound when the basic underlying cause of the bleeding is functional.

The other common cause for bleeding of this degree is hypothyroidism. Suspicion is aroused when the patient indicates that she has abnormal sensitivity to cold, constant fatigue despite adequate rest, and a weight problem. In addition, she may find herself dull, apathetic and unable to concentrate.

On physical examination, the patient may have coarse, dry hair and dry, waxy skin.

When the bleeding is profuse in this age group, it is also well to remember that pregnancy and its complications are still possible explanations. As long as a woman remains productive, there is always the chance that the abnormal bleeding pattern may be secondary to retained products of gestation, miscarriage, ectopic pregnancy or abortion, whether threatened or real.

While a patient rarely bleeds abnormally from abdominal pelvic infection, she may still bleed irregularly from intrauterine sepsis. It is well known that many patients date the onset of abnormal bleeding from the time of a previous miscarriage or abortion. The explanation may lie in the retention of placental fragments or polyps, but it is far more likely that inflammatory changes have occurred in the epithelium and the patient has a chronic endometritis.

Profuse and prolonged uterine bleeding can be due to leukemia, aplastic anemia, thrombopenic purpura or iron deficiency anemia. For example, a vicious circle may develop wherein excess blood lost at menstruation produces a chronic iron deficiency which, in turn, creates further and more intensive bleeding. Proper therapy calls for iron supplements and the correction of the deficiency, not an operation. When blood dyscrasias are suspected, a smear and complete blood study often pinpoints the source while it establishes the degree of anemia. Abnormalities in clot retraction and bleeding time may point to thrombopenic purpura. Too many hysterectomies have been done for excessive uterine bleeding from this cause. The treatment is blood transfusion and splenectomy, not hysterectomy.

Less often, systemic disease may explain a persistent bleeding pattern. This is why a general physical examination is so important. Hypertension and cardiovascular disease, particularly when they manifest themselves by cardiac decompensation and chronic passive congestion, are the most common constitutional causes. In still rarer instances, cirrhosis of the liver may account for abnormal bleeding at the time of the monthly period.

In recent years, more and more attention has been paid to the patient's psyche and emotional state when bizarre forms of menstrual bleeding are encountered. A real effort must be made, when obtaining the history, to uncover any suggestion of emotional stress which might adversely influence the normal endocrine function.

Finally, there is the possibility that the departure from the normal bleeding pattern may be due to malignant disease. Malignant tumors occur infrequently in this age group, but they appear frequently enough so that the possibility of their presence must be excluded before a benign explanation of the cause can be accepted.

Carcinoma of the endometrium is relatively rare, but cancer of the cervix in early age groups is being diagnosed more often, and papillary carcinoma of the ovary may appear at any age. It is well to keep in mind that, excluding functional tumors of the ovary, a neoplasm of the ovary rarely alters the menstrual pattern.

The treatment of abnormal bleeding depends on the underlying cause. When systemic disease, psychiatric causes, metabolic disturbances and blood dyscrasias are excluded, the correct diagnosis lies within two possibilities: endocrine dysfunction and organic pathology within the uterus.

It is possible to obtain considerable helpful information from an endometrial biopsy taken in the office. When taken in the latter half of the cycle, a pathologic report of a proliferative endometrium, when it should be secretory, suggests that ovulation has not occurred. The patient then has an endocrine balance in which estrin is unbalanced by progestin. Substitution therapy designed to replace the missing progestin should correct the bleeding defect. Unfortunately, it is only a sample of the endometrium, and in an obscure functional bleeding problem the response of the endometrium may not be uniform.

The final diagnosis is best established by curettage performed under anesthesia, because it provides the best means of detecting gross pathologic lesions within the uterus while it permits the pathologist to review the histology of all of the endometrium. To obtain the maximum amount of information, the curettage should be performed in the latter half of the cycle.

Hormone therapy should provide the ideal treatment for women in this age group because menstrual and reproductive function can be preserved. In the past, hormone therapy was rather disappointing. It was effective only when bleeding was anovulatory in nature and there was a progestin lack. In this age group, it is not uncommon to find bizarre forms of abnormal endometrium. In very recent years, the sequential type of hormone therapy has been more successful in converting an unusual type of endometrium into a more normal pattern.

Curettage is the most logical and practical method of correcting the abnormal bleeding problem. Not only is it diagnostic, but it is curative as well. When intrauterine pathology is present, such as endometritis, polyps or retained products of pregnancy, curettage removes the cause. It is also the only means of detecting a submucous fibroid. The complete evacuation of all the endometrium goes a long way toward curing the patient with abnormal histologic patterns. A single curettage may be all that is necessary to control cystic or adenomatous hyperplasia. This is important because approximately 10 per cent of patients with adenomatous hyperplasia later develop endometrial carcinoma.

Occasionally, biopsy reveals an endometrium in which secretory changes are noted, when one would normally expect to find reparative proliferative endometrium. The cycles tend to be of normal interval but are apt to be excessive and prolonged. This is termed "irregular endometrial shedding." To obtain the maximum effect from curettage, it should be performed within the first five days of the cycle.

In rare instances, curettage is ineffective. While most patients with functional bleeding respond to curettage, this is not universally true. The abnormal bleeding pattern may recur even after the most meticulous curettement. It is also possible that a flat, sessile polyp may be missed when the endometrial cavity is scraped. Likewise, some submucous leiomyomata may escape detection.

When repeated regimens of hormonal substitution have been ineffective and the patient continues to have an abnormal bleeding pattern after two or three curettements, hysterectomy is indicated. This is far better than intrauterine radium or external radiation, because this can only control the bleeding at the price of castration. Intrauterine radiation has a bad reputation when employed for benign conditions. It is contraindicated in the presence of a submucous fibroid because it can only create slough and sepsis, which simply aggravate the bleeding problem. Moreover, more uterine cancers develop after intrauterine radiation than can be attributed to chance. When hysterectomy is performed, normal ovarian function can be preserved.

CARCINOMA IN SITU OF THE CERVIX

Carcinoma in situ is the earliest form of cancer arising in the uterine cervix. In this phase, it has all the characteristics of malignant disease without the important element of invasiveness. When detected and treated properly, one should expect 100 per cent cure. In recent years, the attention of the medical profession has focused sharply on the problem of detection of cervical cancer at a time when it can be both prevented and cured. Recent statistics from the data of large insurance companies and state boards of health indicate that the incidence of invasive cancer has declined appreciably.

Clinical invasive cancer of the cervix most often occurs in patients in their forties, but the noninvasive type appears most commonly between the ages of 30 and 40 years. Recently, there appears to have been a pronounced increase in the number of instances of invasive cancer seen in the 20-year age group.

DEFINITION. Carcinoma in situ is a pathologic entity established only by microscopic examination of material obtained from biopsy, curettage, a surgical specimen removed for other cause, or by colpomicroscopy. It produces no pathognomonic symptoms and has no characteristic gross appearance.

Carcinoma in situ commonly arises as a local intraepithelial growth, primarily at the squamocolumnar junction between the stratified exocervical epithelium and the glandular epithelium which lines the endocervical canal and its crypts or ducts. It may also arise from the squamous epithelium of the exposed exocervix. Approximately 15 per cent of these carcinomas in situ develop within the endocervical canal itself. Primarily a phenomenon of surface epithelium, the process spreads to the epithelium lining the glands. The first indication that the morphologic epithelial changes are progressing in the direction of true, clinical carcinoma comes when the stroma is invaded.

SIGNS AND SYMPTOMS. The most common symptom of early invasive carcinoma of the cervix is postcoital or intermenstrual spotting. Although only 25 per cent of patients in the 30 to 40 age group, who are proved to have carcinoma in situ, have such a bleeding pattern, it should arouse suspicion whenever it is encountered. All too frequently, carcinoma in situ is discovered in the course of an examination for sterility, or when the uterus is removed for other cause.

There is nothing on gross inspection or palpation to indicate that the epithelium has departed from the normal growth pattern. Most such patients have had children, so it is not surprising that the majority of them who have carcinoma in situ also have laceration and erosions of the cervix. The cervix may bleed easily to light trauma, but the majority do not. In roughly 15 per cent, the surface epithelium is smooth to touch and no break in the surface continuity can be observed. Since more than 10 per cent of carcinoma in situ arises within the endocervical canal, where it can neither be seen nor felt, biopsy specimens should be taken from this area in any patient in whom the suspicion of carcinoma in situ has been raised.

DIAGNOSTIC AIDS. Since there are no pathognomonic signs or symptoms associated with the presence of carcinoma in situ, the physician is forced to rely on the excellent diagnostic tools available for making a diagnosis. They should be employed routinely, whether suspicion has been aroused or the patient is simply undergoing a prophylactic screening examination.

The vaginal smear is a basic part of the vaginal examination. There can be no question but that the incidence of cervical cancer is being materially reduced by routine yearly checkups consisting of a vaginal examination and smear, even in the absence of symptoms. Approximately 1 per cent of normal women have a suggestive smear at some time, and one-half of these show positive findings on repeated examination of the smears.

The chief value of the smear is to alert the physician to the possible presence of malignancy. The test involves a cytologic diagnosis based on the known fact that cancer cells are constantly being shed into the vaginal secretion. The smear may be taken in a number of ways. The simplest and quickest method of collection is to aspirate the secretion pooled in the vaginal fornix with a suction pipette. This should be done as the first step in the vaginal examination, before any lubricant is used. Its chief advantage is its simplicity, plus the fact that the pooled secre-

tions represent the accumulation of cells cast off over a longer period of time. More painstaking techniques involve scraping the entire circumference of the cervix in the area of the junction of the cervical epithelium and the endocervical canal with the sharp edge of instruments especially designed, or if not available, a broken tongue depressor. The material obtained is placed on a slide and immediately immersed in a bottle containing equal parts of 95 per cent ethyl alcohol and ether, which fixes the secretion.

Although no special training is required to take the smear, a high degree of competence is required to interpret properly what is seen under the microscope.

Papanicolaou has classified smears as Class I, benign; Class II, showing some atypical cells; Class III, benign but atypical; Class IV, some atypical cells but not conclusive for cancer; and Class V, malignant neoplastic cells present.

No matter how accurate or competent the cytologist may be, definitive therapy cannot be based upon the findings of the vaginal smear alone. The vaginal smear is but one in a series of tests which must be made before the diagnosis of cancer can be established. It is axiomatic that a positive smear must be confirmed by histologic review of material obtained by biopsy before any treatment is outlined. If the smear continues to be positive in the face of negative pathologic findings from the initial biopsy, the investigation must continue. The accuracy of the vaginal smear, interpreted by competent authority, is such that it is the responsibility of the surgeon to prove that the patient does not have cervical cancer.

If the biopsy is to be meaningful, it must be taken from the proper place. The Schiller test helps to pinpoint the areas which should be biopsied.

After inspection of the cervix and gentle cleansing, Schiller's solution (one part iodine to 300 parts of water), is painted over the cervix. If there is glycogen present in the squamous epithelium covering the cervix, the tissues stain a deep mahogany color, with gradations from bright to light yellow depending on the amount of glycogen present. Cervical epithelium which contains cancer has little or no glycogen.

The suspicious areas are those which fail to take the stain and continue to have the same appearance they had before the Schiller test. This does not mean that the patient has cancer. Only a few patients will actually have carcinoma in situ, but it is a fact that all who have carcinoma in situ fail to take the stain. The test simply tells the surgeon the best area for the biopsy.

Since a negative biopsy means only that no tumor was present in the specimen taken, it is important that the surgeon give the pathologist enough tissue to permit an adequate evaluation, and that the biopsy be taken from several areas. One may have carcinoma adjacent to an area which appears normal in the biopsy specimen, or perhaps invasive carcinoma impinging on an area of carcinoma in situ. Particular attention should be paid to the patient who has a suspicious vaginal smear but an apparently normal cervix upon inspection and palpation. The endocervical canal should be carefully evaluated.

The biopsy may be taken in one of two ways: punch biopsies from four quadrants in the external cervix and in the endocervical canal, and surgical conization. The former can be carried out as an office procedure; the latter requires hospitalization and anesthesia.

Surgical conization should be taken with a knife and not an electric current scalpel, because heat coagulates the specimen and makes histologic interpretation extremely difficult. It should include not only the outer border of any erosion but the full extent of the endocervical canal to include any sulci which may be present because of lacerations acquired at childbirth. Proper performance of a cold knife surgical cone requires experience and accurate technique.

The pathologist is faced with two questions: is cancer present; and are the morphologic changes those of true carcinoma in situ or of invasive carcinoma?

To be called carcinoma in situ, the microscopic picture must involve the entire thickness of the squamous epithelium and it must have all the criteria of malignancy minus evidence of invasion beneath the basement membrane.

There is a tendency to over-diagnose such lesions as squamous metaplasia and atypical basal cell hypertrophy as carcinoma in situ, and treat them as though they were cancer. The decision regarding invasion becomes a problem when the carcinoma in situ involves the cervical glands, particularly when the glandular involvement is extensive and there are fewer normal endocervical glands to

compare. Whether stromal invasion has taken place cannot always be determined with certainty. It has been said that one-third of the specimens believed to have questionable stromal invasion will actually have it when multiple sections are reviewed.

TREATMENT. When a definite diagnosis of invasive carcinoma of the cervix has been established, immediate drastic therapy is imperative. Carcinoma in situ, on the other hand, can be treated much less radically. There appears to be rather a slow progression in the growth pattern of carcinoma in situ, both in the intraepithelial phase and from that phase to stromal invasion. There is some evidence that ten years may elapse before carcinoma in situ becomes invasive.

There is, therefore, no overpowering need to rush the patient to the operating room for immediate therapy. The surgeon can afford to take the time to carry out a thorough pathological and clinical appraisal, especially when an element of doubt appears as to the accuracy of the diagnosis or the degree of invasion. This is particularly true when the problem arises in a young woman who has had no children and wants to have some, or desires to preserve her menstrual function. There is less concern about the older woman who has completed her family, since a total hysterectomy with preservation of ovarian function is a happy solution for her. One might prefer to take a calculated risk and remove the area under suspicion with a surgical cone rather than subject the young patient to hysterectomy. This presupposes that the patient will be scrupulous about reporting for checkup examinations at regular intervals. If the surgeon is unlikely to receive this type of cooperation, he should perform a hysterectomy regardless of the patient's age or desire to have offspring.

FIBROMYOMATA OF THE UTERUS

Single or multiple solid encapsulated tumors growing in the muscular walls of the uterus are usually fibromyomata. It has been estimated that one out of five women over the age of 30 has fibroid tumors. The growth pattern seems to be linked to the functional capacity of the ovary, since they are common in the most active reproductive age groups, but rarely are seen in adolescence, and rarely continue to grow after the menopause. Individual tumors are classified in terms which reflect the point of origin within the uterus. The majority appear in the walls of the uterus and are called intramural fibroids. The size of these tumors varies, and they may be single or multiple. The subserous fibroid grows outward from the wall, pushing the peritoneal cover with it. The contour of the uterus becomes irregular and nodular. Continuing this growth pattern, the tumor becomes pedunculated when the only attachment to the uterus is a pedicle which contains the blood supply. The submucous fibroid juts into the endometrial cavity. This tumor may occupy a position anywhere in the endometrial cavity. Unless the submucous fibroid develops a pedicle, dilates the endocervix and appears in the vaginal canal, physical examination will give no indication of its presence. In rare instances, the fibroid arises in the cervical area. It may grow laterally and compress the lower end of the ureter, or in the midline and produce pressure on the urethra. Occasionally, the subserous fibroid retains a wide base as it expands into the broad ligament where it becomes an interligamentary or broad ligament fibroid.

The fact that the blood supply is peripherally placed explains a variety of complications which may develop within the tumor. The amount of blood reaching the central portion of the myoma becomes less as the tumor becomes larger or more pedunculated. Hyaline degeneration is a common finding in most fibroids. At times, this becomes so massive that the tumor becomes cystic. Necrosis occasionally appears in the central portion of a large tumor, or in the periphery of a pedunculated subserous or submucous fibroid which has undergone torsion of the pedicle. As a result of necrosis and fatty degeneration, the leiomyoma of the post-menopausal patient frequently calcifies.

SYMPTOMS. The symptoms commonly associated with fibroid tumors within the uterus are vaginal bleeding, discharge, localized abdominal pain, pressure symptoms, and presence of a palpable abdominal mass or enlargement. It is possible for a patient to have a fibroid tumor for years without her being aware of it, only to develop symptoms when the blood supply to the tumor changes.

Vaginal bleeding is the most common symptom. The location of the tumor is important because the mechanism of bleeding differs. A patient with large, multiple intramural or subserous fibroids may have no intermenstrual bleeding or alteration of the menstrual pattern. If she does have abnormal bleeding, it is due to the fact that there is a hormonal imbalance in which estrin is unopposed by progestin. The submucous fibroid, however, bleeds heavily in gushing fashion because the endometrium thins out over its surface. In addition, the blood loss cannot be arrested by normal contraction of the uterine muscle. A patient may have profuse hemorrhage from a small submucous fibroid, but a normal menstrual period in the presence of a large intramural or subserous fibroid. It may be categorically stated that a submucous fibroid is the only fibroid which is the direct cause of abnormal uterine bleeding.

There are many explanations of the cause of vaginal discharge in the patient with a fibroid uterus. Except for the submucous fibroid, some cause must be sought other than the fibroid. A necrotic, sloughing submucous fibroid produces a vaginal discharge which is thin, watery, brown and malodorous.

The uncomplicated fibroid does not produce pain. It may create discomfort through pressure, due to its position and size, but not pain. The venous return from the extremities may be obstructed to the point where varicosities or hemorrhoids appear, but there rarely is pain. Malfunction of the bladder, ureter, rectum or stomach may occur because of the pressure of the extrinsic mass, but it is not accompanied by pain other than low backache or heaviness in the upper thighs.

When the patient with a leiomyoma complains of pelvic pain, one of five factors is usually present. Primarily, one suspects that something has happened to the tumor itself, particularly when tenderness is present together with pain. The location of the pain depends on the position of the fibroid within the uterus. The basic cause is usually necrosis within the tumor due to faulty blood supply. Second, if the tumor is intramural, red degeneration or infection may be the explanation. A degenerating leiomyoma in most instances produces a temperature elevation and sudden, severe pain localized over the lower abdomen. This gradually subsides, leaving the patient with a dull, steady, grinding "pelvic toothache." Third, when the pedicle of a pedunculated fibroid twists, shutting off the blood supply and producing obstruction to venous return, leading to necrosis and hemorrhage in the tumor, the patient has the severe, colicky, prostrating type of pain which

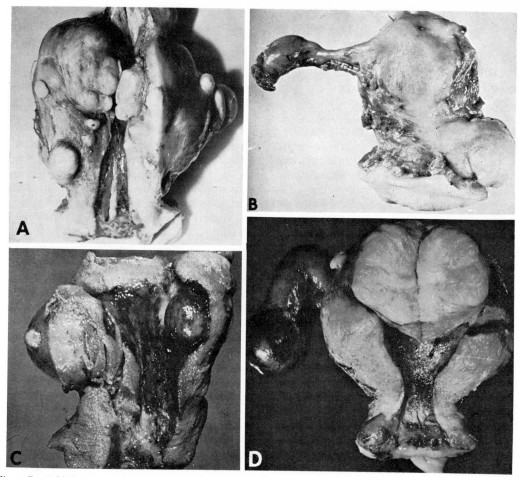

Figure 5. *A,* Multiple uterine leiomyomata of various sizes protrude from the cut surfaces of the myometrium. In this uterus, some of the fibroids are subserous, others intramural or submucous. *B,* Cervical fibroid tumor, which may be a cause of difficult delivery. *C,* To the right is a submucous leiomyoma bulging into and distending the endometrial cavity. *D,* A fibroid tumor of the uterine fundus is protruding from the cut surface in the characteristic way. It also has the typical white, whorled appearance of a leiomyoma. A pyosalpinx is present.

is associated with infarction of a hollow viscus. Fourth, cramplike pain, such as that experienced during labor, usually means that the uterus is trying to dilate the cervix and expel a foreign body, such as a submucous fibroid or fibroid polyp. Fifth, severe lower abdominal pain which follows a blow to the lower abdomen may be due to the rupture of veins lying on the surface of a fibroid. The accompanying symptoms are those of intraperitoneal hemorrhage.

PHYSICAL FINDINGS. The majority of leiomyomata are discovered by palpation. This is true of all but the submucous fibroid, which can only be diagnosed by curettage, endometrial biopsy or interpretation of a hysterosalpingogram.

It is unwise to rely solely on abdominal examination, even in the presence of a large abdominal tumor. If smooth-walled, it may not be possible to estimate accurately its consistency. It may, therefore, be a distended bladder or perhaps a large ovarian cyst which, through partial twist of its pedicle, has come to rest in a midline position. Many large leiomyomata are so placed in the pelvis that they cannot be felt on abdominal examination. By bimanual palpation, the examiner has the best chance of determining the size, contour, location, consistency, degree of fixation and areas of tenderness. It is also the best method of evaluating the extent of associated disease. For example, the palpation of tender, shotty nodules on the pelvic floor or uterosacral ligament suggests that there is an additional element of endometriosis. Generalized thickening of the pelvic floor raises the suspicion of the presence of a concomitant pelvic inflammatory process. It is often difficult to differentiate between pregnancy, adenomyosis and a uterus symmetrically enlarged by an intramural fibroid. It is practically impossible to differentiate a pedunculated, or laterally placed subserous fibroid growing out into the broad ligament from a solid tumor of the ovary.

TREATMENT. There are three basic methods of treating a patient with a myomatous uterus. The patient is observed at regular intervals and definitive therapy is deferred; the patient is operated upon, and either a myomectomy is done or the uterus is removed; the patient receives either radium or roentgen ray treatment.

The decision for or against definitive treatment depends on whether the patient's symptoms are important enough to require treatment; whether the growth pattern and the location of the tumor represent a threat to the continued health and well-being of the patient; and whether the associated disease is extensive or troublesome enough to warrant operative interference independent of the presence of the fibroid. All these factors are, in turn, modified by the age of the patient, her general health and the desire to have children.

Naturally, in the young reproductive age group, the surgeon wishes to be conservative in his therapeutic approach. If there is no indication that the patient has any pelvic pathology other than the fibroid, if the fibroid is small and asymptomatic, or is located in a position that will not interfere in any way with the patient's becoming pregnant or maintaining a pregnancy, the patient should be left alone except for observation at regular intervals to check the growth pattern.

The factors which might influence the surgeon in considering operative interference are the location of the tumor, its growth pattern and the severity of the symptoms. A fibroid growing in the region of the cervix may interfere with the patient's becoming pregnant, or interfere with the conduct of labor if she does. A large tumor may encroach on the endometrial cavity and interfere with the maintenance of pregnancy. The same can be said for a submucous fibroid. Both may undergo degeneration. Pedunculated fibroids are prone to undergo torsion and become necrotic. They may be located in such a position or be of such size as to interfere with the mechanics of labor. A rapid change in size should suggest the possibility of sarcoma or degeneration in a tumor, and call for immediate abdominal exploration.

Myomectomy is the procedure of choice in any woman under the age of 40 who wants to have children. The location of the fibroid is an important consideration, but multiple myomectomies are compatible with conception and the successful maintenance of pregnancy, even though it becomes necessary to enter the endometrial cavity to remove a fibroid. If the main consideration is the establishment and maintenance of pregnancy, only the tumors located within or encroaching on the endometrial cavity should be regarded as the possible cause of sterility. If the tumors are located elsewhere in the uterus and the patient is infertile, it is unlikely that they are making her so. It is far more likely that functional reasons or associated pathology are the true explanation.

Myomectomy should not be done unless the rest of the uterus and adnexae are in a healthy state and there is a reasonable chance for pregnancy to follow. Because this cannot always be determined preoperatively, the patient should be warned that hysterectomy may be required.

After the age of 40 years, the decision for or against treatment and the choice of therapy are predicated on the severity of symptoms plus the importance of associated disease. Many symptoms attributable to the leiomyoma are actually due to other pelvic disease entities such as endometriosis, pelvic inflammation, ovarian tumors and uterine cancer. It is important to evaluate the symptomatology very carefully.

As the patient approaches the time of the menopause, the chances of malignant disease increase markedly. The same is true of the lateral wall leiomyoma in this age group. Too frequently, tumors in this location are indistinguishable from solid ovarian tumors, which are highly lethal.

The symptoms of abdominal enlargement, lower abdominal pressure and interference with the function of the bladder, rectum or ureter must be judged on their severity and the inconvenience to the patient. Any change in the symptomatology or increase in size of a fibroid tumor which is under observation should serve as an indication for operation, since leiomyomata quiescent for years may suddenly degenerate or develop sarcomatous change.

The operation of choice in older patients is total removal of the uterus. Supravaginal hysterectomy should be performed only when great technical difficulties are encountered. Because of the likelihood of associated pathology, the abdominal approach is preferred. In every instance, total hysterectomy should be preceded by a curettage to rule out the possibility of malignant disease within the endometrial cavity or endocervical canal. Whether healthy normal ovaries are left undisturbed at the time hysterectomy is performed depends on the individual preference of the surgeon and his belief about the ability of the ovary to secrete estrogen when menstrual function has ceased.

Irradiation is reserved for the patient past the childbearing age who is too poor a risk to withstand the demands of surgical intervention. Radiation causes no immediate mortality and little morbidity. It should not be used in younger patients if it can be avoided, because any improvement in the symptomatology can only be acquired at the expense of castration.

Irradiation may be administered either as a local instillation of radium within the endometrial cavity or in the form of external radiation by roentgen rays. Intercavitary radiation is preferred, for it makes it necessary for the surgeon to examine the patient under anesthesia and permits him to do a curettage. In this manner, there is less chance that an occult cancer will be overlooked. Radium is contraindicated in the presence of a submucous fibroid. A sloughing effect upon the tumor follows direct contact with the radium applicator; bleeding is increased and infection further complicates the problem.

EXTERNAL ENDOMETRIOSIS

Widespread dissemination of ectopic endometrium, consisting of stroma and endometrial glands, beyond the confines of the endometrial cavity, is called endometriosis. It is an unusual pathologic entity, in that the endometrial implants actually have the power to invade normal tissue, despite the fact that endometriosis is a benign process. These implants respond to cyclic hormone stimulation by proliferation in much the same fashion as normal endometrium.

The five most common sites for ectopic implants, in order of frequency of their occurrence, are the serosal surface of the uterus, the ovaries, the posterior cul-de-sac, the

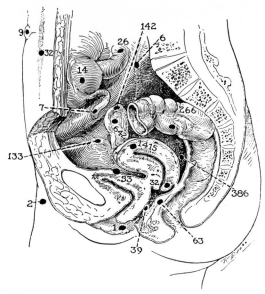

Figure 6. Sites of endometriosis, with the number of instances observed at each. The five most common sites in order are uterus, ovaries, pouch of Douglas, rectosigmoid colon and fallopian tubes. (From Masson and Cariker.)

rectosigmoid colon and the fallopian tubes. Less often, implants may appear in the round ligament, anterior cul-de-sac, cervix, bladder, sigmoid, terminal ileum and appendix. Implants never appear above the level of the umbilicus and are rarely found on the anterior abdominal wall, unless there has been a previous abdominal operation. After operative procedures, they may arise in the abdominal incision, in amputation stumps or in scars in the perineal area and vulva.

The ectopic implants which are found on the posterior surface of the uterus, uterosacral ligaments and pelvic peritoneum appear as blueberry-like spots surrounded by a puckering scar which tends to draw adjacent tissues and organs into it. At times, individual implants coalesce to form solid nodules, particularly on the pelvic floor and uterosacral ligaments.

Approximately 60 per cent of patients with external endometriosis have some form of ovarian involvement. The lesions vary in size from small areas resembling blood blisters to large cysts measuring 20 cm. or more in diameter. Almost invariably, they are found on the lateral and undersurfaces of the ovary.

The typical gross appearance is that of bilateral ovarian cysts of varying size, characteristically filled with a thick, tarry, chocolate-colored fluid. The terms "chocolate cysts of the ovary" and "endometriosis" are commonly used synonymously. The diagnosis of endometriosis cannot be made on the basis of the fluid alone, because the same type of material can be found in an old corpus luteum or lutein cyst.

In the earlier phases of development, a depressed, scarred, puckered, blue-black area appears on the surface of the ovary and seems to communicate with a somewhat larger cyst within the substance of the organ. Since the endometrial lining of the cyst responds to the cyclic stimulation of the pituitary hormones, it tends to swell to the point that it ruptures. The contents are irritating to the peritoneum, which reacts by setting up a local chemical peritonitis. An immediate protective fibroblastic tissue response occurs, which tends to seal the defect in the ovary by fixing it to the posterior leaf of the broad ligament. Because of the inflammatory peritoneal reaction set up by either the initial or recurring episodes of spillage, the ovary may either fix against the back of the broad ligament, or the lower pelvis may become full of dense, fibrotic adhesions which cannot be separated easily. There are no cleavage planes such as one finds in pelvic inflammation. Great care must be taken in separating the endometriotic lesion from the normal tissue of the functioning bladder, rectum or small intestine, to avoid the possibility of tearing into them.

When the rectovaginal septum is invaded, the growth process continues in such a way as to penetrate the vaginal fornix, where it can be seen on direct inspection of the vault, or to invade the serosal surface of the rectal wall and produce a firm, dense mass binding the cervix and rectal wall together.

Gross lesions in the sigmoid and rectosigmoid can hardly be distinguished from carcinoma. Unlike carcinoma, endometriosis invades the serosal surface and burrows deep into the muscular and submucosal layers and extends for varying lengths in the long axis of the bowel. The extent of the invasion may be enough to occlude the lumen and produce varying degrees of intestinal obstruction, but the mucosal layer is rarely, if ever, invaded either grossly or microscopically.

The outline of the mucosal pattern upon a roentgenogram is significant. The bowel is tender at the point of fixation and a long, inconstant filling defect with sharp irregular borders can be seen, but the mucosa is intact.

In the small intestine, endometriosis tends to appear in younger people and may be present without widespread dissemination of pelvic endometriosis or chocolate cysts in the ovary. The scarring and puckering of the serosal surface are readily observed, but there is far less muscle penetration. Intestinal obstruction tends to occur because of the kinking and angulation produced by the serosal lesion rather than because of narrowing of the lumen by tumor growth.

Endometriosis of the urinary tract is relatively uncommon. When it does appear, the bladder is usually involved; the mucosa is rarely implicated. Implants are often seen on the peritoneal surface overlying the bladder, but they are incidental findings and do not contribute to the symptomatology. A number of implants, however, may coalesce and form a tumor which can be palpated in the muscular wall of the bladder. Cystoscopy performed at the time of the menstrual period shows an edematous but intact mucosa pushed forward by the tumor in the muscle wall beneath.

At times, the ureter becomes surrounded, but is rarely ever invaded, by the fibrosis created by endometrial implants to the point that the outflow of urine is impeded and a hydronephrosis develops. The patient may then have intermittent flank pain which becomes more pronounced at the time of menstruation. In the presence of pelvic floor endometriosis, an intravenous pyelogram may demonstrate the ureteral block.

Isolated endometriosis outside the pelvis is usually the result of the transplant of endometrium to the site at the time of operation. Endometriotic implants may be found in abdominal or perineal scars.

SYMPTOMS. Pelvic pain which bears a direct relation to the menstrual period is the most common symptom associated with endometriosis. The small pelvic implant often produces more pain than the larger endometrial cysts of the ovary. Extensive ovarian involvement may be present with very little discomfort.

The patient who has a small implant experiences pain because the endometrial lining is surrounded by a dense fibrotic cover which develops from the intermittent rupture and spillage of the cystic contents on the sensitive peritoneum. As the scar becomes thicker, it is less likely to yield to the periodic pressure created by the hormonal stimulation. Distention of these small cysts invariably produces pain which becomes more severe with each menstrual cycle. In ovarian endometriosis, the constricting element is absent. The patient has pain only to the degree to which the cyst distends and in proportion to the rapidity with which this occurs.

Acute, excruciating pain may appear suddenly if the cyst ruptures and its contents spill on the sensitive pelvic peritoneum. The nature of the pain is similar to that of an ectopic pregnancy, or ruptured corpus luteum cyst. The symptoms are those of intraperitoneal hemorrhage and are not pathognomonic.

The most common type of pain occurs in the lower abdomen and varies in severity. It may be vague and hard to locate. It is usually described as a bearing-down pain which comes on just before the menstrual period and tends to localize in the low abdomen, back and thighs. If the patient has bowel endometriosis, she may have increasing constipation and tenesmus, but rarely passes blood. There is a widespread misconception that endometriosis is a common cause of rectal bleeding at the time of the period. Rarely is this true. If the bladder is involved, the patient may experience dysuria, but hematuria is extremely rare.

The patient may experience dyspareunia and backache due to the widespread dissemination of implants on the pelvic floor and uterosacral ligaments, which tend to fix the uterus. Any motion of the cervix tends to produce pain.

The most significant symptom is dysmenorrhea, which becomes increasingly severe with each passing period. It usually begins before the period and builds up in severity. Any patient who begins to have dysmenorrhea for the first time between the ages of 25 and 35 years may well have endometriosis. The important factor, however, is not that the patient has cramps, which she had not had before, but that the pain, once acquired, increases in severity with each menstrual period.

PHYSICAL FINDINGS. The most difficult problem the physician encounters in establishing a diagnosis of endometriosis by physical examination is the fact that it is frequently associated with other pelvic pathology, such as pelvic inflammatory disease and fibroids. The physical findings have greater meaning when a suspicion of endometriosis has been entertained because of the history of acquired dysmenorrhea of increasing severity, dyspareunia and relative infertility.

The most significant finding is the palpation of a shotty, nodular thickening of the uterosacral ligaments and pelvic floor upon rectal examination. These nodules are usually very tender to the touch. When combined with a fixed uterus which cannot be dislodged, and masses in the adnexal area, the diagnosis can usually be made with a reasonable degree of accuracy.

TREATMENT. The emphasis on therapy today is on the side of conservatism. In the past, the surgical attack was often far too radical. The main object in therapy of endometriosis in younger patients is to relieve pain, correct menstrual irregularities, improve fertility and prevent further destruction of tissue when the ovaries are involved.

The physician may elect to treat the patient with estrogen or the newer progestational agents, since it is recognized that the growth factor, as well as the symptoms, can be held in abeyance when the periods become anovulatory or when pregnancy is established. The lesions of patients who receive such hormone therapy are said to become smaller and atrophic, while the pelvic floor becomes softer and more pliable.

The primary aim is to produce an amenorrheic state for an interval of three to six months. While this can be established by using estrogen of various types, the newer progestational agents seem to be more effective for they not only inhibit ovulation and produce an amenorrhea, but they also create a decidual response in the implant similar to that induced by a true pregnancy.

Operation is indicated when the patient's symptoms increase and the palpable lesions progress while the patient is under observation on medical therapy; when there is extreme fixation of the uterus and pelvic floor and nodular masses are felt in the uterosacral ligaments or rectovaginal septum; when fixed ovarian cysts are palpable on one or both sides; when the symptoms of rectal tenesmus or hematuria appear cyclically in a patient who has a tender mass in either the rectovaginal septum or bladder base; when the patient has a fertility problem in the presence of pelvic disease which gives the clinical impression of endometriosis; when dysmenorrhea and low abdominal pain, associated with palpable abnormalities, become increasingly severe with each monthly period; when blue-domed cysts are encountered in the vaginal vault, vulva, perineum, round ligament or umbilicus; and when acute abdominal pain appears suddenly in a patient who has fixed adnexal lesions.

Modern surgical therapy calls for preservation of menstrual and ovarian function, but it must be kept in mind that a 30-year-old patient with extensive endometriosis may have to be treated more radically than one, aged 40, who has less disease. A conservative operation means the excision of all gross endometriosis wherever possible, with preservation of as much ovarian tissue as possible. There is no problem when the implants are superficial.

The problem is more complicated when invasion of tissue is present. In many instances, it is necessary to remove the uterus as well as the obvious implants, leaving as much ovarian tissue as possible. If the uterus is not removed, because the patient is young and wants to have a family, the surgeon must carefully weigh the patient's chances of achieving pregnancy against the possibility of disabling discomfort in the future.

In some instances, it may be possible to dissect endometrial implants out of the muscle wall of the sigmoid or from the rectovaginal septum. If the surgeon is unwilling to take the risk and remove the endometriosis in the bowel wall, he need feel no urgency about removing ovarian tissue. In many instances, endometriosis has reached its end stage and will progress no further even though functioning ovarian tissue is present. It is even possible to leave a nodule in the intestinal wall and preserve functioning ovarian tissue. When the tumor is of sufficient size to produce bowel obstruction in a young patient, it is preferable to resect the sigmoid and reconstruct it with an end-to-end anastomosis rather than remove ovarian tissue which is not hopelessly involved. The same attitude may be taken toward the bladder and ureter, where segmental resection of the bladder may be done, or the ureter may be dissected from a bed of endometriosis without removing all ovarian tissue. In an older patient with extensive endometriosis, it may be advisable to castrate the patient rather than resect the bowel.

There is a far greater chance to preserve ovarian tissue than is generally believed. While endometriosis does invade adjacent tissue in other areas, it rarely does so in the ovary. Large chocolate cysts can be shelled out of the ovary, leaving normal ovarian tissue behind. When one leaves ovarian tissue, in the presence of known endometriosis,

there is a calculated risk that there will be further progression. The history of the disease amply justifies the assumption of the risks. This is far better than carrying out castration in every age group.

OVARIAN TUMORS

Three basic problems confront the surgeon in dealing with an adnexal enlargement: whether the enlargement is an abnormal physiologic development; whether the tumor is truly a neoplasm; and, if it is a neoplasm, whether it is benign or malignant. The distinction between a physiologic cyst and a neoplasm must be made. A neoplasm requires immediate operative intervention, whereas a physiologic cyst should be left alone and kept under observation. The majority of these cysts rupture spontaneously and disappear.

The two most common physiologic enlargements are follicle cysts and corpus luteum cysts. While physiologic cysts may alter the menstrual pattern, neoplasms do not do so as a rule. If the functional tumors of the ovary are excluded, less than 5 per cent of ovarian neoplasms exert any noticeable effect on the rhythm or the character of the menstrual periods. On the other hand, a follicle cyst may be responsible for shortened cycles, which may be persistent and profuse, and a corpus luteum cyst may cause delay in the onset of menstruation.

FOLLICLE CYSTS. Follicle cysts are frequently multiple and rarely grow any larger than 1.5 cm. Cysts larger than this are apt to be single, simple retention cysts full of clear serous fluid. In most instances, such cysts absorb, although they may rupture spontaneously. This may explain the sharp pain which patients sometimes experience in the lower abdomen, for which no apparent cause can be detected. The pain is due to the irritation of the peritoneum produced by the escape of the cystic content. Residual soreness persists for 24 to 48 hours, and is followed by complete recovery.

Follicle cysts may disappear spontaneously. Far too often, an otherwise normal ovary is removed because it has a few cysts in it. The ovary is normally a cystic organ. In many ways, it is the most abused organ in the body, largely because it is bilateral and hidden within the abdominal cavity. On the other hand, there does come a time when even a benign follicle cyst should be removed. If the cyst is larger than 5 cm. and does not disappear after two or three menstrual periods, the patient should be operated upon because a neoplasm and not a physiologic cyst may be present, and the cyst has become a space-occupying tumor. At this stage, it is an easy matter to excise the cyst and preserve normal ovarian tissue.

CORPUS LUTEUM CYST.   The corpus luteum cyst is a less common finding, but it does have surgical implications. Such cysts tend to delay the onset of the menstrual cycle and are apt to grow to larger size than follicle cysts. They are filled with blood so that, when they rupture, the symptomatology is inclined to be more dramatic and more serious.

Inasmuch as the corpus luteum cyst can cause amenorrhea, develop as an adnexal mass, and either regress slowly or rupture suddenly, the surgeon may be unable to determine whether a simple rupture of a corpus luteum cyst or a more serious rupture of an ectopic pregnancy is present. The history and physical findings are nearly identical. If suspicion is aroused, an Ascheim-Zondek test will help to make the diagnosis.

Occasionally, theca lutein cysts of the ovary, which are usually bilateral and associated with a hydatidiform mole or chorio-epithelioma, are encountered. Inflammatory cysts develop after an attack of pelvic peritonitis secondary to appendicitis, gonorrheal salpingitis, or streptococcal pelvic infection. These are frequently indistinguishable from physiologic cysts of the ovary. Chocolate cysts of the ovary secondary to endometriosis often present the same symptomatology, physical findings and gross appearance as a tarry lutein cyst of the ovary.

PRIMARY NEOPLASMS OF OVARY.   Neoplasms of the ovary can be either benign or malignant and may be either cystic or solid. The more solid the tumor, or the more solid portions appear in an otherwise cystic neoplasm, the greater is the malignant potential. Unlike a physiologic cyst, ovarian neoplasms tend to persist or increase in size. They may be large or small, but are usually mobile and displaceable from their position unless hemorrhage or necrosis has occurred, setting up an inflammatory reaction, or unless the tumor is enormous. They are unilateral, although certain tumors such as the serous cystadenoma or dermoid may be present bilaterally.

The great majority of neoplasms produce no pathognomonic symptoms and do not interfere with the normal menstrual pattern. The exceptions are the so-called functional tumors of the ovary, such as theca granulosal cell tumor, which produces estrin, and arrhenoblastoma, which is androgenic. These tumors change the character of menstruation, either by creating anovulatory periods with a prolonged flow and shortened cycle, or amenorrhea when the hormone produced is androgen. The important fact to remember is that benign and malignant neoplasms, in the early stages of development, produce the same train of symptoms.

Benign tumors, either cystic or solid, occur most frequently just before the menopause, but inasmuch as malignancy can occur in the ovary at any age and the history and physical findings are similar, one must always consider cancer as the primary diagnosis until it has been excluded. At present, seven of every 100 women will develop neoplasms at some time in their lives, and one of the seven neoplasms will be malignant. The growth pattern varies because the ovary has the potential to create a wide assortment of neoplasms. Some are more amenable to treatment than others. As a rule, malignant ovarian tumors carry a poor prognosis. It is said that only 20 per cent of patients with all types of malignant tumors of the ovary survive longer than five years.

SYMPTOMS.   In general, the patient is unaware of the presence of an ovarian neoplasm, however large, until some complication occurs within the tumor to direct attention to it. The symptoms are enlargement of the abdomen, a sense of fullness and bearing-down discomfort in the abdomen and pelvis, pressure on adjacent organs such as the bladder and rectum, and varicosities and edema of the lower extremities secondary to obstruction of the venous or lymphatic return. Pain is rarely a symptom of ovarian neoplasm, as long as the growth pattern of the tumor is not changed and free expansion is possible.

Early neoplasms tend to be unilateral, lie free in the abdominal cavity and obtain their blood supply through a pedicle. Torsion of the pedicle is a common complication, particularly in moderate-sized cysts of the ovary, which have a relatively thin pedicle. The small cysts drop into the pelvis and do not have weight enough to twist, while the large cysts are too heavy and too fixed in the pelvis to move to any extent.

When the twist is incomplete, only the venous return is affected. The veins become engorged and hemorrhage occurs within the cavity, causing it to enlarge and produce the type of pain one expects from distention of a hollow viscus. Grossly, the cyst becomes dark purple and the serosal surface loses its shine and becomes dull. With further degrees of torsion, the arterial supply is damaged and necrosis takes place. The pain becomes more severe because ischemia is added to the distention factor. The viability of the cyst wall becomes impaired, and the excellent culture medium produced by the necrosis within the cyst provides an excellent opportunity for the cyst to become infected. The cyst may rupture either because the hemorrhage within it occurs too rapidly, or because the wall becomes necrotic.

The patient's response depends on the reaction of the peritoneum to the contents of the cyst. Nothing much happens if the cyst contains only the thin serous fluid of a cystadenoma, but violent symptoms and peritonitis may follow when the gelatinous material of a pseudomucinous cyst, or the fatty, hairy content of a dermoid cyst contaminates the pelvic peritoneum.

The severity of the symptoms varies according to the extent of pathologic change within the cyst. There may be no symptoms if only a partial twist occurs, but acute and severe pain appears with dramatic suddenness when the obstruction is complete and occurs rapidly.

PHYSICAL FINDINGS. The physical findings in cystic ovarian neoplasms vary with the size of the tumor, its position and whether the cyst is bound by adhesions. Small cysts are best felt by rectum. As they enlarge and

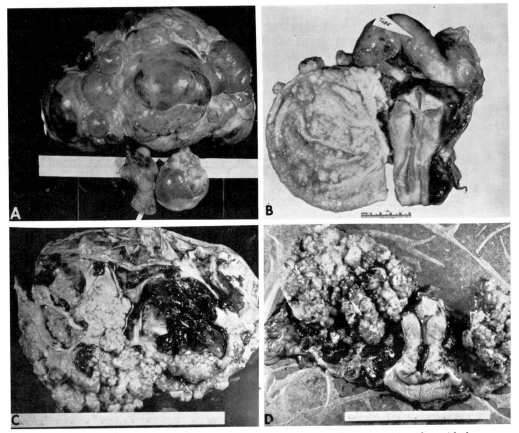

Figure 7. A, Multilocular serous cystadenoma about 15 cm. in diameter of one ovary, together with the uterus and a smaller contralateral serous cystadenoma. The shining outer capsules and translucent walls of the lobules favor benign neoplasms. B, When multiple granular papillomas cover the internal surface of a serous tumor, it is likely to be locally invasive and malignant. Microscopically, this was a papillary serous cystadenocarcinoma. If not ruptured, removal of such a carcinoma may be curative. C, Papillomatous masses both within and growing on the external surfaces of a serous ovarian tumor might be benign, but most of them, as in this case, are papillary serous cystadenocarcinomas. D, Sometimes papillary adenocarcinoma is so extensive, perhaps involving both ovaries as in this patient, that its origin from papillary serous cystadenocarcinoma is obscured.

grow on a pedicle, their weight causes them to gravitate into the cul-de-sac, where they can be felt as a tense, elastic swelling. They can be displaced without discomfort, unless they are trapped by adhesions, in which case palpation produces pain. Because the cysts grow on a pedicle, it is not always easy to tell from which side they arise. A cyst palpable in the left vault may arise from the right ovary. The larger cysts may be felt on abdominal examination, usually in one flank or the other, but occasionally they assume a midline position. The majority descend into the lower pelvis, where the lower border can be felt by vaginal or rectal examination. Whether the cyst be large or small, the palpation of any solid portion should arouse a strong suspicion that malignant disease is present.

When percussion of a distended abdomen is resonant, the cyst does not have an accompanying ascites; but when a fluid mass is present and the flanks are dull to percussion, one should suspect free fluid. Ascites in itself is not a pathognomonic sign of malignant disease, because it may appear with some benign solid and cystic tumors, but it does appear frequently when cancer is present. It is often difficult to distinguish between a large cyst which occupies a flank position and a moderate cyst with ascites.

DIFFERENTIAL DIAGNOSIS. There is no problem in differentiating between benign and malignant lesions when papillary excrescences appear on the peritoneal surface of a cyst, or wide dissemination is noted throughout the lower peritoneal cavity. Otherwise, the only way that the differentiation can be made is by sectioning the cyst after its removal. The fluid content and inspection of the inner surface of the cyst cavity provides the correct diagnosis. The character of the fluid is a helpful indicator. The two most common types of cystic ovarian tumor are the serous cystadenoma and the pseudomucinous cystadenoma. Because it is a papillary tumor, the former has seven times the malignant potential of the latter, occurs bilaterally in 33 per cent of patients, and appears at any time in the reproductive life of a woman.

When the cyst is opened, a clear serous fluid present in a serous cystadenoma should alert the surgeon to the possibility of carcinoma more than the sticky, thick, gelatinous fluid found in a pseudomucinous cyst. Both can have malignant components in their internal structure, but the serous cystadenoma is more likely to be malignant.

The internal surface of the walls of most cystic ovarian neoplasms is predominantly smooth, gray and glistening, whether the cyst is unilocular of multilocular. If the papillary projections are resilient, rubbery or fibrous, they are probably benign. If they are hard, gritty or fixed, carcinoma is likely to be present. Should the papillary process extend into or through the wall, and appear to be invading it, they are almost invariably malignant. It is a general observation that the more solid the tumor, the greater the chance of malignancy and the worse the prognosis. If cancer is present, it will be found in the firm, hard areas at the base of the papillary projections into the cystic cavity.

SOLID TUMORS. The malignant potential of a solid ovarian tumor is far higher than its cystic counterpart. All but fibroma of the ovary have a malignant connotation. They are more dangerous, because the salvage rate is appreciably less following the same type of therapy than with cystic tumors. In addition, it should be kept in mind that all metastatic tumors of the ovary, from breast, stomach, gallbladder, colon or endometrium, are solid growths.

There are no pathognomonic symptoms or characteristic physical findings which help to distinguish between benign and malignant solid tumors of the ovary. Since the differentiation is so difficult, and the incidence of malignancy is so high, it is imperative that all solid ovarian neoplasms should be regarded as malignant until proved benign by section and histologic review of the tissue removed.

Malignant neoplasms are prone to have abdominal effusions in association with them. Ascites should not be considered as a pathognomonic sign of malignant disease, because benign fibromas produce the greatest amount of free abdominal fluid, and not infrequently hydrothorax.

TREATMENT. The primary problem in the treatment of ovarian neoplasms is to be sure that the growth is truly benign. If it is malignant, the uterus and other ovary should be removed. The woman in her late thirties or forties who has completed her family will be best treated in similar fashion. The majority of benign tumors of the ovary tend to appear in the 40 to 50 age group.

In the younger woman, the surgeon may wish to preserve menstrual and reproductive function and remove only the tumor on the involved side, if he has sufficient reason to believe that the tumor is benign. Because some of the benign neoplasms, such as the dermoid cyst and the serous cystadenoma, tend to appear bilaterally, the surgeon runs the risk of having the patient develop another neoplasm in the retained ovary.

The likelihood of a second neoplasm developing years after a single neoplastic ovary has been removed is something less than 10 per cent. There is little chance of malignancy when the primary tumor is a dermoid, benign teratoma, simple cystoma, pseudomucinous cystadenoma or fibroma. Serous cystadenomas are so variable and unpredictable that it is unwise to preserve the uterus and other ovary in any but the younger woman who desires to have a family.

The risk of a new tumor appearing in the opposite ovary is reduced if the apparently normal ovary is bisected in situ and its interior is inspected. Most ovarian carcinomas are developmental in origin. If they have not manifested themselves in the early forties, they are unlikely to do so in the years to follow. The surgeon may then preserve the uterus and opposite ovary in a woman in her early forties, particularly when it is evident that the patient will be disturbed if all ovarian tissue is removed. The advisability of adopting this course declines sharply as the menopause approaches.

The basic treatment of cancer confined to the interior of the ovary is total hysterectomy with removal of both tubes and ovaries. The uterus should be removed because of the extensive intercommunication of the lymphatic pathways between the ovary, tube, uterus and opposite ovary. The other ovary should be removed because many ovarian neoplasms arise primarily in both ovaries and because it may become involved by lymphatic spread from the affected ovary.

As long as the cancer has not broken through the serosal surface, there is probably little reason to carry out an extensive dissection of the pelvic lymphatic channels or even a pelvic lymphadenectomy, because regional lymph node metastases are unlikely to occur. The spread tends to be to the retroperitoneal lymph chain of nodes that lie along the aorta, renal veins and celiac axis. Similarly, with the cancer limited to the interior of the ovary, the omentum may be left intact.

There are few times when the surgeon should consider the possibility of leaving the uterus and other ovary untouched in the face of known malignant disease. A calculated risk may be taken when only a microscopic focus of invasion exists, particularly if the cancer happens to be a pseudomucinous cyst adenocarcinoma, or one of the endometrioid type, which have less lethal potential. The decision to leave the uterus and other ovary would have greater validity when a granulosal cell tumor is encountered in infancy or when a dysgerminoma is found at puberty.

Should the surgeon underestimate the lethal nature of the tumor and the pathologist report a more extensive degree of invasive carcinoma after examining the specimen removed by simple oophorectomy, it is imperative that a second operation be performed to remove the uterus and remaining ovary.

The problem of effective management of ovarian cancer would be relatively simple if the growth were confined to the ovary itself. In the normal process of growth, cystic ovarian carcinoma does begin within the trabeculated portions of the cyst, gradually filling the entire cavity as the tumor proliferates. Unfortunately in the early stages, the benign neoplasm not only has the same growth pattern but actually is indistinguishable from a malignant tumor on gross inspection. This is why the surgeon should avoid tapping a cyst prior to its removal. There is too much danger of disseminating tumor cells throughout the pelvic cavity. If the tumor is so large and heavy that it cannot be dislodged, the surgeon may be forced to balance the risk involved in tapping the cyst against the likelihood of rupture and spillage that may follow attempts to remove it.

The growth pattern of ovarian cancer is so insidious that four-fifths of the malignant ovaries discovered have already extended beyond the confines of the ovary when they are first encountered. After filling the interior of the cyst cavity, the cancer progresses and invades the cyst wall. Only on rare occasions does the cancer arise from the epithelial lining of the cyst. Following invasion of the wall, cauliflower-like excrescences appear on the peritoneal surface, break off and seed throughout the abdominal cavity. Metastatic implants are usually found on the pelvic peritoneum in the cul-de-sac of Douglas. It is not uncommon to find plaques of tumor on both anterior and posterior abdominal walls spreading along the lateral gutter as far as the superior surface of the liver and under the surface of the diaphragm. In widespread ovarian cancer, the omentum is apt to contain tumor nodules in varying amounts and implants are often present in the mesentery of the small intestine.

Frequently, the abdomen is distended by the presence of both tumor and accompanying ascites. The ascites suggests, but is not proof of, widespread dissemination of tumor. For example, the only solid tumor of the ovary, the fibroma, frequently produces an excessive amount of peritoneal fluid. A fibroma ascites and a right hydrothorax constitute the basic findings in the so-called Meigs syndrome. In the presence of ascites, there is a place for paracentesis as a preliminary step to exploration. It performs two functions. The distinction between a large ovarian cyst and a solid plaque of omentum is made easier after the fluid is withdrawn. An examination of the fluid for tumor cells can be done either by the Papanicolaou technique or by histologic study of paraffin blocks made from the centrifugally spun sediment. The presence of tumor cells confirms the diagnosis.

In the face of widespread dissemination of ovarian cancer, the surgeon is faced with a more serious problem in therapy. The patient should be operated upon when irregular fixed tumor masses are felt in the cul-de-sac and a large tumor is present in the abdomen, even though a paracentesis shows the presence of tumor cells. The uterus, both ovaries, the omentum, and as much of the peritoneal extension as possible should be removed, even though the surgeon realizes that he has been unable to remove all the cancer the patient may have. Patients have been known to live for years after incomplete removal of the tumor, when roentgen ray treatment is used in conjunction with surgery. Chlorambucil and other chemotherapeutic agents are now available for use in addition to x-ray therapy. Both x-ray and chemotherapeutic agents have a greater chance of being effective if the primary tumor and its metastatic extensions are removed.

Mature surgical judgment is needed to decide how much of the widely disseminated tumor should be removed. It is not generally recognized that metastatic deposits on the peritoneal surface may grow in large blocks of tissue but have little subperitoneal extension. They seem to heap up on the peritoneum rather than invade it. Basically, they consist of more fibrous tissue than tumor cells. The omentum may be a solid mass of tumor deposit, yet the muscle wall of the adjacent transverse colon is rarely invaded.

It is possible to remove many of these metastatic implants without much difficulty for they have little blood supply.

On the other hand, little will be gained by pelvic lymphadenectomy and it is the rare patient who profits from either partial or total exenteration of the pelvic organs. It would be illogical to attempt to resect the sigmoid even though it was completely surrounded by tumor, if there were such widespread dissemination of tumor throughout the abdomen that the chances of successful therapy of any type were minimal. It would be wiser to perform a colostomy in anticipation of almost certain intestinal obstruction and rely on whatever chemotherapy or x-ray treatment has to offer. Similarly, tumor masses in the small bowel mesentery should not be excised unless they are sharply localized and represent the only tumor deposits in the area.

Roentgen ray therapy has little to offer when the tumor is entirely confined to the ovary, or when the disease has spread diffusely to the upper abdomen. The newer high-voltage roentgen ray machines, cobalt units and linear accelerators are capable of delivering effective cancerocidal radiation to tumor areas deep in the abdomen and pelvis without producing damage to the skin or interfering with the normal function of important viscera. Treatment is started two to three weeks after the operation has been completed. Some patients will be made worse, but the five-year survival of 20 per cent of patients who receive roentgenotherapy for ovarian cancer left behind at operation is enough to justify employing it.

The newer alkylating agents, antimetabolites and antibiotics, whether administered by infusion, by mouth, or by arterial perfusion, have not had the dramatic success hoped for them. The main problem is that tumor effect seems to be linked to drug toxicity. The agents which have had the most favorable effect on ovarian carcinoma are hemisulfur mustard and triethylenethiophosphoramide. Recently, chlorambucil has been employed with encouraging results. Two-thirds of the patients are said to have shown a favorable response to therapy as shown by diminution in the size of palpable tumor masses. The best effects have been noted in the treatment of patients with either abdominal or pleural effusions. The necessity for repeated tapping has been materially reduced.

Problems in the 40 to 50 Age Group

ABNORMAL BLEEDING

In younger patients, the explanation of the cause of abnormal bleeding is apt to be hormonal imbalance. Beyond the age of 40 years, any abnormal bleeding pattern should be regarded with suspicion, because approximately 10 per cent of patients in this group have vaginal bleeding due to cancer.

It is important that a complete account of the character of the period be obtained. This applies particularly to the degree, duration and timing of the flow. The physician should ask the patient when any departure from the accustomed pattern of flow was first noted; whether there have been similar episodes in the past; whether the interval has been constant; what the nature of the flow is; whether the spotting or bleeding occurs in the intermenstrual period and whether it follows intercourse or the use of a douche nozzle; and whether the patient has been taking estrogen, or any other hormone, and on what dose schedule.

PHYSICAL FINDINGS. The external genital tract must be both felt and inspected. Any suspicious lesion around the vulva or in the vaginal canal should be biopsied. The same applies to any abnormal-appearing area on the external portion of the cervix. It is well to remember that some cervices which appear entirely normal on direct inspection and palpation actually have carcinoma in the endocervix.

The size, contour and fixation of the uterus and adnexae are not helpful in establishing the cause for the abnormal bleeding. The patient who has an unusual bleeding history in this age group is likely to have palpable uterine fibroids, adenomyosis, polyps, external endometriosis or pelvic inflammatory disease. Examination may also reveal atrophic changes in the vaginal epithelium, caruncles or cervical polyps.

When no gross pathology is evident on examination, bleeding is probably due to either endometrial hyperplasia, a persistently proliferative endometrium, irregular ripening or shedding of the endometrium, or chronic endometritis. Approximately 25 per cent of patients have hyperplasia of the endometrium. The relation of this form of endometrium to endometrial cancer is not invariable, but it occurs often enough to make such a patient a suspect in this age group.

The important practical point is that obvious benign pelvic pathology should not be accepted as the explanation for the cause of bleeding until cancer of the cervix and endometrium is ruled out.

INVESTIGATIVE MEASURES. The three most important tools to employ in investigating the cause of abnormal bleeding from the genital tract are the Papanicolaou smear, biopsy of the cervix and endocervix, and curettage of the endometrium.

Since the most important explanation for abnormal bleeding in this age group is carcinoma, the pathologist should have the opportunity to review histologic sections from all of the endometrium. This is why curettage is preferred to an endometrial biopsy. To give the maximum amount of information on which to base therapy, the endometrial cavity and the endocervical canal must be independently curetted.

Curettage is not wholly accurate, because a small focus of carcinoma may be present in the cornua of the endometrial cavity, or cancer may be hidden behind a submucous polyp or fibroid. Any reappearance of bleeding calls for either a second curettage or a hysterectomy.

Most patients in this age group bleed abnormally because estrogen stimulation of the endometrium is unbalanced by progesterone. It may be difficult to determine when the bleeding is actually abnormal, since disturbances in menstrual rhythm occur frequently at this time of life. It may be considered as abnormal when the pattern repeats itself in a woman whose periods previously had a regular cycle. Shortened cycles are less likely to have an organic cause than profuse bleeding with menstruation or spotting between periods.

When there is true histologic evidence of a lack of progestin, substitution therapy usually regulates the menstrual flow. If it does not do so, curettage and hysterectomy are indicated.

Cervical and endometrial polyps are commonly the cause of prolonged and excessive bleeding as well as intermittent spotting.

The cervical polyp, because of its exposed position, is readily traumatized and usually produces intermittent spotting. The endometrial polyp, on the other hand, may be the sole explanation for bleeding of hemorrhagic proportions. The polyps may be either single or multiple. Not infrequently, a polyp which has origin high in the uterine fundus will protrude out through the cervical os. The length of the pedicle varies. Some polyps simply heap up on a broad base and are not pedunculated.

Rarely do malignant changes appear in either a cervical or endometrial polyp. When they do, this almost invariably takes place at the base of the polyp. The surgeon may by justified in removing a cervical polyp as an office procedure if he can be sure that he can adequately remove the base, and that there is no suspicion of carcinomatous change in the endometrium. The polyp may grow on a long stalk from a primary source high in the endometrial cavity, or the cervical canal may not be sufficiently dilated. Under these conditions, the surgeon cannot be sure that he has removed the base. Some polyps have such a broad base that the technical problems, particularly bleeding, may be enough to demand hospitalization and excision under anesthesia.

Leiomyomata, endometriosis, adenomyosis and pelvic inflammation may be associated with departures from the normal pattern of menstruation. The decision whether they deserve treatment and the type of treatment to be employed depend on the nature and severity of the symptoms produced. Vaginal bleeding is only one factor in this decision.

SARCOMA OF THE UTERUS

About 3 per cent of all malignant tumors of the uterus are sarcomas, with the ratio of sarcoma to carcinoma being about 1 in 40. Sarcoma may arise in either the myometrium or the endometrium, but the former is the more common site. In the myometrium, it usually appears in diffuse form.

When sarcoma diffusely involves the myometrium, a differential diagnosis between normal pregnancy and degenerating cellular fibroid, which occupies all of the uterine fundus, may be difficult. The presence of moist, edematous tissue suggests the possibility of sarcoma. The exact diagnosis is established when the uterus is examined following its removal. The cut surface is soft and friable, with the appearance of raw pork. Large venous sinuses and dilated vessels are present. Characteristically, sarcomas invade blood vessels and embolize to the lungs and other distant areas. Although sarcoma usually arises within the myometrium, smooth polypoid masses may jut into the endometrial cavity.

SIGNS AND SYMPTOMS. Primarily, sarcomas involve the fundal portion of the uterus. Bleeding and discharge are not pathognomonic, but they have significance when they

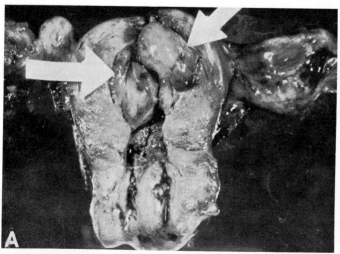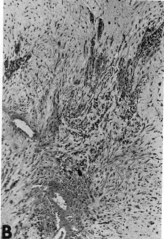

Figure 8.   *A*, Mixed mesodermal tumors have rounded tumor masses that bulge into the endometrial cavity from either the fundus, as in this patient, or from the lower uterine segments. Note the smooth surfaces of the sarcomatous nodules. *B*, Variegated histologic features of mixed mesodermal tumors include undifferentiated sarcoma, foci of malignant smooth or striated muscle, and other connective tissue types.

are considered together with palpation of a rapidly enlarging uterus. The rapidity of the growth makes the uterus feel soft, and its symmetrical contour creates the impression that the uterus contains a pregnancy.

As muscle wall invasion increases, the patient begins to bleed irregularly in small amounts, although occasionally the bleeding reaches hemorrhagic proportions.

Early in the course of the disease, the patient is apt to have a thin, watery discharge. This changes to a malodorous, sanguineous type as the growth progresses. Later, necrotic particles appear in the discharge.

When the tumor begins to grow rapidly in the myometrium, the patient usually has uterine pain. With further progression, anemia, weakness, cachexia and weight loss appear. Because the tumor often becomes necrotic and infected, temperature elevation may be expected.

TREATMENT. In the absence of physical evidence of metastases, the basic treatment is total hysterectomy and bilateral salpingo-oophorectomy.

As supplementary therapy, particularly when the sarcoma has involved the uterine wall, the surgeon may choose to give external radiation therapy in amounts up to 3000 gammas of tumor dose. Radiation should also be considered when the sarcoma has recurred locally in an area in which further surgical excision would interfere with the function of normal organs such as the bladder and rectum. The response to external radiation cannot be predicted.

CANCER OF THE CERVIX

Although the incidence of cancer of the cervix appears to be declining, it is still one of the most common forms of cancer. It has been estimated that 23 out of every 1000 women develop cervical cancer. Prophylactic treatment of precancerous lesions, proper attention to tell-tale symptoms, and universal use of the vaginal smear and biopsy are important reasons for decrease in the incidence of cancer of the cervix.

Cancer of the cervix tends to remain confined to the cervix and the areas immediately adjacent to it. Metastases do occur in the nodes along the external iliac vein and obturator areas, but for the most part the patient with extensive carcinoma of the cervix dies from uremia or hemorrhage, with the cancer localized in the pelvis.

Cancer of the cervix usually appears as a cauliflower-like growth which may spring from one or both lips of the cervix. The size varies widely, but at times it expands to fill the entire upper vagina. Not infrequently, the tumor spreads out over the cervix and extends to the epithelium of the vaginal fornix. Eventually, the deeper tissues are invaded either from the point of its origin into the cervical stroma, or into the paravaginal tissues when the tumor has extended to the surface epithelium of the vaginal vaults. Almost invariably, this type of growth is an epidermoid carcinoma.

Less often, the primary cancer arises in the endocervical canal and may appear in either the proliferative or ulcerating form. When it exfoliates and expands into the vaginal canal, it cannot be distinguished clinically from a tumor which arose from the portio of the cervix. A histologic differentiation is important because endocervical carcinomas may be adenocarcinomas, which are often considered to be less responsive to radiation therapy.

The ulcerative form of cervical cancer occurs less frequently. If the surrounding epithelium is dull red, if the undermining edges of the ulcer are firm and resistant to touch, and if the granulating base bleeds readily, there is an excellent chance that the lesion is cancer and not an erosion of the cervix.

In the past, treatment was outlined and prognosis evaluated on the histologic grade of the tumor. Today, there is more interest in the extent of the disease. The grade of the tumor depends on the individual cell characteristics, while the stage of the disease is a clinical estimate of the amount of cancer present. The two terms should not be used interchangeably, since they refer to different factors in the growth pattern.

METASTASIS. Cancer of the cervix spreads from the primary site by direct infiltration of the adjacent supporting tissues; by following the tissue planes and the line of least resistance along the parasympathetic nerves or blood vessels; by lymphatic embolization directly to the regional lymph nodes; or by blood vessel invasion.

One of the most striking facts about cancer of the cervix is its tendency to remain localized to the cervix and the immediately adjacent paracervical and paravaginal tissues. The tumor tends to spread out in a lateral and an anteroposterior direction. The bladder anteriorly and the uterosacral ligaments posteriorly are often implicated. If it extends far enough laterally from the cervix, the ureter may become occluded to such an extent that the patient has hydroureter or hydronephrosis. Uremia is the most common cause of death. As the disease advances, the growth may become fixed to the side wall of the pelvis.

The regional lymph nodes become involved either by the permeation of tumor cells along lymphatic channels or through embolization. In order of frequency of appearance, the lymph nodes most commonly involved lie in the chain beneath and lateral to the external iliac veins; in the obturator spaces, bounded by the obturator nerve below the side wall of the pelvis laterally and the external iliac vein above; along the internal iliac or hypogastric arteries, particularly at the junction with the external iliac arteries; and in the sacral areas at the promontory, just medial to each common iliac artery and vein.

The true incidence of nodal involvement cannot be established with certainty by palpation. Attempts are now being made to determine by lymphangiography whether metastases are present in the nodes. The studies are too recent, and the data too small to evaluate properly these observations at this time. From the Wertheim procedure, combined with pelvic lymphadenectomy which is performed for disease confined to the cervix or the tissues immediately adjacent to it, we know that positive nodes are found in about 20 per cent of patients.

It would be reasonable to expect a sharp increase in the number of nodes encountered as the patient develops more extensive disease, but this is not the case. When exenteration operations are performed in advanced stages of the disease to remove all the pelvic organs, including the bladder and rectum, the incidence of positive nodes is approximately 35 per cent. This is far less than one might anticipate, but it tends to confirm the impression that cancer of the cervix, unlike many other forms of cancer in the body, prefers to maintain a local pattern of growth.

An international classification of the extent of cervical carcinoma has been established to present a better evaluation of the results of the various types of therapy commonly employed for cervical cancer. It is also a useful guide to use in the selection of therapy.

CLASSIFICATION OF CANCER OF THE CERVIX

Stage 0: Carcinoma in situ; also known as intraepithelial or noninvasive cancer.

Stage I: The carcinoma is strictly limited to the cervix. It may arise from one or both lips and be either exophytic or ulcerative.

Stage II: The carcinoma has extended beyond the cervix:

(a) To involve a small portion or all of the upper part of the vagina, but not the lower third.

(b) To infiltrate the entire broad ligament on one or both sides, but not involve the side wall of the pelvis. The ureters may be occluded and the patient dying of disease but still be classified Stage II.

(c) To involve the endometrial cavity from a primary focus in the endocervix.

Stage III: The carcinoma has invaded the side wall of the pelvis.

(a) This may be by direct cancerous infiltration on one or both sides. No free space can be felt between the tumor and the pelvic wall.

(b) The side wall may also be invaded by isolated pelvic metastases from a small growth in the cervix itself. This suggests embolic spread.

The carcinoma involves the lower third of the vagina.

Stage IV: The carcinoma has invaded adjacent viscera or has spread beyond the pelvis to distant organs or nodes. Carcinoma involves the bladder by direct extension. Vesicovaginal fistulas may be present. The spread may be posterior through the vaginal fornix or rectovaginal septum to involve the rectum.

TREATMENT.   Basically, there are two forms of therapy for cervical cancer; radiation and surgery. They may be used singly or in combination. In selecting one or the other, the extent of the disease and the competence of the roentgenologist and the surgeon in their respective fields must be considered.

The basic aim of surgery is to encompass all the local disease as well as the areas immediately adjacent to the primary site and the regional nodes. The primary objective of radiation is not simply to kill tumor cells, but to alter the tumor bed so that active tumor cell growth cannot be sustained. This presupposes that the supporting tissue as well as the organs in the immediate proximity will not be damaged. The problem is not

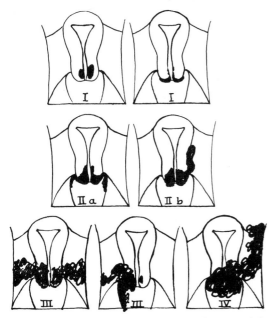

Figure 9. Diagram to show examples of cancer of the cervix in Stages I, IIa and IIb, III and IV. Sometimes such drawings are a useful part of the patient's clinical chart to help determine the best therapy.

whether radiation or operation offers the highest percentage of cure for all patients, but what is best for the individual patient. Both radiation and surgery have a logical place within the scope of individualized therapy.

In general, the patient who has cancer confined to the cervix and the immediately adjacent vaginal and paracervical tissues, or both, may be treated with either operation or radiation. Approximately one-third of the patients have a cancer sufficiently localized to permit a choice. The remainder have too much disease to hope that operation will encompass the entire process, and are best treated by radiation.

The patient should have a reasonable chance of cure when the disease is confined to the cervix and the tissues in close proximity to it, whether the therapy be radiation or operation.

There are many factors concerned with a favorable response other than the histologic nature of the tumor and the extent of its spread. All therapists are disappointed when a patient with a relatively small amount of tumor fails to respond to therapy, and are equally surprised by the patient with a bulky tumor who survives. Among the factors influencing the survival rate are a lack of radia-

tion sensitivity, an acquired radiation resistance, the biologic nature of the tumor growth, the host resistance, and the immunologic variables. These elements should be assessed if the best possible therapy is to be selected for the individual patient. Although the ideal yardstick is not yet available, a number of tests have been devised and are now being used as a guide to therapy.

In an attempt to determine whether the patient is sensitive to radiation, biopsies may be taken from the growing edge of the carcinoma at weekly intervals during the course of radium treatment. It has been reported that a favorable response may be anticipated when the tumor cells show an increase in the number which show differentiation and when there is a disappearance of mitoses, with more resting cells.

Great interest has been created in the use of vaginal smears to detect the response to radiation. Changes in cells are present in the vaginal smear after a trial dose of 1000 milligram-hours of radium; a yellowish brown stain in the cytoplasm; enlargement of the cells and nuclei; vacuolization of the cytoplasm; increase in the number of nuclei; and derangement of the chromatin. A favorable result may be anticipated when more than 75 per cent of the cells show a good response to radiation. A buccal rather than vaginal smear may be used, because the oral epithelium is less subject to hormonal influence and the postradiation changes in the cells are easier to interpret.

It is well recognized that radiation cures a high percentage of patients who have cervical cancer. Surgery is not advocated as a substitute for radiation, nor is radiation the only form of treatment available. Unfortunately, discussions of the relative merits of radiation and surgical therapy have become so tinged with emotion that many physicians have no clear-cut idea when either should be used.

The reasons for consideration of an operation as the definitive treatment for Stages I and IIa carcinoma of the cervix are based on several facts. There have been too many local recurrences of cancer after radiation therapy, and clinical evaluation of the extent of the disease is often inaccurate. The tumor may have extended to the paracervical and paravaginal nodes, or to the regional nodes, and may be undetected. There is a question about the effectiveness of roentgenotherapy to cure cancer in these nodes. Some cancers are radiation resistant. Pelvic inflammation, fibroids, ovarian tumors and pregnancy complicate the clinical evaluation of the extent of the disease, and increase the risks appreciably when radiation therapy is selected.

The Wertheim operation and pelvic lymphadenectomy, often termed a radical hysterectomy and node dissection, and the radical vaginal hysterectomy or Schauta-Amreich operation, are commonly performed for carcinoma of the cervix, Stages I and IIa. Both are adequate operations when the disease is confined to the cervix or the immediately adjacent paracervical and paravaginal tissues. The Schauta-Amreich operation is less well known in this country, but is popular elsewhere. While the Wertheim operation removes the vaginal nodes as an integral part of the primary operation, a second operation is necessary when the radical vaginal procedure is done.

The indications for the Wertheim procedure are sharply drawn. The patient must be in good condition, not too old and preferably not too obese. The disease must be confined to the cervix and the immediately adjacent paracervical and paravaginal tissues.

The operative mortality is approximately the same for both procedures and should not be higher than 1 to 3 per cent. Because the Schauta-Amreich operation is performed through the vagina, it may be more suitable for an obese patient. The operability rate for the radical vaginal operation is approximately 75 per cent, as opposed to 60 per cent for the Wertheim operation performed through an abdominal incision. To extend the operative indications to include the patient with more extensive cancer is to run the risk of having a recurrence, as well as the chance of increasing the likelihood of ureterovaginal and vesicovaginal fistulas. In too many instances, the Wertheim hysterectomy and pelvic lymphadenectomy are employed when the patient has too much disease to hope that this operation can cope with it. When this operation is employed for Stages I and IIa cervical cancer, a five-year survival rate of 80 per cent may be expected, including a 50 per cent survival rate when the patient has regional metastases. The percentage of cures drops appreciably, and the morbidity increases, when the Wertheim is used for Stages IIb or III carcinomas.

It is recognized that the presence or absence of metastases to the regional nodes is one of the most important factors in estimating prognosis. The regional nodes should be dissected. One of the reasons why operation has gained favor in recent years is the fact that approximately 20 per cent of the group of patients who are considered to be good candidates for the Wertheim procedure combined with pelvic lymphadenectomy have regional node metastases. There is a considerable amount of doubt on the part of many that external radiation can cure these patients. On the other hand, 50 per cent of patients who have positive nodes in Stages I and IIa will be alive at five years, if the nodes have been removed and an adequate dissection has been done in the region of the primary growth in the cervix. Over 80 per cent of patients in these classifications survive five or more years when the nodes are negative.

As the disease becomes more extensive in the areas remote from the primary tumor, the number of patients who have regional nodes increases. Approximately 30 per cent of the patients in Stage IIb have positive nodes, and only 20 per cent of these will be cured.

In considering the influence of node dissection on the total survival, it is important to remember that, although a 50 per cent survival can be expected when the nodes are positive in Stages I and IIa, at best one-third of the patients are in this category and only 20 per cent have positive nodes. It is obvious that the node dissections should be done, but the emphasis in surgical therapy should be on the primary tumor.

The five-year survival figures reported by surgeons who subscribe to the more extensive pelvic dissections support the contention that the Wertheim procedure should be restricted to cervical cancers in the category of Stages I and II. The figures reported by Meigs, who was largely responsible for the present trend toward radical surgery, indicate an 82 per cent survival for Stage I lesions, but only 62 per cent for Stage II. Approximately 35 per cent of patients who had positive nodes in these two categories lived five or more years.

There is increasing evidence that the Wertheim operation achieves the maximum benefits when it is restricted to Stages I and IIa. A 65 per cent salvage figure for Stage II appears to be very satisfactory. However, when the Stage II category is broken down into the early IIa and the more extensive IIb, it seems obvious that the Wertheim procedure is satisfactory for the former but not the latter.

COMPLICATIONS. Inasmuch as meticulous dissection must be carried out in the region of the ureters and bladder base, a radical operation carries a morbidity factor which is its major disadvantage. There is the possibility of ureterovaginal and vesicovaginal fistulas, and of bladder atony and consequent dysfunction. Other complications are traceable to sepsis, wound disruption and pelvic thrombophlebitis.

The most undesirable sequelae of the extended abdominal procedures for cancer of the cervix are the ureteral and vesicovaginal fistulas. They are less common following the radical vaginal procedure. Together with ureteral obstructions and pyelonephritis, they are the most frequent complications.

A ureterovaginal fistula often heals spontaneously, if full bladder drainage is constantly maintained by use of an inlying catheter draining into a thigh urinal. If the fistula does not heal after three months, the surgeon has the option of implanting the ureter into the dome of the bladder, or performing a nephrectomy. Nephrectomy is preferred if there is any element of obstruction or pyelonephritis.

Atony of the bladder is unavoidable if an adequate dissection has been done. It may take several months before the bladder tone returns to normal. Some patients never regain the ability to tell when their bladder is full. These patients are instructed to void at regular intervals whether they experience the urge or not.

Since a large part of the vaginal canal is removed forming a vaginal canal with a point at the apex, traction of the posterior wall of the vagina tends to pull down the neck of the bladder, thereby reducing the normal posterior angle. At times, the Marshall-Marchetti procedure is necessary to restore continence. Before resorting to surgery for correction, the muscle-setting exercises of Kegal should be tried.

Because of the wide pelvic dissection, it is not surprising that a few patients develop pelvic abscesses or cellulitis, particularly if the drainage factors are inadequate. Rarely is thrombophlebitis a complication. Antibiotic therapy, coupled with transfusions, usually corrects the infection.

RADIATION THERAPY. Within the scope of individualization in therapy, radiation may be chosen as the sole definitive therapy for the early stages of cervical cancer. It is the only treatment which can be offered for Stages III and IV by all but the most accomplished pelvic cancer surgeons.

The basic aim in irradiation is to destroy cancer at the primary site as well as in the area within the pelvis to which it may have spread. The area of potential dissemination is an extensive one. Unfortunately, the actual amount of disease can be determined only with the examining finger with some help from intravenous pyelograms. The actual direction of spread cannot be determined with accuracy. Disease may be present in tissue spaces and lymphatics on the side which shows the least induration on palpation. It has also been shown that approximately 15 per cent of Stage I lesions have regional node metastases which cannot be felt. Since the amount of disease is only a clinical estimate, the combined dose of radium and x-ray must be uniform throughout the pelvis and lethal for cancer cells wherever encountered. Moreover, the dosage must be delivered at the tumor site without damaging adjacent organs. The effect on the supporting tissues must be considered as well for if they are devitalized by too intensive radiation some of the actual resistance to cancer invasion may be lost. The optimal dose of radiation is not far below the tolerance dose for normal tissue.

Radiation of cervical cancer cells may be accomplished by the use of a combination of radium applied to the cervix itself and to the cavity of the uterus, and external roentgenotherapy. The radium is expected to destroy cancer in the cervix and the areas adjacent to it, while roentgenotherapy is counted on to destroy tumor which is more laterally placed. To prevent overconcentration of ionizing radiation at any one point, the amount of external irradiation must be carefully balanced with that from the intrauterine source. It is of the utmost importance that the dosage at the tumor site be measured physically. The cancerocidal dose is placed roughly at 6000 to 7000 r delivered at the tumor site.

The relative apparent recovery rate in 30,000 patients with Stages I and II carcinoma of the cervix treated by radiation, and reported from 105 institutions, was 73 per cent for Stage I and 51 per cent for Stage II. These figures compare favorably with those obtained by surgical treatment.

Complications of radiation therapy. Although the mortality from the use of irradiation is a minimum, there are complications which follow its use. The organs most likely to be damaged are the bladder and the rectum. The likelihood of damage to the intestine increases when there is associated pathology such as pelvic inflammation, or when a previous laparotomy has been performed, since the small intestine may be adherent and the mesentery may be overly radiated. Progressive endarteritis may result in necrosis years after the initial therapy. The effect on the bladder and rectum is more direct since the epithelium of both structures is very sensitive to the effects of radiation.

Rectal injuries occur more frequently and are more distressing to the patient than bladder damage. Although most of the complications are caused by external radiation, the chances of injury from intrauterine radium increase when the uterus is fixed in retroversion or the disease extends to the posterolateral fornix of the vagina. The symptoms of early damage are diarrhea, tenesmus and bloody stools. Unfortunately, they tend to appear only after treatment has been under way for two or three weeks. Months or years later, the patient may develop a rectovaginal fistula or a stricture. This is due to the progressive endarteritis and thrombosis of the vessels in the mesentery.

The bladder damage is usually due to the effects of radiation produced by the intrauterine source. Although the bladder epithelium is less sensitive than that of the intestine, the patient may frequently experience some degree of dysuria or even hematuria during the course of treatment. The late results of radiation damage to the bladder are very distressing. The frequency and extensive dysuria are secondary to small ulcerations on the bladder floor and the decrease in bladder capacity.

Other complications such as radiation sickness and skin reactions are distressing at the time but have less serious consequences. They may be troublesome enough to interfere with the progress of therapy. Such complications are materially reduced when the higher energy units are employed.

COMBINATION OF RADIATION AND OPERA-

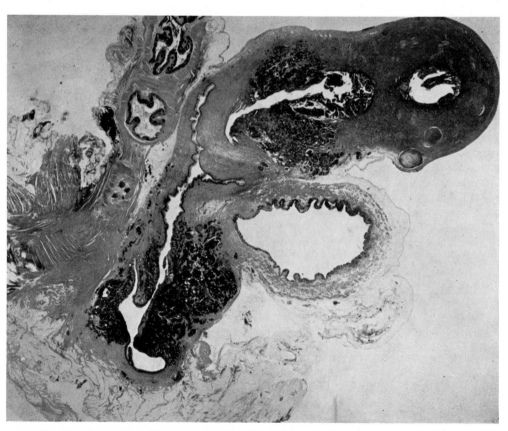

Figure 10.   Giant histologic paramedian section showing, from left to right, the rectum, vagina and a tangential section of uterus. The bladder is demonstrated below the uterus. The dark-stained nodules in the vaginal walls and lower uterine segment are cervical carcinoma, not susceptible to cure by radium therapy because of the depth of invasion.

TION. In many clinics, a combination of radiation and operation is being used for Stages I and II carcinoma of the cervix in the hope that the best features of both will be preserved while the complications are minimized. The combination therapy has been employed in a number of different ways. First, a preliminary trial dose of radiation may be given, followed by a radical hysterectomy and node dissection when either the smears or biopsy show an unsatisfactory response to radiation. Second, a planned course of local radium therapy may be given to the local tumor, followed in six weeks by a radical hysterectomy and lymphadenectomy. Approximately one-half the usual dose of radium employed when radiation is the sole therapy is the dosage usually used. Third, a complete course of radiation may be followed by a radical abdominal operation. Or, fourth, bilateral pelvic lymphadenectomy may be performed either before or after radiation. It may be done transabdominally or through a retroperitoneal approach, in the inguinal region. The rationale is based on the assumption that irradiation does not destroy malignant disease in the lymph nodes.

The twelfth annual report on the results of treatment of carcinoma of the uterus, with 105 institutions reporting from 23 countries, records 15,160 of 49,235 patients, or 31 per cent, classified as Stage III, and 3336, or 6.8 per cent, as Stage IV. The relative apparent five-year recovery rate was 26.7 per cent for Stage III, and 7.8 per cent for Stage IV.

Radiation is indicated for the treatment of Stages III and IV cancer of the cervix in the majority of instances. These patients have too extensive disease to expect that the Wertheim operation can encompass it.

PELVIC EXENTERATION. Partial or total removal of the pelvic contents, coupled with a variety of methods of creating urinary diversion, is called partial or total exenteration. Total exenteration is an en bloc excision of uterus, adnexae, bladder, rectum, vagina and vulva, together with bilateral pelvic lymphadenectomy. The anterior or partial exenteration removes all of these organs but leaves the rectum undisturbed. In both procedures, it is necessary to redirect the urinary stream. This may be done by constructing a new bladder out of an isolated segment of ileum and transplanting the ureters into it; by performing a ureterointestinal anastomosis with the sigmoid colon, with or without the creation of a transverse colostomy; or by establishing skin ureterostomies.

These are formidable operations which place a great strain on the resources and abilities of all concerned with the patient's care before, during and after the operation. The postoperative problems can prove as troublesome and exhausting as any encountered during the operation. This is not a procedure to be undertaken lightly. It does have a place, however, in the treatment of extensive cancer of the cervix. Although the operative mortality, measured in terms of a 28-day hospitalization, runs as high as 15 per cent, the patients can survive, and live happy and useful lives for long periods of time. It has been reported that 33 per cent of patients so treated are living without disease five or more years after operation.

The rationale of these extensive procedures is based on the fact that cancer of the cervix is primarily a local disease. It is surprising how many of these patients have negative lymph nodes, despite their advanced stage of disease. When the nodes are negative, the long-term survival rate is 62 per cent.

TREATMENT OF RECURRENCE. When a previous course of radiation has been adequate, there is little to be gained from a second if cancer persists or recurs. Since lethal amounts of neoplastic disease may be present in the pelvis without any spread to remote areas, or even to the regional lymph nodes, there is a place for a radical operation in the treatment of persistent or recurrent disease. The likelihood of success increases if the cancer has spread anteriorly or posteriorly to involve bladder and rectum, rather than laterally. In our experience with pelvic exenteration, totaling nearly 200 patients, metastases to the regional nodes have been found in only 42 per cent. Although the operative mortality, measured in terms of the failure of the patient to recover regardless of the time after operation, runs as high as 15 per cent in the postradiation cases, 25 per cent are living after five years, and seven of 37 are active after ten years.

These operations have a restricted place in the treatment of cervical cancer. They may be offered to patients who have failed to respond after radiation therapy, developed vesicovaginal or rectovaginal fistulas as a result of either persistent disease or radiation, and have recurrences after an inadequate operation. The surgeon should expect a reasonable chance to cure the patient before offering the procedure. It should not be done simply because the patient has an extensive amount of disease in the pelvis.

LACERATIONS OF THE PELVIC FLOOR

Acute lacerations of the vulva, vagina and perineum occur from a variety of causes. In this age group, the late manifestations of injury are of prime importance. The injuries result from either a traumatic instrumental delivery or a spontaneous delivery of an oversized infant through a relatively small or unprepared vaginal canal. The results of trauma may have been present for years, but the threat of further pregnancies is enough to delay attempts to repair the damage. The majority of reconstructive operations are performed in the 40 to 50 age group.

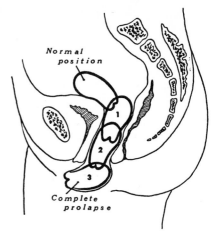

Figure 11. Diagrammatic representation of first- and second-degree prolapses and procidentia of the uterus.

The significance of the laceration depends on the extent of the trauma to the levator ani muscles. There are three degrees of perineal laceration.

FIRST-DEGREE TEAR. Overdistention of the lower portions of the vaginal wall may produce a tear in the posterior fourchette, overlying skin and posterior vaginal wall. When the laceration is confined to this area, and the underlying fascia and levator ani muscles are undamaged, the patient has a first-degree tear. On rare occasions, the perineal body may be severely damaged without any outward evidence of trauma. The perineum may appear to be intact, but other lacerations in the pelvic floor may have taken place farther up the canal.

SECOND-DEGREE TEAR. This injury extends beyond the midportion of the perineum. The anterior components of the levator muscles and the rectovaginal fascia, which provide the lateral support of the vagina, are torn on one or both sides. The extent of the damage can be evaluated by inserting one or more fingers in the vagina and pulling the posterior vaginal wall down and forward while the thumb exerts counter pressure on the perineal body in the midline just above the anus. Depending on the extent of the trauma, a deep sulcus can be felt on one or both sides of the midline of the posterior vaginal wall. Occasionally, scar tissue simulates the presence of muscle tissue which actually is not there. As one looks directly at the perineum, the vaginal introitus tends to gape open, exposing either a cystocele or a rectocele prolapsing through the defect in muscle and fascial support.

THIRD-DEGREE TEAR. The damage in a third-degree tear involves the entire perineum, including a tear through the sphincter ani muscles. The anus is totally or partially incompetent, and the rectal mucosa pouts out through the defect. The examiner can identify the separated ends of the sphincter by observing dimpled areas in the skin on either side of the anal opening.

Naturally, the best time to repair these defects follows immediately upon their recognition at the time of delivery. The descent of the bladder and rectum through the anatomic defect becomes more pronounced with the passage of time. If they are not recognized at delivery, the repair of all but the damage to the external anal sphincter should be delayed until the chance of pregnancy is minimal.

REPAIR OF SPHINCTER ANI. It is important to recognize damage to the external anal sphincter, since incompetence in its function produces distressing complications. The longer repair is delayed, the harder it is to correct the defect.

Under normal conditions, shallow folds of skin can be seen radiating outward in all directions from the central opening. When the sphincter is divided, the folds which should be seen anteriorly between the upper border of the anal opening and the posterior vaginal wall disappear, though they are still present posteriorly and laterally. A fibrotic band of scar tissue replaces the muscle, and the divided ends can often be felt through the dimpled areas of the skin seen lateral to the anus.

PELVIC HERNIATIONS. There are three well-recognized types of prolapse of the pelvic organs which accompany pelvic lacerations damaging to the levator ani muscles and the pelvic fascia. Weakness of the muscles or fascial support which allows the bladder, urethra, rectum, uterus or vaginal vault to descend into the vagina becomes more pronounced as the patient becomes older. They occur uncommonly before the age of 40 years, despite the fact that the obstetric trauma which produced them occurred years before the hernia.

The nature of the prolapse reflects the degree of damage to the pelvic supporting structure. In most instances, they appear in various combinations although they can occur individually. The prolapse is recognized by the appearance of a cystocele, which is a herniation of the posterior wall of the bladder through a defect in the fascial and muscle support of the anterior vaginal wall. When the deficiency occurs in the lower anterior vaginal wall, the floor of the urethra descends and a urethrocele is present. A defect in the supporting structures in the more distal portions allows the rectum to bulge outward into the vaginal canal, and a rectocele is created. Weakness in the muscle and fascial support of the upper vaginal canal allows the posterior cul-de-sac, which often contains small intestine within the hernial sac, to descend. An enterocele is formed in this fashion. With more serious damage, the entire uterus descends and a uterine prolapse develops.

With extensive degrees of prolapse, the uterus, bladder and rectum all descend outside the introitus and a so-called "procidentia" is present. It is not uncommon in view of the intricate anatomic attachments of bladder and uterus to have a cystocele along with a prolapsed uterus in the absence of a rectocele.

SYMPTOMS AND PHYSICAL FINDINGS IN CYSTOCELE AND URETHROCELE. The chief complaint of the patient who has a cystocele is a sense of fullness and bulging in the vagina, coupled with a feeling that the pelvic organs are about to drop out. The symptoms vary with the extent of the cystocele. Many patients who have a small cystocele are unaware of it. The patient with a large cystocele definitely feels the lack of support and experiences bearing down discomfort to a greater or lesser degree. This feeling is aggravated by exertion, or long hours in a standing position. If the prolapse is extreme, she may be uncomfortable on either sitting or walking.

Urinary symptoms are common but the chief problem is difficulty in completely emptying the bladder. Retained urine becomes infected so that the patient often has cystitis, which may produce frequency and dysuria.

It is important to remember that the patient who has a cystocele rarely has stress incontinence, while this is the presenting complaint with a urethrocele.

There is no particular problem in identifying either a cystocele or urethrocele, because in both instances a pronounced bulge is noted in the anterior vaginal wall which increases appreciably when the patient is asked to cough or strain. If there is any doubt, these observations will be accentuated when the patient is examined in the standing position. In addition, the patient with a urethrocele is unable to control the flow of urine which spurts out as the patient coughs.

The only reasons for repairing small or moderate-sized cystoceles in a young patient are that the cystocele is becoming larger and producing increasing discomfort, and the patient has recurrent bouts of cystitis due to inability to evacuate the bladder completely. Large lesions should be repaired unless the patient plans to have more children, or unless there are contraindications such as intercurrent disease or advanced age.

In a patient who is an unsuitable candidate for surgical repair or is too young to warrant it, much can be accomplished by the use of a pessary. The choice of the type of pessary is important. The ring type, which is useful when the patient has a true prolapse, is not effective for a cystocele. It is better to use the Hodge type in a younger patient and a doughnut pessary in the older patient.

Age should not be the sole contraindication to operation. The young patient who has so much prolapse that she needs the constant support of a pessary should be operated on. Likewise, the older patient who has no constitutional disease may prefer to have an operation rather than wear a pessary which does not entirely relieve her discomfort.

RECTOCELE. Although a cystocele may appear in a nulliparous patient, this is rarely true of the patient with a rectocele. For a rectocele to appear, there must be a fascial defect which usually follows childbirth. It is usually found in association with a cystocele and some degree of uterine prolapse.

The symptoms of rectocele are rarely severe enough to warrant surgical repair or the use of a pessary. It is usually the associated elements in the prolapse, such as the cystocele or uterine descent, which account for discomfort. On the other hand, it may become so large that the patient experiences difficulty in completely evacuating the bowel. Occasionally, the bulge is so extreme that the patient has to compress it with her fingers in order to defecate. In this situation, surgical repair is definitely indicated. Usually, the rectocele is repaired as a part of the reconstructive procedures designed to correct other perineal defects.

ENTEROCELE. The so-called "high" rectocele is apt to be an enterocele. This is a true hernia. In the congenital type, there is an actual hernial defect lined with peritoneum lying deep in the cul-de-sac with its opening found between the attachments of the uterosacral ligaments on the back of the uterus. In its descent, it passes between the anterior rectal and the posterior vaginal walls. In the acquired type, the cul-de-sac of pelvic peritoneum, often called the pouch of Douglas, elongates under the stress of obstetric delivery and descends along with the uterus. Both types are apt to increase in size and fill with small intestine and omentum under the stimulus of increasing intra-abdominal pressure. It is possible for a patient to have both types of enterocele.

Unless the enterocele is recognized, the surgeon may repair the pelvic floor either with or without a vaginal hysterectomy only to find that the vaginal wall still protrudes and the patient has the same symptoms she had before the repair. A well-established enterocele can often be seen as a bulge in the posterior vaginal wall behind the cervix. It tends to expand and contract as the patient breathes, suggesting that there is some connection between it and the abdominal cavity. From within the abdomen, a fingerlike downward extension of the peritoneum may be seen through an opening which lies between the uterosacral ligaments, but anterior to the rectum.

Unfortunately, the surgeon may recognize only the rectocele when the patient is examined in the lithotomy position. He should beware of interpreting his findings as a high rectocele because an enterocele is probably present. If there is any doubt, the patient should be examined in the standing position. A rectocele and enterocele frequently coexist. They may be differentiated by placing a finger in the rectum and a thumb along the posterior vaginal wall. The rectal finger enters the saclike cavity formed by the rectocele, but it cannot enter the thickened area on the vaginal wall above the rectocele since this is the enterocele sac.

It is extremely difficult to distinguish between an enterocele and the prolapse of the upper part of the vagina after a total hysterectomy. The location of the scar at the apex of the vagina is of some assistance in differentiating between the two. If the scar is in normal position high up in the vaginal canal, the presenting bulge is an enterocele. A vaginal prolapse is present if the operative scar is felt well down in the vaginal canal.

Unless the enterocele is fairly large, it will cause little in the way of symptoms. It should be repaired at the time of any operation done to reconstruct the pelvic floor. The sac is dissected free from the rectum and vagina and the neck closed before excising the redundancy. The neck of the sac is then sutured to the uterosacral ligaments on the back of the uterus, or to the broad ligament if a vaginal hysterectomy is done. At times, it may be advisable to open the abdomen and obliterate the posterior cul-de-sac with multiple purse string sutures.

UTERINE PROLAPSE. It is unusual for a cystocele or rectocele to appear without some degree of abnormal uterine descent. The underlying anatomic defect, like that of the cystocele or rectocele, is a weakening of the normal supporting structures of the uterus and vagina due to the strain put upon them during childbirth. On rare occasions, prolapse of the uterus is found in nulliparous women. Palpable evidence of lack of support may not appear following delivery, but it becomes increasingly apparent as the tissues lose their supple character through aging.

Prolapse of the uterus is usually classified according to the degree to which it descends. In first-degree prolapse, the uterus comes down but not out through the introitus. In second-degree prolapse, the cervix elongates at the expense of the fundus and appears outside the vaginal outlet as a whole or in part. A complete descent of the uterus with eversion of the vaginal canal is classified as a third-degree prolapse, which is commonly called a procidentia.

Since the relaxation of the supporting structures takes place slowly over a number of years, the patient rarely has any discomfort before the age of 40. From then on, she becomes increasingly aware of the lack of pelvic support, which manifests itself as a bearing-down discomfort, a sense of fullness in the vagina, or a feeling that the womb is dropping out. If there is a true procidentia, the patient may have to push the uterus back in the vagina to be able to sit or walk with ease. Urinary difficulties are common. Because of the abnormal position of the bladder and the strain placed on the ureters, due to the downward pull of the prolapse, residual urine accumulates in the bladder, which predisposes toward cystitis, and the ureters angulate and cause obstruction. Thus, the patient may not only have difficulty in emptying the bladder, but have cystitis and pyelitis as well. It is, therefore, advisable to determine the amount of residual urine and whether it is infected, and examine for any element of ureteral obstruction with an intravenous pyelogram before evaluating the severity of the symptoms and advising surgical procedures for correction.

The best form of treatment for a young patient with moderate prolapse, minimal symptoms and the desire to continue having children is a supporting pessary. The same treatment applies to the older patient who has so much constitutional disease that surgery carries too great a risk.

If the young patient has too much relaxation to expect that a pessary will provide an adequate support, and if the symptoms are sufficient to make her miserable, she should be operated on. Surgical correction should follow a conservative pattern. The cystocele and rectocele may be repaired per vagina, and the uterus suspended through the abdominal approach. Subsequent normal vaginal deliveries are possible after this type of correction; cesarean section is not mandatory. When the prolapse is more extensive, the bladder is freed from the cervix and the cervix amputated at the level of the internal os. The divided ends of the cardinal ligaments are sutured together in front of the amputated cervix and the cystocele and rectocele are repaired. This is the so-called Manchester-Fothergill operation. Following the operation, the surgeon must assure himself that the canal is patulous by dilation of the cervix when the patient returns for her first postoperative visit. In an older patient, a vaginal hysterectomy should be performed and the cystocele and rectocele repaired whether or not there are symptoms.

REPAIR OF VAGINAL PROLAPSE AFTER HYSTERECTOMY. The surgeon is confronted with a real problem if the vaginal vault prolapses after the uterus has been removed in the young patient. The prolapse must be corrected and a patent vaginal canal preserved. Some means must be found to support the sagging vaginal canal. If there is enough resiliency left in the round ligaments, they may be resutured to the lateral and posterior walls of the vagina. When this is not possible, the abdomen is opened and strips of Mersilene gauze are used to suspend the vagina to the posterior bony pelvic wall. In an older patient, the vagina should be obliterated by removing the vaginal epithelium and suturing the pubococcygeus muscles in the midline after repairing the cystocele. A perineorrhaphy completes the operation.

MINOR DEGREES OF UTERINE MALPOSITION. Normally, the adult uterus lies in a position midway between the bladder, which is placed anteriorly and slightly below it, and the rectum, which is located posteriorly. With the patient in the upright position, the uterus lies in a horizontal plane at right angles to the long axis of the vagina. The anterior surface of the uterus rests lightly on the fundus of the bladder. The uterus is kept in this position by the pressure exerted on it by the overlying intestine. Normally, the uterus is not fixed. It is, therefore, possible to displace it in a variety of ways.

Malpositions of the uterus are chiefly in a forward or backward direction. Anterior displacements rarely require any surgical attention because they produce few derangements in function, and only rarely do symptoms appear. The two chief symptoms are dysmenorrhea and sterility. The treatment is hormonal. In rare instances, dilation of the cervix may be indicated to assist in correcting the sharp angulation of the fundus on the cervix. Its chief value is disruption of the nerve endings which concentrate in a plexus on the posterior wall of the cervix at the level of the internal os. Dysmenorrhea is sometimes corrected by this surgical procedure.

In retrocession, the uterus drops back into the hollow of the sacrum. In retroversion and retroflexion, the uterus angulates backward.

Approximately 20 per cent of patients have retroversion normally. Most of them have no symptoms and have no difficulty in becoming pregnant. If the patient does have difficulty in becoming pregnant, other causes for infertility are probably present. The only indication for performing any surgical procedure to improve fertility might appear in the patient in whom repeated investigations have been negative and retroversion is the only abnormal finding.

Every possible means should be employed to try to replace the uterus and keep it there with a pessary before resorting to operation.

Unless the uterus is fixed in a posterior position by pelvic adhesions, it can usually be replaced in a normal position. This is done with the patient in the lithotomy position. With the index and middle fingers in the vagina, pressure is exerted on the posterior vaginal wall behind the cervix in an upward direction. With the uterus dislodged from its posterior position, further pressure by the left hand in the vagina against the cervix applied in an upward and backward direction will direct the uterus forward. The right hand on the abdominal wall above the symphysis assists in guiding the uterus into the forward position. It may be held there by a pessary.

In considering symptoms from an uncomplicated retroversion, the surgeon will be well-advised to consider carefully whether retroversion is a cause of backache. If the uterus is fixed in this position, the patient may well have backache, but the explanation of the cause in patients who simply have a retroverted uterus should be sought in the bony skeleton or its muscular supports.

When the uterus is fixed in retroversion, the symptoms are usually due to the pathologic entity which produced the fixation. Low pelvic pain and backache, dyspareunia, dysmenorrhea and abnormalities in the menstrual bleeding pattern may be present, but the symptoms are not primarily due to the fact that the uterus is in retroverted position.

URINARY INCONTINENCE

The inability to control the evacuation of urine can be a most distressing symptom regardless of the degree to which it exists. If it is slight, the patient is never sure when evacuation will happen, and the uncertainty is enough to make her miserable. If it is moderate, but not enough to wear a protective pad, the patient is miserable because her underclothing is soiled and wet a large part of the time. When it becomes severe and constant, requiring numerous pads or rubber pants, the patient undergoes a personality change and tends to become asocial.

Complete loss of urinary control is usually due to the presence of a fistula. An intermittent loss is usually due to a defect in the action of the group of muscles which combine to form the internal sphincter of the bladder. Fistulas can be identified and appropriate surgical procedures can be taken to repair them. Stress incontinence, wherein the cutoff mechanism is faulty, is much harder to diagnose and at times is more difficult to cure.

A careful history should be taken to identify accurately the cause, because an ill-planned operation is destined to fail. The exact cause may be spinal cord damage or possibly a spina bifida. Stress incontinence may be a manifestation of diabetic neuropathy, multiple sclerosis, tabes dorsalis or tumors of the central nervous system. It is important to discover the patient's voiding habits prior to the development of the loss of control. Some patients void very infrequently from force of habit, and may be spilling over from an excess of urine held in the bladder. If she laughs or sneezes, the patient is bound to leak a small amount of urine. This is overflow, not stress incontinence. This patient is not cured by operation, but by correcting a long-established habit.

It is important to distinguish between true stress incontinence and the so-called "urgency" incontinence. Some patients have an irritable bladder and cannot avoid urinating when a sudden urge to empty the bladder arises. Trigonitis, cystitis and urethritis play a role as a cause of irritability. The symptoms are aggravated by vaginitis or endocervicitis, and are magnified by emotional states.

STRESS INCONTINENCE. Primarily, stress incontinence appears in an older patient who has suffered damage to the muscular support of the base of the bladder at the time of obstetric delivery. The symptoms are magnified by the fact that estrin production is on the wane. The loss of hormonal stimulation produces changes in the epithelium of the urethra and bladder neck. The tissues are far less resistant to bacterial invasion, and low-grade infections increase the irritability of the bladder neck.

The involuntary loss of control occurs only when the patient is in an upright position. Usually, patients who have stress incontinence are dry at night. Stress incontinence is aggravated by any act that increases intravesical or intra-abdominal pressure. The symptoms are brought on by sneezing, coughing, laughing or carrying heavy bundles.

The degree of urinary loss is directly related to the extent of muscle damage. The urethra moves downward and backward, away from its normal position under the pubis. The extent of the damage can best be evaluated by roentgenograms, following the placement of a metallic beaded chain in the bladder to mark the course of the urethra, and the injection of a radiopaque solution into the bladder cavity. Anteroposterior and lateral films are taken with the patient lying and sitting while straining to void, and while resting. Lateral views taken of the patient voiding while in an upright position are the most informative. The patient with stress incontinence shows a rotational descent of the bladder and funneling of the bladder neck, a loss of the normal posterior urethrovesical angle, and a change in the inclination of the course of the urethra.

Obstetric trauma responsible for the formation of a cystocele is in contrast with that which produces stress incontinence. Trauma which creates a cystocele takes place farther posteriorly along the bladder base, rather than anteriorly in the region of the supporting structures of the urethra and bladder neck. The posterior urethrovesical angle is not disturbed in the presence of a cystocele. Stress incontinence, however, is common in the presence of a urethrocele. Stress incontinence is rarely present in the patient who has a procidentia or a large cystocele. The extreme descent of the bladder creates its own angle between the base of the bladder and the urethra. It is important to remember that the same change may be present in the muscles which make up the internal sphincter. When the bladder is replaced in a new position, incontinence may appear when none was present before, unless attempts are made to correct the posterior vesical angle at the time of repair.

A complete physical examination, including a neurologic examination, must be done. Vaginal and rectal examination should exclude pelvic tumors or inflammatory masses which might be responsible for irritability of the bladder through pressure on it. Varying degrees of prolapse of the uterus and bladder are usually present. One of the most constant and distinctive findings appears when one notes the anatomic position of the urethra. Normally, the female urethra points straight out, but the urethral meatus of the multiparous woman who has stress incontinence flattens and is directed toward the ceiling. Beneath it, one frequently finds a bulging area in the posterior wall of the proximal urethra.

There are two practical methods of testing for stress incontinence. The best test is to have the patient strain while in the act of voiding. The anterior vaginal wall in the region of the bladder base can be seen to bulge outward. Urine will usually spurt out from the urethra. The outflow of urine can be abruptly stopped by placing the tips of two fingers in the vagina, one on either side of the urethra near the bladder base. Upward pressure of the finger tips should stop the flow of urine even though the patient strains forcibly, if the patient has stress incontinence. Or, instead of using the two fingers, Allis clamps are placed on the bladder neck at the site of the anterior wall bulge. When traction is applied in a downward direction, urinary loss occurs which promptly ceases when the clamps are pushed upward.

Before operation is attempted, the patient should be catheterized after voiding, to detect whether there is residual urine. The specimen should be examined microscopically and cultured to determine the presence of infection. Cystoscopic examinations should be routine to rule out the presence of fistulas, polyps, calculi, trigonitis, cystitis and urethritis. A cystometrogram should be performed to test the tone of the bladder musculature and the degree of intravesical pressure required to initiate the urge to void. The most important test is the urethrocystogram.

Before the physician advocates surgical repair of the damaged bladder neck and internal sphincter, the patient with a moderate degree of urinary loss should be given an opportunity to correct the situation by nonsurgical means. Several approaches can be tried. Estrin therapy may restore normal epithelium in the vagina, urethra and trigone of the bladder. This reduces the irritability by eliminating low-grade infection. Hypotonic muscular action can be improved by giving pressor drugs such as Urecholine chloride. Bladder infections can be eliminated by appropriate antibiotic drugs. A weight-reduction program is helpful, because it gives the patient a better chance to use her own muscle control and because it will put her in better condition should operation be necessary. A great deal can be accomplished in re-training the pubococcygeus muscles which have atrophied and function inadequately. The muscle-setting exercises of Kegel consist of simply contracting the buttock muscles and holding them in that state for a few seconds. This maneuver carried out repeatedly eventually re-educates and strengthens the muscles.

In severe degrees of stress incontinence, or when all other methods have failed, operation may be necessary. Repair of the cystocele, reconstruction of the bladder neck, and reducing the size of the urethral canal may be carried out as a vaginal procedure. Or, suspension of the bladder neck may be performed through an abdominal incision by employing either the Marshall-Marchetti procedure, or one of the various sling operations which utilizes abdominal wall fascia.

Problems of the 50 to 60 Age Group

CANCER OF THE ENDOMETRIUM

The life history, growth pattern, diagnosis and treatment of carcinoma of the endometrium differ materially from that of cancer of the cervix despite the fact that the two tumors arise in the same organ. Cancer arising in the fundal portion of the uterus appears to grow less rapidly and is less lethal than cancer of the cervix. In the fourteenth annual report of the results of treatment in carcinoma of the uterus, 42 world institutions recorded 14,796 patients with an apparent five-year recovery rate of 62.6 per cent. While this is 12 per cent better than the results reported for treatment of cervical carcinoma, it is not as high a percentage as most surgeons believe they are salvaging.

In the past, ratio of incidence of cancer of the uterine fundus to cancer of the cervix was approximately 1 to 8. In recent years, there has been a pronounced change, so that today the ratio is nearer 1 to 2. Since more women are now living to an age at which they may develop endometrial cancer, the incidence may be expected to increase rather than decline.

Seventy-five per cent of all endometrial cancer occurs in the years after the menopause. Although cancer of the cervix is now found in increasing numbers in women 20 to 30 years of age, only 2 per cent of endometrial cancer appears in this age group. Another 5 to 8 per cent occurs in the 30 to 40 age group. The remainder occurs in patients beyond the ages of 40 and 50.

Cancer of the endometrium grows less rapidly than cervical cancer, and the majority of instances are confined to the epithelial lining of the endometrial cavity, without invading the musculature. As soon as the myometrium becomes involved, or if the point of origin lies in the endocervical canal, endometrial cancer has the same lethal potential as cervical cancer. In some clinics, carcinoma of the corpus and cervix is classified as a separate entity. They behave more like cervical than endometrial carcinoma. When the cancer has spread beyond the confines of the uterus, it is more deadly than cancer of the cervix because there is a greater tendency for it to metastasize to the lungs, liver and bone.

The frankly invasive carcinoma of the endometrium may be either circumscribed or diffuse. The epithelium of the circumscribed type piles up in a local area to form flat, velvety, polypoid masses which vary in size but are usually sharply demarcated from the rest of the mucosa. The cancer may directly invade the myometrium at the point of origin and infiltrate the muscle without implicating the adjacent endometrium, or it may spread superficially to involve the rest of the epithelium lining the cavity.

The majority of instances of endometrial cancer are of the diffuse type in which the growth, in its early phases, spreads throughout the endometrium without involving the muscle wall. Eventually, the muscle is involved, depending on the length of time the cancer has been present and the growth rate of the tumor. The prognosis is directly referable to the extent of muscle wall infiltration. The lymphatic channels run horizontally from the cavity to communicate with a longitudinal network which extends from fundus to cervix. Further extension occurs when these pathways drain into lymphatic connecting channels, which form along the lateral sides of the uterus beneath the serosa. It is evident then that cancer of the endometrium is actually a disease of the entire uterus, and is not solely confined to its fundal portion.

Extension of endometrial carcinoma beyond the confines of the uterus takes place rather late in its course in the lymphatics, fallopian tubes, blood stream, and peritoneum. The pathway of spread depends largely on the location of the primary source of the tumor. A tumor arising in the upper portion

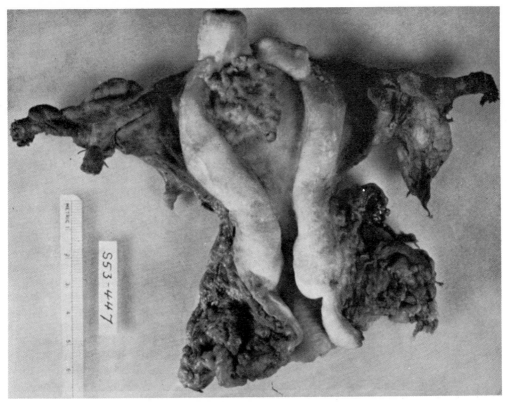

Figure 12.   A localized polypoid carcinoma of the fundus is invading the myometrium at its base.

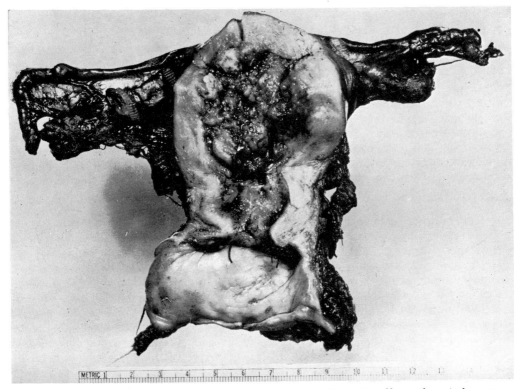

Figure 13.   Diffuse endometrial carcinoma, with polypoid foci and areas of necrosis and hemorrhage, is the most common gross type of uterine adenocarcinoma.

of the body of the uterus is most likely to spread to the tube, ovary or round ligament. Most often, it follows the distribution of the ovarian artery and vein, and metastasizes to the nodes along the side of the aorta and inferior vena cava, and from there to the epigastric and mediastinal areas.

When the tumor arises in the central or lower portion of the cavity, the spread, once the myometrium is involved, is similar to that of cervical cancer. Metastases may be found in the regional nodes along the external iliac vein and in the obturator area. The expectancy of such nodal involvement has been placed as high as 25 per cent, but the figure of 15 per cent is more nearly correct.

One of the most interesting modes of dissemination occurs in a retrograde manner. It is a constant observation that the metastases to the vaginal canal almost invariably appear beneath the epithelium of the anterior vaginal wall. The frequency of such metastases varies from 6 to 12 per cent.

The fallopian tubes become involved through direct spread from an endometrial source or by lymphatic permeation. The latter is more common, but the former occurs frequently enough to advise clamping the tubes as the initial step when the uterus is to be removed.

Recently, tumor cells have been found in the circulating blood at the time of curettage for endometrial cancer. This may be the explanation for the frequency of metastases to distant areas. The mere finding of such cells does not mean that metastases will develop, or that they will be lethal if they do. Many of the tumor cells are destroyed. To form a metastasis the cells must implant, develop a nutritional bed and propagate. There are many well-documented instances of metastases in lung and liver following the removal of the primary growth in the uterus, which have remained static for several years.

Once endometrial cancer has grown through the uterus to reach the peritoneal surface, it becomes very lethal. The subserosal extension of the carcinoma is evident when multiple, firm, white nodules are seen and felt on the surface of the uterus. From these, widespread dissemination occurs throughout the pelvic cavity involving the peritoneum, bladder and rectum.

SYMPTOMS. Except for bleeding, the patient with endometrial cancer has minimal symptoms and negligible physical findings. The two major factors in symptomatology are bleeding and discharge. Anemia occurs infrequently and weight loss is rarely present except in the neglected patient.

If the diagnosis of endometrial cancer is to be made sufficiently early to offer the patient the best chance of cure, it is of the utmost importance that a high index of suspicion be developed toward an abnormal bleeding pattern, particularly in the age groups immediately preceding and after menopause. Bleeding in some form is present in nearly all patients, and appears as the first symptom in approximately 80 per cent.

Most of the patients who bleed abnormally in the 40 to 50 age group do so because of hormonal imbalance, but the most important cause is cancer. Cancer of the cervix is at its peak at this time, and 25 per cent of all endometrial cancer occurs in the years before the menopause. Carcinoma must, therefore, be excluded before a benign explanation can be accepted.

In the postmenopausal age, vaginal spotting is by far the most common symptom. It may be of no great quantity and occur intermittently. Although it often appears after straining at stool or on voiding, it rarely is aggravated by coitus or douches. Should the latter occur, one should be immediately suspicious of cervical, not endometrial cancer. This is important because treatment of the latter is not adequate for the former. Although sudden gushing of blood has little clinical significance in the premenopausal woman, it is highly suspicious in the postmenopausal patient.

There are many explanations of postmenopausal bleeding other than carcinoma. A patient may bleed because she has a cervical polyp, urethral caruncle or hypertension, or because she has been taking hormones for the relief of menopausal symptoms. Because the bleeding is small in amount and often infrequent, the patient is apt to think little of it and neglect to consult her physician. He in turn tends to explain away the symptoms rather than investigate the cause, despite the fact that two-thirds of the patients who have vaginal spotting one or more years after the menopause will have carcinoma. It is imperative that any patient having such a history should be curetted to rule out carcinoma either in the cervix or endometrium.

There is nothing pathognomonic about the appearance of vaginal discharge in either the pre- or postmenopausal patient. Some significance can be attached to a clear, watery discharge, particularly when it assumes a brownish, or blood-tinged appearance. Watery discharge sometimes occurs in spurts, particularly when the patient bends over or is in the act of voiding or defecating.

It is almost impossible to place any emphasis on pain in the diagnosis of endometrial cancer. Cramps do occur in the presence of pyometra or hematometra as the uterus tries to expel its contents. In the majority of instances, however, the pain is due to the association of other pelvic pathology. Even an extensive carcinoma of the endometrium may be present with no pain at all.

PHYSICAL FINDINGS. There are few physical findings which are of material value in establishing a diagnosis of endometrial cancer. The diagnosis is made when a high index of suspicion appears in the mind of the physician, who then confirms his doubts by obtaining endometrial samplings for histologic review. He may do this by an endometrial biopsy or by curettage. Since endometrial cancer takes origin from a site which can be neither seen nor felt, little useful information can be elicited from a pelvic examination.

One might expect that uterine size would give some indication of the amount of disease present. Any attempt to make a prognosis of endometrial cancer on the basis of uterine size alone is actually impossible. When combined with histologic interpretation of the endometrial samples, there may be some correlation. It is true that a patient with undifferentiated carcinoma will do less well than one with a well-differentiated tumor, but this is so regardless of the size of the uterus. In all probability, it is the depth of the endometrial cavity rather than the overall size of the uterus that should be correlated with the histological findings when an attempt is made to stage the extent of the disease, and measure the effectiveness of the different modes of therapy.

One cannot interpret the finding of a large, fixed uterus as endometrial cancer which has spread beyond the confines of the uterus to involve the parametrial tissues. It is far more likely that the disease is confined to the uterus and that the fixation is secondary to a coexisting pelvic inflammation or endometriosis.

Palpation and inspection of the vaginal canal and cervix can produce useful information. The presence of a blue, moist, succulent vaginal epithelium in a postmenopausal woman who has abnormal bleeding heightens the suspicion. It suggests estrin stimulation, which is linked to the etiology of endometrial cancer. The presence of subepithelial nodules along the anterior vaginal wall, which may or may not be ulcerating or fungating, suggests that the patient has extensive endometrial cancer and that the lymphatic pathways beyond the confines of the uterus are involved.

For some reason, the external portion of the uterine cervix is rarely implicated in endometrial cancer. The tumor is usually confined to the endometrial cavity above the level of the internal os. If the cervix does show tumor in its walls, or papillary tumor can be seen projecting into the endocervical canal, the patient has either myometrial invasion or an extensive amount of tumor within the cavity.

The general physical examination is of importance in outlining therapy for the individual patient. These patients are in an older age group and are prone to obesity. One may expect to find hypertension, cardiac pathology and diabetes. Since endometrial cancer is hormone-dependent, it is not surprising that 4 per cent of patients who have it also have a concomitant carcinoma of the breast or ovary.

The patient with endometrial cancer tends to be obese, broad-chested, and have small hands and feet. Large, rounded buttocks make her appear more obese then she really is. This is the body build which is so frequently associated with hypertension and diabetes. The patient is likely to have had episodes of abnormal bleeding which required therapy. The menopause tends to be delayed well beyond the time when it might be expected to occur. These patients frequently continue to have periods well into their fifties. There is a far higher infertility rate in patients who have endometrial cancer than in those who have cervical carcinoma. Less than 10 per cent of cervical cancer patients are nulliparous; it is as high as 33 per cent in cancer of the body of the uterus.

The final diagnosis can only be made after samples have been obtained from the endometrial lining. Despite the fact that this is well known, it is amazing that 70 per cent of the patients in a large series reported never had a curettage.

Unlike cervical cancer, in which the vaginal smear gives definite evidence of its presence, the interpretation of the smear in endometrial cancer is far less accurate. A diagnostic error of 25 per cent is generally noted in cancer of the endometrium, when the material is taken from the vaginal pool.

It will be less if aspirations are taken from the fundus, but few physicians have the equipment to carry out this procedure.

Endometrial biopsy can be carried out in the office, without anesthesia, by any physician. It is particularly useful in the premenopausal patient who is having an abnormal bleeding pattern. Much of the bleeding in this age group is due to functional cause, but the patient should not be treated with hormones until a sample of the endometrium is obtained. It is true that the material obtained is only a sample. If the bleeding persists, despite the negative biopsy and the institution of hormone therapy, the patient must have a curettage.

In the postmenopausal patient, an endometrial biopsy is not adequate because the cause of the bleeding is far more likely to be carcinoma and the material is only a sample. The accuracy of the biopsy is about 93 per cent, and if it can be determined before hospitalization that the patient actually has carcinoma, therapy can be planned more accurately. Endometrial biopsy is a very useful procedure and it has a definite place among diagnostic aids, but it should not be regarded as a substitute for diagnostic curettage.

Curettage is the most important factor in establishing the diagnosis of endometrial cancer. It must be done gently and methodically. Gentleness is essential, for there is a danger of perforating the uterus with the dilator or curette; of forcing malignant cells though the fallopian tube by the plunger action of the dilator; and of causing tumor cells to escape into the general circulation by overenergetic manipulations.

The curettage must be methodical because it is important to determine as far as possible the site of origin of the cancer, as well as the anatomic arrangement of the cavity. The size, depth and contour of the cavity are important considerations in the proper administration of radium. In addition, there is the possibility of missing an area of carcinoma. This is most likely to happen when the cancer arises in the cornu of the uterus, or when a flat, polypoid growth is present. It is excellent practice to explore the endometrial cavity with common duct forceps in order to pick up an occasional polypoid growth that has rolled away from the curette.

The curettage must be fractional, because the bleeding may be due to carcinoma of the endocervical canal and not to endometrial cancer, and because the endometrial cancer may involve both the fundus and the cervix, the so-called carcinoma of fundus and cervix. In either case, the treatment should be that employed for cervical, not endometrial, cancer. After the endocervical canal has been thoroughly scraped and the samples separately labeled, the surgeon proceeds with curettement of the endometrial cavity. All curetted material, however small, should be saved for histologic examination.

In most instances, the pathologist will have no difficulty in making the diagnosis of endometrial carcinoma on frozen section, provided the surgeon gives him enough material to review. If there is any doubt about the diagnosis, it is best to delay any further surgical procedure until the pathologist has a chance to examine the permanent paraffin sections. If he is still in doubt, it is better to err on the side of suspicion of cancer and remove the uterus and adnexae.

The most common pathologic entity which is likely to be misinterpreted is atypical hyperplasia. The "Swiss cheese" type of endometrium and mild degrees of hyperplasia rarely cause any trouble, but glandular hyperplasia often does. These abnormal areas of proliferation may occur in localized foci, or be uniformly distributed throughout the endometrial lining. They appear rather commonly in patients who are approaching the menopause, particularly in the patient who has been given hormone therapy.

Like carcinoma in situ of the cervix, there appears a type of proliferative endometrium composed of heaped up collections of cells which vary in size and shape, which pathologists term "carcinoma in situ of the endometrium." The factors which distinguish carcinoma in situ from true invasive cancer are that it tends to occur in localized layers with glands which are not actually back to back as they are in invasive carcinoma, and the basal membrane is intact and no stromal invasion is present. In patients who have been shown to have carcinoma in situ, progression to invasive carcinoma has been documented. The latent period is roughly three to five years.

There are three main types of carcinoma which arise in the endometrium. *Papillary adenocarcinoma* tends to appear when the superficial endometrium undergoes proliferation. *Adenomatous adenocarcinoma* is more solid, less like the normal endometrium and involves the glands. When squamous epithelium is scattered through the malignant gland pattern, it is called *adenoacanthoma*. The various types of endometrial adenocarcinoma are classified as Grades I through IV, with 60 per cent falling in Grades I and II. The degree of clinical malignancy is correlated directly with the maturity of the cancer cell and inversely with the extent of its undifferentiation. Thus, the more highly differentiated carcinomas are Grade I, while the more anaplastic tumors are classified as Grades III and IV. Although the best clinical results appear in Grades I and II, there is altogether too much difficulty in accurately grading adenocarcinoma, due to local variables in the rate of growth, to use the grade of the tumor as a guide to therapy. Recently, an attempt has been made to link the size of the uterus with the degree of histologic differentiation. More experience with this type of correlation may be a valuable contribution. At present, there is no way of knowing where the tumor arises in the endometrial cavity, the nature of its spread or the degree of invasion.

TREATMENT. The end results of therapy of cancer of the endometrium reflect the uncertainties of histologic differentiation. Approximately 60 per cent of the tumors are the superficial type, with little tendency to invade the myometrium. The annual report of the results of treatment in carcinoma of the uterus suggests, on the basis of 6000 patients, that five-year results in the range of 71 to 72 per cent may be expected. This drops to 45 per cent when any degree of invasion is noted. It descends to 22 per cent in the group who may be classified as unfavorable for operation because of the spread of disease beyond the uterus or associated medical complications such as obesity, hypertension and diabetes.

The accepted forms of therapy for carcinoma of the endometrium are operation, radiation and a combination of radium and operation. The proper choice of treatment must consider the age and size of the patient, coexistent systemic disease and associated local disease, as well as the pathologic nature of the cancer.

The ideal type of treatment for the good risk patient is generally considered to be radiation, followed within ten days to six weeks by total removal of the uterus, bilateral removal of the adnexae and removal of a large segment of the upper vaginal canal. Radiation is given from sources inserted into the endometrial cavity, but in some clinics external radiation is given in lieu of the intercavitary radium.

Radiation is given in an attempt to render the tumor cells nonviable, to reduce the bulk of the tumor and to block the adjacent lymphatics. It is supposed to reduce not only the number of parametrial and vaginal vault metastases, but also distant metastases which might have appeared through dissemination of the tumor incidental to handling of the uterus.

Because of the frequency of such metastases, even when radium is given before the uterus is removed, many surgeons apply radium applicators to the apex of the vagina approximately two weeks after operation. The radium dosage approximates 3000 milligram-hours, which provides a dose of 4500 r at the tumor site at 0.5 cm. depth. Roentgen ray treatment following operation has been used instead of radium with good effect in the prevention of metastases at the vault. It is less effective in the obese patient.

Because the surgeon has little idea of the point of origin of the tumor, the nature of its spread and the degree of penetration of the wall, a cancerocidal dose of radiation must be delivered blindly to the entire cavity. This is not easy to accomplish because this cavity is frequently distorted in its shape by the presence of polyps, submucous fibroids or intramural leiomyomata. There may also be a small carcinoma in a large uterus.

The chief advantage of using preliminary external radiation lies in the fact that the uterus receives no manipulation other than that necessary to make a diagnosis. Thus, there is less danger of disseminating tumor cells. The main disadvantages are that many of the patients are obese, and nearly a month has to elapse before definitive removal of the uterus can take place, because it takes that long to give sufficient lethal radiation to the tumor site.

The reason for removal of the uterus is that there is no way of knowing how and where the disease has spread until the organ is removed. Except in the hands of a few who are thoroughly familiar with the application of the intercavitary radium capsule, there will be a high percentage of patients who show residual cancer when the uterus has been removed, despite the preliminary use of radium. Kottmeier, in a large series, reports only 4 per cent of residual tumor, but others suggest that the incidence ranges from 28 to 65 per cent.

The reason the ovaries and a large segment of the upper vagina are removed is because metastatic cancer is found in these areas in 6 to 12 per cent of patients. The time chosen for the removal of the uterus and adnexae following radiation is usually six weeks.

Cancer of the endometrium is a disease of the entire uterus, not the corpus alone. There is no place for supravaginal hysterectomy, except possibly in the obese patient who is a poor surgical risk. The abdominal approach permits greater freedom of action; it is simpler to remove the ovaries, and the surgeon has an opportunity to explore the rest of the abdomen.

It may be debated whether a pelvic lymphadenectomy should be performed as a routine procedure in patients with endometrial cancer. The incidence of external iliac and obturator nodal involvement has been reported as 10 to 25 per cent. When the tumor arises in the lower uterine segment and involves the endocervical canal, the chances of regional node metastases are approximately the same as cervical carcinoma. But, when the cancer grows as a superficial exfoliating tumor, the likelihood of node metastases is negligible.

If the disease is confined to the fundus alone, the five-year survival figure should approach 90 per cent. There are so many variables, however, that a five-year cure rate of 70 per cent following the use of radium and supplementary hysterectomy is generally accepted. When the endometrial cancer extends to the cervix, the figure drops to 40 per cent. The operability rate is approximately 70 per cent, and the mortality figure in the range of 4 per cent.

Ionizing radiation is used as the only form of treatment in cancer of the endometrium if the physician has the firm conviction that radium can cure as many patients, without the associated morbidity and mortality, as either operation alone or operation combined with radium; if the patient cannot be operated upon because of obesity or associated medical complications; or if the cancer is too widespread.

Some of the reports of the results obtained from intercavitary radiation as the sole form of therapy are comparable to the best obtained by operation. The advocates of radium therapy believe that operation should be reserved for patients with carcinoma of the corpus and cervix and those who have not responded to radiation.

For the patient who has a recurrence in the vaginal apex or in the lung following initial attempts to cure by operation, radiation or the combination of the two, hormone therapy offers palliation and in approximately one-third of the patients appreciable prolongation of life. The best results are recorded in the patient who has a well-differentiated tumor and has experienced a fairly long period without evidence of recurrence. The hormone used most effectively is intramuscular Delalutin in dosages ranging between 1000 and 2000 mg. per week.

When the recurrence is extensive, but still confined to the lower pelvis, the total exenteration of all pelvic viscera, with diversion of the urinary tract into an isolated segment of ilium or sigmoid, offers some hope for survival, but not in the 25 per cent one expects when the same operation is done for cervical cancer. The reason for the discrepancy lies in the slower, more local growth pattern of cervical carcinoma.

MIXED MESODERMAL TUMORS

The symptoms of these unusual tumors are essentially the same as those of endometrial cancer. The discharge is apt to be somewhat more watery and often has a foul odor, because these tumors frequently undergo necrosis. The diagnosis depends on histologic interpretation of the endometrial tissue removed on curettage. The prognosis is almost invariably bad. Little help can be gained from the physical examination, although the uterus of the patient with mixed mesodermal tumors is as a rule larger than the uterus containing adenocarcinoma.

These tumors exhibit a bizarre mixture of all manner of growth patterns. The simplest type is the carcinosarcoma, composed of epithelial elements as well as stromal and myometrial components. Many of the tumors are classified as rhabdomyosarcomas, chondrosarcomas, osteosarcomas, myosarcomas or fibrosarcomas.

The only form of treatment which provides any chance of success is a radical Wertheim hysterectomy with bilateral pelvic lymphadenectomy. The tumors are not radiosensitive.

LESIONS OF THE VULVA

In the older age group of patients, there are many entities which produce distressing symptoms referable to the vulva and perineal area. Pyogenic organisms are prone to infect hair follicles in the anogenital region because of the difficulty in keeping this area dry, particularly when the patient is obese. Vulvar folliculitis, furunculosis and carbuncles occasionally arise. Pruritus vulvae is an unpleasant symptom, which usually has a complicated etiology with a high psychosomatic component. Only rarely is operation indicated.

The two most common degenerative diseases of the vulva are *kraurosis* and *leukoplakia*. Both are associated with atrophy. In the beginning, leukoplakia actually represents hyperplasia rather than atrophy. The skin of the vulva hypertrophies and becomes dry, thick and swollen. The labial folds then flatten and assume an opaque white aspect. The introitus shrinks. In contrast, the skin layer in kraurosis is unusually thin and parchment-like. Shrinkage of the introitus is apparent, as the subcutaneous fat disappears and the labial folds fade away.

It is important to distinguish between the two because leukoplakia is a precancerous lesion, while kraurosis is not. This can only be done by a histologic interpretation of a biopsy specimen, since they often coexist. Many feel that they are actually the same condition in different stages.

With a diagnosis of leukoplakia established, a total vulvectomy is indicated because of the frequent association of leukoplakia with epidermoid carcinoma. The majority of surgeons believe that 50 per cent of all carcinoma develops on a background of leukoplakia. There is, therefore, no place for a prophylactic excision. If the biopsy fails to show evidence of leukoplakia, a variety of medications may be used to relieve the intolerable itching. The basic factor in therapy is keeping the area cool and dry. Cotton rather than rayon or nylon underwear should be worn because the latter tend to keep the area moist. Hydrocortisone lotion, 2.5 per cent, is often useful, together with a mild sedative at night.

CARCINOMA OF THE VULVA. Primary carcinoma of the vulva is relatively uncommon when compared with cancer of either the cervix or fundus. It usually makes its appearance in the postmenopausal age group. If for any reason ovarian function fails in the young woman, or she is rendered castrate, atrophy of the vulva tissues which follows creates the substrate on which cancer of the vulva develops.

Cancer of the vulva is almost invariably an epidermoid carcinoma. The customary site of origin is on the lateral margin on the lower half. Less often, the cancer arises in the midline in the region of the clitoris or fourchette. More often, they become involved by extension of the lateral growth. Rarely, except in the advanced stages, are the vaginal epithelium and urethra involved.

The earliest form of carcinoma in this area is called Bowen's disease, intraepithelial carcinoma or carcinoma in situ. The outward manifestations are red, raised plaques which have a granular surface. Less often, the lesions appear as shallow ulcerations. Although the lesions often arise on one side only, a biopsy of tissues on the contralateral side will show similar pathologic changes, but less far advanced.

The true invasive lesion in its earliest phase appears as a simple fissure or shallow ulceration which does not heal, or a small lump which does not go away. When fully developed, the carcinoma may grow either as a papillary fungoid growth with overlapping edges and a strawberry-like surface, or as an indurated ulcer which may be either superficial or deep. The area of ulceration spreads to involve all of one side of the labium. The opposite side is in-

Figure 14. The pattern of lymphatic drainage from the vulva is primarily to the superficial inguinal lymph nodes, from there secondarily to the deep femoral nodes and to the external iliac nodes. From the clitoral region, drainage is to the deep femoral lymph nodes.

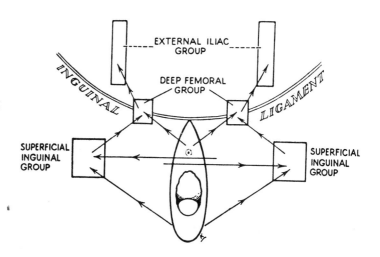

cluded as the disease crosses the midline, usually in the region of the clitoris.

Metastases occur by embolization to the regional nodes freely and early in the course of the disease, due to the free lymphatic anastomoses. This is true regardless of the degree of differentiation of the tumor or the size of the primary tumor. The nodes involved are found in the superficial inguinal and femoral regions, both above and below Poupart's ligament. The deep nodes above Poupart's ligament are usually involved by direct extension, although it is theoretically possible to have metastases from a primary lesion arising in the midline near the clitoris without passing through the superficial inguinal nodes.

Although metastases to the regional nodes occur early in the course of the disease, they may remain there for relatively long periods of time. They are apt to break down and ulcerate without further extension. The patient, untreated, may die a miserable death from invasion of local structures before metastases to distant areas occur. Extension to the lymph nodes along the aorta or vena cava occurs infrequently.

The predominant symptom is intense itching. If the malignant process has developed on a background of leukoplakia, this symptom has been present for some time. The patient has usually tried a variety of medications of her own choosing before she sees a physician. The next most common complaint is the discovery of a lump that fails to disappear. When this nodule ulcerates, or the process begins as an ulcerated fissure, the patient has severe burning after micturition. Following ulceration of the tumor, the local area becomes tender and the patient may have a foul discharge. Cancer of the vulva is one of the few malignant tumors which is tender and painful.

The diagnosis can be made only by biopsy and histologic examination of the tissue. There are few lesions that can be confused with carcinoma of the vulva, but even a trained dermatologist will not attempt to make a diagnosis without a biopsy, because the manifestations of infections in the vulva area are so bizarre.

The failure to biopsy is the chief reason for the marked delay in making the diagnosis. Oncologic teaching suggests that most malignant lesions are nontender. In general this is true, except for the lip and vulva. The fact that these lesions are tender should not deter the physician from injecting a drop of Novocaine into the suspected area and taking a biopsy. Any ulceration or tumor in this area should be biopsied, regardless of the age of the patient or size of the lesion.

The accepted form of therapy for cancer of the vulva is radical surgical removal of the local lesion by vulvectomy, with an en bloc dissection of the regional lymphatics. Since the substrate is basically defective, and there may be multicentric points of origin, there is no place for a hemivulvectomy or local excision of the primary lesion even though it be unilaterally located. Furthermore, radium therapy, whether applied locally, by infiltration of radium needles or by roentgen ray treatment, has no place in the treatment of cancer of the vulva except for the patient who is totally unsuited for operation.

Because of the age factor, the patient and her family are often reluctant to undergo a radical operation, despite its local nature, and try to influence the surgeon to delay adding the node dissection to the radical removal of the vulva. The surgeon may fall into this trap and delay the groin dissection until he can palpate nodes in these areas. This is wrong except for the extremely poor risk patient. There is a 30 per cent error in the clinical appraisal of inguinal nodes by palpation. Furthermore, little useful information is obtained by evaluating the size of the nodes. Approximately 20 per cent contain metastasis when the nodes are less than 1 cm. in size. Nearly 30 per cent are positive when no nodes are felt.

Little can be gained by biopsy of the suspicious nodes. Since the tumor may by-pass one or more nodes in a group, a negative biopsy means nothing. In doing the biopsy, there is an excellent chance of making the subsequent dissection more difficult, as well as a theoretical chance of disseminating tumor.

It is important that the groin dissection be done on both sides despite the apparent unilateral location of the tumor. Bilateral spread occurs in 20 per cent, when the tumor arises on one side only, and in twice this number when the cancer encroaches on or arises in the midline.

There is some reason for debate when the problem of dissection of the nodes above Poupart's ligament arises. Actually, the deep nodes along the side of the external iliac vein and in the obturator space are rarely involved unless the superficial chain is implicated.

This observation is frequently made when the superficial inguinal nodes have actually progressed to the point of ulceration. The survival statistics suggest that the deep nodes should be dissected. A recent report records an 83 per cent salvage when the nodes above Poupart's ligament were removed, compared with a 40 per cent figure when only the superficial inguinal and femoral nodes were removed.

MALIGNANT MELANOMA. There is a distinct tendency for malignant melanoma to occur in and around the vulva. Metastases may appear early, late, or not at all. Regardless of size, they should not be taken lightly, for the small ones may be as lethal as the large. Once metastases have taken place, the prognosis is not good. The best method of dealing with any pigmented lesion of the vulva is to excise it with wide margins, regardless of its size. In this instance, excision is far better than biopsy.

Pathologic interpretation of the specimen is extremely important. If the nevus is not malignant, and the margins given the growth are adequate, nothing further need be done except to observe the patient at periodic intervals. If it is malignant, then the decision must be made about removing the regional nodes.

With the diagnosis of malignant disease established, melanoma of the vulva should be treated by vulvectomy and superficial inguinal node dissection without delay. It is true the melanoma may spread by blood vessels as well as lymphatics, but statistics indicate a difference in survival of 17 to 39 per cent when the lymph nodes are dissected.

CARCINOMA OF THE VAGINA AND URETHRA

Cancer appears in the vaginal canal in the form of primary growth arising in the vaginal epithelium itself, or in the urethra. It is also a favorite place for metastases to appear from a primary tumor in the uterus, ovary, kidney or gastrointestinal tract.

PRIMARY CANCER OF VAGINA. Cancer of the vagina may arise anywhere in the vaginal canal, but it is commonly seen in the postmenopausal patient on the posterior lateral wall near the cervix. It is generally a papillary growth, although indurated tumors may be found. Why the tumor appears in this location is not known but it may have something to do with the prolonged use of a pessary and the irritation produced by it.

Symptoms are identical with those produced by cervical cancer. A thin, bloody vaginal discharge is a common complaint. On physical examination, the examiner may encounter a tender, ulcerating tumor or an exfoliating type of lesion. In general, a superficial widespread ulceration is noted.

Because the results of radiation, whether given in the form of a local applicator, interstitial needles or roentgen rays, have been discouraging, there has been some support for radical surgical removal of the vagina combined with pelvic lymphadenectomy. When the bladder or rectum has been involved, a posterior exenteration may be done. The radical surgical procedures should be performed only on selected patients, because it is a formidable procedure in an older patient.

CARCINOMA OF URETHRA. Carcinoma of the urethra is a relatively rare type of tumor. If the tumor arises in the paraurethral glands, it is an adenocarcinoma which extends down alongside the urethra as a subepithelial growth which may ulcerate in spots. Epidermoid cancers are more common and appear at the urethral meatus as a friable papillary tumor resembling a caruncle or prolapse of the urethral epithelium, an ulcerating lesion with undermined edges or an indurated subepithelial tumor.

Symptoms appear when the cancer ulcerates and produces bleeding and discharge. Only then does the patient have bloody and painful micturition. If the primary site is at the bladder neck, the first indication of its presence may be obstruction to the outflow of urine from the bladder due to encroachment of the tumor on the urethra.

The diagnosis must be confirmed by biopsy of the local tumor. Cystoscopy and direct vision of the urethra gives useful information in planning a course of therapy.

It is customary to treat the ulcerating lesion at the meatus with interstitial platinum needles containing radium. A total dosage of 2500 milligram-hours frequently controls the growth without producing irreparable damage to the urethra and loss of urinary control. The regional lymph nodes should be dissected, because 20 per cent of these tumors metastasize to the superficial inguinal and femoral region.

When the tumor arises at the neck of the bladder, the only treatment which can be expected to give a reasonable chance of cure is radical surgical removal of the bladder and vagina together with a pelvic lymphadenectomy and urinary tract diversion.

CARCINOMA OF THE FALLOPIAN TUBES

Carcinoma of the fallopian tubes is rare. The diagnosis is often missed because the gross appearance is similar to a unilateral hydrosalpinx. Since the latter is a rare finding, the surgeon should be alert to the fact he may be dealing with one of the most lethal of pelvic neoplasms. The five-year survival rate, despite improvements in surgical and roentgen therapy, is somewhere in the range of 5 per cent.

Because these patients are often obese, the tumor cannot be palpated with any accuracy. Primarily, it is a tumor which appears in postmenopausal women, although it has been reported throughout the reproductive age group.

Although the majority of patients who have this form of cancer complain only of vague lower abdominal pain and soreness, a careful history may bring out a few symptoms which are almost pathognomonic. All patients who have carcinoma of the tube in the postmenopausal age group give a history of a sudden onset of vaginal bleeding which thereafter is continuous. Pain and vaginal discharge are common symptoms. One of the interesting observations obtained from the history is the association of an intermittent colicky pain with a sudden gush of a watery discharge which is apt to be serosanguineous. Following this episode, the pain and the one-sided adnexal mass, which is usually present, disappears. This has been called hydrops tubae profluens. It occurs because the tube periodically tries to empty itself.

Cancer of the tube should be considered when no adequate cause can be found for the bleeding on curettage, particularly when there is a palpable adnexal mass and the endometrium is atrophic or absent. Cancer of the ovary rarely produces uterine bleeding unless the tumor is of the functional type, in which case the endometrium would be hyperplastic.

In treatment, the mistake commonly made is to assume that the gross findings are those of benign disease. The minimum treatment is total hysterectomy and removal of the adnexae with supplementary roentgen ray therapy. If the growth is extensive but still local, total exenteration of the pelvic viscera may be offered as a method of therapy. Chlorambucil given orally has proved to be effective in a few instances in the treatment of a recurrence.

READING REFERENCES

Allen, E. D.: Examination of the genital organs in the prepubescent and in the adolescent girl. Pediat. Clin. North America 5:19, 1958.

Ariel, I. M., and Pack, G. T.: Malignant melanoma of the vagina. *In*, Pack, G. T., and Ariel, I. M. (eds.): Treatment of Cancer and Allied Diseases. Volume VI. Tumors of the Female Genitalia. New York, Hoeber-Harper, 1961, p. 119.

Arneson, A. N.: Symposium: Continuing evaluation of endometrial carcinoma. Am. J. Obst. & Gyn. 81:1006, 1961.

Barnes, A. B., and Ulfelder, H.: Septic abortion. J.A.M.A. 189:919, 1964.

Brunschwig, A., and Barker, H. R. K.: Treatment of carcinoma of the cervix. Obst. & Gyn. 27:21, 1966.

Brunschwig, A., and Murphy, A. I.: The rationale for radical panhysterectomy and pelvic node excision in carcinoma of the corpus uteri; clinical and pathological data on the mode of spread of endometrial carcinoma. Am. J. Obst. & Gyn. 68:1482, 1954.

DeAlvarez, R. R.: Adolescent gynecology. Clin. Obst. & Gyn. Vol. 9, No. 3, 1966.

Durfee, R. B.: Management of genital prolapse. Clin. Obst. & Gyn. Vol. 9, No. 4, 1966.

Fricke, R. E.: Treatment of carcinoma of the female urethra. *In*, Pack, G. T., and Ariel, I. M. (eds): Treatment of Cancer and Allied Diseases. Volume VI. Tumors of the Female Genitalia. New York, Hoeber-Harper, 1962, p. 315.

Gardner, H. L., and Kaufman, R. H.: Tumors of the vulva and vagina. Clin. Obst. & Gyn. 8:938, 1965.

Goldstein, D. P., and Gore, H.: Gestational trophoblastic tumors. Clin. Obst. & Gyn. Vol. 10, No. 3, 1967.

Green, T. H., Jr.: Symposium on endometriosis. Clin. Obst. & Gyn. 9:271, 1966.

Green, T. H., Jr.: Development of a plan for the diagnosis and treatment of urinary stress incontinence. Am. J. Obst. & Gyn. 83:632, 1962.

Hertig, A. T., and Sheldon, W. H.: Hydatidiform mole: a pathologic clinical correlation of 200 cases. Am. J. Obst. & Gyn. 53:1, 1947.

Hodgkinson, C. P., and Wong, S. T.: Voiding time pressure event phenomenon in voluntary voiding in females. Am. J. Obst. & Gyn. 94:791, 1966.

Ingersoll, F. M.: Symposium on the fallopian tube. Clin. Obst. & Gyn. 5:853, 1966.

Ingersoll, F. M., and Ulfelder, H.: Pelvic exenteration. New England J. Med. 274:618, 1966.

Jeffcoate, J. N.: Principles governing the treatment of stress incontinence in the female. Brit. J. Urol. 37:633, 1965.

Kimbrough, R. A. T., and Israel, S. L.: Treatment of neoplasms of the genital organs complicated by pregnancy. *In*, Pack, G. T., and Ariel, I. M. (eds.): Treatment of Cancer and Allied Diseases. Volume VI. Tumors of the Female Genitalia. New York, Hoeber-Harper, 1962, p. 330.

Kistner, R. W., Griffith, C. T., and Craig, J. M.: Use of progestational agents in the management of endometrial cancer. Cancer 8:1563, 1965.

Kottmeier, H. L. (ed.): Annual Report on Results of Treatment in Carcinoma of the Uterus 1945–1954. Volume XII. International Federation of Gynecology and Obstetrics.

Krieger, J. S., and McCormack, L. T.: The individualization

of therapy for cervical carcinoma in situ. Surg. Gyn. & Obst. *109*:328, 1959.

Lund, C. J.: Symposium on urinary incontinence. Clin. Obst. & Gyn. *6*:123, 1963.

Masterson, J. G., and Nelson, J. H., Jr.: The role of chemotherapy in the treatment of gynecologic malignancy. Am. J. Obst. & Gyn. *93*:1102, 1965.

Mattingly, R. F.: Symposium: radical pelvic surgery. Clin. Obst. & Gyn. *8*:705, 1965.

McArthur, J. W., and Ulfelder, H.: The effect of pregnancy upon endometriosis. New England J. Med. *274*:648, 1966.

McCall, M. L.: Malignancy associated with pregnancy. Clin. Obst. & Gyn. Vol. 6, No. 4, 1963.

McLane, C., Miller, N. F., and Aldridge, A. H.: Indication for hysterectomy. Am. J. Obst. & Gyn. *72*:534, 1956.

Meigs, J. V.: Surgical treatment of cancer of the cervix. *In*, Pack, G. T., and Ariel, I. M. (eds.): Treatment of Cancer and Allied Diseases. Volume V. Tumors of the Female Genitalia. New York, Hoeber-Harper, 1962, p. 159.

Meigs, J. V.: Fibroma of the ovary with ascites and hydrothorax (Meigs syndrome). Am. J. Obst. & Gyn. *67*:962, 1954.

Nash, A.: Lesions of the vulva in the elderly. Am. J. Obst. & Gyn. *95*:356, 1966.

Novak, E. R.: Postmenopausal bleeding. *In*, Plotz, E. J. (ed.): Symposium: The climacteric and the postmenopause. Clin. Obst. & Gyn. *7*:464, 1964.

Parsons, L.: Endometriosis. *In*, Conn, H. F., Clohecy, R. J., and Conn, R. B., Jr. (eds.): Current Diagnosis. Philadelphia, W. B. Saunders Company, 1966, p. 656.

Parsons, L.: Symposium on ovarian tumors. Clin. Obst. & Gyn. *4*:769, 1961.

Parsons, L., and Friedell, G. H.: Radical Surgical Treatment of Cancer of the Cervix. Fifth National Cancer Conference Proceedings, 1964, pp. 241–246, 1965.

Radman, H. M., and Karmen, W.: Mixed mesodermal tumors of the uterus. Am. J. Obst. & Gyn. *80*:1115, 1960.

Riley, G. M.: Endocrine patterns in polycystic ovarian disease. Int. J. Fertil. *10*:349, 1965.

Rosenblum, J. M., Dowling, R. W., and Barnes, A. C.: Treatment of tubal pregnancy. Am. J. Obst. & Gyn. *80*:274, 1960.

Rutledge, F. N.: Cancer of the vulva and vagina. Clin. Obst. & Gyn. *8*:1051, 1965.

Sampson, J. A.: Perforating hemorrhagic (chocolate) cysts of the ovary, their importance and especially their relation to the pelvic adenomas of endometrial type (adenomyoma of the uterus, rectovaginal septum, sigmoid, etc.). Arch. Surg. *3*:245, 1921.

Smallbrask, J.: Trophoblastic Growths; A Clinical, Hormonal and Histopathologic Study of Hydatidiform Mole and Chorioepithelioma. Amsterdam, Elsevier Publishing Company, 1967.

Southam, A. L., and Richart, R. M.: The prognosis for adolescents with menstrual irregularities. Am. J. Obst. & Gyn. *94*:637, 1966.

Stein, I. F.: The Stein-Leventhal syndrome. New England J. Med. *259*:420, 1958.

Way, S.: Carcinoma of the vulva. Am. J. Obst. & Gyn. *79*: 692, 1960.

Whitelaw, M. J., and Nola, V. F.: Accuracy of immunologic pregnancy test in early pregnancy and abortion. Obst. & Gyn. *27*:69, 1966.

Chapter 31

THE MUSCULOSKELETAL SYSTEM

by
WILLIAM A. LARMON, M.D.

WILLIAM ALEXANDER LARMON was born in the Santa Clara Valley of California, the son of a father engaged in the fruit-canning industry. He attended San Jose College and Stanford University, but it became necessary for him to go to work upon the death of his father and mother. Accepting the advice of a Northwestern University alumnus, a friend of his father, he enrolled in and was graduated in medicine from Northwestern. Because he is modest and quiet-spoken, the great force of his teaching talents is not always apparent at first sight. His presentations are simple, logical and basic. He has written and produced a series of color motion pictures for the Veterans Administration for teaching the principles of the treatment of fractures, and these are classic examples of the goal to be sought in instructional visual methods. He has followed the same method of exposition in this contribution, emphasizing principles and leaving the details for more comprehensive books upon the bones and joints. Dr. Larmon is an Associate Professor of Orthopedic Surgery at Northwestern University, and has devoted a great deal of his time and energy to the affairs of the Board of Certification in that surgical specialty.

Injuries to Bones and Joints

The complex of bones, joints, muscles, tendons, ligaments, bursae, nerves, blood vessels, subcutaneous tissue and skin make up the musculoskeletal system. The composition of this system determines an individual's form and figure. The development, growth and function of these parts determine posture, locomotion and purposeful movements necessary to the daily tasks of living.

The surgeon must understand the normal anatomy and physiology of the musculoskeletal system if he is to restore maximum function when the system is affected by disease or injury. The pathology of fractures, dislocations, sprains, tissue injuries and disease must be recognized in order to plan a logical course of treatment. The surgeon must realize that injury to the spine or extremities affects the entire body, not just the part, and his efforts to restore function should be based upon this broad concept of trauma.

A fracture, dislocation or sprain is a painful, frightening experience. The distraught patient needs assurance and gentle, thought-ful care. Many injuries demand prolonged treatment, and the worry of permanent disability, the loss of earning power and the inconvenience of immobilization all play a role in the emotional reaction of the patient to injury. The doctor must realize this and treat the person as well as the injured part.

PATHOLOGY OF FRACTURE

When a bone breaks, a chain of reactions follows, which must be understood by the surgeon to treat the injury intelligently. First, bleeding occurs at the fracture site, from the bone as well as from the associated soft tissue injury. The amount of hemorrhage varies; it may be severe and life-endangering, or moderate. Shock may develop rapidly from loss of blood.

Bleeding may be internal, into the soft tissues about the fracture, or may be external, from associated wounds. In fractures of the femur, two pints of blood may be lost into the thigh muscles without local external signs of hemorrhage. This hidden bleeding must be recognized and blood volume restored before definitve treatment of the fracture is undertaken. When the bleeding stops, a hematoma is formed about the fracture. This hematoma later becomes an important part of the healing process (Fig. 1).

The second event in a fracture is loss of skeletal stability, often followed by obvious deformity. The lack of stability of the skeleton and the degree of deformity may be marked in long-bone fractures, but very little with the small bones. The type and location of the fracture determines the degree of deformity and loss of stability of the part.

The third reaction is temporary loss of nerve function at the fracture site. Following the initial sharp pain of the break, the part may become numb and the surrounding muscles flaccid. This condition has been termed local shock. During this period, which may last for a few minutes to half an hour, fractured bones may be reduced easily and with little pain. In a short time, however, pain sensation returns, and with it spasms and contractions of the surrounding muscles. Any movement of the part then becames painful.

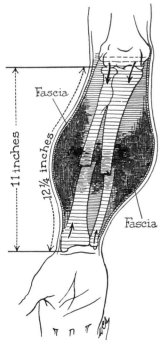

Figure 1. Typical condition following a fracture. A hematoma has formed. There is deformity and loss of skeletal stability, and the fascial compartment of the extremity is distended.

THE HEALING PROCESS OF FRACTURE

When a fracture is reduced and immobilized, the repair process begins immediately. An aseptic inflammatory reaction occurs at the fracture site, often accompanied by a fever and local increase in temperature. The white blood cells increase in number in the blood stream. The blood vessels near the fracture dilate and produce an active hyperemia. Permeability of the vascular bed increases, allowing edema fluid to accumulate in the soft tissues. This edema and the hematoma produce varying degrees of swelling and ecchymosis. Within 48 hours, the products of the inflammatory exudate begin to organize. The adjacent muscles and ligaments lose elasticity and become indurated and firm. If reduction of the fracture has not been accomplished before this period, the resulting inelasticity of the soft tissues may make reduction extremely difficult or impossible.

Local chemical changes take place rapidly. The pH of the fluids about the bone ends becomes slightly acid for the first ten days to two weeks. This acid environment forces calcium salts into solution about the bone fragments, so that some absorption of bone takes place. Fibrin strands form in the hematoma; invasion of the blood clot and damaged tissue by white blood cells begins; and the debris of injury is absorbed. New capillaries grow into the hematoma from the surrounding soft tissues and bone ends. Fibrous tissue is laid down, as in all wound healing.

After ten to 14 days, the local pH becomes alkaline, and the concentration of alkaline phosphatase increases at the fracture site. Bone-forming cells become active. Calcium salts form in the remains of the hematoma, and osteoid tissue is elaborated by bone-forming cells from the periosteum and endosteum, or possibly by metaplasia of other soft tissue cells. In some instances, the fibrous tissue cells which unite the bone fragments may undergo changes resembling cartilage. These cells may calcify, be invaded by new blood vessels, absorbed and new bone laid down by the bone-forming cells. All of these processes of new bone formation may take place in the same fracture area. This process is called callus formation and is the method by which bone heals (Fig. 2).

After the fracture has been bridged by

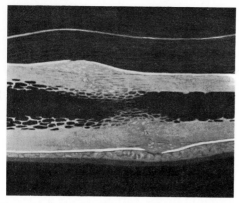

Figure 2. Callus has formed, healing the fracture. Remodeling of the trabecular pattern of the bone will follow.

callus, remodeling of the bone begins. The architecture of the trabecular pattern of the particular bone is re-established by the process. Excess callus is absorbed and new bone is laid down in the predetermined trabecular pattern. This internal structure of bone is determined by Wolff's law, which states that all changes in the function of a bone are reflected in its internal structure.

REHABILITATION OF SOFT PARTS

When the fracture has healed, the soft tissues must be rehabilitated. Inevitably, some scar tissue remains in damaged muscles, ligaments and associated structures. Scar tissue is inelastic, binding muscle to bone and ligaments to joints; since scar tissue contracts in any wound-healing process, deformities may occur. The more scar tissue that is formed, the greater the impairment of function. Muscles long immobilized atrophy and, in some instances, shorten, losing power and tensile strength.

Muscles not only act to move the levers of the skeleton, but also by contraction aid in the dynamics of blood circulation. The careful restoration of muscle, ligament and joint function is essential for movement of the body parts, but is also necessary for proper circulation in the extremities.

Broken bones, torn ligaments, muscles and disrupted joints heal with the maturation of granulation tissue, as do all wounds. The property of bone to re-form to heal a fracture is a specialized variation of this process. Muscles and ligaments do not regenerate, but heal by scar formation.

PRINCIPLES OF FRACTURE TREATMENT

Treatment of musculoskeletal injuries follows logically once the underlying pathology of injury and repair is understood. When a bone breaks, sharp fragments are produced. Movement of these fragments lacerates periosteum, muscle and ligaments, and may damage blood vessels and nerves. Since more damage means greater blood loss, greater shock and eventually more scar tissue, damage must be minimized by proper immobilization of the fragments as soon as possible.

"Splint 'em where they lie" has become a cliché in writings about fractures. However, the principle is as good today as when it was first stated. Picture the damage that is done if a person with a fracture of the tibia is picked up without support for the leg, and placed in an automobile for a wild ride to the nearest hospital. The leg angulates at the fracture. The tibial fragments slice into the muscles, nerves and blood vessels. Additional bleeding occurs. The sharp pieces of bone may lacerate the skin, producing an open wound. Contamination of this wound may lead to infection and osteomyelitis, with further destruction of tissues. The major blood vessels and nerves may be severed, placing the survival of the extremity in jeopardy. What might have been a simple fracture thus becomes a catastrophic injury to the extremity.

In contrast, if a patient has an adequate splint applied before movement, minimal damage is done. Simple reduction and immobilization procedures then suffice, and the healing time of the fracture and residual disability are kept to a minimum. Fractures should be immobilized immediately to avoid additional trauma.

IMMOBILIZATION. Adequate immobilization of a fracture varies with the type and location of the break. Some fractures are stable and require little additional support; others are unstable, tending to shorten, angulate and rotate with any motion of the part. When capillary buds are attempting to grow into the fracture, and collagen strands are organizing to unite the wound, any movement tears these delicate structures. Bleeding takes place and the new, minute hematomas must repeat the entire process. The result of this added trauma is increased scar formation. Complete immobilization of the fracture area promotes the repair process and minimizes damage and scar formation.

REDUCTION OF FRACTURE. Adequate reduction varies with the type and location of the fracture and the age of the patient. The closer the bone ends are approximated, the less will be the gap for repair. Bone ends may be placed side-to-side or end-to-end, as long as good contact is made between the fragments. Several factors may prevent direct bone contact, such as marked angulation or distraction, or interposition of muscle, fascia and other soft-tissue parts. All of these factors widen the gap between the bones and slow or prevent bone healing.

When reduction of a fracture is delayed, organization of the inflammatory exudate reduces the elasticity of the soft tissues. Distention of the fascial envelope shortens the length of the extremity, and this, along with the spasmic pull of the muscles, produces shortening by overriding of the fragments. When the tissues are inelastic and reduction of the fracture is accomplished, soft tissues must tear. This adds to the injury. Muscle fibers are further damaged or ligaments are torn, and new bleeding takes place. The organizing hematoma is disrupted, and the entire process of repair is disturbed; damage to all parts is increased. Early reduction of a fracture, while structures are still pliable and muscles are not in spasm, lessens the trauma of reduction. The development of scar tissue will be minimal and better function will be ultimately restored.

BLOOD SUPPLY. Adequate blood supply to the fractured part is essential, as in all wound healing. Without proper circulation, the destroyed tissue cannot be removed and the building blocks for reconstruction of damage cannot be brought to the site of injury. Because of the limited blood supply to some bones, the fragments may not receive adequate nourishment for quick repair after injury. Knowledge of the limitations of the blood supply to certain areas of the skeleton allows the surgeon to anticipate delayed healing in some fractures without worry: for example, the lower third of the tibia.

Swelling about a fracture is often accepted as part of the normal pathologic process. However, uncontrolled swelling of an injured extremity creates many unnecessary problems. Hematoma and edema fluid make up this swelling for the most part, although deformity of the bones or joints may add to

it. Inflammatory exudate confined by fascial compartments compresses blood vessels. This always occurs to some degree; however, if an unsupported, dilated vascular bed is allowed to pour out edema fluid without control, the fascial compartments and subcutaneous tissues confined by the envelope of the skin may become overdistended. Blood vessels are compressed and circulation to the part may become dangerously impaired. Control of edema is imperative. Elastic compression supports the vascular bed, and minimizes edema fluid and hemorrhage; it should be applied as soon as possible after injury. Elevation of the part increases return circulation by the aid of gravity, thus lessening dilation of the vascular bed.

Although immobilization of the fracture and the damaged soft parts is essential, all uninvolved structures should be allowed to function as normally as possible. Use of undamaged muscles and ligaments prevents atrophy of these structures, maintains strength and tone, and aids circulation. Only those parts necessary to maintain reduction and stability should be immobilized.

Exercise of uninvolved parts should be begun early in the course of treatment. Rehabilitation of the injured extremity or part should be started as soon as it is consistent with the maintenance of reduction of the fracture or dislocation.

Fractures and joint injuries do not heal ideally in a debilitated patient. Fever, weight loss, a negative nitrogen balance and other systemic reactions point to the general body response to trauma. Support to this systemic reaction is needed. Adequate fluid and food intake must be maintained. Abnormalities of metabolism, deficiencies of the general circulation and any existing unrelated disease must be corrected whenever possible.

THE MECHANISM OF FRACTURE

Fracture may be produced by direct or indirect violence. Fractures produced by direct violence result from a direct blow or crushing force. Often, there is considerable soft tissue damage over the fracture site and the bone has a tendency to shatter or crush. Indirect violence fractures are the result of forces transmitted through the bone to an area of weakness where fracture typically takes place. Thus, a fall on the outstretched hand

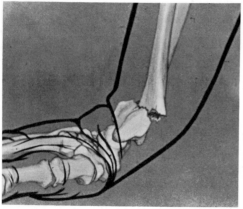

Figure 3. Indirect violence fractures are produced by force transmitted through the bone to an area of weakness, in this instance the distal radius.

transmits compression force through the bones of the extremity from hand to shoulder. The radius may break at the distal metaphysis, along the shaft or at the neck of the bone. If the force is continued, the ulna may break (Fig. 3).

Fractures may also be produced by violent contractions of muscle. An example of this is the fracture of the patella produced by the sudden contraction of the quadriceps muscle.

The position of the part at the time force is applied determines, to a degree, the area which may fracture or dislocate. The force is often complicated. For instance, there may be the element of shearing or rotatory stress, which adds to the complexity of the fractures.

TYPES OF FRACTURE

Fractures may be open or closed. A closed fracture does not communicate with the outside air, although adjacent wounds of the skin may be present. An open fracture is accompanied by a wound which communicates through the skin or mucous membrane to the air. The latter is usually a much more serious problem, because the danger of infection of the wound and bone is present. The wound may be produced by the direct force which produces the fracture, or the bone ends may create the wound by lacerating the skin. When closed fractures are operated upon, they become open fractures.

Simple fractures have only one fracture line and produce two fragments, while comminuted fractures have more than one break and produce more than two distinct fragments. Different types of bone break in char-

acteristic ways, and the fractures of childhood differ in some ways from those in the adult.

Cancellous bone may crush, producing a compression or impacted fracture, usually with comminution. In the vertebral bodies, for example, the two opposing surfaces or cartilaginous plates may be driven toward each other, compressing the trabeculae of bone between them.

An impacted fracture is one in which the bone ends are driven together by the force producing the fracture, so that they are firmly united. This happens most often at the areas where cancellous bone and cortical bone come together near the metaphysis or epiphysis. A typical fracture of this type occurs in adults at the surgical neck of the humerus (Fig. 4). Here the cortical bone of the shaft is driven into the softer cancellous bone of the head. The union of the two major fragments—the shaft and the head—may be quite firm, requiring little, if any, immobilization. A variation of this fracture occurs when compression force buckles the thin cortex of bone near the metaphysis. This buckling of the cortex occurs outwardly, producing a bump on the surface of the bone without displacement of the fracture fragments. This type fracture is called a torus fracture, from the Greek word meaning "to buckle."

Cortical bone of the diaphysis may break transversely, or may be oblique or spiral when rotatory or shearing force plays a role in the mechanism of fracture (Fig. 5).

Fractures of the shaft or diaphysis of the bone in children may be produced by bend-

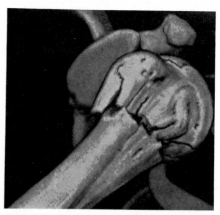

Figure 4. A typical impacted fracture occurs at the surgical neck of the humerus, where the hard cortical bone of the shaft drives into the soft cancellous bone of the head. The impaction is usually quite firm.

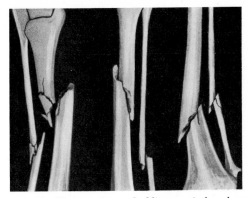

Figure 5. Various types of oblique, spiral and comminuted fractures occur in the tibia when the forces applied to it are complicated. Shearing, rotary forces combined with direct and indirect violence produce the many different varieties of fracture.

ing force. The bone of a child before puberty is more pliable and is surrounded by a tougher, heavier periosteum than that in the adult. Bending or compression force applied to this type bone may produce a greenstick fracture. In this fracture, the convex side of the bone pulls apart while the concave side compresses, but does not break completely. The descriptive term "greenstick" likens this fracture to the break occurring in the limb of a growing tree.

Spontaneous fatigue, or march, fractures occur from repeated trauma of a force which is insufficient to cause fracture as an isolated injury, but which can break a bone when repeated often enough. It is thought that when bone is "overloaded" for a sufficient period, the crystalline structure alters and produces a weak spot in the bone. These fractures can occur in any bone, but most commonly happen in the metatarsal bones of the foot after walking long distances, carrying a heavy load: thus, the term "march fracture."

Pathologic fractures are those which occur in a diseased part of the bone. Most frequently, this happens in areas of cancer metastasis, but can take place in Paget's disease, fragilitas ossium, osteoporosis or osteomalacia.

Epiphysial fractures or separations take place through the epiphysial plate of the growing bone. These injuries are usually caused by shearing force. The epiphysis is displaced from the metaphysis by disruption of the cartilage of the epiphysial plate. The damage produced to this structure may arrest or alter the growth of the bone. The prognosis is uncertain, and the parents of the injured child should always be warned that growth disturbances may occur.

For more precise definition, fractures are described by their anatomic location. Fractures within joints are called intracapsular fractures. Fractures of the metaphysis of the bone adjacent to the joint, but not entering it, are termed extra-articular fractures.

The anatomic area of the bone involved is also designated. For example, fractures of the femur may occur in the neck, intertrochanteric region, shaft and supracondylar area.

FRACTURE DEFORMITY

Displacement and deformity of fracture fragments occur from the force producing the fracture and the pull of muscles after the fracture. The amount of deformity varies, depending upon the force applied, the region of the bone involved, the type of fracture produced, the age of the bone, and the strength and balance of surrounding muscles. The bone may shorten when fracture fragments slide past each other. This deformity is usually increased by pull of muscles in the long axis of the extremity. The deformity is called shortening or overriding.

Angulation of the fragments may occur due to bending force or unequal muscle pulls. Fractures of the midshaft of the tibia characteristically angulate forward due to the bowstring pull of the triceps surae group of muscles along the posterior aspect of the bone. The angulation is termed anterior,

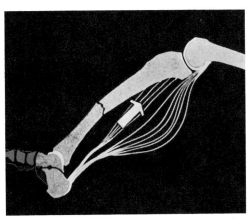

Figure 6. Anterior angulation of the tibia is produced by the bowstring-like pull of the triceps surae muscles. The apex of angulation is anterior.

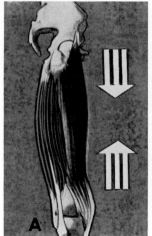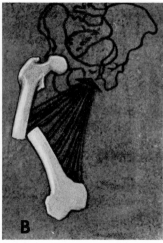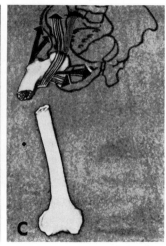

Figure 7. *A*, Shortening of the shaft in fracture of the femur is produced by the hamstring and quadriceps muscles. *B* and *C*, Angulation and rotation are produced by the adductor, abductor and external hip rotator muscles. The proximal fragment cannot be controlled by the surgeon.

posterior, medial or lateral, depending upon the position of the apex of the triangle produced by the deformity. Thus, in anterior angulation of the tibia, the apex of the triangle formed by the two fracture fragments is forward or anterior (Fig. 6).

Rotational deformity occurs when the fracture fragments rotate out of their normal longitudinal axis. This may happen with rotational strain producing the fracture, by gravity, or by the unequal pull of muscles attached to the fragments of the fracture.

Fractures of the middle one-third of the femur characteristically combine the three elements of displacement. Shortening takes place from the pull of the hamstring and quadriceps muscle groups. Lateral angulation takes place because the adductor magnus pulls the distal end of the distal fragment medially, while the abductor muscles attaching to the greater trochanter abduct the proximal fragment. The external rotator muscles are stronger than the internal rotators of the hip, and all are attached to the proximal fragment; thus, the proximal fragment assumes a position of external rotation (Fig. 7).

CORRECTION OF FRACTURE DEFORMITY

To obtain maximum functional restoration of a bone or joint, these deformities must be corrected. The degree of correction necessary for proper function varies with location of the fracture and the age of the patient. Moderate degrees of angulation and shorten-ing may be acceptable, but rotational malalignment must be corrected as fully as possible.

The growing bones of the child will, in many instances, correct angular deformity by the normal remodeling process of growing bone. In the adult, this does not take place, so that the degree of angulation acceptable after reduction of the fracture varies with age. An infant suffering a 45-degree angular deformity of the humerus may remodel this bone in the course of growth in a few years to a normal-appearing bone. The same deformity in an adult would produce extreme disability.

Shortening of a bone of minor degree may be acceptable and, in many instances, is even desirable in both the adult and child. In some fractures, good bone contact cannot be maintained without slight shortening. It may be necessary to accept this deformity if union of the bone is to be obtained.

When fractures occur in children, the hyperemia of healing usually causes stimulation of longitudinal growth. If the fracture is reduced with the fragments in end-to-end apposition, this stimulation of growth may produce a bone longer than normal after healing. This epiphysial stimulation stops after the fracture is healed, and varies with the bone involved and the location of the fracture. Fractures of the midshaft of the femur in children under five years of age may result in overgrowth of the femur by 1 inch. It is acceptable and desirable to reduce these fractures with some overriding, or side-to-side apposition, so that the overgrowth of bone will eventually produce legs of equal length. Rotational deformity is never corrected by growth and is unacceptable in either the child or the adult.

Fractures of joint surfaces are always serious injuries. Malaligned joint surfaces block motion and produce excessive wear of the articular cartilage. Inevitably, some damage is done to the cartilage cells. This eventually leads to traumatic arthritis. Every effort must be made to restore joint surfaces by perfect reduction.

Often associated ligament injuries are not recognized. Failure to restore damaged ligaments may produce an unstable joint. Although the fracture heals, the instability of the joint may be quite as disabling as a poorly aligned joint.

MALUNION

When a fracture unites in poor position, it is termed a malunion. Depending upon the degree of residual deformity, function of the part is altered. This may be severe and disabling, or slight and only of cosmetic significance.

The disability may be apparent immediately following healing of the fracture, or may be slowly progressive over the span of several years. Rotatory malunion of the forearm bones immediately limits pronation or supination, but may not affect wrist or elbow motion, and there may be no increase in the trouble over the years. Moderate angulation of a healed fracture of the shaft of the femur may produce no immediate disability; however, the alteration of the weight-bearing line through the knee joint may cause stress and strain, which eventually leads to traumatic arthritis in the knee and destroys the joint. The surgeon must be mindful of these factors which influence the short and long-term functional results of fractures.

METHODS OF REDUCTION

Reduction of fractures is accomplished by closed or open methods, and fractures are held in reduction by external or internal fixation devices.

Reduction is accomplished by manipulation or traction, or both. When a bone is angulated, but the fragments remain in end-to-end contact, the simple manipulation of straightening the bone may be all that is necessary. However, if the bone ends are displaced and overriding, traction is necessary to restore length and possibly overcome angulation. In addition, manipulation may be necessary to approximate the fragments as closely as possible.

A fundamental principle of reduction is to align the fragment which can be controlled with the fragment which cannot be controlled. A fracture of the femur in the upper one-third produces a characteristic deformity from muscle action. The proximal fragment cannot be controlled and assumes a position of flexion abduction and external rotation. The distal fragment, however, can be controlled by the surgeon by grasping the leg and foot. He aligns this fragment with the proximal one by placing it in flexion abduction and external rotation.

When satisfactory reduction cannot be accomplished by closed manipulation and traction, an open surgical procedure may be necessary. In this instance, the fracture is exposed through an appropriate incision and the bone fragments are approximated under direct vision by traction and manipulation with instruments applied directly to the bone.

CAST FIXATION. Reduction of the fragments is maintained by some type of fixation device. This may be a simple splint or plaster cast, suspension traction or screws, plates and rods applied directly to the bone. As a general principle, a joint proximal and distal to the fracture must be immobilized in order to maintain reduction by the cast method. With cast fixation of the fracture, it may be necessary to immobilize a joint in partial flexion to prevent rotation. If a cast is applied to a fracture of the shaft of the tibia with the knee fully extended, rotary displacement of the fragments may take place. This occurs because the cast is a cylinder surrounding in effect another cylinder made up of the soft tissues about the bone. One cylinder then may rotate within the other. If the knee is bent moderately and the cast is applied from the toe to above the knee, the lower tibial fragment can no longer rotate upon the upper.

A cast not only helps to hold the fragments in reduction, but applies uniform compression of the soft tissues. Elasticity of this compression dressing is supplied by padding placed between the cast and the part. The compression must be uniform and not constricting. Points of undue pressure embarrass circulation, and pressure necrosis of the soft tissue may occur. This is most likely to occur over bony prominences where there is scant subcutaneous fat, such as the posterior aspect of the heel, the malleoli and head of the fibula in the lower extremity. Adequate padding between the cast and the bony prominence usually prevents this complication. If a fracture angulates inside of a cast, a bony prominence may be created at the fracture site. This area is susceptible to similar point pressure which may be excessive. If soft tissue necrosis occurs, the fracture becomes in effect an open fracture with all of the associated hazards.

It must be remembered that a cast applied shortly after a fracture occurs may not be large enough in a few hours to accommodate the inevitable swelling of the parts. When swelling occurs inside of a cast which is too tight, the major blood vessels may be compressed to the point that circulation is inadequate. There is then danger of necrosis of the entire part, with catastrophic damage. The peripheral circulation must be watched carefully after the application of a cast until this danger has passed. Elevation of the part helps to prevent excessive swelling by aiding return blood flow with the help of gravity.

Should the circulation become inadequate, the parts exposed at the end of the cast may become cold, cyanotic or pale and anesthetic. Pain at first may be severe. If an artery in the distal part of the extremity can be palpated, the pulse may be diminished or absent. This condition demands immediate relief before permanent damage occurs. The cast may be split to allow for expansion, or it may be necessary to remove it and apply another of adequate size.

TRACTION FIXATION. Another method for the maintenance of reduction is traction. Traction is a force applied distal to the fracture in the long axis of the bone and always demands countertraction, or a force in the opposite direction proximal to the fracture. Enough force must be applied to create sufficient traction to reduce the fracture and maintain reduction. Traction with countertraction accomplishes several things in reduction and the maintenance of reduction. First, the shortening is overcome by counteracting the contraction of muscles. Second, the displacing or angulating force of muscles is neutralized. This may be aided by placing the part in a position which lessens the deforming force of the muscles. For example, in a spiral, unstable fracture of the shaft of the tibia, traction overcomes the shortening caused by the pull of all of the leg muscles. The angulating force of the gastrocnemius is partially overcome as well, but, by flexing the knee and foot, the pull of the muscle is reduced, thus creating less angulating force.

There are several methods of applying traction to a limb. The most common is skin traction. Adhesive plaster strips are applied directly to the skin distal to the fracture. These strips are attached to a spreader board distal to the end of the extremity. A rope attached to this board runs through appropriate pulleys to weights which exert the necessary pull. When this method is used, the skin must be inspected frequently for irritation, constriction and cutting by the adhesive tape.

If prolonged or heavy traction is needed, skeletal traction may be more useful. This is accomplished by drilling a wire or pin through the bone distal to the fracture. The wire is then fitted to a traction bow, which, in turn, is attached to the rope pulleys and weights. Traction is, thus, made directly through the bone.

When traction is used to maintain reduction, the part must be either suspended in an appropriate supporting splint, or a traction and countertraction device must be incorporated in a cast to maintain the traction force.

A Thomas splint, or a modification of it, is frequently used in emergency transportation of fractures of the lower extremity, as well as for suspension traction. The splint consists of metal bars which run down each side of the leg and connect at the bottom. At the top, the bars insert into a padded metal ring. When the leg is placed through the ring with the splint is proper position, countertraction is made by the ring against the perineum and ischial tuberosity. Traction is then made on the distal fragment by skin traction or an appropriate hitch placed about the ankle and tied to the end of the splint. By means of a Spanish windlass, traction is exerted on the long axis of the leg. When the splint is used for suspension, the leg is held in the splint by slings placed under the extremity and attached to the splint or by incorporating the whole in elastic bandages. The splint holds the leg suspended from the bed by ropes, pulleys and weights attached at the upper and lower ends. Traction may then be made on the leg through another set of ropes and weights with skin or skeletal traction. Raising the foot of the bed creates an inclined plane, and the weight of the body thus creates the necessary countertraction. When this method is used, frequent checks of the apparatus are necessary to make sure that it is functioning properly. X-ray films must be taken at appropriate intervals to ensure maintenance of reduction (Fig. 8).

If too much traction force is applied, the bone ends will be pulled apart, causing a gap in the fracture. This condition is termed distraction and is a contributing factor in delayed union and nonunion.

Occasionally, it may be desirable to use the principle of traction and countertraction in an ambulatory patient. This may be done by placing traction pins through the bone proximal and distal to the fracture, and, while traction and countertraction are applied, the extremity is placed in a cast incorporating the pins. When the plaster cast hardens about the pins, they are held separated by the same amount of force that was applied at the time of reduction.

INTERNAL FIXATION. Internal fixation devices consist of screws, plates, rods, pins, wires and bands designed to hold the fracture in reduction by direct application to the bone. An open operation is necessary in most instances for the application of these devices. The hazard of increased damage to bone and soft parts as well as potential infection of the wound must be carefully considered by the surgeon before the operation is done. These difficulties must be weighed against the inadequacy of reduction by other methods. If adequate function of the part cannot

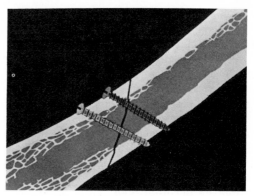

Figure 9. Open reduction with internal screw fixation of a fracture of the shaft of the tibia.

ultimately be achieved by other methods, then open reduction with internal fixation should be considered. For example, a widely separated, transverse fracture of the patella which disrupts the extensor mechanism of the knee cannot be reduced or held in adequate reduction by external forces, and an open operation with internal fixation of the two fragments in apposition is mandatory (Fig. 9).

Although open reduction may be necessary to salvage a damaged part, there are penalities associated with this procedure which must be considered. Infection after opening a fracture is a hazard, but the danger can be minimized by careful preparation and technique. Blood supply to the fracture site is always further disrupted by open reduction, particularly if the periosteum and soft tissues must be stripped extensively from the bone. This usually leads to slower union of the fracture.

Open reduction of fractures in children is rarely indicated, and internal fixation is almost never needed. Unnecessary operations on growing bones should be avoided. The incidence of infection and nonunion is greatly increased by these procedures in children. If, in the exposure of the fracture, the periosteum about the epiphysial plate is disturbed, growth disturbances are likely. Except for a few rare injuries, open reduction, particularly with internal fixation, should be avoided in children under 13 years of age.

PROSTHETIC REPLACEMENT OF BONE. Occasionally, parts of certain fractured bones are replaced by metal prostheses. This may be necessary when the bone is completely destroyed, or when other factors enter into the problem. The intracapsular fracture of the neck of the femur is the site of the most

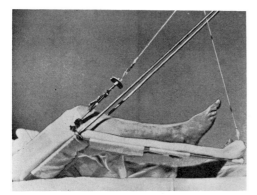

Figure 8. The Thomas splint with Pearson attachment used for suspension while skeletal traction is applied through the wire and traction bow at the lower femur.

frequently used prosthesis. In older people, the osteoporotic head of the femur may not hold the usual internal fixation devices securely, leading to nonunion. Aseptic necrosis of the head of the femur may demand prosthetic replacement. When healing of the fracture is certain to be prolonged to the point where the life of the patient is jeopardized, prosthetic replacement of the damaged head allows early return to function of the hip.

Occasionally, a portion or all of a bone may be excised if adequate restoration of the bone cannot be accomplished. This may be done with a shattered patella, where no amount of reconstruction can produce a smooth articular surface with the femur. The extensor tendon mechanism, however, must be restored.

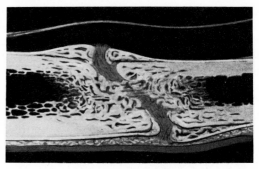

Figure 10. Established nonunion produces rounded fracture ends; there is interposition of fibrous tissue, and the medullary canal is blocked by bone.

DELAYED UNION AND NONUNION

The time necessary for healing a fracture varies with the age of the patient, the location of the fracture, the degree of tissue damage, the amount of movement of the fragments, the presence or absence of infection, the blood supply to the part and the gap between fragments.

Although average times of healing of fractures can be determined for different age groups, there is always some variation. If the healing time is considerably longer than normally expected, the condition is termed delayed union. This does not mean that the bone will not eventually heal, but does mean that this may take many weeks longer than usual. The reason for the delayed union may not be readily apparent. In some instances, inadequate local chemical response to the fracture may play a part.

Economic problems may arise for the patient if the condition is prolonged. In addition, prolonged immobilization may cause excessive muscle atrophy and stiffness of joints. When these conditions exist, attempts may be made to stimulate the healing process. Many methods have been tried. Partial weight-bearing on the lower extremity may stimulate union if this does not create shearing force. This method is only helpful if compression force is exerted on the fracture. If shearing force is produced, the problem may be compounded by deformity, and nonunion may be produced.

Other methods which have been tried are drilling holes in the fracture fragments; repeated insertion of needles into the fracture area to create bleeding; production of repeated minute trauma by pounding the fracture area; and intermittent vasodilation by constricting devices or by the use of shortwave diathermy. None of these methods of treatment produces uniformly good results, and often the results are unpredictable.

Nonunion of a fracture exists when the repair process comes to a complete halt. Many of the factors producing delayed union may have an effect on producing nonunion. However, the two most common causes are absence of adequate blood supply and, more important, failure to immobilize the fracture properly. Although some callus may form, the process stops before the gap in the fracture fragments has been bridged. The fragments are united by mature, inactive fibrous tissue scar. A false joint, or pseudoarthrosis, may develop (Fig. 10).

When x-ray films are made, an established nonunion shows certain characteristics. The sharp edges of the fragments become blunted and rounded. The bone ends may show varying degrees of sclerosis or increased density. This, coupled with the obvious gap between fragments, usually means a nonunion is present. As in delayed union, bone grafting is usually the method of choice to re-create the conditions for healing in nonunion.

BONE GRAFTING

There is considerable clinical and experimental evidence that a bone graft does not grow of itself. In reality, the majority of the graft may die, as it is deprived of its blood supply; a few surface bone cells may, however, remain alive. The significance of bone grafting to obtain union lies in the fact that the repair process is stimulated. The graft brings the building blocks of calcium and phosphorus to the fracture site. In addition, the graft forms a lattice, or network, through which new bone may grow once the repair process has been restarted. Slowly, the graft is resorbed and new bone is laid down in its place. If the process continues, the fracture heals and the graft is remodeled with the new bone.

Two types of grafts are used: homogenous and autogenous. In either case, the bone may be primarily cortical or cancellous bone. The supply of autogenous graft material is, of course, limited. Cortical graft may be taken from any of the long bones; however, the tibia and fibula are the most frequently

used. Cancellous bone is usually obtained from the ilium and ribs.

Homogenous bone is useful because it may be stored in a bone bank. It may be essential when large skeletal defects must be bridged; however, homogenous bone grafts do not "take," or resubstitute, quite as well as autogenous grafts. Therefore, autogenous grafts are preferred when feasible.

Osteoperiosteal grafts include the periosteum as well as the bone. There is thought to be some advantage to this type autogenous graft, as the bone-forming cells of the periosteum are included. Cortical grafts are stronger, at least temporarily, than cancel-

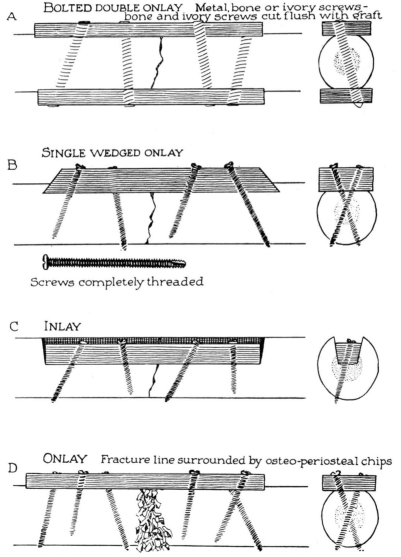

Figure 11. Various methods of bone grafting may be used to create stability at the fracture and provide a building-block for union. (From Magnuson: Orthopedic Subjects. Saunders Military Manuals. National Research Council, 1942, p. 22.)

lous grafts. They may be used to help stabilize the fracture as an internal fixation device as well as to supply new bone. They are, however, more slowly invaded and replaced by the repair process. Cancellous bone is spongy, and the trabecular spaces allow for more rapid resubstitution and incorporation of the graft in the healing process. Many times, it is necessary to use both types of bone, packing pieces of cancellous graft about the fracture to fill a gap, and adding cortical grafts for stability.

There are several common techniques for grafting. Sliding, inlay, onlay, barrel stave, chip, intramedullary and dual bone grafts are used. In addition, grafts may be combined with internal fixation devices for better immobilization of the fracture (Fig. 11).

There are those who believe all scar tissue should be removed from the bone ends, the medullary canal opened and fresh bone exposed at the site of nonunion. This extensive procedure may be necessary in some instances; however, removal of all scar tissue may produce undesirable instability of the fracture or devitalize bone fragments. Some judgment must be used in determining the type and extent of surgery performed.

If deformity is present, it should be corrected when the bone grafting is done. The prerequisites for healing must be present if the graft is to be successful. The postoperative care is the same as for a fresh fracture.

OPEN FRACTURE

An open fracture is an emergency. Whether it is a finger or major leg bone, the open wound presents problems which demand immediate care. It must be assumed that an open fracture is contaminated to some degree, and the bone and surrounding tissues are exposed to possible infection. Infection destroys tissue and delays healing; it may lead to crippling or death when uncontrolled.

In addition to the bone injury in open fractures, there may be extensive damage to the nerves, blood vessels, muscles and tendons. Often, there is serious loss of skin.

Excessive blood loss may be encountered. Crushing, tearing and laceration of the soft parts may produce profound shock. Often, the violent force of high-speed automobile accidents produces multiple fractures and serious injury to other systems.

The course of the patient's ultimate recovery, or survival, is often determined by the quality of first-aid rendered at the scene of the accident. The doctor or ambulance attendant should have a routine of conduct in mind. Is the patient conscious? Is he breathing properly? What is the rate and quality of his pulse? Is there serious external bleeding? These are the vital signs which determine the general physiologic state of the patient, and can be determined rapidly and without moving the patient.

An obstructed airway produces anoxia rapidly and usually complicates or produces shock. Obstruction may be from the tongue in the unconscious patient, from damage to the larynx or trachea, or due to accumulation of blood or secretions in the tracheo-bronchial tree. Occasionally, multiple rib fractures produce a flail chest, which is incapable of proper respiration. The simple maneuver of pulling the tongue forward may relieve obstruction to the airway. Turning the patient carefully face down may allow secretions to drain sufficiently to temporarily save his life. Occasionally, immediate tracheostomy may be necessary if the trachea or larynx has been crushed. Stabilization of a flail chest is best treated in the hospital. Oxygen may be necessary.

Serious bleeding from a wound can usually be controlled by the application of a pressure dressing. Rarely is a tourniquet needed or advisable. Too often, a tourniquet is applied with only enough tension to obstruct the venous flow of blood, thus increasing blood loss.

Splinting the damaged extremities or spine is essential before the patient is transported to the hospital. The unconscious patient should be moved as little as possible, and his spine must be protected until damage to the vital axial skeleton can be determined. If he must be turned, the trunk and extremities must be moved as a unit to avoid injury to the spinal cord. He may be placed on a board, door or stretcher which does not allow the spine to sag.

All wounds should be covered, preferably with sterile gauze dressings, but clean cloth will suffice. Elastic bandages should be used when they are available. Firm pressure helps control hemorrhage and edema. Not only does covering the wound help control bleeding, but it also protects it from increased contamination. The most common sources of pathogenic organisms are the noses and throats of by-standers. Breathing, talking and coughing over the wound may add organisms that are far more dangerous than those on the skin of the patient or ground into the wound from the street.

If the patient is in shock from blood loss, plasma may be given on the way to the hospital.

The arm may be splinted to the body with a triangular sling and swathe bandage about the chest. The forearm, wrist and hand may be splinted with two padded boards applied to the flexor and extensor surfaces and bound in place. A triangular sling may be used in addition for comfort.

Fractures of the lower extremity are best immobilized with a traction splint of the Thomas type. This may be slipped under the leg while manual traction is made at the foot. A clove or Collins hitch is applied to the padded ankle. The ends of the bandage are tied over the distal end of the splint and tightened by twisting them with a stick of wood—the Spanish windlass principle. Countertraction is supplied by the ring of the splint against the ischium. The entire splint may be wrapped with elastic bandages for support and pressure. The part should be elevated moderately to aid return circulation, particularly if shock is present (Fig. 12).

On arrival at the hospital, a more thorough examination must be made, and the patient's condition evaluated before x-ray films are taken. The blood pressure and pulse rate must be determined at frequent intervals. The airway must be cleared and maintained by whatever measures are required. The condition of the heart and lungs must be evaluated. If proper splints and wound coverings were not available previously, they should be applied in the emergency room. The abdomen must be checked for injury to its contents. A neurologic examination should be carried out when the patient's condition warrants it. The urine must be examined if the patient is able to void. If not, a soft rubber catheter should be passed to obtain a urine specimen. Difficulty or inability to insert the catheter into the bladder may indicate disruption of the urethra. Blood in the urine may indicate damage to the bladder and kidneys. The wounds should be evaluated by inspection, without removing the splints. The integrity of the nerve and blood supply to the extremity can usually be determined by inspection and examining sensation and motor function.

Antibiotic therapy should be started promptly. A booster injection of tetanus toxoid should be given if the patient has been pre-

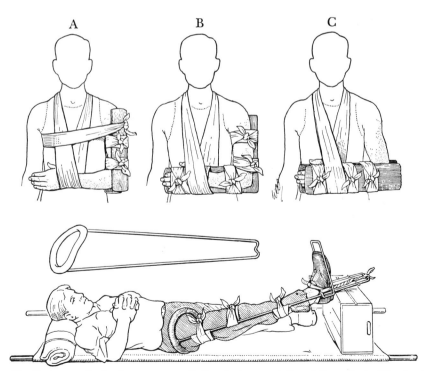

Figure 12. Various methods of emergency splinting for transportation of the patient with a fracture.

viously immunized. If immunization has not been previously obtained, a skin test with tetanus antitoxin should be performed and tetanus antitoxin administered. A blood count, hemoglobin and hematocrit, as well as typing and cross-matching, should be done immediately. Restoration of the circulating blood to normal volume may be necessary, and transfusion of whole blood is indicated. If shock is profound, plasma or plasma expanders may be used until blood is available, but there is no substitute for whole blood when excessive blood has been lost. Only after the blood pressure has been stabilized and the physiology of respiration and circulation has been restored may the patient be considered for x-ray examination.

The physician should accompany the patient to the x-ray department, and should supervise all handling of the patient while the films are taken. Moving the patient from the emergency cart may not be necessary to take adequate survey films; however, if it should be necessary, the physician must supervise the move. Aides and technicians should not be required to assume the responsibility for handling the patient.

When x-ray films are made of the damaged bones, the entire bone should be x-rayed, including the joints proximal and distal to the injury. Too often a fracture at the opposite end of the bone from the open one is missed because of incomplete roentgenographic examination.

Only after thorough evaluation and stabilization of the patient's physiology should definitive surgery of the open fracture be attempted. The primary objective of surgical treatment is to convert a contaminated wound into one that is surgically clean. Success depends upon performing debridement before bacteria have invaded the tissues. Ideally, no more than six hours should elapse between injury and operation. Traction must be maintained, either manually or by one of the devices attached to a fracture operating table, while preparation for debridement is carried out.

As the first step, the area around the wound is cleaned superficially. The wound is covered with sterile sponges while the skin is washed with soap and water and shaved. Following the shaving, a more thorough scrubbing of the skin is carried out with soap and water for at least ten minutes by the clock. During the scrubbing, the skin should be rinsed frequently with sterile water; the wound should remain covered with sterile sponges. Soap and surgical detergents should not be allowed to enter the wound. The wound, however, can be irrigated with sterile physiologic saline solution after the skin has been thoroughly cleansed. A pneumatic tourniquet should be applied to obtain a bloodless operative field for debridement.

After the patient has been draped, the wound is explored. Devitalized or damaged skin edges are cut away, conserving as much skin as possible. It may be necessary to enlarge the wound for adequate inspection and debridement. This may be done by an appropriate incision at each end of the wound. Irrigation with physiologic saline is carried out. A syringe with a blunt tip is placed in the depths of the wound so that the flow of saline is from the depths outward. The stream should be forceful enough to carry away debris, dirt and blood clots. The wound must be painstakingly searched for contaminated tissue, debris and blood clots. More important, however, is removal of devitalized tissue, which is a potential breeding ground for bacteria. Tissue deprived of blood supply cannot be reached by the body defenses, and bacteria thrive on it. The infection which results inevitably destroys surrounding healthy tissue.

Excision of devitalized tissue must be done carefully to avoid removing viable tissue and vital structures. Particularly, muscle must be removed when devitalized, as it is the most likely source of gas bacillus infection. Damaged but viable muscle and soft tissue should be saved. Devitalized muscle does not contract or bleed when cut; this may be a helpful criterion in debridement. Dirt ground into bone may be removed by irrigation and curettage. All bone fragments attached to viable soft tissue must be preserved; however, small detached fragments may be removed. Occasionally, a large, completely detached bone fragment is encountered. Removal of such a fragment may produce an unacceptable gap at the fracture site which cannot be adequately bridged by callus. Such a fragment may be removed from the wound, thoroughly cleaned and then replaced.

Nerves, tendons and blood vessels exposed in the wound should be inspected and damage to these structures estimated. Rarely, it may be necessary to replace or repair a damaged major blood vessel, if the viability of the extremity is jeopardized. Damaged nerves must be preserved. When debridement is complete, the surgeon must decide whether to repair several nerves and tendons immediately or defer this procedure. If these structures are repaired in the absence of complete immobilization of the fracture, movement of the fracture fragments may disrupt the sutures, causing additional scarring of the nerve and tendon ends. If infection develops, the suture material may act as a focus for abscess formation in the nerve or tendon, thus adding to the damage to these structures. Therefore, nerve and tendon repair may be deferred until the threat of infection is past and the bone has healed sufficiently for adequate stability.

If internal fixation of the fracture is desirable, the surgeon must know that he has converted the wound into a surgically clean one before this is done. Internal fixation should not be used if there is actual or potential infection. Screws, plates and rods act as foreign bodies about which bacteria concentrate because of the devitalization of the bone they produce when applied. Osteomyelitis is the result of bacterial invasion of bone about these devices.

Lastly, the surgeon must decide whether to close the wound primarily or secondarily. When infection develops in a closed wound, several serious complications occur. Septicemia may develop, endangering the patient's life. Infection always means destruction of bone as well as soft parts; healing is delayed and more scar tissue is formed, impairing function. If the surgeon is certain the wound is surgically clean, that bacteria have not invaded the tissue and that he will have adequate opportunity for postoperative observation, he may elect to close the wound immediately. However, if the surgeon believes that these conditions are not met, wound closure may be delayed until the threat of infection has passed, usually in three to seven days. The wound is packed open with a loose petrolatum gauze pack to allow adequate drainage should infection develop. Drainage of the wound prevents invasion of the deeper structures and confines the infection to the exposed surfaces of the wound. The body defenses can overcome this type of infection more easily and quickly. The wound is closed later if no infection develops. This is called delayed, or secondary, closure and is the safest procedure.

Finally, a pressure dressing is applied to prevent edema and hemorrhage, and the fracture is immobilized in a cast or by suspension traction. Immobilization must be adequate for the bone as well as the soft tissues. Rest promotes healing and helps to prevent infection.

Three to seven days later, the wound should be ready for secondary closure. Until a wound is closed with adequate skin and subcutaneous tissue, there is danger of secondary infection. Exposed bone, tendons and nerves dry out and become necrotic. If a large gap in the skin must epithelize, more scar tissue is formed, limiting function. In the absence of adequate subcutaneous tissue, a thin, adherent scar is formed which is vulnerable to minor trauma. It is, therefore, necessary to close the wound with adequate tissue early.

The wound is inspected and any remaining necrotic or excessive granulation tissue is removed. In order to ensure healing, the wound must be closed without tension, and dead space must be eliminated. To do this, the surgeon must liberate the skin and subcutaneous tissue by freeing these tissues from the underlying fascia by dissection. This procedure mobilizes skin and subcutaneous tissue from the muscles so that the wound edges may be drawn together. Occasionally, loss of skin at the time of injury may prevent this method of closure. In such instances, one of the plastic surgical procedures may be necessary to allow closure. In any case, the wound must be closed without tension. Tension interferes with blood supply to the healing structures; necrosis of the skin edges takes place, and the wound opens or fails to heal, again exposing the underlying tissue to infection.

Cavities, or dead space, in the soft tissue, created by loss of tissue, allow body fluids to accumulate in these areas and serve as incubators for bacteria. Adequate closure and pressure dressings tend to eliminate dead space and lessen the danger of infection after secondary closure. If it appears likely that fluids will accumulate in the depths of the wound, drainage should be established for a few days to allow the fluids to escape. A drain is inserted to the depths of the wound at the time of closure, but must be removed in 48 to 72 hours. If it remains longer, a tract may be created through which bacteria can invade the area.

After the wound has been closed, either primarily or secondarily, it should not be disturbed by frequent dressings and inspections. Most postoperative complications are reflected in the patient's general condition, and this should be followed carefully. Unnecessary cast changes and dressings disturb the wound and fracture, and only delay healing.

FRACTURES AND DISLOCATIONS OF THE UPPER EXTREMITY

When treating fractures of the upper extremity, the surgeon must be mindful of its specialized functions. The bones, joints and muscles of the shoulder girdle, arm and forearm are designed to place the end organ—the hand—in multiple positions for use. These movements must be smooth, coordinated and stable. Slight malalignment of the shaft fragments may not alter this function greatly; however, limitation of joint motions of these lever arms may reduce the effectiveness of the hand to a marked degree.

THE HAND

The hand possesses the ability to perform a myriad of functions, including sensory perception. The fine tolerances of the bones, joints and tendons demand anatomic reduction of fractures whenever possible to ensure maximum function. Soft tissue injuries to nerves, blood vessels, tendons, skin and subcutaneous tissues must receive as much consideration and care as the fracture or dislocation. Perfect reduction of fractures of the bones of the hand may be meaningless if skin coverage is inadequate, if sensation is lost, or if joints and tendons cease to function. Fractures and dislocations of the hand should be treated as an injury to the whole organ, not as isolated bone or joint injuries.

When the hand is held in the position of function, the arrangement of the fingers and thumb is similar to that of a hand holding a baseball. The metacarpophalangeal and interphalangeal joints are moderately flexed, and the thumb is slightly flexed, abducted and opposed so that the tip of the thumb and index finger may be brought together by slight flexion of the index finger at the metacarpophalangeal joint. This position should be maintained whenever possible if the hand must be immobilized for the treatment of injuries. If motion of the fingers or thumb is impaired after injury, this position allows maximum function. Restoration of maximum flexion and extension of the fingers and rotatory motions of the thumb is more easily accomplished from this position than any other.

FUNCTIONAL ANATOMY OF THE HAND. An understanding of the anatomic structures of the hand which are subject to injury, produce deformity and affect re-establishment of

function is necessary for intelligent management of these fractures and dislocations. The fingers contain three phalanges with two interphalangeal joints. The joints, because of their configuration, allow flexion and extension but no rotation. They are stable from side to side because of the collateral ligaments. These ligaments lie on each side of the joint and are taut in flexion and relaxed in extension; they are subject to sprains and contusions. If the finger is immobilized in extension too long, the collateral ligaments shorten and prevent flexion. This must be borne in mind when it is necessary to immobilize an interphalangeal joint in extension. Fractures of joint surfaces may result in abduction or adduction of the finger at the joint. Deviation of this type causes serious disturbance in relation to the other fingers, and must be corrected.

The distal phalanx is flexed by the flexor profundus tendon running through the split insertion of the flexor sublimis at the base of the middle phalanx. The two tendons in their sheaths lie in intimate contact with the palmar surface of the phalanges. The tendon sheaths and their supporting ligaments fit the tendon and bone closely, allowing little tolerance for abnormal alignment. Angulation of bone fragments may seriously interfere with the gliding motion of the tendons, and the inflammatory reaction of the injury may produce adhesions and scar tissue within these structures, thus limiting function. The fingers are extended at the interphalangeal joints by the action of the interosseous and lumbrical muscles inserting into the extensor tendon mechanism. The angle of pull produces a characteristic palmar angulation of the fragments of the proximal phalanx when this bone is fractured. Avulsion fractures of the tendon attachments produce varying degrees of loss of flexion and extension of the distal phalanx.

The metacarpophalangeal joints allow flexion and extension and, in addition, abduction and adduction of the fingers. Preservation of these motions is essential to the normally functioning hand.

Digital nerves and blood vessels are frequently injured in conjunction with bone injury. The status of circulation and sensation must always be evaluated along with the bone injury.

The metacarpal bones form a stable base from which the fingers move. These bones are straight on the dorsal surface and concave on the palmar surface. Their bases articulate with the distal row of carpal bones to form stable joints in which little motion occurs. The metacarpals, thus, form a long arch to accommodate the palmar muscles, tendons and nerves. The ability of the fingers to form a cone along with the thumb is due to the presence of a transverse arch in the metacarpal bones, coupled with the ability of the fifth metacarpal bone and thumb to rotate toward the other fingers. Loss of these arches by fracture deformity limits the ability to flex the fingers and may cause irregularities in the palm, which make grasp painful and difficult. The interosseous muscles lie between the metacarpal bones and, because of their pull, produce a characteristic dorsal angulation to these bones when fractures occur.

The thumb is made up of two phalanges. The first metacarpal acts in a similar fashion to the proximal phalanges of the fingers; however, it is more stable to lateral motion at the metacarpophalangeal joint. The ability of the thumb to abduct, adduct, rotate and oppose is the reason the hand can perform its myriad functions. This motion takes place at the articulation between the first metacarpal and greater multangular bone. This is a saddle-shaped joint which allows these motions to take place by action of the thenar muscles and the long flexor, extensor and abductor muscles in the forearm. Disruption of this joint, if improperly repaired, leads to serious disability of the thumb.

The median nerve at the wrist is in a vulnerable position for injury, lying superficially to the flexor tendons and confined in the close-fitting carpal tunnel. Extension injuries to the hand at the wrist may stretch or contuse the median nerve, leading to serious impairment of the thenar muscles.

When treating fractures and dislocations of the hand, the injury must be considered in relation to the functional anatomy. Skin and subcutaneous damage must be evaluated, and circulation appraised, the status of the nerve supply established, and an assessment made of the damage to tendons, joints, ligaments and bones. Nowhere in the body is repair of soft tissues along with the bone more important than in the hand.

Fractures and dislocations of the hand are produced by direct and indirect violence, as in other parts of the body. Direct violence, often accompanied by serious soft tissue damage, accounts for the majority of these fractures. This is so because in industry and daily living the hands are frequently placed in hazardous situations.

FRACTURES OF THE PHALANGES. **Distal phalanx.** Fractures of the distal phalanx are of two types: those involving the tuft and shaft of the bone, and those involving the joint and tendon attachments. Crushing injury, such as striking the finger tip with a hammer, is the usual mechanism of tuft and shaft fractures. The fracture is often comminuted, but usually not greatly displaced. Subungual hematoma and soft tissue contusion and laceration are common. Fibrous tissue bands from skin to bone, running through the fat pad of the finger, prevent marked displacement. Prevention of infection of the subungual hematoma or lacerations is imperative. The finger should be prepared with soap and water scrubbing, as in compound fractures. If the finger nail is almost completely avulsed, it may be gently removed. If it is intact, the subungual hematoma should not be disturbed. A pressure dressing of sterile fluff gauze and elastic bandage may provide adequate protection and immobilization. After a week, this may be replaced with a protective metal splint to hold the finger in the position of function for two weeks longer. Firm, painless, fibrous union is usually present by this time, and, although fracture lines may show on the x-ray films for many weeks, the fingers can be used.

BASEBALL FINGER. If the distended distal phalanx is struck and forced into flexion when the extensor tendon is taut, an avulsion fracture of the attachment of this tendon occurs, or the tendon ruptures. The distal phalanx droops in flexion and cannot be actively extended. This deformity is sometimes called mallet, or baseball, finger. Pain and swelling are found over the dorsum of the joint at the tendon attachment. Lateral x-ray films reveal an avulsion of the dorsal lip of the joint surface of the distal phalanx when a fracture is present. If the extensor tendon has ruptured, no fracture is found.

The treatment for both injuries is the same. This is one of the few instances in which the finger joint must be immobilized in hyperextension until there is no tendency for the distal phalanx to droop. This may be done with a plaster or metal splint. If the splint can be securely fixed to the finger, it is necessary to immobilize only the distal phalangeal joint, allowing movement in the remaining joints. Immobilization varies from a minimum of three weeks to usually a maximum of six weeks.

Middle phalanx. Fractures of the middle phalanx involve the condyles of the distal joint, the shaft or the proximal joint. One or both condyles may be fractured by a blow to the extended finger. The usual fracture line is similar to an inverted **V**. The condyles split off at an angle to the shaft and displace medially and laterally. This is due to the wedgelike action of the articular surface of the distal phalanx when compressed against the condyles. The same mechanism and joint configuration produce a similar fracture at the proximal interphalangeal joint. Angulation of the finger distal to the fracture is the important deformity to correct, as well as the restoration of smooth joint surfaces. Since the pull of the flexor and extensor tendons forces the distal phalanx against the fractured condyles, perpetuating the deformity, it may be necessary to apply continuous traction to the distal phalanx to counteract this force while the fracture is healing. At the same time, angulation is corrected. The pull through the joint capsule and ligaments tends to bring the fragments into position. This is aided by molding the fragments by manipulation. Traction may be applied through the finger nail or the distal phalanx, with a small Kirschner wire through the bone. Traction is supplied by a rubber band attached to the wire and a splint extended distally. Countertraction and additional immobilization are provided by a forearm cast, ending at the distal palmar crease and supporting a splint for the finger. The finger is placed in the position of function in this splint. The splint is easily made by bending a wire coat hanger in the shape of a long **U**. The base of the **U** is notched to receive the rubber band, and the arms of the **U** extending along each side of the finger are incorporated in the volar surface of the cast. Cross strips of adhesive tape form a bed for the volar surface of the finger. This splint may be used for all unstable finger and metacarpal fractures which require traction (Fig. 13).

Within three weeks, fibrous union will hold the fragments in reduction. The traction is removed and gentle motion is started. Between exercise periods, it may be necessary to protect the finger from injury with a curved metal splint for another two weeks.

Fractures of the shaft of the middle phalanx may angulate volarward or dorsalward, depending upon the relation of the fracture to the insertion of the sublimis tendon. Fractures distal to the insertion angulate volarward. This is due to the unopposed action of

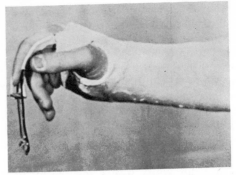

Figure 13. For all unstable finger and metacarpal fractures, traction is made on the flexed finger.

the extensor mechanism pulling the distal fragment into extension while the sublimis tendon pulls the proximal segment into flexion (Fig. 14).

Fractures proximal to the flexor sublimis tendon insertion angulate dorsalward. The extensor tendon, which inserts into the base of the proximal fragment, holds this fragment in extension. The flexor tendons flex the distal fragment.

If the fracture is stable, correction of the angulation by manipulation is done. Immobilization of the finger is accomplished by a curved metal or plaster volar splint. This position usually corrects both types of fractures. Comminuted, oblique or spiral fractures, which are unstable, may require traction in the position of function to maintain length of the finger.

Avulsion fractures at the base of the middle phalanx occur on the volar surface in hyperextension injuries. The volar joint capsule is pulled tight by this mechanism and may avulse a small fragment of bone. Displace-

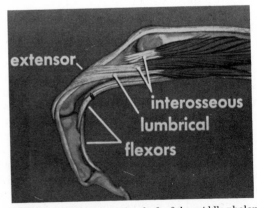

Figure 14. Fractures of the shaft of the middle phalanx angulate in relationship to the insertion of the flexor sublimis tendon.

ment is slight and the fragment tiny, so that immobilization for two weeks on a curved splint is usually all that is necessary while the capsule of the joint heals.

Hyperextension injuries frequently tear the volar joint capsule, allowing the middle phalanx to dislocate dorsally on the proximal phalanx. Occasionally, the condyles of the proximal phalanx are trapped by the capsule or sublimis tendon, making closed reduction impossible; however, in most instances, straight manual traction on the finger will reduce the dislocation. The finger is then splinted in the position of function for two or three weeks while the capsule reattaches and the traumatic synovitis of the joint subsides.

Proximal phalanx. Fractures of the proximal phalanx of the finger occur in three locations: at the condyles of the joint, in the shaft and at the base of the bone. The mechanism is often a direct blow, but fracture may be produced by compression force applied to the phalanx or by medial or lateral angulating forces.

Fractures of the condyles are similar to those in the middle phalanx, and are treated the same way. Fractures of the shaft of the bone assume a characteristic volar angulation. The pull of the lumbrical and the interosseous muscles inserting into the extensor mechanism of the finger extends the interphalangeal joints and flexes the metacarpophalangeal joints. This force acts as a bowstring across the fracture site and forces the fragments into volar angulation. The deformity must be corrected because distortion of the flexor tendon tunnel limits flexion of the distal joints of the finger. Reduction is obtained by traction and manipulation. Immobilization in the position of function is necessary to counteract the deforming pull of the extensor tendons (Fig. 15).

Occasionally, more flexion of the finger is

required to maintain reduction. This is most easily accomplished by bandaging the finger over a roll of one-inch gauze bandage. Immobilization should continue for three weeks. After this time, support should be supplied between exercise periods for an additional two weeks.

Fractures of the base of the phalanx are often impacted with medial or lateral angulation. This angulation is a result of the force producing the fracture; however, the flexor and extensor muscles tend to perpetuate the deformity once it has occurred. The fingers overlap on flexion if this deformity is allowed to persist. The fracture must be disimpacted by traction and manipulation before reduction can be obtained. Immobilization is similar to that used in other fractures of this phalanx. Comminuted and unstable fractures of the phalanx may require continuous rubber band traction. It is important to recognize and correct rotation deformity in all finger fractures. Rotation of the bones in the long axis of the finger results in overlapping of fingers when they are flexed.

FRACTURES OF THE THUMB. Phalangeal fractures. Fractures of the phalanges of the thumb are similar to those in the fingers, except that the extensor mechanism is different and does not produce the volar angulation to the marked degree found in the fingers. Phalangeal fractures are treated in the same manner as those in the fingers.

METACARPOPHALANGEAL DISLOCATIONS. Dislocation of the metacarpophalangeal joints in the hand occurs most frequently in the thumb, and is the result of hyperextension injury to this joint. Since the joint in the thumb does not allow as much hyperextension as do the metacarpophalangeal joints of the fingers, it is more readily dislocated by this mechanism. The volar joint capsule tears, the proximal phalanx dislocates into the dorsum of the first metacarpal, and the head of the metacarpal protrudes through the rent in the volar capsule. If the capsule splits longitudinally, the head of the metacarpal may protrude through the capsule as though through a buttonhole. When traction is made to reduce the dislocation, the buttonhole tightens about the metacarpal head and neck, preventing reduction. Similarly, subluxation of the flexor profundus tendon over the head of the bone may present an obstruction to the reduction (Fig. 16).

Longitudinal traction is made on the thumb. If reduction of the dislocation does not occur

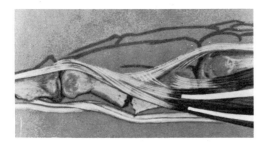

Figure 15. The insertion of the lumbrical and interosseous muscles into the extensor tendons of the finger causes palmar angulation of fractures of the proximal phalanx.

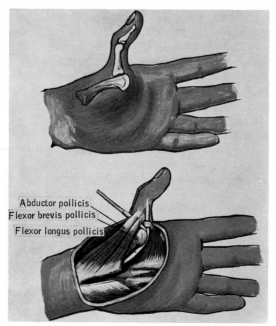

Figure 16. Dislocation of the metacarpophalangeal joint of the thumb may result in the flexor tendon or joint capsule trapping the metacarpal head and prevent reduction by closed methods.

This deformity, if uncorrected, produces a painful lump in the palm upon gripping, and the shortening of the bone places the finger out of line with the others, making grasp difficult. Swelling may obscure the deformity, so that x-ray films should always be made if there is any likelihood of fracture.

It would seem logical that hyperextension of the finger would reduce this fracture. However, the volar joint capsule is lax and allows considerable hyperextension before the capsule becomes taut enough to pull the metacarpal head back into position. For this reason, reduction must be done by forces applied directly to the head of the bone. The finger is flexed to 90 degrees at the metacarpophalangeal joint. Traction is exerted on this finger in the long axis of the metacarpal bone. While traction is applied, pressure is applied over the dorsum of the shaft and the flexed finger is forced dorsalward, carrying with it the distal metacarpal fragment. Following reduction, rotation must be checked carefully with the fingers closed into a fist. Faulty reduction causes the finger to overlap or rotate away from the other fingers. A serious disability results if this deformity is not corrected (Fig. 17).

The position of flexion, with pressure dorsalward on the head and volarward on

easily, the thumb is hyperextended while traction is continued in the long axis of the metacarpal. This maneuver may allow the phalanx to be levered over the head of the metacarpal into flexion. If the manipulation fails, open reduction is necessary. The thumb is immobilized for three weeks in a forearm cast or padded dorsal splint, holding the thumb in 30 to 45 degrees of flexion at the metacarpal phalangeal joint to prevent re-dislocation. Metacarpophalangeal dislocations of the fingers are produced by a similar mechanism and are treated in the same way as those in the thumb.

FRACTURES OF THE METACARPALS. **Metacarpal neck.** Fractures of the metacarpals occur at the neck, shaft and base of the bone, and are produced by direct or indirect violence. Fractures involving the neck are most commonly produced by striking a blow with the clenched fist. Since the fourth and fifth metacarpal bones are smaller and more mobile than the second and third, they are more commonly broken in this area. Compression force drives the metacarpal head toward the palm. When the fracture occurs, the head is carried into the palm along with the finger. Often the fracture is impacted. Frequently, the angulation of the head into the palm of the hand is 45 to 90 degrees.

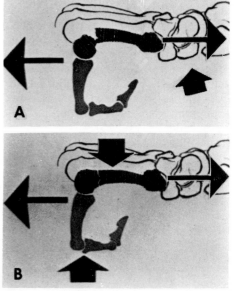

Figure 17. *A*, Traction is made on the long axis of the metacarpal with the finger flexed. *B*, While traction is maintained and pressure is applied over the shaft, the metacarpal head is forced dorsalward. Rotation should be checked following reduction. The fingers must not overlap or spread excessively.

the shaft, is maintained by a molded plaster splint for not longer than three weeks. Prolonged immobilization in this position leads to stiffening of the joints of the finger, as well as the metacarpophalangeal joint. The splint must be padded with felt to prevent necrosis of soft tissues over the pressure points. After three weeks, the plaster splint is replaced by a removable metal splint which holds the finger in the position of function for two more weeks. Active joint motion is started during this period.

Metacarpal shaft. Fractures of the shaft of the metacarpal bones angulate dorsally because of the bowstring-like pull of the interosseous muscles. This deformity causes shortening and malalignment of the distal fragment in the palm of the hand, and produces disability similar to the metacarpal neck fracture. In addition, angulation on the dorsum of the hand interferes with function of the extensor tendons (Fig. 18).

Transverse stable fractures may be reduced by simple manipulation, forcing the distal fragment dorsalward while counterpressure is made at the apex of angulation. A snug-fitting plaster cast is applied, extending from the metacarpal heads to just below the elbow. Immobilization continues for six weeks. X-ray films must be made weekly to ensure against undetected recurrence of the deformity.

Unstable spiral oblique and comminuted fractures of the metacarpal bones shorten as well as angulate, because of the pull of the interosseous muscles and the long flexor and extensor muscles of the fingers. Reduction and maintenance of reduction must be accompanied by continuous traction to overcome the constant pull of these muscles. This is most easily accomplished by the use of rubber band traction applied to the finger and incorporated in a snug-fitting forearm cast. The period of traction is usually three to four weeks, with cast immobilization continuing for another two weeks.

Metacarpal base. Fractures of the base of the metacarpal bones are usually the result of direct violence to the hand. Often, crushing injuries produce comminution of the fragments. There is little tendency for displacement, because the bases of the metacarpal bones are bound firmly to the distal row of carpal bones, and to each other by heavy ligaments. In many instances, reduction of the fracture is not necessary; simple splinting or cast immobilization for four weeks is often all that is needed.

BASE OF FIRST METACARPAL. Fractures at the base of the metacarpal bone of the thumb differ from those of the fingers. The bone is much more mobile because of the saddle-shaped articulation with the greater multangular bone. Two major types of fractures are common, and both are most often produced by indirect compression force. A fall on the rigid thumb is the usual mechanism.

The bone may break transversely or obliquely near the base, or the fracture may involve the joint surfaces. When the joint surfaces are not fractured, the deformity is usually one of dorsal angulation because of the pull of the thenar flexor muscles. If the fracture is stable, reduction by hyperextension of the thumb followed by cast immobilization is done. When the fracture is unstable and there is a tendency for shortening, traction may be necessary.

Fracture of the carpometacarpal joint of the thumb can cause serious disability of the hand. Compression force drives the curved articular surface of the metacarpal bone against the greater multangular bone. The fracture occurs through the ulnar palmar aspect of the joint. A small fragment in this area remains attached to the multangular bone. As the force continues, the dorsal ligaments rupture and the metacarpal bone dislocates dorsal and radialward on the greater multangular bone. The displacement produces a prominence at the base of the metacarpal on the dorsum of the hand. Active extension and abduction of the thumb are lost. The displacing pull of the short thenar, long flexor and extensor muscles of the thumb maintains the displacement (Fig. 19).

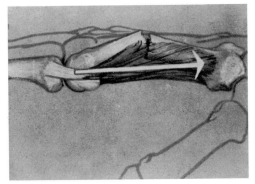

Figure 18.   The bowstring-like action of the interosseous muscles produces volar angulation of fractures of the metacarpal shaft. The head of the bone is forced into the palm and the dorsal angulation interferes with the extensor tendons.

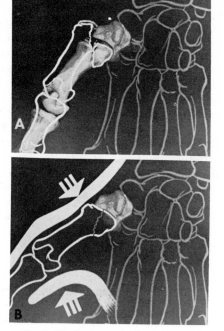

Figure 19. *A,* Displacement in fracture of the base of the first metacarpal, with involvement of the joint surface, is shown superimposed on the normal anatomy. *B,* The forces applied in reduction of this fracture, together with longitudinal traction, are illustrated; the molding of the cast is shown in white.

Reduction of the fracture-dislocation is accomplished by traction and hyperextension of the metacarpal, with pressure applied over its base in a palmar and ulnarward direction. A cast which maintains this position and pressure point is applied from the distal interphalangeal joint of the thumb to just below the elbow. Often, the dislocation will recur in the plaster cast. Frequent follow-up x-ray films are necessary. If the reduction cannot be maintained in nearly an anatomic position, continuous longitudinal traction is applied to the thumb. This is most conveniently done by skeletal traction through the proximal phalanx, allowing active flexion and extension exercise of the distal joint to prevent stiffness. As in all articular fractures, rough joint surfaces may in time produce a painful traumatic arthritis, necessitating further treatment. Occasionally, fractures and dislocations of the hand cannot be reduced or retained in reduction by these closed methods, and open operation with internal fixation may become necessary.

THE WRIST

Any bone in the wrist may be fractured by direct trauma; however, the navicular and lunate bones are the most commonly injured, usually by indirect violence. The carpus is made up of eight small bones, four in the proximal row and four in the distal row. The distal row of bones is less mobile, being firmly attached to the metacarpal bones. The proximal row, containing the navicular and lunate bones, is highly mobile, allowing motion between the two rows of carpal bones as well as at the radiocarpal joint. Because of this mobility, and, because they articulate with the radius, these two bones are subject to greater stresses and strains than the other bones of the carpus.

The lunate bone seldom is fractured, but frequently is dislocated. The navicular bone is seldom dislocated but is often fractured. The two bones may be injured simultaneously (Fig. 20).

FRACTURES OF THE NAVICULAR BONE. The usual mechanism of injury is a fall on the outstretched hand. The hand is forced into hyperextension at the wrist; the navicular bone is trapped between the carpal bones and the radius and is fractured. One of two anatomic areas in the bone is most frequently injured: the tubercle or the waist. The majority of the bone is covered by cartilage, except for these two areas. At the tubercle, carpal ligaments attach and, when they are pulled taut, the tubercle of the bone may be avulsed. At the waist, nutrient vessels enter the bone, producing an area of weakness. Fractures through this area are usually transverse with little or no displacement. This fracture is much more serious, as nonunion is likely. In addition, the blood supply to the bone may be damaged, depriving one of the fragments of nutrition with subsequent necrosis (Fig. 21).

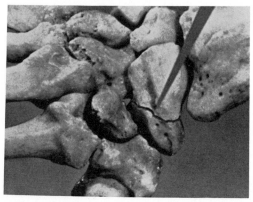

Figure 20. Fracture through the waist of the navicular bone. Note the small holes through which nutrient vessels enter the bone, creating an area of weakness.

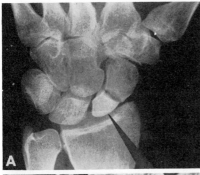
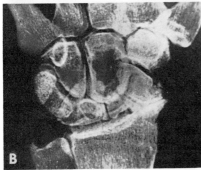

Figure 21. *A,* Necrosis of the proximal fragment in nonunion of the navicular bone is illustrated. *B,* Traumatic arthritis with destruction of the carpus following nonunion of the navicular is the result of neglect in diagnosis and treatment.

All too often, the fracture is not diagnosed. This is due frequently to a hairline fracture, which does not appear on the x-ray film, or to improper visualization of the bone. Whenever tenderness is present on pressure over the snuffbox area of the wrist, or longitudinal compression of the thumb produces pain in this area, a fracture of the navicular bone must be suspected. Swelling may be minimal and pain may be of mild degree. The tendency is to diagnose the injury as a sprain and neglect treatment. This error can lead to nonunion and eventual traumatic arthritis of the wrist. All sprains of the wrist should be treated as fractures of the navicular bone until proved otherwise.

The wrist and thumb should be immobilized in a plaster cast from the distal phalanx of the thumb and palmar flexion crease of the fingers to just below the flexion crease of the elbow. The fingers are allowed free movement, but the thumb must be completely immobilized in the position of function.

After three weeks, the cast is removed and a second x-ray examination is made. This must include oblique views of the wrist to visualize the bone fully. Three weeks after injury, bone will have been absorbed from the fracture, and a previously undiagnosed fracture may be easily seen. If a fracture is found in the waist of the bone, unremitting immobilization must continue for a minimum of three months. The bone heals slowly and may take six to nine months, or a year, to heal. The plaster cast must be changed often enough to maintain maximum immobilization. Nonunion of the bone may require bone grafting. Necrosis of one of the fragments may require bone grafting, or excision of all or part of the bone.

Fractures of the tubercle usually heal rapidly and immobilization for six to eight weeks is usually sufficient.

INJURIES TO THE LUNATE BONE. The lunate bone, like the navicular, is almost completely covered by cartilage, except for the small ligament attachments on the dorsal and volar aspect of the bone. For this reason, the bone is seldom fractured through the body; however, avulsion fractures at the ligament attachments may occur. Displacement of these tiny fragments is usually minimal, and splint immobilization of the wrist for three weeks is all that is necessary.

Anterior dislocation of the lunate bone may occur when the wrist is forcefully hyperextended in a fall. The lunate rotates forward, rupturing the dorsal ligaments and, in some instances, the volar ones, dislocating into the carpal tunnel. The flexor tendons of the fingers and the median nerve are compressed, and flexion of the wrist is blocked. Diffuse swelling of the wrist makes palpation of the displaced bone difficult. Lateral x-ray films of the wrist show the dislocation most clearly, but oblique views must be made to evaluate the navicular bone, which may be broken (Fig. 22).

Close reduction of a dislocated lunate is possible if done within the first few days after injury. Strong, steady traction is made while the wrist is dorsiflexed. This is done to open as widely as possible the space formerly occupied by the lunate. The bone is then pressed into position as the wrist is flexed while traction is maintained. If the wrist flexes completely, the reduction has usually been accomplished. X-ray examination is carried out before the wrist is immobilized in flexion. The ligaments usually heal within three weeks when gentle active wrist motion may be started.

If closed reduction fails, an open operation must be performed to replace or remove the bone. If the blood supply to the bone has been completely disrupted, the bone should be removed. Immobilization following open

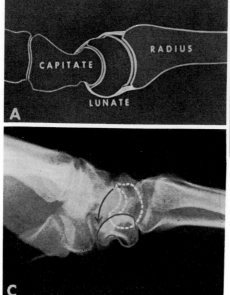
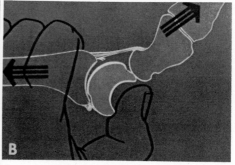

Figure 22. *A,* Ligamentous attachments to the almost completely cartilage-covered lunate bone are shown. Avulsion fractures of these ligaments may occur. *B,* Reduction of anterior dislocation of the lunate is accomplished by traction, dorsiflexion and direct pressure. *C,* Lateral roentgenograms are essential for diagnosis.

reduction is similar to that used following closed manipulation. X-ray examination should be made at three-month intervals for at least a year, because necrosis of the bone may develop due to blood vessel damage.

PERILUNAR DISLOCATION. Perilunar dislocation is a rare but serious injury to the wrist joint. The mechanism is one of hyperextension of the wrist. The volar carpal ligaments rupture and all of the carpal bones along with the hand dislocate dorsally, with the exception of the lunate, which maintains its normal relationship to the radius. The deformity may resemble the "silver fork" deformity of the Colles fracture.

Reduction of this dislocation is accomplished by traction plus hyperextension to engage the head of the capitate bone with the lunate, followed by flexion. The reduction is usually stable and the hand and wrist are placed in a short forearm cast in the position of function for three weeks.

If either lunate or perilunar dislocation is not diagnosed, fibrosis of the wrist joint capsule occurs, limiting motion to a few degrees. The flexor tendons of the fingers cannot function properly and the median nerve may undergo degenerative changes, leading to pain and crippling of the hand.

COLLES' FRACTURE. One of the most common of all fractures, Colles' fracture occurs at the distal radius, usually as the result of a fall on the extended hand. Since the flaring end of the radius is cancellous bone covered by a thin, fragile cortex, it is an area of weakness in the bone. As the wrist and hand are hyperextended, the volar carpal ligaments are pulled tight. The bone is compressed dorsally by the carpal bones and pulled apart ventrally by the tight volar carpal ligaments. The fracture occurs typically about one-half to three-quarters of an inch above the articular surface. The distal fragment is displaced dorsally, and the articular surface is tilted toward the back of the hand. Normally, this articular surface should face slightly toward the palm. This displacement limits flexion at the wrist, and produces the typical "silver fork" deformity of this fracture (Fig. 23).

A second major displacement occurs as the force producing the fracture continues: this is shortening of the radius with displacement of the distal fragment to the radial side of the wrist. This displacement disrupts the distal radio-ulnar joint, either tearing the triangle cartilage or avulsing the ulnar styloid to which it attaches. This displacement, if uncorrected, prevents normal pronation and supination at the disturbed radio-ulnar joint. Finally, the displacement in Colles' fracture may injure the median nerve as it is pressed against the sharp edge of the proximal fragment. Numbness and paresthesia of the thumb, index and middle finger are produced, and there may be weakness of opposition of the thumb (Fig. 24).

Careful and accurate reduction of a Colles'

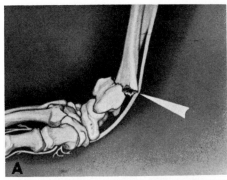

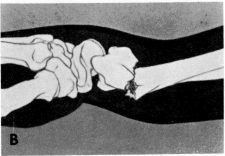

Figure 23. *A,* In Colles' fracture, the distal fragment is tilted and displaced dorsally; normally, the articular surface of the radius tilts 20 degrees palmarward. Note how the median nerve is pulled against the proximal fragment. *B,* The typical "silver fork" deformity of Colles' fracture is produced by the dorsal displacement and tilting of the distal radial fragment of bone.

fracture is important if function is to be restored. The first step is to break up the impaction usually found in these fractures. The surgeon applies traction and bends the patient's wrist backward, at the same time pressing downward and forward on the distal fragment. Straight traction ordinarily will not free the impacted fragments. However, the combination of hyperextension, traction and cross-pressure will usually succeed. Once the fragments are disengaged, pressure with the thumb on the distal fragment will correct the posterior displacement. The surgeon may then complete the reduction. While the surgeon maintains traction and pressure with the thumb, the patient's hand is brought into flexion and ulnar deviation. In this maneuver, traction is exerted on the radius chiefly through the dorsal radiocarpal ligament and through the radial collateral ligament, which is tensed by the ulnar deviation. Therefore, traction is exerted mainly on the radial side of the wrist as the patient's hand is forced into flexion and ulnar deviation. To make sure there are no rough edges projecting, the surgeon should explore the fracture with his finger tips (Fig. 25).

Friction of tendons riding over sharp edges of bone may lead to synovial inflammation or actual rupture of a tendon, usually the extensor pollicis longus.

An estimate of the reduction can be made by comparing flexion of the injured hand with the normal hand. The radial styloid process should be found on palpation, about one-half inch distal to the tip of the ulna if length has been restored.

The wrist is immobilized in flexion and ulnar deviation. This position is best maintained by either a sugar-tong splint or a posterior molded plaster, extending from the elbow to a point on the back of the hand opposite the palmar crease, leaving the fingers free to move.

As a final check on the accuracy of the reduction, x-ray films are taken in two planes. The lateral film should show that the radial articular surface has a normal volar tilt. The anteroposterior film should show the normal slant of the articular surface of the radius and restoration of the radio-ulnar articulation.

To minimize swelling and disabling stiffness in the fingers, the hand should be elevated for the first three or four days after reduction. The patient should be made to understand that, if full function of his hand is to be regained, he must actively exercise his fingers from the moment the plaster is dry and throughout the healing period.

Sufficient healing usually takes about six weeks. If the hand is immobilized in flexion for that length of time, full extension may never be regained, especially in older patients. Therefore, it is suggested that the

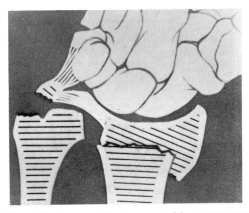

Figure 24. A second displacement of fragments occurs in Colles' fracture. The radius is shortened and the distal fragment is displaced radialward, avulsing the ulnar styloid or tearing the triangular cartilage, and disrupting the distal radio-ulnar joint.

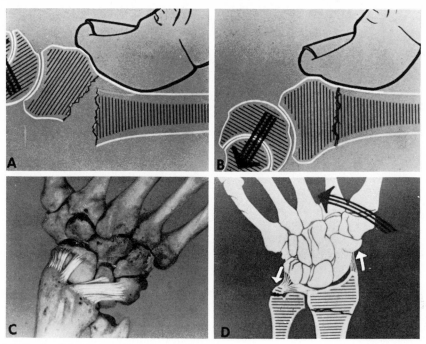

Figure 25. *A*, Following disimpaction of the fracture, the surgeon creates pressure on the distal fragment with his thumb in order to force it plantarward while longitudinal traction is maintained. *B*, When the distal fragment has been moved forward, the wrist is flexed, tensing the dorsal carpal ligaments. *C*, Traction through these ligaments tilts the articular surface palmarward. *D*, Ulnar deviation of the hand lengthens the radius and replaces the ulnar styloid process or reduces the radio-ulnar joint disruption by traction through the radial collateral ligaments.

cast be changed after two or three weeks, putting the hand in a more neutral position.

DISPLACEMENT OF THE DISTAL RADIAL EPIPHYSIS. In the growing child, forces which produce the Colles fracture in the adult often caused displacement of the distal radial epiphysis. The deformity is the same; the displacement takes place through the epiphysial plate. This is a serious injury because the growth from the epiphysial plate may be arrested, resulting in a short radius. The parents of the child should be warned about the possibility of arrested growth of the bone. Fortunately, this complication does not often occur.

The reduction is performed by traction and pressure over the epiphysis. It is done gently to avoid further damage to the epiphysial plate. The immobilization is like that used for Colles' fracture, and should continue for four to six weeks.

SMITH'S FRACTURE, OR REVERSE COLLES' FRACTURE. Smith's fracture, or reverse Colles' fracture, is a fracture of the distal radius caused by a fall with the hand in volar flexion. The displacement is almost the direct opposite of Colles' fracture. The distal fragment is displaced volarward and angu-

lated so that the articular surface faces into the palm. Reduction is accomplished by manipulation similar to that used for the Colles fracture, but in the reverse direction, placing the hand in dorsiflexion and ulnar deviation. Occasionally, the fracture line splits the articular surface of the radius. The fracture line extends from the dorsal articular surface upward and volarward, splitting off a triangular volar fragment.

This fracture is unstable and often cannot be maintained in reduction without continuous traction on the hand. The traction exerted in the long axis of the forearm pulls the fragment into position through the volar joint capsule and counteracts the longitudinal pull of the forearm muscles which displace the fragment. Traction may be applied through a Kirschner wire drilled transversely through the proximal portion of the second and third metacarpal bones and attached to a traction bow. Suspension of the arm through the traction bow by weights and pulleys supplies the traction, and the weight of the hanging arm supplies the countertraction. The fracture is stabilized by plaster splints applied to the flexor and extensor surfaces of the forearm from the elbow to the distal palmar flexion crease. The fingers are allowed to move immediately.

A fixed type of traction may also be used by placing a traction wire transversely through the upper ulna in addition to the wire placed through the metacarpal bones. Traction and countertraction are exerted through these wires, and the arm encased in a plaster cast which incorporates the wires. When the cast dries, traction is maintained by the force exerted through the wires by the cast. This method of fixation traction may be used in comminuted, unstable fractures of the Colles type as well.

In the treatment of all fractures of the wrist and hand, several basic essentials should be kept in mind.

First, fractures of the hand and fingers should be immobilized in the position of function. Should serious stiffness develop, the patient would at least retain the ability to grasp objects with the hand and the thumb would still be in a position of apposition to the fingers.

Swelling should be kept under control by compression and elevation of the injured part. Early and consistent motion of the fingers not immobilized will help prevent stiffness of the hand. If the arm is immobilized in a sling, there is the additional danger of a stiffening of the shoulder. This should be counteracted by exercises for the shoulder.

Following removal of the splint or cast, the joint must be mobilized and the muscle power restored. Soaking, massaging and exercising the wrist and hand in warm, soapy water several times daily helps to restore function.

THE FOREARM

In treating fractures of the forearm, restoration of the normal relationship of the radius and ulna is essential if maximum function is to be achieved. The ulna may be regarded as a downward extension of the arm. The strong hingelike joint with the humerus makes for stability, allowing primarily flexion and extension. The radius, however, is functionally an upward extension of the hand. By rotating about the ulna, the radius carries the hand into pronation and supination, motions vital to the dexterity of the hand. Although the ulna does not rotate in this action, it does deviate slightly medially and laterally during pronation and supination. However, its primary function is to provide stability for the rotation of the radius about it.

The two bones articulate at the proximal and distal radio-ulnar joints. The integrity of both joints is essential for normal rotation. The two bones are bound together by the interosseous membrane and the strong ligaments of the proximal and distal joints. Flexibility of the interosseous membrane and these ligaments is essential for normal movement.

It is obvious that, if one bone in the forearm breaks and angulates or shortens, these joints must be disturbed. Restoration of these joints must be accomplished if proper function is to be achieved.

The complex motions of the forearm and hand require a complex muscle structure. First, there are the two pronators: the pronator teres and the pronator quadratus. They both attach to the lower two-thirds of the radius and rotate it into pronation.

The muscles which rotate the radius outward are the supinator brevis and the biceps. Both of these muscles insert on the upper third of the radius.

When the hand is in full pronation, the brachioradialis also serves as a supinator. However, its principal function is to flex the forearm. The biceps and pronator teres also have a flexor action on the elbow, as well as that of rotating the radius.

Directly opposing the biceps and other flexors is the triceps. Attaching to the olecranon process of the ulna, it extends the forearm.

In addition to these flexors and rotators, with their crosswise pull, the surgeon must contend with the muscles that exert a longitudinal pull between the elbow and wrist. The carpal and digital extensors form one group, and the carpal and digital flexors another group.

The brachioradialis pulls nearly parallel to the bones. These longitudinal forces tend to produce shortening and overriding in all forearm fractures. However, it is the action of the pronators and supinators which causes the greatest difficulty. They pull in directions more or less transverse to the long axis of the bones (Fig. 26).

This fundamental problem—muscles pulling crosswise against the bone—is basic to all fractures of the forearm. The muscles

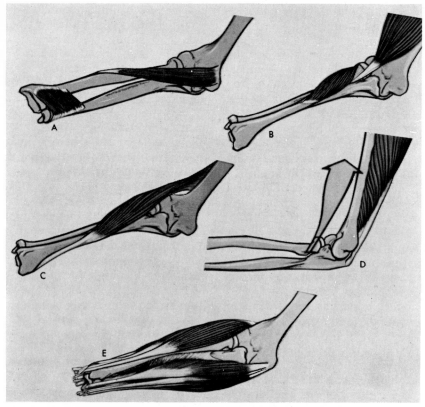

Figure 26.   *A,* The pronator teres and pronator quadratus attach on the lower two-thirds of the radius and rotate it into pronation. *B,* The supinator brevis and the biceps muscle insert on the upper one-third of the radius and rotate it into supination. *C,* The brachioradialis muscle acts as a supinator of the radius with the arm in pronation. *D,* The triceps muscle attaching to the olecranon process extends the forearm. *E,* The digital flexor and extensor muscle groups pull in the long axis of the forearm bones and cause shortening when both bones are fractured. It is the combined forces of the forearm musculature which produce the deformities which are characteristic of the various types of fractures in this area.

of the forearm are extremely active and will produce great deformity unless immobilization is maintained until the fracture heals.

It is obvious that even a slight deformity may interfere with normal functioning of the forearm and hand. Therefore, it is important that the greatest care be exercised in reduction and maintenance of reduction.

FRACTURES OF THE ULNA.   Fractures of the shaft of the ulna are often the result of direct violence, while fractures of the radius are more commonly caused by indirect violence. A blow against the ulna may cause a fracture in any portion of the bone. Since the bone is subcutaneous along the extensor surface of the forearm, the injury may produce an open fracture rather easily. Angulation of the fracture is usually toward the radius, because the elasticity of the interosseous membrane tends to pull the two bones together. The triceps muscle tends to extend the proximal fragment, causing dorsal angulation. Since the rotator muscles of the forearm attach primarily to the radius, there is less tendency

for rotational displacement in ulnar fractures than in fractures of the radius. Angulation may be difficult to correct, more so if comminution of the fragments is present. Traction and manipulation are attempted and, if successful, the arm and forearm are immobilized in a cast extending from the distal palmar flexion crease to just below the axilla with the elbow flexed to 90 degrees and the forearm in midpronation and supination (Fig. 27).

Recurrence of angulation in the cast occurs frequently. Re-examination by x-ray films must be done in a few days and thereafter at regular intervals during the healing process. If the angulation cannot be corrected or recurs in the cast, open reduction with internal fixation must be done. This is most easily accomplished with an intramedullary rod placed through the entire length of the bone. The fracture usually heals in eight to ten weeks. This method should not be employed in children while the bones are still growing. Slight angulation of the

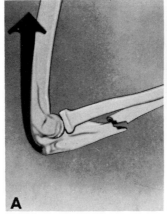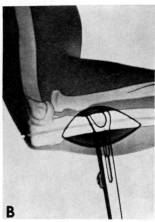

Figure 27.   *A*, The pull of the triceps muscle tends to extend the proximal fragment and may produce dorsal angulation of the fracture. The cast must be molded carefully along the ulna to counteract the angulation force of the triceps muscle. *B*, When the ulna cannot be held in reduction by a cast, open reduction must be performed. An intramedullary rod is used for fixation.

ulna in the growing child will correct with growth of the bone.

FRACTURES OF THE SHAFT OF THE RADIUS. Any fracture in the shaft of the radius, accompanied by shortening of the bone, involves the distal radio-ulnar joint. The distal fragment of the radius, together with the hand, is displaced upward. The brachioradialis, attaching to the lower end of the radius, and the other long muscles of the forearm are active in this displacement. Since the ulna remains stationary, the ligaments are stretched or torn and the distal articulation is disrupted. The hand is displaced laterally, and the lower end of the ulna becomes abnormally prominent on the medial side (Fig. 28).

Unless the normal relationship is re-established between the articular surfaces of the

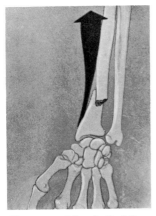

Figure 28.   Fractures of the shaft of the radius disrupt the distal radio-ulnar joint. The radius is displaced proximally on the ulna by the pull of the brachioradialis and long forearm muscles. The elastic interosseous membrane tends to pull the ends of the fractured radius toward the ulna, and the brachioradialis and pronator quadratus tend to angulate the radius toward the ulna.

radius and ulna, pronation and supination will be limited. To avoid such disability, it is essential to restore the radius to normal length. In addition, lateral pressure should be applied at the wrist so that the damaged ligaments may heal in normal position.

In all fractures of the radial shaft, the interosseous membrane tends to draw the ends of the fragments toward the ulna. When the fracture is low in the shaft, this type of angulation is greatly aggravated by the cross-pull of the pronator quadratus, assisted by the brachioradialis. To counteract this displacement, traction should be exerted mainly on the radial side of the hand, and the hand should be in ulnar deviation when the arm is immobilized.

The rotational displacement in fractures of the shaft of the radius depends upon whether the fracture is above or below the insertion of the pronator teres. When the fracture is above the insertion of that muscle, the proximal fragment is held in supination by the biceps and supinator brevis. The two pronator muscles, however, pull the distal fragment into pronation (Fig. 29).

Since the proximal fragment cannot be controlled in this instance, it is necessary to supinate the distal fragment in order to align the two and effect a reduction.

When the fracture occurs below the insertion of the pronator teres, that muscle serves to counteract the supinators, so that the proximal fragment is held in a position midway between pronation and supination. In order to align the fragments, the distal fragment must be rotated to midposition (Fig. 30).

If a fracture of the radius is transverse, it can usually be reduced without operation.

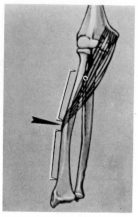

Figure 29.   The displacement in fractures of the radius and of both bones of the forearm depends upon the location of the fracture in relation to the insertion of the pronator teres muscle.

The patient's forearm is suspended from looped bandages attached to an overhead bar. The pull is applied through the index and middle fingers, so that the traction is mainly on the radial side of the hand. A weight hanging from the upper arm provides the required countertraction. Traction must be strong enough to restore the radius to normal length.

The two fragments can then be aligned to the same degree of rotation. Since the proximal fragment cannot be controlled, the surgeon moves the distal fragment until it, too, is in the neutral position, midway between pronation and supination. It is in this position that it must be held during the healing period (Fig. 31).

Before the cast is applied to a fractured radius, the damaged radio-ulnar ligaments

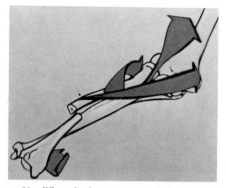

Figure 30.   When the fracture occurs below the insertion of the pronator teres, the pronator teres tends to counteract the supinator, and the proximal fragment remains in midpronation and supination. When the fracture occurs above the insertion of the pronator teres, the proximal fragment is held in supination by the biceps and supinator brevis muscles.

should be supported by felt pads over the distal ends of the radius and ulna. The pressure at the wrist is applied laterally so that there is no impairment of circulation. The cast, on the other hand, avoids lateral pressure and is molded to the flexor and extensor surfaces of the forearm in order to force the shafts of the radius and ulna apart during the healing period. The arm is immobilized with the elbow at a right angle, which helps relax the pull of the biceps.

In many fractures of the lower radius, it may be impossible to prevent angulation and overriding by closed methods, particularly if the fracture is oblique or comminuted. If this occurs, open reduction with internal fixation is required to maintain reduction. Plate and screw fixation is particularly suitable for the radius when it is important to prevent rotary movement of one fragment upon the other. The plate allows the fragments to rotate as a single unit.

FRACTURES OF BOTH BONES OF THE FOREARM. When both bones of the forearm are fractured above the pronator teres insertion, just as when the radius alone is fractured at that level, the upper fragments are held in supination by the biceps and supinator brevis. The lower fragments, controlled by the two pronators, move into the pronated position. The pull of the extensors and flexors for the hand and wrist produces pronounced overriding. If uncorrected, these forces always cause permanent disability. Hemorrhage and edema distend the fascial envelope of the forearm and increase the shortening. Organization of this inflammatory exudate makes the tissues inelastic in a few days; therefore, it is important that the fracture be reduced early (Fig. 32).

The method of reduction is similar to the one used for reducing a fractured radius. With the flexed arm suspended from an overhead bar and countertraction provided by weights, the surgeon's hands are free to manipulate the bones back into alignment. Traction must be strong enough to restore the full length to both bones. The fragments are then manipulated to end-to-end apposition. The distal fragments are rotated into full supination to restore the proper rotational alignment with the proximal fragments, which are held in this position by the biceps and supinator brevis muscles. The cast is applied from the distal palmar flexion crease to the axilla with the elbow flexed to 90 degrees (Fig. 33).

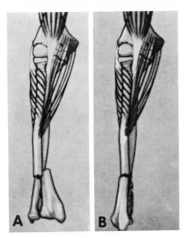

Figure 31.   The distal fragment of the radius, which can be controlled, is rotated to midpronation to align it with the proximal fragment, which cannot be controlled.

If the fracture occurs below the pronator teres, the general principles of treatment are similar. However, the pronator teres and the supinator muscles balance each other, so that the proximal fragment remains in neutral position. The distal fragment is pronated (Fig. 34).

To reduce the fractures, the surgeon restores the distal fragments to a position of midpronation and supination so that they are aligned with the proximal fragments. The entire forearm is then immobilized in this position midway between pronation and supination. Closed reduction of these forearm fractures is usually successful when the fractures are transverse.

It is important to examine the alignment by x-ray films at least once a week for the first few weeks. There is a tendency for

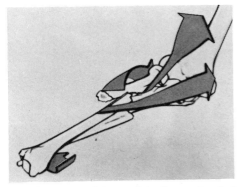

Figure 32.   When both bones of the forearm break above the insertion of the pronator teres, the proximal fragments are held in supination by the supinator brevis and biceps muscles. The pronators hold the distal fragments in pronation. The pull of the flexor and extensor muscles causes shortening.

angulation to occur in the cast, and this must be promptly corrected because forearm bones will not rotate properly when angulated.

If the fractures are comminuted, or unstable, cast immobilization will not hold the fragments in reduction and internal fixation is required. Frequently, an intramedullary rod is used to fix the ulna, since the bone is relatively straight and has little tendency to rotate. Plates and screws applied to the radius maintain fixation and prevent rotation (Fig. 35).

Other methods of internal splinting include the use of two plates, or a combination of plate and bone graft. Whatever the means of internal fixation, it should always be supplemented by an external cast until the fragments unite.

All forearm fractures should be immobilized with the dressing extending above the flexed elbow and below the wrist. Unless this is done, the forearm bones will not remain in the proper rotational relationships as the fracture heals.

A circular dressing which extends only from the hand to the elbow does not prevent rotation of the forearm, but, if the dressing extends above the flexed elbow, it is apparent that the arm will remain in the position of pronation or supination in which the surgeon has placed it.

The cast should be molded along the flexor and extensor surfaces of the forearm to prevent lateral pressure on the bones, which tends to force the radius toward the ulna. Synostosis of the radius to the ulna is an ever-present danger in forearm fractures. Molding the cast along the flexor and extensor surfaces forces the muscle masses between the bones throughout the length of the forearm and tends to prevent this complication (Fig. 36).

MONTEGGIA'S FRACTURE-DISLOCATION. A fracture of the shaft of the ulna with dislocation of the head of the radius at the elbow was described by Monteggia. The fracture-dislocation may occur as a result of a direct blow warded off by the forearm, with the elbow flexed. The force of the blow fractures the ulna and carries through to the radius. Although the radius is not fractured, it is torn loose from the orbicular ligament and dislocates upward and forward. More often the fracture results from indirect violence caused by a fall on the extended hand in which violent pronation force is applied to the forearm. With

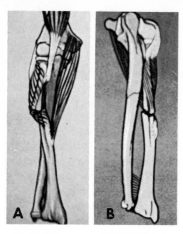

Figure 33.   *A,* Proximal fragments of the radius and ulna are held in full supination. *B,* Distal fragments are rotated into supination to align them with proximal fragments.

Figure 34.   When both bones of the forearm break below the insertion of the pronator teres, the proximal fragments are held in midpronation, while the distal are held in full pronation. The distal fragments are rotated to midpronation to effect reduction.

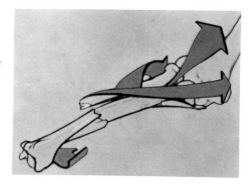

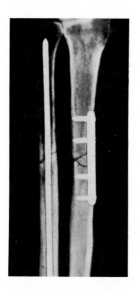

Figure 35.   Unstable forearm fractures cannot be held in reduction by cast fixation. An effective method of internal fixation of forearm fractures is illustrated.

Figure 36.   A cast applied with lateral pressure forces the forearm bones toward each other, and in this position, synostosis is likely. However, pressure made along the flexor and extensor surfaces of the forearm forces these muscles between the bones and tends to separate them, which lessens the danger of synostosis.

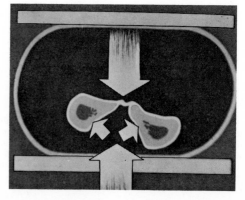

the hand fixed to the ground, the force of the falling body twists the forearm to extreme pronation. The radius reaches the maximum degree of pronation and lies across the shaft of the ulna in the midforearm. The ulna acts as a lever forcing the head of the radius forward or laterally. The orbicular ligament ruptures and the head of the radius dislocates forward. The displacement is increased by the pull of the biceps muscle. The support of the radius is lost, and the force is transmitted to the ulna which fractures usually in the middle or upper one-third of the bone. The characteristic displacement results from the pull of muscles around the elbow. The biceps exerts an upward pull on the radius and the distal fragment of the ulna. The triceps pulls the proximal fragment of the ulna in the opposite direction. The long muscles of the forearm produce overriding and shortening and alteration of the carrying angle. However, it is the opposing pulls of the biceps and triceps muscle that make it difficult to maintain these fractures in reduction (Fig. 37).

The displacement of the radius may injure the motor branch of the radial nerve as it passes through the supinator brevis muscle. The median and ulnar nerves and the brachial artery and its branches may be injured. It is important to examine carefully the neurovascular condition of the forearm and hand.

In treating this injury, the surgeon should first attempt a closed reduction. Longitudinal traction is applied with the arm in extension. Once the ulna has been reduced, the head of the radius is pressed back to its normal position, and the arm flexed beyond

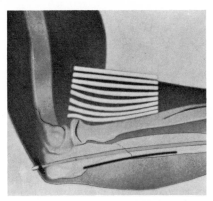

Figure 38. Reduction of the head of the radius is maintained by flexion of the elbow. The ulna requires firm splinting to prevent angulation by the triceps muscle. Internal fixation of the ulnar fragments with an intramedullary rod may be necessary to maintain reduction.

a right angle. This flexed position holds the radial head firmly in reduction. However, such flexion places a pull on the triceps, which tends to angulate the ulna. This bone, therefore, requires firm splinting. A posterior molded plaster splint is applied to hold the ulna in reduction. The circular plaster cast maintains the flexed position, thus holding the radial head in place. Since, in most instances, even the firmest splint will not prevent angulation of the ulna, this reduction must be watched closely until the fragments are united (Fig. 38).

When this injury occurs in children, the reduction is usually stable because of the partially intact sleeve of tough periosteum about the ulna. In the adult, however, often the ulna can be maintained in position only by internal fixation. An intramedullary pin inserted through the olecranon is one satisfactory method of holding this fracture in reduction.

FRACTURES OF THE FOREARM IN CHILDREN. Fractures of the forearm in children are commonly caused by indirect violence. In young children, the most common site is in the distal one-third of the forearm, usually an inch or two above the wrist. The mechanism of production and the displacement are similar to the Colles fracture in the adult. Usually, both bones break at about the same level. Reduction is accomplished by traction, increasing the angulation and by pressure of the surgeon's thumb over the dorsum of the fracture site while the fingers make counter-pressure over the volar surface. The angulation is straightened while this pressure is applied. This maneuver engages the fracture ends which may then be levered

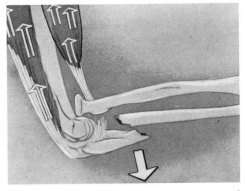

Figure 37. Monteggia's fracture is characterized by fracture of the ulna with dislocation of the head of the radius. The biceps muscle pulls the radius upward while the triceps extends the ulna. The long forearm muscles produce overriding and shortening.

straight. The reduction must be done as early as possible, because after a few days, thickening of the heavy periosteum of the child may make reduction impossible. Perfect apposition is not necessary, but angulation should be corrected as much as possible. Rotational deformity must be fully corrected. Moderate angulation will be corrected promptly by growth in the young child. Rotational deformity will persist. Side-to-side apposition of the fragments is acceptable if rotation and angulation have been corrected, as remodeling of the growing bone rapidly corrects this deformity. The accuracy of reduction is much less critical in the growing child than in the adult.

In the middle one-third of the forearm, greenstick fracture of the radius, ulna or both bones is a common injury. The mechanism may be from a direct blow, but more often is the result of indirect violence of a fall on the outstretched hand. The fracture is incomplete, usually with volar angulation and no rotational deformity. Less frequently, the angulation is dorsalward if the child falls on the flexed rather than the extended hand.

Correction of this type fracture requires reversal of the angulation to the point of overcorrection. This necessitates completing the fracture through the intact cortex by overcorrecting the angulation until a distinct snap is heard or felt by the surgeon. Care should be exercised to prevent displacement after the fracture has been completed. If the greenstick fracture is not converted to a complete fracture, angulation inevitably recurs in the plaster cast.

Recurrence of deformity in the cast is frequent in children. X-ray examination should be repeated at weekly intervals. If angulation in the cast increases, the cast should be changed rather than wedged. In the growing child, fractures heal rapidly and correction of recurrent deformity must be done early. After a week or ten days, the consistency of the fracture is such that angulation may be corrected as though bending a lead pipe with little danger of displacement. In the adult, healing is slower and wedging the cast is less likely to cause displacement when correcting angulation because the fracture is less stable. In the child, however, the "lead pipe" consistency of the fracture produces excessive soft tissue pressure if wedging is attempted, and pressure necrosis of the soft parts is a real danger.

The circulation of the arm must be watched carefully for the first 24 hours. If the child is not admitted to the hospital for observation during this period, the parents must be instructed in the signs of impaired circulation. Pain, cyanosis or pallor, and paralysis of the muscles are the cardinal signs of impaired circulation. Pain is the most consistent early sign. After reduction of a fracture in a child, pain should be minimal, requiring only mild sedation such as aspirin. If any of the signs of circulatory impairment occur, the cast must be opened promptly to relieve pressure on the blood vessels. A few hours delay may result in the permanent damage of Volkmann's ischemic contracture.

THE ELBOW

In treating fractures about the elbow, the surgeon must recognize the mechanics of joint function and must realize the importance of the related soft tissue anatomy. The bones involved are the lower end of the humerus, the upper end of the radius with its cup-shaped head, and the upper end of the ulna, terminating in the olecranon.

At the point of articulation, the humerus has two condyles: medially the trochlea, which articulates with the ulna in a hinge joint, and laterally the rounded capitellum, upon which the radius rotates. The radius also articulates with the ulna at the radial notch.

On the humerus, the points of attachment for important muscle groups are the lateral and medial epicondyles, and just above the epicondyles the lateral and medial supracondylar ridges.

One of the important characteristics of the elbow is the angle at which the forearm bones meet the humerus when the elbow is extended. This carrying angle, as it is called, is normally about 16 degrees. With the arm at the side and the elbow fully extended, this angle throws the hand away from the body, thus facilitating the carrying of bulky objects. If, after a fracture is healed, the patient has the deformity of an increased carrying angle, there is excessive strain on the elbow and wrist when he carries a weight (Fig. 39).

In addition, the ulnar nerve, which crosses the elbow joint, is stretched around this abnormal angle, and ulnar nerve palsy may follow. If the carrying angle is decreased or

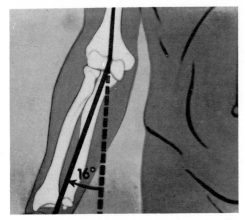

Figure 39. The normal carrying angle at the elbow is approximately 16 degrees. Alteration of this angle following fracture of the humeral condyles causes varying degrees of disability.

reversed, not only is there an added strain on the elbow, but on the shoulder as well, and the deformity is unsightly. For these reasons, it is important that the carrying angle be carefully checked before a fracture may be considered reduced.

A second mechanical factor must be considered when treating fractures about the elbow. As the elbow joint functions in flexion and extension, the two forearm bones move together as one unit, describing parallel arcs. This is possible because the two condyles of the humerus have a common axis.

If a fracture is allowed to heal with the condyles malaligned, the radius and ulna no longer move about a common axis. Efforts to flex and extend the arm meet the resistance of ligaments twisted and overstretched by the bony obstruction. This effectively blocks the range of motion in the joint. Accurate realignment of the joint surfaces, therefore, is essential if normal function in the elbow is to be restored.

The muscles attached about the elbow also play an important role in producing the deformities in fractures about the elbow. Attached to the medial epicondyle through a common tendon is the group of flexor muscles for the hand and wrist. Their displacing effect on the condyles depends on whether the elbow is flexed or extended and the pull is along the forearm toward the wrist. In flexion, these muscles pull the epicondyle forward; in extension, the fragment is pulled downward and outward. A similar force is exerted on the lateral condyle by the extensors for the hand and wrist. They attach to the lateral epicondyle and the supracondylar ridge just

above it. Arising from the medial supracondylar ridge, the pronator teres crosses obliquely to insert on the lateral margin of the radius. The diagonal pull of this muscle tends to rotate a fractured trochlea forward and inward toward the radius. Overlying the extensor is the brachioradialis, which attaches high on the lateral supracondylar ridge. In certain fractures of the capitellum, the brachioradialis has a tendency to rotate the fragment forward at its upper end (Fig. 40).

The muscles of the arm also affect fractures about the elbow. The brachialis, a flexor of the forearm, pulls upward on the ulna. Through the humero-ulnar articulation, this upward force is transmitted to the trochlea, tending to cause upward displacement of the trochlea when it is fractured. The biceps muscle, which flexes and supinates the forearm, pulls upward on the radius at the capitellum, through the humeroradial joint, and causes similar upward displacement of the capitellum. On the back of the elbow, the surgeon is chiefly concerned with the triceps muscle. It inserts into the olecranon, exerts an upward pull and extends the forearm. This pull is important in all fractures of the olecranon, since the force separates the olecranon process from the ulna.

The ulnar nerve is endangered by certain fractures. The nerve rounds the elbow behind the medial epicondyle, where it lies directly on the bone. Displacement of the medial condyle or angulation of the elbow may stretch or contuse the nerve at this point. The median nerve crosses over the medial condyle in front of the elbow while the radial nerve crosses over the front of the lateral condyle. The nerves are flanked by the radial and ulnar arteries arising from the brachial artery, which lies on the anteromedial aspect of the elbow joint and lower humerus.

These structures are confined by the tight, deep fascial envelope about the elbow, and may be compressed by excessive swelling in this compartment. Displaced fracture fragments may contuse or lacerate either the blood vessels or nerves, or both. If the elbow is fixed in acute flexion after injury, these structures in the cubital space may be subject to excessive pressure. Any of these factors may produce paralysis or circulatory impairment. Circulatory inadequacy may lead to Volkmann's ischemic contracture or gangrene.

SUPRACONDYLAR FRACTURES OF THE HUMERUS. A supracondylar fracture of the hu-

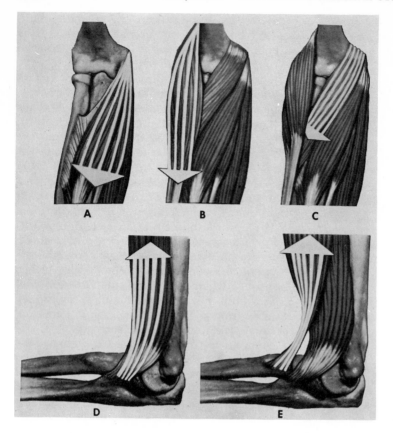

Figure 40. *A*, Flexor muscles of the hand arise on the medial epicondyle, and pull the condyle downward and forward when it is fractured. *B*, The extensor muscles of the hand, along with the brachioradialis, arise on the lateral epicondyle and supracondylar ridge, and tend to pull fragments of the fractured lateral condyle downward and rotate it forward. *C*, The pronator teres muscle tends to pull fractures of the medial condyle in toward the radius and forward. *D*, The brachioradialis muscle pulls the trochlea upward when the medial condyle is fractured. *E*, The biceps muscle pulls the capitellum upward when the bone is broken.

merus, which occurs frequently in children, is caused by a fall on the hand with the elbow flexed. The force is transmitted upward along the radius and the ulna, and strikes the lower end of the humerus anteriorly. The falling body directly opposes this force. The fracture occurs at the thinnest part of the humerus, from front to back just above the condyles. The force of the fracture displaces the condyles posteriorly. The triceps, biceps and brachialis contract and hold the fragment in this displaced position and draw it upward. Medial or lateral shearing force may displace the condylar fragment inward or outward. Rotational forces may rotate the condyles medially or laterally to a moderate degree. The jagged end of the proximal fragment projecting into the anterior cubital space threatens the median nerve and the brachial artery. Before reduction is undertaken, the surgeon should examine the patient to make sure that the fracture has not damaged these structures. The radial pulse is felt and the patient is asked to close the fingers, then to open them and to oppose the thumb and the little finger in order to determine if the median nerve is undamaged. The

radial nerve is examined by having the patient extend the fingers and wrist, and the ulnar nerve by spreading the fingers apart and bringing them back together. Sensation of the fingers and hand should also be evaluated (Fig. 41).

As with all fractures, reduction should be undertaken as soon as possible. The patient is given a general anesthetic and placed supine upon the operating table. Countertraction is provided by a sheet or padded bandage passed under the patient's axilla on the injured side and tied to the table at the opposite side. In the case of a child, since little force is required, traction is made manually. First, the elbow is extended, relaxing the triceps. With countertraction provided, traction is applied longitudinally. The fingers of one hand are placed on the anterior surface of the arm, and the thumb on the posterior surface, beneath the lower fragment of the humerus. When the fragments have been drawn past each other, the surgeon uses his thumb and fingers to press the fragments into alignment. With the other hand, the surgeon angulates, rotates, flexes or extends the arm as necessary. The thumb and fingers of one hand then force the

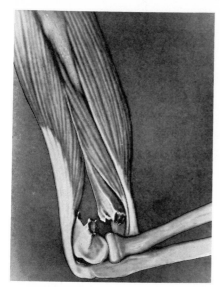

Figure 41. The force of the fall displaces the humeral condyles posteriorly, where the triceps, biceps and brachialis muscles hold the fragment.

fragments into anterior posterior alignment. The other hand manipulates the forearm from side to side to achieve medial and lateral as well as rotational alignment. The elbow is then flexed to 105 degrees. This stretches the triceps and locks the fragments in place (Fig. 42).

After the reduction is complete, the surgeon checks it by gently flexing the forearm. His thumb stays in position against the posterior surface of the lower fragment to prevent recurrence of the backward displacement. If the elbow easily flexes to 105 degrees, anterior-posterior alignment has been achieved. At this point, the pulse is again palpated to make sure that the radial artery is undamaged. The arm is then fully extended and an estimate made of the carrying angle and the rotational alignment of the lower fragment with the upper.

A final evaluation of the reduction can be made by fully supinating the hand and placing the arm in as much flexion as swelling will allow. The forearm should come into alignment with the upper arm. If there is an inward rotation of the fragment, the forearm falls into a position medial to the upper arm. On the other hand, if there is outward rotation, the flexed forearm falls in the lateral position. If the fracture has been reduced correctly, the index finger will point approximately to the tip of the shoulder (Fig. 43).

The fracture heals with the elbow flexed at a 105-degree angle. In this position, the triceps tendon locks the fragments in place. The arm can be immobilized by one of several devices. A posterior molded plaster splint applied from the axilla to the palm is a simple and effective method for maintaining position.

The surgeon must watch with the greatest care for signs of impaired circulation in the forearm and hand during the first few days after reduction. There is always a threat of a Volkmann's contracture following a supracondylar fracture. If the radial pulse disappears or if the signs of circulatory failure appear, the extremity must be extended at the elbow immediately. Often this change of position allows decompression of the blood vessels with return of adequate circulation. It may be necessary to suspend the arm in Dunlop's traction if the swelling is excessive to maintain the reduction as well as the circulation. This method applies moderate traction

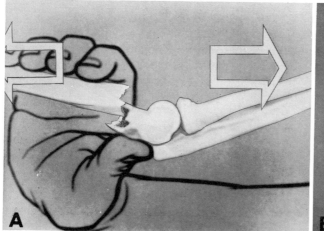
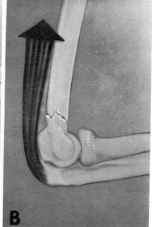

Figure 42. *A*, Reduction of supracondylar fractures of the humerus is accomplished by traction and manipulation. *B*, With the elbow flexed, the taut triceps muscle holds the reduced condyles in position.

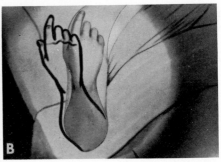
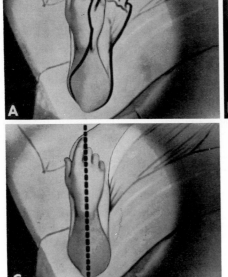

Figure 43. To check the rotational alignment and carrying angle after reduction, the surgeon flexes the fractured arm at the elbow. *A,* If there is inward rotation, the index finger will point medial to the shoulder. *B,* If outward rotation is present, the finger will point laterally. *C,* When reduction is correct, the finger tip will point toward the tip of the shoulder.

in suspension with the elbow only slightly flexed, relieving pressure in the blood vessels. The position may be maintained until the swelling subsides or until union of the bone is firm, usually three or four weeks. If the circulation does not return immediately, the deep fascia of the forearm and elbow must be incised to decompress the blood vessels. As soon as the fracture is healed, the patient is allowed to re-establish motion with his own muscles without forceful manipulation.

CONDYLAR FRACTURES OF THE HUMERUS. **Fractures of the capitellum.** Fractures between the condyles may break off either the trochlea or the capitellum, or the condyles may split from the shaft of the humerus, forming a Y- or V-shaped fracture. The mechanism of fracture is usually indirect violence. A fall on the outstretched hand with the elbow in extension drives the forearm bones against the condyles of the humerus. If the force angulates the elbow medially, the radial head is driven against the capitellum, which is displaced upward. The pull of the biceps muscle holds the fragment in this position, and the carrying angle is increased. In addition, the fragment is rotated outward and often forward by the downward pull of the extensor muscles of the forearm which originate from the lateral epicondyle.

The arc of motion in flexion and extension is blocked by such fractures; therefore, it is necessary to obtain exact alignment of the capitellum with the trochlea, so that function will be restored. The fractures can be reduced by straight traction on the arm, with lateral pressure over the medial condyle. Angulation of the forearm against this fulcrum increases the traction on the capitellum through the radial collateral ligament, pulling the fragment down. The fingers are used to mold the fragments into accurate position. With the fingers still holding the fragment in position, the arm is then flexed to 90 to 110 degrees. Pressure with the thumb completes the alignment. X-ray films taken from proper angles will help determine whether the fragment has been restored to its normal position.

Often, because of the pull of the extensor muscles, the fragment is rotated outward 90 degrees or more. The articular surface then lies against the fractured surface of the trochlea and manipulation fails to correct this rotary displacement. It is important to recognize this deformity in the adult, but more so in the child. The distal humerus in the young child is mostly cartilaginous, and only the small center of ossification of the epiphysis of the capitellum may be visible on the x-ray film. As in all fractures in children, both extremities must be x-rayed in comparable positions so that an accurate estimate of displacement can be made. If this rotational deformity is not corrected and the fracture reduced accurately, nonunion is almost certain. In the child, marked growth disturbance occurs, characterized by angulation at the elbow, which increases the carrying angle and slowly produces ulnar nerve palsy.

Open reduction should be performed promptly in either the child or adult if the deformity cannot be corrected. The fragments are fitted together under direct vision and held in reduction by two small pins driven through the capitellum into the humerus. The pins are removed when the fracture heals.

Occasionally, the capitellum in the adult is split off from the humerus in the frontal plane. This fracture displaces the anterior half of the capitellum upward. Since there are no soft tissue attachments to the fragment, it lies free in the joint and usually cannot be manipulated into position by closed methods. If, at open operation, it is found that the fragment is completely devoid of blood supply, it should be removed. If soft tissues are still attached, the fragment may be replaced and held by appropriate internal fixation.

FRACTURES OF THE MEDIAL CONDYLE AND TROCHLEA OF HUMERUS. Fractures of the trochlea and of the medial condyle of the humerus are produced by a mechanism similar to that of the lateral condyle, except that the angulating force is lateral. The ulna transmits the force to the trochlea, which splits away from the capitellum and is displaced upward. The carrying angle is decreased or reversed. The upward displacement is maintained by the pull of the brachialis and triceps. The fragment is rotated forward by the flexor muscles of the wrist and hand, as well as by the pronator teres, which originates on the medial epicondyle. There is less tendency for the fracture to rotate medially away from the humerus because of the hingelike connection with the ulna, which stabilizes the fracture in this plane.

Y AND T FRACTURES OF THE CONDYLES. Y and T fractures of the condyles of the humerus are combinations of the two previously mentioned fractures, and usually occur in adults. Comminution of fragments frequently makes reduction difficult. Since the stabilizing influence of one intact condyle is lost when both break from the humerus, some type of continuous traction is necessary to maintain reduction. This may be supplied in suspension traction, or by the weight of a hanging cast. This cast, applied from the axilla to the palm with the elbow in 90 degrees of flexion, is suspended from the wrist by a bandage looped about the neck. The cast, thus, is supported only at the wrist, and the weight of the cast at the elbow produces the traction when the patient is standing or sitting. This traction is made through the joint capsule and ligaments. Since the capsule is sleevelike, this pull tends to mold the fragments together. Although this method of treatment allows the patient to be ambulatory, he must sleep in a semi-sitting position for the cast to maintain traction. Open reduction with internal fixation is occasionally required if the fragments cannot be molded into position by traction applied through the joint capsule (Fig. 44).

FRACTURES OF THE OLECRANON PROCESS. Either direct or muscular violence may cause a fracture of the olecranon process. Such fractures occur in a transverse direction and extend into the joint. The triceps, which is attached to the olecranon, pulls the proximal fragment upward. Flexion of the elbow separates the fragments farther. Since it is extremely difficult to overcome the pull of the triceps by any closed method, fracture of the olecranon can best be reduced by operation, if complete asepsis can be assured. Since the fracture occurs in the joint, the consequences of infection are particularly serious.

Internal fixation may be obtained by suturing the fragments together with wire, or by an intramedullary rod placed through the olecranon into the medullary canal of the ulna. Because joint surfaces are involved, accurate restoration of these surfaces is paramount for ideal function. When marked comminu-

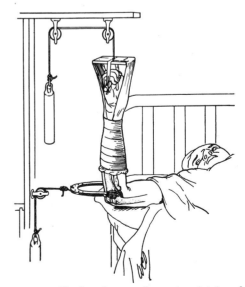

Figure 44. If a hanging cast does not maintain reduction of condylar fractures, skeletal traction may be applied through the olecranon. The forearm is held by suspension.

tion of the olecranon fragment prevents accurate reduction, it may be necessary to excise the fragments and suture the triceps tendon to the ulna. A compression dressing and sling are used for a week while reaction from the trauma and surgery subsides. Then gentle active motion is begun to avoid stiffness and adhesions within the joint.

FRACTURES OF THE HEAD OF THE RADIUS. Fracture of the head of the radius occurs as the result of a fall on the outstretched arm, with the elbow in slight flexion. The force is transmitted upward along the shaft of the radius to the head, driving the head against the capitellum. Sometimes, this type of injury results in very minor damage, producing simple longitudinal fissures in the head. Also, the fracture may occur through the neck, just below the head. Such fractures are usually impacted, and there may be very little displacement. When a fracture in this area results in very little angulation or displacement, it can be treated conservatively with splinting. Motion may be started within a week. However, if the head of the bone is angulated so that the articular surface does not fit the capitellum, or the radio-ulnar joint is disrupted, reduction must be done. Failure to correct marked angulation will result in faulty flexion and extension, as well as limited pronation and supination. Since the head of the radius is devoid of ligamentous attachment, traction and manipulation by angulation have little effect upon it. Direct pressure with the thumb over the radial head accompanied by pronation and supination may correct angulation; however, open reduction is often necessary (Fig. 45).

In the child, moderate angulation will be corrected by growth and may be accepted. A mechanism similar to that which produces the radial neck fracture may cause the proximal radial epiphysis to slip. The displacement may be lateral, forward or backward. Closed manipulation reduction should be attempted. If the displacement is great, open reduction may be done gently, forcing the fragments into alignment under direct vision. The radial head must never be removed in a growing child because serious growth disturbance in the forearm will result.

Often, in the adult, the fragile rim of the radial head is broken into several fragments. When the injury is severe, it seriously interferes with the rotation of the forearm. These fragments cannot be manipulated back into position, and they serve as irritants in the joint. Therefore, it is advisable to remove the head of the radius. In the adult, this may be done without serious loss of function. It is essential, however, to start motion in the elbow within a few days after the operation to prevent adhesions. Since in this procedure the support for the radius against the capitellum is lost, the radius tends to shorten, throwing strain on the distal radioulnar joint. This may produce pain at the wrist for a time; however, the joint eventually compensates for this strain and the pain usually disappears after several months.

PULLED ELBOW. In children from one and a half to about four years of age, the confusing injury termed "pulled elbow" occurs. During this period, the head of the radius is little, if any, larger in diameter than the shaft of the bone. The orbicular ligament may partially

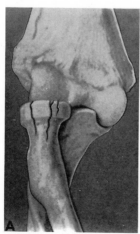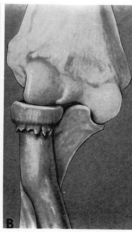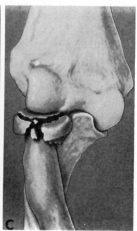

Figure 45. *A,* Longitudinal fissure fractures may occur in the head of the radius without displacement. *B,* The head of the radius may be impacted on the neck, with varying degrees of displacement. *C,* Fractures with marked displacement of fragments may require removal of the entire radial head.

subluxate over the radial head with longitudinal traction, limiting elbow motion, and pronation and supination of the forearm. The injury is usually produced by the parent by jerking the toddler up onto a step or curbing by the extended arm. The child cries out and holds the elbow slightly flexed with the forearm in pronation. The symptoms of pseudoparalysis are present, and the child cries with any manipulation of the upper extremity. The x-ray studies are normal, adding to the confusion of diagnosis. The history of the injury is important for diagnosis, although the child may also produce the injury by catching the arm in the slots of a crib without the parents' knowledge.

Reduction is accomplished by flexing the elbow to 90 degrees, followed by abrupt full supination. Usually, a snap is felt and the child cries out. Shortly thereafter, the child begins to use the arm normally. The arm should be immobilized in a sling for a week to prevent recurrence, and the parents should be instructed to avoid repeating the injury.

Several basic principles apply in the treatment of most of these fractures about the elbow. One is to so reduce the fracture that the normal carrying angle at the elbow is maintained. Another is to align the fragments so that in flexion and extension, the radius and ulna move in concentric arcs. Just as important as proper alignment is the maintenance of smooth joint surfaces. If, after repair, the component parts of a joint do not fit together properly, there will be friction, and ultimately the pain and impaired motion of traumatic arthritis. Circulatory impairment and nerve damage are ever-present dangers, and must be evaluated and cared for properly.

Finally, it should be kept in mind that the elbow joint is prone to stiffness after fracture or operative procedures. Motion should be started as early as possible, but such motion should not be strenuous. It is best to let the force of the patient's own muscles provide the required resistance. Forceful manipulation and rigorous therapy should be avoided, but the joint should be put in motion.

THE HUMERUS

The glenohumeral joint is constructed to allow maximum motion in all planes. For this reason, it is a loose joint. The ball-like head of the humerus rests against the small shallow saucer of the glenoid fossa, and the two structures are approximated by the flexible joint capsule. It is obvious that stability of the joint must come from the synchronous action of the complex shoulder girdle muscles. Fractures and dislocations of the humerus, thus, are influenced to a great extent by these complex muscle actions. Characteristic deformities occur with fractures of the bones of the shoulder girdle because of these muscles. It follows logically that maximum restoration of function depends upon the integrity of the muscles, tendons and ligaments of the area, and that early restoration of function of these parts in treatment is essential.

These muscles may be divided into two main groups. On the anterior aspect, there are the adductor–internal rotators. This group is composed of the teres major, which arises posteriorly from the scapula and inserts into the bicipital groove; the subscapularis, inserting into the lesser tuberosity of the humerus, and the latissimus dorsi, winding about the teres major from the back, inserting into the bicipital groove. The powerful pectoralis major completes the adductor group. It arises on the chest wall and crosses the axilla to insert on the lateral margin of the bicipital groove. The pectoralis major, teres major and latissimus dorsi rotate it inward and adduct it. The subscapularis rotates the arm inward (Fig. 46).

On the posterior aspect of the shoulder are located the abductor–external rotator muscles. In this group are the supraspinatus, the infraspinatus and the teres minor. Arising from the scapula, these muscles insert into the greater tuberosity of the humerus through a common tendon, the external rotator cuff. The external rotator cuff muscles fix the head of the humerus against the glenoid and aid in abduction. All three muscles rotate the humerus externally. Overlying these muscles is the deltoid, the strongest of the relatively weak abductor–external rotator group. Arising from the shoulder girdle, it inserts on the humerus just above the middle of the shaft. It provides the main force for raising the arm.

The most important single factor in the distribution of muscle pull is the uneven power of the abductors and external rotators compared to the adductor–internal rotator group. The abductors exert their power over the head of the humerus. This limits their leverage in lifting the weight of the arm. The stronger adductors, however, exert a much greater force. They are assisted by gravity and have the advantage of better leverage.

This unequal power is even more important

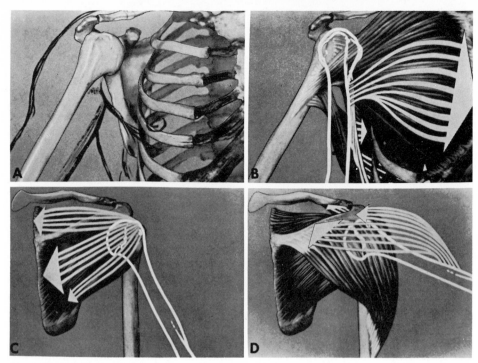

Figure 46.   *A*, The ball-like head of the humerus fits against the shallow saucer of the glenoid. For stability, the gleno-humeral joint depends upon the shoulder girdle muscles rather than any bony contact. *B*, The pectoralis major, aided by the teres major, subscapularis and latissimus dorsi, adducts and internally rotates the arm. The subscapularis is the primary internal rotator of the arm. *C*, The abductor—external rotator group of muscles is composed of the supraspinatus, infraspinatus, teres minor and deltoid muscles. These muscles, with the exception of the deltoid, arise on the scapula and insert on the greater tuberosity of the humerus. The external rotator group fixes the head of the humerus against the glenoid to aid in abduction. Externally, these muscles rotate the arm. *D*, The deltoid muscle, arising on the scapula and clavicle, inserts on the humeral shaft and is the primary abductor of the arm.

in the healing process than in reduction. Consider the hazards of permitting a fracture of the upper humerus to heal with the arm at the side and the forearm across the chest. If the arm is immobilized in this position for any length of time, the strong adductors are relaxed and allowed to shorten. On the other hand, the weaker abductors are stretched, thereby weakening them further. This arm-at-the-side position also tends to force the head of the humerus upward against the acromion, and stretches the deltoid and the external rotator cuff tendon tightly over the greater tuberosity. The subdeltoid bursa is compressed. With the inflammatory reaction of healing of fractures in this area, these structures may become adherent to each other. The gliding action of tendon and muscle over bone is lost and with it shoulder motion.

Ideally, fixation of fractures of the humerus should be in abduction and moderate external rotation. This ensures contraction of the weak abductors and protects the bursae and other structures from adhesion at the shoulder joint. In treatment, this ideal position is not always practical.

A second anatomic factor of great importance is the presence of neurovascular structures in the axilla and upper arm. These nerves and vessels are endangered particularly by fractures of the surgical neck of the humerus and fractures of the shaft just below the insertion of the deltoid. The major vascular structure in this area is the axillary artery and its continuation as the brachial artery. Finally, there is the brachial plexus. As the plexus traverses the clavicular area and the axilla and emerges into the upper arm, five main nerves arise. These nerves may be damaged by displaced fracture fragments. The most vulnerable is the radial nerve, which lies in close approximation to the shaft of the humerus. It winds about the humerus posteriorly to emerge on the lateral aspect, and is particularly prone to injury with fractures of the shaft of the bone.

FRACTURES OF THE SHAFT OF THE HUMERUS. Fractures of the shaft of the humerus are divided generally into those occurring below the deltoid insertion and those occurring above it. The area may be further divided into fractures above and below the pectoralis major, but above the deltoid insertion. Such fractures may be caused by the indirect force of a fall or the direct force of a blow to the humerus.

There is little displacement in the typical fracture below the deltoid insertion, in which the adductors as well as the abductors are attached to the upper fragment. They serve to balance each other. The distal fragment is controlled principally by gravity and by the long muscles of the arm – the triceps and biceps. Since their pull is upward, parallel with the bone, they have very little displacing effect except to produce shortening. The amount of traction used should be determined carefully, because these muscles are easily overstretched, and fractures of this type are subject to distraction. On the other hand, too little traction presents the danger of angulation, especially when the arm is not properly immobilized. Since the elbow is held at a right angle, the biceps is relaxed. The triceps produces anterior angulation by acting like a bowstring along the back of the humerus. The brachioradialis may also contribute to anterior angulation by pulling the lower fragment forward. Another hazard occurs when the patient moves his body and tenses the shoulder muscles. This tends to abduct the proximal fragment, causing lateral angulation, particularly if the traction is not enough to overcome the upward pull of the long muscles (Fig. 47).

Another complication in fractures just below the deltoid insertion is injury to the radial nerve. The winding course of the nerve around the bone at the level of the fracture predisposes it to injury. This nerve may be damaged either by sharp fragments of the bone, or by the trauma which originally caused the fracture. Involvement of the radial nerve can be detected by examining the function of the hand and wrist. Extension of the wrist is lost, and there is inability to extend the fingers at the metacarpophalangeal joints.

Sometimes, no involvement of the radial nerve is evident when the fracture is examined originally, but becomes apparent much later, as a gradual weakening of extension of the hand and fingers. This means that the nerve has been damaged subsequently by growing callus or angulation. Callus may be abundant surrounding the nerve, squeezing it and causing a slowly progressive

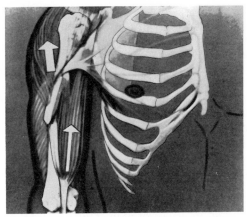

Figure 47. Fractures which occur from below the deltoid muscle insertion to above the humeral condyles exhibit similar deformities. The long muscles of the arm cause shortening. The fracture may angulate laterally or medially, as the proximal fragment remains in neutral position. Since the biceps is relaxed with the elbow flexed, the triceps muscle may act as a bowstring posteriorly, producing moderate anterior angulation.

paralysis. When this happens, the nerve must be freed from the callus by neurolysis. If radial nerve palsy is found immediately or develops later, the wrist and fingers must be supported to prevent overstretching of the paralyzed forearm extensor muscles. This may be done by incorporating into the hanging cast an out-rigger over the dorsum of the hand. The fingers and thumb are then supported by slings suspended from the out-rigger by rubber bands. This allows active motion of the hand and prevents the wristdrop deformity from overstretching muscles while the damaged nerve recovers.

The hanging cast is used to supply suspension traction as it is in fractures above the deltoid insertion. In either fracture, if medial angulation occurs, it may be corrected by placing a pad of soft material between the body and the cast. This acts as a fulcrum over which the traction of the cast tends to correct the angulation. Anterior angulation may be corrected by shortening the bandage loop which suspends the wrist from the neck. Lateral angulation is difficult to correct, as additional traction to correct this may cause distraction of the fragments and produce delayed union or nonunion. It may be necessary to maintain the distal fragment in some abduction in a shoulder spica cast or airplane splint to correct lateral angulation. Suspension traction may be necessary in fractures which cannot be maintained by splints or casts. The arm may be suspended from an overhead frame placed over the bed while traction is applied through a wire placed through the upper ulna. Traction may be supplemented with molded plaster splints to prevent angulation.

Occasionally, reduction cannot be accomplished by closed methods. This is usually due to interposition of muscle between the bone fragments. If the separation of fragments is excessive, open reduction with internal fixation with screws and plates, or intramedullary rod is done.

When the fracture occurs above the pectoralis major insertion, the strong adductor muscles hold the distal fragment in adduction and internal rotation. The weak external rotator–abductor muscles exert very little counterpull, and the proximal fragment remains in neutral position. At the same time, the distal fragment is pulled upward by the triceps, biceps, coracobrachialis and deltoid. The deltoid also exerts a slight lateral pull and acts as a fulcrum about which the adductor muscles displace the proximal end of the distal fragment inward toward the body. The characteristic displacement is medial angulation and displacement of the distal fragment on the proximal, with moderate shortening and overriding.

Since the long muscles of the arm are easily tired, little traction is required for reduction and maintenance of reduction of the fracture. A lightweight, hanging cast may be used if the fracture is checked frequently by x-ray examination. This type of cast stabilizes the elbow and forearm, but does not immobilize the fracture, since its upper margin may not even cover the fracture site. Its sole function is to provide traction. It does this by suspension traction which allows both fragments to move as a unit. The elbow is flexed to 90 degrees, with the forearm in neutral position midway between pronation and supination. The cast is applied over generous padding of sheet wadding, from the axilla to the flexion crease of the palm. A wire loop is incorporated in the cast at the wrist, through which the cast is suspended from the patient's neck by a narrow bandage. The rest of the cast must be unsupported so that continuous traction is made in the long axis of the arm by the weight of the cast. The patient must sleep with the trunk in an upright position so the traction is uninterrupted 24 hours a day. Finger function is encouraged. After a few days, pendulum exercises are started. The patient leans forward and to the side of the fracture, and, with traction maintained by the cast, gently swings the arm in circumduction. The arc of motion is limited to prevent angulation at the fracture site. The hanging cast allows circumduction, but all other exercise should be deferred until the union is firm, usually in four to six weeks.

Fractures between the insertion of the pectoralis major and the deltoid muscles present the opposite deformity. The strong pull of the pectoralis major overcomes the abductor muscles, and the proximal fragment is angulated medialward. The deltoid and long muscles of the arm produce shortening and slight outward displacement of the distal fragment. Usually, a hanging cast will effect and maintain reduction; occasionally, however, open reduction and internal fixation are necessary (Fig. 48).

FRACTURES OF THE SURGICAL NECK OF THE HUMERUS.   Fractures of the surgical neck of the humerus are usually caused by indirect

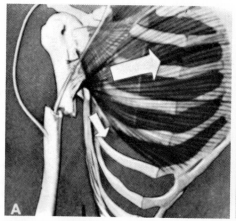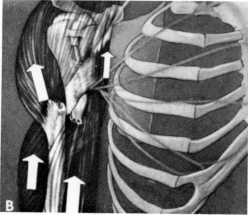

Figure 48. *A,* Fractures below the insertion of the pectoralis major but above the deltoid produce medial angulation of the proximal fragment, because the pull of the adductors is stronger than the force of the abductors. *B,* The long muscles of the arm cause shortening, and the deltoid may pull the distal fragment outward.

violence. They frequently occur as the result of a fall on the outstretched arm. The force is transmitted up the shaft of the humerus, to the surgical neck, where the fracture occurs. Such fractures are frequently comminuted, since the force, as it drives the head of the humerus against the glenoid, is dissipated in many directions. Because the fracture occurs in an area of cancellous bone, the fracture is often impacted.

After the fracture occurs, the upper fragment is held in abduction and slight forward flexion by the supraspinatus. This, in effect, tips the head of the humerus so that the articular surfaces face backward and medial. The rotators, however, are fairly evenly balanced, so that this fragment is held midway between external and internal rotation. The strong abductors pull the distal fragment inward and somewhat forward. If the distal fragment is displaced medially far enough, the sharp edge of the bone may damage the nerves and blood vessels (Fig. 49).

In effecting reduction, the principle is followed of aligning the distal fragment, which can be controlled, with the head of the bone, which cannot. During reduction, countertraction must be provided. It may be obtained by placing a sheet across the patient's chest, under the axilla on the affected side, and attached to the opposite corner of the table. The traction may be applied with a bandage looped about the patient's wrist and then passed around the operator's shoulder. This allows steady, nonvibrating traction with the weight of the surgeon's body as he leans backward in the bandage loop. The traction is made toward the foot of the table with only a small amount of abduction, not more than 25 degrees. If the abduction is greater than this in the early stages of the reduction, the sharp edges of the distal fragment may injure the structures in the axilla. Abduction may be increased after the traction is in force and the fragments have been disengaged. The free hands of the operator then manipulate the shaft and head fragments into alignment.

To maintain reduction, various splints or casts may be applied. A useful device is the airplane splint which is adjusted to hold the arm in 30 to 60 degrees of abduction. The elbow should be in moderate external rotation and moderate flexion. In order to decrease the forward and inward pull of the pectoralis major, it is sometimes necessary to place the arm in forward flexion of 45 to 60 degrees. In addition to relaxing the pectoralis major muscle, this rotates the upper end of the distal fragment backward, and reduces the danger to the brachial plexus (Fig. 50).

Fortunately, most fractures of the surgical neck of the humerus are impacted in fairly good position. It is better to accept a moderate amount of deformity and start early motion of the shoulder than to attempt anatomic reduction. Since the joint is a loose one, and the head of the humerus contacts the glenoid of the scapula over a small area, malalignment has very little effect on ultimate function. However, prolonged immobilization with the arm at the side does produce marked disability through adhesions and shortened muscles.

The shoulder is immobilized by placing the extremity in a sling and bandaging the arm to the side by a swath dressing about the chest. This is maintained for three to five days, until the acute pain has subsided. Gentle pendulum exercises are then started. The arm is removed from the sling and allowed to hang with the elbow extended. The patient leans forward and to the affected side. This brings the arm away from the body, and the weight

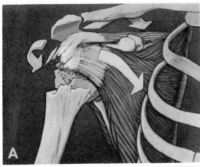
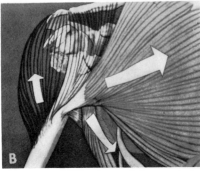

Figure 49. Because the bone of the surgical neck of the humerus is cancellous, fractures in this region are often comminuted and impacted. *A*, The head of the bone is held in neutral rotation, but is tipped medially and backward by the pull of the external rotator and abductor muscles. *B*, The distal fragment is displaced medially by the adductor muscles, and may threaten the neurovascular structures.

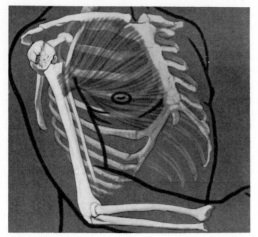

Figure 50. When the forward pull of the pectoralis major displaces the shaft, it may be relaxed by moderate forward flexion of the arm, aligning the·shaft with the head fragment.

of the arm provides gentle traction. The extremity is allowed to swing as a pendulum in abduction, adduction, flexion, extension and circumduction. This exercise provides active muscle exercise, prevents adhesions of the shoulder joint capsule and contraction and shortening of the strong adductor–internal rotator muscles. The exercise program is gradually increased over several weeks to active abduction and internal and external rotation. The fracture usually heals in six weeks. If a well-controlled program of exercise has been instituted early, the patient should have fairly good shoulder motion by this time. However, it may take many months of active exercise to obtain maximum function.

On rare occasions, when the fracture is unstable and the distal fragment projects deep into the axilla, suspension traction may be necessary for several weeks until the fracture stabilizes (Fig. 51).

EPIPHYSIAL DISPLACEMENT. Epiphysial separation of the head of the humerus may occur in an infant following the trauma of delivery, or in growing children from indirect violence. Since the ossification center is not present in the humeral epiphysis at birth, x-ray films fail to reveal the nature of the injury. In the growing child, the injury is rare from the age of infancy until about the eighth year. After this, until about 13 years of age, epiphysial separations and fractures are more common. X-ray studies after the ossification center appears in the humeral head readily reveal the injury.

In the infant, the symptoms are pseudo-paralysis of the arm coupled with swelling

and obvious pain when the part is handled. The infant is irritable. The condition is often confused with birth palsy. Occasionally, crepitation can be elicited on manipulation. X-ray films made a week after injury reveal proliferating callus about the upper humerus. Simple immobilization with a swath about the chest and arm is usually all that is needed in the infant. The minor displacements are usually corrected by growth.

Rarely, the epiphysis is rotated completely around so that the epiphysial plate faces into the glenoid. This injury is only manifested later by disturbed growth of the humerus when it is too late to restore the bone. Fortunately, the injury is rare. It is, however, almost impossible to diagnose early, and a short humerus always develops from the growth disturbance.

In older children, the epiphysial separation is often coupled with fracture of the metaphysis in the subtrochanteric region. The head of the humerus is often rotated inward with the distal fragment angulating laterally and upward. Reduction is accomplished by downward traction and maintained with a hanging cast. Occasionally, suspension traction is necessary, placing the humerus in 90 degrees of flexion and abduction in neutral or external rotation to align the fragments properly. Anatomic reduction is unnecessary because growth will correct the deformity in time. The younger the child, the greater the deformity that may be accepted.

FRACTURES OF THE NECK OF THE HUMERUS WITH ANTERIOR DISLOCATION. This fracture-

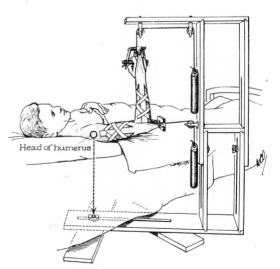

Head of humerus

Figure 51. Suspension traction may be necessary for any of the fractures of the humerus.

dislocation is a result of violence with the humerus abducted posteriorly. The force of the fall and the extreme abduction drive the greater tuberosity against the acromion process. As abduction of the humerus increases, the acromion acts as a fulcrum; the head of the humerus is forced out of its position in the glenoid, stretching and tearing the capsule. This dislocation is increased by the downward and forward pull of the pectoralis major. As the force of the fall exerts its full impact, the head is trapped under the pectoralis major and a fracture occurs through the surgical neck. It is this combination of fracture and dislocation which makes the injury so difficult to treat (Fig. 52).

If closed reduction is attempted by traction and manipulation of the arm, the shaft is usually pulled away from the head completely. This interrupts the blood supply from the shaft to the head. The capsular blood supply to the head has already been seriously impaired by the dislocation so that even though the head is later replaced surgically, the damage has been done. Necrosis of the head of the bone may follow, resulting in permanent disability. Because of the dangers resulting from closed manipulation of this type of fracture-dislocation, open reduction is often advisable. Because of the additional damage done to the blood supply when the shaft is pulled away from the head by manipulation, all dislocations of the shoulder should be examined by x-ray before reduction is attempted.

After open reduction, or careful closed reduction of fracture-dislocation of the humerus, the arm is immobilized with the sling

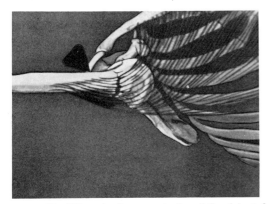

Figure 52. When the humerus is forcefully abducted, the acromion process acts as a fulcrum, forcing the head of the humerus downward and forward, rupturing the anterior inferior joint capsule. The head is trapped under the pectoral muscle, which causes the neck of the humerus to fracture.

and swath bandage for a few days. Exercise is then started similar to that used for fracture of the neck of the humerus.

DISLOCATION OF THE GLENOHUMERAL JOINT WITHOUT FRACTURE. Dislocations of the humerus at this joint are among the most common dislocations in the body. Most dislocations take place anteriorly and inferiorly; less commonly, the dislocation occurs posteriorly. The mechanism is similar to that producing the fracture-dislocation of the humerus.

Frequently, the injury occurs in the teenage group or in young adults engaged in vigorous athletics. Often, the dislocation in this age group occurs with apparently little force applied to the abducted, extended arm. This may happen when there is a defect in the joint capsule, such as deficient or absent glenohumeral ligaments or an excessively relaxed joint capsule. When the head of the humerus is forced out of the joint, the capsule usually tears away from the rim or labrum of the glenoid. The head of the humerus is trapped under the pectoralis major and held there by contraction of the pectoralis major, subscapularis and latissimus dorsi. Deformity of the shoulder is usually obvious, and the elbow cannot be approximated to the side of the body. Active abduction of more than a few degrees is impossible. Pain is usually severe. The circulation and integrity of the nerves of the extremity must be determined and an x-ray examination should always be made before reduction is attempted.

Several methods of reduction are available to the surgeon. One of the simplest methods is to place the patient prone with the arm hanging over the edge of a table. With adequate sedation, the traction supplied by the weight of the arm relaxes the spasm of the muscles holding the head in the dislocated position. Reduction may occur spontaneously after ten or 15 minutes, or additional traction may be necessary, supplemented by gentle internal and external rotatory manipulation.

If this method fails, it may be necessary to apply more traction. The patient is placed supine and, with adequate sedation or a general anesthetic, traction is made on the arm in 30 degrees of abduction. Countertraction is supplied by the surgeon's foot placed against the side of the chest just below but not in the axilla. It is obvious that this form of countertraction should not be used if ribs are fractured on the side of the dislocation. Gentle internal and external rotatory movements are done while the steady, nonvibrating traction is maintained. Reduction of the dislocation is often sudden, signified by an audible, dull thud, accompanied by disappearance of the deformity. Passive movements of the gleno-humeral joint return to normal.

The joint is immobilized with the arm at the side and the forearm across the chest with the humerus internally rotated to allow the torn joint capsule to approximate the glenoid. Although this position allows the strong ad-ductor–internal rotator muscles to shorten, it is the only position in which the anterior joint capsule is relaxed. Adequate circulation and nerve function should be verified following reduction.

The position is maintained for six weeks in patients under 35 years of age. The teenage and young-adult groups are more prone to de-velop recurring dislocations of the shoulder; for this reason, the immobilization must be uninterrupted for this period. Motion is re-gained slowly following this time by grad-ually increasing shoulder exercise. After the age of 35, recurrent dislocation of the shoulder is much less likely, and immobilization for three weeks is usually enough time for heal-ing. Some slight loss of abduction and ex-ternal rotation may persist in patients in the older age groups; this is more marked if im-mobilization is prolonged.

FRACTURES OF THE GREATER TUBEROSITY AND HEAD OF THE HUMERUS. When the pa-tient falls on the outstretched arm the hu-merus is driven upward against the glenoid and acromion process. The external rotator cuff tendon, composed of the supraspinatus, infraspinatus and teres minor tendons, is stretched. The muscles of this tendon con-tract, attempting to hold the head of the hu-merus down. One of two injuries result from this combination of forces. Either the rotator cuff tendon tears, or the greater tuberosity, where it attaches, is avulsed from the hu-meral head. Active abduction is impossible, as the head of the humerus is no longer fixed against the glenoid by these muscles. Point tenderness is elicited on pressure over the area and pain is increased by attempted abduction (Fig. 53).

When x-ray examination fails to reveal a fracture of the tuberosity, a tear of the rota-tor cuff tendon must be suspected. If this is complete, serious permanent disability to the shoulder will result unless the tendon is restored. Suture of the tendon is indicated as soon as possible.

When x-ray examination reveals a frac-

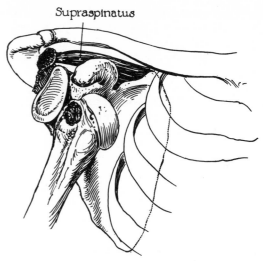

Supraspinatus

Figure 53. Complete avulsion of the external rotator cuff tendon with the greater tuberosity may occur with or without dislocation of the shoulder. These muscles pull the tuberosity fragment upward under the acromion process.

ture of the tuberosity, there may be varying degrees of displacement of the fragment. Often the avulsion is incomplete and the tuberosity remains in contact with the head of the humerus. Simple support with a sling may be the only immobilization needed. Cir-cumduction pendulum exercises are started within a few days. The incomplete avulsion fracture heals within six weeks; however, damage to the fibers of the external rotator cuff may limit full motion for many months.

When the tuberosity is completely avulsed from the humeral head, the supraspinatus, infraspinatus and teres minor muscles pull the fragment upward and backward under the acromion process. The fragment may be approximated by abducting and externally rotating the arm until this is achieved. Stereoscopic x-ray examination of the shoul-der is necessary to evaluate the reduction properly. The arm must be held in this posi-tion with a shoulder spica cast or an air-plane splint, until union is firm in about six weeks. If accurate reduction cannot be achieved by this method, open reduction must be done. The fragment of tuberosity with the attached rotator cuff is sutured to the head of the humerus. Motion is started within a few days and gradually active ab-duction is encouraged after three weeks.

A less common fracture occurs occasion-ally with extremely violent compression of the head of the humerus against the glenoid or acromion. This is a fracture involving the greater and lesser tuberosities as well as the humeral head. The force splits the tuberosity away from the head, which is then driven onto the shaft of the humerus. The fracture of the humeral head usually takes place through the surgical neck, and comminution of the fragments may be marked. The head may be rotated laterally so that the articular surface points upward, laterally or backward.

This injury usually requires open reduction with reapproximation of the tuberosity fragments to the shaft and replacement of the head to a more normal position. Internal fixation by sutures is necessary. The prognosis is indefinite as disturbance to the blood supply of the head of the bone may produce aseptic necrosis later. Motion is started as early as possible to prevent stiffness.

FRACTURES AND DISLOCATIONS OF THE CLAVICLE

Fractures of the clavicle are one of the most common fractures from infancy through the first three decades of life, but may occur at any age. This crank-shaped bone, although short and dense, breaks rather easily. It is the only bony connection between the upper extremity and the body, helping to hold the shoulder girdle backward and upward. The S-shaped curve of the bone is designed to clear the first rib and protect the brachial plexus and subclavian vessels in all positions the shoulder may assume. Because of this close relationship to these vital structures, fractures of the clavicle may cause injury to them.

The sternoclavicular joint is the base and pivot from which the derrick-like arm of the clavicle swings forward and backward and up and down with shoulder motion. In addition, the clavicle rotates at this joint on abduction of the arm. The stability of the joint depends upon the strong but flexible capsule and the attachment of the sternomastoid and subclavius muscles. The sternomastoid muscle tends to pull the proximal part of the bone upward when this joint is dislocated or the clavicle breaks. The scapula is suspended from the clavicle distally by the acromioclavicular joint and the coracoclavicular ligaments. These ligaments are short and strong, but allow 'the scapula to rotate during circumduction of the arm while

holding the bones firmly together. The anterior fibers of the deltoid muscle and the pectoralis minor arise on the anterior distal one-fourth of the clavicle; acting with gravity, they tend to pull the clavicle downward and forward. The trapezius inserting superiorly at the distal end hoists the derrick arm of the clavicle upward in elevation of the shoulder and abduction of the arm. Limitation of motion at the acromioclavicular or sternoclavicular joint following injury will limit shoulder motion.

Most fractures of the clavicle are caused by the compression force of a fall on the outstretched arm, but occasionally are the result of a direct blow to the bone. Because of the structure of the bone, it most frequently breaks in the middle one-third and, fortunately, buckles and angulates upward and away from the subclavian vessels and brachial plexus. When the fracture is completely through the bone, overriding and shortening occurs. The proximal fragment is held upward by the sternomastoid muscle while gravity and the pectoral muscles pull the distal part downward and forward. Reduction of the fracture is accomplished by bracing the shoulder girdle backward and upward accompanied by manipulation of the bone ends.

The type of fracture varies with the age of the patient. From infancy to about the age of ten years, the fracture is usually of the greenstick type. From adolescence through the next two decades, the fracture is complete and often simple. In the older age groups, the fracture is often comminuted.

Fracture of the clavicle occurs occasionally during the manipulation of the baby during delivery. The newborn infant is fretful and cries when handled. The extremity on the side of the fracture hangs limp as though paralyzed. The condition is often confused with birth palsy of the upper extremity. It may be also difficult to distinguish this fracture from separation of the upper humeral epiphysis and greenstick fracture of the humerus. There is no crepitation on examination and little if any, deformity; however, palpation of the parts causes the infant to cry out. X-ray examination is necessary to determine the cause of the pseudoparalysis. If the fracture is not overriding and the angulation is not great, nothing need be done. The fracture in the newborn heals with abundant callus in a week or two. The pseudoparalysis disappears in a few days. If, rarely, the fracture is complete and displaced, a soft figure-of-eight bandage will hold the shoulders back while the fracture heals.

Children ten years of age and younger with greenstick fractures usually do not require reduction of the fracture. The shoulder is immobilized for comfort with a figure-of-eight bandage. Growth will correct the angulation, and, in instances where the fracture is complete and displaced, even bayonet apposition of the fragments results in a normal bone after a few years by the remodeling process.

Older children and adults require reduction of the fracture if there is overriding or marked angulation of the fragments. This is most easily done under a local anesthetic injected into the fracture hematoma. With the patient sitting on a stool, the shoulders are braced backward. The ends of the bone are manipulated into position. A figure-of-eight bandage is applied with adequate padding in the axillae. The bandage must be tightened each day. Since it is impossible to immobilize clavicular fractures completely by any type of external fixation, slight movement occurs which produces abundant callus. This lump of callus may be quite noticeable as the fracture heals, but absorbs slowly in children after a year or two. Remodeling of the callus is less complete in the adult, and some slight deformity may be noticeable permanently.

Occasionally, the fracture in the adult cannot be held in reduction, particularly if comminution is present. If the deformity is objectionable or symptoms of pressure on the nerves and vessels are present, open reduction with internal fixation with an intramedullary rod may be necessary.

Most fractures of the clavicle in adults heal sufficiently in four to six weeks to allow removal of the figure-of-eight dressing. Stiffness of the shoulder is usually not a problem, as the arm has been used during the healing time.

Rarely, nonunion of the clavicle follows fracture. This condition is treated by intramedullary rod fixation and appropriate bone grafting.

DISLOCATION OF THE STERNOCLAVICULAR JOINT. The sternoclavicular joint is occasionally dislocated by a fall on the arm or shoulder. Since the joint is shallow and saucer-shaped, stability depends upon the ligaments of the joint capsule. Compression force applied in the long axis of the clavicle coupled with forward or backward displacement ruptures the capsule, and the clavicle skids off the shallow joint surface of the sternum. Most often the dislocation is anterior. The sternomastoid tends to pull the clavicle upward while the weight of the shoulder and pectoral muscles displace it medially. Occasionally, dislocation takes place backward behind the sternum. This displacement may force the end of the clavicle against the trachea or great vessels, and cause difficult breathing or interfere with circulation. It may require immediate reduction. In either displacement, reduction is accomplished by bracing the shoulders backward; however, the reduction cannot be maintained by closed methods because of the unstable joint surfaces. Open reduction with repair of the ruptured joint capsule must be done soon after the injury. The repair may be reinforced with strips of fascia lata. Temporary wire fixation may be necessary while healing of the capsule takes place.

Neglected or old dislocations of this joint do not need treatment if the condition is painless. However, the deformity is noticeable, and many patients request something to be done for cosmetic reasons. The proximal two inches of the bone may be resected without interfering with shoulder function. This procedure is usually more satisfactory than late reconstruction of the joint.

DISLOCATION AND SUBLUXATION OF THE ACROMIOCLAVICULAR JOINT. This dislocation, or partial dislocation, results from a fall on the joint of the shoulder. The shoulder and arm, fixed to the ground by the weight of the body, pull the arm downward. The momentum of the falling body carries the trunk and thus the clavicle upward. The joint capsule is torn and the main stabilizing ligament, the coracoclavicular ligament, either partially or completely tears. The degree of rupture of this ligament determines whether the dislocation is complete or partial (Fig. 54).

When the patient stands, the distal clavicle is prominent above the acromion, which is pulled downward by the weight of the arm. When the patient lies down, the dislocation may reduce and show no deformity on inspection of the shoulder. For this reason, x-ray examination must be made with the patient upright, preferably holding a weight of 5 pounds in the hand, which accentuates the deformity.

Upward pressure on the bent elbow in the

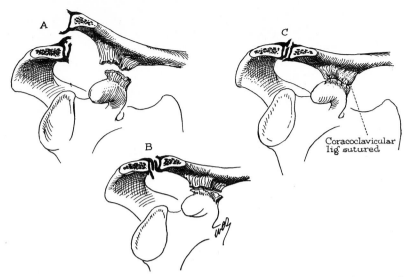

Figure 54. *A*, Complete rupture of the joint capsule of the acromioclavicular joint and the coracoclavicular ligament must occur before the joint can dislocate completely. *B*, The joint capsule may fold into the joint and prevent reduction. *C*, The coracoclavicular ligament must be repaired to maintain reduction of the dislocation.

long axis of the humerus effects reduction, while downward pressure is made on the clavicle. Various methods of strapping have been devised to maintain reduction by continuous exertion of these forces. Unfortunately, the force needed to maintain reduction by this method may produce skin necrosis over the elbow or clavicle, and the method is generally unsatisfactory. Recent injuries are best treated by open reduction with repair of the coracoclavicular ligament and joint capsule. Often, the joint capsule is found folded into the joint, preventing adequate closed reduction. Some type of internal fixation is needed while the ligaments are healing. This may be accomplished by wiring the clavicle to the coracoid process, or the clavicle may be held in reduction by transfixing the acromion and clavicle with multiple wires across the joint. These are removed after the ligaments have healed in four to six weeks.

Old complete dislocations are rarely painful. Partial dislocation or subluxation, however, may lead to painful traumatic arthritis. If the patient does not object to the appearance of the shoulder, and it is painless, the complete dislocation may be accepted, without serious impairment of shoulder function. However, if pain or deformity is to be corrected, either in complete or partial dislocation, the distal 1 to 1½ inches of clavicle may be resected. Elimination of the joint relieves pain, and the resection reduces the deformity without interfering with shoulder

function. The functional result is better than reconstruction of the joint for old injuries.

FRACTURES OF THE SCAPULA

The scapula is a triangular flat, thin, bone divided posteriorly into supraspinous and infraspinous portions by the spine of the scapula. Two other processes, the acromion and the coracoid, also rise from the scapula. The spine of the scapula, the acromion and the coracoid processes serve as the origin of several muscles. The glenoid is a saucer-like, articular surface which provides support for the head of the humerus. It is connected to the body of the bone by the neck of the scapula. The scapula is completely covered by muscles except at the glenoid, where the joint capsule arises.

The scapula is suspended on the posterior thoracic wall by a complicated group of shoulder girdle muscles and by the clavicle. It may be moved by these muscles through a wide range; it may be elevated, depressed, rotated, and displaced forward or backward about the thoracic cage.

The mobility of the bone provides for absorption of shock during falls on the upper extremity. For this reason, the body of the bone is seldom fractured by indirect violence. The mechanism of fracture of the body of the scapula is usually a direct blow, and the fracture is often comminuted, resembling the breaks in the shell of a hard-boiled egg. Since the bone is covered by muscles, the fragments are seldom displaced. However, the force necessary to produce the fracture is considerable and related injuries to the thorax and upper extremity are common.

Fractures of the neck, glenoid, acromion and coracoid processes may be produced by direct or indirect violence. Occasionally, the acromion process is fractured and displaced downward by a fall on the point of the shoulder, which is similar to the mechanism producing acromioclavicular joint separation. Rarely, the coracoid process may be avulsed by violent contraction of the coracobrachialis muscle, which displaces the avulsed fragment downward.

Occasionally, an impacted fracture of the neck of the scapula is produced by the indirect violence of a fall on the outstretched arm. The articular surface of the glenoid may be tipped in any direction; displaced by the direction of force producing the fracture. Rarely, the glenoid margins may be fractured by this same mechanism, or by dislocation of the head of the humerus.

The treatment for most fractures of the scapula is simple immobilization with a sling and swath bandage about the chest until the acute pain subsides. After a few days, gentle circumduction exercises are begun; gradually, shoulder girdle motion is regained. As in all shoulder injuries, early active use is necessary to prevent adhesions and muscle contractures.

Rarely, a portion of the body or spine of the scapula is displaced. If this displacement interferes with the gliding mechanism of the scapula on the thorax, it may be reduced by direct manipulation, or by removal of the fragment.

If the acromion process is depressed enough to interfere with scapulohumeral motion, it may be manipulated by upward compression of the humerus while the body of the bone is fixed against the thorax by the surgeon's hand. However, it is difficult to maintain reduction because the weight of the arm pulls the fragment downward through the origin of the deltoid muscle. Often, it is simpler to remove the displaced fragment and reattach the deltoid origin to the remaining structures.

Avulsion of the coracoid process is usually treated conservatively by immobilization for a short period, followed by active exercise. Reattachment by open reduction is seldom necessary.

Moderate displacement of the articular surface of the glenoid by fractures of the neck of the scapula seldom requires reduction. The joint is a lax one allowing a wide range of motion. As with fractures of the neck of the humerus, displacement has little effect upon motion between the humerus and the scapula.

In all fractures of the shoulder girdle, an early active motion must be carried out to secure maximum function and to prevent adhesions and muscle contractures.

FRACTURES AND DISLOCATIONS OF THE LOWER EXTREMITY

The primary functions of the lower extremities are weight-bearing and locomotion. For this reason, the bones, joints, muscles and ligaments are more massive in construction than in the upper extremity. Since stability is necessary for walking, running, standing and squatting, the motions of the major joints are more limited. While the motion of the knee joint is similar to the elbow, allowing primarily flexion and extension, the motions and construction of the hip and ankle joints differ from the shoulder and wrist joints to provide the required stability.

The deep cup of the acetabulum holds the ball-like head of the femur securely. The strong, thick capsule and ligaments of the joint bind the two together, making a much more stable joint than the shoulder. This stability is obtained by sacrificing motion. The same factors are present in the ankle joint when compared to the more mobile wrist joint.

The foot is an organ of balance and propulsion. Strength and elastic shock-absorbing qualities are required for this function. Again, mobility of the joints is sacrificed for these qualities when compared to the intricate, fine movements of the hand.

Since the center of gravity of the body is located in the midline at the second sacral segment, while the hip joints lie lateral to this point, the femur slants toward the midline in its downward course to compensate for this. The tibia and fibula with the foot, thus, lie closer to the central weight-bearing line of the body. A slight knock-knee effect is produced by this alignment. Since the knee and ankle cannot abduct or adduct to compensate for deformities from fractures which produce medial or lateral angulation, disturbances of this weight-bearing alignment are critical. In the lateral plane of the body, the weight-bearing line of the body passes almost directly through the hip joint. The alignment of the femur and tibia is, thus, almost in a straight line to the foot. Anterior or posterior angulation is less critical because the deformity may be compensated for by flexion and extension at the hip, knee and ankle (Fig. 55).

Rotational deformity always throws one or more joints out of alignment, and cannot be accepted if proper function is expected. Fractures of the lower extremity which heal with shortening or malalignment produce abnormal stress and strain on the joints. In time, traumatic arthritis develops in the hip, knee or ankle.

Shortening of one extremity produces a pelvic tilt. The spine then articulates with the sacrum at an angle. A compensatory scoliosis must develop in the spine to bring the trunk back to the midline. This produces strain in the joints involved, and may lead to backache and traumatic arthritis.

Because of the forces placed upon the joints on weight-bearing, fractures deforming joint surfaces produce wear-and-tear changes in the joints much more rapidly than in the upper extremity. Usually, a painful traumatic arthritis results.

Since the movements of the lower extremity, while walking, running and standing, are less intricate than the movements of the function-

ing hand, stiffness of joints may still be compatible with function. Although some disability is produced, an individual with a completely ankylosed hip, knee or ankle in the proper position may get about with minimum difficulty. However, every effort should be made to re-establish normal joint motion following fractures in the lower extremity.

When a joint has been destroyed by trauma, occasionally surgical ankylosis is deliberately done. An ankylosed weight-bearing joint is painless, while a rough, unstable joint may be impossible to walk upon.

Rehabilitation of the muscles of the lower extremity is imperative if normal function is to be achieved following injury. Muscles atrophy and may shorten with prolonged immobilization. Characteristic deformities develop. At the hip, the strong adductor and flexor muscles tend to shorten, producing a flexion adduction contracture. At the knee, flexion contracture is produced by shortened hamstring muscles while contracture of the calf muscles produces equinus deformity in the foot and ankle. Strength of the atrophied opposing muscles must be rebuilt while the shortened muscles are stretched through appropriate exercises. Failure to strengthen the muscles causes limping at the hip and buckling and instability of the knee.

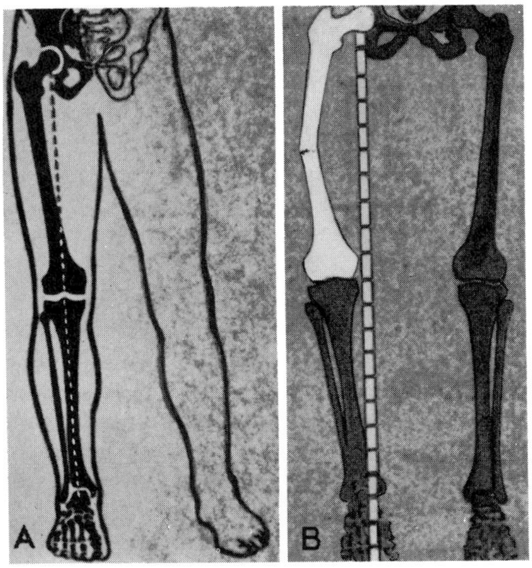

THE HIP JOINT

Fractures about the hip joint are classified as intracapsular and extracapsular. To treat the special problems which arise in dealing with these fractures, the anatomy peculiar to the hip must be understood.

The hip is a ball-and-socket joint, allowing motion in all planes except hyperextension. The weight-bearing portion is on the superior surface of the acetabulum and head of the femur. Inferiorly, the socket is shallow and the bony rim about the acetabulum is incomplete. This space is filled with a fat pad, the haversian gland and the ligamentum teres, running from the inferior acetabulum to the central part of the head of the femur. The ligament carries blood vessels to the head of the femur which are abundant in the child but scanty in the elderly (Fig. 56).

About the rim of the acetabulum is a fibrocartilage, the labrum acetabulae, which, in effect, deepens the socket without limiting motion, thus increasing stability of the joint.

The joint capsule is the strongest and

Figure 55. *A,* The weight-bearing line passes through the center of the hip, knee and ankle joints. *B,* Malunion of the leg bones throws the weight-bearing line out of alignment, and in time produces stress and strain at the hip, knee or ankle which may produce traumatic arthritis in these joints.

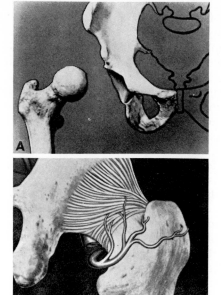

Figure 56. *A*, The bony anatomy of the hip joint is demonstrated, with the femur dislocated from the acetabulum. *B*, The configuration of the fibers of the hip joint capsule prevents hyperextension of the joint, but allows all other motions. The principal blood supply to the head of the femur is from the posterior circumflex artery through the posterior joint capsule. The intramedullary blood vessels and a small vessel in the ligamentum teres augment the capsular blood supply to the head of the femur.

thickest in the body. It arises about the rim of the acetabulum and inserts about the base of the neck of the femur. The anterior fibers arise superiorly on the acetabulum and wind outward and downward to insert on the inferior neck and intertrochanteric line. This special arrangement of fiber is called Bigelow's ligament. The fibers tighten as the femur is extended, preventing hyperextension but allowing all other motions.

The neck isolated from the femur by the joint capsule is covered by the visceral capsule inserting about the rim of the ball-like head. The cavity created by the parietal and visceral capsule is lined with synovial membrane, providing lubrication for the joint.

The blood supply to the head of the femur comes from three sources: through the medullary vessels of the neck, through the ligamentum teres and through the visceral capsular vessels. The visceral capsular vessels come from the posterior circumflex artery and lie primarily on the posterior surface of the neck of the femur. It is important to remember that the blood supply to the neck of the bone is meager and dwindles as it approaches the head.

Fractures of the neck of the bone disrupt the nutrient vessels of the medullary canal completely, and may damage or tear the capsular vessels. The nourishment of the head of the bone is then left to the inadequate resources of the artery of the ligamentum teres. In the aged, this artery may be completely occluded. Bleeding into the tight confines of the joint capsule may produce a tamponade effect and further impair the circulation to the head. When the blood supply to the head is completely cut off, this fragment undergoes necrosis. Dead bone does not aid in the healing process and must be replaced by the process of creeping substitution. In this process, dead bone is absorbed and new laid down. The process is slow and may be incomplete. Nonunion and destruction of the head of the bone is the plague of the surgeon and the patient.

The neck of the femur progresses outward and downward at an angle of 140 to 145 degrees, placing the shaft of the femur lateral to the joint. This lateral placement of the shaft in relation to the joint may produce shearing force on intracapsular fractures, delaying or preventing healing. The angle of the fracture through the neck in relation to the horizontal plane determines the amount of shearing force. Fractures which are more vertical are subject to more shearing force than those which approach the horizontal.

The muscles surrounding the hip produce characteristic deformities following fractures in the region. Shortening is produced by the longitudinal pull of the rectus femoris and gluteals, adduction and shortening by the adductor group of muscles, and abduction and shortening by the abductors, depending upon the location of the fracture in relationship to the insertion of these muscles. The short external rotator muscles lying posteriorly arise on the pelvis and, inserting into the greater trochanter, produce external rotation aided by the iliopsoas. Since the internal rotators of the hip, the tensor fascia femoris and the adductor group work at a mechanical disadvantage, they are overcome by the external rotators and gravity. Thus, the leg assumes a typical deformity of shortening and external rotation in fractures of the femur about the hip (Fig. 57).

Fractures in this region are classified by location. A general classification divides fractures into two main groups, intracapsular and extracapsular. Those fractures occurring within the capsule are termed "subcapital" when they occur at the junction of

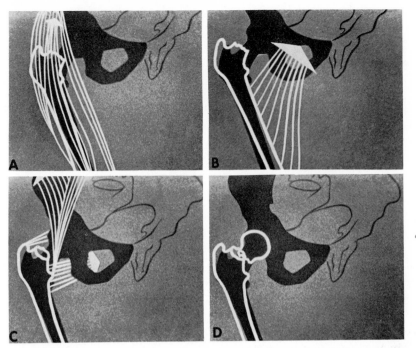

Figure 57. *A,* Shortening of the bone in fractures of the hip is produced by the long thigh muscles, the rectus femoris, sartorius and hamstrings. *B,* The adductors produce adduction and shortening. *C,* The abductor muscles and external rotator muscles, aided by the iliopsoas, tend to abduct, externally rotate and flex the distal fragment in certain hip fractures. *D,* Fractures about the hip result in shortening, adduction and external rotation as the result of muscle contractions and gravity.

the head and neck, "midcervical" when they occur in the midportion of the neck, and "base of the neck" when they occur at the junction of the neck and shaft.

Because shearing force plays such an important role in healing, these fractures have been classified by Pawles by the angle of the fracture to the horizontal. If the fracture line through the neck is nearly horizontal, impacting force may be exerted by the pull of the thigh muscles. However, as the fracture line becomes more vertical, more shearing force is exerted by these muscles and the prognosis for healing becomes progessively worse (Fig. 58).

Fractures outside of the hip joint capsule may involve either the greater or lesser trochanter as avulsion-type fractures. More frequently, however, the fracture line runs between the greater and lesser trochanter— the intertrochanteric fracture. Fractures of the shaft of the femur at the lesser trochanter are called subtrochanteric fractures.

Fractures about the hip are produced by direct or indirect force; in addition, stress or march fractures may occur in the neck of the femur. A fall directly upon the side of the trochanter may produce an impacted fracture of the neck, an intertrochanteric fracture, or a comminuted fracture of the trochanter or upper shaft of the femur. Indirect force, such as a twist of the body on the leg, may produce fractures of the neck or intertrochanteric region. Adduction and abduction forces may also produce fractures. Stress fractures in the neck of the femur may occur from the repeated minute trauma of walking. The fragments may then come apart with a minor twist, the patient falling after the fracture has occurred.

INTRACAPSULAR FRACTURES.   Subcapital fractures may be impacted, or complete and displaced. The fracture impacted in good position may show no deformity and, although painful, may allow considerable motion at the hip joint. Indeed, the patient often walks upon the leg for a variable period until the pain forces him to seek medical help.

If the head is in valgus position, impacted upon the neck, and there is no anterior or posterior displacement of the neck-head relationship, the fracture may be treated by non-weight-bearing without immobilization or fixation. Muscle tension tends to promote the impaction. If the head fragment is in

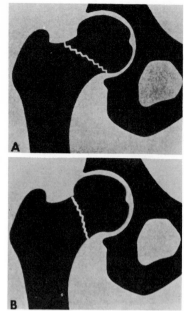

Figure 58. *A*, Horizontal fracture lines in the neck of the femur promote impaction and healing. *B*, Vertical fracture lines tend to produce shearing forces, which delay or prevent healing.

varus position, or the head is tipped forward or backward, the impaction is insecure, and, with absorption of bone during healing, the fracture may displace completely. In this instance, reduction and internal fixation should be done.

Complete and displaced fractures of the femoral neck present the typical deformity of shortening and external rotation of the leg. All motion is painful and may be accompanied by spasmodic contractions of the thigh and hip musculature. The degree of shortening varies. If the joint capsule is torn, the neck fragment may displace upward to a greater degree than when the capsule remains intact, holding the fragments within the joint. The greater trochanter may lie above Nealton's line. This line is drawn from the anterior superior spine of the ilium through the ischial tuberosity. Normally, the upper border of the greater trochanter lies on or below this line.

External rotation is usually more than the normal leg exhibits, but not as great as in intertrochanteric fracture. Gravity plus the pull of the external rotator muscles of the hip account for the deformity. The neck fragment displaces upward and the fractured end of the neck faces almost directly anterior. The head fragment may remain in its normal position, but may rotate in any direction, held in place only by the liga-

mentum teres and the suction-like grip of the acetabulum.

The fracture line may be sharp and clean, but often there is slight comminution of the thin cortex of the neck. Occasionally, a sharp spicule of bone breaks away from the neck and remains attached to the head. These factors, coupled with almost complete loss of control of the head fragment, make reduction difficult.

The head fragment may spin about in the acetabulum like a billiard ball in a cup when the fracture occurs, limited in excursion only by the loose, confining rein of the ligamentum teres. The principle of fracture reduction of placing the fragment which can be controlled in apposition with the one which cannot holds true with this fracture. Obviously, the head cannot be controlled; the neck fragment must be brought into alignment with the unstable head. When this is accomplished, it is still almost impossible to maintain the reduction except by internal fixation. The more vertical the fracture line is through the neck, the more difficult this becomes, because the thigh muscles pull the neck upward. Unless the neck can be placed under the head, converting the shearing force to an impacting one, fixation of any type will fail in a great number of fractures.

Reduction of subcapital and midcervical fractures. Reduction is accomplished by traction and countertraction with the leg in external rotation and neutral or slight abduction. The traction is most easily accomplished on a fracture operating table which ensures accurate, stable control of the leg. Countertraction is applied against the perineum by a post placed between the legs and attached to the table. As traction is applied, the forward-facing neck fragment is brought downward to the level of the head, or slightly below it. The leg is then internally rotated completely, usually about 45 degrees. This maneuver brings the forward-facing neck back to its normal position in relation to the head. If the posterior visceral capsule is still intact, this tightens and pulls the head and neck together, acting as a fulcrum from which the anterior gap between neck and head can be closed. The leg is then brought from slight abduction to almost neutral position to place the neck under the head. Traction is reduced to allow the fragments to come together (Fig. 59).

Excessive traction or distraction must be

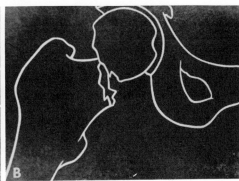

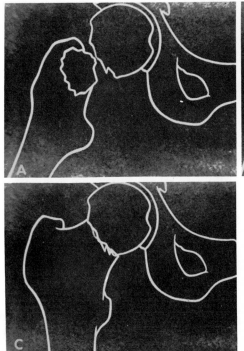

Figure 59. *A*, Traction is made on the leg to bring the forward-facing and shortened neck down to the level of the head or slightly below it. *B*, The femur is internally rotated 45 degrees to bring the fractured neck under the head. *C*, Traction is then reduced to allow the head and neck to come together.

corrected quickly, because this places undesirable tension on the capsular vessels, further impairing the blood supply to the head. This effect, coupled with excessive pressure of blood and fluid in the joint, is like a tourniquet about the blood vessels entering the head. A few hours under these conditions will surely produce necrosis of the head.

Accurate x-ray examinations in the anteroposterior and lateral views are essential to control reduction and for the application of internal fixation. Many fracture operating tables have fixtures to hold the x-ray films in the proper positions, while portable x-ray equipment is used for the x-ray examination. This equipment must be placed in position, and the surgeon must be sure that it is functioning properly before the operation is begun.

A variety of nails, screws and pins have been devised for internal fixation of femoral neck fractures. They are all designed to hold the head fragment securely to the neck of the femur. The number and variety attest to the variability of success in accomplishing this. The most popular nail at present is the cannulated, triflanged Smith-Petersen nail. The three blades of this nail prevent rotation of the fragments and provide strength with minimum cross-sectional area (Fig. 60).

The nail is driven from the lateral cortex of the femur through the neck into the head under x-ray control. Several landmarks serve as guides for placement of the nail. The head of the femur is located one inch distal to the midpoint of a line joining the anterior superior iliac spine and the pubic tubercle. Distal to the greater trochanter the tendon of the gluteus maximus inserts into the linea aspera. Exposed through a lateral incision, the upper border of this tendon marks

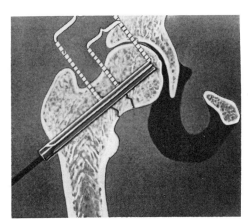

Figure 60. A Smith-Petersen nail is driven through the neck of the femur into the head, fastening the fragments together. The nail is effective in holding fractures in reduction from the subcapital level to near the base of the neck.

the point for insertion of the nail. A hole is drilled in the bone at this point and a guide wire is inserted through the neck into the head, using these landmarks. If the femur is fully internally rotated, the neck of the femur should lie parallel to the floor. The guide wire follows this parallel course through the neck into the center of the head. If x-ray examinations reveal that the guide wire is in the center of the neck and head, a cannulated Smith-Petersen nail of appropriate length is threaded onto the wire and driven into place. X-ray films are again made to confirm the accuracy of fixation of the fracture.

When spicules of bone prevent accurate reduction by closed manipulation, surgical exposure of the fracture site may be necessary to approximate the fragments in an acceptable position. If the fracture through the neck of the femur is almost vertical, fixation is difficult to maintain because of shearing force. The bone softens about the pin because of this force and fixation is lost. It may be necessary to place the head and neck in valgus position by osteotomy of the femur just above the lesser trochanter. This angulation of the neck into a more vertical position brings the fracture line into a more horizontal plane and converts the shearing force into an impacting one.

Since the osteotomy disconnects the shaft from the neck and head, the new relationship of these structures must be maintained by a plate connected to the nail and secured to the femoral shaft.

Since the majority of subcapital and midcervical fractures occur in the elderly, these patients do not tolerate prolonged bed rest or inactivity. Complications involving the lungs, genitourinary system and circulatory system are common if the patient is not made active as early as possible. Internal fixation, while securing immobilization of the fracture, also allows early non-weight-bearing ambulation and exercise. Exercise of the leg is started immediately to prevent contracture and muscle atrophy. The patient should be instructed in the use of a walker, which provides purposeful exercise, but weight must not be borne upon the leg until union is complete. Healing rates vary, and may be as short as three months or as long as a year.

If the fracture line is unfavorable for healing, or, if the survival of the head is questionable, in the elderly patient, the surgeon may elect to replace the head of the bone with a prosthesis. Several types of prosthetic devices are available. They employ the principle of replacing the head of the femur with a metal ball which is connected to the remaining neck and shaft by an intramedullary stem. Weight is then borne by the neck of the femur, transmitted through the prosthesis to the acetabulum. To function properly, the metal head must fit the acetabulum accurately, and the stem must be firmly seated against the neck and within the medullary canal. If the fit is not accurate the acetabulum is subjected to excessive pressure, the cartilage wears and the bone may be eroded. If the stem does not fit against the neck and within the medullary canal properly, bone absorbs about the stem, allowing the prosthesis to wobble; instability and pain are the result.

FRACTURES OF THE BASE OF THE NECK OF THE FEMUR. Fractures of the base of the neck of the femur are characterized by shortening, external rotation of the leg and varus angulation of the neck. The same muscles which cause the deformity of subcapital and midcervical fractures produce this deformity.

The prognosis for healing and survival of the head of the femur is good because the major capsular vessels are not destroyed in this fracture. Reduction is performed as for the other intracapsular fractures. However, fixation by nail must be supplemented by plate fixation to the shaft, as the short segment of bone through which the nail passes in the distal fragment is not sufficient to hold the nail securely.

INTERTROCHANTERIC FRACTURES. Three major types of intertrochanteric fractures are encountered: undisplaced, displaced and comminuted. The prognosis for healing is good in all, but the instability produced by the comminuted type often leads to deformity and permanent disability.

The injury is serious when displacement occurs, because the blood loss may be considerable. Shock is often present. Since the fracture is frequent in the aged and often in the debilitated patient, the mortality is greater than with intracapsular fractures.

Displacement is produced by the long thigh muscles and the external rotator muscles of the hip. Shortening may be marked with extreme external rotation; the lateral border of the foot lies flat against the bed. The neck and head are forced into varus position by the upward displacement of the shaft. If the major part of the greater trochanter is attached to the neck, this deformity is increased by the upward pull of the abductor muscles. The fracture opens anteriorly and the shaft fragment may be displaced backward by gravity and the pull of the gluteus maximus. The neck fragment may also angulate posteriorly by the force of gravity, or by the pull of the external rotator muscles when they are attached to this fragment (Fig. 61).

Undisplaced fractures require no reduction, but are often treated by internal fixation to insure against displacement while healing. Displaced, and particularly comminuted, fractures may be easy or extremely difficult to reduce. Reduction is performed by a method similar to that used in intracapsular fractures, except that internal rotation only to the neutral position is required and abduction is maintained. If the extremity is internally rotated completely, the fracture line closes in front but opens in back, and the neck may be forced into more posterior angulation. If abduction is not sufficient, coxa vara may persist.

Maintenance of reduction may be provided by the continuous suspension traction of Russell or by internal fixation. Undisplaced fractures heal rapidly, usually within two months by any method of treatment. Displaced and comminuted fractures may heal in this time, but often require three or four months. If traction is used, it must be maintained until healing is complete, otherwise soft callus permits recurrence of the coxa vara deformity with shortening. Often, it is undesirable to keep elderly patients in bed for the time necessary for healing. For this reason, open reduction with internal fixation is more commonly done (Fig. 62).

A pin and plate must be used to maintain reduction. The pin is placed as it is for the intracapsular fractures, but in order to prevent medial migration of the shaft fragment, the nail is placed so that it impinges along the lower cortex of the neck. When comminution is severe, firm fixation of the fragments may be impossible to achieve and a certain degree of deformity may slowly recur (Fig. 63).

Nonunion is rare and is usually due to inadequate fixation or interposition of soft tissue. The condition is treated by bone grafting.

DISLOCATION OF THE HIP JOINT. Traumatic dislocation of the hip is produced by extreme indirect violence. Usually, the hip and knee are flexed when the force is applied to the distal end of the femur. This force is often produced in automobile accidents, when the victim's knee strikes the dashboard as the body is thrown forward. The force is transmitted through the head against the posterior capsule and rim of the acetabulum. If the femur is in adduction, the head may be forced laterally out of the socket, tearing the ligamentum teres and the capsule. The head then dislocates posteriorly. If the femur is in a more neutral position, or abduction, the force is exerted against the posterior acetabular rim which may be fractured and driven backward, allowing the head to dislocate. The dislocated head of the femur may displace upward on the ilium, or, if the hip is flexed to a greater degree, it may fall into the sciatic notch of the pelvis injuring the sciatic nerve.

Posterior dislocation usually produces shortening, internal rotation and adduction of the femur. The muscles which produce

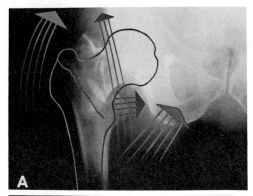

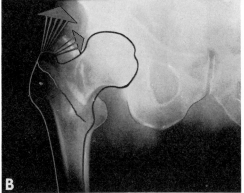

Figure 61. *A*, Intertrochanteric fractures produce varus deformity of the neck coupled with external rotation, because of shortening and rotation by the thigh and hip musculature. *B*, The head and neck fragment may be pulled upward and backward if the abductor and external rotator muscles remain attached to it.

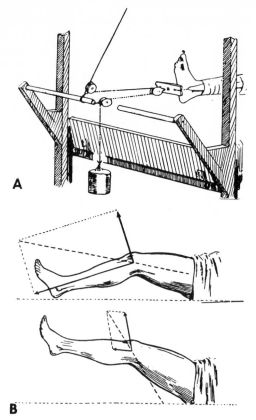

A

B

Figure 62. *A*, The Russell traction apparatus. *B*, Diagram of the parallelogram of forces which produces traction on the flexed hip in the long axis of the femur.

shortening are the long thigh muscles: adductors, flexors and extensors. The adduction is produced by the adductor muscles and the internal rotation by the position of the head and neck against the posterior ilium or sciatic notch.

Less frequently, anterior dislocation is produced by a violent twisting injury with the thigh in extreme abduction. This mechanism forces the head over the shallow inferior rim of the acetabulum and through the joint capsule. Rotational force then dislocates the head forward, where it may come to lie in the obturator foramen or be displaced upward onto the pubis. The leg is usually externally rotated and abducted, but shortening may be absent.

The final resting place of the head determines the classification of the dislocation. Thus, the dislocation may be posterior iliac or sciatic, and anterior pubic or obturator. Central dislocation occurs when the floor of the acetabulum fractures and the head of the femur is driven into the pelvis. Tearing of muscles always accompanies this serious injury. Bleeding may be serious and shock is common. Injury to the sciatic nerve by stretching often complicates the dislocation.

Reduction is accomplished by reversing the forces which produced the dislocation. Several manipulative procedures have been described by Allis, Bigelow and Stimson. The method of Allis is most commonly used and is performed with the patient supine. The hip and knee are flexed and the thigh adducted. Longitudinal traction is made behind the bent knee. Gentle internal and external rotation movements are performed until the head of the femur slips into the acetabulum. When no fracture is present, the reduction is usually accompanied by a snap and is stable. When the posterior rim of the acetabulum is fractured, the head of the femur may slide easily into the acetabu-

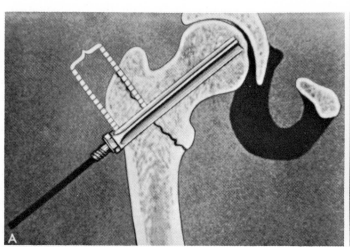
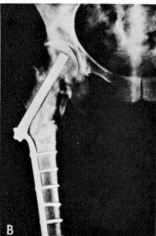

Figure 63. *A*, The trochanteric fragment does not offer enough holding surface for a nail. *B*, A plate must be attached to the femur with screws to secure adequate internal fixation.

lum, and it may be difficult to tell when the dislocation is reduced. The hip is then extended and abducted and externally rotated moderately. A plaster hip spica cast is applied to prevent redislocation and is maintained for three weeks or longer. If the acetabular fragment cannot be replaced and the hip is stable, the dislocation is treated similarly. However, if the dislocation is unstable, it may be necessary to fasten the fragment in position with screws during open reduction. Rarely, a fragment of the head of the femur is broken off and remains in the acetabulum. Reduction is blocked by this fragment and open reduction with removal of the piece of bone must be done (Fig. 64).

Anterior dislocations are reduced by traction in a similar position of flexion at the hip and knee. The femur is slowly abducted to near 90 degrees. This brings the head of the femur downward near the inferior acetabular notch. Internal rotation is performed gently when the thigh is adducted and extended, forcing the head of the bone through the inferior rent in the capsule.

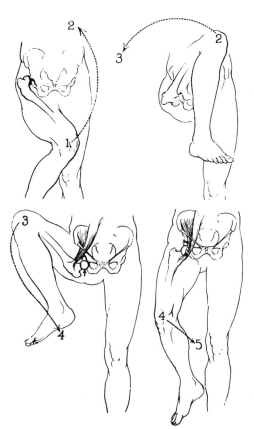

Figure 64.   Bigelow's maneuver for reducing dislocation of the hip.

Immobilization may be accomplished by strapping the legs together to prevent abduction and external rotation for three weeks.

Following reduction and immobilization of either anterior or posterior dislocation, the patient should be placed on crutches for at least two months from the time of dislocation. Active exercise of the hip, thigh and leg should be done regularly to rehabilitate the muscles and regain joint motion.

Aseptic necrosis of the head of the femur follows this injury all too frequently. Damage to the blood supply to the head of the femur is more likely when the rim of the acetabulum is fractured. For this reason, the patient should remain on crutches for two months following the dislocation. During this time, disuse atrophy of the adjacent bone may reveal the relative increase in density of the head of the femur, indicative of aspect necrosis on x-ray examination. When necrosis of the head of the femur is established, bone grafting is done to re-establish the blood supply. A tibial bone graft is inserted through the neck of the femur into the head to aid in the resubstitution of the dead bone. Additional reconstructive procedures may be necessary if necrosis continues, or if it occurs later with the development of arthritis of the joint.

Recovery of the sciatic nerve is variable. Complete return of function may occur in a few weeks or may take a year or longer. Often, there is some permanent residual impairment of sciatic nerve function.

THE FEMUR

FRACTURES OF THE SHAFT OF THE FEMUR. Fractures of the shaft of the femur are classified by location, since the displacing pull of muscles, and thus the deformity produced, varies with the level at which the fracture occurs. These areas are the subtrochanteric, or upper one-third of the femoral shaft, the middle segment, and the supracondylar and condylar area of the bone.

The abductors, flexors and external rotator muscles are unopposed when the femur breaks in the upper one-third, and the proximal fragment assumes this position of abduction, flexion and external rotation. The distal fragment is pulled medially and angulates laterally by the action of the adductor magnus inserting along the entire medial femoral shaft. The quadriceps and hamstring muscles produce shortening.

Fractures in the midportion of the bone have a similar deformity but the external rotation and abduction of the proximal fragment is less, since more of the adductor musculature is attached to this fragment.

Supracondylar fractures are influenced primarily by the gastrocnemius muscles, which pull the distal fragment posteriorly. The long thigh muscles attaching below the knee cause shortening.

The principal blood supply is provided by the femoral artery. Because of the relatively abundant blood supply, necrosis of the bone seldom develops following fractures of the femur. However, as there may be tearing of muscle, or tearing of the perforating branches of the femoral artery, there is invariably a large effusion of blood into the surrounding tissues. Shock from blood loss often accompanies these fractures. Both the vessels and nerves lie close to the bone along its lower portion, and may be injured in supracondylar fractures (Fig. 65).

The femur is a massive bone, and usually extreme violence is necessary to produce fractures of the shaft. The force often is a twist from indirect violence; however, a direct blow to the bone may also produce the fracture.

FRACTURES OF THE UPPER AND MIDDLE THIRDS OF THE FEMUR. Problems relating to fractures of the upper and middle thirds of the femur are similar in many respects. In fractures of the upper third of the femur, the two fragments are subject to characteristic deformities from the pull of strong muscle groups. The proximal fragment is abducted by the gluteal muscles, flexed by the iliopsoas and rotated by the external rotators; it assumes a flexed, externally rotated and abducted position. At the same time, the adductor muscles, assisted by the hamstrings and quadriceps muscle group, cause shortening and medial displacement of the distal fragment. The reduction is accomplished by traction on the distal fragment with the knee flexed to relax the hamstring muscles. The distal fragment is abducted to align it with the proximal fragment and externally rotated as much as necessary to effect proper alignment (Fig. 66).

If the fracture occurs in the middle of the shaft, there is frequently a similar angulation and shortening. However, the displacement of the proximal fragment is less since more of the adductor muscles are attached to it. The fracture is reduced in the same manner as one occurring higher on the femur.

The problem of reducing these fractures is of small moment compared with the problems of maintaining the reduction. Immobilization in a plaster spica is advocated by some surgeons. However, the thickness of the muscles surrounding the fragments is such that angulation may occur inside the cast and immobilization may be inadequate. In any case, immobilization is unsatisfactory for oblique fractures, which tend to override.

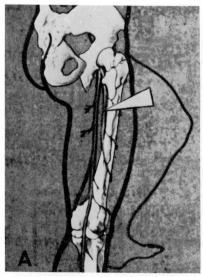 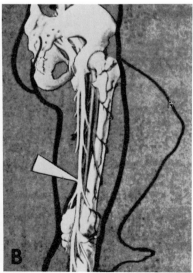

Figure 65.   *A,* The principal blood supply to the femur is from the femoral artery and the profundus femoris. Damage to these vessels may cause profound hemorrhage and shock. *B,* The sciatic nerve lies close to the lower femur, and may be injured by supracondylar fractures.

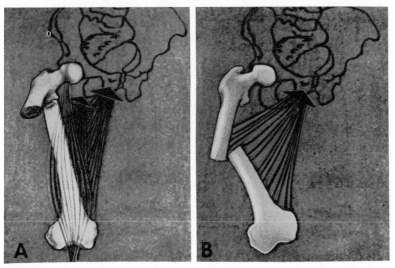

Figure 66. *A*, The proximal upper one-third fragment of the femur is abducted, externally rotated and flexed by the action of the abductor, external rotator and iliopsoas muscle groups. The distal fragment of the femur is adducted and shortened by the action of the adductor and hamstring muscles, as well as the rectus femoris. The distal femoral fragment must be abducted, flexed and externally rotated to align it with the proximal fragment. *B*, Fractures of the midshaft of the femur angulate and shorten, as do fractures of the upper one-third; however, abduction of the proximal fragment is less, since part of the adductor muscle system remains attached to this fragment.

Probably, the most useful device for maintaining reduction is the Thomas splint with the Pearson attachment. The Thomas splint with its attached sling acts as a cradle for the thigh. The Pearson attachment and its sling support the lower leg. It allows knee joint motion, an important consideration later in postoperative care. A foot board may be used for the comfort of the patient and to prevent contracture of the plantar flexors of the foot. Countertraction is supplied by the weight of the patient's body on the bed. Traction is frequently skeletal. A pin or wire through the upper end of the tibia, or through the distal end of the femur, allows traction to be made by pulling directly on the bone (Fig. 67).

When a wire is to be used in the femur, the placement is important. If it is inserted too high on the shaft, it may endanger the femoral vessels. If it is inserted in cancellous bone of the condyles, there is danger that the wire will cut through the bone, since the pull must be sustained for a number of weeks. It should be placed proximal to the condyles where the thicker cortical bone is better able to sustain the weight of traction. The wire must also avoid the suprapatellar pouch to

Figure 67. The Thomas splint with Pearson attachment is used for suspension of femoral fractures. Skeletal traction is made through the upper tibia.

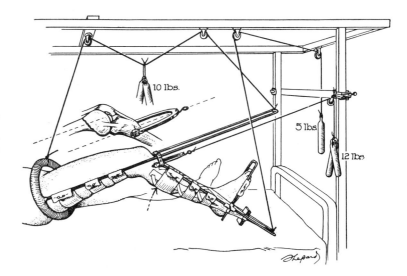

lessen the danger of adhesions. A safer area for skeletal traction is through the upper tibia. Traction is then made through the ligaments of the knee joint.

In addition to providing suspension and traction, the apparatus can be adjusted to control abduction, flexion and rotation. When this method is used, x-ray examinations must be made frequently to ensure that the reduction is maintained. The apparatus must be checked daily to be sure that it is functioning properly.

These fractures usually require at least ten to 12 weeks for healing. Because of this prolonged time in bed, open reduction with internal fixation is often done. The method that has become popular since World War II is the Kuntscher intramedullary rod. Properly applied, the method immobilizes fractures of the midportion of .the bone well, and allows early ambulation and mobilization of the joint.

The intramedullary rod must fit the medullary canal tightly to prevent rotation. It must be long enough to ensure good fixation of both the proximal and distal fragments. This method of fixation, however, cannot be used with fractures just below the trochanters, because the proximal fragment is too short to provide holding power for the rod. Better fixation is provided by the nail and plate used for intertrochanteric fractures. The plate must be long enough to fasten the distal fragment securely to the proximal.

COMMINUTED FRACTURES OF FEMUR. Comminution occurs not infrequently as a result of direct violence, and it may present additional problems. Management in suspension with traction is usually advisable. But sometimes, when enough traction is applied to maintain the alignment of the major fragments, distraction occurs, the distal fragment commonly being separated from the middle pieces.

Occasionally, angulation of a middle fragment may resist all efforts at reduction. This is usually due to penetration of the fragment into muscle or fascia, the interposed soft tissue preventing reduction. Operation may be necessary to clear the muscle and reduce the fracture.

When the fragments of a comminuted fracture are small, open reduction is usually not necessary. Suspension traction will allow union of these fragments.

If immobilization is continued long enough,

callus should ultimately fill what appears to be large gaps. The surgeon can then treat any unattached fragments or gaps that remain. Bone grafts may be used to allow the bone to complete the healing process.

SUPRACONDYLAR FRACTURES OF FEMUR. Supracondylar fractures present a different set of problems from those occurring higher on the femur. They are uncommon, but important because of the difficulties they present. The distal fragment is usually pulled backward by the force of the gastrocnemius and hamstring muscles. At the same time, the contraction of the quadriceps, which is attached to the tibia, tends to make the fragments override (Fig. 68).

The bone ends may threaten the popliteal nerves and vessels with resulting paralysis or massive hemorrhage. Accordingly, the surgeon must watch for signs of damage to these structures.

Reduction demands relaxation of the gastrocnemius muscle. To accomplish this, the knee is flexed 90 degrees and the foot plantar flexed. Traction is then made in the long axis of the femur. The bone ends are manipulated by direct pressure of the surgeon's hands.

The maintenance of reduction is best accomplished by suspension skeletal traction. The extremity is placed in the Thomas splint and Pearson attachment, and suspended by appropriate ropes and weights. Skeletal traction is made by a wire placed through the upper tibia (Fig. 69).

Occasionally, the posterior angulation may persist even with adequate traction. A second wire may be placed through the femoral

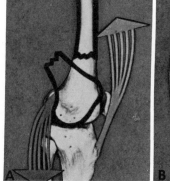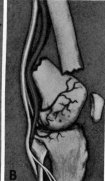

Figure 68. *A,* The distal fragment of supracondylar fracture of the femur angulates posteriorly because the gastrocnemius muscle arises upon the condyles and pulls the fragment backward. *B,* The displacement of the distal fragment may damage the popliteal nerves and blood vessels.

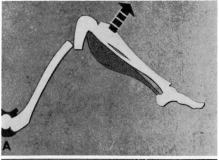

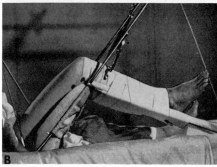

Figure 69. *A*, Reduction of supracondylar fracture is accomplished by flexing the knee to 90 degrees to relax the pull of the gastrocnemius muscle, and applying traction in the long axis of the femur. *B*, Traction is made through the tibia while the extremity is supported in the Thomas splint and Pearson attachment, with the knee in 90 degrees of flexion.

condyles and traction applied at a right angle to the femur pulling the distal fragment anteriorly. This method of traction must be used with caution since the wire in the condyles is close to the fracture. Infection along the tract of the wire may involve the fracture site with disastrous results.

Open reduction with internal fixation is occasionally necessary. The same principle that is used for internal fixation of the trochanteric region of the femur applies. The short distal fragment must be held by a nail or blade plate placed transversely through it and secured to the shaft by the plate and screws.

These fractures usually heal in ten to 12 weeks. Knee motion should be started early in the course of treatment to prevent adhesions within the joint.

FRACTURES AND EPIPHYSIAL DISPLACEMENT OF THE FEMUR IN CHILDREN. Fractures of the femur in children are classified as upper, middle and lower one-third injuries. Slipped or displaced femoral epiphyses may involve these structures at the proximal or distal end of the bone. Injuries of the upper one-third of the bone, including the head and neck, are less common than injuries of the middle and lower one-third of the bone in infancy and young

children. At puberty, slipping and displacement of the epiphysis of the head of the femur is a definite and not uncommon syndrome. Fractures of the neck of the femur are rare in children.

Displacement of the head of the femur through the epiphysial plate may occur with a single acute, twisting injury, but often the process is slow and insidious. The condition occurs most often in obese male children at or about puberty. At this stage of development of the child, the epiphysial plate may undergo changes preparatory to closure, or hormonal changes may weaken the structure. The exact cause of gradual slipping is not understood.

Characteristically, the head of the femur rotates backward and downward while the neck rotates forward. In the acute injury, pain and limitation of motion are obvious, and x-ray examination readily reveals the displacement. When gradual slipping occurs, the only symptom may be a painless limp, and meticulous x-ray films may be necessary to detect the beginning displacement. The degree of displacement in either case determines the details of treatment.

The acute, traumatic, slipped, proximal femoral epiphysis should be replaced by traction and internal rotation in moderate abduction. The reduction may be maintained by a spica hip cast, or by internal fixation with pins of small diameter. Often, the epiphysial plate closes following the injury and growth ceases. When this does not occur, the hip must be protected from weight-bearing for months or recurrence of the deformity is common. Frequent x-ray films are necessary to detect the recurrent deformity.

Gradual slipping of the proximal epiphysis is called adolescent coxa vara. The etiology is not clear. The symptoms may be minimal. The condition is often bilateral. The surgeon must watch the opposite hip carefully for signs of displacement until the epiphysis has closed. The treatment may be conservative or surgical, and the choice depends upon the degree of deformity and the stage of development when the condition is discovered. If the slipping is minimal, but acute, internal fixation and multiple small-diameter pins may be done to prevent increasing deformity. Larger pins and triflanged nails are not suitable. Driven into the hard bone of the head of the femur, these devices may completely disrupt the epiphysial plate and produce marked deformity. When the deformity is found later, the epiphysial plate may be closing. Traction or protection from weight-bearing may be all that is needed. The small deformity is accepted. It may be necessary to correct more pronounced deformity by osteotomy of the neck or subtrochanteric region, followed by appropriate internal fixation. Weight must not be borne until the epiphysis closes.

FRACTURES OF THE FEMORAL NECK IN CHILDREN. Fractures of the neck of the femur are rare in children. The prognosis is poor, as it is in the adult. Nonunion, coxa vara and aseptic necrosis are frequent complications. Reduction with internal fixation with small pins is usually necessary, and is one of the few instances when internal fixation is indicated in the child. Healing may require many months, and weight-bearing cannot be resumed until union is firm.

FRACTURES ABOUT THE TROCHANTERS AND UPPER THIRD OF THE FEMUR IN CHILDREN. Fractures between the trochanters, or at the level of the lesser trochanter, are usually oblique or transverse. The deforming pull of the muscles produces coxa vara. It must be remembered that deformity produced by fractures above the lesser trochanter does not correct with growth. Any deformity which results from the fracture is permanent. Every effort should be made to correct the coxa vara deformity.

Russell traction, or the Thomas splint with the Pearson attachment, is a useful method for reduction and maintenance of extracapsular upper one-third fractures in older children. The spica cast with the leg placed in wide abduction may be used in younger children in high upper one-third fractures, but x-ray examination at frequent intervals is necessary to detect recurrent deformity in the cast.

FRACTURES OF THE MIDDLE THIRD OF THE FEMUR IN CHILDREN. Fracture of the middle third of the shaft of the femur occurs in all age groups of children, and this is the common location of femoral fractures in infancy. The mechanism is direct or indirect violence, and in young children the fracture line tends to be transverse or oblique. Comminution is unusual. As the child approaches puberty, the fractures tend to resemble those in the adult, particularly those fractures occurring after the age of 13 years. Comminution of fragments is found more often after this age. The deformity produced is similar to that in the adult, except that the proximal fragment may, on occasion, assume an adducted position.

Reduction and maintenance of reduction is best done by continuous traction. Rotational alignment must be accurate, but slight angulation may be acceptable in younger children, because it corrects with growth. Shortening, or side-to-side apposition, is desirable in younger children. Stimulation of longitudinal growth always takes place following this fracture, and end-to-end apposition always results in a longer leg, which is just as undesirable as one too short. The fracture also heals more rapidly and union is stronger with side-to-side apposition of the fragments.

From infancy to the age of four years, Bryant's overhead suspension traction is often used. The child should not weigh over 40 pounds if this method is employed. Both legs must be suspended by skin traction from an overhead frame. Sufficient traction is applied to lift the buttocks just off the bed. A restraint is used about the trunk to help maintain alignment. Sufficient traction is usually produced to overcome angulation, but allows some overriding of the fragments. A centimeter or a little more overriding is desirable, since stimulation of longitudinal growth of this amount is expected. When Bryant's traction is used, it must be watched carefully for signs of skin irritation and circulatory embarrassment. Circulatory impairment seems to occur more readily in the unfractured leg, and can lead to Volkmann's contracture or catastrophic gangrene. This tragedy can be avoided by hourly inspection of the suspended legs. Should signs of circulatory embarrassment develop, the constriction must be removed immediately (Fig. 70).

Children over the age of four years and weighing over 40 pounds are best treated in the Russell suspension traction. Suspension and traction must be maintained until union is firm. In the infant, this time may be as short as three weeks, but becomes longer in older children. Angulation can be corrected by manipulation when the callus is soft and reaches the "lead pipe" consistency. However, it must be remembered that the more manipulation of the healing fracture the more will be the stimulation to overgrowth of the bone.

Open reduction of shaft fractures of the femur in children is practically never indi-

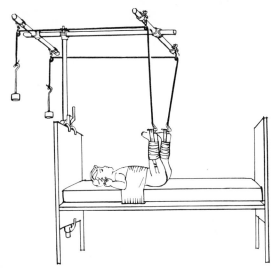

Figure 70. When Bryant's traction is used for treatment of fractures of the femur in childhood, both legs should be suspended. In addition, skin traction should not encircle the leg, as this may contribute to strangulation of the circulation. Volkmann's ischemic contracture can result when traction is applied improperly. Catastrophic circulatory failure may occur if the patient is not watched every hour. (From Schmeisser: Clinical Manual of Orthopedic Traction Techniques.)

cated and internal fixation is to be condemned. Interposition of soft parts at the fracture is of no consequence in children, and is not an indication for open reduction. Muscle fibers interposed in the fracture are readily incorporated in the callus and moderate angulation is corrected by growth and the remodeling process.

FRACTURES OF THE LOWER THIRD OF THE FEMUR IN CHILDREN. Fractures in the lower one-third of the bone may require traction with the extremity placed in 90 degrees of flexion of the hip and knee to prevent posterior angulation. This may be accomplished by modified Russell traction. Care must be exercised to prevent injury to the peroneal nerve. As in the adult, the deformity is produced by the pull of the gastrocnemius muscle.

SLIPPED LOWER FEMORAL EPIPHYSIS IN CHILDREN. Slipping of the lower femoral epiphysis is usually produced by forces which hyperextend the knee. The epiphysis displaces and angulates forward on the metaphysis. Medial or lateral displacement may accompany this major deformity. As in the case of supracondylar fractures in the adult, the displacement may damage the popliteal vessels and nerves. Prompt manipulative reduction is needed. Traction is made on the bent knee while pressure is made backward on the epiphysis and forward on the metaphysis. If the manipulation is unsuccessful and circulatory failure is impending, open reduction with gentle replacement of the epiphysis is warranted. The periosteum must not be stripped from the bone near the epiphysial plate during the process, as growth arrest may result.

If the injury is found after several days, it may be impossible to reduce. The leg is placed in a plaster cast following reduction with the knee in moderate flexion and maintained in this position for three or four weeks. If the displacement cannot be corrected when the injury is found after several days, open reduction should not be done, because at this stage, forceful manipulation will only increase the danger of growth arrest. The knee is immobilized and growth of the bone is allowed to correct the deformity.

Partial growth arrest of the epiphysis may result in knock-knee or bow-leg deformity. In young children, it may be necessary to correct this by repeated osteotomy. In older children, when most of the growth of the extremity has been obtained, completion of the closure of the epiphysial plate with correction of the deformity may be done surgically. A slight amount of shortening is acceptable, but the remaining growth potential in the opposite leg must be carefully estimated before this is done.

THE KNEE JOINT

The stability of the knee depends upon an intricate set of ligaments, functioning synchronously with the activating muscles. These ligaments allow the hingelike action of flexion and extension, but prevent forward, backward and side-to-side movement. The surrounding muscles and their tendons provide stability in varying degrees of flexion and extension.

The rounded condyles of the femur, resting upon the two saucer-like plateaus of the tibia, provide minimum bony contact, ensuring friction-free movement. These saucers are deepened slightly by the semilunar cartilages. The patella, articulating with the femur between the condyles, acts like a pulley, increasing the power of the extensor muscles. The gastrocnemius muscle, originating on the femoral condyles and the medial and lateral hamstring muscles inserting on the tibia, produce active flexion, but also act as a check rein, stabilizing the knee in extension.

Intimately associated with the joint posteriorly are the major blood vessels and nerves to the leg.

Normal function depends upon the synchronous action of all of these parts. Injuries to any one of the components affects the others. The major ligaments which provide stability are the tibial collateral, the fibular collateral and the cruciate ligaments. The broad tibial collateral ligament arises from the medial condyle and inserts some distance below the joint line on the tibia. The fibers in this ligament are arranged so the part of the ligament is always taut in flexion or extension. The fibular collateral ligament, a cordlike structure, arises on the lateral femoral condyle and runs backward and downward to insert on the head of the fibula. This ligament is tight on extension, but relaxes with flexion. These two ligaments prevent angulation and side-to-side displacement of the tibia on the femur.

The anterior and posterior cruciate ligaments arise in the intracondylar notch, wind about each other and insert on the tibial spines. Like the tibial collateral ligament, they remain taut in all phases of flexion and extension. They prevent forward or backward displacement of the tibia on the femur. All of these ligaments help to prevent hyperextension when the condyles of the tibia and femur have a normal configuration. All of them allow slight rotary motion of the tibia on the femur.

The joint capsule posteriorly fits tightly when the knee is extended, but relaxes in flexion, and helps stabilize the extended knee.

Anteriorly, the joint capsule is made up of the retinaculum of the extensor muscles inserting into the tibia and the patella, and is part of the extensor mechanism. Fibers of the rectus femoris tendon insert into the upper border of the patella and progress over the anterior surface to blend with the patellar tendon below, which inserts into the tibial tubercle. These structures, coupled with the retinaculum, transmit the power of the quadriceps muscles to the tibia, providing extension and adding additional stability to the knee. Fractures of the patella may disrupt this extensor mechanism.

The femoral artery and its extension, the popliteal artery, lie close to the lower femur and the joint posteriorly, and are vulnerable to injury in fractures of the condyles of the tibia or femur.

The tibial and peroneal nerves, arising from the sciatic nerve, are similarly vulnerable to injury; the tibial nerve by fractures of the condyles and the peroneal by fractures and injuries of the lateral tibial plateau and head of the fibula.

The weight-bearing line, or mechanical axis of the lower extremity, passes through the center of the hip, knee and ankle joint. Because the shaft of the femur at the upper end is set out laterally by the neck, it must slant medially as it progresses downward to meet this line. Thus, the femoral condyles meet the tibia at a slight angle. However, the joint line is level when standing; this is accomplished by a slightly larger medial femoral condyle. The weight is equally distributed through the medial and lateral condyles of the femur and tibia.

Fractures about the knee which produce the deformity of knock-knee or bow-leg throw the weight-bearing line medially or laterally. Weight is then borne more on one condyle than the other. Strain is created at the hip, knee and ankle joints and wear of the joints is excessive. Fatigue, pain and eventually traumatic arthritis is the end-product of abnormal weight-bearing. Fractures of either the femoral or tibial condyles may produce these deformities.

FRACTURES OF THE FEMORAL CONDYLES. Fractures of the femoral condyles are produced by indirect compression force transmitted up the leg, or from force causing lateral or medial deviation, or by direct violence. One or both condyles may break. The fracture line usually runs from the superior portion of the condyle downward into the intracondylar notch; when both condyles are fractured, the fracture line may be Y or T shaped. When one condyle is fractured, it is usually driven upward and outward by the force producing the fracture. This produces a knock-knee or bow-leg deformity, depending upon which condyle is broken. The fragment is then rotated backward by the downward pull of the gastrocnemius muscle arising posteriorly. If the force continues, the leg deviates to such a degree that the collateral ligaments are damaged by stretching. The origin of the cruciate ligaments in the intracondylar notch may be disturbed. The popliteal nerves and vessels may be endangered by sharp fragments of bone displaced into this area. Circulation and the status of the nerves must be determined before reduction is attempted.

Since the ligaments and joint capsule remain attached to the fragment, these structures are used to exert traction on the condyle in reduction. The opposite condyle acts as a fulcrum, as force is applied deviating the leg to correct the deformity. If the lateral femoral condyle is fractured, the medial one serves as the fulcrum. The tibia is angulated toward the midline of the body while pressure is exerted laterally against the medial lower femur. This manipulation pulls the displaced condyle downward. If the fragment remains laterally displaced, widening the condyles, it is forced back into position by compressing the condyles with the surgeon's hands or a C shaped clamp. The knee is then flexed to relax the pull of the gastrocnemius, and by direct manipulation the backward displacement is corrected. Fractures of the medial condyle are reduced by the same method, with the forces applied in the opposite direction.

Since the femoral condyles are not spheres but are elongated from front to back, and the medial one is larger than the lateral, accurate replacement of the fracture is essential if the joint is to function properly. Backward rotation of one condyle disturbs the axis of flexion and extension, and some of the motion will be lost.

Immobilization in a long-leg cast, molded to maintain the leg in the corrected position, may hold a stable fracture in position. The unstable fracture may require suspension traction or operation securing the fragment to the femur with screws.

INTRACONDYLAR FRACTURES. More often, both condyles are fractured from the shaft of the femur. Considerable force is necessary to produce the fracture and comminution of the bone is commonplace. The force producing the fracture drives the condyles upward. The bone splits at the intracondylar notch. The fracture lines then run upward or transversely to form a Y or T. As the force continues, the condyles are displaced upward; the shaft of the femur acts like a wedge forcing them apart. The pull of the quadriceps and hamstring muscles maintains the shortening. The gastrocnemius may rotate the fragments posteriorly. The neurovascular structures are threatened.

Reduction is accomplished by traction and manipulation making use of the intact ligaments and joint capsule. Traction is made in the long axis of the femur with the knee flexed to relax the gastrocnemius. As the fragments are pulled downward by the traction exerted through the collateral ligaments, they are molded together by compression.

Maintenance of reduction must be obtained by suspension skeletal traction through the upper tibia. The Thomas splint and Pearson attachment suspend the leg while traction is maintained by a wire placed through the upper tibia. The knee must remain flexed as in the treatment of supracondylar fractures.

When severe comminution is present, the knee may resemble a bag of bones. Suspension traction is the method of choice because the joint capsule tends to mold the fragments together. Attempted open reduction may devitalize fragments, and it may be impossible to secure adequate fixation. When comminution is not severe, open reduction may be done when the fracture cannot be accurately reduced by closed methods. The condyles are bolted together and attached to the shaft of the femur by a blade plate or another appropriate device.

These fractures heal in eight to 12 weeks, but weight-bearing must not be allowed until the union is complete. Motion, however, must be started as early as possible.

FRACTURES OF THE PATELLA. A patella can be fractured by indirect or by direct violence. In a fall, the patient may have the good fortune to land on his feet. He is betrayed, however, by a tensed quadriceps muscle acting on a partially flexed knee. The indirect force of the muscle contraction causes the fracture. If the force is continued, the retinaculum tears and the patellar fragments separate. The extensor mechanism is disrupted. The pull of the quadriceps muscle maintains the separation of the fragments. The patella may survive this hazard, to be fractured by the force of the direct blow as the knee strikes the ground. There may be a simple fracture with little displacement of the fragments if the anterior capsule is not torn. Often, however, there are varying degrees of comminution in the fractures caused by direct violence.

Transverse fractures are most frequent and may occur in the upper, middle or lower one-third of the bone. Occasionally, longitudinal fractures occur at the margins or central portion of the patella.

Treatment is directed toward the re-establishment of the extensor mechanism and the creation of a smooth, anatomically accurate, articular surface for the patella.

When the fracture is transverse or longitudinal without separation, the extensor mechanism remains intact through the retinaculum. This situation can be treated conservatively. The leg should be kept in full extension. A posterior splint will provide the needed immobilization. Ice bags may be applied to reduce the swelling.

Almost all fractures of the knee are accompanied by an effusion of blood and synovial fluid into the joint. Aspiration under local anesthesia not only contributes to the patient's comfort, but also minimizes the danger of degenerative changes in the articular cartilage, since blood in the joint is an irritant to the cartilage.

If a cast is applied, it should extend from the ankle to the groin and be snug enough at both ends to provide complete immobilization. The patient whose leg is thus immobilized may start weight-bearing as soon as the cast is applied. Though this cast will give the patient some freedom, it does not allow proper exercise of the quadriceps muscle. The cast is bivalved within a week, and active flexion and extension exercises are begun.

When there is separation of the two major fragments of the patella, the damage can be repaired only through operative treatment. The bone injury is incidental to the rupture of the extensor retinaculum which must be restored before the patient can regain the ability to extend his leg. The patella and retinaculum are exposed through an appropriate incision, allowing the knee joint to be inspected and blood clots and debris to be removed. The patella is fitted accurately together and held by a wire suture placed through or around the fragments. The retinaculum is repaired. Following repair, a cylinder cast or posterior molded splint is applied. Weight-bearing may be started as soon as the patient is comfortable. Active motion is started as soon as the wound has healed, usually within a week or ten days. However, the posterior splint is used for at least three weeks while the tendon and retinaculum heal (Fig. 71).

The fall which damages a patella may cause such comminution that the fragments cannot be repaired surgically to produce a smooth articular surface. It may be advisable to excise the patella entirely. After the fragments have been removed, the patellar tendon is sutured to the quadriceps tendon. This procedure impairs the function of the knee less than the presence of a badly damaged patella.

FRACTURES OF THE TIBIAL PLATEAU. These fractures may involve one or both condyles of tibia; however, the most frequent is the fracture of the lateral plateau.

In fractures of both condyles, a blow to the lateral side of the leg forces the knee into valgus or knock-knee position. The medial collateral ligament and cruciates may rupture. If they hold, they produce a fulcrum upon which the lateral femoral condyle acts as a wedge against the lateral tibial plateau,

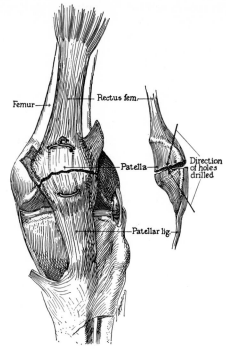

Figure 71. Separated fractures of the patella must be reduced by open methods and held by internal fixation. The extensor retinaculum must be repaired.

forcing it downward. A larger or smaller fragment is split off and displaced laterally and downward. The articular surface is almost always involved. The central weight-bearing portion may be depressed into the cancellous bone for a considerable distance or only slightly. Usually the head or upper part of the fistula is fractured.

Less frequently, a similar fracture occurs in the medial tibial condyle, usually the result of a fall with the knee in the varus or bowed position.

With a fall from a height, the tibia is driven upward against the femoral condyles, the flaring tibial articular surface is compressed. The fracture develops near the tibial spine and slants outward and downward in each condyle if the force is equally distributed. The shaft of the tibia driven upward between these fragments forces them apart. Comminution may be severe. If the force bends the knee medially or laterally, one condyle is depressed and the knee assumes a valgus or varus position. Occasionally, the fracture lines may resemble an inverted T. The condyle splits near the tibial spines while a transverse fracture develops at the junction of the shaft with the condyles.

All of these fractures produce some damage

to the articular surface of the tibia and medial or lateral instability with disturbance of the weight-bearing line. Often, there is some damage to the collateral or cruciate ligaments and, frequently, the semilunar cartilages are torn and displaced. Treatment must re-establish as level and smooth an articular surface as possible, free from internal derangement.

When a single large fragment is present, reduction may be accomplished by forcing the knee into the opposite position from the deformity. If the lateral condyle is split off and displaced downward and laterally, the medial intact tibia and femur are used as a fulcrum. Pressure is made laterally against the medial side of the knee while the leg is adducted on the thigh. The joint capsule on the lateral aspect is, thus, pulled tight and, since it is attached to the fragment, draws it upward. The laterally-displaced fragment is then forced medially by compression with a C shaped clamp. The leg is immobilized in a long-leg cast from the uppermost thigh to the toes. The force of reduction is maintained as the plaster sets (Fig. 72).

If the fragment cannot be maintained in reduction, the fracture site should be opened and internal fixation used to hold the fragments securely. This can often be accomplished with a bolt placed transversely through the tibial condyles. Fractures of a similar nature of the medial condyle are reduced by similar methods, but with the force applied in the opposite direction.

Often the central articular surface of the lateral tibial condyle is depressed into the cancellous bone. This cannot be corrected by external manipulation, since this area is devoid of soft tissue attachments through which traction forces can be applied. If the depression is slight, it may be wiser to accept the slight deformity. The knee is aspirated of blood and immobilized with a voluminous pressure dressing from the toes to the upper thigh and a posterior molded splint. In a few days, when the acute reaction to the injury has subsided, the splint and dressings are removed and active non-weight-bearing exercise is started.

With more severe depression and disruption of the joint surface, open reduction may be necessary to create stability. The articular cartilage is always damaged; however, an attempt should be made to elevate the depressed pieces back to as normal a position as possible. The joint is opened anteriorly over the involved condyle. If the semilunar cartilage is damaged, it should be removed. Often, it is necessary to remove this structure to visualize the articular surfaces properly. A window is then made in the anterior tibia a little below the joint line, and the fragments are levered upward. A gap is then left in the cancellous bone beneath the articular surface, which must be filled to maintain the fragments in position. Bone chips or blocks are obtained locally from adjacent parts of the tibia, or from the ilium and packed into this area. If a fracture line separates the lateral margin of the condyle from the tibia, it may be drawn back into position after reduction by a bolt placed through the condyles. Motion must be started early to prevent intra-articular adhesions; however, the joint should be im-

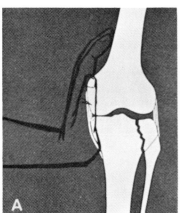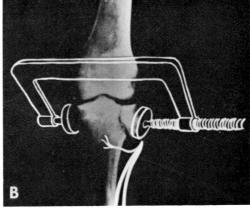

Figure 72. *A*, When a large single fragment of the tibial plateau is depressed, it may be reduced by using the medial condyle as a fulcrum. Pressure is made on the medial aspect of the knee while the tibia is deviated medially. The joint capsule is pulled tightly, drawing the condyle upward. *B*, The laterally displaced fragment is then forced medially with a C shaped clamp.

mobilized in extension for two or three weeks in a cast or splint to allow the reaction of the operation to subside and the fragments to be stabilized with fibrous tissue. Weight-bearing cannot be allowed until firm union is present, or compression of the condyle will cause recurrence of the deformity. A minimun of three months in usually required before union is secure (Fig. 73).

DISLOCATIONS OF THE KNEE JOINT. Dislocations of the knee joint are produced by extreme direct or indirect violence. Since the stability of the knee depends upon the integrity of the ligaments, dislocations always disrupt these vital structures.

The dislocations are classified by the displacement of the tibia on the femur; thus, anterior, posterior, medial and lateral dislocations describe the location of the tibia in relationship to the femur. The medial, lateral, collateral and cruciate ligaments, along with the joint capsule, must be torn to allow dislocation. It is the permanent damage to these structures which accounts for the frequent instability of the joint following dislocation of the knee. Tearing and displacement of the semilunar cartilages may accompany the injury, producing symptoms of internal derangement of the joint following reduction. The popliteal nerves and vessels may be damaged by any dislocation of the knee as may the peroneal nerve. The status of the nerves and blood vessels must be determined before reduction is attempted. Impairment of circulation demands immediate reduction. Occasionally, torn joint capsule or displaced

hamstring tendons may fold into the joint or catch in the intracondylar notch and prevent reduction.

Reduction of posterior and medial, or lateral dislocations is usually best accomplished with the knee flexed to relax the hamstring muscles. Traction is made on the tibia in the flexed position. Anterior dislocations usually require longitudinal traction in extension. The dislocations are usually easily reduced, but are unstable because of the torn ligaments. Immobilization by a long-leg cast in the most stable position follows reduction.

In recent years, immediate surgical repair of the torn ligaments has been advocated for damage to these structures by sprains, subluxations and dislocations of the knee. The end results have been more stable, useful knees when immediate ligament repair is done.

When joint capsule or other structures fold between the joint surfaces, reduction cannot be accomplished except by operation. When this is done, the ligaments should be repaired at the same time.

Cast immobilization for three weeks is followed by vigorous, active exercise to reestablish motion and restore the power of the muscles. The integrity of the quadriceps muscle is most important. It must be brought to maximum efficiency to provide stability of the knee through early, active exercise.

Internal derangements of the semilunar cartilages producing symptoms after repair of dislocations or ligamentous injuries are usually treated by excision of the offending cartilage.

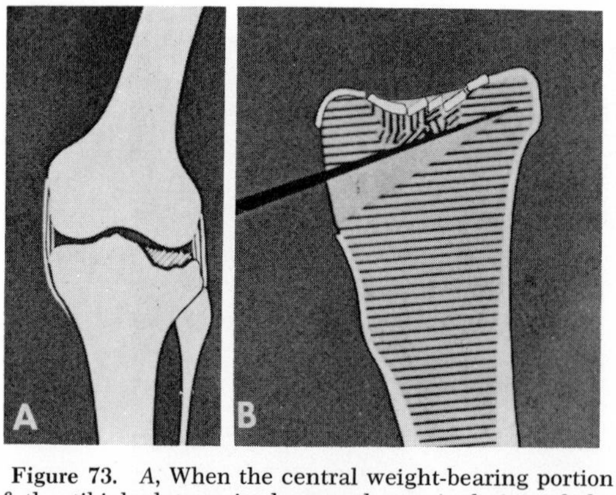

Figure 73. *A*, When the central weight-bearing portion of the tibial plateau is depressed, manipulation of the knee cannot correct the deformity, as there are no ligamentous attachments to this area. *B*, Open reduction of depressed tibial plateau fractures may be necessary in order to lever the depressed articular surface into position with appropriate instruments. The gap created in the cancellous bone is filled with bone chips.

THE TIBIA AND FIBULA

FRACTURES OF THE SHAFT OF THE TIBIA AND FIBULA. The shape and subcutaneous location of the tibia in the leg makes this bone particularly vulnerable to injury. It is triangular in shape from just below the condyles to the lower one-third of the bone where it becomes rounded and more quadrilateral in cross section. This change in shape produces an area of weakness in the bone, and fractures at the junction of the middle and lower one-third of the tibia are common. The bone on the anteromedial surface is covered only with skin and subcutaneous tissue. Direct trauma or angulation easily produces open fractures.

All of the body weight is transmitted through

the tibia. The fibula transmits no body weight and serves primarily as an area for muscle attachments. It also forms the lateral malleolus of the ankle and provides the attachment of the lateral collateral ligament at the knee. The two bones are bound together by strong ligaments proximally and distally, and by the tough interosseous membrane.

The tibia is well supplied with blood near the knee and ankle. The bone in these areas is cancellous and surrounded by a thin cortex which is penetrated by many nutrient vessels. The blood supply to the midsection of the bone, however, is scanty. Muscles arising from the posterior and lateral surfaces supply a few nutrient vessels in the upper one-half of the bone. However, the cortex is thick and relatively avascular. The distal one-third of the bone lacks muscle attachment, and is surrounded primarily by areolar tissue, tendons and subcutaneous fat. The main nutrient artery enters the medullary canal proximally, and this blood supply dwindles as it approaches the ankle. The precarious blood supply to the distal one-half of the shaft of the tibia makes for slow healing. The incidence of delayed and nonunion is high.

As in the forearm, the muscles are confined within tight fascial compartments. Hemorrhage and swelling within these compartments may compress the blood vessels and endanger the circulation to the foot. Volkmann's ischemic contracture is an ever-present danger and occurs much more frequently than is realized. The anterior tibial artery perforates the interosseous membrane just below the condyles to run distally to the foot. It is the sole blood supply to the dorsiflexors of the foot and toes. The blood vessel is easily damaged by fractures near the point of penetration through the interosseous membrane. The result is necrosis of these muscles. Fortunately, this complication is uncommon.

The other major blood vessel, the posterior tibial artery, lies in the posterior compartment of the leg and is less easily damaged, although it is subject to compression by swelling.

The peroneal nerve, winding about the proximal end of the fibula, lies superficially covered only by subcutaneous tissue in close proximity to the bone. It is easily injured by a direct blow, by bony spicules from the fibula and by stretching from angulation. Paralysis of the foot and toe dorsiflexors and peroneal muscles is the result of trauma, producing a foot drop.

The muscles of the leg lie parallel to the bone on the posterior and lateral aspect. They produce shortening and slight anterior angulation of the fracture fragments of the tibia. The interosseous membrane tends to draw the bones together as it does in forearm fractures. Gravity tends to rotate the distal fragment externally and displace it posteriorly when the patient lies supine (Fig. 74).

Fractures of the tibia and fibula may involve one or both bones. The force may be indirect violence such as a twisting injury, or a fall from a height, or direct violence such as that encountered when an automobile bumper strikes the leg. Indirect-violence fractures are usually coupled with a twisting force, producing a spiral or oblique fracture of the bone. Direct-violence fractures may be simple, transverse, or comminuted and segmental fractures. If only one bone breaks, the other acts as an internal splint, and shortening is minimal; however, angulation of an objectionable degree may occur.

X-ray examination must include the knee and ankle joints as well as the entire length of the bone. Often a fracture of the lower one-third of the tibia is accompanied by a fracture in the upper part of the fibula. The second fracture may be missed if the x-ray examination is incomplete.

FRACTURES OF THE FIBULA. Isolated fractures of the fibula usually occur from a direct blow, or from injuries associated with the ankle joint. Since the bone does not transmit body weight, and since it is firmly bound to the tibia by the interosseous membrane, shaft fractures are usually displaced only a little. When the stability of the ankle joint is not impaired, treatment of the fracture is simple.

Reduction is seldom necessary. The bone

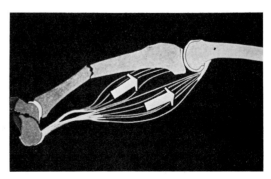

Figure 74. The triceps surae group of muscles lies posterior to the tibia and produces anterior angulation of the fragments. Flexing the knee and foot helps to relax this muscle and lessens the angulating force.

ends are usually in contact, and union occurs readily. Even with comminuted or segmental fractures of the fibula, it must be remembered that this bone serves only as a muscle attachment in the midportion. Displacement of these fragments does not affect function if the upper and lower ends remain in place. Indeed, the midpart is often removed for use as a bone graft without impairing leg function. Simple manipulation under local anesthesia may be done. However, if the approximation is not accomplished, there is little need for worry. An Ace bandage and crutches are all that is needed until the pain subsides, when full weight-bearing may be resumed.

Fractures which involve the peroneal nerve at the upper portion of the bone are usually stable. The damage is done at the time of injury and treatment of the bone has little effect upon nerve recovery. The dorsiflexor and peroneal muscles, however, must be protected from overstretching with a dropfoot brace while the nerve recovers.

Occasionally, when a patient cannot manage crutches or a walker, a walking cast may provide some stability and comfort, and allow the patient to get about.

FRACTURES OF THE UPPER THIRD OF THE TIBIA. Fractures involving the shaft of the tibia may occur at any area of the bone, from just below the condyles to just above the ankle. Fractures just below the condyles are often caused by direct violence. The modern automobile bumper is ideally suited to produce this fracture. Displacement depends upon the direction of the force administered to the bone. Comminution of the fragments is common and open wounds often accompany the injury. The fracture is often stable if marked comminution is not present. Usually, the force which fractures the tibia also breaks the fibula. This force may damage the peroneal nerve directly or angulation may stretch the nerve to cause paralysis. The status of the nerve should be established by testing the power of the dorsiflexors of the foot and toes before reduction is attempted. Reduction is usually accomplished by traction and manipulation followed by long-leg cast immobilization.

Since the fracture occurs at the junction of cortical and cancellous bone, where there is adequate blood supply, the prognosis for healing is usually good.

FRACTURES OF THE MIDDLE AND LOWER THIRDS OF THE TIBIA. Fractures of the middle and distal third of the bone are classified for purposes of treatment as stable or unstable fractures. When the fibula remains intact, an internal splint is present. This usually prevents shortening, but angulation and displacement may be present. When both bones break, the fractures may still be stable if the fracture is transverse or there are jagged edges on the tibial fragments which may be engaged during reduction to provide longitudinal stability. Typically, the tense interosseous membrane angulates the tibial fragments laterally, drawing the bones together. The closer the fracture is to the ends of the bone, the greater will be the effect of the angulation joint alignment. Thus, a fracture 3 inches above the ankle may angulate to a much greater degree than one in the midshaft with a similar displacement. This principle is true for all long-bone fractures (Fig. 75).

If longitudinal stability is present, or can be created by end-to-end reduction, shortening of the bone is not a problem. However, angulation and rotation must be corrected by manipulation. The patient lies supine upon a table; the leg is flexed at the knee and allowed to hang over the edge of the table. In this position, gentle traction can be made at the foot while the edge of the table under the knee provides countertraction. Traction may be made by an assistant or by weights suspended from a bandage looped about the ankle. When reduction has been accomplished, a plaster cast is applied from the toes

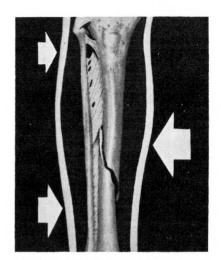

Figure 75. When the fibula remains intact, it acts as an internal splint. However, the elasticity of the interosseous membrane may allow the tibia to angulate. Cast immobilization for stable fractures will correct this angulation by pressure at appropriate points.

to just below the knee. Rotational alignment is then checked by extending the knee to 145 degrees. A line drawn from the anterior iliac spine through the patella to the foot should pass between the first and second toes. The cast is then extended above the knee to the upper thigh, with the knee in 165 to 145 degrees of extension. Rotational alignment can only be maintained in the long-leg cast with the knee bent, as is true in forearm fractures, where the cast must extend above the bent elbow.

The immediate postreduction x-ray films are followed in a few days by another x-ray examination to determine whether the deformity is recurring in the cast. If angulation has recurred, it may be possible to correct it by wedging the cast.

UNSTABLE FRACTURES OF THE TIBIA AND FIBULA. Unstable fractures of the tibia and fibula are usually spiral, oblique, comminuted or segmental. One reduction of these fractures followed by plaster cast immobilization may be tried. If the reduction cannot be maintained, some form of traction or internal fixation may be necessary (Fig. 76).

Skeletal traction through the os calcis or lower tibia may be used in conjunction with a cast suspended in a Thomas splint and the Pearson attachment. A cast stabilizes the fracture, aiding in the prevention of angulation, while the traction prevents shortening and overriding. Frequent x-ray examinations must be made to detect distraction and angulation.

A form of fixed traction may be obtained by placing two traction pins transversely through the proximal fragment and two through the distal. While traction is applied, the pins are incorporated in the cast. Two pins are necessary in each fragment to prevent anterior-posterior angulation.

Open reduction, when necessary, may be done. However, exposure of the bone further impairs blood supply and healing is almost always slower. Plates and screws and a special intramedullary rod may be used for internal fixation. Since healing is slow and nonunion is frequent in mid- and lower one-third fractures, many surgeons add bone grafts obtained from the ilium at the time of open reduction. The healing rate varies considerably, and in the adult may be as short as three months or longer than a year. Nonunion is not uncommon and is treated by appropriate bone grafting.

TIBIAL FRACTURES IN CHILDREN. Fractures of the tibia in children vary with the age of the child. From infancy to about six years, the most frequent fracture is spiral in nature in the mid- or lower one-third of the bone. The injury is produced by a twist to the bone and may occur from catching the foot between the bars of the crib. The fibula usually is not broken and provides an internal splint. Displacement is usually minimal and cast immobilization for a few weeks may be the only treatment required. From six to about 13 years of age, the fractures tend to be transverse, caused by direct violence. Both bones may be broken. Reduction and cast immobilization usually produce satisfactory results. If the fracture is spiral or oblique, overriding of one centimeter may be allowed and slight anterior bowing may be accepted, as growth will correct these defects. However, medial, lateral and rotational malalignment must be corrected as fully as possible. Open reduction before growth ceases is not necessary, and should not be done.

After puberty, the bones become more brittle and the tough periosteal sleeve which stabilizes most children's fractures becomes more like the adult. Fractures in this age group tend to comminution, and instability is much more frequently encountered than in younger children. Skeletal traction through the os calcis may be necessary to secure and maintain alignment; however, open reduction should not be done until the epiphysial plates have closed and growth ceases.

THE ANKLE

The ankle joint is one of the most frequently injured areas of the body. Since it is the con-

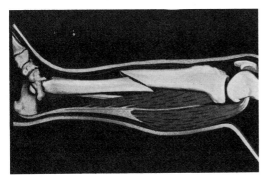

Figure 76. Unstable fractures shorten and angulate because of the pull of the triceps surae muscles. Continuous traction may be necessary to neutralize the muscle pull.

necting link between the stable leg bones and the mobile foot, it is subjected to a great variety of forces in walking, running and standing. Abnormal or excessive forces produce injuries to the bones and ligaments usually by indirect violence.

The talus, fitting into the mortise of the tibial and fibular malleoli allows dorsi- and plantar flexion but no medial, lateral or rotational motion. These latter motions are the property of the joints of the foot. The tibial malleolus forms the medial buttress of the ankle mortise and lies slightly anterior, while the fibula forms the lateral and lies slightly posterior. The axis of joint motion is, thus, in about 15 degrees of external rotation. The two malleoli grasp the talus between them. The articular surface of the tibia is quadrangular and concave and is slightly wider in front.

The tibia and fibula are bound firmly together by the interosseous ligament and the anterior and posterior tibiofibular ligaments. The fibers of these ligaments run outward and downward to the fibula. This arrangement of fibers allows the fibula to move proximally on the tibia and rotate slightly when the foot is dorsiflexed.

The convex articular surface of the body of the talus is slightly wider in front, corresponding to the articular surface of the tibia, fitting it accurately when the foot is in the neutral position. This wedge shape helps to prevent backward displacement of the talus on the tibia. When the foot is dorsiflexed, the wider anterior articular surface of the talus is forced between the malleoli. The ankle mortise widens slightly by allowing the fibula to move upward and rotate outward. In plantar flexion, when the narrower position of the articular surface is in contact with the tibia, the fibula descends to its normal position and rotates inward to maintain the firm grasp on the talus.

The talus and the os calcis are attached to the tibia and fibula by strong medial and lateral collateral ligaments. These ligaments are divided into three parts: anterior, middle and posterior. The anterior and posterior divisions run forward and backward downward from the malleoli to insert into the talus, while the middle courses directly downward to insert in the talus and os calcis. This arrangement of fibers prevents forward and backward displacement of the foot on the leg, and prevents tipping of the talus medially or laterally while allowing dorsi- and plantar flexion (Fig. 77).

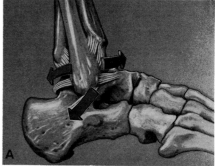

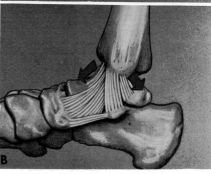

Figure 77. Anterior and posterior tibiofibular ligaments bind the two bones together at the ankle. *A*, Fibers of the fibular collateral ligament run forward, backward and downward. *B*, The fibers of the deltoid ligament at the medial malleolus do the same. This arrangement of fibers creates stability while allowing dorsiflexion and planatar flexion.

The joint capsule is necessarily lax anteriorly and posteriorly to allow this motion. The posterior capsule tightens in dorsiflexion while the anterior capsule tightens in plantar flexion. Some portion of the collateral ligaments is always taut in dorsi- or plantar flexion of the foot to ensure stability.

Since the body of the talus is almost completely covered by cartilage, except where ligaments attach, it is a particularly strong bone and seldom breaks. The neck portion of the bone, however, is weakened by the penetration of nutrient blood vessels and occasionally is the site of fracture. Since the major blood supply to the body of the talus enters through those blood vessels, injury to them may deprive the body of the bone of nutrition. Necrosis of the body of the talus may follow injuries to the neck of the bone.

The lateral malleolus is well supplied by blood vessels and heals readily. The medial malleolus, however, may be deprived of part of its blood supply when the medial malleolar artery is torn. This vessel arises from the anterior tibial artery and courses medial and downward to enter the malleolus anteriorly and is torn with most fractures which displace the malleolus. Although blood vessels enter the tip of the malleolus through the deltoid ligament, they are scanty and the decreased blood supply may account for the slower healing of medial malleolar fractures.

Nonunion of the medial malleolus is common when the fragment is displaced. Frequently, fibers of the deltoid ligament and periosteum fold into the fracture, preventing adequate bone contact after reduction.

The malleoli act as pulleys for the tendons which pass behind them on their way to insertion in the foot. The peroneal tendons pass behind the fibular malleolus, while the tibialis posterior and flexor hallucis longus pass behind the medial. Since these tendons plantar flex the foot, the pull of their muscles, along with the triceps surae, tends to displace the foot backward when the malleoli are fractured. Displacement of fragments may interfere with the normal function of these tendons. All of the leg muscles tend to cause shortening when the articular surface of the tibia is comminuted.

The talus acts as a wedge between the malleoli and against the articular surface of the tibia when fractures are produced. Fractures are most often produced by indirect violence. In a fall from a height, the foot may be violently displaced on the leg, or, when the foot is fixed to the ground, a twist of the leg, as in falling, may displace the leg on the foot.

Fractures about the ankle are classified according to the force that produces them. The talus may be rotated medially or laterally, inverted or everted, pushed backward or forward, medially or laterally, or compressed directly upward. A combination of these forces may take place, producing a variety of fractures, dislocations and sprains. Since the malleoli are attached to the talus by the joint capsule and collateral ligaments, the fragments follow the displacement of the foot on the leg bones.

An understanding of the mechanism of the fracture and the anatomy involved is essential for intelligent management of these injuries. Reduction is based upon reversal of the forces which produced the fracture.

External rotation fractures of the lateral malleolus are among the most frequent ankle fractures. In a fall, the talus is rotated on its long axis laterally or the leg bones are rotated medially. The lateral anterior border of the talus impinges against the anterior articular surface of the fibula. The fibula is twisted in its long axis by this force. The deltoid liga-

ment is stretched while the anterior tibio-fibular ligament is torn. The fibula then breaks in a spiral manner at the malleolus. The fracture line progresses from anterior to upward and posterior. The posterior tibio-fibular ligament remains intact as does the interosseous membrane. The shaft of the fibula maintains its relationship to the tibia while the malleolar fragment follows the foot into external rotation. If the force continues, the deltoid ligament may rupture allowing the talus to displace laterally on the tibia (Figs. 78 and 79).

If rotatory force is coupled with lateral displacement of the talus, the ligaments binding the fibula to the tibia along with the deltoid ligament may tear without fracture of the malleoli. This mechanism produces a diastasis between the tibia and fibula, widening the ankle mortise.

Reduction is accomplished by applying the reverse of the force that produced the fracture. The foot is internally rotated on the long axis of the tibia and displaced medially. Since the lateral collateral ligament attaches the distal fragment to the talus, it pulls the fragment into position as the talus is replaced in the ankle mortise.

Frequently, the deltoid ligament stretches, but does not tear completely. When this occurs, spontaneous reduction may take place when the force producing the fracture abates. X-ray examinations in this instance reveal the fracture of the fibular malleolus without displacement. The fracture may be quite stable.

Immobilization is accomplished with a cast

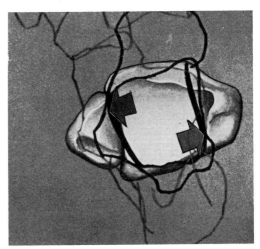

Figure 78. External rotation of the talus in the ankle mortise forces the lateral border of the talus against the lateral malleolus.

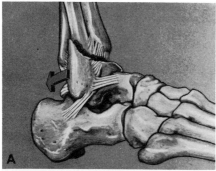

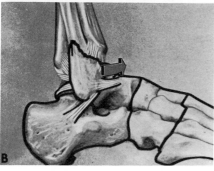

Figure 79. *A,* As the external rotation force continues, the fibula breaks in a spiral manner and is rotated outward. If the force continues, the deltoid ligament ruptures and the talus may displace laterally. *B,* Reduction is accomplished by medial rotation of the talus. The collateral ligament attaching to the talus pulls the fragment into position.

extending from the toes to the knee if the fracture is stable, but, if, on examination, the fibular fragment rotates easily into the displaced position, the cast should extend above the bent knee to prevent this rotation. Weight may be borne on a walking heel as soon as the pain subsides. The fracture usually heals sufficiently in six weeks to allow removal of the cast.

Eversion or abduction fractures are produced by forces which displace the foot in this direction or displace the leg bones in the opposite direction on the foot fixed to the ground. The talus, tipping in the ankle mortise, is forced against the lateral malleolus, which breaks transversely, usually near or above the joint line. The deltoid ligament may rupture, allowing the foot to displace laterally. If it remains intact, traction on the medial malleolus by the ligament may produce a transverse avulsion fracture of the medial malleolus at or below the joint line. Such a fracture is called a bimalleolar fracture. If the force continues, the talus may dislocate completely from the tibia, carrying the fracture fragments with it. When this occurs, it is obvious that the joint capsule has been completely disrupted. The tendons of leg muscles follow the foot and tend to hold the foot in the displaced position (Fig. 80).

Reduction is accomplished by longitudinal traction to overcome the shortening produced by the muscles of the leg. The foot is then forced medially and inverted. If the medial malleolus has remained intact, or is fractured below the joint line, the talus is forced against this buttress of bone, reducing the lateral displacement. Inversion of the foot pulls the lateral malleolar fragment downward and inward through the intact collateral ligament. The ruptured deltoid ligament usually falls into position. However, if the tibial malleolus has been fractured, it must be forced upward by the hands of the surgeon to secure reduction. The foot is held in neutral dorsi- and plantar flexion.

If the fracture of the medial malleolus occurs at the joint line, the buttress of bone is lost, and the talus may be displaced too far medially. This is an unstable fracture and may require internal fixation of the

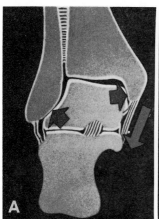

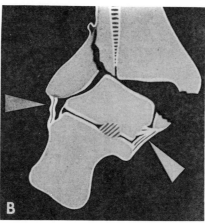

Figure 80. *A,* Eversion or abduction fractures are produced by the wedging action of the talus against the malleoli. *B,* The talus forced against the lateral malleolus produces the fibular fracture, while traction on the deltoid pulls the medial malleolus from the tibia. If the force continues, the talus may dislocate.

medial malleolus to re-establish stability. A cast extending above the flexed knee is molded to maintain the force of reduction. Since the medial malleolus heals more slowly than the lateral, immobilization is necessary for eight to twelve weeks (Fig. 81).

Often a fold of periosteum and ligament is interposed into the medial malleolar fracture. This tissue prevents accurate replacement of the malleolus. Open reduction is then necessary, as nonunion almost always occurs. The fracture is exposed and the fold of tissue removed. A screw is then placed through the malleolus securing it to the tibia. The periosteum and ligament are then sutured over the fracture. Cast immobilization is then employed for the time required for healing.

The same mechanism of abduction fracture when coupled with posterior and upward displacement of the talus may cause a fracture of the posterior lateral articular surface of the tibia in addition to the malleolar fractures. The fragment is displaced upward and posterior. It is often called a trimalleolar fracture. Varying amounts of the tibial articular surface are involved. It may be only the posterior lip of the bone or a third or more of the posterolateral articu-

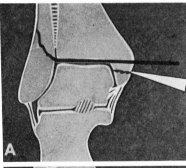
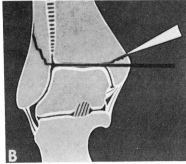

Figure 81. *A*, If the medial malleolus is fractured below the joint line, the remaining portion acts as a buttress for stable reduction. *B*, If the fracture is above the joint line, the buttress effect is lost and the reduction may be unstable.

lar surface. The amount of bone and the degree of displacement dictate the treatment. If less than one-fourth of the posterior articular surface is involved in the fracture, there still remains an adequate stable weight-bearing surface on the tibia. However, if more than this amount of bone is displaced, accurate replacement is essential, as instability and an irregular joint surface will eventually cause traumatic arthritis (Fig. 82).

Following reduction of the malleolar fractures, the foot is pulled forward and placed in dorsiflexion. Since the posterior joint capsule is attached to this fragment, traction is made on the fragment by the joint capsule as the reduction is carried out. This position must be maintained during the immobilization period. When more than one-fourth of the articular surface is fractured and cannot be anatomically replaced, open reduction with internal fixation is necessary.

Inversion or adduction fractures are produced by forces which force the foot into this position, or the leg bones laterally on the inverted fixed foot. The talus acts as a wedge against the medial malleolus and produces a fracture, usually at the joint line. The fracture line runs upward and medially. The foot is displaced in this direction, depending upon the degree of force. The lateral collateral ligament stretches, ruptures or avulses the lateral malleolus, usually below the joint line. Dislocation may be complete. Contraction of the leg muscles maintains the displacement (Fig. 83).

As in other fractures about the ankle, reduction is accomplished by reversal of this force. Traction is made in the long axis of the leg while the foot is displaced laterally and everted. If the fibula fracture is below the joint line, it will afford a stable lateral wall against which the talus may be fixed. However, if it fractures above this point, the reduction will be unstable and the medial malleolus may require internal fixation to maintain reduction. Accurate replacement of the medial malleolus is essential. Since the fracture is oblique, maintenance of reduction may be impossible by external means. Open reduction is, thus, often necessary and should be done whenever the medial malleolus cannot be maintained in position.

Fractures of the anterior and posterior articular surface of the tibia are caused by extreme dorsi- or plantar flexion of the foot, coupled with forward or backward displace-

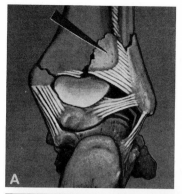

Figure 82. *A*, A triangular fragment of bone may be fractured posterolaterally from the tibia. *B*, The fragment is displaced backward and upward as the talus is pulled backward by the triceps surae. *C*, The foot is pulled forward and dorsiflexed to make traction on the fragment through the joint capsule.

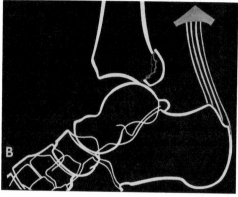

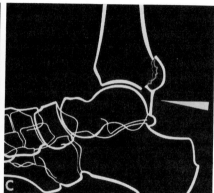

ment of the talus on the tibia. The fracture fragments are triangular with the base of the articular surface. The fracture line runs upward and forward in anterior fractures and upward and backward with posterior fractures. The fragment is displaced in a like manner, along with the talus. Stability of the ankle joint depends upon the amount of articular surface involved in the fracture. Fractures which involve less than one-fourth

of the articular surface are usually stable and are reduced by traction produced through the joint capsule.

Anterior fractures are reduced by plantar flexion of the foot accompanied by posterior displacement of the talus. The reverse maneuver is used to reduce posterior tibial articular fractures. When more than one-fourth of the joint surface is fractured, open reduction with internal fixation is often necessary to ensure stability and restoration of a smooth articular surface. Immobilization in a below-knee plaster cast is necessary for eight weeks, or until definite evidence of healing is present.

Direct compression forces, such as a fall from a height, produce comminuted fractures of the articular surface of the tibia. The talus acts as a wedge, forcing the articular surface of the tibia upward and the malleoli apart. Comminution is often extreme, as though an explosion had taken place within the joint. The foot may be displaced in any direction. Since the major force is directly upward against the tibia, the joint capsule remains, for the most part, intact.

Reduction is accomplished by traction on the foot with appropriate manipulation to align the major fragments. Often, central

Figure 83. Adduction fractures are produced by forces which tip the talus against the medial malleolus. *A*, Fracture of the medial malleolus occurs at the joint line and runs upward. *B*, The fibular collateral ligament may rupture, or may cause the fibula to fracture.

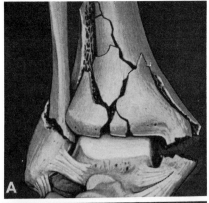

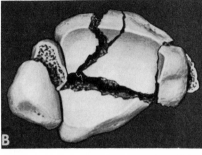

Figure 84. Compression fractures of the tibial articular surface usually produce marked comminution and damage to the joint. *A,* Lateral view. *B,* Inferior view.

articular fragments are driven upward and impacted in the cancellous bone of the tibia. No amount of traction or manipulation can bring these isolated fragments into alignment, and a rough joint surface is inevitable in many instances.

Since the pull of the muscles is in the long axis of the leg, the traction must be

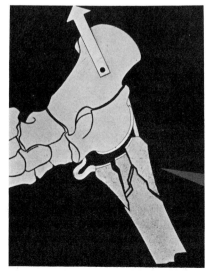

Figure 85. Traction is made through the joint capsule and must be maintained while union occurs. A central fragment may remain displaced.

maintained until union is sufficient to prevent redisplacement, usually two months.

Traction through the os calcis by skeletal means is usually necessary. This may be maintained by suspension in a Thomas splint, supplemented by a cast or splints, or by pins placed through the os calcis and proximal tibia and incorporated in a plaster cast. Immobilization is usually necessary for three months and weight must not be borne upon the joint until union is complete in three to six months.

It is surprising how often a joint which has been destroyed by this fracture may function well for varying periods. Eventually, however, traumatic arthritis produces a painful joint, and arthrodesis is often necessary.

THE FOOT

FRACTURES OF THE BODY OF THE TALUS. Fractures of the talus may involve the body or neck of the bone. Since the majority of the body is cartilage covered, this adds strength to this part of the talus, and fractures are not common. However, falls from a height may occasionally compress the bone between the os calcis and the tibia, producing vertical or longitudinal fractures. There is usually little displacement with this type fracture; however, with extreme violence, the posterior fragments may be squeezed backward out of the ankle mortise.

Reduction is accomplished by heavy traction on the foot in neutral position with the knee flexed to relax the triceps surae muscles. The posterior fragment may be manipulated by direct pressure accompanied by slight dorsiflexion of the foot to open up the posterior joint space. If anatomic reduction cannot be achieved and the fracture involves two large pieces of bone, open reduction with internal screw fixation should be done.

Comminuted fractures of the body of the talus are rare as isolated injuries. Extreme violence or a crushing injury may produce this unusual fracture. The articular surface of the talus is damaged, and the bone is compressed and deformed. Attempts at reduction are usually unsuccessful, since the only ligamentous attachments are about the margins of the bone. Traction with the foot in neutral position with dorsi- and plantar flexion movements may mold the fragments into better configuration. However, the damage to articular surfaces is usually profound and a painful joint with marked limitation of motion is often the result of this fracture. Arthrodesis of the appropriate joints is usually done later to provide a stable, pain-free ankle and subtalar joint.

FRACTURES OF THE NECK OF THE TALUS. Fractures of the neck of the talus are usually the result of a fall in which the foot is forced into extreme dorsiflexion. The anterior lip of the tibia acts as a fulcrum on the neck as maximum dorsiflexion is reached. The force shears the neck vertically from the body of the talus and displaces the head of the bone upward. Displacement may be minimal; however, the consequences of this fracture may be serious. The major blood supply to the bone enters through a series of nutrient arteries at the neck. The fracture deprives the body of the talus of its major blood supply. As in the navicular bone at the wrist, aseptic necrosis of the bone may follow this damage to the blood supply.

Reduction is accomplished by plantar flexion of the foot with manipulation of the foot to align the fragments. Cast immobilization is usually sufficient to hold the reduction with the foot placed in plantar flexion. Although healing of the fracture takes place in two or three months, the necrosis of the body of the bone may be evident within this time. Relative increased density of the bone on x-ray examination usually heralds this unfortunate event. Weight-bearing cannot be allowed until revascularization of the body of the talus has occurred. This may require many months. During this period, active foot and ankle exercises should be carried out to prevent stiffness of the joints and atrophy of the muscles. If revascularization of the bone is incomplete, some deformity of the bone may occur when weight-bearing is resumed. Eventually, a painful arthritis develops in the ankle and subtalar joints, requiring arthrodesis of these joints.

SUBTALAR AND TALONAVICULAR DISLOCATION. Dislocation of the foot from the talus is an unusual injury produced by extreme twisting violence. The talus remains in the ankle mortise while the foot usually displaces laterally at the talocalcaneal and talonavicular joints. Minor avulsion fractures about the margins of these joints may complicate the dislocation. The deformity of the foot is obvious and inversion and eversion cannot be performed, although dorsi- and plantar flexion may be possible to a limited degree. The prominence of the head of the talus in the dorsum of the foot may impair the circulation to the skin, demanding immediate reduction.

Reduction is accomplished by traction on the heel and forefoot in the long axis of the leg, accompanied by pressure on the os calcis directed medially. The dislocation is usually reduced without difficulty. Occasionally, interposition of soft tissue prevents reduction by manipulation, and an operation must be performed to clear this obstruction.

Immobilization in a plaster cast extending from the toes to the knee is necessary for four to six weeks. Following this time, weight-bearing may be gradually resumed in a shoe which supports the long arch of the foot. Some loss of motion and pain can be expected from fibrosis about the subtalar joint for many months.

FRACTURES OF THE OS CALCIS. Fractures of the os calcis are usually caused by a fall from a height in which the heel strikes the ground and absorbs the major force. Since the os calcis is cancellous, the bone compresses and comminution of the fragments with impaction is usually the result. However, a variety of fractures occur. If, in falling, the patient lands on the forefoot and the tense triceps surae pulls upward on the bone at the attachment of the Achilles tendon, splitting the bone longitudinally, a "duckbill" fracture is produced. If the heel is forcefully inverted or everted, the sustentaculum may be sheared off or the anterior part of the bone may be avulsed by the interosseous ligament. Occasionally, a vertical fracture occurs which shears off the medial or lateral tuberosity of the calcaneus without other involvement of the bone. These forces, coupled with adduction or abduction of the forefoot, may drive the cuboid bone against the articular surface of the os calcis, producing fractures into the calcaneocuboid joint (Fig. 86).

Although healing of the bone occurs within two or three months, the prognosis for normal function of the foot is poor. Months of disability often follow the injury and some permanent disability is usual. Several factors contribute to this dismal prognosis. When the main body of the calcaneus breaks, the tuberosity of the heel is driven upward flattening the arch of the foot. The talus, acting as a wedge, drives the articular surface of the subtalar joint downward into the os calcis. Inevitably, damage is done to the joint surfaces.

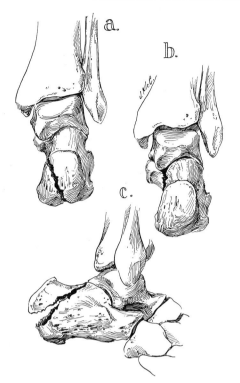

Figure 86. A, Vertical tuberosity fracture of the os calcis. B, Fracture of the sustentaculum. C, Duckbill fracture of the os calcis.

Painful fibrosis or arthritis of the subtalar joint follows. Often, the calcaneus is split longitudinally, the fracture line running from medially below obliquely upward and outward through the lateral aspect of the subtalar joint. The large lateral fragment is displaced upward and outward beneath the lateral malleolus, impinging against it and compressing the peroneal tendons. This impingement and disturbance of the peroneal tendons may produce pain in walking and standing.

The damage to the subtalar joint and peroneal tendons, loss of the long arch and widening of the os calcis with impingement against the lateral malleolus all contribute to the disability. Secondary to these changes, chronic irritation in the subtalar joint and ligaments produces reflex spasm of the peroneal muscles. This reaction produces a painful, spasmodic flat foot. When the fracture extends into the calcaneocuboid joint, deformity of the joint surfaces may lead to fibrosis and traumatic arthritis. This problem, however, is much less common than the disturbance in the subtalar joint.

Injuries to the os calcis produce rapid swelling in the foot. Distention by hemorrhage and edema produces bleb formation in the skin, with the hazard of infection. This complication can often be avoided by the prompt application of a compression dressing and elevation of the foot. Uniform compression is accomplished by applying multiple layers of sheet wadding and elastic bandage from the toes to the knee. The sooner this is done following the injury, the better.

Vertical fractures of the tuberosity which do not involve the subtalar joint and fractures of the sustentaculum tali often are undisplaced and require no reduction. Similarly, avulsion fractures of the attachment of the interosseous ligament are slightly displaced and require no reduction. The application of a compression dressing for a few days followed by a short-leg cast for six weeks may be all that is necessary to produce satisfactory healing.

"Duckbill" or beak fractures of the tuberosity may require reduction if the pull of the triceps surae has separated the fragments. The foot is placed in equinus position with the knee flexed to relax the gastrocnemius and soleus muscles. A pin is driven through the soft tissues just above the os calcis. Traction is made against the upper fragment, forcing it downward and closing the open beak. The foot and leg are immobilized in a plaster cast in this position for six to eight weeks. If the reduction cannot be maintained, open reduction with screw fixation is performed to reattach the insertion of the Achilles tendon.

When the major body of the os calcis is fractured, the tuber joint angle is often lost, producing the flattening of the arch of the foot. This angle is the one made by the tuberosity in relation to the subtalar joint. Normally, the angle is about 45 degrees; however, as the tuberosity is driven upward by the force of the fracture, the angle is lost and the long arch of the foot is flattened (Fig. 87).

The upward displacement of the tuberosity, in effect, lengthens the Achilles tendon, reducing the power of the triceps surae. Loss of the long arch of the foot reduces the shock-absorbing quality of the foot and reduces the effectiveness of the forefoot lever in the push-off phase of walking. Uncorrected, these two factors produce a shuffling, flat-footed limp.

Widening of the os calcis causes impingement against the lateral malleolus and pinching or fibrosis of the peroneal tendons and sheaths. Derangement of the subtalar joint leads to painful fibrosis and traumatic arthritis with loss of the ability to invert and evert

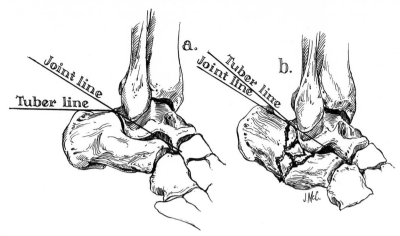

Figure 87.   *A*, The tuber joint angle of the os calcis measures about 45 degrees. *B*, When the os calcis fractures and the subtalar joint is crushed, the tuber joint angle is reduced, lost or reversed.

the foot, and produces pain on walking on uneven surfaces.

Reduction of this fracture is directed to restoring the normal configuration of the bone, reducing the widening, re-establishing the tuber joint angle and long arch of the foot and correcting the deformity of the subtalar joint as much as possible. Practically, this is almost impossible to accomplish.

Since the fractures are almost always impacted, the impaction must be broken up before the fragments can be molded into position. This is done by manual eversion and inversion of the heel with the surgeon's hands. The maneuver may require considerable force, and, if unsuccessful, may demand hammering of the os calcis with the soft tissues protected by appropriate padding. When the fragments are mobilized, a heavy traction pin is placed through the soft tissues just above the tuberosity and forward from the Achilles tendon. Downward traction is made on the tuberosity and forefoot while countertraction is made against the midtarsal region. This force re-establishes the tuber joint angle and the long arch of the foot. The widened bone is compressed by a clamp placed just below the malleoli. The heel is inverted to raise the depressed lateral portion of the subtalar joint through the pull of the joint capsule.

A long-leg cast is applied with knee flexed and the foot in moderate plantar flexion, and is molded snugly about the os calcis. The cast is changed when swelling subsides, to maintain the accurate fit of the plaster about the os calcis. Weight-bearing cannot be permitted until healing is complete, usually a minimum of three months.

When the depressed articular surface of the subtalar joint cannot be reduced, open reduction in some instances is warranted. If there appears to be a major lateral depressed fragment, this may be levered upward after exposure of the lateral surface of the os calcis. The elevated surface is maintained in reduction by a bone graft placed beneath it similar to the method employed for depressed fractures of the tibial plateau.

The complication of a painful subtalar joint is the usual cause of the prolonged disability. If fibrous ankylosis becomes complete, the pain on weight-bearing gradually subsides, but this may take a year or more to occur. If the joint is damaged beyond repair and pain is persistent, subtalar arthrodesis is necessary. Since the subtalar, calcaneocuboid and talonavicular joints act as a unit, arthrodesis of one produces strain on the others. Arthritic changes slowly develop in the joints not fused. For this reason, many surgeons advocate arthodesis of these three joints, particularly in younger people. Because of the prolonged disability following reduction and cast immobilization, some surgeons ignore the deformity of the fractured os calcis and rely on early mobilization to prevent fibrosis. A compression dressing is applied and the leg elevated until the pain and swelling subside. Exercise of the foot and ankle is then started, and the patient is allowed to bear partial weight with crutches as soon as this can be tolerated. The eventual result of this treatment is uncertain. In some instances, the disability time is shortened; in others, the usual complications arise, necessitating arthrodesis or removal of bone beneath the lateral malleolus.

FRACTURE AND DISLOCATION OF THE MIDTARSAL BONES. Fractures and dislocations of the navicular, cuboid and cuneiform bones are usually caused by direct, crushing violence, although a fall from a height may produce dislocations in this area. Since the complex of these bones is bound together by a strong envelope of ligaments, displacement is minimal. Often the fractures are mere avulsions of small fragments of bone at ligament attachments. Since little motion takes place in this area of the foot, even severely crushed and deformed bones in the midtarsal complex cause little permanent difficulty.

Reduction by direct molding of the fragments to eliminate sharp prominences on the dorsum of the foot is all that is necessary in most instances. A compression dressing for a week or two with non-weight-bearing, followed by heat, massage and exercise is the usual treatment for these fractures.

Dislocations may take place between any of these bones. The most common dislocation occurs between the talonavicular and calcaneocuboid joints with lateral displacement of the forefoot. With the heel fixed to the ground, torsion on the forefoot may produce the dislocation, or a fall from a height may produce shearing force medially or laterally, resulting in the displacement.

Reduction is usually easily accomplished by traction on the forefoot accompanied by medial or lateral pressure. Maintenance of the reduction may be difficult and may require temporary pin fixation traversing the joints for a few weeks. Weight-bearing cannot be allowed until the torn ligaments heal, about four to six weeks.

Dislocation of the midtarsal and metatarsal bones is an uncommon injury resulting from direct crushing violence. The displacement is usually lateralward and may spare the first metatarsal cuneiform joint. Accurate reduction may be hindered by interposition of the joint capsules and ligaments. The reduction is often unstable. Open reduction with removable pin fixation across the joints is often required.

FRACTURES OF THE METATARSAL BONES. Fractures of the metatarsal bones may take place at the base, shaft or neck, and articular areas of these bones, and are produced by direct or indirect violence.

A common fracture takes place at the base of the fifth metatarsal bone. This fracture is produced by the indirect violence of turning the forefoot inward while the foot is in equinus position. High-heel shoes are frequently the source of this mechanism, and the fracture is more common in women for this reason. The attachment of the peroneus brevis tendon and the joint capsule hold a triangular fragment of the bone to the cuboid bone, while the shaft of the bone is angulated medially. The fracture takes place through the triangular prominence of the base of the metatarsal. Displacement is minimal and no reduction is necessary; the remaining ligaments hold the fragments together.

A compression dressing and walking with crutches is necessary for a few days until the pain subsides. Weight-bearing may be resumed in a well-fitted oxford as soon as it is tolerated. The fracture line may be visible for many months on the x-ray films, although nonunion is not frequent. However, firm fibrous union takes place, and the foot is serviceable even when nonunion occurs.

Fractures of the shaft of the metatarsal bones are usually due to direct crushing injury. The interosseous muscles bind and hold the bones firmly together so that displacement is usually not great. Theoretically, the displacing pull of the muscles is similar to that affecting fractures in the hand metacarpals; practically, angulation and shortening is less serious.

Simple manipulation by direct pressure followed by a compression dressing or cast usually results in reasonably good reduction. Marked angulation must be corrected to allow proper weight-bearing in the metatarsal heads. Non-weight-bearing is followed until the pain and swelling subside, usually for three to six weeks.

Fractures of the metatarsal necks angulate and displace into the plantar aspect of the foot, producing an objectionable prominence on the weight-bearing surface. The displacement must be corrected by manipulation or a painful callus will develop over the bony prominence. Cast immobilization may be necessary to hold the fragments in reduction, and rarely traction on the toes with rubber bands may be required similar to that used in the hand. The fractures are stable in four to six weeks, when weight-bearing may be resumed. Undisplaced fractures may be treated by a compression dressing and crutches.

FRACTURES OF THE TOES. Fractures of the toes are produced by crushing or stubbing injury. The proximal phalanx of the small toes is most frequently broken. The most common deformity is lateral displacement of the fifth toe. The injury is painful but not serious. Reduction of any deformity is accomplished with traction and manipulation. Immobilization is most easily accomplished by strapping the toe to the adjacent one, which provides a convenient splint. Weight-bearing in a cut-out shoe is permitted immediately. Subungual hematoma often accompanies the fracture, and should be protected from contamination by an appropriate sterile dressing.

FRACTURES OF THE PELVIS

The pelvis, composed of the two innominate bones and the sacrum, is a rigid bony ring, containing the hip joints and housing the pelvic viscera. The two halves of the pelvis are joined by strong ligaments at the symphysis pubis and at the two sacroiliac joints. These ligaments, although preventing motion, lend some elasticity and shock-absorbing properties to the otherwise rigid bony ring. The major portions of the bones serve as muscle attachments which control the trunk and lower extremities.

The hamstring muscles arising about the ischium tend to pull fractures of this bone downward. The adductor muscles attaching to the pubic bone near the symphysis may rarely avulse small portions of the bone downward. The sartorius and rectus femoris muscles attach to the superior and inferior iliac spines, producing avulsion fractures of these bones and displacing them downward. The abductor muscles of the hip arise over the broad wing of the ilium and at the crest of the bone. The downward pull of these muscles is counteracted by the flank and abdominal muscles, which arise on the iliac crest and pull upward. However, when one-half of the pelvis is detached from the sacrum and the other half of the pelvis, these flank muscles tend to pull the detached half upward.

The pelvic viscera, including the bladder, ureters and urethra, the rectum and sigmoid colon, and the great vessels and nerves, may be injured by fractures in this area.

Fractures are classified as avulsion fractures of muscle attachments, fractures of the ring of the pelvis without displacement, fractures of the ring of the pelvis with displacement, fractures of the acetabulum and fractures of the sacrum and coccyx.

AVULSION FRACTURES. Avulsion fractures of the pelvis are caused by the indirect force of muscle contractures. The other fractures of the pelvic bones are usually caused by direct-violence forces from blows, falls or crushing injuries, or by indirect forces transmitted through the femur to the acetabulum. Avulsion fractures most often occur at the ischium and anterior, superior or inferior iliac spines. Occasionally, avulsion of a small piece of bone occurs at the crest of the ilium or near the symphysis pubis.

These injuries are caused by the sudden contraction of the muscle and most frequently occur in athletic endeavors. The ischial tuberosity is the most common site. Sudden contraction of the hamstring group of muscles arising from the bone pull a fragment of bone or the apophysis downward. Reduction of the fragment is usually not necessary, since the displacement is small and union takes place readily. Rest in bed for a few days, followed by the application of heat to the buttock, often eases the pain. Weight-bearing can begin in a week or two.

Open reduction is not necessary, and does not produce a better result than closed methods. The fracture heals with some prominence of the ischial tuberosity, and the area may be moderately uncomfortable to sit upon for several months.

Avulsion fractures of the superior and inferior iliac spines are pulled downward by the sudden forceful contraction of the sartorius or rectus femoris. Confining fascia and ligaments prevents marked displacement.

Avulsion fractures of the crest of the ilium and near the symphysis are less common injuries, but are treated in a conservative manner.

PELVIC RING FRACTURES WITHOUT DISPLACEMENT. Fractures of the pelvic ring without displacement can occur through any portion of the bones, but most often involve the pubic or ischial rami. The injury is common in older people, the result of a fall which compresses the pelvic ring. Slight comminution of the fragment may be present. Since the sacroiliac joints are not disrupted or the symphysis pubis separated, the fracture is stable and the weight-bearing function of the pelvis is not altered (Fig. 88).

Injury to the urinary tract is uncommon with this type of fracture; however, a urine specimen must be obtained and examined for blood. Occasionally, extravasation of blood and edema fluid into the perineum may make urination difficult, but usually this requires no treatment.

Bed rest for a week or two until the pain subsides may be followed by walking with full weight-bearing as soon as this is toler-

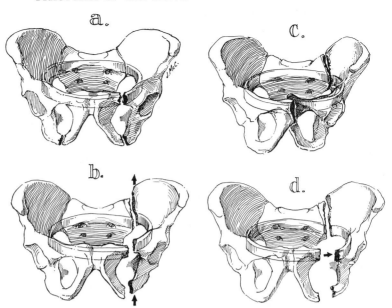

Figure 88. *A,* Stable fractures of the pelvic ring involve only segment of the bone. No displacement is possible if the remainder of the ring remains intact. Weight may be borne as soon as pain subsides. *B,* Unstable fractures of the pelvis involve two segments of the pelvic ring. The flank muscles tend to pull the fragment upward. *C,* When the fracture is due to compression force, the pelvic ring may be constricted. *D,* When the force tears the pelvic bones apart, the pelvic ring opens.

ated. A binder or belt about the pelvis during this time may give the patient some comfort.

PELVIC RING FRACTURES WITH DISPLACEMENT. Fracture of the pelvis with displacement must involve at least two areas of the pelvic ring before deformity occurs. Usually, considerable violence is necessary to produce these fractures. Shock is frequent and may be severe. Hidden blood loss in the retroperitoneal spaces may be considerable, and injury to the pelvic viscera is common. The displacement may alter the shape of the pelvis to a degree that is incompatible with proper weight-bearing. In the female, distortion of the pelvis may preclude the normal delivery of children.

In all pelvic fractures with displacement, the bladder and urethra must be investigated for injury. If the patient cannot void, passage of a soft rubber catheter into the bladder should be attempted. If it is difficult or impossible to catheterize the patient, a tear of the urethra is likely and must be treated promptly. If blood is found in the voided specimen of urine, or that obtained by catheterization, rupture of the bladder must be considered. When these injuries are not recognized, urinary extravasation occurs. Untreated, this complication can result in death. Prompt diversion of the urinary stream to the outside must be done.

Possible injuries to the rectum and sigmoid colon must be investigated. Sharp spicules of bone may penetrate or tear these structures. A rectal examination should be done. Blood on the examining finger following the examination requires careful and immediate investigation of the damage to the bowel. Shock must be treated by blood replacement and other appropriate therapy before reduction of the fracture is attempted.

SEGMENTAL FRACTURES OF THE ANTERIOR PELVIS. Segmental fractures of the anterior pelvis most often involve the superior and inferior pubic rami on each side of the symphysis. The main bony ring of the pelvis is undisturbed, but this anterior section displaces upward because of the pull of the rectus abdominis muscles. The urethra and bladder are frequently injured and must be treated first.

Displacement is usually not great, but the pull of the rectus abdominis muscles must be relaxed by placing the patient in a semisitting position in bed. In this position, the weight of the abdominal contents tends to hold the fragment downward. Rest in this position until fibrous union and stability are obtained is the usual treatment. Slight displacement does not influence weight-bearing, and, if the sacroiliac joints are intact, weight-bearing can begin as soon as stability of the fragment is obtained, usually within three or four weeks.

SEGMENTAL FRACTURES INVOLVING ONE-HALF OF THE PELVIS. More serious disruption of the pelvis occurs when the bone fractures through the rami of the pubis and at or near the sacroiliac joints. This section of the pelvis containing the hip joint may displace inward, outward, upward or rotate anteriorly. If the force compresses the pelvis, the anterior fracture may override, because the posterior fracture or disruption of the sacro-iliac joint acts like a hinge. If the force is outward on this half of the pelvis, the reverse deformity occurs. The pelvis opens anteriorly like a clam shell on the hinge of the posterior fracture. In either instance, the flank and abdominal muscles tend to pull this half of the pelvis upward.

If, in the mechanism of injury, the thigh is hyperextended, the rectus femoris and hip joint capsule rotate this half of the pelvis forward, and this displacement may be combined with any of the others.

Fractures which open the pelvic ring are reduced by traction to counteract the upward displacement by the flank and abdominal muscles, then closed by compression force. The reduction may be done by several methods. The least traumatic reduction is achieved by placing heavy, continuous suspension traction on both legs. This may be effectively applied with Russell's traction. Countertraction is supplied by the patient's body on the inclined plane of the bed, which is raised at the foot. Forty or 50 pounds of traction may be necessary on the affected side to pull the displaced half of the pelvis downward. This amount of force usually requires skeletal traction through the lower femur or upper tibia.

Compression force may be necessary to close the opened pelvic ring by a sling suspending the pelvis. A broad, padded, canvas sling, or one made of felt, is placed about the pelvis. Each side of the sling is sus-pended by balanced suspension from an overhead frame. Compression force is regulated by the degree that the sling is opened or closed over the patient. This method of suspension traction allows the necessary nursing care with minimum discomfort to the patient (Fig. 89).

When reduction has been confirmed by bedside x-ray examination, the weight is reduced to maintain the reduction. Ten to 15 pounds of traction may be all that is necessary to hold the reduction. Suspension traction is continued for six or eight weeks. The patient remains in the apparatus, but the traction is released at this time and x-ray examinations are made at frequent intervals. If there is any tendency for upward displacement of the fragments to recur, traction must be reinstituted and the patient must remain in bed until there is no tendency for recurrence of the deformity. Union is usually complete in three months, when weight-bearing with crutches may be gradually resumed.

An alternate method of reduction makes use of gravity as an aid. The patient is placed on the unaffected side. A folded sheet is placed between the legs at the perineum and attached to the table for countertraction. Using general anesthesia, strong traction is made on the leg of the affected side by an assistant or with the aid of a fracture table. The surgeon grasps the crest of the ilium and forces it downward and inward. The weight of the thigh with the patient in this position aids in closing the open pelvic ring. Following reduction, the patient is placed

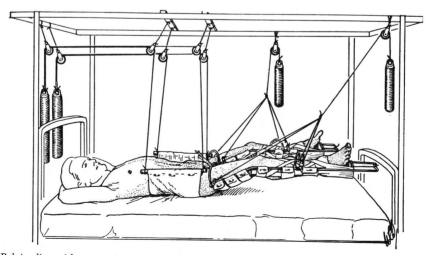

Figure 89.   Pelvic sling with suspension traction may be necessary to maintain reduction of unstable pelvic fractures.

in suspension traction or a spica cast, using the well-leg traction method of Hoke to maintain the reduction.

When the fractures produce compression and overriding of fragments, narrowing the pelvis, traction is again used to pull the fragments downward, but force must be applied to open the pelvic ring. To accomplish this, the intact portion of the pelvis must be fixed to the table. The patient is placed supine on the operating or fracture table. A sheet placed between the legs at the perineum is attached to the table for countertraction. The unaffected leg is then placed in 90 degrees of flexion and abduction at the hip and held against the table by an assistant. This position immobilizes the intact half of the pelvis by the tense hip joint capsule and adductor muscles.

The surgeon then brings the affected leg into abduction, flexion and external rotation to a similar position. Pulling the legs apart in this manner tends to open the pelvis through traction on the hip joint capsule if the overriding is anterior. Lateral and downward traction may be made as necessary to correct upward displacement. Following reduction, the patient is placed in suspension traction with the affected leg in 45 degrees of abduction. If the pelvis tends to collapse inward or override, lateral traction may be made with skeletal traction through the trochanter or by a broad sling placed about the thigh.

When there is no upward displacement, it may be possible to close or open the pelvic ring by placing the legs in long-leg casts with a bar connecting the casts at the knees. This bar is a fulcrum, and, by forcing the lower ends of the casts together or apart, the upper portions of the casts force the hips together or pull them apart. This force, transmitted through the hip joints, opens or closes the pelvis. Longitudinal traction may be made when it is necessary by placing the casts in suspension traction.

FRACTURES OF THE ACETABULUM. Fractures which involve the acetabulum are serious injuries, because the weight-bearing function of the hip is usually deranged. A fall directly upon the trochanter transmits force to the thin floor of the acetabulum through the head of the femur. The head, acting like a ramrod, fractures the floor of the acetabulum and displaces it inward. The displacement may be minimal or the entire head of the femur may penetrate into the

pelvis. If there is no displacement, and the head of the femur remains in normal contact with the superior weight-bearing portion of the acetabulum, no reduction is necessary. The leg is placed in Buck's extension or suspension traction until the acute reaction to the injury has subsided. Active exercise of the hip is started when the pain abates. Weight-bearing is not allowed until union is firm, in about eight weeks.

When the head of the femur is displaced inward, reduction must be attempted to place the head in proper relationship with the weight-bearing surface of the acetabulum. As with all joint fractures, the articular surface must be reconstructed as perfectly as is possible.

The displacement may be moderate when the ischium breaks along with the central portion of the acetabulum, or the head of the femur may penetrate into the pelvis. Closed reduction is attempted in suspension traction. Strong longitudinal traction with the leg abducted to 45 degrees may reduce the displacement. However, if this fails, the degree of abduction is reduced to neutral and lateral traction is added, either with skeletal traction through the trochanter or by a sling placed about the thigh. This combination of downward and lateral traction must be continued until the fractures unite, or displacement will recur.

Occasionally, satisfactory reduction cannot be obtained by traction alone. The floor of the acetabulum is attached to the femoral head only by the ligamentum teres arising from the inferior notch. The remainder of the bony structure is attached to the femur by the joint capsule only at the rim of the acetabulum. The fragments of bone comprising the floor of the acetabulum may be unaffected by traction. Open reduction may be necessary by exposing the inner aspect of the ilium, and under direct vision the fragments are pried into position. A metal plate, placed over these fragments and attached to the ilium by screws, may be necessary to hold them in place. Traction should continue until union is complete.

Following central protrusion of the acetabulum, the blood supply to the head of the femur may fail and aseptic necrosis of this bone may produce trouble later. Incongruous joint surfaces may lead to traumatic arthritis.

After union is obtained, weight-bearing is started gradually with crutches while active exercise is done to rehabilitate the hip musculature and re-establish motion.

FRACTURES OF THE SACRUM AND COCCYX

SACRUM. Fractures of the sacrum are usually transverse through the lower segments of the bone, and are produced by direct forces. Longitudinal fractures at the sacroiliac joint may accompany pelvic fractures which are segmental and displace upward.

Transverse fractures are most often produced by a fall on the buttocks, and frequently are undisplaced and difficult to identify on x-ray films. When more force is applied, the lower fragment is angulated into the pelvis. If displacement is present, it may be corrected by direct manipulation. The surgeon places his finger in the rectum and pries the fragment backward into position.

A binder placed about the pelvis may give the patient comfort, and heat applied locally after the first few days may help ro relieve pain. The patient cannot sit comfortably for several weeks, and this should be avoided when the fracture has been displaced.

Rarely, the sacrum is shattered by direct crushing force, damaging the cauda equina and sacral nerves. If the manipulation of the fragments does not relieve pressure on these vital structures, surgical decompression of the sacral canal may be necessary. Permanent bowel and bladder dysfunction may follow the injury.

COCCYX. Fractures of the coccyx are produced by falling upon the bone or by manipulation at childbirth. More often, pain is produced in the region by a sprain of the sacrococcygeal ligaments and the joints of the coccyx. Coccygodynia, or pain in the coccygeal region, may persist for many months following injury. The configuration of the coccyx varies so greatly that it is difficult to tell when an actual displacement of the bone has occurred. Gentle manipulation by the surgeon's fingers may reduce actual displacement or dislocation rather easily. The normal irregular configuration of these bones is unaffected by manipulation.

Sprains, dislocations and fractures of the coccyx should be protected from the pressure of sitting for many weeks. It is the constant reinjury of strain upon the ligaments

in sitting which may produce coccygodynia. A girdle or binder which draws the buttocks together may protect the bone. The patient should be taught to sit forward on the ischial tuberosities to relieve pressure on the coccyx. Occasionally, an inflated ringlike cushion may allow sitting without pressure on the injured structures.

Persistent coccygodynia is a distressing symptom, and may be due to arthritic changes in the coccygeal joints, painful scar tissue in the ligaments or the constant, repeated injury of sitting. Many types of treatment have been advocated attesting to the variability of successful results. Manipulation, injection of steroid drugs, diathermy and coccygectomy are among the variety of methods used. Coccygectomy should be done only after other methods of treatment fail, and when the surgeon is certain that the pain is arising in the sacrococcygeal joints.

FRACTURES AND DISLOCATIONS OF THE SPINE

The spine is composed of 33 vertebrae: seven cervical, 12 thoracic or dorsal, five lumbar, five fused sacral and four fused coccygeal vertebrae. These vertebrae articulate with each other through the intervertebral disks and apophysial joints, except for the first and second cervical vertebrae and the sacrum, which are specialized structures. The strength and flexibility of the spine depend upon the integrity of the apophysial joints, a variety of heavy ligaments connecting the vertebrae, the shock-absorbing resilience of the intervertebral disks, and a finely coordinated muscular system. These structures, working synchronously, permit the individual to maintain an upright posture while allowing the necessary motion of flexion, extension, rotation and lateral bending of the head and trunk involved in daily activities. Contained within the protecting bony spinal canal are the spinal cord and the cauda equina, and emanating from it are the segmental peripheral nerves. Each vertebra is composed of a number of parts having special functions which vary with the three major regions of the spine. Because the construction and function of the vertebrae differ in the various regions of the spine, certain injuries are characteristic of each area.

Except for the first cervical, each vertebra is composed of a body and a neural arch. The body, roughly cylindrical in shape, is primarily cancellous bone contained in a thin sheath of cortex. It is reinforced by a cartilage plate above and below, and is joined to the adjacent vertebra through the intervertebral disk. The disk is composed of an outer ring of tough fibrous tissue, the annulus fibrosus, and a center section softer in consistency, the nucleus pulposus. The disk is attached firmly superiorly and inferiorly to the vertebra through the cartilaginous plate. Because the disk is compressible, it acts like a shock-absorber and permits bending and a limited amount of rotary motion between the vertebrae. The anterior and posterior longitudinal ligaments connect the bodies of the vertebrae from the occiput to the sacrum.

The major weight of the head and trunk is transmitted to the pelvis through the bodies of the vertebrae and the disks. The bodies of the vertebrae become progressively larger from the cervical to the lumbar region, to accommodate the increasing weight.

Since the bone of the vertebrae is cancellous, it is prone to compression and impacted fractures. Since the disks are soft-tissue structures, they may undergo degenerative changes which predispose them to tearing, rupture and displacement in injuries of the spine.

The neural arch projects posteriorly from the bodies and is composed of the pedicles, lamina, spinous process and articular processes. These structures form a protective bony ring through which the spinal cord passes. This bony tube serves well in its protective function for the cord in the normal spine. However, when injury occurs and the neural arch is displaced by fracture or dislocation, the spinal cord or cauda equina may be compressed and injured.

The vertebrae articulate posteriorly through the apophysial joints. The inferior articular process, overlapping the superior one of the vertebra below, prevents forward and lateral displacement. They are true joints covered by articular cartilage, lined with synovial membrane and possess a ligamentous joint capsule. They are subject to all the ills and injuries of true joints, including fractures and dislocations.

The lamina forms a bony arch over the spinal cord and is connected to the corresponding lamina above and below by the elastic ligamentum flavum. Projecting back-

ward from each lamina is a spinous process which is connected to the adjacent processes by the interspinous ligament. These processes serve as muscle attachments and as levers to strengthen the spine through their connecting ligaments. It is the elasticity of the interspinous ligament and the ligamentum flavum which permits the spine to bend in various directions. These ligaments may be torn when the spine is injured.

Projections of bone laterally from the vertebra, the transverse processes, serve as muscle attachments and levers for movement and stability. In each region of the spine, they serve a special function. In the cervical area, they are perforated, forming a protective canal for the vertebral arteries. In the thoracic region, the transverse processes articulate with the ribs, stabilizing the connection between the spine and thorax. In the lumbar area, they are larger and act as levers through which the balancing muscles of the spine act. The spinous and transverse processes are subject to avulsion fractures by muscle contractions, and the pull of tense ligaments when the spine is injured.

When viewed from front or back, the spine is straight. When viewed from the side, it is convex, being forward in the cervical and lumbar regions and backward in the thoracic and sacral regions. These curves place the contents of the thorax near the central weight-bearing axis of the body and maintain the head directly over it.

The entire column of vertebrae is maintained in the erect position and moved by the complex group of perispinal neck and trunk muscles. Injuries to the spine may strain, tear or rupture these controlling muscles.

Movements of the spine are complex and vary with each area. The head articulating with the ringlike atlas or first cervical vertebra may nod, rotate or bend laterally at this joint. The primary motion, however, is nodding.

The second cervical vertebra, through the upward projection of its odontoid process, articulates with the ring of the atlas. The odontoid process is held in position in the forward confines of this ring by the transverse ligament; the spinal cord occupies the posterior portion. The primary function of this joint is rotation of the head.

The remaining cervical vertebrae permit flexion and extension, lateral bending and a moderate amount of rotation. However, the primary motion is flexion and extension, which becomes more limited as the thoracic spine is approached.

Because the head is a heavy object, rapid acceleration or deceleration of the body may throw the head backward, forward or to the side on the whiplike cervical spine. The cervical spine motions have been likened to a whip, since the upper four cervical vertebrae are more mobile than the lower three. The upper four form the lash, the lower three the handle of the whip. The junction of these two areas is subject to excessive strain in this mechanism of injury, and is frequently the site of fractures and dislocations as well as sprains.

The thoracic spine is stabilized by the rib cage and motion is limited, although some flexion, extension, lateral bending and rotation is allowed. The lowermost segments become more mobile as they join the highly mobile lumbar spine. It is at this junction of high mobility and relative fixation that injuries are likely to occur, as in the cervical spine.

The lumbar spine, curving forward, permits considerable flexion and extension with moderate rotation and functions to balance the body above the pelvis. It is a highly mobile area, as is the cervical region.

Alterations of the spinal curves and loss of mobility produce deformity and cause stress and strain in the spine following injury.

When a vertebral body is crushed, the mechanism of fracture is usually forced flexion of the spine. A wedge-shaped deformity of the vertebra is produced with the apex of the wedge forward. This deformity in the upper lumbar and thoracic region increases the normal curve of this area, and is called a kyphosis or gibbus. When the deformity occurs in the cervical and lower lumbar region, the normal forward curve is decreased. Because alterations in the curves of the spine in one area shift the center of gravity of the body forward or backward, other areas automatically compensate for this by increasing or decreasing their curves. Thus, an increase in the thoracic curve of the spine is compensated by an increase in the lumbar lordosis. When this is excessive, strain is produced on the ligaments and joints, and pain may develop in the compensatory area of the spine as well as at the fracture site.

A similar mechanism occurs if the vertebra is wedged on one side. Compensatory curves above and below the deformity occur to bring the spinal axis back over the center of the sacrum, and the condition is called compensatory scoliosis.

When the spine is immobilized in the treatment of fractures and other injuries, the controlling muscles atrophy and weaken. Since these muscles hold the spine erect and move it, they must be rehabilitated.

Muscles and ligaments may contract and shorten in the position of immobilization, and spinal motion may be limited after the injury heals. The mobility and strength of joints, ligaments and muscles must be reestablished by an appropriate program of exercise if the spine is to function properly.

Every patient who complains of pain in the neck or back following injury must be considered to have a fractured spine until proved otherwise. The reason for this rather rigid principle is to prevent injury to the spinal cord by careless handling of the patient. Until the injury is evaluated, the patient must be handled with care to prevent any movement of the spine which might damage the spinal cord.

Most spinal fractures and dislocations are caused by indirect violence which forces the spine into extremes of flexion, extension, rotation or lateral bending. The most common injuries are produced by flexion. These flexion injuries often are caused by falling from a height, landing on the feet, or by slipping and falling in a sitting position, or by the forced flexion of rapid deceleration of an automobile accident. Less frequently, the spine is injured by falling or diving on the head or shoulders.

When the spine is forced into extreme flexion, the body of the vertebra crushes anteriorly, producing a wedge-shaped deformity. The most common site is the lower dorsal—upper lumbar area; next in frequency, the mid- and lower cervical region. These areas are near the junctions of high and low mobility of the spine, and, thus, are more easily injured.

Usually, the superior aspect of the vertebra is driven downward by the vertebra above, compressing the upper half of the vertebra into the lower half. The ligamentous structures of the posterior elements about the neural arch are pulled tight and are often strained. If the force stops at this point, the fracture is stable and there is no danger to the spinal cord. The wedge-shaped deformity of the vertebral body alters the curves of the spine, depending upon the degree of compression. If one-third or less of the height of the anterior body is lost, no correction is necessary. If more deformity than this exists, it may be necessary to reduce the fracture to prevent painful compensatory strain in other areas of the spine from developing. However, the age of the patient and the location of the fracture determine the course of treatment. When the fracture occurs in the elderly patient, osteoporosis may be a predisposing factor. Frequently, minor trauma may produce the injury in postmenopausal women with osteoporosis, or the fracture may occur spontaneously if the body weight exceeds the capacity of the softened bone. Spontaneous collapse of the vertebral body often occurs when the bone has been destroyed by metastatic malignant lesions.

Whenever the body of the vertebra is fractured, bleeding occurs from the bone, forming a hematoma about the spinal column. If the fracture is the common wedge-shaped compression, the bleeding takes place anteriorly away from the spinal canal and the cord is not usually endangered. However, the sympathetic ganglionated trunk, located on the anterolateral surface of the vertebra, is disturbed and a paralytic ileus may result, which may cause more immediate trouble than the fracture (Fig. 90).

When this type fracture occurs in the cervical region, the hematoma and associated edema accompanying the strain and tearing of the ligaments of the neural arch

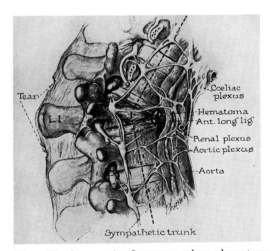

Figure 90. Compression fractures produce a hematoma about the vertebra, disturbing the sympathetic nervous system. This damage may produce paralytic ileus.

may slowly compress the spinal cord. These patients must be observed carefully for signs of central nervous system involvement.

If the force producing the compression is in the long axis of the spine, a bursting type fracture is produced. The body of the vertebra is squashed and expands in diameter, pancake fashion. Comminution and impaction of the fragments may be marked. With this type compression fracture, the spinal canal may be distorted by bone or hematoma and pressure may be exerted upon the spinal cord, demanding decompression.

Treatment of simple wedge-shaped, compression fractures, following evaluation of the injury, requires placing the patient supine on a firm bed. Mild sedation may be given, and the pain usually subsides when the patient is quiet. Movement may produce momentary sharp pain which is not eliminated by narcotics; but, since the pain is momentary, it is usually tolerated without their use.

When the fracture is in the cervical region, traction is applied to the skull by tongs for immobilization and reduction. If the deformity is slight, a cloth head halter may be applied and 6 to 10 pounds of continuous traction made with the neck in moderate hyperextension, although it is not as effective as tong traction. Turning movements of the head may be eliminated by placing padded sandbags on each side of the head. This method of treatment makes use of the intact anterior longitudinal ligament of the spine in reduction. Since this ligament is attached along the anterior surface of the vertebral body, it buckles but does not tear as the compression force produces the wedge-shaped fracture. When the posterior elements of the vertebra are intact, the apophysial joints act like a hinge when the spine is extended. This maneuver tightens the anterior longitudinal ligament which in turn pulls the compressed anterior body apart. The deformity is, thus, reduced, and, if the vertebra is maintained in this position, new bone fills in the gap created anteriorly in the body.

In the cervical area, traction may be continued for four to six weeks after reduction, when a cervical collar or brace may be applied to maintain the neck in extension for an additional three months. Superimposed weight is borne by the posterior elements of the spine during this time. When the fracture occurs in the thoracic or lumbar region, the same principle of hyperextension of the spine is used for reduction; however, traction is not necessary. Reduction may be accomplished slowly by placing the fracture site in the spine over the apex of a triangle created in the mattress. This may be done by putting the patient in the hospital bed so that his head is at the foot of the bed, then slowly raising the knee rest. Another method is to place a 2-by-4-inch plank transversely beneath the mattress and slowly raise it by jacks to produce hyperextension of the spine.

When the pain has subsided and paralytic ileus and other injuries have been controlled, the patient may be placed in a body cast or brace to maintain the hyperextended position. He may become ambulatory as soon as he is comfortable. The cast or brace may be used for four to six months while the fracture site fills in with new bone. Often, some deformity of the vertebra recurs, even with perfect anatomic reduction and adequate immobilization.

Reduction may be accomplished by manipulation in younger people, if it is not accomplished by traction. The patient is placed face down on a strip of canvas suspended from a fracture table. The canvas strip forms a shallow hammock upon which the patient lies prone. As tension on the strip is released, it sags, hyperextending the spine. The surgeon may aid the reduction by making sharp, downward thrusts with his hands over the fracture site, increasing the hyperextension at this point.

Hyperextension of the spine may also be created by placing the patient prone on a table and hauling his legs upward to an overhead support by means of slings and ropes. Following reduction of the fracture, a body cast is applied to maintain the position.

Older people do not well tolerate manipulative reduction, prolonged bed treatment or massive body cast immobilization. Bladder, bowel and lung functions are disturbed and complications arise more readily in these systems in older patients. It is better to place the patient in bed for a few days until the pain subsides, accept the deformity and begin ambulation in a supporting corset as soon as possible. Although some deformity may be present, if the spinal cord is not involved and the fracture is stable, it will heal with minimum complications with early ambulation and rehabilitation of the spinal muscles.

FRACTURE WITH FORWARD DISLOCATION OF THE SPINE. If the flexion force which produces the wedge compression continues, the ligaments of the apophysial joints and neural arch may rupture. This allows the intact vertebra to dislocate forward on the fractured vertebra below. The inferior facet of the cephalad vertebra slips forward over the superior facet of the lower vertebra and may lock in this position. This deformity distorts the spinal canal and the cord or cauda equina may be injured. The fracture-dislocation is unstable and unprotected movement of the patient may increase the deformity and further damage the central nervous system. It is for this reason that all patients with suspected fractures of the spine must be handled carefully until the injury is determined to be stable or unstable.

The cervical region is most frequently involved in this injury. The lumbar region, similar in mobility to the cervical region but stronger, is less often the site of fracture dislocation. The thoracic region is more rigid and the configuration of the neural arch, along with the supporting thorax, prevents fracture-dislocation except with extreme violence. The spinal cord, nerve roots and cauda equina may escape damage, or damage may be minimal, if the displacement of the vertebra is minor. With pronounced displacement, damage to these structures may be severe, permanent and life-endangering. Continued pressure on the spinal cord or cauda equina, whether by displaced fragments or hematoma and edema, must be relieved as soon as possible.

In the cervical region, the injury is treated by heavy skull tong traction with the head and neck in neutral position. Extension and flexion and rotation must be avoided, as the fulcrum of the posterior elements of the spine is lost. Flexion may allow the vertebra to slip forward, increasing the deformity of the spinal canal. Extension forces the lamina of the upper vertebra to move forward against the cord or cauda equina like a guillotine. Rotary or lateral displacement may produce impingement on the central nervous system by distortion of the neural canal.

The amount of traction needed in the cervical region to effect reduction may be 25 pounds or more. The jaw and temporomandibular joints will not tolerate this amount of traction by a halter, so that skeletal traction through the skull by appropriate tong devices must be used. The tongs are inserted through the outer table of the skull under local anesthesia, with the head and neck carefully supported. Heavy longitudinal traction is then applied to pull the apophysial joints apart. When the inferior facet has been unlatched from its anterior position with the superior facets of the vertebra below, the neck may be carefully extended and the traction reduced to allow the joints to engage. Moderate extension then maintains the reduction until the ligaments heal, usually in four to six weeks.

Occasionally, unilateral or bilateral forward dislocation of the cervical apophysial joints occurs without fracture. Bilateral joint dislocations are produced by extreme flexion. The body of the vertebra does not break, but the posterior longitudinal ligament and intervertebral disk part, along with the joint capsules, ligamentum flavum and interspinous ligament. The anterior body of the vertebra is the fulcrum as the soft tissues of the posterior elements tear. If the force continues, the intervertebral disk is disrupted, and, as the facets lose contact, the vertebra slips forward. When the force abates, the inferior facets lock beneath the superior facets of the vertebra below.

Unilateral joint dislocation is produced by flexion and lateral deviation of the head coupled with rotation. The intact apophysial joint acts as a pivot as the opposite one dislocates forward. The head is held in rotation to the right if the left apophysial joint dislocates, and in the opposite direction when the right joint dislocates.

Unilateral dislocations may be reduced by manual traction and manipulation by the surgeon in the absence of abnormal neurologic findings. With the patient anesthetized, the surgeon makes traction on the chin and occiput, deviating the head away from the side of the dislocation, and flexes the neck moderately. When the head can be rotated back into normal position, the facets have disengaged and traction is reduced while the head is brought into extension. X-ray examination confirms the reduction. Halter neck traction of 6 pounds is used for a week or ten days while the reaction of injury subsides. A cervical collar or brace is used for three months while the ligaments heal.

Bilateral apophysial joint dislocations are best treated by skeletal skull tong traction, since the dislocation is unstable and manipulation may damage the spinal cord. The general method of treatment is the same as that used for fracture-dislocation of the cervical spine.

Occasionally, unilateral or bilateral dislocations cannot be reduced by closed methods. If, after a few days of traction, x-ray examination shows a persistent dislocation and the patient's condition has stabilized, open reduction may be done. Tong traction is applied to the skull for stability and traction during the operation. The posterior elements are exposed, and, under direct vision, the vertebra may be levered back into position. Partial resection of the apophysial joints may be necessary to accomplish the reduction.

FRACTURES AND DISLOCATIONS OF THE ATLAS AND AXIS. The joints of the atlas and axis are flat and almost horizontal, allowing the atlas a considerable degree of rotation on the odontoid process of the axis. When extreme rotary force is applied to the head, the apophysial joint on one side may be disrupted. The facet of the atlas slides forward over the facet of the axis and locks in this position. The transverse ligament of the atlas remains intact. Sudden death may occur if the upper cervical cord is compressed sufficiently. However, the cord may escape compression and there may be no abnormal neurologic findings. Reduction is accomplished by traction through the skull followed by cast or brace immobilization to prevent turning of the head while the joint capsule heals, as in other cervical dislocations.

Fractures of the odontoid process are extremely serious injuries. The mechanism of fracture is usually violent, acute flexion of the head from a fall on the back of the head or by striking the head in a driving accident. The atlas remains in normal relationship to the occiput. The odontoid process, attached to the atlas by the transverse ligament, is displaced forward on the body of the axis because the fracture usually occurs at the base of the odontoid process. Stability between the two bones is lost, and the head may slide forward, backward or to the side, producing varying degrees of cord pressure. The displacement may reduce spontaneously. The neurologic lesion may be minimal or severe.

The surgeon may suspect a fracture of the

odontoid process, in the absence of neurologic findings, if the patient complains of a feeling of marked instability of the head on the neck. The patient usually supports the head with his hands and is reluctant to release this support at any time. The diagnosis can only be made by adequate x-ray examination. During the examination, the head must be supported, since any shift of the head or neck may compress the spinal cord and cause sudden death.

If the patient survives the injury, and there is no displacement, he may be placed in head-halter traction with sandbag immobilization for a short period. However, the fracture should be immobilized in a Minerva jacket as soon as possible. The plaster cast extends from the head to the pelvis to secure adequate fixation. The plaster jacket should be used for four to six months.

If displacement is present or a neurologic deficit exists, skull tong traction should be used until the damage to the spinal cord is stabilized. When the patient's condition will allow it, plaster cast immobilization is done.

Nonunion of the odontoid process is not uncommon, and may follow an undiagnosed or even an adequately treated fracture. The fracture may be missed on the original examination, as the fracture may be hairline. Later, following absorption of bone at the fracture site, the fracture may be easily detected by x-ray examination. Many years may elaspse before minor signs of spinal cord compression are evident to the patient. Nonunion of the odontoid process should be treated by fusion of the occiput to the second cervical vertebra to prevent spinal cord damage by slow displacement or subsequent injury.

FRACTURE-DISLOCATIONS OF THE LUMBAR SPINE. Flexion force, which continues after compression of the vertebral body has occurred, may result in fracture or dislocation of the posterior elements of the spine in the thoracolumbar region. Since these structures are stronger in the lower spine than in the cervical region, greater violence is needed to produce the displacement, and complicating injuries to the thorax and abdominal contents are common. The lower spinal cord or cauda equina is frequently injured. The area of contact of the apophysial joints is greater in the lumbar and lower thoracic region than in the upper spine; thus, slipping forward of one facet upon the other is usually accompanied by fractures of these elements. Two major types of injuries occur when vertebrae are displaced in this region of the spine. The inferior facets may break or the fracture may occur through the pedicles. In either case, the spinal canal is distorted and the spine is unstable, endangering the cauda equina and spinal cord.

Forward displacement of the vertebra may be complicated by lateral or rotational deformity if shearing force is coupled with flexion. Displacement occasionally takes place posteriorly, the upper vertebra dislocating backward on the lower. The degree of displacement varies from minor to major, but any malalignment of the posterior border of the vertebra with the adjacent vertebrae indicates damage to the posterior elements of the spine, and thus instability. This finding on x-ray examination always contraindicates hyperextension during treatment, because further damage may be done to the contents of the neural canal.

When a major neurologic deficit is found, surgical decompression of the cord or cauda equina is usually indicated. When major displacement has occurred, it may be impossible to reduce the deformity. Spinal fusion may be necessary to create stability.

If abnormal neurologic findings are minimal, or, if complications prevent laminectomy, the patient should be placed on a Bradford frame, or a posterior plaster shell or bed should be applied. This provides enough stability to allow nursing care while the problems are evaluated and resolved. When the physiologic processes of the patient have stabilized, it can be determined if laminectomy and spinal fusion is needed, or whether a cast will afford sufficient immobilization. It may be wiser to accept some deformity in the absence of neurologic impairment to allow the fracture to heal, and fuse the spine later if pain should arise from the altered mechanics.

FRACTURES OF THE TRANSVERSE PROCESSES. Fractures of the transverse processes as isolated injuries are most often found in the lumbar spine. Occasionally, fractures of the thoracic and cervical regions occur, but they are usually associated with other fractures of the vertebrae. The lumbar transverse processes serve as muscle attachments for the psoas and perispinal muscles. When these muscles suddenly contract, the transverse processes may be avulsed. The injury often involves a series of transverse processes. The avulsed portion of bone may be displaced a considerable distance from the vertebra by the muscle pull. However, when little displacement occurs, the fracture may be overlooked in the x-ray films. The injury is not serious but is painful. All spine motions produce pain and are restricted. Muscle spasm may distort the normal curves of the back. Lifting the leg on the involved side produces pain by tensing the psoas muscle. No reduction is necessary. The muscles reattach and, although nonunion is common, it does not produce symptoms.

Treatment is simple. Bed rest with heat and sedation lessen muscle spasm. When the pain subsides, the patient is fitted with a supporting corset and allowed to be ambulatory. Back-strengthening muscle exercises are started early in the healing process. Disability from the injury should not exceed two or three months.

FRACTURES OF THE SPINOUS PROCESSES. Fractures of the spinous processes result from direct force or from traction of the inter-spinous ligament when the spine is flexed. A direct blow to the spine may fracture any of the spinous processes; however, avulsion by the interspinous ligament most frequently affects the cervical vertebrae. Treatment is similar to that for transverse process fractures: rest and support until the pain subsides is followed by exercise.

REHABILITATION OF THE MUSCLES CONTROLLING THE SPINE. All injuries to the spine affect the muscles which control the spine. Rehabilitation of these muscles must be instituted following the injury if maximum comfortable function is expected. Muscles atrophy and shorten when they are not used. Bed rest or cast-and-brace immobilization promotes the atrophy of disuse. Weak muscles fatigue and ache, and shortened muscles prevent motion. When the spine fracture is stable, exercise should be started as soon as pain subsides. If the fracture is unstable, the exercise program must be delayed until sufficient healing has stabilized the spine.

Amputations and Limb Substitution

A multitude of conditions demand amputation of parts of the extremities in order to maintain life or imporve function. These problems arise in all age groups. The infant born with defective limbs, the child and adult with malignant tumors or irreparable trauma, and the elderly suffering from vascular failure may all require removal of parts of the extremities. The surgeon must know the conditions which can benefit from amputation, and the details of technique which ensure the most efficient use of the remaining parts.

The surgeon's responsibility to the patient does not end with the removal of deformed or diseased tissue. He must be prepared to restore the person to maximum efficiency through the use of appropriate prosthetic devices. In addition to the knowledge of these factors, he must support the patient through the period of emotional adjustment to the loss of a part and the adaptation to an altered way of life.

Amputations may be required when there is irreparable damage from trauma or its sequelae, failure of circulation from peripheral vascular disease or embolic occlusions, tumors, infection, trophic changes secondary to neurologic disease and congenital or acquired deformities.

In the child, the most frequent reasons for amputations are congenital defects, trauma and malignant bone tumors. In the adult, the usual reason for amputation is trauma, infection or malignancy, while in the elderly, peripheral vascular failure is the most common problem.

When amputation is not an emergency, the surgeon must discuss the problem in detail with the patient. He must explain the need for the operation, the postoperative care and the final function which can be obtained through the use of an appropriate prosthesis. The improvement in prosthetic devices in recent years has been remarkable, and, in most instances, substitutes for the missing part can achieve a considerable measure of usefulness.

TYPES OF AMPUTATION

Two major types of amputation are performed: open and closed. Both are accomplished with tourniquet control, except in peripheral vascular disease, when tourniquet pressure may injure diseased blood vessels.

OPEN OR GUILLOTINE AMPUTATION.   When spreading infection is established or is a potential hazard, open amputation is indicated. The amputation allows adequate drainage of damaged tissue until the danger of spreading infection is passed. Since this operation is performed at the most distal level of viable tissue, and the scar after healing will not tolerate a prosthesis, secondary revision of the stump is practically always necessary.

The amputation is performed by a circular incision about the part, thus the term "guillotine amputation." When the skin and subcutaneous tissue is incised, it is allowed to retract. The deep fascia and muscle are incised in progressive layers as the muscle retracts. The bone is sectioned at the level of final muscle retraction. Nerves and major blood vessels are ligated and sectioned at this same level. Because the retraction of tissue occurs in layers, as the limb is sectioned by progressive circular incision, the end of the stump resembles a cone with the apex at the bone level.

Postoperatively, the wound remains open while skin traction is applied to prevent further retraction of the soft tissues. A sheath of Stockinet is glued to the skin, dressings are applied to the open surface, and continuous traction is made on the Stockinet sleeve. As the wound granulates and heals, the skin edges are drawn toward the bone end by scar contraction. A circular scar adherent to the bone with inadequate soft tissue cover is formed, necessitating revision of the stump.

Revision of the stump need not wait until healing is complete, but the granulating surface must be clean and healthy before the final amputation is done. If complete healing of the wound is desired before definitive surgery is undertaken, it may be hastened by applying split-thickness skin grafts to the granulating surface. The purpose of reamputation, or stump revision, is to provide adequate soft tissue coverage for the bone at a level practical for the use of a prosthesis. When reamputation at a higher level is not practical, local revision of the scar is done. The scar tissue must be completely excised. Usually, the bone must be resected at a slightly higher level. The soft tissues are then closed to provide adequate bone cover with a minimum scar at the end of the stump.

CLOSED OR FLAP AMPUTATION.   When infection is not a hazard, primary closure of the wound may be performed. The best available site for the amputation is chosen. The incision is made to produce two flaps of skin and subcutaneous tissue resembling an open fish mouth. Usually, the flaps are of equal length, but special problems may demand unequal flaps to bring the scar anterior or posterior to the bone end. After reflection of the flaps, the deep fascia is incised at a similar level; the muscle is divided by a circular cut, and in most instances allowed to retract. The periosteum is incised and the bone sectioned transversely at the level of the retracted muscles. Periosteal tags are removed to prevent spur formation, but the periosteum is not stripped from the bone end, as was once advocated.

The major blood vessels are separated and ligated individually to prevent the formation of arteriovenous fistulae. The nerves are pulled downward, sectioned, and allowed to retract above the level of the cut muscle. This is done to prevent the nerves from adhering to the terminal scar, where they may be subjected to pressure and tension. Severed nerves heal by the formation of a neuroma. If the neuroma forms in the scar tissue of the distal stump, it may be painful. Local or phantom limb pain may prevent the use of a prosthesis. When the neuroma forms above the distal scar in its normal compartment, it is usually painless.

The wound is closed by approximating the deep fascia over the bone and remaining muscle, avoiding excessive muscle tissue over the bone end. Suturing the deep fascia pulls the muscle downward sufficiently to allow proper attachment to the bone and helps to prevent muscle ends from adhering to the skin. Muscles which become attached to the scar of the flaps distort the stump when the limb is moved. Friction is produced within the socket of the prosthesis, and skin problems may arise from this complication. The subcutaneous tissue is closed with a minimum number of sutures. The skin should be closed under normal tension except in peripheral vascular disease, when no tension should be present.

Drains are inserted in the corners of the wound to allow escape of serum from the sectioned structures. Even in the presence of careful hemostasis, a certain amount of serum accumulates, and, if not drained, interferes with wound healing. The drains are removed after 48 or 72 hours.

A voluminous pressure dressing is used to

supply uniform compression over the stump except in peripheral vascular disease. Amputations for vascular problems are dressed loosely to prevent strangulation of tissues with a precarious blood supply.

POSTOPERATIVE CARE. Dressings are changed infrequently after removal of the drains; however, the outer elastic bandages should be adjusted as often as needed to ensure uniform pressure. Amputation stumps heal slowly, particularly in peripheral vascular disease. The skin sutures should remain in place for at least two weeks. Primary healing of the wound is desirable to minimize scar tissue. Wound breakdown or separation must heal by secondary intention, producing a scar which may be fragile and subject to irritation when the prosthesis is used. Splints may be applied during the healing time ro prevent flexion contractures, particularly in peripheral vascular disease. Proper bed posture is an aid in preventing contractures, particularly with lower extremity amputations. Patients who have had amputations below the knee tend to keep the knee flexed to lessen the pull on the severed gastrocnemius muscle. This must be counteracted by a splint until the wound heals and the irritation of the muscle subsides. Following removal of the splint, the patient must straighten the knee completely numerous times during the day to prevent a flexion contracture.

Patients who have had amputations above the knee tend to flex and abduct the thigh. Short stumps are more prone to develop this deformity. These people must lie face down several times a day to stretch the thigh into complete extension at the hip. They must not use a pillow to elevate the distal stump for comfort, and they must not sit in bed with the hip flexed for long periods. They must be taught to adduct the thigh actively and maintain it against the other leg most of the time to prevent abduction contracture.

When the skin has healed, the process of shrinking the stump begins. After amputation, the subcutaneous fat and muscle atrophy, and the stump shrinks in circumference. This process must be completed before the prosthesis is fitted. Proper bandaging must be done to speed this process, prevent the accumulation of edema and aid in shaping the amputation stump. Elastic bandages are used, and the patient must be instructed in the correct method of wrapping the part. The bandage must be reapplied several times during the day to maintain firm pressure. The process of shrinking usually takes about three months.

Exercises to strengthen and prevent contracture of the muscles controlling the stump may be started when the wound has healed. Massaging the stump serves no useful purpose and may irritate sensitive neuromata; it should not be used in the postoperative care. Pounding the stump with the assumption that this process toughens it is to be condemned. Only damage to healing tissue is produced by this antiquated custom.

Ambulation should begin early. The upper extremity amputee may be out of bed in a few days if other injuries permit it. The lower extremity amputee should begin ambulation in a walker after the wound has healed, if his general condition will allow it. Dependency of the amputated upper or lower extremity should be avoided until the wound has healed; for this reason, assisted walking is delayed in lower extremity amputees until this is accomplished.

AMPUTATIONS OF THE LOWER EXTREMITY

Amputations of the lower extremity alter to varying degrees the ability to stand, walk and run. The lower extremities are a system of bony levers articulated at the ankle, knee and hip joints. The levers activated by muscles assume the necessary positions for balance and ambulation almost automatically. These muscles, bones and joints, acting synchronously, provide shock-free movement of the body from place to place. Loss of any part of this mechanism interferes with balance, propulsion and stability. Prosthetic devices have been evolved to substitute for the various missing parts. The degree of successful use of these devices depends upon the level of amputation and the skill of the surgeon and prosthetist.

AMPUTATION OF TOES AND FOREFOOT. Amputation of one or more toes has little effect on ambulation except for a slight loss of push-off power. Balance is usually not affected and the gait is usually unaltered. The amputation is performed through a racquet-shaped incision. Any part of the toe may be amputated, or more commonly the toe is disarticulated at the metatarsophalangeal joint (Fig. 91).

Amputations through the metatarsal bones affect push-off power in walking to a moderate degree; however, balance of the foot is maintained and minimal disability is encountered.

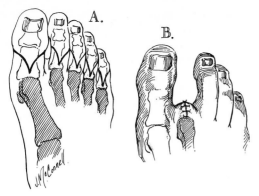

Figure 91. Amputation of all or part of a toe is performed with racquet-shaped incisions.

Whenever possible, the metatarsal bones should be sectioned transversely, all at approximately the same level. The plantar flap is made longer than the dorsal one if possible to produce a dorsal scar. Although a terminal scar is satisfactory, a plantar scar should be avoided (Figs. 92 and 93).

Satisfactory amputations which maintain balance of the foot may be performed to the level of the base of the metatarsal bones. Little power or balance is lost in walking or standing, and a limp is usually not evident. A prosthesis is not necessary, but the shoe must be fitted with a sponge material to help preserve the contour of the shoe.

MIDTARSAL AMPUTATION. For many years, amputation through the midtarsal joints was condemned because imbalance in the remaining muscles produced an equinovarus deformity of the hindfoot and an unsatisfactory stump. Since the peroneal tendons are sectioned and the tibialis anticus is usually detached, the triceps surae muscles of the calf produce the equinus deformity of the remaining foot. Ankle motion is, thus, unopposed plantar flexion. Inversion and eversion at the subtalar joint is usually lost. The tibialis posticus muscle may remain active if the navicular bone is present, pulling the heel into varus. In this position, weight is borne on the end of the irregularly shaped stump. Invariably, the stump is painful and breakdown of the skin is a common complication.

In recent years, an attempt has been made to salvage this amputation by arthrodesis of the ankle joint. The talus is fused to the tibia in 5 to 10 degrees of dorsiflexion. In this position, a full weight-bearing stump is created. The balancing levers of the foot, however, are lost, and there is no active push-off phase on walking. A high shoe with a filler in the fore-

foot is used to create a substitute forefoot lever.

AMPUTATION AT THE ANKLE: SYME'S AMPUTATION. When the major portion of the foot must be removed, the Syme's amputation is preferred. The amputation demands a heel flap free from infection and scarring, possessing adequate sensation and circulation. A transverse anterior incision is made at the ankle joint to the malleoli. A vertical incision is then made directly downward from the anterior tip of the medial malleolus around the bottom of the foot, then upward to the tip of the lateral malleolus. The talus is disarticulated from the tibia, and the talus and os calcis are dissected from the heel flap. The malleoli and articular surface of the tibia are then resected at the level of the joint line.

When the wound edges are brought together, the scar lies anteriorly and the heel flap forms a cushion over the end of the bone. This is a true end-bearing stump with only slight loss of leg length. The patient is able to walk barefoot without a prosthesis when necessary. The normal shock-absorbing and propulsive force provided by the foot and ankle is lost with this amputation. The prosthesis must, in some measure, substitute for this loss if near-normal standing and walking are to be achieved. The socket of the prosthesis encases the leg to just below the knee and is molded to the crest of the tibia to prevent rotation of the artificial foot. Since the space for the ankle joint in the prosthesis is limited, a complete hinge joint cannot be used. Shock-absorbing properties are provided by a special foot with a rubber heel and an ankle joint recessed into the foot. This joint allows a slight amount of dorsi- and

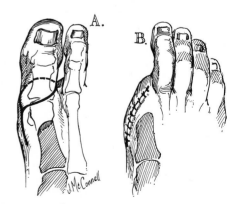

Figure 92. When the great toe is amputated with the metatarsal head, a modified incision is used to reduce the prominence of the remaining bone.

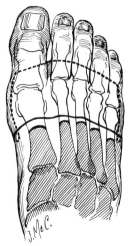

Figure 93. A longer plantar flap is used when amputations are made through the metatarsal bones. The foot remains balanced, and no prosthesis is necessary.

plantar flexion. The forepart of the foot is flexible and dorsiflexes passively at the push-off phase of walking.

During the swing and stance phase of walking, the lower extremity rotates internally and externally on its long axis. When the foot is fixed to the ground, this rotary action of the leg is absorbed in the subtalar joint. With the Syme's amputation and those at a higher level, this action of the subtalar joint is lost. The stump tends to rotate within the socket of the prosthesis. A loose-fitting socket allows excessive rotation, producing friction and skin irritation. Thus, the socket must fit the stump accurately to minimize this problem. A properly aligned and accurately fitted prosthesis should permit smooth, pain-free walking and standing.

AMPUTATIONS THROUGH THE LEG. When amputation is demanded above the ankle, the site of election below the knee is chosen. This amputation should produce a stump 5 to 7 inches long below the knee joint. Stumps longer than 7 inches are difficult to fit with a prosthesis and are subject to circulatory failure. Stumps shorter than 5 inches are less powerful in operating the prosthesis because the lever arm of the stump is reduced; however, amputations as short as 2 inches below the knee can be fitted successfully with a prosthesis (Fig. 94).

Flaps of skin and subcutaneous tissue are made of equal length anteriorly and posteriorly. The length of the flaps can be estimated as two-thirds to three-fourths the radius of the leg at the site of amputation. After the flaps are reflected, the bone and muscle are sec-

tioned at the base of the flaps. The fascia covering the gastrocnemius muscle is preserved to the level of the skin flap. The anterior crest of the tibia is beveled to eliminate this sharp point of bone. The fibula is resected 1 to 1½ inches higher than the tibia. When the tibia is less than 3 inches in length, the distal end of the remaining fibula tends to angulate outward, as there is insufficient interosseous membrane remaining to hold it in position. This angulation produces pressure against the side of the socket which is difficult to relieve. The head of the fibula may be removed, but the lateral collateral ligament and the biceps tendon must be reattached to the tibia. The peroneal nerve should be sectioned above the knee joint.

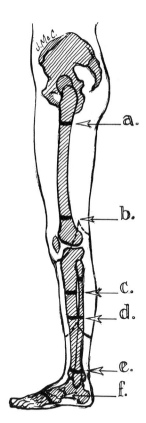

Figure 94. Disarticulation of the hip can be fitted successfully with the Canadian hip prosthesis. (a) Amputation in the upper thigh must produce a stump at least 2.5 to 3 inches below the perineum to allow fitting with a suction-socket prosthesis. All length to this level should be saved. (b) Supracondylar amputation is done just above the flare of the condyles. (c) All length to a level 2.5 inches below the insertion of the hamstrings should be saved. (d) The site of election of amputation below the knee should produce a stump 5 to 7 inches long; however, stumps as short as 2 inches below the knee can be fitted with a prosthesis. Knee-joint disarticulation and Gritti-Stokes amputations produce an end-bearing stump. (e) The level of the Syme amputation at the ankle joint. (f) The level of midtarsal amputation.

Removal of the head of the fibula reduces some of the resistance to rotation of the stump in the socket and, for this reason, is objectionable. In recent years, attempts have been made to retain the head of the fibula in its normal position by creating a bony bridge between the fibula and tibia.

When the amputation is completed, the fascia of the gastrocnemius muscle is sutured anteriorly over the tibia and the skin flaps closed. The scar is terminal or slightly posterior.

Several types of prosthetic devices are used for below-knee amputations, depending upon the length and condition of the stump. The conventional prosthesis consists of a foot articulating through a hinged ankle joint to the shank or shin piece which contains the socket. Attached to the socket are two metal side bars which connect to hinges at the knee joint. The hinges are connected to a leather thigh corset through additional metal side bars. The stump is retained and stabilized in the socket by this harness. To aid in active extension of the knee, an elastic band may be attached to the front of the skin piece and stretched to a belt about the patient's pelvis. This elastic band reinforces the action of the quadriceps muscle in extending the knee.

Weight is borne by the flaring tibial condyles, not the end of the stump. Since this is an area not normally adapted for weight-bearing, the socket must fit accurately to distribute the weight over the largest area available. The stump must be firmly supported by the socket, but the blood vessels posteriorly must not be constricted. Pressure in the popliteal space produces edema in the end of the stump, which may cause breakdown of the skin.

The usual socket is made of willow wood, which is hard and unyielding. In order to provide some cushioning for the stump, soft liners have been made of various materials. Prosthetic sockets of this type are called soft sockets, and are particularly useful when bony prominences are difficult to fit. The exceptionally short stump is difficult to retain in the socket when walking. The hamstring muscles attaching to the tibia below the knee joint tend to lever the stump out of the socket when the knee is flexed. This action produces intolerable friction between the stump and socket. To counteract this tendency, the slip socket has been devised. This mechanism consists of a socket suspended within the shank by a spring or elastic bands from the side bars. The socket, thus, remains more firmly attached to the stump while the up-and-down excursion is absorbed by the suspension mechanism within the shank. Occasionally, the below-knee stump will not tolerate full weight-bearing. When this occurs, the thigh corset may be extended upward and an ischial seat attached to it, to transfer some of the body weight to the ischium.

If a short stump has become deformed by flexion contracture, the leg may be fitted with the knee flexed to 90 degrees in a kneeling, end-bearing socket. Although active control of knee flexion and extension is lost, the stump may be more comfortable than that of the above-knee amputation. Even a short-knee stump is invaluable in transmitting proprioceptive joint sense so necessary for balance. Whenever possible, the knee joint should be conserved, particularly in the bilateral lower extremity amputee.

Fitting and alignment of all parts of the prosthesis must be done accurately to minimize shock, friction and excessive pressure. When this is accomplished, the patient should be able to walk comfortably without limping.

Amputation through the knee joint or lower femur. Disarticulation through the knee joint has been performed for many years. Certain advantages and disadvantages have made this site for amputation controversial. The advantages are a longer lever controlled by musculature which is relatively undamaged and a fully end-bearing stump. The disadvantages are a bulbous stump, at times difficult to fit to a prosthesis and the more distally placed knee hinge.

The amputation is performed through flap incisions made longer and wider than usual. The anterior flap must extend to the tibial tubercle. The patellar tendon and joint capsule is reflected with the anterior flap. The hamstring tendons are clamped and sectioned individually. The vessels and nerves are treated as in other amputations. The hamstring tendons are then sutured to the patellar tendon in the intracondylar notch and the deep fascia and skin closed.

Weight is borne on the end of the stump through the patella. The socket for the prosthesis is usually made of leather treated to prevent absorption of moisture. The socket extends up the thigh as a laced corset. Metal sidebars connect the corset to the knee hinges and shank. Because of the bulbous nature of the stump, it may be possible to suspend the prosthesis from the thigh corset without pelvic-band suspension. Alignment of the knee joint is difficult, as the hinges must be located at the sides of the prosthesis. Stability and control of extension is accomplished by placing the hinges slightly posterior to the weight-bearing line. Elastic bands may be used to control flexion and extension.

A modification of the knee-joint disarticulation is the Gritti-Stokes amputation. Originally, the amputation was devised to prevent the spread of infection into the thigh. The incisions are similar to the knee joint disarticulation except that the posterior flap is shorter. The femur is sectioned transversely at the flare of the condyles. The articular surface of the patella is removed and the patella is placed in contact with the end of the femur. The tendinous and ligamentous structures are closed to hold the patella against the femur. If union of the patella to the femur occurs, a satisfactory end-bearing stump is produced. However, the patella often slips off the end of the femur and fails to unite. The irregularity produced at the end of the stump may be unsuitable for weight-bearing. To avoid this complication, the procedure has been modified by removing the patella and suturing the tendon over the bone. Although full end-bearing may not be obtained by this method, a partial ischial and end-bearing stump may be produced.

THIGH AMPUTATIONS. The site of election for thigh amputation is from the supracondylar region to 10 to 12 inches below the tip of the greater trochanter. Above this level, all length possible should be saved. Long thigh stumps are more powerful than short ones; muscle balance is maintained and control of the prosthesis is positive. When the thigh lever is short, power is lost in the adductor and hamstring muscles. The short thigh stump tends to flex and abduct. Although stumps as short as 3 inches from the perineum can be fitted with a thigh prosthesis, the control of the prosthesis is much more difficult than with a long stump. Conserve as much thigh length as possible above the supracondylar level.

The anterior and posterior flap incisions are made of equal length. The length of the flaps is estimated as two-thirds the radius of the thigh at the level of amputation. The deep fascia is incised with the flaps and reflected upward; the muscles are sectioned near the base of the flaps and the bone sawed transversely at the level of muscle retraction. The

blood vessels and nerves are treated in the usual way. The deep fascia is closed over the end of the bone, anchoring the sectioned muscle at this level. The skin and subcutaneous tissue is closed under normal skin tension.

This type amputation demands ischial weight-bearing. Two major type prostheses are used: the suction socket and the conventional pelvic-band suspension socket. The suction socket is quadrilateral in shape to accommodate the muscle groups of the thigh and to provide an ischial seat. The limb is held in place by negative pressure or suction created by a valve mechanism located in the lower end of the socket. The conventional socket is more conical in shape, but in recent years has been modified to a more quadrilateral shape. The socket is secured to the stump by a thigh hinge suspended from a pelvic band or shoulder harness.

Since the suction socket is applied directly to the thigh stump, proprioceptive sensation and muscular control is better than with the conventional pelvic-band leg. In addition, there is less piston action and friction between the stump and the socket. However, some people cannot tolerate the negative pressure in the socket. Edema and breakdown of the distal stump may occur.

In either the conventional or suction socket, the weight is borne primarily on the ischium. Since the ischium lies posterior to the hip joint, there is some tendency to tilt the pelvis forward, producing a compensatory lordosis. The pelvic tilt and lumbar lordosis is exaggerated if the stump is contracted in flexion and is then forced into a vertically aligned prosthesis. This position may lead to excessive fatigue and backache. When the stump is contracted in flexion, the socket must be fitted in flexion, and the remainder of the prosthesis adjusted to compensate for the deformity.

Since the center of gravity of the body is medial to the hip joint, the pelvis must be stabilized by the abductor muscles of the hip in walking and standing on one leg. These muscles, arising on the ilium above the hip joint and inserting laterally on the trochanter, act as guide wires to hold the pelvis level. If the foot were not fixed to the ground, this same force used to stabilize the pelvis would abduct the leg. This occurs in the amputation stump in walking and standing; the abduction is counteracted by pressure of the stump against the lateral wall of the socket when the prosthesis is in contact with the ground. If the stump is long, the pressure is distributed over a wide area. If the stump is short, the pressure is concentrated near the end of the bone. Thus, a long thigh lever not only is stronger but pressures against the stump in walking are less. When the thigh is flexed, it tends to rotate inward. If the prosthesis is not properly aligned, excessive friction occurs at the ischial seat because of this internal rotation.

The socket usually made of willow wood is attached to a knee block, which contains the knee joint hinge and a braking mechanism to control knee-joint motion. When the amputation is through or above the knee joint, balancing, propulsive and shock-absorbing action of the knee joint is lost. The limb substitute must provide controlled, stable knee motion. Obviously, active flexion and extension and propulsive power cannot be obtained from the prosthesis. The control of these actions must be obtained from the remaining thigh and hip musculature.

Many mechanical knee joints have been devised. None of them fulfills all of the functions of the human knee. In normal walking, two major events happen in the knee. During the stance phase, as the heel strikes the ground, the knee flexes slightly as part of the shock-absorbing mechanism. It continues to flex slightly until the foot is flat to the ground. As the heel rises and the foot dorsiflexes, the knee straightens through the push-off phase of walking. As the toes leave the ground, the knee is again flexed. The knee of the artificial limb cannot maintain stability and allow flexion during the stance phase of walking; otherwise the knee would buckle and the patient would fall. Thus, the knee hinge must be placed posterior to the weight-bearing line of the prosthesis, and the knee must remain extended during the stance phase of walking. The loss of this shock-absorbing power must be compensated for by the ankle joint and foot mechanism.

As the toes leave the ground, the hip and knee flex to allow the toes to clear the ground as the leg swings forward. Normally, the knee flexes to about 65 degrees and is checked by contraction of the quadriceps muscle. At this point, the quadriceps extends the knee gradually during the forward swing of the leg. Just before the heel strikes the ground, the hamstring muscles contract to slow the knee action to prevent it from snapping into extension. This action is lost in above-knee amputations, and the smooth flexion and extension of the prosthetic knee must be ac-

complished mechanically. As the thigh stump is flexed, the mechanical knee must flex easily and smoothly to allow the foot to clear the ground. As the thigh continues to flex, the prosthesis swings forward. When flexion of the thigh ceases, the pendulum-like action of the prosthesis below the knee continues until full extension of the knee is reached. A braking mechanism must be incorporated in the mechanical joint to slow the extending leg smoothly, duplicating the action of the hamstring muscles. The prosthetic foot and ankle are designed to provide a stable, yet flexible, shock-absorbing base for the artificial leg.

In standing, the center of balance passes forward of the ankle joint to the midtarsal region. To prevent the foot from dorsiflexing in standing, the gastrocnemius muscle contracts periodically to maintain balance. In walking, the gastrocnemius contracts at the push-off phase, lifting the body by plantar flexing the foot. In the amputee, this action of the gastrocnemius muscle is lost. It is simulated by limiting dorsiflexion of the artificial foot with a compressible rubber bumper placed anterior to the ankle joint hinge. This compressible bumper, plus a resilient forefoot, aids in the push-off phase of walking, simulating the action of the gastrocnemius muscle. When the heel strikes the ground, the anterior tibial muscles contract momentarily to prevent the foot from slapping against the ground. This action is duplicated in the prosthetic ankle by a compressible bumper placed posterior to the ankle joint.

In the normal foot, balance is aided by inversion and eversion movements in the subtalar and midtarsal joints. This action cannot be successfully duplicated in the prosthetic foot, because it produces instability. Thus, the motion in the prosthetic foot and ankle is essentially flexion and extension. Proper adjustment and alignment of the parts of the artificial foot and ankle is essential for successful action of the entire prosthesis.

HIP DISARTICULATION. Hip disarticulation amputation is usually performed for malignant lesions, or irreparable high-thigh trauma. Fortunately, the operation is not indicated frequently, since lack of a thigh stump makes control of a prosthesis difficult. Two major types of incisions are used; both avoid scars about the ischium.

The first is a racquet-shaped incision. The handle of the racquet centers over the anterior iliac spine and curves medially and downward about 5 cm. below the perineum.

The incision is carried across the posterior thigh to about 8 cm. below the greater trochanter, then upward to join the racquet handle. The femoral artery is ligated and the leg elevated to empty it of blood. Following this, the femoral vein is ligated. The adductor, hip rotators, rectus femoris, iliopsoas and sartorius are all sectioned at their tendinous attachments. The femoral, obturator and sciatic nerves are pulled down and sectioned. Some surgeons believe these nerves should be injected with local anesthetic before section to lessen shock. The fascia lata is sectioned below the insertion of the tensor fascia lata muscle. The gluteus maximus is divided from its insertion on the linea aspera. Sectioning all muscles through tendinous areas lessens blood loss.

The hip joint capsule is then sectioned about the acetabular rim. The head of the femur is dislocated and the leg completely detached. The wound is closed by approximating the gluteus maximus tendon to the adductor muscle origins. The deep fascia is sutured and the skin is closed to produce a vertical anterior scar.

The second type of incision results in an anterior transverse scar. This incision begins over the femoral vessels about 1 inch below the inguinal ligament. The incision then curves medially 4 inches below the pubic tubercle and sweeps posteriorly to create a long posterior flap, then forward to the point of origin. The general steps in completing the disarticulation are essentially the same as for the racquet incision.

Before the development of the Canadian hip prosthesis, the tilting table and saucer-type prosthesis were used. These prostheses were conventional above-knee limbs attached

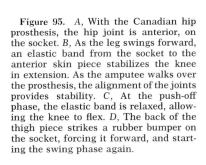

Figure 95. *A*, With the Canadian hip prosthesis, the hip joint is anterior, on the socket. *B*, As the leg swings forward, an elastic band from the socket to the anterior skin piece stabilizes the knee in extension. As the amputee walks over the prosthesis, the alignment of the joints provides stability. *C*, At the push-off phase, the elastic band is relaxed, allowing the knee to flex. *D*, The back of the thigh piece strikes a rubber bumper on the socket, forcing it forward, and starting the swing phase again.

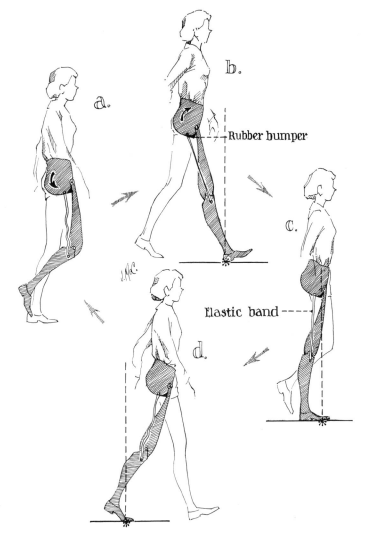

by a hinge to a saucer or bucket suspended from the patient by shoulder and pelvic straps, the stump balanced on the saucer or fitted into the bucket of the tilting table prosthesis. The hip was locked in extension while walking and unlocked to sit. A very awkward gait was almost always found. The patient moved the prosthesis forward by elevating the pelvis and rotating it forward. After the heel contacted the ground and the knee was extended, he vaulted over the prosthesis. Considerable effort was required to operate the artificial leg and instability was always a problem. Over-stressed hinges at the hip joint produced frequent mechanical failures.

The Canadian prosthesis socket is made of plastic and encases the pelvis as well as the stump. Three points of fixation are obtained: the ischium and both iliac crests. This provides firm fixation of the socket to the patient and positive control of the socket by the pelvis. The thigh piece is hinged anteriorly on this socket. An elastic band from the bottom of the socket attaches to the anterior skin piece. When the leg swings forward, this elastic band tightens, extending the knee and preventing excessive hip flexion. As the patient walks over the prosthesis, the hip and knee are stable. When the push-off phase of walking is reached, the posterior aspect of the thigh piece contacts a rubber bumper on the socket, preventing hyperextension. This bumper is compressed, starting the forward swing of the leg again. Since the elastic band controlling knee-joint extension is relaxed in this position, the knee automatically flexes, allowing the toe to clear the floor. The inertia of the forward swinging leg then extends the knee before heel contact. The gait is smooth and little effort is required to swing the prosthesis. Instead of lifting the pelvis and rotating it violently forward to swing the leg, the patient simply tilts the pelvis backward. The bumper on the socket contacts the thigh piece and the leg swings forward more nearly simulating the normal gait (Fig. 95).

AMPUTATIONS OF THE UPPER EXTREMITY

Amputation of the upper extremity is usually necessitated by trauma, occasionally by malignant lesions and, rarely, by peripheral vascular disease. The upper extremity consists of an end organ, the hand, moved about by a system of jointed levers: the forearm, arm and shoulder.

As the levers and joints of the upper extremity are lost at higher levels, the problem of activating and placing the terminal device in positions for function are increased. Lever arms must be incorporated in the prosthesis and joints must be provided which the amputee can control. It is apparent that higher amputations compound the problems of terminal device function. The terminal device must be secured to the remaining parts of the arm by a socket suspended by a harness. The harness, usually placed about the shoulders, is used to activate the hook or hand by appropriate cables. Depending upon the function needed, the cable may be pulled taut by arm or shoulder-girdle movements. For example, the hook in the below-elbow prosthesis may be opened by arm flexion at the shoulder. When the amputation is above the elbow, the mechanical elbow joint is controlled by a second cable attached to the shoulder harness. By shrugging the shoulder up and down, this cable may flex or extend the elbow or lock or unlock it in the desired position. Another cable is then used to open or close the terminal device by arm or shoulder motion. Many harnesses have been devised and the successful use of an upper extremity prosthesis depends upon a proper harness. The harness must be comfortable and transmit forces to the prosthesis efficiently through the appropriate cables (Fig. 96).

AMPUTATION OF HAND. The primary functions of the hand are sensory perception and prehension. Use of the hands to express and transmit feelings of emotion is a secondary function. The organ is a complex miracle of mechanical perfection. Loss of sensation, movement or parts of the hand always produces disability. Loss of the entire hand is catastrophic, as there is no adequate substitute. Every effort must be made to preserve any functional part of the hand. Amputation of the entire hand is reserved for irreparable lesions.

When the hand is lost, many of its functions cannot be replaced by any prosthetic device. The primary loss which cannot be replaced is sensory perception. Knowing this, the surgeon must attempt to replace prehension as efficiently as possible. This function is provided by a terminal device, usually a split hook or hand. Six basic types of prehension are defined by Schlesinger. These are cylindrical, spherical, hook, tip, palmar and lateral grasp. Cylindrical grasp is used in holding the handle of a shovel. Spherical grasp is used to

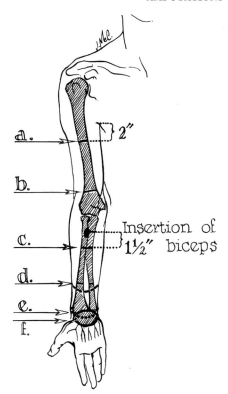

Figure 96. Amputation levels through the upper extremity are illustrated. (a) It is possible to fit a stump as short as 2.5 inches below the axillary fold with an above-elbow prosthesis. (b) Supracondylar amputation provides an adequate lever for control of the prosthesis. Above this level, all length possible should be saved. (c) Amputation through the site of election in the forearm is in the lower one-third of the forearm. (d) Above this level, all length possible must be saved, although amputation as short as 1.5 inches below the biceps insertion can be fitted with a forearm prosthesis. Disarticulation through the elbow joint helps prevent rotary displacement of the socket. (e) Disarticulation of the wrist through the radiocarpal joint produces an excellent stump, and preserves maximum pronation and supination. (f) Above this level, transcarpal disarticulation may occasionally be useful.

hold a large ball. Hook grasp is used in carrying a suitcase. Tip grasp is used in holding and threading a needle. Palmar grasp is used in holding a pen or pencil. Lateral grasp opposes the thumb against the side of the index finger, as in tearing a page from a magazine.

Coupled with these basic types of prehension is the ability to vary the pressure applied and the rapidity of opening and closing. For example, the force required to hold and swing a golf club is entirely different from that used in holding a paper cup. The carrying of a suitcase requires only stationary hook grasp, while sorting small items requires rapid opening and closing motions.

In attempting to substitute these motions, voluntary opening or voluntary closing terminal devices are used. By using the remaining levers of the upper extremity to activate the device, the patient may elect to use a device which he can close voluntarily, regulating to a degree the pressure applied. He may find it better in particular functions to be able to open the device voluntarily, while closing is performed by a spring mechanism which exerts uniform pressure.

The cosmetic hand with less function but a more natural appearance than the split hook may be desirable in certain conditions.

The type of terminal device must be adapted to the age, coordination and functional demands of each patient. The selection of this important replacement part needs thoughtful study by the patient, doctor and prosthetist.

AMPUTATION THROUGH THE WRIST. When the major portion of the hand must be amputated, the surgeon must determine the site for amputation, dependent upon available skin coverage and maximum function which can be obtained from the stump. When adequate palmar skin is present, all or part of the carpal bones may be retained. This amputation demands a long palmar flap and a short dorsal one to ensure a proper, tough cover over the carpal bones. The hand may be disarticulated at the metacarpocarpal joints or through the carpus. The flexor and extensor tendons of the fingers are resected and allowed to retract. The flexor and extensor tendons of the carpal bones must be retained or reattached if function is to be preserved. The nerves and blood vessels are treated as in all amputations. After closure, the scar is dorsal and the end of the stump is covered by tough palmar skin. Carpal bones allow some flexion and extension of the distal stump, and this may be useful when a prosthesis is not used. Pronation and supination of the forearm are preserved. When the stump has good cover, it may be fitted with a terminal device attached to a forearm plastic socket. The terminal device is activated by a cable attached to a shoulder harness.

WRIST DISARTICULATION. Although amputation through the carpal bones has occasionally been possible, it is not often that this is practical. Disarticulation at the radiocarpal joint is the much more common site for total hand amputation. For many years, this site was thought unfavorable because of poor stump coverage, circulatory failure, breakdown of skin and difficulty in fitting a prosthesis. Since World War II, improved surgical technique and prosthetic development have made this area of amputation desirable. When the stump can be covered by good palmar skin, the amputation has many advantages. When the end of the stump cannot be covered adequately, the amputation is useless.

A long palmar flap is fashioned, beginning at the snuffbox area of the wrist and ending $1/2$ inch below the ulnar styloid process. The dorsal flap is shorter, ending at the same point. The flexor and extensor tendons are sectioned and allowed to retract. The carpus is disarticulated at the radiocarpal joint. The triangular cartilage connecting the articular surface of the radius and ulna is preserved to maintain the integrity of the radioulnar joint. The nerves are pulled down and sectioned, including the fine branches of the radial nerve on the dorsum of the wrist. The vessels are ligated. The radial and ulnar styloid processes are removed to round out the bony configuration. The subcutaneous tissue and skin are closed. The resulting scar is slightly dorsal. Full pronation and supination is preserved by this amputation, and the forearm lever is strong. A simple short socket of laminated plastic encases the stump. Because of the flaring end of the radius, the fit is usually secure and about two-thirds of the available pronation and supination is transmitted to the terminal device. When necessary, flexible hinges may be attached to a cuff about the arm above the elbow. The cable activating the terminal device is attached to a shoulder harness.

FOREARM AMPUTATION. If the wrist disarticulation cannot be done, the site of election in the forearm is the junction of the lower and middle one-third of the elbow. This level of amputation creates an adequate lever and preserves about two-thirds of the available pronation and supination. The stump is long enough to fit the socket securely without interference of flexion at the elbow by the socket. From this level upward, amputation may be done to within $1/2$ inches of the insertion of the biceps tendon. As the stump becomes shorter, leverage and pronation and supination are lost progressively. The socket for the short prosthesis may interfere with flexion by impinging against the biceps tendon. All length must be preserved above the site of election compatible with good amputation technique.

Anterior and posterior skin flaps of equal length are made. The deep fascia is incised in a similar manner and reflected upward from the muscles. The muscles are sectioned by a circular incision about $1/2$ inch below the intended level of bone resection. After the radius and ulna have been sectioned transversely, the ends of the bone are tapered to reduce the sharp bony prominence medial and laterally. The nerves and blood vessels are treated in the usual way. The deep fascia is closed over the bone ends and the skin is sutured. A terminal scar is formed. A terminal device with an adjustable wrist fixture is fitted to the plastic forearm socket. The socket is attached to a cuff about the arm above the elbow by metal elbow hinges to hold the stump in place. Attempts have been made to supply active pronation and supination by fitting the socket inside a cylindrical forearm piece which attaches to the elbow hinges and cuff. The socket is attached to the terminal device by a housing which allows the socket to rotate inside of the cylinder forearm piece; thus, capacity for pronation and supination is transmitted to the terminal device. The strength of the prosthesis may be reduced by the procedure, and the prosthesis may be subject to mechanical failure. If this type of prosthesis is impractical, a coupling is placed at the terminal device, which may allow the patient to predetermine the angle at which the hook operates.

SHORT BELOW-ELBOW AMPUTATION. When most of the forearm must be sacrificed, the elbow joint should be saved if possible. However, the most proximal useful stump measures $1/2$ inches below the insertion of the biceps tendon. The amputation is performed like the amputation in the lower one-third of the forearm. The biceps tendon, however, is freed from its attachments to increase the relative length of the stump. The prosthesis for this stump must be short to allow elbow flexion, yet long enough to hold the stump securely. This may be accomplished with a special prosthesis. A socket is fitted to the stump, and, in turn, this small socket is attached to a forearm piece by a gear mechanism incorporated in the elbow hinges. When the stump moves one degree, the forearm piece moves two degrees. Thus, it is possible to flex the forearm piece fully while flexing the stump half this distance. Power is lost, however, by this gear mechanism, and it may be necessary to reinforce this by a cable from the shoulder harness.

ELBOW DISARTICULATION. When the forearm is disarticulated at the elbow or the amputation occurs at a higher level, a mechanical elbow joint is required to place the forearm and terminal device in useful positions. This device must allow free voluntary flexion and extension activated by the shoulder harness. It should also provide positive locking in multiple degrees of flexion for stability.

For many years, the amputation through the elbow joint produced a stump too long to fit the standard elbow-joint mechanisms. In recent years, external locking elbow joints have become available, making the amputation practical.

An advantage to elbow-joint disarticulation is that the flaring humeral condyles provide some rotational stability for the above-elbow socket. A disadvantage is the problem of adequate skin coverage and padding of bony prominences. Flaps are made of equal length when skin is available, but may be fashioned in any way which will allow proper cover. Ideally, the posterior flap begins at the epicondyles and curves to one inch below the tip of the olecranon. The anterior flap curves to one inch below the biceps insertion. The biceps and brachialis tendons are sectioned at their respective insertions. The forearm flexors are sectioned at the medial epicondyle. The brachial artery is ligated, and the median and ulnar nerves are pulled down and severed. The forearm extensors are sectioned about two inches below the lateral epicondyle along with the radial nerve. The capsule is incised and the elbow disarticulated. The triceps tendon is detached from the olecranon process.

The triceps tendon is sutured to the biceps and brachialis muscles over the joint surface. The lateral extensor muscle stump is trimmed to form a thin pad when it is drawn across the front of the joint and sutured to the medial epicondyle. The skin flaps are then closed.

SUPRACONDYLAR AMPUTATION. Although amputation may be done through the condyles of the humerus, the most frequent site is about 2 or 2½ inches above the joint line. Equal skin flaps are made. The triceps tendon is sectioned as low as possible. The flexor muscles are incised about ¾ of an inch below the level of the bone section. The nerves and blood vessels are treated as in other amputations. The wound is closed by suturing the triceps tendon over the end of the bone to the fascia

of the biceps muscle. The skin flaps are closed with interrupted sutures.

SHORT-ARM STUMPS. Amputation may be carried out to within 2½ inches of the anterior axillary fold. Above this level, the conventional above-elbow socket will not retain the stump; a shoulder cap must be used, which limits effective arm motion.

As much length as possible should be preserved in amputations above the supracondylar level. The technique is similar to amputations lower in the arm. The triceps muscle is tapered from front to back to provide a thin musculofascial cover for the bone.

The prosthesis for arm amputations contains the usual forearm and terminal device but provides a mechanical elbow attached to the socket. Many joints have been designed. Essentially, these joints allow full flexion and extension but no pronation or supination. Flexion is controlled by a cable attached to the shoulder harness. Extension is usually activated by gravity. A positive locking mechanism is provided, either by a shoulder cable or locking lever. The elbow must be locked to permit the cable to act on the terminal device.

Shoulder joint disarticulation should be avoided whenever possible. The head of the humerus helps to round out the shoulder and reduces the bony prominence of the acromion process. Amputations which must be done above 2½ inches distal to the axillary fold are fitted with a prosthesis suspended from a plastic shoulder caplike socket. Arm motion at the shoulder is lost, and use of the prosthesis is limited. However, elbow flexion and extension is possible by shoulder motion, as is activation of the terminal device. Scapulothoracic motion may also help position the terminal device.

Stump socks of wool are used by most amputees, except those using the suction socket. The sock absorbs perspiration, lessens friction between the stump and prosthesis and provides a cushion. The sock must fit the stump without wrinkles and must not constrict the circulation.

Careful hygiene of the stump must be followed to prevent skin problems. Stump socks must be washed frequently. The stump should be washed with an antimicrobial soap daily and thoroughly dried. Any skin lesions or abrasion must be treated promptly.

Infections of the Bones and Joints

Infection of bone consists of two major types: hematogenous and exogenous. Hematogenous osteomyelitis is produced by bacteria carried to the bone by the blood stream. Exogenous osteomyelitis is produced by direct contamination of the bone through a wound. The courses of the two types of infection are different, as are the prognosis and treatment.

Since the introduction of chemotherapy and antibiotic drugs, the course and prognosis of bone and joint infections has changed. Before these therapeutic tools were available, bone infection was a serious malignant disease; crippling and death were commonplace. Today, the prognosis is brighter; crippling is less frequent and death occurs infrequently. However, to maintain this present prognosis, the surgeon must be alert to prevent infection when he can, diagnose it promptly, and treat bone infection intelligently when it occurs.

Hematogenous osteomyelitis is primarily a disease of infancy and childhood; it is rare in the adult, while exogenous osteomyelitis may occur at any age. The anatomy and blood supply of the growing skeleton accounts for the difference in age distribution of the disease.

ANATOMY OF BONE. Growing long bones are made up of an epiphysis, epiphysial plate, metaphysis and diaphysis. The epiphysis is separated from the metaphysis by the cartilaginous, avascular epiphysial plate, from which the diaphysis grows in length. The epiphysis and metaphysis are made up of spongy cancellous bone surrounded by a thin layer of cortex. In the infant the metaphysial cortex is very thin and fragile. As the child grows, this cortical layer thickens and becomes stronger. The diaphysis is primarily thick cortical bone.

The blood supply to the epiphysis and metaphysis is separate and distinct. Three major vascular systems supply the growing bone. The first is composed of nutrient arteries entering the diaphysis. These blood vessels enter the shaft of the bone, divide and progress upward and downward to supply the metaphysis and diaphysis. In the metaphysis, the arteries become arterioles and finally, capillary loops adjacent to the epiphysial plate. At the capillary loop, the blood flow is slowed to nourish the developing bone produced by the epiphysial plate. The blood from these capillary loops is collected in venous sinuses which empty into the veins of the medullary canal.

A second set of blood vessels enters the bone through the periosteum by the haversian canal system. These vessels anastomose with the intramedullary vascular system through very fine blood vessels penetrating the cortex of the bone.

A third set of blood vessels nourishes the epiphysis. These blood vessels are carried about the capsular reflections of the joint and are independent from the metaphysial vessels. They enter the epiphysis, form a network of fine capillaries adjacent to the growing cartilage which surrounds the epiphysis, and emerge through venous sinuses and veins at the margins of the joint. A tough, heavy layer of periosteum surrounds the diaphysis and metaphysis. The periosteum is firmly attached at the epiphysial plate, but may extend onto certain parts of the epiphysis. The attachment of the periosteum to the diaphysis and metaphysis is less firm than at the epiphysial plate.

In the adult, when bone growth has ceased, these anatomic entities are blended into a single unit. The blood supply becomes confluent at the epiphysis and metaphysis as the epiphysial plate turns to bone. The capillary loops are eliminated, the blood supply to the bone diminishes, the cortex of the metaphysis and epiphysis thickens, and the periosteum of the metaphysis thins and blends with that of the epiphysis. These changes account for the different types of bone infection in infancy, childhood and adult life.

OSTEOMYELITIS

PATHOLOGY OF ACUTE HEMATOGENOUS OS-TEOMYELITIS. Hematogenous osteomyelitis is produced when bacteria carried by the blood stream lodge and grow in bone. The bacteria which circulate in the blood arise from active foci of infection in other parts of the body. These foci may be produced by many types of bacteria and any system of the body may be involved. Furuncles, infected tonsils, and bowel and urinary tract infections may produce bacteremia. Exanthematous lesions, such as scarlet fever, may also liberate bacteria into the blood stream.

When bacteria enter the blood stream, they are carried by the current of arterial blood to all parts of the body. As the flow of blood slows in the capillary beds, the bacteria settle into the tissues as sediment in a stream settles to the bottom in the quiet areas of a river. Undisturbed, these bacteria grow, establish a new colony and proceed to destroy the surrounding tissue.

The anatomy of the growing bone provides ideal conditions for this chain of events. A large volume of slowly flowing blood is present in the capillary loops and venous sinuses of the metaphysis, and in the quiet area of blood flow bacteria can settle and grow. For this reason, osteomyelitis of the metaphysis is most common in infants and children, in whom this particular anatomic condition occurs.

When bacteria begin to grow, they feed upon the surrounding tissues. In this process, tissue is destroyed. The products of this metabolism, coupled with the inflammatory reaction of the body, produces an abscess or cellulitis. Enzymes and chemicals formed in this process influence the pathologic and clinical course of the disease. Some bacteria are easily killed by the body defenses; others are resistant and proceed to multiply under the most adverse conditions. Some bacteria produce toxic substances which affect the whole body; others produce lytic materials which dissolve and destroy tissue locally. As infection becomes established, a general systemic reaction follows. The temperature is elevated, the white blood cells multiply and the sedimentation rate rises. There may be chills, malaise and nausea and vomiting. The patient may become rapidly dehydrated.

A local reaction in the bone also takes place. As the products of bacterial growth and tissue destruction accumulate, the body attempts to isolate the process by building a wall of inflammatory cells. As this occurs, pressure is built up within the bone and pain becomes present in the area. Localization of the pain near a bone end is an important sign in the early recognition of the disease.

When pressure builds up in the unyielding bone, the blood supply to the area is strangled. The blood in the capillary loops and venous sinuses clots, and eventually the arterioles are thrombosed. Bone, thus deprived of its blood supply, dies. This dead bone is called a sequestrum. The size of the sequestrum varies, depending upon the degree of vascular damage. It may be a small area in the metaphysis or the entire shaft of the bone may be affected.

If the infection is controlled by the body, an abscess is formed, containing dead bone and bacteria. The repair process starts with the growth of new blood vessels into the area. The debris is absorbed and capillaries invade the dead bone. Osteoclasts remove the devitalized bone and osteoblasts lay down new bone. However, if the body defenses are inadequate, the destructive process continues. Pus formed in the abscess under pressure ruptures through the cortex, elevating the periosteum from the bone. For a time, the tough periosteum contains the inflammatory secretions and bacteria; however, bacteria may invade the bone through the haversian canals of the diaphysis as the periosteum is progressively stripped from the bone. New foci of infection are thus created and the entire shaft of the bone may become infected. Eventually, the periosteum ruptures, liberating pus into the soft tissues. In the infant, the cortex of the metaphysis is fragile and the periosteum is less firmly attached to the epiphysial plate. When rupture of the abscess occurs, the infection may spread into the joint. Rapid destruction of the joint and epiphysial plate follows. In older children, this is less likely to occur, because the metaphysial cortex is thicker and the periosteum more firmly attached to the epiphysial plate. The infected material usually burrows through fascial planes to the skin. The skin eventually breaks down, allowing discharge of the pus on the surface of the extremity. A sinus tract is thus formed.

Although the periosteum is stripped from the bone, the periosteum remains viable. New bone is formed by the periosteum surrounding the dead bone of the metaphysis and diaphysis. This new bone surrounding the sequestrum is called involucrum.

Small pieces of sequestrum may be discharged through the sinus tract; however, larger pieces of dead bone are trapped and held by the involucrum. Bacteria continue to grow in this focus of dead bone, slowly destroying the sequestrum. At this stage, osteomyelitis becomes chronic. Infection with discharge of pus through the sinus tract may continue for many years. Pathologic fractures may occur in areas of weakened bone. Periodically, new abscesses in the bone may cause intermittent acute attacks of osteomyelitis during this phase. Bacteremia may arise from the continued infection and produce abscesses in other bones or organs.

Pathology of hematogenous osteomyelitis in the adult. In the adult, hematogenous osteomyelitis is not common. When it occurs, the infection is usually less fulminating than in the child. Since the anatomy of the mature bone is different from that of the growing bone, the infection may arise in any part of the bone. The abscess is often walled off early in the course of the infection and contained usually within a small area of cancellous bone. This abscess may, in time, become sterile, but continues to produce pain by pressure and inflammatory reaction. This type of abscess in bone of the adult is often called Brodie's abscess.

PATHOLOGY OF EXOGENOUS OSTEOMYELITIS. Exogenous osteomyelitis most often occurs following open fractures. The infecting organisms are introduced into the soft tissues and bone through the wound. If an abscess forms, the bone fragments may become devitalized, forming sequestra. Since the tract of the original wound offers a path for exit of secretions, a sinus usually forms in the wound. If drainage is insufficient, bone and soft tissue destruction continues and a systemic reaction may occur. Spread of the infection is by direct continuity, and is usually confined to the devitalized bone ends. Intact bone and periosteum of the adult has great resistance to infection, and, even though exposed, may not become infected. However, when the bone breaks, this resistance is lost at the damaged bone ends. The bone infection is thus usually confined to this area. When internal fixation devices have been used, the infection may spread about these foreign materials; however, the infection is usually not as extensive as in hematogenous osteomyelitis.

ORGANISMS PRODUCING OSTEOMYELITIS. The organism most commonly involved in producing hematogenous osteomyelitis is *Staphylococcus aureus*. Next in frequency is *Staphylococcus albus* or hemolytic streptococci; however, any organism may invade the bone. The clinical course of the infection depends upon the invasiveness and toxigenic characteristics of the invading organisms. Staphylococci and streptococci may produce severe systemic toxic reactions as well as rapid local destruction of bone, while tuberculosis may produce little systemic reaction and slower, more quiet destruction of tissues.

DIAGNOSIS OF ACUTE HEMATOGENOUS OSTEOMYELITIS. Acute hematogenous osteomyelitis presents varying symptoms and physical findings in the infant, child and adult. All exhibit some evidence of general systemic reactions. Fever and chills with nausea and vomiting may be the first signs of infection in the infant and child. In the adult, the systemic reaction may be mild. The white blood cell count is elevated.

Local manifestations of infection are different in each group early in the course of the disease. In the infant, the infection is often fulminating. Pseudoparalysis of the part develops rapidly. The joints adjacent to the infection are usually held in flexion. The infant is irritable and cries out when the part is moved. Local pressure applied along the course of the bone may produce evidence of discomfort. With these findings, accompanied by the systemic reaction, osteomyelitis must be suspected, and treatment started promptly if serious destruction of the bone is to be avoided.

X-ray films of the part are usually normal in the infant for the first three or four days. If the disease is untreated until the bone shows destructive change and periosteal reaction on x-ray examination, the damage has already been done.

The thin cortex of the metaphysis and the loose periosteal attachment allows rupture of the abscess into the adjacent joint within the first few days of infection. The joint and epiphysial plate are rapidly destroyed and growth disturbance of the bone is inevitable. Permanent disability is always expected when this occurs.

The child one year of age and older usually can help localize the process in the bone. Swelling and local heat may be absent at the onset of the infection; however, tenderness about the bone involved is usually present. Tapping the superficial bone with the examining finger helps to localize the area of maximum tenderness. In deeper bones, pressure may still elicit local tenderness near the bone ends. As the disease progresses, swelling and local heat develop. The adjacent joint may develop an effusion. The joint is usually held in flexion. Although some active and passive motion remains in the joint, the patient may resist attempts to move the part. Muscle spasm may further limit motion. X-ray examination is usually normal for the first week or ten days.

The adult usually presents milder, ill-defined symptoms. He may complain of aching pain in the involved area of infection. Swelling may develop slowly. Any part of the bone may be infected. Effusion and limitation of motion of the adjacent joints are often absent.

TREATMENT OF ACUTE HEMATOGENOUS OSTEOMYELITIS. To be effective, treatment must be instituted early. Blood cultures should be made promptly in an attempt to identify the infecting organism. Any focus of infection in the skin, nose and throat, or other areas should be cultured and sensitivity tests made. X-ray films of the suspected part should be made for comparison with those which should be made later.

Antibiotic or chemotherapy should be started immediately. Formerly, penicillin was the antibiotic of choice; however, many staphylococci and streptococci have become resistant to this drug. The tetracycline antibiotics may be given promptly in large doses at least 75 to 100 mg. per kilogram of body weight.

These broad-spectrum antibiotics may be used until the organism is identified and sensitivity tests indicate a more specific antibiotic. Intravenous fluids and blood may be necessary to maintain hydration and combat anemia. Electrolyte balance must be watched carefully, particularly if the patient is vomiting.

The involved part may be put at rest with a posterior plaster molded splint to immobilize the adjacent joint.

If the infection is controlled early, there may be minimal tissue destruction, and the bone may recover promptly. Antibiotic therapy should continue for three to four weeks after the temperature is normal to ensure sterilization of the bone.

X-ray examination of the bone ten to 14 days after the onset of symptoms may show a destroyed area of bone in the metaphysis. The periosteum may be stimulated to produce new bone if it has been separated from the bone. This new bone may be seen on the x-ray film.

If the blood supply to the bone has been damaged, a sequestrum may form even though the infection has been controlled. The x-ray examinations over a period of time will then show the changes associated with the repair process. An involucrum forms about the sequestrum. The sequestrum is slowly absorbed and new bone is produced to replace the dead bone.

Occasionally, an abscess in the bone may rupture into the soft tissues while the antibiotic therapy finally controls the infection.

This soft tissue abscess may be sterile. Aspiration and culture of the abscess may reveal that the infection is controlled. Aspiration removes the debris of infection and allows the repair process to proceed more rapidly. This should be done in most instances if the soft tissue sterile abscess is a large one.

Surgical drainage of such an area is usually not necessary if the surgeon is sure that the abscess is sterile. Open drainage in this circumstance permits entrance of new bacteria with the danger of secondary infection. When the infection is not completely controlled, or bone destruction is excessive, surgical treatment may be mandatory. Decompression of the bone and soft tissues may be necessary to prevent continued destruction. Dead bone which harbors bacteria must be removed to allow healing of draining sinuses.

If an abscess forms and the infection remains active in spite of adequate antibiotic therapy, surgical decompression of the infection is demanded. Incision and drainage of the bone is performed by removing a window of cortical bone over the infected metaphysis. The wound is packed open with petrolatum gauze and the part is immobilized in an appropriate plaster cast. The defect is allowed to close by granulation tissue growing from the depths of the wound. When a major part of the bone is sequestrated, removal of this dead bone may disrupt the continuity of the skeleton. It is necessary to wait until an adequate involucrum has formed before this is done. Drainage is established to prevent added destruction; then the surgeon waits until enough new bone has formed to support the part before the sequestrum is removed. This may take several months. When adequate new bone is formed, the sequestrum is removed and the cavity in the bone opened completely. This operation is termed saucerization because the bone cavity is made as shallow and broad as possible by the surgeon. This is done to eliminate overhanging edges and pockets in the bone which might harbor growing bacteria. The wound may be packed open until it is evident that the infection has been controlled; then the cavity is closed with split-thickness skin grafts applied to the granulating bone. Occasionally, it may be possible to remove the dead bone and close the soft tissues immediately. This procedure can be done when infection is inactive and the cavity can be filled with soft tissue to eliminate dead space. Muscle and fat may be used to fill the bone cavity. If the cavity in the bone cannot be filled with soft tissue, the wound must be left open and closed later to prevent growth of bacteria in this cavity.

TREATMENT OF EXOGENOUS OSTEOMYELITIS. Exogenous osteomyelitis can be prevented by adequate care of open fractures and wounds involving the bone. The proper debridement and cleansing of open fractures is essential to prevent infection. When the wound has been invaded by bacteria because of delayed debridement, the area must be packed open to prevent accumulation of the products of infection. Adequate drainage prevents destruction of bone and soft tissue if infection occurs.

When an open fracture is closed and infection develops, it must be opened promptly to establish drainage. Antibiotic therapy must be instituted. Rest for the part is essential. Appropriate splinting must be continued. When the infection is controlled, dead bone and foreign material must be removed to allow healing of the wound. The wound is usually packed open after sequestrectomy and closed secondarily when the infection is eliminated.

SEPTIC ARTHRITIS

Septic arthritis, or pyogenic infection of a joint, occurs when bacteria invade the joint and grow. The bacteria may reach the joint by the blood stream by extension from the surrounding tissue, or by direct implantation through a wound into the joint.

The most common bacteria causing the infection are the various staphylococci and streptococci; however, any organism may produce joint infection. The condition occurs most frequently in infants and children.

The blood supply to the growing joint is independent of the circulation to the shaft of the bone. The epiphysis and metaphysis, separated by the epiphysial plate, further isolate the joint and shaft of the bone. Blood vessels enter joints through the capsular attachments about the margins of the joint. These vessels divide, some entering the epiphysis while others form a fine capillary network throughout the synovial membrane. In this capillary bed, bacteria may be trapped. If the local defenses of the body are inadequate, infection occurs.

When the bacteria are introduced into the joint by direct penetration, or by extension from osteomyelitis, the bacteria begin to grow on the surface of the synovial membrane. The synovial membrane becomes thickened and an inflammatory reaction stimulates the synovial membrane to form more joint fluid and an effusion develops. The leukocyte content of the joint fluid increases markedly in response to the infection.

As bacteria begin to invade and destroy the tissue of the joint, proteolytic enzymes are liberated which dissolve the cartilage of the articular surface. This dissolution of cartilage is most marked where the articular surfaces are in contact.

Pressure within the joint rapidly increases. Heat, redness and swelling of the joint become obvious. A generalized systemic reaction accompanies the joint reaction. Pain is severe. Any motion of the part is resisted, and even shaking the bed may be extremely painful. Muscle spasm holds the joint flexed. If the condition is treated promptly, the damage to the joint may be minimal. However, if unrecognized or inadequately treated, the joint will be destroyed. The cartilage of the articular surfaces is rapidly dissolved, exposing the underlying bone which, in turn, is infected and destroyed. If the process continues, the distended joint capsule may rupture, discharging the abscess into the surrounding tissues. Sinus tracts may form and communicate with the joint.

Since hyaline cartilage cannot regenerate, it is replaced by scar tissue or fibrocartilage. Dependent upon the degree of cartilage destruction, the joint surfaces are damaged in variable amounts. Minimal surface damage may produce no permanent loss of joint function. However, when the deeper layers are involved, some permanent roughness of joint surfaces is inevitable with some loss of joint function. When bone is exposed, scar tissue forms across the joint surfaces. This scar tissue may produce a fibrous ankylosis of the joint, limiting motion and function. The scar may eventually become bone, completely ankylosing the joint. All of these changes occur rapidly in the joint, demanding prompt diagnosis and treatment if the joint is to be preserved.

Broad-spectrum antibiotics must be started at once. The joint is aspirated and the material sent to the laboratory for culture and sensitivity tests. Microscopic examination of the joint fluid shows a tremendous number of leukocytes. Bacteria may be found in the joint fluid and this may help to establish the type of infection. Treatment cannot wait, however, while the organism is identified by culture.

The part should be splinted to prevent all joint motion. If the aspirated fluid is cloudy but still resembles synovial fluid, the infection may subside with splinting, repeated aspiration and massive doses of broad-spectrum antibiotics. If the aspirated material is thick pus, the joint should be opened surgically and the pus evacuated. The joint is then irrigated with normal saline solution to remove mechanically the debris of infection. The synovial membrane is closed loosely with interrupted plain catgut sutures, and the wound is packed open. Loose closure of the synovium allows drainage but prevents exposure of the cartilage to the outside environment. This surgical drainage removes the proteolytic enzymes so damaging to cartilage. Reduction of intra-articular pressure restores circulation to the synovial membrane and allows the antibiotics to enter the joint more effectively.

When the organism has been isolated, sensitivity tests may indicate that a specific antibiotic drug may be more effective. This drug should then be used. As in osteomyelitis, drug therapy should continue for three or four weeks after the temperature returns to normal. During the active phase of treatment, the joint should be splinted in the position which will allow maximum function, should ankylosis or loss of joint motion occur. When the temperature has returned to normal and the drainage has stopped, gentle active and passive joint motion may be started. If there is any evidence of reactivation of the infection, splinting of the part must be reinstituted and the joint maintained at rest. Use of the part should be restricted for weeks until the tissues return to as nearly normal as possible.

TUBERCULOSIS OF THE BONES AND JOINTS

Tuberculosis of the bones and joints, an extremely destructive disease, has decreased in frequency in the United States in recent years. The pasteurization of milk, better living conditions and early diagnosis of pulmonary tuberculosis, along with the development of specific drug therapy, have all contributed to this decline in this joint disease. This once common problem has now become rare as a cause of joint infection.

Tuberculosis affects primarily the epiphyses and joints rather than the metaphyses.

The infection differs from pyogenic infection. While pyogenic infection stimulates a walling-off process, tuberculous infection is primarily destructive with little defense reaction in the surrounding tissues. The infection is secondary to a primary focus elsewhere in the body. This primary infection may be in the lung, bowel, lymph glands or other organs. The tubercle bacilli are carried to the joint or epiphysis by the arterial circulation. The bacilli lodge in the end arteries of the epiphysis, or in the synovial blood vessels. Tuberculous abscesses are formed in the bone or synovial membrane. The local reaction to the infection is limited. The course of the disease is usually quite destructive of the involved parts. The process is primarily a lytic one, and new bone is rarely formed.

When the infection becomes established in the epiphysis, bone is destroyed until the abscess communicates with the joint. Discharge of this material into the joint produces synovial infection. The infection may start in the synovial membrane and spread to the bone of the epiphysis by direct erosion and pannus formation. Either method of infection eventually destroys the joint if treatment is delayed or is inadequate.

Frequently, tuberculous pus ruptures through the joint capsule and forms soft tissue abscesses. The pus dissects through fascial planes and the abscess may appear some distance from the infected bone or joint. If the tuberculous infection is controlled by the body, these distant abscesses may become isolated from the original focus of infection. The abscess may calcify slowly and become inactive. If the infection is not controlled, the abscess may, in time, rupture through the skin. A sinus forms and pyogenic bacteria may invade the bone or joint through this tract. This mixed infection adds to the destructive process and complicates treatment.

Although any joint in the body may be infected by the tubercle bacillus, the spine is the most frequent. The joints of the lower extremities are next most frequently infected, while those of the upper extremity the least often involved.

A positive diagnosis of tuberculosis depends upon isolation of the organism from the infected area. Acid-fast staining and microscopic examination may be helpful. The guinea-pig test is the most reliable method for establishing the diagnosis.

TREATMENT. The treatment of bone and joint tuberculosis is both systemic and local.

Infection at the primary site must be controlled, as well as that of the joint. Prior to the introduction of the combined drug therapy of streptomycin, para-aminosalicylic acid and isonicotinic acid, there was no specific treatment for tuberculosis. Rest of the part and the patient was the essential method of treatment, plus arthrodesis of the joint. Although rest is still essential, the combined drug therapy controls the infection much more rapidly and completely.

Casts and splints and occasionally traction are used to immobilize the joint. Abscesses are aspirated if they are in danger of rupturing. When the infection is controlled, signified by return of the temperature and sedimentation rate to normal, definitive treatment of the joint may be undertaken. Usually, arthrodesis of the joint is performed. In the spine, this may involve several vertebrae. Although function is limited by this procedure, it is the surest way to prevent recurrence of the infection in the joints. Occasionally, synovectomy has been performed, with debridement of the joint, to salvage some function. However, this excision of the focus of infection cannot always be accomplished completely and reactivation of the infection is a potential hazard. Arthrodesis is still the safest method of treatment. Isolated abscesses are aspirated and, occasionally, they can be completely excised, if they no longer communicate with the original point of infection. Observation of the patient must continue for years to allow prompt treatment of any reactivation of the disease.

Tumors of the Musculoskeletal System

The musculoskeletal system may be affected by tumors arising in any of the component tissues or by metastatic lesions from other organs. Tumors involving the skeleton may occur in primary bone cells or in the hematopoietic elements of bone, in cartilage and in the fibrous and synovial components. Other tumors may arise in muscle, nerve, blood vessels and the fat of the musculoskeletal system. These tumors may be benign or malignant. The surgeon must understand thoroughly these pathologic processes to treat these patients intelligently.

Through the years, numerous classifications of these tumors have evolved as knowledge about them increased. The classification of bone tumors is necessary for a clear understanding of the pathological changes that are possible within the system. The classification devised by Louis Lichtenstein is based upon the origin of the tissue involved, and is the most popular one at present (Table 1).

The accurate diagnosis of these tumors is essential because treatment is primarily a surgical problem. The nature of the tumor determines the extent of the surgical procedure, varying from simple excision to radical amputation.

TUMORS OF CARTILAGE CELL OR CARTILAGE-FORMING CONNECTIVE TISSUE

OSTEOCARTILAGINOUS EXOSTOSIS OR OSTEO-CHONDROMA. The most common type of benign tumor arising from precartilaginous tissue is the single or multiple osteocartilaginous exostosis or osteochondroma.

Because these tumors arise from aberrant foci of cartilage, as precartilage cells on the surface of the bone, they may be regarded as congenital anomalies.

The tumor arises most often on the metaphysial surface of the long bones, but may be found on the flat bones, ribs, vertebrae and small bones of the hands and feet. The tumors are usually found before the age of 20, and affect males and females about equally.

Symptoms are usually minimal. The patient often becomes aware of a painless mass near a joint by accidental palpation. Occasionally, a painful bursa develops over the exostosis when the mass is subjected to pressure by muscle or tendon action or by weight-bearing.

The tumor may be sessile or pedunculated and may vary in size from a small protuberance on the bone to a large, cauliflower-like mass. The mass is composed of a cartilage cap covering an extension of cortex from the parent bone surrounding a center of spongiosa continuous from the spongiosa of the involved bone. The entire tumor is covered by a layer of periosteum. Areas of calcification of the cartilage cap may be evident in the roentgenograms of the tumor.

The microscopic appearance of the tumor is characteristic. The cartilage cap is composed of columns of chondrocytes arranged perpendicular to the underlying cortex. In the growing tumor, a zone of enchondral ossifica-

Table 1. Classification of Primary Tumors of Bone*

	BENIGN TUMORS OF BONE	MALIGNANT COUNTERPART (IF ANY)	MALIGNANT TUMORS OF BONE (ARISING THROUGH MALIGNANT CHANGE OR INDEPENDENTLY)
Of cartilage-cell or cartilage-forming connective tissue derivation — Peripheral	Osteocartilagenous exostosis (multiple exostosis)	Peripheral chondrosarcoma	Chondrosarcoma
Central	Enchondroma (skeletal enchondromatosis)	Central chondrosarcoma	
	Benign chondroblastoma	(Not known)	
	Chondromyxoid fibroma	Mesenchymal chondrosarcoma	
	Poorly differentiated chondroid tumors	Chondroblastic sarcoma	
Of osteoblastic derivation	Osteoma	(Not known)	Osteogenic sarcoma — Central / Parosteal
	Osteoid-osteoma	(Not known)	
	Benign osteoblastoma	(Osteogenic sarcoma)	
Of nonosteoblastic connective tissue derivation	Desmoplastic fibroma	(Not known)	Fibrosarcoma
	Nonosteogenic fibroma	(Not known)	
	Least aggressive giant-cell tumors→	More aggressive and malignant giant-cell tumors→	Frankly malignant giant-cell tumors
Of mesenchymal connective tissue origin	——		Ewing's sarcoma
Of hematopoietic origin	——		Multiple myeloma / Chronic myeloid leukemia / Acute leukemias — Reticulum-cell sarcoma / Malignant lymphoma — "Lymphosarcoma" / Hodgkin's disease
Of nerve origin	Neurofibroma / Neurilemoma / Ganglioneuroma	(Malignant schwannoma)	
Of vascular origin	Hemangioma / Hemangiopericytoma (glomus)	(Hemangioendothelioma)	Hemangioendothelioma
Of fat-cell origin	Lipoma		Liposarcoma
Of notochordal derivation		——	Chordoma
Of adamantine or possibly basal-cell derivation		——	So-called adamantinoma

*From Lichtenstein, L.: Bone Tumors. St. Louis, C. V. Mosby Company, 1965.

tion is present on the surface of the cortex similar to that found in the epiphysis of a growing bone. The spongiosa may contain hematopoietic, fatty or fibrous marrow. Rests of the cartilage cells may be found scattered throughout the tumor. When the involved bone ceases to grow, the tumor becomes quiescent and the cartilage cap may slowly involute.

In about 2 per cent of tumors of the solitary type, malignant transformation may occur, whereas the incidence of this complication may rise to 11 per cent in multiple osteocartilaginous exostosis. Chondrosarcoma is the usual malignant transformation of the benign tumor. Rapid growth or increasing calcification of the cartilage cap may herald the malignant change; thus, roentgenographic records of the benign tumors should be kept. These changes may occur at any time, but are more likely after the age of 30.

Complete excision of the tumor and periosteal covering flush with the surface of the long bones or section of the tumor with its base from the flat bones is the treatment of choice. Because the incidence of malignant transformation is low, routine resection is not indicated unless the tumor is painful, unsightly or interferes with function; however, careful periodic roentgenologic studies should be made of the tumor. Recurrence of the tumor is rare, but should alert the surgeon to the possibility of malignant change or to the possibility of a primary chondrosarcoma.

CHONDROMA (ENCHONDROMA OR ENCHONDROMATOSIS). Chondromas are benign tumors usually found in the interior of the small bones of the hands and feet, although the tumor may arise in the metaphysis of the long bones or the flat bones of the thoracic cage. When they are centrally located, they are called enchondromas. The lesional cell resembles hyaline cartilage. Often areas of calcification or bone formation are found in the interior of the tumor. Usually, the surrounding cortex is thin, and the tumor may expand the bone to form a fusiform swelling. The tumor is usually found between the ages of ten and 50 years, and is often manifested by pathologic fracture through the weakened cortex or by a painless, firm swelling of the bone. There is no predilection for either sex.

The gross appearance of the tumor is usually pearly-white and firm with small, scattered areas of yellow, gritty, calcified cartilage. At times, the tumor is rather soft and granular.

The microscopic findings reveal usually uniform cartilage cells with a single, small nucleus. Areas of degeneration and calcification are found scattered throughout the tumor in varying degrees. Irregular and multinucleated cells may indicate early transformation to a malignant phase; although rare in the small bones, the larger tumors in the long bones occasionally undergo the change.

Treatment is usually curettement of the lesions of the small bones followed by bone-graft replacement. The ribs, sternum and long bones may require resection of the involved bone followed by reconstructive procedures in the long bones.

MULTIPLE ENCHONDROMAS OR ENCHONDROMATOSIS. These may affect multiple bones, causing varying degrees of deformity. When confined to one side of the body, the condition has been called Ollier's disease, and, when associated with multiple hemangiomas of the skin, Maffuci's syndrome. Removal of multiple lesions is usually impossible, and treatment is directed toward correction of deformity created by growth disturbance. Rarely, these tumors may undergo transformation to malignant chondrosarcoma, demanding radical resection or amputation.

BENIGN CHONDROBLASTOMA. Chondroblastoma is usually a small benign tumor derived from chondroblasts, and is usually located in the epiphysis of the long bones, but, with growth, may extend into the metaphysis. The size of the tumor varies from a few millimeters up to 6 or 7 cm. in diameter. Often, it is eccentrically placed in the epiphysis, and may lie just beneath the articular cartilage without destroying it. Radiographically and microscopically, the tumor is often confused with benign giant-cell tumor of bone.

The most common sites for the tumor are the femur and tibia at the knee joint and the upper end of the humerus, although the tumor may arise in any epiphysis.

The tumor is usually found in patients between the ages of ten and 20 years, and is more common in males. The ratio is approximately three male patients to one female.

The symptoms are usually pain and swelling about the adjacent joint, frequently of several months' duration.

The roentgenographic appearance is fairly characteristic. An area of rarefaction is found in the epiphysis, eccentrically located, surrounded by a thin area of sclerotic bone. Trabeculae may traverse the tumor, and flecks of calcified tumor are practically always observed. With growth, the tumor may extend into the metaphysis and produce thinning of the cortex.

Grossly, the tumor is firm and grayish-pink, with areas of hemorrhage and necrosis and areas of gritty calcification.

The microscopic picture is varied, consisting of areas of chondroblasts, which are clear, distinct cells with oval or round nuclei. The nucleus is often indented. Scattered in areas of the tumor are multinucleated giant cells, which are usually smaller and fewer in number than in the typical giant-cell tumor of bone, and occur in areas of hemorrhage. Chondroid material is found in varying amounts, and is a distinctive feature of the tumor. Degeneration of cartilage cells leads to calcification similar to the degenerative change found in cartilage during osseous transformation. These areas may show absorption, hemorrhage and replacement by connective tissue and collagenous plaques.

The treatment is curettage followed by replacement with bone grafts. When the location allows resection without loss of function, this may be done. Local recurrence is rare, and malignant changes have been reported only in two instances in which roentgen therapy was used.

CHONDROMYXOID FIBROMA. Chondromyxoid fibroma is derived from cartilage-forming connective tissue. The tumor is usually found in the metaphysial region, eccentrically located, and is rare compared to the frequency of other bone tumors. The majority of tumors occur in the second and third decades of life, and there is no predilection for either sex. More than half of these tumors have been reported in the tibia, with the lower femur second, although the small bones of the hands and feet, pelvic girdle, ribs and scapula may be affected.

Pain and swelling of the metaphysial area of the bone of several months' duration is the usual complaint of the patient.

Roentgenographically, the appearance of the tumor in the long bones is fairly characteristic. An eccentrically placed, circumscribed, rarefied defect, often involving the cortex, is found in the metaphysis at varying distances from the epiphysis. If the cortex is completely destroyed, a thin shell of periosteal new bone may cover the tumor which does not invade the surrounding soft tissues. A thin zone of sclerotic bone confines the tumor in the medullary portion of the bone. In the small bone, the rarefied area may appear lobulated and expand the cortex.

Grossly, the tumor is firm and distinctly lobulated, and white or yellow-tan in contrast to the bluish-white of chondromas. Microscopic sections of the tumor reveal spindle-shaped cells arranged loosely in a matrix of myxoid, intercellular substance. At the periphery of the tumor lobules, the cells may be more densely packed. As the tumor matures, areas of myxomatous matrix may show collagenization or chondroid formation.

The tumor is apparently completely benign, and cure is usually effected by complete curettage with bone grafting or local resection.

CHONDROSARCOMA OF BONE. Chondrosarcoma may arise centrally in the bone or peripherally from the cartilage cap of osteocartilaginous exostosis. The central lesion may arise from an enchondroma by malignant transformation, or may arise as a primary tumor.

The peripheral chondrosarcomas are usually made up of actively growing, mature hyaline cartilage, whereas the central tumors may show less differentiation.

The long bones are primarily affected—the femur, tibia and humerus particularly; however, the ribs, scapula and innominate bones are frequently the site of this tumor. It is rare for malignant transformation to occur in single enchondromata of the bones of the hands and feet. The condition is much more likely to occur when multiple enchondromata are present.

These tumors have a slight predilection for males—about 60 per cent. The majority of tumors appear between the ages of 30 and 60. This history often reveals that the patient has been aware of a painless swelling of a long bone or the presence of an osteocartilaginous exostosis for a considerable period of time. The patient may have noticed the mass slowly enlarging or becoming mildly painful.

However, the time interval of pain and swelling may be relatively short in rapidly developing central tumors. In general, however, the tumors are slow growing, and do not produce much discomfort. Metastasis occurs late in most chondrosarcomas, but local extension into blood vessels is common. These lesions growing into the larger vessels may grow along the interior of the vessel for great distances from the primary tumor, eventually reaching the heart and lungs by this route. Metastasis to the periphery of the lungs can occur in late stages of the disease or in the highly malignant tumors. Metastatic lesions to the lymph nodes are rare.

Physical examination may indicate the presence of an osteocartilaginous exostosis, or may simply indicate an enlarged long bone. The mass may be mildly tender, but the skin is not red or warm. When the tumor is near a joint, the joint may be swollen with some limitation of motion.

The roentgenologic findings in the central tumors usually show irregular mottling with calcification and fuzzy destruction of the cortex. If the cortex has been perforated by the tumor, the extension of the tumor into the soft parts may produce an abnormal shadow overlying the bone.

Roentgenographs of the peripheral chondrosarcoma show much more blotchy densities than in the benign osteochondromas, and the areas of calcification in the cartilage may extend away from the tumor in irregular, stringy patches.

The histologic appearance of chondrosarcoma may be subtle, but malignancy is indicated when many cells contain plump nuclei, more than an occasional cell contain two such nuclei, and giant cartilage cells with one or more nuclei are found. In the more advanced tumors, frank sarcomatous changes are evident.

Because metastasis generally occurs late in this tumor, wide resection of the lesion or amputation may effect a cure. Central tumors of small size may be resected widely, followed by reconstructive procedures; however, if it appears that complete eradication of the tumor cannot be accomplished by this method, amputation should be performed.

Peripheral chondrosarcoma arising from osteocartilaginous exostosis should be resected widely, including the soft tissue over the tumor, as well as resection of the bone containing the base. Inoperable tumors may be treated with roentgen therapy, but the tumor is radio-resistant, and the results have been disappointing.

TUMORS OF OSTEOBLASTIC DERIVATION

OSTEOID-OSTEOMA. This tumor of bone is composed of a small, oval or round nidus of osteoid tissue and new bone deposited within a bed of highly vascularized, osteogenic connective tissue. The tumor may occur in medullary or cortical bone, and is most often found in the bones of the lower extremities, but may occur in any bone.

For many years, the origin of this lesion was controversial, but it is now regarded by most authorities as a true neoplasm of bone. There is a slight tendency for the tumor to occur more frequently in males. The age distribution is from five to 30 years, with the preponderance of lesions occurring in adolescents or young adults.

Symptoms are primarily pain, most noticeable at night and relieved to a degree by aspirin. Occasionally, slight heat or redness may be noted. Characteristically, the lesion is quite painful to pressure.

The roentgenographic evidence of the tumor is characteristic, but varies with the location of the tumor in cancellous or cortical bone. When the lesion occurs in cancellous bone, an area of rarefaction with a central area of dense bone may be seen, surrounded by a thin zone of sclerosis. When the lesion is in the cortical area, dense sclerosis extends in the cortex for a considerable distance from the nidus. The nidus often lies on the inner aspect of the cortex, and is observed as a rarefied area with or without a dense central area. In cortical bone, laminographs may be necessary to distinguish the nidus in the sclerotic bone. The radiographic appearance may be confused with bone abscess or chronic sclerosing osteomyelitis.

Grossly, when the specimen can be removed intact, the lesion stands out as a reddish, circumscribed area in the bone with surrounding sclerosis and adjacent periosteal reaction. Microscopically, the lesion appears to be a circumscribed area of osteoid with areas of calcification and atypical bone formation within a vascular background of osteoblastic connective tissue.

Surgical removal of the lesion is the only effective treatment. The relief of symptoms is immediate and lasting. If the nidus is incompletely removed, pain recurs and a secondary operation becomes necessary.

BENIGN OSTEOBLASTOMA. This benign tumor, composed of osteoblasts and osteoid tissue in avascular stroma, has been called by various names – osteogenic fibroma and giant osteoid-osteoma. There is some resemblance to osteoid-osteoma; however, the tumor is usually larger, and there is less tendency to form sclerotic bone. The lesion is often expansile, enlarging the bone and thinning the cortex.

The limb bones are most commonly affected in the shaft or metaphysial regions, and the vertebrae and skull may also be affected. Usually, the neural arch of the vertebra is involved rather than the body.

There is no great difference in the incidence of the tumor in male or female. The majority of these lesions occur in teen-agers or children, and the remaining one-third occur in adults.

Symptoms are usually pain in a slowly enlarging bone of months' or several years' duration. When the lesion occurs in the spine, pain and neurologic deficit may be evident as the tumor encroaches on the spinal cord.

The roentgenographic appearance is usually a radiolucent area within an expanded, thin cortex without periosteal new bone formation. There may be a thin wall of sclerosis surrounding the tumor in the medullary portions. Calcification or dense areas of bone may be seen in the interior of the lesion.

Grossly, the tumor appears reddish, is gritty and quite vascular. The microscopic appearance is quite variable, but consists primarily of osteoid and proliferating osteoblasts with calcification of osteoid in patches. The stroma may often consist of highly vascular, fibrocytic tissue. Giant cell macrophages may be found in relation to newly formed, mineralized matrix. The lesions may be confused with giant-cell tumors or osteogenic sarcoma. Because the lesion is benign, care in microscopic interpretation must be exercised to prevent inadvertent radical surgery in the mistaken belief that one is dealing with an osteogenic sarcoma.

Thorough curettement or resection of accessible lesions is the preferred treatment. Decompression of the skull and spinal cord must be done as completely as is necessary to relieve the symptoms. When the tumor cannot be removed completely, roentgen therapy is of value.

OSTEOGENIC SARCOMA. Osteogenic sarcoma apparently arises from primitive bone-forming mesenchyme. Of the malignant tumors of bone, it is second only to myeloma as the most common malignant neoplasm. The tumor is made up of anaplastic connective tissue forming tumor osteoid and bone, but may also form tumor cartilage, which, in turn, ossifies. The tumor may be primarily osteolytic or osteoblastic, depending upon how much tumor bone is formed. These tumors are highly malignant, metastasizing to the lungs by way of the blood early in their development. Five-year survivals after treatment average only about 10 per cent.

The tumor seems to affect males more often than females. The most frequent occurrence of the tumor is between ten and 25 years of age, but it may occur at any age. The older people afflicted with osteogenic sarcoma are most frequently the victims of malignant transformation of Paget's disease, and the incidence of this change may be as high as 10 to 15 per cent.

The most common locations for this tumor are the lower end of the femur, upper tibia and upper end of the humerus, but other bones may be affected as well.

The usual presenting complaint of the patient is pain and enlargement of the affected part. When the tumor is growing rapidly, weight loss, anemia and elevated alkaline phosphatase blood levels may be found. Usually, the patient is aware of trouble for a few weeks to several months before seeking treatment.

Usually, the tumor arises in the interior of the bone, but rapidly destroys the cortex, elevating the periosteum, which may form nontumorous new bone where it is stripped from the shaft. Tumorous bone then forms about the shaft of the bone. Upon perforating the periosteum, the tumor invades the surrounding muscle, or may invade the adjacent joint.

The roentgenographic appearance is not always characteristic, but perforation of the cortex and formation of tumorous bone beneath the periosteum should indicate the possibility of the serious tumor. The degree of sclerosis or osteolysis depends upon the amount of new bone and bone destruction that is taking place.

The gross appearance of the tumor varies with the degree of osteoblastic or osteolytic activity. When the tumor is primarily osteoblastic, the interior of the bone may be very sclerotic; however, if the tumor is actively growing outside the cortex, it may be softer and more vascular. The osteolytic tumors are usually softer and cystic with areas of hemorrhage and necrosis. In the medullary cavity, the tumor may extend for a considerable distance, and may be patchy in distribution, occupying areas of normal bone. Thus, it may be difficult to determine the extent of the tumor roentgenographically.

The histologic appearance varies considerably. The criteria for diagnosis of osteogenic tumor are the presence of a sarcomatous stroma and the direct formation of tumor osteoid and bone. Tumor cartilage undergoing ossification may or may not be present.

When the diagnosis has been confirmed by biopsy, treatment is radical amputation. The level of amputation should be well above the tumor, and should be done between tourniquets placed above the tumor. Hindquarter and forequarter amputation may be necessary for tumors extending into the upper femur and humerus. The value of roentgen therapy or chemotherapy is still not determined.

OSSIFYING PAROSTEAL SARCOMA. This tumor arises on the surface of the bone in contradistinction to osteogenic sarcoma, which arises centrally. The neoplasm apparently arises from slow-growing bone and cartilage-forming periosteal and parosteal connective tissue. The most frequent site of this tumor is the posterior aspect of the femur near the knee joint. Although the tumor is malignant, it is slow growing, but may eventually perforate the cortex and invade the medullary canal. Metastasis to the lung occurs late in the course of the tumor.

Block resection of the tumor is recommended, except when the tumor is recurrent; amputation should then be performed.

TUMORS OF NONOSTEOBLASTIC CONNECTIVE TISSUE

NONOSTEOGENIC FIBROMA OF BONE. This lesion, consisting of spindle-cell connective tissue, has also been called nonossifying fibroma, metaphysial fibrous defect and fibrous cortical defect. It occurs in the shafts of long bones of the extremities, seemingly sparing the other bones of the skeleton. It occurs usually between the ages of ten and 20, but may occasionally be found in younger children. There seems to be no sex predilection.

Symptoms are minimal or may be absent.

The lesion is often found accidentally when roentgenograms are made of an extremity following trauma. Occasionally, pathologic fracture may bring the condition to the attention of the surgeon.

The roentgenographic appearance is characteristic in most instances. The lesion usually appears as a sharply delineated, eccentric, lobulated area of rarefaction, usually involving the cortex. The cortex may bulge outward on the surface, but new bone formation is not evident. The lesion may occupy the entire width of the smaller tubular bones. Calcification in the interior of the lesion is lacking.

Grossly, the tumor is yellow or yellow-brown and of rather rubbery consistency. Microscopically, there are whorls of spindle-shaped connective tissue cells with occasional areas of small, multinucleated giant cells and foam cells.

Surgical excision is elective unless the lesion is painful or likely to cause pathologic fracture. Curettage of the lesion followed by bone grafting is usually all that is necessary to effect a cure.

GIANT-CELL TUMOR OF BONE (OSTEOCLAS- TOMA).   Giant-cell tumors of bone arise from the non-bone-forming, supporting connective tissue of the marrow. They may be benign or malignant. It has been stated that 50 per cent of these tumors recur after excision and 15 to 30 per cent are malignant or undergo malignant transformation. Thus, the tumor must be regarded as a potentially dangerous one.

The tumor typically arises in the epiphysial end of the long bones; the lower femur, upper tibia and lower radius are the most frequent sites in that order. The lesion may arise in any bone, but it is rare in the innominate bone, ribs and skull.

These tumors affect females twice as often as males. The greatest incidence of the tumor is between 15 and 40 years, but the tumor may occur in older patients. It is rare in young children.

The roentgenographic appearance of giant-cell tumors is not always characteristic, but the location of the tumor in the ends of the bone is significant, as these tumors always arise in this location. The lesion produces rarefaction, and is often eccentrically located with thinning and expansion of the cortex withour periosteal new bone formation. Eventually, the cortex may be destroyed.

The gross appearance of the tumor varies with the amount of necrosis, degeneration and hemorrhage within the lesion. Early, the tumor is dark red or reddish-brown. As hemorrhage occurs, patches of bright red or black appear and cystic areas develop. The tumor is destructive of bone, and may perforate through the periosteum, but the cartilage of the articular surface is not destroyed, although it may be distorted by loss of bony support or fracture.

The microscopic appearance of the tumor varies with the amount and degree of hemorrhage and degeneration. In unaffected areas, the tumor is made up of spindle-shaped stromal cells which are moderately vascularized with multinucleated giant cells and collagen fibrils interspersed throughout the tumor cells. In areas of degeneration, osteoid trabeculae and new bone may be found. The more cellular and atypical stromal cell type, the more likely the tumor is to recur or metastasize.

The treatment of choice is total excision of the tumor; however, the size and location of the tumor and the cytologic picture may warrant thorough curettement and replacement by bone grafts. When the tumor appears frankly malignant or has recurred several times, amputation may be the only method of controlling the lesion. The results of roentgen therapy are debatable.

FIBROSARCOMA OF BONE.   Fibrosarcoma of bone is a malignant fibroblastic tumor which does not form osteoid or bone. The tumor is usually less malignant than osteogenic sarcoma, as indicated by a five-year survival rate of 25 per cent. The tumor is less frequently found than osteogenic sarcoma or chondrosarcoma. It is primarily a bone-destructive lesion.

There is no sex predilection, and the age of occurrence is from the second through the sixth decades of life. Thus, the tumor occurs in a much older group of patients than primary osteogenic sarcoma.

The most frequent locations are the interior of the ends of long bones, primarily the femur, tibia and humerus.

There is no characteristic roentgenographic appearance of the lesion, except for bone destruction.

Symptoms are pain or pathologic fracture and a slowly enlarging swelling. The symptoms may be present for a few months to many years.

Grossly, the tumor appears to be made up of fibrous tissue that is destroying bone, and may be confused with nonossifying fibroma or fibrous dysplasia of bone.

The microscopic appearance varies from

rather mature fibroblasts to rather anaplastic fibroblasts. There is no true osteoid or bone formation, although occasionally calcification may be found.

When the diagnosis has been established by biopsy, radical amputation is indicated. Although these tumors grow at varying rates and exhibit varying degrees of malignancy, they are all potentially life endangering, and should be treated as such.

TUMORS OF MESENCHYMAL CONNECTIVE TISSUE ORIGIN

EWING'S SARCOMA. Ewing's sarcoma of bone is a highly malignant, multicentric, small round-cell sarcoma. The origin of the cell is not clearly defined, but it may be of undifferentiated mesenchymal origin. Clinically and cytologically, the lesion is easily confused with reticulum cell sarcoma, neuroblastoma and metastatic cancer. The lesion is primarily bone destructive; however, periosteal new bone formation is a common feature of the lesion as it perforates the cortex of the bone. Either multiple primary foci of tumor, or early metastatic spread to other bones, produces multiple lesions of the skeleton. The solitary lesion may be confused with the inflammatory reaction of osteomyelitis as reflected by bone destruction and periosteal new bone formation.

The tumor may appear to originate in any bone, but is common in the trunk bones and long bones. The lesion arises in the metaphysis or more toward the center of the shaft, but apparently excludes the epiphysis.

The neoplasm is more common in males, and the age distribution is from infancy to about 25 years.

Pain is the usual symptom localized to the area of the tumor. When the pelvic girdle is involved, referred pain in the distribution of the sciatic nerve may occur. Local tenderness to palpation is usual. There may be visible swelling of the part, and occasionally dilated veins are found in the skin over the tumor. Local increase in temperature of the area is common. Weight loss, fever, anemia and leukocytosis with an elevated sedimentation rate may confuse the clinical picture with osteomyelitis. When these findings predominate, the likelihood of a rapidly fatal course is increased.

The radiographic findings reveal mottled bone destruction with extensive involvement of the shaft of the long bones. Periosteal new bone may occur in layers, producing an onion-peel-like picture, which was considered pathognomonic of the disease, but is now recognized to occur in other conditions and only occasionally in Ewing's sarcoma. Multiple bone involvement is almost inevitable.

Grossly, the tumor is gray-white, glistening, and, in many instances, soft to almost liquid in consistency. Hemorrhage, degeneration and cyst formation in the tumor are common findings. At the time of biopsy, the liquid portion of the tumor may resemble pus, further misleading the surgeon that he may be dealing with osteomyelitis; however, careful biopsy should rectify this confusion promptly.

The microscopic findings reveal cellular tumor with little intercellular stroma. Fibrous tissue strands may separate the tumor cells into rather large compartments. The nucleus of the lesional cell is oval or round. The cytoplasm is slightly granular and scanty with indistinct cell outlines. Mitotic figures are numerous. Periosteal new bone may form where the periosteum has been elevated by the tumor.

The results of treatment either by roentgen therapy or amputation are uniformly poor. Relief of symptoms may be obtained by roentgen therapy for varying periods of from a few months to a year. Eventually, metastasis to lungs and other organs leads to a fatal outcome.

TUMORS OF HEMATOPOIETIC ORIGIN

PRIMARY RETICULUM CELL SARCOMA OF BONE. Primary reticulum cell sarcoma of bone is derived from the reticulum cells of bone marrow. The cell type is similar to that of the reticulum cell sarcoma of lymph nodes; however, the course differs in that solitary lesions of bones accessible to surgical excision have a fairly favorable prognosis when this treatment is accompanied by roentgen therapy.

When it occurs in long bones, the tumor tends to occur in the end or shaft of the bone. The lesion is primarily bone destructive, and may perforate the periosteum and invade the surrounding tissues. Metastasis to regional lymph nodes is common. There is a predilection for males in the ratio of three to two. The tumor may occur at any age, but is rare in very young children.

There is no characteristic roentgenographic picture. Mottled destruction of bone and areas of sclerosis and cortical destruction with minimal periosteal new bone are the general findings.

Pain with pathologic fracture is the common symptom.

Grossly, the tumor is friable when it invades the soft tissues, and has the appearance of malignant lymphoma.

The predominant lesional cell is the reticulum cell; however, lymphocytes and lymphoblasts may be found in varying amounts in the tumor. There is a tendency for the cells to be in alveolar groupings, separated by the reticulum framework of the tumor. Special stains for reticulum cells may be helpful in differentiating the tumor.

When it has been determined that the lesion is solitary, surgical and roentgen therapy offer a good possibility for a survival rate of 40 to 50 per cent in these patients. Roentgen therapy has been shown to arrest the tumor, but it has not been determined whether amputation in conjunction with this treatment increases the survival rate. The regional lymph nodes should be irradiated.

The other tumors arising from the hematopoietic system include multiple myeloma, chronic and acute leukemia, lymphosarcoma and Hodgkin's disease. None of these tumors are amenable to surgical treatment as they involve the skeleton in its entirety.

TUMORS OF NERVE ORIGIN

The types of tumors arising from nerve tissue are neurofibroma, neurilemoma and malignant schwannoma. These tumors rarely involve bone, except for neurofibromatosis or von Recklinghausen's disease.

NEURILEMOMA. Neurilemoma is usually a solitary, encapsulated, benign tumor produced by proliferating Schwann cells. When the nerve is small, the tumor surrounds the nerve, and attempts to remove it may destroy the nerve. In large nerves, the tumor is usually located eccentrically, and it may be possible to remove the tumor without destroying the nerve.

The tumor consists of two types of tissue; one is composed of proliferating masses of Schwann cells arranged in twisted cords, the stroma being reticular, and may resemble tactile corpuscles. The second type is composed of Schwann cells arranged at random in a mucinous reticular stroma.

MULTIPLE NEUROFIBROMATOSIS. Multiple neurofibromatosis is characterized by neuromas involving skin, nerve and bone. When the bone is involved, it is most often by invasion from a subperiosteal nerve. Growth of the tumor may erode the bone and elevate the periosteum, which forms new bone. When the bone is invaded and extensively involved, cystic areas develop within the bone which may become expansile. Gross deformity of the extremities is not uncommon. Involvement of the spine often produces scoliosis.

Excision of accessible masses may be done; however, correction of deformity in involved bones is the most common surgical procedure.

MALIGNANT SCHWANNOMA. Malignant schwannoma is a rare tumor, difficult to diagnose because of the variety of tissues that may be formed from the parent cell. Amputation is the treatment of choice as the tumor appears to be highly malignant.

TUMORS OF VASCULAR ORIGIN

HEMANGIOMA AND MALIGNANT HEMANGIOENDOTHELIOMA. Hemangiomas may involve an entire limb, including the bone and soft tissues, or may be an isolated lesion in either. These tumors may be primarily capillary or cavernous hemangiomas. Isolated lesions may be excised when accessible; however, vertebral lesions, when producing symptoms of nerve or spinal cord compression, are probably best treated by irradiation followed by decompression when necessary.

Malignant hemangioendothelioma is a lesion of varying aggressiveness. The tumor is rare. When bone is involved, the tumor tends to destroy bone and expand the cortex. The course of the tumor is unpredictable. At present, resection or amputation is indicated for accessible lesions. The value of radiation therapy is debatable.

TUMORS OF FAT CELL ORIGIN

LIPOMA AND LIPOSARCOMA. Lipoma is one of the common tumors of the soft tissues, but is rare within the bone. The tumor consists of an accumulation of adult fat cells confined by an extremely thin fibrous capsule. The tumor is benign and need be excised only when it becomes unsightly or interferes with function.

Liposarcoma is rare in bone, but not uncommon in the soft tissues. The tumor usually occurs in the fat of the buttock, thigh, lower leg or the back and shoulder regions. The tumor rarely occurs before the age of 30, and is more common in the fifth decade. It usually grows slowly, producing few symptoms except for local tumefaction. Metastasis tends to occur late in the course of the tumor, although recurrence after resection may be as high as 50 per cent.

The tumor is composed of adult and embryonic fat cells scattered throughout a sarcomatous stroma. Giant cells may be found.

Wide excision of the tumor should be performed. The percentage of five-year survival may be as high as 85 per cent with adequate resection.

CHORDOMA. Chordoma is a rather uncommon tumor arising from neoplastic proliferation of notochordal remnants. It is of low grade malignancy, but of high recurrence rate, affecting the spine and base of the skull. The tumor is primarily destructive of bone, and has a predilection for the ends of the spine and the sacrococcygeal and spheno-occipital regions. The condition affects males twice as often as females. The tumor is uncommon before the age of 30.

The symptoms are usually pain, but encroachment on the central nervous system may produce a variety of symptoms and physical findings.

The roentgenographic appearance is one of midline bone destruction, often accompanied by a soft tissue mass.

Grossly, the tumor is a soft, friable, grayish mass. It appears encapsulated except in the areas of bone destruction.

Microscopically, the tumor may be composed of cavities lined with cuboidal cells resembling epithelium; however, cords, lobules and sheets of vacuolated cells in a mucinous matrix may predominate.

Wide excision of sacral tumors should be attempted, although recurrence from incomplete removal is common. Inaccessible tumors or recurrent tumors may be treated by high-voltage irradiation.

TUMORS OF MUSCLE ORIGIN

RHABDOMYOSARCOMA. Rhabdomyosarcoma is the most common tumor affecting striated muscle. Three types have been described: the orthodox, the alveolar and the embryonal. All are malignant tumors; however, survival rate of the orthodox type may approach 50 per cent whereas the alveolar and embryonal types are uniformly fatal.

The orthodox type of rhabdomyosarcoma rarely occurs before the age of 50, whereas the other two types occur in children and young adults. The tumor commonly occurs in the thigh, but may occur in any skeletal muscle. Disparity in cell size and type is characteristic in the orthodox tumor. Elongated, strap-like cells, which often contain more than one nucleus, are diagnostic, particularly when cross-striations are found. Spider cells, which are large, clear cells traversed by thread-like processes, are helpful in the diagnosis when they are found.

The alveolar tumor is composed of embryonic muscle cells divided by fibrous trabeculae.

The embryonal tumor is composed of short, spindle cells arranged in interlacing bands mixed with cells resembling lymphocytes.

Metastasis is usually by way of the blood to the lungs.

Wide resection or amputation is the treatment of choice. The tumor is radioresistant.

TUMORS OF SYNOVIAL ORIGIN

MALIGNANT SYNOVIOMA. Malignant synovioma is a true neoplasm arising from elements of the synovial membrane. Although of rather benign gross appearance and slow growing in many instances, the tumor is highly malignant. Local recurrence following resection is commonly followed by metastasis to the lungs.

The tumor arises most often in the knee joint or joints of the lower extremity; occasionally the upper extremity is involved.

Grossly, the tumor may appear as fleshy masses in the synovial membrane.

Two main types of cytology are seen microscopically. The sarcomatous type is composed of spindle or fusiform, uniform cells with little fibrous supporting structure. Slit-like spaces usually occur lined with tumor cells. In the second type, cells are more cylindrical and are arranged radially about the slits or spaces, forming a pseudoacinar pattern.

Treatment has been unsatisfactory, and long-term survivals are rare. Amputation or radical resection followed by roentgen therapy has not appreciably lowered the mortality rate.

CONDITIONS SIMULATING BONE TUMORS

Many conditions occur in the skeleton which may simulate bone tumors. Careful roentgenographic studies, appropriate blood studies and biopsy material usually determine the diagnosis of the true lesion.

The common lesions simulating bone tumors are metastatic carcinoma, fibrous dysplasia of bone, bone cysts, histiocytosis, aneurysmal bone cyst, Paget's disease and the skeletal changes of hyperparathyroidism. All these conditions must be considered in the differential diagnosis of bone tumors.

READING REFERENCES

Advisory Committee on Artificial Limbs: Artificial Limbs. National Academy of Sciences, National Research Council, Washington 25, D.C. January, May and September, 1954; January, May and September, 1955.

Aegerter, E., and Kirkpatrick, J. A., Jr.: Orthopedic Diseases. 2nd ed. Philadelphia, W. B. Saunders Company, 1963.

Aitken, G. T., and Frantz, C. H.: Management of the child amputee. The American Academy of Orthopaedic Surgeons. Instructional Course Lectures *17*:246, 1960.

American Academy of Orthopaedic Surgeons: Orthopaedic Appliances Atlas. Artificial Limbs. Volume II. Ann Arbor, J. W. Edwards, 1960.

Bado, J. L.: The Monteggia Lesion. (Ponsetti, I. V., trans.) Springfield, Illinois, Charles C Thomas, 1962.

Blanche, D. W.: Osteomyelitis in infants. J. Bone & Joint Surg. 34-A:71, 1952.

Blount, W. P.: Fractures in Children. Baltimore, The Williams & Wilkins Company, 1955.

Bosworth, D. M., and Levine, J.: Tuberculosis of the spine: an analysis of cases treated surgically. J. Bone & Joint Surg. 31-A:267, 1949.

Buchman, J.: Osteomyelitis. American Academy of Orthopaedic Surgeons. Instructional Course Lectures *16*: 232, 1959.

Buchman, J.: The rationale of the therapy of chronic osteomyelitis. American Academy of Orthopaedic Surgeons. Instructional Course Lectures *8*:125, 1951.

Cave, E. F.: Fractures and Other Injuries. Chicago, Illinois, The Year Book Publishers, 1958.

Cave, E. F.: Tuberculosis of the spine in children. American Academy of Orthopaedic Surgeons. Instructional Course Lectures *5*:114, 1948.

Chandler, F. A.: Tuberculosis of the lower extremity. American Academy of Orthopaedic Surgeons. Instructional Course Lectures *5*:121, 1948.

Charnley, J.: The Closed Treatment of Common Fractures. 3rd ed. Baltimore, The Williams & Wilkins Company, 1961.

Clark, J. M. P.: Modern Trends in Orthopaedics. Third Series: Fracture Treatment. Washington, D. C., Butterworth, Inc., 1963.

Clark, J. M. P.: Modern Trends in Orthopaedics. Fourth Series: Science of Fractures. Washington, D.C., Butterworth, Inc., 1964.

Committee on Prosthetic Research and Development: The Geriatric Amputee. Publication 919. National Academy of Sciences, National Research Council, Washington, D.C., 1961.

Committee on Trauma, American College of Surgeons: The Management of Fractures and Soft-Tissue Injuries. Philadelphia and London, W. B. Saunders Company, 1960.

Conwell, H. E., Reynolds, F. C.: Key and Conwell's Management of Fractures, Dislocations and Sprains. 7th ed. St. Louis, The C. V. Mosby Company, 1961.

Dahlin, D. C.: Bone Tumors. 2nd ed. Springfield, Illinois, Charles C Thomas, 1967.

DePalma, A. F.: The Management of Fractures and Dislocations: An Atlas. Volumes I and II. Philadelphia and London, W. B. Saunders Company, 1959.

Dobson, J.: Tuberculosis of the spine. J. Bone & Joint Surg. 33-B:517, 1951.

Duchenne, G. B.: Physiology of Motion. (Kaplan, E. B., trans.) Philadelphia, J. B. Lippincott Company, 1949.

Geschickter, C. F., and Copeland, M. M.: Tumors of Bone. Philadelphia, J. B. Lippincott Company, 1949.

Hampton, O. P., Jr., and Fitts, W. T., Jr.: Open Reduction of Common Fractures. New York and London, Grune & Stratton, 1959.

Jaffe, H. L.: Tumors and Tumorous Conditions of the Bones and Joints. Philadelphia, Lea & Febiger, 1958.

Klopsteg, P. E., and Wilson, P. D.: Human Limbs and Their Substitutes. New York, Toronto and London, McGraw-Hill Book Company, Inc., 1954.

Larmon, W. A.: Amputations and prostheses. S. Clin. North America 29:223, 1949.

Lichtenstein, L.: Bone Tumors. St. Louis, The C. V. Mosby Company, 1965.

Magnuson, P. B., and Stack, J. K.: Fractures. 5th ed. Philadelphia, J. B. Lippincott Company, 1949.

Orr, H. W.: The treatment of acute osteomyelitis by drainage and rest. J. Bone & Joint Surg. 9:733, 1927.

Pack, G. T., and Ariel, I. M.: Tumors of the Soft Somatic Tissues. New York, Paul B. Hoeber, 1958.

Prosthetic Research Board: Artificial Limbs. National Academy of Sciences, National Research Council, Washington 25, D.C. Vol. 3, No. 1, 1956; Vol. 4, No. 1, 1957; Vol. 5, No. 1 and No. 2, 1958; Vol. 6, No. 1, 1961; Vol. 6, No. 2, 1962; and Vol. 7, No. 1, 1963.

Public Health Service Cooperative Investigation: Evaluation of streptomycin therapy in a controlled series of ninety cases of skeletal tuberculosis. J. Bone & Joint Surg. 34-A:288, 1952.

Robertson, R. C.: Acute infectious hematogenous osteomyelitis. American Academy of Orthopaedic Surgeons. Instructional Course Lectures *5*:136, 1948.

Slocum, D. B.: An Atlas of Amputations. St. Louis, The C. V. Mosby Company, 1949.

Watson-Jones, R.: Fractures and Joint Injuries. 4th ed. Volumes I and II. Baltimore, The Williams & Wilkins Company, 1957.

Wiles, P.: Fractures, Dislocations and Sprains. Boston, Little, Brown & Company, 1960.

Chapter 32

THE HAND

by
JOHN L. BELL, M.D.

JOHN LOUIS BELL received his education at Duke and Northwestern universities. He is an Associate Professor of Surgery at Northwestern University. He has devoted his special talents to the surgery of the hand, and represents the third generation of the school of surgeons, originated by Kanavel, interested in surgery of the hand. The meticulous and thorough efforts characteristic of the surgical teachings of this group to create closed, clean wounds out of open, dirty, destructive injuries and to restore function of the hand have been multiply repaid by shortening the convalescent period and returning the patient to an independent social and economic position.

Historically, surgery of the hand has evolved from a consideration of infections into a broad field encompassing the most complex phases of repair and reconstruction for an infinite variety of injuries, diseases and deformities. The care of these conditions demands techniques employed in orthopedics, plastic surgery and neurologic surgery, as well as expert knowledge in the handling of wounds. In the past, hand injuries were usually entrusted to the least experienced, whereas it is now recognized that optimal functional results stem from skilled attention at the onset of treatment.

An epoch-making advance in surgery of the hand was the publication of Kanavel's book, *Infections of the Hand,* the first edition of which appeared in 1907, and the seventh edition, at the time of the author's death, in 1938. It is difficult to estimate the influence which this book has had in the development of surgery of the hand. In the experimental and clinical observations contained in this volume, a sound anatomic basis was laid for an understanding of crippling and baffling infections involving the hand. A firm knowledge of infections soon led to paying greater attention to the care of wounds and to the surgical treatment of other disabilities of the hand.

INFECTIONS

Infections of the hand may result in crippling disabilities, particularly if treatment is late or inept. Hand infections vary in severity according to bacterial virulence, anatomic site of inoculation, pathways of spread and the kind of tissue involved. In addition to these local factors, the clinical course is influenced by the health of a patient prior to the onset of an infectious process. A thorough knowledge of the relevant surgical anatomy is necessary to diagnose and treat correctly any infection involving the hand.

Most infections on the dorsum of a hand are similar to those occurring in skin and subcutaneous tissues in other parts of the body. In volar wounds of the hand, however, the consequences of infection are different. A puncture wound of the thick skin quickly seals, allowing bacteria to propagate under ideal anaerobic conditions. On the volar aspect, early egress or surface localization of an infectious process is unusual due to the barrier of thick, tough skin. An infection may extend either into deeper tissues, which offer less resistance to invasion, or may spread along fascial planes. If flexor tendon sheaths or subfascial spaces are inoculated primarily with bacteria, a widespread infection can develop in a few hours following a seemingly trivial wound.

Consequently, it is necessary to know anatomic pathways to understand the possible course of an infectious process. Should surgical drainage be indicated, it is equally important to apply knowledge of the pertinent surgical anatomy to avoid operative injury of nerves, tendons and specialized tactile areas.

Some estimate of the virulence of an infection is essential to plan intelligent care. In an infirm or debilitated patient, infection may spread rapidly and lead to serious complications. Similarly, when a virulent bacterium is involved, as from scratches with autopsy knives or pinpricks while dressing patients with infections, a fulminant process may develop in a few hours in otherwise healthy persons. In the preantibiotic era, many surgeons, pathologists and nurses suffered severe infections, and not a few lost their lives from hand infections. It is important to know if infection is being brought under control by body forces: if it is being localized, or if bacteria are multiplying and extending into surrounding tissues and lymphatic channels. When localization has occurred, surgical drainage can be instituted. On the other hand, if the process is diffuse and spreading, particularly if there is evidence of lymphatic invasion, the problem is more serious. All efforts must be directed toward favoring localization and increasing the patient's resistance. Furthermore, manipulation of the part or incision prior to localization must be avoided. Fortunately, antibiotics are of value in bringing spreading infections under control. Nevertheless, even under antibiotic coverage, too early active surgical treatment is perilous.

Identification of the bacteria responsible for an infectious process should be made whenever possible; culturing, both aerobic and anaerobic, will lead to better care. The development of chemotherapeutic and antibiotic agents has served to emphasize the need for accurate knowledge, not only of the infecting organism, but also of its sensitivity of these drugs.

General Principles of Care

Certain general principles of care apply to all types of hand infections.

An early decision must be made about the site of the process, and whether it is spreading or is localized.

Only by knowing the anatomic location of an infection can adequate and proper drainage be carried out and the possible course of extension be predicted. The need for determining whether body immune processes have succeeded in localizing infection is of great importance. In an adequately localized process, prompt drainage is indicated. In acute spreading processes, or in any infection in an

early stage before its spread has been stopped, surgical intervention is contraindicated. In acute spreading infections, surgical intervention during the stage of spread may lead to serious extension of the process, increased tissue injury and delay in healing.

The proper treatment for an infection should be started at once. Delay in care may lead to serious sequelae such as tenosynovitis, felon and spreading infections. Prompt care does not necessarily mean immediate incision; on the contrary, it may mean strict avoidance of incision.

Rest of the part is an integral element of treatment of any infection. In an infection of the hand, proper splinting is a necessary feature. The extent to which splinting is carried out, and the means of obtaining immobilization, vary with the location and severity of infection. In infections involving one digit, such as a paronychia or felon, it may be necessary to put only the digit at rest. In more extensive processes, the hand and forearm must be immobilized.

Whenever the hand, or any of its parts, is immobilized because of infection, it is essential that it be splinted in the posture which was called by Kanavel "the position of function" (Fig. 1). This is a position of grasp, not of rest. The wrist is dorsiflexed 45 degrees, the metacarpophalangeal and interphalangeal joints are flexed to 30 degrees and the fingers are separated from each other. The thumb is abducted and rotated so that its pulp faces the pads of the fingers.

The advantages of this position are several. If any stiffness results from infection, the hand will be capable of some use even with a minimum of motion. Also, with a hand in this position, restoration of function is easier. The ligaments of the joints are at maximum length when the hand is in a grasping position. Hence, if they become involved, they do not restrict motion. If the joints are in an ex-

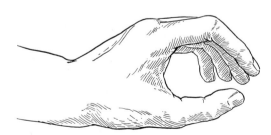

Figure 1. The position of function. An important milestone in the development of surgery of the hand was the establishment by Kanavel of the importance of this position in immobilization of the hand.

tended position, the ligaments shorten. If they become fibrosed, they hold the joints stiffly in extension, so that restoration of mobility is difficult, if not impossible (Fig. 2). With the wrist in moderate extension, the grasping power of the digits is greatest, but it diminishes as the wrist is straightened and flexed.

This position of function is applicable, likewise, if only one or two digits or the wrist is to be immobilized. Fingers should be splinted in slight flexion, the thumb in rotation and apposition, the wrist in extension.

Operation to drain an infection is done with the same care accorded any elective operative procedure. As a rule, except for an early paronychia in which incision may be made without anesthesia, general anesthesia is preferred. Local anesthetic infiltration is hazardous in an infected area, and injection about the base of a digit may be followed by gangrene of the finger. Incisions should be made in a bloodless field. Hasty incisions within an area obscured by bleeding are certain to cause trouble. Especially is this true of incisions for tenosynovitis or palmar space infections where nerves, blood vessels and tendons are subject to injury.

Drainage is secured by adequate incision and not by use of drains. When an incision has been made, it is advisable to insert a strip of petrolatum-soaked, fine-mesh gauze into one corner of the wound to keep the skin edges from becoming agglutinated. The strip

is left in the wound not over 48 hours. Stiff drains that press against nerves and tendons are to be avoided, as are through-and-through drains.

After-care is as important as incision. Following incision, moist packs are used for two or three days, or until it is evident that the process is receding. This is manifested by recession of swelling and reappearance of normal skin creases. As soon as recession begins, mobilization in all joints not directly involved must be started. This is accomplished by reducing splinting to only those digits affected. It is necessary to stimulate the patient in the use of uninvolved fingers which may have become stiff. Warm soapy baths are instituted, once or twice daily.

As long as the possibility of adding secondary contaminants obtains, an infected hand should be accorded aseptic care. Every precaution is taken to preserve asepsis while removing and applying dressings.

Antibiotics should be considered only as part of the treatment of an infection. In most instances, before the offending organisms have been identified, it is customary to administer antibiotic therapy. The gradual emergence of penicillin-resistant strains of staphylococci has posed a real problem. On the other hand, many patients have developed sensitivity to penicillin, in which case some other antibiotic should be given. As soon as the bacterium causing an infection has been identified, sensitivity tests should be made to determine which antibiotic is most effective.

TYPES OF INFECTION

FOLLICULITIS. This relatively minor infection involves only the dorsal surface of the hand, which alone is supplied with hair follicles. It responds to simple care; usually, it is enough to cover it with a small dressing. The temptation, however, is for the patient to pick or squeeze the inflamed area. Not infrequently such action leads to extension of the infection, usually staphylococcal in nature, into deeper tissues.

FURUNCLE. The furuncle, or boil, frequently stems from a follicular infection. It starts as a small, reddish, painful swelling. In early stages, the process may subside if covered with a dressing, and if the part is put at rest. Sometimes, injection of penicillin parenterally will bring about subsidence. More often, however, the process leads to

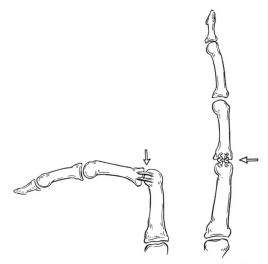

Figure 2. When the joints of the digits are flexed, the collateral ligaments are lengthened; when the joints are extended, these ligaments are shortened. Hence, when a joint is put at rest in a straight position, the ligaments are shortened. Flexion may be difficult or impossible if immobilization is prolonged.

necrosis of subcutaneous tissues, and a core of necrotic material, will require release. Moist dressings may produce spontaneous evacuation of the necrotic plug; if not, an incision is required.

DORSAL SUBCUTANEOUS ABSCESS. Folliculitis, or a furuncle, may give rise to a deep abscess on the dorsum of a finger, usually on the proximal phalanx (Fig. 3). This process overlies the tendon and may spread subcutaneously over the entire dorsal surface of the phalanx. Operative drainage is indicated and must be done in a bloodless field, with the patient under adequate anesthesia.

CARBUNCLE. This entity occurs on the dorsum of the hand, usually on its ulnar side, or over the dorsal surface of the proximal phalanx. It may start as a follicular infection, and, frequently, there is a history of trauma. This infection should make one immediately suspicious of diabetes. If diabetes is present, control measures should be started. Parenteral antibiotic therapy should be instituted without delay. With the patient at bed rest and his hand immobilized in a moist dressing, the carbuncle may drain and evacuate spontaneously. If this does not occur, incision is required. It is seldom necessary to consider a 'cruciate incision, usually required in the past, because immobilization, plus antibiotic therapy, tends to minimize spread and favor localization.

COLLAR-BUTTON ABSCESS. The skin on the palmar surface is thick. It is subject to minute trauma; small cracks, puncture wounds and blisters are frequent. These favor deposit of bacteria beneath the thick epidermis. A small abscess may form which spreads beneath the cuticular layer to form a purulent blister, or *subepithelial abscess*. Such a blister causes few serious symptoms, and usually subsides if it is unroofed. However, the blister may represent a subcuticular accumulation of pus which has found its way from beneath the corium into the subcuticular area. Arriving at the epidermis, which is thick and impenetrable, it spreads, raising the surface covering (Fig. 4). In a similar fashion, a simple subcuticular abscess, unable to rupture to the surface, may perforate the corium and form a deeper abscess (Fig. 4). In either case, the subcuticular blister is simply the superficial manifestation of a more deeply lying process. Such infection is known as a collar-button abscess, since there are two lakes of pus connected by a narrow neck passing through the derma vera.

Collar-button abscesses occur typically at the distal end of the palm, usually in the region between the metacarpal heads. They may lie, however, directly over the flexor tendons at the base of the digits (Fig. 5). The deep portion of the abscess lies in the web space, from which it may extend to the dorsum and also into the subcutaneous tissues of the proximal phalanx.

Treatment of such a process consists in drainage not only of the purulent blister, but of the deeper process as well. When opening a purulent blister, it is necessary, even if there are no signs suggestive of a deep abscess, to inspect its floor to be certain that there is no sinus leading to a deeper cavity.

PARONYCHIA. This infection starts between the nail and cuticle at the base of the nail. It is also called "run-around" because it tends to spread under the cuticle. If it is seen early, pain may be relieved and the process halted by means of an incision in the nail wall, or by lifting the cuticle over the base of the nail with a blunt instrument (Fig. 6).

If a paronychia is neglected, a more serious extension takes place. The pus finds its way under the nail, separating it from the nail

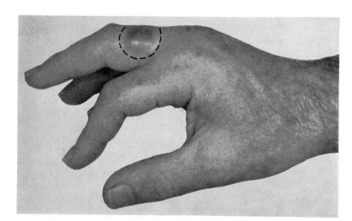

Figure 3. The dorsal subcutaneous abscess on the finger usually starts as a follicular infection which spreads over a much larger area than the superficial process would seem to indicate.

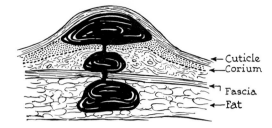

Figure 4. Any subcutaneous abscess on the hand may rupture through the corium and lead to subcuticular accumulation of pus. Drainage of this alone will not adequately evacuate the deeper pocket.

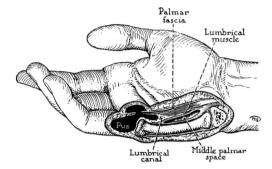

Figure 5. The frog felon or collar-button abscess is a typical bilocular abscess occurring at the base of the digits. A superficial subcuticular accumulation of pus simply indicates a deeper pocket. (Mason, M. L.: Infections of the hand. *In,* Sajous: System of Medicine, Surgery and the Specialties. J. B. Lippincott Company.)

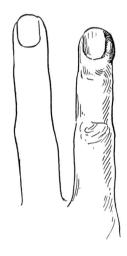

Figure 6. In its early stage, paronychia starts as a tender swelling in the nail wall, which may usually be unroofed easily with a sharp scalpel or scissors without employing an anesthetic.

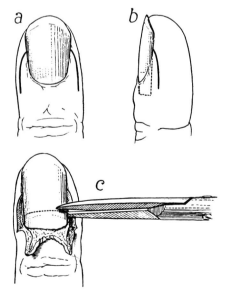

Figure 7. When the paronychia has extended beneath the nail, it is necessary to raise the eponychium and excise the overlying nail to secure adequate drainage.

bed. The cavity is drained by making incisions to either side of the nail base, and lifting the cuticle and turning it proximally (Fig. 7). The nail is inspected and, if it is undermined, it is removed. Care must be taken to remove all nail that has been undermined. Sufficient nail should be removed so that when the eponychium drops back, it does not overlie the distal portion of the nail and create a closed pocket. Following incision, the hand is put at rest on a splint in a voluminous warm moist pack for 24 hours, until acute symptoms have subsided. Thereafter, light dressings are applied. The nail will regenerate satisfactorily, provided surgical drainage has not been too long delayed. At first the nail is likely to be quite rough and irregular, but as it grows it becomes smoother, and eventually is a satisfactory nail.

The neglected paronychia, which has been allowed to persist for weeks or months without adequate drainage, presents one of two conditions. The nail may have been partly destroyed, so that an exuberant plug of granulating tissue protrudes from the nail fold, covered with purulent discharge. Or, the eponychium may be raised, red and swollen, and an occasional drop of pus may be expressed. In either instance, adequate drainage is necessary, and the classic incision with nail removal should be carried out.

Chronic ulceration or exuberant granulations involving the nail bed may not be chronic paronychia, however, and a careful history should be taken.

A carcinoma of the nail bed may occur, usually following an injury which has refused to heal after many months. A malignant melanoma of the nail bed is suggested by black pigmentation, especially around its border. Rarely, a subungual exostosis elevates the nail and leads to granulation tissue.

SUBUNGUAL ABSCESS. This process, as distinguished from subungual infection which occurs with paronychia, is usually seen as the result of a splinter or needle prick which enters beneath the nail. Not infrequently, a small bit of foreign material is imbedded, or a splinter breaks off. A painful infection develops which soon leads to an abscess that can be visualized beneath the nail. It subsides rapidly when the process is unroofed by excising a small triangular slip of nail overlying the abscess. This may often be done without anesthesia, although it is sometimes so painful that brief general anesthesia is required.

FELON. A felon is a staphylococcal infection involving the resilient cushion which covers the volar surface or pad of the finger tip. Examination of this pad will show that it is uniquely adapted to the functions which it subserves, namely, grasp and fine touch. The finger pad enables one to pick up or cling to large or small objects, giving a firm grip with tissues which do not slip or slide. Stereognostic sense enables one to distinguish size, shape, consistency and texture of various objects. This pad, or cushion, occupies the distal two-thirds of the tip of the finger and is made up of a tough meshwork of connective tissue fibers attached on one side to the corium of the overlying skin and on the other to the volar surface of the distal phalanx. This latter insertion ends just distal to the point of attachment of the flexor profundus tendon. The anterior closed space is not connected with the tendon sheath of the finger.

The digital vessels and terminations of the digital nerves run through this space, and are quickly compressed when inflammation occurs. This leads to early severe pain and, if tension is not soon released, to interference with the blood supply.

A felon usually starts from a puncture wound of the finger tip, which leads to throbbing pain within 24 to 48 hours. Along with pain, tenderness and tension occur in the pad, which can swell only moderately. The pain becomes progressively severe, and it is usually after a sleepless night that the patient sees his physician.

Examination will show the pulp to be slightly swollen, tense, hard and tender. There will be little redness, and the original puncture wound may be invisible.

Treatment should be started at once, since the combination of a closed infection, interference with blood supply, and a necrotizing invading organism soon leads to necrosis of the soft tissues and involvement of the bone. This is probably the most frequent cause of osteomyelitis in the hand. If the patient has reported early for care, it may be permissible to apply a splint, continuous warm moist packs overnight and to administer an antibiotic. The infecting organisms are usually staphylococci. In an occasional patient, the process may subside under conservative management. If, however, the symptoms are no better, or are worse after such a regimen, incision should be carried out.

Immediate incision is called for in the patient seen late or if severe, acute symptoms are present. The incision should divide the fibrous tissue bands or retinacula which bind the skin to the anterior surface of the distal phalanx (Fig. 8). It should be placed along the lateral side of the phalanx midway between the anterior surface of the bone and the volar skin. After incising the skin, the knife enters the closed space parallel to the bone surface and sweeps across the space dividing the retinacula. It is not necessary to incise the skin on the opposite side of the phalanx. Caution should be exercised not to carry the incision too far proximally lest the tendon sheath be opened and infected.

Following incision, a strip of petrolatum gauze is placed in the wound to prevent agglutination of the edges. The hand is then placed on a splint in the position of function in continuous warm moist dressings. The originally administered antibiotic is continued unless sensitivity tests indicate that another is more efficacious.

If drainage has been adequate, the process subsides fairly rapidly. If, however, a large necrotic plug has formed, this may take a considerable time to separate. If there is involvement of bone, a conservative attitude is indicated. If drainage has been adequate, dead bone will slowly sequestrate or absorb; if drainage is not adequate, further incision of soft tissues is required.

OSTEOMYELITIS. Osteomyelitis is seen particularly in the distal phalanges following a felon or, occasionally, in association with other infectious processes. It may occur following severe wounds which have become infected. It is practically never seen as a hematogenous infection. As a sequela to a felon, it is evidenced by persistent drainage and a granulomatous plug coming from an incision or from a sinus tract. Early x-ray films may show rarefaction in the distal phalanx, which may be mistaken for osteomyelitis. However, while it is important to make the diagnosis early, the treatment of this condition is the same as that for felon without osteomyelitis. Under no circumstances should the bone be attacked surgically. The soft tissues must be adequately drained, but the bone must not be curetted or otherwise tampered with. Following soft tissue drainage, the part is immobilized and sequestrum formation awaited. As soon as the dead bone is discharged, the wound closes. Occasionally, in children, bone reforms, but this seldom, if ever, occurs in adults.

TENDON SHEATH AND FASCIAL SPACE INFECTIONS. In order to understand tendon sheath and fascial space infections, a knowledge of the anatomy of these spaces is necessary (Fig. 9).

The flexor tendons of the hand are enclosed over a greater part of their extent by synovial tendon sheaths. These structures are long, closed sacs which are invaginated by tendons in such a way that the tendon is covered by a layer of sac, much as the bowel is covered by peritoneum. The sheath is folded back on itself to line the space in which the tendon lies. Along the area through which the tendon invaginates the synovial sheath, there is a structure through which blood vessels pass. This is often stretched out to form a wide membrane similar to the intestinal mesentery (Fig. 10). It has been called the mesotendon. In the digits, mesotendon is reduced in the region of the joints to ligament-like structures known as the vincula longa et brevia.

The tendon sheaths of the index, middle and ring fingers extend from the insertion of the flexor profundus tendon into the palm. They end just proximal to the metacarpophalangeal joint, which lies at the level of the distal palmar crease. Within the digit, the tendon and its synovial covering lie within a dense osteofibrous tunnel formed by a fibrous tendon sheath on the volar surface.

The little finger sheath does not terminate in the palm, but proceeds proximally beneath the transverse carpal ligament into the lower

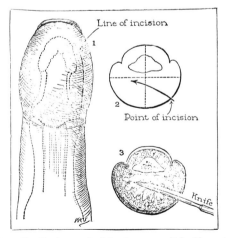

Line of incision

Point of incision

Knife

Figure 8. Drainage of a felon is accomplished by a single hockey-stick incision along the side of the phalanx, which is designed to divide the fascial septa. Care must be taken not to carry the incision too far proximally, lest the tendon sheath be opened. (Koch, S. L.: J.A.M.A. 92:1171, 1929.)

forearm. As it passes through the carpal tunnel, the sheath invests the tendons of the ring, the middle and the index finger. This compartment is known as the *ulnar bursa.*

The sheath surrounding the thumb flexor continues through the carpal tunnel to end in the lower forearm. This prolongation is known as the *radial bursa.* It usually connects with the ulnar bursa as the two pass side by side through the carpal tunnel.

Three fascial spaces lie deep to the tendon sheaths, and their relationship to each other is of importance. Two spaces are in the palm in relation to sheaths of the index, middle and ring fingers; the other lies in the lower forearm in relation to the radial and ulnar bursae.

In the palm (Fig. 11), a sheet of fascia from the palmar aponeurosis attaches to the middle metacarpal bone along the point of origin of the adductor pollicis muscle. On strictly

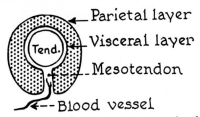

Figure 10. A cross section of a sheath-enclosed tendon shows the synovial sac which encloses it and also the thin membrane which forms the mesotendon, through which pass the blood vessels nourishing the tendon.

anatomic grounds, such a sheet is difficult to demonstrate but, from a clinical standpoint, the presence of such a barrier is unquestioned. The retroflexor space to the radial side of this fascia is known as the *thenar space,* and in its roof lie the flexor tendons to the index finger. The space to the ulnar side of the sheet of fascia is known as the *middle palmar space,* and in its roof lie the flexor tendons of the middle and ring fingers. The proximal ends of the digital tendon sheaths, therefore, lie in the roof of the two spaces.

The *retroflexor space* in the lower forearm lies just above the wrist beneath all the flexor tendons, and in direct relation to the ends of the radial and ulnar bursae (Fig. 12).

Infections starting in a tendon sheath tend to travel throughout the whole length of the sheath (Fig. 13). In any of the three central digits, the infection is confined to the one digit until the synovial sheath ruptures. When it ruptures, it does so as a rule through the least protected area, which is its proximal end, in the palm. The fascial space in relation to the sheath is then involved. This means that, if the index finger is involved, the *thenar space* will be invaded. If the middle or ring finger is implicated, the *middle palmar space* is involved. Occasionally, infection in the middle finger sheath will lead to infection of the *thenar space.*

The situation with regard to the *ulnar* and *radial bursae* is different. When these bursae are infected, the process extends into the lower forearm. Since the radial and ulnar bursae are usually connected with each other at the wrist, involvement starting in one is almost certain to affect the other. When either the radial or ulnar bursa ruptures, the process extends into the *retroflexor space* in the lower forearm.

ACUTE TENOSYNOVITIS. This infection starts usually from a puncture wound, most often at the site where the sheath is nearest the surface on the volar surface of the finger,

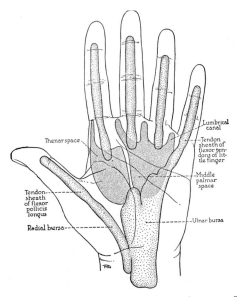

Figure 9. The tendon sheaths and fascial spaces of the volar surface of the hand and forearm form definite pathways for the spread of infection. When infectious organisms gain entrance into a tendon sheath, the process soon spreads throughout the whole sheath. When any of the three central digits is involved, the process comes to a momentary halt in the palm. If drainage is not soon provided, the process then ruptures into one of the fascial spaces in the palm: the middle palmar space if the middle or ring finger is implicated, the thenar space if the index finger is the original site. The pathway from the ulnar bursa on the side of the little finger, however, ends in the lower forearm, and an infectious process originating in this bursa ruptures into the retroflexor space here; similarly, a process from the radial bursa extends into the lower forearm. The radial and ulnar bursae usually communicate with each other and, hence, when one is primarily involved, the other is quickly invaded. (Mason, M. L.: Infections of the hand. *In,* Sajous: System of Medicine, Surgery and the Specialties. J. B. Lippincott Company.)

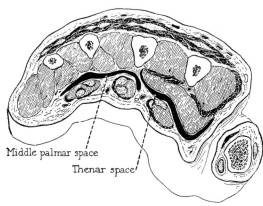

Figure 11. The relationship of the tendon sheaths to the fascial spaces in the palm.

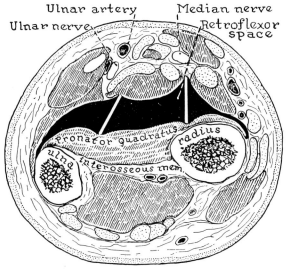

Figure 12. The relationship of the radial and ulnar bursae to the retroflexor space in the lower forearm.

Figure 13. The spread of infection through the various tendon sheaths and fascial spaces of the palm and forearm is shown diagrammatically.

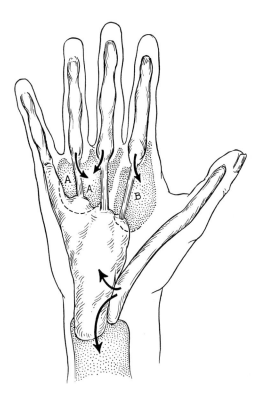

at the proximal or distal interphalangeal joint crease. Once in the sheath, the infectious organisms quickly set up a reaction, and the whole sheath is soon the site of inflammation. The sheath forms a channel through which infection may spread.

As the process develops and fluid accumulates in the sheath, tension increases and, since the synovial sheath is surrounded by a dense, fibrous vaginal sheath, expansion is impossible. This is an example of the phenomenon of the closed-space infection. Extrinsic pressure upon tiny vincula which supply blood to the tendons leads to blockage of vessels and, if not soon relieved, to necrosis of tendon. Since rupture of the synovial sheath is retarded by the vaginal sheath, the synovial outpocketing in the palm or lower forearm bulges and ruptures. Thus, infection is introduced into one of the three retrotendinous fascial spaces, depending upon which tendon sheath is involved. In case of the index, middle or ring digits, fascial spaces in the palm are involved. The process from the index finger invades the *thenar space*, that from the middle finger ruptures into the *middle palmar*, or the thenar space, and that from the ring finger into the *middle palmar space*. If the radial or ulnar bursa is involved, the retrotendinous space of the lower forearm is invaded.

In case of radial or ulnar bursa invasion, the course of events is more extensive. It should be recalled that these bursae are closely associated at the wrist, where both pass through the carpal tunnel. In most instances, the bursae communicate, and consequently, an infectious process starting in one is quickly transmitted to the other. The extent of area involved is greater than that of the digital sheaths of the index, middle and ring fingers. The retrotendinous involvement in radial-ulnar infection is in the forearm; in index, middle and ring sheaths, in the palm.

The recognition of acute suppurative tenosynovitis is not difficult if one remembers the nature of the process, and if one keeps in mind the four cardinal symptoms (Fig. 14). The patient with acute suppurative tenosynovitis usually reports early to his physician because of pain and inability to secure relief from simple home remedies, and because he feels sick. It is apparent to the patient that something seriously is wrong with the finger or hand.

Upon questioning, the patient usually gives a history of a minor injury to the volar surface

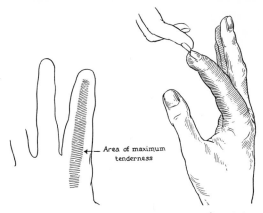

Figure 14. Cardinal signs and symptoms of acute tenosynovitis: the finger is uniformly swollen; it is held slightly flexed at all its joints; any attempt to extend the finger passively causes exquisite pain; and the area of maximum tenderness maps out the anatomic outline of the sheath.

of the digit 24 to 48 hours previously. Aching pain will have begun in the finger the night following injury, and will probably have been severe enough to interfere with sleep.

On examination, it will be noted that the patient is protecting the finger, that he holds it slightly flexed and that the wrist likewise is flexed; the forearm is supinated and supported on the opposite forearm. Jarring, motion and dependency of the part are avoided. The patient is reluctant to permit any except the gentlest examination. The finger is swollen and this swelling involves the whole finger, which assumes a sausage-like shape. Attempts to straighten the finger passively lead to marked pain. Finally, if the examiner gently tests the digit for an area of maximum tenderness, he will find this to coincide with the anatomic extent of the involved sheath.

These symptoms and findings hold true for all tenosynovitis; however, there are additional features in case of infection of the radial and ulnar bursae. The bursae almost always communicate; hence, while initial symptoms and findings occur in the bursa first affected, it is not long before the other is involved. Thus, with suppurative tenosynovitis of the radial bursa, the thumb is swollen, flexed and resistant to passive extension. There is a typical tenderness, which extends from the distal phalanx of the thumb upward into the wrist and above the transverse carpal ligament. Added to this will be evidence of ulnar bursa invasion.

Kanavel pointed out that the earliest sign of ulnar bursa invasion is an area of maximum tenderness in the palm at the point where the flexor tendon sheath of the little finger comes closest to the surface. This point lies in the palm where the distal flexion crease crosses the hypothenar eminence. Gentle pressure at this point leads to pain if the ulnar bursa is infected.

If infection starts in the little finger and involves the ulnar bursa, the chain of events is just the opposite. There will be maximum symptoms and findings on the ulnar side of the hand and, later, evidence of radial bursa invasion.

The general symptoms associated with acute suppurative tenosynovitis are those associated with other types of surgical infections. However, the rapid extension of the process within a closed space with relatively large surfaces of absorption often causes symptoms out of proportion to the small wound of entrance.

The treatment of acute suppurative tenosynovitis must be prompt and efficient if tendons are to be saved and extension prevented. Penicillin, or another antibiotic, is started at once, and preparation is made for immediate drainage. Only in exceptional circumstances should drainage be delayed 12 to 24 hours.

As with all hand infections, incision is made in a bloodless field. The incision is made with all the care of an anatomic dissection, since nerves, tendons and uninvolved spaces of the hand must not be damaged (Fig. 15). Incision on the digits must be made on the lateral side of the finger and, since the fingers are swollen, it is often difficult to know where the true lateral side is located. As landmarks, the surgeon takes the terminations of the transverse creases of the skin which appear at the joints. It is a rule never to cross perpendicular to flexion creases in incisions of the hand. Without following these guides, incision on the side of a swollen digit will be found to lie close to the midline when swelling subsides. Such incisions lead to contracture scars which produce flexion deformities of the finger.

Incision on the index, middle and ring fingers extends from the base of the distal phalanx to the proximal flexion crease of the digit (*a* in Fig. 15). It does not extend into the palm. The proximal cul-de-sac of the sheath of these fingers is drained by a transverse incision in the palm at about the level of the distal flexion crease in the palm. Since this incision passes directly across nerves (*e* in Fig. 15), vessels and tendons, it is obvious

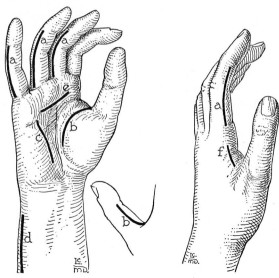

Figure 15. Incisions for drainage of the tendon sheath and fascial spaces must be made with the care of an anatomic dissection in a bloodless field. The incision in the digit is made on the midlateral side and, since the finger is swollen, it may be difficult to place this incision correctly. The proper location of the incision is indicated by the ends of the transverse creases on the digits, which are never obliterated, regardless of the degree of swelling. (Mason, M. L.: Infections of the hand. *In,* Sajous: System of Medicine, Surgery and the Specialties. J. B. Lippincott Company.)

that a bloodless field permitting clear vision is necessary.

After the finger is opened, edematous fat will bulge into the field. The surgeon must have assistance to keep this fat retracted so that he can identify the digital nerve and vessels. Passing volar to these structures, the tendon sheath is exposed and opened throughout its length in the digit.

When incisions have been made and culture taken for identification and sensitivity tests, moist compresses are held in the wounds and the pneumatic cuff is released. After a few minutes the incisions are inspected for bleeding vessels, which are ligated. A petrolatum gauze strip is laid in the wound to prevent agglutination of its edges, and a voluminous moist pack is applied with the hand placed on a splint in the position of function.

More extensive incisions are required if the radial and ulnar bursae are involved. Drainage of the palmar and forearm prolongation of the bursae may be required. The palmar portion of the ulnar bursa is opened by an incision which parallels the hypothenar eminence (*c* in Fig. 15). Proximally, this incision ends at the level of the transverse carpal ligament. The forearm portion of the ulnar bursa is drained by an incision (*d* in Fig. 15) about 3 inches long placed anterior to the ulna.

The palmar portion of the radial bursa is drained by an incision which parallels the ulnar border of the thenar eminence (*b* in Fig. 15). It extends from the region of the proximal flexion crease of the thumb to within a thumb's breadth of the transverse carpal ligament. It must stop there; otherwise, there is danger of dividing the motor branches of the median nerve. In fact, this portion of the incision of the radial bursa is difficult since the sensory rami of the median nerve to the thumb also cross the tendon sheath and must be visualized.

The proximal, or forearm, portion of the radial bursa is opened along the radial aspect of the wrist by an incision about 3 inches long, made anterior to the radius. Usually, if the ulnar bursa is to be drained at the same time, the ulnar incision will suffice for drainage of the proximal ends of both bursae.

Usually, the middle palmar space is involved by extension from a digital sheath. The thenar space is primarily involved more often.

Evidence of middle palmar involvement may be surmised if, in association with tenosynovitis of the middle or ring fingers, there is brief relief from pain followed by exacerbation of both local and general symptoms. Locally, the normal palmar concavity is lost, and the palm becomes flat, tense, hard and gray. The tenderness, which at first was confined in its maximum intensity to the tendon sheath, becomes localized in the center of the palm. The general symptoms increase in intensity; pain becomes more severe, and the swelling of the hand increases.

The thenar space infection produces similar, but usually not quite such severe, symptoms. The swelling is typical. The hand looks as if a golf ball had been inserted in the soft tissues between the metacarpals of the thumb and index finger. The thumb is pushed away from the hand and the whole area is markedly edematous. Maximum tenderness is in the first interosseous space, particularly in the palm. Early drainage of these spaces is indicated. If the associated tendon sheath is infected and requires drainage, the fascial space is drained at the same time.

The middle palmar space is opened through the same incision which drains the proximal cul-de-sac of the sheath (*e* in Fig. 15). Forceps are inserted beneath the tendon and passed proximally to enter the space. To drain the thenar fascial space, an incision is made on the dorsal surface of the web space between the first and second metacarpals, on a line joining the metacarpal heads and proximal to the border of the web (*b* in Fig. 15). A hemostat is passed over the first dorsal interosseus muscle, posterior to the flexor tendons of the index finger, into the thenar space.

LYMPHANGITIS AND ACUTE SPREADING INFECTIONS. Most infections of the hand begin as a small diffuse process, which soon becomes localized to certain areas of the hand or lower forearm. Many require a longer or shorter period of rest and immobilization. Often, the use of warm moist packs is permissible to favor adequate localization before drainage. The one exception to this is suppurative tenosynovitis, which demands early incision.

Acute lymphangitis and acute spreading infections are caused by highly virulent organisms which spread rapidly in lymphatic and tissue spaces before body resistance can combat them.

The hand is richly supplied by lymphatic vessels, especially on the palmar surface (Fig. 16). Lymphatics from the palm drain roughly in two directions. Those on the proximal portion of the palm, drain along the volar surface of the forearm toward the elbow and axilla, following the main venous channels. The remainder of the lymphatics of the palm, and those of the digits, pursue the shortest course to the dorsum of the hand and then pass to the axilla, some passing through the epitrochlear nodes. Some skip both axillary and epitrochlear nodes to empty directly into lymphatic channels in the neck.

Kanavel pointed out that the lymphatics of the ring and little fingers pass through the epitrochlear nodes before reaching the axilla, and that those of the thumb and index finger pass directly to the axilla. Those from the middle finger may skip both sets of nodes and pass directly into the neck. It was for this reason that the middle finger was known as the "dangerous finger," since lymphangitis starting there quickly leads to systemic infection unless brought under early control.

Acute spreading infections start as lymphangitis, which quickly leads to diffuse involvement of soft tissues of the extremity.

The source of infection for an acute spreading process is usually a minor injury, frequently one whose treatment has been neglected. There usually is lymphangitis, which is manifested by red streaks in the areas of drainage of the involved part. Soon, this

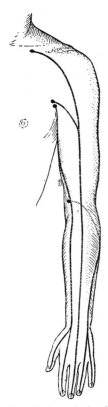

Figure 16. The lymphatics of the hand pursue the shortest course to the dorsum, where they form into a number of channels which pass up the forearm and arm. The drainages from the thumb and index finger usually skip the epitrochlear nodes and empty into the axillary nodes. Those from the ring and little finger pass first through the epitrochlear nodes before emptying into the axillary nodes. Those from the middle finger may miss both sets of nodes and drain directly into the lymphatic vessels in the supraclavicular area. (Mason, M. L.: Infections of the hand. *In,* Sajous: System of Medicine, Surgery and the Specialties. J. B. Lippincott Company.)

treatment is started early, no localization whatever may occur. There will be the streaks of lymphangitis, and the nodal areas will show swelling and tenderness, but the process subsides, often as rapidly as it began, without abscess formation. This latter course is the one usually seen, now that antibiotics are available and promptly administered.

These infections, which were once ranked with peritonitis as a cause of death of victims, have tended to disappear since the advent of antibiotics. While it is true that antibiotic agents are used much too promiscuously, it cannot be denied that their use has forestalled lymphangitis, with a life-threatening infection.

The therapy for acute spreading infections must be aggressive but conservative. Measures must be instituted at once to combat the process. The process must be handled with the greatest gentleness, and all temptations and attempts at persuasion to operative intervention must be firmly resisted. Operative intervention before the process has been brought to a standstill is certain to lead to disaster. In the preantibiotic days, some patients lost their lives and many patients became hand cripples from the sudden and uncontrollable spread which followed ill-advised active intervention.

The patient with a spreading infection must be immobilized immediately in a hospital, and measures instituted promptly to favor localization of the process. The hand,

process is complicated by a much more diffuse and tense swelling, particularly of the dorsum of the hand and forearm. Localization of infection follows certain predictable patterns, depending upon the site of inoculation (Fig. 17).

If inoculation occurred on the volar surface of a finger, the lymphatics in passing from volar to dorsal surface lead to a tenosynovitis of the digit. The infection not infrequently becomes localized on the dorsal surface of the hand and wrist. In fact, in many instances, localization occurs over the dorsum of the wrist, and is associated with extensive necrosis of subcutaneous tissues and sloughing of overlying skin.

Such extensive invasion and local necrosis do not always develop. There may be marked lymphangitis and inflammation of epitrochlear and axillary nodes, which may occasionally break down into abscesses. When

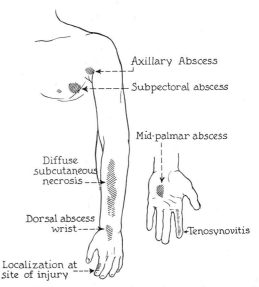

Figure 17. The acute spreading infections show several quite definite patterns of spread and localization as described by Koch.

forearm and arm are placed on a splint, enclosed in a voluminous, warm, moist pack and kept at rest. This prevents motion, the consequent milking of lymphatics, and the breakdown of whatever barrier is being laid down by body defense processes. Fluids and sedatives for pain should be given. Antibiotics are given in large doses from the start. If material is available for bacteriologic identification and study of sensitivity, the appropriate agent is given.

This regimen is maintained until the process has been brought under control, which may occur in 24 hours or may require several days. The subsidence of the process is evidenced by disappearance of local signs of lymphatic inflammation and diminution of general symptoms. In many instances, no localization occurs and the findings and symptoms subside completely over a period of several days. If localization occurs, the involved area, usually over the dorsum of the wrist, suddenly softens; the overlying skin may show areas of necrosis and, when these are opened, copious discharge of necrotic subcutaneous tissue and pus takes place. If an infection had its onset on the volar surface and a suppurative tenosynovitis has been present, its presence will have been evident and the severe pain associated with it will have subsided.

At this time, drainage should be instituted if necessary. Drainage is needed when suppurative tenosynovitis has been present. The dorsal subcutaneous processes often drain spontaneously, although incisions will hasten recovery. Following drainage, warm moist packs and splints are maintained for two or three days, following which they may be discontinued and dry dressings or dressings moistened with saline solution are instituted.

HUMAN BITE INFECTIONS. Injuries to the hand from contact with the teeth of a human opponent are not infrequently encountered. If these wounds are not recognized for what they are when first seen, or if an individual neglects to seek help, serious infections may occur. Most often the wound is received when one person strikes another, his knuckles coming in contact with his opponent's teeth. The skin and tendon are tightly stretched over the metacarpophalangeal joint and are easily perforated, leading to direct contamination of the joint cavity. At the same time, several other spaces are entered above and beneath the extensor tendon. As the joint straightens, tissues slide back in layers and effectively seal the wound. Suppurative arthritis, sub-

fascial and subtendinous infection may develop and, if the process lasts long enough, infection may pass into the palm via the lumbrical canals.

The tissues are not just perforated, but crushed, and hence are less resistant to infection. The organisms introduced into the tissues are extremely virulent and immediately invasive. Both aerobic and anaerobic streptococci and staphylococci, as well as various spirochetes and numerous other organisms, will be found on smear and cultures. These lead to immediate development of infection characterized by production of foul-smelling pus. Unless brought under control, a severe acute spreading infection supervenes and may lead to a fatal process. Locally, the process invades and destroys bones and joints.

When these injuries are seen early, they should be widely opened, excised and irrigated. Under no circumstances should these wounds be closed. The extensor tendon, which is not infrequently divided, should not be repaired. The hand should be splinted in the position of function and a voluminous warm, moist dressing applied.

Antibiotics should be started at once in large doses. Bacitracin, applied locally, has proved of great service in these patients. As soon as bacteriologic studies have been completed, it may be necessary to change the antibiotic therapy.

The further management consists in securing proper drainage, when and if required. There is a temptation to attack bones surgically when osteomyelitis appears. It must be remembered that the roentgenologic findings may simply represent calcium absorption and not actual destruction. The osteomyelitis is managed, as in the case of felon, by watchful waiting and maintaining adequate soft-tissue drainage, and removing sequestra when they appear.

TUBERCULOUS TENOSYNOVITIS. This disease should be suspected whenever chronic swellings involve tendon sheaths and bursae of the hand and wrist (Fig. 18). Such synovial lesions are commonly called compound ganglia. Absolute proof that the process is tuberculous depends upon isolation of the organism by culture or guinea-pig inoculation from material removed at operation.

Other foci of active tuberculosis, such as pulmonary or renal lesions, may be present. However, in many patients there is no clue as to the source of synovial disease. Direct inoculation of the tendon sheath is a rare

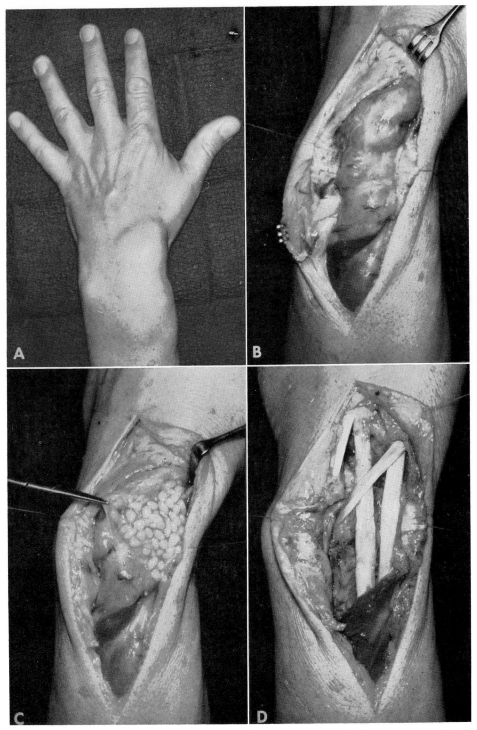

Figure 18.   A, Tuberculous tenosynovitis of the dorsum of the hand and wrist. B, The synovial sheaths are markedly thickened. C, Rice bodies are often contained within diseased tendon sheaths. D, In this instance, the completed excision shows tendons without gross evidence of invasion.

possibility. Usually, the disease is unilateral, but bilateral involvement does not exclude the possibility of tuberculosis. It is imperative to examine the patient carefully for evidence of pulmonary and bone or joint involvement.

The radial and ulnar bursae of the hand are the most frequently involved; next in frequency are the dorsal tendon sheaths of the hand; then the digital sheaths of the index, middle and ring fingers. The radial and ulnar bursae are almost always infected together, but their distal prolongations into the thumb and little finger may remain free from disease.

The sheaths may be slightly thickened and injected, and contain a moderate amount of yellow serous fluid. More often, however, both parietal and visceral layers are thick and shaggy. The enclosed tendons are gray and lusterless, while in the small amount of yellow fluid are fibrin flakes and rice bodies. There may be extensive formation of granulation tissue with caseation and destruction, with or without rice-body formation. As the disease progresses, tendons are invaded and whole segments of tendon are destroyed or so fragmented as to require removal. In late cases, bones, joints and muscles are invaded and cold abscesses form, with their attendant danger of secondary infection. The median nerve, though compressed and swollen, is never infiltrated.

The rice bodies, or melon-seed bodies, are small, grayish, ovoid or kidney-shaped masses, varying in length from 1 to 15 mm., and in number from one to many hundreds. They are probably the result of mechanical action of moving tendons on villi and fibrin-encrusted products of necrosis of the tendon sheath.

The disease is characterized by insidious development of a slowly progressive, painful or painless swelling over the anatomic area of involved sheaths. Usually, the swelling is preceded by sensory or functional disturbance, such as pain, tingling, numbness or prickling sensations, or by stiffness in one or more fingers. These premonitory symptoms may persist for weeks or months before actual swelling appears. A leathery crepitus may occasionally usher in the process.

The swelling often appears as a sudden diffuse edema which responds to rest, only to be replaced by a more localized, persistent swelling. With involvement of the radial and ulnar bursae, swelling begins at the wrist and extends slowly into the palm, whence it may proceed distally over the volar surfaces of the thumb and little finger. With involvement of digital sheaths of the index, middle and ring fingers, the swelling first appears over the proximal phalanx and then extends proximally into the cul-de-sac of the sheath. In cases of long standing, the disease spreads beyond the limits of the sheaths and leads to swelling in the middle palmar space, thenar space or fascial spaces of the forearm.

Pain is often mild or absent. In some patients, however, a severe burning or throbbing pain occurs which radiates over the extremity and is increased by use of the hand. It may occur only at night or in early morning hours, and leads the patient to seek relief by application of heat or cold. After persisting for several months, the pain usually subsides even though the swelling slowly increases.

In early stages of the disease, the patient has good use of the part except for pain. Stiffness, weakness and difficulty in closing the fist soon develop, while later on, swelling interferes mechanically with movements, and destruction of tendons leads to its actual loss.

If the disease is allowed to progress, bone and joint destruction may render the hand useless, and the formation of cold abscesses or secondary infection may necessitate amputation.

Tuberculous tenosynovitis produces a fusiform swelling which in its early stages may not be apparent unless compared with the sound side. The swelling at the wrist is divided into a proximal and distal half by the transverse carpal or dorsal carpal ligament. On the dorsum of the wrist, the several longitudinal compartments can be discerned, corresponding to the dorsal tendon sheaths. Disease of the digital sheaths produces a swelling resembling spina ventosa. If rice bodies are present, they give a sensation resembling lead shot in a leather bag, and produce a peculiar crepitus when the patient is asked to move his fingers. A moderate amount of atrophy of associated muscles occurs. There is little or no increase in temperature of the part, and the skin appears normal unless cold abscesses, sinuses or secondary infection are present.

Tuberculous tenosynovitis must be differentiated from other forms of chronic tenosynovitis and from tumors of tendon sheaths.

Chronic traumatic tenosynovitis, most often on the dorsum of the hand, is diagnosed by the history of an acute onset following unaccustomed strenuous use and a rapid response to immobilization.

Rheumatoid arthritis frequently involves the tendon sheaths, and the gross operative findings may be indistinguishable from tuberculous tenosynovitis.

Chronic nonspecific tenosynovitis cannot be differentiated except by cultures and microscopic section examinations.

Syphilitic tenosynovitis is rare but may so closely resemble tuberculosis that differentiation is difficult. An acute or subacute inflammation may occur in the secondary stage, and the syphilitic hygroma and chronic gummatous type in the tertiary stage. A diagnosis is established by the presence of associated lesions, a positive serum reaction and response to specific therapy.

Gonorrheal tenosynovitis occurs most often in males. The onset is acute, with rapidly developing pain and loss of function. A tender swelling is produced over the course of the tendon sheath but there is little or no change in the overlying skin. Aspiration of the swelling yields a cloudy, serofibrinous or even purulent fluid.

The common dorsal ganglion produces a tense, circumscribed swelling on the dorsum of the wrist, most often on the radial side.

Xanthomatic tumor, or villinodular synovitis, of tendon sheaths may occasionally lead to confusion when it occurs as a diffuse tumor at the wrist instead of a nodular swelling of a

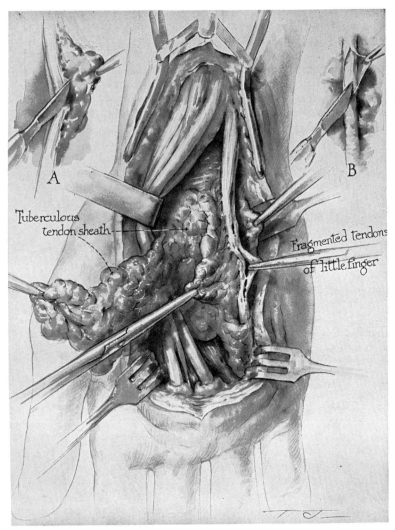

Figure 19.   Details of operative treatment of tuberculous tenosynovitis. After the median nerve has been carefully retracted, each tendon is taken in turn, as in *A*, and the tuberculous tissue removed. Great care must be exercised to remove the visceral layer of the sheath, as in *B*.

finger. It is firmer and more nodular than tenosynovitis, and fluctuation is absent.

Extrasynovial lesions are rarely confused with tuberculous tenosynovitis. A roentgenogram of the hand and wrist should be made to determine the presence of bone or joint involvement.

The prognosis for tuberculous tenosynovitis is good. Few patients are found with active tuberculosis elsewhere, and unless neglected, the local process should not threaten life. If the condition is treated early, a cure should be obtained in the majority of patients, but repeated operations will be necessary in a few. The functional results are good. In an occasional patient, amputation of a digit or an extremity may be necessary.

Management should be directed both toward the local lesion and toward the general state of the patient. The treatment of choice for the local lesion is surgical excision of the diseased tissue. The operation is performed under general anesthesia, in a bloodless field. Appropriate incisions are made, avoiding midline incisions and incisions perpendicular to flexion creases. Great care is taken to identify and isolate important nerves and blood vessels. The tendon sheath is opened, and each tendon in turn is carefully stripped of diseased tissue (Fig. 19), after which the parietal portions of the sheath are excised. Fragmented and diseased portions of tendons must be removed, and it may be necessary to repair tendon defects by means of suture or tendon graft.

Other, less radical, procedures are not recommended. Partial excisions, simple drainage, simple removal of rice bodies and injection of various medicaments have not proved successful.

Following operation, it is advisable to give a course of antituberculous drugs, since it is doubtful if even the most meticulous dissection removes all diseased tissue.

RHEUMATOID ARTHRITIS

Rheumatoid arthritis is a systemic disease affecting mesenchymal tissues. In the hand and wrist, this disease produces an infinite variety of disabling deformities. Surgical treatment has assumed an increasing role in the correction and prevention of deformities resulting from the rheumatoid diathesis. To achieve the best results, however, the combined talents of the surgeon, rheumatologist and physiatrist are needed.

Early in the course of the disease, it may be difficult to establish a diagnosis of rheumatoid arthritis of the hand by clinical and roentgenologic examination. Helpful aids in confirming the clinical impression are an elevated sedimentation rate, a positive agglutination test for rheumatoid factor, tissue biopsy, and analysis of joint fluid.

Tendon sheaths, as well as synovia of joints, frequently are involved in rheumatoid arthritis, and this involvement may long precede any evidence of joint damage. Rheumatoid disease eventually leads to destruction of articular cartilage and subchondral bone. When rheumatoid tenosynovitis is present, tendons may be invaded and destroyed by the disease process.

Many of the deformities produced by rheumatoid arthritis involve the soft tissues alone and result in defects similar to those occurring after injury or other diseases. Some of these are mallet finger, boutonniere deformity, stenosing tenosynovitis, carpal tunnel syndrome, intrinsic contractures, and rupture of the flexor or extensor tendons. Several of these conditions may be present concomitantly in the same hand.

It is now recognized that is is neither necessary nor advisable to postpone surgical procedures until this crippling disease has become quiescent or has run its course of devastation. In fact, early surgical intervention, such as radical synovectomy, may result in lasting local benefit and avoid the development of deformities which are either difficult or impossible to correct by any measures. It has been reported repeatedly that arrest of the systemic rheumatoid process has been achieved following excision of the evident local disease in a hand, foot or other major joint regions.

When small joints of the hand have been destroyed, many variations of arthroplasties of metacarpophalangeal and proximal interphalangeal joints have been described and are useful in selected patients. The status of artificial joint prostheses, however, is still in an experimental phase and should not be undertaken without strict reservations.

INJURIES

Countless accidents in industry, homes and farms involve the forearm and hand. The injuries vary from simple lacerations or contusions to extensive mutilations. The management of hand injuries is based upon certain principles of care which apply to all wounds. After any trauma, it is essential to establish a working diagnosis and a plan of care before proceeding with operative treatment of the wound. If preliminary details are neglected, important injuries of deep structures may be overlooked.

It would be difficult and impractical to contrive a classification of wounds to cover all the complexities of diagnosis, treatment and prognosis. Because of important differences in management and healing, however, it is essential to determine the cause, nature and circumstances of every hand injury. Mechanical injuries are caused by either cutting or crushing forces. Regardless of the anatomic structures involved, any open injury is readily classified as either a tidy or an untidy wound.

Typically, *tidy wounds* are caused by broken glass, knives or other sharp objects (Fig. 20). In these cutting or slicing injuries, tissue damage is confined closely to the path of the wounding agent. In an instant, tendons and nerves may be divided.

Untidy wounds are encountered frequently in accidents resulting from industrial or farm machinery, power tools, explosives and gunshots (Fig. 21). In such injuries, crushing or tearing forces may cause extensive tissue damage which extends far beyond any obvious external wound. Multiple fractures, dislocations, amputations and degloving injuries are commonly observed. In any case, proper initial care should be either definitive or, at the least, should pave the way for early reconstruction.

The chance for an optimal return of function is impaired unless wounds heal by primary intention with little residual scarring. Mobility of soft parts and stability of the bony framework are imperative for securing satisfactory results. The scope of initial treatment depends not only on the type of injury but on many other factors, both local and general.

FIRST AID. First aid for open injuries in-

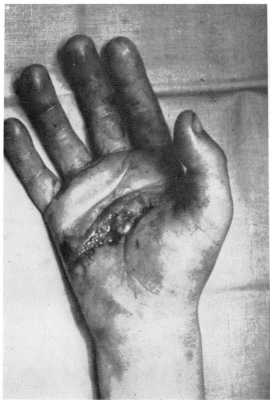

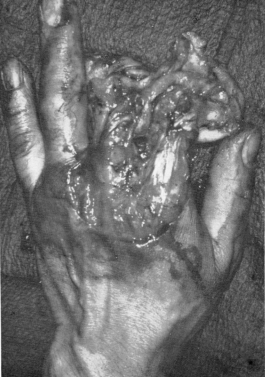

Figure 20   Figure 21

Figure 20.   Tidy wounds are those produced by sharp implements which result in clean-cut injuries. Division of nerves and tendons is determined by clinical examination before proceeding with operative care.

Figure 21.   Untidy injuries, due to crushing forces, are associated with extensive tissue damage, loss of covering skin and devitalization to tissues. Fractures are commonly present. Final assessment of the degree of injury is determined only after careful exploration at the time of operative care of the wound.

cludes measures to control hemorrhage, prevent further bacterial contamination and avoid additional trauma. Wounds should be covered with a sterile dressing, if available, or by a clean cloth until a proper dressing can be applied. Adequate wound dressings serve the dual purpose of avoiding secondary contamination and controlling hemorrhage.

Application of a resilient compression dressing, and elevation of the hand above heart level, usually controls bleeding until the time of operative care. An injured hand or digit should be positioned carefully on a padded splint. In applying the dressing, bony prominences should be protected by padding and gauze placed between digits to prevent constriction of the blood supply and local pressure necrosis. Care should be taken to avoid folding or angulating skin flaps because of the danger of further compromise to their blood supply.

In hand injuries, a tourniquet is rarely indicated as a first aid measure; its use by inexperienced persons is not without danger. Bleeding is accentuated when venous circulation is obstructed, but arterial flow continues unchecked. Constriction without regard to the degree of pressure on the arm can produce severe damage to neurovascular structures underlying the site of a tourniquet.

ASSESSMENT OF ACUTE HAND INJURIES. From an intelligent assessment of information obtained in the history and the examination, a proper plan of management can be outlined. Certain details must be known about the patient as well as the injury. A proper history of trauma should include facts relating to the cause and circumstances of injury, first aid and subsequent care prior to definitive treatment. An estimate of the degree of contamination and the probable severity or extent of tissue damage can be made by correlating these data.

The time lag following injury is important, since it is known that bacteria introduced into wounds require a certain amount of time to propagate and invade tissues. Generally, the latent period is assumed to be six to eight hours. After this interval has lapsed, the extent of reparative surgery permissible is limited to certain necessary elements of wound care.

The manner in which an injury was produced affords some clue to the severity and extent of tissue damage that may be encountered during treatment. Frequently, sharply lacerated wounds are amenable to extensive primary repair. On the other hand, crushed tissues heal poorly and those which may be expected to survive have a reduced capacity for combating contamination.

Some wounds are inoculated with such highly invasive bacteria that deep repair and even primary wound closure are contraindicated. Injuries contaminated initially by oral or intestinal micro-organisms are to be regarded with proper awareness of the danger of severe infection developing in spite of early, thorough wound care. Wounds contaminated with barnyard or street dirt must always be suspected.

Although there may be little primary contamination in many home and industrial accidents, severe secondary contamination can occur from inept first aid or injudicious interference with the wound. The most serious source of secondary contamination is from human oronasal bacteria.

The patient's age, occupation and status of health have an important influence on treatment. The possibility of complications due to diabetes and other serious systemic disease cannot be overlooked. It is particularly important to inquire about drug sensitivity, allergy or untoward past experience with any form of anesthesia. The patient's status regarding tetanus immunization should be ascertained.

Preoperative examination is concerned principally with function of the hand and not with the minute details of the wound. Regardless of the location or appearance of a wound, it must be assumed that deep structures are severed until their integrity is established by either clinical examination or operative intervention. Any inspection of an open wound should be carried out with aseptic precautions. A wound should not be manipulated or probed to try to determine damage to deep structures. Diagnosis of nerve or tendon division is made by performing a few simple tests. Suspected bone and joint injuries have to be confirmed by roentgenologic examination.

In acute injuries of the hand and forearm, elicitation of gross sensory loss provides the most reliable evidence of nerve division. If a patient can cooperate, there is no excuse for overlooking a nerve injury in a tidy wound. Testing for motor reactions of nerves should be done, but in acute injuries it must be remembered that voluntary movements may be restricted because of the pain associated with injury.

A diagnosis of sensory nerve division may be secured by touching the patient's finger tips gently with a wisp of cotton (Fig. 22). It should be remembered that not only must the examiner test for the median and ulnar nerves, but, when injuries involve the palm and digits, each side of every digit must be tested. The common digital or lateral digital nerves may be involved.

Motor functions of the median nerve may be tested by asking the patient to rotate and appose the thumb to the tip of the little finger. This tests the integrity of the motor branch of the median nerve to the thenar muscles. A complete median nerve lesion may be present in the forearm and still the thenar muscles may not be paralyzed, because of crossed innervation from the ulnar nerve. The motor function of the ulnar nerve may be tested by requesting the patient to form a cone with the tips of the fingers. This function is never taken over by the median nerve.

By and large, the sensory findings are by far the most important, since, if the tests are carefully made and the patient is cooperative and intelligent, the findings are unequivocal. In children, the examination is quite difficult and conclusions as to nerve division must often be made on probability.

Examination for tendon division is made by testing the action of the fingers against slight resistance (Fig. 23). The patient is directed to flex each joint. It is sometimes difficult to make the diagnosis of sublimis tendon division in the presence of an intact profundus tendon, although it will usually be noted that the initiation of flexion may be somewhat delayed. The metacarpophalangeal joints, flexed by the interosseus and lumbrical muscles, may act normally even if the tendons are divided, provided the median, and, particularly, the ulnar nerves are intact.

It is possible to have median and ulnar nerve division at the wrist and still have flexion of the digits, if tendons are intact, since innervation of the sublimis and profundus muscles comes from nerve trunks in the forearm well above the wrist. The superficial position of the median nerve, just beneath the palmaris longus tendon, renders it susceptible to injury and, if tendons have been divided at the wrist, it is almost certain that the median nerve is involved.

Any hand with a crushing wound should have a roentgen ray examination, as should one with a saw cut or deep laceration.

Examination should not stop with the hand, but a general examination of the patient must be carried out. Blood and urine tests are essential, especially if a general anesthetic is

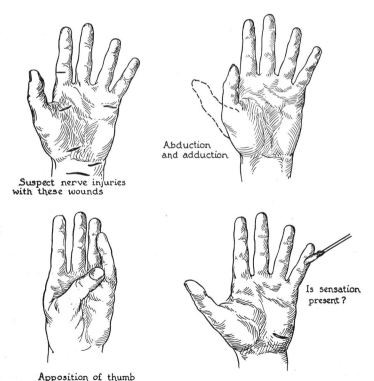

Figure 22. Diagnosis of nerve damage in acute injuries may be made by testing for light touch with a sterile cotton applicator, and testing for motion of the intrinsic muscles. Nerve damage must be suspected and carefully sought for when wounds are present over the course of any of the nerves of the hand.

Suspect nerve injuries with these wounds

Abduction and adduction

Apposition of thumb

Is sensation present?

to be administered. It must not be forgotten that the patient may have other wounds which may take priority over the wound of the hand. It is rare for a wound of the hand to lead to sufficient hemorrhage to cause shock; however, this possibility should be kept in mind.

OPERATIVE CARE. The logical fundamentals of wound care of injuries of the hand are to protect the hand from further injury and bacterial contamination; evaluate the injury thoroughly before embarking upon any treatment; select anesthesia that will be adequate for the scope of any operative procedure; transform the open wound into a surgically clean wound; excise devitalized tissue methodically, but not en bloc; reduce fractures and dislocations to obviate further procedures for stabilization of the skeletal framework of the hand; repair nerves and tendons only as conditions permit; close wounds either primarily or purposely delayed with tissues of unquestionable viability, and immobilize the injured part in the position which favors healing without tension or subsequent deformity.

With the diagnosis made and all other other necessary factors under control, operative care of the wound itself may be undertaken.

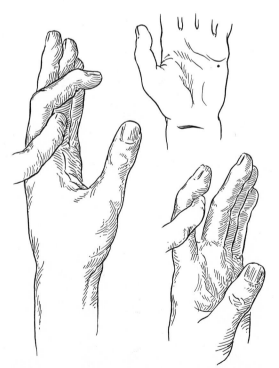

Figure 23. Diagnosis of tendon injury is made by testing motion of the fingers and wrist against slight resistance.

The treatment of open hand injuries, even the most simple, should be carried out under operating room conditions. This does not mean that all the equipment of a major operating room is always needed, but that the wound must be accorded the same aseptic care wherever it is treated. If a correct working diagnosis has been attained, the experienced surgeon does not attempt an extensive reparative procedure in an ill-equipped operating area.

The selection of anesthesia depends upon many factors. For operations on extensively damaged hands, general anesthesia or brachial plexus block anesthesia is preferred. For some injuries, blocks of the median, ulnar or radial nerves are sufficient. Superficial wounds may be treated under local infiltration anesthesia.

A bloodless field is essential during many operations for hand injuries, and is obtained readily by application of a blood-pressure or pneumatic cuff to the arm. In normotensive patients, a pressure of 280 mm. Hg is safe and sufficient to enable accurate identification of nerves and tendons encountered during the procedure. To avoid venous congestion and backflow, the hand should be elevated for at least one minute prior to rapid inflation of the pneumatic cuff to a pressure which prevents arterial bleeding.

For tidy injuries, in which nerves and tendons are involved, it is essential to employ a bloodless field to identify the injured structures. On the other hand, in untidy or crushing injuries a proper assessment of the viability of damaged tissues may be jeopardized further by injudicious use of any type of tourniquet. Finally, it is important to detect any detrimental color changes in skin flaps which are being sutured into place.

Proper preparation of the operative field is an integral part of any surgical procedure. For most hand injuries, the entire hand and forearm must be cleansed. It is often necessary to anesthetize the patient before cleansing can be carried out, particularly in extensive injuries. It may be necessary to have the pneumatic cuff inflated during wound cleansing, since washing may loosen clots and cause bleeding to begin again.

After the patient has been anesthetized, the forearm and dorsum of the hand are shaved. The fingernails are cleaned and trimmed, and sterile gauze pads are placed in the wound while a ten-minute washing with soap and water removes oil, dirt, grease and carbon from the skin of the forearm and hand. This cleansing is performed gently, using large cotton pads and copious amounts of soapy water. The hand is rinsed with sterile water, or isotonic saline solution.

A second sterile field is prepared to re-wash the hand and forearm and to cleanse edges and surfaces of wounds. This procedure requires another ten to 15 minutes. Antiseptic solutions are not applied to skin surfaces or wounds in preparing a hand for operation.

After proper cleansing, the hand is draped with sterile towels and sheets and the limb is positioned on a sturdy armboard which extends at a right angle to the operating table. The surgical team should sit comfortably with their feet braced firmly, and should rest their forearms against the edge of the armboard. This position is not tiring and permits concentration with a minimum of effort and movement.

The first step is wound excision or debridement, which must be carried out in an orderly manner (Fig. 24). Debridement is an exploratory procedure extending into all depths and recesses of the wound to remove debris and blood clots, to ligate torn or divided vessels and to remove devitalized tissues. Wound excision for a crushed hand is a complex procedure, but in most tidy injuries all that is necessary is removal of blood clots and foreign bodies, and ligation of bleeding vessels. For untidy wounds, the first part of debridement involves exploration, and the second concerns removal of devitalized tissues or tissues likely to become necrotic.

Injured and divided structures are identified as they are encountered during exploration, and severely displaced fractures are placed in better alignment. Edges of torn joint capsules are tagged with fine suture material for later identification. Damage to muscle, nerves and tendons is noted. Usually, a bloodless field is used to accomplish the cleansing and exploration of wounds.

After preliminary exploration and estimation of damage, excision of devitalized tissues is the next consideration. Before this can be started, the pneumatic cuff apparatus is deflated to allow return of circulation to the hand. For three to five minutes following release of the pressure, gentle compression is applied by means of moist laparotomy pads to wound surfaces which bleed briskly because of an intense, active hyperemia.

After about five minutes' compression, the pads are carefully removed from the wounds

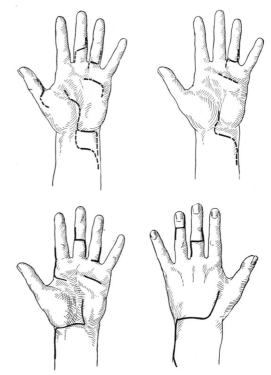

Figure 24. Certain general principles apply to the location of incisions on the hand. Incisions should avoid the midline; they should not cross flexion creases, but should parallel them as closely as possible and should be planned so as to produce flaps of skin and subcutaneous tissue to overlie the operative area. The same principles apply to enlargement of accidental wounds, which should be incorporated as well as possible into the general pattern of ideal incisions. (From Surg. Gyn. & Obst. 70:392, 1940.)

and a thorough examination is made to assess the viability of tissues. Each type of tissue in the hand must be evaluated. Removal of completely avascularized tissues is not a problem, but correct assessment of less severely damaged tissues may be difficult.

Skin, the first tissue encountered, often is the most difficult to evaluate. Flaps of skin with distally based pedicles, or those torn loose as cuffs, cannot be replaced with any degree of assurance that they will survive, no matter how well the flaps fit into position. Eventual necrosis of a major portion of skin so replaced is almost a certainty. Survival of skin pedicles depends upon adequate venous circulation as well as efficient arterial supply. Severely crushed flaps whose vessels are thrombosed should not be retained.

Removal of an appreciable amount of skin from the hand requires some kind of replacement to close the wound. Frequently, joints, tendons, nerves and bones are exposed in areas where coverage with skin and subcutaneous tissue is difficult to accomplish. Needless removal of skin adds to the problem of wound closure; hence, every viable skin tag should be saved at the time of debridement for possible use later. However, there should be no hesitation in excising obviously devitalized skin, regardless of extent.

The tourniquet blush test aids in determining the viability of skin. Return of circulation to the skin of the hand is observed after release of the pressure on the arm. Because of active hyperemia resulting from the sudden inflow of arterial blood, viable skin turns pink but areas deprived completely of arterial supply remain pale. In some instances, however, blanched skin flaps may change gradually to pink after several minutes. When viability is doubtful, it is well to wait for five to ten minutes before removing the skin.

Skin which gradually assumes a purplish hue, indicating impairment of venous return, is difficult to evaluate. When venous return is cut off, the subsequent congestion in the skin often leads to necrosis. In some patients, a compression dressing may save a doubtful flap. To determine the benefit from compression, one should apply firm, gentle pressure to the wound by means of a moist, folded pad and observe the color of the flap after a few minutes. A return to normal color is encouraging, but the skin should be excised if it remains dusky despite the compression.

Viability of muscle is determined by inspection and by testing its contractility. Viable muscle is red, its cut surface bleeds and contraction occurs when it is stimulated by touch. Muscle suffused with dark blood and showing no evidence of active bleeding or contraction is not viable and should be excised. In some injuries, muscles are squeezed from the thenar and hypothenar compartments and protrude through bursting wounds of the skin. A portion of such muscle has to be removed to a point where color is normal and active bleeding is observed from cut surfaces.

Nerves should not be excised unless amputation is necessary. In most crushing injuries, nerves are not severed, but when division is encountered, a fine suture should tag each end of the nerve through perineural tissue to facilitate its identification later.

Tendons are subjected to minimal excision. Although immediate repair may not be possible, any remaining tendon must be covered with viable subcutaneous tissue and skin to avoid eventual necrosis.

Bone fragments without any remaining soft tissue attachments are removed, but bone fragments should not be needlessly sacrificed if there is any connection whatsoever between the fragment and soft tissue. Many extensively comminuted fractures, particularly around joints, may be molded into good position after surrounding soft tissues have been repaired.

In extensive crushing injuries involving multiple digits, the only absolute indication for amputation of a part is complete lack of blood supply. The less definite indications for primary amputation vary considerably. Sound surgical judgment is required before a decision is made concerning removal of a seemingly hopelessly damaged digit. When several fingers are about equally injured, every effort is made to salvage as much as possible of each, since even a crippled finger is better than none.

After debridement, a decision must be made concerning the feasibility and extent of repair of deep structures. It is during this phase of treatment that the cause and circumstances of an injury and sound surgical judgment influence the course. Fractures and dislocations should always be reduced, but primary repair of tendons and nerves requires more consideration.

It is seldom advisable to repair flexor tendons under the conditions encountered in crushing injuries. Frequently, tissues surrounding the site of proposed tendon suture are too extensively damaged to offer any hope for return of the gliding mechanism and active motion. Accessory incisions necessary to expose retracted ends of flexor tendons may interfere with the circulation of skin flaps whose viability is already doubtful. Open fractures associated with injuries of flexor tendons preclude any possibility for tendon repair. Reduction of a fracture and maintenance of its position take precedence over restoration of tendon continuity.

In contrast to flexor tendons, extensors may often be approximated over metacarpal or phalangeal areas, even in the presence of an underlying fracture. Extensor tendons do not retract very far and the cut ends are secured without the need for extensive accessory incisions. Usually, it is possible to cover the site of extensor tendon repair with areolar tissue and skin by shifting a rotation flap. Suture of most extensor tendons will not disturb maintenance of reduction of an accompanying fracture.

Even in tidy injuries, management of flexor

tendons within the digital sheaths presents a special problem. The area between the proximal portion of the fibrous sheath in the palm and insertion of the sublimis tendon on the middle phalanx is commonly called "no-man's land." In this zone, the two sublimis slips and the profundus tendon are encased in a smooth fibrous tube. The results of primary repair are poor in this critical area, and until the problem is solved, treatment is best limited to cleansing, debridement and skin closure. Initial failures at repair jeopardize the chance for functional return even if secondary tendon grafting is carried out.

If performed correctly, excellent results may be anticipated after initial repair of flexor tendons neatly severed in the palm, wrist or lower forearm (Fig. 25). At these sites, an excellent blood supply and abundance of areolar tissue favor healing with minimal adhesions to surrounding tissues. If the line of suture lies beneath the volar carpal ligament, sublimis tendons should be excised and only the profundus tendons repaired. Attempts to approximate both sets of tendons fail because of the development of a dense cicatrix at the site of repair. Results of primary tendon suture in the wrist and in the forearm are superior to secondary reconstruction, for muscle retraction is difficult to overcome after a few weeks have passed.

Results following primary nerve suture in incised wounds, whenever possible, are better than after delayed repair. There is little doubt that return of function, following a carefully performed initial end-to-end suture of the motor branches of the median and ulnar nerves, cannot be surpassed by a delayed secondary procedure after neuromas have

developed, and must be resected, thus producing a continuity defect. Digital nerves should be repaired whenever possible. In the proximal palm and wrist, primary suture of the median and ulnar nerves should be performed if at all permissible.

To obtain the most favorable result, fractures in the hand should be aligned, reduced and stabilized at the time of the primary operative procedure. Overlying soft tissue wounds must heal primarily and fractures must not become displaced during the healing process. Open joints should be closed and covered with living tissue.

The simplest methods possible are recommended for reduction and stabilization of fractured bones in the hand. A guiding principle in treatment is to place an injured part in the position of function. In many instances, an extensively fractured hand may be maintained in the position of function by molding it over a universal splint. However, many open fractures are unstable and become displaced unless some type of internal fixation is used. According to many experienced surgeons, open fractures of the hand can be treated as if they were not compounded, provided that debridement has been adequate and wounds can be closed with viable tissues. Small-caliber Kirschner wires, or stainless steel sutures, may be employed for internal fixation of unstable open fractures. Skeletal traction for maintaining reduction of fractures of multiple digits is not generally satisfactory, and skin traction cannot be used if soft tissue damage in a digit is extensive. One should never use a banjo splint with traction on a digit held in an extended position. This leads to severe shortening of collateral ligaments of joints, and the resultant stiffening often is irreversible.

Following whatever deep repair is indicated, the next step is closure of the wound. If possible, closure should be accomplished with local skin of the hand, for which there is no substitute. Lacerations and wounds in which there has been minimal skin loss may be closed by suture. In crushing injuries, however, despite salvage of every viable skin tag, it is often necessary to provide some type of skin replacement.

If wound closure cannot be accomplished by suture of available local skin, there is recourse to several procedures: free skin grafting, rotation pedicle flaps and distant pedicle flaps. The choice depends mostly on the surface to be covered and the size of the defect.

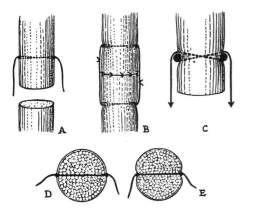

Figure 25. Tendon repair is carried out with the finest possible nonabsorbable sutures; the tendon is handled with extreme care to avoid traumatizing the delicate tissue.

If the recipient site is vascular, and composed of viable areolar or subcutaneous tissue, free skin grafting is the method of choice. Partial-thickness skin grafts suffice for a permanent coverage in most instances.

When bones, tendons or joints are exposed and devoid of overlying areolar tissue, some type of pedicle is required to salvage or preserve some function of these structures, which will become necrotic if they are not covered. One must resist the temptation to replace traumatized flaps so extensively damaged that there is little chance for their survival. Occasionally, it may be possible to shift adjacent areolar tissue over bared structures and close the wound with a free skin graft, but more often a pedicle flap of skin and subcutaneous tissue is necessary. If possible, a rotation flap should be used. Over the dorsal surfaces of the hand and fingers, rotation flaps can be fashioned without difficulty. The flap is rotated to cover the traumatic defect, and its donor area is closed with a partial-thickness skin graft.

When the use of local flaps is not possible, pedicle flaps from more distant areas are required. The cross-finger flap is a most practical means of covering denuded flexor surfaces of digits. Skin on the dorsal surface of fingers is well vascularized, and generous flaps can be raised primarily and transferred to an adjacent digit. The donor site is closed by a partial-thickness graft.

A final method for skin coverage of exposed bone or tendon is application of a pedicle flap from the chest or abdomen. This procedure should be used only if absolutely necessary, particularly in the presence of fractures, since it is difficult to maintain reduction with the hand attached to a flap. At times, however, such flaps may be the only alternative for salvage of the deeper structures, particularly when the defect is extensive.

Following closure of the wound, the hand or part is placed in the position of function and covered by a voluminous compression dressing on a splint. In instances of nerve or tendon repair, however, the functional position cannot be employed, since it provides no means of removing tension from the suture lines.

A compression dressing properly applied deters venous congestion and tends to minimize swelling. It helps to deter accumulation of blood from capillary oozing, but is not a substitute for accurate hemostasis. Compression dressings serve to obliterate dead spaces and prevent accumulation of excess serous fluid in the interstitial spaces. There must be no areas of constriction or excessive pressure on bony prominences. An improper dressing may ruin an otherwise well-performed procedure.

FINGER TIP AMPUTATIONS. Preservation of the length of digits is important in preserving function of the hand. A common injury is an amputation of a segment from the tip of a finger. Since it is not possible to close these wounds by suture, the temptation is to amputate the bone higher up in order to procure flaps to cover over the tip. This produces a good stump, but necessitates sacrifice of length. If there is adequate subcutaneous tissue overlying the bone, the preferred procedure is to cover the amputated tip with a partial-thickness skin graft, usually taken from the volar surface of the forearm, a procedure which can be done with the patient under local anesthesia and without special equipment. When the bone is exposed, a free skin graft will not provide adequate padding to the tip. In these instances, a pedicle flap raised from the dorsum of an adjacent digit will provide a satisfactory covering over the bone. These cross-finger flaps also are useful to cover an amputated thumb tip. Donor sites of the pedicles are closed with partial-thickness skin grafts.

EXTENSIVE CRUSHING INJURIES. These present some of the most difficult surgical problems. At first glance, many look as if nothing could be done in the way of repair and, if a pessimistic attitude is assumed, needless sacrifice of tissue may result. It is not possible to assess these injuries until the hand has been cleansed and the obviously nonviable tissue has been excised. Great care is taken in excision to retain all viable tissue, even though it may appear that much of it will be useless. When complete excision has been accomplished, the surgeon then reviews what is left and tries to fashion from the viable remnants as functional a hand as the tissues left by trauma will permit.

The approach to the problem is to restore function, not appearance. To make the decision on function, the surgeon must understand what the essential functions of the hand are. The finer functions and motions may eventually be restored, but effort is first made to restore basic sensation, grasp and pinch.

If these principles are followed in crushing injuries, it follows that, in most, nerve repair should be carried out, since a hand without sensation is almost useless. Restoration of grasp and pinch may seen hopeless, especially in the presence of multiple tendon injuries. Loss of skin may be extensive and repairs of tendons must await not only wound healing, but also application of a pedicled flap under which tendon repair may be undertaken. Multiple fractures and loss of bone and digits may leave a poor framework and little to work with. However, the surgeon should remember that molding the hand or its remnants into the position of function will give the part the best chance for function. Molding will bring fractures into alignment and digits, or their remnants, into the grasping position. With the hand in this position, the surgeon will be able to visualize functional possibilities of the remnants and can utilize flaps to the best advantage. If no more than closure can be accomplished, with fractures reduced and the hand in the position of function, a great step will have been achieved.

Later, flaps of skin may be applied to replace skin grafts and to make a suitable bed for tendon repair. If such are needed, a hand in the position of function makes the best possible starting point.

TENDON INJURIES. Repair of divided or ruptured tendons of the hand is based upon a knowledge of tendon healing, an appreciation of the delicate structure of the tissues to be dealt with, and a willingness to follow a strict and careful technique in handling these tissues. It is not a question of simply obtaining union of tendon to tendon, or tendon to bone. This will occur quite readily if these structures are kept in contact for a sufficiently long time. It is a matter of obtaining union where it is wanted and free gliding along the remainder of the course. It is a matter of obtaining primary healing at all stages of surgery, and of maintaining mobility of joints, which rapidly stiffen when they are kept immobile. It is a matter of knowing when to start motion, and how and when to encourage active and purposeful use.

When severed tendons are first brought together, or when tendons are sutured to bone, a definite healing process begins which may conveniently be divided into four phases (Figs. 26 and 27). The first, or exudative, phase of union is characterized by an outpouring of body fluids at the site of union. This exudate soon coagulates into fibrin, which glues the ends of the tendons together rather weakly, so that they can be separated

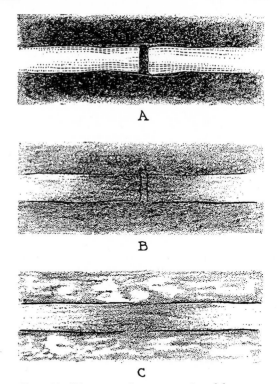

Figure 26. Diagrammatic representation of the manner of healing of a tendon. *A,* First week: proliferation of peritendinous and intratendinous connective tissue. *B,* Second week: tendon cell proliferation and obliteration of gap. *C,* Third to fourth week: consolidation of gap tissues and beginning stages in adaptation of surrounding tissues to subserve gliding function. From the fourth week on, and for many months thereafter, the union undergoes slow changes of maturation resulting in reduced cellularity, an increase in collagen and an increase in tensile strength.

by very slight pull. Soon, however, this fibrinous area is infiltrated by fibroblasts which come from various sources, more especially at the onset by fibroblasts from the surrounding tissues and sheath elements of the tendon.

This fibroblastic union forms the second phase of repair and, while it is much stronger than the fibrinous phase, it is still quite weak and reacts to motion by becoming more and more prolific, and may produce heavy callus which may be palpable. Obviously, if such callus lies near to bone or fibrous tissue, it will become adherent to it and the subsequent gliding of the tendon is seriously jeopardized or even completely prevented.

Toward the end of the third week, the callus begins to soften about the tendon, while that part which lies between the tendon ends becomes more dense and organized; its cells and collagen fibers tend to line up in the direction of tendon pull. At this time, the union has become quite strong and will withstand

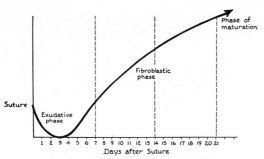

Figure 27. Diagrammatic representation of tensile strength of sutured tendons following suture. When first sutured, the tendons are held together by the sutures only. However, very soon the tendon ends soften in the process of repair, and the sutures tend to pull out. Union during this phase is due only to fibrinous exudate. Not until the seventh day, when fibrous proliferation has started, has the line of union approached in tensile strength that equal to the holding power of sutures alone. From then on, a gradual increase in strength occurs and by the nineteenth to twenty-first day is sufficient to permit some active but guarded use. Thereafter, increase in strength, as a process of maturation, continues over a period of many months.

a fair pull without rupturing. It would seem, at this phase of the healing process, that some motion is helpful and tends to strengthen the union.

The final phase of healing begins at this time and is known as maturation. At the start, motion and use must be restricted for a week or ten days. Strenuous use and sudden forceful tensions are best avoided until the end of the fifth or sixth week after repair. Maturation lasts for many weeks or months, until the site of union has become as strong as or stronger than the normal tendon.

Relaxation of the sutured tendon is necessary to prevent separation of the tendon ends during early stages of repair, since union at this time is weak and easily separated. During the second ten days following suture, strenuous use will lead to separation, while even mild motion without much force may lead to increase in the size of the tendon callus and its consequent firm adherence to surrounding tissues. Following tendon repair, the parts are splinted in relaxation for a period of three weeks, permitting no motion of any sort until the end of that time.

In case of the flexor tendons, the wrist is held flexed at about 30 degrees and the involved fingers in what approximates the position of function: slightly flexed, more so at the metacarpophalangeal joints than at the interphalangeal joints.

At the end of three weeks, the wrist is kept flexed on a splint and the fingers are provided with check reins which permit flexion but prevent more than just slight extension. This small splint and the check reins are worn for a week to ten days, during which time the patient is permitted to flex the digits and mobilize them actively. After about ten days of this restricted motion, the splint is removed entirely and the patient is permitted and encouraged to use his hand in his daily life activities. Strenuous duties are, however, not permitted for another couple of weeks.

When dressings and splints have been removed, the patient is instructed in "daily soaks." These are not just soaking of the hand in warm water, but consist in warm soapy hand washes, using a cloth or simply washing one hand against the other for four to five minutes, four or five times daily. Both hands are washed, since it is the motion of the fingers and intrinsic muscles of the hand which act on the vessels to pump the blood though the tissues and into the forearm veins. It must be stressed to the patient that perfunctory fluttering of the fingers and waving them in the air is not accomplishing anything. The patient is told to feel the flexor muscles of his forearm, and to make them hard by contracting them forcefully.

Splinting following repair of extensor tendons is, of course, just the opposite of that for flexor tendons. In this instance, the wrist is dorsiflexed about 40 degrees and the fingers are extended. However, one must avoid hold-in the metacarpophalangeal joint out to complete extension, since this joint stiffens quickly at complete extension of hyperextension, and correction is difficult. The finger joints, likewise, are seldom splinted in complete extension, unless the tendon division has occurred over the phalanges. In case of the thumb, the digit is abducted and usually extended fully.

Immobilization of the extensor tendons is carried out three and one-half to four weeks for complete immobilization, and another week with restricted motion. Following this, the patient is fitted with a padded splint with straps which he wears at night for a few weeks. The night splint is necessary for extensor tendons since constant flexion, often strong, which occurs during sleep may lead to stretching of the site of union and loss of a certain amount of extension.

RUPTURE OF EXTENSOR POLLICIS LONGUS TENDON. Rupture of this tendon was described many years ago as "drummer's palsy," since it was seen so frequently in drummers in the German army. After years of drumming, these men would suddenly lose the power of extension of a thumb. The condition would come on painlessly but completely, and no amount of conservative therapy would cure it. It was assumed for some time that it was an isolated paralysis of the extensor pollicis longus muscle of unknown cause. However, it was discovered that the condition was actually a rupture of the tendon in an area of attrition along that part of the tendon which moved back and forth over the lower end of the radius, obliquely transverse across the wrist and, finally, distally to the thumb. Age seems to be of some significance in the development of spontaneous rupture, since the circulation of the tendon becomes less as the tendon ages.

Similar rupture of this tendon is seen infrequently following Colles' fracture. It comes on suddenly in the second or third week and is thought to be due to irritative damage to the tendon as it passes over the site of fracture. It is a condition inherent in the fracture and has nothing to do with the reduction or manipulation. It may occur in instances in which reduction is perfect, and has been accomplished with little trauma.

The findings are typical of loss of function of the extensor pollicis longus tendon. The thumb droops forward in flexion at the metacarpophalangeal and interphalangeal joints and the patient is unable to extend it. Although the extensor brevis and abductor longus are functioning, the great significance of the extensor pollicis longus in all motions having to do with extension and abduction is clearly revealed in this injury. When there is doubt as to the diagnosis, the crucial test is extension of the distal phalanx, which is not possible in loss of the extensor longus.

Treatment of the condition is operative. No amount of splinting will restore function. Suture of the tendon is seldom possible or feasible. The ends are degenerated and repair is impossible. It is quite possible to insert a tendon graft between the distal stump at the base of the metacarpal, thread it through the proper tunnel and then attach it to the proximal stump. However, this is a formidable procedure. The proximal stump is difficult to find and requires an extensive dissection in the forearm. Besides these disadvantages, the tendon graft would have to run through a tortuous tunnel with rigid walls and stands a good chance of being stuck therein.

A procedure which fortunately works out well because of availability of tendons is that of tendon transfer. Either the extensor indicis

proprius, or common extensor tendon of the index finger, may be used to provide motor power for the disrupted extensor pollicis longus. The substitute motor tendon is divided proximal to the second metacarpophalangeal joint. It is tunneled subcutaneously to attach to the distal portion of the extensor pollicis longus in the proximal portion of the first metacarpal area.

After-care for tendon transfer consists in splinting of the thumb in the position of abduction and extension for three weeks; then, a removable splint is applied which the patient takes off for a few hours a day for the next two weeks and wears at night for another two weeks. Any vigorous use of the thumb is prohibited for at least six weeks.

BASEBALL FINGER (DROP PHALANGETTE; MALLET FINGER). The insertion of the extensor tendon into the base of the distal phalanx of the finger is extremely thin and is frequently torn when the extended tip is forcibly flexed. The tendon may rupture, usually at the level of the joint, or an avulsion fracture may occur with the bone of insertion being fractured by the pull of the tendon. It is essential to secure x-ray examination to determine if there has been a fracture.

Regardless of cause, there is a typical deformity (Fig. 28). The distal phalanx is flexed and cannot be actively extended. It can be extended passively but drops immediately into a flexed position as soon as the support is released.

Treatment varies with the pathologic condition present, with the probable extent of the damage, and with the time elapsed since the

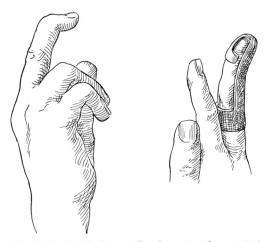

Figure 28. Baseball, or mallet, finger is a characteristic deformity due to rupture or avulsion of the extensor insertion into the base of the distal phalanx.

injury. When there has been avulsion of the tendon with a chip of bone from the phalanx, healing often occurs satisfactorily following splinting of the distal phalanx in hyperextension. This must be maintained for at least five weeks. The patient will have to wear a splint at night for several weeks longer.

For rupture of the tendon without bone avulsion, splinting is often successful, especially if the patient is seen quite early after the injury, and if he wears the splint continuously for a period of five weeks, and at night for a further two to three weeks. The tendon heals quite rapidly; however, it is tissue-paper thin at the site of rupture and the thin callus stretches easily so that even though a full extension may be present early the tip will droop later. It is sometimes difficult to prevent a certain amount of dropped tip even under the best of conditions.

When the condition is seen late, an open repair may be necessary since the gap between the torn ends of the tendon fills quickly with callus, and splinting in extension cannot be expected to shorten this callus. The open procedure consists in tendon shortening or, rather, callus shortening, since the distal stump is short and thin. The callus is divided obliquely in a longitudinal fashion and then, with the finger in maximum extension, the two flaps are overlapped and tacked together with a few fine sutures. The essential step is to maintain the hyperextension, since the sutures themselves serve little function after the first day. At times, it may be indicated to put a tendon graft into the digit to secure more stable union.

After-care following operation is the same as the treatment of acute injury, namely, continuous uninterrupted extension of the finger for a minimum of five weeks, and a splint at night for a further two to three weeks.

BUTTONHOLE DISLOCATION. This term applies to the deformity following the division of the central slip of the extensor, usually just distal to the proximal interphalangeal joint. In order to understand the deformity produced by this division and to rationalize its treatment, it is necessary to understand the anatomic arrangement obtaining with regard to the insertion of the extensor tendons on the digits.

The common and proper extensors of the index, middle, ring and little fingers originate in the forearm and, after passing through synovial sheaths on the dorsum of the wrist, reach the region of the metacarpophalangeal joints. Certain fibers attach to the base of the proximal phalanx, where they serve as extensors of the joint. The capsule and these tendon slips form what is known as the extensor hood. Approaching the hood from the sides are the tendons of the lumbrical and interosseus muscles, which form the lateral slips of the extensor aponeurosis. These slips become attached to the central slip, or that portion of the extensor aponeurosis coming from the common extensor tendons, distal to the metacarpophalangeal joint, passing along the side of the proximal phalanx and proximal interphalangeal joint to reach the dorsum of the finger. The lateral slips come together distal to the proximal interphalangeal joint and proceed as a single band distally to insert in the base of the distal phalanx. The central slip in the meantime has inserted into the base of the middle phalanx where the majority of its fibers stop.

This arrangement accounts for the fact that the lumbrical and interosseus muscles act as flexors of the metacarpophalangeal joint and extend the interphalangeal joints. It accounts for the fact that the central slips coming from the common and proper extensors extend the metacarpophalangeal and proximal interphalangeal joints, but do not extend the distal interphalangeal joint unless the whole extensor expansion is put under tension by flexion of the wrist and flexion of the metacarpophalangeal joints. When the central slip of the extensor aponeurosis has been divided, the proximal interphalangeal joint drops down into flexion and the extensor communis retracts. At the same time, the lateral slips become tense and exert pull on the distal phalanx to draw this joint into extension. With the central slip divided, the lateral slips dislocate forward, thus accentuating flexion of the proximal interphalangeal joint. A typical deformity is thus produced. The proximal interphalangeal joint tends to become more acutely flexed and the distal joint eventually becomes hyperextended. This deformity is called buttonhole dislocation since the joint, while not actually dislocated, projects dorsally between the lateral slips of the extensor aponeurosis.

Repair of this injury entails repair of the divided tendon, which is not simple since the situation is usually not seen early, and contracture has already occurred. It is usually necessary to relocate the lateral slips as well as repair the central slip. For this procedure, tendon grafts are often necessary.

It is sometimes possible early to secure satisfactory healing by splinting of the proximal interphalangeal joint in extension. A splint should permit some flexion of the distal interphalangeal joint. If a patient is seen late, this same splinting should be carried out to correct the deformity before operation. In some instances, even when the patient is seen late, this splinting may correct the condition.

RUPTURE OF FLEXOR TENDONS. Flexor tendons rarely rupture. In certain types of injuries, the tendon may pull out along with a digit, tearing through at the musculotendinous junction. Rarely, a flexor profundus will rupture through the insertion into the distal phalanx. When it does so, it will retract variable distances up the sheath, often restricted by the vincula. Symptoms are those one would expect from loss of the proper flexor of the distal phalanx. Repair usually entails a tendon graft since, except soon after injury, it will be impossible to bring the stump distally and reinsert it into the distal phalanx.

BURNS

While the principles of care are the same wherever a burn may occur, there are certain special features in burns of the hand which require emphasis.

It cannot be stressed too strongly that, from the very start of care, it is important to place the hand in the position of function and maintain it on a splint under a compression dressing until healing has been secured. The hand goes so easily into a vicious position, if great precautions are not taken to prevent it, that this must be a constant care of the surgeon attending a patient with a burned hand. A compression dressing is of importance for, although this does not entirely prevent the formation of swelling and edema, it does tend to minimize it. Much of the stiffness of the hand which occurs after burns is due to the organization of the exudate which comes with burns. If this exudate can be reduced in amount, and if the hand can be kept in the position of function, much of the disability following burns will be avoided.

A good result following care of a burned hand depends on securing early healing. The longer sloughs are allowed to remain and the longer raw surfaces are allowed to stay open, the greater will be the scar.

Many deep second degree burns of the hand become converted into third degree burns by infection. Hence, every means possible should be taken to prevent the development of infection.

Burns of the dorsum of the hand especially, even if not full thickness, tend to heal with thick keloid scars which contract and form an armor-like covering which seriously interferes with function.

Full-thickness burns of the hand should be excised early and the raw surface covered with split grafts. These grafts will seldom be the definitive cover for these areas, probably because it is not possible to carry out a complete excision in depth and in extent of the burn. However, they secure early healing and minimize deep scarring. Later, it will be possible to excise these areas and apply more suitable grafts.

Dorsal burns of the hand, especially when the fingers are affected, tend to expose the tendons and the interphalangeal joints, especially the proximal joints. This unfortunate condition may result when the burn, originally perhaps deep second, becomes converted into third degree or full-thickness loss from infection. It is, therefore, especially important to get rid of slough or destroyed areas as early as possible, and to secure healing.

Maintenance of the position of function is not as easy to accomplish as it may seem when deep burns and massive destruction are present. It is, however, not enough to keep the hand in the position of function. Unless the surgeon also secures early coverage, splinting the hand is of no avail, since the raw surfaces pile up granulations and the scar becomes thicker and more contractile.

Further care of the deep destructive burn with loss of tendons, joint fusions and severe contractures consists in the provision of adequate covering tissue, in securing the position of function and in providing as much motion to the hand as the contracture permits.

VOLKMANN'S ISCHEMIC CONTRACTURE

This crippling condition, when fully developed, is characterized by necrosis, followed by fibrous replacement of the flexor muscles of the forearm and wrist, with subsequent contracture that leads to flexion deformity of the wrist and hand. Associated with it are varying degrees of nerve involvement, particularly of the median but also of the ulnar nerve. It is most frequently seen following supracondylar fractures, particularly those treated in flexion with tight casts, but may occur without these etiologic factors. A similar muscular condition may occur in the small muscles of the hand alone, often due to constricting bandages and leading to a typical contracture deformity from shortening of the interosseus muscles.

The pathogenesis of the condition is not clear. In most instances, it would appear that swelling due to hemorrhage and edema in an extremity, which cannot expand because of tightness of fascial compartments or tight dressings, or both, is the prime factor. However, in those instances in which tight dressings are not present, and in which the mechanical factor of compression does not obtain, it is thought that arterial damage over the fracture site or arterial spasm is present to account for the necrosis due to lack of blood supply. Considerable experimental work has failed to explain the condition satisfactorily.

In some instances, the median and ulnar paralysis recovers gradually while the patient is undergoing conservative treatment. In other patients, exploration of the forearm has shown the nerves to be reduced to scarred cords for a considerable area. In some, the median nerve at the elbow is actually divided or compressed by bone fragments, or is constricted by scar involving the pronator teres. The nerve condition, however, is not the cause of the necrosis, but rather part of, or secondary to it.

The brachial artery may be impinged on bony fragments at the elbow and its flow stopped. The significance of this in causing true Volkmann's contracture is likewise not clear. Certainly, arterial blockage is more likely to lead to gangrene than to Volkmann's contracture.

The significance of compression is real, as evidenced by the beneficial effects of release of compression by division of the cast and straightening of the elbow.

The onset of Volkmann's contracture is ushered in by severe pain in the forearm and hand. The radial pulse disappears and the hand becomes swollen and blue. If the situation is recognized early, if tight dressings are removed, and if the flexed elbow is straightened, the initial symptoms may subside, the pulse return and the pain disappear. If these symptoms are ignored, however, or if the patient is not under hourly surveillance, irreparable damage results. The pain will slowly subside after reaching a peak; the fingers gradually contract into flexion and

swelling recedes. When the cast is finally removed, areas of necrosis of skin and subcutaneous tissues of the forearm will usually be found. When this process has cleared, the typical deformity will be present.

When fully developed, the deformity produces an unmistakable picture. The forearm is markedly atrophic, especially the volar aspect. The fingers are thin and atrophic and flexed at the interphalangeal joints. The wrist is flexed and the thumb tightly adducted to the side of the hand. The fingers can usually be straightened if the wrist is flexed, but when one attempts to extend the wrist, the fingers flex tightly into the palm. The forearm is pronated and attempts to supinate it meet with resistance.

Sensation may be absent over the median and ulnar nerve distributions. Growth of the forearm and hand almost ceases and, since the condition is seen particularly in youngsters, it is not long before this difference in size is noticeable. The hand becomes an almost useless appendage. There may develop a modicum of flexion, but the range is limited and extension is restricted by the contracted flexor muscles.

Treatment depends upon the stage in which the condition is encountered. When the premonitory symptoms occur, immediate steps must be taken to release all constricting casts or dressings and to readjust the elbow to the point where the radial pulse returns. It may be necessary to attempt some other means of controlling the fracture. At the moment, the most serious problem is that of combating the threatened Volkmann's contracture.

If conservative measures fail, the surgeon must consider releasing tension under the forearm fascia, by wide splitting of the fascia, leaving it open, although the skin may usually be closed. At this time, opportunity should be taken to inspect the brachial artery which may be damaged or in spasm. The spasm may release spontaneously or infiltration of Novocain in the area may effect release. The median nerve should be inspected.

When the contracture has become established, treatment is long and tedious. Corrective tension-splinting should be started early. This is designed to prevent or correct the flexion contracture by exerting constant but gentle pull of the fingers and wrist into extension, to hold or pull the thumb into abduction and extension, and rotate the forearm into supination. Numerous ingenious splints have been devised to accomplish this end.

None is perfect and all require constant watching and attention. The pressure must be accurately adjusted and inspection must be frequent lest the patient develop pressure areas.

Splinting and physical therapy may restore a hand to considerable function. However, much depends upon the extent to which muscles and nerves have been damaged. Obviously, if there are no living muscle fibers in the flexor group, one cannot hope for return of function. If, however, some motion can be detected in them, there is a chance that, with use, a fair amount of function can be developed.

If it is not possible to bring digits into a functional position, and there appears to be a fair amount of muscle present which is too short, some means of compensating for this discrepancy may be considered. Several possibilities present themselves, such as detaching the flexor group at its origin and advancing it an inch or so distally on the forearm. Another possibility is to shorten the forearm by removing segments of the radius and ulna. It has been suggested to remove one row of carpal bones. The general principle is to shorten the forearm or lengthen the tendons, so as to permit the digits to be extended.

In patients in whom sensory and motor recovery does not occur after a reasonable time, it is advisable to explore the median and ulnar nerves. This may or may not be successful. When no motor function can be detected in the entire flexor group, the only remedy is to attempt transfer of functioning tendons into the nonfunctioning flexors. Usually, the extensors of the wrist are functioning and may be utilized for this purpose.

DUPUYTREN'S CONTRACTURE

This tumor-like proliferation of the palmar aponeurosis is called Dupuytren's contracture or palmar fibromatosis. In 1822, Sir Astley Cooper wrote about flexion contracture due to chronic inflammation of the palmar fascia. Ten years later, Baron Guillaume Dupuytren of Paris described in detail an anatomic dissection of a cadaver's hand with digital flexion deformities caused by thickening of the palmar aponeurosis. Since that time, Dupuytren's name has been associated with this disease of unknown cause.

Dupuytren's contracture is a condition involving the palmar aponeurosis and its pro-

longations and connections, leading to the formation of hard fibrous nodules and bands in the palm, interdigital clefts and digits, and producing contractures of the skin and fingers (Figs. 29 and 30).

To understand Dupuytren's contracture, the anatomy of the fascia of the hand, particularly the palmar fascia which is the structure involved in the disease, is essential (Fig. 31).

The palmar aponeurosis is a triangular plaque of fascia beneath the subcutaneous fat of the palm. Proximally, it begins at the level of the transverse volar carpal ligament. From the apex of the fascial triangle, the palmar aponeurosis broadens as it passes to the distal part of the palm. Distally, the fascia is composed of four prominent pretendinous bands with transverse interconnections. These bands are not attached to the flexor tendons. As the pretendinous bands approach the fingers, the separate like ribs of a fan and pass into the fingers to blend into the superficial digital fascia. At the web spaces, transverse fibers pass from one band to another. These transverse fasciculi are called natatory ligaments.

From the deep surface of the palmar fascia, vertical septa pass between the flexor tendons to attach to the fascia covering the metacarpal and interosseus muscles. Secondary vertical septa envelop the neurovascular bundles in the palm. In Dupuytren's contracture, the pathologic process involves both the triangular portion and the vertical ramifications of the palmar aponeurosis.

The cause of this disease is unknown. Many theories have been proposed, but none has

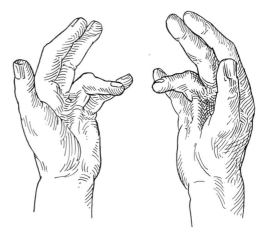

Figure 29. Typical Dupuytren's contracture: flexion of the ring finger, moderate flexion of little and middle fingers and a hard, fibrous band beneath the palmar skin.

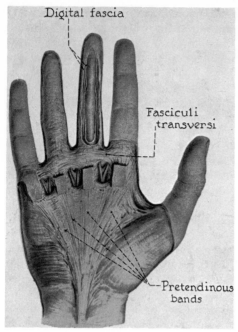

Figure 30. The superficial palmar fascia or palmar aponeurosis. This is the tissue involved in Dupuytren's contracture.

found universal acceptance. Most investigators agree on certain predisposing factors, but no single factor is predominant.

Among the accepted predisposing factors are age, sex and heredity. The majority of persons with Dupuytren's contracture are 50 to 60 years of age, but it is also observed in younger persons. The condition is encoun-

tered in males more frequently than in females. The usual ratio reported is 8 to 1.

The factor of hereditary influence has been demonstrated in about 30 per cent of patients in many series of studies. This, while not universal, has been more consistent than any other. It is found not infrequently in a family for two or three generations.

As far as trauma as an etiologic agent is concerned, this seems to have the strongest support. However, the evidence is equivocal and circumstantial. The history of trauma is by no means universally present, not even in an overwhelming majority of individuals afflicted. The hands obviously are the most subject to trauma of any part of the body, so that one would be hard put to find a patient who could not give a history of some sort of trauma to the hands. Usually, the condition begins in one hand, often the right. The patient may give a definite history of an acute injury years before or of excessive use of the hand with repeated trauma to the palm. This seems to fit the condition quite well until several years later the same condition develops in the opposite hand, or is discovered there by the examining surgeon. Nor does Dupuytren's contracture occur only in individuals who do manual labor. It is seen quite frequently in persons whose severest work is the use of pen and pencil.

The gross pathologic state of the condition shows the pretendinous bands to be thickened and shortened. Often, in the region volar to the metacarpophalangeal joints, thick

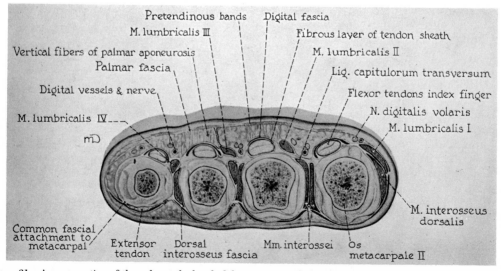

Figure 31. A cross section of the palm at the level of the metacarpophalangeal joints shows the relationship of the pretendinous bands of the palmar fascia to the underlying tendons. The perpendicular sheets from the undersurface of the fascia are shown passing deeply to either side of the tendons to become attached to the deep transverse metacarpal ligaments.

nodules 1 to 2 cm. in diameter can be seen in the hands. Similar thick nodules are found in the volar surfaces of the digits when these are involved. As these bands shorten, they pull the overlying skin into folds and dimples.

The fascia is intimately attached to the undersurface of the skin. Separation is difficult and, in some instances, impossible, so that sacrifice of the skin is required.

As the fascia is pulled away from the underlying tendons, the vertical septa passing dorsalward to either side of the tendons are thickened and, as the fascia is followed distally, the neurovascular bundle becomes enclosed between two sheets. This portion of the fascia may be involved and, when this obtains, the nerves are drawn out of their course, often to the midline of the digit.

The joints and tendons are not primarily involved in the process. Some compensatory shortening may occur. If the joints have been held for a long time in acute flexion, the capsules may contract and a mild subluxation may be present.

Occasionally, the patient will have pads on the dorsal surfaces of the proximal interphalangeal joints. These knuckle pads are not frequently seen, nor is it generally realized that they are part of Dupuytren's contracture. Likewise, in a small percentage of patients, a nodular thickening of the plantar fascia will be found similar to that seen in the hand. In extremely rare instances, plaques of similar nature will be found in the fibrous septum of the penis: Peyronie's disease.

Microscopically, the thickened fascia is made up of dense fibrous tissue, scanty in blood vessels and nuclei. There are scattered areas of increased vascularity and round cell infiltration. Skoog thinks these areas represent healing of microscopic tears in the fascia. On this finding, he bases his contention that Dupuytren's contracture is due to trauma in the form of tiny repeated fascial tears which, upon healing, lead to scar formation with its attendant thickening and contracture of the fascia. There is no evidence that the condition is a tumor, although many contend that the process is a type of fibroma.

The condition begins as a nodular thickening in the palm in the region of the distal palmar crease, generally over the fourth metacarpophalangeal joint. The digits involved are, in order of diminishing frequency: ring, little, middle, index and thumb. Similar thickening also may occur in the web spaces. It is unusual for it to begin as nodules or bands in the digits.

The nodule becomes more prominent, and a thickened hard cord may be felt to extend proximally and often distally, mistaken by the uninitiated for the tendon. Soon, as this band thickens and shortens, the proximal phalanx of the finger is drawn into flexion; at first, flexion is slight, but, as the condition progresses, the finger becomes more flexed at both the metacarpophalangeal and the proximal interphalangeal joints. This may draw the finger down until the tip lies in the palm. The distal interphalangeal joint tends to remain extended, or even hyperextended, because of involvement of the dorsal expansion.

There are few subjective symptoms other than the inconvenience caused by the contractures. Patients complain that it is difficult to shake hands, to hold a golf club or grasp a hammer. Occasionally, one will complain of vague discomfort, rarely of actual pain.

Examination reveals the contractures and thickening in the palm and digits. Early, there may be only the nodule in the palm. However, careful palpation often reveals the thickening of the pretendinous band. It can often be more easily demonstrated if the fingers are passively hyperextended. When this is done, the nodule becomes slightly more prominent and the pretendinous band becomes evident.

The treatment of Dupuytren's contracture is surgical, and in general, there are three types of operative procedures used. In order of increasing frequency they are fasciotomy, limited fasciectomy and radical fasciectomy. The selection of any of the procedures requires careful evaluation of the patient.

Fasciotomy, the simplest of the procedures, usually is performed as an operation preliminary to more extensive excision of the diseased fascia. In subcutaneous fasciotomy, there is danger of cutting blood vessels or nerves in the palm. Most surgeons restrict fasciotomy to those patients in whom more extensive operations are contraindicated.

Limited or partial fasciectomy denotes excision of contracted bands and nodules which have caused an impairment of function. Uninvolved portions of the fascia in the palm or digits are not removed. Partial fasciectomy is done with the realization that other contractures may occur, and if so, another local excision is carried out. In contrast to more extensive excision of the fascia, the convalescence

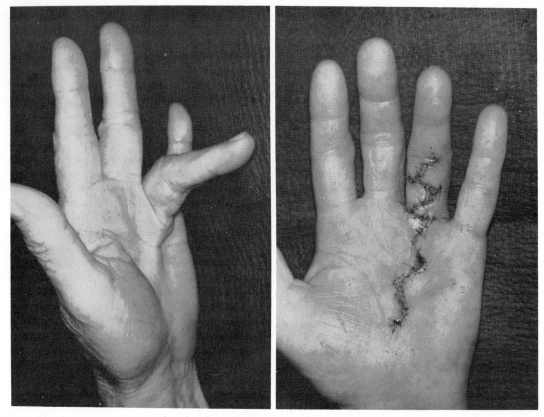

Figure 32. A zig-zag incision combined with transposition flaps heals rapidly without subsequent scar contracture.

following limited fasciectomy is briefer and attended by fewer complications.

In otherwise healthy persons with widespread involvement and evidence of steady progression of the process, a more complete fasciectomy may be indicated. Radical fasciectomy is best reserved for young individuals who have involvement that is progressive and who give a history of an extensive hereditary process.

Fasciectomy, partial or complete, requires use of a bloodless field during dissection, since it is imperative to visualize the nerves, blood vessels and tendons. It is important to use incisions which heal without subsequent scar contractures.

Care is taken to avoid incisions made perpendicular to flexion creases. To obtain adequate exposure, a Z-shaped incision is useful and heals without deformity following transposition of the triangular skin flaps (Fig. 32). There must be complete hemostasis in the wounds. Prior to wound closure, it is essential to evaluate the viability of skin flaps. Skin of questionable viability should be excised and the wound closed by application of a partial-thickness or full-thickness skin graft.

The most serious complication to follow operation is the formation of a hematoma in the palm. This lifts the already poorly vascularized palmar skin, and necrosis is certain to follow. The postoperative course is unduly prolonged and the recovery poor. To avoid this complication, the palmar dressing is applied firmly with large amounts of resilient gauze.

The hand should not be dressed in complete extension following the operation. Complete extension of the fingers puts a great deal of tension on the palmar suture line, and this may lead to necrosis. Full extension also prevents the skin from being pressed firmly into the palm so that hematoma formation is more likely to occur. If held for some time in complete extension, the fingers tend to develop joint capsule changes, so that full flexion is seldom regained.

STENOSING TENOSYNOVITIS

The fibrous sheaths which hold the flexor tendons in position over the metacarpophalangeal joints, and the sheath enclosing the abductor pollicis longus and extensor pollicis brevis alongside the styloid process of the radius, may become thickened and inflamed (Fig. 33). When they do so, they constrict the tendons beneath them, interfering with their action. In the digits, the constriction may cause actual indentations on the tendons. When the patient attempts to flex the finger, it comes down to a certain degree of flexion where it appears to stick. Only with real effort and with pain can the patient complete the flexion. This release may occur suddenly, often with an audible snap, always with a palpable snap. For this reason, this condition is usually called "snapping finger." When an attempt is made to straighten the finger, the process is reversed. The patient is unable to extend the finger actively, and must assist it with the opposite hand. It is a troublesome condition which is a handicap and the patient hesitates to use the painful finger.

Snapping thumb appears both as a congenital and an acquired condition. It is seen in children at birth, or is recognized shortly afterward, since the child refuses to use this digit. In adults, snapping thumb often appears to be an occupational injury, since it occurs in persons who strike the base of the thumb frequently against some object or tool with which they are working.

Stenosing tenosynovitis over the radial styloid is known as de Quervain's disease. Usually it affects one hand, but it may be bilateral, and is most often seen in females. It

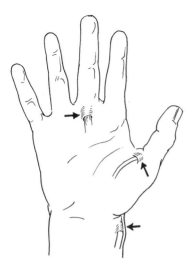

Figure 33. Stenosing tenosynovitis occurs typically in two locations on the hand: in the fibrous sheaths of the flexor tendons over the metacarpophalangeal joints, where it causes snapping finger and snapping thumb, and over the radial styloid where it is called de Quervain's disease.

would frequently appear to be due to trauma, usually to blows over the area, or to wringing actions of the wrist.

The pathologic appearance of snapping tendon and de Quervain's disease is quite similar. When the fibrous sheath is uncovered, it will be found to be thick, tight and constricted about the tendons. Since the patient is usually operated upon under local anesthesia, one can request him to move the affected digit and can actually see the tendon snap in and out beneath the constricted sheath. The tendon itself may present an actual constriction. Occasionally, there may seem to be an actual thickening or nodule in the profundus tendon. Rarely, a tumor, such as a ganglion, may lie within the tendon and cause the trouble. When the thumb is involved, the surgeon more often finds a definite constriction of the flexor pollicis longus tendon.

In de Quervain's disease, the pathologic appearance is similar, except that tendon constriction leading to snapping is not seen and there is usually a moderate inflammatory reaction of the synovial lining. Not infrequently, there is an increase in the fluid content. Microscopically, the tissues show a chronic inflammatory process with fibrosis, and moderate round cell infiltration.

The symptoms and findings in snapping tendon in the digits differ from those of de Quervain's disease. When the digits are involved, the patient usually complains of moderate pain which is referred to the proximal interphalangeal joint. This may persist for some time before actual blocking of tendon movement occurs. Palpation of the proximal end of the sheath in the palm will show that there is thickening and tenderness. If the surgeon palpates this region while the patient flexes or extends the finger, the tendons will be felt to snap back and forth beneath the thickened sheath. Watching the process of flexion and extension will show the temporary stoppage which occurs just before the finger finally "snaps" into full flexion or is brought back, often by use of the opposite hand, into complete extension.

In de Quervain's syndrome, or tenosynovitis over the radial styloid, there is greater pain, and interference with motion is due more to pain than to mechanical block. X-ray examination will reveal no abnormality of the bone, but will show the soft tissue swelling. A sign which is almost pathognomonic of the condition is that adduction of the thumb with ulnar deviation of the wrist is extremely painful.

Treatment of snapping tendon and de Quervain's disease consists in division of the fibrosed sheath. Usually, it is best to excise the roof of the thick tunnel, although this is not absolutely necessary. Incisions for approach to the fibrosed sheath are made transversely at right angles to the tendons, nerves and blood vessels. The operation may be easily done with the patient under local anesthesia, but must be done in a bloodless field. The incision in the palm lies at the level of the distal palmar crease. The sheath is uncovered, care being taken not to damage the neurovascular bundles which lie to either side. The sheath is then split longitudinally to permit free motion of the underlying tendons, which may be tested by asking the patient to move the affected digit. The whole roof of the proximal half of the sheath may be excised without leading to functional disturbance. In the thumb, the approach is the same; however, the surgeon must be extremely cautious, since the digital nerves lie to either side of the flexor tendon quite close to the surface. They are easily injured if not visualized during operation.

In de Quervain's disease, the approach to the sheath or compartment is made transversely across the wrist at the level of the radial styloid. This incision lies directly across the sensory fibers of the radial nerve. Deep dissection should be in a longitudinal direction and the nerve must be identified. The sheath is exposed and divided longitudinally and the interior is inspected. There may be

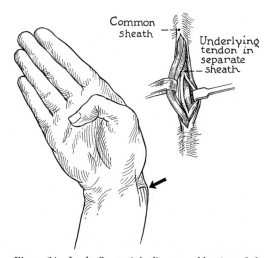

Figure 34. In de Quervain's disease, adduction of the thumb and ulnar adduction of the wrist cause exquisite pain. The tunnel containing the extensor pollicis brevis and adductor pollicis longus may be divided into several compartments, which must all be opened at the time of operation.

more than two tendons passing through this tunnel. In fact, the extensor pollicis brevis, abductor pollicis longus, or both, may be represented by two or three slips each. One or several of these slips may lie in separate tunnels in the wall of the main tunnel (Fig. 34) and, unless these tunnels are also opened, the pain will not be relieved.

TUMORS

A great variety of tumors occur on the hand. Their accessibility and ease of examination should lead to early diagnosis and proper therapy. The vast majority are benign and are amenable to successful surgical removal. Malignant tumors comprise only about 10 per cent of all tumors of the hand and, of these, nearly 90 per cent are carcinoma, most of which arise as the result of irradiation dermatitis. Malignant tumors should be diagnosed, or at least suspected, early and the cure rate should be high.

The anatomy of the hand is such that removal of the superficial tumors frequently entails the necessity of skin replacement, since there is little laxity of cutaneous tissues, particularly on the digits and palmar surface. Deep tumors present their problems in demanding a careful anatomic dissection lest important nerves and tendons be damaged during removal of the tumor mass. Extensive and, particularly, neglected growths may require major reconstructive procedures. Their treatment should not be attempted without adequate experience with this type of surgery.

One-third of all tumors of the hand are ganglia. Another one-third is made up of four other types of tumors in approximately equal numbers: xanthoma, epidermoid cyst, angioma and carcinoma arising from irradiation dermatitis. The remaining third may be divided into two approximately equal groups. One group, or one-sixth of the whole, are carcinoma not due to irradiation, lipoma, fibroma, neuroma and enchondroma in approximately equal numbers. The remaining sixth comprises rare tumors of the hand. Among these are synovioma, glomus tumor, fibrosarcoma, giant cell tumors of bone, osteosarcoma, osteoma, Ewing's tumor, osteoid osteoma, lymphangioma, sweat gland carcinoma, myxoma, leiomyoma and metastatic tumors.

It is customary to group tumors according to the tissues from which they are considered to arise. Thus, there are tumors arising from the skin, from fibrous subcutaneous tissue, from fatty tissues, bones and joints, joint capsules, tendon sheaths and tendons, nerves, blood vessels, lymphatics, smooth and striated muscle. Some growths classified as tumors may very well not be tumors in the real sense of the word. Tumors arising from nerves and fibrous tissue may be confused, and their true status may frequently be in doubt.

Tumors of skin. Subungual wart. The subungual wart is a nuisance, since it forms an unsightly mass at the finger tip, partly under the edge of the nail, and is difficult to keep clean. Removal demands excision of part of the distal nail bed and, not infrequently, a tiny skin graft is needed. The surgeon is inclined to be timid and to leave part of the wart behind and the mass promptly regenerates.

Keratoses. Keratoses and hyperkeratotic lesions are frequently seen on the dorsum of the hand in older people, particularly those who have exposed the skin to wind, sun and weather. They present themselves as slightly raised light brown plaques, rough on the surface and not tender. They should be excised since they may be the forerunners of malignant disease.

Squamous papillomas. These may occur on the hand as well as elsewhere. They resemble soft warts, are quite benign and may be removed surgically under local anesthesia.

Epidermoid cyst. Epidermoid cyst, often referred to as implantation cyst, occurs on the palm and volar surfaces of the digits. It is thought to be due to implantation of small bits of epithelium into the subcutaneous tissues by pricks of thorns or other penetrating types of injury. These cysts differ from sebaceous cysts in that they are derived from the epithelium only, and not from the sebaceous glands. The contents of the cyst consist of desquamated epithelial cells and other cutaneous debris. They are harmless tumors, but occasionally become infected. They may be confused with ganglia and with xanthomas. The treatment is surgical removal, usually under local anesthesia. These cysts show no tendency to recurrence.

Sebaceous cysts. These occur rarely on the hand; when they do, it is on the dorsum. They are treated, as similar cysts elsewhere, by complete removal.

Pigmented nevi. These are rather infrequently seen on the hand. Since the hand is frequently traumatized and exposed, it is wise to excise them to forestall any possibility of their injury. Fairly wide and deep excision should be carried out. Under no circumstances should they be irradiated, fulgurated or cauterized. Nevi should be either left alone or excised widely.

Carcinoma. Carcinoma is the most frequent malignant lesion to occur in the hand, and accounts for 90 per cent of all cancer of the hand.

An interesting feature of carcinoma of the hand is the frequency with which some irritative factor can be discovered in the patient's history (Fig. 35). Because of this frequency,

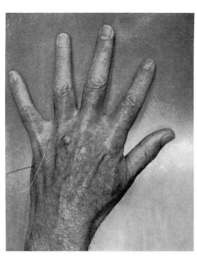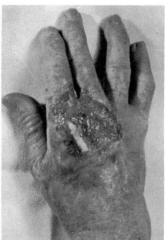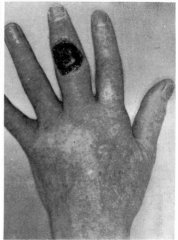

A	*B*	*C*

Figure 35. *A*, Carcinoma of the dorsum of the hand associated with exposure to sunlight. *B*, Carcinoma of the dorsum of the hand arising from a wart. *C*, Carcinoma arising from area of chemical irritation.

it is possible to group carcinomas of the hand into seven categories, depending upon the type of irritation: exposure to sun and weather, irradiation with x-rays and radium, chemical irritation, burn scars, internal medication, chronic infection, and irritation of previously benign lesions. The 30 per cent or less of carcinomas of the hand arising from previously normal skin appear to be the most malignant of cutaneous carcinomas.

Hand cancer occurs with greater frequency in persons whose skin is exposed for long years to the vicissitudes of the sun and weather. A similar higher percentage of carcinoma of the skin of the face is noted in sailors, farmers, ranchers and others who spend much time in the great outdoors.

It is not generally appreciated that irradiation with x-rays and radium is so frequently the cause of carcinoma of the hand. The majority of carcinomas of the hand are due to changes in the skin subsequent to exposure to x-rays or radium. In the overwhelming majority, the exposure has been unnecessary or unwise.

Carcinoma most often results from exposure to small, frequently repeated doses or minute daily exposure over a long time. Thus, when x-rays were first introduced into clinical medicine, their dangerous potentialities were unknown and few or no precautions were taken to guard against the rays.

Later, precautions were taken to prevent or minimize direct exposure. However, it was then realized that even minute exposure to infinitesimal amounts of x-radiation, if kept up day after day, will eventually cause a skin reaction which is persistent. This skin reaction may not become manifest for several years after exposure has been initiated. It persists even if the individual stops exposing himself to irradiation. Not only this, but often as much as 25 years later, the original dermatitis may break down into areas of carcinoma.

At the onset of this type of chronic irradiation dermatitis, the skin becomes dry, atrophic and shiny; the hair may disappear or become sparse on the backs of the hands; the nails become rough and ridged. The cutaneous vessels in the area become apparent as telangiectases. The dry skin is easily traumatized and bothersome to the patient, who treats it with various oils and ointments. Soon, however, numerous areas of keratosis and roughening appear. Areas of skin, which at first appear normal, begin to show changes of dermatitis. Possibly because of a minor injury, or because of exposure to intense sunlight or other irradiation, an area of keratosis may break down into an ulcer. This ulcer may be exquisitely tender, so that the patient hesitates to permit anyone to examine it.

Pain is more frequent and severe in relatively acute ulcers than in the chronic ones. The development of an ulcer in chronic dermatitis usually, though not always, indicates malignant disease. In many instances, the malignant lesion develops in situ, often in several areas of the skin. If numerous sections are taken from a segment of skin which has been excised in treatment of the dermatitis, early changes in the epithelial cells in numerous areas, which indicate early malignant change, may be found.

The therapy of irradiation carcinoma, therefore, must be considered in three phases: first, prophylaxis of irradiation dermatitis; second, prophylaxis of carcinoma in irradiation dermatitis; and third, treatment of irradiation carcinoma once it has developed.

With regard to the prophylaxis of irradiation dermatitis, it should go without saying that one should avoid needless exposure to irradiation from any source. Roentgenologists now take adequate precautions against the repetitious exposure to which they are subjected. However, the nonprofessional who uses x-rays, especially in diagnosis, is not so careful and may expose himself frequently to x-rays. The dentist is inclined to be thoughtless in exposing himself to irradiation while taking dental films. Techniques have now been developed which do not entail exposure to irradiation. Many surgeons expose themselves to irradiation while nailing fractured hips. Foreign bodies in the hand, if radiopaque, are easily seen in the fluoroscope and the temptation is great to search for them with forceps through a small skin incision. However, this has often led to serious acute radiation dermatitis both in the patient and the surgeon.

Professional exposure is not the only cause of chronic irradiation dermatitis of the hands. One of the most frequent types of exposure is therapeutic, incurred in the treatment of various chronic recurrent skin diseases. Eczema, ringworm and psoriasis are often treated by irradiation. The evil of this treatment is that the dermatologic condition may clear, either spontaneously or as a result of x-rays, only to recur. The patient returns for more treatment. If it is refused, the patient frequently seeks help elsewhere and often does not inform the other physician of the previous x-ray treatment. Such a performance may be repeated several times, until the patient has received a large dose of x-rays delivered over a period of years. Since the rays are those which especially affect the skin, the damage produced is serious.

Carcinoma is almost always of a squamous cell type and occurs not just in one spot, but in many. Numerous theories have been promulgated as to the mechanism by which this irritant gives rise to carcinoma, especially so many years following its discontinuance. One theory long held has been that the effect the irradiation has upon the circulation of the skin leads to chronic oxygen deprivation, and that this eventually leads to nutritional disturbances which end in carcinoma. Another theory, somewhat similar in nature, has likewise to do with the effect of the irradiation on the vascular system. Dermatitis and telangiectatic vessels occur about the periphery of areas of irradiation. From time to time, these vessels thrombose and the thrombus lying beneath the thin skin forms a dark black speck, known as a "coal spot." The theory is that these spots signify areas of tissue irritation and devitalization, and that they stimulate the epithelium to repeated efforts at regeneration. Eventually, from such irritative stimulation, carcinoma develops.

The treatment of this type of carcinoma may be considered separately from carcinoma arising from apparently normal skin. The prognosis, if the lesion is properly treated at the start, is good. Prophylactic measures may be taken both to prevent the development of the dermatitis and to prevent the occurrence of carcinoma in skin already affected by dermatitis. Likewise, even if carcinoma has developed in the skin, the prognosis is quite good if the initial operation is thorough. If there has been delay in treatment, and invasive carcinoma with lymph node involvement is present, a 25 per cent mortality can be anticipated.

It is wise to excise the involved skin and to replace it at once with grafts. It is not always possible to determine accurately the true limits of the skin involvement at the first observation. An apparently adequate excision may prove later to have been incomplete, since skin which at first appears normal may later show evidence of dermatitis about the borders of the grafts. Why this is so is difficult to explain. The gross appearance of the skin suggests no trouble; however, there must be significant basic changes in the cells, which are latent but which inexorably manifest themselves as time goes on. For this reason, persons who have such lesions should be examined periodically and new manifestations treated. The surgeon will often be surprised when the pathologist reports areas of carcinoma in situ in what appears to be only moderately involved skin.

When carcinoma is present it is treated, as is cutaneous carcinoma elsewhere, by wide excision. If it is attacked early, there will probably be no deep invasion, since the dense fibrosis of corium and blockage of lymphatics tend to hold the process localized. However, once these barriers have been passed, x-ray and radium carcinoma metastasize, as do other squamous cell lesions. Fortunately, the great majority are of low-grade malignancy. However, the roll of roentgen ray martyrs stands as evidence of the malignant possibilities. Lymph node invasion may well occur, and is present in about 50 per cent of the patients in whom enlarged nodes can be felt. Epitrochlear and axillary dissections are indicated if enlargement is felt; otherwise, such dissections do not appear necessary. With deeply invasive carcinoma, in which amputations are needed to effect removal of the local lesion, lymph node removal is advisable regardless of the findings.

Chemical irritation has long been recognized as leading to the development of carcinoma of the skin of the hands. Among the chemical irritants used commercially, of particular importance are coal tar and its derivatives, aniline, oils and greases, paint and coal soot. These are important only when the hands are constantly exposed over long periods. Certain industries are particularly hazardous in this respect; this has been recognized and measures are taken to avoid or minimize exposure.

It is well known that burn scars of long duration, especially those of deep third degree burns with marked keloid formation, may break down into carcinomas. The thin epithelium overlying the dense scar beneath is frequently traumatized, breaks down easily into ulcers, cracks in usage and is frequently infected. Many years, often as many as 60, may elapse between the burn and its breakdown into carcinoma.

Internal medication may be responsible for carcinoma of the hands. Fortunately, the use of Fowler's solution has been curtailed, since this medication used over a period of years often led to arsenical keratosis, which eventually broke down into squamous cell carcinoma. The lesions occur especially on the palms and soles, but may be found wherever there is squamous epithelium, and have been seen in the larynx. The condition is especially treacherous, since not one but multiple carcinomas develop on many regions of the body and continue to do so over a long time, until metastases and a fatal outcome occur.

Chronic infection may be associated with carcinoma of the hand. At one time, areas of cutaneous tuberculosis were irradiated and these occasionally developed carcinoma in association with the tuberculous lesion. Carcinoma may develop in chronic osteomyelitic sinuses on the hand, down which epithelium has grown.

Irritation of previously benign lesions may be responsible for carcinoma of the hand. The ordinary wart, if irritated sufficiently by picking and shaving, or by overdoses of irradiation, may occasionally break down into carcinoma.

Carcinoma of the hand is almost always on the dorsal surface. Why the dorsal skin should more frequently develop carcinoma is not known, although it is tempting to speculate on the possibility of greater exposure of this area to various types of irradiation. Certainly, the palm is more subject to mechanical trauma than is the dorsum and, if mechanical trauma were a factor, here is where carcinoma should occur. Possibly, the histologic difference between palmar and dorsal skin is the reason.

If recognized early for what it is, the lesion is seldom found to be invasive, although it has the same malignant, locally invasive potentialities and tendency to lymphatic spread as do any cutaneous carcinomas. Early wide excision, if there is no deep extension, is frequently sufficient. When invasion has occurred, more extensive procedures are called for and often partial amputations of a metacarpal and its digit will suffice. The extensive lesions involving wide areas of the palm or dorsum, however, require amputation of the hand.

Dissection of the nodes draining the hand should be carried out in all patients in whom these nodes are enlarged or deep invasion has taken place. Whether or not routine axillary and epitrochlear dissection should be carried out in every patient rests on the judgment of the surgeon. Axillary and epitrochlear dissection is not necessary in patients with superficial lesions without deep invasion. However, in all whom there is deep invasion or palpable nodes, dissection should be carried out.

Malignant melanoma. Malignant melanoma of the hand is most often seen involving the nail bed. It was first clearly described by Hutchinson, who pointed out that these lesions are most often treated as chronic paronychia. He also pointed out that these lesions show a pigmented border even if their central portions do not show any pigment. Their apparent innocuousness in early stages may be misleading, and the lesion may be deeply invasive when its surface appears innocent. Nothing should be done to irritate the area. Biopsies are out of the question unless the surgeon is prepared to carry out at once the initial operation. In malignant melanoma of the nail bed, amputation of the digit should be performed. One widely accepted course of action is to carry out an axillary and epitrochlear dissection some four to six weeks later. Whether this is logical or the best treatment has not been determined. On grounds of analogy and logic, dissection starting at the axilla and extending down along the supposed line of the lymphatics would seem more reasonable. It does not appear that mutilating forequarter amputations have offered much better prospects in regard to prognosis than have less extensive procedures.

TUMORS OF FIBROUS TISSUES. **Fibroma.** Fibromas occur in many locations in the hand. They are usually subcutaneous and produce superficial masses which are frequently diagnosed as neurofibromas, implantation cysts or early xanthomas. They may be pedunculated, and hang from the skin by a thin pedicle. The early nodules of Dupuytren's contracture are usually diagnosed by the uninitiated as fibroma of the palm, and only as the fascial bands become more evident is the true identity suspected. Deep fibromas are seen in or on the tendons, where they may cause symptoms of blockage due to mechanical interference with gliding. The fibroma is quite benign and does not recur after removal.

However, a peculiar fibroma does develop on the hand which does recur and usually is more extensive at each operative procedure. The microscopic appearance of this recurring fibroma may suggest nothing unusual. After several postexcisional recurrences, however, its structure may change somewhat. This type of tumor probably should be included in the sarcomas.

Sarcomas. There are many varieties of sarcomas of the hand (Figs. 36 and 37). Many probably take their origin from nerve sheaths, and are neurofibrosarcomas. They may, however, arise from any of the soft mesodermal

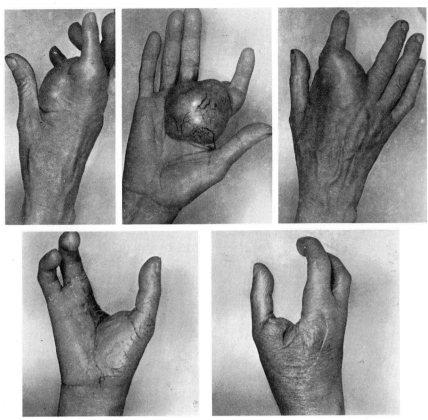

Figure 36.   Fibrosarcoma.

tissues, and vary from hard fibrous tumors to cellular masses containing only slight amounts of stroma. They may begin as tiny nodules in the lower layers of the skin or subcutaneous tissues, but can arise deeply from any fibrous tissue as hard, usually painless, masses. They become fixed early to surrounding tissues and may cause pain. They may grow slowly for months or even years before their malignant nature becomes apparent. On the other hand, some of them develop very rapidly, become invasive, and lead to early metastases and death. They may be composed of round cells, spindle cells or a mixture of the two, and present a varying amount of stroma.

There is a variety which, while not peculiar to the hand, appears as a recurring fibroma

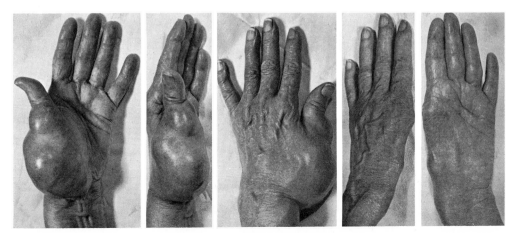

Figure 37.   Malignant xanthosarcoma.

that involves the overlying skin. This tumor is usually excised quite easily and apparently well beyond its limits. The defect left by the excision often requires a skin graft. Several months or even longer afterward, following an apparent cure, the tumor reappears in or along the border of the previous excision. A second, and often a third or fourth excision, each wider than the preceding, will fail to lead to a cure. Careful study of microscopic sections may show nothing incompatible with a diagnosis of fibroma. After numerous recurrences, however, it will become apparent that nothing but very wide excision or amputation will suffice. Often, at this time, the microscopic characteristics become more compatible with a diagnosis of sarcoma. Despite this, however, distant metastases are seldom encountered.

Lipoma. Lipoma is a fairly frequent tumor of the hand, where it forms a rather typical soft mass. Usually, it is lobulated, particularly if crossed by tendons or other dense structures. A superficial lipoma may be mistaken for an epidermoid cyst or xanthoma; however, the characteristic consistency is usually a clue to its nature. Deep lipomas may arise within muscle bellies, about nerves, on or about tendons and within tendon sheaths.

One variety of lipoma, known as an arborescent lipoma, occurs within the tendon sheaths, where it spreads throughout the involved sheath and produces an appearance quite similar to that seen in chronic teno-

synovitis. Its removal entails an extensive dissection. It may be confused preoperatively with tuberculous tenosynovitis, xanthoma of the tendon sheath or villonodular tenosynovitis. The prognosis for lipoma is good as far as recurrence or malignancy is concerned.

TUMORS OF JOINT CAPSULES AND TENDON SHEATHS. Ganglia. The most frequent of these tumors is the ganglion (Fig. 38). It is held by many to be due to trauma and is said to occur especially in persons who subject their hands to frequently repeated motions, such as pianists, typists, violinists, and others whose work entails use of the fingers and wrist for long periods of fine coordinated activity. Clinical observation does not seem to bear this out, since this tumor is seen in persons with all types of occupations.

Microscopically, ganglia are made up of a basal tissue, which is fibrous joint capsule or tendon sheath containing cellular areas within which may often be seen tiny cystic spaces. The cystic mass is continuous with this and consists of a thin-walled unilocular or multilocular cyst. The large cysts come about by the enlargement and coalescence of the smaller cysts which originate in the basal tissue. It would appear that recurrence of ganglia is due to basal tissue which was not excised. This concept of origin may explain the frequent recurrence which follows simple rupture or aspiration.

Ganglia occur in a number of typical locations on the hand. Most frequent are those on

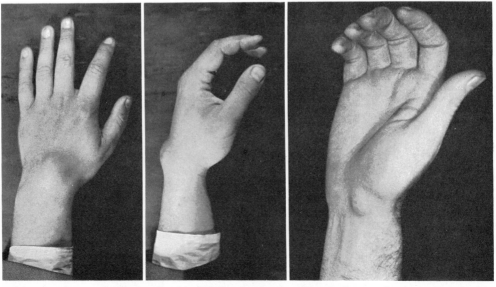

Figure 38.   Ganglia of the hand: dorsal carpal and volar carpal.

the dorsal surface, which take origin from the joint capsule at the base of the second metacarpal and protrude between the common digital extensor and the radial extensor tendons. Another dorsal site is in the anatomic snuff box, where they originate from the joint capsule at the base of the thumb and from adjacent tendon sheaths. A volar carpal ganglion is seen on the wrist at the radial side, in connection with the joint capsule at the base of the thumb and the fibrous sheath tissue about the radial carpal flexor. These latter ganglia are in intimate association with the radial artery, which is liable to injury during excision of the ganglia and must be visualized at all times.

Ganglia also arise from the fibrous tendon sheath of the flexor tendons over the proximal phalanges of the fingers, usually the index, middle and ring fingers, just distal to the proximal digital crease.

The symptoms of ganglia are mainly due to the presence of a hard mass in the tissues, which causes either a lumpy cosmetic blemish or pain when the mass is pressed against underlying tissues. At times, the development of the dorsal carpal ganglion may be heralded by pain and tenderness at the base of the second metacarpal, which may be present for weeks or months before the actual tumor appears. The recurrence of a ganglion may be predicted by similar pain and tenderness.

Treatment of ganglion is surgical excision. The basal tissue, from which the ganglion originates, is difficult to distinguish from normal joint capsule, and only the presence of tiny cysts within it gives evidence of its identity. The ganglion should be dissected to its base and a generous segment of capsular tissue should be excised with the ganglion. It is imperative that the procedure be carried out in a bloodless field. Local infiltration anesthesia usually suffices, although there are certain advantages to removal with the patient under general anesthesia so as to avoid obscuration of tissue detail by infiltration with fluid. The volar digital ganglion is excised in toto with an underlying square of tendon sheath. There is no clearer demonstration that ganglia are not herniations of tendon sheath than these tiny tumors.

A transverse incision is always indicated. The incisions which run transversely across the lines of nerves, blood vessels and tendons must be made with great care to avoid injury to these structures. Following operation, the wrist or finger is splinted in a functional position for about ten days to permit healing.

Other methods of treatment yield a high percentage of recurrences. Crushing the tumor by directing a heavy blow upon it with a book may sometimes effect a cure, although the surgeon who employs this treatment is not likely to know the final results. Injection or aspiration and injection usually are unsatisfactory.

Mucous cyst. The mucous cyst which occurs on the dorsum of the distal phalanges near the base of the nail resembles a ganglion in appearance and in the gelatinous character of its contents. The location over the base of the nail often leads to a depressed deformity of the nail. It recurs promptly after removal, unless the underlying skin and cyst are excised together. This would seem to indicate that these tumors originate from the lower layers of the corium. Removal, therefore, necessitates covering the defect with a tiny skin graft. These cysts must not be mistaken for Heberden's nodes.

Xanthomas. Xanthomas, or giant cell xanthomatic tumors, occur as isolated tumor masses on the hand, in contrast to the multiple xanthomatic processes which are seen in association with a metabolic disturbance. There does not appear to be any cholesterol disturbance in the instance of the isolated tumors, and their exact nature is somewhat of a mystery. They are probably synovial tumors arising from tendon sheaths and joint capsules.

Study of a single section will not give a true picture of the histologic structure. The tumor is made up of four elemental areas intermixed in varying proportions from tumor to tumor. Foreign-body type giant cells are a striking characteristic. Intermixed with the giant cells is a stroma of spindle-shaped epithelioid cells. There are areas of variable size and shape made up of foamy cells with small nuclei and bubbly cytoplasm filled with cholesterol. Dissolved in the cholesterol is xanthine, which gives the tumor its yellow color; the cholesterol itself is colorless. Scattered throughout the tumor are hemosiderin deposits which some believe to represent hemorrhages indicative of trauma.

The tumor is benign and is amenable to local removal. This must, however, be very thorough. The recurrence rate is high because the tumor takes origin from deeper tissues and the superficial mass may be only the surface manifestation of a long stalk, which passes into the tendon sheath of a digit. If the stalk is not removed, the tumor re-forms. Recurrences are not true recurrences, but simply growth of the portion of the tumor mass which has been left behind. In rare instances, following several removals, the tumor may assume malignant characteristics.

Xanthomas occur particularly on the digits, where they may be confused with epidermoid cysts. These latter are usually unilobular, in contrast to xanthomas which are usually multilobular. Either may be mistaken for the other. Xanthomas do not involve the overlying skin, but are firmly attached in the depths and, hence, are not movable. They are occasionally seen in the palm or the wrist, where they assume the characteristics of villonodular synovitis.

Treatment is surgical removal. Every trace of the tumor must be removed to ensure against recurrence. The digital nerves and vessels will be found coursing across the tumor mass, usually in a deep groove which separates one lobule from another. Great care must be taken to follow the tumor throughout its entire course, and not be content with removing simply the large lobulated more superficial mass. A tail of the tumor will often be found to enter the tendon sheath and to run for a variable distance in it. This may be the origin of the tumor and must be removed. When the tumor presents itself at the wrist, it may be very extensive and involve the whole of the radial or ulnar bursa, or both, and require as extensive a dissection as does tuberculous tenosynovitis.

The prognosis for xanthoma is good as far as malignancy and metastases are concerned, but the recurrence rate tends to be high unless special care is taken in the primary removal. In occasional instances, the tumor may be so extensive on a digit as to replace large areas of the digital fatty tissue and to compromise the blood supply so seriously that a finger may have to be amputated.

Malignant synovioma. The term "synovioma" has become attached to a particular malignant variety of these tumors which fortunately is rarely seen on the hand. These lesions occur near the joints as painless, slow-growing, rather indefinite masses. They form encapsulated or diffuse masses, often butter-yellow in color. They may be solid or fleshy and often are not easily distinguishable from the surrounding tissues. They appear to spring from the joint capsule, and in early stages do not involve bone. Following simple removal, prompt recurrence is to be

suspected and metastasis may be anticipated if amputation of the digit is not soon carried out.

TUMORS OF BLOOD VESSELS. All of the varieties of vascular tumors met with elsewhere on the body occur on the hand and forearm. Whether or not they are true tumors is often to be questioned.

The only malignant blood vessel tumor resembles the angioblastic phase of vascular development. Other blood vessel tumors suggest the stage of capillary plexus formation; some, the retiform stage; and still others, arrest in the stage of stem formation. The diffuse arteriovenous aneurysms with multiple arteriovenous communications would certainly seem to represent arrests in intermediate stages of vascular tree development.

While arrest in development of blood vessels may represent the origin of the tumors, their continued growth may be a manifestation of the effects of arteriovenous communications and the effect of the abnormal circulation upon neighboring vessels. A specific blood vessel tumor may not always be of a certain type but may contain various mixtures of capillary and cavernous and vessel types of angioma.

Capillary angioma. The capillary or telangiectatic type of angioma is present familiarly as the port-wine stain or strawberry mark, and has usually been manifest since the birth of the patient. It is usually elevated and soft, of bright color and nonpulsatile. It may occupy only the under layers of the skin, but there may be cavernous spaces beneath it. Occasionally, it will disappear during the first year of life. From a small beginning, the tumor may grow, extending over larger and larger areas until its eradication presents a difficult problem. Early removal seems indicated if the mass is of any size, and especially if it shows any tendency to growth. It may be necessary to replace the excised skin area with skin grafts.

Cavernous angioma. The cavernous angiomas are occasionally seen on the hand, particularly in the palm, where they seem to take over the venous elements of the circulation. Large thin-walled venous lakes extend along nerves and tendons, into muscles and, not infrequently, from palm to dorsum. Extensive involvement is almost the rule and, although the arteries are not involved per se, it is often impossible to remove the angioma without damaging the normal vessels. Hence, a staged operation is frequently required.

In not a few instances, these cavernous lakes involve the bones, usually of one or two digits, a fact which is indicated by x-ray examination.

Congenital arteriovenous aneurysms. The congenital arteriovenous aneurysms, as they occur on the hand, frequently affect the vessels of one or two digits. They are characterized by extensive pulsating vascular tumors, enlargement of the involved digits or of the whole hand, and venous dilatation over the hand and forearm. The arteriovenous communications in these instances are multiple, in contrast with the traumatic arteriovenous aneurysm. The tiny vessels in the skin become dilated; the skin becomes thin over them and hemorrhage may occur following a trivial injury.

Treatment of the angiomas consists in surgical eradication. Although the capillary type is sensitive to irradiation, this must be given in such destructive doses to effect cure that the skin is involved with irradiation dermatitis. When irradiation has been carried out, subsequent excision of the skin followed by grafting is often required. Such therapy seems contraindicated in youngsters since epiphyses may be damaged and serious growth disturbances result.

Capillary angiomas may be excised and satisfactory results obtained. The need for skin replacement at the time of excision will depend upon the size of the area removed. Cavernous angioma may be excised, although it presents a more difficult problem than does the capillary type. The tumor may be so extensive that complete removal may be impossible and the surgeon must be content with partial excision of the most troublesome area. At times, the procedure must be staged for fear of compromising the blood supply to one or more digits, if excision of the tumor involves the blood supply too seriously. These tumors only rarely develop arteriovenous communications; hence, partial excision may be successful.

Congenital arteriovenous aneurysms present one of the most difficult problems in surgery of the hand. Theoretically, one should be able to approach and ligate the arteriovenous communication. Practically, this is seldom possible, except in a limited sense. The communications are multiple, often affecting vessels over a large area, on both volar and dorsal surfaces, and one usually finds that after supposedly adequate excision and ligation the tumor promptly grows again, often to a greater proportion than previously. If the vessels of a single digit are involved, amputation of that digit is indicated. Unfortunately, the process is seldom confined to one finger. The surgeon may offer some chance of cure, or at least of amelioration, by local attack on the tumor, plus ligation in stages of the blood vessels to the hand, allowing sufficient time between ligations to permit collateral circulation to develop.

Telangiectatic granuloma. Telangiectatic granuloma may or may not be a true tumor. It is most frequently called a pyogenic granuloma and the implication is that it is an infectious granuloma. It appears as a small mushroom-like growth, frequently located near the finger tip, but may be in any location on the hand. The stalk of the growth protrudes through a small opening in the skin which forms a thin collar about it. Microscopic study shows it to be made up of myriads of capillary vessels, resembling a capillary angioma. Some think it is, in fact, an angioma which has burst through the skin. It is quite amenable to simple excision with closure of the defect. This seems to be the preferred treatment. The tumor does not recur after removal.

Glomus tumor. This tumor originates from the neuromyoarterial glomus, a structure associated with the autonomic nervous blooded animals and is especially developed in the feet of ducks. Glomera are essentially arteriovenous communications made up of arterioles connecting directly with venules forming the canals of Sucquet-Hoyer. The vessels are surrounded by cells resembling epithelioid cells, which are thought by many to be modified smooth muscle cells. No nerve cells are found in the glomus; however, there are many myelinated and nonmyelinated nerve fibrils in it, and these give evidence of its close association with the neurovegetative system. Glomera are found scattered over the body, and tumors arising from them have been reported in bone and other deeper structures. They are especially abundant in the palmar skin and in the nail bed. The vast majority of glomus tumors are reported as occurring on the hand, although these lesions have been reported in practically every region.

The tumor is frequently 5 mm. or less in diameter but may attain sizable proportions, measuring up to 1 inch in diameter. Multiple tumors have been reported.

Glomus tumors give rise to a pathognomonic chain of symptoms. Starting insidiously, they develop into painful nodules or painful areas which may not be palpable as nodules. If they occur in the nail bed, they may be visible as reddish or purplish tumors, a few millimeters in diameter, which do not perforate the overlying nail. Sometimes, they are especially painful when cold, in other instances when warm. They are always painful to touch and may be so exquisitely tender that the patient protects the part by placing his hand in his pocket. They often give rise to paroxysmal attacks of pain which radiate up the forearm and arm, or even into the neck. The patient usually presents himself with a long history of an undiagnosed painful spot which has made life generally miserable.

Diagnosis is usually suggested by the history and the findings of a tender, subcutaneous or subungual nodule. The tumor under the nail may be visible and the nail itself may be pushed up and rounded by the underlying mass. An x-ray examination of the finger tip may reveal a depression in the distal phalanx due to the pressure of the tumor.

Treatment consists in simple excision of the tumor. Because of pain and apprehension on the patient's part, operation may often have to be accomplished under a general anesthetic. A bloodless field is essential, since the tumor may suddenly constrict and what was a pink or red tumor mass may become invisible. This is especially liable to occur when the patient is under local anesthesia. Recurrence is rare unless the tumor is missed. These tumors do not become malignant.

Lymphangiomas. Lymphangiomas are extremely rare. They are seen as congenital lesions leading to enlargement of parts or all of the hand, forearm and arm. They may produce a type of gigantism. Excision is usually difficult because of their extent.

Tumors of bone. Enchondroma. Except for enchondromas, tumors of the bones of the hand are rare. Enchondroma is, however, not at all infrequent. It is seen particularly in the shafts of the metacarpals and proximal phalanges. It may be multiple, and both hands should be x-rayed when a suggestive bony swelling is present.

Enchondromas develop as slowly growing, hard tumor masses in the tubular bones, usually near the head of a metacarpal or base of a proximal phalanx. Occasionally, the patient complains of dull pain, but more frequently there are no symptoms until a trivial injury leads to a fracture which prompts an x-ray examination which discloses the tumor. There is seldom gross displacement of the fracture, probably because the injury has been so trivial or because the solid tumor helps support the bone. X-ray examination shows a well-defined vesicular area of rarefaction within the shaft of bone, which has expanded and thinned out the cortex but does not perforate it.

Treatment consists in unroofing of the tumor and thorough curettage of its contents. If the patient presents himself with a fracture, the bone should be splinted and allowed to heal before the tumor is attacked. Healing of the fracture can be anticipated to take place satisfactorily.

Exostoses. These tumors appear infrequently on the hand, usually in the region of tendon insertions, and are occasionally multiple. They are larger on palpation than x-ray examination indicates, since they are capped with cartilage, and are properly called cartilaginous exostoses. They may rarely develop in the nail bed as Dupuytren's exostoses. They erode through the nail, leading to a granulomatous lesion. These tumors are not malignant and respond to simple local removal.

Osteoid osteoma. Osteoid osteomas are easily confused with other rarefying bone lesions, such as osteomyelitis, bone abscess and syphilis, and must be differentiated from them as well as from osteochondritis dissecans, xanthoma or even bone callus. The tumor appears roentgenologically as a small translucent area in the bone, either in spongy bone or the cortex, surrounded by an area of increased density or sclerosis. Pathologically, it is made up of a center of osteoid tissue surrounded by sclerosed bone.

The most prominent symptom is chronic pain, nagging in character rather than severe, and increasing especially at night. However, the pain responds to mild sedation with aspirin. Study of the x-ray film, with these facts in mind, makes the diagnosis certain.

Treatment consists in removal of the tumor. Great care must be taken to remove the nidus or center of osteoid tissue since, if any of this remains, recurrence is certain.

Giant cell tumors. When they occur on the upper extremity, giant cell tumors are usually seen in the radius near the wrist. They are slow-growing tumors. Their presence is characterized by boring pain, usually severe and worse at night. They may appear a great deal like enchondroma on x-ray examination but usually appear more like soap bubbles. The severe pain tends to differentiate them from enchondroma which is painless.

Treatment of the giant cell tumor consists in its complete removal, which may be more difficult and more extensive than the procedure required for enchondroma. Frequently, a segment of bone must be excised and a bone graft inserted although, occasionally, thorough curettage of the currant jelly-like contents may suffice.

Bone cysts, myxomas, osteomas, fibromas, hemangiomas and Ewing's tumors. These may occur in the bones of the hand. They resemble giant cell tumor and enchondroma on roentgen examination. Only microscopic study will determine the diagnosis.

TUMORS OF NERVE. Tumors of the peripheral nerves are actually tumors of the sheath elements. They are nodular, diffuse, spindle-shaped enlargement of the nerves, or a plexiform thickening of all the nerves of an area, as in von Recklinghausen's disease.

The nodular types of neuromas, neurinomas or neurofibromas (Fig. 39) are usually subcutaneous nodules, single or occasionally multiple, in the subcutaneous tissues, in connection with subcutaneous sensory nerves. They are derived from the connective tissue elements of the nerve sheath and present a typical histologic picture. Their removal occasions no disturbance in nerve function.

The fusiform neuromas develop along the course of the major nerves of the hand, usually the median, less often the ulnar nerve, and may extend over large distances of the trunk. There is usually such an interwoven complex of nerve fibers and tumor that sep-

aration proves impossible. The tumors are benign, but one must always suspect multiple occurrence in other parts of the body. Many of these may well be manifestations of von Recklinghausen's disease.

Plexiform neuroma. This condition is characterized by diffuse thickening of a nerve or group of nerves. A single finger, several digits or even the whole hand may be involved. The thickening involves not only the main nerve trunk, but the fine terminal twigs and even the skin. Associated with this is general thickening of the skin and subcutaneous tissues; the fingers become thick, soft and long. Grotesque enlargement may take place. When it is marked, it is known as elephantiasis neuromatosa. It is impossible in many instances to remove all involved tissue without complete sacrifice of parts of the hand. However, it is usually possible to improve the condition from a cosmetic standpoint by partial excision and skin grafts.

Neurosarcoma or neurofibrosarcoma. This tumor may appear as a nodular mass which grows back slowly after apparently adequate excision. The tumor may give all the appearance of being benign, even on microscopic section, and only its prompt reappearance gives a clue as to its identity. Often, its course may extend over many years; eventually amputation of the extremity may be required. On the other hand, some of the neurosarcomas are extremely malignant, metastasizing early and leading to death in 12 to 18 months. As with any sarcoma, the initial operation is the most important. It should be radical and extensive.

METASTATIC TUMORS. The hand is occasionally the site of a metastatic tumor, usually lodging in the bone. In rare instances, they may be the only manifestation of the primary tumor. The source is usually the lungs, prostate or testes.

CONGENITAL DEFORMITIES

Although congenital deformities of the hand tend to follow certain patterns, these are only roughly definite and there is no general pattern of deformity such as is seen, for example, in harelip and cleft palate. Except in a general way, no two cases are exactly alike and, except for such conditions as syndactylism, it is not possible to devise standard operative procedures.

Many and various theories have been put

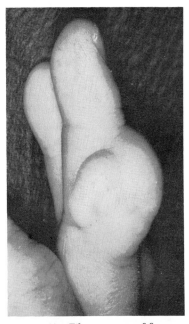

Figure 39. Fibroneuroma of finger.

forth to explain the origin of congenital deformities. External influences and intra-uterine accidents have been suggested. However, in most instances it would seem that actual changes in the germ plasm, often of an inherited nature, are to blame. Experiments with irradiation indicate that this modality might lead to gonadal damage, and the latter may cause the development of inheritable deformities in offspring.

Despite difficulties in classifying these deformities, better understanding is gained if one attempts to place them in certain groups, depending on certain general characteristics. Kanavel concluded that deformities could be grouped into three types: those showing hypoplasia and aplasia, those showing disorientation of tissue, and those showing hyperplasia.

The hand and forearm may be divided into ulnar and radial divisions, separated by a fibrous partition attached to the middle metacarpal bone. The vascular and nerve supplies suggest a close relation of the little, ring and middle fingers to the ulnar division, and a less close association of the index finger. The thumb is radial alone. Functionally, the thumb acts alone, the three ulnar digits together and the index finger in association with the ulnar digits. The fourth and fifth digits are frequently involved together and, not infrequently, the middle finger is involved with them. The index finger is seldom involved with other digits, while the thumb is usually involved alone. In congenital absence of the ulna, the thumb and index are usually preserved. In lobster-claw hand, the middle finger is usually the one absent, while the thumb, the index, ring and little fingers are preserved.

In a study of congenital deformities of the hand, the surgeon is inclined to think only of configuration of the bones, as evidenced by x-ray examination, and gross morphologic changes, as evidenced by examination of the hand. One sees absence of bones, bones reduced in size, fused to each other or actually duplicated. On examination of the hand, the fusion of digits, webbing and rudimentary or extra digits are easily seen and recorded. What is not so often considered is the fact that these changes affect the whole fabric of the forearm and hand. There may be absence not only of the bones, but of nerves and tendons as well. Fusion may affect deep soft tissues, as well as hard tissues and skin. Attempts to correct these deformities operatively must not be approached as simple

problems of bone and skin surgery; attention to the nerve, vascular and tendon supply is equally significant. It must be remembered that, although certain types of deformities may be discussed as entities, they are seldom present alone. Thus, syndactylism, or fusion of adjacent fingers, is frequently combined with fusion or absence of joints, with shortening or absence of digits, with absence of a phalanx in a digit, or even with an accessory digit.

CONGENITAL AMPUTATIONS. Congenital amputations are now thought to be due to actual factors in the germ plasm, or to the effect of noxious factors such as irradiation, on the developing embryo (Fig. 40).

When there is absence of a part, surgery can do little about it. Constricting bands, however, can often be corrected or helped. Thus, deep constricting bands may seem almost ready to amputate a digit at its base and it would hardly seem possible that there is space for blood vessels to enter. Such bands may often be released by a Z-plasty, and considerable improvement in appearance and function can be secured.

HYPOPLASIA AND APLASIA. The group of deformities classed as hypoplastic and aplastic have in common the element of tissue destruction ascribed to injury to the germinal anlage, or to damage to the growing embryo. Parts of the extremity may vary in evidence of this destructive factor from simple diminution in size to complete absence or loss. In about 50 per cent of instances of congenital deformities of the hand, the most serious defects fall into this group.

The severity varies from such anomalies

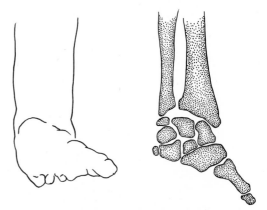

Figure 40. Congenital amputation. This was long thought to be due to amniotic bands and adhesions, but is now recognized to be due to defects in the germ plasm. (Kanavel, A. B.: Arch. Surg. 25:1, 1932.)

as shortness of a digit to its complete absence; from diminution in size of the hand to complete loss; from shortness of arm and forearm to their absence, with the hand coming directly off the shoulder, to absence of the whole upper extremity. Nor are anomalies single; they are often multiple and are associated with other defects due to disorientation of tissue. The hypoplastic and aplastic deformities show marked hereditary tendency to development of similar anomalies in succeeding generations.

Congenital absence of the radius is bilateral in almost one-half of reported instances. The radius may be completely or partially absent (Fig. 41). If it is partially absent, the upper end may be missing with a rudimentary diaphysis; the lower end may be missing with varying amounts of diaphysis, or the diaphysis may be absent with upper and lower ends present. The ulna is usually thick, short and curved to the radial side. Other deformities of the hand may be present, such as absence or atypical forms of the carpal bones, absence of the first metacarpal and absence of, or rudimentary, thumb. The other digits are usually normal. The elbow may be ankylosed. The muscles and nerves of the forearm may be disoriented, atrophic, fibrotic and contracted. The hand is deviated to the radial side, thus producing the radiopalmar clubhand, and may be small, but is usually potentially functional.

Absence of the ulna occurs much less frequently than does absence of the radius, probably in the ratio of about 1 to 5. It is a complementary picture to that of radial absence in that the forearm is short, the radius is curved and there is ulnar deviation of the hand. The elbow, however, is usually dislocated and there are more likely to be deformities and destruction of the digits and carpal bones. The loss of digits often makes these hands less functional than does the radial type of deformity. The little, ring and middle fingers are the ones usually absent. Loss, atrophy and fibrosis of muscles, nerves and vessels usually accompany the deformity in varying degrees. The defect is frequently bilateral. If the hand has not taken part in the process, function is good. If, however, the hand is involved, the functional loss is often very great.

Hypoplasia affecting the hand produces a multiplicity of deformities which do not follow any definite pattern. The involvement may start at the wrist and the whole hand may be implicated. Only the medial digits may take part in the condition, or the thumb bud may be the most affected. Individual bones may be shortened or lost. There is seldom hypoplasia alone; usually more than one extremity is affected and a hereditary tendency is very frequently noted.

Hypoplasia of the elements which make up the middle finger produces a picture out of proportion to the general importance and, because of its redness, lobster-claw hand has been accorded a prominent, easily-remembered spot among congenital deformities of the hand. In this condition, the middle finger with all or most of its metacarpals is missing, and the hand is cleft down the center into two halves, each bearing two digits, presumably the ring and little fingers to the ulnar side and the thumb and index finger to the radial side (Fig. 42).

Treatment for median hypoplasia attempts to restore the digits to a functional and more cosmetic position. It must be remembered that attempts to restore cosmetic appearance should not interfere with the use of the hand which the patient already has or may develop. The deformed hand is the only hand the patient has known and he learns to use it remarkably well despite its bizarre appearance. In some cleft hands, it may be possible to unite the two halves of the hand after removal of remnants of the third metacarpal and to correct the syndactylism which obtains following it. Release of contracting bands, physical therapy and traction splinting are often valuable in eventually improving function. However, left to his own resources, the patient will usually secure a most functional member from a seemingly hopeless situation.

Hypoplasia and aplasia of elements of the

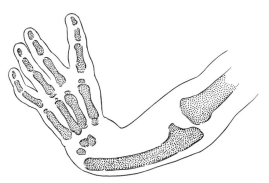

Figure 41. Congenital absence of the radius. (Kanavel, A. B.: Arch. Surg. 25:1, 1932.)

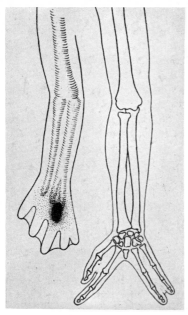

Figure 42. Lobster-claw hand. (Kanavel, A. B.: Arch. Surg. 25:1, 1932.)

hand and wrist are many and varied. There may be shortening of digits, due to short metacarpals or short or absent phalanges, in various combinations. There may be flexion deformities and deviations of the digits, occasionally with disorientation of epiphyses.

FUSION OF HAND AND ARM ELEMENTS. Fusion of the various parts of the hand, wrist and forearm may vary from simple webbing of the digits to actual fusion of bones in whole or part in all degrees. In the forearm, radio-ulnar synostosis is a definite entity. The union usually occurs at the proximal end of the bones and is often associated with anterior dislocation of the head of the radius. The forearm is usually in pronation. There is often little functional disturbance due to this lesion in itself, supination being carried out by movement of the shoulder. If the disability is severe, some motion may often be secured by osteotomy of the radius below the point of union.

SYNDACTYLISM. Syndactylism is a common condition, often part of other congenital deformities of the hand. It consists in fusion of two or more digits (Fig. 43). The fusion may be complete from base to tip, or may extend only a short distance from the web space. There may be only fusion of skin, or there may be many degrees, ranging from fusion of distal phalanges to fusion of all phalanges. The soft tissues may partake of this fusion, so that tendon, nerves and vessels may be

reduced to a single set between fused bones. Any group of fingers may be involved, although the most frequent are the ring and middle fingers.

Several factors are to be considered in the indications for operation and in the technique. As to whether operation is indicated, it must be remembered that, as far as use is concerned, the patient uses the hand quite well despite the uncosmetic and unusual anatomy. In some patients, the webbing may be so severe and the distortion of the digits so grotesque as to render the hand useless. The surgeon must study each hand most carefully to learn as much as possible about nerve and tendon involvement in the process and the condition of the bones and joints. When it would appear that only one tendon serves two fused digits, the wisdom of separating them, except for cosmetic reasons, is questionable. The age at which separation is indicated is important. Parents bring their children soon after birth and the request for surgery is often quite urgent. It must be remembered that these operations usually require skin grafting and much after-care; that the little hand can be immobilized only with difficulty; and that grafts are displaced by wiggling fingers. Unless there is gross distortion, or longer digits are being distorted by the shorter ones, it is best to delay operation until the child has reached the age of four or five years, or even older.

Separation of the fingers is a plastic procedure based on a few definite principles. The first lesson the surgeon must learn is that it is seldom if ever possible to fashion flaps

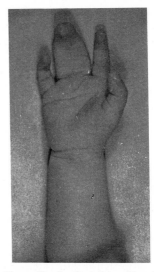

Figure 43. Syndactylism of hand.

of skin from the webs to cover the defects left by separation of digits. There is never enough skin to cover the raw surfaces, and suture lines under tension heal with scar contracture.

Occasionally, in a young child in whom digital distortion is occurring, early operation is justified to release digits which are being pulled into deviation, or in which the tips of the fingers and thumb are fused. In early operation, grafts must be used and since they seldom keep pace with the growth of the hand, they must be replaced later.

In all other instances, the surgeon must start by realizing that a free full-thickness skin graft will be required. A tongue or flap of skin should be fashioned from the web, either anteriorly or posteriorly, to fill the web space between digits. This skin flap is brought volarward or dorsally and forms the base of the web. After it has been formed, the remainder of the web is divided in a wavy line and the digits are separated. This procedure leaves triangular defects on either side, which are covered with free full-thickness grafts.

An alternate procedure is to excise the whole of the web and fill it with a free full-thickness skin graft shaped somewhat butterfly fashion. Care is taken that the lines of suture on the digits are zigzag, not straight; otherwise, contractile scars will develop.

POLYDACTYLISM. Polydactylism, or duplication of digits, is a condition which is often symmetrical and usually has a hereditary history; it is frequently associated with deformities of the feet. It ranges from simple dichotomy of a digit to a so-called mirror hand. The digits most often involved are the little finger, the middle and ring fingers, the thumb or the index finger, in that order of frequency.

In the case of the little finger, the extra digit may be represented by a flabby nubbin of skin and subcutaneous tissue, or there may be two complete digits. In the case of the middle and ring fingers, the situation is usually complicated by syndactylism (Fig. 44), the polydactylism being unsuspected until x-ray examination reveals duplication of parts of the phalanges.

Various degrees of polydactylism of the thumb are seen; as many as three thumbs on one hand have been recorded. There may be associated syndactylism, triphalangeal thumbs (Fig. 45) and extra metacarpals.

Double major bulbs produce the mirror

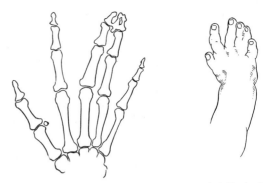

Figure 44. Polydactylism of hand. (Kanavel, A. B.: Arch. Surg. 25:282, 1932.)

hand. In this condition, there may be two ulnar elements with absence of the radial element. The sets of fingers are set at an angle to each other in such a way that they appear to be the mirror image of each other.

Treatment of polydactylism in its various forms may be simple or complex. The tiny, flabby nubbins not infrequently seen in the newborn may be snipped off without any qualm. When more serious deformities are met, the problem becomes one of determining the muscle and tendon attachments of apparently accessory digits. It may be wise in some instances to leave the hand alone, since function is more important than cosmetic appearance. Bifid digits may often be improved in appearance if such an operation does not destroy function.

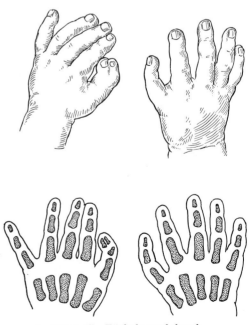

Figure 45. Triphalangeal thumb.

RECONSTRUCTIVE SURGERY

The problems which are encountered by the surgeon who carries out reconstructive surgery of the hand are many and varied. These range from the correction of scar contractures through nerve and tendon reconstruction, bone replacement, tendon transferences and digital reconstruction and transference.

The surgeon who undertakes this work must first of all have a concept of the functions of the hand and an appreciation of the basic motions. He must be able to visualize the anatomic structure of the part, and have the diagnostic acumen to detect the basic loss and to recognize the potentialities of what is left. He must be able to plan a series of procedures, often requiring months or even years of effort and several stages, to restore even minimal use to a hand. He must appreciate that function and not cosmetic appearance is the end result to be secured.

It must be remembered that only in a certain percentage of patients is a single element of difficulty present; frequently more than one problem is present and these must usually be solved individually.

The sine qua non for any reconstructive surgery of the hand is intact, healthy, pliable skin. As the result of burns, crushing wounds, infection and other causes, the skin may be lost or seriously damaged, so that when the patient presents himself for care there are serious contracted scars which interfere with use of the part. Burns on the dorsum may have resulted in hypertrophic scars which prevent proper flexion of the digits. A similar scar between the thumb and second metacarpal may draw the thumb into extreme adduction. Scars on the volar surface may hold one or more or all digits in acute flexion.

These scars may be the only element leading to disability; the structures beneath them may be undamaged. In such instances, it will only be necessary to correct the cutaneous scar by some type of skin replacement to restore the hand to use.

If, however, along with the damage to the skin there is damage to nerves, tendons and bones, the skin replacement must be such that the surgeon can subsequently lift it along one side and carry out surgical repairs. In such instances, a free graft will not be satisfactory and a pedunculated flap of skin with subcutaneous fat will be necessary.

Also, if excision of scar contracture of the skin entails uncovering of bones, joints,

nerves and tendons, it is usually necessary to apply a pedunculated flap to replace the skin excised. Determination of whether such a flap will be needed often requires critical judgment, and the surgeon must be prepared to use whichever seems indicated at the time of operation.

At times the functional loss may be due to loss or division of tendons or nerves, or both. The first problem is to determine the extent of damage; that is, a diagnosis of the tendons and nerves involved must be made. The second problem is to determine how repair may be carried out.

The first essential is to assure that the covering through which surgery must be carried out is satisfactory. This may require, therefore, that before any nerve and tendon repair can be carried out, a pedicled flap will have to be applied.

Joints which are to be moved by newly repaired tendons must be mobile. Mobilization of joints may in itself require long periods of dynamic splinting, physical therapy and open operation before the tendon repair can be undertaken.

Lastly, some decision must be reached as to tendon suture, tendon graft or tendon transfer. The first problem is that of nerve and tendon division in the palm. The problem is not simple, but there are probably fewer factors to be considered than, for instance, in division within the digits. If the patient is seen early and there has been no infection, no unsuccessful attempts were made at repair at the time of injury, the factor to be considered is the amount of tendon retraction. Under ideal circumstances, retraction in a few weeks will not have been very great. In all probability, a suture of tendons can be carried out, certainly of the profundus tendons, and the nerves may likewise be repaired. The important factor is the amount of retraction which the proximal stumps have undergone.

If, on the other hand, the tendon injury occurred six months or a year previously, the forearm muscles will have retracted a good deal and, under such circumstances, it is quite likely that tendon grafts will be needed.

Another factor is introduced when one comes to consider late repair of tendons in the digits. Whether immediate repair was either not carried out or was attempted and failed, there is only one answer to the problem and that is the introduction of a tendon graft. There is only one possible exception to this rule, which does not often obtain, and that is profundus tendon division alone. If division has occurred close to the distal joint, the amount of tendon retraction may be so minimal that a secondary suture may occasionally be feasible. Usually, however, the proximal retraction will be so great that a tendon graft will be required.

Division of the flexor pollicis longus may or may not demand a tendon graft. The proximal stump frequently "snaps" up into the lower forearm, becomes bulbous and shortened, and its distal end may degenerate.

Division of the flexor tendons in the wrist and lower forearm, unless immediately repaired, presents one of the most unfortunate situations to correct. The median nerve is usually divided, and often the ulnar nerve. A useless hand results which is not only without motion, but also without sensation. The forearm muscles retract with alarming rapidity; the hand assumes a position which is difficult to prevent, even with splinting, and the most careful of repairs promise but mediocre improvement. It is for this reason that primary suture of nerves and tendons should be undertaken whenever possible.

Secondary repair of the nerves and tendons above the wrist may require tendon grafts; not infrequently five grafts will be necessary, four for the profundus tendons of the fingers and one for the flexor pollicis longus.

Division of tendons over the dorsum of the wrist presents a similar problem in that the proximal tendon stumps retract into the forearm and, within a short time, it is not possible to carry out secondary suture. Tendon grafts are often required.

The extensor pollicis longus is usually best repaired by tendon transfer. The course of the tendon through its tunnel on the dorsum of the wrist is so irregular that suture within it is certain to end in failure. Therefore, a neighboring tendon, preferably the extensor indicis proprius, is used.

Division over the dorsum of the metacarpus may be repaired secondarily by suture unless there has been too great a loss of tendon substance. The paratendon through which the tendons pass in this portion of their course tends to prevent too great retraction.

Injuries of tendons over the dorsum of the fingers present complex problems varying from phalanx to phalanx. Division over the dorsum of the metacarpophalangeal joint is usually amenable to suture, even when seen late. The attachment of tendon to joint capsule prevents too great separation, and the

gap between the divided capsule and tendon ends fills with tendon callus. It is usually possible to excise this callus, freshen the tendon ends and carry out satisfactory suture.

Tendon transfers are frequently required when paralytic conditions cannot be remedied by nerve repair. The most common condition met with requiring transfers is in patients having median and radial paralyses. In median nerve paralysis, the intrinsic muscles of the thumb may fail to recover after median nerve suture. This makes it impossible for the patient to rotate the thumb about into the position of apposition for grasping. The thumb lies back against the side of the hand and can grasp only against the side of the index finger. It is advantageous in this condition to transfer a tendon, frequently the sublimis flexor of the ring finger, from the lower forearm subcutaneously across the thenar eminence to the thumb in the region of the metacarpophalangeal joint. This tendon will then pull the thumb out in abduction and apposition to face the other digits (Fig. 46).

In radial nerve paralysis, in which for some reason or other repair of the nerve is not possible, it is customary to transfer one or both of the carpal flexors onto the dorsum of the wrist, and insert it or them into the common digital extensors and into the extensor of the thumb.

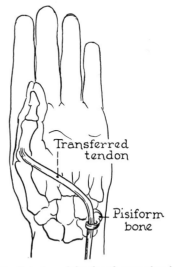

Figure 46. Rotation of the thumb may often be secured by transfer of a tendon, usually the sublimis flexor of the ring finger, to the region of the metacarpophalangeal joint. The transferred tendon is led through a fascial loop about the flexor carpi ulnaris, or may simply be passed beneath the flexor carpi ulnaris so that the line of pull is from the region of the pisiform bone. This is a very valuable procedure when the motor function of the median nerve has not returned and the small muscles of the thenar eminence are paralyzed.

One other transfer which is occasionally carried out is valuable in ulnar paralysis in which, despite nerve repair or when repair is not possible, the interosseus muscles fail to regenerate. The sublimis tendons of two fingers are divided at their insertions and slips are led around the sides of the finger to be inserted into the lateral slips of the extensor expansion. If transfer is successful, these slips will extend the interphalangeal joints.

Many other tendon transfers are practiced. In most instances, individual indications obtain in each case and the surgeon must determine what motions are most important and which motors are present to make those motions possible.

Problems with regard to the bony framework of the hand likewise occur. If they are present, they take precedence over every other repair except that of the skin, which must be satisfactory to permit deep repairs on the bones. Correction of malunions, consolidation of nonunions and bone replacement by bone graft may be needed to restore satisfactory framework.

It may be obvious that active motion can never be secured in certain joints, and that it would be better to fuse them in a functional position. Thus, it may be indicated to place the thumb into a position of abduction and apposition to face the pads of other digits and fix it there by means of a bone block between the first and second metacarpals. Occasionally, the interphalangeal joints may be so badly damaged that active motion is not likely to be restored. In these instances, it may seem wise to fuse them in a slightly flexed position, thus permitting the digits to be flexed as a whole at the metacarpophalangeal joints.

The hand has three simple functions: grasping, feeling and pinching. These three functions should be the minimum which the surgeon should strive to restore. However, this does not mean to imply that finer and more complicated actions should not be restored if the possibility exists. Thus, it may be possible to restore individual flexion and extension of the digits by various tendon transferences or tendon grafts. Abduction and adduction of the fingers, so necessary in certain fine movements, may be partially or completely restored by certain operative procedures.

The loss of the thumb, which renders grasp impossible, is disabling, and many procedures have been devised to provide a functional substitute. In some patients, it may be possible to restore grasp, provided the metacarpal and a bit of proximal phalanx are left, by deepening the cleft between the first and second metacarpals. This will render the thumb remnants more mobile, and will often make a most satisfactory buttress against which the fingers can grasp objects. In instances in which a fair remnant of the thumb is left and the index finger is gone, the cleft may be further deepened by removal of the second metacarpal.

If there is no thumb remnant left, or if what little is left is too short to be serviceable, various procedures have been carried out to devise a new thumb. These have consisted essentially in formation of a tubular graft of skin into which a bone or rib cartilage graft is inserted to give stability. Sensation is provided by the transfer of a neurovascular island pedicle to the volar aspect of the substitute thumb.

In a few instances, surgeons have successfully reported the grafting of a toe to the hand to replace a lost thumb. The procedure would be applicable only in youngsters who could withstand the long period of awkward and tiring immobilization necessary for such a graft to take. Likewise, the tissues must be young and well vascularized to withstand such procedures.

A more ingenious procedure was devised by Hilgenfeldt, and later popularized by Littler. This consists in transferring another digit of the same hand to the location of the thumb. To be successful, it is necessary that some of the base of the metacarpal be present, into which the metacarpal of the transferred digit is fixed. The digit to be transferred is isolated along with its nerve, vascular supply and flexor tendons intact, and set onto the thumb metacarpal.

Before procedures of this sort are undertaken, the surgeon must make sure that the patient will benefit from them and that he cannot carry on satisfactorily without a thumb. Hilgenfeldt has advised that patients be permitted a trial of use without the thumb for about a year before the procedure is contemplated.

While there is no doubt that the thumb is a most valuable digit, there may be some question as to the exalted position it is given. Certainly, the surgeon must make every effort to save all length possible and to restore to every possible function whatever remnants there are of the thumb. However, when this digit is irretrievably gone, there is some question as to whether its loss is as great a handicap as we have been prone to think.

If there is a good thumb on the opposite hand, the indications to restore the thumb are much less urgent than in instances in which the thumb has been lost bilaterally.

Age and occupation of the individual should be taken into account, as well as those other factors which the surgeon must consider, when starting off on a long series of operations or a course of treatments which will require the fullest cooperation of a willing and honest patient. Many patients are reduced to dependent loafers by apparently justifiable attempts to restore a moderate increase in function to an already fairly useful hand.

READING REFERENCES

Allen, H. S., and Mason, M. L.: A universal splint for immobilization of the hand in the position of function. Quart. Bull. Northwestern Univ. M. Sch. *21*:218, 1947.

Bailey, D. A.: The Infected Hand. London, Harper and Row, Publishers, 1963.

Barsky, A. J.: Congenital Anomalies of the Hand and Their Surgical Treatment. Springfield, Illinois, Charles C Thomas, 1958.

Boyes, J. H.: Bunnell's Surgery of the Hand 4th ed. Philadelphia, J. B. Lippincott Company, 1964.

Brand, P.: Tendon grafting. J. Bone & Joint Surg. *43-B*:444, 1961.

Brown, J. B., and McDowell, F.: Skin Grafting. 3rd ed. Philadelphia, J. B. Lippincott Company, 1958.

Brown, J. B., McDowell, F., and Fryer, M. P.: Surgical treatment of radiation burns. Surg. Gyn. & Obst. *93*: 385, 1951.

Clarkson, P., and Pelly, A.: The General and Plastic Surgery of the Hand. Philadelphia, F. A. Davis Company, 1962.

Felländer, M.: Tuberculous tenosynovitis of the hand treated by combined surgery and chemotherapy. Acta chir. scandinav. *111*:142, 1956.

Flatt, A. E.: The Care of Minor Hand Injuries. 2nd ed. St. Louis, The C. V. Mosby Company, 1963.

Flatt, A. E.: The Care of the Rheumatoid Hand. St. Louis, The C. V. Mosby Company, 1963.

Flynn, J. E.: Hand Surgery. Baltimore, The Williams & Wilkins Company, 1966.

Furlong, R.: Injuries of the Hand. Boston, Little, Brown & Company, 1957.

Hilgenfeldt, O.: Operativer Daumenersatz. Stuttgart, Ferdinand Enke, 1950.

Iselin, M.: Atlas of Hand Surgery. New York, McGraw-Hill Book Company, 1964.

Kanavel, A. B.: Infections of the Hand. 7th ed. Philadelphia, Lea & Febiger, 1938.

Kanavel, A. B.: Congenital malformations of the hands. Arch. Surg. *25*:1; 282, 1932.

Kaplan, E. B.: Functional and Surgical Anatomy of the Hand. 2nd ed. Philadelphia, J. B. Lippincott Company, 1965.

Koch, S. L.: Injuries of the parietes and extremities. Surg. Gyn. & Obst. *76*:1; 189, 1943.

Koch, S. L.: Acute rapidly spreading infections following typical injuries of the hand. Surg. Gyn. & Obst. *59*: 277, 1934.

Larsen, R. D., and Posch, J. L.: Dupuytren's contracture. Surg. Gyn. & Obst.; Internat. Abst. Surg. *115*:1, 1962.

Littler, J. W.: The hand and upper extremity. *In*, Converse, J. M.: Reconstructive Plastic Surgery. Vol. IV. Philadelphia, W. B. Saunders Company, 1964.

Mason, M. L.: Tuberculous tenosynovitis of the hand. Surg. Gyn. & Obst. *69*:363, 1934.

Mason, M. L.: Tumors of the Hand. Surg. Gyn. & Obst. *64*: 129, 1937.

Mason, M. L., and Allen, H. S.: Rate of healing of tendons. Ann. Surg. *113*:424, 1941.

Mason, M. L., and Shearon, C. G.: The process of tendon repair. Arch. Surg. *25*:615, 1932.

Milford, L.: The hands. *In*, Campbell's Operative Orthopaedics. 4th ed. St. Louis, The C. V. Mosby Company, 1963, Vol. I, Chap. 4, p. 139.

Nichols, H. M.: Manual of Hand Injuries. 2nd ed. Chicago, Year Book Publishers, 1960.

Peacock, E. E., and Hartrampf, C. R.: The repair of flexor tendons in the hand. Surg. Gyn. & Obst.; Internat. Abst. Surg. *113*:411, 1961.

Pimm, L. H., and Waugh, W.: Tuberculous tenosynovitis. J. Bone & Joint Surg. *39-B*:91, 1957.

Rank, B. K., and Wakefield, A. R.: Surgery of Repair as Applied to Hand Injuries. Baltimore, The Williams & Wilkins Company, 1960.

Robins, R. H. C.: Injuries and Infections of the Hand. Baltimore, The Williams & Wilkins Company, 1961.

Skoog, T.: Dupuytren's contracture with special reference to etiology and improved surgical treatment; Its occurrence in epileptics; Note on knuckle-pads, Acta chir. scandinav. (Supp. 139) *96*:1, 1948.

Teloh, H. A., Mason, M. L., and Wheelock, M. C.: Histopathological study of radiation injuries of the skin. Surg. Gyn. & Obst. *90*:335, 1950.

Chapter 33

THE FOOT

by

WILLIAM A. LARMON, M.D.

WILLIAM ALEXANDER LARMON also contributed the chapter on the Musculoskeletal System for this textbook. He has brought the same clarity of presentation to this chapter, emphasizing the basic principles underlying the afflictions of the foot which have surgical importance.

The surgeon must be mindful of the complex relationships of the foot to the rest of the body. The foot is the connecting link with our terrestrial environment, balancing the body in the upright posture and propelling it about. Proper function of the foot depends upon the integrity of the musculoskeletal and nervous systems for balance and movement, the circulatory system for nourishment and the skin and subcutaneous tissues for protection and covering. Pathologic changes in any of these systems may affect the foot and alter or limit the ability to stand, walk or run.

FUNCTIONAL ANATOMY

MOTION AND POSITIONS OF THE FOOT. To treat pathologic conditions of the foot successfully, the surgeon must understand the normal anatomy and physiology of the lower extremity.

Movements and positions of the foot are traditionally described with the foot off the ground and unencumbered. When the dorsum of the foot is brought toward the anterior surface of the leg, the movement is dorsiflexion and the position of the foot is termed calcaneus. The opposite movement is plantar flexion and the foot is in the equinus position. These motions take place at the tibiotalar joint. When the heel is inclined toward the midline of the body, it is inverted and in varus position. The opposite is eversion and valgus position. This motion takes place in the joint between the talus and the os calcis or subtalar joint. When the forefoot is brought toward the midline of the body it is adducted. The opposite movement and position place the

forefoot in abduction. These motions take place in the calcaneocuboid and talonavicular joints, as well as in the joints of the other tarsal bones.

The subtalar, calcaneocuboid and talonavicular joints work as a unit, producing supination of the foot when the plantar aspect is directed toward the body midline. Pronation of the foot is found when the sole of the foot is directed away from the midplane of the body. Varus and valgus positions of the foot are synonymous with supination and pronation.

When the toes are brought toward the plantar surface of the foot, they are flexed, and when in the opposite position, they are extended.

The cardinal positions of the foot are calcaneus, equinus, varus and valgus. Various combinations of these terms describe the positional deformities that occur in the foot. Thus, talipes equinovarus points out the abnormal position of clubfoot.

ARCHES OF THE FOOT. The act of standing demands stability and balance in the structures of the foot; walking and running require mobile, elastic, shock-absorbing properties. The architecture of the foot fulfills all of these functional requirements.

The hindfoot, composed of the talus and the massive os calcis, is adapted to support body weight. The midtarsal bones, the metatarsal bones and the phalanges are more mobile and are adapted to the function of balance and propulsion.

The medial and lateral halves of the foot are also designed for special purposes (Fig. 1, *B*). The os calcis, cuboid and fourth and fifth metatarsal bones with their phalanges

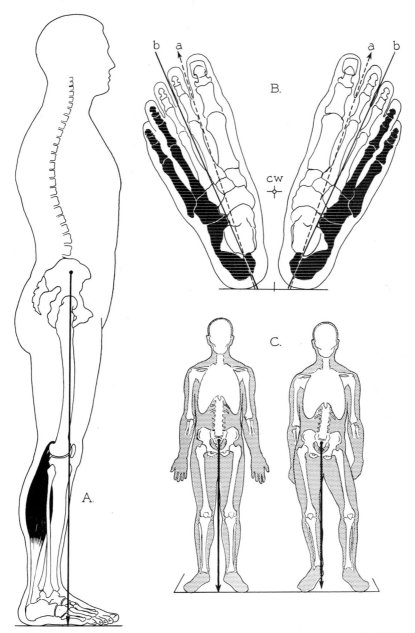

Figure 1. *A*, The center of gravity of the body is located at the second sacral vertebra. The weight of the body falls between the feet at the level of the navicular bone (point CW in *B*). When standing, the body sways forward periodically. Contraction of the triceps surae muscle (*A*) pulls the tibia posteriorly on the foot to maintain balance. *B*, The medial half of the foot is mobile, while the lateral half is a stable platform. *C*, Ligamentous strain in the foot is relieved by frequently shifting the body weight from one foot to the other. The axis of leverage in walking is line *a*. The axis of medial and lateral balance is line *b*. (Redrawn from Morton, D. J.: The Human Foot. Columbia University Press.)

form a stable platform in contact with the ground. The medial half of the foot, composed of the talus, navicular and cuneiform bones, and the first, second and third metatarsal bones and phalanges form an arched, elastic and mobile structure necessary for balance and propulsion.

The arches of the foot have been likened to a stone bridge, the fit and shape of the bones

of the foot maintaining a rigid arch. Such is not the case (Fig. 2, *A*). The medial longitudinal arch is composed of bones with curved articulations which in no way resemble the keystone shape of the stones in a bridge. These curved joints, held together and supported by strong ligaments, tendons and muscles, provide elasticity and mobility necessary for the function of the foot. The

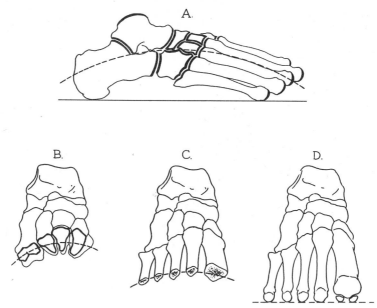

Figure 2.   *A*, The longitudinal arch of the foot is made up of bones with curved articular surfaces adapted for complex movements. Ligaments must maintain the relationships of these surfaces to preserve the arch. *B*, The transverse arch is well-defined at the base of the metatarsal bones. The articulations are wedge-shaped and stable. *C*, The transverse arch flattens in the midmetatarsal area. *D*, No arch is present at the head of the metatarsal bone. Body weight is carried by all of the metatarsal bones. When one bone becomes prominent in the sole of the foot, more weight is borne by the involved bone and pressure symptoms occur.

longitudinal arch of the foot is more accurately described as a bow or spring. The plantar structures, composed of fascia, ligaments, tendons and muscles, are the bow strings.

The transverse arch of the foot exists at the metatarsal cuneiform joints but gradually flattens as the heads of the metatarsal bones are approached (Fig. 2, *B*, *C* and *D*). All of the metatarsal heads in the normal foot make equal contact with the ground when weight is borne, and no true arch exists at this point. The transverse arch is stable at the metatarsal cuneiform joints as these bones more nearly resemble the keystones of the stone bridge. The configuration of these joints provides stability.

LIGAMENTS OF THE FOOT. The bones in the foot are joined by ligaments, which are thickened areas in the joint capsules. In addition to the ligaments of the individual joints, there are two major ligaments and the plantar aponeurosis which act as bow strings to aid in maintaining the arches (Fig. 3, *A*). One of these—the calcaneonavicular ligament—arises near the sustentaculum tali on the calcaneus and inserts into the plantar aspect of the navicular bone. This ligament passes under the head of the talus as a sling, providing support but not restricting motion of the talonavicular joint. It prevents the

talus from excessive plantar flexion at the midtarsal joints, thus preserving the longitudinal arch.

The second important ligament is the long plantar, arising near the tuberosities of the calcaneus and inserting into the cuboid and the base of the metatarsal bones (Fig. 3, *B*). This ligament supports the midportion of the longitudinal arch, approximating the metatarsal bases to the calcaneus, and is a second string in the bow.

The third structure—the plantar aponeurosis—arises at the tuberosities of the os calcis and inserts into the toes on the plantar aspect (Fig. 3, *C* and *D*). When the toes are extended, the plantar aponeurosis, passing over the rounded metatarsal heads, tightens. This mechanism shortens the plantar aponeurosis, approximating the metatarsal heads toward the heel, maintaining the longitudinal arch. This action can be likened to the mechanics of the windlass: the toes are the handle and the metatarsal heads the drum of the windlass; the plantar fascia is the rope pulled over the drum, shortening the distance between metatarsal heads and the heel, raising the longitudinal arch. This takes place when most needed at the point of push-off in walking when maximum strain is thrown on the arch of the foot.

MUSCLES OF THE FOOT.   The intrinsic mus-

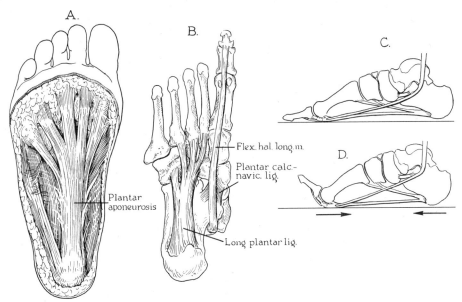

A.

B.

C.

D.

Flex. hal. long. m.

Plantar calc.-
navic. lig.

Plantar
aponeurosis

Long plantar lig.

Figure 3. *A*, The plantar aponeurosis aids in support of the longitudinal arch. *B*, The long plantar and the calcaneo-navicular ligaments support the midpart of the arch. The calcaneonavicular ligament acts as a sling under the head of the talus. The pulley-like arrangement of the tendons on the plantar aspect of the foot running beneath the malleolus produces active support for the arch. *C* and *D*, The heads of the metatarsal bones act as a pulley for the plantar aponeurosis when the toes are dorsiflexed. This shortens distance between the metatarsal heads and the condyles of the os calcis and raises the arch. This mechanism supports the arch at the point of "push-off" in walking. (*C* and *D* redrawn from Hicks, J. H.: Mechanics of foot; the plantar aponeurosis and the arch. J. Anat. 88:25, 1954.)

cles of the foot lend active support to the ligaments in standing and walking. They are arranged to aid in supporting the elastic arches (Fig. 3, *C* and *C*). Medially, the abductor hallucis, arising on the os calcis and inserting into the great toe, adds another string to the bow. The central muscle group, composed of the quadratus plantae, the flexor brevis of the toes and the lumbricales, maintains the central portion of the arch.

The long muscles arising in the leg provide the motor power for the gross movements of the foot necessary for balance and locomotion.

The triceps surae, or calf group of muscles, composed of the gastrocnemius and soleus muscles, is the prime lifter of the body in walking, through plantar flexion of the foot at the tibiotalar joint. In addition to this action, this muscle group inverts the heel at the subtalar joint in plantar flexion (Fig. 4, *A*). This inverting action is prevented by the balanced action of the peroneus longus muscle, which contracts synchronously in walking (Fig. 4, *B*). The pulley action of the peroneus longus tendon, passing from the lateral side of the foot at the cuboid bone to the base of the first metatarsal bone, everts the foot in plantar flexion. It also depresses the distal end of the first metatarsal against the ground

in walking and standing, thus elevating the arches of the foot and aiding in propulsion.

The dorsiflexors of the foot are the strong tibialis anticus and the weaker extensor digitorum longus. The tibialis anticus inserting into the medial aspect of the foot inverts and supinates the foot, elevating the arch, while the extensor digitorum longus, passing lateral to the axis of balance of the foot, tends to evert the foot in dorsiflexion (Fig. 5).

The tibialis posterior, passing beneath the pulley of the medial malleolus and inserting into the plantar aspect of the navicular bone, inverts the foot and adducts the forefoot. The peroneus brevis, passing beneath the lateral malleolus and inserting into the base of the fifth metatarsal, balances this action of the tibialis posterior and produces eversion of the foot and abduction of the forefoot.

The action of these muscles can be likened to three sets of reins attached to a bridle in providing medial and lateral stability for the foot. The triceps surae and peroneus longus balance each other in plantar flexion. The tibialis posterior and peroneus brevis balance the foot in neutral position, and the tibialis anticus and the extensor digitorum longus balance in dorsiflexion.

Any disturbance in the function of these muscles and tendons results in foot imbal-

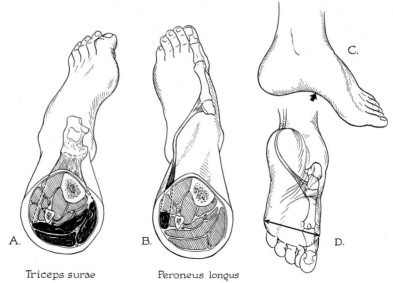

Triceps surae   Peroneus longus

Figure 4. *A*, The triceps surae muscles produce plantar flexion and inversion, equinovarus position. *B*, The peroneus longus counteracts the inversion by the triceps surae in plantar flexion. *C* and *D*, Acting alone it everts the foot in plantar flexion: valgus position. It also depresses the distal end of the first metatarsal bone, raising the arch and fixing the bone to the ground in walking during the push-off phase.

ance and produces static and dynamic deformities and disturbances in walking.

STANDING AND BALANCING.   When we stand in the normal position, the feet are moderately separated and the toes point outward. In this position, the body weight is equally divided between the feet. The center of gravity of the body may be assumed to be at the center of the second sacral vertebra (Fig. 1,

A and *B*). A plumb line dropped from the center of gravity falls midway between the feet at the level of the navicular bone. Thus, the body is supported by two pillars with the center of gravity falling between them. These two pillars are supported on the lever arms of the foot, which extend forward of this center of gravity as the forefoot and backward as the heel. Thus, stability is insured through

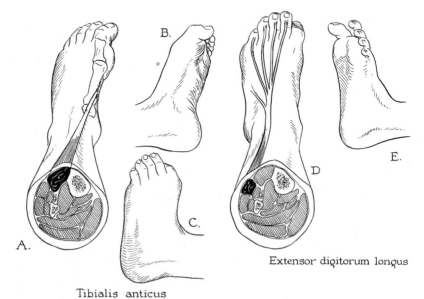

Extensor digitorum longus

Tibialis anticus

Figure 5. *A, B* and *C*, The tibialis anticus dorsiflexes and inverts the foot and elevates the first metatarsal bone: calcaneovarus position. *D* and *E*, The extensor digitorum longus is a weak dorsiflexor of the foot as well as the toes. The tendons pass lateral to the axis of balance of the foot, and produce eversion of the foot in dorsiflexion: calcaneovalgus position. The two muscles balance each other in pure dorsiflexion of the foot.

these lever arms forward, backward and from side to side.

Balance is maintained by a minimum expenditure of muscle power. The muscles contract periodically to correct swaying of the body, but the majority of the time they are at rest (Fig. 1, A). There is a rhythmic forward sway of the body which is counteracted by periodic contraction of the triceps surae muscles and the toe flexors. This forces the forefoot lever against the ground. Since the foot is fixed to the ground, the effect of this force is to pull the tibia backward, bringing the center of gravity back to the normal position. The act of balancing can be clarified if we consider the foot as fixed to the ground. The muscles then act on the leg to maintain its position over the foot. Attempts to plantar flex the foot pull the tibia backward. When one attempts dorsiflexion, the tibia is pulled forward. Inversion force pulls the leg medially and eversion force on the foot pulls the leg laterally.

While this balancing is taking place, the weight passing through the feet is supported by the ligaments. However, these ligaments are not strained because we shift position frequently (Fig. 1, C). It has been found that the standing person shifts his position about every 30 seconds from one foot to the other and forward and backward on both feet. Seldom does a person stand still for a full minute. This economy of muscle power and shifting of body weight to various ligaments accounts for our ability to stand for long periods without fatigue.

Weight transmission through the feet while standing has been determined by many investigators. When the center of gravity falls opposite the navicular bone, equal weight is supported by the forefoot and heel. The heel bears half of the body weight; the metatarsal bones bear the other half. The division of weight through the metatarsal heads, however, is not equal. The first metatarsal bone

supports one-third of the weight borne by the forefoot, and the lateral four metatarsal bones share equally the remaining two-thirds. Thus, it is apparent that there is no transverse arch or weight bearing at the level of the metatarsal heads. Any disturbance in transmission of this load through these structures produces static problems in the foot. The typical callus on the plantar aspect of the foot over the distal end of a metatarsal bone signifies a disturbance in weight bearing and indicates overloading of that metatarsal.

This distribution of weight in the long axis of the foot has been termed the *axis of leverage* by Morton (Fig. 1, B). However, in balancing, the functional axis of the foot falls between the second and third metatarsal bones, each half bearing equal weight. This has been termed the *axis of balance*.

WALKING. The act of walking is accomplished by shifting the center of gravity of the body forward. This is accomplished by inclining the body forward and propelling it upward by plantar flexion of the foot (Fig. 6). Gravity pulls the center of gravity forward and downward. The forward-swinging opposite leg and foot catch the falling body. The momentum of body weight carries the trunk over the leg. The process is then repeated; the center of gravity is raised and propelled forward as the triceps surae contracts, forcing the foot into plantar flexion. Thus, muscle contractions raise the center of gravity and incline it forward; gravity then supplies the acceleration necessary to carry the body over the advanced leg. This mechanism conserves muscle power. The muscles in the leg and foot act only for short periods in the swing and stance phase of walking; gravity supplies part of the force necessary for locomotion.

Other muscles in the leg and foot contract briefly at various phases of the step. Following the forward propulsive force of the triceps

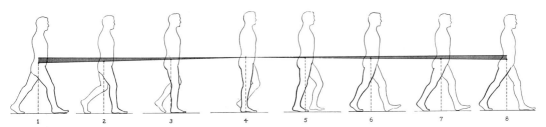

Figure 6. In walking, the center of gravity falls forward and is caught by the advancing foot (*1*). The forward momentum carries the body over the foot, raising the center of gravity (*2-3-4*). During the push-off phase, plantar flexion of the foot inclines the center of gravity forward and propels it forward (*5*). The center of gravity then falls forward, advancing the body, to be caught by the opposite foot (*6-7-8*). (Adapted from Morton, D. J.: The Human Foot. Columbia University Press.)

surae and toe flexor muscles, the quadriceps muscle group contracts briefly to straighten the knee (Fig. 7). As the leg swings forward, the hamstring muscles contract for a short period just before the leg is completely extended. This action of the hamstring muscles prevents the leg from snapping into extension at the knee. The dorsiflexor muscles contract as the heel strikes the ground to prevent the foot from sudden plantar flexion. These various muscle contractions supply no forward propulsion but control the forward-swinging leg and make for a smooth rhythmic gait.

Disturbances of the muscle control of the leg and foot in the swing and stance phases of walking produce dynamic changes in the foot, a source of limping and abnormal strain.

The joints of the foot and leg not only are concerned with the up-and-down oscillations of the body, but also take part in other actions. Because of the configuration of the hip and knee joints, the femur internally rotates at the hip and the tibia at the knee as the lower extremity swings forward and the knee is extended. As the heel strikes the ground and weight is borne on the foot, the tibia and femur externally rotate. Since the foot is fixed to the ground, the external rotation of

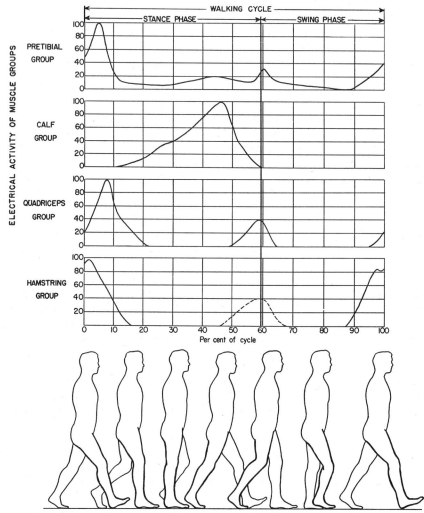

Figure 7. Electromyographic tracings of muscle activity during the stance and swing phases of walking indicate the economy of muscle power. As the heel strikes the ground, the pretibial muscles (the dorsiflexors of the foot and toes) contract to prevent the forefoot from slapping the ground. The quadriceps muscles contract briefly to straighten the knee. The hamstring muscles have already contracted to slow the forward swing of the leg at the knee, acting as a brake. As the body advances over the foot, there is little muscle activity in the leg until the push-off phase, when the calf muscles contract forcefully to propel the body forward. During the swing phase, the pretibial muscles contract to dorsiflex the foot enough to clear the ground. Just before the heel strikes the ground, the hamstring muscles contract to slow the forward swinging leg. (Redrawn by permission from Klopsteg, P. E., and Wilson, P. D.: Human Limbs and Their Substitutes. McGraw-Hill Book Company, Inc.)

these bones is taken up in the subtalar joint. This produces torque to the foot similar to that applied in skating, aiding in forward propulsion.

When there are disturbances in the alignment of these joints, normal function is com promised and abnormal strains are imposed on the ligaments and joint surfaces.

The weight borne by the foot during the stance phase passes through the center of the talus to the os calcis as the heel strikes the ground. As the body swings over the foot, the weight progresses into the midtarsal region. A part of this is transmitted to the navicular and cuneiform bones to the first two metatarsal bones and part through the cuboid and lateral three metatarsal bones. The weight with the foot flat to the ground is thus divided between the medial and lateral halves of the foot along the axis of balance between the second and third metatarsals (Fig. 1, *B*). As the push-off phase of the step is reached, the weight of the body is transferred to the leverage axis of the foot between the first and second metatarsal bones. Strong plantar flexion of the great toe at this point adds further forward propulsive force.

Abnormalities of this weight-bearing transmission through the foot will produce abnormal strains on bones, joints, ligaments, tendons and muscles and abnormal pressure on the protecting covering of skin and subcutaneous tissue.

DISEASES OF THE FOOT

Diseases of the foot may be classified as congenital and acquired. Congenital deformities include skeletal defects, absent or supernumerary parts, defects in muscles and tendons, defective joints, circulatory and lymphatic system defects and defects of the nervous system producing abnormalities of the leg and foot.

Acquired defects include postural strains, static and dynamic deformities, diseases of the nervous system producing paralysis or spasticity of muscles, circulatory diseases, tumors, infections, injuries and generalized systemic disease.

Congenital Diseases of the Foot

Congenital defects of the foot are many and varied. Some of them have a tendency to transmission to succeeding generations.

CONGENITAL TALIPES EQUINOVARUS. Congenital talipes equinovarus, or clubfoot, is a serious deformity which occurs once in every 700 to 1000 births (Fig. 8). The defect in varying degrees encompasses 75 per cent of the congenital anomalies of the foot. Frequently, it is bilateral, and it is found twice as often in boys as in girls.

Clubfoot is a combination of three distinct deformities in the foot and ankle. The forefoot is adducted and supinated, the heel is inverted and the foot is in equinus at the ankle. The degree of deformity varies from a mild, flexible one to a severe, rigid defect. There is no bone deformity at birth, but the relationship of the joints is abnormal. The metatarsal bones are adducted at the metatarsal-tarsal joints. The first metatarsal bone may be shorter than normal. The cuboid and navicular bones shift medialward, producing widening laterally at the calcaneocuboid joint. The navicular bone lies on the medial surface of the head and neck of the talus.

The normal relationship of the talus and the calcaneus is disturbed. When viewed from above, the long axis of the talus is directed forward and medially while the axis of the calcaneus is directed forward and laterally (Fig. 9). The intersection of these axes forms a V with the opening forward. The clubfoot heel is inverted and the os calcis appears to lie directly under the talus, their long axes being parallel.

The soft tissues are contracted on the medial and plantar aspect of the foot, accompanying the varus deformity.

The calf muscles are short, holding the foot in equinus position, and the insertion of the Achilles tendon appears to lie more medially on the os calcis.

The etiology of clubfoot is not clear. Several theories are applied to explain the deformity. Arrest or anomalous development of the germ plasm concerned with development of the foot in the first trimester of pregnancy may explain the defect in some

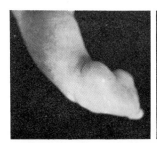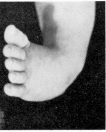

Figure 8.   Talipes equinovarus, or clubfoot, in infancy.

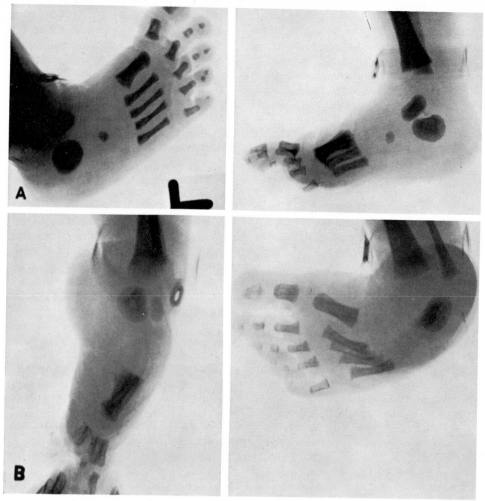

Figure 9. *A*, Relationship of bones in the normal foot. *B*, Abnormal position of bones in clubfoot. The adduction of the forefoot is marked. The talus lies directly over the os calcis in the anteroposterior view and the foot is plantar flexed at the ankle.

instances. During fetal development, the limb bud first is in the equinovarus position, but gradually the limb rotates to the normal position. Failure of rotation may account for clubfoot.

Biopsy material has shown degenerative changes in the muscles, and there may be anomalous insertion of the tendons in the foot.

In infancy, since the deformity is produced by soft tissue contractures, stretching of these structures should be begun as soon as possible, often within the first week of birth, and continued until complete overcorrection is obtained.

Three definite steps are followed to correct the deformity. Adduction and supination of the forefoot are gently changed into abduction and pronation. The inverted heel is everted and the equinus is corrected by dorsi-

flexion of the foot. The overcorrection must be maintained until the affected muscles recover, which often may require many months. There is frequently a tendency for recurrence of the deformity. The child must be observed until growth is completed, and any recurrence treated immediately.

To correct the deformity, the foot is gently stretched manually by the surgeon and a well-padded cast applied from the toes to above the flexed knee, with the forefoot abducted. The cast is changed every two weeks. When full abduction of the forefoot is obtained, the heel is gradually everted. Dorsiflexion of the foot must not be attempted until this has been accomplished.

Failure to correct fully the adduction of the forefoot, the talonavicular joint and the inverted heel before dorsiflexing the foot will result in a rocker-bottom foot. The foot dorsiflexes through the midtarsal joints; the talus and calcaneus remain in equinus. This deformity may be as disabling as clubfoot. When this occurs, the entire procedure must be started over.

When clubfoot is fully corrected, the surgeon should be able to approximate the little toe to the lateral side of the leg.

Following cast treatment, in order to maintain the correct position, the baby wears prewalker clubfoot shoes and a Denis Browne splint until walking is begun.

When the foot is rigid or treatment is started late, wedged casts may be necessary (Fig. 10). Occasionally, soft tissue contractures on the medial side of the foot are released surgically. The joint capsules are incised to allow correction of the forefoot adduction and heel inversion. Excessive stripping of the structures from the bone is avoided, as the scar tissue which forms is inelastic and may cause recurrence.

The Achilles tendon may be lengthened when there is persistent equinus in order to prevent a flat-top talus. The talus held in prolonged equinus develops a flat tibial articular surface which blocks dorsiflexion. However, some weakness of the leg results from lengthening of the Achilles tendon and the

procedure should be reserved for resistant clubfeet which fail to respond to stretching.

When the peroneal muscles function poorly or do not develop, even a well-corrected clubfoot will recur. When the child walks, the peroneal muscles fail to contract and the foot swings into inversion. Transferring the tibialis anticus to the cuboid bone tends to balance the foot and prevent the deformity.

Older children who have not been treated, or who have been allowed to develop recurrent clubfoot, may have abnormally shaped bones in the foot. If wedged casts fail to correct the deformity, resection of the deformed bones may be necessary. This is most conveniently done by removing appropriate wedges of bone from the subtalar, talonavicular and calcaneocuboid joints and fixing these joints in the proper position by arthrodesis (Fig. 11). The operation must not be done before the age of ten years because disturbance of growth of the foot follows.

CONGENITAL METATARSUS VARUS OR ADDUCTUS. Two types of congenital metatarsus varus are found in the newborn. The first type exhibits adduction and inversion of the metatarsal bones with the heel in the valgus position. This foot deformity is rigid and diffi-

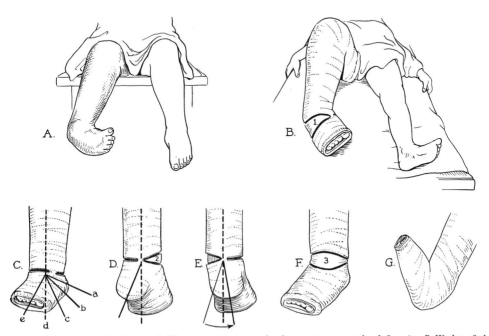

Figure 10.   A, Recurrent and resistant clubfeet may require wedged casts to correct the deformity. B, Wedge of plaster is removed laterally to allow gradual stretching of the adducted forefoot. C, The wedge closed and the forefoot abducted. D, The heel viewed posteriorly is forced into eversion by removing a wedge of plaster laterally just above the subtalar joint. E, The wedge closed and the heel everted. F, The equinus deformity is corrected by removing a plaster wedge from the cast at the level of the ankle joint. G, The fully corrected position of the foot in the plaster cast.

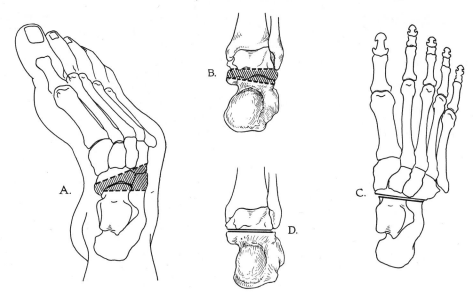

Figure 11. *A,* Bony deformity of clubfoot demands resection of bone to place the foot in the normal position. Arthrodesis of the talonavicular and calcaneocuboid joints is done to prevent recurrence of the adduction deformity. (Redrawn from Speed, J. S., and Smith, H.: Campbell's Operative Orthopaedics. 2nd ed. The C. V. Mosby Company.)
B, Wedge of bone is removed from the subtalar joint to place the heel in slight eversion. *C* and *D,* The corrected foot.

cult to correct and recurrence is the rule. Fortunately, the condition is rare.

The second type is flexible; the forefoot is adducted and the heel is in neutral or slight varus position (Fig. 12, *A* and *B*). This type has been increasing in frequency in recent years. Fortunately, the deformity is easily corrected and recurrence is uncommon. The forefoot is adducted and inverted and the longitudinal arch is higher than normal through the action of the tibialis anticus muscle. The lateral aspect of the foot at the base of the fifth metatarsal bone is prominent. The hindfoot is normal, and the foot can be readily dorsiflexed.

In mild deformities, stretching the fore-foot in abduction and eversion is done by the mother each time the baby's diaper is changed. This may be the only treatment necessary. Prewalker clubfoot shoes attached to the Denis Browne splint in external rotation may correct more severe deformity. Occasionally, casts are used as in the first part of the correction for clubfoot.

Untreated, the deformity may persist and increase in severity. Older children who fail to respond to use of a wedged cast require osteotomy of the base of the metatarsal bones (Fig. 13, *A* and *B*). Following union of the bones, outflare shoes are worn for several months.

CONGENITAL CALCANEOVALGUS. The con-

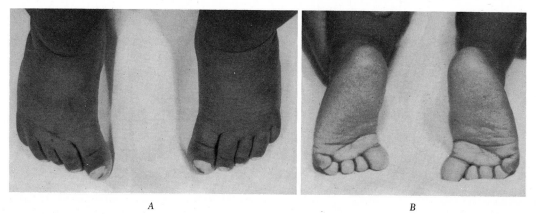

| A | B |

Figure 12. *A,* Metatarsus varus deformity. *B,* The deformity is increased and perpetuated if the infant sleeps with the legs internally rotated.

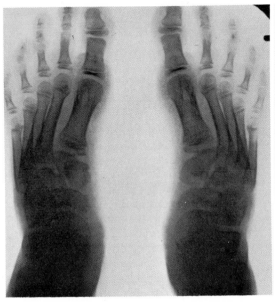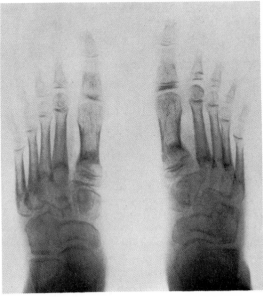

A

B

Figure 13. *A,* Roentgenogram of bilateral metatarsus varus. *B,* Healing after osteotomy near the base of the metatarsal bones, correcting the varus deformities.

genital calcaneovalgus foot is the direct opposite of talipes equinovarus. The etiology is thought to be an abnormal intrauterine position of the foot.

The bones of the foot are normal. The foot is in dorsiflexion; the heel points downward in valgus position and the forefoot is abducted and dorsiflexed. The fifth toe may be easily approximated to the anterolateral aspect of the leg. Usually, the foot is quite flexible and may be partially plantar flexed and inverted without difficulty.

The deformity is easily corrected by repeated gentle stretching, and there is little tendency toward recurrence. The mother is instructed to stretch the foot in plantar flexion, inversion and adduction each time the baby's diaper is changed. Denis Browne splints may be used if the deformity is resistant to stretching. The feet are internally rotated and inverted by the splint. Rarely is cast correction indicated.

When the child begins to walk, the foot may tend to assume a valgus position on weight bearing. The child should be fitted with a one-eighth inch inner heel wedge on the shoe during this period.

SYNDACTYLISM. Syndactylism may occur in two or more toes. The deformity tends to be a familial one. The toes may be webbed completely or partially from the base to the tip. The soft tissues only may be affected, or the deformity may have a bony bridge between the phalanges. Little if any functional disability results from the defect. Separation of the toes by operation is seldom necessary as the foot functions well and shoe-fitting problems are unusual.

If, for cosmetic reasons, the toes are separated surgically, x-ray films must first be made to determine the degree of bone involvement. When the bones are joined near the epiphysial plates of the phalanges, the operation should be deferred until spontaneous closure of the epiphyses has taken place. If the operation is done too early, unilateral closure of a portion of the epiphysial plate will cause angulation and deformity of the toes with growth.

POLYDACTYLISM. Polydactylism in the foot is a condition characterized by the presence of supernumerary toes. The deformity is usually familial. The extra digit may be completely formed and normal in both appearance and function, or it may be misshapen, rudimentary and functionless. Reduplication of a part of the toe, such as the distal phalanx, is a variation of the deformity. Shoe-fitting problems are frequently encountered, demanding amputation of the extra toe or plastic reconstruction of reduplicated phalanges. Amputation of a complete toe can be done at any age; however, resection of portions of duplicate phalanges must not interfere with the epiphysial plate. X-ray films should be made to determine the degree of deformity and involvement of the epiphysis.

AGENESIS. Agenesis of part or all of the foot may result from faulty limb bud development and be the source of profound disability. The forefoot is most frequently the site of deformity. Parts of toes and metatarsals may be absent. Abnormal insertion of tendons and absence of bones may produce considerable distortion of the foot. Occasionally, tendon transference, plastic operation, or stabilization of the joints of the foot is necessary to correct deformity.

MACRODACTYLISM. Occasionally, a foot is encountered which exhibits one or more giant toes. The overgrowth of the part may be due to vascular or neurotropic lesions or to some defect in the growth capacity of the toe. Amputation of the toe, or reduction of the size of the toe by plastic surgical procedures, is usually necessary to permit the wearing of matched shoes.

ACCESSORY BONES. Accessory bones of the foot occur in many locations, but most do not produce symptoms and are found incidental to x-ray examination of the foot. The recognition of these bones as accessory bones and not fractures is of medicolegal importance. The accessory bone has a complete cortex surrounding the bone, while the recent fracture shows an absence of cortex at the fracture line.

The most common accessory bones in the foot are the os trigonum, found near the posterior aspect of the talus, and the os vesalianum, at the base of the fifth metatarsal bone. These bones do not produce symptoms or weaken the foot, but they are often confused with fractures.

The accessory navicular bone located at the medial aspect of the parent bone produces a prominent mass. A bursa and painful callus may form over the medial aspect of the foot at this site from shoe pressure. The longitudinal arch of the foot may be weak and flat because the tibialis posterior tendon is abnormally inserted.

Symptoms are usually pain and swelling of the bursa over the bony prominence, and fatigue and aching in the midtarsal region because of faulty support for the longitudinal arch. When the symptoms cannot be relieved by supports to the arch of the foot, surgical correction of the deformity is necessary. The accessory navicular bone is removed and the tibialis posterior tendon is inserted under the navicular bone.

PES PLANUS OR FLATFOOT. Pes planus may be either congenital or acquired (Fig. 14). Flatfoot may also be associated with congenital calcaneovalgus deformity and the accessory navicular bone. Other congenital defects may be etiologic factors in the development of flatfoot. Hypermobile flatfoot with a short Achilles tendon and coalition of the tarsal bones producing peroneal spastic flatfoot are examples.

Pes planus may be acquired as a result of excessive strain in the obese with weak ligaments, neurologic lesions affecting the muscles and ligaments, trauma or infection producing bone, joint or muscle abnormalities, and disease of muscle.

Not all flatfeet are painful. Like the shape of noses, the height of the arches of the foot varies and may follow familial patterns. The small child beginning to walk may appear to have no arch at all. A fat pad occupies the plantar area at this age and may obscure the arch which is readily revealed when weight-bearing x-rays are taken.

Pain develops in flatfeet when the ligaments are subjected to abnormal strain. Continued use leads to synovitis of the joints of the foot and later traumatic arthritis. In the growing child, the tarsal bones develop abnormal shapes. The patient suffering from painful flatfoot rotates the foot and leg externally while walking. In this position, the anterior lever of the foot is shortened; the push-off is from the medial side of the first

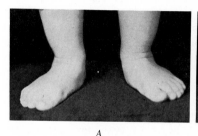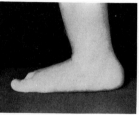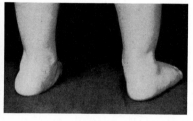

A   *B*   *C*

Figure 14.   *A*, Pes planus; flat medial arch with abduction of the forefoot. *B*, Complete flattening of the longitudinal arch. *C*, Valgus position of the heels.

metatarsal head and great toe. The stride is shortened, producing a shuffling gait.

The calcaneus is in valgus position at the subtalar joint. The talus points more medialward and the head of the bone tips downward. The longitudinal arch is flattened by angulation plantarward at the talonavicular or cuneiform-navicular joints, or at both joints. These bones rotate medialward and down, carrying the base of the metatarsal toward the plantar surface of the foot. The metatarsal bones abduct and the joints on the medial aspect of the foot open and compress on the lateral side (Fig. 15). The calcaneonavicular and long plantar ligaments are stretched and relaxed.

SHORT TRICEPS SURAE MUSCLES. When the Achilles tendon and triceps surae muscles are short, dorsiflexion of the foot is limited and increased strain is placed on the anterior lever arm of the foot. If the supporting ligaments stretch with weight bearing, the longitudinal arch flattens. The talus and calcaneus remain in equinus and the forefoot dorsiflexes through the midtarsal joints. The condition may occur because of congenital shortening of the muscle group, or may be secondary to the contractures of spastic paralysis or other neuromuscular afflictions.

Treatment is directed toward lengthening the Achilles tendon and calf muscles, and

supporting the arch in the normal position until the muscles and ligaments recover. The triceps surae muscles in the child are stretched with wedged casts. The foot must be inverted and the forefoot adducted during this procedure to prevent further stretching of the medial plantar ligaments and increasing the deformity.

When the calf muscles cannot be stretched, the Achilles tendon or the musculotendinous junction can be lengthened surgically. The foot and leg are immobilized in a plaster cast with the foot inverted and dorsiflexed for three to six weeks. A supporting shoe with an extended rigid counter, Thomas heel and medial heel wedge is used postoperatively to support the repositioned arch.

HYPERMOBILE FLATFOOT. Hypermobile flatfoot with short Achilles tendon occurs secondarily to a congenital defect in the relationship of the talus to the os calcis. Characteristically, the foot is flat only on weight bearing, assuming a normal-appearing arch when weight is removed. A history is obtained usually of asymptomatic flatfeet during childhood followed by aching, easily fatigued feet in adolescence or early adult life. Occasionally, pain develops in childhood. Symptoms vary in intensity.

The primary etiologic factor is inadequate support for the head and neck of the talus by

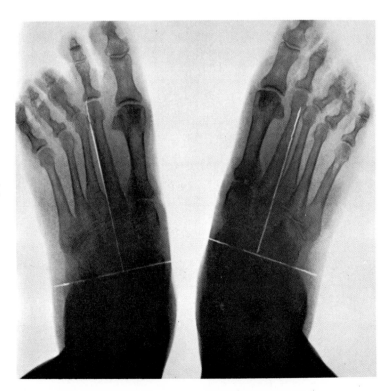

Figure 15. Abduction of the forefoot with separation of the anterior relationship of the talus and os calcis: adult flatfoot.

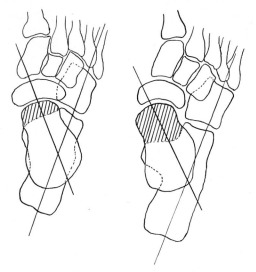

Figure 16. *A,* The normal relationship of the bones is shown for comparison. *B,* Relationship of the talus to the os calcis in hypermobile flatfoot. The talus is displaced medially and the long axis of the bones diverges anteriorly. The head and neck of the talus project farther forward and the sustentaculum tali is narrow, offering less support for the talus. (Redrawn by permission from Harris, R. I., and Beath, T.: Hypermobile flatfoot with short tendo achillis. J. Bone & Joint Surg. *30-A:*116, 1948.)

the os calcis. The triceps surae muscles are short, but this finding is secondary to the bone anomaly. The head and neck of the talus are displaced medially and the bone forms a more divergent angle with the long axis of the calcaneus (Fig. 16). The talus appears to project farther forward on the os calcis, and the sustentaculum tali is underdeveloped, slanting

and more posterior on the calcaneus than normal. This lack of bony support under the head of the talus allows it to plantar flex. Coupled with this defect, the midtarsal joints are more mobile than normal, allowing the forefoot to abduct and dorsiflex to a greater degree. The calcaneus assumes a valgus position on weight bearing and, since the calf muscles are short, the forefoot dorsiflexes and abducts to produce the flatfoot.

Treatment is directed toward support for the talus and relieving the pull of the short triceps surae. Since the degree of anatomic abnormality and the severity of symptoms vary, so must the treatment. In children, it may be necessary only to support the foot with adequate shoes and arch supports. A heel lift may be used to lessen the pull of the calf muscles. This same treatment may continue into adult life if the condition is mild and the symptoms easily controlled.

When the symptoms and anatomic deficit are severe, the subtalar and midtarsal bones must be stabilized by arthrodesis in the correct weight-bearing position. This may be accomplished by triple arthrodesis after growth of the foot is complete (Figs. 17 and 18).

PERONEAL SPASTIC FLATFOOT. Peroneal spastic flatfoot is a painful rigid foot associated with spasm and contracture of the peroneal muscles. It is due to congenital coalition of the tarsal bones. Complete or partial bony bridges form between one or more tarsal bones. This coalition of tarsal

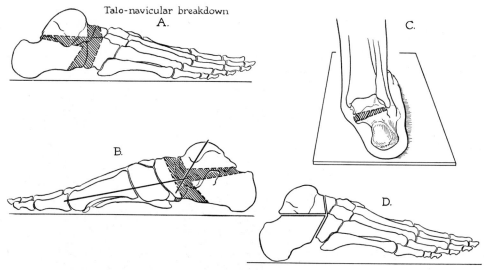

Figure 17. *A* and *B,* Triple arthrodesis of the subtalar, talonavicular and calcaneocuboid joint is performed to correct and stabilize the hypermobile flatfoot when the major angulation is at the talonavicular joint. The procedure may be used in any type of flatfoot. *C,* A wedge of bone is removed from the subtalar joint with the base medial to correct the valgus of the heel. *D,* Diagram of end result.

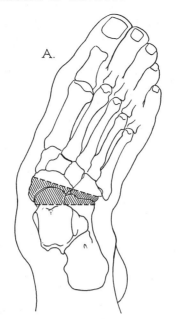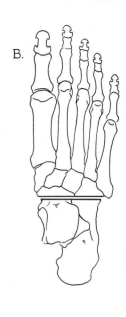

Figure 18. *A* and *B*, The forefoot abduction is corrected by removing a wedge of bone with the base medial, stabilizing the talonavicular and calcaneocuboid joints.

bones limits motion between the involved bones. Since the subtalar, talonavicular and calcaneocuboid joints act as a unit, limitation of motion in any joint throws additional strain on the remaining mobile ones. This strain eventually produces irritation in the joints and ligaments. The irritation, in turn, produces reflex spasm of the peroneal muscles which forces the foot into eversion. As the irritation continues with weight bearing, pain develops in the midtarsal and subtalar joint areas, often beneath the lateral malleolus.

The patient cannot voluntarily invert the foot. Attempts by the surgeon to do this produce immediate pain, and the peroneal muscles involuntarily contract. Similar clinical symptoms may occur when irritation and limitation of motion are present in the damaged subtalar joint following fracture of the articular surface of the os calcis.

The most frequent coalition is between the anterior os calcis and the navicular bone. The bones fuse by either a complete or partial bridge of bone at the medial anterior portion of the os calcis and the lateral inferior portion of the navicular bone. This bridge of bone limits inversion and eversion in the subtalar joint. Routine anteroposterior and lateral roentgenograms fail to reveal the abnormality. Oblique x-ray films are necessary to show the coalition.

Other bony or cartilaginous bridges form between the os calcis and talus. One may occur posteriorly through the os trigonum, the other in the region of the sustentaculum

tali. The latter can only be visualized by special x-ray technique. The patient should be placed on the x-ray table with the knees flexed. The x-ray beam is directed from the posterior, downward and forward between 35 and 45 degrees to correspond to the angulation of the articular surface of the sustentaculum.

The calcaneus may coalesce with the cuboid bone through a bridge of bone through the os peroneum. Other fusions of bone take place between the cuboid and navicular bones, and the talus and navicular bone. Rarely, massive fusion of several tarsal bones is found.

Injury may precipitate the original pain in the ligaments followed by the syndrome of peroneal spastic flatfoot.

Treatment is directed toward relief of irritation and muscle spasm. Rest, elevation and heat are prescribed, followed by gentle manipulation of the foot to the inverted position. The foot and leg are immobilized in a plaster cast with the foot inverted for six weeks. Weight bearing in a walking cast is resumed at the end of three weeks. If the symptoms subside, the patient is fitted with an orthopedic shoe to support the longitudinal arch and hold the heel slightly inverted.

Recurrence of the symptoms and deformity is the rule, and surgical correction is often necessary. Arthrodesis of the tarsal joints eliminates motion and the irritation which produces the peroneal muscle spasm. Following this procedure, inversion and eversion of the foot are lost, but the foot is stable in the proper weight-bearing position and is painless.

Triple arthrodesis of the subtalar, calcaneocuboid and talonavicular joints is useful in correcting flatfoot deformities which do not respond to conservative supportive measures (Figs. 17 and 18). The operation is indicated in peroneal spastic flatfoot, hypermobile flatfoot, arthritic flatfoot and in flatfoot when the main deformity occurs at the talonavicular joint.

Some flatfeet exhibit the primary plantar angulation at the naviculocuneiform joint. Children or young adults with symptomatic flatfeet which do not respond to conservative measures may require correction and fusion of this joint with the first metatarsal-cuneiform joint (Fig. 19). Following operation, the

foot is immobilized in inversion and plantar flexion to raise the arch until arthrodesis occurs.

CONGENITAL VERTICAL TALUS. The deformity of congenital vertical talus produces a rigid rocker-bottom foot. The longitudinal arch is nonexistent or reversed. Although the etiology is considered congenital, the high incidence of this deformity associated with arthrogryposis suggests a definite relationship to this disease.

The forefoot is dorsiflexed; the heel is in equinus and deep creases may be present over the anterior ankle. Eversion of the heel and abduction of the forefoot are not present at birth, but develop later. Rigidity of the foot is a characteristic finding. The posterior os calcis does not touch the ground when standing. The first metatarsal is dorsiflexed, and a

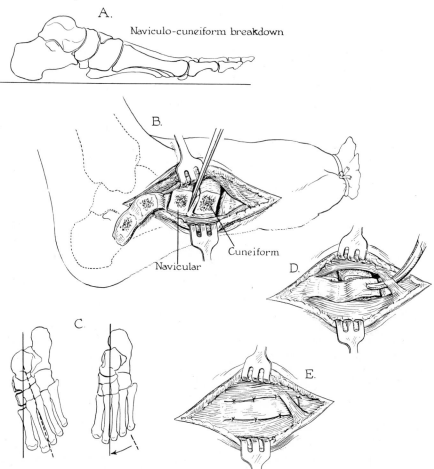

Figure 19. *A*, Painful flatfoot with the major plantar angulation at the naviculocuneiform joint is stabilized by arthrodesis of the naviculocuneiform and cuneiform-metatarsal joints. *B*, A flap of joint capsule and bone is raised from the navicular and cuneiform joints. The cartilage and subchondral bone are removed. *C*, The abduction and eversion of the forefoot are corrected. *D* and *E*, The flap of ligament and bone is sutured under the tibialis anticus tendon, and reefed to hold the new position of the arch. While fusion takes place, the foot is immobilized in inversion with the arch molded by a plaster cast. (Redrawn by permission from Miller, O. L.: A plastic flatfoot operation. J. Bone & Joint Surg. 9:84, 1927.)

flexion deformity may be present at the metatarsal-phalangeal joint of the great toe. The calcaneus is narrow and beak-shaped anteriorly, and the talus resembles an hourglass. The navicular bone dislocates dorsally and laterally, and articulates with the talus at the neck of the bone.

The disability is profound. Shoes are difficult to fit and pain develops in the foot. The rigidity of the foot defeats conservative corrective measures. Triple arthrodesis at an appropriate age may place the foot in a better weight-bearing position, but the result is never perfect.

TALIPES CAVUS. Pes cavus, or clawfoot, is the opposite deformity of flatfoot. The longitudinal arch is higher than normal. Usually, the hindfoot is near normal; the os calcis may be slightly inverted. The high arch is due to plantar flexion of the forefoot through the tarsal and metatarsal joints (Fig. 20).

Mild deformities may not affect the toes and are asymptomatic. With more severe deformity, the toes become flexed at the interphalangeal joints and hyperextended or dorsally dislocated at the metatarsal-phalangeal joints. The plantar fascia becomes shortened and the metatarsal heads are prominent in the ball of the foot. Calluses develop over the metatarsal heads and corns appear over the proximal interphalangeal joints of the toes. The foot may be in moderate equinus position associated with contracted calf muscles.

The deformity may be idiopathic or secondary to diseases of the nervous system or the muscles. It frequently follows poliomyelitis, myelodysplasia, spina bifida and muscular

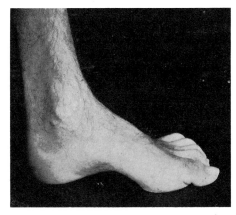

Figure 20. The arch is elevated in the cavus foot. The dorsum of the foot is prominent. The deformity is primarily due to plantar flexion of the forefoot with the heel in normal position. In this patient, the toes are contracted into the clawfoot deformity.

dystrophy. The intrinsic muscles of the foot are insufficient and may be contracted. Failure of these muscles to maintain extension of the interphalangeal joints of the toes creates imbalance. The unopposed long extensor muscles produce hyperextension at the metatarsal-phalangeal joints, and the long flexor muscles promote flexion of the interphalangeal joints.

Conservative treatment in the mild condition consists in elevation of the depressed heads of the metatarsal bones and stretching of the tight plantar structures. This may be done with a transverse metatarsal bar placed on the sole of the shoe just proximal to the metatarsal heads. A similar method may be used in which a metatarsal arch support is placed in the shoe. This raises the metatarsal heads and relieves pressure on the plantar calluses by transferring the weight more proximally in the foot. The elevation of the metatarsal bones tends to straighten the contracted toes.

When more severe deformity is found, operative correction may be necessary to relieve the symptoms. Since the plantar aponeurosis is short, it may be lengthened by section of the attachment to the os calcis. The foot is stretched and immobilized in the corrected position in a plaster cast for three weeks. When the toes are in the claw position, the metatarsal heads are depressed and the toes do not function. Arthrodesis of the interphalangeal joints so they are straight permits the long flexor muscles of the toes to act at the metatarsal-phalangeal joints, holding the toes in proper weight-bearing position.

If the deformity is progressive or the foot is rigid, more extensive operative procedures are demanded. In addition to arthrodesis of the toe joints, the extensor tendons of the toes are resected with the dorsal joint capsules. The dorsally dislocated toes can then be reduced. The extensor digitorum longus tendons are transferred and inserted into the neck of the metatarsal bones. This aids in elevating the distal metatarsal bones, reducing the forefoot drop and prominent metatarsal heads.

Wedge resection of the naviculocuneiform joints and the cuboid bone, coupled with the foregoing procedures, may be necessary to correct severe deformity. The base of the removed wedge of bone is dorsal (Fig. 21). When the osteotomy site is closed and the base of the metatarsal bones is displaced plantarward, the longitudinal arch is lowered.

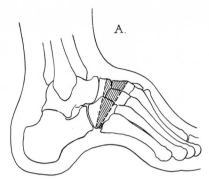 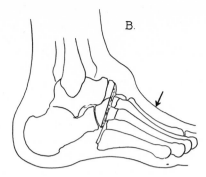

Figure 21.   *A,* The high arch of cavus deformity is lowered by resecting a wedge of bone through the talocuneiform joints and the body of the cuboid bone. The triple joints of the foot, the talonavicular, calcaneocuboid and subtalar joints, are preserved and retain normal motion. *B,* When the wedge defect is closed, the forefoot is displaced plantarward at the osteotomy site and dorsiflexed to lower the longitudinal arch. Dorsal wedge section is useful when the heel is in neutral position.

This is feasible only when the relationship in the hindfoot is normal. If the heel is inverted and the forefoot adducted, triple arthrodesis with removal of appropriate wedges of bone from the subtalar, talonavicular and calcaneocuboid joints is necessary to correct the deformity. These operations on bone should be deferred until the foot is well developed. Before the age of ten years, the ossification of the bones is incomplete and growth of the foot is retarded or arrested when the operation is done. The operative procedures on the soft tissues can be done before this time and may help prevent more serious deformity.

AFFLICTIONS OF THE FOREFOOT AND TOES

HALLUX VALGUS AND BUNION.   One of the most common and distressing deformities of the forefoot and toes is hallux valgus and bunion (Fig. 22). The great toe points laterally, producing a prominence on the medial aspect of the head of the first metatarsal bone. Shoes create pressure on the bony prominence and a painful bursa develops. When the deformity is pronounced, the great toe overlaps or underlaps the second toe, forcing this toe dorsally or plantarward. The second toe may dislocate (Fig. 23, *A* and *B*).

The cause is usually an abnormal varus angulation of the first metatarsal bone. Occasionally, the condition occurs with metatarsus latus or splayfoot, which produces a similar angulation of the first metatarsal bone. The space between the distal end of the first and second metatarsal bones and toes is exaggerated. The adductor of the great toe deviates the toe laterally and the extensor hallucis longus tendon subluxates

laterally. The flexor hallucis brevis with the lateral sesamoid bone and the flexor hallucis longus become similarly displaced. The abductor hallucis subluxates plantarward and the corrective influence of the muscle is lost. The tendons in the laterally displaced position increase the angulation of the great toe. The condition is usually slowly progressive.

When the deformity is mild and inflammation of the bursa periodic, a wide shoe made of soft kidskin is worn to minimize pressure on the bursa. The longitudinal arch of the foot and first metatarsal bone is supported

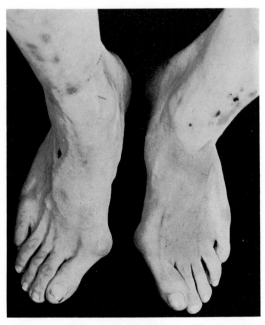

Figure 22.   Hallux valgus and bunion. The great toe is deviated laterally; the first metatarsal bone is angulated medially. The prominent medial aspect of the head of the metatarsal bone is the site of a painful bursa.

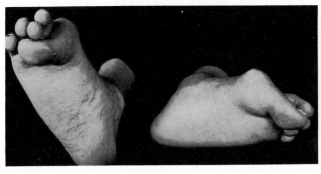
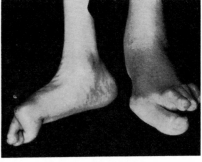

A   *B*

Figure 23. *A,* Severe hallux valgus with plantar flexion forces the small toes dorsally. *B,* The second toe is dislocated dorsally at the metatarsal-phalangeal joint.

with pads or a corrective shoe. To prevent increasing splayfoot, the metatarsal arch is elevated with a pad.

Since the deformity is progressive, the metatarsal head becomes more prominent. The inflamed bursa stimulates the bone and an exostosis forms medially beneath the bursa and joint capsule. Osteoarthritis is prone to develop in the metatarsal-phalangeal joint. The push-off action of the great toe is lost as the deformity progresses.

Surgical treatment is indicated when conservative measures fail. Numerous operations have been devised to relieve the distress of bunions. The objective is to correct the valgus position of the great toe, remove the prominence of the head of the metatarsal bone and correct the deforming pull of the muscles.

The metatarsus primus varus or metatarsus latus can be corrected in young people to prevent recurrence. The presence of osteoarthritis in the joint demands remodeling of the joint surfaces.

Three general types of operative procedures are available to the surgeon. The choice of operation depends upon the patient's age, the state of his circulation, the degree of deformity and the presence or absence of arthritis in the joint. Mild deformities require only removal of the exostosis and the prominent bone (Fig. 24, *A*). Correction of the toe is obtained by shortening the medial joint capsule and, in some patients, sectioning the lateral joint capsule and adductor tendon. When the deformity is greater, the adductor tendon may be reinserted into the metatarsal bone to remove the deforming influence and to help correct the metatarsus primus varus. The abductor tendon may be repositioned over the medial aspect of the joint.

If osteoarthritis is found, arthroplasty or remodeling of the joint must be done in order to prevent pain and stiffness (Fig. 24, *B*). This is most simply done by excision of the proximal third of the proximal phalanx of the great toe. The malposition of the toe is easily corrected as relaxation of soft tissues follows removal of the segment of bone. Pseudoarthrosis develops at the metatarsophalangeal joint, which is pain free and mobile.

Young adults or older patients who have excessive metatarsus varus may require a more extensive operation to correct the deformity and to prevent its recurrence (Fig. 24, *C*). Adequate circulation in the foot is a prerequisite. The objective is to correct the metatarsus varus as well as the hallux valgus. Osteotomy or wedge resection, at or near the base of the first metatarsal bone, is performed and the bone realigned. Arthrodesis of the first metatarsal base to the second as well as the metatarsal-cuneiform joint may be necessary to maintain the position.

Metatarsus latus, or splayfoot, may be corrected by a similar procedure combined with the creation of a plantar sling of tendon from the fifth to the first metatarsal heads, pulling the metatarsal bones together.

HALLUX RIGIDUS OR HALLUX NONEXTENSUS. Hallux rigidus, as the name implies, is characterized by painful limitation of extension at the great toe joint.

The etiology is not always clear; however, an exostosis develops over the dorsal articular margin of the metatarsal-phalangeal joint. Extension of the toe is blocked to varying degrees and osteoarthritis frequently accompanies this change. A bursa may develop over the dorsum of the joint. The foot is turned outward when walking to avoid dorsiflexion of the toe. A callus may form on the

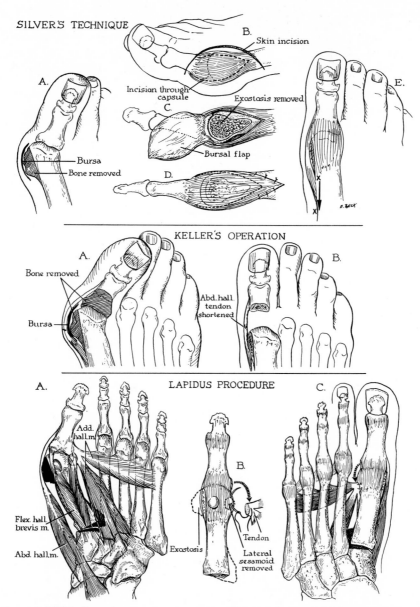

Figure 24.   *Upper: A,* Mild hallux valgus may be corrected by Silver's technique. *B,* The joint capsule is reflected, exposing the exostosis of the head of the metatarsal bone. *C,* The excess bone is removed. *D* and *E,* The toe is straightened by shortening the joint capsule when it is sutured. Occasionally, the lateral joint capsule is incised to relax the joint and allow correction. (Redrawn with permission from Silver, D.: The operative treatment of hallux valgus. J. Bone & Joint Surg. 5:225, 1923.)

Middle: Keller's operation is used when the deformity is pronounced or the metatarsal-phalangeal joint is arthritic. *A,* The exostosis is removed from the metatarsal head, and the proximal third of the phalanx of the great toe is resected. *B,* The toe corrects easily and a painless pseudarthrosis forms. The toe is shortened but functions well. (Redrawn from Keller, W. L.: Further observations on the surgical treatment of hallux valgus and bunions. New York M. J. 95:696, 1912.)

Lower: The Lapidus procedure corrects the metatarsus varus and hallux valgus. *A,* The exostosis is removed from the metatarsal head. The cuneiform-metatarsal joint is resected to correct the metatarsus varus. *B,* The adductor tendon is resected from the proximal phalanx and sutured to the first metatarsal. *C,* The deformity is corrected, and the base of the first metatarsal bone is stabilized to the cuneiform bone and the second metatarsal bone to prevent recurrence. (Redrawn from Lapidus, P. W.: Operative correction of the metatarsus varus primus in hallux valgus. Surg. Gyn. & Obst. 58:183, 1934.)

plantar aspect of the interphalangeal joint secondary to hyperextension of this joint.

Conservative measures are limited to the use of a stiff-soled shoe to prevent dorsiflexion force on the toe, and removal of pressure on the bursa when it is present.

The dorsal exostosis may be removed surgically and the proximal third of the phalanx of the toe resected. Following operation, the patient must be taught to walk with the foot pointing forward to lessen arch strain.

DIGITUS QUINTUS VARUS, OR BUNIONETTE. Varus position of the fifth toe with bunion formation is less common than hallux valgus. The bursa forms over an exostosis or prominence of the head of the fifth metatarsal bone on the lateral aspect of the foot. The little toe may exhibit little or marked varus deformity angulating toward the medial side of the foot. It may overlap the fourth toe or lie beneath it.

Conservative treatment is designed, as for hallux valgus, to lessen pressure on the bursa and to straighten the fifth toe. Stretching the shoe over the bursa and placing a felt pad between the fourth and fifth toes often is all that is necessary to relieve the symptoms.

Resection of the exostosis, combined with shortening or reefing the lateral capsule of the metatarsal-phalangeal joint, straightens the toe and removes the irritating prominence. When the fifth toe is in extreme varus position over or underlapping the fourth toe, osteotomy of the base of the first phalanx will correct the position of the toe.

When the fifth toe is held in dorsiflexion and varus by a contracted extensor digiti quinti longus tendon, the tendon is sectioned at the ankle. The tendon is withdrawn through a second incision at the base of the toe. A tunnel is created by blunt dissection medially and plantarward about the base of the phalanx, and the tendon passed through the tunnel and terminated laterally. It is sutured into the abductor tendon and muscle of the fifth toe, converting the tendon to a flexor abductor pulling the toe down and out.

HAMMER TOE. Hammer toes are similar in appearance to claw toes, but lack the extreme hyperextension of the metatarsal-phalangeal joints. The proximal interphalangeal joint is flexed and the distal joint flexed or extended.

Symptoms are produced when the toe rubs in the shoe. A callus is formed over the plantar pad of the distal phalanx, and a corn is found over the dorsum of the flexed interphalangeal joint. Shoes with a boxlike toe may give the toes room and relieve the pressure symptoms. Padding beneath the metatarsals tends to straighten the toes when they are flexible.

Straightening the toes by resection or arthrodesis of the proximal interphalangeal joint produces a comfortable foot, eliminating the points of pressure and friction.

PLANTAR CALLOSITIES AND PROMINENT METATARSAL HEADS. The heads of the metatarsal bones may be depressed into the sole of the foot by a variety of abnormalities. The involved bone then carries more weight. Friction and pressure lead to hyperkeratotic skin changes. Pain on weight bearing is the usual complaint.

Treatment is directed toward correction of associated foot deformity and redistribution of weight through the metatarsal bones. Transverse metatarsal bars and arch supports elevate the metatarsal bone and relieve the abnormal pressure. With relief of excessive pressure, the callus disappears.

Plantar warts, thought to be virus infections, may be found in the callus. These lesions may disappear when excessive pressure is relieved. Some plantar warts, however, are persistent or recurrent. Salicylic acid adhesive plaster is applied to the area for 48 hours. The callus and wart may be carefully trimmed after the skin softens.

X-ray therapy supervised by a roentgenologist is warranted when plantar warts do not respond to this treatment. Care must be exercised to prevent excessive radiation.

Occasionally, pressure of a prominent metatarsal head cannot be relieved with arch supports. After the other associated defects in the foot are corrected, one or two metatarsal heads, with the exception of the first, may be resected without weakening the foot. Removal of the head of the first metatarsal bone produces a serious defect in the weight-bearing mechanism of the foot.

INTERDIGITAL NEUROMA. Neuroma of the common digital branch of the plantar nerves produces characteristic symptoms, which have been called Morton's toe (Fig. 25, A). Lancinating pain in the region of the third and fourth toes and metatarsal bones occurs periodically while walking. Pain may radiate to the anterior surface of the leg, and the toes may be drawn into the claw position. Relief is obtained by removing the shoe and massaging the foot.

Examination may reveal a normal-appearing foot, or the common forefoot deformities may accompany the condition (Fig. 25, B).

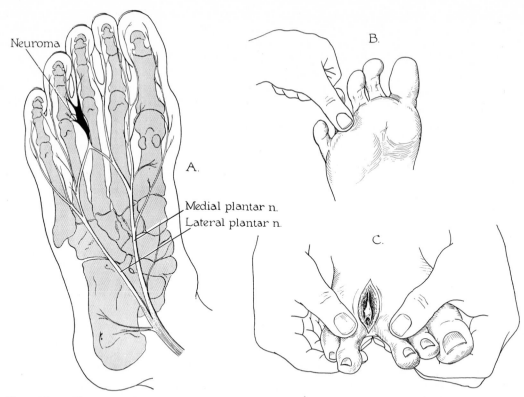

Figure 25.   *A,* The medial and lateral plantar nerves join between the third and fourth metatarsal bones. The common digital nerve is fixed at this point. The most frequent site of interdigital neuroma is between the third and fourth toes. *B,* The typical symptoms of Morton's toe are produced by pressure between the heads of the metatarsal bones. *C,* A web-splitting incision and blunt dissection expose the tumor mass between the metatarsal bones. The entire mass is excised.

Pressure exerted by the examining finger between the base of the third and fourth toes often reproduces the typical attack of pain. Occasionally, a firm tender mass can be palpated between the metatarsal bones. The sensation of pain and temperature is usually diminished on the adjacent surfaces of the toes.

The medial and lateral branches of the plantar nerve form an arch in the forefoot, joining at the fourth common digital nerve. Traction or pressure on the nerve at this fixed point is thought to be the etiologic factor producing the neuroma. Inflammatory reaction about the nerve stimulates the formation of fibrous tissue in the nerve, forming the tumor mass. Occasionally, a small bursa filled with clear yellow fluid surrounds the neuroma.

During the early stages of the syndrome, symptoms may be relieved by a transverse metatarsal bar on the sole of the shoe to minimize pressure on the third and fourth metatarsal bones. If the symptoms recur or persist, the area about the tumor is injected with local anesthetic and 25 mg. of compound F.

Symptoms which have been present several months and do not improve with conservative measures usually require excision of the tumor. This is done through a web-splitting incision between the toes (Fig. 25, *C*). Identification of the tumor mass just proximal to the bifurcation of the proper digital nerves is easily accomplished by blunt dissection. The common digital nerve is sectioned proximal to the mass and the tumor removed.

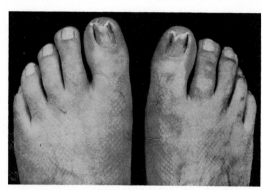

Figure 26.   The ingrowing toenail is abnormally curved, predisposing to encroachment on the soft tissues at the margin of the nail.

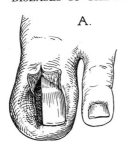

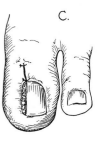

Figure 27.   Resection of ingrowing toenail. *A*, Eponychium incised and reflected to expose the base of the toenail. *B*, Wedge-shaped resection of the nail and toenail bed. *C*, The eponychium is closed and the remainder of the wound packed with petrolatum gauze.

The lesion is found less frequently in the other toes, but it may occur in any of the digital nerves.

INGROWING TOENAILS. Ingrowing toenails develop secondary to injury, infection or pressure (Fig. 26). The edge of the nail cuts into the adjacent soft tissue, injuring the skin. Bacteria invade the area and an abscess or chronic granuloma results. Periodic recurrent episodes of pain and swelling occur as the nail grows. Injury to the nail bed or a fungus infection may deform the nail. Pressure of the shoe on the soft tissues about the nail margin can produce the condition.

During the acute infection, the principles of rest, heat and the establishment of adequate drainage are applied. The offending portion of the nail is removed and the nail margin packed away from the skin with cotton. Packing with cotton is continued to form a gutter through which the nail may grow without pressure on the skin. Frequent changes of cotton, application of fungicides and removal of keratotic skin are carried out until the nail has grown past the distal skin margin of the toe. The toenail is then trimmed straight across.

Recurrent episodes of infection are treated by resection of the margin of the nail and destroying the nail bed from which it grows (Fig. 27).

CLAVUS OR CORNS. Pressure and friction by shoes on the toes produces localized keratotic lesions in the skin called clavus or corns. The lesions occur typically at the flexed interphalangeal joint with claw-toe deformities. The lateral dorsal surface of the fifth toe is the most frequent site. When pressure and friction are excessive, a small, painful bursa develops beneath the layer of keratotic skin. Eliminating pressure with a soft leather, low-heel shoe with adequate room for the toes may relieve the symptoms. The toes can be straightened if they are clawed. The corn over the lateral aspect of the fifth toe is due to prominence of the lateral condyle of the proximal phalanx. Excision of the bony

prominence along with the bursa is usually successful.

AFFLICTIONS OF THE HINDFOOT

Afflictions of the hindfoot involve primarily the heel and adjacent structures. Bursitis of the os calcis on the plantar aspect and Achilles tendon posteriorly is a frequent source of pain in the heel. Spurs about the origin of the plantar aponeurosis were at one time thought to be a source of pain. Removal of these spurs seldom gave relief and the procedure is now done infrequently.

Symptoms of bursitis in the plantar surface of the os calcis are localized to that area. Tenderness to pressure and weight bearing is confined to the condyles of the os calcis over which the bursa forms. Plantar fascitis producing similar symptoms is more diffuse and follows the course of the plantar aponeurosis into the foot.

Bursitis about the attachment of the Achilles tendon may be deep or superficial. The deep bursa is located between the upper margin of the os calcis and the tendon. The superficial one lies between the subcutaneous tissue and the insertion of the Achilles tendon. Irritation of these bursae results from pressure of the shoe coupled with a prominent posterior border of the os calcis. Hyperkeratotic skin forms over the protruding bone or bursae. Cracks or blisters in this skin lead to infection. Reduction of pressure at the inflamed bursa is necessary to bring about relief of symptoms. On the plantar surface, sponge rubber pads are placed in the heel of the shoe to cushion the bursa. Posteriorly, felt pads are placed on each side of the heel to relieve pressure on the Achilles tendon insertion. It is sometimes necessary to cut out the counter of the shoe.

Injection of local anesthetic and compound F into the bursae frequently relieves the inflammation. Operation is seldom necessary. Excision of the plantar bursa of the os calcis is often followed by the formation of painful scar tissue. Resection of the prominence of bone about the Achilles tendon insertion narrows the os calcis and relieves the pressure.

PARALYTIC DEFORMITIES

Poliomyelitis and other neuromuscular afflictions are the etiologic factors in many disabling deformities of the foot. Since these diseases frequently occur in childhood during the growth period, muscle imbalance and contractures produce profound changes in the foot. Growth disturbance in the paralyzed leg may result in unequal leg length and foot size.

Obviously, countless combinations and grades of muscle weakness and paralysis can take place following poliomyelitis. The major deformities, however, follow the pattern of the cardinal positions of the foot: equinus, calcaneus, varus and valgus (Fig. 28). Combined deformities are usual. The high arch, or cavus, or flatfoot may accompany these deformities. Frequently, cavus and equinus or cavus and calcaneus deformities are combined. Pes planus and valgus, or cavus and varus, also occur in combination.

These deformities result from muscle imbalance. The development of deformity follows a pattern. First, dynamic muscle imbalance appears, which is exaggerated by use of the part. Static deformities appear, accompanied by contractures. Alteration of bone configuration occurs with growth. These changes lead eventually to fixed deformity.

The deformities of the foot may be classified according to the loss of power in the major groups: dorsiflexors, evertors, invertors, intrinsic and plantar flexor muscles.

As in all paralytic disorders, prevention of deformity by preventing contractures and developing maximum muscle power in the remaining muscle fibers is essential to rehabilitation. Physical medical measures consisting of active exercise, stretching of contracted muscles, supporting braces and corrective shoes are aids in the prevention of deformity. However, when gross muscle imbalance is present, deformities will develop in the growing child and to a lesser degree in the adult. Restoration of muscle balance and power is necessary to correct the deformity and provide maximum function. Often, it is impossible to obtain sufficient power from other muscles to substitute effectively for those paralyzed. Stabilization of foot joints to provide a firm, stable base for walking and standing is then necessary. When deformities are established, the deformity must first be corrected; then, the foot must be balanced and stabilized. This may demand stretching of contractures with wedged casts, surgical lengthening of soft tissues or resection of deformed bones to reestablish proper weight bearing.

PARALYSIS OF DORSIFLEXOR MUSCLES. When the tibialis anticus and long toe extensors are functioning, the foot assumes the equinus position because of the unopposed power of the triceps surae. If the peronei and tibialis posticus are normal, the foot is usually balanced medially and laterally. If the calf muscle group is regularly stretched in walking, fixed equinus may not occur and little deformity is present. In walking, it is necessary to raise the leg higher to clear the ground when swinging the plantar flexed foot forward. A lightweight footdrop brace may be all that is necessary to provide a practically normal gait.

If the calf muscle group has been allowed to contract so that a fixed equinus position

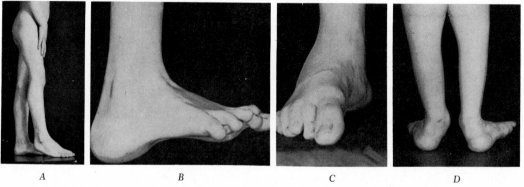

| A | B | C | D |

Figure 28.   *A*, Equinus position of the foot. *B*, Calcaneus position. *C*, Varus position. *D*, Valgus position.

of the foot is present, the muscle may be stretched with wedged casts, forcing the foot into dorsiflexion. In exceptional instances, it may be necessary to lengthen the Achilles tendon; however, this should be avoided if possible as inevitably some weakness of plantar flexion and push-off in walking results (Fig. 29).

PARALYSIS OF EVERTOR MUSCLES. When paralysis of the peroneus longus and brevis muscles occurs, the primary evertors are lost, except for the rather weak evertor action of the long extensors of the toes. The peroneus longus acts as a depressor of the first metatarsal bone as well as an evertor. The unopposed dorsiflexor invertor action of the tibialis anticus elevates the first metatarsal and inverts the foot. The tibialis posterior inverts and adducts the forefoot. The weak action of the long toe extensors, acting as evertors, is insufficient to overcome this tendency and the foot gradually assumes the position of varus of the heel, adduction of the forefoot and elevation of the first metatarsal. The great toe flexes in an attempt to contact the floor. With growth, the bones adapt to this position and the deformity becomes fixed (Fig. 30, A).

The foot may be balanced by transferring the tibialis anticus tendon from the normal insertion on the cuneiform and first metatarsal to a more lateral position on the dorsum of the foot in the middle or lateral cuneiform, or the second or third metatarsal. The strong invertor action is thus eliminated and, when done early, may be all that is required. If deformity of the bones and marked contracture of the soft tissue on the medial side of the foot are present, wedge resection of the bone with triple arthrodesis of the talonavicular, calcaneocuboid joints and the subtalar joints may be necessary, reshaping the foot to a normal weight-bearing position (Fig. 30, B and C).

PARALYSIS OF INVERTOR MUSCLES. Paralysis of the tibialis anticus and posticus muscles allows overaction of the peroneals, forcing the foot into valgus or eversion (Fig. 31, A) with complete loss of the longitudinal arch and a completely flat foot with an everted heel (Fig. 28, D). If the calf muscle is allowed to contract, an equinovalgus deformity develops. If the long extensor tendons of the toes are lost, dorsiflexion of the foot is lost as well. The peroneus longus and brevis may be transferred to the dorsum of the foot to remove the deforming evertor action and to produce dorsiflexion of the foot (Fig. 31, B and C). Since medial and lateral stability is lost, triple arthrodesis is necessary to stabilize the

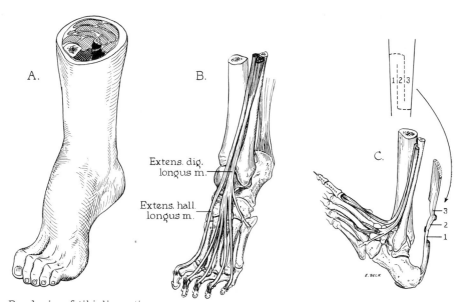

A. B.

Extens. dig. longus m.

Extens. hall. longus m.

C.

1 2 3

3
2
1

E. BECK

Paralysis of tibialis anticus

Figure 29.   A and B, Paralysis of the tibialis anticus muscle with the remaining muscles balanced often produces equinus deformity by contracture of the calf muscles. The extensor longus tendons of the toes produce claw toes, and cavus deformity may occur. C, To convert the long extensor muscles of the toes to dorsiflexors of the foot, the Achilles tendon is lengthened or stretched. The extensor hallucis longus is transferred to the neck of the first metatarsal, and the extensor digitorum longus to the base of the middle metatarsal bones or cuneiform bones.

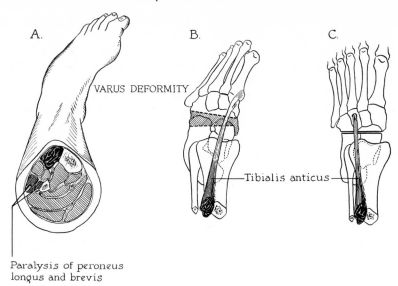

A.

VARUS DEFORMITY

B.

C.

Tibialis anticus

Paralysis of peroneus
longus and brevis

Figure 30.   *A*, Paralysis of the evertor muscles, the peroneus longus and brevis, allows the tibialis anticus (*B*) to invert the foot and elevate the first metatarsal bone. *B*, Triple arthrodesis to stabilize the foot is combined with (*C*) transfer of the tibialis anticus to the middle of the tarsal region.

foot or to correct fixed deformity. If the foot is in equinus, this must first be corrected by wedged casts or Achilles tendon lengthening.

Paralysis of the tibialis anticus, with normal posterior tibial and peroneals and strong long toe extensors, may result in a cavovarus deformity. In this instance, the tibialis posterior may prevent the valgus deformity of the heel. The peroneus longus depresses the first metatarsal and the extensor hallucis longus forces the toe into cock-up position,

further depressing the first metatarsal. A paradoxical situation arises; dorsiflexion of the foot causes the foot to evert through the action of the long extensors of the toes. On weight bearing, however, the fixed depression of the first metatarsal head forces the foot into varus position.

Transferring the long extensor of the great toe to the neck of the first metatarsal helps to elevate the metatarsal and eliminates the dorsiflexion of the toe. Transfer of the pero-

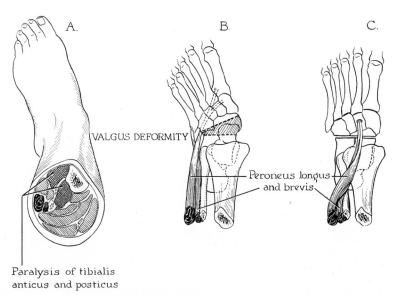

A.

B.

C.

VALGUS DEFORMITY

Peroneus longus
and brevis

Paralysis of tibialis
anticus and posticus

Figure 31.   *A*, Paralysis of the invertor muscles, the tibialis anticus and posticus, produces valgus deformity by the action of the peroneal and toe extensor muscles. *B*, Stabilization of the foot by triple arthrodesis. *C*, Transfer of the peroneal muscles to the middle tarsal region.

neus longus tendon to the dorsum of the foot in the region of the base of the second metatarsal eliminates the depressor effect on the first metatarsal and aids in dorsiflexion.

INTRINSIC MUSCLE PARALYSIS OF THE FOOT. Cavus deformity with claw toes may be produced by intrinsic paralysis of the muscles of the foot. Loss of the lumbricales, interossei and short flexors of the toes, which normally produce extension of the interphalangeal joints, allows hyperextension of the toes at the metatarsal-phalangeal joints. The long flexors of the toes produce flexion of the interphalangeal joints. This deformity depresses the metatarsal heads and, coupled with soft tissue contracture of the plantar structures, results in cavus deformity.

Before fixed bony deformity develops, transfer of the long extensor tendons to the necks of the metatarsals eliminates the dorsiflexion of the toes and aids in elevation of the metatarsal heads. Interphalangeal joint fusion of the great toe is usually necessary to prevent excessive plantar flexion at this joint. Plantar fasciotomy may be necessary to correct a mild cavus deformity. Often coupled with this defect is insufficiency of the tibialis anticus, producing an equinocavus deformity. The calf muscles, or Achilles tendon, are first stretched or lengthened to correct the equinus deformity (Fig. 32). The above procedure is performed, or the extensor digitorum longus is transferred to the base of the third metatarsal to produce greater dorsiflexion power.

When fixed cavus deformity has occurred, dorsal wedge section through the cuneiform-navicular joints and through the body of the cuboid is demanded. The high arch is further depressed by plantar displacement of the distal lever of the foot.

PARALYSIS OF PLANTAR FLEXOR MUSCLES. Paralysis of the triceps surae, or calf muscle group, produces one of the most serious disabilities in the growing child, the calcaneus or calvaneocavus foot (Fig. 33, A). In bilateral paralysis, which may occur in poliomyelitis or spina bifida with myelodysplasia, the disability may be profound.

The forward sway of the body in balancing while standing is normally counteracted by the strong calf muscles. When paralysis of the calf muscle group takes place, this effect is lost and such patients cannot balance well without external support. When walking, the normal push-off is lost and the foot is forced into dorsiflexion. When the pull of the triceps surae is lost on the growing calcaneus, the unopposed intrinsic muscles of the foot, along with the plantar aponeurosis and the flexors of the toes, tend to approximate the heel toward the metatarsal heads. The os calcis grows vertically, producing an abnormally high arch. The weight-bearing surface of the heel becomes a peg and provides less bearing surface. Valgus or varus of the heel may also be coupled with the deformity when there is weakness of the invertors or evertors.

Since the calf muscle group is more powerful than all of the other long muscles to the foot combined, it is almost impossible to re-

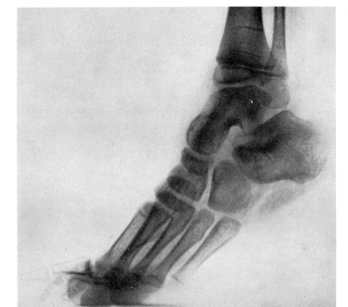

Figure 32. Prolonged equinus position of the foot secondary to either paralysis or clubfoot produces a flat tibiotalar articulation. This deformity of the bone prevents dorsiflexion.

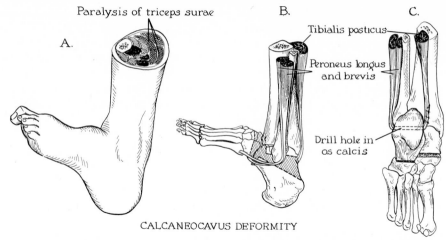

Figure 33. A, Paralysis of the triceps surae muscles prevents active plantar flexion. Unopposed dorsiflexor muscles pull the foot into dorsiflexion. The long and short muscles of the plantar aspect contract to compensate for the triceps surae in walking and produce cavus deformity. B, The deformity of the os calcis and midtarsal bones is corrected and the foot stabilized by triple arthrodesis. C, The tibialis posticus tendon and the peroneal tendons are transferred to the os calcis to provide limited plantar flexion and counteract the deforming pull of the plantar muscles.

produce normal plantar flexion power by tendon transference to the heel. However, every effort should be made early in the development of the deformity to prevent progressive changes.

Long-leg braces should be used to prevent hyperextension at the knees, and a check-rein at the ankle should be incorporated in the brace to prevent excessive dorsiflexion. Plantar fasciotomy may lessen the pull on the metatarsals and os calcis, and lessen the bowstring effect. Early transfer of available active muscles to the os calcis is essential. When the peroneal and posterior tibial muscles are normal, they may be transferred to the os calcis and the foot will remain balanced medially and laterally and the forefoot depression is lessened (Fig. 33, B and C). If maximum power is required, the tibialis anticus may be transplanted posteriorly into the heel through the interosseous membrane. If the calf muscle group is completely paralyzed, the transferred muscles will not produce enough power to allow tiptoe walking; however, they tend to counteract the vertical growth of the os calcis and eliminate some of the excessive dorsiflexion power. Practically all feet affected with this deformity require some bone correction, either dorsal wedge section to correct the forefoot drop or triple arthrodesis, with removal of appropriate bone wedges, to correct the deformity and stabilize the foot. The bone procedures must await the time when the foot is more mature, and are seldom done before the patient is ten or 12 years of age.

When the foot is completely flail, there is little tendency to progressive or fixed deformity other than flatfoot. To secure a stable base for walking or standing, it may be necessary to perform arthrodesis of the ankle joint along with the subtalar and calcaneocuboid and talonavicular joints.

SPASTIC PARALYTIC DEFORMITIES. Spastic paralysis of the lower extremity may produce similar changes in the foot. However, the most frequently encountered deformity is equinus due to spasticity and contracture of the calf muscle group. Tendon transfer in spastic paralysis is much less useful than in flaccid paralysis, because normal muscles are usually not available to transfer and the deformities result from overactive abnormal muscles.

Lengthening of contracted muscles and soft tissues is useful, either by stretching casts, by surgical lengthening of tendons or by section of fascia and soft tissue. Occasionally, a deforming muscle pull may be weakened by partial denervation of the muscle. The often encountered equinus deformity tends to be recurrent, particularly during periods of rapid growth. The use of splints worn at night is helpful in preventing the deformity. These splints hold the foot in dorsiflexion, preventing contracture of the calf muscle. Gait training is essential. The child is taught the importance of making the heel contact the ground in walking.

If the deformity progresses, wedged and stretching casts are useful. The stretching cast is applied below the flexed knee with the foot in maximum dorsiflexion. An anterior heel is incorporated in the cast. When the knee is straightened in walking, the gastrocnemius muscle originating on the femoral condyles is stretched. If the soleus muscle is not excessively contracted, this method of treatment will re-establish dorsiflexion in walking. However, the procedure must be repeated as the child grows. If excessive spasticity of the calf muscle group prevents maintenance of the corrected equinus, section of the motor nerves to the gastrocnemius muscle is done in the popliteal space. This lessens the power of the muscle group and may prevent recurrence of the equinus. When the equinus recurs after this procedure, the musculotendinous junction of the triceps surae is lengthened. This procedure consists in making chevron-like incisions on alternate medial and lateral aspects of the junction of the Achilles tendon and the muscle, thus lengthening the muscle as well as the tendon.

If the Achilles tendon alone is lengthened, a small misshapen calf muscle results and muscle function is lessened.

Flatfeet are frequently encountered with the short, contracted calf muscle group. Orthopedic shoes with rigid extended counters tend to preserve the arch after overcoming the contractures. Rarely, triple arthrodesis may be required to correct excessively deformed flatfeet.

OSTEOCHONDRITIS

Osteochondritis of the growing foot usually occurs in three locations: the second metatarsal head, the navicular bone and the apophysis of the calcaneus. The etiology of the condition is not clear, but the progressive changes noted in x-ray examinations of the bones suggest interference with the blood supply of the bone with necrosis, followed by substitution of new bone. Local metabolic, toxic or traumatic factors may have a place in the etiology of the disturbance.

The osteochondritic lesions occur during the periods of rapid growth between four and 13 years of age in the case of the calcaneal apophysis and navicular bone, and near the age of closure of the epiphysis at 18 years in the second metatarsal bone.

The symptoms are pain on weight bearing, swelling and local tenderness to pressure over the involved bone. The onset of symptoms may be acute or gradual and the disease is self-limited but may be symptomatic for weeks to months.

X-ray films show irregular density of bone, fragmentation and at times abnormal growth of bone.

When the condition occurs in the region of the second or third metatarsal head, it is called Freiberg's infraction. The symptoms are pain and swelling about the involved joint, particularly at the push-off phase of the step. Enlargement of the head and distal shaft of the bone, flattening and widening of the joint surface, irregularity of the epiphysial plate and increased joint space between the proximal phalanx of the toe and the metatarsal head characterize the lesion. Degenerative arthritic changes in the joint occur later and may produce symptoms in adult life.

During the acute, painful stage of the disease, weight bearing should be relieved with crutches. Hot packs to the foot may be applied several times daily. Usually the acute distress is of short duration, a week or two. Following relief of the acute pain and swelling, the foot should be fitted to a stiff-shank, low-heel shoe with a stiff leather sole to protect the metatarsal head. A felt pad is placed in the shoe just back of the metatarsal head to relieve pressure on the head and joint, and a transverse metatarsal bar is placed on the sole of the shoe.

Alteration of growth of the metatarsal joint surface may lead to chronic degenerative arthritic changes in adult life which, if not relieved by pads and arch supports, may require resection of the proximal third of the phalanx of the toe to form a painless pseudarthrosis. Excess bone about the head of the metatarsal may be removed at the same time if the bone is prominent.

When the condition occurs in the navicular bone, it is termed Köhler's disease and is found in patients between the ages of four and ten years. Pain and swelling about the navicular bone on weight bearing are the usual symptoms. Non-weight bearing during the acute phase may be necessary; however, the symptoms are usually mild and padding the shoe with felt may relieve the strain on the longitudinal arch.

X-ray examination reveals a progressive narrowing of the navicular bone between the talus and cuneiform bones. The bone increases in density and may project dorsally above the level of the adjacent bones. Substitution of bone takes place slowly, but in several years the navicular bone is usually completely restored with little, if any, residual deformity.

Calcaneal apophysitis occurs in the apophysis of the os calcis. On weight bearing, pain is present at the prominence of the heel and about the attachment of the Achilles tendon. The symptoms frequently appear between the ages of seven and 13 years. X-rays show increased density of the calcaneal apophysis with fragmentation and irregularity of the epiphysial plate. Non-weight bearing with crutches may be necessary for several weeks followed by limited weight bearing with a built-up heel and sponge rubber pad in the shoe to lessen the pull of the Achilles tendon and to cushion the heel. Healing takes place over several months with no residual deformity.

RHEUMATOID ARTHRITIS

Rheumatoid arthritis occurs in the foot in varying degrees, and characteristically affects the peripheral joints. The toes and metatarsophalangeal joints are frequently involved; however, any and all parts of the foot may be involved.

During the acute phase of rheumatoid arthritis, the inflammatory process may be confined to the interphalangeal joints or may progressively affect the metatarsophalangeal joints, the midtarsal, subtalar and ankle joints. The tissues swell and there is increased local heat. Weight bearing is often impossible. Frequently, the heel pad becomes painful over the plantar aspect and about the margin of the heel. The plantar fascia may become tender, as may the Achilles tendon. Rheumatoid nodules may form over the dorsum of the foot in the bunion areas about the heel and, occasionally, on the plantar aspect of the foot. Bursae filled with fibrin-flecked yellow, cloudy fluid may form over the metatarsal heads. Later in the course of the disease, debris and fibrin may form cottage cheese-like deposits in these bursae.

As the disease progresses, the joint surfaces are destroyed by a synovial pannus and fibrous ankylosis may take place in the joints of the foot and toes. Contractures of the toes may develop early. The usual deformity is one of dorsal dislocation and hyperextension of the proximal phalanx and flexion of the interphalangeal joint. All of the toes may deviate laterally. As the subtalar joint is destroyed, lateral motion is lost and the foot becomes more rigid. Destruction of the joint capsules and loss of elastic tissue in the ligaments may lead to flatfoot deformity. When the toes contract, the metatarsal heads become promi-

nent in the sole of the foot and the fat pad in the ball of the foot atrophies. Weight bearing results in callous formation over these pressure areas.

During the acute phase of the disease, the patient is placed at bed rest and no weight bearing is allowed. Since contractures develop early, equinus deformity is prevented by placing a padded footboard at the bottom of the bed. The weight of the bed clothing is removed from the feet and the feet are kept in neutral position with the sole of the foot supported by the board. Often, the heels are tender and pain is produced when they are rested on the mattress. A small pillow under the calf of the leg lifts the heel off the mattress and relieves the pressure. Hot, moist packs applied for one hour several times a day help relieve the pain and prepare the feet for mild, active exercise.

Muscles atrophy rapidly in rheumatoid arthritis, and joints tend to stiffen quickly. To minimize this, the patient is instructed in active exercise of the foot without weight bearing. The toes should be flexed and extended, the foot inverted and everted and plantar flexed and dorsiflexed several times following use of the hot packs. Vigorous massage, whirlpool baths and stretching aggravate the condition and should not be employed during the acute phase of the disease. Administration of steroid and salicylate drugs, and the general supportive measures for the treatment of rheumatoid arthritis, should be started.

When the pain, heat and swelling subside, weight bearing may be started on a very restricted schedule, walking only a few minutes of each hour or several times a day. A low-heel, well-fitted Oxford must be used, not a soft bedroom slipper, because the weakened ligaments demand support. Usually, rigid arch supports and metatarsal bars are not tolerated. Felt pads placed in the shoe and, occasionally, a foam-rubber insole help to support the arches and cushion the weight-bearing surface of the foot.

Rheumatoid nodules and bursae may be excised if they persist and are subject to pressure. Injection of compound F into joints and bursae has been disappointing.

When deformities have occurred, they usually involve the forefoot. If relief of contracted toes and plantar calluses is not obtained with arch supports, operative correction becomes necessary. Since the joint surfaces are destroyed, the extensor tendons of the toes are contracted and the metatarsal heads are prominent, the proximal phalanx of the lateral four toes is resected. This allows the toes to fall into a more normal position and shoes can be fitted more comfortably. The Keller type resection of the proximal third of the proximal phalanx will relieve pain in the metatarsal-phalangeal joint. The prominent metatarsal heads are shaved flat, parallel to the plantar surface of the foot. This converts the rounded marble-like head into a flat spatula. Adjacent remaining fat tends to cover the partially resected bone and a fairly effective cushion at the ball of the foot is re-established. Arthrodesis of other painful joints may be done. Following operative correction of deformities, an adequate supporting low-heel Oxford with transverse and long flexible arch supports should be used permanently.

OSTEOARTHRITIS

Osteoarthritis frequently follows trauma to the joints of the foot. The trauma may be massive, producing fractured joint surfaces, or it may be minimal and often-repeated, occurring with abnormalities of weight bearing. Degeneration of cartilage and the production of osteophytes about the margins of the joint is a slow process, and symptoms may not develop in the foot until the changes are far advanced or the foot is suddenly traumatized or strained by unusual activity. Pain is often confined to one joint. The subtalar joint following fracture of the os calcis is frequently the site of painful osteoarthritis. The great toe joint degenerates in time when hallux valgus or rigidus is present. Pain usually is produced by chronic synovitis secondary to the destruction of joint surfaces. When acute synovitis is present, rest, heat and elevation of the foot are necessary and weight bearing should be eliminated. Usually, the symptoms subside quickly. The foot is then fitted with a supporting Oxford with appropriate arch supports. If the foot is flat and fairly rigid because of the joint changes, radical raising of the arch should not be attempted. Fixed joints do not tolerate extensive position changes. Pads should be built up gradually in the transverse and long arches until comfortable weight bearing is obtained.

Occasionally, injection of compound F into the osteoarthritic joints will give relief of pain for varying periods. Salicylate drugs are helpful.

Arthrodesis of the subtalar joint may be necessary in the younger patient with adequate circulation. Extensive operative procedures in the elderly are not warranted. The Keller bunionectomy is useful for relief of the damaged metatarsophalangeal joint of the great toe.

GOUT

Gout is a metabolic disturbance of uric acid metabolism. Greater amounts of uric acid are formed in the body periodically. Attacks of acute arthritis develop. The metatarsophalangeal joint of the great toe is a characteristic area for the lesion. The sudden pain, heat, redness and swelling resemble cellulitis, and fever and leukocytosis may add to the confusion. The serum uric acid level should be determined to confirm the diagnosis. The pain is intense and weight bearing is impossible. The maximum area of tenderness is usually along the medial side of the joint. The discoloration has a cyanotic tone rather than the brighter red of infection. Symptoms subside rapidly with use of colchicine and uricosuric agents and little, if any, residual change remains. Ten per cent of patients who have gout have deposits of urates in the skin, subcutaneous tissue, tendons, ligaments, bones and joints. These tophi are destructive. Severe crippling of the foot can take place if the disease is inadequately treated. Proper therapy to prevent destruction by tophi demands the routine continued use of uricosuric agents. These drugs increase excretion of uric acid by blocking tubular resorption in the kidney. The most effective agent at present is probenecid, although salicylates have long been used. Colchicine is an ancient drug, specific for relief of pain in gout; however, it

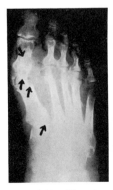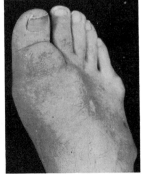

Figure 34. Chronic tophaceous gout. Massive deposits of urates destroy bones and joints and produce deformity of the foot. (Reproduced by permission from Larmon, W. R., and Kurtz, J. F.: The surgical management of chronic tophaceous gout. J. Bone & Joint Surg. 40-A:743, 1958.)

has no effect on the serum uric acid level. The two drugs should be combined in the management of gout.

When tophi form in the foot, they should be removed surgically when they cause pressure, interfere with tendon movement, ulcerate, or destroy bones, joints and tendons (Fig. 34). Because the deposits of urate are infiltrative, special surgical techniques are required to preserve vital structures.

LEDDERHOSE'S DISEASE

Dupuytren's contracture of the hand is a familiar affliction. Contracture of the palmar fascia with the formation of nodules and cords producing fixed flexion of the fingers is well known. Microscopically, the fascia is more cellular than normal and shows increased collagenous elements. A similar affliction occurs in the plantar fascia of the foot, and may be associated with Dupuytren's disease of the hand. The condition in the foot is called Ledderhose's disease.

Painful nodules develop in the plantar fascia of the foot. The nodules slowly increase in size, and pain on weight bearing is complicated by burning pain at rest, particularly at night. The disease must not be confused with Volkmann's ischemic contracture of the foot or the fibrous contractures which follow cast immobilization for fractures of the lower extremities. These conditions may produce tight plantar fasciae and deformed toes, but the nodules typical of Ledderhose's disease do not develop.

The plantar fascia should be resected when the painful masses do not spontaneously regress. The fascia may be excised through a medial plantar incision, avoiding the weight-bearing areas of the sole of the foot. Weight bearing must be delayed until the wound is completely healed in order to avoid excessive scar formation, usually three weeks.

TUMORS OF THE FOOT

Tumors of the foot are uncommon lesions when compared to the many other lesions which affect the foot. The classification of tumors of the hand applies equally well to the foot with the exception of irradiation carcinoma. This lesion in the foot usually follows excessive radiation in the therapy of plantar warts, but is of rare occurrence. Tumors of the foot usually demand attention when they occur on the weight-bearing surface of the

foot and produce pain. When they occur on the dorsum of the foot, or produce enlargement of the foot, shoe fitting is difficult.

The principles of treatment are similar to those in the hand. However, there are several differences. The plantar, or weight-bearing, skin must be avoided in the excision of tumors of the foot, to prevent painful scars. If radical excisions which involve supporting ligaments, tendons or bone are necessary, stabilization of the foot by appropriate arthrodesis may be required.

Partial amputations for tumors of the foot must preserve adequate balance and painless weight bearing. If this cannot be done, amputation at a higher level in the leg is mandatory.

INFECTIONS OF THE FOOT

Infections in the foot, fortunately, are usually superficial and may be caused by Streptococcus, Staphylococcus, fungus or other inhabitants of the skin. Deeper infections of the fascial spaces, tendon sheaths and bones and joints are uncommon. The plantar skin is thick and affords good protection for the deeper structures, except in the case of penetrating wounds or from extension of infection from the toes.

The most common sources of infection are blisters, bursae, corns and ingrowing toenails. Blisters usually occur over the heel near the insertion of the Achilles tendon or at the dorsum of the toes, from friction of shoes or tight stockings.

Bursae over the first and fifth metatarsal heads, secondary to corns, may become infected through cracks in keratotic skin. Usually, the infections are localized; however, infection in the toes may drain through the lymphatics of the superficial dorsal tissues of the foot, creating spreading cellulitis and lymphangitis. Infections about the heel drain through lymphatics on the posterior aspect of the leg to the popliteal lymph nodes. The cardinal signs of infection are present: heat, redness, swelling and pain. Since the skin is loosely applied to the dorsum of the foot, any infection in the foot may produce swelling over the dorsum.

Weight bearing must be eliminated immediately. The foot should be elevated, and warm, moist, sterile packs applied. The foot should be splinted with a well-padded, molded, metal splint. Excessive heat should not be applied, particularly in the elderly when vascular impairment may be present. In a leg and foot with considerable arterial insufficiency, excessive heat may precipitate gangrene.

If a wound or lesion is open, a culture should be obtained and sensitivity tests made for the various antibiotic drugs. If the infection is spreading after the culture is obtained, broad-spectrum antibiotics may be administered until the specific antibiotic is determined by the sensitivity tests. The wounds should be dressed as often as necessary to maintain cleanly care and remove toxic bacterial products.

When the infection originates in a paronychia, or ingrowing toenail, adequate drainage may be instituted by incision through the eponychium and removal of the offending portion of nail.

If an abscess develops on the dorsum of the foot, it should be incised through a longitudinal incision, the wound packed open with moist gauze, and the warm, moist, sterile saline packs and splinting continued. When the drainage has stopped and necrotic tissue separated, the wound may be allowed to close.

Occasionally, the deeper tissues may be involved. Infection introduced through puncture wounds in the sole of the foot, or spreading along the tendons from the toes, involves the fascial spaces of the foot. Pus may accumulate beneath the plantar aponeurosis or in the deep median, central or lateral plantar fascial spaces located between the short plantar muscle groups. Incision and drainage of this area of the foot are done, either medially or laterally, at the junction of plantar and dorsal skin. Incisions should never be made through the plantar skin or from the dorsum of the foot for drainage of the deep spaces. Incisions through plantar skin usually leave a painful scar in a weight-bearing area, and adequate drainage cannot be secured through the dorsal approach, resulting in a chronic draining sinus.

Occasionally, a collar-button abscess originates in a plantar callus or wart. The infection forms a localized collection of pus beneath the adjacent metatarsal head, or may burrow between the metatarsal heads to produce swelling on the dorsum. Pyogenic arthritis involving the metatarsophalangeal joint or osteomyelitis invading the metatarsal shaft and head may occur. This is a serious complication which usually demands surgical drainage and, occasionally, excision of the affected joint and metatarsal head. The approach is through the web space, where blunt dissection is carried out until the abscess is evacuated. In chronic draining osteomyelitis or pyogenic arthritis, the metatarsal head and joint may be excised by extending the incision onto the dorsum of the foot. The wound may be partially closed and a drain inserted in the web space for 72 hours. The original wart or callus is treated locally.

Osteomyelitis may be of pyogenic, fungus or tuberculous origin. Whenever possible, the organism must be identified. Pyogenic osteomyelitis is treated as elsewhere in the body. Rest and splinting of the part and massive doses of appropriate antibiotics are used. Saucerization of involved bones may be necessary when draining sinuses develop, along with excision of sinus tracts. Often, joints are destroyed and spontaneous bony or fibrous fusion takes place. Therefore, it is essential to maintain the foot in weight-bearing position while treating the infection. This may be done with splints or casts.

Tuberculous arthritis and osteomyelitis involving the foot are extremely serious, as are the fungus infections. Before the advent of antibiotic therapy and chemotherapy appropriate for these infections, amputation was the usual result. The outlook is now more hopeful with the availability of these drugs. However, the old principle of immobilization in tuberculosis still applies. Cast fixation may be necessary with non-weight bearing for many months and surgical fusion of infected joints may be necessary to permanently arrest the lesion.

Superficial skin infections in the foot are commonly caused by fungus or yeast organisms. The condition is known as dermatophytosis. The common causative organisms are the Epidermophyton, Trichophyton or *Candida albicans*. These organisms are normal inhabitants on the skin. They require moisture, warmth and an alkaline medium for growth. In the presence of these conditions and lowered resistance of the skin, infection can take place. A frequent area of invasion is between the toes, particularly the fourth and fifth toes which fit closely together, and the plantar surface of the foot and toes. The lesions produce maceration between the toes in which cracks may occur, allowing secondary invading bacteria to cause spreading cellulitis. Lesions on the plantar aspect may resemble the lesions of ringworm, or they may be vesicular, filled with clear or milky fluid. Occasionally, numerous small lesions coalesce or large bullous lesions develop. The bullae may rupture, followed by crusting and peeling of the superficial layers of the skin. The disease tends to be chronic or recurrent.

Treatment is directed at cleanly care of the feet, reduction of moisture, conversion of the alkaline to an acid medium and the use of fungicides.

The feet should be washed daily and dried thoroughly. Application of undecylenic acid compounds night and morning changes the skin to an acid medium. Nystatin, a potent fungicide, may be applied daily in resistant infections. Allowing the shoes to dry thoroughly by changing shoes daily reduces the moisture content. Clean stockings should be used daily.

VASCULAR DISEASE OF THE FOOT

When peripheral vascular disease is known to be present, prophylaxis of complicating lesions in the foot should be the concern of the surgeon as well as the patient. Since the foot is the farthest point from the heart in the area of the peripheral circulation, manifestations of failure or impairment may occur early or be precipitated by acute failure.

The primary objectives of prophylactic care are to prevent pressure and friction, to guard against exceeding the circulatory capacity, and to avoid excessive heat or cold. Any of these factors may precipitate circulatory failure. Trauma is an important factor. Trimming toenails or calluses to the point where the skin is damaged may permit bacteria to invade the tissues, increasing circulatory demands through infection and thus precipitating gangrene.

Toenails must be kept free from debris under the margins. Lubricating the skin with lanolin prevents the accumulation of keratotic skin which may crack or cause pressure on the underlying skin, leading to necrosis. Careful removal of this material with an orangewood stick is helpful. Trimming the nails so that ingrown nails do not occur is important. Calluses and corns must be carefully trimmed. When the skin is broken by excessive or careless trimming, infection frequently supervenes in the devitalized tissues. Pumice stone or an emery board may be carefully used to reduce the thickness of calluses and corns. Salicylic acid should not be used, as the devitalizing effect on already impaired tissues may allow infection to develop. Shoes and stockings should be carefully fitted to prevent friction and pressure. Excessive moisture or drying should be counteracted by appropriate measures.

READING REFERENCES

Bechtol, C. O., and Mossman, H. W.: Club-foot. An embryological study of associated muscle abnormalities. J. Bone & Joint Surg. 32-A:827, 1950.

Betts, L. O.: Morton's metatarsalgia: neuritis of the fourth digital nerve. M. J. Australia 1:514, 1940.

Bohm, M.: The embryologic origin of club-foot. J. Bone & Joint Surg. 11:229, 1929.

Duchenne, G. B.: Physiology of Motion. Philadelphia, W. B. Saunders Company, 1959 (translated and edited by E. B. Kaplan).

Elftman, H. A., and Manter, J. T.: The evolution of the human foot with especial reference to the joints. J. Anat. 70:56, 1935.

Grodinsky, M.: Study of tendon sheaths of foot and their relation to infection. Surg. Gyn. & Obst. 51:460, 1930.

Grodinsky, M.: A study of the fascial spaces of the foot and their bearing on infections. Surg. Gyn. & Obst. 49:737, 1929.

Haines, R. W., and McDougall, A.: The anatomy of hallux valgus. J. Bone & Joint Surg. 36-B:272, 1954.

Hauser, E. D. W.: Diseases of the Foot. Philadelphia, W. B. Saunders Company, 1950.

Jones, F. W.: Structure and Function as Seen in the Foot. Baltimore, The Williams & Wilkins Company, 1944.

Jones, R.: The soldier's foot and the treatment of common deformities of the foot. III. Hammer toe. Brit. Med. J. 1:782, 1916.

Keller, W. L.: Further observations on the surgical treatment of hallux valgus and bunions. New York M. J. 95:696, 1912.

Klopsteg, P. E., and Wilson, P. D.: Human limbs and their substitutes. New York, McGraw-Hill Book Company, 1954.

Larmon, W. A., and Kurtz, J. F.: The surgical management of chronic tophaceous gout. J. Bone & Joint Surg. 40-A:743, 1958.

Mayer, L.: The physiological method of tendon transplants reviewed after forty years. American Academy of Orthopaedic Surgeons. Vol. XIII. Ann Arbor, Michigan, J. W. Edwards, 1956.

McCarroll, H. R.: Foot deformities resulting from irreparable nerve lesions. In, Reconstructive Surgery of the Extremities. American Academy of Orthopaedic Surgeons. Ann Arbor, Michigan, J. W. Edwards, 1944.

Morton, D. J.: Mechanism of the normal foot and of flat foot. J. Bone & Joint Surg. 6:368, 1924.

Murphy, D. P.: Congenital malformations. A study of parental characteristics with special reference to the reproductive process. 2nd ed. Philadelphia, J. B. Lippincott Company, 1947.

Willis, T. A.: Orthopaedic anatomy of the foot and ankle. In, Regional Orthopaedic Surgery and Fundamental Orthopaedic Problems. American Academy of Orthopaedic Surgeons. Vol. I. Ann Arbor, Michigan, J. W. Edwards, 1947.

Chapter *34*

PHYSICAL MEDICINE AND REHABILITATION

by

WILLIAM J. ERDMAN, II, M.D.

and

EMERY K. STONER, M.D.

WILLIAM J. ERDMAN is a Philadelphian by birth and was educated in the Germantown Friends School and Swarthmore College, two noted Quaker institutions. He spent a year at the Virginia Polytechnic Institute before serving as an army infantryman and entering the School of Medicine at the University of Pennsylvania. His entire professional career has been spent in physical medicine and rehabilitation to which he has made fundamental valuable contributions. He is Professor and Chairman of the Department of Physical Medicine and Rehabilitation at the University of Pennsylvania.

Associated in the writing of this chapter is EMERY K. STONER, a native Pennsylvanian, and a graduate of the University of Pennsylvania and its School of Medicine. He has made valuable basic contributions in tissue temperature studies and is Associate Professor of Physical Medicine and Rehabilitation and Clinical Director of this department at the Hospital of the University of Pennsylvania.

Physical medicine is that division of medicine which uses heat, cold, massage, light, water, electricity and mechanical means in the diagnosis and management of disease and injury. Rehabilitation is the restoration of the handicapped individual to his maximal usefulness physically, emotionally, socially and economically.

Rehabilitation requires the integrated efforts of various medical specialists as well as personnel such as physical therapists, occupational therapists, rehabilitation nurses, speech therapists, psychologists, social workers, recreational therapists and rehabilitation counselors.

There is a tremendous and growing need for the services of physical medicine and rehabilitation. The programs seek to restore the patient to his maximal degree of independence. This does not mean that he must do things normally or without aids, but every effort is made to help him to make maximal use of the abilities he has left.

A marked increase of interest in the concepts of rehabilitation as performed in rehabilitation centers or rehabilitation wards of general hospitals has occurred in the past two decades. The thrust for development of these facilities has come from increased interest on the part of government, labor, voluntary health agencies, insurance companies and other third parties, and, to a lesser extent, from the medical profession itself. The rehabilitation center affords a common meeting ground where all the interested medical specialists may bring their skills to play in the total restoration of an individual physically, socially, emotionally and vocationally.

Too frequently, rehabilitation has been considered a process employed after usual medical specialty care had produced the limit of improvement. There has been too little consideration of rehabilitation as a process which begins at the onset of illness or accident and is not completed until the individual has reached his maximal potential.

Physicians are frustrated frequently by an apparent lack of motivation on the part of the patient, by the obvious secondary gains achieved through his illness, or by his passive dependent personality, and turn in desperation to the use of the facilities of the rehabilitation center. The center affords an excellent meeting ground for the special expertise

1233

1234 Chapter 34 PHYSICAL MEDICINE AND REHABILITATION

of medical groups and the paramedical groups previously listed.

The positive stimulating effect of the group dynamics of one patient upon another should not be minimized. When most of the seriously disabled are making heroic efforts toward independence, those not so inclined are caught up in this enthusiasm. Additionally, there are distinctive advantages in nursing care provided to patients undergoing rehabilitation in comparison to the customary medical or surgical service, in that the nursing personnel are specifically trained and oriented in helping the patient make maximal use of his remaining capabilities, rather than in doing things for him in a most efficient fashion for the nursing service. This may be more time consuming but in the end it develops a degree of independence and self-care which the other procedure fails to achieve.

HEAT AND COLD

Heat is one of the oldest and most generally used forms of treatment. Its use is still rather empirical but its beneficial effects are unquestionable. Cold is simply the absence of heat, or low thermal energy. Because heat is a form of energy, a given amount of heat should appear when a given amount of energy is dissipated, when a given amount of work is done, or when a given quantity of electrical energy is consumed. The sources of heat are chemical, electrical and frictional.

The transfer of heat is primarily by conduction, convection and radiation. In clinical practice, mass transfer of heat energy is used in heat transport along with conduction. An example would be heating the skin with a hot pack, conduction, and distributing it throughout the body by means of the circulating blood, mass transfer.

PHYSIOLOGICAL RESPONSE TO HEAT AND COLD. Man is a self-regulating machine made up of cells and organs. The effects of heat and cold can be subdivided into those acting at the cellular level, the organ level, or the total self-regulating mechanism. Effects at all three levels occur simultaneously and are more or less interrelated.

The rate of metabolic processes increases with slowly rising temperatures, at first exponentially, and as higher temperatures are reached the increase in rate diminishes. After reaching a maximum, the rate decreases with

further increase in temperature until at a certain temperature the metabolism ceases completely. Typical activity temperature curves have been found not only for protozoa, bacteria, leukocytes and erythrocytes, but also for isolated enzyme systems in vitro. In complex activity such as nerve conduction velocity, the ascending part of the activity temperature curve more or less resembles a straight line. This indicates that the activity increases proportionally to the temperature increase.

In man, cardiovascular, hormonal and nervous control are involved in so-called temperature regulation. This is the sum of all the complicated regulating mechanisms which enable man to maintain a fairly constant body temperature despite considerable variation of environmental temperature.

What we call body temperature represents only the temperature of the "core" of the body. Even in the core there is no uniform temperature throughout because the temperature of each organ, in the end, depends on the temperature of the blood flowing through it and the relative level of the metabolism of the organ. The "shell" of the body has a much lower mean temperature. There is a temperature gradient from core temperature down to skin temperature. The body loses heat from its surface by conduction, convection, radiation and evaporation. The skin temperature will increase or decrease quickly to a level at which the blood loss balances heat production. Some heat loss is caused by evaporation from the skin as insensible perspiration or is connected with sweating, and partly from the lungs. Although the absolute temperature difference between core and skin is regulated according to the need of the heat balance, the slope of the temperature gradient in the shell depends on where the heat is primarily liberated and the heat transport from the core to the skin. Circulation can be regarded as a cooling system for the core and as a heating system for the shell.

EFFECTS OF HEAT AND COLD APPLIED TO RESTRICTED BODY AREAS. Locally, heat increases and cold decreases skin blood flow by local as well as reflex mechanisms. If enough heat is applied externally and the skin temperature in that area becomes greater than that of the core temperature, the gradient in this case becomes reversed and the increased blood flow helps to distribute the added heat uniformly throughout the body. If we apply cold to a restricted area, the resulting decreased blood flow diminishes heat transport from the core to the skin and enhances the direct cooling effect.

Remote effects. Heat vasodilatation and cold vasoconstriction spread to adjacent areas and with higher intensities to remote areas. The latter is often called the consensual heat vasodilatation or cold constriction. Thus, when heat is applied to one arm the effect can become evident in the other arm and, in time, in the legs.

Applying external heat or cold to the abdomen has the opposite effect on bowel blood flow. Externally applied heat decreases intestinal blood flow, decreases intestinal motility and decreases acid secretion in the stomach. Cold application has the opposite effect.

Deep heating. With the use of short wave diathermy, microwave diathermy and ultrasound, muscle blood flow increases, but much less than a comparable increase in the skin temperature and increase in blood flow. At best, deep heating doubles muscle blood flow. This is a rather small increase as compared to muscle blood flow after exercise or electrical stimulation of the muscles.

The effects of heat and cold on blood flow and the secondary processes elicited by blood flow changes are the only physiologically reasonable well-understood effects of heat and cold. Therefore, clinically, it is assumed that these changes are the main rationale for the use of heat and cold therapy.

The sensation of pain is decreased by mild heating, whereas it is increased with the use of mild cold. However, the prolonged use of cold produces an anesthesia.

Heat has a relaxing effect on pathologic tonic activity of skeletal muscles. Heat decreases tonic activity leading to diminished pain. Work with the effects of heat and cold on the muscle spindles and gamma fibers remains to be clarified.

APPLICATION OF HEAT AND COLD. There are numerous methods of applying heat clinically. Hot water bottles, heating pads, hydrocollator packs, whirlpool, paraffin baths and infrared generators have in common the effects of surface heating, with heat entering the body by conduction and being dissipated by means of the circulation. The choice of the method is dependent on the part to be treated, the availability of equipment, patient comfort and preference, and the nature of the disorder being treated. Actually, heat is

heat and the difference is merely one of quantity and the location of the heating, whether it is surface or deep. Hot packs are more comforting to some patients, whereas to others the weight of the pack itself is unpleasant. Hot water is the one method of heating with which the degree of heat being applied can be determined. Other methods rely on the sensation of the patient as a guide to dosage. Hydrocollator packs are a convenient and comfortable way of using heat both in the hospital and at home.

Deep heating can be produced by short wave diathermy, microwave diathermy and ultrasound. In diathermy and microwave applications, electromagnetic waves are converted into heat in the tissues. In the case of ultrasound, mechanical waves are transformed into heat at interfaces. Much has been written about the specific effects of diathermy and ultrasound but, as used clinically, heat appears to be the only effect.

Cold has been given by cold packs, massage with ice cubes, cold bath immersions, or by the use of ethyl chloride spray. There are enthusiasts for each method, and each appears to have his own system of application. Cold has a counterirritant effect as well as an anesthetic result. It is most useful in acute and subacute conditions.

The important fact to be kept in mind is that heat and cold are adjuncts to other modalities, usually as a preparation for exercise and functional use of the part. A prime indication for use of heat or cold is for relief of pain which will in turn permit function.

MASSAGE

Massage consists basically of palpation, rubbing, and kneading. It is one of the oldest analgesics known, but today its true value is not appreciated fully.

Systematized massage consisting of stroking, kneading, percussing, and vibrating brings about improvement of the circulation, increase of warmth to the skin, more rapid removal of waste, dissolution of soft adhesions, reduction of swelling in induration of tissues, loosening and stretching of contracted tendons, and soothing of the peripheral nerves as well as the central nervous system.

Massage is traditionally preceded by some sort of heat and is usually followed by exercise. Ideally, massage should be done by the physician himself, but he rarely has the time or the skill to do it and delegates it to a therapist. The simplicity of massage has led to its disregard in favor of more intricate treatments.

TRACTION

Traction may be defined as a force applied to the body along its length or to any portion of the spine in such a way as to separate or attempt to separate vertebral and spinal structures. It is most easily applied to the cervical and lumbar spine.

Traction is prescribed to produce rest by immobilization, to overcome muscle spasm and to separate bony surfaces. Probably all that is achieved by the low tractive force applied to the pelvis or legs for patients with acute back pain is immobilization.

Experimentally, it has been shown that traction is useful to stretch muscles and ligaments, to stretch the whole or a segment of the spine, widen disc spaces that have been narrowed by disc degeneration, separate vertebral bodies, and stretch and separate apophyseal joints.

Application of traction may be made by manual force or by mechanical means. Traction may be continuous for several days, sustained for hours on a traction table, or intermittent for short periods. The position of the patient may be vertical, horizontal or tilted. The magnitude of the force required varies considerably but the lowest force required to produce symptomatic relief should be used.

Traction is ordinarily quite safe, but its use should be avoided in the presence of infection or malignancy of the spine, or if there is evidence of cord compression.

EXERCISES

Of all the methods used in physical medicine and rehabilitation, exercise is the most useful and universally used. It is unequaled by any other physical modality in its ability to alleviate and even to cure many infirmities of the body. Rest has its advantages in acute illness, but the abuse of rest is more hazardous than that of exercise.

PHYSIOLOGY. The physiology of exercise involves the function of muscles, nerves, bones and joints. Other systems are intimately involved, such as the cardiovascular and pulmonary systems.

The contractile molecule of skeletal muscle is a protein, myosin. This myosin molecule can shorten by about 40 per cent. Contraction in intact muscle occurs only in the presence of adenosine triphosphate. Contraction is a coupled chemical and mechanical phenomenon in which the terminal high energy phosphate bond of adenosine triphosphate is removed, supplying the energy for the mechanical shortening of myosin. Proper concentration of calcium, magnesium and potassium is of importance in the reaction.

The motor unit is made up of a motor nerve cell, its axons and branches and all the muscle fibers which it innervates. The all-or-none law applies to this group of fibers. Smooth contraction of the muscle is produced through asynchronous contraction of active motor units. By varying the number of active motor units and, perhaps, by increasing the frequency of nerve firing, graded strength of muscular contraction is accomplished.

There are four qualities of muscle to be considered in therapy. They are strength, endurance, speed and coordination.

Strength is the ability to develop tension. It is related to the size of the muscle in cross-section and to the number of motor units which can be activated by voluntary effort. Exercises at higher tensions require principally strength. Repeated efforts against maximal or near maximal loads leads to the ability of muscle to develop greater tension on effort. Probably, the first change is the recruitment of a larger proportion of the motor units in voluntary efforts, because increased strength occurs before hypertrophy is seen. Hypertrophy is a fundamental adaptation to the increased use of a muscle. Isometric or isotonic maximal contractions both effectively build up strength. In practice, exercises are usually not designed just for maximal strength but also for other effects.

Endurance or stamina has the connotation of sustained work capacity. Stamina, power and work capacity refer to similar qualities and mean work per unit of time. Endurance is related more to circulation and metabolic changes than to the size and strength of muscle. The blood vessels to muscles are affected most profoundly by local metabolic products. The number of open capillaries in muscles is increased several times in exercises. Strenuous and sustained exercise is most effective in increasing the local blood flow through the muscle and enhancing the metabolism. The muscle adapts by increasing its ability to produce work. This adaptation consists of increasing the circulation and building up stores of metabolites. Muscle exercise increases the capacity for anaerobic as well as aerobic work. When the lactic acid of the tissue fluids approaches 10 mEq. per liter in the muscles of an untrained man he may be unable to continue work; but with training, a level near 20 mEq. per liter may be tolerated.

Practically speaking, exercises in the area of maximal work should be those requiring tension less than half of maximum and should be continued for a period of time sufficient to develop metabolic stress. Usually, more than five minutes of continuous exercise is needed.

Speed in muscle action depends on both muscle and the central nervous system. Speed is related to the load and skill. The greater the load, the lower the speed. Skill involves the number of motor units brought into action at the proper time and the appropriate inhibition of antagonist muscles.

Skill is a comprehensive term which describes a function of the central nervous system rather than any one quality of muscle. It is the ability to control muscle action precisely in a progression of motion in order to accomplish a specific physical task. Coordination is very similar to skill.

Coordination might be more properly termed coordinated function. It encompasses skill and balance. Balance appears to be a special form of skill requiring use of the proprioceptive system. Exercise in the range of low tension has little effect but does demonstrate coordination or skill. Repetition is the key to developing coordination and skill.

An important therapeutic goal in exercise is range of motion. Maintenance of full motion in joints and periarticular tissues may accompany exercise and may be the therapeutic goal. Active exercise is usually the safest and most convenient method of retaining or restoring joint motion.

SYSTEMIC EFFECTS OF EXERCISE. Almost every system of the body responds to the changes effected by exercise. Circulatory changes are the most prominent ones seen outside the neuromuscular system. In normally functioning hearts, the cardiac output increases with even mild exercise. In athletes, it may increase to seven or eight times normal. Owing to vasodilatation in muscle the blood pressure shows only minor changes in all but the most severe exercise. Elevations of 10 to 20 mm. Hg in systolic pressure and less in diastolic pressure are usual.

Hyperpnea is an outstanding response to exercise. However, except for pulmonary invalids, circulatory capacity is the limiting factor in exercising and not pulmonary function.

Leukocytosis may be observed even in moderate exercise. Strenuous exercise leads to hemolysis of the older red cells. The body temperature rises to a level dependent upon the severity of the exercises.

The overall result of an exercise program is to improve the metabolic capacity of working muscle. The general effects are most striking when muscle groups are involved in exercise for a period of time sufficient to induce metabolic and circulatory distress. Therefore, the severity of the exercise must be adjusted continually and increased as training progresses. Individual bones as well as the entire skeleton may be modified by muscular exercise. It has been shown that regular exercise increases the density of bones. There is evidence that elderly patients, debilitated persons and convalescents respond favorably to a graded exercise program much in the fashion of normal persons.

MUSCLE TESTING. Manual muscle testing is useful in disorders of the peripheral nerves and of the muscles themselves. It is of limited value in upper motor neuron derangement. Muscle testing reveals the muscles needing muscle-strengthening exercises. In addition, muscle testing is helpful in diagnosis, such as the weakness of proximal musculature seen in myopathies, or weakness of the toe extensors as found in an L5 root lesion.

TYPES OF EXERCISES. Exercises may be labeled passive, active, active assistive and resistive. Actually, exercises should be done actively if at all possible. Assistive motion may be needed if weakness is profound or in order to complete full range of motion. To be precise, all active motion is resistive in type. Resistance may only be gravity or even the internal resistance of the muscle itself, but it is giving the muscle work to do. Gravity may be eliminated as a source of resistance to a given motion but still it may be heavy resistance for that particular muscle.

Re-education of muscle action is a term carried over from the treatment of poliomyelitis and from the days of numerous tendon transplants. Today, the tendency is to re-educate or to re-establish patterns of movements rather than concentrate on individual muscles. This does not hold true for peripheral nerve injuries in which separate muscles may require training.

THE GOAL OF EXERCISE. Exercises of all types have in common the development, restoration or preservation of function of the individual. In most instances, there is need for exercising more than just the affected part.

It can be inferred that the type of exercise needed depends upon the development of strength, improvement of endurance, promotion of coordination or increase of range of motion.

The amount of resistance given depends upon the initial power of muscle. It should be kept clearly in mind that to increase strength, the resistance must be near maximum with few repetitions; to increase endurance, the resistance should be in the range of less than half of maximum and the repetitions continued for at least five minutes so that metabolic stress is developed. Coordination is best obtained by frequent repetition, in the range of minimal tension. The goal is increased function of the individual.

ENERGY COSTS. In order to have an idea of the stress imposed on a patient by exercises and activities, studies of oxygen consumption have been done. Energy costs are expressed in calories per minute with basal metabolic rate being unity. A list of common activities with their energy requirements is shown in Table 1.

The increase of energy requirement in using a bedpan as compared to a bedside commode is well known. A surprise is the metabolic demand for taking a shower. Showering is usually a brief activity but in some cases the demand is too great. This could be minimized by helping the patient into the shower and having him sit on a shower stool.

The best known simple test of functional capacity is the Master two-step test. This

Table 1. Common Activities and Their Energy Requirements

ACTIVITY	CALORIES/MINUTE
Rest – supine	1.0
Sitting	1.2
Standing – relaxed	1.4
Eating	1.4
Using bedpan	4.7
Bedside commode	3.6
Dressing	3.6
Showering	4.2
Walking (2.5 m.p.h.)	3.6
Walking downstairs	5.2
Occupational therapy	1.2–2.0

effort involves a caloric expenditure of 8.5 calories per minute. For handicapped persons, this energy cost may be much greater for a given activity. For instance, a paraplegic patient walking slowly with crutches and braces may be expending energy at the rate of eight times basal. This soons leads to exhaustion. This also explains why so many patients prefer using a wheelchair.

Energy expenditure decreases with age. This has been determined to be approximately a 3 per cent decrease for each decade over 35 up to the age of 55.

ELECTROTHERAPY

Interest in the use of electricity in medicine has fluctuated since its discovery. Overenthusiasm in its use has often been followed by neglect. Equipment used in electrotherapy is often spoken of as "low voltage generators." This terminology is used to differentiate it from the high frequency machines such as diathermy generators.

The effects of electricity can be explained on the basis of physics and physiology. Like other physical agents the effects can be both local and remote. The result may be stimulating or depressing to the vascular, motor and sensory systems. All electrical currents cause some heating of the tissues. This is especially true for currents with a frequency over 10,000 per second. Rapid changes in current flow cause muscular contractions. This fact is used in treating or testing muscles with damaged nerve supply.

Electrical currents may be direct or alternating. Excluding diathermy, the currents used in electrotherapy are direct current and low frequency current.

The direct current represents an uninterrupted constant and unidirectional flow at low voltage. It produces positive and negative polarity effects when passed through an electrolyte.

When a direct current passes through body tissues, the chlorine ion migrates to the positive pole and when its electric charge neutralizes it reacts chemically with water in tissues to form hydrochloric acid. If concentrated, this strong acid can harden tissues. The sodium ion goes to the negative pole where its charge is neutralized and sodium hydroxide is formed. This strong alkaloid tends to soften tissue. For practical purposes, the passage of direct current to the body as used clinically produces only mild changes under the electrodes and no real caustic or acid effects.

The introduction of ions in the tissues for therapeutic purposes is known as ion transfer. If positive ions are to be utilized, the positive pole is used, whereas if negative ions are concerned, the negative pole is used, as like charges tend to repel each other.

It has been observed clinically that the positive direct current produces sedative effects and that the negative direct current increases irritation. We can conclude that counterirritation is present at both the positive and negative electrodes, but if the current flows at an appreciable length of time, more irritation will be felt at the negative electrode. Vasodilatation is produced at both positive and negative electrodes. The tissue between electrodes tends to become warmer during the passage of electric current. This is assumed to be due to the impedance that the tissues offer to the flow of the electrical current.

A normal muscle can be stimulated to contract by making and breaking a direct current if the current flow is of sufficient magnitude. Less current is needed to produce a minimal contraction when a normal muscle is in contact with the negative electrode. The direct current is used for medical galvanism, ion transfer, surgical galvanism and electrical testing. Surgical galvanism is the use of caustic polar effects of direct current for the removal of superfluous hair and the destruction of small warts and moles.

The sudden make or break of a direct current of sufficient strength over muscular tissues or motor nerves acts as a stimulus to bring about a muscle contraction and a sensory sensation of slight shock.

The most important use of electrical stimulation is in the treatment of peripheral nerve lesions such as Bell's palsy, axillary nerve damage and peroneal palsy. It must be kept in mind that muscles are treated in order to preserve them in as good a condition as possible while the nerve is regenerating. There is no evidence to show that electrical stimulation of a muscle makes any difference in the rapidity of reinnervation or its quality. As soon as any voluntary control is regained, exercise is the most important procedure and electrical stimulation is discontinued.

Stimulation of muscles in spasm by a suitable tetanizing current often results in marked relief of spasm and pain.

PAIN AND PAIN RELIEF

One of the objectives of physical medicine is to relieve pain. Pain is of primary importance to the individual for his protection. With its loss in disease such as in leprosy, repeated injuries occur and major losses ensue.

Pain receptors are widespread and evidence is preponderant that naked nerve endings are the only pain receptors. A given nerve fiber may supply a skin area of 50 square cm. However, many similar nerve fibers may also share that same area so that there is much overlapping.

Two types of fibers carry pain, the A delta and C fibers, and also mediate other sensations. The A delta fibers are those of 2 to 4 microns in diameter which conduct at a speed of 15 to 20 meters per second. They are relatively thinly medullated and make up about one-third of the total number of medullated fibers in mixed peripheral nerves. When the ending of such a fiber is tetanized with electric shocks, clear pricking pain is felt. The C fibers are small nonmedullated fibers about 1 micron in diameter and conducting at 1 to 2 meters per second. In a somatic nerve trunk the C fibers comprise as much as 20 per cent of the fibers. The threshold for C fibers is one hundred fold for that of the A delta fibers.

Pain messages that come along A delta fibers enter the cord and run up the dorsal column on the same side, primarily in relatively large fibers, in speeds of 50 to 80 meters per second. Those messages that come via C fibers travel in the crossed ventrolateral columns in the thin fibers at low speeds. The two systems of pain afferents continue to be separate as far as they can be traced.

These systems are antagonistic in some ways and complementary in others. When the A delta system is active there is a clear awareness of sharp, cutting, pricking pain but this does not cause great suffering.

However, when the C system is active it leads to suffering. It facilitates the responses of cortical neurons to other pain impulses and adds to the pain experience involved. The A delta system and other fibers, such as for touch and pressure, tend to suppress the C fiber type of pain.

The essential point is that there is a distinct difference between awareness of pain and suffering from pain. This tolerance for pain must not be confused with the threshold for pain. The final difference between individuals consists in a variance in tolerance for pain in spite of the fact that their sensory threshold may be identical. Therefore, a drug that may increase tolerance for pain may not affect the pain threshold.

There is no objective way of measuring pain. The simplest and most reliable index of pain is a verbal report of the patient. The visible and measurable changes resulting from acute pain, such as increased pulse rate, palmar sweating, alteration in skin resistance and motor reaction, are not particularly useful in the study of pain and its relief. For instance, hypnosis may be used to relieve pain but it does not alter the body response to pain.

Pain relief may be approached by decreasing the sensory input, increasing pain receptor threshold, increase in A delta stimulation and a central action.

Some aspects of placebo effects must be considered. It has been found that a placebo is ten times more active in relieving severe pain than in relieving experimental pain. In an arthritis outpatient clinic, 60 per cent of an oral preparation of placebo was found to be effective. Severe pain has been relieved in up to 70 per cent of patients by placebos.

Many patients are placebo reactors and respond favorably with pain relief whether the treatment is in the form of a drug or as physical therapy. This is fortuitous for physician and patient, but it makes the evaluation of pain relief difficult.

Pain receptors are chemoceptive and not nociceptive. Pain is not produced simply by increasing the intensity or frequency of stimulation of any somesthetic receptor. Chemical agents, acids, alkalis, concentrated salt solution and bradykinin peptides, are most active in producing pain without injury. The normal uninjured pain receptor is chemosensitive. Injury of tissue leads to vasodilatation, by injury itself or by liberation of histamine and serotinin, which in turn induces accumulation of erythrocytes and leukocytes with the formation of bradykinin-like peptides by action of a trypsin-like enzyme on alpha-2 globulin in serum. This in turn causes further vasodilatation and increased vascular permeability with leakage, edema, inflammation and pain. H^+, K^+, amines and peptides excite pain receptors. The receptor sites are negatively charged and algic agents positively charged.

Non-narcotic antipyretic analgesics act peripherally by blocking the generation of impulses at the chemoreceptors for pain. It appears that they block the action of bradykinin. A simple explanation is that they cause reduction of local edema with resulting pain relief.

The narcotics do not raise the threshold of pain receptors to peripheral stimulation or block transmission of impulses. The messages enter the nervous system as before, but they no longer seem as important as before.

Turning to the use of physical measures in the relief of pain, certain observations have been made. For instance, vibrations applied to the skin raise the threshold to touch, temperature and pain. The effects of vibration have not been thoroughly studied, especially with regard to changing its amplitude and frequency.

Heat is used almost universally for pain relief. In some methods such as hydrocollator packs and whirlpool, pain relief is likely from decreasing the sensory input by decreasing edema, increasing local circulation and removal of pain-producing substances. Other heat modalities such as infrared may help by counterirritation to stimulate A delta fibers and inhibit C fiber activity.

The various forms of electrical stimulation causing mild tingling sensation without motor contraction interfere with the perception of pain accompanying certain diseases. The stimulation of large myelinated fibers inhibits the suffering type of pain.

Modalities used in physical medicine, including heat, light, water, electricity, massage, mechanical devices and exercises, can be used for the relief of pain. They act by decreasing the sensory input, increasing the pain receptor threshold or by A delta stimulation. Certainly, physical measures can be most effective in pain relief and can be applied locally, repeatedly and safely. Very few individuals have reactions or hypersensitivities to physical measures.

It behooves all physicians to remember that the tremendous psychotherapeutic benefit of the doctor-patient relationship outweighs the importance of drugs or treatments.

ELECTRICAL TESTING

Electrical testing has become very useful in determining the presence of minimal disease of the lower motor neuron, the location, severity, and timing of the damage and the earliest evidence of recovery. It is helpful in differentiating between myopathy and neuropathy. Defects of transmission at the neuromuscular junction may be demonstrated.

Electrical testing commonly includes nerve trunk stimulation, strength duration curves, chronaxie testing, conduction velocity of motor nerves and electromyography.

The motor unit consists of a single neuron with all the muscle fibers that it innervates. The number of fibers supplied by each neuron varies considerably from hundreds of fibers for the quadriceps muscle to a few for the frontalis muscle.

NERVE TRUNK STIMULATION. Stimulation of peripheral nerves by an electrical current is useful in testing for damage of peripheral nerves. Electrodes are placed on the skin over the chosen nerve and brief stimuli are applied while the response of the muscles innervated by that nerve is observed. Contractions may be seen or palpated. The current used is one millisecond or less in duration with an intensity greater than that required for a maximal contraction of the muscles.

A normal contraction of muscles innervated by the nerve under study indicates that it is conducting the impulse and that the cause of paralysis, if present, is proximal to the point stimulated. If there is damage of the lower motor neuron proximal to the point of stimulation, a normal response indicates that wallerian degeneration has not occurred. This may follow from pressure ischemia or in neuronitis where only a functional block of conduction may be present. This has been termed neuropraxia. However, the damage may be severe but so recent that wallerian degeneration has not been completed. After an acute injury, the nerve may remain responsive to electrical stimulation for about three days.

Absence of response or a weak response may be due to impaired nerve conduction distally, abnormality of the nerve at the level of stimulation, damage of some nerve elements proximally or inability of the muscle fibers to contract.

In facial palsy, stimulation of the nerve is helpful early in determining the severity of the damage. If, after three days the muscles supplied by the involved facial nerve contract upon stimulation of the nerve trunk, then wallerian degeneration has not taken place and recovery should be rapid.

STRENGTH-DURATION CURVES. In normal muscles, the nerve is the most sensitive component to electrical stimulation. Stimulation with a current of one millisecond or less in duration requires little strength of stimulus to produce a response. However, if the muscle is denervated, the strength of stimulation needed to produce a response with a current of one millisecond duration is appreciably increased. This difference in threshold to excitation by electric currents between innervated and denervated muscles has been used to detect degeneration of nerves by such procedures as the galvanic-faradic test, chronaxie determination and strength-duration curves. Plotting of the strength-duration curves has been found to be the most reliable of these tests.

Although electromyography is more sensitive in evaluating the status of the lower motor neuron, these tests often provide earlier evidence of denervation following nerve injury because abnormalities may appear in ten to 14 days, whereas electromyographic evidence may not be detected until 18 to 21 days after injury.

To plot a strength-duration curve, an electrical stimulus is applied to the muscle at its motor point, the most excitable point. Using a pulse of long duration, about 300 milliseconds, the strength of current necessary to provide a minimal visible or palpable contraction of the muscle is found. This value is called the rheobase. The duration of the pulse is shortened successively and the strength of current to produce a minimal response is determined. These values are plotted to become a curve relating the strength and duration of the stimulus required to produce minimal contractions.

In normal muscles, little or no increase in strength of stimulus is needed to get a response with a current of one millisecond duration than for one of 100 milliseconds. In denervated muscle, the curve rises steeply as the pulse duration becomes less than 30 milliseconds. The strength of stimulus needed for a response with a pulse duration of one millisecond may be two or more times that required for one of 100 milliseconds. With a galvanic current or with pulses of long duration, the contraction of denervated muscle is slow and prolonged.

In partially denervated muscles and during the reinnervation of muscles, irregularity of the curve may be found. These have been called discontinuities and they represent a mixture of responses from denervated fibers and innervated fibers.

Chronaxie is the duration of the pulse required to produce a minimal response using a current of twice rheobase strength. For normal muscle, the chronaxie value is one millisecond or less, and more than one millisecond for denervated muscle. The chronaxie is just one point on the strength-duration curve.

The procedure for strength-duration curve may be modified by using values determined at 100, ten and one millisecond. If the strength doubles from ten to one millisecond, the curve is considered to be abnormal.

CONDUCTION VELOCITY OF MOTOR NERVES. Certain diseases affecting peripheral nerves result in slowing of conduction velocity. This can be demonstrated in the electromyograph by studying the response to nerve stimulation. This may result in an increase in conduction time from the point of stimulation to the muscle or a prolongation of the action potential of the muscle or both. Increased duration of the action potential is due to an increased temporal dispersion when the rate of conduction is not slowed uniformly in all nerve fibers.

Conduction velocity may be greatly slowed in Charcot-Marie-Tooth disease, Guillain-Barré syndrome, neuropathies and during regeneration of nerves after nerve injury or neuritis. Conduction velocities are generally within the normal range in polymyositis, progressive muscular atrophy, amyotrophic lateral sclerosis and muscular dystrophy.

ELECTROMYOGRAPHY.   Electromyography is a study of the electrical activity produced by muscles. It does not give a clinical diagnosis but aids in arriving at a final diagnosis. Normally, there is electrical silence with the muscle at rest. On voluntary effort, action potentials of motor units are detected. In disease of the motor unit, electrical activity may appear in a muscle at rest, and on activity the action potential may have abnormal forms and patterns of activity.

The essential components for electromyography are needle electrodes, an amplifier, cathode oscilloscope and a loudspeaker. A tape recorder and a camera are often included. The needle electrodes may be unipolar, coaxial or double coaxial. The variations in voltage are picked up and amplified about one million times. The rates of fluctuation are in the audible range and thus may be changed to sound waves. The characteristic sounds produced are often more helpful than the visual display. Permanent records may be made by a camera or by storing the signal by using a tape recorder.

Clinical procedures.   The case history and a neurological examination are prerequisites for planning and interpreting the electromyograph. In this way, those muscles probably most affected by the disease may be examined first and then other muscles studied, if necessary, to establish the distribution of the disease.

With the patient in a comfortable position, the needle electrode is inserted into the muscle and the electrical activity in response to this needle insertion and movement is noted. Observations are made during minimal and maximal effort. The needle is advanced to several depths and in several directions in a single muscle.

Observations.   In normal muscle at rest the motor units are inactive and no electrical activity is noted. During voluntary contraction, all the muscle fibers innervated by a single lower motor neuron "fire" off together and their small action potentials summate to produce the action potential of the motor unit – normally, diphasic or triphasic waves of three to 15 milliseconds in duration and 0.2 to 2.0 millivolts in amplitude. They produce a thumping sound over the loudspeaker. As voluntary effort increases, the rate which a motor unit fires increases and other motor units are recruited to increase the strength of contraction. During a strong contraction, the action potentials which are firing rhythmically and independently are indistinguishable from one another, thus forming an "interference pattern."

In normal muscles, insertion of the needle electrode results in only a brief period of electrical activity. However, some abnormal muscle fibers respond with prolonged repetition activity. This is true of denervated muscle fibers, muscle fibers in myotonia and muscle fibers in early degeneration. Two types of potentials are seen. One is a spike of short duration and the other a larger potential called a "positive sharp wave." The potentials evoked in denervated muscles by needle insertion are indistinguishable from those appearing spontaneously. However, abnormal insertion potentials may be seen earlier after nerve injury than the spontaneous fibrillation potentials.

In myotonias, prolonged trains of spikes and positive sharp waves are seen. These discharges occur at high frequency, up to 120 per second, and are characterized by waxing and waning in frequency and amplitude. Bizarre high frequency discharges are sometimes seen in progressive muscular dystrophy and polymyositis.

Fibrillation potentials have a duration of 0.5 to 1.5 milliseconds, and amplitude of 25 to 100 microvolts and recur two to ten times per second. They sound like rain on the roof, or the crumpling of tissue paper.

Degeneration of the lower motor neuron results in fibrillation potentials. The lesion may affect the anterior horn cells, nerve roots or peripheral nerves. Simple disuse atrophy does not result in denervation fibrillation; neither do upper motor neuron lesions.

Fibrillation potentials were once considered pathognomonic of lower motor neuron disease. However, potentials are found commonly in polymyositis and dermatomyositis which look like fibrillation potentials. Sometimes, they are found in myopathies. Other abnormalities of the electromyogram and clinical observations help differentiate neuropathic from myopathic diseases.

Fasciculations represent the spontaneous contraction of a bundle of muscle fibers and are accompanied by potentials resembling those of the motor unit. Fasciculation potentials are not evidence of degeneration of the lower motor neuron unless accompanied by evidence of other abnormalities.

Motor unit action potentials are studied during minimal voluntary effort. Random study of a large number of potentials is needed to see if there is any abnormality in duration, amplitude and shape of the potentials. Differentiation between neurogenic and myogenic lesions usually depends on this part of electromyography.

Normal motor unit potentials are usually diphasic or triphasic. However, about 5 per cent of potentials may have four or more phases and are called polyphasic potentials. Polyphasic potentials are the result of temporal dispersion of the action of the fibers of the same motor unit, likely due to differences in conduction times along the branches of the lower motor neuron.

In primary muscle diseases, polyphasic potentials may be seen with a reduction in the mean duration and amplitude of motor unit potentials. On maximal effort, many motor units are brought into action but the interference pattern is low.

In neuropathic diseases, polyphasic potentials may be demonstrated which show an increase in the duration and amplitude of motor unit potentials. This is most marked in diseases of the anterior horn cells such as amyotrophic lateral sclerosis, poliomyelitis, syringomyelia and Charcot-Marie-Tooth disease.

In recovery from peripheral neuropathies, the action potentials of the immature motor units are of low amplitude and brief duration and they are polyphasic in configuration. They may resemble those seen in myopathies. After reinnervation from a severe nerve injury, large potentials may be seen.

Because whole motor units are lost or inactive in disease affecting the lower motor neuron, on maximal effort the interference pattern is not full although the amplitude may be high. In severe cases, the activity of single motor units may be observed during strong efforts.

In a normal muscle, fatigue during a voluntary contraction is not associated with a significant decrease in the size of action potentials, but the number of active motor units decreases. In myasthenia gravis, a progressive decline in amplitude of potentials occurs, along with a decrease in the number of fibers responding.

Peripheral nerve injuries. Nerve injury may be followed by degeneration of the nerve. Immediately after the injury, the electromyograph is normal except for the lack of motor unit activity during voluntary effort. The earliest evidence of degeneration is failure of the nerve to react to electrical stimulation below the site of injury three days after the damage. On electromyography, insertion fibrillation potentials may be seen in ten to 14 days. Abnormal strength duration curves, elevated chronaxie values, may be detected in ten to 14 days. By 18 to 21 days spontaneous fibrillation potentials may be prominent. As reinnervation occurs, fibrillation potentials decrease and small voluntary potentials appear. Serial examinations are needed to follow reinnervation and electromyographic evidence of recovery may precede clinical signs by many weeks.

Electromyographic localization of nerve lesions depends on finding abnormality only in those muscles supplied by a particular nerve root or portion of a plexus. However, abnormalities may be widespread, such as in polyneuropathy or degenerative disease of the cord. Also, changes may be found to be predominantly in distal musculature or in proximal groups.

Clinically, electromyography is useful in detection of diseases in the motor unit, in the diagnosis of primary muscle disease, in detection of defects in transmission of the myoneural junction and in diagnosis of disease of the lower motor neuron.

ORTHOTICS

Bracing has come a long way from the old appliance maker who made hernia trusses, abdominal belts and limb braces. Progress has meant longer training, more research, improved technology and higher status. The brace maker is called an orthotist and the field, orthotics.

To qualify as a certified orthotist the candidate must have had at least four years of acceptable experience and must pass written, oral and practical examinations by the American Board in Orthotics and Prosthetics, Inc. The tendency today is for the orthotist to be a college graduate in engineering so that his knowledge of physics, materials and mechanics will be of help in the rehabilitation of the sick and injured.

The indications for bracing are relief of pain; rest of a part; support of weakened muscles; prevention of contractures; provision of joint stability; improvement of body alignment, and functional improvement. The primary goal of all bracing is improvement of function. This might be in a baby with congenital dislocation of a hip or in an old person with a hemiplegia.

Certain principles must be considered in prescribing a brace and in making certain that it fits and operates properly. Any pressure or weight bearing surface of an appliance must have adequate surface areas to minimize pressure per unit area. Any joint should be in the correct position. The brace should be contoured and fitted so that pain and constriction are avoided. The part should be held in the desired position of function. In addition, the brace should have good appearance, be easy to apply and be as simple and light as possible. Little maintenance should be necessary.

After receiving a brace that has been prescribed, it should be checked carefully by the surgeon to inspect its fit, alignment and appearance. If acceptable, the patient should be taught how to put on and take off the appliance and be trained in its use. This training is usually carried out in the course of physical or occupational therapy. Regardless of how well informed a physician may be, he needs to work closely with the orthotist to obtain the best possible device for his patient.

A good way to name a brace is according to the task it is intended to accomplish. This may be termed a functional nomenclature. However, many eponyms have appeared in the literature and are most confusing. There are over 100 named back braces and many of these do not warrant distinctive names. Here again, the surgeon must work closely with the orthotist. He knows the problem and what he wishes to accomplish; the orthotist knows what types of devices and materials are available and how to fit them to the patient.

SPINAL CORD INJURIES

Paraplegia and quadriplegia are conditions that result from injuries to the spinal cord through disease or accident. Injury at the thoracic or lumbar area leads to paralysis of the lower extremities, whereas damage in the cervical region results in paralysis of all extremities. Poliomyelitis, cerebral palsy, spina bifida, multiple sclerosis, and other diseases, as well as trauma, may lead to cord damage. Fortunately, some spinal injuries are not complete and recovery may take place.

The rehabilitation of quadriplegic or paraplegic patients is long and difficult. Each patient is different and requires different management. Most of the problems revolve about the care of the skin, bowels and bladder and achievement of locomotion and activities of daily living. These must receive consideration from the onset of the paralysis.

After the initial acute care of four to six weeks, which usually takes place in a general hospital, the patient should be transferred to a rehabilitation center. There the neurological, urological, surgical and psychiatric problems can be considered in conference and treatment carried out accordingly.

Just being in a rehabilitation center provides hope for a patient. Nearly every paraplegic patient can become independent with the use of braces and crutches. The quadriplegic patient is usually confined to a wheel chair but he can develop an appreciable degree of independence.

New ideas, devices and procedures are being developed constantly. Most of them have to do with skin and bladder problems.

Skin breakdown can be prevented only by the most meticulous nursing care. The patient must be turned every two hours without fail throughout the day and night. The patient must be impressed with the importance of his skin care because sooner or later it will be his personal responsibility.

The bladder problem remains a permanent one. Each patient should be followed at regular intervals by a urologist. Studies have shown that if damage to the kidney parenchyma secondary to infection and recurrent decubitis is avoided, the renal circulation and tubular functions are well preserved for at least 15 years.

Surgical procedures have been devised to help with spasticity; tendon transplants, tenodeses and skin grafts are often indicated. Lesions at the C6-7 level may be aided by appropriate tendon transplants. Above C6 tendon transplants are not helpful and below C7 they are not needed.

The diagnosis of an "acute abdomen" in cord-damaged patients is difficult. Shoulder pain, shock, alteration in spasticity and free air in the abdomen are helpful signs.

The time spent in treatment of the paraplegic or quadriplegic patient varies considerably. It all depends on the complicating factors such as decubiti, bladder infections, surgical procedures and motivation.

Although it is impossible to prognosticate the future of a quadriplegic or paraplegic patient, one principle is certain — treatment in a rehabilitation center offers him the best opportunity for reintegration into society.

REHABILITATION OF THE AMPUTEE

Proper management of the amputee requires an integrated rehabilitation program including adequate medical and surgical care; postsurgical care of the stump; preprosthetic training; fitting with a modern comfortable prosthesis; prosthetic training; psychological aid to the patient; prevocational and educational training, and proper job placement. Education, training and job placement are not needed for a great majority of the patients with amputation.

Responsibility for rehabilitation of these patients is not that of the physician alone. Members of several professions are involved. Success can be achieved only through a team approach, in which each member of the team realizes his own function and sees clearly the role of each of the other members. The basic rehabilitation team should be comprised of the physician, the physical therapist, the occupational therapist, the prosthetist and a rehabilitation counselor.

The chief duties of the group are to study each patient and to initiate each indicated step at the appropriate time: prescription, fitting, training, evaluation and follow-up. It has been clearly demonstrated that amputees under the direction of clinical teams become far more better adapted to return to

their place in society than those who do not receive such care.

It must be remembered that the amputee has a psychological problem which may become more disabling than the amputation itself. This problem must be recognized and faced early. The emotion experienced at the removal of a limb has been compared to the grief one feels at the loss of a loved one. Part of the responsibility of the physician is to allay the apprehension and fears that develop. The patient must be brought to the point of accepting his physical loss, of preparing for return to his home, family and friends and of overcoming his feeling of inferiority.

POSTOPERATIVE PROGRAM. The care of the amputee following surgical treatment is undergoing rapid change. The use of a rigid, plaster dressing immediately postoperatively with early mobilization of the patient may well minimize the problem of contractures, edema and generalized deconditioning of the patient.

Positioning the upper extremity of the amputee infrequently offers a problem postoperatively. He seldom requires a splint or prolonged immobilization in bed. Aftercare of the leg amputee begins with a pressure dressing using elastic bandages. In the above the knee amputee, the hip is extended while the patient is in bed. In the below the knee amputee, a bulky dressing or a plaster splint is used to immobilize the knee and it should be dressed in extension if possible.

Soon after amputation the patient should be instructed to lie face down part of the day to keep his stump parallel with the center of his body and to avoid propping his stump on a pillow.

After wound healing, the stump should be wrapped with an elastic bandage to minimize edema and promote shrinkage of the stump. The bandage must be changed several times daily. Bandaging should be continued every day until the prosthesis is obtained. For several months thereafter, the stump should be wrapped when the prosthesis is not worn.

Systematic body exercises should be carried out several times daily, starting as soon as postoperative pain permits and continuing until the patient has learned to use his prosthesis. Stump exercises can be started as soon as swelling and pain have subsided. In the upper extremity, full motion in the shoulder girdle and strengthening of the muscles about the upper back and shoulder are important for control of the prosthesis. In below the elbow amputees, full motion and strength of the elbow in flexion and extension and forearm rotation are emphasized. In the lower extremity amputee, the muscles of the trunk and hip on the normal side as well as the stump must be strengthened. Special effort must be made to develop hip extension, adduction and rotation in the above the knee amputee. Flexion contractures of the hip cause serious difficulty in fitting and training. A below the knee amputee should maintain full extension at the knee and develop good strength in the quadriceps muscle.

During the preprosthetic period, the lower extremity amputee is instructed in crutch walking. He is concurrently trained in activities of daily living as needed. By the time the sutures are removed, many amputees are ready to go home independent in self-care, ambulatory on crutches, more or less skilled in wrapping the stump properly and faithful in carrying out a daily exercise program.

It is important in lower extremity amputees to teach stump hygiene and foot care. After healing has occurred, the stump may be washed daily with soap and water. Ordinarily, there is no need for the use of alcohol or other agents to toughen the skin. Instructions in foot care are those which would be given in diabetic and vascular clinics.

The stump is ready for fitting when swelling and soreness have subsided, flexion contractures relieved and muscle strength built up. Today, studies are being made of immediate fitting and early weight bearing. The application of a rigid dressing immediately after surgery has the advantage of preventing edema and leads to early relief of discomfort and prompt healing. The temporary prosthesis should have a conventional foot and knee motion should be allowed when walking.

Prescription of the prosthesis should be a joint effort of the clinic team, taking into consideration factors such as the site of amputation, the condition of the stump, the age of the patient and his general physical condition, medical complications and his occupation. After the prescribed prosthesis is completed, its fit, alignment and appearance are checked out by the clinic team. Necessary adjustments are made at this time and training is started.

The major problem in training a lower extremity amputee in using his prosthesis is balance. The ability to balance properly on the artificial leg in its stance phase is of primary importance. The initial step in prosthetic training is learning how to put the limb on properly. After this comes supervised practicing, balancing, forward and backward steps, side steps and walking between the parallel bars. As skill improves, practice is given in negotiating curbs, stairs and ramps. Younger patients are taught how to fall safely. All patients should be instructed in getting down to the floor and up again without help.

In the beginning, the amputee patient tires quickly and needs frequent rest periods and short training sessions. The use of crutches and canes depends to some extent upon the ability of the patient, the level of his amputation and the condition of his remaining leg.

Bilateral below the knee amputee patients do not offer a great problem in training. Instruction proceeds as in the unilateral amputee and progress is generally satisfactory. However, the loss of both knee joints presents a great challenge to the amputee. The energy cost in most patients, except for the young, is overwhelming and ambulation with prosthesis is soon abandoned. In the patient with the loss of one leg below the knee and the other above the knee, the outcome is more hopeful in training and subsequent practical use of the prostheses.

Upper extremity amputee training is carried out by the occupational therapist. The patient first becomes familiar with the parts and function of his prosthesis and after learning how to put it on he practices how to use it functionally. A hook still remains the most functional terminal device, although advances are being made in the function and appearance of artificial hands.

The number of training sessions required in using a prosthesis depends upon many factors and varies greatly. Ordinarily, it is expected that the unilateral below the knee amputee will require no more than 12 training sessions and the unilateral above the knee amputee, 18 periods of instruction. The hip disarticulation amputee usually learns to use his limb quickly but seldom has a good gait. Instruction of the unilateral arm amputee requires only a few hours but skill in the use of the prosthesis comes only with persistent practice.

It must be remembered that the stump is only part of the individual and that the rest of his body is subject to all kinds of disease, injury and degenerative changes. Those working with amputees should remember to consider these other problems concurrently with prosthetic guidance.

As in all rehabilitation, the psychological aspects are of utmost importance. Adverse psychological reactions can become a major additional handicap. Counseling before operation and especially postoperatively may help to minimize this problem.

Walking requires that work be done. As patients grow older, they become less efficient and the energy cost of walking increases. When amputation of a leg requiring the use of crutches is added to this, the energy cost is multiplied. Training the body by preprosthetic exercises helps the body meet these demands. For learning to walk, a pylon probably makes the least energy demands, even less than walking with crutches. A prosthesis with a locked knee is less tiring to use than a leg with a swinging knee. The use of a rigid pelvic band appears to assist lateral stability to an appreciable extent and thus conserves energy.

The stump itself may be a source of difficulty. Normally, the patient has phantom sensation of the amputated part. Gradually the sensation fades, especially with early prosthetic fitting. It does not disappear entirely. Occasionally, it becomes persistently painful and interferes with rehabilitation. The mechanism of phantom pain is probably a peripheral stimulus from the stump and a central perception and response. In time, the response becomes increasingly prominent, and may be closely related to the personality of the patient. Physical therapy, including exercises of the stump and of the missing part, may give relief.

Divided nerves normally heal by neuroma formation. In some patients, the neuroma may become hypersensitive and interfere with wearing a prosthesis. Ultrasound therapy and use of electrical currents have been helpful in giving relief.

Bone spurs, local edema, cyanosis and pigmentation are encountered at times. Furunculosis, dermatomyosis, contact dermatitis and eczema interfere with the wearing of a prosthesis. Each must be treated in a logical manner.

Occasionally, a blind person has an amputation of a leg. It is surprising how well the blind do in ambulating with a prosthesis.

Deafness should not interfere with prosthetic training, but it has been found that the deaf person does not progress in learning to use his prosthesis as rapidly as the amputee with normal hearing.

A more difficult problem is the amputee, usually a diabetic patient, who has a severe peripheral neuropathy. This person likely had difficulty in ambulating prior to amputation and after surgery is faced with a formidable task in learning to walk with a prosthesis.

LOW BACK PAIN

The majority of instances of low back pain are caused by mechanical conditions which yield to conservative treatment. These lesions include congenital defects, unequal leg lengths, abnormalities of posture and pathological changes in the intervertebral discs. Local lesions such as infections, tumors, trauma and visceral lesions with referred pain must be considered.

Pain is the result of stretching or pressure upon the ligamentous structures resulting from defects of posture, or from an abnormal disc pressing against a ligament. Pain can also accompany pressure on the nerve roots by a herniated nucleus pulposus with radiating pain and sensory symptoms in a leg. Narrowing of intervertebral discs may lead to subluxation of the articular facets and to pinching of the synovium. Acute or chronic back pain from mechanical conditions responds well to a flexion program. This includes exercises, supports and bed rest, producing a flattened lumbar spine in the patient. Flexion of the lumbar spine leads to an enlargement of the intervertebral foramina, thus relieving root pressure and correcting overriding of the facets. The posterior longitudinal ligament is tightened, tending to push the degenerative disc forward.

Exercises for low back pain are designed to strengthen lumbar flexor muscles and stretching of the low back muscles and soft tissues. The principal exercises are pulling the knees to the chest while in the supine position and raising head and shoulders at the same time; sitting in a chair with knees bent and thighs apart and allowing the head and shoulders to drop down until the head is between the knees, then pulling erect to the sitting position; sit-ups from the supine position with the knees flexed, and alternate hip extension in the prone position.

Exercises should be done three times a day for a period of ten to 15 minutes. The use of a supportive corset or brace can be helpful while muscles are being strengthened. Electromyography has shown that the abdominal muscles do not come into play on lifting or straining if abdominal support is given by an appliance. Many patients with low back pain can be treated on an ambulatory basis without the necessity of bed rest. Heat, massage and exercises are the basis of treatment.

READING REFERENCES

Advisory Committee on Artificial Limbs: Artificial Limbs. Vol. 10. Washington, D.C., National Academy of Sciences, National Research Council, 1966.

Bryce, M.: Physical Therapy After Amputation. Madison, Wisconsin, University of Wisconsin Press, 1954.

Frost, A.: Handbook for Paraplegics and Quadriplegics. Chicago, The National Paraplegia Foundation, 1964.

Gordon, E. E.: The use of energy costs in regulating activity in chronic diseases. A.M.A. Arch. Indust. Health *16*:434, 1957.

Klopsteg, P. E., and Wilson, P. D.: Human Limbs and Their Substitutes. New York, McGraw-Hill Book Co., Inc., 1954.

Krusen, E.: Handbook of Physical Medicine and Rehabilitation. Philadelphia, W. B. Saunders Company, 1965.

Licht, S.: Electrodiagnosis and Electromyography. 2nd ed. Baltimore, Waverly Press, Inc., 1961.

Licht, S.: Orthotics Etcetera. Baltimore, Waverly Press, Inc., 1966.

Licht, S.: Therapeutic Exercise. 2nd ed. Baltimore, Waverly Press, Inc., 1961.

Licht, S.: Therapeutic Heat and Cold. 2nd ed. Baltimore, Waverly Press, Inc., 1965.

Lim, R. K. S.: Pain Mechanisms. Anesthesiology *28*:106, 1967.

Mayo Clinic and Mayo Foundation: Clinical Examination in Neurology. 2nd ed. Philadelphia, W. B. Saunders Company, 1963.

Melzack, R., and Wall, P. D.: Pain Mechanism: a new theory. Science *150*:971. 1965.

National Academy of Sciences, National Research Council: The Geriatric Amputee. Publication 919. Washington, D.C., 1961.

Rusk, H. A.: Rehabilitation Medicine. 2nd ed. St. Louis, C. V. Mosby Company, 1964.

Whitelock, O.: Non-narcotic drugs for the relief of pain and their mechanisms of action. Ann. New York Acad. Med. *86*:1, 1960.

Chapter 35

THE VASCULAR SYSTEM

The Arteries and Veins

by
HAROLD LAUFMAN, M.D.

HAROLD LAUFMAN was born in Wisconsin and educated at the University of Chicago and Rush Medical College. His graduate education in surgery was pursued at Northwestern University where he became a Professor of Surgery. He has made important research contributions to surgery in several areas of study. He is presently Director, Institute for Surgical Studies, Montefiore Hospital and Medical Center and Professor of Surgery, Albert Einstein College of Medicine. Dr. Laufman's talents as an artist have won recognition among that group of surgeons who have unusual artistic gifts in addition to their surgical talents.

The Arteries

In recent years, the surgeon's interest in the arterial system has expanded from one dealing with the control and prevention of hemorrhage to one related to the establishment and maintenance of arterial flow to tissues. The lesions of the peripheral arteries which are amenable to surgical treatment include occlusive diseases, vasospastic disorders, aneurysms and arteriovenous fistulas.

Although the surgeon often is able to reconstitute disturbed arterial flow by operative methods, his contribution to the care of patients with arterial disease is not always surgical. Just as important as his knowledge of which reconstructive procedure to perform and when to perform it, is his knowledge of which patients to operate upon and which patients not to operate upon. He must know something of the natural history of vascular lesions; he must be aware of the physiologic responses of blood vessels to various stimuli and diseases, and he must be acquainted with the body's expected tolerance or intolerance to interruptions in arterial flow. Wide variations in these phenomena occur in health as well as in disease.

GENERAL PRINCIPLES
OF DIAGNOSIS

HISTORY. The history of patients with peripheral arterial disease varies considerably with the type of lesion. In general, it is related to one or all of three phenomena: pain, change in skin color and breakdown of tissue. An important feature of the history of pain is its suddenness of onset, as well as its character, distribution and severity. Typical of chronic occlusive arterial disease is the tendency for pain to occur after a certain amount of muscular activity.

In the lower extremities, a common symptom of arterial occlusive lesions is intermittent claudication. The patient relates that he can walk comfortably for a certain distance, usually measured in city blocks, until he must stop because of pain, aching, cramping or a sense of sudden fatigue, usually in the calf muscles. After a few moments of rest, the pain disappears and the patient is able to resume walking for a similar distance. This type of pain is due to the relative anoxia of muscles whose actions demand an increase in blood supply with exercise. The blood supply may be adequate for muscle metabolism at relative rest, but inadquate to meet the oxygen demands required by exercise. The distance such a patient can walk before he must stop has been designated as his "claudication distance." Intermittent claudication can occur in the hip, thigh and foot, as well as in the calf, and may also occur in the forearm and hand in conjunction with occlusive lesions of the brachial artery. Also of significance is the occurrence of pain at rest, and the presence or absence of pain associated with ischemic neuritis, ulceration and gangrene.

The suddenness of the occlusive process is of considerable prognostic and therapeutic importance, and should be elicited in the history. Sudden onset of pain, pallor and palsy in an extremity of a patient with auricular fibrillation is prima facie evidence of embolism until proved otherwise.

A history of extreme pallor of fingers or toes in response to psychic stress, mild cold or some unknown exciting factor is a clue to one of several vasospastic responses of arteries, commonly referred to as Raynaud's phenomenon.

Rate of nail growth can be elicited by questioning. Slow growth is indicative of poor blood supply.

A history of the patient's general health is mandatory, with special reference to diabetes, cardiac and renal status, and cerebrovascular symptoms. A history of trauma, arthritis, rheumatic fever, and smoking and drinking habits should be obtained.

PHYSICAL EXAMINATION. There is no need for elaborate instruments in the examination for peripheral vascular disease. Only after a tentative diagnosis has been made is it sometimes necessary to employ special tests such as arteriography.

Observation provides valuable diagnostic information when there is an obvious color difference between the two extremities, or when both appear grossly different from the normal. After acute major arterial occlusion, a limb appears extremely pale, with or without bluish mottling. It is not swollen. With gradual occlusion, there is often no gross color change when the legs are in a horizontal position, but raising the limb causes an extreme pallor, and lowering it leads to a deep burgundy color. In more advanced occlusive disease, one may see the paradoxical "ischemic rubor" due to an anoxic dilatation of metarterioles of the skin, and even

some edema due to persistent dependency and inactivity of the limb. In the presence of bilateral edema, one must differentiate between arterial and venous disease and the remote causes for ankle edema.

The presence of ischemic ulceration requires differentiation between ulcers caused by arterial insufficiency and those which accompany the postphlebitic syndrome. Occasionally, leg ulcers are due to combined causes. The examiner must be prepared to differentiate between ulcers due to syphilis, fungi and infection, and those due to ischemia. Excessive callus and ulcer formation on the toes or sole of the foot is common in diabetes. Infections in and about the nail beds are not infrequent in advanced arterial occlusive disease.

Gangrene is diagnosable on sight. It may be "wet" or "dry," depending upon whether saprophytic invasion has taken place, and whether its onset was rapid or slow. If peripheral gangrene exists in the presence of palpable pulsations in the regional blood vessels, it is due to small blood vessel occlusion. If pulses are not palpable, gangrene may be due to large and small vessel occlusion.

Palpation provides valuable diagnostic information. The examiner palpates for arterial pulsation in the usual sites, and for changes in temperature of the skin. In addition, he palpates for the presence of masses, unusual pulsations, tenderness and pitting edema.

Whether ischemic symptoms are present or not, palpation of arterial pulsation should be part of every general physical examination. In the lower extremity, the pulses commonly palpated are those of the femoral artery in the groin, the popliteal artery behind the knee, the posterior tibial artery behind the medial malleolus, and the anterior tibial or dorsalis pedis artery on the dorsum of the foot just lateral to the extensor hallucis longus tendon. In the arm, the pulses are the subclavian artery behind the clavicle, usually palpable only in the presence of aneurysm, the axillary in the axilla, the brachial in the upper arm and the radial at the wrist. The ulnar artery is rarely palpable. In the abdomen, one palpates the aortic pulsations and contour of the abdominal aorta. In the neck, pulsations of the carotid arteries are palpated up to their bifurcations (Fig. 1).

In palpating for arterial pulsation, certain deviations from the normal character can be ascertained, many times providing as much diagnostic information as the presence

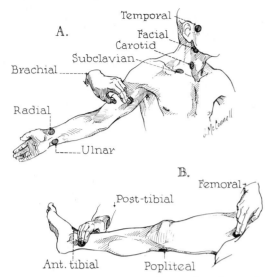

Figure 1. *A*, Usual points of palpation for pulses in the head, neck and upper extremity. *B*, Usual points of palpation for pulses in the lower extremity.

or absence of the pulse itself. With some experience, it is possible to determine the relative fullness of the pulse, especially when it is compared with its fellow on the opposite side. Also palpable are bruits and thrills, the former indicative of partial occlusion and the latter of arteriovenous fistula.

Palpation of skin temperature and moisture usually provides adequate information for diagnostic purposes without resorting to special measuring devices. As a rule, differences between the surface temperatures of paired extremities are obvious to touch. Excessive coolness denotes lack of blood supply. If the skin is unusually moist, one should suspect a vasospastic element due to sympathetic stimulation. This may be present with or without organic arterial occlusion. If the skin of one limb is excessively warm in the presence of a palpable thrill or auscultative murmur over regional vessels, one may well suspect arteriovenous fistula, especially when there is a history of penetrative trauma. In young people, excessive growth and warmth of one extremity may be indicative of congenital arteriovenous fistula.

Auscultation may reveal a systolic bruit over a segmentally or irregularly narrowed artery. This is a softer sound than the loud mechanical bruit usually heard over an arteriovenous fistula.

Venous filling time is the length of time it takes for superficial veins to fill when the limb is lowered after elevation. Normally, this takes about five seconds. In the presence

of arterial insufficiency, venous filling time is prolonged. In the presence of varicose veins, this observation may be unreliable.

Capillary filling time is the length of time it takes for a blanched area of skin to resume its color after fingertip pressure. This test may be of value in determining viability of tissue in limbs critically deprived of blood supply, and may aid in making a decision for surgery.

Leg raising and lowering tests the phenomenon of reactive hyperemia. Although a normal limb tends to blanch with elevation and become somewhat hyperemic with dependency, a limb deprived of a major portion of its blood supply blanches rather remarkably upon elevation and becomes violaceous or deep red with dependency. The small collateral vessels supplying the skin are unable to carry their nonpulsatile flow against gravity, resulting in an almost total emptying of their lumina and corresponding diminution in their caliber when the leg is raised above the horizontal position. After lowering the leg below the horizontal position, the red response, a reactive hyperemia occurs. In an arterially insufficient limb, the reactive hyperemia becomes evident very slowly, but once it occurs, lasts considerably longer than in a normal limb.

If pulses are difficult to palpate because of obesity or edema, it is advisable to use the oscillometer. This instrument consists of a blood pressure cuff attached to a manometer. When the cuff is applied to the calf or thigh, and inflated to just above diastolic pressure, one can observe the magnitude of the pulse by oscillations of the needle. In a normal limb with the cuff placed on the thigh, the oscillations of the needle usually cover a swing of four or more units on the dial. In the calf, the normal oscillation is 4 to 8 units. The reason for the increased pulse volume below the knee is that the combined pulsations of the two major channels in this area provide a wider swing of the needle than the single pulse of the femoral artery in the thigh. When there is partial or complete occlusion of the arterial stream proximal to the cuff, the oscillations are proportionately lessened. Complete occlusion of major arteries results in an almost total absence of oscillation, and yet the limb may remain viable because of the abundance of collaterals which form with slow occlusions.

The plethysmograph is no longer used in the average clinical examination, and is reserved only for special studies. It is a time-honored method of assessing the increase in volume of a limb or digit after sudden occlusion of the venous return. The accumulation of trapped venous blood is roughly equal to arterial flow distal to the venous occlusion. In addition to being cumbersome, the plethysmograph is inaccurate when local blood pressure is low. Whereas the oscillometer requires the presence of gross pulsations of large vessels and records pulse amplitude in terms of millimeters of mercury at various pressures, the plethysmograph records changes in volume per cubic centimeter of tissue which occur during each cardiac cycle, and does not depend on gross pulsations of large arteries.

ARTERIOGRAPHY. Since the advent of arteriography, many ancillary tests of circulatory status have been eliminated. Visualization of blood vessels by the injection of contrast media and roentgenography is unquestionably the most precise way of defining pathologic anatomy of the vascular tree. The term "arteriography" refers to the visualization of arteries only, whereas "angiography" implies the visualization of arteries or veins by variations in timing after an intra-arterial injection. Intravenous arteriography is the visualization of arteries by means of an intravenous injection under great force.

There is almost no area in the human body that cannot be studied by angiography. Improvements in technique and in contrast media have made angiography highly useful in diagnosis, prognosis and therapy. However, certain hazards still exist, and should be known in order to avert complications.

Methods. Depending upon which part of the arterial vascular tree one wishes to visualize, there are a variety of techniques of arteriography. The goal is to obtain the best visualization with minimal risk to the patient.

An artery may be injected by direct percutaneous insertion of a needle, by surgical exposure of the artery, by passage of a catheter from a distant vessel to the desired site, by noncatheter injection against the arterial stream and by forceful intravenous injection.

Translumbar aortography is fraught with dangers, the most important of which is paraplegia. Nonetheless, this technique is widely used, and in experienced hands carries a satisfactorily low complication rate. The advantages of visualization far outweigh the risks of ill effects.

A promising technique for visualizing any vessel in the body is the recently developed percutaneous noncatheter brachial angiography. Right brachial injection gives excellent visualization of the innominate, right vertebral and right common carotid arteries, as well as the right cerebral vessels. Injection of the left brachial artery gives visualization of the left vertebral, thoracic and abdominal aorta, renal arteries, and iliac and femoral arteries. One of the main reasons for the success of this method is the development of a low viscosity contrast medium, meglumine iothalamate. A rapid cassette changer or a continuous roll film unit is used to make multiple exposures.

Intravenous aortography is carried out by injecting highly concentrated contrast medium with great force simultaneously into both antecubital veins. The success of this maneuver depends upon accurate timing and trained personnel.

For sharp visualization of arteries of the lower extremities an aortogram or femoral arteriogram produces the best results. It is rarely necessary to do an aortogram in the presence of normal pulses in both femoral arteries in the groins. A percutaneous femoral arteriogram will serve the purpose under these circumstances. Because arteriography is ordinarily performed in the presence of occlusive disease, in anticipation of performing direct reconstructive surgery, and because this type of surgery is not usually successful below the popliteal bifurcation, there is usually no practical reason to perform an arteriogram if pulsations are bilaterally present in the popliteal arteries or below.

Arteriography should be employed only when it is essential to the formulation of the operative plan, or when the decision for or against operation cannot be made by clinical examination. Arteriography should not be employed as a routine diagnostic procedure, nor should it be performed casually by untrained physicians or technical personnel. It is a specialized procedure carrying a certain amount of risk and often requiring general anesthesia. Complications include thrombosis and its occlusive consequences, hemorrhage, hematoma, dissecting aneurysm and renal shutdown. In many instances, it is possible to perform arteriography in the operating room prior to, or during the actual operative procedure, where minimal amounts of contrast medium can be used under well-controlled circumstances.

OCCLUSIVE DISEASES

ACUTE ARTERIAL OCCLUSION

Except for external compression or trauma, sudden blockage to the flow of arterial blood is due to embolism or thrombosis, or both. Sudden deprivation of arterial circulation is more critical to the survival of the part than is gradual occlusion. In sudden occlusion, intense spasm may occlude or narrow collateral channels both proximal and distal to the occlusion. Thrombosis distal to the occlusion may be extremely rapid, thus further preventing collateral circulation.

ARTERIAL EMBOLISM. An embolus is any abnormal particle carried by the blood from one anatomic location to another, and which becomes lodged in a vessel too small to permit its passage. When lodgment takes place, embolism is said to occur.

Arterial embolism may result from a clot which has been liberated from elsewhere in the arterial system, or it may result from other substances, such as amniotic fluid, air, tumor, atherosclerotic plaques, valve vegetations, fat, bacteria, bile or missiles. The commonest source of clot embolism is the lining walls of the cardiac chambers. Auricular fibrillation, due to any cause, tends to build up clots within the left atrial appendage because of turbulence, and these clots may be thrown off into the arterial system. Other intracardiac causes are myocardial infarct with mural thrombosis, mitral and aortic valvulitis, and heart failure. Intraventricular thrombi have also been known to develop in hearts with no demonstrable functional or pathologic abnormality. Thromboses may arise on the endothelium of main arteries outside the heart, and when broken off, travel distally as embolic bodies. Arterial mural thrombi may arise in aneurysms or may be the result of arteriosclerosis, trauma or inflammation. Arteriosclerotic plaques of the aorta may become loosened through trauma, ulceration or degeneration, finally becoming detached and traveling as emboli. So-called paradoxical embolism arises in the venous system but passes through a patent foramen ovale to lodge in the arterial system. By far the most common cause of arterial embolism is chronic auricular fibrillation, with or without accompanying congestive heart failure.

ARTERIAL THROMBOSIS. Exactly why thrombotic arterial occlusion occurs suddenly in some patients and gradually in others is not altogether known. One predisposing cause of acute thrombotic occlusion of arteries is arteriosclerosis, in which thrombi tend to form on a roughened intima or in a slowed blood stream within a narrowed channel. Injuries such as gunshot wounds and compression are frequent causes. Acute thrombosis may follow a narrowing or kink induced by a long-standing lesion, such as aneurysm. Hematogenic causes of thrombosis include polycythemia vera, thrombophilia and cryoglobulinemia.

Long-standing shock due to any cause may result in intravascular thrombosis, either as a disseminated phenomenon, or localized to an area of pre-existing narrowing, or other lesion.

Repeated vibrational trauma, as occurs in men operating pneumatic tools, may precipitate arterial thrombosis in vessels of the hand. Sudden arterial thrombosis may also occur in severe infections, such as septicemia, pneumonia, peritonitis, intractable diarrhea, ulcerative colitis and carcinomatosis, but more often these conditions are accompanied by venous thrombosis. Not infrequently, segmental arterial thrombosis occurs in the presence of other arterial diseases, such as thromboangiitis obliterans, as well as in any condition causing a fall in blood pressure, such as following trauma or during operation. Such thromboses usually occur in vessels narrowed as a result of chronic atherosclerotic disease. Depending upon where the acute occlusion occurs, there is almost invariably a severe local spasm set up in the branches both proximal and distal to the area of the occlusion.

SIGNS AND SYMPTOMS OF ACUTE ARTERIAL OCCLUSION. In most patients, the onset of an acute occlusion is accompanied by sudden, severe pain distal to the point of occlusion. However, the symptoms sometimes may come on gradually, with the pain progressing as the occlusion persists. In general, the part distal to the occlusion is pale and cold, and the veins are empty. There is no pulsation in the arteries. Motor and sensory disturbances are obvious, and tend to progress to paralysis and numbness. The diffuse vasospasm may lead the examiner to an erroneous conclusion as to the site of the occlusion.

It is sometimes impossible to distinguish between acute arterial thrombosis and embolism. In general, if the patient has known heart disease with fibrillation, and his occlusive episode is sudden, with no previous signs or symptoms, the presumptive diagnosis of embolism is logical. On the other hand, if the patient has a recent history of coronary thrombosis, followed by a sudden ischemic episode in an extremity, it need not necessarily mean that a mural thrombus has been detached from the left ventricle. This patient might have suffered an acute myocardial infarct with shock, and, during the acute hypotensive period, a stenosed atheromatous distal artery may have become occluded suddenly by local thrombosis induced by slowed flow and increased coagulability. In fact, instances have been reported of "silent" coronary occlusions, in which the first and only demonstrable signs were those of peripheral arterial thrombosis or embolism. It is less important to argue the possible cause of the acute occlusion than it is to diagnose the exact location and institute proper treatment in order to save the distal part. Time is of great importance in achieving a successful result in reconstituting arterial flow in an occluded artery.

The clinical diagnosis and localization of an acute thromboembolic arterial occlusion is usually not difficult, and ordinarily requires no special instruments. Emboli usually lodge at bifurcations. Occasionally, there is tenderness over the region of the occlusion. If the occlusion is in a palpable area, it is obvious that pulsation is absent distal to the occlusion and may even be bounding just proximal to the occlusion. However, if the area of occlusion cannot be palpated, the best means of locating it is by observing the level of temperature change in the skin of the distal part. Acute occlusion at the aortic bifurcation is usually accompanied by an obvious temperature change at the mid- or upper thigh. An acute occlusion at the bifurcation of the common femoral artery results in a temperature change at or just above the level of the knee. An occlusion of the femoral artery, as it emerges from Hunter's canal, results in a line of temperature demarcation at midcalf. Occlusion of the upper popliteal artery usually results in a temperature demarcation line at the lower level of the calf. If the occlusion is in the low popliteal artery, the line of demarcation is at or just above the malleoli. Occasionally, a low popliteal occlusion results in a temperature line in the foot. Variation in these levels depends, to a large extent, upon the degree of accompanying vasospasm in the branches

about the occlusion. Similar relationships between the location of the embolus and the line of sudden change in temperature of the skin are observed in the upper extremity (Fig. 2).

As the occlusion persists, the motor power distal to the occlusion diminishes, and numbness supervenes, regardless of accompanying pain. These phenomena usually occur distal to the line of temperature change. When arteries are paired, as in the arm and lower leg, occlusion of one of the paired arteries usually does not result in marked change in peripheral circulation, but there is tenderness and pain in the region of the occlusion, persisting for a variable period of time. Under these circumstances, minimal or negligible changes in temperature, color and other phenomena may be present.

Occasionally, it is expedient to use the oscillometer to aid in the location of an embolus or thrombus. By application of the cuff at various levels on the extremity, the area of occlusion can be demonstrated. The error of interpreting transmitted pulsations as true pulsations is inherent in the use of this instrument, as it is in the use of the palpating finger.

Spasm and distal thrombosis combine to aggravate the effects of acute arterial occlusion. The spasm accompanying acute arterial occlusion is probably more responsible for the acuteness and the severity of the

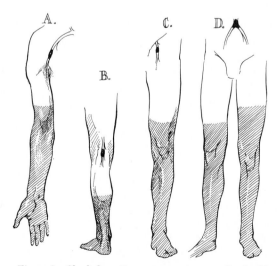

Figure 2. Shaded portions represent areas of palpable coldness of skin in sudden occlusions of major arteries. *A*, Axillary artery occlusion; *B*, popliteal artery occlusion; *C*, common femoral artery occlusion; and *D*, aortic bifurcation occlusion. Note that in each instance the cold level is well below the level of occlusion.

symptoms than is the actual occlusion. The extent of the spasm is highly variable, and is mediated through the sympathetic nerves. It may well be accentuated by local chemical changes, since sudden ligation or pressure occlusion of a vessel does not result in spasm of the severity usually noted in an acute embolic or thrombotic occlusion. As the occlusion persists, whether it was originally an embolus or a thrombus, there is propagation of thrombosis distal to the occlusive agent, and there may be a moderate amount of proximal thrombosis as well. The rate at which thrombosis propagates distal to an embolus is not predictable. In some patients it proceeds with great speed, spreads into many branches and causes rapid onset of gangrene, whereas in others the propagation is very slow. As the occlusion persists, the distal part becomes white and, occasionally, shows some blue mottling, depending upon the amount of blood trapped in the extremity. Actual gangrene ordinarily does not supervene until at least three or four days after an acute occlusion in a critical vessel is allowed to persist without removal. However, tissue ischemia reaches a stage of irreversibility much more rapidly, in some instances within six to ten hours. In other instances, return of viability has been obtained by removal of the occlusion as long as 36 hours after the initial episode. Spontaneous recovery occurs after some hours when an embolus lodges in an uncritical area, and the initial vasospasm is released, either spontaneously or through treatment.

TREATMENT OF ACUTE ARTERIAL OCCLUSION. Before recent advances in direct arterial surgery, it had been customary to put a patient through a rather discomforting diagnostic procedure, including several attempts at conservative management, in an effort to release the initial spasm and to avert surgical intervention. Recently, there has been more and more agreement on the advantages of early surgical intervention. Even in extremely poor risk patients, it is possible to operate under local anesthesia and remove the embolus or thrombus.

As soon as the diagnosis of acute arterial occlusion is made, the patient should be given an intravenous injection of 5000 units of aqueous heparin. Occasionally, this measure alone will cause the embolus to pass onward to an uncritical location in the vascular tree, and the result will be a return of viability of the part. Recently, the intravenous admin-istration of low molecular weight dextran has been reported to cause resumption of arterial flow in a vessel occluded by a recent embolus. In the event that such measures fail within a few hours, further delay should be avoided. The patient is then taken to the operating room, and the operation is performed under local anesthesia, in the presence of heparinization. The heparin is administered in order to prevent propagation or thrombosis from the occluding area. It may be argued that release of vasospasm is much more important than the prevention of thrombotic propagation. However, the trauma associated with turning the patient and attempting a sympathetic block, as well as the poor success attending this procedure in obviating surgery, has virtually removed sympathetic ganglionic block from the present management of acute arterial occlusions located in or above the femoral artery.

When an occlusion appears to be at the popliteal artery level or below, the first step is to proceed with a lumbar sympathetic ganglionic block using 1 per cent procaine, provided the condition of the patient permits it. Often, occlusions at this level allow survival of the limb without operation, provided that vasospasm in alternate arteries is released and peripheral thrombotic extension can be arrested. Heparin is withheld until after a paravertebral sympathetic block is performed. Shortly after it is performed, the first dose of intravenous heparin is given. A common error at this stage of therapy is to wait a given number of hours after performing these measures before deciding upon surgical intervention. More important is the time interval from the moment of occlusion, since the eventual survival of the limb depends more upon the total period of ischemia than upon any arbitrary period after treatment is begun. It is best not to delay surgical intervention beyond six hours following the occlusive episode, regardless of what other treatment is instituted. The longer one waits after this period, the greater the risk of permanent residual nerve damage, even though circulation may be restored.

In our experience, the use of fibrinolytic agents has met with no success in the effort to dissolve arterial emboli or clots, no matter how soon after the initial occlusion they have been used, and no matter whether they have been injected directly into the artery above the occlusion or into the systemic circulation.

The operative removal of an arterial embolus or thrombus, properly performed and without turning the patient, is in our opinion more conservative, yet more successful, than most of the conservative nonoperative measures.

For saddle emboli, at the aortic bifurcation, embolectomy can be done by exposing both common femoral arteries in the groin and using Fogarty balloon catheters to extract the embolus (Fig. 3). An ill-timed laparotomy on a poor risk patient is accompanied by a high mortality rate. It is good practice to subject the patient to the least amount of turning and surgical trauma in the removal of an embolus or a thrombus.

The removal of an embolus in a peripheral artery is technically simple and follows a definite series of maneuvers. Proximal control is obtained by anatomic exposure of the vessel proximal to the embolus, and a tape or soft rubber tube is slung under it. The same procedure is done distal to the embolus. A noncrushing arterial clamp is placed at the site of the proximal sling, and the vessel is opened with a vertical incision directly over

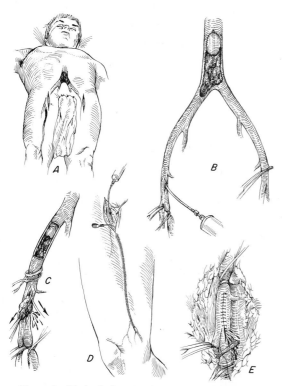

Figure 3. Method of removal of aortic saddle embolus without laparotomy. *A,* Incisions over both common femoral arteries in groin. *B,* Fogarty catheter inflated after being passed proximal to embolus. *C,* Extraction of embolus and attached clot. *D,* Small Fogarty catheter inserted distally to remove distal thrombi. *E,* Closure of femoral arteriotomy site.

the embolus. If the thrombus does not extrude itself under the impetus of the blood flow, the "tail" or distal thrombus is aspirated first. A distal noncrushing clamp is placed on the artery only after good backflow is obtained. Ten cubic centimeters of a dilute heparin solution, made with 5000 units in 200 cc. saline, is injected into the artery peripheral to the distal clamp. The bulging embolus is then carefully removed without traumatizing the intima. The proximal clot, if present, will either be forced out by the arterial stream, or can be aspirated until the arterial stream escapes with full force. The proximal clamp controls the flow of blood while the open vessel is washed out with heparin solution. The arteriotomy incision is closed with a continuous suture of fine silk and the clamps are removed. No further injections of heparin are used postoperatively.

The removal of an acute arterial thrombus differs from that of an embolus only in the added maneuvers necessary to remove a considerably longer thrombotic tail. These maneuvers consist of passing the Fogarty catheter into the lumen distally as far as possible and withdrawing it after distending its balloon. This maneuver will usually cause the withdrawal of long clots. Another maneuver is to open the vessel at some distance below the occlusion, and to wash out the clot by injecting heparin solution proximally under pressure.

When there is previously existing atherosclerotic disease distal to an acute occlusion the return of distal pulsations cannot be expected since they were not there before the acute occlusion. The reactive hyperemia after removal of the clot may persist somewhat longer than it would in a person with previously normal vessels. Under these circumstances, one may perform an arteriogram on the operating table by injecting the artery distal to the arteriotomy in order to determine the presence, configuration and location of the previously existing atherosclerotic occlusions. It is usually inadvisable to proceed with a formal endarterectomy or other angioplastic procedure under these circumstances. Occasionally, it may become necessary to perform a limited endarterectomy or to employ a patch graft at the site of arteriotomy, if the linear flow of blood appears to be impeded with simple closure of the vessel.

Postoperative care consists of horizontal positioning of the limb, with neither elevation nor dependency. Movement is encouraged.

As a rule, heparin is not used postoperatively unless there appears to be some evidence of reocclusion. In most instances, however, this is not necessary, and may lead to wound hematomata or other evidence of tissue oozing.

CHRONIC ARTERIAL OCCLUSION

A chronic arterial occlusion is one which develops slowly, usually over a period of years, and is often conducive to acute thrombotic occlusion. Most chronic occlusions of major vessels occur as a result of arteriosclerotic thickening of the intima. Other causes include musculofibrous thickening such as occurs in renal arteries, and pressure from without. Occasionally, aneurysms cause occlusion because of thrombosis or kinking at the proximal or distal extremity of the aneurysmal dilatation. Certain individuals tend to develop partial or complete atherosclerotic occlusions more readily than do others.

Knowledge of the pathologic behavior of atherosclerosis underlies the modern advances in arterial surgery. Although atherosclerosis is considered a generalized disease, an appreciation of the segmental nature of its obstructive or aneurysmal lesions forms the basis for reconstructive surgery. The decision for or against surgical intervention depends, among other things, upon evaluation of the distribution of the disease throughout the body, and the possible effects of disseminated lesions on vital organs remote from the symptomatic part. A patient may suffer occlusive symptoms in only one area despite generalized atherosclerosis. The location of the prime occlusive process may be in any artery of the body, most commonly the abdominal aorta, the iliac, femoral and popliteal arteries, the coronary arteries, the carotid arteries, the renal arteries, and less commonly the superior mesenteric artery and the subclavian, innominate and brachial arteries. Extremely localized atherosclerotic occlusive disease occurs occasionally with no evidence of the disease elsewhere. This phenomenon is unexplained, and points to the possibility that local factors such as trauma, selective spasm or local inflammatory disease are just as important in the etiology and pathogenesis of the disease as are the more popularly accepted metabolic, dietary and degenerative factors. In certain clinically recognizable disease states, the process is more or less limited to small vessels and may or may not extend to larger arteries. This is especially true in the atherosclerosis associated with diabetes, with many vasospastic diseases and with certain inflammatory diseases of the arteries.

Typically, an atherosclerotic plaque begins with an irregular thickening of the intima, which is rich in fatty acids and cholesterol. Growth of the plaque leads to narrowing of the lumen. Roughness of the surface of the thickened intima may cause deposition of platelets and blood cells from the passing arterial stream. Disturbance of the linear flow may lead to thrombosis or to dilatation of the vessel distal to the partial occlusion. Thrombosis, under these circumstances, may be the result of high viscosity which accompanies slow or turbulent flow. As the plaque ages, and as other local and general factors contribute, a plaque may become partially or completely calcified. The vessel loses its elasticity, and portions of a calcified plaque may become fractured. Such defects may allow blood to dissect into the wall of the vessel and between its layers, causing a dissecting aneurysm. Weakening of the wall and fragmentation of muscular fibers in the media may lead to overstretching with each systolic thrust and inability to return to the original caliber with diastole, resulting in a true aneurysm. Occasionally, a portion of a plaque becomes disconnected from its mooring and is carried distally as an embolus. Acute occlusion superimposed on a chronic atherosclerotic process may also occur with excessive narrowing. Gradual occlusion is the rule in most instances of atherosclerotic narrowing of arteries, and the actual moment of complete occlusion may not be discernible. Symptoms are usually in direct proportion to the degree of occlusion, but vary widely with the rate of occlusion, the caliber of the vessels involved, and the location of the occlusion.

Many variations on the basic pathologic picture occur. One curious variant is known as Mönckeberg's sclerosis, which affects mainly the femoral arteries. It is characterized by sclerosis and calcification of the media, with some narrowing of the lumen but without actual occlusion. This type of arteriosclerosis is generally considered to be a distinct pathologic entity, unrelated to the usual type of arteriosclerosis.

Ordinarily, the amount of calcium seen in

vessels viewed on scout roentgenograms has no bearing on either the location or extent of arterial occlusions. It is not unusual to see extensive calcification in the walls of arteries in patients with no clinical evidence of occlusive disease. In contrast, many of the most severe occlusive processes are unassociated with calcium deposition.

Chronic Arterial Occlusion in the Lower Extremity

SYMPTOMS. The pain of vascular occlusive disease of the lower extremity may assume a variety of forms. Most common is the pain of intermittent claudication, which may reach severe proportions long before any changes are noted in the skin. Claudication pain may come on gradually, as a result of slowly progressive obliteration of arteries, or abruptly, when a thrombosis forms upon partially occluding atherosclerotic plaques. The nature and severity of the pain depend upon the location and extent of the occlusion. When intermittent claudication is the only symptom, there are sufficient collaterals to supply the tissues at rest. As more severe ischemia develops, the pain may persist even at rest. Intermittent claudication and rest pain are usually the result of a single or several segmental obstructions in a large vessel. When the viability of the distal tissues of an extremity becomes endangered in chronic occlusive disease, it is more likely to be the result of diffuse disease with combinations of lesions in the aortoiliac, femoropopliteal and smaller distal arteries.

As a rule, intermittent claudication begins unilaterally, but may become bilateral. This symptom may exist for years and be the only subjective manifestation of the disease. As the claudication distance shortens, the patient usually seeks the advice of a physician. The most common site for the pain of intermittent claudication is the calf muscles. It may also occur in the foot, or as high as the thigh, and occasionally in the hip or lower back. Hip claudication pain is invariably associated with aortoiliac occlusion, whereas calf claudication pain may result from either aortoiliac or ileofemoral occlusion. Foot claudication pain follows femoropopliteal or tibial artery occlusion.

Claudication distance tends to be shorter when the patient walks at a fast pace, or with long strides or on a hard pavement. It is made worse by psychic tension. An ex-

ample of the effect of psyche on claudication distance is the remarkable improvement which follows the injection of a placebo of sterile water. This type of response has made the objective evaluation of therapy difficult.

When typical intermittent claudication occurs in a patient in the arteriosclerotic age group, the diagnosis of arteriosclerosis obliterans is presumed. When it occurs in younger individuals without a history of trauma, the presumptive diagnosis is thromboangiitis obliterans.

Rest pain occurs typically in the calf or foot. It appears most commonly at night, and is characterized by a severe, persistent ache which interferes with sleep. Rest pain is worse after excessive activity during the previous day. It rarely occurs in patients who have palpable distal pulses, and is assumed to be the result of interference with blood supply to nerves.

The pain of ischemic neuropathy may coexist with rest pain, or with the pain of ulceration and gangrene, but usually extends the entire length of the leg. The pain may be steady or paroxysmal. There may be sensations of electric shock with periods of numbness, deadness, coldness or burning at various times. The pain of ischemic neuropathy is more common in diabetics than in nondiabetics, and may disappear spontaneously after months or years as numbness ensues, with or without the breakdown of tissue.

The pain of ulceration and gangrene is localized either in the region of the lesion or proximal to it. The paradoxical combination of numbness and pain is evident in these lesions. Some patients with severe ischemic ulceration and gangrene have remarkably little pain, whereas others experience excruciating pain, often difficult to control with opiates. The pain is worse at night, and the patient often seeks to lessen it by holding the limb in a dependent position. Unfortunately, this leads to edema, venous congestion and further embarrassment of the small artery circulation.

Other symptoms of occlusive disease of the arteries of the legs depend upon the progression and distribution of the disease. The Leriche syndrome consists of the triad of bilateral intermittent claudication, absence of both femoral pulsations and sexual impotence. It is due to arteriosclerotic occlusion of the aortoiliac bifurcation (Fig. 4).

Osteoporosis and muscular atrophy of disuse are seen in advanced arterial insuffi-

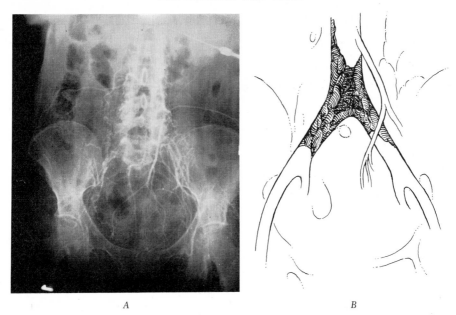

A   B

Figure 4. *A*, Arteriogram of patient with Leriche syndrome: occlusion at the aortic bifurcation, accompanied by bilateral intermittent claudication, absence of both femoral pulsations and sexual impotence. *B*, Diagram of typical occlusive lesion at aortic bifurcation in Leriche syndrome.

ciency. Atrophy of the skin and subcutaneous tissue is usually accompanied by sensitivity to touch. Hyperesthesias of this type are sometimes severe enough to prevent the wearing of shoes. Diabetic patients tend to experience hypesthesia, often disproportionate to the degree of arterial insufficiency. In such patients, care must be taken not to injure the skin. Minor cuts, blisters and other disruptions may become gangrenous. Patients with arterial insufficiency must never be subjected to a vein cutdown in the legs, lest gangrene ensue. Sensitivity to cold is not uncommon. Weakness of muscles is a symptom difficult to evaluate, since it may be due to a variety of causes. Stiffness of joints may be caused by the ischemia or by underlying hypertrophic arthritis or gout, both common in patients in the older age group.

Ischemic rubor is a paradoxical finding in some patients with small vessel occlusions, especially diabetics. The skin of the foot, gradually deprived of its blood supply, may undergo a variety of unusual changes besides actually ulcerating or becoming gangrenous. The redness of ischemic rubor is one example. It is probably the result of loss of reactivity of the small vessels of the skin, causing an agonal dilatation. Despite its red color, the skin is cold to touch, and regains its color very slowly if blanched by finger pressure. Another manifestation of small

vessel disease is known by the descriptive term "purple toes." In this condition, some or all the toes exhibit a cyanotic purple mottling in sharp contrast to the normal color of the remaining skin of the foot. This condition remains stationary for a considerable period of time if untreated, but the purple color changes to blue as viability disappears. It is usually accompanied by severe pain.

Other evidences of small vessel occlusive disease, especially in diabetics, include excessive callus formation, skin fissures occurring in the skin lines, paronychia and skin ulcers at pressure points between toes. Any of these phenomena may become severely infected and tend to burrow rapidly, leading to abscesses and osteomyelitis (Figs. 5 and 6).

DIAGNOSIS. In order to institute the most appropriate form of therapy, and to determine operability and the most suitable operative approach, it is necessary to determine the nature of the occlusive process.

Local examination determines the presence and character of arterial pulsations in the usual locations. When only intermittent claudication is present, one must be particularly careful to rule out discogenic disease, sciatica, rheumatic pains and lumbar spine lesions. These processes may be present in addition to arterial occlusive disease. A good diagnostic test is one which notes the height

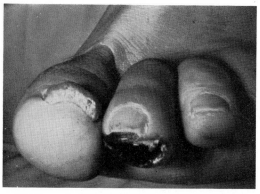

Figure 5. Gangrene of great and second toes following paronychia of great toe and blister of second toe due to ill-fitting shoes in patient with arterial occlusive disease.

to which the foot must be raised to obtain blanching.

Auscultation for systolic bruits in the region of the aortic bifurcation, common iliac bifurcations and common femoral arteries is highly useful in determining distribution of the disease.

Functional significance of partially occlusive lesions can be determined by measuring distal arterial pressures. This can be done with an ordinary blood pressure cuff or with the oscillometer cuff. When distal pulsations are diminished, a normal blood pressure may be present distal to the occluded site when the patient is at rest. Examination after the symptoms have been brought on by exercise will reveal an arterial hypotension distally, and the peripheral pulses may disappear.

Arteriography is indicated if an operative approach is considered. Except for aortic aneurysmal disease, in which it should not be

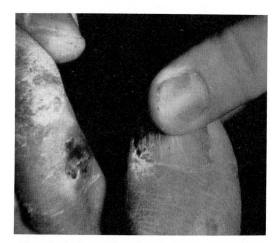

Figure 6. Ischemic ulcer on medial aspect of second toe in patient with arterial occlusive disease.

performed, arteriography is the one clearest way of defining the architecture of an occlusive arterial pathologic process. Although physical examination may locate the lesion, arteriography provides information about its extent and distribution, in addition to the presence and quality of arterial outflow tracts distal to the occlusion. With proper timing, the contrast medium reaches the outflow tract by means of collateral vessels to demonstrate the distal runoff. This knowledge is of utmost importance in planning the operative approach and procedure.

MEDICAL MANAGEMENT OF CHRONIC ARTERIAL OCCLUSION. Despite many recent advances in the knowledge of the nature of the atherosclerotic plaque, there is no known treatment, either preventative or curative, for atherosclerosis. On the other hand, a general plan of medical and surgical management has evolved which can be applied for the relief of symptoms. Patients with mild involvement may require nothing more than general medical care and advice. Such patients should be followed closely to watch for progression of disease, either locally or generally.

Nonoperative measures. In general, medical measures for the care of chronic arterial occlusive disease of the legs are directed toward two goals. One is the reduction of the work load on the legs, the other is an effort to enhance peripheral circulation. Reduction of work load can be accomplished in several ways. If the patient is overweight, weight reduction should be seriously undertaken as a therapeutic measure and not as a casual effort. Next, quantification of effort by grading the effects of cadence, pace and length of step on claudication distance is useful. This can be done by the use of a treadmill, or a chronometer and stop watch, or it can be done less exactly by using a long hallway with more crude devices, such as timing by command. Such tests not only provide the examiner with some quantitative data, but may serve a therapeutic purpose by showing a patient how much farther he can walk if he slows his cadence and speed, and shortens his step.

Another general measure is good foot hygiene and protection from injury. Aside from great care in the avoidance of infections and minor trauma, the patient should be instructed in the care of minor skin conditions, such as intertrigo and fungus infections, which may lead to gangrenous change in the presence of reduced arterial supply. Itching lesions are treated with rest and local steroid ointments, as well as with protective dressings.

Diabetes, either overt or occult, must be treated. If the fasting blood sugar level is within normal limits, a glucose tolerance test should be made to determine the presence or absence of occult diabetes. Gout should be tested for by determining the blood level of uric acid.

If hypertension is present, its etiology should be sought. In patients with arteriosclerotic involvement of the lower extremity, the renal arteries may also be narrowed by the same disease. Similarly, the efficacy of the coronary circulation must be evaluated. This is particularly important in the consideration of reconstructive surgery, not only with respect to tolerance of the patient for a major surgical procedure, but with respect to the possibility of exceeding cardiac reserve by increasing walking distance with successful surgery.

The rapidity of progression of symptoms is an important facet in the general plan of management. If a patient finds that his claudication distance has shortened rather rapidly, say, from three city blocks to a half block within a year or two, he is a more likely candidate for surgical intervention than a patient whose progression of symptoms is much slower.

Medical measures to reduce vasospasm are carried out, but, in general, do not yield gratifying results. An ostensibly successful measure is the cessation of cigarette smoking. Cigarette smoking is usually considered to be harmful in sensitive individuals, because it causes spasm of small arteries, which carry collateral blood supply in the presence of a major vascular occlusion. Heavy smokers should be advised to give up smoking altogether, not merely to reduce the number of cigarettes smoked per day. It is often psychologically advantageous to demonstrate to the patient the changes in surface temperature readings of the great toe before and after a cigarette is smoked. One can usually demonstrate a reduction of more than one degree with the smoking of a cigarette.

Drug therapy. Vasodilator drugs tend to produce dilatation of vessels which are capable of dilating. The paradox of the situation is that the patients who most need the vasodilating effects react poorly to them. A patient with normal peripheral arteries will show a gratifying vasodilating effect after taking a vasodilating drug, whereas a patient whose arteries are rigid and partially occluded will not react to such drugs, and may actually show a reversal of effect. The blood normally flowing through a diseased area is actually diverted away by dilatation of normal vessels in parts of the body distant from the diseased area.

In our experience, none of the presently available vasodilating drugs has been of any lasting therapeutic value in patients with peripheral arterial occlusions, whether these occlusions involve the larger vessels or the smaller ones. Alcohol is perhaps as useful as any, but it also tends to lose its effect as time passes. The subjective relief purportedly obtained by patients with arterial occlusive disease who take vasodilator drugs may often be categorized as psychic, since we have never been able to demonstrate increased blood flow after administration of these drugs to patients with occlusive lesions. The effort to find a useful drug may involve switching from one drug to another over a prolonged period of time, and thus valuable time may well be lost from a more useful approach.

Pain medications with or without tranquilizing drugs usually are part of the palliative care until definitive therapy is carried out.

Physical measures. Physical measures can be subdivided into physical therapy and reduction in activity. Physical therapy for peripheral arterial occlusive disease at one time included many gadgets, such as oscillating beds, alternate hot and cold water sprays, various massage measures, intermittent compression and hydrotherapy.

In our experience, the only measure which has proved even temporarily helpful is indirect heat, that is, heat applied to the lower abdomen. If heat is applied directly to the legs or feet, it tends to raise the metabolic demand of tissue deprived of its major blood supply, and thereby may precipitate gangrene. Moreover, a burn of such tissue is likely to degenerate into a gangrenous ulcer. Indirect heat unquestionably raises the temperature of the skin of the legs temporarily by releasing vasomotor tone, if it is present. However, we have found that benefits from this method are not lasting, and symptoms are not appreciably alleviated (Fig. 7).

An interesting use for indirect heat, not widely employed, is as a preliminary test for the advisability of sympathectomy. We do not usually perform a paravertebral sympathetic

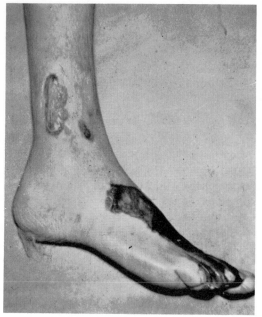

Figure 7. Gangrene following local heat treatment for thrombophlebitis in patient with peripheral arterial insufficiency. Amputation above the knee was necessary.

block as a preliminary test before undertaking sympathectomy, because of the unreliability of the test and because in most situations, the decision for or against sympathectomy can be made without the block. However, a rise in skin temperature of the legs following application of indirect heat to the lower abdomen indicates the presence of vasospasm and, therefore, is a fairly reliable test if one wishes to use it in making a decision for sympathectomy.

Certain patients whose disease is far advanced but whose skin tissues still retain integrity and viability, and who are sufficiently comfortable at rest to allay the need for amputation, constitute a group for whom bed rest has been advocated. If operation is contraindicated, or if it has already been performed to no avail, the patient may be put to bed with the feet horizontally placed, neither elevated nor dependent. Under these conditions, the legs are in a position of minimum metabolic demand; that is, the available blood supply will not have demands put upon it above its capacity. A minimum period of six weeks at rest often leads to the alleviation of pain and results in the healing of ischemic ulcers, provided they receive proper local care. Minimal graded exercises and gentle massage can be applied to the joints to prevent stiffness. The risk of atrophy of disuse must be run under these circumstances. Nonetheless,

many patients on this regimen are relieved of their ischemic rest pain, and remain relatively comfortable after carefully graded activity is resumed.

The rationale of this type of treatment is akin to that of the six weeks of bed rest prescribed for patients with severe coronary artery occlusion. Its purpose is to promote collateral circulation while permitting ischemic tissue to heal, and to place a minimal load on the available vascular supply.

There is some difference of opinion about the amount of exercise a patient with arterial insufficiency should be allowed. One school of thought holds that patients should be encouraged to exercise beyond the point of pain with the hope of extending this point, thereby encouraging collateralization by increasing the demand. The other school of thought believes in keeping exercise within the bounds of comfort, even to the extent of advocating bed rest when necessary. Clinical improvement with this regimen has been repeatedly demonstrated by the healing of ischemic ulcers, the ability to walk short distances without pain after a period of bed rest, and a lessened need for medication for the relief of ischemic pain.

Some physicians recommend a slightly dependent position for the legs, accomplished by placing four-inch blocks under the head of the bed. A footboard is used to prevent sliding and to permit the patient active motion of the feet against resistance.

Precautionary measures. In addition to measures designed to protect an arterially deficient limb against trauma and temperature extremes, certain other measures pertaining to precautionary care are valuable.

Intravenous infusions in the veins of the foot or leg with or without a cutdown are strongly contraindicated. Rapidly developing gangrene may follow such maneuvers (Fig. 8).

A patient who is bedridden, especially one who has undergone unilateral amputation, should wear a loose, heavy sock to prevent linen friction on the heel. Nurses should be advised against urging an amputee to push on the heel of the intact limb in order to change position in bed. Blisters caused by this action often become gangrenous. So-called cotton doughnuts rarely protect the heel and require an absence of activity if they are to stay in place.

Meticulous cleanliness of the feet is important. Pressure points between toes or maceration in the digital webs should be treated by placing cotton between the toes. Patients with dry skin, especially following sympathectomy, should be instructed in applying lanolin cream or ointment to the feet at least once daily.

Bedridden patients should be spared the pressure of sheets and blankets on the toes. Tightly made beds may be the pride of the nursing service, but they are anathema to the vascular surgeon who wishes to relieve pressure points on the ischemic feet of his patient. A simple metal bedspan, usually consisting of a single heavy wire, may be attached over the foot of the bed to hold the sheets above the toes, Metal cradles are to be avoided; they limit motion and may be struck by moving feet, thereby causing injury.

Heavy calluses and corns may be pared by the surgeon or by an experienced, conservative chiropodist. Special care and attention should be paid to the fitting of shoes in ambulatory patients with arterial insufficiency. This measure tends to prevent calluses and corns. The overzealous chiropodist who does not appreciate the hazards involved may be responsible for nonhealing, often gangrenous, ulcers developing at the site of a too-radical corn removal (Fig. 9).

Patients with a plantar corn over the head of the second metatarsal with long second toe, and patients with osteoarthritic spurs on the head of the second metatarsal bone, tend to develop an ischemic ulceration on the sole of

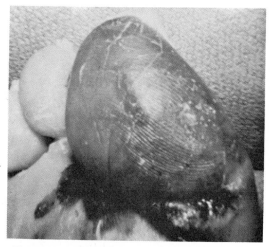

Figure 9. Gangrene of great toe following paring of callus, leaving ulcer seen at base of toe.

the foot at the site of maximum pressure. This may be prevented by various measures, including a metatarsal bar on the sole of the shoe, and careful corn paring. Once such an ulcer has occurred, it is extremely difficult to heal, often requiring bed rest for weeks, or surgical removal of the bone if osteitis or osteomyelitis ensues.

SURGICAL TREATMENT OF CHRONIC ARTERIAL OCCLUSION. Surgical therapy for arterial disease of the lower extremity consists of indirect procedures for the release of vasospasm; direct operation for the re-establishment of arterial flow, and for the resection and replacement of diseased arteries; and ablative surgery for the removal of parts which have lost their viability. Often, a combination of these approaches is advisable in the same patient. A number of adjunctive surgical procedures are performed to supplement these main approaches, including such procedures as patch grafts and other angioplastic reconstructions.

Indirect surgical therapy. The only indirect surgical procedure which has survived the test of time is sympathectomy. Such measures as Achilles tendonotomy, unroofing of Hunter's canal, neurotomy and arteriectomy have not proved of sufficient value to be retained.

The indications for lumbar sympathectomy have come into sharper focus over the years. For 25 years, lumbar sympathectomy was the only procedure of any value to be offered to a patient suffering from occlusive arterial disease of the lower extremity. Because it was applied to patients with every variety and

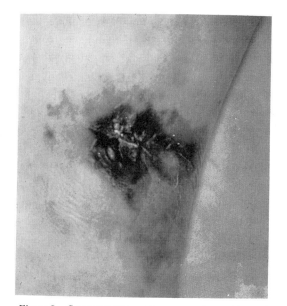

Figure 8. Gangrene of a cutdown wound at ankle made to administer intravenous fluids. Spread of gangrene required amputation above the knee.

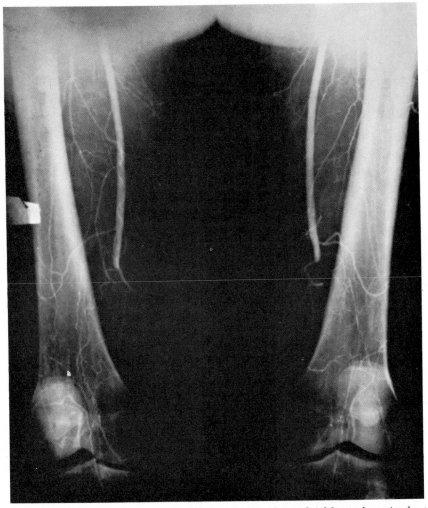

Figure 10.   Arteriogram showing almost symmetrical total occlusions of superficial femoral arteries due to emboli from intracardiac mural thrombus in a patient who recently had suffered a myocardial infarct.

stage of arterial disease, its success was somewhat limited. Sympathectomy, properly employed, is a valuable surgical procedure, not only as a definitive method of producing dilatation of a vascular bed in spasm, but as an ancillary measure to complement reconstructive arterial operations. When reconstructive procedures cannot be carried out, because of the absence of an adequate channel peripheral to an occlusion or for other reasons, sympathectomy is the only means of improving small vessel circulation to the part. The value of thoracic and lumbar sympathectomy in the treatment of arterial insufficiency of the upper and lower extremities is so generally accepted that most vascular surgeons usually perform a sympathectomy prior to, or in combination with, one of the direct reconstructive procedures. It is believed that

sympathectomy enhances the success of direct reconstructive operations by obviating postoperative vasospasm and by permitting a broader area of small vessel bed to accept the new blood flow.

There has been an unfortunate tendency to compare lumbar sympathectomy with arterioplastic operations for the treatment of all types of occlusive arterial lesions of the lower extremity. The two procedures should not be placed in competing positions, for they accomplish different purposes. Sympathectomy can only be expected to dilate small vessels and collateral channels in an extremity; yet this is usually sufficient to raise the total blood flow to an extremity enough to eradicate the pain of intermittent claudication, or to permit healing of ischemic lesions of the skin and tissues. It has been suggested that

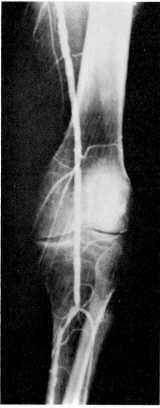

Figure 11. Arteriogram of patient who complained of foot claudication. Note narrowing at bifurcation of popliteal artery. Occlusion at this site may require only lumbar sympathectomy, or later, regional endarterectomy and patch graft if symptomatic relief is not satisfactory.

spasm from all small vessels, regardless of what tissues they supply. Thus, roughly 50 per cent of patients who have been subjected to sympathectomy obtain significant relief from intermittent claudication. Furthermore, there is an unmistakable tendency for sympathectomy to increase the rate of development of collateral arterial supply in many patients. The effects of lumbar sympathetic ablation are in direct proportion to the dilatability of the small vessels. It is obvious, therefore, that a number of patients will not benefit from sympathectomy.

Temporary sympathetic procaine block is not a useful measure to predict the reaction to sympathectomy. The test is relatively unreliable, since one cannot be sure of the efficacy of the block. Testing the patient's ability to walk without pain after a procaine sympathetic block is not reliable, because the diffusion of the procaine to sensory fibers may relieve pain and give a false positive. Moreover, an unsuccessful block may be falsely interpreted as a negative result. Therefore, if sympathectomy is to be considered at all, and there are no true contraindications, it should be performed, either as a therapeutic procedure in itself, or as preliminary or complementary to a reconstructive procedure. If femoral arterial pulsations are present, a bilateral percutaneous femoral arteriogram can be done under the same anesthesia at the time of the sympathectomy. The arteriographic findings then serve as a factor in the decision for or against later direct arterial surgery.

Many patients subjected to sympathectomy, as a preliminary to a reconstructive procedure, obtain sufficient clinical improvement to obviate the need for any further operation. Many such patients have remained symptom-free for life.

sympathectomy alone may be the procedure of choice in most patients with atherosclerotic segmental femoropopliteal occlusion, reserving direct arterial reconstruction for patients with the most severe claudication and the most advanced ischemic changes, and patients whose livelihood depends on resuming sufficient function.

Sympathectomy cannot be expected to remove an occlusive lesion in a main artery, and, therefore, cannot compete directly with a successful reconstructive operation which restores full pulses to the distal part. Sympathectomy is especially indicated in the types of occlusive disease which involve the smaller arteries and which are not amenable to reconstruction. It is also valuable for patients with inflammatory arterial diseases with a vasospastic element and in diabetic patients.

There has been a good deal of confusing literature indicating that sympathectomy increases only the blood supply to the skin, at the expense of that to the musculature. However, the procedure tends to release vaso-

Direct reconstructive surgical procedures. Currently employed operations for the reestablishment of arterial blood flow include resection and replacement of a diseased arterial segment accompanied by graft replacement; insertion of a by-pass graft around an obstructive lesion without resection; thrombectomy; embolectomy; and endarterectomy.

The current techniques of vessel grafting had to await the discovery and purification of heparin, the advent of arteriography, the invention of noncrushing arterial clamps, information on the behavior of various grafting materials, knowledge of the physiologic responses to prolonged occlusion of major arteries, and improved techniques of physiologic monitoring.

This body of knowledge grew on a foundation of general surgical advances which was being built independently: the safer use of blood and electrolyte replacement, improved anesthesia, antibiotic therapy, and the therapeutic application of hypothermia and extracorporeal circulation.

Advances have been so rapid that today more is known of the mechanical correction of the effects of atherosclerosis than of the etiology and pathogenesis of the disease. Technically, it is possible to rehabilitate patients with occlusive disease of the extremities, kidneys, abdominal viscera, brain and lungs. A growing body of information is accumulating on the long-term prognosis and consideration of weighing the prospects for rehabilitation against morbidity and mortality of the surgery, as well as against the natural history of the disease.

MATERIALS USED IN ARTERIAL GRAFTING. Autogenous veins are especially suitable for reconstructive grafting procedures in the extremities. The saphenous vein is used for bypassing, replacing or patching the femoral and popliteal arteries. When it is normal, its accessibility is a great advantage. However, it is not always available in sufficient length for a by-pass operation. The first autogenous vein graft was performed by Kunlin in 1951, who used it to by-pass a femoral artery occlusion. Today, long-term results in operations for femoropopliteal arterial occlusions strongly favor autogenous grafts over plastic woven prostheses in operations distal to the inguinal ligaments. In our experience, the late occlusion rate of 20 per cent is considerably less than that following plastic grafts (Fig. 12).

When used to replace or by-pass femoral artery occlusions, the vein must be inserted upside down so that its valves will not interfere with the arterial flow.

Autogenous saphenous vein grafts are ideally suited for popliteal artery substitution after resection of popliteal aneurysm and to repair femoropopliteal defects caused by trauma. An advantage of autogenous vein grafts is their maintenance of pliability, a feature of importance when bridging joints (Fig. 13).

Small segments of saphenous vein are conveniently used as patch grafts to close arteriotomy openings made in conjunction with several types of arterial operations such as

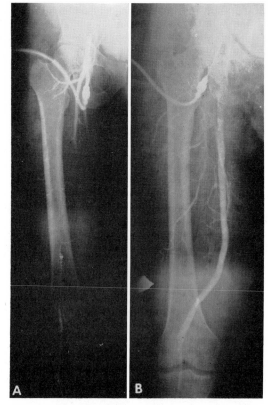

Figure 12. *A*, Femoral arteriogram showing arteriosclerotic occlusion of almost entire length of superficial femoral artery with only fair popliteal runoff. *B*, Re-establishment of circulation with reversed autogenous vein by-pass graft.

embolectomy, thrombectomy and endarterectomy.

Arterial homografts have been extensively used since Gross and his associates in 1947 investigated techniques for preservation of these vessels. Preservation by lyophilization, introduced in 1951, permitted long-term storage by vacuum packing. Arterial homografts, ideal to handle and suture, and literally made to order, enjoyed wide popularity in replacement operations for aneurysms and in by-pass operations for occlusions at many anatomic sites, especially the aortoiliac and femoropopliteal areas.

Evidence began to accumulate in 1956 that homografts were far from ideal. It was found that arteriosclerotic changes, leading to thromboses and aneurysms, developed much more rapidly in homografts than in the parent vessels. It was learned that thoracic aorta homografts underwent the least change with time. Abdominal aorta bifurcation homografts have been, for the most part, satisfactory for at least a decade. Femoral artery

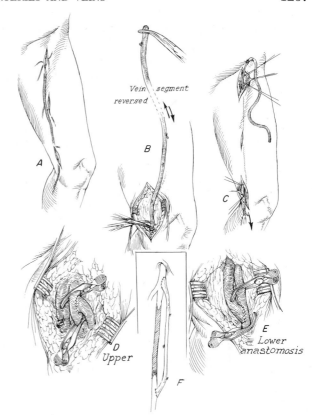

Figure 13. By-pass femoropopliteal graft for femoral artery occlusion, using reversed saphenous vein.

homografts were found to degenerate in three to five years in most patients. As a result of this, homografts are rarely used today in reconstructive arterial operations.

PLASTIC ARTERIAL PROSTHESES. At the turn of the century and shortly thereafter, surgeons attempted to suture rigid or semi-rigid tubes of various impermeable materials into severed blood vessels of animals and man. It was soon learned that no matter how smooth or nonwettable the tube, a high incidence of thrombosis and separation followed implantation. Although the perfect artery substitute is probably not yet available, many thousands of successful artery grafts have been performed since 1952. The modern era of blood vessel grafting was ushered in by Voorhees, Jaretski and Blakemore who employed Vinyon N cloth in animals and in man. Many materials, including cotton, silk, compressed Ivalon and nylon have been tried through the years. Today, Dacron and Teflon woven prostheses are the most widely used. It is now known that the material must be porous to permit ingrowth and the development of pseudointima. The crimping principle was introduced in 1955 by Edwards to add flexibility without kinking.

In aortic or iliac artery grafts, the plastic prostheses are generally considered highly satisfactory. However, in vessels the caliber of the femoral artery or smaller, there is some dissatisfaction with woven artificial grafts. Nonetheless, many of these grafts have been notably successful, and are used when autogenous vein is not available. The problem with woven grafts of femoropopliteal caliber in a moving limb is their tendency to become rigid and encased in inelastic scar tissue. This leads to kinking or deformity at the anastomosis upon flexion of a joint (Fig. 14).

When elasticity is not required, woven grafts of smaller caliber have yielded gratifying short-term success in areas such as the renal and superior mesenteric arteries.

Thromboendarterectomy. Endarterectomy is the removal of the thickened, obstructing intima, literally a process of routing out the vessel. If there is an attached or contained thrombus, the procedure is termed thromboendarterectomy. Leriche, Kunlin and dos Santos originated this technique, and Wylie, Barker and Warren developed and refined it.

A distinct line of cleavage can usually be

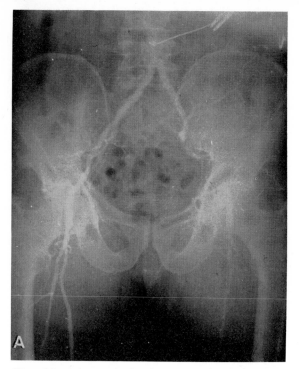
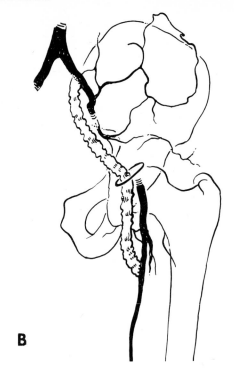

Figure 14.   *A*, Aortogram showing segmental occlusion of the iliac artery. *B*, Diagram of iliofemoral Dacron by-pass graft.

found between the diseased intima and the musculofibrous coat of a vessel, making it possible to strip away the intima and restore the lumen of an artery. The remaining muscle lining rapidly develops a new intima, much the same as that which develops in plastic prostheses. The neointima is at first thick and velvety, and later becomes thin and almost indistinguishable from normal intimal lining.

An endarterectomy of a short obstructed segment is performed through an arteriotomy incision made the length of the obstruction. For longer segments, a loop stripper may be passed after the cleavage plane has been developed. Two or more arteriotomy incisions may be made (Figs. 15 and 16).

Failure of an endarterectomized vessel to remain patent is usually due to occlusion by clots which form on shaggy shreds of tissue left behind after the stripping. It is important that all such shreds be removed during the procedure.

Since thromboendarterectomy was introduced in 1947, it has been alternately condemned and condoned. Today, properly applied and skillfully performed, it has a place in the technique of vascular surgery. It is often combined with grafting procedures in the same patient. The greatest success is

found in endarterectomies of the larger arteries, although operations of this type may be successful in vessels the size of the popliteal and even the posterior tibial artery.

An important technical detail is that of tacking down the intima at the distal end of the endarterectomy procedure. This is necessary to prevent dissection by the blood stream between the remaining intima and the mus-

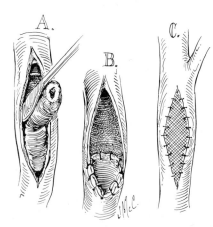

Figure 15.   Endarterectomy through single arteriotomy incision. *A*, Dissection of intimal core from musculofibrous coat with spatula. *B*, Suture of intima to artery wall at distal end of endarterectomy. *C*, Closure of arteriotomy wound with patch graft of either autogenous vein or plastic woven material.

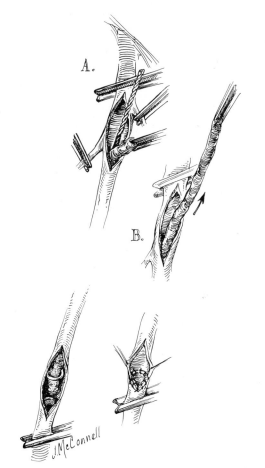

Figure 16. Thromboendarterectomy. *A*, Stripping of occluding core through proximal and distal arteriotomy incisions. *B*, Removal of core and suture of distal intima to artery coat to prevent dissecting aneurysm or occlusion at this point.

cular coat. Another technical advance which has enhanced the success of endarterectomy is the use of the patch graft at the site of arteriotomy, especially in vessels in which the lumen may be compromised by linear closure of the arteriotomy incision.

Follow-up studies indicate a 24 per cent thrombosis rate during the first year after initially successful femoral endarterectomy. However, this rate of failure apparently does not increase appreciably over the next two years. Late failures have been ascribed to progression of the occlusive process just proximal or distal to the endarterectomized segment, and may be due to trauma from occluding clamps at the time of operation.

When closure of an arteriotomy incision tends to compromise the lumen of a vessel, it is expedient to employ an elliptical patch of autogenous vein or woven plastic material.

This maneuver is especially valuable in vessels the caliber of the femoral, popliteal, renal and carotid arteries.

Results of surgical treatment. In order to judge the results of any treatment, the expected natural history of the disease, the expected longevity of the population involved, early and late mortality due to operation, and late complications must be known. The value of a surgical procedure depends not only upon whether worthwhile relief is obtained, it also depends upon an acceptable operative mortality and a comparison of late prognosis with that of other forms of therapy. Published results of such data, unfortunately, are not easily available for chronic occlusive arterial disease of the lower extremity, because of great variations in methods of reporting. The results of vascular operations should be reported in a manner similar to those of operations for cancer, that is, in terms of three-year or five-year results.

RESULTS IN AORTOILIAC OCCLUSION. In chronic aortoiliac occlusion, claudication of one type or another exists in 90 per cent of patients, impotence in 40 per cent of males, and severe ischemic phenomena in only 10 per cent. Systemic hypertension coexists in about 25 per cent, and disseminated atherosclerosis, either visceral or peripheral, with associated symptoms, in 25 per cent.

About 35 per cent of patients with aortoiliac occlusion are suitable for or require surgical treatment. Of all the areas of the body in which reconstructive operations have been done, by far the best results, both immediate and late, are obtained in aortoiliac occlusive disease. If one or both limbs of a graft must pass the inguinal flexion crease, the success rate falls to approximately that of femoropopliteal surgery.

In isolated aortoiliac occlusions, thromboendarterectomy or prosthetic by-pass grafts yield an excellent early result in over 95 per cent of patients, with a surgical mortality rate of 2 per cent or less. Two years after operation, there is a 2 per cent failure rate, but this decreases thereafter. However, within three to five years, occlusive disease distal to this area can be expected in at least 25 per cent of the patients. When homografts were used, at least one iliac limb occluded within three years in 40 per cent of patients.

If aortoiliac disease is associated with occlusive processes of the coronary or femoral vessels, the operative mortality rises to 12 per cent, and the initial success rate falls to

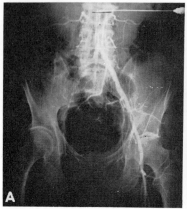
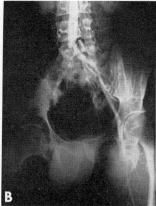
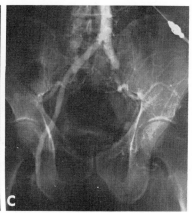

Figure 17. Aortograms showing three varieties of complete common iliac artery occlusion due to arteriosclerosis. *A*, Patient treated by aortofemoral by-pass graft. *B*, Patient treated by iliac endarterectomy. *C*, Patient treated by insertion of iliofemoral Dacron graft by end-to-end anastomosis above, and end-to-side anastomosis below.

under 70 per cent, with a proportionately higher rate of late failures and mortality. In view of such statistics, the surgeon must weigh the mortality and morbidity of major amputation in this group of patients against the risk of a direct operation.

Because ambitious reconstructions from aorta to popliteal artery can be done only on exceptionally good-risk patients, and because of the high incidence of late failures in this group, some surgeons believe in re-establishing continuity only as far as the deep femoral artery, even when there is occlusion distally. Limited operations of this type, especially when accompanied by lumbar sympathectomy, are often rewarded by healing of ischemic ulcerations and occasionally, by restoration of pedal pulses.

RESULTS IN FEMOROPOPLITEAL OCCLUSION. The average age of patients with symptomatic arteriosclerotic occlusive disease of the lower extremities is 63 years; 80 per cent are males, and 15 to 30 per cent are diabetic. Life-table statistics of this group reveal that 50 to 60 per cent of the diabetics, and some 70 to 80 per cent of the nondiabetics, survive five years; that is, they escape death from any cause for this period of time, if at the time of examination they were free of coronary vessel disease and hypertension.

In nondiabetic patients with untreated occlusive disease of the femoral artery, gangrene develops at some time in 10 per cent, and eventual amputation is necessary in about 7 per cent. These figures are somewhat lower than one would expect, and may be used to formulate an opinion on the need and the urgency of surgical intervention when only mild symptoms of claudication

are present. In diabetic patients, gangrene may occur in 40 per cent, for which amputation is required in 25 to 30 per cent. Over 90 per cent of patients with mild intermittent claudication, if not operated upon, experience no progression of symptoms over a five-year period; some in this group report spontaneous improvement. From these data, it is clear that the surgeon should feel no sense of

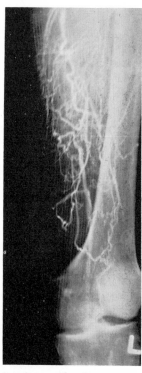

Figure 18. Arteriogram showing segmental occlusion of superficial femoral artery with extensive collateralization and excellent distal runoff. An autogenous vein by-pass graft relieved the symptoms.

urgency for surgical intervention when only mild claudication exists without a history of progression of symptoms. When symptoms are progressive, or when they are combined with other ischemic phenomena, the surgeon must choose surgical candidates from this group in accordance with expected relief from symptoms and salvage of extremities.

Of patients with progressively symptomatic occlusions in the femoropopliteal region, about 40 per cent are suitable for a surgical procedure. When combined aorto-iliac and femoropopliteal disease occurs, the operability rate falls to 25 per cent. Only the severely disabled patient with combined disease of this type should be considered for surgical intervention.

For segmental occlusions of the femoral artery, a by-pass procedure utilizing the saphenous vein probably offers the best long-term results. If a suitable saphenous vein is not present, a prosthetic by-pass graft is inserted. Thromboendarterectomy, in some hands, offers about as good results as the by-pass procedures. The initial success rate with by-pass procedures approaches 90 per cent, and endarterectomy of the femoral artery is successful in about 75 per cent of the patients. However, results after two years indicate that 25 to 40 per cent of saphenous vein by-pass grafts of the femoropopliteal artery become occluded, whereas 30 to 50 per cent of prosthetic by-pass grafts and 25 to 40 per cent of thromboendarterectomies in this area are reoccluded at this time. Good results after four years are proportionately reduced. One possible advantage of endarterectomy is that late occlusion is usually gradual following endarterectomy, while it is more likely to be acute following late failure of a by-pass, and may cost the patient his leg. Despite these statistics, it should be noted that some by-pass grafts and endarterectomized femoral arteries are functioning normally after ten years.

If acute occlusion becomes superimposed upon a chronically diseased artery, the long-term statistics assume less importance in favor of the immediate prospects of saving a limb by reconstructive arterial procedures. If arteriography reveals a patent distal channel in such a limb, the prospects of obtaining a good result by a reconstructive procedure are gratifyingly high. By-pass procedures are easier to perform and can be done faster than extensive endarterectomies. However, when a distal channel must be created, endar-terectomy necessarily becomes at least part of the procedure.

This type of endarterectomy, performed to save a limb otherwise destined to be amputated, has been called a "desperation endarterectomy." These operations are tedious and trying on the surgeon, but surprisingly well tolerated by the patient. The mortality rate is under 5 per cent, and the initial success rate in our experience is 60 per cent. If there is any doubt about the patency of a long endarterectomy of the femoral artery, the vessel may be split for most of its length and a strip graft of autogenous vein sutured on to provide a wider lumen. Many times, an operation performed to save a limb results in long-term success, and if the channel becomes reoccluded slowly enough, only minor amputation may eventually be necessary. In all of these procedures, it is our policy to perform preliminary or concomitant sympathectomy, for we believe it enhances both the immediate and late success rate. It tends to obviate spasm in the early postoperative period, and provides a greater collateral bed subsequently.

Limb salvage. Although lumbar sympathectomy alone may have considerable value in the palliative treatment of occlusive arterial lesions of the legs, it is apparent that direct restoration of blood flow in major vessels, when applicable, is more effective for limb salvage. However, by-pass techniques currently employed are not practicable when arteriosclerotic involvement of the distal popliteal artery causes marked narrowing or occlusion of this vessel, sufficient to prevent construction of an adequate distal anastomosis.

Patients who have inadequate distal run-off are usually poor risks for restoration of circulation. Rather than consign such patients to a painful, useless existence until amputation is inevitable, an effort has been made to broaden the indications for reconstructive arterial surgery by offering extensive or desperation endarterectomy to such patients. When the arteriogram shows little or no filling of the popliteal artery, or when the distal popliteal artery is found at the time of operation to be occluded, the procedure is to be considered.

Before an extensive operation of this type is planned, one must realize that in the event of failure, amputation may be hastened to a certain extent. Therefore, the procedure is applied only to limbs which are either functionally useless or are to some extent a hazard to health. The indications are irreparable gangrene to a part of the foot and intractable pain. Under these circumstances, risking loss of the limb from surgical failure is the price of possible restoration. In general, the procedure is applied only to patients who are destined to amputation and, therefore, it can be considered a last resort, or desperation procedure. In our experience with 75 such patients, circulation has been restored in 46. Through the use of extensive endarterectomy, it is possible to prevent what appear to be inescapable amputations, and to rehabilitate the patient to a symptom-free period of usefulness.

Extensive endarterectomies are rarely applied to limbs which might otherwise be restored by other procedures. The risk of failure is just as important as the possibility of salvage, and, therefore, the procedure is reserved only for limbs otherwise destined for amputation.

Limb salvage operations may also be performed with the by-pass technique, using autogenous saphenous vein or knitted Dacron tubes. In some of these operations, the lower anastomosis is located well below the knee, occasionally just above the ankle. Onlay grafts and patch grafts, with or without endarterectomy, are also employed.

Microsurgical procedures. Reconstructive operations upon vessels less than 4 mm.

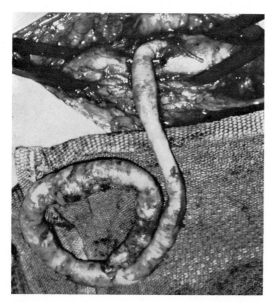

Figure 19. Limb salvage endarterectomy: atheromatous intima core removed from femoral artery through arteriotomy in proximal portion of popliteal artery after using endarterectomy stripper.

in diameter were formerly considered largely unsatisfactory because of technical difficulties. A number of nonsuture cuff methods have been devised, employing rings and coupling devices, but these all require leaving a foreign body at the operative site. Other methods employ the use of an acrylic tissue glue known as Eastman 910. The techniques employing this substance are handicapped by handling difficulties and by postoperative tissue reaction, which may lead to constriction and thrombosis. Stapling devices have been successfully employed for small vessels in accessible anatomic areas.

At present, the most successful method of small blood vessel suture is that of Jacobson, in which small vessels are sutured in the same manner as large ones, except that the operation is done under magnification and the instruments and suture materials are miniaturized. A dissecting microscope is used. Special holding instruments steady the small vessel ends, and an 8-0 silk suture is employed.

PERIPHERAL ARTERIAL DISEASE IN DIABETIC PATIENTS. Patients with diabetes are subject to all varieties of arteriosclerotic occlusive disease, but tend to be affected at a somewhat earlier age than nondiabetic patients. In addition, a number of manifestations of arterial occlusive disease are peculiar to diabetic patients. In general, small vessels tend to become more severely affected. The small vessel disease of diabetes differs from that of arteriosclerosis obliterans in that both the media and intima are thickened in diabetes, whereas only the intima is thickened in the absence of diabetes.

Often, gangrene of the toes is found in the presence of palpable dorsalis pedis and posterior tibial arteries. Patches of subcutaneous hemorrhage may be found on the feet and lower legs. Any of these patches may become gangrenous. The cause of these lesions is thought to be increased capillary fragility aggravated by local pressure or minor trauma. A variety of neurotropic lesions are found, including anesthesia, ulceration, painless erosions, clawfoot and painless, distorted joints similar to Charcot's joints.

Peculiarly, intense local pain may be felt subjectively, whereas palpation or instrumentation of the lesions is altogether painless. Large, thick calluses are common. Minor infections tend to lead to abscess formation and osteomyelitis with surprising rapidity. Inflammatory reactions include lymphangitis, cellulitis and phlebitis.

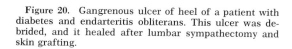
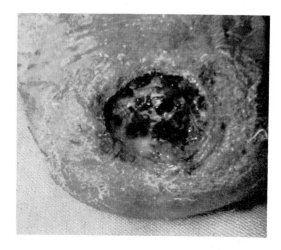

Figure 20. Gangrenous ulcer of heel of a patient with diabetes and endarteritis obliterans. This ulcer was debrided, and it healed after lumbar sympathectomy and skin grafting.

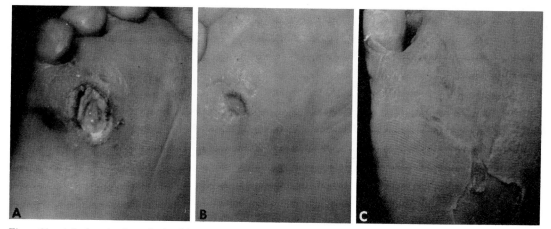

Figure 21. *A*, Ischemic ulcer of sole of foot in diabetic patient, before debridement. *B*, Appearance after two weeks of bed rest and careful diabetic management following initial debridement. *C*, Healed appearance after four weeks.

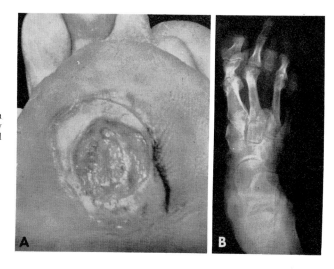

Figure 22. *A*, Large, draining ischemic ulcer on sole of foot in diabetic patient. *B*, Healed x-ray appearance after surgical removal of metatarsal bone; patient walks without pain or limp.

The general principles of local treatment in diabetic patients are essentially those of other patients with arterial disease, except that minor amputations and other procedures are more often necessary in diabetic patients. Meticulous diabetic control is essential to all local care. Often, eroded or gangrenous areas heal by careful local management (Fig. 21). Multiple toe amputations are possible, as well as debridement and skin grafting of ulcerations. The wide excision of gangrenous ulcers and the removal of infected metatarsal bones and phalanges often lead to bizarre distortion of the shape of the foot, but the patient is able to walk on such feet with surprising comfort, without a limp (Fig. 22). Lumbar sympathectomy is often performed to enhance small vessel circulation in diabetic patients, but yields salutary results in only about 50 per cent.

In the treatment of large vessel occlusive lesions in diabetic patients, the same principles are employed as in nondiabetic patients with these lesions, except, of course, for the medical control of the diabetic state.

HYPERTENSIVE ARTERIOLAR LESIONS. Arteriolar necrosis of the skin of the calves may be found in hypertensive patients between the ages of 50 and 70 years. Typically, this lesion occurs on the lateral or posterior surface of the lower third of the leg and is often surrounded by a purple halo. After ulceration, it shows pale, glassy granulations with minimal secretions and adherent gangrenous crusts.

Histologically, there is a marked subendothelial hyalinosis, a thickening of the wall and a diminished lumen in the vessels. This lesion has been likened to a cutaneous infarct, although the actual occluding thrombi are usually not seen. It occurs more frequently in diabetics and in patients with thromboangiitis obliterans and hypertension, but it has also been found in the presence of normotension. It is difficult to understand why these lesions should occur in the calves, unless minute trauma is a contributing factor.

Chronic Arterial Occlusion in the Upper Extremity

In contrast to the ease with which chronic occlusive arterial disease of the legs may be diagnosed, it is often difficult to make an accurate diagnosis without arteriography when the upper extremity is involved. Arteries of the arm are far less commonly af-fected by chronic atherosclerotic occlusive disease than are those of the legs.

Athletes, such as baseball pitchers and jai alai players, who repeatedly exert an arm violently, occasionally suffer arterial thrombosis of the axillary or brachial artery. Treatment of such patients follows the same principles as that of atherosclerotic occlusive disease except for the factor of urgency.

SYMPTOMS. The symptoms consist of severe aching in the arm, especially when it is in motion. The fingers are intolerant to cold, and the arm muscles tend to cramp easily. The difficulty in ascribing these symptoms to arterial occlusion lies in the fact that a relatively normal radial pulse is usually palpable. If arthritis or bursitis are also present, the symptoms are often erroneously ascribed to these afflictions.

The usual site of partial or complete occlusion is at the subclavian or innominate artery, or less often at the level of the axillary artery. Collateral channels are present to compensate for the occlusion, and are responsible for carrying pulsatile flow to the radial artery. It is rare for a thrombus to propagate distally from the primary occlusive site. As a result, severe ischemia is only seen in the arm following acute arterial occlusions due to emboli and primary thrombi.

Thromboendarterectomy of the short occluded segment near the aortic origin results in full symptomatic relief. Upper thoracic sympathectomy will provide better flow through collateral channels, but is less effective for large vessel occlusions than for small vessel disease. It must be remembered that occlusive lesions of the arteries of the arms may be associated with generalized atherosclerosis, including the vessels of the cerebrum. The latter may contribute to weakness and other symptoms, and the presence of cerebral ischemia must be weighed against the advisability of performing an operation on the great vessels.

Acute ischemia of the entire arm, besides being due to embolic disease or trauma, may be caused by ascending arterial thrombosis secondary to some blood dyscrasias. It may also follow occlusion of the brachial artery secondary to catheterization and perfusion procedures.

PULSELESS DISEASE (TAKAYUSU'S DISEASE). A proliferative stenosing process of unknown etiology affects major branches of the aortic arch. It is known as pulseless disease because it obliterates the pulsatile flow of blood to the head and arms. Arteriosclerotic occlusion of the origins of vessels from the aortic arch gives the same symptoms and, therefore, could also be considered as manifestations of pulseless disease. Takayusu, however, described the disease in young women who would not be suspected of having arteriosclerotic occlusion. Takayusu's lesion may be similar to the fibromuscular hyperplasia occurring in renal arteries of young people. Symptoms of carotid artery occlusion include dizziness, headache, syncope and hemiplegia. Subclavian or innominate artery involvement prevents pulsatile flow to the arms, but ischemic symptoms of the arms are absent. The disease is suspected when blood pressure is unobtainable in either arm and pulses are absent at the wrist. The leg vessels are usually unaffected. A by-pass operation or endarterectomy is recommended in suitable patients.

OCCLUSION OF ARTERIES TO THE BRAIN

Symptoms of cerebral ischemia may vary from fleeting or recurrent attacks of dizzi-ness, headache and other signs of transient cerebral ischemia, to those of hemiplegia.

It is estimated that roughly one-third of all patients with symptoms of cerebral ischemia have occlusive lesions of the extracranial vessels to the brain which are sufficiently isolated to be operable.

Because the incidence of multiple atherosclerotic occlusive lesions is high, arteriographic visualization of both carotid artery bifurcations and vertebral artery origins is necessary. In addition to atheromatous narrowing, arteriosclerotic tortuosity and buckling are often seen. Both types of lesions are amenable to reconstructive operations. When vertebral artery narrowing is due to scalenus muscle pressure, relief may be obtained by cutting the muscle without resorting to an arterial procedure. The diagnosis of this lesion depends upon the coexistence of the scalenus anticus syndrome in the arm and signs of cerebral ischemia.

The most common lesion of the extracranial vessels is a partially or completely occluding atheroma at the bifurcation of the common carotid artery with extension of the

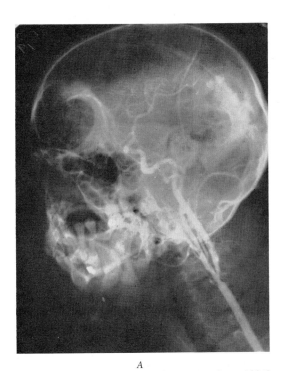

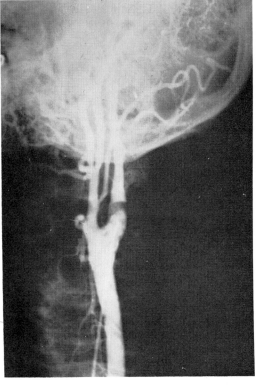

A   *B*

Figure 23. *A*, Arteriosclerotic narrowing of carotid bifurcation, involving both internal and external carotid arteries. Lumen was reconstituted by endarterectomy and patch graft. *B*, Arteriogram showing partial arteriosclerotic occlusion of internal carotid artery an inch above bifurcation of common carotid artery.

lesion for a short distance into the internal or external carotid arteries (Fig. 23). The presence of a bruit at the carotid artery bifurcation, or reduction in measured retinal artery pressure on the affected side, is a good clinical indication of partial occlusion at the carotid bifurcation. Obstructions of the larger arteries emerging from the aortic arch are evidenced by changes in common carotid artery pulsations and arm pressures. Aortography confirms the diagnosis, localizes the lesion and reveals the dissemination of the disease.

The category of patients best suited for reconstructive operations is the group with only transient attacks of cerebral arterial insufficiency, who are otherwise intact neurologically. Some 90 per cent of such patients have reparable lesions of the extracranial vessels. Surgical mortality rate with carotid reconstruction is extremely low, varying between 0.3 and 5 per cent, but when the great vessels must be reconstructed, the mortality rate rises to about 20 per cent. Once the procedure is successful, some 70 to 80 per cent of the survivors are reported free of symptoms after operation.

In sharp contrast with these figures, only some 45 per cent of patients with acute, progressively developing neurologic deficit have an obstruction susceptible to surgical repair. Reconstruction may be of value in arresting and allowing subsidence of the neurologic signs. Although complete return to a symptom-free state cannot often be expected in such a patient, some surgeons claim to have achieved this state in 40 to 80 per cent of patients in whom the circulation was restored.

In the presence of an old established hemiplegia, vascular operations are of no value. When the operation is performed during fugitive symptoms of cerebral ischemia, successful re-establishment of circulation with disappearance of symptoms is possible in about two-thirds of the patients. Results are difficult to evaluate because of the tendency for spontaneous recovery in a certain number of these patients. Although comparable data in patients treated nonsurgically are not abundant, it is known that untreated extracranial occlusions of the internal carotid artery carry an early mortality rate of some 35 per cent, and complete recovery from paralysis occurs in only 12 per cent.

When surgical attack is possible on a sudden thrombotic or embolic occlusion of the

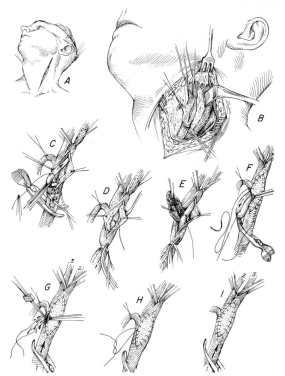

Figure 24.   Carotid artery endarterectomy. *A*, Incision. *B*, Retraction of jugular vein and carotid arteriotomy. *C*, Insertion of tubular stent to maintain flow during operation. *D* and *E*, Steps in endarterectomy. *F*, Application of dacron patch graft and removal of stent. *G*, *H* and *I*, Steps in removal of clamps.

internal carotid artery, it has resulted in dramatic disappearance of major hemiplegia, provided the operation is performed within hours of the onset, before secondary distal thrombus propagation or brain swelling occurs. This finding has cast new light upon the surviving tendencies of central nervous system cells. It appears that collateral flow, though inadequate to maintain function, is sometimes adequate enough to permit survival of central nervous system cells well beyond the few minutes of life that they are known to have with total ischemia. Re-establishment of circulation has proved possible in about 50 per cent of acutely thrombosed carotid arteries (Fig. 24). It is agreed that acute hemiplegia deserves to be considered an urgent surgical emergency, until extracranial vascular occlusion cannot be proved.

SUBCLAVIAN STEAL SYNDROME

In an editorial appearing in a 1961 issue of the New England Journal of Medicine, the graphic term "subclavian steal syndrome" was coined to describe cerebrovascular insufficiency due to subclavian artery occlusion. Although correlation of absent arm pulses with cerebrovascular insufficiency had been suspected as early as 1839, the clinical symptoms were first described in 1944 by Martorell-Otzet and Fabre. As angiography developed, more exact diagnosis became possible, and surgeons began to become interested. The first successful case of subclavian reconstruction with relief of neurological symptoms was reported by Davis, Grove and Julian in 1956. After Contorni in 1960 discovered that vertebral artery flow was actually retrograde in this syndrome, Reivich and coworkers in 1961 published intraoperative flowmeter recordings in two patients to demonstrate the siphoning of blood from the brain to the arm in the presence of subclavian artery occlusion.

The syndrome typically is found in patients in their late fifties. Men and women seem to be about equally affected. Dizziness is the most common symptom, but transient blurring of vision, occasional syncope, lateralizing motor or sensory signs, aphasia and dysarthria also occur. Transient blindness or diplopia is more rare. Characteristically, symptoms are precipitated by suddenly arising or turning the head to one side. Aching

and weakness tend to occur in the affected arm upon exertion.

Physical examination usually reveals a weak or absent radial pulse in the involved limb, although only a pulse lag may be present. Systolic pressure may be considerably lower or altogether undetectable in the arm. Bruits about the clavicle may be discerned in the presence of partial occlusions.

Demonstration of the lesion by angiography is best accomplished by transfemoral insertion of a Seldinger catheter. Retrograde vertebral artery flow can be demonstrated in about half the cases.

Surgical correction is achieved by subclavian thromboendarterectomy and reconstruction. A gratifying bonus of a successful operation is the disappearance of memory loss, mental dullness, and inability to concentrate which are often attributed to old age by patients (Fig. 25).

OCCLUSION OF THE RENAL ARTERY

Ever since Goldblatt showed that hypertension may be caused by gradual occlusion of the renal artery, it has been suspected that many instances of so-called essential hypertension in man are in fact due to the "Goldblatt kidney." Although this suspicion was confirmed by postmortem studies, it remained for the advent of arteriography to make possible the discovery of these lesions during life and the application of reconstructive arterial surgery to their cure.

Many different tests have been employed to determine whether one or both kidneys are affected. These include urographic evidence of decrease in kidney size, delay in excreting radiopaque media, split function tests, asymmetry in the radioactive iodopyracet renogram, the urea-insulin test to demonstrate decreased plasma flow and increased water absorption, and angiotensin assays. Although all these tests may be helpful, the ultimate diagnosis must come from arteriographic studies, which not only demonstrate the presence of bilateral lesions but are necessary for planning the surgical attack.

Several clinical entities have been reported, and appropriate surgical techniques for dealing with them have been delineated. Atheromatous narrowing at the origin of the renal artery is the most common lesion in the older age group and may be treated by end-

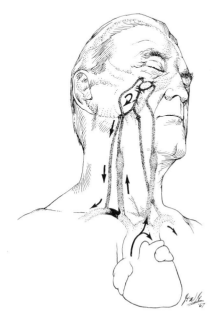

Figure 25. Subclavian steal syndrome; cerebrovascular insufficiency due to subclavian artery occlusion. Circulation to arm provided by means of reversed arterial flow through vertebral artery.

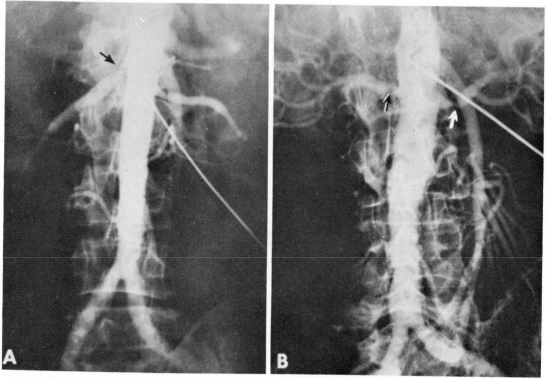

Figure 26.   *A,* Aortogram showing narrowing of right renal artery. *B,* Bilateral renal artery narrowing. (Courtesy of Dr. O. H. Trippel.)

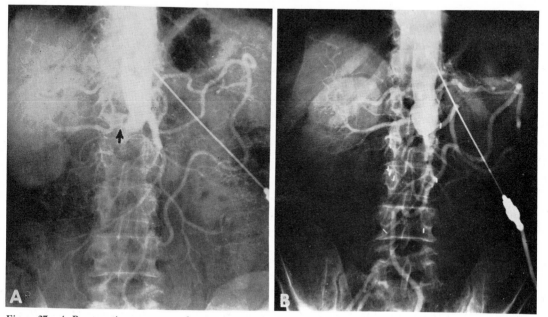

Figure 27.   *A,* Preoperative aortogram showing narrowing of right renal artery and total occlusion of aorta just below level of renal arteries. *B,* Postoperative aortogram showing reconstruction of lumen of left renal artery. Aorta was not operated upon at this stage. Silver clips remain after bilateral lumbar sympathectomy. (Courtesy of Dr. O. H. Trippel.)

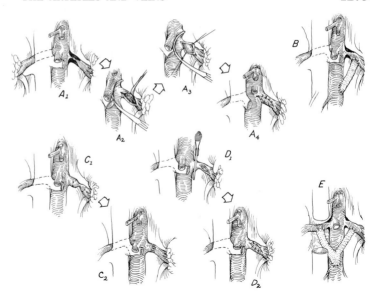

Figure 28.   Methods of restoring renal artery flow. A, Renal endarterectomy with or without patch graft. B, Aortorenal by-pass using Dacron graft. C, Excision of stricture with end-to-end anastomosis. D, Bilateral by-pass using Dacron bifurcation graft.

arterectomy and patch graft, or by a by-pass graft. Reduction in blood pressure in these patients may be obtained in about 80 per cent, although it may require a period of several weeks or even months to be seen. Achievement of a normotensive state is reached in only about 50 per cent of the patients.

Renal artery aneurysm is a less frequent cause of hypertension, and the blood pressure responds to repair of such aneurysms much as it does in instances of atheromatous occlusion. This tends to confirm the proposition that damping of pulse pressure may be more important in the genesis of hypertension than actual obstructive reduction of flow per se (Figs. 28 and 29).

In young adults, a lesion of the renal artery known as fibromuscular hyperplasia tends partially to occlude the vessel. This is a proliferative lesion of the deeper layers of the renal artery which appears as a long, irregular narrowing of the lumen, commonly extending to the trifurcation, or as a short, sharp narrow band. Since it does not lend itself to endarterectomy, it is best treated by by-pass graft or resection and reanastomosis.

In children, hypertension associated with coarctation of the abdominal aorta is accompanied by narrowing at the orifice of the renal arteries. This has been treated by by-pass grafting and by enlargement of the narrowing segment by a patch graft. The narrowing at the orifice of these aortic branches may sometimes be relieved by the release of constricting fibrous periadventitial tissue. The expected growth and life ex-

pectancy of children tends to be a contraindication to the use of grafting materials. When grafting materials must be used in these circumstances, the use of saphenous

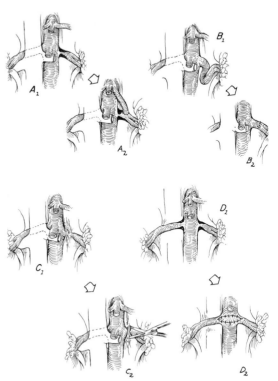

Figure 29.   Methods of restoring renal artery flow. A, Use of splenic artery for by-pass. B, Excision of kinked redundancy with end-to-end anastomosis. C, Dissection of retroperitoneal fibroplasia. D, Transaortic renal endarterectomy with aortic patch graft.

vein, either for patch or by-pass grafts, appears indicated in all young patients.

OCCLUSION OF MESENTERIC ARTERIES

Narrowing of the superior mesenteric and celiac arteries by atherosclerosis is common and is usually asymptomatic. Such lesions are found in some 33 per cent of routine autopsies. Occlusion of the superior mesenteric artery may occur acutely, as in embolic disease, or it may become critically narrowed, or gradually occluded by atherosclerotic disease. Acute occlusion superimposed upon chronic narrowing occurs when thrombosis suddenly occludes an already narrowed passage. The latter situation may result from lowering of the blood pressure due to any cause, or spontaneously when the lumen is sufficiently narrowed.

Symptoms of acute occlusion are those of intense abdominal pain, constant and unremitting between cramps, and out of proportion to abdominal findings. The abdomen may be soft or doughy to palpation. Bowel sounds are somewhat altered, but may not be absent. As the lesion progresses, the leukocyte count increases sharply and the abdomen may become more distended. Roentgenograms may be noncontributory early in the disease, but after some hours may reveal distended small intestinal loops as the abdomen becomes silent. If such a group of symptoms occurs in a patient who is fibrillating, the diagnosis of superior mesenteric artery embolism must be strongly considered. When these symptoms appear in a patient in the arteriosclerotic age group, often with evidence of occlusive disease elsewhere the diagnosis of acute occlusion or vasospasm superimposed upon chronic occlusion of the superior mesenteric artery should be entertained.

Gradual or chronic occlusion of the superior mesenteric artery, if it is symptomatic, produces symptoms consistent with a malabsorption syndrome together with postprandial pain, which has been called intestinal angina. Patients with this problem lose weight rapidly, and neoplastic disease is often suspected. The pain lasts for about an hour and disappears until the patient eats another meal. Pain may also be aggravated by emotional stress or any other stimulus of the sympathetic nervous system, for the mesenteric vessels are strongly reactive to sympathetic vasoconstrictor stimuli. Moreover, if cardiac output should become diminished for any reason, the pain may appear, and augur actual infarction of the intestine.

When the syndrome of chronic occlusion of the superior mesenteric artery occurs, arteriography may be carried out to confirm the presence of atherosclerotic narrowing. Almost invariably, the occluding plaque is found at or near the aortic origin of the vessel.

Treatment depends upon the suddenness of the occlusion and the findings at laparotomy. If the onset has been sudden, or if there is other presumptive evidence of embolism, a relatively easy surgical maneuver should be attempted. No matter how gangrenous the bowel may appear, the superior mesenteric artery is opened and a Fogarty catheter is directed proximally into the aorta. Upon distention of the small balloon at the tip of the catheter and withdrawing the catheter, the superior mesenteric flow can often be gratifyingly reconstituted as the clot is delivered. This maneuver saves an extensive dissection

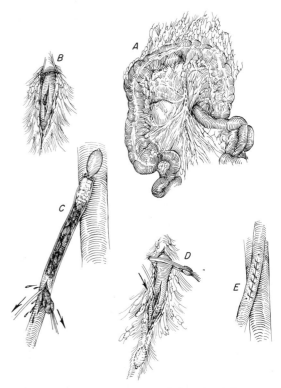

Figure 30. Mesenteric artery embolectomy. *A*, Exposure of superior mesenteric artery through mesocolon. *B*, Mesenteric arteriotomy. *C*, Cutaway diagram showing extraction of embolus and clot by distended Fogarty balloon catheter. *D*, Maneuver for removing distal thrombus. *E*, Closure of arteriotomy.

if it is successful (Fig. 30). Resection of bowel is not done at this procedure unless it is ruptured or obviously irreversibly gangrenous. As a rule, when arterial flow is resumed, the entire bowel takes on a burgundy, hyperemic appearance, and it is difficult to distinguish viable from nonviable bowel. The proper procedure is to close the abdomen and reopen it 12 to 24 hours later, at which time necessary intestinal resections can be done. Chronic occlusions of the superior mesenteric artery may be corrected by planned endarterectomy, or, occasionally, by aortomesenteric by-pass.

ANEURYSMS

When an artery progressively stretches to abnormal dimensions because of degeneration of elastic tissue in its wall, a true aneurysm results. The loss of elasticity prevents the vessel from returning to its normal size following each systolic thrust of the arterial stream. An aneurysm may be fusiform, with relatively symmetrical enlargement, or it may be saccular, with one side of the vessel wall ballooned as a bulbous protrusion.

Most true aneurysms are associated with arteriosclerosis, but they may also be caused by trauma, congenital abnormalities or syphilis. Pyogenic infections and periarteritis are infrequent causes of aneurysms. Lodgment of bacterial emboli in the wall of an artery has been known to weaken the wall and lead to aneurysmal dilatation. Since the advent of arterial reconstructive surgical procedures, another cause of aneurysms is the weakening at the suture line of end-to-side anastomoses, which may occur after several years.

The turbulence created at the periphery of the arterial stream causes deposits of platelets, fibrin and cells on the wall of the dilated channel. As a result, an aneurysm is typically lined with a laminated clot, usually leaving a flow channel not much wider than the normal channel.

A false aneurysm is a pulsating hematoma, confined by nonarterial tissue of laminated clot and endothelial cells. It is usually caused by trauma.

Arteriosclerotic aneurysms are typically fusiform, whereas syphilitic aneurysms tend to be saccular. Almost any major artery of the body may be affected by arteriosclerotic aneurysms. In the periphery, they are observed in the carotid, axillary, brachial and popliteal arteries. Intra-abdominally, they may be found in the mesenteric, renal and hepatic arteries, and in the aorta with or without involvement of the common iliac arteries. The two most frequent sites for arteriosclerotic aneurysms are the abdominal aorta and the popliteal arteries. Syphilitic aneurysms occur for the most part in the thoracic aorta.

ABDOMINAL AORTIC ANEURYSM. At the turn of the century, abdominal aortic aneurysms were rarely reported. Current statistics indicate that the incidence of abdominal aneurysm has increased both in relative and absolute frequency, with a 2 to 1 ratio in favor of abdominal aneurysm. Two reasons are offered for this finding. As syphilis has been controlled, thoracic aneurysms have decreased in frequency; and as our population has aged, the incidence of arteriosclerosis and its complications has increased. Virtually all abdominal aortic aneurysms are arteriosclerotic, and are most common in the seventh decade of life. Men are affected ten times as frequently as women.

It is not known why over 95 per cent of abdominal aneurysms are found distal to the renal arteries. A likely explanation is that turbulence distal to the celiac, superior mesenteric and renal arteries is responsible for stress upon the aortic wall, leading to degenerative changes and stretching. A tendency toward aneurysmal disease is intimated by the frequent simultaneous occurrence of abdominal, iliac, femoral or popliteal artery aneurysms.

Extension of the aneurysmal dilatation distally is somewhat variable, but it usually involves one or both common iliac arteries. Rarely does the distortion extend distal to the level of the hypogastric branch of the iliac artery. Typically, the aortic dilatation is accompanied by the pantaloon appearance of iliac artery dilatations of unequal length.

Despite the lining by a thick laminated clot, all aneurysms tend to expand in size. The rate of enlargment varies considerably, but rupture is inevitable if the patient survives long enough.

Some abdominal aneurysms grow to huge size with few or no symptoms; others cause severe pain before they have become greatly enlarged. The average symptomatic aneurysm of the abdominal aorta is over 15 cm. in diameter.

Pain may be caused by pressure on surrounding structures or by stretching of the aneurysmal wall. Another source of pain is the slow leakage of blood, causing retroperitoneal pressure. Stretching of the mesenteric root by an expanding aneurysm is excruciating, and may be accompanied by digestive symptoms. Erosion of vertebrae may occur if the aneurysm grows to large size. Low back pain varies from mild to almost unbearable severity. Pain in the presence of a palpable abdominal aneurysm and a soft abdomen can usually be taken as evidence of stretching of the aneurysmal wall, and should be looked upon with a sense of urgency because of the possibility of impending rupture.

One or both iliac arteries may become partially or completely occluded because of thrombosis or kinking at the lower end of the aneurysm, and may lead to ischemic symptoms of the legs such as intermittent claudication.

Some patients with abdominal aneurysm have referred pain in the hips or legs, often interpreted as arthritic pain. Distal embolization may be the first sign in a few patients. Occasionally, a patient discovers the pulsating mass but reports no other symptoms.

Obstruction of the third portion of the duodenum with nausea and vomiting may occur as the aneurysm gradually extends upward, compressing the duodenum against the ligament of Treitz. Other gastrointestinal symptoms may be caused by pressure on the mesenteric root. The inferior mesenteric artery becomes gradually occluded as the aneurysm grows. This ordinarily does not lead to symptoms pertinent to the left colon, except occasionally some loss of colon motility and severe constipation.

Patients with abdominal aneurysms frequently have other evidence of cardiovascular disease, most often hypertension, and commonly, a history of coronary occlusion or cerebrovascular accident.

Palpation of the abdomen confirms the presence of a pulsating mass, usually predominantly to the left of the midline, but occasionally to the right. Small aneurysms, especially in obese patients, may not be palpable. A bruit is occasionally discernible over the mass. Not all aneurysms are tender when palpated.

X-ray scout films taken in the anteroposterior and lateral planes usually confirm the diagnosis by revealing the calcific wall of the aneurysm (Fig. 31). Direct aortography is contraindicated because of the danger of initiating leakage, and is noncontributory to the management in any event.

If a patient with an abdominal aneurysm does not die from some other cause, he will

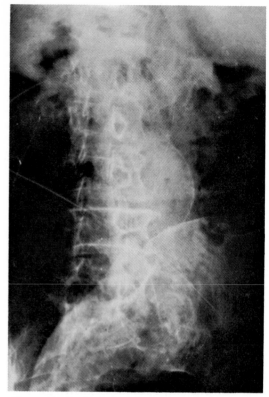

Figure 31. Configuration of abdominal aortic aneurysm with calcified wall as shown in oblique x-ray scout film.

inevitably succumb to rupture of the aneurysm. Thus, rupture is the most serious and the most common complication. The life expectancy in patients who harbor nonsymptomatic abdominal aneurysms is one year for about half of them, and there is a predictable mortality rate of 90 per cent within five years. Yet, patients have been known to harbor an almost symptomless abdominal aneurysm for up to 15 years.

When rupture is threatened, the abdominal and back pain may become excruciating, but asymptomatic rupture has been known to occur. Rupture of an abdominal aortic aneurysm need not necessarily lead to prompt exsanguination and death. Depending upon the location and extent of the leak, rupture may occur in one of several ways. If the leak is tangential and retroperitoneal, it may be controlled by tamponade of surrounding structures for a number of hours or days. The patient may not go into shock at any stage of the rupture. If the leak is anterior and near the upper portion, rupture may occur into the retroperitoneal duodenum with massive melena, shock and death. Rupture into the free peritoneal cavity also leads to rapid exsanguination. Occasionally, rupture into the vena cava creates a large arteriovenous fistula, which may be diagnosed by the loud bruit and signs of heart failure.

Operations upon aneurysms have been performed for a sufficiently long period of time to permit acceptable postoperative survival statistics to be compared with those of patients not operated upon.

Among patients with untreated aneurysms who die within five years, approximately two-thirds succumb to rupture of the aneurysm, and the remaining third to coronary occlusion, strokes and tumors.

The five-year survival rate of patients treated by elective resection and graft replacement is about 65 per cent, a figure closely approaching that of patients without abdominal aneurysms. The mortality rate following surgical intervention is now as low as 10 per cent, and in some institutions, lower. If emergency operation is done after the aneurysm has leaked or ruptured, the mortality rate is about 40 per cent, representing a significant salvage of patients with otherwise hopeless disease. From these data, it is obvious that operative intervention is indicated upon discovery of an abdominal aneurysm, whether the lesion is symptomatic or not. The only instances in which the operation may not be justified are those in which the patient has unrelated disease of such severity that prognosis is hopeless.

The operative treatment of abdominal aortic aneurysm consists of resection of the lesion and replacement of the removed portion of aorta and iliac arteries with a prosthetic graft of woven Teflon or Dacron (Fig. 32).

Resection and graft replacement of abdominal aneurysm was introduced by DuBost of Paris in 1940. Prior to this time, a number of surgical palliative procedures had been tried. These included ligation above the aneurysm, as practiced by John Hunter, the introduction of coiled wire to stimulate clot formation within the aneurysm, gradual occlusion of the aorta by polythene film wrappings, and surrounding the aneurysm with various fibroplastic materials to reinforce the wall. None of these methods was definitive, and at best, they provided only temporary cessation of growth of the aneurysm with some relief of symptoms.

In the early days of resectional operations for aneurysm, homologous aorta was used as

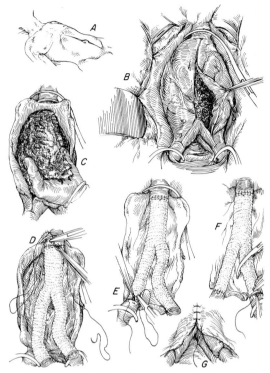

Figure 32. Resection of aortoiliac aneurysm and replacement with Dacron prosthesis. *A*, Incision. *B*, Exposure of aneurysm and incision into lumen after placement of arterial clamps. *C*, Removal of laminated clot and atherosclerotic material. *D*, Proximal anastomosis after intraluminal suture closure of lumbar artery ostia. *E*, and *F*, Distal anastomoses. *G*, Closure of aneurysm wall and posterior peritoneum over graft and suture lines.

the replacement graft. Because of the tendency toward rapid arteriosclerotic degeneration of such grafts, and the incidence of late rupture, homologous material has now given way to the exclusive use of the plastic woven prostheses.

Today, many thousands of aortic resections have been carried out. Operative hazards include hemorrhage during operation, acute occlusion of the leg arteries by thrombi or emboli, and hypotension which may lead to cardiac arrest or anuria. In our experience, gradual intermittent release of the aortic clamp after completion of the proximal anastomosis, and one iliac anastomosis, prevents profound hypotension and has made it unnecessary to administer a vasopressor drug prior to release, as has been recommended. Also, the administration of intravenous mannitol during the operation is helpful to prevent water reabsorption and thereby encourage diuresis.

Almost every surgeon who has performed a

large number of aortic aneurysm resections has encountered an occasional instance of ischemia of the descending colon after clamping and severing the inferior mesenteric artery during the resection. Often, this vessel may be sacrificed without difficulty. When ischemia occurs at surgery, it may become manifest immediately by cyanotic discoloration of the colon, necessitating resection, or it may be indiscernible, only to become evident several days after operation. In the latter case, chronic ulceration and stricture formation may ensue, with symptoms of tenesmus and melena. Ordinarily, the marginal vessel of Drummond, and the somatic retroperitoneal blood supply are sufficient to supply the left colon. Only when these vessels are absent or occluded will ligation of the inferior mesenteric artery lead to embarrassment of the vascular supply of the left colon.

Late suture line failure has been reported, especially in patients in whom arterial homografts were used. Rupture of the proximal suture line with exsanguination into the third portion of the duodenum is ascribed to insufficient interposition of soft tissue between the suture line and the duodenum. Late aneurysm formation in the graft has not been reported since the abandonment of the use of homografts.

Another rare complication of aneurysm surgery is paraplegia resulting from sacrifice of lumbar vessels arising from the aneurysm.

POPLITEAL ARTERY ANEURYSM. Most popliteal aneurysms are caused by arteriosclerosis. When a popliteal aneurysm becomes demonstrable, the patient discovers it by noting a pulsating area, or pulsating mass, behind the knee. It is associated with some discomfort and annoyance, particularly when the patient crosses his legs. Popliteal aneurysm is prone to produce some obstruction to blood flow, not only because it disturbs the pattern of flow, but because the elongation produces kinking, usually at the lower end. This may lead to intermittent claudication of the calf muscles. Pain also may be produced by compression of adjacent nerves. A long-standing popliteal aneurysm may result in a flexion deformity of the knee, because of the difficulty in extension (Figs. 33, 34 and 35).

Two main complications of popliteal aneurysm tend to occur. These are acute thrombosis and rupture of the aneurysm. When acute thrombosis occurs, it causes sudden ischemia of the extremity with rapid onset of gangrene, unless emergency treatment is successful. When rupture occurs, there is a tremendous increase in swelling because of bleeding into the tissues. The blood dissects its way in both directions: upward through Hunter's canal, filling the fascial compartments in the thigh, and downward into the calf, in the spaces between the fascia and the gastrocnemius muscles. Because the structures are firm, exsanguination rarely occurs; however, the arterial supply to the limb is embarrassed because of compression of the vessels.

Stretching and compression of the popliteal vein by the aneurysm may result in swelling and venous congestion of the lower leg, with or without arterial insufficiency.

The history of the treatment of popliteal aneurysm occupies a prominent place in every book on the history of surgery. John Hunter discovered that if surgical ligation was done above the aneurysm only, and not below, gangrene did not always ensue, since it allowed collateral channels to remain open. Early in the twentieth century, Rudolph Matas opened directly into the aneurysm, evacuated the contained clots, and sutured the inlet and outlet from within. This procedure, known as endoaneurysmorrhaphy, preserved collateral channels and further reduced the incidence of gangrene to 10 per cent. Later, Matas described a technique which restored arterial continuity by folding down the trimmed aneurysmal wall and suturing it in place to leave a lumen. The next advance in treatment consisted of combining complete resection of the aneurysm with lumbar sympathectomy. Lumbar sympathectomy is performed to improve the blood-carrying capacity of the collateral channels and to prevent spasm of adjacent arteries. There have been several series reports of combined resection and lumbar sympathectomy resulting in an incidence of zero for gangrene.

Since the advent of grafting procedures, the method of treatment has been excision of the aneurysm, followed by end-to-end implantation of a suitable prosthesis. This may consist of a vein, artery or prosthetic graft. Autogenous vein is the preferred material, because it remains pliable and does not degenerate. When resection and grafting are done, lumbar sympathectomy is considered a good ancillary procedure.

MYCOTIC ANEURYSM. Although mycotic aneurysms have not been seen in any profusion in recent years, they still occur occasionally and cause both diagnostic and therapeu-

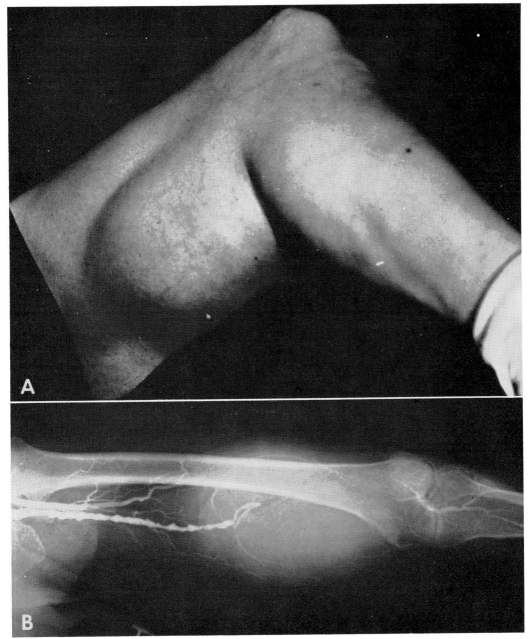

Figure 33. *A*, Clinical appearance of large popliteal aneurysm. *B*, Arteriogram of same patient, showing complete occlusion at inlet.

tic problems. The arterial wall is weakened by a bacterial infection which is carried to it by small emboli arising from vegetations on heart valves, usually associated with endocarditis. Mycotic aneurysms have been found in many locations, especially in the lower extremities. The brachial artery is most frequently involved in the upper extremity. Mycotic aneurysms have also been described in the mesenteric arteries. Special character-

istics are the extreme pain and the inflammation in the surrounding structures.

Treatment of mycotic aneurysms consists of resection and restoration of blood flow and implantation of a graft, if a major vessel is involved. Attempts should be made to discover the causative agent, if possible. However, ideal timing for surgical intervention cannot always be carried out if an extremely painful, expanding lesion is present. A culture of the removed lesion often leads to identification of the causative microorganism. Therefore, after removal of a mycotic aneurysm, cultures should be taken before the specimen is placed in preservative solution.

SYPHILITIC ANEURYSM. Syphilitic aneurysms are commonly saccular and tend to occur in the upper thoracic aorta, usually in or near the arch. They grow to compress and erode adjacent structures. Symptoms depend for the most part on pressure effects on the surrounding areas. Pain, cough, hoarseness and dysphagia are common symptoms. Dyspnea is usually due to aortic regurgitation rather than to compression of the trachea. The superior vena cava syndrome is due to impingement upon the superior vena cava by the aneurysm. This syndrome consists of plethoric cyanosis of the arms and head, with great congestion due to elevated venous pressure, especially upon bending. The pulsating mass can often be palpated through the intercostal spaces and in the sternal notch. Upper extremity pulses are usually unequal. Paralysis of one vocal cord, usually the left, and deviation of the trachea are common signs. Horner's syndrome may be present because

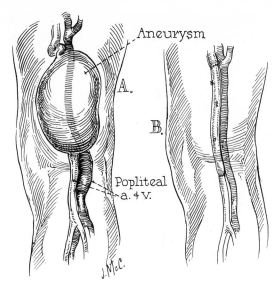

Figure 35. Typical features of large popliteal aneurysm. *A,* Note kink occlusion at proximal limb of aneurysm and dilatation of popliteal vein below aneurysm caused by pressure. *B,* Resection of aneurysm and re-establishment of continuity by end-to-end reversed vein graft.

of pressure on the upper dorsal sympathetic ganglia.

X-ray appearance of thoracic aneurysm is sometimes obvious, but must often be differentiated from mediastinal tumors. The pulsatile nature of these aneurysms is usually not marked. The x-ray findings may be complemented by angiocardiography.

Resection of all or a part of the diseased vessel wall is the only direct curative approach. There is a relatively high mortality rate in operations for syphilitic aneurysm. The best procedure is that of lateral aneurysmectomy, which consists of removal of the lateral expanded wall of the saccular aneurysm. This is done by clamping the aneurysm at its base without interfering with blood flow, and oversewing the edges left by the resection. Resection of the entire length of the involved aorta and replacement with a graft has been successfully carried out, but the procedure carries an extremely high mortality rate.

ARTERIAL INJURIES

Much knowledge was gained during World War II on the general care of a patient with a major vascular injury. During the Korean conflict and the Viet Nam military action, much more had been gained in the techniques of specific repair of arterial injuries, so

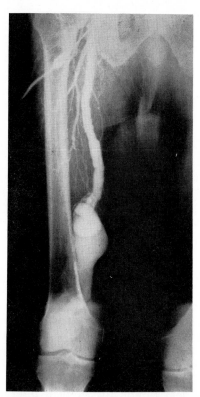

Figure 34. Arteriogram showing arteriosclerotic popliteal aneurysm with partial occlusion at inlet due to buckling.

that the combined experience to date has culminated in knowledge of proper systemic care, as well as reconstruction of arteries damaged by trauma in civilian injuries, as well as war injuries (Fig. 36).

The first goal, as with any injury, is the preservation of life, but in the presence of arterial injury, it may be necessary to consider emergency surgical intervention an integral part of resuscitation. If shock is not relieved by the administration of blood and the correction of other deficits, continuing hemorrhage must be checked by direct means. It is no longer sufficient to save the life of patients with vascular trauma. With currently available techniques, the reconstitution of normal vascularity is possible in virtually any area of the body, providing that life can be maintained until the repair is made. Special techniques of vascular repair and restoration of circulatory dynamics are applicable to different areas of the body and to different types of trauma.

INCISION OR LACERATION. An incision or laceration of a vessel without complete transection is an injury which leads to extensive bleeding, because a vessel not completely transected tends to bleed from the gape held open by retraction of the vessel. A completely transected vessel, on the other hand, is drawn back into the tissues, and its ends tend to contract. Both the tamponade and the contraction of the cut ends are factors which control bleeding.

PERFORATION. Perforations occur when a sharp instrument or a high-velocity missile transgresses the vessel. Usually, these injuries are accompanied by minimum damage to surrounding tissue, and often with only a small opening on the skin. Ordinarily, very little outside bleeding occurs. This is the type of injury which leads to pulsating hematoma and arteriovenous fistula.

CONTUSION. Contusion of an artery is caused by a blunt crushing or grinding force, or a perforating foreign body which is traveling at low speed. These injuries occur by impinging an artery against a fractured bone or some other firm object. Crushing injury damages all the coats of the wall, so that bleeding occurs between the layers of the vessel, and, as the hematoma grows, compression of the lumen follows, with obstruction and thrombosis which may extend the entire length of the lumen.

If bleeding dissects into tissue spaces or in the body cavities or viscera, the amount will depend on the tightness of the tissue and the amount of tamponade. An artery may bleed into a vein if both are perforated. It may also bleed into its own vessel wall, causing an intramural hematoma, with an absence of frank hemorrhage. Therefore, the diagnosis of arterial injury cannot depend entirely on the presence or absence of outside bleeding. For example, the only evidence of arterial injury may be ischemia of a limb, as may occur when an intramural hematoma occludes the lumen.

When an artery and a vein are injured together, a fistulous opening from the artery to the vein is established. Early diagnostic signs include a machinery-like murmur audible through a stethoscope, and a thrill palpable

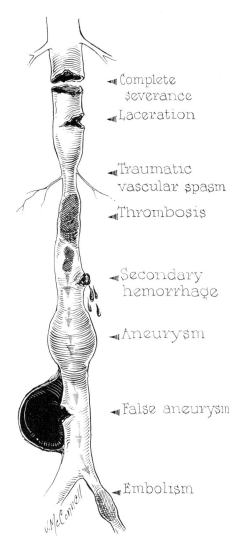

Figure 36. Composite illustration of acute lesions of arteries causing hemorrhage or occlusion.

over the site of the injury. The latter may or may not be present. Examination for palpable pulses in a region normally supplied by the artery tends to confirm the continuity of the vessel wall. Swellings, whether pulsatile or not, and the presence or absence of hemorrhagic shock, aid in the diagnosis of arterial injury.

TREATMENT OF ARTERIAL INJURIES. The treatment of arterial injuries may be divided into three stages. The first deals with control of the local bleeding by adequate pressure dressings, and the general treatment of the patient for shock. In many patients, rapid transfusion combined with immediate operation is the only practical means of treatment. Pressure dressings may be difficult to apply in areas such as the groin, axilla, base of the neck and abdomen, making early surgical intervention mandatory (Fig. 37).

The second stage of treatment consists of the restoration of blood volume, once the bleeding has been controlled. This may be done as an emergency measure by the use of plasma, dextran, gelatin or other blood substitutes. There is, however, no fully adequate substitute for whole blood. Blood transfusion should be instituted as soon as typing and cross-matching can be done.

The third stage of treatment involves definitive care of the arterial lesion. Lacerations may be repaired. It is always important to use heparin solution locally, and to use it generously in order to prevent propagation of thrombosis at the site of the repair. Patch grafts or segmental grafts are often essential in order to re-establish continuity.

Certain general principles apply to the treatment of arterial injuries and must be followed for successful results. Adequate anesthesia is used for proper muscular relaxation. Because of the possibility that delayed infection may disrupt an otherwise satisfactory suture line, infection must be prevented in every possible way. Skin preparation must be most meticulous, and the aseptic precautions taken during the operation are of great importance. Since tourniquets are seldom of any value in such procedures, the principle of control of the major vessel proximal to the site of injury must be carried out. Often, this requires an incision at some distance from the bandage before the bandage itself is removed. Usually, this is accomplished by slipping a length of cotton tape under the artery and constricting the vessel against the finger sufficiently to produce stoppage of flow. The second step consists of gaining the same type of control beyond the lesion, although this is not always essential. The wound is then unbandaged and dissected out carefully, and once the type of injury is determined, repair is carried out.

Repair may consist of simple suture of the laceration or resection and end-to-end anastomosis of the transected vessel, or it may consist of correcting any type of defect by the use of grafts. Complicated lacerations are often resected and substitute grafts inserted. The choice of grafts usually depends on what is available. Commonly used arterial substitutes are veins and prosthetic woven grafts. In most patients, the long saphenous vein is expendable and makes a very satisfactory graft substance, both for patches and for lengths of continuity. Dacron and Teflon may be used for patches, but are not usually recommended for tubular grafts below the inguinal ligament because of their tendency to stiffen. Arterial prostheses of woven plastic yarn are a great advance, but they must be used with an understanding of their properties and limitations.

When implanting a vein for continuity, it is

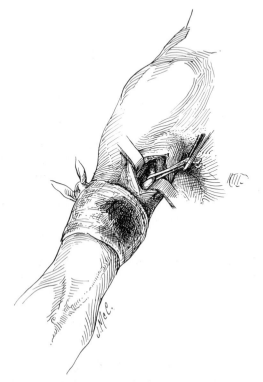

Figure 37. Proximal control of main artery before removal of hemostatic bandage in case of injury to the vessel.

important to turn the vein upside down, so that the valves will not interfere with the flow of arterial blood.

POSTTRAUMATIC REFLEX SYMPATHETIC DYSTROPHY

Posttraumatic reflex sympathetic dystrophy may occur following injury, or occasionally following operation upon an extremity. Thoracic outlet injuries following extension-flexion trauma of the neck, or avulsion trauma of the arm, often produce the symptoms.

In addition to pain, the symptoms and findings include coldness, burgundy-colored hyperemia and later, pale cyanosis and atrophy of skin. Many patients with this affliction exhibit mild edema, stiffness or palsy of digits, hyperesthesia and paresthesia. Often, trigger points can be found which, when touched, set off an exacerbation of symptoms. If allowed to persist for weeks, the syndrome may be associated with osteoporosis of bone, known as Sudeck's atrophy.

The condition cannot be correlated with the severity of the trauma, but is prone to occur in patients with a tendency toward vasomotor instability.

Treatment of milder forms of the syndrome consists of warmth, encouragement, graded exercise and physiotherapy measures such as whirlpool baths, gentle massage, and passive and active exercises.

Vasodilating drugs are said to be useful, but their effects are difficult to evaluate in the presence of other therapeutic measures. The most definitive and lasting therapeutic procedure is regional sympathetic ganglionectomy.

FALSE ANEURYSM (PULSATING HEMATOMA)

When an artery is perforated by a high speed missile or a sharp instrument, a pulsating hematoma, or false aneurysm, forms. If the surrounding tissues are resistant enough to control the extravasation of blood, a cavity is formed outside the vessel which is walled off and actually becomes surrounded by a layer of endothelium. The blood pulsates into this cavity during systole and leaves it during diastole. Occasionally, blunt injuries and tears may also cause a pulsating hematoma. A mass can usually be palpated. A thrill can usually be palpated under the examining finger, and a variety of sounds are audible with the stethoscope. These are commonly called bruits, but they have a softer swishing sound which is quite characteristic, and somewhat different from the machinery-like murmur of an arteriovenous fistula.

Surgical treatment is indicated upon discovery of the pulsating hematoma. If it remains long enough, dilatation of the artery above and below the lesion tends to occur and forms a new, extensive collateral arterial bed. It was formerly advocated that operation be delayed until collateral channels formed. However, the current method of treatment is excision and the replacement, if necessary, with a vessel graft. If the pulsating hematoma is allowed to remain, pain caused by pressure on adjacent nerves, and pressure necrosis of adjacent tissues may occur. If one has waited about a week after the initial injury, it is better to delay operation a considerable period longer, because at one week the reaction to the injury results in softening and edema of the artery wall, making the operation virtually impossible, except for wide resection and long graft insertion. For unimportant arteries, the pulsating hematoma can be removed between ligations above and below. When more critical vessels are involved, the lumen should be preserved by excision and direct repair either by end-to-end anastomosis or by interposition of a graft.

ARTERIOVENOUS FISTULA

Several types of arteriovenous fistula are recognized. The type most amenable to surgical repair is that due to trauma. When the fistulous channel is associated with a true or false aneurysm, it is known as an arteriovenous aneurysm (Fig. 38).

Congenital arteriovenous fistulas often have literally thousands of communications. These may appear as a hemangioma or as a large, warm, pulsating area on a limb with a palpable thrill or audible bruit. Congenital arteriovenous fistulas ordinarily are not amenable to surgical care, except by amputation. New channels form perpetually, even after radical resection.

Traumatic arteriovenous fistula is usually the result of penetrating injury by a high speed missile or by a stab wound. It also may occur due to rupture of arteriosclerotic aneurysm into an adjacent vein to which it has be-

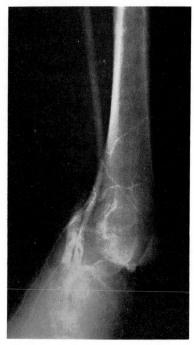

Figure 38. Late phase arteriogram showing direct filling of popliteal vein from arteriovenous fistulous connection with popliteal artery.

come adherent. A traumatic arteriovenous fistula often does not lead to much external hemorrhage. The fistula often becomes active shortly after the injury. The fistula is established when there is some organization of adjacent tissue, and a thrombus either becomes absorbed or washed away by the stream, thus freeing the opening between the artery and the vein.

Occasionally, surgical trauma will produce fistulas. This is known to occur in thyroidectomies and nephrectomies, when an artery and a vein are sutured together. Under such circumstances, a ligature erodes through the two vessels and establishes the communication. Arteriovenous fistulas have been reported occurring between the common iliac artery and the inferior vena cava following operation for herniated nucleus pulposus, when a curette is used and penetrates the annulus fibrosus anteriorly, injuring the artery and vein.

DIAGNOSIS. A continuous, machinery-like murmur can be heard through the stethoscope placed over the lesion. This murmur is caused by the continuous flow of blood from artery to vein, in which a turbulence and vibration are set up. The murmur is described as machinery-like because the pitch of the murmur is increased during the systolic phase of the pulse as the blood flows from the artery

into the vein. When this phenomenon is palpable, it imparts a buzzing sensation to the examining finger, described as a thrill.

Certain physiologic disturbances are known to accompany arteriovenous shunts. Once the shunt is well established, the venous return to the heart is increased. The pressure within the right atrium is raised and ventricular filling time is shortened, thus accelerating the pulse rate. This sequence of events can be altered by pressure directly over the fistula or proximal to it. This maneuver stops the flow through the fistula, and the pulse rate will drop immediately, producing the Branham-Nicoladoni sign.

Visible venous dilatation results from the abnormally high pressure flow from the artery into the vein. The increased flow from the arterial side produces a warming of the skin in the region of and distal to the fistula. However, at some distance distal to the shunt the skin is usually cool because of diminished pressure in the artery. Other findings are increased cardiac output and increased blood volume. Arterial blood pressure is diminished, and both the systolic and diastolic pressures tend to fall. In due course, the systolic pressure regains its former level and may even rise from there, whereas the diastolic pressure remains low, causing increased pulse pressure.

Ultimately, the increased cardiac output, increased blood volume and rapid pulse produce heart strain and consequent hypertrophy of the left ventricular wall. With patients who have had a previously normal heart, this strain does not frequently cause heart failure. However, if an arteriovenous fistula occurs in a patient who has had previous valvular heart disease or coronary occlusive heart disease, heart failure ensues quite rapidly following the establishment of the arteriovenous fistula.

TREATMENT. Two modern techniques are utilized in the treatment of arteriovenous fistula. Of these, excision with re-establishment of the circulation is the superior. The other consists of four-point ligation to exclude the fistula from the circulation (Fig. 39).

From a physiologic as well as an historical point of view, the previous methods of surgical treatment are of some interest. Matas and others discovered that, when the artery is ligated proximal to an arteriovenous fistula, severe ischemia develops in the extremity. This is due to the fact that all of the blood enters the artery from collaterals distal to the fistula, and this lower-pressure blood, flowing proximally in the distal segment, is completely

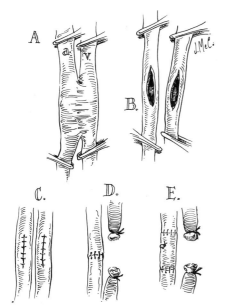

Figure 39. Reconstructive surgery of arteriovenous fistula. *A*, The lesion. *B*, Severance of arteriovenous communication with four-point control. *C*, *D* and *E*, Optional methods of repair, showing continuity repair of both artery and vein, end-to-end anastomosis of artery with ligation of vein, and vein graft to span artery defect.

diverted into the vein through the fistula, thus depriving the tissues of arterial blood supply. If distal ligation alone is performed, the amount of blood which is shunted into the vein is increased and thus the degree of heart strain is increased, leading to early heart failure. When both proximal and distal ligations are done, the physiologic results are somewhat diminished, but there may still be enough collaterals present between the ligations to shunt the arterial blood into the venous system. The ligation of the four ends of the fistula rarely produces ischemia, particularly if it is delayed for three months or more after the occurrence of the fistula. Nonetheless, because the artery is deprived of its ability to carry arterial blood to tissues, there is some disability following this procedure, depending upon the anatomic location.

Certainly, resection of the fistula and graft replacement of the artery is the preferred procedure. It is usually best to precede replacement with arterial resection in order to prevent recurrence of the fistula through collateral channels.

THROMBOANGIITIS OBLITERANS (BUERGER'S DISEASE)

Thromboangiitis obliterans is an inflammatory disease involving primarily the arteries and secondarily the veins and nerves. It is characterized by an acute phase, during which the inflammatory nature of the process is evident, and a quiescent phase in which only residual atherosclerosis is evident. Because the disease is often found in its quiescent phase, the pathologic features have often been confused with arteriosclerosis. In fact, some investigators believe that thromboangiitis obliterans is merely a premature form of arteriosclerosis obliterans. However, its inflammatory characteristics differentiate it sharply from the degenerative and metabolic characteristics of arteriosclerosis.

The condition is found most often in young men, although women are known to acquire the disease as well. Characteristically, its symptoms begin between the ages of 20 and 40 years. Primarily, it involves the lower extremities, but is also found in the arms. It may also involve vessels of the mesentery, brain and heart. It usually involves medium-sized arteries, such as the anterior and posterior tibial and the ulnar and radial, but it may also involve digital arteries.

Although Leo Buerger's name is applied to this condition, his description in 1908 was not the first. Thromboangiitis was described by von Winiwarter in 1879.

ETIOLOGY. The specific etiology is unknown, but certain possible etiologic features have been observed. Because of Buerger's classic description, it was assumed for many years that the disease had a predilection for Jewish people and people of the Mediterranean races. However, it has since been found in people of all races and types. Patients with Buerger's disease appear to have extreme sensitivity to tobacco, as well as to certain ingested foods which may induce vasospasm, including rye and certain herbs.

SYMPTOMS. The predominant symptoms of Buerger's disease are those which result from the inflammatory reactions of the condition, and are related to intense pain of nerve ischemia and the associated thrombophlebitis. It is rare for a patient with Buerger's disease to complain of claudication, as would a patient with arteriosclerosis obliterans. This is probably because the disease does not affect major channels as readily as it does the smaller vessels. It is not unusual for extensive gangrene to occur without the patient ever complaining of claudication. Acute thrombophlebitis of short segments of superficial veins of the legs, particularly those below the knee, is characteristic. The red painful lumps may migrate, healing in one place after some weeks and cropping up in another. The usual sites for these attacks of segmental thrombophlebitis are over the anterior portion of the lower extremities; less often, they occur in other parts of the body and the arms. When migrating phlebitis of this type is present, careful search for Buerger's disease should be made. This type of phlebitis is also said to occur in the presence of hidden carcinomas, usually those of the lung and pancreas.

PATHOLOGY. The microscopic appearance of the lesions of the acute stage of Buerger's disease differs sharply from those of arteriosclerosis obliterans. In the early stage, the arteries exhibit a panarteritis involving all layers in an inflammatory reaction. The early appearance of diffuse distribution of multinucleated giant cells is characteristic. The intima thickens progressively and fairly rapidly, until the lumen becomes occluded by a thrombus. From this stage on, organization and fibrosis of the entire artery proceeds, and in the end stage, the entire artery may be represented by only a fibrous cord, containing many small vascular channels. If a leg with Buerger's disease is biopsied in a number of places, many different stages of acute, subsiding and healed lesions may be demonstrated. The lesions of the superficial thrombophlebitis do not show the histologic change characteristic of the acute stage, as occurs in the arteries. Thrombosis of the veins is present without a great amount of phlebitis. However, perivascular inflammation may be extensive and may involve an entire neurovascular bundle. This accounts for involvement of sensory nerves and the production of the severe pain.

DIAGNOSIS. Arterial obliterative disease in a patient in his early forties or younger should make the examiner suspicious of Buerger's disease rather than of arteriosclerosis obliterans. Diabetes may tend to lead to premature arteriosclerosis, but this type of arterial disease does not lead to the distinctive symptoms characteristic of Buerger's disease. In patients with diabetes, the characteristic findings are those of lesions of the feet, such as excess calluses, ulcerations and osteomyelitis, whereas in Buerger's disease, the thrombophlebitis and the acuteness of the pain are more characteristic. Occasionally, one finds Raynaud's phenomenon in a patient with Buerger's disease. Typically, a patient with Buerger's disease exhibits erythema of the feet, together with a coolness of the skin, which is evidence of the special type of vaso-

spastic phenomenon accompanying this disease. The extreme pain in the acute stage is typical. The course is rather unpredictable. If the disease progresses to involve larger arteries, it is rare that a direct arterial operation can be performed because the smaller vessels beyond large vessel obstruction are also involved. The intensity of the vasospastic phenomena accompanying the acute stage may be so severe that psychic stress, cold or trauma anywhere in the body may lead to spasm, thrombosis and death of tissue. Even under good management, the disease may progress and terminate in gangrene. In other instances, regardless of treatment, the acute process subsides, and the patient is left with a variable degree of arterial insufficiency.

TREATMENT. The tendency to treat the superficial phlebitis without knowledge of the status of the arteries is a common error. Typically, the superficial phlebitis of Buerger's disease responds only poorly to elevation and treatment with heparin, in contrast to ordinary thrombophlebitis. Actually, elevation is quite painful because of the arterial insufficiency. It is important to discontinue all forms of tobacco in patients with this disease, because of their known hypersensitivity to it. Supportive care includes the treatment and prevention of infections anywhere in the body, prevention of exposure to cold, and proper rest.

During the acute stage, it is necessary that the patient be kept at bed rest with sufficient sedation to relieve the pain. Patients usually insist on keeping the leg in a dependent position, with the result that edema develops. This edema, of course, enhances the opportunity for infection to progress and healing to be slowed because of the stasis of the fluid in the tissues. The horizontal position is the optimal one. Reflex vasodilatation from a heat cradle over the lower abdomen may be of some help. Antibiotics are not useful. The acute stage appears to be greatly influenced by the psyche; therefore, every effort should be made to keep the patient in a quiescent mood and away from stress situations. Often, this requires preventing the family from visiting the patient during the acute stage. Vasodilators have not been found to be beneficial. Occasionally, amputation is required in the acute phase for patients who cannot otherwise be relieved of their ischemia and agonizing pain.

The typical appearance of a patient with acute Buerger's disease is that of one who sits in bed rocking back and forth, gently rubbing his leg between his hands. Despite the extreme degree of suffering of these patients, it is difficult to get them to stop smoking. As a matter of fact, when they do not smoke in the ward, they may be found smoking surreptitiously in the bathroom. We have seen an acute spastic phase with gangrene of both lower limbs occur following relatively minor stimuli, such as a small skin incision to biopsy a thrombosed vein in the leg.

Only the acute process subsides; the degree of insufficiency remaining must be estimated and treatment decided upon. Usually, the only treatment of any avail is lumbar sympathectomy, and, when gangrene is present, amputation. It is rare for a below-the-knee amputation to be successful in a patient with Buerger's disease. If sympathectomy is done in the acute stage, it is often followed by recurrence of symptoms after a variable period of relief. It is possible that many of the so-called reversals of effect following sympathectomy occur in patients who undergo the operation during the acute stage of Buerger's disease.

TEMPORAL ARTERITIS

This unusual affliction occurs in elderly patients and is characterized by signs referable to inflammation of one or both temporal arteries. Histologically, the artery shows granulomatous changes and evidence of granulomatous arteritis. Although the etiology of this type of arteritis is unknown, it has a predilection for branches of the carotid artery, particularly the temporal artery. Local symptoms include throbbing headache, with extreme tenderness and swelling, and often nodularity of the temporal and occasionally occipital arteries, with erythema of the overlying skin and pain in neighboring organs, such as the eyes and temporomandibular joints. Occasionally, the disease is unilateral, but it usually becomes bilateral.

Excision of the involved segment of artery usually is definitive treatment, since it relieves the local pain and is effective if the pain is localized. The combination of surgical excision plus corticosteroid therapy is considered the treatment of choice. When the disease spreads to the retinal vessels, treatment is extremely difficult, since anticoagulants, vasodilating drugs and stellate ganglion block do not seem to affect the course of the disease.

NEUROVASCULAR DISEASES

In 1862, Raynaud published a paper "On the Local Asphyxia and Symmetrical Gangrene of Extremities." He considered this condition to be a specific entity due to vasospasm alone, without a pathologic lesion. Although he included a number of patients with pathologic disease of the arteries, in addition to vasomotor disturbances, he did not recognize that the arterial disease was present.

The present-day classification of patients with hyperreactive vasoconstrictor responses places them into three main groups: those with exaggerated vasomotor responses but no primary arterial pathologic lesion; those with an underlying arterial lesion; and a group of patients who present an abnormal vasomotor response because of a traceable etiologic factor, such as scleroderma, trauma, lesions of the nerves, and poisonings with drugs such as ergot or metals such as lead. The first group has retained the name Raynaud's disease. Patients in the second and third groups are said to have Raynaud's phenomenon, attributed to arterial disease or to one of several specific etiologic agents.

In the hands and feet, the vasomotor control of blood vessels is greatest. Therefore, these areas present the most severe aberrations of the vasomotor phenomena. There is a definite sequence to these phenomena when they occur. The skin becomes white due to arteriolar and capillary spasm, and then goes through a series of changes ranging from blueness to burgundy, and finally returns to normal. This group of changes appears to be self-limited. Although the time sequence cannot be explained, the course of events is always the same. For example, why one psychic stimulus should cause dead-white blanching of parts or all of certain fingers and not others, cannot be explained; nor can the length of time the blanching remains until reactive hyperemia sets in. The theory describing the sequence of events begins with a diffuse arteriolar spasm which produces the white appearance. This, then, causes an ischemic paralysis of the arteriolar musculature, and the anoxic exhaustion leads to a state of dilatation. The venous end of the capillary bed tends to dilate first, and this allows backfilling and gradual opening of capillaries, causing the initial cyanotic color. Then, as the arterial blood is admitted from the arterioles, the dilated capillaries are flushed with red blood, and the burgundy rubor results. After a few more minutes, the capillary walls become well oxygenated and normal tonus is re-established.

RAYNAUD'S DISEASE. At least 80 per cent of patients with this disease are young women between puberty and 40 years of age. These patients are frequently emotionally labile and tend to be rather intelligent but usually sexually frustrated. The sequence of vasomotor responses usually is seen first in the hands. When exposed to cold or emotional stress, the hands, fingers or parts of the fingers go through the changes described above.

Early in the disease, a part of one finger may be involved, and later on more parts, until, occasionally, the entire hand may be blanched with the vasomotor response. In contrast to Raynaud's phenomenon, Raynaud's disease is strongly bilateral and rather symmetrical. When the blanched stage appears, there is numbness in the part and a feeling of deadness. Between attacks, the parts are quite normal, and the condition progresses until the series of events occurs more frequently. Actual ischemic necrosis does not make itself evident until years after the affliction has been present. When necrosis occurs, it is in the form of black dots the size of pin heads or match heads at the tips of the fingers. As the areas heal, they become depressed scars. Pain is present while the ischemic and necrotic areas are present. Typically, all palpable pulses of the extremities remain undisturbed. As the years progress, skin of the fingers and hands becomes excessively dry and coarsened. The finger tips acquire a tapered appearance as the subcutaneous fat at the tips atrophies, and the finger nails grow very slowly. The skin also acquires a waxy appearance, similar to that of scleroderma.

The general management of patients with Raynaud's disease may well fall into the area of psychotherapy. However, results have not been satisfactory with this mode of therapy. Avoidance of exposure to cold is important. All of the usual vasodilator drugs have been used and have not been found to be of any lasting value. It might be thought that removing the anatomically applicable sympathetic ganglia would be curative. In some 40 per cent of the patients in whom regional sympathectomy has been employed, dramatic permanent relief has resulted. Lack of complete cure by sympathectomy indicates that some local vascular sensitivity is responsible for the condition. As a result, sympathectomy is reserved for patients with severe symptoms, particularly those with the small areas of necrosis at the tips of the fingers. No cure is known.

RAYNAUD'S PHENOMENON. Exactly the same series of events occurs in this condition as is seen in Raynaud's disease, except that the phenomenon can occur in any type of person. It may be unilateral, and it is usually traceable to a specific cause. It may occur in people of all ages, depending upon the inciting lesion. When Raynaud's phenomenon occurs in one extremity, it is obviously differentiated from Raynaud's disease. However, occasionally, it occurs bilaterally, and then the cause must be determined. Some of the more frequent causes are arteriosclerosis and trauma. Other causes are scalenus anticus syndrome, food or drug poisonings, blood dyscrasias, cervical arthritis, and cervical disk syndrome. Loss of pulses and, perhaps, more extensive evidence of gangrene indicates that the causative agent is arterial disease. Pain is usually a more prominent symptom of Raynaud's phenomenon than it is of Raynaud's disease. Scleroderma as a primary disease frequently is accompanied by Raynaud's phenomenon. This has led to some confusion on the relationship between Raynaud's disease, Raynaud's phenomenon, and scleroderma, especially since sclerodermatous changes may follow long-standing Raynaud's disease. Thus, sclerodermatous change in Raynaud's disease is a late feature; when it occurs before or during the edematous stage, it is considered to be part of Raynaud's phenomenon.

Patients with Raynaud's phenomenon respond specifically to upper thoracic sympathectomy. Every effort should be made to determine and eradicate the etiologic agent.

SCLERODERMA

Sclerodermatous changes in the skin of digits may be a late sequel to Raynaud's phenomenon and Raynaud's disease. But primary scleroderma of either the localized or generalized type may occur as an initial disease in which the skin becomes waxen and taut, the subcutaneous tissue becomes atrophic and the blood vessels exhibit characteristic changes. Thickening and hyperplasia of intimal cells and thickening of the fibrous tissue component of the arterial wall may become severe enough to cause occlusion. Thrombi are also noted. The vessels chiefly affected are those of the digits.

Early in the disease the sclerodermatous changes are gradual, with only tenseness and stiffness in the fingers. If Raynaud's disease or Raynaud's phenomenon are part of the syndrome, the blanching phenomenon may occur in relatively warmer environments than without scleroderma. The course from this point on determines the prognosis. The sclerodermatous changes may progress to involve the dorsum of the hands and forearms, and eventually the face and chest. In severe cases, the sclerosis of the skin and subcutaneous tissues extends to the toes, feet and legs, and later may involve the entire surface of the body, including some mucous membranes. The bland, expressionless facies of scleroderma, with thin puckered lips, leads to baring of incisors due to contraction of the lips.

Gangrene of finger tips is more extensive than in Raynaud's disease, involving part or all of the distal phalanx, or more. Internal changes depend upon the length of survival. These changes include esophageal shortening and stiffening with dysphagia, pulmonary fibrosis and other organ involvement. Typically, death is caused by aspiration pneumonia and heart failure.

Treatment with cortisone and adrenocorticotropic hormone has been used, and temporary improvement reported. Sympathectomy may yield temporary relief early in the disease.

THORACIC OUTLET SYNDROME

The symptoms caused by cervical ribs are induced by pressure on the subclavian artery and trunks of the brachial plexus. Short ribs are more likely than others to cause pressure on the brachial plexus, while long ones produce compression on the subclavian artery. Actually, the artery is caught between the scalenus anticus muscle and the cervical rib causing the compression.

The symptoms with or without cervical rib can be divided into those due to irritation and compression of the brachial plexus and those secondary to disturbed physiology of the subclavian artery and its peripheral branches. The most common and characteristic symptoms are pain and paresthesia in the involved extremity. Later, muscular atrophy, motor weakness, disturbances in sensation and

symptoms of circulatory insufficiency may develop. There may be uncomfortable tingling, with severe lancinating pain. Usually, supraclavicular tenderness is pronounced on pressure over the scalenus anticus muscle, which causes extension of pain down the ulnar side of the arm. The pain frequently is aggravated by turning the head toward the affected side, with the neck extended, and by deep inspiration. Vascular manifestations consist of diminution of the pulse on the affected side, decrease in surface temperature, numbness, coldness and formication. Sympathetic stimulation may be responsible for these vasomotor disturbances. Early vascular changes are best determined by oscillometrigrams with the Tycos recording sphygmomanometer. Determinations should be made on both arms and forearms before and after block of the cervicothoracic sympathetic nerves with procaine.

Simple sectioning of the scalenus muscle through a small incision above the clavicle relieves pressure on the artery, and in many patients relieves all of the symptoms. How-

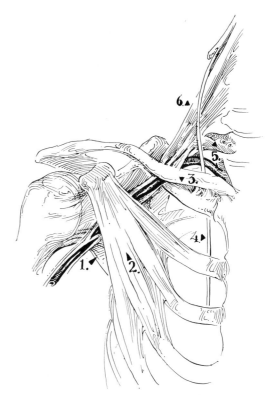

Figure 40. Structures participating in the thoracic outlet syndrome: *1*, subscapularis muscle; *2*, pectoralis minor muscle; *3*, clavicle; *4*, phrenic nerve; *5*, first thoracic rib or seventh cervical rib; and *6*, scalenus anticus muscle. (Adapted from Hughes, E. S. R.: Brit. J. Surg. 36:155, 1948.)

ever, a certain percentage of patients suffer from an aneurysm distal to the point of constriction. Some of these patients require resection of this aneurysm and graft replacement. When an aneurysm occurs, thrombi are formed within it and are cast distally as emboli. Occasionally, it is necessary to perform embolectomy or thrombectomy, in addition to a grafting operation at the site of the resected aneurysm. Also, it is sometimes necessary to perform a cervicothoracic sympathectomy, combined with anterior scalenotomy, because of the existence of marked vasospasm in the arteries of the extremities, or because of marked arterial insufficiency.

CAROTID SINUS SYNDROME

Pressure on the area of the carotid artery bifurcation causes dizziness, faintness and convulsions in susceptible people. If the pressure is strong enough to obliterate the pulse momentarily, the syndrome can occur upon release of pressure and activation of the carotid sinus by the sudden distention of the resuming flow. In normal persons, pressure at this point causes only a slight bradycardia and a fall in blood pressure of less than 10 mm. Hg. Hyperactivity of the reflex can be produced by drugs such as digitalis and opiates. More often, a unilateral hyperactive carotid reflex becomes manifest by turning the head suddenly, hyperextending the neck or wearing a stiff collar.

The carotid sinus is a plexus of nerve fibers receiving afferent branches from the ganglion nodosum of the vagus nerve and the glossopharyngeal nerve, and receiving efferent fibers from the superior sympathetic ganglion.

The full-blown syndrome may appear with or without the presence of a tumor of the carotid body. The tumor, when present, can usually be palpated in the area of the carotid bifurcation. Several patients have been reported in whom carotid body tumors gave evidence of being malignant, insofar as they metastasized to the mediastinum.

Treatment of a hyperactive carotid reflex consists of a trial with atropine or its derivatives. If this does not afford relief of attacks, carotid sinus denervation is carried out under local anesthesia. Postural hypotension may follow bilateral procedures. Removal of carotid body tumors, identified as chemodectomas, can usually be done without damage to the carotid artery or its branches. If the tumor is firmly attached to the vessel and the vessel is opened, arterial repair, usually with patch graft, is recommended rather than ligation.

ERYTHROMELALGIA

The term erythromelalgia, first suggested by S. Weir Mitchell, indicates a red, painful extremity. The direct cause of the spontaneous attacks of burning distress appears to be vasodilatation. Increased blood flow, however, is only an indirect and not an integral part of the mechanism causing the distress. Erythromelalgia primarily affects children, but adults of both sexes are also affected. Although the distress may be localized in a small portion of the foot, usually both the hands and feet are involved. The distress comes on either while the patient is walking or after he has gone to bed at night and is under the covers. The distress is usually aggravated by warmth and is especially noted during the summer months.

Primary erythromelalgia occurs in an otherwise healthy person without detectable organic disease of the nerves or vascular system. Secondary erythromelalgia usually is a symptom of vascular disease, occurring particularly with hypertension or polycythemia vera. It may also occur in gout, neurologic disease or metal poisonings.

Relief is obtained by exposing the affected part to cool air or by immersing it in cool or ice water. Various methods of treatment have been advocated, including Dibenzyline and injection of epinephrine. When simple measures fail, it may be necessary to section or crush the posterior tibial, peroneal or sural nerves.

ACROCYANOSIS

Painless, persistent coldness and cyanosis of the hands or feet, or both, is termed acrocyanosis. It occurs at ordinary environmental temperatures. In contrast to Raynaud's phenomenon, there are no episodes of blanching, nor do trophic changes, scleroderma or gangrene occur. Edema may occur in cold environments, accompanied by some tenderness.

The etiology and pathology of this syndrome are obscure. The venules appear dilated and the metarterioles constricted, but these findings are inconstant. Excessive sympathetic tone has been implicated as a likely etiologic factor.

An interesting observation of Day and Klingman is that, during sleep, the skin re- turns to a normal color and responds nor- mally to changes in external temperature. If the symptoms become severe, sympathectomy is indicated, with prospects of an excellent result.

The Veins

When man assumed an upright posture his venous system, at best a relatively inefficient conduit system, became subject to added burdens. The veins serve as little more than channels to return blood to the heart. Pro- pulsion of blood through veins depends pri- marily upon what force remains after arterial blood has passed through the capillary bed. Venous flow is assisted by such auxiliary measures as the sucking action of respiration, skeletal muscle contraction, the valves and gravity, except in the lower portion of the body where gravity hinders venous flow. These aids to venous circulation have not prevented the venous system of man from falling heir to the consequences of stagnant flow. When extraneous influences such as injury, infection and obstruction to flow are superimposed, the veins and the spent, poorly oxygenated blood they carry become ready ground for pathologic alteration.

Although the most common surgical opera- tions for the treatment of diseases of veins continue to be vein ligations and strippings for varicose veins of the legs, technical de- velopments of the past decade have resulted in a variety of rehabilitative and lifesaving operations on veins. These include venous thrombectomy, vena caval ligation or plica- tion, and pulmonary embolectomy. Still in an experimental stage are venous grafting and construction or replacement of venous valves.

ANATOMY AND PHYSIOLOGY

In the extremities and mesentery, the veins are more or less paired with the arteries. This relationship is not constant throughout the body, for in the liver, cranium and chest, the veins and arteries run independent courses. The muscular coat of veins is considerably thinner than that of arteries, and possesses neither the contractile power nor strength of artery muscle. Consequently, spasm in veins, though it does occur, is not extreme. Disten- tion may become marked with moderate in- creases in venous pressure. Persistently elevated venous pressure can overstretch and attentuate the muscular coat of vein walls to such an extent that the muscle loses its homeostatic ability to resume normal tonus. The result may be irreversible ballooning and tortuosity. Alterations in the vein wall itself may weaken its structure.

The veins of the extremities contain valves, whereas those of the abdomen, thorax and cranium do not. Venous valves are arranged in such a way that blood flows past them to- ward the heart. They are cupshaped, with their concave face pointing proximally. Their function apparently is to prevent backflow under sudden increases in venous hydro- static pressure, and to aid in the directional flow of blood when venous pressure falls to low levels. Valves are located rather irregu- larly along the main stem veins, but invari- ably occur at the branching sites between deep and superficial vein systems in the ex- tremities.

The deep and superficial sets of veins in the leg bear special consideration, since their differences and their relationship with each other may be the background for disabling disease. The superficial, saphenous system lies between the deep fascia and skin, sur- rounded only by weak superficial fascia and a variable amount of subcutaneous fat. The deep femoral vein system is housed in muscu- lar compartments, or fascial spaces. The two systems connect at two main points, in the groin, and in the popliteal space. Valves exist at these junctions. The two systems are also connected by a number of perforating, or communicating veins, each containing valves, as well as by many smaller anasto- motic veins. Thus, blood flowing from the toes to the heart has many alternate routes of flow. Communications between the deep and superficial venous systems of the leg are most numerous in the foot, less in the calf and least in the thigh.

The great saphenous vein runs the entire length of the leg from foot to groin. Its course is along the medial aspect of the leg at the ankle, anterior to the medial malleolus; it ascends posteromedially behind the medial condyle of the femur, then directly to the fossa ovalis of the superficial fascia inferior to the inguinal ligament. It dips medially and deep to join the femoral vein. Branches at or near the saphenofemoral junction are of surgical importance, since all must be recognized and divided in order that excision of the great saphenous vein for varicosities will not be followed by recurrence of the condition. As a rule, five branches with or without variations are seen. These are the superficial inferior epigastric vein, which ascends from the junction to run in a cephalad direction; the superficial circumflex iliac vein, which takes an obliquely lateral course; the superficial external pudendal vein, which runs medially; and the medial and lateral femoral cutaneous veins, which take an obliquely downward course. Variations on this basic anatomic pattern may be extreme, and as many as 12 or more branches may be found.

The lesser saphenous vein collects superficial venous drainage from the lateral malleolar area and posterolateral region of the calf and ascends to the popliteal space, where it dips below a strong layer of the superficial fascia to join the popliteal vein.

Neither the great nor the lesser saphenous vein is accompanied by arteries.

The deep veins of the leg, on the other hand, are paired with arteries. The anterior and posterior tibial veins approach the midline as they ascend in the leg and join approximately in the posterior midline to form the popliteal vein behind the knee. The popliteal vein perforates the adductor magnus muscle to reach the adductor canal, at which point it is known as the femoral vein or superficial femoral vein. The femoral vein and artery are closely associated in the remainder of their cephalad course, the vein lying lateral and posterior to the artery in the lower thigh, and medial to it at the inguinal area.

The profunda femoris, or deep femoral vein, collects blood from the deep thigh muscles and emerges to join the superficial femoral vein about an inch and a half below the inguinal ligament. The profunda femoris vein has generous anastomotic connections with the branches of the inferior gluteal vein above and popliteal vein below.

Above the juncture of the deep and superficial femoral veins, the common stem is known as the common femoral vein. As it dips behind the inguinal ligament, it becomes the external iliac vein. In the pelvis, it is joined by the internal iliac or hypogastric vein to form the common iliac vein. The latter joins its opposite fellow to form the inferior vena cava.

Normally, venous pressure in the lower extremity is highest upon standing and lowest when the legs are elevated. Under normal circumstances, after an initial slight rise, it drops precipitously during walking. The motion undoubtedly has a milking effect which aids in emptying the veins. In the presence of incompetent valves, the standing pressures are higher than normal and walking causes no drop or only a moderate drop. Actual reversal of flow has been demonstrated in some individuals with varicose veins.

The two main diseases of veins are varicosities and thrombophlebitis. It is of more than passing interest that these diseases often occur together as interdependent cause-and-effect entities, although they may appear independently.

VARICOSE VEINS

Varicose veins appear as tortuous, dilated distortions of otherwise relatively straight veins. Varices may appear in several areas of the body. The commonest types, aside from those of the lower extremities, are esophageal varices, usually resulting from portal hypertension; varices of the spermatic veins; dilatation of the inferior hemorrhoidal veins; varices of the broad ligament, urinary bladder and prostatic venous plexus; and varices of the central nervous system.

INCIDENCE. Various estimates of the incidence of varicose veins have been made. In general, it probably can be said that about 10 per cent of all adults over 35 years of age have some degree of varicose change in their saphenous venous system.

ETIOLOGY. The fundamental defect responsible for varicosities in the legs is probably incompetence of the valves in the connecting veins between the superficial and deep venous systems (Fig. 41). When incompetent, the valves no longer prevent backflow and thus allow blood with a greater than normal pressure-head to fill the superficial system. Important factors in the etiology of varicose veins are heredity, increased postural strain, trauma, compression or constriction of veins and phlebitis of the deep venous system.

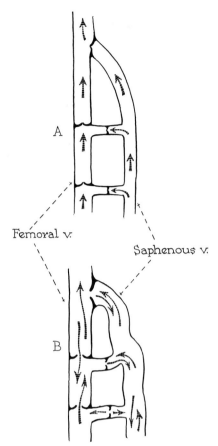

Figure 41. Schematic representation of venous blood flow in superficial and deep veins of the legs. *A*, Normal relationship. Competent valves permit blood to flow only proximally and only from superficial to deep veins. *B*, Incompetent valves allow reversal of flow, from deep to superficial veins, causing the latter to dilate and become tortuous. Valves in deep vein may remain competent.

Congenital weakness of veins appears to be a familial tendency. One can often find the same defect in one or both parents. The offspring of parents with varicosities tend to develop varicosities at a young age. In addition to familial, or perhaps congenital, weakness of vein walls, other etiologic factors may be endocrine, or even chemical, changes.

Prolonged standing is said to produce enough undue strain to cause varicosities. However, examination of people who might be predisposed by their occupations does not show a higher incidence of varicose veins in this group than in any other segment of the population.

Other factors tending to increase venous pressure in the legs include constricting garters, enlarged lymph nodes and pelvic tumors. The relatively high incidence of symptomatic varicose veins during pregnancy has aroused curiosity regarding a possible rela-

tionship. Occasionally, the most severe symptoms occur in the early stages of pregnancy, long before the growing uterus reaches its greatest size. This observation has led to the speculation that an endocrine factor may produce weakness of the vein walls. However, the congestion within the pelvis during the early stages of pregnancy may more than offset the relatively small size of the uterus as a pressure phenomenon.

The superficial venous system of the leg is less able to cope with the stress of increased hydrostatic pressure than is the deep system, since it lies relatively unsupported in the subcutaneous tissue. Venous flow through the deep system is aided by the support of relatively strong tissues, such as muscle and fascia, and by the contractions of the muscles. Undue increases in hydrostatic pressure tend to follow paths of least resistance. Increased femoral vein pressure is transmitted through communications to the superficial veins of the leg. The valves at these junctions give way and become incompetent, and the disproportionately high pressures in the poorly supported saphenous system may lead to tortuosity.

So-called secondary varicosities may follow by months or years the development of deep vein thrombophlebitis. A greater load of venous blood than is normal is shunted into the superficial venous system following blockage of the deeper veins and the ensuing incompetence of their valves after recanalization.

PATHOLOGY. Microscopic examination of the dilated, tortuous, thinned-out veins reveals areas of muscular hypertrophy interspersed with areas of remarkable thinning of the vein wall. Fibrosis is widespread. Low-grade inflammatory changes are frequent. Phlebosclerosis, with actual calcium deposition as a sequel to fibrosis, is a rather common finding, even in relatively young patients.

Occasionally, the venous stasis is carried into the tiny intradermal radicals. When this occurs, so-called spider burst or spider web varicosities are seen in the skin. Microscopic examination reveals these areas to be tortuous enlargements of the subpapillary plexus of intradermal veins.

Arteriovenous fistulas, particularly of the minute multiple type, are often associated with varicosities and have been ascribed an etiologic role in certain cases.

SYMPTOMS. Great disparity often exists between the clinical appearance of varicose veins and the symptoms they produce. Thus, patients with minimal varicosities might have severe symptoms, while some with markedly tortuous veins have minimal or no symptoms. As a rule, the early symptoms are heaviness, drawing sensations and cramping, particularly in the region of veins, and especially while standing. Pain is a variable symptom and most often occurs in conjunction with localized areas of thrombosis. However, it may occur in the absence of thrombosis and may be accentuated by pressure or by the presence of a cluster of varices. The most severe symptoms are due to the complications of varicose veins such as dermatitis, ulceration and superficial thrombophlebitis. Curiously, symptoms may be more severe in the earlier, developmental stages of varicose veins than later.

DIAGNOSIS. Because patients with varicose veins often have other infirmities of middle age, symptoms are often erroneously ascribed to the veins. On examination, static deformities, arthritis, sciatic neuritis, myositis and arterial system symptoms may be the actual cause of the symptoms present in a patient who has varicose veins. Patients often express great disappointment when symptoms do not disappear upon removal of the varicose veins. Thus, careful history taking and physical examination are important. A complete physical examination should accompany every local examination for varicose veins to search for constitutional diseases, infectious diseases, peripheral arterial disease and abdominal tumors.

Observation of the legs should begin with the patient standing. Once the extent and location of the varicose veins have been determined, it is traditional to perform the Trendelenburg test and Perthes' test.

The Trendelenburg test is made to determine the location of incompetent valves in the saphenous and communicating veins (Fig. 42). With the patient sitting or lying, the leg is elevated above the level of the pelvis so that the superficial veins empty by gravity, assisted by upward massage by the examiner's hand. Compression is then made over the fossa ovalis in the groin, either by the examiner's fingers or by a tourniquet, in order to compress the saphenofemoral junction. The patient is then asked to stand. If the saphenofemoral valve is the sole source of the incompetency, the veins will remain empty for a minute or two before filling slowly from below. Removal of the compressing fingers or tourniquet before complete filling permits rapid filling from above. Rapid filling from below in

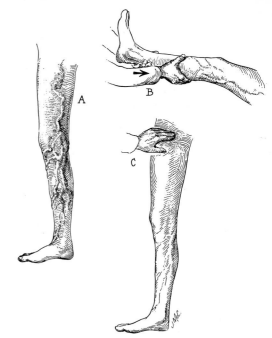

Figure 42. Trendelenburg test. *A*, Incompetent great saphenous vein with marked varicosities. *B*, Leg elevated above level of pelvis to empty veins. Emptying aided by gentle upward massage. *C*, Occlusion of saphenofemoral junction by examiner's fingers; veins remain relatively empty when patient stands; refill rapidly from above when hand is removed.

the presence of the pressure indicates incompetence of one or more perforating veins below the level of the constriction. The site of the incompetency can be found by repeating the maneuver with the tourniquet placed at various lower levels. The short saphenous vein may be a contributing, or the sole source of the varicosities. Incompetency of the valve at the junction of the short saphenous and popliteal veins can be tested by a similar method at that level.

Perthes' test is performed in order to determine the patency of the deep venous system. The test is carried out by constricting the saphenous trunk in the thigh by use of a tourniquet. The patient is asked to exercise his leg by kicking it vigorously back and forth, or by walking about the room. With exercise, blood normally is routed into the deep veins, causing the varicosities to empty. If the deep veins are not patent, or if there is increased hydrostatic pressure in the deep veins, the varicosities will not diminish in size. Perthes' test is not of much practical value in most instances because the deep veins are almost never blocked so completely that some channel will not be available for the flow of venous blood.

Several other tests have been devised to locate the position of incompetent perforating veins. However, most of these tests are of little more than academic interest to the surgeon. In the present-day surgical approach to the problem, the entire main stem is usually eradicated by stripping. Thus, all perforating branches are interrupted where they join the great saphenous vein and their exact location is not crucial.

COMPLICATIONS. So-called varicose ulcer occurs characteristically in the lower third of the leg or in the area of the malleoli. Almost without exception, a varicose ulcer appears directly over a vein. For this reason, its pathogenesis has been ascribed to periphlebitis which occurs as a sequel to localized phlebitis. The inflammatory reaction about the vein is said to choke off the nutrient blood supply to that portion of the skin. When such an area of skin is irritated by trauma, it does not heal normally. Instead, the tissue may break down and ulcer formation results. Therefore, varicose ulcer is not due to varicose veins alone, for, if it were, ulcers would occur in other areas of the legs where varicosities may be more extensive. Nor is stasis alone responsible, since ulcers rarely occur on the foot. The relatively poor blood supply to the skin in the area above the malleoli and the characteristic location of an ulcer directly over veins in this area are factors responsible for the phlebitis concept. As a rule, varicose ulcers occur more readily in limbs which have been previously afflicted with deep vein thrombophlebitis, complicated by chronic circulatory changes in the skin.

Although edema is not always a characteristic sequel to otherwise uncomplicated varicose veins, it occurs in a large number of the patients. The examiner must be careful to exclude the possibility of systemic causes of ankle edema if the condition is bilateral. Edema which occurs with otherwise uncomplicated varicose veins tends to be accentuated toward the end of the day and to subside with elevation of the limb. If the edema is associated with pain and with shiny skin and tenderness of tissue, one should suspect deep vein occlusion or thrombophlebitis.

Rupture of varicosities may take place with loss of considerable blood. This may occur without warning, particularly in patients who have superficially placed varicosities. In such individuals, the veins have a deep blue color and are covered only by a thinned layer of dermis. Such simple activities as crossing the legs may result in bleeding, first noticed by a surprisingly large flow of blood down the leg, without pain. Such bleeding is usually easily controlled by elevation of the limb and the application of a pressure bandage.

Thrombophlebitis is a relatively frequent complication of varicose veins. Local areas of thrombophlebitis of the superficial veins are probably more the result of stasis and trauma than of bacterial invasion. The usual clinical appearance is that of a painful, red, tender area of the skin overlying a firm segment of vein. Such involvement may vary from a low-grade inflammatory reaction to a severe suppurative type of lesion with systemic septic phenomena. As a rule, inflammatory types of thrombophlebitis in superficial veins do not produce embolism.

Varicose dermatitis varies from the leathery, scaly discoloration so often seen in patients with long-standing varicose veins to an acutely inflammatory, red, itching, burning type of lesion. The dermatitis is usually located over the lower third of the limb. The lesion has been termed varicose eczema, and may be due in some cases to allergic phenomena. Secondary pyogenic or fungal invasion is not uncommon.

TREATMENT. The treatment of varicose veins can be divided into nonoperative and operative measures. The nonoperative treatment is reserved for patients who for some reason cannot withstand operation and for those whose involvement is minimal. When operation cannot be undertaken, wearing elastic stockings from toes to groin offers symptomatic palliation. They compress the superficial veins and shunt venous flow through the deep veins. When the veins are minimal and consist only of an occasional small, tortuous twig in the absence of a positive reaction to the Trendelenburg test, such a small segment can usually be obliterated by the injection treatment.

Injection treatment consists of the injection of a sclerosing solution directly into the vein. This mode of treatment is usually temporary. There are some definite contraindications to injection treatment. Veins which are large, distended and extensive either become extremely tender, red, and painful after injection, or do not respond at all. Injection treatment should not be carried out in the presence of an acute upper respiratory infection, uncontrolled diabetes, local ulcers or inflammation or advanced arterial disease of the legs. It should be avoided if the patient has a history of cardiovascular accident. A few deaths from embolism following the injection treatment of varicose veins have been reported. An obvious criticism of this form of treatment is that it only obliterates the immediately visible segment, and there is no assurance that the obliterated vein will not become re-canalized. In the presence of a positive reaction to the Trendelenburg test, the sclerosing treatment of veins is of no value, since the main stem is incompetent. Also, when the varicosities are secondary to deep vein disease, this type of treatment is worthless.

Today, the greatest usefulness of the injection treatment lies in the postoperative period, at which time small remaining varices may be obliterated if they persist after main-stem stripping.

A wide variety of solutions have been used, including hypertonic glucose solutions and alkaline soap solutions, such as sodium morrhuate, sodium ricinoleate and sodium tetradecyl sulfate. They act by producing a local thrombus.

Injections are made with the patient standing and with no tourniquet on the leg. Care must be exercised not to allow any of the irritating solution to reach the perivenous tissues. If this occurs, a painful irritation may be set up, which may lead to sloughing of the skin. Injections are usually made no more often than a week apart.

Surgical treatment for varicose veins consists in the ligation and separation of the great saphenous vein at the saphenofemoral junction, ligation and severance of all the branches arising from this area of the saphenous vein, and removal of the entire length of the great saphenous vein from the groin to the ankle. If indicated, the lesser saphenous vein at its juncture with the popliteal vein behind the knee is similarly ligated and stripped. Separate incisions may have to be made to remove clusters of veins which are only indirectly connected with the main stream. Only by such a complete maneuver can one expect to remove most of the involved veins as well as the main, incompetent channels. An electrical coagulator can be used during a stripping operation to obliterate extensive branchings. If new, small varicosities should appear in the months following, these may be injected or excised. Despite this radical type of treatment, a few patients, particularly those with secondary varicosities pursuant to deep vein thrombophlebitis, will have recurrences.

A most important feature of surgical treatment is patient, long-term follow-up, so that new varicosities may be treated appropriately.

PHLEBOTHROMBOSIS AND THROMBOPHLEBITIS

As the name implies, thrombophlebitis is a composite disease consisting of thrombosis of blood within a vein and inflammatory involvement of the vein wall. A wide variety of types exists, depending upon degree of severity, extent of involvement, anatomic location and amount of inflammatory reaction.

The problem of thrombophlebitis is an important one, not only because of its local effects, but because of the propensity for portions of the venous clot to break off and travel back to the heart and into the pulmonary artery. The result may be pulmonary infarction or death from pulmonary embolism. This phenomenon, known as thromboembolism, unfortunately is still as prominent a cause of death today as it was before the advent of modern advances in treatment and prevention. The inability to recognize the existence of bland thrombosis in the lower limbs early enough and the ever-increasing success in operations upon poor-risk patients probably keep the incidence high. Bland thrombosis, or "silent" thrombosis, originally described by Homans in 1934, has been termed phlebothrombosis by Ochsner and DeBakey. The most usual site for this type of thrombosis is the deep veins of the legs.

ETIOLOGY AND PATHOGENESIS. In the earliest stages of bland thrombosis, a fresh clot appears in a vein which otherwise may exhibit no obvious changes. Many theories have been devised to explain this occurrence, some based upon sound experimental or clinical evidence, others deduced from known applicable facts.

Most instances of venous thrombosis in the lower extremities occur without a demonstrable precipitating factor. Possible causative factors may be divided into three main groups: local vessel changes, such as intimal damage; venous stasis; and changes in the coagulating properties of the blood.

It is plausible to suspect that intimal damage due to local injury or disease in the vein wall is a likely cause of bland thrombosis (Fig. 43). While extensive studies of the veins of patients dying of thromboembolism do not appear to bear out this concept, experimental thromboses can be produced by deliberate intimal damage.

Venous stasis has long been suspected as an etiologic influence in phlebothrombosis. Supportive evidence for this relationship has been provided by close examination of fresh,

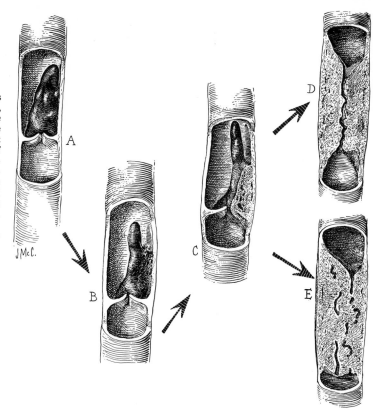

Figure 43. Natural history of venous thrombosis in lower extremity. *A,* Fresh clot forming on proximal surface of valves. *B,* Retraction of clot (more pronounced in anemia) and attachment to vein wall; beginning involvement of vein wall in reactive process. *C,* Further organization of clot and involvement of vein wall (note valve structure not easily discernible from organized clot, on section); propagation of fresh "tail" clot on thrombus (this portion may be swept away as an embolus). *D,* Recanalization of organized clot with one main channel. *E,* Recanalization of organized clot with several smaller channels. Note in sketches *D* and *E* that vein wall and organized thrombus appear almost indistinguishable from each other. (Adapted from Hussey.)

small thrombi seen to originate in areas where stagnation is maximal: in the cul-de-sacs formed by the proximal surfaces of venous valves. As the clot grows and becomes organized, this localization becomes less and less obvious because of propagation and involvement of the entire contiguous vein wall.

Changes in the coagulative properties of the blood have been found postoperatively in some patients, but studies on blood fibrinogen, antithrombin, fibrinolysin and platelet counts have been unfruitful. Under certain circumstances, such as following splenectomy, increased platelet counts do parallel an increased tendency to thrombosis.

Many clinical conditions seem to predispose to venous thrombosis. These include surgical operations, injuries, burns, infectious diseases, pulmonary and pancreatic cancer, dehydration, shock, heart failure, myocardial infarction, polycythemia vera, anemia, advancing age, bed rest, obesity, pregnancy and the puerperium. A perusal of this list reveals that slowed circulation or stagnation is common to most of the conditions, that hypoxia prevails in others and that perhaps some enzymatic change in the circulating protein moieties of the blood may be held responsible

in certain instances, as in cancer of the pancreas and lung.

Bland thrombosis usually originates in the deep veins of the legs, although occasionally other sites may be involved. The more inflammatory types of thrombophlebitis, which may vary from low-grade nonbacterial inflammation of the vein to full-blown suppurative lesions, are best known to occur in superficial veins of the legs, in pelvic veins, in the appendiceal vein and in veins accompanying the arteries in thromboangiitis obliterans.

Microscopic examination of the site of clinically bland phlebothrombosis reveals that after 48 to 72 hours, this lesion is indistinguishable from actual thrombophlebitis (Fig. 44). Thus, strictly speaking, the term phlebothrombosis applies only to lesions of perhaps less than four days' duration.

Suppurative thrombophlebitis may occasionally follow postpartum or postabortal sepsis. So-called migratory thrombophlebitis usually involves only the superficial veins and usually does not give rise to emboli. Thrombophlebitis occurring in an uninjured limb of an otherwise healthy person may be the first clinical indication of thromboangiitis obliterans. This happens in 40 per cent of patients

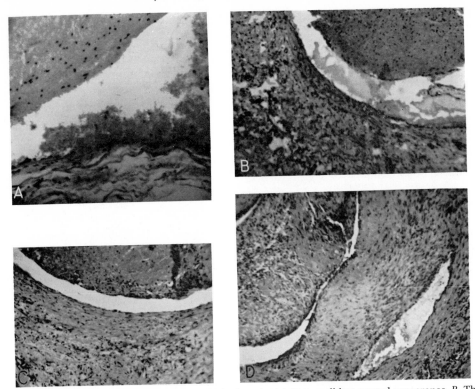

Figure 44. *A*, Thrombosis of 24 hours' duration (phlebothrombosis). Vein wall has normal appearance. *B*, Thrombosis of three days' duration. Note beginning involvement of vein wall (thrombophlebitis). *C*, Thrombosis of four days' duration. Clot shows early organization and covering by endothelial cell layer. Vein wall thickened. *D*, Thrombosis of seven days' duration. Organized clot almost indistinguishable from the greatly thickened vein wall. Beginning recanalization.

with thromboangiitis obliterans, and as an occasional first sign of carcinoma of the pancreas or lung, or of certain blood dyscrasias. The occurrence of otherwise unexplained thrombophlebitis is reason enough for careful search for undetected neoplastic or systemic disease.

Surgeons have long held the impression that major, time-consuming abdominal operations, especially those involving great blood loss or those producing hypotension, are more liable to be followed by venous complications than are the more superficial or shorter operative procedures. Acutely ill patients appear to be more susceptible than do many chronic invalids. Bed rest is certainly not the only precipitating cause, as evidenced by the extremely low incidence of thrombotic disease among chronically bedridden patients.

Partial obstruction to return flow from the lower limbs may result from tumors of the pelvis, unusual positioning during operation, abdominal distention and pregnancy. Stagnation and thrombosis may result.

SITES OF THROMBOSIS IN LOWER EXTREMITIES. It has been supposed that thrombi originate predominantly in the smaller, deep veins of the calf. However, meticulous postmortem dissections reveal the distribution of clots to be extremely widespread and their location appears to bear little relationship to antemortem local symptoms. In 40 per cent of the patients, thrombi occur bilaterally in the lower extremities. The deep femoral venous system of the thigh contains thrombi oftener than does the superficial femoral venous system in the thigh and the calf, including the so-called deep veins of the calf. The internal iliac veins contain thrombi in only 6 per cent of patients. Thus, it would appear that phlebothrombosis actually is more common in the deep femoral vein branches of the thigh than in the calf veins, although clinical symptoms are more readily detectable when it is in the calf (Fig. 45).

It has been suggested that thrombi in the legs begin during operation, although they may not become clinically evident for several days, or perhaps not at all.

INCIDENCE. Despite all the therapeutic and diagnostic advances in recent years, the incidence of phlebothrombosis, thrombophlebitis and thromboembolism has not changed appreciably. Failure to recognize a bland

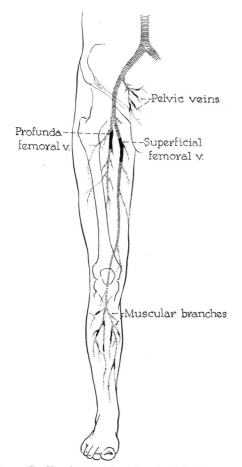

Figure 45. Usual sites of origin of phlebothrombosis in the lower extremity and pelvis.

attention for diagnosis and prophylactic treatment.

Among hospitalized patients, 60 of every 100 patients with pulmonary embolism are on medical services, the remaining 40 coming from surgical services. In 20 to 25 per cent of the patients, the first embolus is the fatal one. From 53 to 94 per cent of patients who die of pulmonary embolism, or who exhibit pulmonary embolism at postmortem examination, were not known to have had any thromboembolic disease. In one series, the first signs of thrombosis were recognized in 74 per cent of patients only after massive pulmonary embolism.

It is obvious from these figures that significant numbers of patients have thrombotic disease without its being recognized. Therefore, the true incidence of phlebothrombosis is not known. More important is the obvious inability on the part of the clinician to diagnose the condition early enough.

CLINICAL SIGNS AND SYMPTOMS. Superficial thrombophlebitis is ordinarily easy to diagnose because of the readily observed local signs, such as redness, local heat and subjective pain, supplemented by the usual systemic signs of inflammation, such as fever, tachycardia, rapid sedimentation rate and leukocytosis. The systemic signs vary in degree according to the amount of inflammation.

The diagnosis of deep vein thrombosis of the lower extremities is much more elusive and the lesion often goes unrecognized. The diagnosis can sometimes be derived inferentially by an otherwise unexplained occurrence of the systemic signs of thrombophlebitis. When such signs appear, they are usually soon supported by the detection of local signs of venous thrombosis or by those of pulmonary embolism.

The incidence of phlebothrombosis in a given institution is usually proportional to the diligence with which the condition is searched for. If daily examination of the legs is carefully carried out on both the surgical and medical services, the number of detected cases will be higher than if such examinations are not done.

Unless specifically questioned about soreness or discomfort in the legs, at least half of all postoperative patients fail to mention spontaneously aches in the calf muscles or other comparable minor symptoms.

Incipient cyanosis of the skin may not be obvious unless the legs are dependent, as in sitting or standing. Comparison of one leg

thrombus until embolism occurs has no doubt kept the incidence of embolism virtually constant. A review of reports from all over the world, involving over three million operations, showed an incidence of fatal pulmonary embolism ranging from 0.1 to 0.87 per cent, averaging 0.14 per cent, with remarkably little change over the past 50 years. When statistics were based upon autopsy findings, the incidence of death from pulmonary embolism varied from 0.2 to 23 per cent, with an average of 2.8 per cent. In these long-range statistics, there appeared an interesting but unexplained wavelike periodicity, even in the same institution. On a shorter range basis, thromboembolism appears to be more prevalent in the spring and autumn months in temperate climates. Since 95 per cent of all fatal pulmonary emboli are said to originate in the lower extremities, this anatomic site has naturally attracted the most with the other makes for more accurate judgment than examining each leg separately. This test is not reliable in the earliest cases of bland thrombosis.

Measurement of the circumference of the legs at given points in the thigh, calf and ankle and, most important, comparison with preoperative measurements.

Palpation for tenderness in the calf, thigh and foot should be done with only moderate pressure between the bellies of the gastrocnemius muscle, in the popliteal space and along the medial and posterior aspects of the thigh. The knee is moderately flexed during palpation. The examiner must learn to distinguish between the response to abnormal degrees of pain on the one hand, and the discomfort produced by too strenuous palpation on the other. This sign is not very reliable, since other causes for calf tenderness may confuse the problem.

Homans' sign, or dorsiflexion test, consists of dorsiflexing the foot of the patient while the knee is extended. If dorsiflexion of the foot elicits pain in the calf or popliteal area, the reaction to the test is positive. However, as in the palpation maneuver, the test is not pathognomonic for thrombosis.

The pneumatic cuff of the sphygmomanometer is placed about the calf or thigh and slowly inflated. Normally, patients do not register discomfort at pressures below 180 mm. Hg on the calf or thigh. In the presence of thrombosis, the patient complains bitterly of pain at a pressure significantly below the normal. At this point, the cuff is immediately deflated and the test is repeated on the other calf. The patient should not be alerted to the possibility of pain, but should be watched for alteration of facial expression or a withdrawal reaction, such as flexing the thigh. This test appears to be the most sensitive and perhaps the most valuable of the diagnostic procedures available today to detect early bland thrombosis in the legs.

Elicitation of pain on calf muscle rocking is an acceptable clinical test, perhaps somewhat more sensitive than the palpation test, but not as reliable as the cuff test. The knee is slightly bent with the heel resting on the bed. The calf muscle group is rocked back and forth in its relaxed state. Severe pain or discomfort is suggestive of thrombosis.

Local pain on coughing has been claimed to be of some value especially in acute thrombophlebitis.

Search must also be made for signs such as superficial venous congestion, dilated pretibial veins, increased local heat, redness and swelling, cyanotic mottling and similar indications. These may be present when the inflammatory element is pronounced, but as a rule they are absent in most patients with early, bland phlebothrombosis (Fig. 46).

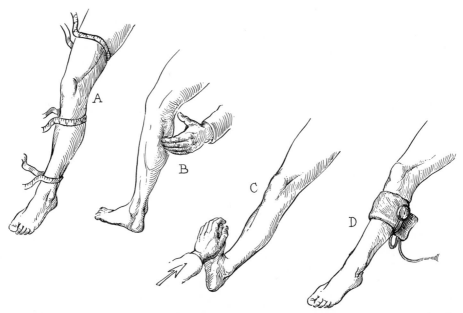

Figure 46. Some useful maneuvers to detect phlebothrombosis. *A*, Circumferential measurements using fixed sites on limbs. *B*, Palpation for tenderness between bellies of gastrocnemius muscle and popliteal area. *C*, Homans' sign or dorsiflexion test. *D*, Sphygmomanometer cuff pain test (Lowenberg) on calf or thigh.

PROGNOSIS OF THROMBOPHLEBITIS OF LOWER EXTREMITIES. Thrombophlebitis may progress along one of three lines:

No residual, detectable lesion. Probably in the majority of the milder cases of thrombophlebitis of the lower extremities, the disease subsides completely in due time, in some patients because of good treatment, in others without adequate treatment. In the latter group are many originally unrecognized cases. In many patients, mild residual edema of one extremity, with or without pain, eventually subsides completely. It must be remembered that one attack predisposes to another, particularly after another surgical operation or injury or recurrent illness, such as heart failure. Consequently, a painstakingly careful history regarding leg symptoms after previous surgical procedures or illnesses is mandatory. Only by such screening can prophylactic measures be properly instituted.

Chronic venous insufficiency (postphlebitic syndrome). In a large percentage of patients, the first indication of postpartum or postoperative thrombosis is the development of a pale, swollen, painful leg as ambulation is resumed postoperatively. This type of limb has been referred to as phlegmasia alba dolens, or, more commonly as milk leg. The lowered surface temperature of such a limb is apparently due to reflex arteriospasm which commonly accompanies venous occlusion. This condition may gradually spontaneously subside or it may persist for life.

If the condition progresses, the venous blockage results in development of other more serious sequelae. Secondary varicosities are usually the result of shunting of the major portion of the venous return to the superficial leg veins. As a rule, this is more often the result of imcompetency of the valvular system of the deep veins than of persistent blockage. As the deep vein thrombus becomes organized, the vein wall and its valves become an integral, inseparable part of the conglomerate thrombus (Fig. 47). In due time, recanalization occurs, often with multiple channels, but the blood in the new channels is no longer aided along its course by valves. As a consequence, a high degree of stasis develops in the lower third of the leg. The skin and underlying tissues become poorly oxygenated, stasis thrombi form in small subcutaneous veins and the skin about the malleoli loses its normal color and consistency. It may become shiny and thinned.

Induration may begin in a small area overlying a perforated vein and involve skin and

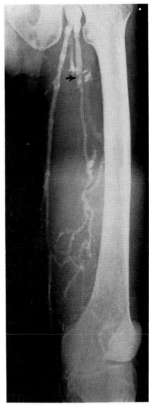

Figure 47. Retrograde phlebogram showing collateralization of deep vein occlusion in patient with postphlebitic syndrome. Arrow points to upper limits of occlusion with resumption of normal channel above.

underlying fat. Fibrosis of the underlying fat either accompanies or follows induration of the skin. The skin gives the appearance of parchment paper under which the fatty layer is atrophic and hard.

The least trauma may result in chronic ulceration. Episodes of acute cellulitis or infected dermatitis may supervene. When associated lymphatic thrombi occur, the skin becomes thickened and leathery and in extreme instances elephantiasis may develop.

The patient unfortunate enough to suffer from chronic venous insufficiency with these symptoms must be resigned to lifelong care of the limb.

In decreasing order of frequency, the postphlebitic leg exhibits edema, pigmentation, secondary varicosities, pain, dermatitis, induration and ulceration. Most of these sequelae can be obviated if proper early treatment is instituted and good care is taken of the leg afterward.

Pulmonary thromboembolism. While death from pulmonary embolism occurs in an extremely small percentage of patients with thrombotic disease of the lower extremities, it is likely to follow bland phlebothrombosis. Since phlebothrombosis often goes unrecognized, pulmonary embolism usually occurs without warning. An overwhelming proportion of patients who die of pulmonary embolism are not known to have had clinically demonstrable thromboembolic disease, nor did they show signs or symptoms requiring therapy prior to the fatal embolism. Not all large pulmonary emboli are fatal. Some of them, particularly smaller pulmonary emboli, may produce pulmonary infarction. However, in 20 to 25 per cent of patients, the first embolus is the fatal one.

Animal experimentation has demonstrated that nonfatal pulmonary emboli do not invariably produce infarcts. Pulmonary infarction following pulmonary embolism apparently depends on the presence of other factors, such as diminished aeration, interference with blood supply and infection. If none of these factors is present, an embolus may organize in the pulmonary vessels and produce no demonstrable effects.

Certain concepts have been developed from the search for factors which may precipitate the embolization of a thrombus. For example, in the presence of anemia, clot retraction following coagulation is known to be greater than normal. It is, therefore, possible that exaggerated clot retraction, if it occurs following thrombosis, might tend to draw the clot away from contact with the vessel walls and permit it to be dislodged by the passing stream of blood. Excessive clot retraction occurs in either chronic anemia or in the anemia following acute blood loss from operation.

Another concept of embolization is based on the nature of thrombus propagation. The oldest portion of the clot adheres to the intima, while the clot propagates by adding a soft "tail" of freshly clotted blood elements. The tail is only loosely attached over a small area to the adherent portion, but its largest surface area, exposed as it is to the stream of venous blood, makes ready ground for deposition of circulating platelets, cells and other clotting elements. The tail of a thrombus may later become attached to the vessel wall. Any sudden increase in venous pressure, as may accompany coughing, sudden motion, straining at stool, or any other physical expression of the Valsalva maneuver, may easily cause the tail to break from its mooring and become an embolus. Similarly, if the tail of the thrombus extends past a branching

vessel which brings blood from a neighboring part, the current from the branch may sweep off a portion of the soft clot.

The classic clinical symptoms of pulmonary embolism are the sudden onset of constricting chest pain, painful breathing, anxiety, shock and cyanosis. In a few patients, hemoptysis or cough with frothy pink sputum may occur. Rib cage tenderness, pleural friction rub and an x-ray shadow suggestive of infarction in the presence of these symptoms of prima facie evidence of pulmonary infarction. Tachycardia, fever and leukocytosis are later sequential phenomena. Early clinical differentiation from acute coronary occlusion may be difficult.

Pulmonary embolism may cause death within a few moments; however, several hours may elapse with the patient in a state of shock, with or without loss of consciousness, before death occurs. In such patients certain therapeutic measures may be tried.

Electrocardiographic findings immediately after an attack are not easily differentiated from those due to posterior coronary vessel occlusion. Later, the changes of acute cor pulmonale are usually demonstrable.

In general, it can be said that a massive pulmonary embolism is usually lethal; smaller emboli usually result in infarction with pleuritis, often with effusion. Many smaller emboli result in no demonstrable pulmonary pathologic process, provided the lung is not previously diseased.

A paradoxical arterial embolism occurs when a venous embolism passes through a patent foramen ovale, from the right to the left side of the heart, and into the arterial system. Such an embolus may lodge in a femoral vessel, cerebral vessel or other peripheral artery.

TREATMENT. No known test or method can accurately foretell whether a patient will or will not have venous thrombosis. The recently introduced antithrombin and heparin tolerance tests have not proved reliable. Nonetheless, there are some measures which can be undertaken to reduce the risk. Also, the realization that thromboembolism may occur under certain circumstances should serve to alert the surgeon to identify and treat phlebothrombosis, if possible.

Since early recognition of thrombosis is the only hope of preventing embolism, daily examination of the legs in all postoperative patients and in severely ill medical patients is mandatory.

Prophylactic measures during operation include prevention of shock and maintenance of effective circulating blood volume when blood loss is great. For patients who must undergo prolonged surgical operations, the simple expedient of elevating the legs on a pillow during the procedure has been shown to encourage venous drainage from the legs as well or better than wrapping the legs with elastic bandages. The rationale behind encouragement of venous drainage is based upon evidence that venous stasis during surgery is an important contributing cause to postoperative thrombosis.

Postoperatively, venous stasis in the legs may be discouraged by such measures as prevention of excessive abdominal distention, avoidance of tight abdominal binders, and by not permitting prolonged periods of immobility or dependency of the legs.

Elastic stockings or bandages compress the superficial veins and tend to cause more rapid flow of venous blood through the deep veins. As a result, this measure is excellent prophylaxis against deep vein thrombosis. If elastic bandages are used, they must be applied carefully and reapplied daily. Elastic compression is particularly useful in patients with varicosities. The elastic stockings or bandages can be applied prior to operation and worn by the patient during and after operation. In the presence of inflammation or ischemia, elastic compression cannot be tolerated by the patient because of the local pain.

Early ambulation after operation is considered to be a preventive measure against thromboembolism. It may not be as important a preventive measure as elevation of the legs during operation. If ambulation cannot be carried out for any reason, a definite routine of leg exercises and periodic deep breathing may be instituted. All such measures are aimed at preventing venous stasis in the legs.

Attempts to prevent thrombosis of leg veins by administration of anticoagulant drugs have led to inconclusive results. Clinical evidence indicates that the best preventive of venous thromboembolism is prevention of venous stasis, especially during operation.

Thrombophlebitis of superficial veins is treated by bed rest, elevation of the limb and the administration of heparin. Within a few days, after periphlebitis has subsided, these veins may be excised.

Inasmuch as the two outstanding features of deep vein thrombosis are pulmonary embolism and disability due to postphlebitic syndrome, therapy is aimed at prevention of each of these complications, once the thrombosis is discovered.

If the diagnosis is deep vein phlebothrombosis or thrombophlebitis, it is customary to wrap the legs in elastic bandages from toes to groin and immediately institute anticoagulant therapy. At this time the legs are neither elevated nor lowered but are kept flat in bed. Jack-knifing the patient to a full sitting position is to be avoided since this may encourage venous pooling or stagnation at the hip level.

Unfortunately, anticoagulant therapy has come to mean a stereotyped program of heparin administration for a day or two with simultaneous coumarin administration until the Quick test for prothrombin time reaches therapeutic levels. In recent years, this program has been found to be less antithrombotic than anticoagulant. Many patients with venous thromboembolic disease may actually bleed from the coumarin therapy while the thrombosis continues to propagate. Investigation of this paradox of coexisting thrombosis and bleeding in the presence of therapeutic dosage of coumarin has been carried out in both laboratory animals and patients. These studies warrant the following conclusions: the Quick test verifies the rapidly reacting clotting factors, including factor VII, but is blind to the slowly responding thromboplastic factors which are best verified by a thromboelastogram; prothrombin time reaches therapeutic levels in 24 to 48 hours with coumarin drugs, but quantitative prothrombin levels require at least five days of therapy for adequate response; coumarin drugs are anticoagulant but not antithrombotic, as proved by animal studies in which thrombus propagation was not controlled even with hemorrhage-producing doses, whereas heparin is antithrombotic and prevents thrombus formation and propagation of an existing thrombus. Because of these facts, many investigators agree that heparin should be used exclusively for anticoagulant therapy in the management of venous thromboembolic disease. It is administered as the aqueous solution, 10,000 units (100 mg.) by deep subcutaneous injection every 12 hours for at least ten days, and is gradually withdrawn.

If embolic phenomena occur despite this treatment, it may be necessary to perform a femoral vein thrombectomy, or a vena cava ligation or plication procedure. (Fig. 48).

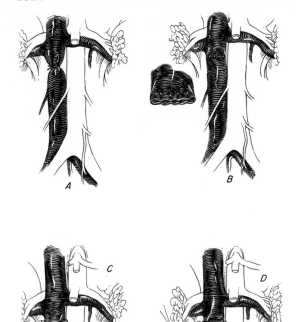

Figure 48. Methods of total and partial vena cava ligation. *A,* Complete ligation using stout ligature or tape. *B,* Spencer method of partitioning by interrupted sutures. *C,* Moretz method of narrowing lumen with Teflon clip. *D,* Miles method of partitioning with serrated Teflon clip. Methods *B, C,* and *D* were devised to permit venous return while preventing passage of large clots from legs to pelvis.

Fogarty has described a method of thrombectomy which has enhanced the safety of the procedure. Prior to attempts to manipulate the thrombosed femoral vein, proximal control of the vena cava is obtained by means of inserting a balloon catheter into the opposite, or unaffected, femoral vein via the saphenous bulb. After this maneuver, the thrombus is removed from the affected side. The added safety of this procedure over all previous techniques has resulted in the unequivocal recommendation of thrombectomy for early deep vein thrombosis without an extensive trial of anticoagulant therapy.

For a number of years in certain institutions, bilateral femoral vein ligation was carried out as the initial procedure upon discovery of thrombosis in the legs. Later comparison of results, however, indicated no significant difference between the incidence of embolism in these patients and that in patients given anticoagulant therapy.

Death from massive pulmonary embolism often supervenes within seconds of the embolization. Some patients may survive several hours or even days. In roughly 50 per cent of patients so afflicted, there is time to apply one or more of the emergency measures.

Since the first of these measures is immediate administration of oxygen by mask, it is always best to have oxygen readily available on surgical wards. The subcutaneous injection of atropine sulfate, 0.0013 gm. is advised to overcome reflex vagal effects if they are present. The intravenous or subcutaneous administration of papaverine, 0.032 gm., has been recommended to overcome bronchial spasm and to conteract ventricular fibrillation. Immediate heparinization is also advised.

Because one cannot predict which patients will survive, no valid statistics are available as to the efficacy of this form of treatment.

The decision for or against pulmonary embolectomy depends upon certainty of the diagnosis and appraisal of the clinical condition. Pulmonary angiography for accurate diagnosis is performed after partial pulmonary by-pass is instituted as a lifesaving procedure. Fibrinolytic enzymes injected into the pulmonary artery have been reported as successful in a few patients, and may be tried if the patient's condition warrants. If the injection of vasopressor drugs is necessary to maintain blood pressure, a pulmonary embolectomy is indicated.

When a patient with deep vein thrombosis is allowed to become ambulatory, he is fitted with elastic stockings from toes to knees to minimize the edema.

If the diagnosis is acute inflammatory thrombophlebitis of the deep or superficial veins of the leg, initial treatment is similar, except that elastic bandages cannot be used immediately because of the discomfort they cause. In the acute stages, these patients usually require much larger doses of heparin than the usual ones in order to elevate their coagulation time to therapeutic ranges.

Another useful measure in the presence of severe pain, usually due to distention of veins in spasm, is to block the sympathetic impulses to the legs. If this is done by paravertebral sympathetic ganglionic block, it is best to begin the block before instituting anticoagulant therapy. Other methods of blocking the sympathetics include continuous caudal block and the use of parenteral ganglionic blocking agents, such as phenoxybenzamine or related compounds. Antibiotics have been used empirically, together with anticoagulants, but their role remains to be evaluated since most of these lesions are not caused by bacterial invasion. If only superficial veins are involved, the affected segments may be excised once the early, acute inflammatory stage has subsided. Pulmonary embolism is not a common sequel to this lesion.

Ambulation is usually not attempted before a week or ten days, or as soon as it is possible to wear elastic stockings.

In rare instances, massive thrombosis occludes practically all the veins of the leg, including the main stems. When this occurs, the entire leg up to midthigh becomes deeply cyanotic and extremely painful and swollen within a few hours. A patient with such a lesion may go into shock from blood loss into the extremity. Treatment consists of thrombectomy as soon as the patient is in condition to withstand surgical intervention. It is done under local anesthesia in the presence of heparinization. The incision is made over the femoral vein in the groin. The clot is removed from proximal and distal veins through a venotomy incision, using a Fogarty balloon catheter.

Such treatment may be rewarded by gradual return of almost normal color to the skin within hours. In an occasional patient, the limb may become gangrenous and require amputation despite good treatment. Sympathetic block is usually of no avail in these patients. Thrombectomy is now applied to patients with early phlegmasia alba dolens, as well as to those with phlegmasia cerulea dolens. In either case, it prevents the life-long sequelae of postphlebitic syndrome, if it is successful.

The chronic sequelae of thrombophlebitis present one of the most difficult therapeutic problems in surgery.

For patients whose skin is not ulcerated, but whose main symptoms are pain on standing and edema with or without skin discoloration, certain precautions must be taken. These individuals are instructed to avoid even minor trauma to the area of the ankles and lower legs; not to stand for a long time; when sitting for long periods, to keep the legs elevated; when walking, to wear elastic stockings; not to rub the skin of the legs too vigorously when drying after bathing; to apply lanolin ointment to the skin of the ankles before retiring at night, and if obese, to go on a strict weight-reduction regimen.

If varicosities are present, the great saphenous vein, and short saphenous if indicated, should be stripped and individual clusters of veins excised. The rationale for this procedure in the presence of chronic deep vein insufficiency is based on the supposition that if the stagnant superficial system is removed, venous return from the legs will be hastened through deep, uninvolved veins as well as recanalized veins.

If ulceration occurs, treatment depends upon the extent of tissue destruction. Superficial, small ulcers usually heal with a few days of bed rest with elevation and sterile saline dressings. However, as ambulation is resumed, the ulcers may recur unless the superficial venous system is stripped or proper elastic compression is applied.

Deep, infected ulcers often present a serious problem in therapy. Local application of antibiotic preparations is usually of no avail unless the basic principles of elevation, compression and cleanly care are applied. Purulent, pseudomembranous granulation tissue can usually be converted into clean, red, flat surfaces without the use of antibiotics, enzymatic debriding agents, or other chemical means. In some patients, a split-thickness skin graft can be applied to such healthy granulations. In others, surgical excision of the ulcerous area and neighboring poor tissue, often including the underlying fascia, may be necessary after attempts to clean the ulcer base have been carried out. It is known that granulation tissue which appears healthy grossly is most receptive to grafting when its pH is over 7.4.

Occasionally, the skin continues to break down repeatedly after healing with or without a graft, despite the measures outlined. Various modes of treatment have been prescribed for such patients, including sympathectomy, ligation of the popliteal vein or femoral vein, and extensive excision of all superficial veins of the leg through long flap incisions. These measures have yielded good results in some patients.

The largest percentage of milder ulcers can be healed, while the patient is ambulatory, by means of weekly or semiweekly application of Unna's paste boot after painting the ulcer with gentian violet or a similar dye. The rationale for this treatment is one of compression, protection and maintenance of moisture and softness in the area. The boot consists of wrapping the leg, from the base of the toes to the knee, with gauze impregnated with zinc oxide-gelatin-glycerin mixture. The method permits healing over a number of weeks or months.

Infected dermatitis pursuant to chronic venous insufficiency is usually best treated by identification and eradication of secondary factors, such as epidermophytosis, sensitization to various allergens, secretions, medication or bacterial invasion. Most patients respond to elevation, cleanly care and, later, compression.

It is important to impress upon the patient that, despite the success of specific immediate therapy, lifelong care of the limb is mandatory.

THROMBOSIS OF THE UPPER EXTREMITIES

Thrombophlebitis of the superficial veins, especially the antecubital vein, commonly follows intravenous infusions. It may be due to hypertonicity or irritability of the solution, contamination, or intimal irritation from the needle.

As a rule, the area is painful and tender. The overlying skin is red and warm. The vein usually can be palpated as a firm cord under the skin. Moist hot packs usually cause the condition to subside in a few days.

Thrombosis of the axillary and subclavian vein may arise from a variety of causes. Direct trauma and prolonged compression are known etiologic factors. So-called effort thrombosis usually follows some unusual physical exertion involving compression of the vein by the subclavian muscle tendon or by the scalenus anticus muscle. In addition, fractures, hematomas, tumor growths and postoperative mastectomy compression have been responsible for axillary vein thrombosis.

The axillary vein may also become involved in phlebitis migrans.

Symptoms are usually ushered in with pain at the site of thrombosis. In 24 to 48 hours, the arm appears somewhat swollen and the skin assumes a burgundy color. Cyanosis of the deep blue variety may occur. Superficial veins become dilated. The arm feels heavy and full to the patient.

Strangely, the incidence of pulmonary embolism following upper extremity venous thrombosis is extremely low. Collateral channels about the axilla and shoulder are rich and soon assume the added burden of venous circulation, becoming visibly dilated.

A diagnostic aid is the injection of radiopaque medium into an arm vein in order to visualize the site of the occlusion on an x-ray (Fig. 49). This should not be done for at least 48 hours in order not to dislodge the clot. Diagnosis without venography is preferred.

Treatment depends upon the location of the thrombosis and the severity of the symptoms. If symptoms are minimal, simple elevation of the arm and anticoagulant therapy for seven to ten days may suffice. Sympathetic and stellate ganglionic blocks with 1 per cent procaine solution may be carried out to minimize spasm, but thrombectomy is to be performed if the occlusion is massive. In chronic occlusion of the axillary vein, without satisfactory recanalizations, scalenotomy may relieve symptoms of pain due to pressure upon the vein. If symptoms persist after many months, sympathectomy may be performed to alleviate both arterial and venous spasm.

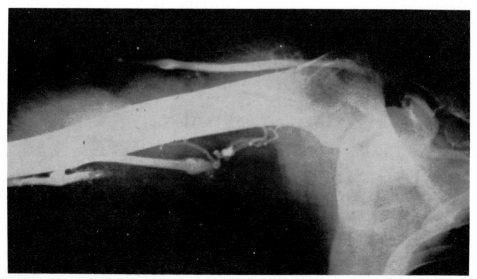

Figure 49.   Venogram showing thrombosis of axillary vein. Note collateral channels about area of occlusion.

READING REFERENCES

Allen, E. V., Barker, N. W., and Hines, E. A., Jr.: Peripheral Vascular Diseases. Philadelphia, W. B. Saunders Company, 3rd ed., 1962.

Beall, A. C., Jr., and Cooley, D. A.: Embolectomy for acute massive pulmonary embolism. Angiology 16:637, 1965.

Buerger, L.: Thrombo-angiitis obliterans: a study of the vascular lesions leading to presenile spontaneous gangrene. Am. J. M. Sci. 136:567, 1908.

Butcher, M. R., Jr., and Hoover, A. L.: Abnormalities of human superficial cutaneous lymphatics associated with stasis ulcers, lymphedema, scars and cutaneous autografts. Ann. Surg. 142:633, 1955.

Cannon, J. A., Barker, W. F., and Kawagami, I. G.: Femoral popliteal endarterectomy in the treatment of obliterative atherosclerotic disease. Surgery 43:76, 1958.

Carrel, A.: Results of permanent intubation of the thoracic aorta. Surg. Gyn. & Obst. 15:245, 1912.

Crauley, J. J., Krause, R. S., and Strasser, E. S.: Chronic venous insufficiency of lower extremity. Surgery 49:48, 1961.

Crawford, E. S., DeBakey, M. E., Blaisdell, F. W., Morris, G. C., Jr., and Fields, W. S.: Hemodynamic alterations in patients with cerebral artery insufficiency before and after operation. Surgery 48:76, 1960.

Crawford, E. S., DeBakey, M. E., Morris, G. C., Jr., and Garrett, E.: Evaluation of late failures after reconstructive operations for occlusive lesions of aorta, and iliac, femoral and popliteal arteries. Surgery 47:79, 1960.

Creech, O., Jr., DeBakey, M. E., Cooley, D. A., and Halpert, B.: Structural alterations in human aortic homografts one to two and one-half years after transplantation. Surg. Gyn. & Obst. 103:147, 1956.

Creech, O., Jr., Schramel, R. J., and Reemstma, K.: Critical evaluation of direct surgical procedures in the treatment of occlusive peripheral vascular disease. Am. Surg. 25:492, 1959.

Dale, W. A., and Mavor, G. E.: Peripheral vascular grafts: experimental comparison of autogenous veins, homologous arteries, and synthetic tubes. Brit. J. Surg. 46:305, 1959.

Dardik, H., Seidenberg, B., Parker, J. G., and Hurwitt, E. S.: Intestinal angina with malabsorption treated by elective revascularization. J.A.M.A. 194:1206, 1965.

Davis, J. B., Grove, W. J., and Julian, O.: Thrombotic occlusion of branches of aortic arch, Martorell's syndrome: report of case treated surgically. Ann. Surg. 144:124, 1956.

DeBakey, M. E.: A critical evaluation of the problem of thromboembolism. Surg. Gyn. & Obst.; Internat. Abst. Surg. 98:1, 1954.

DeBakey, M. E., Crawford, E. S., Garrett, H. E., Beall, A. C., Jr., and Howell, J. F.: Surgical considerations in the treatment of aneurysms of the thoracoabdominal aorta. Ann. Surg. 162:650, 1965.

DeBakey, M. E., Crawford, E. S., Morris, G. C., Jr., and Cooley, D. A.: Surgical considerations of occlusive disease of the innominate, carotid, subclavian, and vertebral arteries. Ann. Surg. 154:698, 1961.

DeBakey, M. E., Creech, O., and Woodhall, J. P.: Evaluation of sympathectomy in arteriosclerotic peripheral vascular disease. J.A.M.A. 144:1227, 1950.

DeBakey, M. E., Henly, W. S., Cooley, D. A., Crawford, E. S., and Morris, G. C., Jr.: Surgical treatment of dissecting aneurysms of aorta: analysis of 72 cases. Circulation 24:290, 1961.

Derrick, J. R., Pollard, H. S., and Moore, R. M.: Pattern of arteriosclerotic narrowing of celiac and superior mesenteric arteries. Ann. Surg. 149:684, 1960.

De Weese, M. S., and Hunter, D. C., Jr.: A vena caval filter for the prevention of pulmonary embolism. A five-year clinical experience. Arch. Surg. 86:852, 1963.

Eastcott, H. H. G.: Reconstruction of the subclavian artery for complications of cervical rib and thoracic outlet syndrome. Lancet 2:1243, 1962.

Estes, J. E.: Abdominal aortic aneurysms: a study of 102 cases. Circulation 2:258, 1950.

Ferguson, F. S., Byrd, W. M., and McAfee, D. K.: Experiences in management of arterial injuries. Ann. Surg. 153:980, 1961.

Fogarty, T. J., Cranley, J. J., Krause, R. J., Strasser, E. S., and Hafner, C. D.: Surgical management of phlegmasia cerulea dolens. Arch. Surg. 86:256, 1963.

Fogarty, T. J., Dennis, D., and Krippaehne, W. W.: Surgical management of iliofemoral venous thrombosis. Am. J. Surg. 112:211, 1966.

Fuller, C. H., Robertson, C. W., and Smithwick, R. H.: Management of thromboembolic disease. New England J. Med. 263:983, 1960.

Glotzer, D. J., and Glotzer, P.: Superior mesenteric embolectomy: report of two successful cases using the Fogarty catheter. Arch. Surg. 93:421, 1966.

Guthrie, C. C.: Blood Vessel Surgery and Its Application. New York, Longmans, Green & Co., 1912.

Haller, J. A., Jr.: Thrombectomy for acute iliofemoral venous thrombosis. Arch. Surg. 83:448, 1961.

Hershey, F. B., and Spencer, H. D.: Surgical repair of civilian arterial injuries. Arch. Surg. 80:953, 1960.

Homans, J.: Thrombosis of the deep veins of the lower leg causing pulmonary embolism. New England J. Med. 211:993, 1934.

Horton, B. T., Magath, T. B., and Brown, G. E.: Arteritis of the temporal vessels: a previously undescribed form. Arch. Int. Med. 53:400, 1934.

Humphries, A. W., Young, J. R., de Wolfe, V. G., and Le Fevre, F. A.: Complications of abdominal aortic surgery. Arch. Surg. 86:43, 1963.

Hussey, H. H.: Venous thrombosis of the lower extremities. GP 10:58, 1954.

Janes, J. M., and Ivins, J. C.: A method of dealing with arteriosclerotic popliteal aneurysms. Surgery 29:398, 1951.

Kampmeier, R. H.: Aneurysms of the abdominal aorta: a study of 73 cases. Am. J. M. Sci. 192:97, 1936.

Laufman, H.: Peripheral arterial occlusive disease: what can the surgeon offer? J. Iowa M. Soc. 52:342, 1962.

Laufman, H.: Surgical management of chronic iliofemoral arterial occlusions. S. Clin. North America 40:153, 1960.

Laufman, H.: Ancillary care in postphlebitic syndrome. S. Clin. North America 39:183, 1959.

Laufman, H., Berggren, R. E., Finley, T., and Anson, B. J.: Anatomical studies of the lumbar arteries: with reference to the safety of translumbar aortography. Ann. Surg. 152:621, 1960.

Laufman, H., Hohf, R., Bernhard, V., and Trippel, O.: End-to-side bypass homograft without resection in segmental arterial occlusion. Arch. Surg. 73:418, 1956.

Laufman, H., Nora, P. F., and Mittelpunkt, A. I.: Mesenteric blood vessels: advances in surgery and physiology. Arch. Surg. 88:1021, 1964.

Lawrence, E. D.: The cough-pain sign in acute superficial thrombophlebitis. J. M. Soc. New Jersey 47:164, 1950.

Lewis, T.: Observations on some normal and injurious effects of cold upon the skin and underlying tissues. Brit. M.J. 2:795; 837, 1941.

Lowenberg, R. I.: Early diagnosis of phlebothrombosis with aid of a new clinical test. J.A.M.A. 155:1566, 1954.

Marshall, T. R., and Ling, J. T.: Direct percutaneous non-catheter left and right brachial angiography. Radiology 80:258, 1963.

Matas, R.: An operation for the radical cure of aneurysm based upon arteriorrhaphy. Ann. Surg. 37:161, 1903.

McKechnie, R. E., and Allen, E. V.: Sudden occlusion of the arteries of the extremities: a study of 100 cases of embolism and thrombosis. Surg. Gyn. & Obst. 63:231, 1936.

McLachlin, A. D., McLachlin, J., Jory, T. A., and Rawling, E. G.: Venous stasis in the lower extremities. Ann. Surg. 152:678, 1960.

Moretz, W. H., Rhode, C. M., and Shephard, M. H.: Prevention of pulmonary emboli by partial occlusion of the inferior vena cava. Am. J. Surg. 25:617, 1959.

Morris, G. C., Jr., DeBakey, M. E., Cooley, D. A., and Crawford, E. S.: Surgical treatment of renal hypertension. Ann. Surg. 151:854, 1960.

Ochsner, A., and DeBakey, M. E.: Therapeutic considerations of thrombophlebitis and phlebothrombosis. New England J. Med. 225:207, 1941.

Paterson, J. C., and McLachlin, J.: Precipitating factors in venous thrombosis. Surg. Gyn. & Obst. 98:96, 1954.

Raynaud, M.: On local asphyxia and symmetrical gangrene of the extremities. Selected Monographs. London, The Sydenham Society, 1888.

Reid, M.: Studies in abnormal arteriovenous communications, acquired and congenital. Arch. Surg. 10:601; 11:25, 1925.

Reivich, M., Holling, H. E., Roberts, B., and Toole, J.: Reversal of blood flow through vertebral artery and its effect on cerebral circulation. New England J. Med. 265:878, 1961. Also: Editorial: New vascular syndrome—"subclavian steal." New England J. Med. 265:912, 1961.

Roach, H. D., and Laufman, H.: Relationship between pulmonary embolism and pulmonary infarction: an experimental study. Ann. Surg. 142:82, 1955.

Shaw, R. S.: Reconstructive vascular surgery. New England J. Med. 266:339, 1962.

Shumacker, H. B.: The use and abuse of diagnostic aids. Surg. Gyn. & Obst. 100:112, 1955.

Spencer, F. C., Quattlebaum, J. K., Quattlebaum, J. K., Jr., Sharp, E. H., and Jude, J. R.: Plication of the inferior vena cava for pulmonary embolism. A report of 20 cases. Ann. Surg. 155:827, 1962.

Spencer, F. C., Stamey, T. A., Bahnson, H. T., and Cohen, A.: Diagnosis and treatment of hypertension due to occlusive disease of renal artery. Ann. Surg. 154:674, 1961.

Stokes, J. M., and Butcher, R., Jr.: Comparison of thrombo-endarterectomy and arterial substitutions using life table method of reporting results. Surgery 48:554, 1960.

Szilagyi, D. E., Smith, R. F., Machsood, A. J., and Whitcomb, J. G.: Expanding and ruptured abdominal aortic aneurysms: problems of diagnosis and treatment. Arch. Surg. 83:395, 1961.

Szilagyi, D. E., Smith, R. F., and Whitcomb, J. G.: The contribution of angioplastic surgery to the therapy of peripheral occlusive arteriopathy. Ann. Surg. 152:660, 1960.

de Takats, G.: Postphlebitic syndrome. J.A.M.A. 164:1861, 1957.

Trippel, O. H., Bernhard, V. M., Hohf, R. P., and Laufman, H.: Considerations in the accuracy and safety of arteriography. Surgery 41:153, 1957.

Trippel, O. H., Bernhard, V. M., and Laufman, H.: Limb salvage in occlusive arterial disease of the lower extremities. Arch. Surg. 81:357, 1960.

von Winiwarter, F.: Ueber eine eigentümliche Form von Endarteriitis und Endophlebitis mit Gangrän des Fusses. Arch. klin. Chir. 23:202, 1879.

Wheeler, H. B.: Surgical treatment of subclavian-artery occlusions. New England J. Med. 276:711, 1967.

Wylie, E. J., and Gardener, R.: Thromboendarterectomy: a clinical appraisal. Surgery 37:415, 1955.

Zimmerman, L. M., Miller, D., and Marshall, A. N.: Pulmonary embolism: its incidence, significance, and relation to antecedent vein disease. Surg. Gyn. & Obst. 88:373, 1949.

The Lymphatic System

by
GERALD H. PRATT, M.D.

GERALD HILARY PRATT was educated at the University of Minnesota and the University of Iowa, and educated in surgery in the South and on the Eastern Seaboard. He had experience in both the Army and Navy Medical Corps during World War II, and there developed his interest in the diseases of the vascular and lymphatic systems. He is an Associate Clinical Professor of Surgery at the New York University School of Medicine.

The lymphatic circulation, like the arterial and venous systems, is one of the fluid components of the human body. It has its own conduits, collecting areas and circulatory system.

PHYSIOLOGY

The lymphatic system has a twofold purpose. One function is defensive. The other is the transport and distribution of fatty lymphatic substances from the intestinal tract to the rest of the body, a digestive function.

The lymphatic defensive system acts against the usual infectious organisms, as well as against foreign bodies and malignant infiltrations. The lymphatic system is able to contain these threats for a time locally; and, as the invaders extend along the lymphatics, it can also stop them, at least temporarily, at lymph gland masses strategically spaced throughout the body. Should these defenses be overwhelmed, the invaders then spread throughout the body, and eventually reach the blood stream, mainly at junctions with the venous system on either side of the neck.

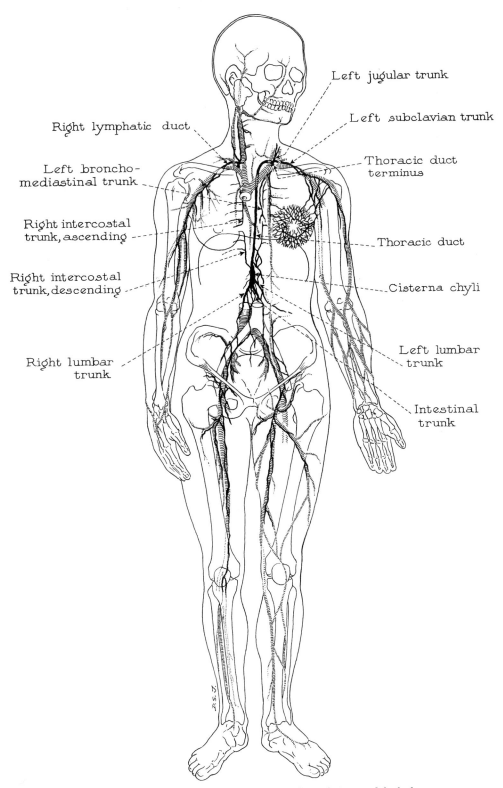

Left jugular trunk

Left subclavian trunk

Right lymphatic duct

Left broncho-
mediastinal trunk

Thoracic duct
terminus

Right intercostal
trunk, ascending

Thoracic duct

Right intercostal
trunk, descending

Cisterna chyli

Left lumbar
trunk

Right lumbar
trunk

Intestinal
trunk

Figure 50. Diagrammatic drawing of the lymphatic drainage of the body.

Thus, the lymphatic system opposes and sometimes dominates the infection, holding its spread through the lymphatics by the resistance of the glands. In like manner, malignancy, particularly of the carcinoma type, may be arrested for a time of indefinite length in the neighboring lymph glands. Suddenly, these lymph glands seem to lose their resistance both to infection and to malignancy, and they pass on these invading forces rapidly, often with seemingly more intense vigor, to reach other areas and the blood stream.

In some respects, this appears to be like a dyke holding back a flooding river which cannot get over the barrier until some weakened area gives way, and the entire water force first puddles and then completely tears out the wall and pours through to inundate and overcome other areas without further resistance. It is upon this temporary stoppage of the spread of infection or malignancy that medical, surgical and radiologic treatment is based. Why some lymph glands can contain, neutralize, or destroy this invasion permanently, or longer in some patients than others, is puzzling, but seems to be an individual characteristic. This disability may be based on biologic and endocrinal factors, genes, stress, general or individual reserve strength, or any of a number of unknown factors.

Once the neighboring glands have been overwhelmed, however, the lymphatic system passes these destroyers on, and even seems to speed them on their way. There may be "skip" areas also, since some of the lymphatics do not enter the localizing glands. In such event, the neighboring nodes are missed in part or all, and other glands are invaded, prior to generalized involvement of near-by or distant areas or organs. At times, lymph-venous shunts rapidly spread lymph pathological materials.

The lymphatic system also collects the fat globules from the lymphatics of the stomach, the intestines, the pancreas, the spleen and the lower and forward part of the liver. This fluid is transported to the collection center, the cisterna chyli, and thus through the thoracic and right lymphatic ducts. This lymph and chyle then are carried into the blood stream.

EMBRYOLOGY

The lymphatic endothelium arises from the venous endothelium in the form of paired and unpaired sacs. The unpaired jugular lymph sacs arise from the jugular veins and extend to the head, neck, thorax and arms. The other paired sacs arise from the iliac veins, with which they unite at the junction of the cardinal veins. These sacs develop in the abdominal wall, the pelvis and the legs. Unpaired lymphatics arise from the vena cava and the mesonephric veins to form the peritoneal lymph sac. These join with veins from the wolffian body and develop the cisterna chyli. The cisterna chyli is both a node and a conduit.

GENERAL ANATOMY

The lymphatic system, like its corollary the venous system, has a liquid component, capillaries, larger vessels which collect fluid from the capillaries, and major or thoracic ducts; it also possesses the lymph glands.

LYMPH. Lymph is a yellowish, thin liquid which is more dilute than blood plasma. Its specific gravity varies with its content, and fluctuates between 1.010 and 1.024, with an average of 1.016. The fluid flows by osmosis, diffusion and filtration from the tissue fluids, but unlike these fluids, it contains lymphocytes and red blood cells.

LYMPH CAPILLARIES. Important lymph capillaries are situated in the connective tissue regions throughout the body, and have a flat pavement-like endothelial lining. The lymphatic capillaries are both continuous and blind, and their anastomoses are made in a peculiar form. There are both superficial and deep lymph systems; the superficial group is in the dermis, and not in the epidermis, a point of surgical importance in lymphedema therapy. The subcutaneous tissue is usually free of capillaries. The skeletal system, including the periosteum, muscles, joints, tendons and such lining membranes as the peritoneum, pleura and pericardium, are richly supplied with lymph capillaries.

The endothelium of the digestive tract has many deep and superficial lymphatic plexuses. Papillae extend into the villi of the small intestines in a blind-end formation. Lacteals arise in the lymph spaces of these intestinal villi and other digestive organs.

The kidney, the spleen, the adrenals, the liver and the salivary glands also have a large number of lymph capillaries; and the respiratory tree from the nose to the bronchi is equally well supplied. The genitourinary tract, including the bladder, ovaries, prostate, testes and uterus, has many lymphatic capillary plexuses. The cardiac system has lymphatics in the endocardium and through the myocardium.

Some parts of the body are not supplied with lymphatics. Among these are the central nervous system, the bone marrow and cartilage system, the eye, the internal ear, striated muscle and the epidermis.

Lymph capillaries have been found to undergo senile changes. These are not the same in all organs of the body, or at the same time of life in different individuals. Illness may bring on senile changes in these lymph capillaries at a much earlier time in life than would be expected.

LYMPH VESSELS. Lymph vessels have three coats, as do the blood vessels. The inner coat is of endothelium placed on an elastic membrane. The middle layer is made of smooth muscle in all but the finer vessels. The external coat consists of a connective tissue covering, the thickness of which depends upon the size of the vessel. A few muscular fibers may be found in the external layer of larger lymph vessels. All lymph capillaries feed into these lymph vessels. The nerve and blood supply to such vessels is provided by nerve fibrils and small vessels which enter the outer and middle coats.

There are valves in the lymphatics similar in construction to those in the veins. The valves increase in number in a vessel just proximal to a lymph node chamber. Lymph vessels are much more numerous than veins, and anastomose more often.

MAIN LYMPHATIC CHANNELS. The cisterna chyli is the collector and chamber for the chyle drainage from the intestines, the pancreas, the liver, the spleen, the lumbar lymphatic trunks from the legs, the pelvis, the kidneys and the adrenal glands. From this

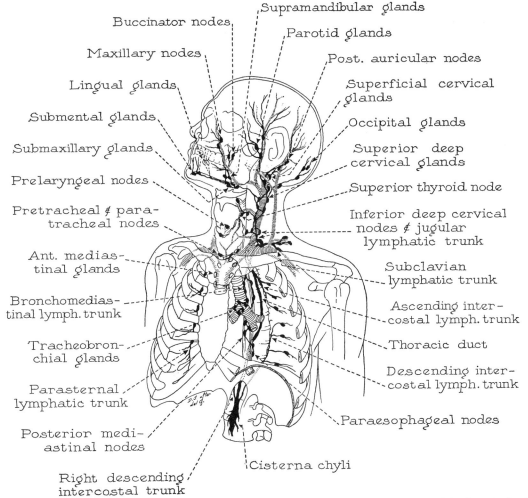

Figure 51. Lymph drainage of the thorax, thoracic duct, neck and head. The early involvement of the thoracic glands by cancer of the lung reduces the possibility of cure in this disease. The large thoracic duct may be injured in its abdominal or thoracic portions. This results in chyle peritoneum or chyle thorax.

collecting chamber, the thoracic duct carries the lymph to its final integration with the venous system in the neck. Except for certain parts of the right side of the body—the heart and the upper part of the liver, the thorax, neck, right arm and right side of the head— the drainage of this lymph is by the thoracic duct. This canal follows the aorta anatomically. After passing through the diaphragm, the duct lies between the aorta and the azygos vein. The left jugular and left subclavian trunks join it. In its upper portion, the duct usually rises from 1 to 2.5 cm. above the clavicle and in front of the subclavian and vertebral arteries and veins. It then opens into the left subclavian vein at its junction with the right internal jugular vein.

LYMPH GLANDS. The lymph glands vary in size from that of approximately a B-B shot or a pea to as large as a small plum. They are round or slightly kidney shaped. In malignant disease, they may become enormous, and may be irregular and deformed in shape. These roundish-ovular structures lie in the channels of the lymph vessels. The afferent lymph vessels enter at the side of the gland, and this lymph passes through tightly massed lymphocytes held in position in the gland by trabeculae from the lymph capsule. Thus, the lymph gland is divided into sinuses. In the center of the cortical sinuses are the germinal centers which divide and thus increase the number of the lymphocytes. The lymph leaves the gland through efferent vessels, which gather the lymph at the hilum of the gland.

DIRECT LYMPHATIC VENOUS COMMUNICATION. The original 100-year-old concept of Virchow that lymph nodes were a barrier or a mechanical filter through which no purulent material or tumor could pass, unless they were assaulted for a long time, has been contradicted. That this thinking was in error has been shown not only clinically, but also by newer methods of study. Direct communication between lymph nodes and the vascular system was suggested 70 years ago. More recent work has shown that there are direct connections between lymph nodes and venous communications through which cells, bacteria and even air can pass. Electron microscopy demonstrates that there are both vascular and lymphatic capillaries in nodes. It is apparent that the sinuses of the lymph nodes are the point of junction between the venous and lymphatic systems. The passage of material from one to the other is often rapid and experimentally occurs as fast as in 22 seconds. Pressure within the two systems is a

factor. The normal lymphatic capillary pressure is lower than that of the venous capillary. Certain physical conditions, such as the injection of air or other substances into the glands, can raise the pressure in the lymphatic capillary. The pathway then of least resistance for flow would be into the venous rather than the lymphatic capillaries. When lymph flow is increased by pressure, there may be a direct invasion of the venous capillaries of material in the gland without its passing through lymphatic capillaries first. Abnormal positions of the glands as in twisting the neck, invasion of the glands by injection or new growth may be the cause of pressure changes and lymphatic venous shunts.

SPECIFIC ANATOMY

HEAD AND NECK. The glands of the neck may be divided into the deep and superficial plexuses and those associated with the salivary glands. There are five or six submaxillary nodes which are in the submaxillary triangle, in close association with the salivary glands. One node lying over the external maxillary artery at the mandible is called "the node of Stahr." These glands drain the upper and lower lip, the gums, the side of the tongue, the cheek and the palpebral commissure, as well as the facial and the submental nodes. From these lymph nodes, the drainage is to the deep cervical nodes. The suprahyoid or submental nodes lie between the bellies of the digastric muscles. They drain the floor of the mouth, the lower lip and the apex of the tongue. They pass through the submaxillary nodes to the deep cervical nodes.

The superficial cervical nodes follow the course of the external jugular vein. These nodes drain the parotid area and the ear, and follow the veins to the superior deep cervical nodes.

The anterior cervical nodes which drain the upper trachea, the thyroid and the larynx, have a superficial and a deep set, the former on the deep jugular vein and the latter in front of the larynx and trachea. They drain into the deep cervical nodes.

The deep cervical glands follow the carotid sheath from the skull to the thorax along the pharynx, trachea and esophagus. The more superficial group run to the sternocleidomastoid muscle, and are near the internal jugular vein. The upper deep cervical nodes drain the ear, the neck, part of the tongue, the nasal cavities, trachea, thyroid and larynx, and nasal pharynx, palate and esophagus, as well as part of the scalp. These glands also drain all the other glands of the neck except the lower deep cervical nodes. They drain to the inferior deep cervical nodes and the nodes around the jugular vein. In the triangle above the clavicle are the inferior deep cervical nodes, which are lateral to the sternocleidomastoid muscle. Anatomically, they are close to the brachial plexus and to the subclavian vein. They drain part of the arm, the pectoral region and the back of the head and neck. Surprisingly, they also drain part of the upper surface of the liver. They accept drainage from the superior deep nodes and they form the jugular trunk, which ends on the right side in the subclavian vein and on the left in the thoracic duct.

The neck skin and muscles drain to the deep cervical nodes. There are retropharyngeal nodes which drain the pharynx and subsequently join the deep cervical nodes. The upper laryngeal lymph drainage is to the superior deep cervical nodes through the hypothyroid membrane. The lower pharyngeal lymph vessels go to the nodes in front of the trachea and larynx, and thereafter to the lower deep cervical nodes and to the paratracheal nodes.

The intricacy of a complete radical neck dissection is emphasized by a consideration of the complexity of the lymph nodes and their afferent pathways as well as the possible skip pathways.

LYMPH CIRCULATION OF THE THORAX. There is in the thorax an anterior and posterior mediastinal group of visceral lymph nodes, as well as the tracheobronchial glands. The anterior nodes lie in front of the aortic arch and along the innominate veins. In tumors with metastases, these glands may become very large and show a widened mediastinum on roentgen examination. They are very adherent to the aorta. The sternum, the pericardium and the thymus glands drain to this group. The bronchomediastinal trunks on the right and left side are formed then by anastomosis of these vessels and the tracheobronchial group. The posterior mediastinal glands follow the esophagus and the descending aorta behind the pericardium. In order, they drain the upper surface of the liver, the diaphragm and the posterior part of the pericardium, as well as the esophagus. The lymph then leaves these glands to join with the thoracic duct or the tracheomediastinal trunk. The lungs, trachea, bronchi and the heart are drained to the tracheobronchial glands, which also drain the posterior mediastinal glands. Lymph from the lung may drain also to the preaortic glands. These lymph vessels, with the internal mammary vessels and the drainage from the anterior mediastinal glands, form the right and left bronchomediastinal trunks. They may enter the thoracic ducts or go directly into the subclavian or jugular veins, a point of surgical importance. This may explain the rapid and widespread dissemination of disease or new growth.

The parietal sternal glands are close to the internal mammary artery, and they may drain the breast, the deep structures of the anterior upper abdominal wall, and part of the upper surface of the liver. Like the other glands, they may drain directly to the subclavian or internal jugular veins, or via the thoracic and right lymphatic duct.

Intercostal glands follow the intercostal vessels, and accept the deep lymphatic drainage from the sides of the chest. They form a descending trunk to the cisterna chyli or thoracic duct. The upper glands drain to the thoracic duct on one side and to the right lymphatic duct on the other.

The diaphragmatic glands have anterior and posterior components. The anterior ones lie behind the xiphoid. They drain the vessels from the diaphragm and liver, and then go directly to the sternal glands. The medial glands may be in the pericardial sac or near the phrenic opening in the diaphragm. The middle diaphragm on the right and the upper part of the liver are thus drained. The lymph from this area goes to the posterior mediastinal glands. These posterior glands then feed to the posterior mediastinal nodes, and are located posteriorly on the crux of the diaphragm.

Breast. The lymphatic vessels of the breast arise in the interlobular spaces and in the walls of the milk ducts. The central vessels form a plexus below the areola and nipple, and pass to the pectoral group of the axillary glands. The lateral and medial parts of the breast drain to the subclavicular axillary glands. The outer part of the breast drains to these same nodes. The medial breast glands pierce the chest wall and drain mainly to the sternal glands, but occasionally may drain to the subclavicular glands. Bizarre arrangement of lymph drainage may occur, and there may be direct connection with the right lymphatic or thoracic duct. The rapid and widespread dissemination of cancer of the breast at times may thus be explained.

Heart. The lymph vessels of the heart are both superficial and deep, the superficial being close to the pericardium, and the deep under the endocardium. These plexuses form a right and left connecting lymph trunk. The left trunk drains both ventricles and begins in the anterior longitudinal sulcus. At the coronary sulcus, it receives the diaphragmatic trunk, and this vessel then drains to the tracheobronchial nodes. The right trunk drains the right atrium and the diaphragmatic side of the right ventricle. It ascends on the posterior longitudinal coronary sulcus and ends in the tracheobronchial nodes.

Lungs. The superficial and deep lymph plexuses of the lungs do not anastomose to any great extent. In the presence of disease or malignant infiltration, these structures may drain directly to each other. The superficial plexus, beginning beneath the pleura, drains to the glands at the hilus of the lung. The deep plexus involves the bronchi and pulmonary vessels, ending in the mucosa or beneath it. These vessels are joined at the hilus, and they drain to the tracheobronchial glands. The surgical importance is that the alveolar walls have no lymph vessels, and there is a lack of anastomoses between the superficial and deep lymph plexuses. The lymphatic venous shunt can change the pattern of lymph drainage markedly.

The lymph from the pleura and the visceral part of the lung ends in the superficial vessels of the lung. The parietal pleura lymph drains to the sternal glands, while the diaphragmatic part involves the diaphragmatic chain. The mediastinal portion ends in the posterior mediastinal glands.

Thymus and esophagus. The thymic lymph vessels drain to the sternal, tracheobronchial and mediastinal glands. The esophageal vessels form a plexus around this organ, and its main drainage is into the posterior mediastinal glands.

ABDOMEN AND PELVIS. The glands of the abdomen and pelvis are placed retroperitoneally, and follow the arteries and veins in the same area, for which they are named. The hypogastric, the epigastric and the circumflex glands all drain the area supplied by those arteries, and are located behind, in front of and beside the aorta. On the right, they are in intimate association with the inferior vena cava, the renal vein and the psoas muscle. On the left, they are associated with the abdominal aorta, and drain to the cisterna chyli. The superior and inferior mesenteric glands, with the celiac glands, form the preaortic plexus; with the retroaortic glands, they drain to the cisterna chyli.

The superior mesenteric glands lie along the main arterial and venous supply in the terminal branches of the mesenteric artery at the secondary vascular loops. They may number from 100 to 200, and they drain into the mesenteric, ileocolic and mesocolic lymph nodes. Normally, there are anywhere from ten to 25 ileocolic nodes around the artery of the same name. They are termed ileo or ileocolic glands, depending upon where they lie, the latter lying behind the cecum and the ascending colon. There is also a single or double node in the appendiceal mesentery, and some along the ascending colon called the right colic glands. The mesocolic nodes are numerous and lie mostly in the transverse mesocolon, particularly at the hepatic and splenic flexures. They drain to the preaortic nodes.

The inferior mesenteric nodes consist of three groups. One is along the left colic and sigmoid arteries; the second is around the superior hemorrhoidal artery; and the third is in and around the muscular coat of the rectum. These drain the sigmoid and descending colon, as well as the upper rectum, and drain to the lower preaortic nodes.

The superior gastric glands have a peculiar anatomic distribution beginning at the base of the left gastric artery, a second part which follows the artery on the lesser curvature, and are placed between the layers of the omentum. There is a third or paracardial group which forms a necklace-like arrangement at the upper part of the stomach near its esophageal junction. The lower gastric glands, numbering five to ten, usually lie between the layers of the greater omentum on the greater curvature of the stomach, mostly on the pyloric end.

The hepatic glands, along the hepatic artery, follow a common viaduct into the lesser omentum. A well-known node called the cystic gland arises at the neck of the gallbladder. The liver nodes, called the subpyloric hepatic nodes, are approximately six in number, and are at the bifurcation of the gastroduodenal artery, and drain the superior and descending parts of the duodenum, the stomach, the liver and the pancreas. All these nodes drain into the preaortic nodes.

The pancreaticolienal nodes are in close contact with the splenic artery on the upper and posterior border of the pancreas. These also drain the pancreas, spleen and the stomach.

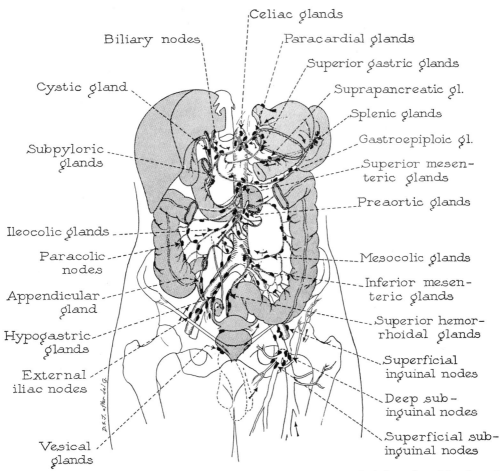

Celiac glands

Biliary nodes

Paracardial glands

Superior gastric glands

Cystic gland

Suprapancreatic gl.

Splenic glands

Subpyloric glands

Gastroepiploic gl.

Superior mesenteric glands

Preaortic glands

Ileocolic glands

Mesocolic glands

Paracolic nodes

Inferior mesenteric glands

Appendicular gland

Superior hemorrhoidal glands

Hypogastric glands

Superficial inguinal nodes

External iliac nodes

Deep subinguinal nodes

Superficial subinguinal nodes

Vesical glands

Figure 52. Lymphatics of the pelvis and abdomen. The lymphatic drainage from both the male and female genitalia and pelvis is superimposed. Note drainage of external genitalia through inguinal glands. The stomach, liver and colon have been divided to show the drainage of these and the other intestinal organs to the lymphatic glands which follow the major vessels. Arrows indicate direction of inguinal drainage. The irregularity of the lymphatic drainage illustrates the difficulty of the cure of malignant disease.

All these lymph vessels follow the course of the blood vessels and drain to the preaortic glands. The delineation is of great importance in the diagnosis of extension and spread of carcinoma or inflammation.

Diaphragm. The abdominal diaphragm is drained in two ways. The diaphragm on the right drains to the glands near the inferior phrenic artery, and the right lateral aortic glands. Those from the left half of this plexus drain to the lateral aortic glands and to the glands near the end of the esophagus.

Stomach. The lymphatic vessels of the stomach join those of the duodenum and the esophagus, and on the left side drain to the superior gastric nodes. The fundus and body of the stomach to the left of the esophageal junction drain to the pancreaticolienal nodes. The vessels to the right of this point drain to the subpyloric nodes via the inferior gastric nodes. Of surgical importance is the pylorus,

which is drained to superior gastric nodes with by-way stops at the hepatic and subpyloric nodes. The complexity of the node drainage from the stomach is of therapeutic importance, and indicates the difficulty of eradicating gastric malignant disease if it was not contained at its original source.

Intestinal vessels. The duodenal vessels drain in front of and behind the organ to the pancreaticoduodenal nodes between the duodenum and the head of the pancreas, and then to the hepatic and preaortic nodes.

Jejunal and ileal vessels are called lacteals and arise between the intestinal villi. Their milklike fluid is carried between the layers of the mesentery of the small bowel to the mesenteric nodes. From these nodes, they empty into the preaortic nodes, and then to the cisterna chyli. The appendix and its neighboring cecum have many lymph vessels, and drain into an anterior and posterior group of local lymph nodes. The anterior go to the ileocolic nodes, and the posterior pass to the back of the cecum.

The lymphatic vessels of the right colon and the transverse colon drain to the mesocolic nodes, and then to the left colic and sigmoid nodes, terminating in the preaortic nodes.

The rectal lymphatic vessels, after passing through the perirectal glands, go to the sigmoid and mesocolon glands and then to the preaortic nodes. The anal lymphatic vessels drain to the superficial inguinal nodes. The vessels of the anal canal proper follow the middle and inferior hemorrhoidal arteries to the hypogastric nodes.

Liver, gallbladder, pancreas, spleen, and suprarenals. The liver has similar superficial and deep lymphatic vessels. The superior portion of the superficial nodes drains the convex portion of the liver. One such vessel draining the right and left nodes passes through the diaphragm with the vena cava, and goes to that vessel's glands. Some lymphatics from the undersurface of the liver go to the hepatic nodes, while one vessel goes directly through the diaphragm to the vena cava nodes. The deep lymphatics form an ascending and descending trunk, the first draining to the inferior vena cava area, and the latter to the hepatic nodes.

The vessels of the gallbladder drain to the hepatic nodes, as do those of the bile ducts. Lymph from the latter may also drain to the pancreaticoduodenal nodes.

The pancreas drains mainly to the pancreaticolienal nodes, but some lymph vessels end in the preaortic nodes.

The lymph vessels of the spleen pass to the pancreaticolienal glands.

The suprarenal vessels drain mainly to the lateral aortic nodes, but may also drain to the posterior mediastinum above the diaphragm.

The lymph vessels of the omentum have a bizarre anastomosis and many valves. They vary in size, but in general are very large.

Urinary tract. The urinary organs are quite complex in their lymph drainage.

There are three plexuses of lymph vessels in the kidney, one just below its capsule, a second in the surrounding fat of the kidney and the third in the substance of the kidney. These all drain through vessels which pass to the hilum, following the renal vein to end in the aortic nodes. Perinephric vessels also drain to these same glands.

The lymph vessels of the ureter depend on the part of the ureter involved. The upper ureter drains into the efferent vessels of the kidney and into the aortic glands. The common iliac glands are the termination of the lymph vessels from the lower portion of the ureter above the brim of the pelvis. The pelvic portion of the ureter drains into the hypogastric glands.

The mucosa of the bladder does not appear to have a lymphatic supply. The intramuscular and extramuscular tissues do have such structures. The anterior surface of the bladder drains into the external iliac glands, and has small glands situated in its course called vesical glands. The lymph vessels of the posterior bladder wall drain to the hypogastric and the iliac glands.

The posterior portion of the prostate has a lymphatic vessel which drains to the external iliac nodes, while the anterior part drains to the same lymph vessel as from the membranous urethra.

The urethral glands and those of the glans penis drain to the subinguinal as well as the external iliac nodes. The membranous and prostatic portions of the urethra in the male and the entire urethra in the female have vessels going to the hypogastric glands.

Reproductive system. The lymph drainage vessels from the ovary and testis are similar, and both have a superficial and a deep plexus. These accompany the spermatic vein in the spermatic cord in the male, and the ovarian vessels in the female, to the lateral and preaortic lumbar glands.

The uterus has superficial vessels under the peritoneum, and another plexus in the uterine wall itself. These lymphatics are tremendous in size during pregnancy. Their course of drainage is through the broad ligaments, continued up to the ovarian vessels and then to the preaortic glands. A few vessels drain via the external iliac collectors to the superficial inguinal glands. The cervix drains to the external iliac glands and the hypogastric glands, as well as to the common iliac glands. The uterine tube drains partly with the ovarian and partly with the uterine vessels.

The vagina drains according to the part of the organ involved. The external iliac glands are the recipients of the vessels from the upper vagina, the hypogastric glands from the middle part, and the iliac glands from the lower part. The extensive anastomosis of the lymphatic vessels of the rectum, bladder, vulva and cervix is of surgical importance. The vulvar lymphatics drain to the superficial inguinal nodes.

THE EXTREMITIES. Upper extremity. As

in other parts of the body, the upper extremity has a superficial and a deep lymphatic plexus, and these follow the veins. The glands are few in number in the superficial system. There are some nodes at the medial epicondyle through which the third, fourth and fifth fingers are drained, while the medial side of the hand and the ulnar side of the forearm drain to the deeper vessels. There are a few pectoral nodes which also drain superficially.

The deep glands follow the brachial, ulnar and radial arteries. There are only a few glands until one approaches the axilla, where there may be from 30 to 40. These are of great surgical importance.

There are five groups which have been described. The anterior group, situated at the lower border of the pectoralis minor muscle and in intimate relation to the lateral thoracic artery, drains to the subclavicular group. The posterior or subscapular glands, which sur-

round the subscapular artery, drain the back of the neck and thorax, and go to the central axillary nodes. The lateral nodes, located behind the axillary vein, drain the whole arm except for the cephalic side. These lymphatics drain into the subclavicular axillary nodes, and the inferior deep cervical nodes. The central or intermediate nodes are deep in the base of the axilla and drain all the other groups of axillary glands and these drain to the subclavicular nodes. The subclavicular or medial nodes may be approximately ten in number, and are under and above the pectoralis minor muscle. Since they drain all the other nodes in the axilla, these glands are of utmost surgical importance, particularly in cancer operations. These glands accompany the cephalic vein, after draining the upper and outer parts of the breast. A subclavian lymphatic afferent vessel is formed by the union of these vessels. This vessel may open directly into the subclavian and jugular veins,

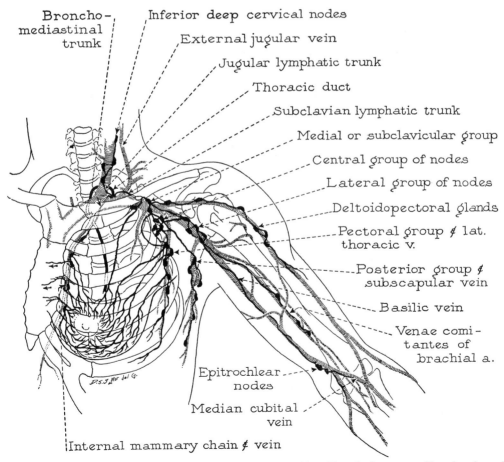

Figure 53.   Lymph drainage of the axilla. Arrows indicate direction of flow. Note the five groups of lymph nodes and their vessels. Drainage of the lymphatic ducts to the neck and mediastinum makes eradication of malignant disease difficult once it has extended to the glands.

or on the left the jugular lymphatic trunk or the thoracic duct.

The lymphatic vessels of the upper extremities form trunks which accompany the cephalic, median and basilic veins. On the ulnar side, a few of the vessels drain to the supratrochlear nodes. The other lymph vessels drain into the lateral axillary nodes. Some may pass by the deltoid-pectoral nodes into the cervical or subclavicular axillary nodes. The deep lymphatic vessels follow the deep blood vessels, and in general drain into the lateral axillary glands.

Lower extremity. There are three sets of lymph glands in the lower extremity: the inguinal, the popliteal and the anterior tibial nodes.

The superficial inguinal glands lie directly below the inguinal ligament, and they are anatomically close to and above the saphenous vein. Their drainage is mainly from the abdominal wall below the umbilicus, the buttocks, perineum, scrotum and penis, and the labia majora and other external portions of the female genital tract. The saphenous vein divides the superficial and deeper groin glands, which have a secondary subdivision. The saphenous vein is again the dividing line between the superficial and the deep gland components.

The superficial subinguinal glands drain the superficial tissues, and also have conduits from the genital areas. The fascia lata is superimposed on the deep subinguinal glands, medial to the femoral vein. The main drainage is from the penis, the clitoris and the superficial subinguinal glands as described.

The anterior tibial glands are on the interosseous membrane. Except for local inflammation, they are of insignificant importance.

The popliteal glands are in close proximity to the popliteal artery and vein, and number generally from five to ten. They drain the area of the lesser saphenous vein and the popliteal vein, but also have drainage from the knee joint. In this latter capacity, they may be of greater surgical importance. The popliteal glands drain those tissues which receive their blood supply from the anterior and posterior tibial arteries.

The lymphatic vessels in the lower extremity are of great importance. These are superficial and deep in type. The superficial vessels have both a lateral or fibular group of vessels, rising from the lateral side of the foot, which accompanies the lesser saphenous vein, and drain to the popliteal glands. The medial, or larger group of vessels follows the

great saphenous vein to the subinguinal group of superficial glands. The deep lymphatic vessels are few in number, and they follow the deep blood vessels to the popliteal glands. There are some lymph vessels which drain to inguinal lymph nodes from the gluteal and ischial regions.

The lymph supply of the lower extremities becomes extremely important in any infection and in malignancy, especially of the epithelial type. The inguinal gland dissection for such malignancy has become an integral part of surgical treatment, and the delineation of these glands and their skip areas by lymphography can be of utmost importance in the therapy of such growths.

The lymph gland vessels of the lower extremities are important in the lymphatic hypertrophy which follows a venous obstruction. In these patients, the lymphatic system, which is a corollary of the venous system, tries to take over the function of the venous system in carrying away waste products and foreign matter, and returning it to the venous system. The lymphatic vessels hypertrophy to large sizes, but because lymph is such a slow-moving substance, it is usually ineffective in taking over the work of the blocked venous system, and lymphedema occurs.

The importance of lymphaticovenous communications or shunts has only lately been recognized with the improvement of lymphangiography. Clinical efforts to use shunts from the venous to the lymphatic system have been made. The thoracic duct has been surgically joined to the systemic veins to relieve ascites from hepatic vein occlusion or hepatic cirrhosis. An anastomosis between the thoracic duct and the pulmonary vein in right heart failure due to various causes has been conjectured.

In an early stage, lymphedema is primarily a mechanical disorder and can be relieved by mechanical means, such as elevation of the part above the heart and neck level, warm packs and adequate support when the patient stands. If the lymph is allowed to remain stagnant, pathologic changes occur; fibrous trabeculae grow between the large lymph spaces, and the lymphedema becomes chronic and persistent.

When the lymph conduits are unable to carry the lymph and their valves fail, a massive lymphedema may occur. This condition may be either congenital or acquired.

The lymphangiographic delineation is of great importance, both diagnostically and in aiding efforts to correct the block surgically or for the glands' radical excision in malignancy.

LYMPHOGRAPHY

Lymphography is a term which includes the contrast visualization of the lymphatic vessels; lymphangiography, which may or may not demonstrate the nodes, and lymphandenography, the direct injection of dye into the lymph nodes. The latter method is becoming important with the more advanced operations for malignancy.

LYMPHANGIOGRAPHY. As early as 1941, dos Santos experimented to develop a technique to determine lymph pathways and their pathology. Homans injected graphite in the skin and as this foreign material was accepted by the lymph vessels, he dissected them and often was able to canalize them. His work was done on patients with elephantiasis. Kinmonth refined the technique and at the present time it is an integral part of a well-directed radiology service. Both water solutions and oils have been used as the vehicle to carry the iodine for lymphangiography. The possibility of oil embolism exists because there are connections between the lymphatics and the venous system. Serious embolism is sufficiently rare as to be a negligible factor if the data derived from the examination are important to the patient's health. If such a lymphatic venous spillover is observed fluoroscopically, the injection should be stopped.

The indications for lymphangiography are abnormal, general or local swelling of the extremity of a congenital or acquired type; to diagnose lymphoma; to determine the spread of malignancy, and to determine whether the lymph blocks are superficial (prefascial) or whether the block is in the deep lymphatics. Although one can eliminate surgically the lymph block in the prefascial area, such an elimination, if the deep lymphatics were blocked, necessarily would make the patient's condition worse.

The contraindications are allergy or intolerance to the drug; infection in the area; dermatitis at the site of injection; acute lymphangitis; arterial occlusive disease; bleeding tendencies, and advanced renal, malignant or hepatic disease.

The same problem of anaphylaxis may occur in lymphangiography as it does in an iodine injection into arteries or veins. Sensitivity tests should always be performed prior to lymphangiography.

There is a febrile reaction in the first 24 hours in approximately one out of three patients. The temperature usually subsides in 24 to 48 hours with the use of acetylsalicylic acid.

Oil emboli may occur from injecting the oily material too rapidly or in too large amounts. They can be avoided by fluoroscopy, noting

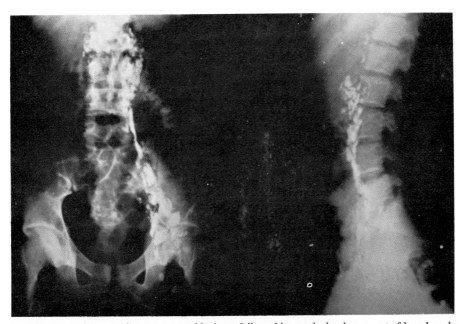

Figure 54.   Lymphogram showing severe blockage followed by marked enlargement of lymph nodes.

the lymphatic venous shunt and stopping the injection if there is a shunt.

There will be some pain at the time of the injection. This is greater if the injection is so forceful as to break the lymphatics.

Infection of the site has occurred but this can be prevented by careful asepsis.

Lymphangitis may occur as a chemical reaction and follow the course of the lymphatics. It subsides with local treatment by packs and elevation.

Ethiodol remains in the glands for many days or weeks. It apparently does not cause fibrosis as Wallace et al. have reported.

Dermatitis of the legs has been observed. It is thought to be a vascular type of reaction to the extravasated ethiodized oil adjacent to lymphatic pathways. It responds to local packs. Topical fluocinolone acetonide aids in rapid recovery.

Technique of lymphangiography. After a complete surgical preparation has been made, a solution of 1 cc. of Sky Blue and 1 cc. of 1 per cent procaine is mixed in the syringe. Although Patent Blue V (11 per cent) or Prontosil Rubrum (10 per cent) has been used, we use only Sky Blue. From 0.1 to 0.15 cc. is injected into the web space between the toes, usually between the first and second toes. In approximately one-half hour in most instances, this dye will have entered the lymphatics and they can be visualized. An incision is then made in the skin in the line of the lymph channel and the dyed lymphatic vessel is isolated. This dye may also be in the venules and the differentiation between a lymphatic vessel and a vein can be made by milking the selected vessel proximally. A vein will empty with this maneuver, but a lymphatic channel will not. Two fine silk sutures are placed around the isolated vessel and the assistant holds these sutures, closing the upper one while the dye is milked into the space between them to distend it. A short beveled needle just large enough to fit into this lymphatic is inserted. A magnifying glass or an eye loop helps in this maneuver. The silk suture is tied around the needle.

Purified iodized ethyl ester of poppy seed oil, each milliliter containing 37 per cent iodine by body weight, is injected very slowly, usually at a rate of between 2 and 3 cc. per hour. The injection is terminated if fluoroscopy shows that there is a lymphatic venous shunt. The injection is stopped also if there is an obstruction to the flow. It is terminated when the lymphatics at the level of the second

and third lumbar vertebrae are visualized. Serial x-ray films of the flow in the lymphatic vessels are made. The lymphatic conduit can be ligated to prevent a lymph fistula and the wound is closed. Several films of the abdomen are made. At 24 hours of elapsed time, films are repeated to show the status of the nodes themselves, because these are rarely shown in the initial films.

Retroperitoneal and pelvic nodes will be shown in many of these delayed films. A lymph node is usually round or slightly kidney shaped. The malignant ones become larger and irregular, often lumped together and there are more of them than normal. A lacy or frosty pattern of dye is quite characteristic of lymphoma.

The technique in the upper extremity is the same as for the lower extremity. There are two separate pathways in the upper extremity for lymph drainage. The ulnar tract drains principally the skin of the third, fourth and fifth fingers and the ulnar side of the hand and forearm. The radial lymphatics drain the skin of the first and second fingers and the radial side of the hand and forearm. To visualize all the lymphatics of the upper extremity, therefore, two injections are necessary. Again the injection is discontinued if there is a lymph shunt to the vein or an obstruction to the flow, or when the axillary area is well visualized. A 24-hour x-ray picture may delineate axillary lymph nodes as well as those along the major vessels in the thorax.

LYMPHADENOGRAPHY. The main purpose of such a study is to determine possible causes of lymphedema and the course and spread of malignant disease. Unidentified masses in the pelvis and abdominal cavity, chest or extremities may be demonstrated through this medium. A surgical procedure for malignancy may be thus outlined or found to be contraindicated. The plan for x-ray or other ray therapy may be altered or guided by this method of study.

The contraindications to lymphadenography are allergy to the drug; inability to palpate nodes; patients in whom a surgical procedure of any type is not indicated; patients with limited pulmonary reserve because of the possibility of pulmonary emboli, and the possibility of spread of tumor. The occurrence of this complication has not been proved or disproved.

The sites of injection are usually the cervical, axillary or inguinal nodes. Retroperitoneal, pelvic or thoracic nodes will be de-

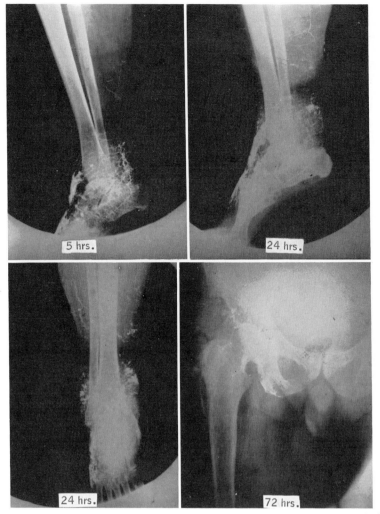

Figure 55. Lymphogram at 5, 24 and 72 hours, showing slow progression of dye in the blocked lymphatics.

lineated through injections in the inguinal, axillary or cervical glands.

Purified, iodized ethyl ester of poppy seed oil, each milliliter containing 37 per cent iodine by body weight, is used. The largest node at the group of glands is selected for the injection. It is thoroughly prepared surgically. One can ascertain that the needle is in the node if the needle moves when the node is moved manually. The use of a solution hyaluronidase injected into the gland before the dye will accelerate the spread of the dye through the glands. This solution is inserted through a 20 gauge needle very slowly. The syringe with the Ethiodol is then exchanged, leaving the needle in situ. Five to 10 cc. of the contrast media is injected, the amount necessarily depending upon the size of the node and the desire to see the other nodes

beyond it. X-rays are then taken in the anterior-posterior and lateral and, at times, in the oblique position. Follow-up pictures are taken at the end of 24 hours.

There have been fewer complications reported from the direct node injection than have followed the injection of the lymphatic vessels. Iodine sensitivity is the ever possible and serious danger. Embolism is possible, but has not been reported as a serious problem as the dye clears through the lung in approximately one week. The possibility of gland breakdown must be considered, especially if the glands are badly diseased. Sepsis should be eliminated technically. The possibility of disseminating a growth by this method of study is worthy of consideration.

The decision to perform direct gland injection again depends on the necessity of the information to be derived and each patient must be individually considered.

Roentgen cinematography has been used in lymphography. This medium has demonstrated valve systems of the lymph tree. It also demonstrated that normally the lymph flow is equal in all lymphatics. The connections between the dye and superficial lymph system have been shown to open only when there is an obstruction to the flow. Because the pressure in the lymphatic capillaries in lymph nodes is less than that of venous capillaries, the flow of the dye taking the path of least resistance will enter the lymph and not the venous capillaries. Severe distortions of the glands by pressure or invasion may increase the lymphatic capillary pressure to above that of the venous capillaries. In such event, the venous capillaries will pick up the dye. Careful fluoroscopy should be observed in patients with distorted glands to prevent a flow into the veins and emboli.

Recently, lymphangiography has been used therapeutically. The catheter is inserted through the needle and the needle withdrawn. Cytotoxic drugs are injected in an effort to destroy the malignant cells which have metastasized to the lymph nodes. The catheter has been left in the lymph canal for as long as six days. The possibilities of this and other similar methods in the future seem encouraging with the thought that the cure of cancer eventually will be biological or chemical.

MECHANICAL INJURIES

Injuries to the lymphatic system may involve the glands or the lymph vessels. Injuries to the vessels are the most important. Large lymph ducts or the small lymphatic vessels may be the site of the injury. Any trauma which breaks the skin necessarily divides lymphatic channels. In healing and particularly in delayed healing of such wounds, scarring may occur with temporary or permanently blocked lymph channels. Edema around the wound and below it is an indication of such blocks. Poorly placed incisions or inadequate coaptation may cause an enlargement of the lymph blocks.

INJURIES TO THORACIC AND LYMPHATIC DUCTS. The thoracic duct, which measures between 36 and 48 cm., runs from the second lumbar vertebra to the root of the neck. It is in intimate association with the vertebrae, and

from the fifth thoracic vertebra upward runs to the left side.

The duct may be injured by an open wound, an indirect bruising wound or, most often, by a crushing wound. In the latter instance, the other associated injuries take precedence in treatment and the lymphatic duct injury may be masked. The duct may be severed in part or entirely during a surgical operation. Burns, x-rays and other rays may also cause duct injuries. The thoracic duct may also be injured in operations upon the posterior triangles of the neck. Two to 4 liters of chyle can be discharged daily. This results in dehydration, starvation, thirst, emaciation and weakness. This accident is fatal in 5 per cent of the patients. The injury to the right thoracic duct is not too serious.

If the lymph wound is an open one, a lymph fistula occurs, causing lymphorrhea. The chyle escapes freely with each respiration. Chyle thorax may be a most serious condition. The diagnosis follows a history of injury and is confirmed by the x-ray appearance of fluid and pressure or by displacment of organs. It may be made certain by thoracentesis. Aspiration often relieves the pressure on other organs, and the laceration in the duct may close spontaneously.

If injured at the time of an operation, the thoracic duct or the right lymphatic duct may be reanastomosed. Repair of the right lymphatic duct may be technically impossible, and a ligature or suture may resolve the pathologic process.

Ligation may stop the flow of lymph from the thoracic duct, and it may continue to carry chyle through collateral lymph vessels or through a spontaneously created anastomosis.

In crushing injuries, immediate treatment should be directed toward the other injuries. Thoracentesis or paracentesis will relieve the chyle pressure and accumulation in the chest or abdomen. The damaged duct often repairs itself as the other wounds heal. Chyle thorax may require surgical intervention because of pressure upon, or displacement of, the lung or heart. If the fluid continues to reaccumulate, or if body depletion from its loss is threatened, it can be repaired surgically through a thoracotomy. If this is impossible technically, the duct should be ligated. The collateral circulation usually will carry the chyle through the opposite duct.

Most injuries to the abdominal portion of the duct heal spontaneously. If an injury continues to drain, or x-rays show pressure on the abdominal viscera, the duct must be repaired or ligated.

Recent studies have shown that cannulation of the thoracic duct may provide information about problems of autoimmunity, hypersensitivity and homograft rejection. Antibody globulin was present in the lymphocytes in patients with cirrhosis or congestive heart failure. When lymph drainage was diverted, a homograft remained viable much longer than when the lymph flow was normal.

INJURIES TO SMALL LYMPHATIC VESSELS. The small lymphatic vessels are injured with any laceration or incision. Usually, extensive operations, and particularly lymph node dissections, divide many lymph vessels. Lymphedema may occur in these patients if a tissue space or cavity remains for lymph accumulation. External pressure will control most of these accumulations unless they are complicated by sepsis or unless the wound is drained. Lymphatic collections and obstructions occur more often in drained than in undrained wounds. If the lymph collection is not infected, it should be evacuated and further accumulation prevented by pressure dressings. It should never be drained.

Injuries to lymph vessels occur also from burns and irradiation. The nuclear explosions at Hiroshima and Nagasaki during World War II caused widespread damage to the lymphatics of the victims, and the healing of the burns resulted in lymphedema and heavy keloids.

Fistulas caused by laceration of lymphatic channels of smaller size than the thoracic duct often close spontaneously. Lymphorrhea may be stopped by a sterile pressure dressing. This applies to lymph drainage after gland resections in the neck, groin or axilla. The accumulation may be erroneously considered purulent, and an attempt may be made to drain the fluid, thus keeping its fistulous nature active. Compression should be maintained by a firm bandage.

LYMPHEDEMA (LYMPH STASIS, ELEPHANTIASIS OR LYMPH OBSTRUCTION)

LYMPHEDEMA IN THE LOWER EXTREMITY. Since the lymphatic system is a closed one, except for the recently recognized lymph venous shunts, any obstruction causes lymph accumulation. Such a collection, by its size and its complications, causes increasing disability. Lymph obstruction always is accompanied by dilatation of the venous drainage system, as it makes an effort to return the fluid from the involved tissues. The lymphatic obstruction, by pressure, causes deleterious skin changes and distention or destruction in the other tissues, often with atrophy or even displacement of the muscles. The lymph vessels involved in lymphedema are those in the dermis, but not the epidermal layer of the skin, since the epidermis does not have lymphatics. The fluid collection extends into the subcutaneous fat and deep fascial layers. The muscle lymphatics usually do not become involved in this process, because of their protected position.

The lymphatic drainage channels may be closed by a congenital valve or vessel defect, or they may become obstructed secondarily by inflammation or internal or external pressure. Lymphedema may be localized, due to a block in the main lymphatics, or it may be generalized with all of the lymphatics of the part obstructed. When the extremity or part is elevated, the fluid will flow by gravity through the subcutaneous tissues to areas where there are no lymphatic blocks, and the lymph then will be drained. This method of drainage occurs only when there is elevation of the part. With dependency, the lymph reaccumulates, since there are no physical pathways for its removal. With failure of lymph drainage, the involved part may become inflamed, by the usual contaminant organisms. Healing after each inflammatory attack causes further scarring and more lymph vessel obstruction. The pathologic process thus recurs and becomes self-perpetuating.

Etiology. Any disease or trauma which directly or indirectly obstructs the lymphatic canals or destroys their valves may cause lymphedema. The causes of this condition are innumerable. A congenital or developmental failure of the lymph vessels or their valves may be responsible for the lesion. In some patients, the lymph stasis may be due to an endocrine dysfunction. A specific or nonspecific infection in the lymphatic system, an injury, a burn and a primary or secondary new growth are the usual acquired causes. Thrombophlebitis, in addition to producing tissue space fluid accumulation, also causes lymphedema.

The originating or precipitating factors in the development of lymphedema have been classified into eight types: specific lymphedema, infectious lymphedema, allergic lymphedema, postthrombotic lymphedema, traumatic lymphedema, congenital lymph collections, malignant lymphedema and essential lymphedema.

SPECIFIC LYMPHEDEMA. Certain organisms have a predilection for invasion and inflammation of the lymphatic channels. Of these, the filarial worm (*Wuchereria bancrofti*), *W.* (or *Brugia*) *malayi*, *Loa loa*, *Onchocerca volvulus* (Africa), *O. caecutiens* (Central America), the tuberculosis organism (*Mycobacterium tuberculosis*) and the *Treponema pallidum*, which causes syphilis, are examples.

A mosquito, the *Stegomyia pseudoscutellaris*, or *Culex fatigans*, picks up the worm, the *Wuchereria bancrofti*. The larvae are deposited and injected by the penetration of the bite of the mosquito. Adult filariae live in the lymph channels and discharge embryos. The dead worms also may cause a lymphatic inflammation. Streptococci and other pyogens frequently cause an associated suppurative infection. The lymph vessels become filled by organisms and inflammatory cells and this causes secondary lymph collections in the tissues. The lymph glands are infected and enlarged. The filariae produce recurrent febrile attacks, each one resulting in an inflammatory reaction with more pathologic changes.

Lymphedema due to filarial worm invasion has had historical implications. The Roman Legions fought natives in Africa who had these grotesque obstructions which caused disfigurement of the limbs and genitalia. The term "elephantiasis" originated in their reports on these natives. Not only the skin resembled that of the elephant, with its thickening and wrinkling, but the affected parts were grotesquely large.

In the American campaign in the Pacific against the Japanese during World War II, certain staging areas, the Samoan and Wallace Islands, for example, used for final training prior to the invasion of the islands had epidemic and endemic filariae-infected natives. In 1943, 6000 trained troops had to be evacuated because of filariasis of the legs or genitalia following lymphatic obstruction. Rigid quarantine dropped this number in one year to 10 per cent of that figure. The Korean and Vietnam wars have presented similar but less numerous patients with lymphedema.

The tuberculosis and syphilitic organisms cause similar invasions, infections and reactions.

INFECTIOUS LYMPHEDEMA. The lymphatic system is both a block to and pathway for the spread of infection. The ordinary contaminant organisms such as the streptococci and staphylococci may increase in virulence and the host's defense may be overcome; these organisms then enter the lymph vessels. They locally inflame these vessels and spread to the regional lymph nodes. These nodes filter out the infection and retain it unless the sepsis overwhelms them. In the latter event, the organisms may pass on to other lymph vessels and eventually to the blood stream. Shunts to the venous system prior to the emptying of the thoracic duct into the subclavian vein may cause an early septicemia. Such infections usually cause localized lymphedema. If the infection is continued or recurrent, fibrosis and scarring within the lymphatics is the end result.

In their invasion, these organisms may cause sufficient inflammation to obstruct the lymphatics and destroy their valves.

Repeated infections invariably cause low-grade changes in the glands. These glands, in themselves, may keep the infection active or recurrent, similar to the situation in tonsillitis.

ALLERGIC LYMPHEDEMA. Some individuals are sensitive to certain pollens, proteins or environmental changes which affect the lymphatics and precipitate lymph blocks. An example is the allergic reaction to exposure to cold. A type of temporary block is due to massive hives. Such diathesis rarely is the cause of permanent lymphedema, but such reactions if extensive can produce lymphedema.

POSTTHROMBOTIC LYMPHEDEMA. Thrombosis of the deep or superficial veins causes edema, which throws an overload on the lymphatic component. There may be a damming back of the lymphatics, with permanent lymphedema. When the major venous vessels are clotted, rarely are there sufficient collaterals to return the fluid. Unless gravity drainage is utilized, a massive swelling must occur. This results in the postphlebitic leg, or milk leg. Even if the veins recanalize at a later date, their valves are defective and they do not function adequately again. The fluid which has accumulated has created a space between the skin and fascia which, if not obliterated, becomes permanent. Fibrous trabeculae form in this space and, in the late stage, while elevation may drain some of the fluid, the heavy, thickened tissue space re-

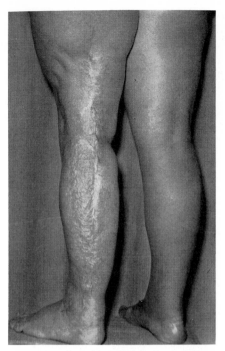

Figure 56. Postthrombotic lymphedema with massive swelling, showing patient after surgical correction.

mains. Early and continued high elevation of the part affected, for a sufficiently long time, will prevent many of the permanent lymphedema changes.

TRAUMATIC LYMPHEDEMA. Lacerations, thrombosis, burns, operation incisions, keloids and the scarring which results from roentgen, radium and radioactive isotope rays may destroy the continuity of the lymph channels. If the injuries are extensive enough, massive lymph collections follow because of the inability of the lymphatics to carry away the lymph fluid. The development of the fluid may be delayed until the scars have contracted, this final scarring obliterating the remaining collateral lymphatics.

CONGENITAL LYMPH COLLECTIONS. Many abnormal lymph collections have been reported. These may be due to lymph rests, cystic hygroma, simple lymph cysts, cavernous lymph collections or lymphangiectasis. Abnormal lymph growths may interfere with obstetric delivery. Bizarre symptoms may develop, depending upon the location, size and extent of pressure.

MALIGNANT LYMPHEDEMA. Just as the lymphatics are the site of the spread of infection, they are a pathway for the spread of malignant disease, particularly carcinoma. The rate of spread varies in different types of growths and in different individuals. There is an inverse ratio of speed of spread to age. The growth spreads along the lymphatics to the regional nodes which contain extensions for a time. The localization does not appear related to the size of the spread, although it is related frequently to the length of time that the primary growth has existed. In some patients, it appears that the regional nodes pass on the growth after their resistance has been overcome. The localization of growths in regional nodes varies greatly. The tumor may involve all the nodes or only one or two. In some instances, there is widespread dissemination with only minimal, or with no involvement of the regional nodes. Some groups of nodes may be skipped with involvement of the others in the same channel. The change in pressure in the lymph capillaries in the lymph nodes owing to the distortion caused by the malignant cells may shunt these cells directly into the venous capillaries in the nodes.

Sarcoma may spread by the lymphatic pathway, although it most often extends by way of the blood stream. Melanoma frequently metastasizes by way of the blood stream. Sarcomas of the tonsil, thyroid or testicle are exceptions. The degree of involvement regionally often determines the size of the lymphedema. Secondary obstruction or overload of the venous drainage complicates the edema problem.

Malignant tumors also may involve the lymphatics primarily; thus lymphosarcoma, Hodgkin's disease (malignant lymphoma) and lymphatic and leukocytic leukemia all may present lymphatic collections and secondary lymphedema.

ESSENTIAL LYMPHEDEMA. Some types of lymphedema are of unknown origin. These collections appear to be hereditary in nature, although most of them do not appear clinically until the time of puberty. The advent of the symptoms with this developmental changing time in life suggests that the maturing endocrine system, or some dysfunction of it, plays a part in precipitation of these lesions.

Some forms of congenital lymphedema also are known as Milroy's disease, originally described as both a familial and congenital disease (Fig. 57). Many of the patients in whom swelling of unknown origin appears at puberty do have a history of similar involvement occurring in other members of the family. Congenital lymphedema has been described as "simple" when the patient is the only one in the family so affected, and "heredi-

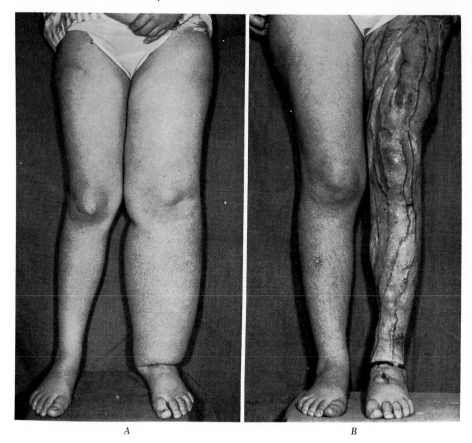

A   B

Figure 57.   *A*, Essential lymphedema of the Milroy type in a 15-year-old girl. Measurements: right calf, 27.4 cm.; right thigh, 56.0 cm.; left calf, 56.0 cm.; left thigh, 66.6 cm. *B*, Postoperative view. Scars can be covered by stocking or cosmetics.

tary" if other relatives are afflicted. There is some anatomic and physiologic defect in these patients from birth. It may be that a congenital swelling present from the day of birth is of such mild degree as to be not noticed until the time of more rapid growth. While the leg or legs are most often involved, the upper extremity may be affected as may the labia, scrotum and other male and female genitalia. The entire retroperitoneal space may be involved. The lymph vessels may be varicosed or may become angiectatic, cavernous or cystic. Some lymph spaces may contain both lymph and venous blood.

Symptoms. The symptoms of lymphedema vary, depending upon the degree of blockage, the age of the patient, the type of tissue involved, the secondary skin changes and whether the part has been subjected to repeated inflammations.

The usual appearance is that of symmetrical enlargement of the extremity. In the leg, the swelling begins in the groin. It may be confined more to the upper or lower part of the limb, but usually both portions are involved as are the foot and toes. In the congenital type, it most often involves one extremity, both legs being implicated in only 25 per cent of the patients. The skin is tight, tense and usually shiny. There may be wrinkled and lobular areas irregularly situated. The larger collections of lymph are in the dependent medial areas. In some patients, the collections are most irregular with overhanging masses of tissue which may obscure the normal contour of the extremity. In the enlargements of the upper extremity, the mass may have involved even the fingers. In some of the massive collections, the normal position of the bones may be displaced.

The shiny skin may become thickened and roughened. It may resemble the skin of an elephant. The pores enlarge and develop a pigskin appearance. There is usually a pigment deposit, particularly in the lower extremity. The color varies from light yellow to all degrees of brown, purple and black. Ulcerations may be present because of the poor vascularity of the overdistended tissue. The associated venous involvement may be evidenced by large veins, dermatitis and ulcers. Dermatitis, especially of the fungus type, is often associated. Often there are weeping and eczematoid changes, particularly around the toes. The skin in such areas will be heaped up and frequently is openly draining. The nails usually show curvature, irregularity and atrophy with associated fungus infection. There may be signs of repeated phlebitis.

The patients are subject to frequent attacks of sepsis. These bouts are characterized by high fever, chills, malaise and general upsets. The local reactions are similar to those of cellulitis, lymphangitis or erysipeloid reactions. The patient often gives a history of having had many attacks of erysipelas. These reactions are due to lack of resistance of the part to the common skin contaminants, the streptococci and staphylococci. The limbs appear to lose their power to resist infection. Some patients have regularly recurring febrile attacks. There may be skip periods of freedom from fever, and some patients may go for years without any septic attack. Such periods usually are associated with a time of excellent general health. Why some patients have innumerable attacks and others none is not explainable. Each recurrence of the reaction increases the pathologic process, closing off more lymph channels. The febrile reactions, while violent, will respond to antibiotics.

Patients who have specific infections, such as syphilis, filariasis or tuberculosis, will show the symptoms of these diseases. The symptoms of lymph collections due to trauma, allergy and malignant disease are self-evident. The symptoms of lymphedema due to the postthrombotic syndrome include those of that syndrome. In addition to the enlargement of the part, there may be all the signs of

thrombotic veins, depending upon the stage of the thrombosis and the recovery from it. Causalgia-like pain is not an uncommon symptom. Repeated attacks of phlebitis are not unusual. Reflex arteriospasm frequently coexists.

Pathology. The epidermis of the skin per se, although thickened, does not contain lymph stasis. The lymph accumulates in the dermis beginning at a depth of approximately 0.5 mm., and shows great thickening. The papillae and sweat glands become obliterated. The edema is condensed and there may be avascularity due to pressure on the blood vessels from the fluid (Fig. 58). The lymph collections within the spaces become enlarged. The pressure of this lymph increases in the subcutaneous and fascial spaces. The lymph walls may be fragmented, and gross lymph will be found in the extralymphatic spaces. Some of the structure of the subcutaneous tissues, fascia and collagens may be broken up. The fat is compressed and may become necrotic. Some of it is replaced by lymph spaces. The lymph channels are fibrosed, although some of them may be widely dilated. The muscles, tendons and even bone will show the effect of pressure and atrophy. The lymph may spread to the fascia, and it often involves the fat below the fascia and within the muscle or around blood vessels. Lymph nodes are enlarged and many of them become chronically inflamed and fibrosed.

In the stage of acute inflammation, the organisms may directly invade the lymphatics or pass through the cellular lining if there is no open lesion. The organisms multiply. The lymph fluid and the vessels react

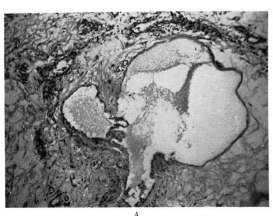
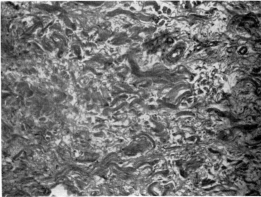

A   B

Figure 58. *A*, Massive lymphedema with pathologic picture of lymph. *B*, Trauma to tissues surrounding lymph collections of collagen fibers.

with an increase in the cellular elements and spread proximally. The edema is a hard, brawny type which indents or pits with difficulty. In the more advanced stage of the affection, suppuration may occur.

With elevation, the lymph flows gravitationally. With dependency, it reaccumulates.

At a later stage, fibrous trabeculae form between the skin and deep layers. These form a skeleton-like framework which then maintains the space in which the lymph collects. The valves in the lymph channels are destroyed.

Treatment. The primary aim of treatment is to eliminate the cause of the condition and to relieve the residual lymph stasis.

In filarial infections, evacuation from the area of infection and avoidance of reinfection usually are all that are required. Lymphangiography should be performed prior to treatment in all cases of doubtful etiology. If the lymphedema is due to secondary infections, cultures should be made from material taken from the inflamed or infected area, and the sensitivity of any organism to standard antibiotics should be determined. Antibiotic therapy should be thorough. When febrile attacks have been recurrent, the time pattern of these attacks should be determined and antibiotics given prophylactically prior to the anticipated time of the fever. Such therapy may have to be continued for months, years or indefinitely to maintain the control of the sepsis, which is of great importance. This program of management of lymphedema due to infection is of help in the prevention of lymphedema due to other causes and has aided in controlling lymphedema seen after radical mastectomy, in which infection and not malignant metastasis is the cause. Allergic lymphedema sometimes responds to desensitization. Antihistamines may be helpful. Patients with lymphedema due to cold exposure may become conditioned by exposure to slowly lowered temperatures. Other patients require a change of climate to warmer areas in order to control the lymphedema. Obstructions due to burns or scars require surgical correction. Lymphedema following irradiation, in the absence of retained malignant disease, is due to burns. Excision of the burned area and various plastic procedures may be helpful.

Lymphedema which follows the postthrombotic syndrome presents a complicated picture and its therapy is difficult. The treatment depends upon the stage of the disease which the patient presents. In the acute stage,

spasm is the most likely causative factor. For the patient with incompetent veins, ligation and stripping of these veins may be helpful. In all these patients, venograms and lymphangiograms should be obtained routinely to determine the actual venous involvement and the adequacy of the remaining veins and lymphatics. For causalgia and the reflex spastic problems, sympathectomy may be successful if paravertebral blocks produce a good clinical result.

The surgical treatment may be a combination of lumbar sympathectomy and a wedge excision of the lymphatic tissue to return the extremity to its natural size and shape (Fig. 59).

In patients with mild residual lymph stasis, elevation of the part when the patient is not using it, and good support when the part is dependent, may be all that is necessary. Such therapy must be applied early and continued for as long as a year. Basically, this therapy is

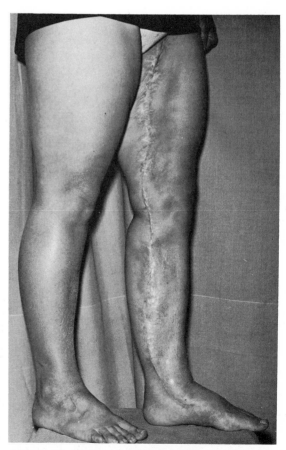

Figure 59. Postthrombotic lymphedema surgically corrected by sympathectomy and a wedge excision of the lymph tissue. Skin excised elliptically and undermined for half the circumference of the limb and skin replaced after excising fat, lymph and fascia directly on the muscle.

planned to remove and keep the lymph fluid from the leg until such time as other lymph collaterals are developed or the lymph spaces are closed. This regimen consists of elevating the limb sufficiently high for gravitational drainage. This should be done each night and every time during the day that the limb begins to swell, as shown by a tightness and discomfort of the bandage. Adequate support requires even application of a well-fitted pressure bandage, reaching from the toes to as far as the swelling extends. The bandage must be removed and replaced each time that the part is elevated. To be effective the elevation must be above the heart level.

Massage, like exercise, causes lymph flow within the lymph channels. It also aids in the movement of extraluminal lymph. The massage should be from the distal to the proximal end of the swelling and should not be traumatic. A simple massage expedient is the walking in water of a lake, river or ocean. This produces mild massage which will empty the lymph.

To these measures must be added antibiotic therapy, care of fungus infection, treatment of any allied ulcers and sympathetic nerve blocks or sympathectomy for those patients in whom there is a large reflex spastic element.

In the moderate types of lymphedema, especially when the postthrombotic syndrome is an etiologic factor, sympathectomy may resolve the process. This operation should be selected as a treatment only if a sympathetic nerve block gives good laboratory and clinical evidence that some of the fluid collection results from a reflex spastic element. In some of the patients with venous involvement, this can be combined with resection of the pathologic veins. In other patients, in whom the lack of good early bandaging has left a residually enlarged leg, the surgical correction by wedge excision has been sufficient to give relief. In this operation, a medial section of skin, subcutaneous tissue, lymph, fat and deep fascia is excised. The width of the skin segment removed is sufficient to reduce the part to normal size, but a segment of subcutaneous and deep fascia wider than the skin segment is excised. The remaining superficial tissue is then mobilized and approximated with a plastic closure.

Surgical measures to develop lymph drainage to other nonblock areas have been tried for nearly as long as surgery has been performed. Originally, Handley placed silk sutures subcutaneously in hopes of developing new lymph channels. Drainage tubes of all types, sizes and materials have been constructed. Tissue bridges with large pedicle grafts have been formed. Testifying to the ingenuity of their originators if not to their surgical success. Techniques using glass needle tubes and various types of metal wires as well as tissue bridges are advocated by some surgeons. Our observed results have been poor.

The omentum has been used in attempts to carry blood supply to other organs such as the heart. An attempt has been made to utilize this structure with its great absorption power to carry away the accumulated lymphs. The omentum has been separated from all but its essential blood supply to obtain sufficient length to reach the lower extremity and also to extend to the axilla. A subcutaneous tunnel is prepared and the omentum is sutured in place, at the proximal end of the lymphatic collection. In the lower extremity, this area is the inguinal gland region and in the upper extremity, it is the axilla. This is an extensive and serious operation and the effectiveness of this method in comparison to the dangers such as slough, infection or even peritonitis would make most surgeons look elsewhere for the relief of the disabling lymphedema.

A therapeutic technique based on the original observation of Kondoleon, that lymphedema is confined to the tissues external to the muscles, has been employed. Kondoleon excised windows in the fascia, hoping that the lymph would flow internally and be absorbed by the muscle lymphatics. This procedure was extended by others and the technique consisted of undermining the skin and excising part, or all, of the subcutaneous and deep fascia. The skin was replaced directly on the muscles. While reduction in size of the part resulted, lymphedema recurred in nearly all patients. The reason for the recurrence is that the nonfunctioning lymphatics in the skin itself were not removed. The value of the operation is temporary and consists in plastic excisions of lymph-swollen tissues. This operation and its modifications have limited value.

Grafts of skin, or skin and subcutaneous tissues, have been pedicled so that their base is proximal to the lymphatic block. The results have not been good. The technical difficulties attending use of these large grafts and the discomfort entailed in their production, and subsequently, have made this type of operation obsolete.

Certain tissues of the body do not contain

lymph. Among these is the epidermis. With the modern electric dermatomes, one can remove skin so thin that only the epidermis is in the graft. All the skin from the involved part is removed in long strips. Our best results have been obtained with skin in 0.35 mm. thicknesses. Repeated biopsies show that the abnormal lymph collections begin approximately 0.5 mm. below the skin surface. After this thin skin excision is completed, all the rest of the skin, the lymph, the fat and subcutaneous and deep fascia are removed. Great care is exercised to remove all the fatty tissue and fascia from the underlying muscles. After hemostasis is secured, the skin previously removed is placed directly onto the muscle. The operation is performed in stages, the front half of the leg from the groin to the toes being operated upon first, and the back half being operated upon when healing of the front graft is complete, approximately in three weeks (Fig. 60).

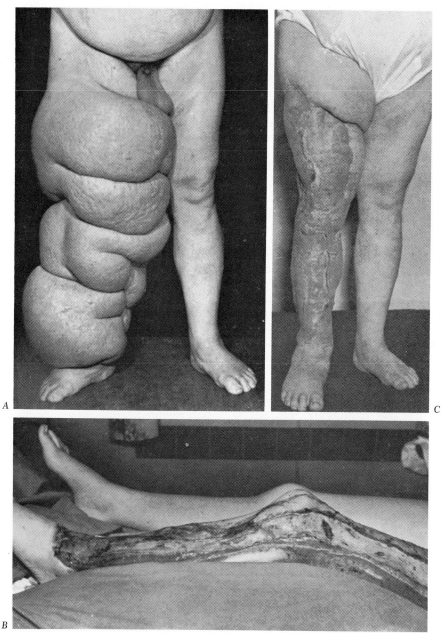

A

C

B

Figure 60. *A*, Grotesque appearance of severe lymphedema. *B*, Immediate postoperative appearance. *C*, Appearance after healing has taken place.

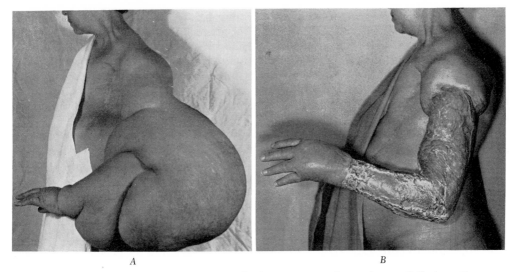

A *B*

Figure 61. *A*, Massive lymphedema nine years after radical mastectomy and x-ray therapy. *B*, Postoperative appearance. Patient had no recurrence of malignant disease 13 years after original operation. Lymphedema has not recurred since the operation was performed in 1954.

SECONDARY KELOIDS AND FUNGUS INFECTIONS. Since the skin is often diseased and subject to fungus infection, disfiguring keloids or fungus collections may appear. In such patients, these lesions should be surgically excised down to red muscle, and the area regrafted and treated with x-ray, beginning immediately after operation to prevent recurrence.

LYMPHEDEMA IN THE UPPER EXTREMITY. Any of the etiologic factors detailed as a cause of lymphedema of the lower extremity may cause such an accumulation in the upper extremity. Most cases of lymphedema of the upper arm, however, follow operations for carcinoma of the breast (Figs. 61 and 62). In one of the last papers written by Halsted, he named the streptococcus as the offending cause for lymphedema of the arm following radical mastectomy.

Swelling of the arm after mastectomy should be considered of possible malignant origin until proved otherwise. There remains, however, a sizable group of patients in whom lymphedema develops and annoyingly persists in the absence of carcinoma. It has been demonstrated not only that lymphedema follows infection, but that the elimination of

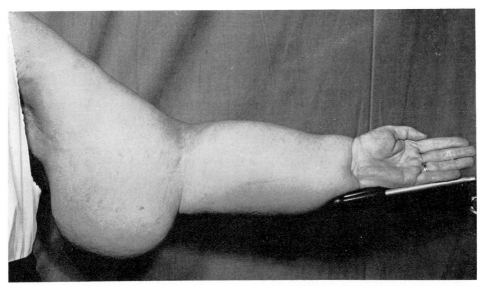

Figure 62. Lymphedema occurring seven years after radical mastectomy for carcinoma of the breast.

this infection by antibiotics controls and sometimes corrects lymphedema. In the absence of malignancy or infection, the cause of the lymphedema of the arm is effective destruction of the lymphatics necessary for cure. Some of the best long-term results in the surgical treatment of cancer of the breast have some lymphedema because the operation was sufficiently radical.

If it is determined that there is no malignant or infectious cause for the lymphedema, surgical eradication of the lymphedema may be performed. If the lymphedema is so massive as to be disabling, the technique as described for the treatment of massive lymphedema of the lower extremity has been satisfactorily applied to nonmalignant massive lymphedema of the arm after radical mastectomy. This operation is reserved only for those in whom the lymphedema is so massive as to be disabling.

Congenital lymphedema in the upper extremity. The cause for this condition is unknown. Some congenital rest, overactivity as in the Milroy's syndrome, or a glandular imbalance may be a factor. The lymphedema may involve the entire extremity or parts of it. Unfortunately, it often involves the digits, causing not only an unsightly aspect but also a mechanical obstruction to function.

The milder conditions may respond to elevation and support. Some of the vasodilator drugs seem to be partially effective.

Treatment of the patients with extensive lymphedema is unsatisfactory. The arm, forearm and hand can be treated effectively. The digits themselves pose a problem both from the general surgical and plastic standpoint. The viability of the graft must be obtained without sacrificing the mobility so necessary to tendon and joint motion. The fact that most of these patients are children adds to the difficulty, since patient cooperation is required for the necessary active motion. Each patient's problem must be individually assessed, and the treatment planned specifically for him.

LYMPHEDEMA OF SCROTUM AND LABIA. The cause for these lymphatic collections is unknown. The lymph stasis may be minimal in amount, or it may develop into a tremendous and grotesque collection. The symptoms may vary from those in which the patient is aware of the enlargement only when tight-fitting clothing is worn, to that typified by the textbook picture of the East Indian sitting on his scrotum. The scrotum may be so large as to

hang below the knees and weigh more than 50 pounds. When lymphorrhea is a complication, the problem may become most severe. Some patients must wear towels or rubber devices to collect the lymph. Secondary sepsis and dermatitis are common. In the female, pregnancy complicates the symptoms markedly.

The treatment of these lymph collections depends upon the extent of the lymph stasis. Antibiotic therapy, hygienic care and elastic support to the genitalia may ameliorate the symptoms. In the extensive and advanced degree of lymphatic obstructions, surgical eradication may be necessary. In the patient with massive lymph labia, partial or complete vulvectomy may be necessary and at times curative. In lymph scrotum, treatment must be individualized. The lymph area may be excised. In others, a new scrotal covering must be constructed by grafts and the skin and all subcutaneous and lymph-bearing tissues surgically excised.

One patient presented a scrotum the size of a volleyball and the penis a near exact replica of a football. Surgical correction in stages was successful. New skin for both these organs was raised with the electric dermatome from the thigh. The skin, subcutaneous tissue and lymph were removed on the scrotum down to the cremaster muscle and the skin plastically placed to cover the organ. In the penis, the skin and the subcutaneous tissue and lymph deposits were excised down to the corpora cavernosa. The glans was circumcised. The skin again was plastically applied. These operations were performed in stages.

LYMPHATIC INFECTIONS

ACUTE LYMPHANGITIS. The most common causative organisms of acute lymphangitis are the Staphylococcus and Streptococcus. Any organism, however, may be the invader. The colon bacillus often is an originator in regions near the rectum or where prolonged bed rest may have permitted fecal contamination. The gas-forming organisms such as *B. welchii* or *B. perfringens* presents a special problem. Usually, the infection gains entrance through some skin break caused by an injury. The entry point may appear innocuous. A small paronychia or an ingrown nail, fungus infection, or puncture wound often is the site of entry and source of infection.

The small lymph vessels or capillaries may be first involved. Usually, there is redness, some heat and tenderness with edema. The condition spreads proximally, involving first the lymph plexus and then the larger lymph vessels.

Once the main channels are involved, a red streak develops from the original site of infection to the focal nodes. In the arm, these may be the epitrochlears. The infection then goes to the axillary nodes, or it may go directly to the veins by shunt. In the lower extremity, the popliteal glands less often are involved. A red streak extending directly from the site of origin of the infection to the inguinal or axillary nodes is the most common.

Usually, there are associated perilymphangitis and cellulitis. Once the glands are involved, there may be all degrees of sepsis from simple inflammation to suppuration and abscess formation. If the infection extends beyond the regional nodes, it invades the blood stream, producing bacteremia and septicopyemia. Abscesses then may occur in any part of the body. There may be shunts to veins before the inguinal nodes are fully involved.

An essential part of the treatment is a search for a point of entrance. Rest and immobilization of the part are primary. Local cultures and blood cultures should be obtained, and the sensitivity of the causative organism to antibiotics should be determined. The correct antibiotic should be given in massive doses. In the absence of a positive culture or until it is obtained, antibiotics can be given empirically. Massive wet dressings should be applied locally and the part elevated. Blood transfusions should augment the antibiotic therapy. The purpose of the blood is not to replace red blood cells. The transfusions are given to replace some defensive factor lacking, at least temporarily, in the patient so afflicted. This defensive factor, when supplied by blood, is used up rapidly and must be replaced regularly, approximately every two days. Regular, repeated small blood transfusions have been decisive in overcoming infections of this type in innumerable patients. Abscesses should be drained wherever they occur. The original site, if it is a blister, broken nail or callus, should be incised only if there is localized suppuration. Surgical intervention in the presence of localized pus is imperative, but without such localization, the best treatment locally is surgical restraint. Such cutting in the absence of pus is bungling

surgery, and will be registered by increased morbidity and possibly mortality.

CHRONIC LYMPHANGITIS. The usual septic organisms may cause chronic lymphangitis if their virulence is not too great or the defense of the host is high. Repeated attacks of acute lymphangitis may also result in chronic lymphangitis. In the absence of a septic cause for chronic lymphangitis, the specific types of infection may be the cause of chronic lymphangitis. The various fungus infections, such as epidermophytosis, occasionally involve the lymphatics, usually in the form of the "tid." Most often the fungus infection is associated with a secondary invading organism. Sporotrichosis, a more rare mycotic disease caused by *Sporotrichum schenckii,* may be the cause. Carcinoma may spread through the lymphatics and cause signs and symptoms not unlike those of an inflammation. The possibility of malignant disease should always be ruled out in any patient with nonspecific lymphangitis.

In nonspecific chronic lymphangitis, there may be recurrent signs of redness and swelling. The degree of lymph obstruction varies from a mild block to lymphedema. The glands are enlarged and their physical size often adds to the lymph obstruction. In many patients, thrombophlebitis is associated. The skin changes depend upon the degree of lymph obstruction and the venous involvement. Often, there is pigskin appearance with enlarged pores. There may be secondary dermatitis or ulcer formation. A duskiness appears in the skin in the later stages of the disease. The edema is of the brawny type which pits with difficulty and persists longer than normal edema. In tuberculosis, the lymphatic channels are cordlike nodules which later break down with caseation necrosis, forming abscesses, and may become secondarily infected. A similar type of nodular change occurs with syphilis, but the lesions are less likely to suppurate. The epitrochlear glands may be involved by both of these lesions. In lymphangitis due to filariasis, the lymphatic inflammation is often caused by the dead worms. Streptococci and pyogenic infection frequently are associated. The dilated lymphatics become thickened and tortuous and the lymph may be clear or turbid.

In chronic lymphangitis secondary to sepsis, the initial site of infection may have to be excised. A small callus, infected nail bed, foreign body or an area of osteomyelitis may be responsible for continuance of the lymphangitis infection until the source is eliminated. Antibiotic drugs should be used and the specific one for the organism cultured should be selected. Tuberculous lymphangitis requires general therapy for the disease. Streptomycin with paraaminosalicylic acid and isoniazid should be utilized. X-ray therapy has had some beneficial results in some patients. A search for the primary site must be made and sometimes its removal is curative. Excision of the involved lymph nodes often is necessary. In each patient, the possibility of malignant disease should be considered and biopsies performed when doubt exists.

LYMPHADENITIS. The cause, course, symptoms and treatment of lymphadenitis in general are similar to those of lymphangitis, and the infections of the glands may be acute or chronic.

The glands enlarge and become tender when the invading organisms are septic in type. The degree of inflammation depends upon the virulence of the organism and the defense of the host. In tuberculosis, the glands enlarge rapidly, become firm and discrete nodules and then break down and caseate. The glands become fused together and suppuration and sinus formation take place. In syphilis, the nodes are universal but discrete. They are painless and do not tend to suppurate. In carcinoma, gland enlargement and secondary reaction depend upon the type of cell and extent of the spread as well as the therapy.

In the treatment of mild inflammation, correctly selected antibiotics with rest, wet dressings and elevation may be all that is necessary. The organism should always be cultured and sensitivity to the routine antibiotics determined. Locally, warm packs may help to resolve the process. If suppuration occurs, surgical drainage is necessary. When doubt as to the cause of the enlarged gland exists, biopsy or excision is necessary and should not be delayed.

The glands most often involved in tuberculous adenitis are the mediastinal nodes which drain the lungs. These nodes may be fibrotic and heal with surrounding calcium deposits. Most persons have such calcified nodes in their lungs or in the mediastinum. At other times, cold abscesses form with caseation. It is likely that from these latter abscesses develops miliary tuberculosis which is disseminated by the blood stream. Inflammation of these glands subsides when the primary disease abates.

Cervical tuberculous glands are visible and palpable and are important in differential diagnosis of cervical adenopathy. At the time of the biopsy, surgical excision is indicated. Most of these glands require excision. Their chronic draining sinuses will lead to secondary suppuration.

Syphilitic adenitis requires specific therapy and operation is indicated for biopsy only.

REPETITIVE SEPTIC ADENITIS. Suppurative adenitis in itself may continue bouts of sepsis. These glands chronically, subacutely and acutely reinfected become sources of the disease. Like repeated tonsillitis which results in frequent sore throat, these glands no longer are defensive. Their radical excision may help the patient. It must be recognized that these glands were placed by nature as a defense mechanism. When they have been reinvaded by organisms, they are containers of, but not defenders from, infections. While their excision removes a natural barrier and this protection is no longer present, the patient often is better after radical surgery.

LYMPHOGRANULOMA INGUINALE. This tropical disease also occurs in temperate climates. Adult male Negroes are most commonly affected. The etiologic factors are intracellular microorganisms called Donovan bodies. They are passed from one person to another most often by sexual contact.

Three to seven weeks after contact, the organisms cause a papule to develop on or near the genitalia. The involved area enlarges and breaks down and gives a thin, white discharge which has a fetid odor. Other nodules may be secondarily affected. The regional lymph nodes are not enlarged in all cases but may be secondarily affected.

The diagnosis is made from the clinical appearance, the demonstration of the organisms, a typical pathologic section or reaction to the complement fixation test. There is no active surgical treatment, although surgery may be necessary for biopsy or plastic repairs. Intravenous injections of tartar emetic have been effective and streptomycin may be of value.

TUMORS OF THE LYMPHATIC SYSTEM

Tumors of the lymphatic system are not too uncommon. Lumb divides the malignant ones into those having lymphocytic differentiation; those with reticular cell characteristics; those with mixed cell types; and those with imperfect cell type differentiation. Benign lymphatic tumors may be primarily lymphatic, or a mixture of lymphatic and blood vessel development.

LYMPHANGIOMA. Most lymphangiomas are of congenital origin. Some are noted in early life, but even these may have been present at birth but not noted. They are usually associated with other congenital anomalies. They have been seen in association with hemangiomas, neurofibromas and undescended testicles.

This type of tumor may develop as an individual growth called lymphangioma simplex. It may be any size from that of a minute nodule to as large as a baseball. These tumors are usually the color of skin, but there may be some discoloration due to venous pressure or venous involvement. Dilated blood vessels, especially the veins, often accompany these growths. They may occur at any place, but are often seen in the extremities. The head, face, neck, shoulders and chest are more unusual sites. They may develop a vesicular or keratotic appearance and, in the latter instance, they resemble warts. When this tumor occurs in combination with blood vessels, it is called lymphangioma cavernosum (Fig. 63). Such a tumor is red to blue in color and is livid. Many of them are considered birthmarks. When they occur around the mouth, they are called macroglossia. Around the lips, they are named macrocheilia.

Grossly, these tumors vary markedly. The large ones are compressible. Histologically, they are found to arise from epithelial cells. The lymphangioma simplex has vesicles, and these distend the epidermis. The proliferation of the epidermis over the vesicles forms keratosis. The vesicles contain coagulated lymph and the interstitial connective tissue is edematous. The cavernosum type shows much larger sinuses, and in these the epithelial lining is well formed.

In the small growths, electrocauterization has been effective. Application of carbon dioxide snow eradicates some of the superficial ones. The larger lesions should be excised surgically. These tumors become malignant on occasion, and this is a valid reason for their excision.

Lymphangioma cysticum. Lymphangioma cysticum appears to be caused by germ rests. In some of the tumors, trauma or chronic inflammation is a contributing factor. They occur most often in the neck and sacrum. They have been seen frequently on the extremities, and more rarely in the internal organs.

These cysts are large, not compressible and cause symptoms depending upon their site

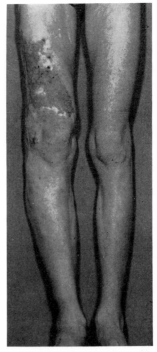

Figure 63. Lymphangioma cavernosum in a boy aged 12 years. There is massive involvement of the right lower extremity which includes both the lymphatics and the venous system.

and size. They may cause distortion or pain by pressure. They are softer than xanthomas. Biopsies may be required for differentiation from other tumor masses.

The cysts are lined with endothelium. The fluid is serous or chylous. The surrounding sac is made of connective tissue and includes muscle fibers.

These tumors should be surgically excised. If they are removed without puncture, a complete cure will be obtained. In children, excision if often difficult. Incomplete excision may leave a persistent lymphorrhea and if the excision if infected, infection may be most severe.

Other lymphangiomas. These small tumors also may be in the form of congenital lymphangiectasis. They may be in the skin (nevus lymphaticus), the lips (macrocheilia), the tongue (macroglossia), the dorsum of the hand (macrocheiria) or the neck (cystic hygroma). They may be lymphatic cysts or hydrocele of the neck, axilla or floor of the mouth. In the neck, the tumor is beneath the deep fascia and may protrude either anteriorly or posteriorly to the sternocleidomastoid muscle. The tumor may be of such size as to interfere with respiration or swallowing.

Surgical treatment is difficult and sometimes dangerous. If the cyst is not too large and does not interfere with swallowing or breathing, conservative therapy may be used. Sometimes, the condition regresses spontaneously. X-ray therapy has been effective. Radium has been used. In some instances, a combination of radium and subsequent surgery has been effective with secondary plastic repair.

LYMPHOSARCOMA. This is the most common of the malignant lymphomas. The tumor starts in the neck, the mediastinum or the axilla, and grows rapidly with infiltration of the surrounding tissues. It also extends to and involves the skin. It may enlarge rapidly because of hemorrhage within it. The early signs may be those due to pressure on nerves or other vital structures. Secondary lymph stasis begins distal to the involved glands. Metastasis occurs by way of the blood stream, particularly to the lung and the liver. The condition must be differentiated from other primary and secondary tumors of the glands, particularly from Hodgkin's disease. Lympho-

sarcoma grows and spreads more rapidly, usually occurs on one side of the body and has ulceration, whereas Hodgkin's disease rarely ulcerates and is slower in its extension (Fig. 64).

Two distinct types of lymphosarcoma are recognized. These are a localized form and a generalized one called lymphosarcomatosis. In the localized form, the tumor may be composed of large, round lymphoblasts (lymphoblastoma). When the cells are small, the tumor is called lymphocytoma. When the tumor cells originate from the reticular cells, the growth is called a reticulum cell sarcoma.

In the generalized form, the sarcoma is in many different parts of the lymphatic system and metastasizes early by way of the blood stream. The tumor may be in the blood vessels or in the blood stream itself. Any organ in the body may be involved.

Surgical excision usually is indicated only for biopsy or to relieve unusual pressure.

Radiation therapy has been used exten-

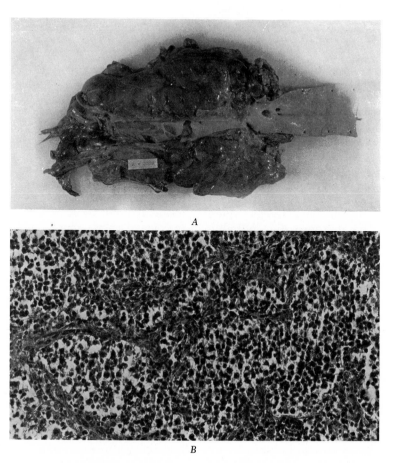

A

B

Figure 64. *A*, Lymphosarcoma arising from the periaortic lymph nodes. Note growth around and into the aorta. *B*, Microscopic appearance of lymphosarcoma with massive infiltration of round cells. (Courtesy of Dr. A. Rottino.)

sively and the results at first are good, but the tumor recurs. Regression can be maintained for some time with radiation therapy. Nitrogen mustard (mechlorethamine hydrochloride) and radiophosphorus have been effective in causing remissions. Mechlorethamine hydrochloride is thought to act by halting mitosis. This substance has been used in conjunction with radiation. If the lesion is localized, surgical excision may be tried and occasionally has been effective.

HODGKIN'S DISEASE (MALIGNANT LYMPHADENOMA). This disease is one of the malignant lymphomas and was described by Hodgkin in 1832. It was also called lymphadenoma without leukemia by Wunderlich, malignant lymphoma by Billroth, and lymphogranuloma by Sternberg.

The cause of Hodgkin's disease is unknown. It attacks males more often than females, and is seen in early adult life.

The lymph nodes rapidly enlarge without pain. Often the enlargement begins in the glands of the neck and progresses in the direction of the lymph flow. The affected glands are discrete, variable in size and elastic. There is usually a high fever. The condition is progressive and fatal, but remissions have occurred.

Enlargement of the glands in the neck or thorax may cause coughing, shortness of breath and difficulty in swallowing. There may be inequality of the pupils and paralysis of the recurrent nerve. Edema of the arm or face with dilated veins occurs. Any type of neurologic symptoms may arise from intracranial or spinal cord pressure.

All of the lymphoid tissue of the body may become involved. The affected glands are round, not adherent and encapsulated. On cut section, they appear gray and nonnecrotic. Microscopic examination reveals giant cells with three or four nuclei, increased endothelial cells having single nuclei, many eosinophils and excessive connective tissue (Figs. 65 and 66). The spleen is enlarged and has gray areas within it resembling lymph nodes. It has been called the "hard-baked" spleen. Lymph nodes also are found in the liver and bone marrow. The blood shows secondary anemia and leukopenia with relative lymphocytosis. Leukocytosis may occur terminally.

The disease has been grouped into the localized; the acute generalized; the Pel-Ebstein syndrome, characterized by alternate periods of fever and nonfever occurring at two-week intervals, and the typhoid type, because of its insidious onset, remittent fever and enlarge-ment of the retroperitoneal and mediastinal glands.

The main lesion from which Hodgkin's disease must be differentiated is lymphosarcoma. Lymphosarcoma occurs on one side of the body primarily, grows more rapidly than does malignant lymphadenoma, and tends to develop skin ulceration. Carcinoma normally has a primary source. Biopsy may be necessary to determine the correct diagnosis. Leukemia is differentiated by the blood count. In tuberculous lymphadenitis, the glands are irregularly nodular, coalesce and caseate. In syphilis, the gland enlargement is generalized, but slight and positive reactions to serologic tests and a therapeutic test will differentiate this disease.

Patients with Hodgkin's disease may live two to four years after the condition becomes manifest. Those having remissions may live five to ten years. These life spans may be extended with new therapeutic regimens.

Operation is indicated for biopsy and occasionally for relief of pressure. The glands respond to radiotherapy, but, unfortunately, this is only temporarily effective. Methyl-bis (β-chloroethyl) amine hydrochloride (mechlorethamine) has been used and there has been some fair response. This substance may be employed in conjunction with x-ray therapy. The radioactive isotopes, particularly phosphorus (P^{32}), are being used in some patients. Triethylenemelamine (TEM) was introduced in treatment in 1951. Some patients have survived ten years after x-ray therapy. It is apparent that no one type of treatment should be tried to the exclusion of all others. With supportive and other therapy, the patient can be made more comfortable and months or years may be added to his life.

Tumors of the lymphatic system have been treated by supervoltage therapy. This can be given by x-ray or cobalt. This latter substance can be given in large dosages and can reach the site of the lesion more readily than roentgen therapy. In addition, the adverse reaction of the patient to the treatment is much less. Both general and local response to supervoltage therapy as administered today is minimal.

CARCINOMA. Since carcinoma is disseminated by the lymphatic system, it is a frequent cause for tumors of the lymph glands. The primary focus usually is apparent. In certain parts of the body, such as the cervical nodes, the primary site may be difficult to demonstrate. Repeated biopsies of the tonsil, pharynx, thyroid gland or bronchus may be

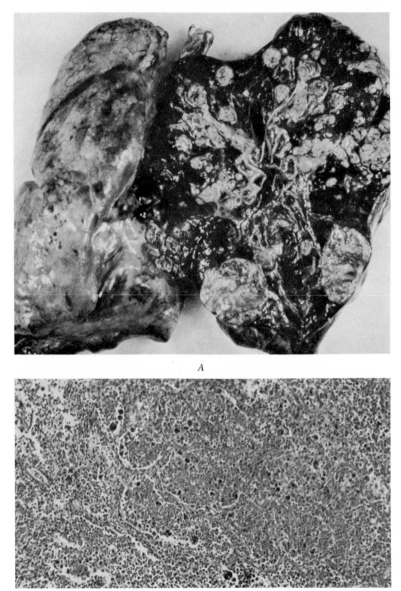

A

B

Figure 65. *A*, Hodgkin's disease invading the spleen. *B*, Microscopic section showing giant cells and single-nucleus endothelial cells.

required when undifferentiated carcinoma is found in the cervical gland. The tendency of some carcinomas to skip certain local glands may add to the confusion.

The so-called occult carcinoma of the lung may have large glandular metastases without the primary site being found by bronchoscopy, sputum test, Papanicolaou stain or even thoracotomy. These patients often are symptomless and the presence of pathologic glands may be determined only on routine chest roentgen films. The mediastinal glands may be quite large and displace structures such as the lung or even the pericardium with

minimal symptoms. X-ray or cobalt therapy may delay their progression in the onset of symptoms for a long time. Enlarged glands in the neck just above the clavicle lead one to suspect carcinoma of the stomach.

Squamous cell carcinoma may present as an abscess in a gland rather than the hard, odd-shaped mass one expects. Persistent discharge after aspiration is a sign. Often a drill biopsy is preferable to excision to avoid the breakdown in the tissue around the excised site.

With the improvement in lymphangiography, the lymphatics have been canalized

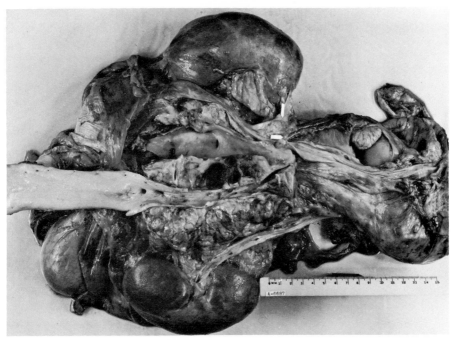

Figure 66. A view of the posterior retroperitoneum. One sees enlarged nodes caused by Hodgkin's disease markedly constricting the aorta and inferior vena cava. The ureters are constricted, producing hydroureter above the constriction.

and cytotoxic drugs injected to try to destroy metastatic cells. These catheters have been left in place for therapy for as long as six days.

SARCOMA. Sarcomas, other than those specific for the lymphatic system, may involve the glands. Unlike carcinoma, however, most of these tumors spread by way of the blood stream. The rapid enlargement of a tumor in a gland may make one suspicious of sarcoma, as these tumors tend to have internal hemorrhages and increase suddenly in size.

ENDOTHELIOMA. Endotheliomas arise within the endothelial linings of the lymph sinuses and the lymph glands and may metastasize. These tumors are rare and are differentiated by biopsy, particularly from secondary carcinoma.

CHLOROMA. Chloroma has been described as a sarcoma of the blood-forming organs. It involves the lymph nodes and spleen. The greenish color, indicated by its name, is thought to be due to blood pigment or the products of fatty cell metabolism. The disease affects young males and is rapidly fatal.

LYMPHATIC LEUKEMIA. This is a disease of the blood characterized by a marked increase in the number of circulating lymphocytes. The lymph glands enlarge, as does other lymphoid tissue throughout the body. Lymph-

atic leukemia may go through an aleukemic stage, at which time diagnosis may be difficult. The relative lymphocytosis and the clinical course suggest the diagnosis even in this phase. Children are usually affected by the acute form, which is rapidly fatal. Their glands enlarge, but are soft and discrete. High fever and weakness as well as the blood picture are characteristic. The chronic form occurs in older persons. The glands are generally enlarged. The nodes are gray and homogeneous. On section, the reticulum is seen to be packed with lymphocytes. Often the larger the lymphocytes, the more rapidly growing is the tumor.

There is no surgical treatment for leukemia. Biopsy is indicated. Nitrogen mustard administered intravenously, urethan, adrenocorticotropic hormone and cortisone have been tried. X-ray therapy will relieve some of the symptoms, and P^{32} has given equivocal results.

LYMPH DIALYSIS BEFORE ALLOGRAFT

The tissue rejection problem is important in present efforts to replace major organs; this includes possibly the heart itself. There have been approximately 1500 kidney transplants performed. When these replacements are between identical twins, the problem has not been an important one as the host accepts the organ. It is in the use of the kidney from non-identical twins or grafts from animals that the rejection problem arises. The hope of the use of artificial internal replant organs lies with the ability to prevent rejection.

Dialysis separates crystalloids and colloids by their difference in rates of diffusion through semipermeable membranes, the crystalloids diffusing rapidly and the colloids slowly or not at all.

In dialysis, it has been noted that there is a marked lymphocytopenia. The lymph is dialyzed against a tap water bath, and the hypotonic lymphocytes are lysed. Grafting tests show that homografts on the forearm of a patient under lymph dialysis remain alive only 90 days before rejection occurs.

Extracorporeal irradiation of lymph as a technique for immunosuppression has been tried and reported. The thoracic duct was canalized, but it was difficult to keep this fistula open owing to hematochylia or infection. Lymphocyte depletion and irradiation were carried out from 30 to 60 days prior to the transplantation of the kidney. The lymph was dialyzed daily against a tap water bath and treated with strontium 90 before reinfusion. The first patient reported in the literature showed no evidence of graft rejection after 50 days. That patient was then maintained on 125 mg. of azathioprine and 10 mg. or prednisone. This technique does not remove the serum immunoglobulin as rapidly as does immunosuppressive drug therapy. The lymphatic system has been accepted as a major factor in the survival of serum immunoglobulin and apparently offers a better chance of success, if it is treated by extracorporeal dialysis combined with irradiation. If this is true in renal transplants, it may be found to be true in other organ transplants, including such organs as the liver and heart.

READING REFERENCES

Abitbol, M. M., Meng, C., and Romney, S.: Anatomic and therapeutic aids of lymphangiography in pelvic malignancy. Am. J. Obst. & Gyn. 93:95, 1965.

Allen, E. V., Barker, N. W., and Hines, E. A., Jr.: Peripheral Vascular Diseases. 3rd ed. Philadelphia, W. B. Saunders Company, 1965.

Arnulf, G.: Lymphatic problems and lymphography. J. Cardiovas. Surg. 5:638, 1964.

Dos Santos, R., Lames, A. C., and Caldas, J. P.: Arteriographie des Membres et de l'Aorta Abdominale. Paris, Masson & Cie., 1931.

Duane, R. J., and Rottino, A.: Constrictive pericarditis caused by Hodgkin's disease. New York State J. Med. 67:288, 1967.

Foley, W. T.: The medical management of lymphedema. Mod. Concepts Cardiovas. Dis. 24:255, 1955.

Gergely, R.: The roentgen examination of lymphatics in man. Radiology 71:59, 1958.

Gergely, R., and Zsebök, Z.: De la lymphangiographie. Presse Med. 64:2200, 1956.

Ghormley, R. K., and Overton, L. M.: The surgical treatment of severe forms of lymphedema (elephantiasis) of the extremities. Surg. Gyn. & Obst. 61:83, 1935.

Gould, H. R.: Personal communications, 1967.

Guttman, R. J.: Role of supervoltage irradiation of regional lymph node bearing areas in breast cancer. Am. J. Roentgenol. 96:560, 1966.

Halsted, W. S.: Swelling of arm after operation for cancer of the breast–elephantiasis chirurgica. Bull. Johns Hopkins Hosp. 32:309, 1921.

Handley, W. S.: Lymphangioplasty: a new method for the relief of the brawny arm of breast-cancer and for similar conditions of lymphatic edema. Lancet 1:784, 1908.

Hartgill, J.: Report at the First International Symposium on Lymphology. Medical Tribune and Medical News, Vol. 7, No. 95, 1966.

Holman, C., McSwain, B., and Beal, J. M.: Swelling of the upper extremities following mastectomy. Surgery 15:757, 1944.

Homans, J.: Phlegmasia alba dolens and relation of lymphatics to thrombophlebitis. Am. Heart J. 7:415, 1932.

Homans, J., Drinker, C. K., and Field, M. E.: Elephantiasis and the clinical implications of its experimental reproduction in animals. Ann. Surg. 100:812, 1934.

Hudack, S. S., and McMaster, P. D.: Lymphatic participation in human cutaneous phenomena; study of minute lymphatics of living skin. J. Exper. Med. 57:751, 1933.

Jdanov, D. A.: On senile changes in lymphatic capillaries and vessels. J. Cardiovas. Surg. 7:108, 1966.

Kenyon, N. M., Soto, M., Viamonte, M., Parks, R. E., and Farrell, J. J.: Improved techniques and results of lymphography. Surg. Gny. & Obst. 114:677, 1962.

Kinmonth, J. B.: Lymphangiography in clinical surgery and particularly in treatment of lymphoedema. Ann. Roy. Coll. Surgeons England 15:300, 1954.

Kinmonth, J. B.: Some problems of the lymphatics and skin. Tr. St. John Hosp. Derm. Soc. 50:121, 1964.

Kinmonth, J. B.: Some general aspects of the investigation and surgery of the lymphatic system. J. Cardiovas. Surg. 5:680, 1964.

Kinmonth, J. B., and Taylor, G. W.: Lymphatic circulation in lymphedema. Ann. Surg. 139:129, 1954.

Kinmonth, J. B., Taylor, G. W., and Harper, R. A. K.: Lymphangiography; technique for its clinical use in lower limb. Brit. M. J. 1:940, 1955.

Kinmonth, J. B., Taylor, G. W., and Janet, G. H.: Chylous complications of primary lymphoedema. J. Cardiovas. Surg. 5:327, 1964.

Kondoleon, E.: Die Lymphableitung, als heilmittel bei cronischen Oedemen nach Quetschung. München. Med. Wchnschr. 59:525, 1912.

Lee, F. C.: The establishment of collateral circulation following ligation of the thoracic duct. Bull. Johns Hopkins Hosp. 33:21, 1922.

Lemmon, W. T., Jr.: Lymphatic stasis induced by chlorophyllated ethiodol. Surg. Forum. 16:116, 1965.

Lumb, G.: Tumours of Lymphoid Tissue. Baltimore, The Williams & Wilkins Company, 1954.

Matas, R.: The surgical treatment of elephantiasis and elephantoid states dependent upon chronic obstruction of the lymphatic and venous channels. Am. J. Trop. & Prev. Med. 1:60, 1913.

Milroy, W. F.: An undescribed variety of hereditary edema. New York M. J. 56:505, 1892.

Poth, E. J., Barnes, S. R., and Ross, G. T.: New operative treatment for elephantiasis. Surg. Gyn. & Obst. 84:642, 1947.

Pratt, G. H.: Lymph node infections. In Gellis, S. S., and

Kagan, B. M. (eds.): Current Pediatric Therapy—3. Philadelphia, W. B. Saunders Company, 1968.

Pratt, G. H.: Complications of procedures on the lymphatic system. Chapter 35 *in*, Artz, C. P., and Hardy, J. D.: Complications in Surgery and Their Management. Philadelphia, W. B. Saunders Company, 1960.

Pratt, G. H.: Definitive treatment of the post-thrombotic syndrome: the use of venograms to differentiate and delineate surgical treatment. A.M.A. Arch. Surg. 80: 112, 1960.

Pratt, G. H.: Panel discussion on cardiac and circulatory diseases. J. Am. Geriatrics Soc. 5:757, 1957.

Pratt, G. H.: Correlation of angiography with surgical treatment of vascular diseases. A.M.A. Arch. Surg. 72:118, 1956.

Pratt, G. H.: Surgical sympathectomy for obliterative vascular disease. New York State J. Med. 24:3357, 1954.

Pratt, G. H.: The pathogenesis and early and late treatment of the post-thrombotic syndrome. (The patient with the post-phlebitic leg.) S. Clin. North America 33:1229, 1953.

Pratt, G. H.: New operative technique for surgical correction of lymphedema. J.A.M.A. 151:888, 1953.

Pratt, G. H.: Surgical management of lymphedema. J.A.M.A. 147:1121, 1951.

Pratt, G. H., and Levine, A. A.: Surgical treatment of lymphedema of the upper extremities. A.M.A. Arch. Surg. 74:183, 1957.

Pratt, G. H., and Wright, I. S.: The surgical treatment of chronic lymphedema (elephantiasis). Surg. Gyn. & Obst. 72:244, 1941.

Pressman, J. J., Dunn, R. F., and Burtz, M.: Lymph node ultrastructure related to direct lymphanticovenous communication. Surg. Gyn. & Obst. 124:963, 1967.

Pressman, J. J., and Simon, M. B.: Experimental evidence of direct communications between lymph nodes and veins. Surg. Gyn. & Obst. 113:537, 1961.

Pressman, J. J., Simon, M. B., Hand, K., and Miller, J.: Passage of fluids, cells, and bacteria via direct communications between lymph nodes and veins. Surg. Gyn. & Obst. 115:207, 1962.

Redman, H. C.: Dermatitis as a complication of lymphangiography. Radiology 86:323, 1966.

Reichert, F. L.: The recognition of elephantiasis: the problem of experimental lymphedema. Arch. Surg. 20: 543, 1930.

Reichert, F. L.: The regeneration of the lymphatics. Arch. Surg. 13:871, 1926.

Ribbert: Ueber Regeneration und Entzundung der Lymphdrussen. Beitr. Pathol. Anat. 6:187, 1889.

Ross, H.: Metastatic squamous carcinoma in lymph nodes with abscess formation. Aust. & N. Z. J. Surg. 35:103 1965.

Rottino, A.: Hodgkin's disease. New York J. Med. 55:794, 1955.

Rottino, A.: Personal communications, 1967.

Ruzicka, F. F., Jr.: Personal communications, 1967.

Schinz, H. R., Baenoch, W. E., Fromhold, W., Glauner, R., Wehlinger, E., and Wellaner, J.; Roentgen Diagnosis. 2nd American ed. New York, Grune and Stratton, 1967.

Schobinger, R. A., Cooper, P., and Rousselot, L. M.: Observations on the systemic venous collateral circulation in portal hypertension and other morbid states within the thorax. Ann. Surg. 150:188, 1959.

Schobinger, R. A., and Ruzicka, F. F., Jr.: Vascular Roentgenology. New York, The Macmillan Company, 1964.

Schumaker, S. V.: Ueber Phagocytose und die Abfuhrwege der Leucocyten in den Lymphydrussen. Arch. Mikr. Anat. 54:311, 1899.

Servelle, M.: Pathologie Vascularie Medicale et Chirurgicale. Paris, Masson & Cie., 1952.

Servelle, M., Bouvrain, Y., Tricot, R., Soulie, J., Turpyn, H., Frentz, F., Cornu, C., and Nadim, C.: Lymphatic circulation in constrictive pericarditis. J. Cardiovas. Surg. 7:182, 1966.

Shanbrom, E., and Zheutlin, N.: Radiographic studies of the lymphatic system. Arch. Int. Med. 104:589, 1959.

Sistrunk, W. E.: Kondoleon operation for elephantiasis. J.A.M.A. 71:800, 1918.

Symposium on Lymphology. Medical Tribune, Vol. 7, No. 96, 1966.

Virchow, R. L. K.: Cellular Pathology. Translated by F. Chance. Philadelphia, J. B. Lippincott Company, 1863, p. 218.

Watson, W. L., and McCarthy, W. D.: Blood and lymph vessel tumors; a report of 1,056 cases. Surg. Gyn. & Obst. 71:569, 1940.

Weissleder, H.: Lymphography. Ergebn. inn. Med. u. Kinderh. 23:297, 1965.

Chapter 36

THE NERVOUS SYSTEM

by
BRONSON S. RAY, M.D.

BRONSON SANDS RAY is an Indianian whose father was also a doctor. He graduated from Franklin College in Indiana and from Northwestern University Medical School. He received his surgical training in Chicago and at the Peter Bent Brigham Hospital in Boston. He has spent his professional life in neurologic surgery at Cornell University Medical School, where he is Clinical Professor of Surgery (Neurosurgery) and Director of Neurological Surgery at The New York Hospital.

The surgical treatment of diseases of the nervous system has become an important specialty within this century. The factors contributing to this progress have been an acceleration in the acquisition of knowledge of functions of the nervous system, the classification of pathologic characteristics of neoplasms, the development of diagnostic methods and the application of increasingly significant improvements in surgical technique, in anesthesiology and in supportive care of the patient.

Cerebrum and Cerebellum

INTRACRANIAL TUMORS

Although tumors constitute only one of the numerous intracranial diseases requiring surgery, they have commanded the principal effort in the development of intracranial surgery and continue to present many unsolved problems. Intracranial tumors are relatively uncommon but are not to be regarded as rare. In one large clinic, a survey showed that 7 per cent of all neoplasms removed surgically were located intracranially. In the same survey, the incidence of carcinoma of the stomach and of the rectum was about 10 per cent, of the colon about 9.5 per cent and of the female breast nearly 10 per cent. Although intracranial tumors occur less frequently in infancy and youth than at other times, no age group is spared. The greatest incidence occurs in individuals between the ages of 30 and 50 years. The sexes are equally affected and, as far as is known, there is no racial variation.

PATHOLOGIC CLASSIFICATION OF INTRACRANIAL TUMORS

Intracranial tumors may be secondary, occurring by metastasis from malignant lesions elsewhere in the body, or they may be primary, in which case they are derived from the brain itself or some of the other intracranial structures such as blood vessels, cranial nerves, the meninges and the hypophysis.

The commonest intracranial tumors, the gliomas, arise from the neurolgia, or supporting tissue of the brain, and make up nearly half of all primary brain tumors. The gliomas are subclassified according to the resemblance of the predominating cells to the various embryonal or adult cells in the brain; the more anaplastic the cells, the more malignant the tumor.

The classification of gliomas proposed by Bailey and Cushing, based on the histogenesis of the brain, has been almost universally employed (Fig. 1). Other classifications have usually been modifications of this system. A classification proposed by Kernohan, Mabon, Svien and Adson is based on the concept that gliomas arise from adult cells still capable of proliferation by a process of dedifferentiation, or anaplasia. These authors suggest that the commonly used names, polar spongioblastoma, astroblastoma and glioblastoma multiforme, be replaced by a gradation of malignancy using the name astrocytoma, Grade 1 to 4, Grade 1 being the least malignant and Grade 4 the most. This has the appeal of simplicity, yet the histogenic classification has the advantage of long use and familiarity.

While the gliomas tend to infiltrate the brain, the meningiomas arising from the meninges displace rather than invade the brain. This obtains in most of the other tumors, such as the neurinomas arising from nerve sheaths, the hypophysial adenomas, the congenital tumors which arise from developmental defects and the blood vessel tumors.

The frequency of the different types of intracranial tumors is indicated in Table 1. The figures are similar to those of compilations from numerous clinics, the slight differences reflecting some particular circumstance which may have attracted more of one type of patient to one clinic rather than another. For example, pituitary adenomas had a high incidence of 17.8 per cent in Cushing's series because of his interest in the pituitary gland, whereas in the series reported here there is a disproportionately high percentage of metastatic tumors because of the proximity of an affiliated neurosurgical service in a hospital for cancer. The variation in the relative frequency of types of glioma in different series, particularly between glioblastoma and astrocytoma and astroblastoma, reflects the different attitudes of pathologists in regard to these tumors.

Table 1. 1905 *Verified Intracranial Tumors (The New York Hospital)*

CLASSIFICATION OF TUMOR		NUMBER	PERCENTAGE
Gliomas		928	48.7
Glioblastoma multiforme	492		
Astrocytoma	258		
Medulloblastoma	52		
Oligodendroglioma	36		
Spongioblastoma polare	15		
Astroblastoma	8		
Ependymoma	36		
Pinealoma	15		
Ganglioneuroma	4		
Neuroepithelioma	3		
Papilloma, choroid plexus	9		
Meningiomas		285	15.0
Pituitary Adenomas		218	11.4
Chromophobe	149		
Chromophil	48		
Mixed	15		
Adenocarcinoma	6		
Acoustic Neurinomas		132	6.9
Blood Vessel Tumors		65	3.4
Hemangioblastoma	23		
Angioma	42		
Congenital Tumors		56	2.9
Craniopharyngioma	35		
Cholesteatoma	5		
Dermoid	3		
Teratoma	4		
Chordoma	9		
Metastatic		198	10.4
Miscellaneous and Unclassified		23	1.2
Cysts	7		
Granuloma	7		
Other	9		

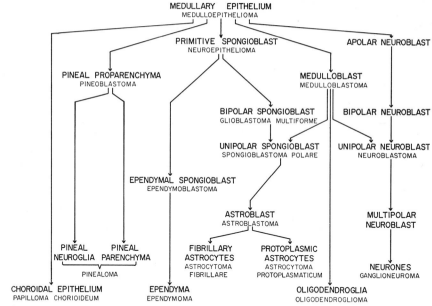

Figure 1.   Scheme to relate types of gliomas according to the predominant cellular constitution of each group (Bailey).

CLINICAL SYNDROMES OF INTRACRANIAL TUMORS

There are certain general effects to be expected from the presence of a tumor in or on the brain, without regard to the pathologic type. There are also distinct clinical aspects and characteristics in behavior that individualize most types of brain tumor. In addition, there are different clinical syndromes which result from the presence of tumors in various areas of the brain.

In children, for instance, the majority of tumors occur beneath the tentorium in the cerebellum and brain stem, and some types of these tumors do not occur in persons of older age. The converse is true in adults, who more commonly have supratentorial tumors, many of which are meningiomas not seen in children. Symptoms indicative of pressure of the optic nerves and chiasm are likely in children to be due to craniopharyngioma, while in adults they are usually due to a pituitary adenoma.

The manifestations of intracranial tumors fall into two classes: those resulting from increased intracranial pressure and those caused by irritative or destructive effects on specific regions of the brain. While it is advantageous to recognize the presence of a tumor before papilledema and significant increase in intracranial pressure develop, tumors in the so-called silent areas of the brain, and those which block the cerebrospinal fluid pathways, may cause only increased intracranial pressure. Supratentorial tumors, by displacing the cerebral hemispheres, may produce herniation of the temporal lobes through the incisura of the tentorium, resulting in a variety of effects including compression of the mesencephalon, narrowing of the aqueduct of Sylvius and occlusion of local blood vessels, any one of which may lead rapidly to irreversible damage to the brain. Infratentorial tumors, in addition to producing direct pressure on the medulla, may cause herniation of the cerebellum into the foramen magnum and additional medullary compression, resulting in vascular and respiratory failure.

As intracranial pressure increases, and before more dire effects develop, there are frequently symptoms of headache, vomiting, failing visual acuity and diplopia, though all of these may not occur. Headache rarely has value in localizing an intracranial tumor, exceptions being the occasional lateralization over a supratentorial tumor and localized suboccipital pain with a tumor of the posterior cranial fossa. In about 15 per cent of the patients having increased pressure, there is no headache at all and, when present, headache is rarely of severe degree; if it does become an excruciating pain there is imminent danger.

Vomiting may at times be secondary to the pain, but more often it is due to irritation of vagal centers in the medulla. Exertion, straining or sudden change in position by further altering the intracranial pressure may enhance the headache or lead to sudden and forceful vomiting. Matutinal vomiting on rising from bed is a common manifestation of posterior fossa tumors, particularly in children.

Some degree of blurring in vision is a common accompaniment of papilledema, which occurs with increased intracranial pressure, though significant loss of acuity is slow to develop. This characteristic is of value when a differential diagnosis must be made between papilledema and optic neuritis, since in the latter there is rapid loss of visual acuity. Diplopia, which sometimes accompanies increased intracranial pressure, results from compression of an abducens nerve, occasionally both abducens nerves, and before a gross squint can be recognized the patient is aware of duplication of objects on the horizontal plane.

The features which make for precise localization of a brain tumor are those that have to do with motor and sensory functions. The development in a local area of the body of a change in muscle function, such as convulsive movements, weakness, rigidity, incoordination, adventitious movements and reflex changes, indicates involvement of motor areas of the brain, the cortex, the tracts or certain cranial nerves. If there are abberations or defects in smell, vision, hearing or of the various tactile senses, these may point to the involvement of specific structures of the brain. Exceptions sometimes exist because of the remote effects of altered intracranial pressure, as exemplified by hemiparesis, or even a lateralized fit which may occur with a tumor that occupies a region of the cerebrum removed from the motor cortex and tracts. But the localizing value of certain sensory disturbances is highly reliable. An uncinate fit in which the patient experiences fleeting episodes of unpleasant odors occurs only when the uncus in one of the temporal lobes is directly affected by tumor. Loss of discriminatory and position sense in an extremity, with preservation of other forms of sensation, indicates direct involvement of the postrolandic sensory cortex or its immediate subcortical connections. A homonymous hemianopic visual field defect results only from direct involvement of the contralateral visual pathway.

Disturbances in speech are of two types: those related to expression and those related to reception. Rarely, if at all, does one type exist without some degree of the other. Aphasia of any degree or type indicates that the tumor lies above the tentorium in the temporal lobe, or in an immediately adjacent region. The early manifestations of aphasia are easily mistaken for psychotic changes, but aphasia is a defect in language and allied functions and is not related to mood or behavior.

Convulsions, when associated with intracranial tumors, indicate that the tumor lies above the tentorium. Fits do not result from tumors in the posterior fossa, with the possible exception of their rare occurrence in a patient with a tendency to convulsions who develops increased intracranial pressure from a posterior fossa tumor. Patients with posterior fossa tumors may develop episodes of rigid hyperextension. These are sometimes spoken of as cerebellar fits, but in fact are manifestations of a decerebrate state and have a serious implication. Fits, usually with focal qualities and more often diurnal than nocturnal, are a fairly common accompaniment of cerebral tumors. They occur in about 45 per cent of all patients with supratentorial tumors, particularly in those with the more benign types of glioma or with meningiomas, with which there is an incidence of fits of about 65 per cent. Convulsions may be the only manifestation for many months of a slowly growing tumor. An adult who develops them for the first time in life should be suspected of having a tumor.

Evaluation of visual symptoms and of funduscopic, pupillary and extraocular signs is of great importance. Reduction in visual acuity, when accompanied by primary optic atrophy rather than by papilledema or its late effects, secondary atrophy, is usually the result of involvement of the optic nerves or chiasm by tumor. Perimetry can be particularly helpful, and although careful testing on a tangent screen is desirable, often much can be learned by confrontation testing with fingers in the initial examination. A defect in the visual field of one eye indicates involvement of the nerve on that side. Bitemporal field defects indicate a chiasmal lesion, while homonymous field defects invariably indicate a lesion in the contralateral visual pathway somewhere between the chiasm and the calcarine area of the occipital lobe.

Diplopia, causing duplication of objects on a diagonal plane, results from palsy of the third or fourth cranial nerve or from a lesion in the tegmentum in the midbrain. This is in contradistinction to diplopia with horizontal duplication due to abducens palsy. Third cranial nerve palsy is evidenced by an enlarged pupil and drooping eyelid on one side, as well as by discernible defects in movements of the involved eye except in lateral deviation. An enlarged pupil due to incomplete oculomotor nerve palsy occurs particularly on the side of rapidly developing tumors of the temporal lobe, causing a shift of the brain stem and compression of the nerve.

Impairment in upward gaze results from a lesion of the quadrigeminal plate or adjacent regions of the midbrain, and is nearly pathognomonic of a tumor in this region. Defects in horizontal movements of the eyes, with preservation of vertical movements, result from a lesion slightly lower in the brain stem; they are seen almost exclusively accompanying gliomas of the brain stem. Nystagmus does not result from a supratentorial tumor, but is primarily the result of a disturbance in the vestibular system and is linked with tumors in the posterior cranial fossa.

TUMORS OF THE CEREBRAL HEMISPHERES. The commonest tumors of the cerebral hemispheres are gliomas. Unfortunately, glioblastoma, which thus far has rarely been cured, outnumbers all others. Astrocytoma, which is a more benign growth and sometimes curable, occurs about half as frequently, while oligodendroglioma, the rarest of these three, is the most slowly growing and most benign. All these tumors occur with about equal frequency in the several lobes of the hemispheres with the exception of the occipital, where there is a relatively low incidence of all types of tumor.

Meningiomas, which affect the brain by compression and not by invasion, occur principally above the tentorium and with about one-third the frequency of gliomas. They are regarded as usually benign, encapsulated and surgically removable, though their location, size and vascularity sometimes may defeat attempts at radical removal. They tend to originate from regions where arachnoid villi are clustered and thus are found along the sagittal sinus—"parasagittal" and "falx" tumors—and along the course of meningeal vessels, where they compress the superior surface of the hemisphere and are sometimes referred to as convexity tumors. Other common locations are along the sphenoidal ridges and the floor of the frontal fossae, particularly in the olfactory grooves, and on the tuberculum sellae. Those on the sphenoidal ridge affect the temporal lobe and adjacent portions of the frontal and parietal lobes.

Those in the olfactory groove encroach on the inferior surfaces of one or both frontal lobes and destroy the olfactory and optic nerves. The syndrome described by Kennedy of anosmia and visual loss on one side, with homolateral primary optic atrophy and contralateral papilledema, is pathognomonic of olfactory groove meningioma. Tumors of the tuberculum sellae may cause compression of the optic nerves and chiasm in the early period of their growth and can be detected by the pattern of visual changes, though sometimes they attain great size and displace the frontal lobes before vision is affected.

Frontal lobe tumors, which invade or compress the brain, cause subtle changes at first. Later, there is more pronounced alteration in personality, with loss of interest, irritability, impaired judgment and memory, and an attitude of facetiousness. Forced grasping can often be demonstrated and if the lesion encroaches on the prerolandic area, there may be convulsions or progressive corticospinal tract signs. Lesions on the left side may also cause aphasia, particularly of the anomial type.

Parietal lobe tumors cause striking motor and sensory changes on the contralateral side of the body. Jacksonian convulsions are a frequent manifestation, particularly in the early phase of the disease. In later stages, there is increasing hemiparesis. Involvement of the sensory cortex results in contralateral astereognosis and loss of discriminatory sense, and lessens the degree of spasticity in hemiparesis. On the dominant side, parietal lobe lesions also produce aphasic defects, especially of the receptive type.

Temporal lobe tumors may be relatively "silent" and attain considerable size before detection, particularly if they occur on the nondominant side. When they are on the dominant side, aphasia is to be expected. Deep lesions involve a part of the optic radiation, sometimes causing visual hallucinations of bizarre forms and usually causing contralateral homonymous upper quadrantanopsia of incongruous type. Uncinate fits, feelings of déjà vu and psychomotor seizures are inconstant effects of temporal lobe lesions, but, when present, they are diagnostically important.

Occipital lobe tumors, in particular, cause visual hallucinations of light and homonymous hemianopsia of congruous type, often without other localizing signs. If the lesion involves the lateral convexity of the lobe on the dominant side, there may be difficulty in reading ability (alexia) and inability to recognize objects by sight (visual agnosia).

TUMORS OF THE CEREBELLUM. The common brain tumor of childhood is the benign cerebellar astrocytoma which has its peak in age distribution at 12 years and is rarely seen in persons older than 20 years. The results of surgical treatment are excellent, which makes it all the more desirable to reach a diagnosis before irreversible changes occur. The symptoms are those of gradual increase in intracranial pressure, accompanied by ataxic movements, dysmetria and hypotonia; nystagmus is an inconstant finding. Particularly in younger children, the significance of unexplained vomiting, the development of a squint from abducens palsy and the moderate enlargement of the head, due to increased intracranial pressure, may go unrecognized for months.

The next most common tumor of childhood is the malignant cerebellar medulloblastoma. It produces much the same pressure effects and cerebellar disturbances as does astrocytoma, but the development of symptoms is more rapid and the peak age of occurrence is several years earlier. Even so, it is usually impossible to be sure of the differential diagnosis without operation. The medulloblastoma, as with few other primary intracranial tumors, tends to spread along the cerebrospinal fluid pathways; occasionally, the tumor will give evidence of its presence in the lower spinal canal before cerebellar signs develop. The tumor is highly sensitive to radiation therapy, sometimes for a number of years, but radiotherapy should not be employed without first identifying the tumor and performing surgical decompression.

Other tumors of the cerebellum which occur with less frequency, though not rare, are ependymomas, papillomas of the choroid plexus and hemangioblastomas. These may occur at any age, but the first two are more common in early life, while the last is the benign cerebellar tumor of adults. A differential diagnosis on the basis of neurologic signs is not usually possible, though there are a few special features which are helpful.

Ependymoma and papilloma tend to become firmly attached to the floor of the fourth ventricle and at times produce facial palsy as a result of invasion of one or both facial nuclei. Because of this firm attachment, it is usually impossible to perform complete surgical excision. Ependymoma, like medulloblastoma, may seed itself along the fluid pathways. Also, this tumor has a tendency to bleed spontaneously, causing the symptoms of acute subarachnoid hemorrhage.

Hemangioblastoma, which has a high rate of surgical cure, may produce any or all of the signs of a cerebellar tumor. But more especially, it should be recognized that this tumor may be accompanied by true polycythemia, is sometimes familial and may be associated with hemangiomatosis elsewhere in the body, most particularly in the retina, in which case the combination of retinal and cerebellar tumor is referred to as von Hippel-Lindau disease.

TUMORS OF THE BRAIN STEM. Tumors of the brain stem are gliomas, usually relatively benign, such as spongioblastoma polare or astrocytoma, but because of their location are not amenable to a radical operation and can be controlled only for a while with radiotherapy. The pons is much more frequently involved than the medulla and the age of incidence is principally in childhood, occasionally in young adulthood.

The characteristic of these tumors is that they produce cranial nerve palsies, usually for some time before long-tract signs or increased intracranial pressure appear. It is remarkable that in many instances the aqueduct and fourth ventricle, though narrowed, are not occluded, and papilledema never develops. Among the various cranial nerve palsies commonly seen are extraocular palsies, dysphagia, dysphonia and facial monoplegia or diplegia, but other cranial nerve palsies may occur. Nystagmus and ataxia in the extremities are also common.

TUMORS OF THE THIRD VENTRICLE. Neoplasms of the third ventricle, for practical purposes, can be divided into anteriorly and posteriorly placed lesions. The pinealoma typifies the latter and characteristically produces increased intracranial pressure by blockade of the ventricle or aqueduct, impairment in conjugate movement of the eyes above the horizontal plane and a variety of pupillary reactions. These tumors are usually not suited to surgical removal, but some type of ventricular shunt is useful to overcome the ventricular block. Some of the several types of tumor which occur in or about the pineal gland can be controlled by roentgen therapy.

The colloid cyst, a benign and curable tumor, occurs in the anterior third ventricle and is so located that it blocks the foramina of Monro, thus causing dilatation of the lateral ventricles and increased intracranial pressure. Except for symptoms and signs resulting from the altered pressure, there are no manifestations. Other tumors, such as gliomas, craniopharyngioma and ectopic pinealoma, sometimes encroach on the anterior third ventricle and are likely to cause hypothalamic disturbances characterized by diabetes insipidus, diencephalic epilepsy, somnolence, obesity and precocious sexual development.

TUMORS OF THE CEREBELLOPONTILE ANGLE. The syndrome, produced by tumors in the cerebellopontile angle, deserves special mention because its recognition can be relied on to identify the presence of the acoustic neurinoma, which is surgically curable. Other tumors which may occur in this region are meningioma and cholesteatoma, the latter being particularly favorable to treatment.

Symptoms of acoustic neurinoma develop insidiously, beginning usually with unilateral tinnitus and progressive deafness. The vestibular response on the same side disappears early in the disease and there may be vertigo and instability in walking, but paroxysms of vertigo, such as occur in Ménière's disease, are not encountered. After many months, involvement of the adjacent trigeminal and facial nerves becomes evident, the former being particularly identified by loss of corneal sensation even before other sensory loss in the face develops. Additional growth of the tumor may cause palsy of other cranial nerves in the posterior fossa and also ventricular block, though the presence of the tumor can usually be recognized by refined audiometric and radiologic tests before it has advanced to this stage.

TUMORS OF THE SELLAR REGION. Tumors of the region of the sella turcica can be separated into intrasellar tumors, which are almost exclusively pituitary adenomas, and suprasellar tumors, which include in order of frequency, craniopharyngioma, meningioma of the tuberculum sellae and gliomas of the optic chiasm.

The tumors of the pituitary usually occur in adulthood and arise from one of three types of cells which make up the anterior lobe of the gland. The commonest is the chromophobe adenoma, derived from the indifferent cells. It produces hypopituitarism as a result of compression of the normal gland, enlarges or "balloons" the sella turcica and compresses the optic nerves and chiasm, causing visual field defects, usually bitemporal hemianopsia, loss of visual acuity and primary optic atrophy. The growth of these tumors may be held in check by radiation therapy, but if there is any significant impairment of

vision, surgical removal of the tumor should not be delayed, for it has a high degree of success.

The chromophil adenoma is derived from the eosinophil cells which are believed to control growth. The presence of the tumor can be easily recognized by the appearance of gigantism during puberty, or of acromegaly after puberty. A relatively small percentage of these tumors enlarge enough to compress the optic nerves and chiasm. Since the tumors are relatively sensitive to irradiation, this has usually been the treatment of choice. But since radiotherapy cannot be relied on always to control the tumor, and because it produces subtle, persistent bodily changes, surgical excision has come to be employed more often. The risk of destroying normal pituitary function by surgical removal of the tumor is no longer a hazard because of the availability of adrenocorticotropic hormone and cortisone for substitution therapy.

The basophil adenoma, derived from basophil cells, is usually of small size and insufficient to give rise to compression of the pituitary gland or adjacent structures. This tumor is believed by some to be the cause of Cushing's syndrome. Most of the tumors of the pituitary found at operation or at autopsy, in conjunction with Cushing's syndrome, are microscopically of the chromophobe type. A few show malignant qualities, invading adjacent structures and even metastasizing to distant organs. Although adrenalectomy is the common method of treating Cushing's syndrome, there are circumstances in which hypophysectomy or irradiation of the pituitary is more appropriate.

In the suprasellar region, the craniopharyngioma is the commonest of the several types of tumors that are found. It may be difficult to differentiate from pituitary adenomas, whose effects it mimics. However, craniopharyngioma is a congenital tumor and often produces symptoms before the patient is 15 years of age. It has a tendency to cause diabetes insipidus, sometimes for transient or intermittent periods, and to show calcification on roentgenograms, findings which are unusual in pituitary adenomas. Meningiomas produce local hyperostosis of the tuberculum sellae and gliomas of the optic chiasm cause infraclinoid erosion, sometimes with enlargement of the optic foramina, which can be identified on roentgenograms.

METASTATIC TUMORS. The most common source of metastatic tumors of the brain is the lung, but malignant tumors of the breast, kidney, gastrointestinal tract, nasopharynx and of many other tissues of the body may give rise to secondary growths in the brain. Malignant melanoma is especially prone to spread to the brain and to produce spontaneous subarachnoid bleeding. Metastases are more commonly found in the cerebral hemispheres and, in a surprising number of instances, there appears to be only one lesion in the brain. The progression of neurologic symptoms and signs is likely to be fairly rapid and may constitute the only complaint or discernible manifestation of the malignancy. The best that can be expected from surgical removal, which is often a relatively simple operation, is prolongation of life and possibly some reversal of palsies and relief of headache. But to many patients and their families, this much is greatly worth while.

Diagnosis of Intracranial Tumors

It would be a serious mistake to assume that the diagnosis of tumors and other diseases of the brain could be made without diligent clinical study, since the combination of an accurate history and thorough physical examination remains the most reliable method. Yet, without the aid of numerous present-day adjuncts, the factor of error in identification and localization would be considerable.

Roentgenograms of the skull yield some type of positive information in about 30 per cent of brain tumors. The changes to be looked for are erosion of the sella turcica; shift in position of the calcified pineal gland; calcific deposits in the neoplasm; alteration in vascular markings of the skull; enlargement of certain foramina; separation of cranial sutures in children; thinning or destruction of the skull in adults, and hyperostotic changes caused by meningiomas.

A roentgenogram of the chest should be obtained in every patient suspected of having an intracranial tumor because of the possibility of metastasis from lung cancer.

Lumbar puncture and withdrawal of spinal fluid cannot be performed without risk in the presence of increased intracranial pressure, though occasionally the risk is justified. The possibility that symptoms of brain tumor may become rapidly worse following withdrawal of spinal fluid emphasizes the need for omitting lumbar puncture, or restricting its use to a time when craniotomy can be performed promptly if need be. Compression of jugular veins sometimes erroneously performed in conjunction with the puncture adds materially to the risk.

In addition to determination of the resting pressure of the cerebrospinal fluid, the other important determinations are the protein content of the fluid and the cell count. The protein content in the fluid is elevated in the majority of, but not in all, patients with brain tumor. The most consistent elevations occur with acoustic neurinomas and meningiomas which exist near the floor of the skull. Occasionally, glioblastomas which encroach on the ventricle, or metastatic tumors, produce pleocytosis in the fluid.

Sometimes, it is possible to identify the presence of neoplastic cells in centrifuged cerebrospinal fluid. In extensive involvement of the meninges by tumor, there may be significant decrease in the sugar content of the fluid. Studies of the transaminase content of cerebrospinal fluid suggest that some information is provided in differentiating vascular and neoplastic diseases of the brain; transaminase is usually increased in the former and less often altered by tumors.

Electroencephalography is found to be useful in identifying the presence and location of a brain tumor in from 50 to 75 per cent of patients, depending on the experience and diligence of the examiner. In particular, infratentorial and deep supratentorial tumors evade detection, and often an abnormal pattern due to vascular disease cannot be distinguished from that of a neoplasm. Even so, the electroencephalogram has value as an adjunctive method of examination.

Radioactive isotopes are employed in the identification of brain tumors, on the premise that the presence of the isotope deposited temporarily in greater concentration in the tumor can be detected by a suitable counting device. The tests made with gamma-emitting radioactive I^{131} and a scintillation counter have shown an efficiency of about 70 per cent in the detection of brain tumors above the tentorium. The results in detection of tumors by this method are at least as good as those obtained by electroencephalography. Improved results in diagnosis have been reported by the use of a positron-emitting isotope and automatic coincidence scanning as compared to single or multiple channel scanning utilizing gamma radiation. Other methods employ photoscanning of isotopes of mercury, Hg^{203} and Hg^{197}, and of technetium, Tc^{99m}.

Angiography performed by the injection of

a radiopaque dye, usually 50 per cent Hypaque, directly or by retrograde methods, into the carotid or vertebral arteries has added significantly to diagnostic procedures and is attended by relatively little risk (Fig. 2). The test is of less use in posterior fossa tumors than in supratentorial tumors, where it can be of considerable advantage in identifying the presence, relative size and vascularity of the lesions, and has about 80 per cent accuracy. With somewhat less accuracy, the type of tumor can sometimes be determined. For the diagnosis of vascular lesions, such as aneurysms and arteriovenous anomalies, the method is ideal. A refinement in identifying vascular shadows is obtained by the subtraction method, whereby the bone is blotted out by a photographic procedure and only the vessels stand out.

Echoencephalography, a recent development, depends on the reflection of ultrasonic echoes from intracranial structures to define the position of the midline of the brain and other intracranial structures as well as the presence of tumors. Thus far its widest use is in identifying a lateral shift of the brain and its use for this purpose is enhanced by the fact that the test is simple, harmless and about 90 per cent accurate. More complicated equipment and less accuracy attend the use of the method for other purposes.

Ventriculography and encephalography, by air injection into the ventricles or spinal sub-arachnoid space, are still the most reliable methods of identifying the presence and the location of a tumor in any part of the brain (Fig. 3). The efficiency of the tests is about 95 per cent. The latter method requires lumbar puncture and is attended by risk in the presence of increased intracranial pressure. But if the air is injected in graduated amounts, without also withdrawing cerebrospinal fluid, the procedure may be used with relative safety, particularly if preparations have been made to proceed immediately with removal of the tumor, or at least for withdrawal of ventricular fluid through a trephine opening in the skull in case the patient's condition should be made worse.

DIFFERENTIAL DIAGNOSIS.   In the diagnosis of an intracranial tumor, there are many other diseases of the brain which require differentiation. Some of these are characterized by increased intracranial pressure alone, such as atresia of the aqueduct of Sylvius, or pseudotumor cerebri, also termed benign increased intracranial pressure. Some conditions present convulsions or various palsies, or both, such as may occur with a variety of degenerative and cerebral vascular diseases. Still others demonstrate increased pressure, as well as various other neurologic signs. Included among these conditions are abscess, parasitic and granulomatous infections, and several kinds of intracranial hemorrhage.

Most of the diseases which require differ-

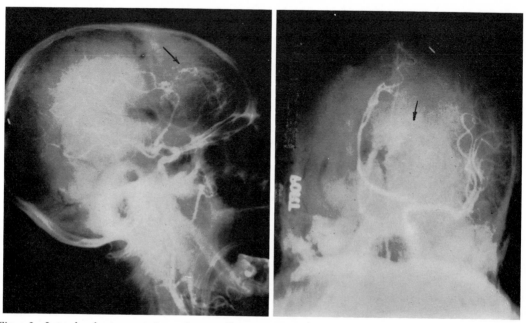

Figure 2.   Lateral and anteroposterior angiograms showing "staining" in a large glioma of the frontal lobe and distortion of regional arteries.

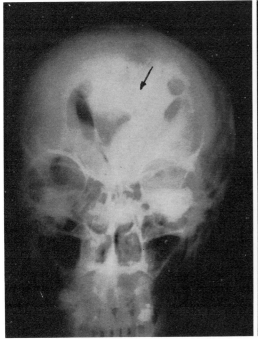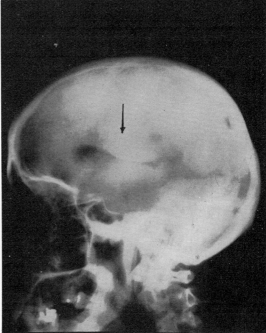

Figure 3. Anteroposterior and lateral ventriculograms showing depression of the body of the ventricle and a lateral shift of the ventricular system caused by a parietal tumor.

entiation can be identified by relatively simple diagnostic measures, whereas a few require time and repeated observations. Some of the diseases are amenable to surgical treatment.

TREATMENT OF INTRACRANIAL TUMORS

SURGICAL TREATMENT. If it were possible, all brain tumors should be surgically removed, but many are confined to vital parts, or have extended to these parts by the time of operation, and defeat any hope of cure by excision. However, even partial removal of most tumors of this kind is repaying in terms of improvement in symptoms and extension of life. Certain tumors, which constitute about 35 per cent of the total number, can be totally removed, or nearly so, and the patients restored to useful life. The tumors included in this last group are meningiomas, pituitary adenomas, acoustic neurinomas, hemangiomas, astrocytomas, craniopharyngiomas, cholesteatomas and a miscellaneous group of less common neoplasms.

The two great adjuncts to neurosurgical technique, strong suction and an electrosurgical unit for control of bleeding, have been used to advantage for over 35 years, but many refinements have been added. Consid-

erable thought has been given to the cosmetic result of cranial operations, and an unsightly wound is now an exception.

The Torkildsen operation of ventricular shunt, by means of a tube passing from a lateral ventricle to the cisterna magna, has been highly useful in certain irremovable tumors such as the pinealoma, and other tumors that block the ventricular system. Other methods of ventricular shunting now in common use in the treatment of hydrocephalus in children are sometimes applicable.

In many clinics, local anesthetics, the use of which was tedious for both the surgeon and the patient, have been replaced by a general anesthetic administered endotracheally. There is a distinct advantage in the protection against respiratory difficulty during operation provided by the endotracheal tube, and operations can be continued for hours without fear of difficulty from this source. Ethyl ether is used and preferred by some surgeons, but halothane (Fluothane) is used by many as the anesthetic agent.

The ready availability of blood for transfusion has simplified the correction of blood loss and has virtually done away with the need for multistage operations that formerly were used in the treatment of some tumors.

Though muscle is probably the best material for use in the control of more brisk bleeding from torn blood vessels in the brain or dura, Gelfoam and absorbable cellulose provide ready means of dealing with the general ooze of blood, which can be such a nuisance to control.

The antimicrobial agents have been a godsend in neurosurgery, for the risk of infection and death from meningitis is now virtually a thing of the past. A tuberculoma can now be removed without the almost inevitable sequence of meningitis and death, thanks to streptomycin and other antituberculous drugs.

Several other developments have added significantly to the facility and safety of operations. One of these is the production and maintenance of a hypotensive state during operation by means of Arfonad, a sympathetic blocking agent which minimizes blood loss, reduces the bulk of the brain, has a complementary effect on anesthesia and yet does not expose the brain to anoxic effects which often occur when blood pressure falls because of blood loss.

A more recent development is the lowering of body temperature to a degree that reduces the metabolic requirements of the brain, thus making it possible to occlude the main blood supply to the brain safely for minutes at a time while dealing with a vascular lesion.

Another development has been the use of hypertonic solutions of either urea or Mannitol, administered intravenously, for reducing intracranial pressure through "shrinking" of the brain. It appears that these agents have advantages which will lead to their replacing other chemical agents used heretofore for this purpose. The administration of steroids, usually in the form of dexamethasone, reduces edema of the brain and is especially useful in the postoperative period, though its use is attended by some risk of inducing gastrointestinal bleeding, or complicating the management of insulin in a diabetic patient.

RADIATION THERAPY. There is a limited place for radiation therapy as a substitute for operation in tumors of the brain. Gliomas of the brain stem cannot be excised, and sometimes are dramatically improved for limited periods by radiation therapy. Pituitary adenomas which have not grown to a size to compress the optic nerves may benefit by x-radiation. Pinealomas and tumors not well suited to direct surgical attack often show favorable effects from such treatment. This

includes certain metastatic tumors, particularly bronchogenic ones.

As a supplement to partial removal of certain tumors, radiation treatment is beneficial, but the results are difficult to evaluate and there is a wide diversity of opinion regarding its use. Some would limit its use postoperatively to a few tumors, such as medulloblastoma and pituitary adenomas, but, at one time or another, claim of benefit from radiation treatment has been made for nearly every type of intracranial neoplasm. Some of these claims are unjustified, but others undoubtedly represent the occasional observation of benefit and thereby emphasize the vagaries in the response of tumors to irradiation. It is sufficient to say that no brain tumor has ever been cured by radiation and the decision to employ this treatment usually depends on a number of factors pertinent to the individual patient.

There has been renewed interest in the use of radiation therapy since the development of the high voltage machine, radioactive cobalt and the activation of boron injected intravenously by exposing the patient in an atomic pile. None of these methods of radiation therapy has shown results thus far which justify enthusiasm.

PSEUDOTUMOR AND ALLIED CONDITIONS

Pseudotumor is a term applied to a condition in which increased intracranial pressure develops without evident cause. The condition has also been labeled serous meningitis, otitic hydrocephalus, toxic hydrocephalus, arachnoiditis and benign increased intracranial pressure.

Clinically, most of the patients have headache, papilledema, increased intracranial pressure by spinal measurement, and occasionally diplopia, transient palsies and convulsions. The patient's feeling of well-being is out of keeping with the potentialities implied by the increased pressure. But for elevation of pressure, the spinal fluid is normal, though the protein content may be relatively low. The electroencephalogram at times shows an abnormal pattern of nonspecific nature and the pneumoventriculogram shows a normal or, perhaps, small-sized ventricular system.

Some of the patients have been found by sagittal sinus venography to have unsuspected thrombosis of the sagittal sinus or of a dominant lateral sinus. The condition is believed to have been present in many of the disorders designated as otitic hydrocephalus associated with mastoiditis and middle ear infections.

In a study of 28 consecutive patients followed for one to five years, it was found that in six of the patients the nature of the illness was not evident until some months had passed, but three patients had neoplasms, one had multiple sclerosis, another had periarteritis and one had an aneurysm of the basilar artery.

In ten of the 28 patients, venous obstruction was conclusively demonstrated as the cause of the increased intracranial pressure. In the remaining 12, no cause could be discovered. The fortunate thing is that most patients with venous obstruction, or without any demonstrable disease, tend to recover in a period of several months without visual loss or other sequelae. A few begin to lose vision, and then it is desirable to resort to decompressive procedures, such as unilateral or bilateral subtemporal decompression. Repeated lumbar puncture is safe and may serve a useful purpose in diminishing the risk of visual loss. Repeated intravenous injection of hypertonic solutions is not an effective therapeutic measure, though daily oral administration of glycerine has sometimes been useful.

In arachnoiditis, there is unexplained thickening of the arachnoid membrane resulting in obstruction to the cerebrospinal fluid pathways. The effect is at times localized about the chiasmatic cistern, causing visual loss, and there are reports of dramatic return of vision after resection of the arachnoid and release of trapped fluid. When arachnoiditis occurs in the cisterna magna and lateral recesses of the posterior fossa, there is ventricular obstruction and increased intracranial pressure. The condition is distinguished from pseudotumor by the fact that the ventricles tend to become dilated in arachnoiditis. Exposure of the cisterna magna by craniotomy and disruption of the arachnoid, together with suboccipital decompression, usually terminates the increased intracranial pressure. If not, then some shunting device is employed.

Symptomatic occult hydrocephalus with normal cerebrospinal fluid pressure is a term applied to a syndrome characterized principally by progressive dementia and unsteady gait, sometimes of severe degree. There is normal or borderline elevation of pressure of the cerebrospinal fluid with dilated ventricles and limited outline of subarachnoid spaces on pneumoencephalography. The condition is presumably due to pathologic changes in the subarachnoid spaces about the brain. Although the differential diagnosis is uncertain, extracranial shunting of the cerebrospinal or ventricular fluid sometimes results in gratifying improvement of symptoms.

INTRACRANIAL ABSCESSES

Localized suppurative infection of the brain, once a relatively common and fearsome disease, has become nearly a rarity, principally because of antimicrobial therapy. Brain abscesses result from extension of infection in adjacent regions of the head or by metastasis from remote foci in the body. Adjacent sources include middle ear and mastoid; the nose and accessory nasal sinuses; the cranium and scalp; and also compound fractures and penetrating wounds of the skull, through which there is implantation of infected material. Of this group, middle ear infection is by far the commonest source in civilian practice. Metastatic abscesses originate principally from lesions in the chest and, less frequently, from endocarditis, osteomyelitis, abscessed teeth, carbuncles, septic endometritis and suppuration in any part of the body. Occasionally, the source of a brain abscess cannot be determined, in which case it is assumed that the infection started in a period of unrecognized bacteremia.

The abscesses which result from direct extension of an adjacent infection are usually solitary, while metastatic abscesses are often multiple. The infecting organisms most frequently found are *Staphylococcus pyogenes* var. *albus* and *aureus*, the hemolytic streptococci and the pneumococci. Other organisms as well as mixtures have also been found, their nature depending on the source of the contamination.

PATHOLOGY. Extension of infection to the brain from adjacent foci in the head may occur by one of two pathways, or possibly at times by a combination of the two. The commonest is the successive infection of intervening structures. Osteomyelitis or localized osteitis first develops, followed by the formation of an epidural abscess which penetrates the dura and invades the underlying brain, passing through the highly vascular cortex to lodge and take growth in the white matter. In the course of progression of the infection, the subdural or subarachnoid spaces may become contaminated, giving rise to a subdural abscess and leptomeningitis, respectively. A part of this process of extension undoubtedly entails thrombosis of blood vessels in the bone, meninges and brain, and this serves to extend the infection as well as to make the tissues more susceptible by devitalization. Brain abscesses arising from frontal sinusitis occupy chiefly the frontal lobes, while those arising from the middle ear and mastoid occupy the temporal lobe or the cerebellum.

The other common mode of extension is by way of the veins draining the structures about the upper portion of the face and head toward the dural venous sinuses. By this means, retrograde thrombosis or septic emboli may carry the infection through tributary veins to any part of the brain, thus accounting for what have been called "distant abscesses." Occasionally, abscesses have resulted from implantation by an exploring brain needle which was passed through an infected area. The location of a metastatic abscess from a distant source of infection is purely fortuitous; and in about two-thirds of the patients, more than one abscess develops. When an abscess results from a penetrating wound, the inciting factors are pulped brain and blood clots, plus retained bone fragments and foreign material, which have carried in bacteria that are largely skin inhabitants of relatively low virulence. Shell fragments are not usually infective even when they are retained in the brain.

Irrespective of what route the infection takes to the brain, the local reaction is always essentially the same. As the infection grows in the devitalized tissues, the clinical symptoms are those of encephalitis. After some days, an equilibrium is reached between the infection and the reaction of the surrounding brain. Regional blood vessels throw off a heavy exudation of leukocytes, constituting the first line of defense. Behind this defense, the blood vessels increase in size and number, and connective tissue cells proliferate, producing a wall, or capsule, for the abscess. From this time on, it is a struggle between the wall and the leukocytes on the one hand and the invading bacteria on the other. If a breakthrough occurs, a secondary or "daughter" abscess may result, or there may be a spreading encephalitis or a rupture into the ventricles, the last two conditions being rapidly fatal.

Although the wall of an abscess begins to form in the first week, it is not firm enough to offer appreciable resistance to an exploratory needle until at least two or three weeks have passed. In some types of infection of strong virulence, particularly in metastatic abscess of pulmonic origin, a wall may not develop and the clinical course is one of fatal, spreading encephalitis from the start.

If surgical evacuation of the abscess is instituted, the wall of the abscess will contract and form a scar. Rarely, an otogenic abscess has been known to discharge spontaneously into the external ear or mastoid wound. Occasionally, spontaneous cures take place, and some abscesses when drained are found to contain sterile pus. But in spite of apparent quiescence, reactivation of even a drained or sterile abscess may take place long after the process has been thought to have subsided.

SYMPTOMS AND SIGNS. The symptoms of a brain abscess vary with the stage of the disease, the virulence of the infection, the degree of increased intracranial pressure and the location of the abscess. Early in the clinical course, it may be difficult to make an accurate diagnosis, even though it may be obvious that infection has reached the brain. Usually, the temperature remains high for the first few days and then takes on a low, spiking contour. The blood leukocyte count may rise to 20,000 or more, but it may decline. The count may be normal from the start or soon afterward, particularly if antimicrobial drugs are given when the patient first develops fever or other signs of illness. Examination of the spinal fluid discloses an increase of pressure, protein content and leukocytes, chiefly of lymphocytes, unless frank suppurative leptomeningitis occurs.

Headache and vomiting develop early and persist. Irritability, or apathy and lethargy reflects the development of encephalitis and increasing intracranial pressure. The neck becomes stiff as a result of the associated meningeal reaction and in time, as the pressure increases, the pulse rate, at first fast, becomes slow, and papilledema appears. These are the general symptoms and signs of the initial stage of the disease, representing the struggle between destructive and reparative forces. If the virulence of the infecting organism is great and the patient's resistance is poor, surgical drainage of the abscess may be useless, and profound coma followed by respiratory failure may ensue.

In more favorable instances, the infection becomes localized and a wall develops around the abscess. Signs of sepsis subside and fever and leukocytosis recede. Edema of the brain abates and all symptoms improve, with the possible exception of localizing symptoms, which will usually have made their appearance some time during the first week of the illness. The patient still appears apathetic and complains of headache, so that the clinical signs and symptoms at this stage may be much like those of an intracranial neoplasm.

The symptoms may continue for months throughout the quiescent stage, until the abscess is evacuated or until the patient dies from rupture of the abscess into the ventricle. More rarely, the abscess resolves spontaneously.

Localizing signs depend upon the size and position of the abscess. The commonest sites for abscesses in the brain are, in the order of frequency, the frontal lobes, the temporal lobes and the cerebellar hemispheres. Less commonly, the parietal and occipital lobes and the brain stem are involved.

Abscesses in the frontal lobe may attain considerable size and still remain relatively silent. Yet, it is unusual if there are not at least a few suggestive signs, such as alteration in mood, contralateral convulsions, muscle weakness or pathologic reflexes, and possibly motor aphasia if the lesion is on the left.

Temporal lobe abscesses may produce homonymous hemianopic defects, paralysis, sensory impairment and pathologic reflexes on the contralateral side, and palsy of the third and sixth cranial nerves on the homolateral side. If the left temporal lobe is involved, aphasia is the earliest and most striking sign. Occasionally, the acute displacement of the brain stem caused by a temporal lobe abscess may cause homolateral corticospinal tract signs due to pressure on the crus cerebri by the margin of the tentorium on the side opposite the abscess. Cerebellar abscesses produce dysmetria in the homolateral extremities, nystagmus and frequently pathologic reflexes on the opposite side of the body. It has occasionally been observed that the patient prefers to lie on the side of the lesion and that turning the head to the opposite side induces vertigo, vomiting and vigorous nystagmus. Another infrequent sign of apparently reliable localizing value is strong conjugate deviation of the eyes toward the opposite side from the lesion. This is in contradistinction to the occasional occurrence of deviation of the head and eyes toward the side of the lesion in abscesses of the frontal or parietal areas.

DIAGNOSIS. In the initial stage, it may be difficult to differentiate a brain abscess from purulent pachymeningitis, or leptomeningitis. The former is a much more fulminating infection than a brain abscess, though obviously difficulties arise if both exist, as may sometimes be the case. Leptomeningitis produces relatively more cellular changes in the spinal fluid and less striking localizing neurologic changes. Differentiation from a brain tumor, when the signs of infection are minimal or are overlooked, may be difficult. Most neurosurgeons have had the experience of accidentally coming upon an abscess when exploring for a tumor. Thrombosis of the lateral venous sinus in association with otitic infections may produce general symptoms like those of the early stages of an abscess, but not localizing neurologic signs. The Tobey-Ayer test of jugular compression to determine lateral sinus thrombosis is potentially dangerous, because jugular compression during the performance of a lumbar puncture in the presence of a brain abscess may lead to medullary compression and rapid respiratory failure.

Electroencephalography, angiography and air studies all have value in diagnosis, though often there is enough evidence of the presence and location of an abscess to make these diagnostic adjuncts unnecessary.

TREATMENT. The treatment of a brain abscess, except possibly when the brain stem is involved, is always surgical drainage. The history of the surgical treatment of brain abscesses is replete with a variety of methods, and even now there is lack of unanimity of opinion regarding the preferable method of evacuation of certain types of abscess.

In the early stages of formation of a brain abscess, hasty operations are usually futile. At this time, reliance must be placed on supportive measures and antibacterial therapy. The opportune time for operation is after the abscess has become walled off, at least two weeks after the onset, and before the patient's condition becomes critical or before irreparable damage to important brain centers has occurred.

Although complete extirpation of the intact abscess wall, or evacuation of the abscess plus removal of its wall, is the ideal treatment, it is not well suited to abscesses of the cerebellum, those deeply situated in the cerebrum, or those occupying the rolandic and speech areas. For abscesses located in these areas, simple drainage or repeated tapping, accompanied by local and systemic antimicrobial therapy, often proves to be effective treatment.

EXTRADURAL ABSCESS (PACHYMENINGITIS EXTERNA)

Localized suppurative infections between the dura and the cranium are usually the result of otitis media and mastoiditis, frontal sinusitis or osteomyelitis of the skull. The infection may travel by contiguity, or by continuity chiefly via veins which drain toward the dural venous sinuses.

The degree of development of the inflammatory process varies between the formation of circumscribed granulation tissue, a thin deposit of fibrin, and the formation of a local collection of thick pus. Extensive lateral spread of the abscess is prevented by adhesion of the dura to the skull. It is rare for an uncomplicated extradural abscess to assume proportions sufficient to cause intracranial pressure. Its importance lies wholly in the necessity for early recognition and drainage before the infection spreads to deeper structures. Occasionally, infection in the petrous tip may result in an extradural abscess and Gradenigo's syndrome, which is characterized by diplopia and pain in the eye on the side of the lesion, symptoms of irritation of the abducens and trigeminal nerves.

Early surgical drainage and sequestrectomy are usually followed by prompt recovery. Complications arise only when there is inadequate debridement and drainage.

SUBDURAL ABSCESS (PACHYMENINGITIS INTERNA)

ETIOLOGY. A subdural abscess is the result of extension of infection from an adjacent focus, principally the middle ear, the mastoid or the frontal sinus. It may rarely follow maxillary sinusitis, septic thrombosis of the cavernous sinus, compound wounds of the skull and evacuation of a brain abscess.

Two possible pathways of infection exist. In one, the infection advances from osteitis to an extradural abscess and thence, through the necrotizing dura, directly to the subdural space. In the other, there is retrograde extension along venous channels leading from the infected mucosa. By this means, infection arising in the frontal sinus may invade the superior longitudinal venous sinus. In otitis media and mastoiditis, the infection spreads to the lateral venous sinus. From the venous sinuses, the retrograde septic thrombosis involves the cerebral veins and the infection comes to lodge in the subdural space which these veins traverse.

The purulent exudate which collects in the subdural space has little tendency to localize. Often, the entire space over one or both cerebral hemispheres will contain 100 cc. or more of pus. Unfortunately, after surgical drainage there is a tendency for isolated collections to become walled off and surrounded by a neomembrane. The remarkable property of the arachnoid to impede the spread of infection to the subarachnoid space accounts for the existence of little more than a mild leptomeningeal reaction and low-grade pleocytosis of the spinal fluid until the last stage of the disease. Thrombosis of the cerebral veins leads to edema of the brain and, not infrequently, to the development of large and small abscesses in the brain.

SYMPTOMS. The symptoms of a subdural abscess at first are not readily distinguishable from the symptoms of acute infection of the frontal sinus or ear. But increasing fever, malaise and headache, usually frontal and on the side of the lesion, should give early warning of the possible existence of a subdural abscess. After a few days, drowsiness increasing to stupor and coma supervenes. At about the same time, focal neurologic signs develop, the most significant being jacksonian convulsions, hemiplegia and, if the lesion is left-sided, aphasia. The profound illness of the patient and neurologic signs distinguish the condition from an extradural abscess. A cerebral abscess can usually be distinguished by its milder initial stages, the more insidious onset of neurologic signs and less febrile reaction.

TREATMENT. It must be kept in mind that usually this is a fulminating disease which rapidly terminates in death if the patient is not treated. With the earliest sign or suspicion of the disease, exploratory trephines should be performed. If pus is encountered, it is drained through this and additional small openings. The space should be treated with an initial instillation of penicillin. Drains are usually useless since the space tends to close rapidly and reliance must be placed on obliteration of the source of infection and systemic treatment with antimicrobial therapy.

VASCULAR LESIONS OF THE BRAIN

The vascular lesions of the brain include aneurysms of the major cerebral arteries, congenital arteriovenous anomalies and carotid artery-cavernous sinus fistulae.

ANEURYSMS. Aneurysms of the circle of Willis and its main branches are believed to be principally congenital, the exceptions being occasional mycotic and arteriosclerotic dilatations. The congenital aneurysms represent remnants of embryonal vessels, or weakness in the angle of juncture of two arteries, resulting in a saccular outpouching. They rarely produce symptoms before adulthood, when they may rupture or attain sufficient size to cause pressure on adjacent structures. Although these lesions are common, interest in them has been greatly increased since the development of angiography and improved methods of surgical treatment. Experience has shown that the majority of cases of subarachnoid hemorrhage result from rupture of aneurysms. Their importance is reflected in the mortality rate of approximately 50 per cent which occurs in untreated patients.

Rupture of an aneurysm is spontaneous and characterized as a rule by sudden severe headache, most intense in the frontal or occipital regions, and by vomiting, collapse and coma in many instances. Stiff neck nearly always ensues. There may be no localizing signs, but the commonest local effects resulting from pressure and irritation of adjacent structures are pain in the eye, diplopia, unilateral dilatation of the pupil, ptosis of the lid and sometimes sensory impairment of the cornea and face. These are the result of involvement of the third and fifth cranial nerves. There may be other signs resulting from compression of the brain by collections of blood in the sylvian fissure, or from subcortical hematomas which occur particularly in the temporal and frontal lobes. From the effects of blood in the cerebrospinal fluid spaces, patients may remain restless and confused for many days. There is often fever, which sometimes confuses the diagnosis with meningitis, and usually there is increased intracranial pressure. Patients surviving the initial hemorrhage are subject to one or more recurrent hemorrhages in the first month and any one of these may be fatal.

The diagnosis of subarachnoid hemorrhage is confirmed by lumbar puncture which reveals grossly bloody fluid. Xanthochromia develops in the spinal fluid within several hours after hemorrhage and persists for ten days or longer.

The precise location of the aneurysm cannot be determined from the clinical features alone. Angiography can be expected to identify the presence and location of an aneurysm in 60 per cent of patients having spontaneous subarachnoid hemorrhage (Fig. 4). There are other possible sources of hemorrhage, such as from neoplasms and arterial rupture in vascular hypertension. Often, when an aneurysm is not visualized by angiography, it is too small to be recognized or has become thrombosed. Fortunately, there seems to be less tendency to recurrent hemorrhages when aneurysms are not demonstrated by angiography.

The main problem pertaining to intracranial aneurysms is not so much their recognition, but the preferred manner of treatment. The most appropriate plan of procedure is to verify the subarachnoid hemorrhage immediately by lumbar puncture and follow this as the patient's general condition permits by angiography. Any theoretical risks attending these procedures are minimal compared to the advantages.

The demonstration of an aneurysm of the vertebral or basilar arteries, or of multiple aneurysms, usually precludes surgical treatment. If the angiogram discloses the presence of a hematoma, it should be evacuated promptly, but it is preferable to delay direct surgical attack on an aneurysm for ten days or so, until cerebral edema and arterial spasm have subsided. In the waiting period, there may be advantage to ligation of the carotids in the neck, particularly for aneurysms of the internal carotid artery, and many times this comparatively safe procedure is all that is employed in treatment. However, this is not a sure safeguard against recurrent rupture of an aneurysm. The most logical approach is to occlude the vessel on each side of the sac, or to occlude the neck of the sac itself.

The commonest place for intracranial aneurysms to be found is on the internal carotid artery, more often in its supraclinoid than in its infraclinoid portion. The next most common place is on the anterior cerebral arteries at their anterior communication.

The serious risks of surgical ablation of an

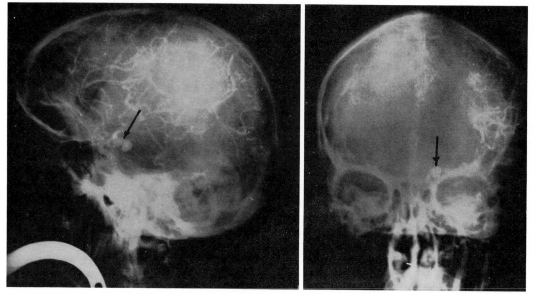

Figure 4. Lateral and anteroposterior angiograms by carotid injection, showing a saccular aneurysm of the internal carotid artery at its juncture with the posterior communicating artery.

aneurysm are related to unmanageable hemorrhage which may occur at the time of operation, and the cerebral damage which may follow occlusion or damage to one of the main arteries.

The employment of controlled hypotension and hypothermia has added significantly to the facility and safety of the direct intracranial attack on aneurysms, but the final evaluation of the surgical treatment remains to be made.

ARTERIOVENOUS ANOMALIES. The lesions, variously referred to as angiomas (Fig. 5), cirsoids, varices, arteriovenous aneurysms and malformations, are believed to be congenital and result from failure of development of the capillaries. In a small number of patients, there are manifestations of the lesions in childhood, but more often they come to attention in adulthood, particularly in the third and fourth decades of life.

The lesions are found most often to involve the middle cerebral artery, but they have been observed in all parts of the brain and in sizes ranging from a small marble-sized nest of racemose vessels to the extensive involvement of a cerebral hemisphere.

Convulsions are a common manifestation of the presence of the lesions in the cerebrum, and doubtless some patients believed to have idiopathic epilepsy have arteriovenous anomalies. In others, the lesion has been overlooked as a cause of retarded development on one side of the body which, instead, is pre-

sumed to be due to birth palsy. Headache is sometimes a symptom, but usually the lesion is discovered when a subarachnoid hemorrhage takes place and an angiogram demonstrates the unsuspected anomaly. A cephalic bruit can be detected in over half the patients, but is not diagnostic since there are other causes for bruit. Recurrent hemorrhage into the subarachnoid space of the brain is common, but fatal hemorrhage is infrequent.

Treatment of arteriovenous anomalies is a

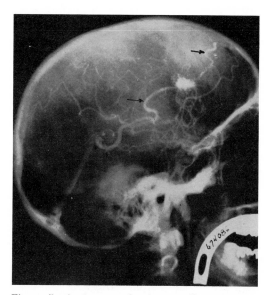

Figure 5. Angiogram showing small arteriovenous anomaly ("angioma"). Note the veins (arrows) connecting the lesion to the sagittal and straight sinuses.

surgical accomplishment which has been aided by exact delineation of the abnormal vessels by angiography, by the use of controlled hypotension during operation and sometimes by hypothermia, which permits temporary occlusion of the carotids while the vessels are being isolated and ligated.

The principal indication for surgical removal of the lesions is spontaneous hemorrhage, but progressive palsies or uncontrolled convulsions may also be benefited.

CAROTID CAVERNOUS FISTULA. The development of a fistula between the intracranial portion of the internal carotid artery and the cavernous sinus is usually the result of a basilar skull fracture. Occasionally it is seen following penetrating wounds, or following spontaneous rupture of the intracavernous portion of the carotid artery which has become sclerotic or aneurysmal.

The classic symptoms and signs include unilateral pulsating exophthalmos, chemosis, edema of the lids and fullness of orbital and retinal vessels. The patient is aware of a bruit, may suffer from considerable pain about the eye and may lose motion and sight of the eye. Occasionally, the other eye also will become involved.

Treatment initially is conservative, since the fistula may close spontaneously. Thereafter, if closure does not take place, the carotid artery in the neck should be ligated, usually in a two-stage procedure, or it should be occluded gradually over a period of days by the use of a specially devised clamp on the artery. If this does not result in closure of the fistula, the intracranial portion of the carotid just above the cavernous sinus should be ligated. It is important to know that double ligation of the carotid in this manner will not cause blindness because of the rich arterial anastomosis with the external carotid artery in the orbit.

Because the fistula cannot always be obliterated by double carotid ligation, another method that has gained favor is to occlude the internal carotid and ophthalmic arteries intracranially and follow immediately with introduction of small fragments of muscle into the internal carotid in the neck. These fragments carried up the artery to the fistula plug the opening and ligation of the carotid in the neck completes the operation.

CAROTID ARTERY OCCLUSION. Carotid artery thrombosis in the neck has only recently been considered in the differential diagnosis of "stroke." Moniz first described occlusion of the cervical portion of the internal carotid artery and brought it to the attention of clinicians. There had been a puzzling lack of evidence of occlusion of the middle cerebral artery in the patient who had died following a "stroke." Investigation of the problem received its greatest impetus from angiographic studies.

The usual cause of obstruction of the common and internal carotid arteries is atherosclerosis with overlying thrombus formation. This is most frequent during the fifth decade. The carotid narrowing is more frequent at the bifurcation in the neck, and occurs less often in the region of the siphon. Because of the frequency of anomalies and variation in size of the component vessels of the circle of Willis, the patency of the carotid-vertebral system is of major importance in normal circulation as well as collateral cross-circulation.

There may be a complete or incomplete obstruction and if it is complete, the thrombus is gray and laminated and may have an attached red thrombus distally. Following complete occlusion, the internal capsule may have areas of softening in the areas supplied by major radicles of the internal carotid artery. There may be multiple areas which show evidence of various stages of softening. There may be extension of the carotid thrombosis into the middle cerebral artery. The incidence of atherosclerosis in the first segment of the internal carotid artery distal to its bifurcation in the neck is second only to that found in the abdominal aorta.

When the carotid artery is occluded, the arterial blood supply to the involved cerebral hemisphere depends on collateral circulation from the opposite carotid system, which shunts blood primarily through the anterior communicating artery; from the external carotid artery on the occluded side; by collateral channels through the facial, superficial temporal and branches of the opthalmic artery, and from the basilar artery through the posterior communicating artery. The collateral circulation to the ischemic hemisphere may be inadequate because of anomalies, such as absence of the anterior or posterior communicating artery, small or incomplete development of an artery, or atheromatous narrowing of a vessel.

Hemiplegia of abrupt or more gradual onset is the cardinal clinical feature of carotid occlusion. There are premonitory symptoms which are described as "stuttering" or "fugitive"; transitory motor weakness of one extremity; temporary dysphasia; paresthesias, or blindness in one eye. A persistent headache behind the eye is often present and initial loss of consciousness takes place in about 10 per cent of patients. A profound hemiplegia accompanied by impaired consciousness is usually accompanied by sensory deficit over the involved side, a homonymous visual field loss, and a permanent mental change. The clinical course may extend over many months with fugitive signs and symptoms, or a massive ischemic event may occur during sleep. Palpation of the carotid arteries in the neck and posterior pharynx may be misleading, but ophthalmodynamometry usually reveals a relative difference in retinal artery pressures.

The definitive diagnosis of carotid artery thrombosis is made by arteriography, which reveals whether the occlusion is complete or partial. This may be performed by direct puncture of the cervical portion of the carotid artery, by retrograde arteriography, through the brachial or femoral arteries.

Experience has shown that consideration of patients with cervical carotid artery occlusion for surgical treatment must be selective to ensure adequate results. Initial loss of consciousness and severe neurologic deficit are usually associated with complete arterial occlusion, which carries a grave prognosis not only for recovery but for life. When occlusion is partial and causes transient neurologic findings, operation may be expected to give a good result. If partial occlusion is associated with a sudden apoplectic onset, owing to distal embolization with infarction, an operation is of little help. The objective of surgical treatment is to restore normal blood flow, to alleviate symptoms, and to prevent further progression of the occlusive process. Two varieties of operation have been used: endarterectomy and the by-pass graft. In well localized and incomplete occlusions, endarterectomy is the procedure of choice.

With local anesthesia and an adequate collateral circulation, the internal carotid artery may be clamped temporarily for five to 30 minutes. If the collateral circulation is inadequate, or there is partial occlusion in the opposite carotid artery, temporary shunts without hypothermia are used when the vessel is clamped.

The principle of endarterectomy involves dissection of the atheroma from the normal outer arterial wall, the two structures being separated by a tissue plane. Without backflow

bleeding from the distal segment of the carotid artery, endarterectomy will have no benefit.

The end-to-side by-pass arterial graft is used when the atheromatous plaque extends over a greater length in the region of bifurcation of the common carotid, or the internal carotid artery in the neck. The end of the graft is anastomosed to the common carotid artery proximal to the point of obstruction.

Results of cervical carotid artery operations should be evaluated not so much on restoration of so-called normal circulation as demonstrated by arteriography, but rather on the return of, or improvement in, neurologic function. The carotid artery and its major intracranial radicles may appear normal on an arteriogram, but the important smaller, perforating branches of the middle cerebral artery may nevertheless be occluded, producing infarction with irreparable neurological deficit. It has been clear that recovery of function with restored cerebral circulation is poor if the patient initially was unconscious and hemiplegic, and that endarterectomy or a by-pass graft is of little value. If the occlusion is partial and the neurologic deficit is transient, or intermittent, restoration of circulation is established and neurologic findings are improved.

CONVULSIVE DISORDERS

Convulsive disorders, more commonly referred to as epilepsy, are symptoms of disease and, strictly speaking, should not be used as a name for the disease. Convulsions are evidence of dysfunction in the brain resulting from the effects of a noxious stimulus which causes a sudden and intense discharge of cells within gray matter of the cerebrum. It is believed that the discharge then spreads into adjacent regions of the cortex or into projection tracts which reach the brain stem, from whence there is a discharge in turn to other parts of the brain. If the discharge remains localized, the nature of the convulsive effects give a clue to the area of the brain from which the impulses arise. If the discharge spreads to adjacent regions, there will be a march of symptoms reflecting in some degree the successive areas that are excited, though often events happen so rapidly that there is a limit to how accurately the spread of excitation can be correlated. If the discharge spreads to subcortical centers, a generalized convulsive seizure usually follows.

In patients said to have idiopathic epilepsy (essential epilepsy, cryptogenic epilepsy), there are none of the elements of localized cortical discharge. The attack is characterized by an immediate generalized response which varies from minor forms, in which there is only momentary suspension of consciousness, or petit mal, to immediate loss of consciousness and violent generalized convulsion, or grand mal. No anatomic substratum or etiologic factor has been discovered for this type of epilepsy, though some congenital abnormality in the brain has been invoked and treatment depends on medical management, which fortunately is adequate to control the attacks in many patients.

Surgical interest in convulsive disorders obtains only in patients who are known or believed to have some localized disease of the cerebral cortex from which attacks are easily incited. Such diseases include intracranial tumors; granulomas; arteriovenous anomalies; abscess; cortical scars with meningeal adhesions which follow inflammation or trauma; localized atrophic lesions of the cortex having numerous causes; and a variety of other lesions including porencephalic cysts, calcific lesions, gliosis, birth trauma, embolic and thrombotic lesions, and tuberous sclerosis. Since every patient with a brain tumor or cortical scar does not have convulsions, it must be assumed that some predilection exists in those who do have convulsions.

In the patients with tumors, arteriovenous anomalies, granulomas and abscesses, the surgical problem is to eradicate the disease, and once this is accomplished the convulsions may subside. But often the seizures do not subside and it can only be assumed that damaged cortex or disease left behind is the source.

Focal epilepsy, a term employed when a demonstrable localized cortical lesion exists, is recognized by the occurrence of initial events in the attack which reflect the site of the lesion. These events include initial unconsciousness, motor phenomena, sensory phenomena, autonomic motor and sensory phenomena, psychic phenomena and miscellaneous phenomena.

Initial unconsciousness has been the most difficult to ascribe to a specific localization. Localization appears in many to reside in the frontal lobes anterior to the motor area. Initial motor phenomena, exemplified particularly by jacksonian seizures, are characterized by turning of the head and eyes usually, though not always, away from the side of the lesion, vocalization and jerking of the muscles of some part or all of the opposite side of the body. Initial sensory phenomena and their corresponding cortical areas of representation are: somatic—contralateral, central or postcentral; visual—contralateral occipital lobe; auditory—either temporal lobe; vestibular—either temporal lobe; olfactory—either temporal lobe. Autonomic motor and sensory phenomena include a variety of visceral sensations and have been found to be related to areas in the region of the fissure of Sylvius and island of Reil. Psychic phenomena have much evidence to support their localization in the temporal lobes.

The clincial study of a patient with focal epilepsy and, in particular, a scrutiny of the pattern of the seizure, is all-important in arriving at a localization of the lesion, but additional evidence is sought from roentgenograms, pneumograms, angiograms and electrograms. Great emphasis has been put on the use of the electrogram in determining the exact epileptogenic focus or firing point, since present-day surgical treatment depends on the assumption that seizures can be alleviated only if the irritable focus is removed. Because of the limitations of the extracranial electroencephalogram, the corticogram taken from the exposed brain has sometimes been employed in the hope of attaining more precise localization.

Those engaged in the surgical treatment of convulsions have usually insisted on the need for the assistance of electrograms, but unfortunately the number of patients who have been relieved of epileptic seizures following excision of suspected cortical foci has not met expectations. The disparity has been accounted for on the basis of practical difficulties in identifying the firing point, incomplete excision of the focus, the probable existence of other unrecognized firing points and the need for limiting the excision to avoid unwanted neurologic deficits. It is only fair to say that some have raised a doubt of the justification of this manner of rationalizing the failures of operation. They have raised, in particular, the question of whether, even with the acceptance of the epileptogenic focus as a primary factor, the site of the focus is revealed by the spike potentials that happen to be recorded by the electrogram.

To add to the difficulties of interpreting results of cortical excision in the treatment of convulsions is the older literature which records many cures and beneficial effects in epileptics following an amazing variety of surgical procedures, many of which seem without the slightest scientific justification.

But even with the recognized uncertainties of surgical treatment of convulsive disorders, it seems important to continue efforts in this direction on selected patients. The indications for operation are generally agreed to include a clinical pattern of seizures that have focal aspects; a relatively long duration of the ailment; frequent, severe seizures; and failure of control of attacks by adequate anticonvulsant measures. Under the present possibilities for benefit from operation, it appears that about 10 per cent of the populace afflicted with convulsions would conform to these indications.

Penfield and his associates, who have been leaders in the effort to treat convulsive disorders in recent years, have reported their results from time to time. The operative mortality has been between 1 and 2 per cent. The evaluation of cortical excision for all types of focal convulsion has been judged to demonstrate that about 25 per cent of the patients have been cured and another 30 per cent significantly benefited in terms of lessening of the frequency and severity of seizures. The results reported by Meyers and associates are less salutary; they estimated about 11 per cent were cured and 25 per cent were improved with an operative mortality of 6 per cent.

Walker summarized the results of cortical excision in 36 patients who had developed convulsions following head injuries sustained in World War II. One year after operation, approximately one-third had had no attacks and another fifth had had only one attack or the isolated aura of their former attacks. The criticism of drawing final conclusions from any report is that the beneficial effects bear an inverse relation to the time of follow-up. At least ten years should elapse before the evaluation is reliable.

There have been impressive reports of beneficial effects resulting from cerebral hemispherectomy, or extensive resection of the abnormal cortex, in children who have had birth palsies resulting in hemiplegia, convulsive seizures and mental retardation. Some of the reports have given convincing evidence not only of cessation of convulsions, but also improvement in mental status which can be assumed to have been secondary to termination of the seizures. Also, a surprising observation has been that limbs previously spastic on the hemiplegic side have lost much of their rigidity and some useful motion and sensation have remained.

Penfield and associates have presented evidence in support of their belief that many epileptics suffer from temporal lobe seizures resulting from birth trauma. The pathologic findings suggest that compression of the lobe by temporary herniation through the tentorial incisura at birth is the mechanism whereby injury takes place. They believe this process was evident in 63 per cent of patients with temporal lobe seizures treated by surgical resection of the temporal lobe.

Spinal Cord

INJURIES

The majority of injuries to the spinal cord are the result of fractures or dislocation of vertebrae which follow violent flexion, extension or torsion. Less often, the injuries are from direct blows or penetrating wounds. Fractures and dislocations are most common in the cervical (C5 and 6) and lumbar (L1 and 5) vertebrae, and least common in the thoracic vertebrae, where the rib cage lends stability and protection. The damage to the cord varies from small discrete hemorrhages

to complete division and, in addition, there are the factors of edema and compression which may contribute to the deleterious effects on the cord.

Cervical cord injuries usually result from falls that may also produce a head injury and, if there is unconsciousness, attention may be directed to the head while an important accompanying cervical injury is overlooked. The midcervical cord injury results in a classic group of neurologic changes: the forearms are held in flexion and biceps reflex is present, while the triceps action and reflex are absent;

the sensory level is at the fifth cervical segment; there is a bilateral Horner's syndrome, and respiration exists only by diaphragmatic movements. A special and infrequent type of fracture or dislocation occurs at the atlanto-axial joint where the odontoid process may fracture at its base or the ligament supporting the odontoid posteriorly is disrupted. This type of injury is the one which takes place in hanging. If the cord is seriously damaged, death occurs shortly. With less pronounced dislocation at this joint, the cord may be partly spared, enough to support respiration and some degree of neurologic function in the trunk and limbs.

Injury to the thoracic cord is unusual except by direct blow or penetrating wounds common in warfare; the resulting neurologic changes correspond to the level of the injury. It must be remembered that in the upper and middle portions of the thoracic cord the segmental levels lie one to two segments above the corresponding vertebrae. All of the lumbar and sacral segments of the cord are between the levels of the eleventh thoracic and first lumbar vertebrae.

Injury to the upper lumbar cord produces motor and sensory paralysis of both lower limbs, though sparing of the first lumbar may preserve some sensation and flexion of the thighs. Injury to the cord of significant degree at any level produces loss of sphincter control as well as spasticity of muscles, exaggerated tendon reflexes, pathologic reflexes and loss of sensation below the lesion. If the injury is in the cervical or thoracic cord, there is loss of sweating and the skin becomes dry and warm below the lesion.

Damage to the cauda equina from spinal injury usually is patchy and incomplete since the nerve roots are less vulnerable than the cord. The resulting paraparesis or paraplegia is of the flaccid rather than spastic type, and reflexes are absent. Loss of sphincter control occurs readily and at times, with incomplete injury to the cauda equina, there may be little other deficit.

Care of patients with cord injuries is of extreme inportance from the initial handling through the prolonged period of rehabilitation. Improper transportation from the place of injury too often adds to the damage of the cord and deprives the patient of the recovery that might otherwise take place. Attention must be given particularly to avoiding flexion positions. Extension position of the neck and back is preferred, but this can be overdone. A flat supporting appliance to which the patient is firmly fixed is safest while he is being transported to a hospital and while being moved after reaching the hospital.

In the hospital, all examinations should be performed with the least manipulation of the patient. Early evaluation of neurologic changes provides a basis for comparing any subsequent changes. Early lateral and anteroposterior roentgenography is imperative, but should be acquired cautiously, reserving special views until a more appropriate time.

In patients with fracture or dislocation of the cervical spine, traction applied to the head is the treatment of choice. There is no justification for attempting blind manipulative procedures for reduction of malalignment. While halter traction may be used as a temporary measure, skeletal traction applied to the skull is far better. Traction is begun with 5- to 10-pound weights and, if necessary for reduction of the deformity, increased to 15 or 20 pounds within 24 hours. Greater weights of 35 or 50 pounds, sometimes recommended, are unsafe and usually not necessary, since with rare exceptions even severe dislocations are realigned with lesser weights.

Compression fractures of the thoracolumbar vertebrae occur principally as a result of hyperflexion of the spine. The anterior surface of the body of the fractured vertebra becomes compressed, causing an acute angulation of the spinal canal. Such injuries are best treated in hyperextension by either bed rest or a body cast.

Surgical treatment of spinal injuries with accompanying trauma to cord or cauda equina in many instances is controversial. In treatment of unreduced dislocations, crush injuries of the laminae and most penetrating wounds, there is unanimity of opinion in favor of exploratory operation, decompressive laminectomy and fusion if necessary. There is less agreement about "closed cord injuries," in which there has been no displacement of vertebrae, or realignment has soon been accomplished by head traction or immobilization of the trunk in hyperextension. The decision becomes important if the degree of paralysis is severe.

The following are the criteria usually accepted in deciding on the need for decompression laminectomy: a progression of neurologic signs; a complete subarachnoid space block as demonstrated by lumbar puncture and manometric studies of the spinal fluid pressures upon jugular compression; and, occasionally, when there is doubt as to the effectiveness of reduction of the vertebral deformity by traction or positioning of the trunk.

While early operation in selected patients may be desirable, a high mortality accompanies hasty surgical procedures performed while the patient is in shock, or having respiratory difficulty from high cervical trauma, or when facilities are inadequate for maintaining traction, proper anesthesia, adequate suction and blood replacement if needed.

Nursing and medical care of the patient with cord injury can be one of the most exacting yet rewarding efforts in medicine. The prevention of skin abrasions and decubitus ulcers requires almost fastidious attention. Such lesions develop quickly but may require weeks and months for healing and, if infected, seem actually to retard recovery of neurologic function. The use of a Stryker frame makes it relatively easy to change the patient's position frequently. A great boon to the prevention of decutibus ulcers has been the development of the air mattress with chambers of alternating pressure.

For care of the paralyzed bladder, an indwelling urethral catheter is introduced immediately and a closed system of intermittent bladder irrigation maintained. It is imperative that all means be taken to prevent or minimize infection of the urinary tract. In some patients, urinary control returns at least in part while some develop a degree of automaticity in evacuation of bladder. In others, the permanent loss of bladder control becomes a major problem in management and a threat to life. These patients present special urologic problems about which there is no general agreement.

Bowel habits, including use of periodic enemas, low residue diets, digital evacuation and self-care, can be taught to the intelligent patient so that loss of anal sphincter control need not be an important problem.

Spasms of muscles of the lower limbs, particularly flexion spasms, at times constitute a serious problem and are aggravated by infections of the bladder and by decubitus ulcers. Sometimes, correction of these inciting lesions will control or minimize the spasms, but if not, it is appropriate to resort to extensive rhizotomy or intrathecal injection of alcohol or phenol to abolish reflex action.

A rehabilitation program should be organized as soon as the patient's condition permits. As a part of the program, a recognition of the need for the patient's social adjustment to his suddenly altered way of living may be the more difficult task. Passive and active exercises together with massage preserve motion at joints and prevent contractures. Braces and various supportive devices help the patient to stand and walk, though efforts in this direction often require great effort by the patient as well as perseverance and the sympathetic direction of one skilled in management. The development of paraplegic training centers since World War II has done much to improve and advance rehabilitation methods.

TUMORS

Tumors of the spinal cord, as a category, are usually meant to include intraspinal tumors of great variety which implicate the cord, its roots and the cauda equina. Such tumors may arise from the cord, itself or from nerve roots, the meninges, the vasculature of or about the cord, the vertebrae or, occasionally, from tissues adjacent to the spinal column. In addition, there may be metastases from tumors elsewhere in the body which spread to the vertebrae, the epidural tissues or, rarely, to the cord and meninges.

The tumors of the spinal canal are classified anatomically as intramedullary or extramedullary, and the latter as intradural or extradural. Also, some tumors are both intraspinal and extraspinal connected by a narrow tube of tumor tissue lying in the root foramen or the interlaminar space (Fig. 6). Such tumors are referred to as hourglass or dumbbell tumors.

INCIDENCE. The incidence of intraspinal tumors is about the same in the two sexes, with a few exceptions. For example, meningiomas, which are one of the two common primary tumors, have a higher incidence in women, while the commonest metastatic tumors occur nearly exclusively in one sex, namely, bronchogenic metastases in males and mammary carcinoma in females. Though tumors are occasionally encountered in children or in the aged, the third to the sixth decades, and most of all the fifth decade of life, are the periods when tumors most often make their appearance. If all types of tumors are included, a survey shows that they are found with about equal frequency in the cervical, thoracic and lumbosacral levels, although their occurrence at the extremes, namely, the uppermost cervical and the sacral regions, is exceptional.

Of the primary intradural neoplasms, nearly 75 per cent are either meningiomas or nerve

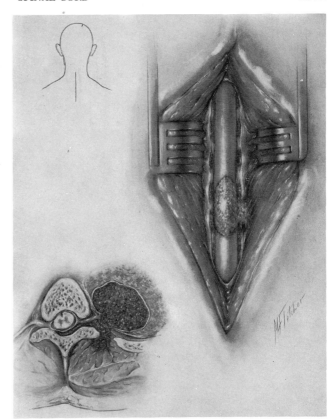

Figure 6. Extradural tumor of the spinal canal extending from the lung and mediastinum.

sheath tumors; both are benign and usually cured by surgical removal. Of all intraspinal tumors encountered at operation, nearly 50 per cent are benign and removable. Meningiomas are variously known as meningothelioma, dural endothelioma, meningoendothelioma, pachymeningioma, leptomeningioma, meningeal fibroblastoma, dural sarcoma, arachnoidal fibroblastoma and psammoma, and by various qualifying terms, such as pigmented, angiomatous and others. Nerve sheath tumors are also referred to as neurilemoma, neurinoma, schwannoma, neurofibroma and perineural fibroblastoma.

Gliomas of the cord arise from the interstitial elements of the parenchyma and comprise 15 per cent of the primary intradural tumors. The commonest type is the ependymona arising, as the name implies, from the ependyma of the central canal or from the vestigial filum terminale. The tumors of the filum terminale may reach large size, virtually filling the lumbosacral canal, but can be removed safely providing they have not invaded the conus medullaris. The ependymomas arising in the cord sometimes extend for many segments and are visible through the widened posterior sulcus of the cord; a few have been successfully removed. Any of the types of glioma occurring in the brain may also be encountered in the cord, but whereas the commonest glioma of the brain is the highly malignant glioblastoma, the commonest in the cord, next to the ependymoma, is the less malignant astrocytoma. These tumors are incurable, but occasionally they can be removed in large part. They often grow very slowly over a period of years, and their growth may be slowed still more by roentgenotherapy.

The term malignancy, when applied to the primary intradural tumors, refers only to the tendency for the tumors to enlarge locally and spread to adjacent parts of the cord; distant metastases do not occur, except rarely with ependymomas.

SYMPTOMS. The symptoms of intraspinal tumors can be conveniently divided into three phases: nerve root symptoms, beginning compression of the cord, and advanced myelitis.

In the first phase, initial involvement of nerve roots causes pain, which may be severe and lancinating, distributed in the corresponding dermatome and often aggravated by various forms of straining which suddenly increase the intraspinal pressure. A feature of the pain is that in many it is worse when the patient reclines, compelling him to seek relief in sitting upright or walking about. In addition to pain, irritation of a sensory root may cause a sense of numbness and paresthesias in the same area while at times the involved area of the skin may become hypersensitive, particularly to the light touch of clothing. Though the patient may experience abnormal sensation in an area of skin corresponding to the nerve root involved by the tumor, there is usually little or no demonstrable sensory loss in the area because there is considerable sensory overlap from adjacent dermatomes. With involvement of the motor fibers of the root, the corresponding muscles develop atrophy, weakness and fibrillations. In the trunk, localized palsies may go unnoticed, but in the extremities, particularly in the hand, the muscle wasting and weakness can be more easily recognized.

The second phase, caused by beginning compression of the cord or invasion of its fibers, is evidenced by symptoms related to changes in the long tracts. The symptoms may make their appearance simultaneously with radicular pain, although occasionally tumors cause progressive myelitis without accompanying pain; this is more likely to be true of intramedullary growths.

Unilateral compression of the cord results in the Brown-Séquard syndrome in which there are homolateral alteration of reflexes; muscle weakness; impaired touch, position and vibratory senses, and contralateral loss of pain and temperature senses below the level of the lesion. Compression of the anterior part of the cord may result in loss of pain and temperature senses with preservation of other functions, while compression of the posterior cord may produce only decreased positional and vibratory senses. Intramedullary tumors, in addition to their relative painlessness, can sometimes be discerned by a bandlike area of loss of pain and temperature senses corresponding to the level of the tumor, and by preservation of sensation in the saddle region in the presence of sensory loss in the trunk and lower limbs. In patients with incomplete myelitis, the upper level of sensory loss does not correspond to the segmental level of the lesion, but can be from several to many segments lower, thus making it impractical to localize the level of the lesion accurately, while in complete myelitis the sensory level corresponds more exactly.

In the third phase, with the advent of complete myelitis, there is loss of all but reflex functions below the segmental level of the lesion. If the myelitis has developed rapidly, even the segmental reflexes may be absent for a while and the muscles become flaccid. But, in slowly progressing myelitis, and in some days or weeks after more acute myelitis, the tendon reflexes become exaggerated, pathologic reflexes develop and muscles become spastic. There is also loss of sweating and of sphincter control. The sensory loss and the presence of muscle inaction predispose to the development of bedsores, ulcerations from pressure, edema and wasting of soft tissues and demineralization of bones, erroneously referred to as trophic changes.

DIAGNOSIS. A comprehensive history of the nature and chronology of the symptoms is of particular importance in detecting intraspinal tumors. The neurologic examination must be complete from head to foot and not just limited to the region under suspicion, since other common diseases of the central nervous system and even brain tumors may simulate, for a while, a cord tumor. A practical knowledge of the segmental innervation of reflexes, muscle groups and sensory areas is invaluable in determining the location of a tumor. A useful accessory test is application of heavy pressure or percussion over the spinous process in the region of a tumor, thereby eliciting local pain and, occasionally, peripheral shocklike sensations.

Some of the common diseases which require differentiation from intraspinal tumors are abnormalities of the intervertebral disks; multiple sclerosis; syringomyelia; amyotrophic lateral sclerosis; subacute combined cord degeneration; myeloradiculitis (Guillain-Barré syndrome); diabetic myeloneuropathy; idiopathic lateral sclerosis; arachnoiditis, and syphilis. All of these diseases produce some symptoms similar to those of tumor, but each has also some distinguishing features which set it apart.

Useful adjuncts to diagnosis include roentgenography of the spine, spinal fluid studies and myelography. Roentgenograms may reveal the presence of a metastatic or other invasive tumor, or disease of the vertebrae. Primary intraspinal tumors present for long periods often produce erosion of bone by pressure, which may be evident particularly in the pedicles of the vertebrae, or by enlargement of interlaminar or foraminal spaces.

Lumbar puncture as a diagnostic aid is particularly valuable. The Queckenstedt test provides positive identification of a complete or nearly complete block of the spinal subarachnoid space. In the majority of patients, the presence of a tumor causes elevation of the protein content in the fluid, while a total block of the canal produces not only an increased protein, at times sufficient to clot the fluid, but also a degree of xanthochromia. It must be remembered that, while the information to be gained by lumbar puncture is important, there is distinct risk of increasing the neurologic deficit through altering the intraspinal dynamics. It is preferable, therefore, that lumbar puncture be performed as one of the last tests, and only when surgical facilities are made ready or available.

Myelography, performed with Pantopaque or a comparable iodized radiopaque agent, is the last test to be used since it is attended by the possibility of rapidly worsening the condition. But, the test may be invaluable in determining the presence and exact location of a tumor.

TREATMENT. Tumors of the spinal canal, with few exceptions, should be treated surgically without needless delay. Postponement of operation for a few hours in rapidly advancing myelitis may make the difference between permanent paralysis and recovery of function. Meningiomas and nerve sheath tumors can usually be removed completely with negligible risk, and the same applies to a number of other less common extramedullary tumors. Intramedullary tumors are less favorable, but occasionally an ependymoma can be totally removed. In many of the other gliomas, benefit results from partial excision, evacuation of cystic formations and decompression through laminectomy and the opened dura. In metastatic tumors, partial excision of the compressing extradural mass and decompression laminectomy followed by roentgenotherapy often restores function and avoids disabling paralysis during the patient's remaining life. An exception to the need for urgent operation for intraspinal tumors is found in the lymphomas, which fairly commonly invade the spinal canal, particularly in the thoracic region, by extension from mediastinal nodes. These tumors respond readily to roentgenotherapy, especially if it is administered in conjunction with nitrogen mustard. Such patients must be closely observed and, if myelitis progresses under treatment, surgical decompression is necessary.

INTERVERTEBRAL DISK

Rupture of an intervertebral disk and protrusion of the nucleus pulposus can occur at any spinal level, but the commonest sites are at the last two lumbar and the fifth and sixth cervical interspaces. Protrusions in the thoracic region are seldom encountered.

The intervertebral disk is made up of several structures: a tough fibrous membrane which corresponds to a joint capsule and is known as the annulus fibrosus; cartilaginous plates which face the surfaces of the opposing vertebral bodies, and the nucleus pulposus, the remnant of the embryonic notochord, which occupies the closed space. Repeated stress may lead to thinning or rupture of the annulus fibrosus, with bulging or actual extrusion of the nucleus pulposus into the spinal canal. The nature of the resulting symptoms depends on the degree and location of the protrusion.

In the lumbar region, the initial symptoms, which often begin simultaneously or soon after some stress on the lower back, are most often pain and limited movement in the lower back. It is believed that this initial pain arises from the torn annulus fibrosus, but the pain is indistinguishable from that which may come from any number of other structures and pathologic processes in the region. Later, the pain extends into a lower limb along the course of the sciatic nerve as the nucleus pulposus compresses adjacent nerve roots. Because of the strong support of the longitudinal posterior spinal ligament, the protrusion of the nucleus is to one side or the other, accounting for the laterality of the symptoms.

The pain characteristically extends from the lower back on one side to the buttock, posterior thigh and calf as far as the ankle. It is aggravated by movements of the back and various forms of straining. In some patients, numbness and paresthesias also occur, particularly in the leg and toes. Tilting of the spine and limping with the painful limb are common. There may be weakness of muscles which control the foot and toes and, rarely, loss of bladder control.

Since it is rare for rupture to occur in lumbar disks other than the last two, the symptoms and signs are attributable for the most part to compression of fifth lumbar roots by the fourth disk, or the first sacral roots by the fifth. Painful limitation of low-back movements and of straight-leg raising are common to both and may be the only demonstrable abnormalities. But differences in location of the symptoms and of elicited neurologic abnormalities usually permit localization of the level of the rupture. For example, rupture of the fourth disk (L4 to 5) and compression of the fifth lumbar root are more likely to cause paresthesias in the great toe, weakness in dorsiflexion of the foot and toes, and diminution of the knee reflex with preservation of the ankle reflex. Conversely, rupture of the fifth disk (L5 to S1) and compression of the first sacral roots more often cause sensory changes in the last toes, weakness in plantar flexion of the foot and toes, and absence of the ankle reflex.

The degree of disruption of the disk and of the symptoms varies widely. The majority of patients recover spontaneously or improve greatly in a period of six to eight weeks aided by relative inactivity and comforted by various forms of symptomatic treatment. Natural recovery depends on shrinkage of the nucleus pulposus and subsidence of reaction in the nerve root.

Repeated recurrences of sciatic pain, which in the beginning is relieved by conservative measures, commonly result in a chronic persistence of symptoms which demand surgical treatment. If pain and disability persist beyond a reasonable time, or if paresis of muscles controlling the foot or bladder develops at any time, surgical removal of the nucleus pulposus is desirable. Some employ myelography for the corroboration of diagnosis and localization. Diagnosis on clinical findings is usually reliable, but atypical symptoms and signs make differential diagnosis uncertain.

The decision to remove a herniated nucleus pulposus should be made only after careful evaluation of the clinical signs and symptoms. In many patients, the clinical history and findings are the most important; in others, the myelogram may be decisive.

The surgical treatment consists of unilateral exposure, excision of the ligamentum flavum, widening of the interlaminar space, retraction of the nerve root and excision of all of the nucleus pulposus. The operation thus performed does not alter the structure of the back and can be regarded as a means of accomplishing what nature has not in removing the offending nucleus pulposus. Some favor fusion of the joint by bone grafting as a part of the operation and at times there may be a need for it, but fusion is not necessary in patients whose complaints and physical findings point to root compression as the source of their complaints.

Following operation, a regimen of rehabilitation is desirable before full activity is resumed and this in turn depends on a number of factors, not the least of which is the patient's emotional make-up and the factor of legal compensation. Some patients who minimize or accept minor discomforts and have a need for return to work do so without delay.

In the cervical region a ruptured disk, by compression of a corresponding nerve root, causes changes comparable to those of a ruptured lumbar disk. The neck is stiff and painful, particularly so on hyperextension. Pain extends from the neck across the shoulder into the arm and forearm, usually not farther than the wrist, while paresthesias and numbness are often present in the fingers. There are accompanying alterations of reflexes and at times weakness of muscle groups. As in the case with ruptured lumbar disks, it is usually possible with clinical findings to localize the source of trouble. Rupture of the fifth cervical disk (C5 to 6) compresses the sixth cervical roots, characteristically causing numbness and paresthesias in the first two or three fingers, impairment of the biceps reflex and weakness in flexion of the forearm. Rupture of the sixth cervical disk (C6 to 7) compresses the seventh cervical nerve roots, causing numbness and paresthesias of the middle fingers, impairment of the triceps reflex and weakness in extension of the forearm.

Lateral protrusions of the nucleus pulposus which compress the nerve roots may also be large enough to compress the spinal cord, particularly in its anterolateral quadrant. The first signs of such compression may be miosis and lid ptosis of the homolateral eye, which constitute a warning of the potential seriousness of the condition. Further compression of the cord may produce a Brown-Séquard type of hemimyelitis, though there is usually preservation of the posterior columns of the cord which subserve positional and vibratory senses. Less laterally placed or centrally placed protrusion of a cervical disk is not so likely to cause nerve root compression, and much more prone to affect the cord.

When the symptoms and signs point to irritation of the nerve roots only, it is appropriate to employ expectant treatment just as in the case of sciatica. Often, light traction on the head will give relief by lending support to the neck and overcoming painful spasm in neck muscles. An immobilizing neck collar is also helpful. Added comfort may follow the use of heat applications, light massage of muscles and analgesic drugs. Spontaneous recovery occurs in the majority as the reaction in the involved nerve root subsides.

Surgical removal of the herniated nucleus pulposus and decompression of the involved nerve roots are indicated in the severe and persistent cases of radiculitis. The operation is performed by means of a posterior unilateral approach between the widened interlaminar space, much the same as in the operation for lumbar disk herniation. Through a similar approach, the larger herniations affecting the cord may also be removed from the extradural space, but, in some, wider exposure through bilateral laminectomy is required.

Cervical disk ridging, or spondylosis, is a condition which simulates herniation of the nucleus pulposus. Often, the two cannot be distinguished except at operation. The ridging consists of unyielding calcified fibrous tissue which constitutes the changes visible on roentgenograms and is referred to as hypertrophic osteoarthritis. The condition develops as a part of the aging process and of degeneration of the intervertebral disk. An exuberance of this tissue in the region of a cervical nerve root foramen may narrow the opening to the degree that the nerve is easily irritated. In other patients, a prominent ridge may extend across the anterior surface of the cord, causing a chronic state of distortion, increased vulnerability of the cord to frequent neck movements and possibly changes in the intrinsic blood supply. The result is the subtle and insidious development of myelitis at this level, which at times has been confused in diagnosis with cord tumor, syringomyelia, amyotrophic lateral sclerosis and other diseases of the cord. The treatment consists of appropriate surgical decompression to alleviate the pressure on cord and nerve roots.

Cranial Nerves

While any one of the cranial nerves may become involved by the many diseases of the central nervous system, only certain nerves may require surgical treatment for either intrinsic disease of the nerves themselves or for relief of disease in areas supplied by them. The trigeminal nerve is by far the commonest nerve requiring some form of surgical treatment, because of the frequency of neuralgia and of painful diseases within the area supplied by it.

TRIGEMINAL NERVE. Trigeminal neuralgia, also called trifacial neuralgia, tic douloureux and Fothergill's disease, is one of the few true neuralgias. It is a disease of unknown origin and is characterized by paroxysms of sudden excruciating pain in the area of the face supplied by the trigeminal nerve. Since there are no physical changes to be demonstrated in the disease, except some transient flushing of the face and the patient's convincing evidence of agony during a paroxysm, the diagnosis is made on the basis of the history. Because of the need for differentiating the disease from the numerous other causes of facial pain, it is imperative that the characteristic properties of the pain be recognized. The salient properties of the pain constitute a triad: the pain is strictly limited to some part, or occasionally all, of the region supplied by the sensory root of the trigeminal nerve; the pain is paroxysmal and of short duration, a single paroxysm rarely lasting longer than 60 seconds; and the pain is induced by stimulation of the nerve endings (trigger zones), such as light touch of the face, talking and eating.

The disease usually makes its appearance between the ages of 40 and 60 years, and rarely develops at earlier or later ages. Men and women are affected equally. Though the etiology is unknown, the appearance of the affliction principally in older ages suggests a relationship to vascular deficiency or some aging process of the nerve. There is a higher incidence of trigeminal neuralgia in patients with multiple sclerosis than occurs in the general populace. Also, occasionally a tumor of the gasserian ganglion or a tumor lying adjacent to the nerve, such as acoustic neurinoma, cholesteatoma or meningioma occupying the cerebellopontile angle, will produce pain difficult to distinguish from trigeminal neuralgia. These accompanying diseases, unlike trigeminal neuralgia, should be evident by the presence of abnormal neurologic signs.

The pain of trigeminal neuralgia never crosses the midline, and bilateral disease is a rarity. Although spontaneous remissions of pain may last for months, the natural history of the disease is one of unrelenting recurrence of pain with shorter and shorter intervals of relief. Rarely, if ever, does the untreated disease fail to recur.

Over the years, many medical treatments have been proposed, but none of them provides more than temporary or partial relief at best. The drug in common use today is Dilantin. A drug under investigation for which preliminary claims of benefit are made has the trade name of Tegretol. The pain can be relieved with certainty only by interruption of the trigeminal nerve somewhere along its pathway.

Injection with alcohol of one or more of the branches of the nerve supplying the painful region of the face is a common means of providing relief, but the effect is temporary, as the nerve always regenerates. The sites of injection, depending on the location of the pain, are at the points of emergence of the nerves from the skull, as the maxillary and mandibular divisions, or the several peripheral branches, as the supraorbital, infraorbital and mental nerves. It must be remembered that it is one thing to infiltrate procaine in the general region of a nerve for anesthesia and another to instill a small amount of absolute alcohol directly into the nerve. The procedure of alcohol injections is sometimes an unpleasant experience for the patient and not without occasional complications. Even so, many physicians feel that relief of the neuralgia by injection of a nerve, though temporary, is worthwhile, and that the facial numbness experienced by the patient is valuable in acquainting him with what he may expect if eventually surgical division of the nerve root is required.

Injection of alcohol or other destructive agents, such as boiling water, directly into the gasserian ganglion via a needle introduced through the foramen ovale has been recommended by a few. The procedure has the advantage of avoiding an operation and, if successful, in preventing regeneration of the nerve, but it has the disadvantage of being a blind procedure not without possibility of complications, and it does not permit the selectivity which can be accomplished by partial surgical division of the nerve root.

Avulsion of the supraorbital or infraorbital nerves at their foramina is a more certain and often more effective procedure than attempts at alcohol injection of the nerves but is useful only when pain is limited strictly to areas supplied by these nerves. The surgical scars are unnoticed since one is within the eyebrow and the other within the mouth.

Rhizotomy, surgical interruption of the sensory root of the trigeminal nerve, is the means by which the pain of trigeminal neuralgia can with certainty be terminated permanently. The root is that portion of the nerve lying between the gasserian ganglion and the brain stem. Regeneration does not take place because the nerve fibers do not have neurilemmal sheaths, as is the case distal to the ganglion. The root is exposed by an opening either in the temporal bone or the occipital bone. In the former operation, the root is exposed extradurally, while in the latter the root is intradural. The choice of surgical exposure is more or less arbitrary, each possessing advantages and disadvantages. But important complications of either operation are relatively few and mortality from operation does not exceed 1 per cent. In about 5 per cent, there is paresis or paralysis of facial muscles on the side of the operation. The most likely cause of this complication in the temporal operation is traction during the operation on the superficial petrosal nerve, a branch to the geniculate ganglion of the facial nerve. Recovery of facial motion is much the same as occurs in Bell's palsy.

If the operation results in corneal anesthesia, precautions must be taken to avoid trauma and ulceration of the insensitive cornea. With reasonable care of the eye, such ulcerations can be avoided. All patients experience some degree of paresthesias in the anesthetic area and, for most, accommodation is no problem. But for a few, particularly the overanxious, there may be considerable unhappy preoccupation over the sensations for which, unfortunately, there is no satisfactory remedy.

Partial or selective section of the sensory root is employed particularly in patients whose pain is restricted to the lower part of the face, in which case nerve fibers supplying the cornea can be preserved, thus obviating the risk of corneal ulceration. The motor root of the trigeminal nerve is preserved if possible, since its loss results in paralysis of masticator muscles on that side. It may not always be possible to preserve the root, but fortunately patients readily adjust to the paralysis.

Section of the descending tract, pain fibers only, of the trigeminal nerve in the medulla oblongata was proposed by Sjöqvist in the hope of avoiding total anesthesia of the face and possibly diminishing the degree of paresthesias that follow rhizotomy. The operation is attended by greater risks, but these might be acceptable if the operation had accomplished what was hoped for. Unfortunately, in about 35 per cent of patients there was recurrence of pain and paresthesias in the same degree as following rhizotomy. For these reasons, tractotomy is now rarely performed for relief of trigeminal neuralgia.

Decompression of the root of the trigeminal nerve was proposed by Taarnhøj. It was his hypothesis that the neuralgia might result from some degree of compression and irritation of the root along its course and that relief might result from dividing the meningeal coverings of the root. A certain degree of success attended the operation, but the uncertainty of the means by which the operation accomplished success has led to a variety of other technical procedures in which the nerve root or ganglion is exposed and lightly traumatized. No doubt, in such operations some of the sensory fibers are interrupted, but the principal claim of advantage made for the operations is preservation of most of the facial sensation. The rate of recurrence of neuralgia following the operations is not established, although it is probably at least 50 per cent.

Patients having trigeminal neuralgia should be made aware that any procedure which accomplishes less than total division of the root, or total destruction of the ganglion, may fail to give permanent relief and necessitate additional operation.

OTHER CRANIAL NERVES. The other cranial nerves which sometimes may be advantageously divided for therapeutic effects are the sensory portion of the seventh, the eighth, the ninth, the sensory portion of the tenth, the eleventh and the twelfth. These nerves all lie, intracranially, in an area which is readily exposed by a suboccipital craniotomy of the type used to expose the trigeminal nerve in the cerebellopontile angle. The seventh, ninth, eleventh and twelfth nerves in their extracranial course lie in general proximity in the superior triangle of the neck.

The facial nerve. The sensory division of the facial nerve is the nervus intermedius of Wrisberg. A rare type of neuralgia comparable in quality to trigeminal neuralgia, but principally localized deep in the ear, is believed to implicate the nervus intermedius. Relief is obtained by division of the nerve intracranially. The principal risk of the operation is damage to the motor division of the facial nerve, with resulting facial paralysis. There is also chance of damage to the auditory nerve which lies in proximity to the facial nerve.

Disturbances of the extracranial portion of the facial nerve are evidenced by either paralysis or paroxysmal spasm of the face. Paralysis is most commonly of the Bell's palsy type, but may result from operations on the parotid gland or mastoid bone and from lacerations of the face, skull fracture through the petrous bone, facial nerve tumors, geniculate herpes zoster, birth injury and congenital maldevelopment. Hemifacial spasm is often the sequel of incomplete recovery from Bell's palsy, but the etiologic factors are usually not evident. The condition is to be distinguished from facial tic, or habit spasm, which is a manifestation of neurosis.

Bell's palsy, a unilateral paralysis of the face, involves all branches of the nerve and is sometimes spoken of as "peripheral" in contradistinction to "central," a supranuclear type of paralysis seen for example in hemiplegias in which the distortion of the face is not so profound and motion in the forehead in unaffected. The cause of Bell's palsy is uncertain, but the facial nerve has been found to be swollen in the narrow facial canal without demonstrable inflammatory lesions or proof of infection. The paralysis develops abruptly, usually within a few hours, and may be accompanied by some premonitory pain in the ear or face, by hyperacusis and by blunting of taste if the nerve damage is proximal to the point of juncture of the chorda tympani. Spontaneous subsidence of the paralysis in about 85 per cent of patients commonly begins in two to four weeks or may be prolonged for several months. The more severe the degree of paralysis and delayed the return of function, the more ikely will be some motor abreactions of the face such as mass movements, twitching and overcontraction. Because of these undesired effects in delayed recovery, surgical decompression of the nerve in the facial canal is recommended, but the merits of this procedure are uncertain.

Trauma to the facial nerve in the facial canal has most often been a complication of mastoid operations, now a rarity since the advent of antimicrobial treatment has minimized the need for mastoidectomy. However, injury to the nerve is greater today from other sources such as automobile accidents and more radical operations both inside and outside the cranium. Whenever possible, anastomosis of the divided nerve is preferable. Nerve grafting within the facial canal has sometimes yielded surprisingly good results and is one of the few instances in which nerve grafting to bridge a defect has been successful. When the ends of the divided nerve cannot be approximated, the method usually resorted to for restoration of facial mobility is anastomosis of the distal end of the facial nerve to the proximal end of a divided adjacent nerve such as the spinal accessory or hypoglossal nerve. The functions of either of these latter nerves may reasonably be sacrificed in exchange for restoration of even partial facial motility.

In hemifacial spasm, the aim of surgical treatment has been to alter the facial nerve by partial selective sectioning of the motor fibers, thereby lessening the degree of facial movements and at the same time preserving some degree of voluntary and involuntary motion. An ideal technique for accomplishing these ends has not been developed, but sometimes the results of the operation are an improvement over the preoperative condition.

An approach to the problem of hemifacial spasm has been offered by Gardner, who believes it to be a reversible pathophysiologic state which is sometimes corrected by exposure and manipulation of the facial nerve in the cerebellopontile angle. Occasionally, the operation produces dramatic and lasting improvement or cessation of the spasms.

The acoustic nerve. The importance of the acoustic nerve is brought to attention particularly in the surgical relief of symptoms designated as Ménière's disease. The disease is characterized by a syndrome which includes paroxysms of vertigo, unilateral tinnitus and loss of hearing. Without the existence of all of these symptoms, the diagnosis cannot be made with certainty. Although paroxysms of vertigo may for a time exist alone, its origin cannot be lateralized until unilateral tinnitus or deafness appears. Various causes of Ménière's disease have been proposed, but all lack convincing proof. It is not established whether the inciting lesion lies in the peripheral endings of the nerve, in the nerve itself or within the labyrinth.

The vertigo occurs characteristically in explosive attacks so severe at times that the patient may be thrown off balance. There is usually associated vomiting and, at times, prostration by the more severe attacks, which may not subside for many hours. Between the paroxysms of vertigo, there exist only the tinnitus and hearing impairment. In some, the vertigo is of mild degree, insufficient to cause concern, and in some there is spontaneous subsidence of the vertigo. A variety of medical treatments have been given credit for benefit, but the occasional patient is so distressed by the severity and frequency of the paroxysms of vertigo that relief is sought in surgical measures.

Relief of the vertigo can be accomplished by either surgical destruction of the labyrinth, or division of the acoustic nerve intracranially on the side of the tinnitus and hearing loss. The results of nerve section are good in terms of relief of the vertigo, but tinnitus is not always relieved and hearing is made worse unless a differential section of the nerve is performed by which the cochlear neurons are preserved. Unless some useful hearing exists at the time of nerve section, it is usually preferable to divide the entire nerve, since a partial section may preserve some of the vestibular fibers and perpetuate the vertigo and, too, there is greater likelihood of terminating the tinnitus if a total nerve section is performed.

The glossopharyngeal nerve and sensory fibers of the vagus nerve. The principal interest in these nerves pertains to glossopharyngeal neuralgia, which in all respects is akin to trigeminal neuralgia except in its location. While the condition is not common, neither is it rare, and sometimes neuralgia of both the trigeminal and glossopharyngeal nerves exists in the same patient. The pain characteristically occurs in sharp, short-lived paroxysms in the region at the base of the tongue and tonsillar fossa on one side. It is usually induced by swallowing or by internal or external pressure in the tonsillar region. Intracranial division of the glossopharyngeal nerve is a satisfactory form of treatment since it can be counted on to relieve the pain and does not result in any demonstrable neurologic deficit. Experience has shown that in a few instances full relief of pain is not obtained unless several rostral sensory fibers of the vagus nerve are divided as well as the glossopharyngeal nerve. For this reason, both nerves are usually divided to ensure the desired relief of pain.

Rarely, the paroxysms of glossopharyngeal neuralgia are accompanied by syncope resulting from cardiac asystole. The phenomenon is explained by the role which the glossopharyngeal nerve serves in the transmission of afferent impulses arising in the carotid sinus. In the investigation of this striking combination of glossopharyngeal neuralgia and syncope from cardiac asystole, the latter effects can be obliterated by atropinizing the patient while the paroxysms of pain persist. Both can be temporarily abolished by cocainization of the region of the tonsillar fossa and permanently abolished by section of the glossopharyngeal nerve.

Occasionally, and particularly in older patients with arteriosclerosis, hypersensitivity of the carotid sinus and syncopal attacks exist in a degree sufficient to constitute a serious threat to the patient's safety. While the condition can be corrected by local resection of the nerves about the involved carotid sinus, intracranial section of the glossopharyngeal nerve can be performed with as much safety and with more assurance of benefit.

Because intracranial section of the glossopharyngeal nerve interrupts afferent fibers from the carotid sinus which influence the cardiovascular reflexes, there is frequently a significant but temporary rise in blood pressure following rhizotomy. The elevation of pressure, if present, rarely lasts longer than a few hours.

Another instance in which the glossopharyngeal nerve may be involved is in the condition known as the auriculotemporal syndrome, characterized by excessive sweating in the temporal region induced by gustatory stimuli. The condition results from an abnormal union of the chorda tympani and the auriculotemporal branch of the trigeminal nerve following penetrating wounds or surgical procedures in the region of the parotid. Section of the glossopharyngeal nerve intracranially interrupts the reflex and causes no untoward effects.

The spinal accessory nerve. This nerve has origin from both cranial and spinal levels and is a motor nerve supplying the sternocleidomastoid and trapezius muscles. It has surgical significance in several circumstances. Injury to the nerve from penetrating wounds or surgical procedures in the neck is relatively common. While the loss of muscle function resulting from the division of the nerve is not seriously disabling and is accompanied by certain compensatory muscular actions, repair of the divided nerve should be performed if feasible. Damage of the nerve should be avoided in operations on the neck.

In surgical treatment of spasmodic torticollis, the spinal accessory nerve is sometimes divided along with several upper cervical motor roots to accomplish deliberate paralysis of the muscles responsible for moving the head and neck. The operation has limited use but has occasionally proved helpful.

A more common practice in which the spinal accessory nerve is divided is in repair of facial paralysis, particularly that resulting from interruption of the nerve in the removal of acoustic neurinomas in the cerebellopontile angle. In the reparative operation, the main trunk of the nerve is divided and its proximal end anastomosed to the distal end of the facial nerve at its site of emergence at the stylomastoid foramen. An additional refinement of the operation is to divide the descending hypoglossal nerve and anastomose its proximal end to the distal end of the divided spinal accessory nerve. This operation provides a degree of innervation for the muscles supplied by the spinal accessory nerve and, in particular, has value for its cosmetic effects in providing tone to the sternomastoid muscle.

The hypoglossal nerve. As an alternate procedure to the use of the spinal accessory nerve for anastomosis to the facial in the alleviation of facial paralysis, the hypoglossal nerve may be used to equal advantage. The choice in use of either nerve for the anastomosis is arbitrary.

Peripheral Nerves

Peripheral nerve injuries in peacetime, even in busy civilian hospitals, are not common. Teaching clinics find a paucity of material suitable for sustaining interest and for demonstrating to students the principles of this important subject. The two world wars produced thousands of these injuries, and it is to the credit of many physicians working under the hardships of war that important advances were made in diagnosis and treatment. Not only was this concerted effort invaluable to the wounded soldier, but it has provided far more understanding of civilian nerve injuries than would otherwise have been possible.

The increased number of injuries from automobile accidents has made most physicians aware of the problems of acute trauma, but the point cannot be overstressed that lacerations, fractures and deep tissue bruises of the extremities are likely also to injure important nerves. Failure to recognize the nerve injuries and institute early care can be a serious oversight. It is especially important to identify the presence of a nerve injury before attempting to reduce fractures or encase an extremity in dressings or plaster.

Besides lacerations and fractured long bones, there are other common causes for peripheral nerve injuries, such as dislocations; retained hematoma; accidental injury by the surgeon's scalpel; compression by tourniquet, splint or cast; aneurysms; sudden stretching; malposition during sleep or while under anesthesia; birth palsies; adjacent callus formation; repeated local trauma, and injury from injection needles.

From United States Army records, Pollock reported the distribution of peripheral nerve injuries in 7050 patients. There is probably little variation from this in civilian patients (Table 2).

PATHOLOGY. A divided or seriously traumatized nerve undergoes wallerian degeneration, characterized by fragmentation and disappearance of myelin and axons of the segment distal to the injury. Regenerative changes soon begin, but in the distal segment are abortive. In the proximal segment, within the first week, protoplasmic bands form pathways along which regenerating neurofibrillae of the segment find their way distally. If the nerve has not been divided, the downward growth of neurofibrillae continues to complete the regeneration. Regeneration occurs only from the proximal segment.

If the nerve has been divided, the ends draw apart and scar tissue fills the interval. As regenerating axons of the proximal segment meet the scar tissues in their downward growth, they are turned back to form a coiled bulbous neuroma. A bulbous enlargement also develops at the end of the distal segment, but is made up of connective tissue and known as a false neuroma. A neuroma may also form on the proximal end of interrupted fibers of an incompletely divided or "notched" nerve trunk, while intraneural injury to an intact nerve may result in a fusiform neuroma

within the nerve sheath, referred to as neuroma in continuity. Scar tissue resulting from injury or infection adjacent to a normal nerve may occasionally compress the nerve and result in a degree of degeneration, but more often the scar in perineural tissue is a part of a traumatic scar in the nerve.

SYMPTOMS. All of the peripheral nerves in the extremities are made up of afferent, efferent and sympathetic fibers. Interruption of a nerve, therefore, results in loss of motions subserved by muscles supplied by that nerve and the muscles become atrophied. Sensation of all forms disappears within an area, the pattern of which with slight variations is fairly constant for each nerve. Loss of sympathetic innervation is evidenced by loss of sweating and a degree of warming and reddening in the corresponding area due to loss of sudomotor and vasomotor control. Not only do muscles atrophy in the area supplied by the divided nerve, but many so-called trophic changes take place, the result principally of disuse and minor trauma to anesthetic tissues. These changes include demineralization of bones, stiffening of joints, atrophy of skin, keratosis, diminution of subcutaneous tissue, ulcerations, overgrowth and ridging of nails and overgrowth of hair. Incomplete severance of a peripheral nerve results in partial loss of the normal functions and tissue changes are less profound. If regeneration of a divided nerve takes place, and in the meanwhile proper care of the denervated tissues is provided, these changes can be kept at a minimum and are in large part reversible with reinnervation.

A variety of unpleasant sensations may accompany interruption of peripheral nerve function. They include principally paresthesias, hyperalgesia, stiff and wooden feelings, coldness and pain. The pain is of two varieties, so-called spontaneous pain and causalgia. The former pain is ill defined and inconstant. Its nature is not fully understood, but it probably represents overresponse to unrecognized stimuli from marginal areas.

Causalgia is a term coined by S. Weir Mitchell at the time of the Civil War. It is characterized by intense, persistent, burning pain radiating diffusely up the injured limb. It is adversely affected by extremes of temperature, light touch and psychologic stimuli to the degree that an afflicted patient will hold the limb immobile and devote his entire attention to avoiding the stimuli, which he soon learns adds to his misery. Causalgia occurs

Table 2. *Distribution of Peripheral Nerve Injuries*

Brachial plexus	139
Median	1376
Ulnar	2261
Radial	997
Musculocutaneous	87
Sciatic	1191
Tibial	252
Peroneal	558
Femoral	21
(and small groups of others)	

only with partial division of nerves and is more likely to result from injuries to the median nerve in the upper limb and the sciatic nerve in the lower limb. In spite of many investigations, the cause of causalgia remains an enigma, for none of the proposed theories accounts for all the facts. Unfortunately, the diagnosis is too often used loosely to include many or all discomforts associated with nerve injury. This error becomes important since sympathectomy will usually alleviate causalgia, whereas sympathectomy is wholly ineffective in other complaints associated with the injury.

DIAGNOSIS. The recognition of common nerve injuries is not difficult if a few simple tests for motor and sensory functions are employed, particularly in the distal parts of the extremities. One need be acquainted only with the major functions of the principal nerves, though once the existence of a nerve injury is recognized more detailed studies are important.

In examining muscle function to determine the possible interruption of nerve supply, there are several factors to consider. One of these is to have in mind the levels at which branches to various muscles leave the main trunk of the nerve. For example, in testing for possible injury to the median nerve from a wrist laceration, one would not conclude that the nerve was intact because the patient could flex the last joint of the index finger. This action is produced by a flexor muscle which receives its innervation from a branch of the median nerve above the wrist.

Other factors to be considered are anomalous or dual innervation of some muscles, such as the flexor and opponens muscles of the thumb, and anomalous muscle action. The latter term is used to describe unusual action of a muscle without reference to its nerve supply. Two types are recognized: supplementary and trick movements. These movements result from tension on paralyzed muscles by their antagonists, as occurs when formation of a fist causes extension at the wrist in the presence of radial paralysis; rebound movements which occur when normal muscles are suddenly relaxed; and movements resulting from gravity. Failure to recognize these accessory movements leads to error in evaluating the presence and degree of a nerve injury.

In sensory tests for determining nerve injury there is also variability. For example, the autonomous sensory zone of the ulnar nerve in the hand usually includes the fifth finger and the ulnar half of the ring finger, but occasionally it is limited to the fifth finger and median nerve sensory fibers overlap the ring finger.

Numerous electrodiagnostic tests have proved to be useful in the study of peripheral nerve injuries both in determining the degree of the injury and in assessing regeneration. These electrical tests refer particularly to the results of stimulation of various strengths of motor nerve, the determination of chronaxie as an index of excitability, and electromyography which measures action potentials of muscles. These refinements in examination of nerve and muscle functions are important and at times of great practical use but not always simple to perform or interpret.

RADIAL NERVE. The intimate relationship of the radial nerve to the humerus makes the nerve particularly vulnerable to injury and, as a result, it is the most frequently injured nerve in the arm. With a lesion in the midarm, the most notable deformity is wristdrop in which there is inability to extend the hand at the wrist or the fingers at the metacarpal joints (Fig. 7). In addition, there is loss of extension and abduction of the thumb and failure of the brachioradialis to contract with forceful flexion at the elbow. It is not possible for the patient to make a firm fist or hold ob-

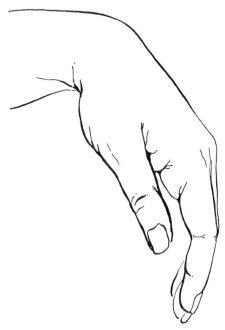

Figure 7. The characteristic wristdrop deformity of radial nerve paralysis.

jects in the hand with the wrist in full flexion. With support to the wrist, such as a splint holding the wrist in midposition or slight cock-up, full strength in grasping is possible. The thumb, deprived of extensor and abduction motions, interferes with flexion of the index finger and patients may hold the thumb aside with the other hand when making a fist.

If the nerve is injured at a high level in the arm, there is loss of triceps action and inability to extend the forearm in addition to the other paralyses. If the branch of the nerve in the forearm is injured, the typical palsies in the hand occur but without loss of extension at the wrist. Injuries of this kind are not uncommon because of the frequency of lacerations of the forearm and of accidents in surgical operations near the elbow such as removal of the head of a fractured radius.

Sensation is lost in a small area in radial nerve lesions (Fig. 8). It is unimportant to the patient and easily overlooked by the examiner, but if present along with motor palsies, it is a fairly reliable sign of the completeness of the nerve injury. The isolated area of anesthesia lies in the region of the dorsal aspect of the

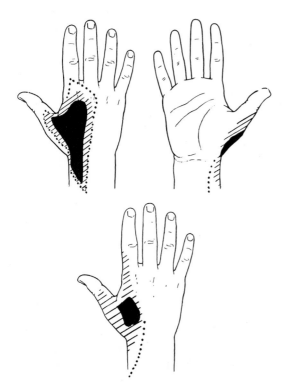

Figure 8.   The sensory loss of radial nerve paralysis is small because of the overlap from adjacent uninjured median and ulnar nerves. The solid black represents loss to all modalities; the dots represent loss to pinprick; and the cross-hatch, loss to touch.

thenar web, adjacent areas of sensory overlap being supplied by the median, ulnar and musculocutaneous nerves.

MEDIAN NERVE.   Although the commonest site of injury to the median nerve is at the wrist, particularly from cuts by glass, the nerve may be injured at higher levels by stab wounds and lacerations of the arm and forearm, or be extensive fractures about the elbow. The most striking changes are in the small muscles in the hand, but with the higher lesions of the nerve, the characteristic loss of flexion of the distal phalanx of the index finger from loss of contraction of the flexor profundus is a highly reliable sign (Fig. 9). This defect is easily demonstrated by having the patient clasp fingers of the two hands in the attitude of prayer, a position which will emphasize the absence of flexion of the index finger. Or, when asked to scratch with the nail of the index finger while holding the hand on a flat surface, the patient will be unable to do so.

The striking changes in the hand from atrophy of the small hand muscles due to median nerve paralysis produce a characteristic deformity referred to as ape hand, in which the thenar eminence becomes flattened and the thumb takes a position in the plane of the palm. The single examination most often used in testing for median nerve paralysis is to have the patient oppose the tip of his thumb to the tip of the little finger to form the letter "O." Care must be taken in the testing, however, since supplementary movements develop readily in median nerve palsy, with the exception of flexion of the distal phalanx of the index finger.

The area of sensory loss is over the radial side of the palm and the palmar aspect of the thumb, index, middle and radial side of the ring finger (Fig. 10). On the dorsum of the hand, the loss is limited to the distal half of the index and middle fingers. Because of extensive overlap from the ulnar and radial nerves, there is considerable variability in the extent and degree of sensory loss except for the distal ends of the index and middle fingers. Even in patients with extensive overlap of sensation, the region of lost sensation imposes a considerable degree of impairment in use of the hand. Because of loss of sympathetic innervation, moisture of much of the palmar skin is lost, resulting in dryness and chapping.

ULNAR NERVE.   The most striking changes in ulnar nerve paralysis are in the hand. The marked degree of wasting in the dorsal aspect of the thenar web and of the interosseous

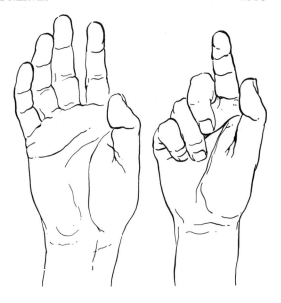

Figure 9. The deformity of median nerve paralysis is characterized by the position of the thumb in the same plane as the palm of the hand, and inability of the patient to flex the index finger as in making a fist.

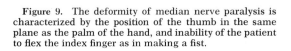

Figure 10. Typical loss of sensation to all modalities, pinprick and touch as a result of a median nerve lesion.

Figure 11. The atrophy of the dorsal interosseous muscles is marked in an ulnar nerve injury, particularly between the metacarpal of the thumb and the index finger.

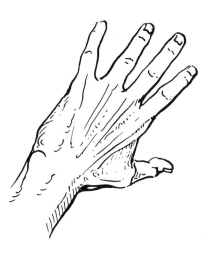

spaces gives the hand a skeleton-like appearance (Fig. 11), and the last two or three fingers assume a clawing attitude which is due to unopposed action of the extensor digitorum communis (Fig. 12).

When the lesion is at the elbow or higher, there is loss of ability to flex the proximal or distal phalanges of the last two fingers; to abduct or adduct the fingers when they are put in extension by placing the hand on a flat surface; to adduct the thumb; to abduct or oppose the little finger; and to contract the flexor carpi ulnaris. In lesions at the wrist, or distal part of the forearm, the flexor muscles of the last two fingers and the flexor carpi ulnaris are spared.

There are a few simple tests well suited to demonstrating the loss of function: inability to bring the fingers together when held in extension; loss of strength in grip in the ulnar side of the fist; inability to hold an object by adduction of the thumb without flexing it; and inability to approximate the tips of the last three fingers in forming a cone (Fig. 13).

Sensation is lost over the little finger, ulnar side of the ring finger and ulnar side of the hand on both the palmar and dorsal aspects (Fig. 14). Occasionally, sensory overlap reduces the area of absolute sensory loss to the fifth finger. The sympathetic paralysis accompanying ulnar nerve lesions causes loss of sweating, dryness of the skin and a violaceous discoloration on the ulnar side of the hand.

COMBINED MEDIAN AND ULNAR NERVE

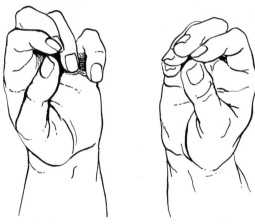

Figure 13. The patient with an ulnar nerve lesion is unable to make a cone with the tips of the fingers and thumb.

LESIONS. It is not uncommon that both the median and ulnar nerves are divided in lacerating injuries at the wrist. Such injuries also divide the flexor tendons to the hand. Serious disability can be avoided only by the most painstaking care in surgical repair of tendons and nerves followed by diligent aftercare. The deformity resulting from the combined nerve injuries represents a composite of the changes seen with each. The simian hand is even more striking than that occurring in median nerve paralysis; the thumb is held in abduction in a plane with the palm, and the last two phalanges are held in moderate flexion. Sensation is absent in the palmar side of the hand, both sides of the fingers and the ulnar side of the dorsum of the hand; the thumb is partly supplied by overlap from the radial and musculocutaneous nerves. Discoloration from loss of vasomotor control, dryness of the skin and trophic changes develop in the entire hand.

BRACHIAL PLEXUS. Lesions of the brachial plexus are usually designated on the basis of the anatomic site or the mode of injury. The plexus arises from the fifth cervical to the first thoracic nerve roots; the roots combine to form trunks and the trunks to form cords. The modes of injury are traction, pressure and laceration.

A common type of traction injury is that which occurs to the child at birth. If by some means the head and shoulder are forced apart, the upper part of the plexus is stretched and the resulting paralysis of the deltoid, biceps and brachioradialis muscles is referred to as Erb's palsy. The same type of injury is encountered postnatally from a great variety of accidents which cause stretching of the head and neck away from the shoulder, sud-

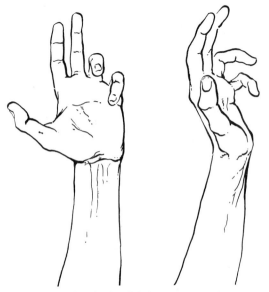

Figure 12. The clawhand deformity of an ulnar nerve lesion.

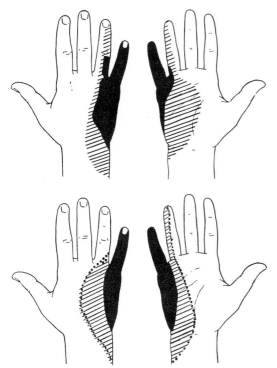

Figure 14.   Loss of all modalities and pinprick and touch sensation in an ulnar nerve lesion.

den forceful depression of the shoulder or violent downward pull on the arm.

If hyperabduction and traction are put on the arm, the injury occurs to the lower part of the plexus and is referred to as Klumpke's palsy. These injuries also occur during childbirth as well as in later years and result in palsies of ulnar or ulnar and median nerve types, often accompanied by Horner's syndrome.

Pressure injuries to the plexus occur in a variety of circumstances, some of the more common being: prolonged dislocation of the shoulder; pressure in the axilla from a crutch; pressure from shoulder braces in prolonged Trendelenburg position; aneurysm of the subclavian artery; and displaced fragments of a fractured clavicle.

Injury to the axillary nerve occurs almost exclusively as a complication of dislocation of the humerus at the shoulder. Usually, the continuity of the nerve remains intact though it may be disrupted. The paralysis is recognized by loss of function of the deltoid muscle and by a small patch of sensory loss over the muscle. The motor deficit requires differentiation from disruption of the cuff of rotator muscles attached to the humerus.

Lesions of the cord of the plexus more often result from penetrating wounds. In their

effects, they simulate the changes which follow nerve injuries more peripherally. Involvement of the medial cord affects areas innervated by the ulnar, lower portion of the median and the medial cutaneous nerves. Lateral cord injuries cause paralysis of the areas supplied by the musculocutaneous and upper portions of the median nerves. Depending on the location of injury in the posterior cord, the thoracodorsal, subscapular, axillary or radial nerves are affected. It is rare that injury to the plexus involves a single component, and recognition of the exact degree of injury is often further complicated by local edema, hemorrhage, traumatic aneurysm or the later development of scar tissue.

SCIATIC NERVE.   Severance of the main trunk of the sciatic nerve from penetrating wounds is a seriously crippling injury since it results in paralysis of all muscles below the knee and loss of sensation over the outer side of the leg and the entire foot, with the exception of the inner border of the arch. Partial injuries of the sciatic nerve, particularly in the lower part of the thigh, may involve one or the other of its two main divisions, the peroneal and tibial nerves.

PERONEAL NERVE.   The peroneal nerve is the most frequently injured nerve in the lower extremity as a result of common fractures of the upper end of the fibula and from pressure by casts, splints, traction devices and under-knee rolls. To this list of causes should be added pressure from the cross-leg position that some people assume for hours while in sitting posture, and resting pressure in emaciated bedridden patients. The deformity is easily recognized by foot drop and alteration in gait characterized by lifting the leg to avoid tripping with the toe. Partial paralysis can be identified by weakness in dorsiflexion of the foot and great toe when an attempt is made to walk on the heel. The sensory loss is over the lateral aspect of the leg and dorsum of the foot to the base of the toes.

TIBIAL NERVE.   Isolated lesions of the tibial nerve are uncommon, particularly from injuries below the knee. The principal motor supply is to the muscles which plantar flex the foot and toes, and the paralysis is identified simply by inability to walk or support weight on the toes. Sensation is lost over the sole of the foot except the inner border of the arch. Traumatic ulceration of the sole is a complication which readily occurs if the patient walks on the foot.

SURGICAL TREATMENT.   It is not possible to determine at the time of nonpenetrating injuries whether a nerve has been anatomically or physiologically interrupted, and there is seldom need for immediate surgery. Recovery often occurs spontaneously, but it is imperative that frequent periodic examinations be made and, if within three to five months recovery is uncertain or not proceeding satisfactorily, there should then be no hesitation about exploring the nerve surgically. Even earlier exploration is sometimes justified, since the attending risks of the operation are negligible; if the nerve is found intact, no harm has occurred. For example, when the radial nerve is caught between the fragments of a fractured humerus, valuable time is saved in healing of both bone and nerve if early exploration is performed. In traction and pressure paralyses of the brachial plexus or some of its branches, such as the axillary nerve, there is so little to be expected from operation that exploration is rarely required.

In the presence of puncture or lacerated wounds, the ideal time for repair of injury to a peripheral nerve is immediately. It is even reasonably safe with the use of antimicrobial therapy to repair a wound as long as 48 hours after its infliction, and carefully repair a divided nerve. Even if infection develops in the wound, the nerve may regenerate or, if a secondary operation and reanastomosis of the nerve are required later, the ends will be approximated and retraction will have been prevented.

In the repair of a divided nerve, the approximation of the freshened ends without torsion and by the use of fine silk sutures in the epineurium is sought. When tension on the nerve is necessary in order to approximate the ends, sufficient relaxation can usually be had by flexion or extension of the extremity and immobilization in that position for six weeks. Transposition of the nerve may afford the needed gain in length for anastomosis. For example, the radial nerve divided in the midarm has a shorter route in the arm if its position is transposed to the opposite side of the humerus. Larger defects in a nerve can be overcome by procedures designed to stretch the proximal segment of the nerve gradually to bring it in approximation with the distal segment. Repair of unreduced gaps with nerve grafts has not been successful in the past, but there may be merit in the use of freeze-dried, irradiated homografts of nerve protected by a Millipore sheath as proposed by Campbell.

When important peripheral nerves cannot be repaired, one has recourse at times to muscle and tendon transplantation or arthrodesis of joints with good functional results. Also, occasional good results follow direct implantation of a nerve end into a muscle.

AFTER-CARE. It is not possible to overemphasize the place of carefully supervised and persistent physiotherapy to the limb following peripheral nerve injury, both before and after surgical repair. The treatment is directed toward preservation of the intact skin and the prevention of fibrosis and atrophy of muscles, and of contraction of joint capsules. The methods should include application of wet and dry heat, massage, passive movement of joints, electrical stimulation of paralyzed muscles and re-education exercises as soon as possible. Mechanical splints help not only in early use of the limb but provide support in the normal position, thereby preventing contraction at a joint or overstretching of paralyzed muscles.

As a part of the after-care, it is important to detect the early evidences of regeneration of the nerve and to follow the progress. One of the oldest and most easily applied tests is Tinel's sign. The test consists of eliciting a tingling or shocklike sensation in the area of sensory distribution of a nerve by tapping gently over the nerve distal to the site of injury. The response is presumed to result from stimulation of regenerating unmyelinated sensory axons. Its accuracy as a test is sometimes questioned but, in practice, it usually proves to be a simple and satisfactory way of following the downward progress in a regenerating nerve.

A highly reliable test which can be utilized when it is important to detect regeneration of motor fibers in a nerve is intraneural stimulation by means of fine wire electrodes introduced percutaneously directly into the nerve.

Electromyography and chronaxie tests, useful means of detecting function in the initial evaluation of the nerve injury, are of equal value in assessing regeneration. The tests can show evidence of reinnervation of a muscle some time before it can be recognized by clinical methods, and thus give early assurance that a nerve suture is intact.

TARDY NERVE PALSY. Occasionally, palsies of peripheral nerves in the upper extremities develop insidiously years after a fracture which has healed either with excessive callus which compresses the nerve, or with a deformity that displaces the nerve and exposes it to easy trauma. Such lesions of the radial or median nerves are not often seen, but tardy ulnar palsy is a well-recognized syndrome which follows injuries about the elbow. There is a gradual loss of sensation, sometimes accompanied by paresthesias, in the ulnar distribution of the forearm and hand, more particularly in the fifth finger at the outset. Palsy of muscles supplied by the ulnar nerve also occurs and is usually evidenced first by wasting of the dorsum of the thenar web and the dorsal interosseous spaces. Later, the little finger assumes an abducted position and cannot be approximated to the ring finger. If the process is permitted to go on untreated, complete ulnar paralysis may occur.

Surgical treatment should be employed just as early as the condition is recognized, since often the best that can be hoped for from operation in chronic palsy is cessation of the progress with relatively little reversal of the neurologic changes. Treatment consists in moving the ulnar nerve from its position in the olecranon groove to a position in the cubital fossa where it is no longer exposed to repeated stretch and easy trauma.

MEDIAN NERVE COMPRESSION IN THE CARPAL TUNNEL. The insidious development of median nerve palsy in the hand has sometimes been found to occur with osseous deformity of the wrist following fractures, and has been appropriately regarded as tardy median palsy. However, the carpal tunnel syndrome of median nerve palsy has come to attention in recent years. The pathogenesis of the syndrome is not entirely understood, but it is believed the nerve somehow becomes irritated and swollen within its tunnel through the volar carpal ligament. The condition is more often seen in patients who have overindulged in some kind of unaccustomed manual work.

Sensory symptoms in the distribution of the median nerve in the hand and fingers constitute the earliest and major disability. Tingling, burning and sometimes painful dysesthesias are usual and, as numbness increases, the patient finds increasing limitation in facile use of the fingers. Motor symptoms and signs are less prominent and may be absent. Moderate wasting and weakness occur in the opponens pollicis and abductor pollicis brevis muscles. A helpful sign in diagnosis is the elicitation of Tinel's sign on tapping over the median nerve at the wrist.

Rest and immobilization of the wrist are sometimes helpful early, but in more advanced lesions, surgical decompression of the nerve by division of the carpal ligament over the course of the nerve has proved to be highly successful.

CERVICAL RIB AND ANTERIOR SCALENE SYNDROME

A cervical rib is a supernumerary rib arising from the seventh cervical vertebra. It is accompanied by a number of variations in anatomic arrangement of the regional structures, including muscles, nerves and blood vessels. A relatively small percentage of those born with cervical ribs develop symptoms and, then, usually not till middle life.

The symptoms and signs resulting from the presence of a cervical rib are due to stretch and compression of the subclavian artery and components of the brachial plexus in the acute angle between the rib and the scalenus anticus muscle. The muscle is a very important part of the arrangement, and this is emphasized by the fact that somewhat the same, though less marked, symptoms, the anterior scalene syndrome, may occur in the absence of an extra rib.

The characteristic symptoms include pain, disturbances in sensation, wasting of muscles and peripheral vascular changes. Paresthesias and sensory loss occur along the ulnar side of the forearm and hand. Pain of variable degree is experienced along the inner aspect of the arm and forearm and occasionally in the suprascapular region. Aggravation of pain occurs on rotation of the neck, depression of the shoulder or overhead stretching movements. The same motions may obliterate the radial pulse.

Motor signs include gradual muscle wasting and weakness in the hand in a pattern comparable to that of ulnar palsy. In more severe cases the muscle changes simulate combined ulnar and median palsy. The peripheral vascular changes due to compression of the subclavian artery are not always present, but can be of such severe degree that gangrene develops in one or more fingers.

Treatment consists of dividing the anterior scalenus muscle at its lowest attachment for alleviation of the anterior scalene syndrome. The same procedure may also be adequate for relief in the presence of a cervical rib, but if the nerves of the plexus and the subclavian artery do not appear to have been fully released by division of the muscle, the cervical rib is resected.

TUMORS

The commonest primary tumor of peripheral nerves is the neurofibroma seen in von

Recklinghausen's disease. In this disease, there are multiple tumors, sometimes hundreds, varying in size and in degrees of malignancy, though they are usually benign. Less often the same type of tumor occurs as an isolated single lesion. Whether these tumors take origin from the neurilemma, perineurium or epineurium is often difficult to determine and has led to confusion in classification as well as many synonyms (perineural fibroma, neurinoma, neurilemmoma, schwannoma, neurofibroblastoma, neurofibrosarcoma and others).

Since the longest course of peripheral nerves is in the extremities, it is understandable that these neoplasms are most numerous there. In the upper limbs, they are somewhat more common on median and ulnar nerves in the forearms, but may arise from small nerve branches even in the fingers. In the lower limbs, they are usually found on the posterior aspect of the thighs and legs. The neck, with its multiplicity of nerves, is a favorite location, and nerve tumors must always be considered in the differential diagnosis of tumors in this region.

Von Recklinghausen's disease is of congenital origin, though the tumors do not usually grow to recognizable or disturbing size till young adulthood. Not only are peripheral nerves involved, but, in many patients, the cranial nerves, spinal nerve roots and sympathetic nerves as well. Associated conditions include scattered areas of pigmentation of the skin producing café au lait spots, abnormalities of bone, cutaneous tumors which are sometimes plexiform or pedunculated, evidence of defective development of the nervous system and other malformations. Any of the tumors may undergo sarcomatous degeneration and become actively invasive in adjacent tissues.

Neurofibromas which involve major nerves and threaten paralysis should be removed, and this can usually be accomplished without sacrifice of the nerve if malignant changes

umors known to be, or malignant should be margin, and residual d at times to respond oy. Rarely, such tumors ases.

ally understood to be its at the ends of di-the course of injured euromas of benign na-found on peripheral and traumatic neuromas in tion stumps assume im-because of pain associ-gical revision of painful ay relieve pain, but more art to psychologic factors. are made up of the end-e together with elements of ls and smooth muscle. They eir presence should be recognized ense pain caused by pressure over th they are usually small, rarely more than a few millimeters in size, and though they have been encountered in the subcutaneous tissues in many parts of the body the majority occur in the subungual region of the fingers. The tumors are benign and curable by excision.

Invasion by malignant tumors adjacent to peripheral nerves is often met with, particularly in the brachial plexus and in the lumbosacral plexus in the pelvis. The malignant tumors of the breast and lung which invade the brachial plexus produce neurologic symptoms and signs referred to as the superior sulcus syndrome or Pancoast syndrome. Initial symptoms are pain in areas supplied by the lower part of the plexus, namely, the inner side of the arm and forearm, and also paralysis of sympathetic fibers in the limb from involvement of the region of the stellate ganglion. With advance of the disease, there are progressive motor and sensory palsies in the limb. Treatment is restricted to appropriate methods of controlling pain.

Autonomic Nervous System

The autonomic nervous system, also known as the vegetative, sympathetic or involuntary system, is composed of the craniosacral outflow, the thoracolumbar outflow and the visceral afferent nerves which traverse these systems (Fig. 15). Parasympathetic fibers arise from the third, seventh, ninth and tenth cranial nerves and the second, third and fourth sacral nerves, while the sympathetic fibers arise from the thoracic and the first two lumbar nerves and possibly the lowest two cervical nerves. Preganglionic

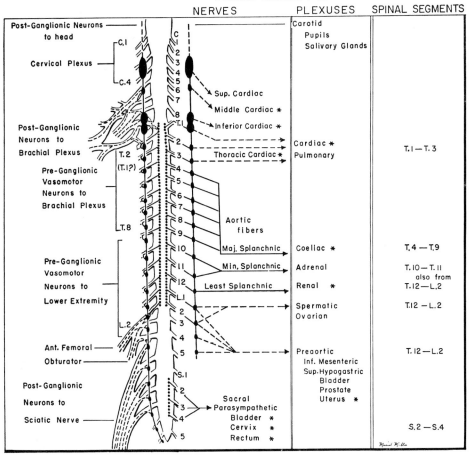

INNERVATION OF   **INNERVATION OF VISCERA**

Periph. Blood Vessels·

Sensory and Motor

* Indicates Conduction of pain

NERVES   PLEXUSES   SPINAL SEGMENTS

Figure 15. The outgoing vasomotor and sudomotor fibers to the extremities from the lateral horn of the spinal cord are illustrated diagrammatically on the left side. On the right side are shown the mixed visceromotor (sympathetic) and viscerosensory (posterior spinal root) fibers, together with the principal visceral plexuses which they supply and the spinal segments from which they are derived. Preganglionic sympathetic axons are indicated by continuous lines and post-ganglionic by interrupted lines. Direct preganglionic connections with the stellate ganglion via the first thoracic nerve are marked by dotted lines. Recent anatomic studies suggest that they are often present, possibly in C8 as well. The asterisk (*) indicates the presence of pain fibers running to the posterior roots.

and postganglionic neurons constitute the efferent system. The synapses are located close to the innervated structures in the case of the parasympathetic system, but have a more central location in the sympathetic system, in which they are found principally in the paravertebral ganglionated chain.

The autonomic nervous system tends to preserve the internal environment of the body. Its nerves innervate smooth muscles, such as are present in the pupil, and the blood vessels, the bronchial and gastrointestinal tracts, the urinary bladder and the sex organs. The nerves also supply the heart and regulate the activity of the various glands of the gastrointestinal tract, the sweat glands

and the lacrimal glands. Together with hormonal influences, they regulate internal secretions of the adrenals, the pancreas and the pituitary. Even though all these visceral structures are influenced by autonomic nerves, their functional and anatomic integrity is independent of the impulses of these nerves, as is demonstrated in totally sympathectomized animals or man.

Strictly speaking, there are no diseases known definitely to be due to pathologic states of the autonomic nervous system. There have been occasional reports of pathologic changes in sympathetic ganglia in exophthalmic goiter, diabetes mellitus and following infectious diseases, but few of the conclusions can be supported. In vasotropic disorders in which there is commonly believed to be a functional relationship with the autonomic nerves, autopsy has not shown abnormalities either in any peripheral or central nervous structures. An example of what is believed to be a functional increase in sympathetic activity is seen in some younger emotionally labile individuals with cold, sweaty, cyanotic hands and feet. It has been pointed out by Lewis that neurogenic vasoconstriction of normal arteries or arterioles does not result in blanching ischemia of a finger. In Raynaud's syndrome, which includes ischemic blanching of digits, it is believed that vasomotor tone is normal, but that a local fault, possibly in the nature of obliterative vascular disease, exists in the arterioles.

SURGICAL PRINCIPLES

Surgical procedures designed for interruption of the autonomic nervous system have had several periods of enthusiastic endorsement, particularly for vasomotor disturbances. At present, there is less use of the procedure, as a result of extensive experience indicating more clearly the limitations of the operations and also as a result of the development of other surgical and medical treatment of some of the diseases for which sympathectomy was formerly performed. Nevertheless, selected operations for interruption of autonomic nerves continue to have a useful place in selected patients. There are but few indications for operations upon the parasympathetic system—vagotomy for the treatment of peptic ulcer being virtually the only one of importance. Sympathectomy, on the other hand, has a much wider application and is employed principally for its effect on the heart, blood vessels and sweat glands, and for interruption of visceral afferent nerves in the relief of certain painful visceral disorders.

Operations on the sympathetic system have for the most part been empiric (Fig. 16). Among the earliest operations performed were those for the relief of epilepsy, migraine, glaucoma, exophthalmic goiter, retinitis pigmentosa and birth palsies; all of which proved worthless and are now discarded. In certain conditions for which sympathectomy has been useful, it is not always evident whether interruption of the efferent or afferent pathways is the more important. For example, the relief of cardiac pain was thought by some to result from interruption of constrictor nerves to the coronary arteries, whereas the

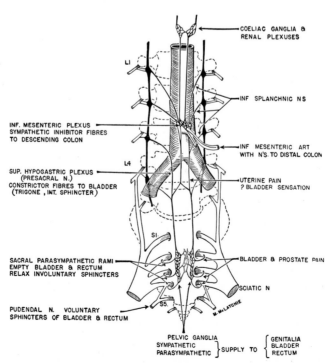

Figure 16.   The nerve supply of the pelvic viscera.

usual explanation for the relief of cardiac pain is the interruption of visceral pain fibers from the heart. A similar difference of opinion exists in the explanation for relief of pain by sympathectomy in pancreatitis.

Much of the surgical literature has been occupied with the problem of how to select patients who may be benefited by sympathectomy, what the extent of the operation should be to interrupt appropriate nerves, and how to gain a more complete and permanent effect. A three-fold dictum commonly employed in evaluating sympathectomy is that the operation, to be successful, should be preganglionic in type, anatomically complete and extensive enough to prevent regeneration. In the light of more recent evidence, the interpretation of the value of each of these has changed considerably.

The concern over hypersensitivity of small arteries to circulating adrenalin following sympathetic ganglionectomy, or interruption of postganglionic fibers based largely on animal experimentation, was thought by many to account for poor clinical results. This led to a variety of operations employed for sympathectomizing the upper limb, all designed to preserve the stellate and other paravertebral ganglia, and thus, the postganglionic neurons. But, ganglionectomy in man does not produce nearly as great sensitization of smooth muscle as in the monkey, and whatever increase in sensitivity occurs temporarily becomes inconsequential with the passage of time. The removal of the stellate and adjacent paravertebral ganglia actually accomplishes a more complete sympathectomy of the upper limb than do the various preganglionic operations which have been devised. Furthermore, removal of paravertebral ganglia provides a safeguard against possible regeneration of divided sympathetic nerves. Postganglionic axons cannot regenerate if their cells of origin are destroyed by excision of paravertebral ganglia, and preganglionic nerves do not develop terminal effector structures.

The desirability of anatomic completeness in a sympathectomy employed to denervate any part of the body is evident, and operations have been based on the belief that the result could be accomplished by a sufficiently extensive resection of the paravertebral ganglionated chain. However, there is ample evidence that some structures of the body are supplied in part by sympathetic nerves which leave the spinal cord to synapse directly with postganglionic neurons accompanying so-matic nerves and do not traverse the paravertebral ganglia. For example, following total paravertebral sympathectomy, from the stellate ganglion to the third lumbar ganglion in man, there is complete and permanent interruption of sympathetic function below the knees but not in the thighs. To attain complete sympathectomy in the thighs, it is necessary to section the anterior roots of the twelfth thoracic and first and second lumbar nerves intraspinally. A similar arrangement exists in the sympathetic supply to the upper limb, where postganglionic fibers appear to pass directly to the brachial plexus from lower cervical segments of the cord without any connection with the stellate ganglion or cervical sympathetic chain. However, there are no accessory fibers to the legs and feet and none have been demonstrated to the viscera. Even in the upper extremities, an anatomically and physiologically incomplete sympathectomy may still be useful.

Still other circumstances may detract from hoped-for results following sympathectomy, the chief of which are the irreversible structural changes of tissues in patients with vascular disease. This, more than any other factor, has made the prediction of the results of sympathectomy difficult. It has been the hope that blocking of the sympathetics would temporarily duplicate what might result from cutting sympathetic pathways, and that various tests devised to demonstrate the state of blood vessels in vascular disease would predict the efficacy of sympathectomy, but all such efforts leave much to be desired. There are certain diseases which, through rationale and experience, can reasonably be expected to be benefited by appropriate sympathectomy, as well as characteristics pertinent to each disease and to each individual, which are useful in deciding to employ sympathectomy. In the last analysis, sympathectomy may often be employed justifiably as a therapeutic test. While the operations require specialized knowledge, they are rarely accompanied by significant risks, the periods of disability are short and the loss of a portion of the sympathetic system does not impose serious untoward effects.

SURGICAL PROCEDURES

Periarterial sympathectomy, once extensively employed, encouraged by the reports of Leriche and others, is no longer in use and the reason deserves explanation. The operation was based on the erroneous assumption that the nerve fibers through which more distal parts of an artery and its branches are innervated extend distally in the periarterial plexus. In fact, however, both the vasomotor and the accompanying afferent fibers which innervate peripheral vessels traverse nearby spinal nerves and join the perivascular plexuses at short intervals along the courses of the arteries. Consequently, more distal innervation of a vessel is not altered by excising periarterial nerves from a proximal segment of an artery.

Cervical sympathectomy refers to total removal or resection of any part of the ganglionated chain in the neck, and may include the stellate ganglion. The operation has been recommended and employed for a number of conditions including migraine, exophthalmos, tinnitus, retinitis pigmentosa, retinal arterial spasm, glaucoma, excessive sweating in the face and neck and cerebral vascular disease, particularly strokes. There is little justification for continuing to employ the operation for any of these conditions. Only occasional use for the operation has been found in two conditions: one is in "malignant" exophthalmos in which the production of ptosis of the upper eyelids aids in better protection of the corneae if decompression of the orbits or hypophysectomy has not been fully effective. The other use is in the occasional patient who, for whatever reason, may have a unilateral Horner's syndrome and prefers the symmetrical appearance of the eyes afforded by bilateral cervical sympathetic paralysis.

Cervicothoracic sympathectomy consists in resection of the upper portion of the paravertebral thoracic ganglionated chain to include the stellate and the lower ganglia of the cervical chain, or division of the communicating rami of the ganglia and section of the chain below to interrupt ascending fibers in the chain. The latter procedure is designed as a preganglionic operation and is performed through a posterior or axillary intrathoracic approach, whereas ganglionectomy including the middle and lower cervical, the stellate and the second and third thoracic ganglia is performed through a supraclavicular approach.

The operations are performed principally for vasomotor, sudomotor and certain painful states in the upper limb, for relief of pain originating in the heart and great vessels of the region, or occasionally to counteract bouts of tachycardia of atrial origin not responding to medical management.

There are sound physiological reasons for preferring ganglionectomy over preganglionic operations in sympathectomizing the upper extremity. In addition, it should be recognized that there is much more frequent complaint of pain from thoractomy wounds than occurs following a supraclavicular operation. However, there are certain circumstances which dictate the way in which the operation might best be performed. For example, in order to produce anhydrosis of the axilla and hand, it is necessary only to divide the rami communicantes of the second thoracic ganglion and the chain below the ganglion. This can most simply be done through a resection of a short portion of the second or third rib posteriorly. In the case of sectioning of the efferent nerves of the heart for control of paroxysmal tachycardia, it is necessary to resect the upper four thoracic ganglia bilaterally. This operation must be done through a posterior rib resection, since it would rarely be possible to perform a resection of the ganglionated chain below the third thoracic ganglion through a supraclavicular operation.

Lumbar sympathectomy consists of resection of segments of the lumbar paravertebral ganglionated chain, principally for the purpose of depriving the legs and feet of sympathetic innervation. There are occasional reports of relief of pain in the lower limbs following the operation in patients with paraplegia resulting from disruption of the lower spinal cord.

To sympathectomize the leg and foot, all that is required is excision of the second and third lumbar ganglia. Though the segmental level in the cord for sympathetic nerve supply to the lower limb is as high as T10, or T11, it is never below the L3 cord segment and all fibers which enter the paravertebral ganglionated chain traverse the second and third ganglia on their way to the limb. While it may not be possible easily to identify the second and third ganglia as such, because of several ganglionic enlargements and numerous rami, an adequate sympathectomy results from the resection of that portion of the chain which readily comes to view just below the attachment of the diaphragm and as far as the pelvic brim. One must divide attachments of the diaphragm in order to expose the first lumbar ganglion. Contrary to the recommendations of some, to remove the first lumbar and even the lowest thoracic ganglia, neither the degree nor the permanency of sympathectomy in the lower limbs is at all altered by extending the operation above the second or below the third lumbar ganglia.

The usual surgical approach to the lumbar

ganglionated chain is   .-
cision, exposing the r   e.
However, in conjunctio   n-
inal repair of atheroscler   lying the lower limbs, it is ‹   e to
perform simultaneous lu   nec-
tomy through the open abd‹

Presacral neurectomy, wh   ists of resection of the superior hypoɩ   plexus, sometimes in conjunction with resection of the lumbar ganglionated chains, has been reported favorably as a means of relieving dysmenorrhea. A similar operation had a passing vogue for relief of bladder pain such as might arise from Hunner's ulcer. The operation now finds little favor because the results have not been uniformly successful and other forms of treatment usually suffice.

Combined splanchnicectomy and thoracolumbar sympathectomy was designed as a means to counteract vascular hypertension through the production of blood vessel dilatation in a large area of the body. A variety of operations have been performed, including resection of splanchnic nerves only, combined resection of the splanchnics with the lower thoracic and upper lumbar ganglionated chain, and total excision of the ganglionated chain from the stellate to the third lumbar ganglia. The operation which came to be most widely used was resection of the splanchnic nerves together with the lower thoracic and upper lumbar chain. The upper limit of the resection was the eighth or ninth thoracic ganglion and the lower limit was the second or third lumbar ganglion. The operation was performed bilaterally through the extrapleural and extraperitoneal spaces. Since visceral afferent nerves were also interrupted, these operations came to be employed occasionally for relief of pain of abdominal viscera such as that occurring with chronic forms of pancreatitis.

In recent years, the development of a number of drugs which lower blood pressure has largely superseded surgical treatment. However, during the time the operations were being commonly performed, it was possible to make numerous investigations of the anatomy and function of the sympathetic system and its accompanying afferent nerves, which had not been possible previously.

The collective experience in the past 35 years with sympathectomy performed for innumerable conditions has lent itself at times to overenthusiasm and false conclusions. Even now, the basis on which successful operation is employed in many patients is largely one of empiricism, or trial and error. Nevertheless, there are certain well-established rules and values for the use of sympathectomy in properly selected patients.

Congenital Anomalies of the Nervous System

Diseases and deformities of the central nervous system which are present at birth may be immediately evident, or become so soon after birth in the neonatal period or at any time in life. They are spoken of variously as congenital, hereditary or familial. Certain anatomic anomalies of the neural axis evident at birth, or in the early years of life, are common and constitute special problems in surgical management. In the majority of children with these anomalies, there is little to indicate whether the condition has resulted from a primary defect in the germ plasma or whether the fetus has been affected in its development by some external agent.

SPINA BIFIDA

Spina bifida is the name given a developmental defect in the vertebral spines and laminae, occurring principally in the lumbo-sacral region, but also in the cervical and occasionally in the thoracic regions. If the defect in the spine is unaccompanied by protrusion of the meninges or neural elements of the spinal canal, it is spoken of as a spina bifida occulta and its presence may not be suspected except by telltale signs in the overlying superficial tissues, such as dimpling, discoloration or hirsutism of the skin, or the presence of a lipoma. The diagnosis is made by roentgenograms. Accompanying neurologic defects vary from mild to severe, and are most evident in deformity of the feet, motor palsies, sensory defects in the lower limbs, and impaired sphincter control. Surgical treatment is not advisable unless there is convincing evidence that neurologic signs are worsening. Even then, surgery must be undertaken with caution for fear of adding to the deficit. At best, the partial removal of lipomatous tissue, division of adhesions or severance of the filum terminale may prevent additional neurologic changes. Fusion of the spine for stabilization or for protection of the neural elements is not indicated.

SPINAL MENINGOCELE AND MYELOMENINGOCELE

Protrusion of the meninges and neural elements from the spinal canal in the presence of spina bifida may exist in several forms (Fig. 17). Although the protrusions are usually posterior and easily identified at birth, occasionally they extend into the thorax, abdomen or pelvis, where they may be mistaken for other lesions.

The term "meningocele" is meant to imply the protrusion only of the meninges. If the sac contains neural elements, the term "myelomeningocele," or "meningomyelocele," obtains. The former usually is accompanied by neurologic disturbances, while the latter is

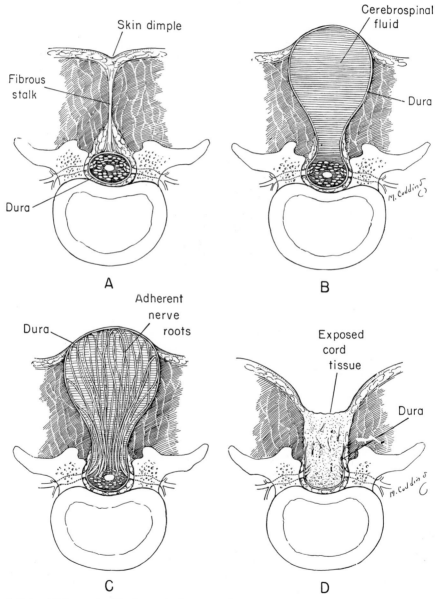

Figure 17. *A, Spina bifida occulta.* The intraspinal contents do not protrude to the surface, although often the site of the underlying bony defect is marked by a cutaneous abnormality. *B, Spina bifida with meningocele.* A meningeal sac containing cerebrospinal fluid protrudes on the surface, but there is no abnormality of spinal cord or nerve roots. *C, Spina bifida with myelomeningocele.* Nerve roots of the cauda equina are atrophic, displaced and adherent to the exposed membranous sac. *D, Spina bifida with rachischisis.* Disorganized and distorted central neural tissue is exposed directly to the surface.

expected to be complicated by varying degrees of motor and sensory abnormalities and sphincter impairment. Exceptions exist when normal neural elements "float" in the meningocele or are attached to the sac by flimsy adhesions, in which case there are no neurologic abnormalities. The size of the lesions varies from small unimportant protrusions to head-sized swellings and their superficial covering may be skin or an epithelized membrane. When disorganized meningeal and neural tissue lacks an epithelial covering, the condition is referred to as rachischisis.

The indications and timing for surgical repair of meningocele and myelomeningocele are often indefinite, but certain principles are of help in guiding decisions.

In the presence of total paralysis of the lower limbs with loss of vesical and anal control, it is questionable whether any reparative operation should be performed even if the defect lacks covering or is leaking spinal fluid. The hopeless crippling and the unpredictable survival should be a deterrent to employing surgery in an attempt to prolong life. If the infant survives with supportive treatment and does not develop hydrocephalus or evidence of other serious congenital defect, it may be justifiable after some months, or even years, to correct the defect surgically, principally for cosmetic reasons and to facilitate the care of a paraplegic patient.

As a rule it is desirable to repair the defect early. There is greater urgency if the covering membrane is thin, macerated or leaking spinal fluid, unless the area is infected, in which case operation must be delayed until the infection is brought under control.

A small or pedunculated lesion can safely be removed soon after birth. Although some prefer and insist on early operation, even in the first 24 hours after birth, delay of some weeks or months often permits toughening of the covering membrane and relative decrease in the size of the defect at the base of the protrusion. Delay also makes it possible to determine whether hydrocephalus is an accompanying defect. Progressive enlargement of the spinal protrusion or enlargement of the head, or both, indicates the presence of hydrocephalus, and probably of an Arnold-Chiari malformation of the hindbrain. If hydrocephalus exists, it is useless to attempt repair of the spinal defect until measures are taken to control the increased cerebrospinal fluid pressure, because healing of the wound will be prevented by the pressure of the fluid.

The purpose of a surgical procedure is to obliterate the protruding mass and provide a tight cosmetic closure of the wound, but not to attempt extensive exploration or dissection of neural elements. To do so accomplishes nothing but possibly to produce or add to a neurologic defect. Except that part to which neural elements are adherent, the meningeal sac should be excised, and closed if possible. For further protection and support, fascial flaps should then be brought together over the defect and the skin closed. Approximation of the skin may be difficult, but the skin can usually be mobilized by undercutting at some distance in the subcutaneous tissue or by releasing incisions made at some distance from the repair.

Thereafter, periodic observations for the possible development of hydrocephalus are essential, together with rehabilitation measures to deal with musculoskeletal deficiencies and training in bowel and bladder control.

ENCEPHALOCELE

A congenital defect in the skull occurring in or near the midline, cranium bifidum, is the counterpart of spina bifida, and the protrusion of the intracranial meninges or brain tissue through the defect morphologically resembles the lesion seen in the spine. The usual site is in the occipital region and, less commonly, in the frontal region. Rarely, the protrusion is into the orbial or nasopharyngeal spaces, where its nature may not readily be recognized and where surgical repair is more complicated. It is common to find accompanying hydrocephalus and various anomalies of brain development. As in the comparable spinal lesions, the cephalic protrusions vary in size, content and covering tissues. Similarly, hydrocephalus must be dealt with if it exists.

Surgical repair of encephaloceles is not indicated when accompanied by obvious gross anomalies of the brain, but in other instances should be performed early. The treatment entails excision of the meningeal sac, and sometimes of brain tissue within it, watertight closure of the sac and approximation of the scalp by whatever plastic repair is required. As in the repair of spinal lesions, healing cannot be expected in the presence of hydrocephalus. Its correction must be accomplished before or at the time of repair of the encephalocele. Large defects in the skull, especially those producing unsightly deformity in the frontal region, should be closed by cranioplasty, but usually at a later date.

DIASTEMATOMYELIA

One type of occult developmental anomaly of the vertebrae is that in which a spicule of bone extends from a vertebral body into the spinal canal, producing a cleft in the canal and thereby not only dividing but transfixing its contents. The condition is termed diastematomyelia, which designates the separation of meninges, cord and roots by the bony partition. The location has been found at various vertebral levels between the mid-thoracic and the lowest lumbar. In most patients, there is some associated neurologic abnormality, while in others there is only an overlying cutaneous deformity. The true nature of the condition becomes apparent in roentgenograms of the spine, particularly in the anteroposterior views which show a vertical line of increased density in the center of the spinal canal and usually in an area of spina bifida. The condition is even more strikingly demonstrated by Pantopaque myelography (Fig. 18).

Fixation by the bony spicule prevents the rostral migration of the cord and its nerve

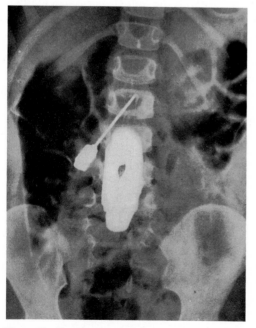

Figure 18. Pantopaque myelogram showing characteristic division of the column of dye around the midline bony spicule and dural septum.

roots which normally occur in a growing child. With correction of the defect, existing neurologic abnormalities are not expected to improve, but the development of additional ones should be prevented. The surgical repair consists of excising the abnormal bone through an opening in the posterior dura and reapproximating this part of the dura.

ARNOLD-CHIARI MALFORMATION

The Arnold-Chiari malformation is a specific deformity in which the cerebellum is abnormally developed and the hindbrain is displaced caudally. The fourth ventricle is partly obliterated and the cisterna magna is replaced by numerous adhesions. Although the condition is occasionally found alone, most often it accompanies a spina bifida with or without the presence of a spinal meningocele or myelomeningocele, and its presence may not be discovered until puberty or even adulthood. The hydrocephalus, usually present, may be in part due to fourth ventricle obstruction, but is more likely to be due to interference with the subarachnoid spaces at the foramen magnum. Surgical decompression of the region of the foramen magnum with lysis of adhesions has not been uniformly successful, probably because of unrelieved subarachnoid obstruction. Third ventriculostomy or another type of ventricular shunt is indicated if the decompressive operation fails.

DERMAL SINUS

In the embryologic development of the brain and cord, failure of the ectoderm to close completely along the dorsum of the embryo results in a persistent defect which takes the form of a sinus tract that may extend to any depth, even to the brain or cord. The common sites of occurrence are the occipital and lumbosacral regions.

Though shallow sinuses are of minor importance, those that extend deeply are potential sources of serious complications and, therefore, any midline tract should be excised. There is a tendency for deep tracts to become infected and to lead to intracranial or intraspinal infection. Blockage of the tract may result in its dilatation by a collection of epithelial debris, sebaceous material and hair, sometimes causing a mass of dangerous proportions in the posterior fossa or the spinal canal. Infection in the tract adds still more to the danger because, in the process of surgical excision, infection of the meningeal spaces can occur where infection did not previously exist.

With intracranial dermal sinuses, a defect in the skull through which the tract passes can sometimes be palpated and more often be identified by roentgenogram. Careful total excision of these tracts is imperative. Prior to the advent of antibiotics, the mortality following the operations was high and even in the present day the risk of uncontrolled intracranial abscess or meningitis either before or following surgical excision is considerable.

NEURENTERIC CYST

A rare embryologic defect of the neural axis is the neurenteric cyst. In a sense, it is the counterpart of a dermal sinus, since the cysts lie anterior to the cord. The condition results from failure of interposition of the mesoderm between the entodermal and ectodermal layers in the primitive embryo.

The cyst, lined by entodermal mucosa, is found in the anterior part of the spinal canal, anterior to the cervical or thoracic cord. A defect in the body of an adjacent vertebra is usually evident on roentgenogram, and an enlargement of the cyst may be found anterior or lateral to the vertebra. Surgical treatment requires excision of the intraspinal cyst, and secondarily of the paravertebral portion in the thorax if it exists.

CRANIOSYNOSTOSIS

Premature closure of one or more of the cranial sutures not only results in a misshapen head, but may seriously injure the growing brain and the optic nerves by compression and distortion. Because most of the growth of the brain takes place in the first two years of life, it is especially important that deficiencies in growth of the skull be identified and repaired early.

The condition is more common in male babies and has a familial tendency. The cause is not well understood, but it is not unusual for other congenital anomalies, particularly syndactylism, to be associated.

The nature of the distortion of the head depends on which of the several sutures of the skull becomes closed (Figs. 19 and 20). By far the most common variety is fusion of the sagittal suture, and closure of the coronal suture is the next commonest. Closure of other single sutures or combinations of sutures, or even closure of all sutures, is less frequently encountered. A small head requires differentiation between closure of multiple sutures and microcephaly, in which the brain is small and the sutures are open.

Although the particular shape of the head and the presence of palpable ridges marking bony closures of a suture often indicate the condition, final diagnosis depends on identification by roentgenogram.

It is of primary importance that a diagnosis be made early and that surgical repair be performed without needless delay, not only to minimize the deformity, but to avoid

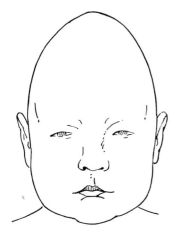
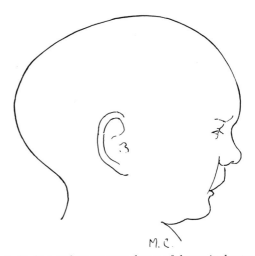

Figure 19.   Anteroposterior and lateral appearance of head of infant with premature closure of the sagittal suture.

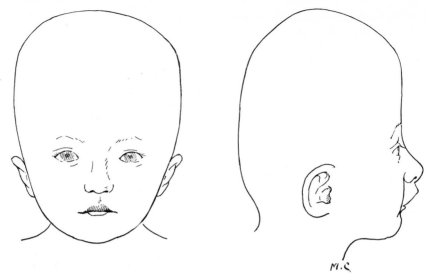

Figure 20. Anteroposterior and lateral appearance of head of infant with premature closure of the coronal suture. Often the orbital and nasal bones are also involved, causing much more deformity of the facial structures than is shown in this illustration.

retardation of growth of the brain. In the first year of life, the operation consists of creating an artificial suture line by excising a groove of bone at the site of the closed suture. Since there is a tendency for rapid reformation of bone in an infant, it is the usual practice to place a cuff of polyethylene film along each edge of the bone to delay their rejoining. Even so, thin bridges of bone grow quickly, and if solid union occurs too promptly the operation should be repeated within the first two years of life. In older, untreated children who develop increased intracranial pressure, surgical procedures are directed toward creating some type of decompression. As a rule operations for correction of premature closure of the sutures after the first or at most the second year of life are unrepaying.

HYDROCEPHALUS

Hydrocephalus is a condition in which there is an excessive amount of cerebrospinal fluid within the cranial cavity. It is characterized by distention of the ventricles by fluid which does not have an outlet to the subarachnoid spaces, or which is obstructed in its passage through the subarachnoid spaces, or which is not absorbed into the venous system. In brief, the condition is one of obstruction in either circulation or absorption of the cerebrospinal fluid, and sometimes both. There is little evidence to indicate that the cerebrospinal fluid is produced in excessive amounts except in rare instances of papillomatous tumors of the choroid plexus.

Though some uncertainty persists about the sites and mechanism of formation and absorption of cerebrospinal fluid, it seems clear that the area of principal origin is within the ventricles and the area of principal absorption is in the blood vessels of the pia arachnoid over the cerebral hemispheres. The circulation of the fluid, sometimes referred to as the "third circulation," is from each lateral ventricle through the foramina of Monro into the third ventricle, through the aqueduct of Sylvius into the fourth ventricle, and thence through the foramina of Luschka and Magendie into the subarachnoid spaces. In the subarachnoid spaces, the fluid extends into the spinal canal to bathe the cord and spinal nerves and through various basal cisterns to ascend over the cerebral hemispheres.

Congenital hydrocephalus is spoken of as either communicating or noncommunicating, depending on whether there is transmission of fluid between the ventricles and the subarachnoid spaces. The question of which condition exists is settled by demonstrating whether air or dye passes from one space to the other. Stenosis or failure of development of the sylvian aqueduct and occlusion of the foramina of the fourth ventricle cause the common forms of ventricular obstruction, while faulty development or prenatal obstruction of the subarachnoid spaces, particularly the basal cisterns, accounts for the communicating type of hydrocephalus. The common association of spinal meningocele, especially myelomeningocele, and hydrocephalus is due to the obstruction of cerebrospinal fluid passages by malformation of the hindbrain at the foramen magnum.

The signs of hydrocephalus may be apparent in the disproportionately large head at the time of birth, but, more often, the gradually enlarging head does not become apparent for some weeks or, rarely, several months. As the head enlarges, the fontanelles enlarge and bulge, the sutures separate, scalp veins become prominent, and there is a downward displacement of the eyeballs. Slowly advancing hydrocephalus is frequently unaccompanied by symptoms, and the infant may be reported by parents to be brighter than their normal children were at the same age. More rapidly developing hydrocephalus may cause vomiting, convulsions, hyperirritability and alterations in respiration and cardiac rate.

In diagnosing the condition, it is recognized that hydrocephalus may be of relatively minor degree or may be spontaneously arrested when the child is brought for examination, necessitating periodic measurement of the head at short intervals and comparison with tables of normal growth. Of great con-

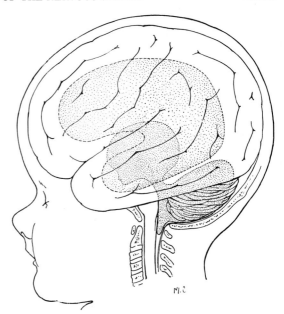

Figure 22. Hydrocephalus due to prenatal obstruction of the foramina of Magendie and Luschka. The fourth ventricle is dilated into a huge cystlike structure filling the posterior fossa and herniating into the upper spinal canal.

cern should be the retardation and permanent mental damage which occurs if progressive hydrocephalus goes untreated. In differential diagnosis, subdural hematoma, papilloma of the choroid plexus and intracranial tumors should be ruled out respectively by aspiration of subdural spaces, by examination of the ventricular fluid for xanthochromia and elevated protein content and by air studies (Figs. 21, 22 and 23). By the same studies, other rarer conditions may also be identified.

A small amount of air injected directly into the ventricle by insertion of the needle through the anterior fontanelle will demonstrate the thickness of the brain and may be helpful in determining the advisability of employing surgery. When the ventricles have become so dilated that the overlying brain is but a few millimeters thick, there is little to be hoped for in the way of benefit even with the successful arrest of the hydrocephalus.

Surgical treatment of congenital hydrocephalus consists of shunting the cerebrospinal fluid from one compartment to another in the normal fluid pathways, or from the cerebrospinal fluid compartments to some other location in the body where the fluid can be either absorbed or excreted. When there is obstruction in the sylvian aqueduct, or at the outlets of the fourth ventricle, one has recourse to third ventriculostomy or a tube

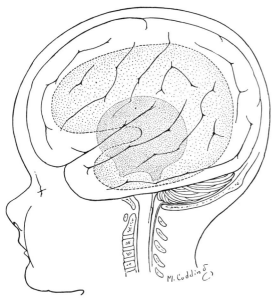

Figure 21. Hydrocephalus due to congenital obstruction of the aqueduct of Sylvius. The lateral and third ventricles are dilated, but there is no demonstrable communication through the midbrain to the fourth ventricle.

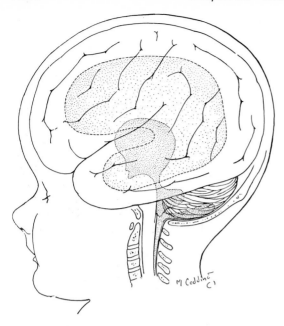

Figure 23. Hydrocephalus due to prenatal obstruction or failure of development of the intracranial surface subarachnoid pathways. There is dilatation of the entire ventricular system and cisterna magna as well.

shunt between the lateral ventricle and the subarachnoid space in the cisterna magna and upper cervical canal. In communicating hydrocephalus, the shunting procedures are those from the ventricle, or some part of the subarachnoid spaces, by catheter to the pleural space, the peritoneal cavity, the ureter or the right cardiac atrium through the jugular vein. Although none of these methods is uniformly satisfactory, they provide the best means of treatment available and are deserving of trial.

Neurosurgical Relief of Pain

Pain is a specific sensory experience which defies further definition. Yet, like other subjective phenomena, "it is known to us by experience and described by illustration." It is recognized as an important warning of danger to the organism and in this respect serves a useful purpose. The recognition of the cause and the means of correction are the principal matters of concern in the science and art of medicine. When the cause cannot be identified or corrected, the continuation of pain serves no useful purpose. Severe and unrelenting pain becomes a serious problem for it soon is accompanied by anxieties which together can lead to both bodily and moral deterioration of the individual. Medicinal management of pain has its place, but also its limitations, since in pain of maximal intensity a reduction of 75 per cent is the most that can be expected with the available agents. Opiates have the advantage not only of an analgesic action, but they reduce anxiety and create a state of detachment. The undesirable effects and the diminishing ability to assuage a patient's complaints by increasing the dosage of opiates are well recognized. Furthermore, numerous drugs developed as morphine substitutes have not provided a solution to the problem.

That severe and unrelenting pain in incurable disease can often be relieved by an appropriate operation on some part of the nervous system is too often overlooked or requested only after drug addiction has occurred or the disease has advanced too far to justify an operation. In cancerous disease, it is usually possible to anticipate the course, at least with respect to the degree in which pain will constitute a major problem in management. If there are months of life expectancy, pain-relieving operations should be employed when it becomes evident that medications will be inadqute. In noncancerous painful states, it is imperative to establish that the complaint is not psychoneurotic, for to impose a pain-relieving operation and its resulting neurologic deficit without relieving pain leads to unhappiness for all concerned.

ANATOMY AND PHYSIOLOGY OF PAIN PATHWAYS

The ability to perceive pain depends on an intact system of nerve pathways from sensory end organs to the highest levels in the brain. Whether or not pain occurs depends upon an appropriate stimulus and the individual's threshold for pain. The reaction to pain must also depend on nerve pathways, but they are little understood and the response is largely a matter of what the sensation means to the individual.

Painful impulses are initiated in special receptors found extensively in skin, in many subcutaneous structures and in viscera. Those arising in somatic structures of the trunk and extremities are transmitted along fibers in spinal nerves to their respective posterior root ganglia, whereas visceral sensation is transmitted to these ganglia directly or indirectly via autonomic nerves and white rami communicantes. The cell bodies of all sensory nerves lie in the posterior root ganglia and the dendrites of those which subserve pain enter the posterior horn of the cord via the posterior roots, where they synapse with a second neuron.

Impulses traversing the second neuron are promptly carried through the anterior commissure to the opposite side of the cord, where they ascend in the lateral spinothalamic tract to the thalamus and thence through additional neurons to the cerebral cortex, where it is believed appreciation and reaction to pain occurs.

Pain impulses arising in the head and neck regions are carried not only by upper cervical spinal nerves, but also by the fifth, seventh, ninth and tenth cranial nerves. These nerves connect with the thalamus by way of secondary neurons, as to the spinal nerves.

The sites at which pain is felt have for the most part a segmental relationship to the areas stimulated. For the skin and supporting structures of the body, the arrangement is beltlike and the patterns of innervation by peripheral nerves and nerve roots are well established. However, there are wide overlaps of innervation, particularly in the skin. For example, division of a peripheral nerve results in total loss of pain sense in only a limited area supplied by the nerve because of a dual innervation in the marginal regions by adjacent peripheral nerves. In the case of spinal nerve roots to truncal areas, the overlap of sensation in the periphery is such that it is necessary to divide at least three consecutive roots before loss of pain sense in the skin is detectable.

Pain arising from visceral structures has a deep aching quality and is poorly localized, in contradistinction to the sharper quality of pain having a more discrete localization when it arises from somatic structures. Visceral pain fibers enter the cord via the same posterior nerve roots as do somatic pain fibers, an anatomic arrangement which accounts for referred pain to the corresponding superficial somatic dermatome. If the noxious stimulus is of sufficient degree, the spread of excitation, through multisynaptic fibers in the spinal cord from either visceral or somatic nerves, may be to adjacent or even remote segments on the same or opposite sides, and may be perceived as "referred" pain in other regions.

What is called "central pain" is not well understood, but the condition occurs in lesions of the cord which partially involve the lateral spinothalamic tracts and in lesions of the brain which involve the thalamus. The condition is characterized by a persistent discomfort and hyperpathia or hypersensitivity to stimuli in the painful areas. Both the cord and the brain appear to be insensitive to pain from any kind of direct stimulus.

SURGICAL PROCEDURES

The principal ways by which pain may be reduced or abolished are by interruption of peripheral nerves, by interruption of sensory nerve roots and by interruption of pain tracts within the central nervous system.

PERIPHERAL AND CRANIAL NERVES. Except for the head region, painful conditions are few for which interruption of the peripheral nerves can be employed to advantage. In painful vascular occlusive conditions involving a lower leg or foot, or more particularly the toes, the anatomic arrangement of nerves is well suited to local nerve section. The sural and saphenous nerves are purely sensory nerves, while the tibial, superficial and deep peroneal nerves, though mixed, have motor fibers of no great importance. By division of all of these nerves, the lower leg and foot can be made totally insensitive, or selected areas of anesthesia can be produced by dividing the appropriate nerves. The use of alcohol or phenol injections into the nerves for their destruction is inadvisable because of possible sloughing of tissues already devitalized by the impaired vascularity for which the procedure is employed. The nerves should be interrupted by direct section or crushing through short incisions in the leg. The obvious disadvantage of the procedure is the resulting total sensory loss which exposes the foot to trophic changes.

Painful neuromas at the ends of divided peripheral nerves are a common source of complaint, and numerous methods are suggested for avoiding the condition when sectioning a nerve. None of them seems to have advantage over sectioning the nerve cleanly and allowing it to retract into surrounding tissues. Sometimes it is useful to redivide a nerve in this fashion proximal to a painful neuroma, but successive operations on a nerve are usually unrepaying. Hyperalgesia frequently accompanies an incompletely regenerated peripheral nerve. The problem arises especially in thoracic or flank wounds, where intercostal nerves are divided. Occasionally, benefit follows temporary procaine block or even proximal division of a nerve or its accompanying root, but the results are by no means uniform. A patient fully informed of the nature of the complaint can usually be induced to accommodate for it.

SENSORY NERVE ROOT SECTION (RHIZOTOMY). Division of spinal nerve roots is performed intradurally and the posterior root is divided between its ganglion and the cord. Since motor roots remain intact, the operation has the advantage of interrupting sensation and preserving motion. In addition, the divided roots do not regenerate. There is limited use for posterior rhizotomy, since in rendering an area of the trunk or extremity anesthetic, it is necessary to sever multiple roots to allow for overlap from adjacent roots. The loss of sensation, including tactile and position senses in an upper limb, renders it largely useless. Occasionally, when the lower part of the brachial plexus is involved by cancer extending from the breast or apex of the lung, division of seventh and eighth cervical and upper thoracic roots suffices to reduce the pain yet leaves the fifth and sixth roots with useful sensation in the thumb and index fingers. In case the entire brachial plexus is involved by tumor, section of all sensory roots

supplying the limb would not result in more disuse of the limb than already existed. Rhizotomy in the treatment of pain following herpes zoster has given disappointing results and should not be recommended. The same is true in cases of painful phantom limb following amputation.

Section of the upper four posterior thoracic roots bilaterally has sometimes been employed successfully for relief of angina pectoris. It has the disadvantage of producing a band of anesthesia in the skin, but it has the advantage over sympathectomy which requires an operation on each side.

By far the most satisfactory use of rhizotomy is section of cranial and upper cervical roots for relief of painful states in the head and neck. Not all of these states are due to cancer; they sometimes result from painful scars of heavy radiation used in the treatment of cancer. Experience with rhizotomy of the trigeminal and glossopharyngeal nerves for major neuralgias has demonstrated its usefulness. The face, nasal passages, internal ear, tongue, mouth and upper pharynx all receive sensory innervation from the trigeminal, sensory component of the facial nerve, glossopharyngeal and rostral fibers of the vagus nerve. Any or all of these nerves can be cut on one side through a single intracranial exposure without concern over important handicap to the patient. Section of the nervus intermedius is attended by the risk of facial palsy and need not be performed except when pain is deep in the ear. An alternative to section of these multiple cranial nerve roots is incision into their descending tracts in the medulla. This operation has a limited use, since it is not consistently successful in producing full loss of pain in the intended areas, and because an incision of adequate extent is attended by unwanted divisions of adjacent nerve tracts.

When the painful lesion borders or straddles the areas of the head and neck supplied by both cranial and cervical nerves, the operation to expose the cranial nerves for section can be extended into the upper cervical canal to permit simultaneous posterior rhizotomy of any or all of the upper four posterior cervical roots.

SPINOTHALAMIC CORDOTOMY. Spinothalamic cordotomy entails division of the spinothalamic tract in the anterolateral portion of the cord. It is best suited for pain in the trunk and lower limbs and is performed bilaterally in the uppermost segments of the thoracic cord (Fig. 24). It is expected that, as a result, pain and temperature senses will be abolished below the middle thoracic levels and that other forms of sensation as well as motor functions of the limbs will be preserved. There is usually impairment of bladder function in the nature of urinary retention immediately after cordotomy, but in most patients, particularly those who are ambulatory, adequate function returns. In males, the operation usually impairs sexual function. The principal concern is over some resulting palsy in the lower limbs, but serious loss of function is rare. Satisfactory relief of pain is expected in at least 70 per cent of patients, and mortality following the operation is ascribable mostly to factors other than the operation itself.

High cervical cordotomy is employed for painful lesions above the thoracic level, particularly for those about the upper chest, shoulder and upper limb, such as cancer of the breast and apical bronchogenic tumor. In these cases, the operation is unilateral on the side opposite the lesion. Bilateral high cervical cordotomy is accompanied by possible respiratory complications. Also, since there is no assurance that the level of analgesia will be high enough for relief of the pain, there is need at times to combine cervical cordotomy with division of several cervical sensory roots. Of late, there is rejuvenated interest in high cervical cordotomy under direct vision, with improved results over those accompanying past techniques.

At present, percutaneous chordotomy is under extensive trial. Several methods of producing destructive lesions of the anterior spinothalamic tract are in use. The various methods employ the transdural introduction into or against the cord of a radioactive strontium needle; a unipolar anodal device for electrolysis; a needle that produces destruction by radio frequency, and a cryogenic probe. The procedures are each performed with the aid of fluoroscopy and have been reported as having a relatively high degree of success but not without occasional complications.

THALAMOTOMY. In view of the increasing familiarity with the use of stereotaxic devices in the surgical treatment of hyperkinetic and hypertonic disorders, it has seemed logical to produce lesions in the thalamus, particularly the caudal ventral lateral nucleus, in the hope of giving relief of pain through interruption of pain pathways at this level. Although in a few scattered instances temporary improvement has been accomplished, the results on the whole have been disappointing and much more experience with the procedure is required in order to evaluate its usefulness.

SENSORY CORTICAL ABLATION. The sensory cortex of the cerebrum in the postrolandic area, and possibly in supplementary areas of cortex, undoubtedly plays some role along with the thalamus in the perception and reaction to pain. Wide resection of the sensory cortex on one, and even on both sides, has been tried, especially when other surgical procedures for the relief of pain have failed. For the most part, such efforts have been

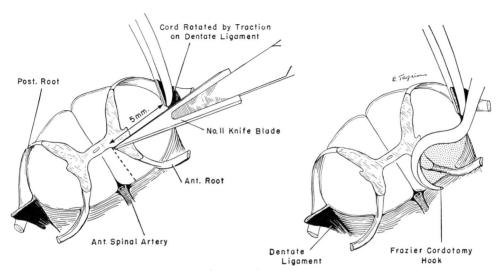

Figure 24. Technique of anterolateral corodotomy at upper thoracic level.

made in cases of phantom limb pain. Few benefits and mostly failures have been reported. It seems unlikely that more success would follow cortical ablation in the treatment of other types of pain. One of the striking observations made on youths who have had cerebral hemispherectomy for the control of convulsive seizures, sometimes including excision of the thalamus as well, has been the limited deficit in sensory perception on the opposite side of the body.

FRONTAL LOBOTOMY. There is little to indicate in theory or experience that frontal lobotomy, which interrupts principally the frontothalamic connections, reduces the perception of pain. Yet, it sometimes dramatically relieves the psychic aspects accompanying pain. The operation is best suited for trial in those patients who have widespread painful cancerous disease not readily controlled by other therapeutic measures and who have a limited time to live. The extensive transection of the white matter in the prefrontal region commonly employed for the treatment of psychotic states is not appropriate in others because of the profound alteration in mood and intellectual functions which may follow. Lesser procedures, in which the operation is performed on one side only, or in which a part of the frontal connections is interrupted on each side, are found to be beneficial. When the operation is successful, not only is the patient less troubled by his sensations, but addiction to opiates ceases to be a problem. In lieu of direct surgical transection of limited areas of white matter, Grantham has proposed destruction of subcortical tissue in the medial inferior area of the frontal lobes by electrocoagulation, increasing the area of destruction in stages to accomplish the desired result. White and Sweet have modified the procedure by using wire electrodes implanted in desired areas of the frontal lobes for coagulation of tissue progressively over a period of a few weeks.

HYPOPHYSECTOMY. The purpose of employing hypophysectomy, or ablation of other endocrine organs, is to alter the hormonal effect on certain types of metastatic cancer, principally mammary and prostatic, in the hope of producing a temporary arrest of the disease. Usually, pain of important degree in these patients reflects the presence of skeletal metastases. The cortical and medullary parts of bone are relatively, if not totally lacking in pain sensitivity, but the periosteum is richly supplied with pain receptors. Unfortu-

nately, there are no tests which will predictably indicate what success may accrue from removing the pituitary. If remission of the disease does follow, one of the first signs of success is relief of pain. The speed with which relief can occur following operation makes it all the more difficult to understand the mechanism by which it occurs, but in these common cancerous diseases of breast and prostate, hypophysectomy has a place in the management of pain.

CHEMICAL BLOCK OF NERVES AND NERVE ROOTS. The injection of procaine in the paravertebral or intrathecal regions for temporary block of sensory impulses has little value in dealing with persistent pain, though the hope is sometimes voiced that by "breaking the circuit" even temporarily, some good will be accomplished.

Attempts to block spinal nerves for long periods by paravertebral injection of absolute alcohol or phenol are highly unsatisfactory even with the aid of radiologic guidance of the needle. It is virtually necessary that the point of the needle be within the nerve for a successful block, and when it is considered that injection of at least several nerves is required to produce even a small area of anesthesia, the limitations of the method are evident. Paravertebral block of viscerosensory nerves traversing the sympathetic ganglionated chain, however, has had somewhat more success. The method has been employed principally in the second and third lumbar ganglia to produce vasodilatation in the lower limbs, and in the stellate ganglia or upper thoracic ganglionated chain to counteract cardiac pain. In patients with coronary disease or peripheral vascular disease, who may be too debilitated to tolerate surgery safely, the injection procedures may be justified, but surgical section of nerves is always to be preferred.

Intrathecal injection of ethyl alcohol to block roots of the cauda equina is a procedure of long use and frequent success in the relief of pain in dermatomes below the first sacral. It is found useful particularly in cancer of pelvic viscera that produces pain over the sacral region and perineum. The procedure consists of slowly injecting 1 cc. of absolute alcohol into the subarachnoid space at the lumbosacral level as the patient lies prone with head lowered and pelvis elevated. Since alcohol has a specific gravity less than that of spinal fluid, the alcohol rises in the caudal sac and bathes the sacral roots of the cauda equina. If pain is more pronounced on one side, the patient is rotated so that the more painful side is uppermost. If one injection is insufficient to relieve pain, successive injections of never more than 1 cc. at a time can be given on successive days. If care is taken, it is unusual to produce any significant or lasting motor weakness in the extremities, though loss or impairment of sphincter control of bladder and bowel at least temporarily is common. If circumstances make it reasonable to accept possible sphincter impairment for relief of pain, the procedure is appropriate.

A fresh 5 per cent solution of phenol in dehydrated glycerine is sometimes used for subthecal injection to block nerve roots of the cauda equina. The procedure is similar to that followed in alcohol injection, except that phenol has a greater specific gravity than spinal fluid and the injection is made with the patient in a sitting position. Advantage is claimed for the use of phenol in that sphincter disturbance is thought to be less than with alcohol, but experience shows there is little difference.

Disorders of Involuntary Movements

A variety of hyperkinetic movements are commonly regarded as evidence of disease of the basal ganglia or of their immediate connections with other centers of the brain. Although the emphasis is often put on tremor or other involuntary movements, there are usually accompanying changes which can assume importance as great as or greater than the tremor, such as weakness, spasticity or hypotonicity, dysarthria, dysphagia and a degree of emotionalism, all of which may occur without any true paralysis or reflex or sensory changes. In certain diseases in which involuntary movements are present, it has been found that destruction of some part of the basal ganglia or their connections may reduce tremor and also hypertonicity.

Parkinson's disease, or paralysis agitans, is characterized principally by hyperkinesis and hypertonicity. This disease, together with similar conditions referred to broadly as "parkinsonism," has most often been treated by surgery. The tremor, which in the hands is characterized as a "pill rolling" motion, occurs at rest and is lessened by voluntary movement. Though it is often the more obvious, it may not be as distressing or as restricting to activity as the associated hypertonicity. General weakness, slowness and poverty of movement are responsible for physical handicap which may progress to near total disability. Other especially distressing symptoms sometimes present are excessive salivation and oculogyric crises. Distinction is made by some between paralysis agitans believed to be degenerative in nature and conditions designated as parkinsonian such as chronic encephalitis or carbon

monoxide poisoning, but tremor and rigidity are common to all.

Although collectively several thousand patients with parkinsonism have had palliative operations for their disease, the treatment is still in the experimental stage. Surgical procedures have utilized resection of the premotor cortex; incision of cerebral peduncle or pyramidal tract in the cord; ligation of the anterior choroidal artery; and destructive lesions of the ansa lenticularis, the medial portion of the globus pallidus, the anterolateral part of the thalamus and several regions of the extrapyramidal system in the brain stem. At present, most operations are directed to the globus pallidus and the thalamus, by means of some stereotaxic device, and destructive lesions are made by a number of methods including mechanical, chemical, electrical, cryogenic, ultrasonic and radiational.

The optimum site of the surgical lesion and the most effective method of producing it are unknown, but most investigators agree that pallidal lesions are more effective in relieving rigidity, while thalamic lesions are more effective in relieving tremor. The results in relieving tremor by operation are better than those for rigidity, and it is well established that patients with poverty of movement are not improved, nor are those with predominantly bulbar symptoms such as dysarthria, dysphagia, drooling or fixed stare. The results are best in relatively young individuals with a minimum of rigidity and with tremor predominant on one side of the body.

Other dyskinesias which are reported as

sometimes deriving benefit from stereotaxic surgery of the basal ganglia are dystonia musculorum deformans, hemiballismus, athetosis, intention tremors and a variety of other less common hyperkinetic disorders.

The mortality rate of these operations is about 2 per cent. Complications, though they have been steadily reduced, include motor palsy, intellectual and psychologic changes, speech difficulty, convulsive seizures, intracranial hemorrhage and infection. The incidence of morbidity and mortality rises if the operation is performed on both sides. Even with the uncertainties and risks attending this type of surgery, benefit is frequently secured in those patients carefully selected for operation.

READING REFERENCES

Adams, R. D., Fisher, C. M., Hakim, S., Ojemann, R. G., and Sweet, W. H.: Symptomatic occult hydrocephalus with "normal" cerebrospinal fluid pressure. J.A.M.A. 273: 117, 1965.

Adson, A. W.: Intraspinal tumors; collective review. Internat. Abstr. Surg. 67:225, 1938.

Bailey, P.: Intracranial Tumors. 2nd ed. Springfield, Illinois, Charles C Thomas, 1948.

Bailey, P., and Cushing, H.: A Classification of Tumors of the Glioma Group on a Histogenic Basis with a Correlated Study of Prognosis. Philadelphia, J. B. Lippincott Company, 1926.

Barr, J. S., Kubik, C. S., Molloy, M. K., McNeill, M., Riseborough, E. J., and White, J. C.: Evaluation of end results in treatment of ruptured lumbar intervertebral discs with protrusion of nucleus pulposus. Surg. Gyn. & Obst. 125:250, 1967.

Brinkman, C. A., Wegst, A. V., and Kahn, E. A.: Brain scanning with mercury²⁰³ labeled neohydrin. J. Neurosurg. 19:644, 1962.

Campbell, J. B., Bassett, C. A. L., and Bohler, J.: Frozen-irradiated homografts shielded with microfilter sheaths in peripheral nerve surgery. J. Trauma 3:302, 1963.

Cooperative study of intracranial aneurysms and subarachnoid hemorrhage, report on (VIII sections). J. Neurosurg. 24:779, 922, 1034; 25:98, 219, 321, 467, 574, 660, 1966.

Crutchfield, W. G.: Skeletal traction in the treatment of injuries to the cervical spine. J.A.M.A. 155:29, 1954.

Dandy, W. E.: Meniere's disease; its diagnosis and method of treatment. Arch. Surg. 16:1127, 1928.

Davidoff, L. M.: Pseudotumor cerebri: benign intracranial hypertension. Neurology 6:605, 1956.

Davis, L., and Davis, R. A.: Principles of Neurological Surgery. Philadelphia, W. B. Saunders Company, 1963.

Earl, K. M., Baldwin, M., and Penfield, W.: Incisural sclerosis and temporal lobe seizures produced by hippocampal herniation at birth. Arch. Neurol. & Psychiat. 69:27, 1953.

French, L. A.: The use of steroids in the treatment of cerebral edema. Bull. New York Acad. Med. 42:301, 1966.

Gardner, J., and Sava, G. A.: Hemifacial spasm—a reversible pathophysiologic state. J. Neurosurg. 19:240, 1962.

Grant, F. C.: Surgical methods for relief of pain in head and neck. Proc. Assoc. Research Nerv. & Ment. Dis. 23:408, 1943.

Grantham, E. G.: Prefrontal lobotomy for relief of pain with a report of a new operative technique. J. Neurosurg. 8:405, 1951.

Green, J. R.: Temporal lobectomy with special reference to selection of epileptic patients. J. Neurosurg. 26:584, 1967.

Guidetti, B.: Tractotomy for the relief of trigeminal neuralgia; observations in 124 cases. J. Neurosurg. 7:499, 1950.

Hamby, W. B.: Carotid-Cavernous Fistula. Springfield, Illinois, Charles C Thomas, 1966.

Heaton, L. D., Coates, J. B., Jr., and Meirowsky, A. M. (eds.): Neurological Surgery of Trauma. Washington, D.C., The Historical Unit, U.S. Army Medical Service, U.S. Government Printing Office, 1960.

Ingraham, F. D., Alexander, E., Jr., and Matson, D. D.: Clinical studies in craniosynostosis, analysis of fifty cases and description of a method of surgical treatment. Surgery 24:518, 1948.

Ingraham, F. D., and Matson, D. D.: Neurosurgery of Infancy and Childhood. Springfield, Illinois, Charles C Thomas, 1954.

Kernohan, J. W., and Sayre, G. P.: Tumors of the Central Nervous System, Washington, D.C., Armed Forces Institute of Pathology, 1952.

Krayenbuhl, H., Maspes, P. E., and Sweet, W. H.: Progress in Neurological Surgery, Vol. I. Chicago, Year Book Medical Publishers, Inc., 1966.

Krynauw, R. A.: Infantile hemiplegia treated by removal of one cerebral hemisphere. South African M. J. 24: 539, 1950.

Lewis, T.: Pain. New York, The MacMillan Company, 1942.

Linton, E.: Peripheral vascular disease. New England J. Med. 260:272; 322; 370, 1959.

Luessenhop, A. J., Kachmann, R., Jr., Shevlin, W., and Ferrero, A. A.: Clinical evaluation of artificial embolization in management of large cerebral arteriovenous malformations. J. Neurosurg. 23:400, 1965.

Mayfield, F. H.: Causalgia. Springfield, Illinois, Charles C Thomas, 1951.

McKenzie, K. G., and Alexander, E.: Restoration of facial function by nerve anastomosis. Ann. Surg. 132:411, 1950.

Merritt, H. H.: Evaluation of surgical therapy of disorders of the basal ganglia. Neurology 6:755, 1956.

Meyers, R.: The surgical treatment of "focal" epilepsy: an inquiry into current premises, their implementation and the criteria employed in reporting results. Epilepsia 3:1, 1954.

Mullan, S., Hekmatpanah, J., Dobben, G., and Beckman, F.: Percutaneous intramedullary cordotomy utilizing the unipolar anodal electrolytic lesion. J. Neurosurg. 22:538, 1965.

Murphey, F., and Simmons, J. C. H.: Ruptured cervical disk: experiences with 250 cases. Am. Surg. 32:83, 1966.

Nathan, P. W., and Scott, T. G.: Intrathecal phenol for intractable pain: safety and dangers of method. Lancet 1:76, 1958.

Olivecrona, H., and Rives, J.: Arteriovenous aneurysms of the brain. Arch. Neurol. & Psychiat. 59:567, 1948.

Penfield, W., and Kristiansen, K.: Epileptic Seizure Patterns. Springfield, Illinois, Charles C Thomas, 1951.

Pollock, L. J., and others: Electrodiagnosis of lesions of peripheral nerves in man. Arch. Neurol. & Psychiat. 60:1, 1948.

Pool, J. L.: Suboccipital surgery for acoustic neurinomas: advantages and disadvantages. J. Neurosurg. 24:483, 1966.

Pudenz, R. H., Findlay, E. R., Hurd, A. H., and Sheldon, C. H.: Ventriculo-auriculostomy; a technique for shunting cerebrospinal fluid into the right auricle; preliminary report. J. Neurosurg. 14:171, 1957.

Ray, B. S.: Sympathectomy of the upper extremity. Evaluation of surgical methods. J. Neurosurg. 10:624, 1953.

Ray, B. S.: Differential diagnosis between ruptured lumbar intervertebral disk and certain diseases of the spinal and peripheral nervous systems. S. Clin. North America 26:272, 1946.

Ray, B. S., and Console, A. D.: Evaluation of total sympathectomy. Ann. Surg. *130*:652, 1949.

Ray, B. S., and Console, A. D.: Residual sympathetic pathways after paravertebral sympathectomy. J. Neurosurg. 5:23, 1948.

Ray, B. S., and Dunbar, H. S.: Thrombosis of the dural venous sinuses as a cause of pseudo tumor cerebri. Ann. Surg. *134*:376, 1951.

Ray, B. S., and Neill, C. L.: Abdominal visceral sensation in man. Ann. Surg. *126*:709, 1947.

Ray, B. S., and Wolff, H. G.: Studies on pain: "spread of pain," evidence on site of spread within the neuraxis of effects of painful stimulation. Arch. Neurol. & Psychiat. 53:257, 1945.

Rosomoff, H. L., Carroll, F., Brown, J., and Sheptak, P.: Percutaneous radiofrequency cervical cordotomy: technique. J. Neurosurg. 23:639, 1965.

Ruge, D., Brochner, R., and Davis, L.: A study of the treatment of 637 patients with trigeminal neuralgia. J. Neurosurg. *15*:528, 1958.

Russell, D. S.: Observations on the Pathology of Hydrocephalus. London, His Majesty's Stationery Office, 1949.

Russell, D. S., and Donald, C.: The mechanism of internal hydrocephalus in spina bifida. Brain, 58:203, 1935.

Scarff, J. E.: Treatment of hydrocephalus; an historical and critical review of methods and results. J. Neuro. Neurosurg. & Psychiat. 26:1, 1963.

Schneider, R. C.: Trauma to the Spine and Spinal Cord; Correlative Neurosurgery. Springfield, Illinois, Charles C Thomas, 1955.

Seddon, H. J. (ed.): Peripheral nerve injuries. Medical Research Council Special Report Series No. 282. London, Her Majesty's Stationery Office, 1954.

Sjöqvist, O.: Ten years' experience with trigeminal tractotomy. Brasil-méd. *10*:259, 1948.

Spurling, R. G.: Lesions of the Lumbar Intervertebral Disc. Springfield, Illinois, Charles C Thomas, 1953.

Taarnhøj, P.: Decompression of the trigeminal root and the posterior part of the ganglion as treatment in trigeminal neuralgia; preliminary communciation. J. Neurosurg. 9:288, 1952.

Tanaka, K., Ito, K., and Wagai, T.: The localization of brain tumors by ultrasonic techniques: a clinical review of 111 cases. J. Neurosurg. 23:135, 1965.

Taveras, J. M., and Wood, E. H.: Diagnostic Neuroradiology. Baltimore, The Williams & Wilkins Co., 1964.

Thulin, C., and Feringer, E. R.: Microfilter sheaths in peripheral nerve surgery. J. Trauma *1*:139, 1961.

Torkildsen, A.: Ventriculocisternostomy: A Palliative Operation in Different Types of Non-Communicating Hydrocephalus. Oslo, Johan Grundt Tanun Forlag, 1947.

Vieth, R. G., and Odom, G. L.: Intracranial metastases and their neurosurgical treatment. J. Neurosurg. 23:375, 1965.

White, J. C., Smithwick, R. H., and Simione, F. A.: The Autonomic Nervous System. New York, The Macmillan Company, 1952.

White, J. C., and Sweet, W. H.: Pain. Its Mechanisms and Neurosurgical Control. Springfield, Illinois, Charles C Thomas, 1955.

Woltman, H., Kernohan, J., Adson, A., and Craig, W.: Intramedullary tumors of the spinal cord and gliomas of intradural portion of filum terminale. Arch. Neurol. & Psychiat. 65:378, 1951.

Woodhall, B., and Beebe, G. W. (eds.): Peripheral Nerve Regenerations; A Follow-up Study of 3,656 World War II Injuries. Veterans Administration Medical Monograph. Washington, United States Government Printing Office, 1956.

Yahr, M. D., and Bering, E. A. (eds.): Parkinson's Disease. Present Status and Research Trends. Bethesda, Maryland, U.S. Department of Health, Education and Welfare, 1966.

Chapter 37

ARTIFICIAL ORGANS

by
CLARENCE DENNIS, M.D.
and
KARL E. KARLSON, M.D.

CLARENCE DENNIS was born in Minnesota and migrated east to graduate with honors from Harvard College and The Johns Hopkins University School of Medicine. He returned to the University of Minnesota for post-graduate work in physiology and surgery in which he earned advanced degrees. Subsequently, he attained professorial rank in the Department of Surgery. He became Professor and Chairman of the Department of Surgery, State University of New York Downstate Medical Center in 1952. He is Surgeon-in-Chief and Director of Surgery and Surgical Specialties at the Kings County Hospital, Brooklyn. His bibliography and society memberships reflect his broad, basic and pioneering interests in the surgical problems of artificial organs.

KARL E. KARLSON was born in Worcester, Massachusetts, where his father was a Baptist Church minister and Professor of Philosophy at Clark University. His parents moved to Minnesota and he received his elementary, college, medical and surgical education at the University of Minnesota. He is Professor of Surgery at the State University of New York Downstate Medical Center.

In the past three decades, rapid advances in medical engineering have permitted the development of apparatus to perform some of the functions of some organs. Heart-lung machines, artificial kidneys, pacemakers, artificial heart valves, and vascular prostheses are examples. Intrathoracic artificial hearts are still in an experimental stage, although some intrathoracic cardiac assist devices have been given clinical trial.

CARDIOPULMONARY BYPASS

In the experimental laboratory, small pumps and oxygenators have been in use for decades for perfusion of individual organs. The first serious attempt to perfuse the whole body was made by Gibbon and his associates before World War II. Gibbon was able to make a pump-oxygenator of sufficient capacity to perfuse a cat during 25 minutes of pulmonary arterial clamping with survival of the animal. His oxygenator consisted of a vertical rotating cylinder upon the inner surface of which blood could be filmed. Following the war, Dennis and associates used an enlarged rotating multiple cylinder oxygenator with diaphragm-type compression pumps and internal valves for successful perfusion of large dogs. Because the capacity of the rotating multiple cylinder oxygenator was inadequate for human application, they devised a vertical rotating screen oxygenator which was used for attempted repair of congenital cardiac defects in two patients in 1951. Concomitantly, Gibbon designed a stationary vertical screen oxygenator (Fig. 1), which in combination with roller pumps was used for the first successful pump-supported open-heart operation, in 1953.

A different type of oxygenator was designed by Anderson, a Swedish engineer, and evaluated by Björk at the Karolinska Institute. This consisted in multiple rotating discs mounted upon a horizontal shaft, dipping into a pool of blood. The design was modified and improved by Kay and Cross, and the so-called Kay-Cross oxygenator (Fig. 2) has been one of the most popular of many film oxygenators in clinical use.

DeWall and his associates developed the first bubble oxygenator to be widely accepted for clinical use. The bubble oxygenator consists of an oxygenating column some 18 inches long and 1 inch in diameter through

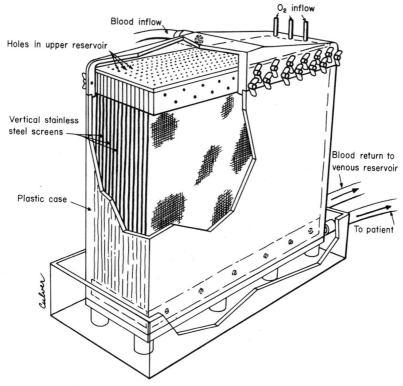

Figure 1.   Vertical screen oxygenator, designed by Gibbon.

which blood rises while oxygen is bubbled through it. The blood and bubble mixture then passes from the top of the column into a de-bubbling chamber containing beads or shredded material coated with a film of anti-foam, a silicone material which is biologically inactive but which lowers surface tension remarkably and thus assists in the removal of bubbles from the blood. This principle has been incorporated into disposable oxyge-nators, in which the entire oxygenating, de-

bubbling, and collecting chambers are con-structed of thin sheets of flexible plastic material (Fig. 3).

Although bubble oxygenators are effective, simple, and economical, they are suspected of introducing microbubbles of gas into the arterial blood, especially in the late stages of prolonged use, and the serious complica-tions therefrom have been well documented. For this reason, and because of changes in serum proteins in the open blood-gas inter-

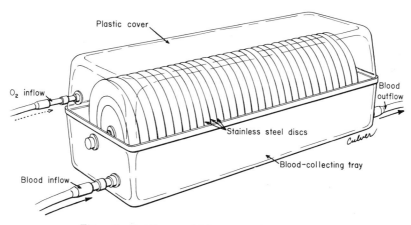

Figure 2.   Kay-Cross multiple rotating disc oxygenator.

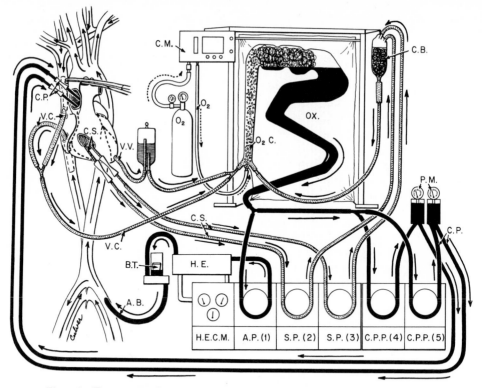

Figure 3.   Extracorporeal circulation apparatus using a disposable bubble oxygenator.

C.M. = control module
O_2C. = oxygenating column
OX. = oxygenator
H.E. = heat exchanger
B.T. = bubble trap
A.B. = arterial blood line
V.C. = vena cava drainage
C.P. = coronary perfusion

C.S. = cardiotomy suction
V.V. = ventricular vent
A.P. = arterial pump
S.P. = suction pump
C.P.P. = coronary perfusion pump
C.B. = cardiotomy suction bag
P.M. = pressure monitors

face, extensive studies have been made of the use of thin membranes, now usually of silicone rubber, to separate the blood from the gas. Such oxygenators have been shown to be effective, and they appear to cause fewer changes in blood proteins than oxygenators with open blood-gas interfaces. Unfortunately, they have been relatively cumbersome to assemble, and the very thin membranes have had a tendency to leak. Recently, a highly successful large capacity membrane oxygenator has been developed for clinical use by Bramson and his associates.

In the most complete form, most heart-lung machines used for open-heart operations are composed of an oxygenator which fills by gravity from the patient, an "arterial" pump for return of oxygenated blood to the arterial system of the patient, a heat exchanger for control of the body temperature, connections and pumps for aspirating blood from the open heart and for perfusing the coronary arteries, and devices for monitoring temperatures,

blood pressures, and sometimes rates of blood flow.

OXYGENATORS. Oxygenators used for clinical purposes must be capable of raising the blood oxygen content from venous levels to normal arterial levels and of removing carbon dioxide at blood flow rates sufficient for total metabolic requirements. At normal temperatures, this blood flow rate has been found to be approximately 2.4 liters per square meter of body surface area per minute. The most commonly used oxygenators are those with open blood-gas interfaces, whether of the bubble type or the filming type. Because of the limitations of duration and blood flow rate imposed by development of microbubbles and alteration of plasma protein observed in such oxygenators, it is likely that development of easily used membrane oxygenators will lead to wide adoption of these much safer devices.

PUMPS. Pumps for clinical use must be capable of delivering necessary flow rates at normal blood pressures, up to 6 liters per minute for an adult. They must be minimally traumatic to the formed elements of the blood. They must be simple to assemble and to operate, and they must be capable of manual operation in the event of power failure. In Europe, a modification of the Dale-Schuster pump, such as that incorporated in the Swedish AGA unit (Fig. 4), is most widely used.

In this country, roller pumps are most commonly used (Fig. 5), for they are simple, relatively atraumatic to blood, and highly maneuverable.

Good pumps produce relatively small amounts of red cell hemolysis, and this is usually the criterion used in selection of the proper pump for any given circumstance.

A small amount of free hemoglobin in the plasma, resulting from such hemolysis, is readily tolerated by the patient. Such hemoglobin in the plasma is either phagocytized

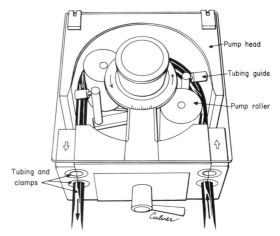

Figure 5. Roller pump. Blood is driven through the tubing in the pump by compression rollers.

by the reticuloendothelial system, excreted by the kidneys, or transformed into methemoglobin. The levels of plasma hemoglobin which result from usual clinical open-heart operations range from 30 to 150 mg. per cent; these are well below the level of 2.4 gm. per cent indicated by Flink as requisite for renal damage on the basis of hemoglobinemia. There apparently is some residual damage to red cells after bypass, because the red cell survival after such operations has been shown to be abnormally short, one-half to two-thirds of normal.

HEAT EXCHANGERS. The perfusion system includes a heat exchanger through which the entire blood flow passes. The exchanger usually consists of two chambers separated by very thin, highly conductive metal. Blood flows through one of these chambers, while water at controlled temperature passes through the other to permit heat exchange between the two fluids. Either normalcy of body temperature may be maintained in this fashion, or the temperature of the patient may be lowered to reduce metabolic demands and to allow somewhat lower flow rates than would otherwise be necessary. Hypothermia is also advantageous if blood flow to any organ is to be interrupted for more than a very few minutes; an example is the clamping of the ascending aorta as a means to arrest coronary arterial flow and thus coronary venous return to the cardiac chambers as a means to visualize intracardiac defects more clearly. It is customary to release the clamp on the ascending aorta for one minute out of every ten minutes in such work, even though such clamping is usually tolerated at 28° C. for as long as 30 minutes.

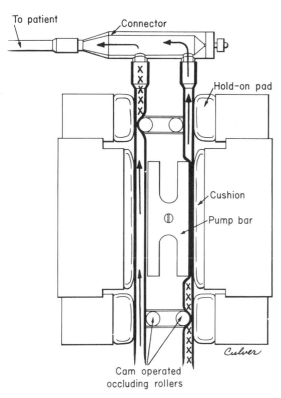

(——— = direction of blood flow,
XX = temporarily stagnant blood)

Figure 4. Compression pump used by Crafoord and Senning. The pump bar oscillates about 100 times a minute so as to compress the flexible plastic tubing alternately against the cushions. Directional flow is provided by properly timed closure of the tubing by the cam-operated occluding rollers. Blood flows upward alternately in both of the pumps.

Body temperature is monitored during such procedures, usually by a temperature probe passed down into the esophagus through the mouth, for temperature recording from this site more accurately reflects the temperature of vital organs than does rectal temperature.

OTHER COMPONENTS. Additional components of the heart-lung machine include suction devices for aspirating blood from the open heart and returning it to the circulation, usually by a junction with the tubing which drains venous blood from the patient to the oxygenator. Commonly, these consist of roller pumps, tubing, and de-bubbling chambers.

During operations in which it is necessary to clamp the ascending aorta for extended periods of time, such as replacement of the aortic valve, it is necessary to perfuse the coronary arteries with arterial blood. Special flexible catheters with olive tips are commonly used for insertion into the orifices of the coronary arteries, where they may be secured by temporary suture in the adjacent aortic wall. A separate pump is commonly used for each coronary artery to provide assurance that a predetermined rate of flow is delivered to each. Pressure monitoring devices located between pumps and coronary arterial catheters are used to indicate obstructive malposition of the catheters and adequacy of perfusion; individual coronary arterial flow rates may be raised or lowered to adjust the pressure for optimal perfusion of the myocardium.

Systemic arterial and venous pressures are also monitored, in these instances with very slender plastic catheters inserted into a peripheral artery and into the superior vena cava. These pressure measurements are essential for proper adjustment of the circulating blood volume during and after bypass.

THE PERFUSION CIRCUIT. Blood is ordinarily withdrawn through large catheters inserted into the superior and inferior venea cavea through the wall of the right atrium. Tubing connections made of transparent, very smooth-walled plastic materials conduct the blood by gravity flow to the oxygenator. Blood accumulates in a reservoir chamber of the oxygenator and is passed from this chamber by the pump through the heat exchanger to a cannula ordinarily placed in the femoral artery of the patient.

Under certain circumstances, the manner of withdrawal of venous blood may be altered. As an example, in operations on the left side of the heart in the absence of septal defects, it is simpler to place a single catheter in the right atrium, pulmonary artery, or right ventricle.

The pattern of return of blood to the arterial tree may also be varied; marked sclerotic change or smallness of size of the femoral arteries may indicate direct cannulation of the ascending aorta or an iliac artery.

PREVENTION OF CLOTTING IN THE CIRCUIT. Until further research leads to development of synthetic surfaces which do not cause the blood to clot, it is essential to render the blood incoagulable whenever it must pass through artificial external circuits. In this country, it is usually done by administration of 1.5 to 2 mg. of heparin intravenously per kilogram of body weight. In the Swedish clinics, approximately twice this amount is ordinarily used. During the course of prolonged perfusions, the heparin concentration in the blood is determined by titration in vitro against protamine, and occasionally more heparin must be added to maintain freedom from clot formation. At the conclusion of perfusion, the heparin remaining in the patient is neutralized with intravenous administration of protamine sulfate. Usually, the amount of protamine required is 1.5 to two times the amount of heparin originally administered. It is customary to check the adequacy of this neutralization by further protamine titrations.

Abnormal bleeding, particularly in the form of oozing, may occur after perfusion. This is due in part to aberrations in the clotting mechanism secondary to passage for long periods through the pump-oxygenator. Destruction of clotting factors occurs chiefly in the oxygenator and is accentuated if insufficient heparin has been employed during the bypass period. Those clotting factors which are concerned with the formation of the thromboplastic complex are most frequently deranged during perfusion. Factor V is most quickly and commonly depleted, with factors VII and X following. Prothrombin concentration is next frequently disturbed. Platelet count and fibrinogen concentrations are less often deranged. Fibrinolysis occurs least frequently. The bleeding time may also become abnormal. Clinically, it appears that unless several clotting factors become deranged, bleeding in the form of uncontrollable oozing does not occur. In perfusions no longer than three or four hours for open-heart operations, uncontrollable postoperative bleeding is uncommon.

MEASURES TO SUPPORT THE FAILING HEART

PUMP OXYGENATORS. Although the principal use of pump-oxygenators has been to substitute for cardiac and pulmonary functions during open-heart procedures, the apparatus has also been used for support in acute heart failure. Clinical success has occasionally been realized in support after acute myocardial infarction, in congestive heart failure, and in the immediate postoperative period after open-heart operations in which the coronary arterial flow has had to be temporarily interrupted.

LEFT HEART BYPASS. In 1958, Senning observed that hearts which failed to recover readily after open operations on the aortic valve, with the pump-oxygenator, responded well if given support for a half hour or more by withdrawal of blood from the left atrium and return of it at normal blood pressures through a femoral cannula. Such left heart bypass has been shown to reduce the oxygen uptake of the left ventricle about 50 per cent and therefore to reduce the work of the left ventricle. It has similarly been found more recently that patients who apparently have been recovering satisfactorily for the first few hours after open-heart operations, and then develop heart failure, benefit greatly by left heart bypass for a period sufficient to correct the metabolic acidosis deriving from an initial low cardiac output. Resuscitation of heart, brain, and kidneys follows adequate flow of oxygenated blood under normal pressure. Elimination of the oxygenator, made possible by withdrawal of already oxygenated blood from the left atrium, permits such by-pass for many hours.

In the patient whose chest is not opened, the simplest and least traumatic approach to the left atrium is accomplished with a special cannula which may be inserted by way of the right internal jugular vein. The tip of the cannula is so fashioned as to permit ready identification of the upper anterior quadrant of the

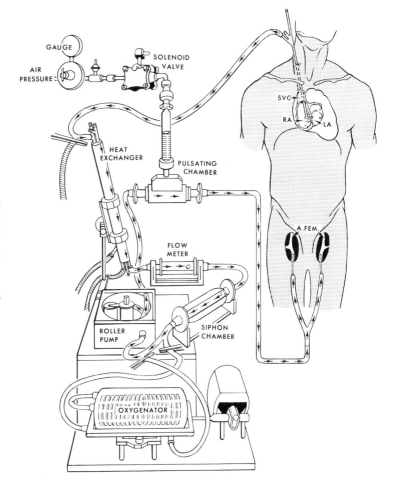

Figure 6. Left heart bypass. SVC = Superior vena cava; RA = right atrium; LA = left atrium; A. Fem. = femoral arteries. The Senning-Dennis cannula draws blood from the left atrium through a heat exchanger and a Senning flowmeter to a flexible siphon chamber. From this point it is pumped by a roller pump through a pulsating chamber synchronized for delivery only when the aortic valve is closed, and to the femoral arteries. An oxygenator can be tied in quickly if needed.

fossa ovalis, through which area the left atrium may readily be entered. The cannula is 7 mm. in internal diameter and readily draws as much as 5 liters of blood per minute (Fig. 6). The residual defect after withdrawal of the cannula is usually smaller than the diameter of the cannula, too small to be hemodynamically significant, and usually heals within three months in the experimental animal. This technique is likely to occasion survival in otherwise fatal clinical coronary arterial occlusion, for experimental occlusion of the circumflex branch of the left coronary artery by pre-placed ligature in the dog almost regularly is followed by survival if the dog is given four hours of such closed chest left heart bypass, whereas the same occlusion is uniformly fatal without it.

COUNTERPULSATION. Counterpulsation is a technique which has been described to support the failing heart. Blood is quickly withdrawn through large arterial cannulas during ventricular systole and rapidly re-injected during ventricular diastole. Thus, the ventricle is permitted to contract against greatly reduced pressures, and systemic perfusion is assured by artificially raised pressures while the aortic valve is closed. In meticulously controlled experiments using bilateral femoral cannulas in which the mean blood pressure is held at fixed levels during both counterpulsation and control periods, counterpulsation has reduced the work of the left ventricle as much as 20 per cent, as measured by the area under the left ventricular pressure tracing. Under similar circumstances, left heart bypass reduces left ventricular work to a considerably greater extent, particularly if the mean aortic blood pressures of both the control and the assist observations fall below 100 mm. Hg. This would indicate that left heart bypass is probably superior to counterpulsation if the blood pressure is depressed. There is experimental evidence, however, that such counterpulsation is strikingly effective in bringing about the opening of collateral circulatory channels in the myocardium.

EXTERNAL COUNTERPULSATION. It has been found that the use of half of a pressure suit so as to bring about precisely timed compression of the hindquarters and lower extremities can extrude from the arterial tree of the compressed area approximately three times the cardiac ventricular stroke volume of blood. With proper timing devices, it has been found possible to reduce the work of the

left ventricle approximately 10 per cent. This technique has not yet had clinical application.

TECHNIQUES TO BYPASS PORTIONS OF THE AORTA DURING RECONSTRUCTIVE OPERATIONS

Resection or revision of the ascending aorta, the arch, or the descending thoracic aorta requires bypass during the period of occlusion for two reasons. In the first place, such viscera as the intestine, liver, kidney, and brain, in that order, tolerate interruption of circulation poorly, and bypass permits continuance of blood flow to them throughout reconstruction of the abnormal aorta. In the second place, left ventricular contraction against the high resistance resulting from limitation of run-off to the coronary arterial system or to that system plus a portion of the branches of the aortic arch, subjects the left ventricular myocardium to abnormally high pressures and therefore distention and strain, which lead to loss of sufficient rhythmicity or contractility to maintain life. Partial bypass permits proper control of the pressure against which the left ventricle must contract. Usually blood is withdrawn by a plastic catheter placed in the left atrium, thus utilizing the lungs of the patient and dispensing with the need of an oxygenator. The pump in the circuit usually returns blood by cannula to a femoral artery (Fig. 7). In special circumstances, such as reconstruction of the aortic arch, total cardiopulmonary bypass is required, and branches of the arterial line from the oxygenator return blood to the major branches of the arch as well. Heparinization is necessary with current apparatus to avoid clotting in the circuit, and if synthetic segments are to be sewed into the aorta, they must either be meticulously preclotted by immersion in previously drawn unheparinized blood of the patient or constructed of nonporous material.

Although such a circuit is less complex than those used for open-heart work, it has nonetheless proved necessary to monitor pressures in the base of the aorta and flow rates to the brain. Only thus can the requirements of protection of the left ventricle from overdistention and of the brain and other organs from ischemia be fulfilled.

In operative procedures requiring temporary obstruction of the descending aorta below the left subclavian artery, bypass is

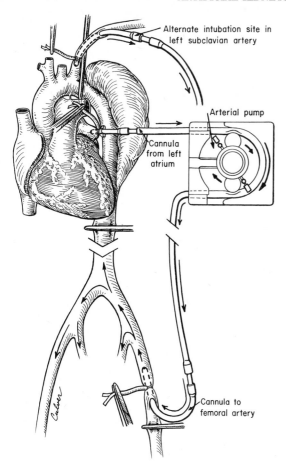

Figure 7. Partial left heart bypass for resection of the descending thoracic aorta.

also essential if the risk of damage to the spinal cord and viscera is to be avoided. A simple plastic tube connection from the left subclavian artery to a femoral artery suffices, no pump being necessary. With currently available tubing, heparinization is needed, but Gott has recently reported the use of shunts with heparin-coated surfaces which preclude the need for heparinization of the patient.

ARTIFICIAL PULMONARY FUNCTION

The heart-lung machine has been used as an adjunct to pulmonary operations in which it is difficult to maintain pulmonary function. Such situations include resection of the carina of the trachea and other massive mediastinal resections in which the airway to the lungs or the vessels to the heart or lungs must be temporarily occluded.

Attempts have been made to maintain ade-

quate arterial oxygen tension in the face of failure of oxygenation of blood in lungs, as in extensive pneumonia, in which it is hoped that support for a number of hours might suffice. Under these circumstances, the blood might be withdrawn from the venous system at a distance from the right atrium and, without opening the chest, passed through a pump-oxygenator, and returned to the right atrium. The intent with this method is to provide oxygenation for extremely desaturated venous blood sufficient that the limited remaining pulmonary function may return oxygen tension to tolerable levels for tissue metabolism. Membrane oxygenators in these circumstances appear to be better tolerated than those with open blood-gas interface. Successful use for a 30-hour period has been accomplished. The method is not yet in general use.

ARTIFICIAL KIDNEYS AND HEMODIALYSIS

The artificial kidney is a dialysis apparatus containing a cellulose membrane which separates blood and rinsing fluid. Two basic designs of hemodialyzers are in general use. In the twin coil hemodialyzer, arterial blood is pumped through cellophane tubing wound in concentric coils separated by fiberglass screening to provide space for circulation of the dialyzing fluid (Fig. 8). In the flat plate design, of which the Kiil kidney is the most popular type, thin sheets of cellulose membrane are laid upon a flat frame and pressed between grooved polypropylene boards (Fig. 9). Connections are so constructed that alternate layers of blood and dialysis fluid are separated by the cellulose membranes. Solutes diffuse through the membrane from the flowing blood to the flowing rinsing fluid or vice versa, according to the concentration gradients existing between blood and dialysis fluid. The fluid currently used with the Kiil hemodialyzer has the following ionic concentration, though calcium and magnesium concentrations may be adjusted according to variation in local water supply:

Sodium	—	132 mEq./l.
Potassium	—	2 mEq./l.
Chloride	—	105 mEq./l.
Magnesium	—	1.5 mEq./l.
Calcium	—	2.5 mEq./l.
Acetate	—	33 mEq./l.
Dextrose	—	200 mg. %

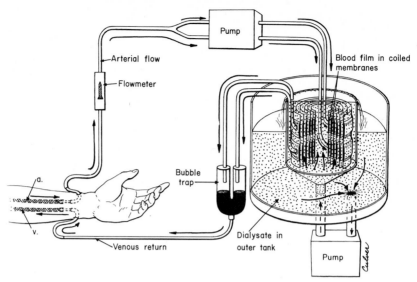

Figure 8. Twin coil (Kolff) dialyzer.

Twin coil dialyzer units are commercially prepared, sterilized, and prepackaged for immediate insertion into a dialysis machine, effecting simple, though somewhat expensive, operation. The flat plate Kiil dialyzer must be completely assembled by hand and then sterilized by flowing acetic acid or benzalkonium chloride solution through the blood compartment.

A twin coil hemodialyzer requires a pump to propel blood through the coils and requires a relatively large volume of blood for filling. The Kiil hemodialyzer has a low resistance and does not require a pump, arterial blood

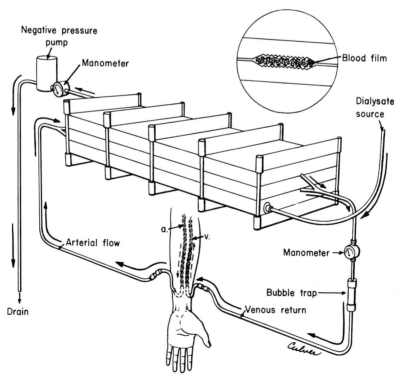

Figure 9. Flat plate (Kiil) dialyzer.

pressure of the patient sufficing to produce a flow of 200 ml. per minute through the dialyzer and back to a vein of the patient. The blood volume contained in a 0.9 square meter Kiil dialyzer and connecting tubing is 225 ml., eliminating blood priming; all except some 20 to 40 ml. of this blood can be returned to the patient at the end of each dialysis. The dialysate is pumped in a reverse direction to blood flow and then discarded. In renal failure, attention is directed primarily toward reducing elevated nitrogenous waste levels and potassium concentrations; these substances pass readily through the membrane and are therefore lowered during dialysis. Because substances can pass either way through the membrane, depending on the concentration gradients, other electrolyte aberrations, metabolic acidosis, and overhydration can be corrected by effective hemodialysis. Hemodialysis has proved lifesaving for occasional surgical patients whose course has been complicated by acute renal shutdown. This complication is unfortunately seen not infrequently following open-heart operations, and the hazard of cardiac arrest secondary to rise in potassium level in the blood can be reduced by dialysis. Prompt institution of conservative medical therapy is essential.

The artificial kidney has been employed principally in the treatment of acute reversible renal failure, although it has been demonstrated that chronic renal failure may be satisfactorily managed for months or years with the help of dialysis two or three times a week and institution of diets low in protein.

Repeated hemodialyses have been made feasible by the use of indwelling silicon rubber and Teflon arteriovenous shunts, usually placed on the forearm. A junction in the arteriovenous shunt may be disconnected to permit attachment of the arterial and venous connections to the kidney. Heparinization is necessary only during the period of actual dialysis, the rapid flow through the arteriovenous shunt sufficing to keep it free of clot at other times.

PERITONEAL DIALYSIS. Peritoneal dialysis is in many ways a simpler technique for treatment of acute renal shutdown in surgical patients. Peritoneal irrigation is accomplished through a slender special catheter inserted by way of a trochar and a 1 cm. skin incision. The normal peritoneum provides rapid equilibration with the extracellular fluid of the patient, and dialysate is withdrawn every few minutes and replaced with fresh dialysis fluid. Sterile dialysis fluid is commercially available in 1- and 2-liter bottles for quick and easy use. The composition of this sterile solution is similar to that of the dialysate for hemodialysis, except that the glucose concentration is varied between $1\frac{1}{2}$ and 7 per cent, the higher concentrations being used for alleviation of overhydration.

Several machines have been designed which automatically pump a predetermined quantity of dialysate into the peritoneal cavity and drain it out again according to an automated cycle (Fig. 10). This apparatus has the further advantage that it may be set up to mix automatically ordinary tap water with quantitative addition of a concentrated

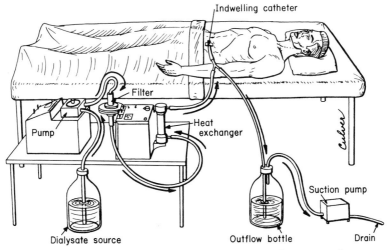

Figure 10. Peritoneal dialysis using an automatic pumping system. The cycling system alternates operation of the two pumps (wiring not shown).

electrolyte solution. The automatic dialysis machine passes the dialysis solution through a Seitz-type filter for sterilization to enhance the convenience and economy of dialysis.

Patients may be carried on dialysis for long periods of time by either the peritoneal or hemodialysis technique. Peritoneal dialysis may be difficult or impossible in patients with extensive intraperitoneal adhesions. Peritonitis was at first thought to be a contraindication, but it has proved to be not only not a contraindication but to be favorably influenced by peritoneal dialysis. Acute pancreatitis appears similarly to be benefited by peritoneal dialysis.

The urea and creatinine clearances effected by the peritoneal dialysis are from 2) to 40 per cent those of hemodialysis. Peritoneal dialysis, however, avoids the need for heparinization, an item which could be of considerable importance in the early postoperative patient.

PROSTHETIC HEART VALVES

Even though intensive work is being done on totally implantable artificial hearts, no totally implantable artificial organs have yet become a clinical reality. On the other hand, prosthetic valves have been designed which are acceptable for replacement of diseased human valves. The first valve to be implanted in a significant number of patients was designed and implanted by Hufnagel. This was a ball valve of methyl methacrylate for insertion into the descending thoracic aorta for the amelioration of severe aortic insufficiency. Experimental valves of ball and socket design or flap design for replacement of the mitral valve were demonstrated to be feasible by Stuckey and co-workers not long after extracorporeal circulation made intracardiac operations possible (Fig. 11, *A* and *B*). These valves functioned acceptably, but implantation of them was complicated by formation of thrombus at the fixation site and in the valve orifice, resulting in death from systemic emboli, failure of valve closure, or obstruction of the orifice. In addition, there was difficulty with fixation of the valve ring to the orifice remaining after removal of the normal mitral valve, and occasionally the ball of a ball valve escaped into the aorta.

The first clinical replacements of valves were substitutions of synthetic fabric, usually

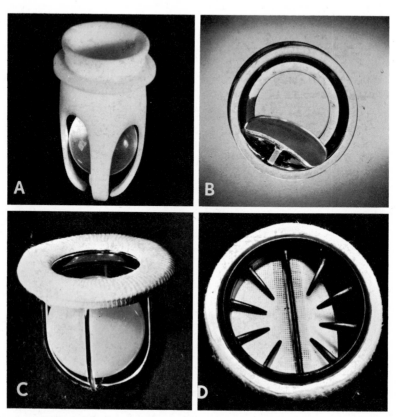

Figure 11.   *A* and *B*, Two of the first experimental heart valves. *C*, Starr mitral valve. *D*, Gott flap valve.

Teflon, for cusps of the aortic valve. Somewhat later, tricuspid aortic valves and bicuspid mitral valves were also fashioned of fabric. Competent valves could be constructed which were initially anatomically and physiologically similar to normal valves, but function was commonly compromised in a few months by increasing stiffness of the leaflets from fibrous tissue infiltration, thrombus formation, and occasionally calcification. Such valves have, therefore, been almost completely replaced by either ball valves or some type of disc valve.

Starr modified the ball valve design of Stuckey and employed it clinically first in the mitral and then in the aortic position (Fig. 11, C). The construction of the ball valve has since been modified repeatedly to reduce the incidence of thrombus formation.

The ball valve has been further modified by others to use a lens-shaped disc rather than a ball, thereby permitting use of a shorter cage and in turn less protrusion into either the left ventricle or the aorta. Protrusion of the mitral prosthesis into the ventricle as far as the ball valve does may impede contraction of the ventricle by rubbing against the septum or may actually damage the endocardium there, with secondary production of emboli. In the aortic position, a large ball valve may take up so much of the cross-section area of the aorta in the open position as to give rise to obstruction of serious degree. In both these positions, therefore, the disc appears to offer distinct advantages quite apart from the lesser weight and volume; it secondarily is thought to displace less blood from the left ventricle and thus increase stroke volume.

Several types of flap valves have also been designed, the most notable being that of Gott (Fig. 11, D). Gott's valve is coated with a combination of graphite, benzalkonium, and heparin to reduce the formation of thrombus upon the surface. An additional valve is that of Wada, in which the disc rotates in the open position to lie parallel with the flow of blood and thus to be constantly swept clean and therefore free of even initial thrombus formation. No true hinge exists, simply a notch on each side of the floating portion which fits into a notch on the ring of the valve (Fig. 12).

An ideal valve must be designed in such fashion that it may be fixed securely in position. Most prosthetic valves have a fabric sewing rim on the periphery of the base, through which sutures are passed in the course of insertion. The valve must allow adequate physiologic flow with minimal pressure gradient in the open position, and closure must be rapid and complete. The construction must be such that thrombi do not form on any part and that failure does not occur from breakage, loss of a moving part, or sticking of a moving part. It has recently been shown experimentally that complete encasement of the metal ring and cage of a prosthetic ball valve with good synthetic fabric greatly reduces the incidence of excessive thrombus formation upon the prosthesis, the surface instead becoming smoothly covered with a layer strongly resembling endothelium. Recent reports have indicated that plastic balls do wear and occasionally break, and, therefore, hollow metal moving parts have also been introduced.

A further problem consists in postoperative infection. Not infrequently, such infection has responded to reoperation with removal of the prosthetic valve and replacement with a fresh one, with long-term apparent cure.

Great attention is currently being given to prevention of excessive turbulence in the blood, such as might occur from faulty design or inaccurate attachment to the surrounding tissues. Such excessive turbulence is productive of red cell damage.

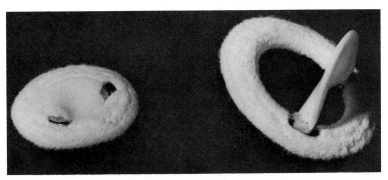

Figure 12. Wada hingeless valve, teflon Breuer covered.

In the past few years, homograft aortic valves have been introduced with remarkable early success. Experience with late rejection has begun to appear, and it is possible that utilization of the patient's own tissues, as Senning has done in fashioning an entirely new aortic valve of fascia lata, may prove to be the best long-term solution to the problem.

VASCULAR PROSTHESES

The first successful prosthetic bridge for a defect in the arterial tree was devised by Hufnagel, who introduced the era of increasingly successful prosthetic replacement of arteries. He replaced a segment of aorta with a rigid solid-walled tube made of methyl methacrylate, which was fastened into the vessel ends with a multiple-point fixation ring. The concept of porous flexible plastic prostheses was introduced by Voorhees, who constructed tubes from a synthetic fabric called Vinyon-N. The demonstration that these tubes were satisfactory blood conduits, at least for a limited time, was followed by exhaustive testing of different fabrics for this purpose. Many fibers have been tested for tissue reactivity, carcinogenic potential, and strength after prolonged periods of implantation. Dacron has become the synthetic fiber of choice in view of low tissue reactivity and durability.

At present, arterial prostheses are manufactured in a variety of diameters and lengths, including bifurcations for replacement of the bifurcation of the aorta. Prostheses in general are fabricated either by the process of knitting or the process of weaving. Exhaustive experimental studies by Wesolowski have emphasized the importance of high porosity in such blood vessel replacements if one is to develop an internal lining layer of tissue which remains smooth, thin, intact, and free of thrombus formation and calcification. His studies appear to have indicated the superiority of the knitted prosthesis and the advantages to be gained from utilization of loosely twisted Dacron yarn with a large number of stitches per inch.

In placement of such a prosthetic graft of the knitted design, it is necessary that it be placed in unheparinized blood of the patient involved in a stretched position to accomplish the process of pre-clotting. The high porosity of the synthetic Dacron graft is thereby prevented from permitting an excessive amount of blood loss after clamps have been removed from the vessel at either end and blood has been allowed to enter. After a prosthetic graft has been sutured into place and the abdomen closed, host tissues begin to grow around and into the interstices of the graft. The graft becomes encapsulated with a thin layer of fibrous tissue both on the outside and on the luminal surface. Ideally, the luminal surface becomes covered with an internal elastic membrane which is thin and smooth and intact, factors which have been shown experimentally by Wesolowski to be dependent upon high porosity of the prosthesis, for only by this means is adequate circulation permitted through the wall of the prosthesis to the internal elastic membrane. Ischemia of the inner capsule, on the other hand, results in areas of necrosis, with sloughing of the lining, precipitation of fibrin on the ulcerated surface, partial or complete occlusion of the graft, or late calcification.

In addition to the type of synthetic fiber and the porosity of the graft, other desirable characteristics are elasticity, pliability, good handling properties during implantation, and ease of suture to the host vessels.

In general, knitted fabrics which are crimped to improve flexibility are most desirable for the majority of clinical applications. If one must use a graft which will be placed while the patient is heparinized, a tightly woven prosthesis appears to be most satisfactory, because it does not leak excessively during the time until the patient can be given protamine, and coagulation time can be returned to normal. This is obviously an unhappy compromise because of the late complications of internal ulceration, thrombosis, obstruction, and calcification.

CARDIAC PACEMAKERS

Electrical stimulation of the heart is an effective treatment for the arrhythmias of atrioventricular dissociation associated with Stokes-Adams attacks or heart failure. The stimuli for ventricular contraction have been commonly applied to the heart through external electrodes on the skin, to wires in the myocardium, or to a long catheter-like electrode passed transvenously to the right ventricular chamber. Apparatus has also been devised which sends signals in the form of radio waves or electrical induction fields through the skin to buried receivers. The system in commonest use today combines a long transvenous endocardial electrode and an implanted subcutaneous pulse generator.

Pacemaker units for external use have manual rate and voltage adjustments and are used for temporary pacing under emergency circumstances until implantable pacemakers can be inserted. In most instances, temporary pacing is done with a long endocardial catheter electrode inserted via an antecubital or external jugular vein. This electrode is removed after the rhythm has returned to normal or a pacemaker has been implanted.

Implantable pacemakers are of three general types. The most common has a fixed rate which is independent of either the spontaneous atrial or ventricular rates. Although the rate may be adjustable, it does not respond to physiologic stimuli. A second type of pacemaker responds to atrial rate and rhythm, and is termed synchronous. The rate of the electronic pacer responds to changes in atrial rate through artificial atrioventricular conduction established by placing a sensor to pick up atrial electrical activity. The third type is the stand-by pacer, which stimulates ventricular contraction only when the spontaneous A-V conduction delay is so long as to yield a ventricular rate of less than a predetermined minimum, such as 70 per minute. This type of pacer may be advantageous in circumstances in which the patient has intermittent A-V dissociation with Stokes-Adams attacks, alternating with regular sinus rhythm.

The following description of apparatus and technique is typical of one type of fixed rate asynchronous pacer, the pacing system most commonly employed currently.

Implantable and external pulse generators provide a rectangular pulse with a duration of 1.5 to 2.0 milliseconds. The pulse is biphasic, a characteristic which reduces polarization of the electrodes, although stimulation of the ventricle occurs in only one phase. The vo tage is 3.8, with a maximum current of 5 milliamps. Current may be adjusted, according to the impedance encountered, to provide a stimulus which, for pacing safety, is twice threshold. The rate of stimulation may be adjusted manually between 55 and 120 beats per minute before or after implantation.

The implantable unit is a mercury-cell-powered, transistorized blocking oscillator with amplifier. It is encased in epoxy resin and covered with silicone rubber. It is im-

planted subcutaneously to energize the stimulating electrodes.

The long electrode leads connected to the pulse generator are composed of two long spring coils which lead to the positive and negative electrodes. These coil leads are encased in a silicone rubber sheath to allow bending and elongation in conformity to body movements. The electrodes designed for suture to the myocardium are fashioned appropriately for penetration of the myocardium and suture fixation to the epicardium, with the two poles being separate for individual implantation. The endocardial catheter-type electrode terminates with two platinum contacts, one at the tip, and the other a short distance proximal to the tip.

Myocardial electrodes are inserted into the wall of the left ventricle near the apex in an avascular area (Fig. 13, B). A left anterior thoracotomy under general anesthesia is necessary to expose the heart, whereas a separate transverse incision in the left upper quadrant is made to form a subcutaneous pocket to accommodate the pulse generator. These are connected with a subcutaneous tunnel through which the electrodes are passed from the abdominal pocket to the chest. The entire unit is thus implanted. Because a thoracotomy is necessary to implant these electrodes, the transvenous endocardial route has recently gained preference.

The transvenous catheter-type electrode is inserted with local anesthesia through a small incision in the cephalic vein below the clavicle or in the external jugular vein (Fig. 13, A). The electrode tip is advanced to the apex of the right ventricle under fluoroscopic control, where it is impinged between trabeculae in a situation in which the threshold

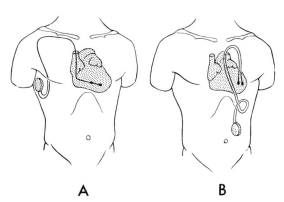

A   **B**

Figure 13. *A*, Implanted transvenous endocardial fixed rate pacemaker. *B*, Implanted fixed rate cardiac pacemaker with leads sutured to the myocardium.

for stimulation is less than 1.5 milliamperes. The catheter is fixed in this position at the point at which it enters the vein. A subcutaneous pocket is then formed in the subclavicular or axillary region to house the pulse generator. After the wounds are closed, the units function without attention by the patient, except for daily counting of the pulse rate. Systemic antibiotic or anticoagulant therapy is generally unnecessary.

Patients without heart failure have an excellent prognosis with an implantable pacemaker. If heart failure is present and this failure is refractory to pacing with a temporary endocardial pacer, prognosis with an implanted pacer is very poor. Late mortality is related generally to progress of arteriosclerotic cardiovascular disease, such as coronary occlusion, stroke, and renal insufficiency.

Complications with pacers include wire breakage, infection, electrode dislodgment, perforation of the ventricle, and generator failure. These complications are occurring with less frequency as apparatus and techniques are improving, and the recent experience with implanted transvenous endocardial pacers has been excellent.

The generators must be changed when the batteries approach the end of serviceable life, some 24 months. This requires a new incision, exposure of the generator, and connection of a new one to the electrodes.

READING REFERENCES

Barratt-Boyes, B. G.: Homograft aortic valve replacement in aortic incompetence and stenosis. Thorax 19:131, 1964.

Björk, V. O.: An artificial heart or cardiopulmonary machine. Performance in animals. Lancet 2:491, 1948.

Bramson, M. L., Osborn, J. J., Main, F. B., O'Brien, M. F., Wright, J. S., and Gerbode, F.: A new disposable membrane oxygenator with integral heat exchange. Jour. Thoracic & Cardiovasc. Surg. 50:391, 1965.

Brown, L., Goldenberg, A. L., and Dennis, C.: Myocardial assist: comparison of left heart bypass with counterpulsation. Surg. Forum 17:152, 1966.

Chardack, W. M., Gage, A. A., Federico, A. J., Schimert, G., and Greatbatch, W.: The long-term treatment of heart block. Prog. Cardiovasc. Dis. 9:105, 1966.

Clauss, R. H., Birtwell, W. C., Albertal, G., Lunzen, S., Taylor, W. J., Fosberg, A. M., and Harken, D. E.: Assisted circulation. I. The arterial counterpulsator. J. Thoracic & Cardiovasc. Surg. 41:447, 1961.

Clowes, G. H. A., Jr., and Neville, W. E.: Experimental and clinical results with a practical membrane oxygenator. Circulation 16:867, 1957.

Craford, C., Norberg, B., and Senning, A.: Clinical studies in extracorporeal circulation with a heart-lung machine. Acta Chir. Scandinav. 112:220, 1957.

Cross, F. S., Berne, R. M., Hirose, Y., Jones, R. D., and Kay, E. B.: Description and evaluation of a rotating disc type reservoir oxygenator. Surg. Forum 7:274, 1957.

Dale, H. H., and Schuster, E. H. J.: A double perfusion pump. J. Physiol. 64:356, 1928.

DeBakey, M. E., Jordan, G. L., Jr., Abbott, J. P., Halpert, B., and O'Neal, R. M.: The fate of Dacron vascular grafts. Arch. Surg. 389:757, 1964.

Dennis, C., Hall, D. P., Moreno, J. R., and Senning, A.: Reduction of the oxygen utilization of the heart by left heart bypass. Circ. Res. 10:298, 1962.

Dennis, C., Moreno, J. R., Hall, D. P., Grosz, C., Ross, S. M., Wesolowski, S. A., and Senning, A.: Studies on external counterpulsation as a potential measure for acute left heart failure. Tr. Am. Soc. Artif. Int. Organs 9:186, 1963.

Dennis, C., Spreng, D. S., Nelson, G. E., Karlson, K. E., Nelson, R. M., Thomas, J. V., Eder, W. P., and Varco, R. L.: Development of a pump-oxygenator to replace the heart and lungs; an apparatus applicable to human patients, and application to one case. Ann. Surg. 134:709, 1951.

DeWall, R. A., Warden, H. E., Varco, R. L., and Lillehei, C. W.: Helix-reservoir pump oxygenator. Surg. Gyn. & Obst. 104:699, 1957.

Flink, E. B.: Blood transfusion studies. III. The relationship of hemoglobinemia and of the pH of the urine to renal damage produced by injection of hemoglobin solutions into dogs. J. Lab. & Clin. Med. 32:223, 1947.

Fries, C. C., Levowitz, B., Adler, S., Cook, A. W., Karlson, K. E., and Dennis, C.: Experimental cerebral gas embolism. Ann. Surg. 145:461, 1957.

Furman, S., Escher, D. J. W., and Solomon, N.: Standby pacing for multiple cardiac arrhythmias. Ann. Thoracic Surg. 3:327, 1967.

Gibbon, J. H.: Application of a mechanical heart-lung apparatus to cardiac surgery. Minn. Med. 37:171, 1954.

Gott, V. L., Daggett, R. L., Koepke, D. E., Whiffen, J. D., Dutton, R. C., and Young, W. P.: Replacement of the canine mitral valve with a graphite coated hinged leaflet valve. Surg. Gyn. & Obst. 123:43, 1966.

Hufnagel, C. A.: Aortic plastic valvular prosthesis. Bull. Georgetown Univ. Med. Center 4:128, 1951.

Hufnagel, C. A.: Permanent intubation of the thoracic aorta. A.M.A. Arch. Surg. 54:382, 1947.

Hufnagel, C. A., and Conrad, P. W.: Comparative study of some prosthetic valves for aortic and mitral replacement. Surgery 57:205, 1965.

Karlson, K. E., Caracci, V. W., Krasnow, N., and Wechsler, B. M.: Electrical pacing of the heart with endocardial and implanted pacemakers. Ann. Surg. 163:339, 1966.

Kay, J. H., Kawashima, Y., Kagawa, Y., Tsuji, H. K., and Redington, J. V.: Experimental mitral valve replacement with a new disc valve. Ann. Thoracic Surg. 2:485, 1966.

Kiil, F.: Development of a parallel flow artificial kidney in plastics. Acta. Chir. Scandinav. Suppl. 253:142, 1960.

Kolff, W. J., and Watschinger, B.: Further development of coil kidney: disposable artificial kidney. J. Lab. & Clin. Med. 47:969, 1956.

Kusserow, B. K., and Clapp, J. F.: Red blood cell survival after prolonged perfusion with a blood pump. Tr. Am. Soc. Artif. Int. Organs 12:121, 1966.

Lee, W. H., Krumhaar, D., Fonkalsrud, E. W., Schjeide, O. A., and Maloney, J. V.: Denaturation of plasma proteins as a cause of morbidity and death after intracardiac operations. Surgery 50:29, 1961.

McDonald, H. P., Jr.: An automatic peritoneal dialysis machine. J. Urol. 96:397, 1966.

Nathan, D. A., Center, S., Chang-You, W., and Keller, W.: An implantable synchronous pacemaker for the long-term correction of complete heart block. Am. J. Cardiol. 11:362, 1963.

Senning, A.: Operativ behandling av angina pectoris. Nord. Med. 60:1455, 1958.

Starr, A., McCord, C. W., Wood, J., Herr, R., and Edwards, M. L.: Surgery for multiple valve disease. Ann. Surg. 160:596, 1964.

Starr, A., Pierie, W. R., Raible, D. A., Edwards, M. L., Siposs, G. G., and Hancock, W. D.: Cardiac valve replacement;

experience with the durability of silicone rubber. Cardiovasc. Surg., Suppl. I to Circulation 33 & 34:115, 1966.

Stuckey, J. H., Newman, M. M., Berg, E., Goodman, S., and Dennis, C.: Design and placement of prosthetic valves to fit in the mitral ring of the dog after excision of the leaflets. Prosthetic Valves for Cardiac Surgery, Merendino, K. A. (ed.). Springfield, Illinois, Charles C Thomas, 1961, pp. 266–276.

Stuckey, J. H., Newman, M. M., Dennis, C., Berg, E. H., Goodman, S. E., Fries, C. C., Karlson, K. E., Blumenfeld, M., Weitzner, S. W., Binder, L. S., and Winston, A.: Use of the heart-lung machine in selected cases of acute myocardial infarction. Surg. Forum 8:342, 1958.

Voorhees, A. B., Jr., Jaretski, A., III, and Blakemore, A. H.: Use of tubes constructed from Vinyon-N cloth in bridging arterial defects. Ann. Surg. 135:332, 1952.

Wada, J., and Kitaya, T.: Prosthetic heart valves and artificial heart. Shindan-to-Chiryo (Diagnosis and Treatment) 55:132, 1967.

Wesolowski, S. A.: Evaluation of Tissue and Prosthetic Vascular Grafts. Springfield, Illinois, Charles C Thomas, 1962.

Young, W. P., Gott, V. L., and Rowe, G. G.: Open-heart surgery for mitral valve disease, with special reference to a new prosthetic valve. J. Thoracic & Cardiovasc. Surg. 50:827, 1965.

Chapter 38

TRANSPLANTATION OF TISSUES AND ORGANS

by

THOMAS E. STARZL, M.D.

and

LAWRENCE BRETTSCHNEIDER, M.D.

The son of a newspaper editor in a small town in Iowa, THOMAS E. STARZL graduated with honors from Westminster College in Fulton, Missouri. He received masters and doctor of philosophy degrees in neurophysiology in addition to his doctor of medicine from Northwestern University. Following his post-graduate education in general and thoracic surgery, he became a Markle Scholar in the medical sciences. Dr. Starzl has been a pioneer in the investigation of the basic principles underlying the transplantation of tissues and organs and his imaginative fundamental research has been recognized internationally. He is Professor of Surgery at the University of Colorado Medical School.

LAWRENCE BRETTSCHNEIDER was born in New Jersey and attended Union College and the State University of New York Upstate Medical College. He is a career officer in the United States Navy assigned to work with the transplantation unit at the University of Colorado. He is a lacrosse player and a devotee of early American history.

INTRODUCTION

Although the prospect of replacing defective organs has intrigued physicians and surgeons since antiquity, there was little evidence until the last few years that this was a realizable objective. Before then, an almost total ignorance of the biologic problems which would be encountered precluded the development of appropriate methods of therapy. As recently as 1940, there was still a widespread belief that application of tissue transplantation needed only the refinement of better surgical techniques, despite the slow accumulation of evidence that this was not the case.

Early in this century, Carrel had appreciated that the fate of transplanted canine kidneys was different when the organs were obtained from another animal than when they were transferred from one location to another in the same dog. Jensen had noted that the behavior of transplanted tumors was markedly influenced by a host reaction against the inoculated neoplasms. He believed that the same phenomenon applied to normal tissues. Loeb explained the nonacceptance of alien tissue by a somewhat confusing hypothesis that all organisms are born with an "individuality differential" present in both cells and body fluids.

The shrewd clinical observations of Holman came close to the truth. He placed small skin grafts upon the granulating wounds of several patients. Permanent takes were obtained when the patients provided their own grafts from other portions of the body. Skin from other donors was ultimately rejected, but the period of viability was longer for those transplants obtained from family members than for those taken from genetically nonrelated sources. Holman observed that a second graft from the same donor was rejected more quickly than the first, leading him to suggest that a state of specific sensitization had developed as a consequence of the initial exposure. At the time, these findings attracted

1424

little attention, and the situation remained obscure for almost another 20 years until the appearance of the first of the studies by Medawar and his colleagues.

Medawar's investigations were conceived and executed under trying circumstances. Questions concerning skin replacement had become more urgent than ever because of the need to treat mass wartime casualties. The answers were provided on the basis of investigations with inbred rodents in which the genetic homogeneity of the donor and recipient animals permitted a high degree of reproducibility of results. The conclusions were precise.

First, skin grafts were rejected after an interval which was essentially invariable for given donor-recipient strain combinations. There was evidence that the repudiation was due to an immunologic reaction of the host to the foreign tissue. The key observation in support of this concept was the fact that a second homograft from the original donor was destroyed in an accelerated fashion, suggesting the acquisition of immunity by the host. The immunity, conferred by contact with the first graft, was permanent or of long duration, and applied to all tissues subsequently transplanted from the same donor. The sensitization was specific inasmuch as grafts from other donor strains were not usually rejected in an accelerated manner. The initial delay before the first set rejection, and the subsequent development of active immunity prompted comparison between these events and those of delayed tuberculin type hypersensitivity.

GENERAL PRINCIPLES

REJECTION. The control problem of transplantation is summarized in Figure 1. Tissue which is transplanted from one location to another on the same person is termed an *autograft*. It is not identified as "non-self" and does not, therefore, evoke a hostile host reaction. The success or failure of the graft is exclusively dependent upon the technical adequacy of the procedure and upon other well-accepted principles of surgical care.

The same applies when tissues or organs are exchanged between identical twins (*isografts*). Because there is total genetic identity of the donor and recipient, the graft is not recognized as foreign and can be expected to have the same life expectancy as that of the

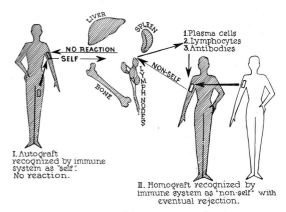

I. Autograft recognized by immune system as "self". No reaction.

II. Homograft recognized by immune system as "non-self" with eventual rejection.

Figure 1. Response of the immune mechanism to autografts (I) and homografts (II). When tissues from one homozygous twin are transplanted to the identical sibling, the situation is analogous to autotransplantation in that there is no rejection.

host. This was first proved in man by Brown with skin transplantation experiments, and later applied by Murray and Merrill to the inter-twin transplantation of kidneys.

Tissues transplanted from nonidentical members of the same species are called *homografts* or *allografts*. A host response follows which is termed rejection. The intensity of the reaction is roughly related to the degree of genetic dissimilarity between donor and recipient, as defined by Snell in inbred rodents. In the outbred canine and human populations, there is a tremendous and as yet unpredictable variability in the vigor of the attack which a homograft will elicit. These observations have led to an intensive search for methods which would allow identification of a favorable donor-recipient combination in advance of clinical transplantation.

When transplantation is from another species, the tissue is called a *heterograft* and the rapidity and magnitude of rejection are even greater than with homografts. However, Reemtsma's studies with chimpanzee to human heterografts have suggested that such transplants can sometimes be tolerated for long periods in recipients who are receiving immunosuppressive therapy.

The mechanism by which homografts or heterografts are rejected is poorly understood. There is abundant evidence that lymphocytes participate in the process in an important way. This can be illustrated by experiments using millipore chambers, in which enclosed fragments of tissue are shielded by a mesh barrier of appropriate size to exclude lymphocytes but through which nutrient fluid can pass. Survival of the transplants is longer than with tissue that is not thus protected. Corneal homografts, which have been used clinically for many years, presumably escape rejection for similar reasons; their nutrition is from a cell-free fluid. If a corneal graft becomes revascularized, it usually fails.

Unfortunately, the way in which lymphocytes contribute to rejection, or to a variety of delayed hypersensitivity reactions, is not known. Presumably, the antigen is brought to lymphoid centers, possibly after an intermediary stage in phagocytosis. Subsequently, there is rapid multiplication of other lymphocytes which are now specifically sensitized against and capable of reacting with the original antigen. The fraction of lymphocytes which undergo this change is probably small, totaling no more than 5 to 10 per cent.

There is reason to believe that the cellular immune response is not the only means by which homograft rejection can occur. In millipore chamber experiments, grafts are quickly destroyed if they are placed in animals previously sensitized to tissue from the same donor, apparently as the result of attack by humoral antibodies. In a small number of well-documented renal homotransplantations, preformed humoral antibodies which were demonstrated in the recipient prior to operation have caused immediate destruction of renal homografts by almost instantly binding to the revascularized kidney tissue. In the serum of patients who have tolerated renal homografts for years, there are often circulating antibodies which can be demonstrated by absorption techniques to react against tissues of the original donor or against the transplanted kidney. Finally, such homografts commonly contain deposits of gamma G, gamma M, and gamma A globulin as well as host complement, suggesting an antigen-antibody reaction with the alien tissue.

Recently, an additional possible mechanism of injury termed allogeneic inhibition was described by Hellström and Hellström and by Möller and Möller. This phenomenon is not dependent upon a classic antigen-antibody reaction, but it is due to differences in the antigenic structure of surface cell membranes. When certain dissimilar cells are contiguously placed in cell cultures, one can destroy the other even if the first has been previously rendered nonviable by irradiation. The significance of this observation in transplantation remains to be clarified.

MANIFESTATIONS OF UNMODIFIED REJECTION. Although a precise explanation of re-

jection is not available, the effects of this process upon various tissues and organs have been thoroughly studied. In the untreated recipient, the end point for each is necrosis but the preceding stages are of interest because changes observed during this time may also be seen despite the provision of host immunosuppression.

After transplantation of a whole organ in which revascularization is established by direct vascular anastomosis, the homograft usually functions well for several days. In dogs whose livers are removed and replaced with those from other animals, there is prompt arousal from anesthesia. The animals may resume a diet. They often appear to be quite normal. After three to four days, however, function begins to deteriorate. There is progressive jaundice as well as changes in serum glutamic oxaloacetic transaminase and serum glutamic pyruvic transaminase which are indicative of hepatic necrosis. At about this time, there is an abrupt fall in total blood flow to the homograft. Death almost always occurs within three or four days. The same events follow renal homotransplantation and can be monitored with appropriate tests of kidney function such as blood urea nitrogen, plasma creatinine and creatinine clearance. For other organs, characteristic syndromes can be defined based upon tests of function of the grafts.

Histologic changes in the various homografts are minimal or absent during the first few postoperative days (Fig. 2). Then, immature and metabolically active mononuclear cells appear at the same time that similar cells begin to be seen in large numbers in host lymphoid organs. Within the graft, these tend to be concentrated around small vessels. In both rejecting renal and hepatic grafts, fusion of these immunoblasts has been noted to the endothelial cells of small vessels.

The number of infiltrating mononuclear cells increases until the entire organ is eventually riddled. In time, their character begins to change; there are increasing numbers of mature lymphocytes and plasma cells and finally, neutrophils. Large areas of parenchymal necrosis develop, which are usually most extensive around the blood vessels; finally extensive destruction occurs (Fig. 2). If the graft is a life-sustaining organ such as the kidney, liver, or heart, the unmodified canine recipient usually dies within seven to 14 days. However, longer survival is occasionally obtained.

These events in the liver and kidney per-

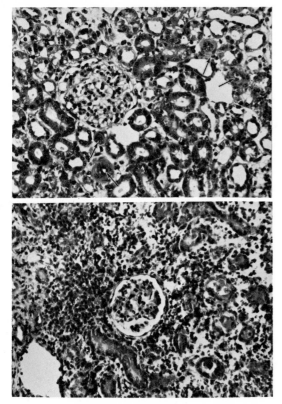

Figure 2. Progressive abnormalities of a canine renal homograft in an untreated recipient. The graft repudiation was less rapid than usual in this dog, apparently because of an accidental good histocompatibility match between the donor and recipient but the ultimate pathologic findings were typical of acute rejection. *Upper,* Biopsy after three days. There is swelling of the endothelial cells lining the arterioles and small arteries (arrows). Otherwise the kidney is relatively normal. *Lower,* The same homograft after 18 days. There is marked cellular infiltration, edema and tubular damage. (H & E × 250.)

tain in a general way to rejection of all organs. There is a delay before host defenses are brought to bear upon the homografts, but following this, the anatomic features of the tissue are distorted, and its blood supply is choked off at the microcirculatory level.

HISTOCOMPATIBILITY. The magnitude of rejection in healthy inbred strains of experimental animals can be more or less well correlated with the degree of genetic dissimilarity between the donor and the recipient. In this kind of investigation, variables other than the genetic differences can be largely eliminated, making it possible to use the homograft reaction itself as the means of classifying those genetic factors which are important in directing the intensity of this process.

In mice, at least 15 histocompatibility loci are known to exist. The gene determinants of several of these are associated together from generation to generation on specific non-sex chromosomes. There is also a weak histocompatibility antigen on the Y chromosome which can be responsible for what is called the Eichwald-Silmser effect, an indolent kind of rejection after placement of male to female skin isografts. In the mouse, the strongest transplantation antigen is found at what is designated as the H-2 locus. The H-2 system involves at least 20 alleles. Its antigens are not only involved in transplantation immunity but also in the elicitation of humoral antibodies such as hemagglutinins and cytotoxins.

In outbred groups including the canine or human populations, it is impossible to categorize antigens on the basis of such genetically controlled experiments. Nevertheless, there is hope that individual specific human antigens can be classified. When this is accomplished, it will be possible to identify in advance of operation the histocompatibility differences between donors and recipients. If the number of distinctive transplantation antigens in man is relatively limited, as now seems likely, some donors could be found who would be superior to others on the basis of their not possessing antigens which are absent in the proposed recipient. Statistically, the chances of meeting this objective would be better by intrafamilial transplantation. However, even with people who have no blood relationship it would also be possible to exclude donor-recipient pairs in which there was incompatibility of strong or multiple transplantation antigens.

The principal hope that this kind of matching will become feasible comes from current studies of human isoimmune antisera. These antisera are obtained from patients who have been accidentally or deliberately sensitized to cell membrane antigens. Typical examples are women who have had several pregnancies, patients who have had multiple blood transfusions, or volunteers who have received skin or lymphoid tissue homografts. The sera from such donors contain antibodies which can be used to determine the antigenic structure of nucleated cells in other people.

For example, the agglutination or cytolysis of test lymphocytes by a given antiserum indicates that the lymphocytes possess the same or similar antigens as those which originally sensitized the serum donor. Failure of the reaction implies the absence of the antigen in the lymphocytes. In various centers in Europe and the United States, large numbers of sensitized donors have been identified and the activity of their sera has been determined against panels of human lymphocytes collected from normal people. The results have been pooled in recent scientific workshops. The conclusions were, first, that the available antisera could identify approximately a dozen different white cell antigens; second, that these antigens by and large were the same as those in other tissues including the kidney; and finally, that an antigenic profile which might be useful for tissue typing could be established for each human.

However, the application of these techniques to tissue typing was not yet assured, because there was as yet no real evidence that the antigens being catalogued were in any way associated with histocompatability. Subsequently, observations in humans after test skin grafting, or therapeutic renal homotransplantation, have provided such evidence. In untreated patients who received skin homografts, the interval before rejection was longest when the donors were shown to have the best antigen match. In the patients who were treated with immunosuppression after receipt of renal homografts, the kidneys were biopsied after two postoperative years. The quality of histologic preservation in these renal homografts was strongly, although not absolutely, correlated with the degree of antigenic compatibility between the donors and their recipients.

These findings, as well as others too numerous to cite, provide reason to believe that a tissue typing method will be part of the future in organ transplantation. The system which evolves will probably be somewhat more complicated than that necessary to type blood. At the moment, it seems unlikely that any single histocompatibility factor will be found in man that has the overriding importance of the H-2 antigen in mice. There will probably be two or three strong antigens and a number of moderate or weak ones. It is highly unlikely that any single histocompatibility antigen will preclude successful clinical transplantation if adequate immunosuppression is used.

MEASURES TO PREVENT REJECTION. For a number of years after the features of rejection had been defined, the not unreasonable assumption was made that this process was one of nature's most powerful and persevering reactions which could be prevented only by relatively complete crippling of the host's immune potential. In view of the evident connection between the capacity to mount an effective rejection and to react forcibly against a variety of other inimical environmental antigens, including those of pathogenic microorganisms, the possibility of achieving chronic graft survival without killing the host was seriously questioned.

The first clue that this might after all be realizable came from the observation that permanent acceptance of adult donor tissue could be induced in fetuses or newborn animals. The initial disclosure was made by Owen, who noted that dizygotic calf siblings, whose circulation in utero communicated freely, had each others' formed blood elements which persisted indefinitely (Fig. 3).

On the basis of this, Burnet suggested that exposure of the fetus to donor tissue might similarly confer protection persisting after birth to subsequent grafts from the same donor but not to those from other donors. The hypothesis was confirmed by Billingham, Brent, and Medawar in rats and later extended to other species. It was soon found that the use of immunologically competent lymphoid tissue for inoculation caused a serious and often fatal disease, termed the "runt syndrome," which was caused by an attack of the mature homograft cells upon the defenseless recipient. In contrast, the transplantation of skin, kidney and liver did not have this complication.

These remarkable events appeared to be the result of exposing the host to donor antigens at a time when its immune mechanism was too rudimentary to recognize the graft tissue as foreign. After maturation of the immune mechanism, neither the graft nor other tissues from the same donor were identified any

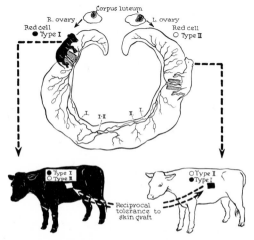

Figure 3. Chimerism in cattle siblings. There is cross tolerance to formed blood elements and to subsequently placed homografts as the result of intrauterine circulatory communication.

longer as alien. Although of no immediate clinical value, the studies were of great importance. They indicated the feasibility of inducing acquired tolerance, and thereby stimulated the search for immunosuppressive agents with which it was hoped that a similar sequence of events could be duplicated in adult recipients. Those agents which have since been effectively used to abrogate rejection do not act by this mechanism of inducing tolerance, but the stimulus that this possibility provided was an important factor in subsequent research efforts.

Total body irradiation was the first kind of therapy which was demonstrated to prolong the life of homografts in adult animals. However, the treatment was dangerous, requiring doses sufficient to cause bone marrow depression. There was a consequent excessive acute mortality. Nevertheless, the two first long-term survivors after clinical renal homotransplantation were treated primarily by this means. These patients, who were at the Peter Bent Brigham Hospital in Boston and the Necker Hospital in Paris respectively, both received kidneys from their fraternal twins more than seven years ago. They are still alive.

For a time, it was hoped that the risks of irradiation therapy could be reduced by transplanting to recipients either lymphoid tissue or bone marrow from the same donor as that from which kidneys, livers or other organs were obtained. The resultant composite subject, termed an *irradiation chimera*, could then have function of the desired organ as well as an endowed means of defense which would not identify the presence of the homograft as abnormal. Unfortunately the irradiation chimera is an unstable preparation in which re-colonization by host elements usually eventually eliminates the lymphoid or hematopoietic graft. Even if this does not occur, the immunologic reactivity is directed by the donor tissues. If these remain in ascendancy, antigens from the defenseless host may provoke an attack by the graft with a consequent graft versus host reaction. This complication, which is comparable to the runt syndrome, has been called secondary homologous disease.

A highly significant subsequent advance was the development of azathioprine, a potentially radiomimetic drug which is a ribonucleic acid inhibitor and possibly a desoxyribonucleic acid inhibitor as well. With this drug, chronic homograft function could often be obtained without the need for doses large enough to cause leukopenia. For the first time, whole organ grafts could successfully be performed in dogs in a standard laboratory environment in which no extraordinary infectious precautions were taken. However, the number of really long-term survivors after homotransplantation of vital organs was still small, because no more than one-fifth of the animals lived for as long as six months.

Similarly, there is at present no single immunosuppressive agent reliable enough to be used as the sole treatment for patients who receive homografts. Fortunately, there are adjuvant measures which can be taken, including the administration of azaserine or intravenous actinomycin C, and the use of local homograft irradiation. With these methods the desired effect upon rejection is relatively feeble and transient.

In contrast, the action of adrenal corticosteroids is a powerful one, and the use of one of the steroid analogues, prednisone, has been a decisive factor in the development of clinical transplantation. Prednisone has a synergistic effect with either total body irradiation or azathioprine. It can either reverse a rejection which has developed in spite of prior therapy with either total body irradiation or azathioprine or, alternatively, it can reduce the incidence of rejection if it is used from the time of transplantation with one of the aforementioned agents.

In the past several years, another immunosuppressive agent, heterologous antilymphocyte serum has received increasing attention. The serum is obtained from animals previously immunized against the lymphoid tissue of the species which is eventually to be treated. For example, horses can be inoculated with human lymphocytes obtained from spleens, lymph nodes, or thymuses (Fig. 4). The resulting antibody response of the horse can be measured by determining the ability of the serum to agglutinate or to lyse human white cells in vitro. After intensive immunization the equine titers may rise to as high as 1:32,000.

The serum collected from an immunized animal is a powerful immunosuppressive agent when given by a variety of routes to members of the lymphoid donor species. Previously established delayed hypersensitivity reactions become negative within a few days. Skin or whole organ grafts have a prolonged functional survival.

Unfortunately, there are certain risks with the administration of foreign protein. In dogs

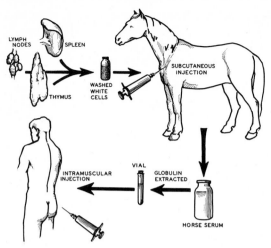

Figure 4.   The preparation in the horse of heterologous antilymphocyte globulin for use in patients.

treated chronically with heterologous anti-canine antisera raised in the horse, there are occasional anaphylactic reactions. Further-more, a significant number of the treated animals develop renal lesions.

The latter complication is a form of serum sickness nephritis which is due, first, to an antibody reaction of the treated animal to the foreign protein; then, to the formation of soluble antigen-antibody complexes by their interreaction; and, finally to the mechanical entrapment of these complexes in the microcirculation of the kidney. There, the complexes evoke a secondary inflammatory reaction.

The undesirable reactions are related in part to the amount of animal protein injected. One way of reducing the dose is to remove and use only the active antibody fractions. This can be done by several biochemical methods. The product obtained is a globulin, which can be sufficiently concentrated to permit intramuscular injections in dogs or humans of volumes as small as 1 to 4 ml. Despite this improvement, renal lesions can still be produced in some dogs treated with the refined horse globulin.

The potential threat of serum sickness nephritis has influenced the way in which derivatives of antilymphocyte serum have been tested clinically. Thus far, they have been used only as adjuvant agents, added to therapy with reduced quantities of azathioprine and prednisone, and with limitation of their administration to the first few postoperative months. The patients who have been so treated appear to have benefited.

ADAPTATION.   Because successful clinical organ transplantation cannot usually be done with a single immunosuppressive agent, various combinations of drugs have been used to prevent loss of the homografts. Azathioprine and prednisone have most often been used together. It was soon learned that the most intensive therapy was required during the early postoperative weeks or months. This was fortunate, for it is highly unlikely that chronic survival could be achieved in any but the rare instance, if the stringency of such early therapy had to be maintained for long periods. The fact that the degree of immunosuppression can often be subsequently relaxed is apparently due to some alteration in the host-graft relationship which transpires during residence of the foreign tissue in its new environment.

This change was called "adaptation" by Woodruff. He originally studied small thyroid homografts which were transplanted to the anterior chamber of the eye in unaltered guinea pigs. In this location, normal rejection does not occur, because the transplants are not revascularized and receive nutrition by diffusion. This favored site is not unlike that which can be artifically created in other locations by the use of millipore chambers.

Woodruff later removed the tissues from the eye, and transferred them to other portions of the body where they were promptly revascularized. Surprisingly, they did not undergo rejection. In contrast, other grafts from the same donor which were then placed in comparable recipient beds were promptly repudiated. Woodruff predicted that an essential goal of clinical therapy would be to prevent destruction of the homograft until there had been time for the adaptation to take place. It was upon this foundation that many advances in clinical transplantation were later based.

The nature of the change in graft-host reactivity is not understood, but much evidence is consistent with the hypothesis that it is the graft which undergoes the most important metamorphosis, as shown by the fact that other subsequently transplanted tissues from the same donor enjoy no special advantage. The alteration is apparently not one of basic genetic structure, because accepted grafts can be later transferred back into the original donor without eliciting any reaction. It is possible that the adaptation is due to some kind of coating of the cells with nonlethal host antibodies and that utilization of available binding sites in this way is itself a long-term protective device.

Whatever its explanation, the importance of changes in the graft-host relationship can be appreciated in almost every successful instance of either experimental or clinical organ transplantation. This is exemplified by the clinical course of a patient who received a kidney homograft from his younger brother. Initial therapy was solely with azathioprine. There was an immediate diuresis and continued excellent renal function which lasted for more than two weeks. During this time, the pre-existing metabolic defects of uremia were completely corrected and the patient felt better than he had for years.

After 17 days, however, the smooth convalescence was interrupted by a rather sudden deterioration of homograft function. The blood urea nitrogen began to increase secondarily. Urine volume diminished. The creatinine clearance fell and protein appeared in the urine in increased quantities. The blood pressure rose, requiring treatment with antihypertensive drugs. There was leukocytosis, and a rise of rectal temperature to almost 40° C. It was a classic rejection crisis which consisted of manifold evidence of homograft failure, plus the manifestations of a systemic immunologic disease.

At this critical time, many of the events which can be documented are identical to those in the nontreated recipient. There is a reduction in organ blood flow. Biopsies from the homografts may be full of mononuclear immunoblasts, and focal areas of necrosis may be present. However, these morphologic changes and the consequent adverse effects are more or less reversible.

Complete functional reversal was almost immediately achieved with the addition of large quantities of prednisone. Later, it became possible to attenuate rapidly the steroid doses, and after five months to discontinue them altogether. Thereafter, the patient had stable renal function while being treated only with azathioprine which at the beginning had been incapable of preventing a moderately serious rejection. A biopsy of the kidney after two years was normal. The patient is in good health after more than four postoperative years.

After all organ transplantations in which survival of more than a few weeks is attained, it is probable that adaptation occurs to some degree. The extent to which it happens determines the subsequent outlook. If it is relatively complete, the ultimate maintenance doses of prednisone may be very small or may not be required at all, in which circum-

stances the patient can be expected to live for years. If the adaptation is minor, the recipient is usually committed to long-term therapy with unacceptably large quantities of steroids and his morbidity both from sepsis and from unstable homograft function is apt to be great.

There is now evidence that the development of adaptation is relatively rapid, and that it is in fact already occurring even during a rejection crisis. In a number of dogs, it has been possible, as early as four months after transplantation of either kidneys or livers, to stop all immunosuppression. Between a third and a half of these animals have then survived for several years. The unpredictability of the outcome after such a drastic step has precluded this practice in patients.

Animal experiments have clarified other features of rejection, its reversal, and the events of adaptation. The value of steroids in reversing rejection is indisputable. However, it has been noted in canine experiments that rejection can sometimes recede without the addition of any additional therapeutic agent.

A dog treated before and for only three weeks after removal of his liver and its replacement with a homograft, had an early rejection as indicated by the appearance of jaundice. This reversed and he has had more than a year of relatively good health, during which he has received no therapy whatever. This kind of observation has led to the conclusion that rejection is not only a phenomenon which can be reversed, particularly with steroids, but also one which tends to be spontaneously reversible.

These observations indicate that the effective control of rejection is not simply a matter of poisoning the host to the extent that he cannot respond to foreign antigens. Instead, an important contributing factor is the development of a dynamic biologic alteration which occurs rather quickly and which is probably not dependent upon any peculiar quality of the immunosuppressive agent being used.

INITIAL HOST REACTIVITY. Some degree of therapeutic specificity is eventually possible even when techniques are used which cause nonspecific depression of immunologic reactivity. A system can ultimately be established in many patients in which the effectiveness of host responsiveness against the antigens of the homograft is selectively attenuated.

The ease with which this can be achieved is influenced by several factors of which the degree of histocompatibility is perhaps the most important. Another critical variable is the capacity for immunologic response with which the host is originally endowed. In uremia, for example, many but not all patients have a reduced ability to mount either a cellular or humoral response to a variety of antigens. The need for heavy iatrogenic immunosuppression is probably thereby correspondingly decreased. Other disease states such as Hodgkin's disease, agammaglobulinemia, thymic aplasia and terminal liver failure are other well-documented illustrations of diseases which are accompanied by immunologic depression.

In patients who have received renal homografts, certain surgical procedures, including excision of the thymus gland and the spleen, have been used with the objective of similarly reducing the intrinsic level of host immunologic competence. The effectiveness of this approach, as an aid to homotransplantation in man, has not been proved. For splenectomy, the rationale is based upon animal experiments which suggest that the immediate responses to intravenous antigens may be partially spleen dependent. However, there is no clear evidence that patients subjected to this procedure have fared better after transplantation than those in which the spleen was not disturbed.

An effect of thymectomy upon the outcome after human renal homotransplantation has also never been demonstrated, despite the strong evidence in animals that this could be anticipated. The role of the thymus in the development of immune competence was first clarified by the studies carried out in rodents by Miller, Good and their associates. They and subsequent workers showed that the presence of this gland was essential for normal maturation of lymphoid tissue throughout the body, probably as the result of the elaboration and release of a thymic humoral substance (Fig. 5). Loss of this influence as the consequence of thymectomy of fetuses or newborn animals resulted in immunologically crippled offspring which had generalized lymphoid hypoplasia, retarded physical development, and a reduced ability to reject skin homografts.

In adult rodents, continuing function of the thymus can also be demonstrated under specific experimental conditions. If mature inbred rats are subjected to sublethal total body irradiation, the degree to which reactivity to skin homografts is eventually restored can be sharply reduced by thymectomy. The same has been reported to be true after therapy

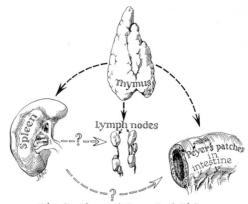

Distribution of Lymph Follicles

Figure 5.   Theoretical considerations in the use of adjuvant thymectomy and splenectomy for the conditioning of recipient patients. The concept of organizer function of the thymus in establishing fetal and neonatal immunologic reactivity is based largely on the work of Miller and Good, and may have no relevance in the adult human. The role of the spleen in controlling response to antigenic stimuli in adult life is suggested by the work of Wissler and his colleagues. The contribution of these ancillary procedures to homograft survival in humans is highly speculative at present. (By permission of Surgery 56:296, 1964.)

with heterologous antilymphocyte serum. More recently, evidence has been reported that a gradual loss of immunologic reactivity follows adult thymectomy in rodents, although at a very slow rate.

The conclusion seems justified that the thymus retains its monitor role in adult life, usually in a relatively unimportant way, but that this function could become highly significant during recovery from a state of immunologic depression such as that induced by iatrogenic immunosuppression. In clinical transplantation, however, it has not yet been possible to detect any difference in the course of patients treated with immunosuppression who have, versus those who have not had, either pre- or post-transplantation thymectomy.

RENAL HOMOTRANSPLANTATION

The application of these concepts to the treatment of human disease has unfolded one of the most fascinating and potentially rewarding chapters in medicine. It has now been possible on several hundred occasions to restore patients to vigorous health who had previously been crippled by the complications of terminal renal failure.

The swiftness with which rehabilitation could be expected was demonstrated by the early experience of Murray and Merrill with identical twin transplants. In most of these patients, good graft function was immediately obtained. There was a brisk or even massive postoperative diuresis, disappearance of anasarca, resolution of heart failure, and rapid return of serum chemistries to normal. Frequently, the recipient patients recovered more quickly than their donors. Most of these same benefits can be expected after homotransplantation, but the course is complicated by the need for constant immunosuppression.

SELECTION OF RECIPIENTS. The initial screening of candidates for homotransplantation is by ordinary medical criteria. The patient should have irreversible renal disease from which life expectancy without definitive therapy is limited to a few weeks.

A highly desirable condition is that he not have major disease of other organ systems. The original disease may itself be responsible for a number of extrarenal complications including neurologic disorders, muscle wasting, pancreatitis, gastrointestinal ulceration, or heart disease. In older patients who have had chronic uremia, it is particularly important to look for evidence of generalized atherosclerosis. A 40-year-old man with a 15-year history of chronic glomerulonephritis may have the blood vessels of a septuagenarian. His chances of dying from a myocardial infarction or a stroke will not be eliminated by a successful renal homotransplantation. In general, the operation is offered only to patients who are less than 45 years old.

A crucial criterion is that the patient be free of all sepsis before immunosuppressive therapy is started. Occasionally, it will be possible to convert an unacceptable candidate to one who is suitable. An example would be a patient with an intractable upper urinary tract infection who could have preliminary nephrectomies.

Providing active infection is not a factor, and if a normal lower urinary tract is present through which to provide drainage, the original cause of the recipient's uremia is usually not an important consideration. The results have been similar in treating patients with chronic glomerulonephritis, burned out pyelonephritis, and polycystic kidney disease. There are exceptions, however. Homografts in patients with congenital oxaluria or certain other inborn errors of metabolism are subject to the same complications which destroyed their own kidneys. The serum of patients with acute glomerulonephritis may

contain antiglomerular antibodies which can damage a homograft. In such patients, preliminary removal of the diseased kidneys may be mandatory before transplantation can even be considered.

THE DONOR PROBLEM. A decision for or against transplantation is inevitably influenced by donor availability. There are three sources: the healthy volunteer who is willing to submit to an elective nephrectomy, the patient who is having a normal kidney excised for some surgical indication, and the recently deceased cadaver. In the first two instances, there is time for complete assessment of the health of the person who is to give, as well as of the kidney which is to be removed. With cadavers, there is a need for haste and such careful evaluation may not be possible.

In any case, it is essential to know the blood types of both donor and recipient. If these are not the same, a judgment must be made concerning the advisability of using the donor-recipient blood group combination which is available. The rules upon which the decision is made are simple (Table 1), and are the same as those which govern transfusion of other than matched blood. They are designed to avoid exposing the red cell antigens, which are the same in the renal tissue as in the red cells of the donor, to circulating hemagglutinins which may be in the plasma of a prospective recipient.

For example, a person with AB blood type does not have circulating anti-A and anti-B hemagglutinins. He could, therefore, receive a kidney from a donor of any blood group. He is a universal recipient. However, because his kidney cells contain both A and B antigen, he could only give to another patient of AB type.

In contrast, the plasma of a patient with O blood type contains both anti-A and anti-B hemagglutinins. Such a person could receive a kidney only from another O patient, but be-

Table 1. *Direction of Acceptable Mismatched Tissue Transfer**

O to non O	Safe
Rh− to Rh+	Safe
Rh+ to Rh−	Relatively safe
A to non-A	Dangerous
B to non-B	Dangerous
AB to non-AB	Dangerous

*O is universal donor. AB is universal recipient.

cause his renal tissue has no A and B antigens, he could serve as a universal donor.

Having determined the acceptability of a donor's blood type, further information is sought. In potential living donors, a complete physical examination is done and a chest x-ray is obtained as well as an electrocardiogram and a glucose tolerance test. Detailed studies of renal function are made, including a blood urea nitrogen and creatinine, inulin, and para-aminohippurate clearances. Multiple urine cultures are mandatory, as are careful urinalyses. An intravenous pyelogram and an aortogram complete the workup. Generally speaking, kidneys are not removed which are shown by aortography to have a multiple arterial supply.

Another factor enters into selection of the donor. There has been an increasing confidence in antigen typing techniques. Although these are imperfect, they do appear to be able to discriminate both very bad and very good histocompatibility combinations. Consequently, matching is probably an important step to take, even in the present state of our knowledge, particularly when several otherwise equally good volunteers are available.

There are a number of volatile social and ethical issues concerned with donor procurement from either living volunteer or cadaveric donors.

PREOPERATIVE PREPARATION OF THE RECIPIENT. Renal homotransplantation is never an emergency. Usually, the condition of the uremic patient is initially too poor to permit a major surgical operation. Very effective resuscitative measures can be instituted.

The most useful of these is renal dialysis. This can either be done with peritoneal lavage or, preferably, by hemodialysis on one of several kinds of artificial kidney. To obtain a substantial improvement in the patient's condition, it is usually necessary to have intensive therapy with dialyses at least two or three times a week for two or more weeks. Excess fluid can be removed, electrolyte abnormalities can be restored toward normal, the bleeding tendency of uremia can be partially corrected, and the patient can be placed back on an adequate diet.

Because a single hemodialysis is almost never adequate, all such patients should be initially managed as if they were entering a chronic dialysis program. Rather than sacrificing peripheral vessels for single hemodialyses, a Scribner-type shunt should be placed either in the upper or lower extremity (Fig. 6).

This provides a high flow arteriovenous connection. At the time of hemodialysis, the shunt can be taken apart and the two ends attached to the inlet and outflow of the artificial kidney. Between treatments the arms of the shunt are reconnected. After transplantation, the prosthesis is removed as soon as it is evident that good homograft function has been obtained. If this objective is not immediately achieved, as is often the case after cadaveric transplantation, the shunt is retained and used for postoperative treatment for as long as is necessary.

The ability to maintain patients on intermittent renal dialysis for months or even years has been a critical factor in the development of renal homotransplantation for reasons other than just resuscitation. It has provided the necessary time to obtain the requisite medical information alluded to earlier concerning blood groups, the etiology of the uremia, histocompatibility data, and the state of the recipient's lower urinary tract. Furthermore, it has allowed patients who did not have volunteer living donors to be kept alive until suitable cadaveric organs could be found.

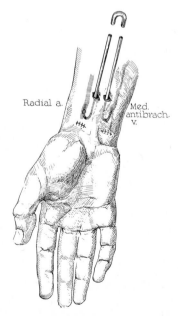

Radial a.

Med.
antibrach.
v.

Figure 6.   External arteriovenous shunt used for chronic hemodialysis. For attachment to the artificial kidney, the connection between the arterial and venous sides is removed. At all other times these two limbs communicate. The high flow through the prosthetic fistula is a crucial factor in the prevention of clotting.

TECHNICAL CONSIDERATIONS. Donor nephrectomy must be performed with attention to important details. The requirements are to avoid trauma to the kidney itself, to obtain adequate lengths of the renal vessels for subsequent anastomosis, and to protect the blood supply of the pelvis as well as a long segment of ureter. To accomplish these things, it is necessary to perform the dissection as far away from the hilum as possible. In some cases, the ureteropelvic blood supply comes from a fine spray of arteries which originate from the main renal artery. These filamentous structures must be preserved.

After its removal, the homograft is without a blood supply for whatever period is required to re-establish its vascular channels in the recipient. Significant protection of the kidney from ischemic injury can be obtained by quickly cooling it. The most efficient method is to perfuse the organ through the renal artery with a cold fluid. If procaine is not added to the solution, afferent arteriolar constriction may occur, making the perfusion difficult. Heparin is used to prevent intraparenchymal clotting during the avascular interval.

Ordinarily the excised donor kidney is transplanted to the contralateral iliac fossa of the recipient, in an extraperitoneal location (Fig. 7). This reverses the normal anteroposterior relationship of the hilar structures. The pelvis and ureter are now in front, the renal arteries intermediate, and the renal vein posterior. The arterial and venous anastomoses are usually made to the hypogastric artery and the external iliac vein respectively.

However, the exact technique of establishing the vascular connections is not important and can be adjusted to meet the requirements imposed by many situations. For example, the presence of atherosclerosis in the lower pelvic arteries may make it necessary to implant the kidney into the common iliac artery or even the aorta. In very small children, the attachment of the renal vessels at this more superior site is usually necessary when adult kidneys are to be placed. Under these circumstances, the operation is done through an intraperitoneal incision.

The rapidity with which the cooled renal homograft can be transferred has an important bearing upon its immediate function. When this can be done with an ischemic interval of 40 minutes or less, excellent urine excretion is almost always observed within two hours. With longer times, good early

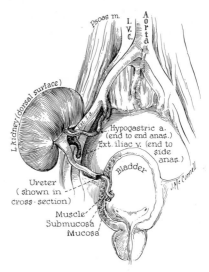

Figure 7. Usual method of renal transplantation. The operation is performed in the extraperitoneal space through an oblique lower abdominal incision. This is a useful technique but there are several alternative ways of revascularizing the organ or of establishing urinary drainage. (By permission of J.A.M.A. *187*:734, 1964.)

function can also often be obtained, but its predictability is progressively diminished with each further increment of time. If kidneys are to be stored for one or more hours, refinements in preservation techniques are necessary.

The methods of restoring a blood supply to the homograft kidney are quite satisfactory. The chief risk of technical complications is from reconstruction of the channels for urinary drainage. This can be done by implanting the homograft ureter directly into the bladder, passing it through a submucosal tunnel in order to duplicate the valve action of the normal ureterovesical junction. With this method, postoperative urinary fistulas are rare, but there is approximately a 10 per cent incidence of late anastomotic stricture.

Alternatively, the homograft ureter may be anastomosed to the distal portion of the recipient ureter, following ipsilateral nephrectomy. This method has important advantages. The ureterovesical junction is, of course, normal. It is not necessary to enter the bladder. Late anastomotic strictures almost never occur. However, the incidence of postoperative urinary fistula is between 5 and 10 per cent and in an occasional patient such a complication eventually leads to death or to loss of the homograft.

PROBLEMS AND COMPLICATIONS OF POSTOPERATIVE CARE. If a technically satisfactory operation has been performed, the immediate beneficial effects can be expected which follow identical twin transplantation. However, continuation of function depends in every instance upon a greater or lesser reduction of the host immune potential. This fact influences almost every decision concerning postoperative management. For one thing, cystostomy drainage is avoided, and when bladder catheters are used they are removed within a day after operation. Usually drains are not employed. These measures are designed to prevent contamination of either the wound or the urinary tract.

At frequent intervals cultures are made of the patient's wounds, skin, urine, sputum, and feces. At the first sign of significant growth of pathogenic bacteria, specific antibiotic therapy is instituted. These antimicrobial measures are far more important than aseptic isolation of the patient. It has been learned that most postoperative infectious complications are due to endogenous pathogenic organisms harbored by the patient himself, and that prophylactic measures are best applied to eradication of these microorganisms rather than to strict avoidance of those in the general hospital environment.

In the long run, however, precautions to prevent sepsis are doomed to failure if excessive immunosuppression is given either by accident, or by the necessity imposed by an uncontrolled rejection. When azathioprine and prednisone were first used together, there were many deaths from bone marrow depression. Most of these tragedies were attributable to the azathioprine. A common sequence of events is shown in Figure 8. The patient received azathioprine both before and for some days after operation. Early renal function was excellent, but a severe rejection crisis developed after ten days, resulting in complete anuria. Following the addition of high dose steroid therapy, urine excretion eventually returned. Just when it appeared that the rejection was reversing, pancytopenia developed, and the patient died of a mixed fungal and bacterial blood infection.

Subsequently, the role of rejection itself in fostering this lethal chain of events has become appreciated. Azathioprine has an important renal pathway of detoxification in that significant quantities of the drug or its breakdown products, including 6-mercaptopurine, are cleared through the kidney. In the event of a severe rejection crisis, this avenue is lost, and the same quantities of azathioprine may have a far more profound effect. It is important to reduce drastically the dose under these circumstances.

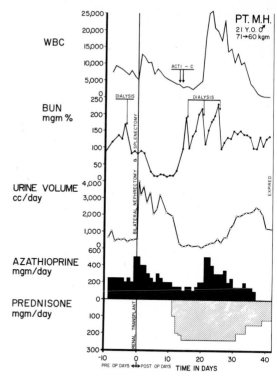

Figure 8.   Typical unsuccessfully treated case. The donor and recipient were brothers, both of A+ blood type. A violent rejection crisis followed good early function, and anuria developed which lasted two weeks. Although the rejection was reversed and a secondary diuresis began, the patient died from drug toxicity, leukopenia and septicemia. Acti C – Each arrow is 200 μg. intravenous actinomycin C. (By permission of Surgery 56:296, 1964.)

The same principle applies if early renal function is defective for other reasons. Cadaveric homografts often must pass through a period of acute tubular necrosis caused by ischemia before they begin to function. During such times of poor or absent urine excretion, the amounts of azathioprine should be correspondingly reduced.

As increased experience with azathioprine was accumulated, the deaths during the first few postoperative weeks from acute bone marrow depression were largely eliminated. Remaining, however, were problems with a more insidious and indolent kind of drug toxicity in which prednisone, not azathioprine, appeared to play the dominant role.

The setting in which the resulting complications developed was almost always the same. It was seen in patients who, after passing through a rejection crisis, were not able to maintain good renal function without chronic administration of high doses of steroids. The quantities required many months after operation were as much as 0.5 to 1.0 mg. per kg. per day or even more.

Eventually, often after an interval of many

months, such patients develop a very evident predisposition to infection despite maintenance of a perfectly normal white count. If the responsible bacteria are of the ordinary pyogenic variety, they can be effectively treated with specific antibiotics. Very often, however, the infecting microorganisms are funguses, viruses, or bacteria which ordinarily have a low virulence. Frequently, specific antibiotic therapy is not available and the patients follow a slow but inexorable downhill course.

The most common location for these ultimately lethal infections is the lungs. Collectively, the resulting infections have been termed transplantation pneumonias. They are caused by a wide variety of opportunistic organisms. However, there is one kind of pneumonitis which has had such a consistent clinical course and typical appearance on chest x-rays that it has been accorded a special position in the transplantation literature. Within the lungs is found *Pneumocystis carinii*, a protozoan which ordinarily causes pneumonitis only in debilitated infants, in patients with naturally occurring immunologic deficiency states, or in patients being treated with cytotoxic drugs. Often there is coexistent infestation of the pulmonary tissue with a cytomegalic inclusion virus.

The clinical syndrome which results usually has a slow onset with the insidious development of progressive pulmonary alveolar capillary block. Cyanosis may become intense, often without any change in blood carbon dioxide. Chest x-rays reveal a quite homogeneous infiltrate involving the middle and lower lung fields. There is no good specific therapy. However, somewhat more than half of the patients recover spontaneously. The prognosis is thus better than with any of the fungus pneumonitides which are almost invariably fatal.

Whatever their bacteriologic etiology, it is tempting to ascribe the various delayed infections simply to the necessity of maintaining heavy immunosuppression with multiple drugs for long periods of time. There may, however, be another important factor. Host reactivity to continuously present renal antigens often is eventually reduced. It is conceivable that a similar specific loss of responsiveness to bacterial antigens could also ultimately occur (Fig. 9).

Renal function is often adequate, although reduced until the time of death. One patient had excellent renal function for the first nine postoperative months. Then a late rejection developed. After this, stable renal function

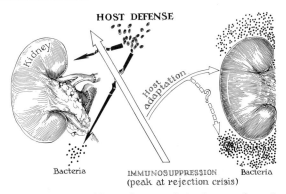

HOST DEFENSE

Figure 9. Possible mechanism of simultaneous loss of host reactivity to specific strains of endogenous bacteria, as well as to the alien renal tissue. (By permission of Surgery 56:296, 1964.)

could not be maintained without prednisone doses of 40 to 100 mg. per day. Two months before death, the patient developed a pulmonary infiltrate and eventually died of respiratory insufficiency. At autopsy, the consolidated lungs were diffusely infected by *Pneumocystis carinii*. There were also several necrotic foci filled with colonies of *Aspergillus fumigatus*.

Although infection is the most serious complication of steroid therapy, particularly when it is used in combination with cytotoxic agents such as azathioprine, prednisone in large quantities causes a number of other side effects. These include cosmetic deformity, arrest of normal growth in children, bone demineralization, polyphagia and consequent obesity, hypertension, steroid diabetes, fatty infiltration of the liver, pancreatitis, and endogenous fat embolization.

THE INFLUENCES OF ANTILYMPHOCYTE GLOBULIN UPON MORBIDITY. Many observers have concluded that azathioprine, when it can be used alone and is not given in excessive quantities, is a relatively safe agent. However, it has also become evident that if the other indispensable drug, prednisone, is required in high doses for long periods, the morbidity is predictably unacceptable. Consequently the use of antilymphocyte globulin as a steroid-sparing device has had unusual appeal.

The guidelines provided by animal experimentation have been incorporated into the therapeutic regimen used for patients. The immune horse globulin was used as an adjuvant agent added to therapy with azathioprine and prednisone. It was started intramuscularly five to six days in advance of surgery, continued daily for ten to 14 days afterward, then every other day for two weeks, two times a week for two months, and once a week for a final month.

The effect of antilymphocyte globulin therapy upon the peripheral white cells was unpredictable during the period of preoperative treatment when only this immunosuppressive agent was being used. The production of lymphopenia was irregular. Nevertheless, a profound effect upon immunologic reactivity was evident. A number of patients previously had positive skin tests to *Candida albicans*, tuberculin, mumps, histoplasmin, and Trichophyton. In each instance, the skin test became negative when redetermined after three or four days of antilymphocyte globulin therapy. Thus, antilymphocyte globulin promptly prevented the expression of preexisting delayed hypersensitivity.

In these patients, the amount of azathioprine given was less than in any previous series of comparable patients. More important was the fact that the amount of prednisone required was sharply reduced during the critical first four months of convalescence. The reduction in dose of the standard immunosuppressive agents was not paid for by the sacrifice of renal function. The blood urea nitrogens and creatinine clearances were better than in any of the earlier series of patients.

Most important, the incidence of septic complications was strikingly reduced. Seemingly, it has thus been possible with the aid of antilymphocyte globulin to improve the protection afforded the homografts and at the same time to less seriously hamper the host's ability to deal effectively with dangerous environmental antigens.

Thus far, there have not appeared to be prohibitively serious toxic reactions with the use of antilymphocyte globulin. The injections are often painful and cause fever. A few relatively minor anaphylactic reactions have occurred but in some patients these have not even necessitated discontinuance of the globulin. The first eight patients treated with globulin therapy had biopsy of their homografts after approximately four months of therapy. In none was there any evidence of serum sickness nephritis.

RESULTS AFTER RENAL HOMOTRANSPLANTATION. Until now, primary attention has been focused upon the problems caused by the slender margin between that therapy which is ineffective and that which is overzealous. Appreciation of these limitations, particularly as they applied in the earlier days of

transplantation, should not obscure the fact that many patients have been rewarded with relatively complete social and medical rehabilitation.

A total of 117 patients have been treated from March 1962 to April 1966, three with kidneys from identical twins, nine with cadaveric homografts, and 105 with homografts from volunteer donors. With the exception of the identical twin recipients, these patients were all provided with various combinations of azathioprine and prednisone, to which irregular administration of intravenous actinomycin C and local homograft irradiation were added. Subsequently, from June to December 1966, 20 more patients were treated, with the addition of antilymphocyte globulin to azathioprine and prednisone. Sequential division of the results from this experience illustrate the influence of several factors upon survival, including various adjustments in therapy and changes in policies of donor and recipient selection.

Identical twin cases. Three patients were 27, 20, and 54 years old when their operations were performed 72, 56, and 23 months ago. All three had glomerulonephritis. They now have normal renal function. Their courses have been completely satisfactory.

First living donor series. These 64 consecutively treated patients were treated from 48 to 64 months ago. Forty-six received kidneys from family members (20 parents, 23 siblings, and three aunts, uncles, or cousins); the other 18 donors were nonrelated. No other effort was made to match biologically donor and recipient pairs other than to ensure against ABO blood group incompatibilities.

Life survival curves of the patients are shown in Figure 10. Thirty-seven lived for one year, 34 for two years, and 32 for three years. Thirty (47 per cent) are still alive. The difference in long-term survival was striking in the recipients of homografts from related as compared to nonrelated donors. In the former subdivision, 28 of 46 (61 per cent) are still alive from more than four to five and one-half years. In the latter group, only two of 18 patients survive to date, one by virtue of a second homograft placed after two and one-half years.

Another important point can be made from this early series, aside from the proof it provides that many patients can be expected to live for a long time after homotransplantation. The disparity in results with essentially randomly selected donors is evident when the

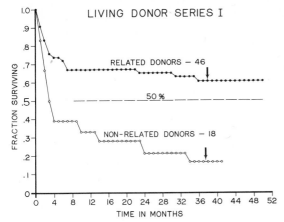

Figure 10. Survival curves of a consecutive series of 64 patients treated with renal homotransplantation from 38 to 55 months ago. Note that the long-term results with the use of kidneys from blood relatives are far superior to those which followed transplantation of genetically non-related kidneys. The arrows show the minimal postoperative follow-up for the most recently operated upon of these patients.

antigen matching. Whenever more than one donor was available, the antigen profile of each, as well as that of the recipient, was determined and the most compatible volunteer was accepted. There were 42 recipients who received homografts from 23 to 41 months ago.

In 25 patients, the donors were blood relatives (15 parents, nine siblings, one uncle). Because the selectivity within most families was limited, the quality of matching was only slightly, and not significantly, better than could have been achieved with random intrafamilial pairing. Of these 25 patients, 14 (56 per cent) are still alive (Fig. 11). The survival of 64 per cent after one year was not significantly different than in the previous series in which selection was not attempted on the basis of antigen matching.

For the nonrelated patients, the use of a donor pool, which at times offered as many as 100 possible selections, permitted a very substantial upgrading of donor-recipient antigen matching, as compared to that which would be expected on a chance basis. Of 17 recipients of these kidneys, nine lived for at least one year and six are still alive from 28 to 40 months after operation.

It was discouraging to note that the use of prospective antigen matching for donor selection did not have more influence upon prognosis. This was not surprising in the consanguineous transplantations because of the

outcome is compared with the use of homografts from intrafamilial and nonrelated donors.

Second living donor series. The antigens detected with human isoimmune sera have a significant relationship to histocompatibility. Such methods might have a clinical application even though they are admittedly still imperfect. The second series was, therefore, undertaken with an attempt at prospective

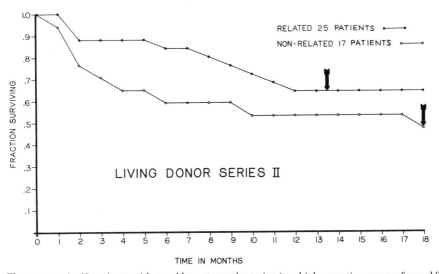

Figure 11. The outcome in 42 patients with renal homotransplantation in which operation was performed from 13 to 31 months ago. The minimal follow-up is indicated by vertical arrows. In this series, an attempt was made to select donors on the basis of the best possible donor-recipient antigen compatibility. In the consanguineous homotransplantations, the results were not improved over those previously obtained with random intrafamilial pairing. However, an improvement was found in the nonrelated patients.

inability to improve selection. For the non-related patients, in which the situation was different, survival was increased but only to the still unacceptable one-year level of 53 per cent.

This did not imply that the use of tissue-typing techniques would play an insignificant role in the transplantation practices of the future. Instead, it suggested that antigen matching could not receive a fair trial with the treatment programs being used widely unless transplantation was performed only between almost perfectly matched donor-recipient pairs. Such an approach would limit consideration to all but a very small number of patients who needed this kind of therapy. Consequently, the alternative approach of using new and hopefully better immunosuppressive regimens was evaluated.

Antilymphocyte globulin series. Twenty patients were operated upon. Kidneys were donated to 19 of the recipients by blood relatives on an essentially random selection basis—parents in five instances, siblings in 13, and a maternal uncle in the other. The twentieth patient received a cadaveric homograft from a donor who was shown to have an extremely poor antigen compatibility with the recipient.

Because of the preponderance of related patients, the mortality was compared to that of three consecutive past series of consanguineous transplantations in which therapy had consisted of azathioprine and prednisone. In the globulin-treated patients, there has only been one death (Fig. 12), the fourteenth patient in the group. The failure was caused by complications stemming directly from a technical accident.

The favorable slope of the survival curve in these patients is evident from Figure 12. These findings indicate that at least the early outlook after renal homotransplantation has been improved by the addition of adjuvant globulin therapy.

Cadaveric transplantations. Ten patients were treated with cadaveric transplantation prior to December 1966. Three of these recipients who received cadaveric homografts in 1963 died after four to 39 days with unrelieved uremia and sepsis. In 1965 and 1966, seven more attempts were made, including one patient who was treated with antilymphocyte globulin. All the kidneys functioned following delays of ten minutes to 23 days after revascularization. Four of the recipients died after three, eight, ten and 12½ months with failing homografts and with sepsis. Three are

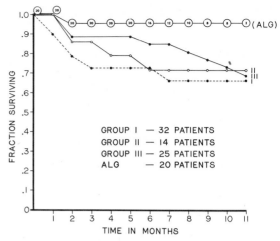

Figure 12. Early mortality in 20 patients treated with adjuvant antilymphocyte globulin (ALG). The number of patients available at each month of follow-up in this series is indicated. For comparison, the death rate is charted for each of three previous consecutive groups of patients in whom transplantation was from genetically related donors.

still alive, one after placement of a second homograft.

The future of transplantation is clearly dependent upon the exploitation of cadaveric organs. In the past, the high incidence of both early and gradual late failure has prevented this objective to more than a very limited degree. Nevertheless, the improvements in immunosuppression and antigen typing, as well as research in organ preservation, should make it possible eventually to limit organ procurement to cadaveric sources.

LIFE EXPECTANCY OF TOLERATED RENAL HOMOGRAFTS. The number of chronically functioning and life-sustaining homografts has been exponentially increasing since 1962. There have been 46, 34, and five patients who have lived for at least three, four, and five years respectively with the aid of a single homotransplanted kidney in our group of patients. Nevertheless, the ultimate functional interval of these organs can only be speculated upon.

Actuarial studies have been published based upon projections from follow-ups that are already available. These suggest that the outlook of a typical recipient of a related homograft is quite good for a number of years, if he reaches the sixth postoperative month without significant complications. The prognosis of homografts from nonrelated donors is far less certain. Whereas few kidneys in the former group have failed in the second and third postoperative years, the attrition in the latter group has continued at a moderately high rate.

Although the functional life of either type of homograft is not accurately known, there is reason to believe that it will not be normal. Many patients have had biopsies of their more or less well tolerated homografts two years or longer after operation. In only a small number were the tissues completely preserved. There was a high incidence of vascular lesions which caused obliterative changes in small, medium, and especially in large vessels (Fig. 13).

In addition, a common finding was the presence of interstitial fibrosis, which could have resulted from healing of an earlier rejection or alternatively from a diminished renal circulation caused by the vascular lesions. Many such homografts contained focal collections of mononuclear cells which were morphologically indistinguishable from the immunoblasts characteristically found in acutely rejecting homografts.

When the spectrum of histologic abnormali-

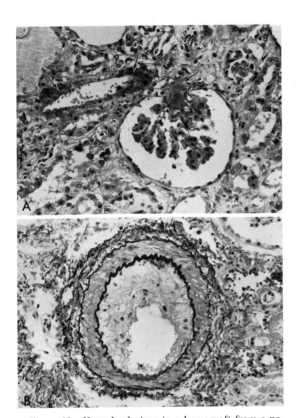

Figure 13. Vascular lesions in a homograft from a patient who died ten months after operation. The donor was nonrelated. *A*, There is fibrinoid necrosis (arrows) of part of the wall of an afferent arteriole with extension of the process into the glomerular tuft capillaries. The tubules are atrophic and the interstitium shows some fibrosis and edema (H & E × 350). *B*, An arcuate artery which has marked fibrous intimal thickening (elastic–van Gieson × 200). (By permission of Ann. Int. Med. *61*:470, 1964.)

ties in late homografts was first described more than three and one-half years ago, it was feared that many of these kidneys would begin to fail in a relatively short time. The view has proved to be overly pessimistic, because during the ensuing three and one-half years there has not been a further loss of function in the majority of patients insofar as could be detected by detailed testing.

At the moment, it must be conceded that the future is uncertain for any patient after renal homotransplantation, even for those who have had normal function for years. This fact has led to the point of view that such therapy should be considered a useful and increasingly effective form of palliation. Any conclusion that transplantation is a curative procedure will have to await a much longer period of observation.

TRANSPLANTATION OF OTHER ORGANS

Efforts have already been made in man to transplant the liver, lung, pancreas, and heart. The possibility has never seemed brighter of treating patients who are dying from isolated failure of these organs, because the advances made with the simpler problem of renal homotransplantation can probably be generally applied.

In the summer of 1967, the first successful orthotopic liver transplantation was performed. The patient is still alive nine months later. In principle, the feasibility of this undertaking had been proved long before because several dogs have now survived for as long as four years after complete excision of their own livers and placement of a homograft in the normal anatomic position (*orthotopic transplantation*). Except for a few details, the techniques of orthotopic liver transplantation in man (Fig. 14) and dogs are comparable in that all major structures entering and leaving the liver are reanastomosed.

Prior to 1967, eight clinical attempts had been made at orthotopic homotransplantation of the liver, in Denver, in Boston, and in Paris. Six of the patients survived the operation, but died from six to 23 days later. The causes of death were similar. Sepsis invariably developed. Gastrointestinal ulceration with hemorrhage, poor early liver function due to ischemic injury to the homograft, and intra- and postoperative abnormalities of blood coagulation were common. In addition, several of the earlier patients had pulmonary emboli which originated from the lower vena cava or

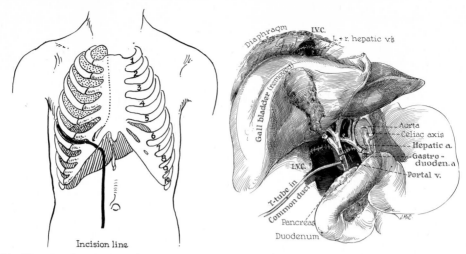

Figure 14. Human orthotopic transplantation of the liver. The diseased liver is removed and replaced with a cadaveric homograft which is revascularized in a normal way. Biliary drainage can be provided for with a choledocho-choledochostomy as shown, or by a cholecystenterostomy. (By permission of Surg. Gyn. & Obst. *117*:659, 1963.)

iliac veins. The complexity of these findings suggested that changes of several kinds would be required before further trials would have a reasonable chance of success. The most evident requisites were to improve both the techniques of immunosuppression, and the means of preserving postmortem homografts. Both objectives were at least partially met, thereby explaining the more encouraging recent results.

With orthotopic transplantation of the liver, immediate life-sustaining function of the homograft is an absolute necessity because there is no instrument analogous to an artificial kidney with which to tide the patient over a recovery period. Consequently, an appealing alternative possibility, particularly for the treatment of nonmalignant disease, would be to transplant an auxiliary liver to some abnormal location without disturbing the patient's own liver. For example, the homograft could be revascularized in the pelvis, the paravertebral gutter, or the splenic fossa.

The latter approach has the important advantage of not eliminating the residual function of the diseased liver, but it also introduces serious problems. The addition of a large extra organ to the abdominal contents may create serious mechanical difficulties. In one such patient, it is known that excision of the autologous liver was ultimately necessary before the incisions could be closed. In addition, it has been established that optimal performance of the homograft can be expected only if its portal venous inflow is derived from the venous effluent of the non-hepatic splanchnic bed. The technical difficulty of connecting the portal vein of a heterotopically placed homograft to the recipient's distal portal bed has led to the evolution of several useful compromise methods in which the venous inflow to the liver is derived from systemic veins. Nevertheless, the results in the laboratory with auxiliary transplantation have been distinctly inferior to those with the orthotopic operation.

Successful orthotopic transplantation of the heart has also been carried out in dogs but with a less consistent success rate. The most useful method is that shown in Figure 15. The recipient heart is removed during circulatory support by a heart-lung apparatus. A cuff of autologous left and right atrium is retained and this is used to suture to the atria and the atrial septum of the homograft. The pulmonary artery and aorta are reconstructed with end-to-end anastomoses.

The clinical application of orthotopic cardiac transplantation will depend upon some very difficult problems of supply. It will be necessary to have an organ which is not badly damaged in the process of donor death, to preserve it for a substantial period, and to have it resume effective pump action quickly after its revascularization.

In addition, this procedure has its own specific complications. The homografted heart does not beat with a normal sinus rhythm. Postoperatively, the impulse initiation is often in the less reliable atrioventricular node. A common cause of death in dogs after heart transplantation is cardiac arrest owing either to asystole or to the development of fatal arrhythmias. When such operations are employed clinically, it will probably be necessary to provide means to control these complications by electrical stimulation during the postoperative period. That such problems do not preclude at least temporary success has been illustrated by the report of a recent patient with a cardiac transplant who has lived more than five months at this writing.

Orthotopic transplantation of the whole lung is a relatively easy procedure which can be done in several ways (Fig. 16). Technically, it is easiest to transfer a piece of donor atrium into which all the pulmonary veins enter. Homografts of lobes can also be readily transplanted by anastomosis of the major lobar structures.

If entire lungs are transplanted in experimental animals, there are problems caused by the necessity for denervation which in turn result in the loss of certain respiratory reflexes. Equally limiting, when either whole lungs or lobes are used, is the fact that only the pulmonary arterial component of the normally double blood supply can be easily reconstructed; the bronchial arteries are too small to permit their successful anastomosis.

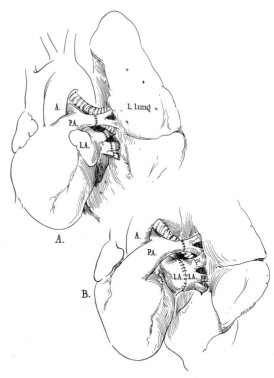

Figure 16. Two techniques for orthotopic homotransplantation of the left lung. In *A*, the pulmonary veins are individually anastomosed. Alternatively (*B*), an atrial cuff with the homograft can be sutured to the left atrium of the recipient. Neither method provides for reconstitution of the bronchial artery supply.

Consequently, the homograft bronchus which must be sutured has subnormal perfusion. This has caused a high incidence of bronchostenosis or anastomotic disruption in animal experiments, particularly in dogs. There is some evidence that this may present less of a hazard in subhuman primates or in man.

Other tissues and organs have been transplanted in humans, including skin lymphoid tissues of various kinds, various endocrine organs, limbs, and living cartilage, to mention only a few.

ORGAN PRESERVATION

With all living grafts, a crucial technical problem is to restore nutrition within the permissible time limits of ischemia. Although the ability to recover from an avascular interval varies with different tissues, the necessity for prompt transfer imposes sharp limitations on all grafting procedures. Several methods can be used either alone or in combination to prolong the viability of extirpated tissues and organs.

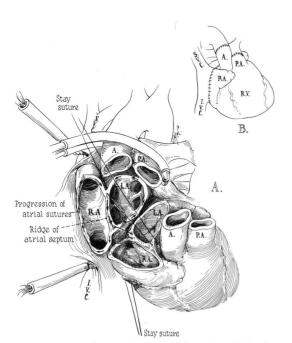

Figure 15. Orthotopic homotransplantation of the dog heart as developed by Shumway and Lower. Note that the atria and interatrial septum of the donor and recipient are sutured. This method makes it unnecessary to anastomose separately the venae cavae and the pulmonary veins.

INHIBITION OF METABOLISM

HYPOTHERMIA. Hypothermia refers to a reduction in temperature which is not below 0° C. It offers perhaps the simplest and most practical method for short-term preservation. Cooling can be accomplished quickly by the intravascular perfusion of excised organs with chilled electrolyte solutions. Within limits, the magnitude of the protection obtained is more or less directly related to the degree of cooling. This is not difficult to understand because it is known that for each 10° C. decrease in temperature, oxidative metabolism is reduced by one-half. At 2° C., it is less than 5 per cent of that at 37° C., and with supercooling it is possible to bring the oxygen requirement to zero. However, this does not necessarily ensure long-term viability because activity of certain enzyme systems cannot be arrested even with temperatures as low as −80° C. In time, these are responsible for cell death by causing autolysis and by other, poorly understood mechanisms.

The usefulness of hypothermia varies with the metabolic characteristics of individual tissues. Those which are ordinarily resistant to anoxia, such as skin, bone, cartilage, and cornea, can be preserved for several weeks in a cooled state. Complex and metabolically active organs, such as the kidney, liver, heart, and lung, all can be kept in a potentially functional state by this means for only a few hours.

SUPERCOOLING. With these techniques, the temperature is reduced to lower than 0° C. Supercooling offers important possibilities for storage sufficiently prolonged to permit establishment of organ banks, because it is probable that all metabolic activity can be arrested at temperatures below −100° C. Organ storage by this means is not yet a practical objective because of damage which occurs as the result of freezing and thawing.

The cause of cellular injury with freezing is still not completely understood. Until relatively recently, it was thought to have a mechanical etiology by which intracellular formation of ice spicules caused perforation of the cell membranes. To some extent this may be true, but it can be avoided by very rapid cooling which promotes the formation of small and nondisruptive ice fragments. Furthermore, it has since been learned that a critical element of the injury is a biochemical one. Ice which is formed, whether it be within or outside the cell, contains little or no solute, and as a consequence the fluid which is left becomes hyperosmolar. It is thought by most authorities that the resulting excessive electrolyte concentrations are responsible for irreversible damage.

Significant protection from these adverse effects of supercooling can be obtained by exposure of some tissues to 10 to 30 per cent glycerol, propylene glycol, or dimethyl sulfoxide. Such substances, which collectively are termed endocellular cryophylactic agents, have in common the ability to freely permeate cell membranes and presumably to bond with water, preventing its crystallization. The use of these agents to preserve red cells, spermatozoa, and bacteria has been spectacularly successful. However, attempts to use them for the conservation of whole organs have not been effective enough to warrant clinical application.

One of the most intriguing possibilities for future investigation is to cool so rapidly that water is frozen into an amorphous glass rather than into crystals. To be able to do this, water must be cooled in one second to at least −130° C. Theoretically, such vitrified water could enter the solid phase without deadly effect.

CHEMICAL PROTECTION. Several agents have been described which, when perfused into the vascular system of excised organs, appear to prolong the acceptable limits of ischemia. These include magnesium sulfate, sodium fluoride, and adrenochrome. The reason for the beneficial effect has not been completely explained because aerobic and anaerobic metabolism continue, although at reduced rates.

It is conceivable that these chemicals have some other unrecognized means of protection such as stabilization of cell membranes. During the past few years the role of intracellular enzyme release in determining the irreversibility of anoxic injury has been discussed. It is known, for example, that the escape of lysosomes from their intracellular envelopes is a lethal development. Both adrenal cortical steroids and chlorpromazine are thought to delay this event. In the future, these and other agents with a similar effect may be of adjuvant value in preservation techniques.

HYPERBARIC OXYGENATION

There have been numerous reports of the benefits of storing organs in chambers containing oxygen under 2 to 15 atmospheres of pressure. The validity of these claims has been challenged, inasmuch as penetration of the oxygen, even under high pressure, can be demonstrated to be relatively limited in tissue slices. At 7 atmospheres with a temperature of 37°, the distance that oxygen can diffuse in heart muscle is only 2 mm.; at 5° C. it is increased to only 6 or 7 mm. Thus, the effect should only be at the surface of kidneys, livers or other bulky organs. Champions of hyperbaric techniques have pointed out that the pessimistic data from tissue slice experiments may not be directly relevant to preservation of whole organs which are immersed in fluid, and which are kept at very cold temperatures under high compression.

COMBINED TECHNIQUES

The limitations of each of the individual methods of organ conservation can often be partially circumvented by using two or more techniques together. An effective method for protecting several organs in the same cadaveric donor is to institute artificial perfusion of all or part of the body with a heart lung machine (Fig. 17). By incorporating a heat exchanger in the circuit, rapid core cooling can be accomplished at the same time as the perfusion. In dogs, immediately functioning

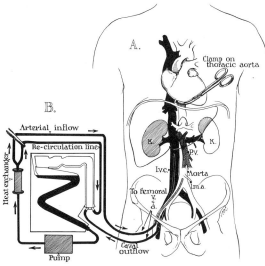

Figure 17. Technique of extracorporeal cadaver perfusion. Catheters are inserted via the femoral vessels into the aorta and vena cava as soon as possible after death. The extracorporeal circuit is primed with heparinized glucose or electrolyte solution to which procaine is added. The cadaver is anticoagulated with the first surge of the pump. Temperature control is provided by the heat exchanger.

renal homografts can always be obtained with this method when they are removed and transplanted 12 hours after the sacrifice of the donor animal.

Some of the combinations are favored by well-accepted physical laws. For example, the inherent value of hypothermia for extending the viability of nonvascularized tissue is not the only advantage of cold. If perfusion at reduced temperatures is carried out with a non-hemoglobin–containing solution, oxygen can be dissolved more readily in the perfusate; furthermore, the rate of flow can be markedly reduced without incurring a metabolic deficit. Similarly the gaseous diffusion through tissues is promoted in hyperbaric oxygen chambers in relation to the degree that the temperature is lowered. With several combinations of these methods, kidneys, hearts, and intestinal segments have been successfully preserved for two to three days.

PREMORTEM INFLUENCES UPON CADAVERIC HOMOGRAFTS

Virtually all research on organ preservation is carried out under ideal circumstances in which a normal circulation of the donor is maintained until the time of homograft removal. When human homografts are obtained from cadavers, these conditions are never duplicated and they are not even closely simulated except for the rare instance in which a patient is rushed to the hospital and dies a few minutes after massive craniocerebral trauma.

For most patients who are considered as potential candidates for cadaveric donation, the events leading to death are less acute and there is a variable terminal period of inadequate tissue perfusion. During this time organs may be damaged, often to an unpredictable degree. In animals, the adverse effects of slow death can partly be circumvented by various measures such as the administration of heparin or large doses of steroids, or by the induction of hypothermia. In humans, the propriety of such actions which are not designed primarily for the treatment of the dying patient has been seriously questioned.

ETHICAL RESTRAINTS IN TRANSPLANTATION

Developments during the past few decades have caused increased and often unwanted attention to be focused upon the medical profession. The public has begun to appreciate the immense power which is potentially in the hands of physicians and surgeons. For example, it has already become perfectly practical to control population growth. Now, there are authorities who believe that more discriminating efforts should be made at genetic control in an effort to improve the future quality of the human race.

It is important to define the distinction between the noble aims of these society-oriented proposals and the humbler but by no means ignoble objectives of the vast majority of practicing physicians and surgeons whose efforts sometimes seem almost to tend in the opposite direction. It is doubtful if many physicians or surgeons who actually care for the sick and the infirm plan their actions on the basis of the predicted effect upon society. Instead, the dominant tradition is for the doctor to provide the best care of which he is capable for those who either seek his services or who are assigned to his responsibility. By and large this is done without regard for the conceivably broader issue of whether or not treatment is justifiable on social grounds. His reasons may include pride, altruism, compassion, curiosity, a spirit of competition, even avarice, or a combination of all these things. Whatever the motives, the reflexes which follow are sure, and respond similarly to the needs of the productive members of the community, the insane and feeble-minded, children with incurable birth defects, condemned criminals, or even soldiers who moments before were members of a hostile army.

The foregoing viewpoint is a narrow one, but there is no reason to believe that it should be abandoned in the face of advancing technocracy. It has shielded the ill from the caprices and the moral judgments of other men through centuries of evolving philosophical, religious, and legal doctrines. It has placed the concept of the sanctity of human life on a practical foundation, because the responsibility of one person for another could not be more clearly defined than through the doctor-patient relationship, irrespective of the reasons for the contract entered into between the two involved parties.

Has this ancient creed of medicine been ravaged by the scientific explosion in which we are now involved? Examination of this question as it applies to organ transplantation is inevitable, first, because of the widespread lay publicity which has accompanied such efforts and, second, because the harsh term "purely experimental" has consistently been applied to these procedures by virtually all workers in the field as well as by interested observers.

The designation of experimental is perfectly correct. Few endeavors have ever yielded such a rich and diversified harvest of both fundamental and practical information, so united basic and clinical scientists in the pursuit of a common goal, and defined and stimulated such large areas of potentially fruitful new research. Nevertheless, the primary purpose in these patients was therapeutic and it is important to realize the degree to which this objective has already been met. Almost from the beginning of combination therapy with azathioprine and prednisone, it was evident that many patients could profit from homotransplantation, at least of the kidney. Unfortunately, it also quickly became clear that an impasse had been reached beyond which further reductions in mortality could not be expected without new immunosuppressive techniques.

This conclusion raised two important philosophical issues. The first concerned the advisability of continuing to provide a standard form of therapy which carried a high and by now relatively predictable failure rate. The corollary question was whether new, clinically untried, and potentially dangerous immunosuppressive measures should be incorporated in the therapeutic regimen. The gain might be a substantial improvement in patient care. The loss in the event of unexpected complications could be the injury or death of patients who might otherwise have had an untroubled postoperative convalescence had it been realized in advance that they were unusually favorable candidates. Eventually, the change in therapy involving the addition of antilymphocyte globulin was instituted.

The growing field of transplantation can be used to illustrate some principles to which most involved investigators have adhered. First, the clinical trial of new therapeutic methods is based more firmly than ever on prior animal experimentation. Virtually all practices in cardiac as well as in transplantation surgery have been transferred, almost without change, from the laboratory to the clinical ward or operating room.

Not infrequently, the transition has been made with haste and with an air of urgency which was fed by the needs and wishes of desperate patients who had the misfortune of not becoming ill at a later and more convenient time. Historically, the decisions to proceed have often been wrong. Nevertheless, they have almost invariably been based on the hope, however fleeting or erroneously conceived, of potential benefit to the individual patient.

Right or wrong, the actions are eventually subjected to implacable scrutiny, principally by other members of the scientific community but also by intelligent and informed outsiders. Inaccuracies in reporting, claims that cannot be reproduced, and procedures which neither relieve suffering nor prolong life are rapidly identified. Harmful practices are snuffed out quickly; homeopathic ones may suffer a lingering death but they also ultimately disappear from the scene. The system is ruthless and impiteous and demands a policy of nonconcealment from those who would innovate in medicine. It is not sufficient to report only successes. Failures must also be fully documented, no matter how painful and humiliating these may be, in order to prevent repetition by others of the same mistakes. In general, such openness has characterized efforts in the field of transplantation.

Until now, some problems of transplantation have been discussed only as they apply to the recipients of potentially life-sustaining organs. The thoughtful trial of a variety of therapeutic variables, in which the risk of adverse effects was borne by the persons who had the most to gain, seems highly defensible both in prospect and retrospect. The involvement in such ventures of persons who may be harmed or who do not stand to derive any direct benefit is not such a simple matter. This practice, as epitomized by the testing of new drugs or procedures in human volunteers, is defined in the Helsinki Declaration (1964) as "clinical research, the essential object of which is purely scientific and without therapeutic value to the person subjected to the research." It adds that the subject must "be in such a mental, physical, and legal state as to be able to exercise fully his power of choice." Because the propriety or even the legality of such experimentation has been questioned, it may now be well to examine in this context the problem of organ donation.

No easy answers are available. When intrafamilial homotransplantation is performed under the proper circumstances, it cannot be reasonably said that there is no value to the donor who usually has been the first to suggest this possibility. His willingness may be based on the extent to which the fullness of his inner life is involved with and dependent upon that of the recipient or because of a variety of other acceptable reasons; to our knowledge, the objective is never the acquisition of scientific data. Progress in medicine confronts him with a decision which may be difficult but which is consonant with the dignity and responsibility of free life.

Quite another situation exists, of course, with the reluctant donor who by arbitration has been selected by the family on the basis of his or her presumed expendability. It is ordinarily not difficult to detect this kind of coercion, particularly if trouble is taken to make the appropriate specific inquiries. The potential victim is excused from further workup on the grounds of some medical diagnosis which will protect him from guilt feelings and from the ostracism of those who were so anxious to volunteer his services.

In a recent symposium on ethics in medical practice, the previously cited matter of free choice as it affected all kinds of clinical investigation became one of the dominant themes of the conference. The ability of minors, prisoners, and even medical students to "fully exercise their power of choice" was seriously questioned and discussed at some length because transplantation donors had already been employed from the first two of these classes of captive populations.

The transplantations from minors had been done in other institutions under exceptionally favorable psychological and medical circumstances involving identical twins. Nevertheless, it was challenged that these accidents of birth should have set the well twins apart, in the eyes of the law, from other minors who would automatically have been disqualified.

The penal volunteers were accepted under conditions which it was thought would fully ensure the protection of their individual rights and permit their complete freedom of choice, objectives which in principle may have been even less realistic than with the identical twin minors. In any event, there is every reason to believe that this practice, however equitably handled in a local situation, would inevitably lead to abuse if accepted as a reasonable precedent and applied broadly. For these reasons, and because the donor motivation which characterizes proper intrafamilial transplantation could not be said to exist except in the most idealized and universal sense, the acceptance of criminal volunteers was permanently discontinued at the University of Colorado two and a half years ago.

The question of organ procurement from living volunteers is perhaps the most sensitive and limiting issue in clinical transplantation. The best prognosis today can be offered to the recipient only with the use of such donors, particularly when these are from within the family. In the future, it is hoped that the need for living donors will be made obsolete by improvements in immunosuppression, antigen typing, and tissue preservation. Then, organs obtained solely from cadavers could be used with a high expectation of long-term survival.

Unfortunately, success will not imply that an ethical panacea will have been found, primarily because the terminal events in a prospective cadaveric donor are of such importance in determining the quality of a subsequently transplanted organ. It is conceivable that this fact could lead to subtle or even major adjustments in care which would be designed for the protection of the organ to be removed rather than for the benefit of its donor.

Examples can be cited. In several centers outside the United States, conventional death has been re-defined, in some patients in the presence of a continuing heart beat, in terms of objective evidence of irreversible injury to the central nervous system. The judgment that death was imminent and unavoidable was made by a panel of expert referees who were not members of the transplantation team, although the need for their mediation was clearly the consequence of the requirements for fresh and uninjured organs. One or both kidneys were then removed from these "living cadavers," with apparent benefit to the recipients; the incidence of immediate urine excretion was very high. That a high degree of social conscience dictated these actions is beyond dispute. What could be questioned is the concept of imposing further trauma upon a dying patient, however apparently hopeless his condition, at a moment when he is the epitome of mental incompetence. The act itself could be construed as an erosion of the historic medical creed of responsibility to the individual patient, at least as this applies to the donor, and the timing as a violation of the principle of free choice.

Perhaps it is not inaccurate to say that the important features of the selection and management of homograft recipients or their donors illustrate some problems of day to day ethics which apply in principle to other forms of clinical investigation and in fact to traditional medical practice. No effort has been made to say that errors have not been made in the development of clinical transplantation nor to imply that new mistakes can be completely prevented from this day forward. It has, however, been suggested that progress in this and other new fields of medicine has been made in a sturdy framework which is ethical, practical, and efficiently policed. There are few surgeons who believe that the traditional responsibility of the doctor for the welfare of his patient has been, or that it should be, lessened by the emergence of new forms of therapy which of necessity must at some time be tried for the first time in man.

READING REFERENCES

Annals of the New York Academy of Sciences, Vol. 129, Article 1, 1966.

Calne, R. Y.: Renal Transplantation. Baltimore, The Williams and Wilkins Company, 1963.

Carrel, A., and Lindbergh, C. A.: The Culture of Organs. New York, Paul B. Hoeber, Inc., 1938.

Ethics in Medical Progress: With Special Reference to Transplantation. London, J. and A. Churchill Ltd., 1966.

Good, R. A., and Gabrielsen, A. E.: The Thymus in Immunobiology. New York, Hoeber Medical Division, Harper and Row, 1964.

Loeb, L.: The Biological Basis of Individuality. Springfield, Illinois, Charles C Thomas, 1945.

Medawar, P. B.: Antilymphocytic Serum. London, J. and A. Churchill Ltd., 1967.

National Academy of Sciences: Histocompatibility Testing. Washington, D.C., Research Council Publication 1229, 1965.

Peer, L. A.: Transplantation of Tissues: Cartilage, Bone, Fascia, Tendon and Muscle. Two volumes. Baltimore, The Williams and Wilkins Company, 1955, 1959.

Russell, P. S., and Monaco, A. P.: The Biology of Tissue Transplantation. Boston, Little, Brown & Company, 1965.

Starzl, T. E.: Experience in Renal Transplantation. Philadelphia, W. B. Saunders Company, 1964.

Welch, C. E.: Advances in Surgery, Vol. II. Chicago, Year Book Medical Publishers, Inc., 1966.

Woodruff, M. F. A.: Transplantation of Tissues and Organs. Springfield, Illinois, Charles C Thomas, 1960.

Chapter 39

THE SURGEON

by
LOYAL DAVIS, M.D.

LOYAL DAVIS was born in Galesburg, Illinois, the son of a locomotive engineer, and attended Knox College. He served for 31 years as Chairman of the Department of Surgery, Northwestern University, from which he graduated. He has been active as a Regent and President of the American College of Surgeons. He is Editor of Surgery, Gynecology & Obstetrics.

Surgery is the application of the knowledge of the basic biological and physical sciences to the care of the patient. Surgery is not an exact science in the narrow sense. In that it is based on accepted and applicable principles of anatomy, physiology, chemistry, bacteriology and related disciplines, it is a science.

Surgery is also an art. The surgeon must translate his knowledge and apply his skills by a series of mental, moral and physical acts into their highest potential for the care of each individual patient under certain circumstances and at a specific time.

EDUCATION OF THE SURGEON

Qualifications of surgeons have changed with advances in surgery but there are basic characteristics of every dedicated practitioner of the healing arts. These are integrity, honesty, humanity, fidelity to responsibility and freedom from avarice. For the surgeon, there must be added the quality of calm judgment and decisive action in sudden crises and the ability of critical self-analysis.

As Susruta noted, surgery is less liable than internal medicine to the fallacy of conjecture. Early surgeons were practical men and this characteristic continues to distinguish them from speculative philosophers. It accounts for their interest in and development of the basic sciences and their application to the treatment of patients.

The pragmatic approach of surgeons was responsible for their low social status until modern times. The knowledge of Latin and Greek was not essential to the use of a knife. One of the attacks upon Ambroïse Paré by the physicians of his day was that he wrote in his native tongue rather than in a classical language.

Perhaps, the most significant advances in surgery in the past few years have been in the preoperative and postoperative care of patients. Competence in these fields distinguishes the surgeon from the operator. The physiological functions of the patient must be fortified against the terrific insults to his metabolism which cannot be avoided in many surgical procedures. The physiological processes must be re-established promptly and maintained.

Surgeons have led the way in research and investigation seeking the solution to these problems. While it is possible for the practitioner of surgery to apply techniques of which he has little or no basic understanding, those who will push forward the boundaries of surgical treatment must have a thorough, applicable knowledge of all the sciences involved in the mechanisms of living tissue. Surgery is no longer a mechanical art; it is the coalition of several sciences and those who contribute to its advancement in the future, and who give their patients the best possible care, must be educated and trained accordingly. To become a surgeon today requires postgraduate education and training. This period of study must be one of teaching, learning, study and training. Too often, the words "residency training" are interpreted as an apprenticeship in techniques.

There are programs available for those who voluntarily wish to devote years of their life and career to become a surgeon. There are no excuses today for short cuts for those unwilling to make all the sacrifices necessary, or

1449

unable intellectually and mentally to accept the disciplined education necessary to become a surgeon.

Regardless of the special field of surgery in which the postgraduate surgical student becomes interested, he should be educated and trained basically in the principles of surgery which apply to all the body. The minimum should be two years, and it is to be hoped that eventually the pendulum may return to a 3:1 or 3:2 proportion, between so-called "general" surgery and a special field of surgery.

A philosophy has developed that if one has an elementary education in diagnosis and examination, and if there is a real interest in research, he automatically is a fully equipped surgeon. This is a completely false assumption, which denies the art of surgery. This is as indefensible as the viewpoint of a surgeon who takes satisfaction in the number of patients he has operated upon that day, without careful thought of their preoperative and postoperative problems, without a study of the pathologic condition found, or a meticulous record which may become part of an enlightening clinical study, and who has no interest in or sympathy with contributions from the research laboratory. Neither one of these individuals is a surgeon.

There are other reasons for a broad, basic education and training in the principles of surgery. Not every young graduate can make a fixed decision in the beginning about a special field of surgery. He may change more than once to his own and his patients' advantage, and he should analyze and keep his mind open as he becomes temporarily a surgical specialist in each field, as he progresses through his program.

Of more importance is the fact that if he decides to live and prosper in a smaller community without a medical school, he should have knowledge in all fields of surgery. He should be able to recognize and confidently deal with an impacted fracture of the surgical neck of the humerus or femur, for example. He must also be professionally and ethically honest, and direct his patient to the orthopedic surgeon for the introduction of a prosthetic head of the femur.

This lack of basic education and training for all surgical residents is one of the weakest areas of many postgraduate programs. Each surgical specialty seeks its own medical school department, autonomous and in many instances unwilling to cooperate in the education and training of surgeons in the true sense.

On the other hand, there are chairmen of departments of surgery who are reluctant to provide places for basic surgical training in their programs for young men who have decided to devote themselves to a particular field of surgery. This separation into compartments of surgery should be stopped, either in the medical school where administration and teaching can be decentralized but coordinated under the department of surgery chairman, or in the hospital, so that residents may receive basic education and training in every aspect of surgery. Ideally, both medical school and hospital staffs should be so organized, not only for the best immediate interests of young men, but for the best surgical care for the patient, the goal which so often is taken for granted in the struggle of men to build their own little empires.

There are at least two facets of present residency programs which are difficult to resolve. One deals with the methodology of education and training, the other with remuneration for the postgraduate student in surgery.

No essential difference exists in the opportunities for education and training of the resident between patients, who pay the attending surgeon and teacher for his services, and those who are unable to pay a professional fee but are, or are not, able to finance their hospitalization costs. That resident can become an envied surgeon who is taught step-by-step the proper technique of the repair of an inguinal hernia and the gentle handling of tissues; the thought which should be devoted to each patient's surgical problem before operation; the critical review of how each operation might have been performed more skillfully and expeditiously, from incision to placement of the last suture and dressing; the art of dealing with the patient's relatives for the protection of the patient, and the discussion of the proper fee based completely upon the patient's ability to pay in relation to the magnitude of the surgical procedure, though his experiences have been confined wholly to so-called "private" patients.

It must be recognized that the resident and his surgical teacher have reciprocal responsibilities to teach and to learn, and a joint responsibility to give the patient the best possible surgical treatment. One surgical chief once said that every young doctor who aspired to become a surgeon should evaluate his inherent ability to use his hands and his brain cooperatively, and the breadth and integrity of his imagination. He did not mean an imagination to conceive new procedures, new operating table attachments, or instrumental gimmicks but the ability to imagine himself, his wife, mother, father, or children as the patient.

Such an aspiring resident, as he sits in a comfortable chair in his quarters, can perform an operation upon an imaginary patient. He should be able to imagine difficulties in finding the appendix, or identifying the cystic duct, and then deal with them successfully, as would Walter Mitty. He should collect many questions for his chief to be asked at the propitious moment, under the proper circumstances, not when the great man is having difficulty in identifying the common duct.

This is not to say that teaching beds supported by endowment, taxes and, in part, insurance hospitalization benefits are unnecessary and superfluous. It is to say, however, that patients who occupy such beds should not be under the complete, sole authority of the senior resident and his assistant residents. The best education and training for surgery require that the professor and his associates assume responsibility for the best possible surgical care and act as the residents' first assistants. This requires energy, time, and dedication to the task of teaching, and it does interfere with the professorial staff's personal interests in surgical practice, laboratory investigations, and peripatetic desires supported by boxes of large and small lantern slides.

It also requires that the patient, admitted to the hospital under these circumstances, be informed and made to understand that the resident will operate and have responsibility, assisted by the surgeon-in-chief or his associates. This, too, requires time and effort, but it prevents the criticism of "ghost" surgery, and ensures the best care for the patient. It may help the resident realize that, regardless of his seniority and his youthful, admirable self-confidence, there will always be something he can learn about surgery and that if he does not have an inner stimulus to continue to learn, he will fail as a surgeon.

With some understanding of the changing social and economic structure of the United States, it remains difficult to reach a satisfactory opinion concerning the remuneration of interns and residents during their postgraduate years of study. It is only fair to accept the premise that biologic urges in men of the same age group were the same 40 years ago as they are now. It is difficult to accept the statement that because the residency applicant is married and has children, some-

one else is responsible completely for his economic security during this period of continued education. It would seem to be a question of whether or not he is providing services to the hospital and its attending staff, or whether he is present primarily to be educated and trained as a surgeon.

Postgraduate students in surgery have been placed at a disadvantage with their college classmates in engineering, and the physical or biologic sciences. They do not receive subsidies for their professional education; their contemporaries earn respectable incomes immediately after graduation from college; the medical school graduate is more certain to give military service, and the postdoctoral years have been assumed voluntarily, without remuneration. All these factors affect the national requirements for the best medical care, the financial burdens of universities and hospitals, and the cost of medical care.

In a voluntarily supported hospital and university, funds to support such an educational program come, in great part, from the hospital bed income. In state or county supported institutions, it is derived from taxes. In either case, it becomes an item in the increased cost of medical care. It is worth the money expended, but the only criterion of evaluation should be whether it provides better surgeons to give the best possible care to the patient. This one goal is often lost in the multiplicity of factors which govern postgraduate education and training.

SURGICAL SOCIETIES AND COLLEGES

In medieval times, certain monks were appointed to perform the tasks of shaving, bleeding, pulling teeth and dressing wounds. In 1163, at the Council of Tours, the activities of the monks were restricted to their religious duties and they were forbidden to leave the monastery to attend the sick and injured. Consequently, elementary surgical practices fell into the hands of military surgeons, barbers, bath-keepers and traveling charlatans, and it became necessary to belong to a guild to practice a craft. Guilds, like unions today, exerted great power. The members had specific religious and civic duties, wore their own livery, participated in processions and contributed to the treasury of the city. Soon, barbers took on more of the duties originally performed by the monks and became barber-surgeons.

The red and white striped pole represented

the blood and bandages of the barber-surgeon's craft. The number of members of the guild trained in anatomy and surgery gradually increased and the guild became a union of barbers and surgeons, which existed a long time mainly for civic and economic reasons. Eventually, the surgeons formed companies of their own, gained authority to train apprentices, conduct examinations, license practitioners and guard the public health. As charters were granted by kings with permission to use the royal favor, these companies became Royal Colleges.

The oldest Royal College is that of Edinburgh, which was incorporated in 1505 by the favor of James IV, who was interested in medicine and tried his skill at surgery. The charter required that each member be acquainted with anatomy, and the company was entitled to receive each year the body of one criminal "efter he be deid" for dissection. The organization had a bath house, a laboratory and a library. In 1695, the surgeons were separated from the barbers and in 1778, the corporation became a Royal College, though it remained a municipal body until 1850.

The chronological development of the Royal College of Surgeons in England was similar: from 1300–1540, there was an incorporated Company of Barbers and the Guild of Surgeons was unincorporated; from 1540–1745, the Company of Barber-Surgeons; the Company of Surgeons from 1745–1800, and the Royal College of Surgeons of London from 1800–1843, when the present name was adopted. Henry VIII granted the charter to the Company of Barbers in 1540 and this is depicted in a famous painting by Holbein. Of the ten identified members, four were barbers, four were surgeons and two were "foreigners." A barber is shown receiving the scroll.

After complete separation of the surgeons and the receipt of their charter in 1800, examinations for Fellowship were initiated in 1883 and today a Fellowship is required to be qualified to practice surgery in England. Each of the Royal Colleges has devoted its efforts to postgraduate education and research to elevate the standards of care to patients.

The American College of Surgeons, founded in 1913, was patterned in many respects after the Royal Colleges in Great Britain. Its primary goal is to improve the care of surgical patients and this has been contributed to by its efforts in improving postgraduate surgical education, elevating the standards of hospitals, and education of the lay public. Gradually, the qualifications for Fellowship have been raised until at present they consist of an education and training which qualify the candidate for examination by the Boards of surgery and its specialties, and evidence of high personal and professional moral and ethical standards.

There are hundreds of medical societies, surgical associations and colleges in the United States. Doctors voluntarily join county medical societies, which entitles them to membership in their state medical society and the American Medical Association. These basic medical organizations require graduation from an approved medical school, a state license to practice medicine, and evidence of good ethical and professional practices. Their activities include the presentation of scientific papers by their members and invited guests, and discussion of problems which influence the practice of medicine. Each state has a medical society, as does each county except in those instances when two or three contiguous small counties have joined together to form one society.

The American Medical Association was founded in 1847 through the efforts of Nathan Smith Davis. It is a confederation of state societies. It has a Board of Trustees which is the policy making body but, in effect, this power lies within the House of Delegates. This body consists of 235 delegates, chosen by each state society in a number proportionate to the number of doctors practicing in the state, who are members of the state society and the American Medical Association; representatives from the scientific sections of the Association, and from the five government medical services.

There is a multitude of more exclusive societies representing specialty areas in the practice of medicine and surgery and still others dedicated to specific diseases or organs of the body. The specialty societies require evidence of proper education and training in the specific field, and the disease and organ societies limit their membership to those who have shown interest by their work and contributions in the particular area.

The American Surgical Association is typical of associations and societies formed by doctors who have an interest in a special area of medicine and is one of the oldest. It was founded in 1881 by a group of surgeons whose leader and first president was Samuel Gross. Objections to it centered around the supposition that a new association was being organized which would usurp the functions of the American Medical Association, and destroy its influence as the representative body of the medical profession. It was argued that all the objectives sought by such an association of surgeons could be accomplished through the section on surgery of the American Medical Association. There had been many discussions of the rights of surgical specialists compared with general practitioners; the economic, scientific and social aspects of specialization were attracting increasing attention.

In his presidential address, Gross met the arguments directly:

"If it be said that we are striking a blow at the American Medical Association, we deny the soft impeachment. On the contrary, we shall strengthen that body by rousing it from its Rip Van Winkle slumbers and infusing new life into it. We can hurt no society now in existence, or likely to come into existence. We can hurt only ourselves if we fail to do our duty. We hope to make the American Surgical Association an altar upon which we may annually lay our contributions to surgical science and so show the world that we are earnest and zealous laborers in the interest of human progress and human suffering."

It is doubtful that any new medical or surgical society has been formed without meeting opposition from the members in an older society. Often, the members of exclusively small, special societies become so conservative that they oppose the admission of younger men. So the younger men band together and form a new society; they, in turn, become older and more reactionary; young, aggressive men rebel and form a society; and so the cycle is repeated. Or, certain geographic areas of the country are not represented in the membership of national societies and thus, directions of the compass designate new associations of surgeons. The ever increasing multiplicity of medical and surgical societies is not bad; it only emphasizes the desire of doctors to meet together, discuss their problems, learn from each other, and indulge their inherently peripatetic personalities, armed with a box full of lantern slides.

ETHICS AND PRACTICES

Surgeons should always be proud of belonging to a profession which stands alone in the enforcement of adherence of its members to a high code of ethical conduct, which guides the relationship between its members and their patients, and which dates back to the Hippocratic oath.

The Principles of Medical Ethics of the American Medical Association contain the code of ethics to which all medical organizations subscribe. However, neither the Principles nor their interpretation by the Judicial Council of the Medical Association have always been clear and precise; violations by the more enterprising members of the profession have been frequent. Therefore, the Board of Regents of the American College of Surgeons, in no way a subsidiary organization of the Medical Association, has made its own interpretation and requires its Fellows to observe a more stringent course of ethical conduct than that specified in the Principles. The Regents have held that the College has the right and responsibility to do this in the interest of the welfare and best professional care of the patient and disciplines its Fellows for infractions.

The most controversial interpretation of the Board of Regents has been the principles governing the financial relations in the professional care of patients. A pledge against fee-splitting has been required of its Fellows since the founding of the College, and was also required of every physician practicing in a hospital approved by the College when it originated and conducted the program of hospital standardization.

It has been well established that the practice of the operating surgeon to return a portion of the patient's fee to the referring doctor, without the patient's knowledge, has not been prevalent in every state of the Union but where it has existed, it has been a serious threat to the advancement of the best care of the patient. The result has been that the patient has been referred for care to the surgeon who proved to be the highest bidder and not necessarily the best qualified surgeon.

Many do not understand the serious implications of fee-splitting; in fact, lawyers make a practice of returning a percentage of a client's fee to the referring firm. Lawyers deal with estates, properties, businesses and not with human lives. Errors by inept attorneys can be judged in money lost, not lives.

When a patient is referred for care and treatment, the surgeon is morally and legally responsible for the preoperative diagnosis; the decision to operate; preoperative care; performance of the operation, and postoperative care as long as the surgical condition of the patient is of major importance. Consultation with and advice from colleagues in other fields of practice should be sought freely and when surgical care is no longer needed, the patient should be referred back to his physician, with a complete and detailed report of the care given and the progress of the patient.

The concept of surgical care as a combined effort of several doctors is important and the patient should be informed that he may be cared for by several individuals working under the direction of the responsible surgeon. The attending surgeon is also responsible for the acts of residents, and to discharge fully this reponsibility to the patient, he must actively supervise operations performed by the resident and so inform the patient. The active supervisory participation provides excellent teaching for the resident, ensures the best possible surgical care, and obviates the charge of ghost surgery, which exists when the patient is unaware of the identity of the operating surgeon.

Discussion between the doctor and the patient or his relatives, prior to submitting a statement for a professional fee, may prevent misunderstandings and the resentment of patients, about a fee which they learn about for the first time when they receive it on the doctor's billhead in the mail. A satisfactory agreement can be reached by a frank discussion of all the considerations involved in determination of a fee. The fee should be commensurate with the services given and the reasonable ability of the patient to pay. The value of the services performed depends upon the nature of the disease and the skill required to treat it, as well as the length of time the patient is ill, in the case of the physician. The surgeon's fee depends upon the nature and extent of the operation, and the special skill required, and should include those services given by him personally, by his employees, or by surgical associates under his direction.

Reasonable ability to pay a fee should be based upon all the expenses incident to the care of the patient, and upon the economic level of the family, regardless of the existence of insurance against the cost of the medical or surgical care. Medical or surgical insurance is not designed to serve as a platform upon which to erect an additional fee not justified by the economic circumstances of the family. To abuse insurance in such a way nullifies the individual's benefits for which he has paid a premium and will quickly destroy voluntary insurance programs.

A surgical assistant, who has no other professional relationship with the patient, may be compensated by the surgeon. The referring physician, or consultant, should submit his individual bill directly to the patient for the services which he performs. Ethically, a surgeon should not pay the referring physician for any services the latter may perform in the care of the patient; nor should he resort to any subterfuge to assist the referring physician to collect an unjustifiable fee, such as permitting him to render unnecessary services.

Combined statements of the fees of two or more doctors should be itemized to show clearly to the patient the services performed by each doctor and the amount each is to be paid. It is far better if separate statements are sent to the patient, or to an insurance carrier. In the submission of statements to patients, clinic groups and formal partnerships are regarded as single contractors and it is ethical and proper to submit one bill for all the services given by individual members of the group clinic or partnership.

Some insurance companies will pay only one physician for the care given by all doctors in the treatment of the patient, stating that multiple bills complicate their bookkeeping practices. This is not an ideal arrangement because it encourages unethical financial practices. If the insurance benefit specifically covers the entire medical care of the patient, and not merely the surgical operation, the surgeon may receive the single check and then pay the fees submitted by other physicians for their services by his own check, if it is made payable jointly to the patient and the doctor.

The sole point at issue is the interests of the patient, which should be the primary responsibility of the physician; referral of the patient for surgical care, or expert care in any special field, should be based only upon the quality of the care expected. Acceptance of any other inducement is a violation of the trust which should exist between the patient and his doctor. The most common unethical inducements are division of the surgical fee between the surgeon and the referring physician, regardless of the source of payment, be it an insurance carrier or the patient; permitting the referring physician to collect the total bill from the patient and pay the surgeon; alternate billing of surgical patients, whereby the surgeon and the referring physician collect and retain the entire fee from alternate patients; disproportionate reduction of the surgeon's fee to enable the referring physician to charge excessively for his services, or payment of office rent on a percentage of professional income, particularly when the owners or lessees of the space can refer patients to the surgeon.

It is also unethical to accept a rebate from a manufacturer or dealer who has supplied a patient with drugs, appliances or any other adjunct to treatment, such as eye glasses, or to accept a rebate or reduction in cost from clinical pathology or roentgenology laboratories for work referred to them.

To avoid abuse of the distribution of benefits of medical care insurance, and innumerable interpretations of what is and is not ethical practice, the benefits should be paid directly to the patient, and the fee for professional services paid to the doctor by the patient, thus strengthening an important part of the patient-doctor relationship, and giving to the policy holder the benefits he is entitled to by the payment of his premiums.

The benefits of medical insurance should be based upon the premium costs of the policy coverage and not upon the name of the operation or disease. Insurance companies have obtained the cooperation of county and state medical societies in setting fee schedules for various types of operations, and many of the designated surgical fees are ridiculously scheduled. Moreover, fee schedules thus established tend to be the fee understood as acceptable to the profession, regardless of the skill and talent required or the economic ability of the patient to pay. It makes a trades union of a profession and encourages the establishment of a level of mediocrity.

SURGEON AND PATIENT

The reputation of a surgeon is more sensitive than that of a member of any other profession and his good name is exquisitely reactive to patients' gossip. The most stimulating, gratifying, and at the same time the most exasperating, experiences in a surgeon's life can be the relations with patients and their families. It is quite simple for a surgeon to become careless and assume that they know as much about their illness as he does; or to become frustrated, after explaining carefully to them in as simple language as he can use, to have them give evidence by their next question that they have comprehended little. It is easy to form the habit of telling them nothing, and to rationalize it by believing this is the best for their psychological state. Many patients learn of their forthcoming surgical treatment only that their operation will be on Friday.

The indications for an operation, what it is hoped can be accomplished, and the extent of the continued follow-up care should be explained in detail to the patient and his family. The most fantastic errors can be encountered in the relay of this information from the patient to his relatives, or from one relative to another, so that sometimes multiple explanations must be given patiently.

These meetings afford another method of learning about the responsibilities of the family, their ambitions and aims; in short, an opportunity to establish a personal relationship of the type enjoyed by the old style family doctor. The less personal the relationship, the more certain it is that the patient and his family will think bitterly in terms of percentage of recovery based upon his condition as a healthy youth, when he is dissatisfied with the results of his surgical operation.

There is, of course, a difference in the patients of today and yesterday; it is too easy to place all the onus for a poor doctor-patient relationship upon changes in the doctor. With some modern patients, a major surgical operation is followed by a minor degree of gratitude. The patient's life may be saved only to have him complain that his sutures stick, the nurses have cold hands, the hospital bed is hard, the coffee abominable, and the hospital bills outrageous. The final summing up consists in the conclusion that the high cost of medical care is due to the surgeon's fee.

Today, the patient may rush off to the law courts following an operation if he wakes up from an extensive life-saving operation and a safety pin is sticking him, or if he develops a backache at his work. If he coughs in front of a jury, or limps into the courtroom on a cane, he gets an award, the size of which is increasing as is, naturally, the fee his lawyer receives. The individual citizen has become more and more security minded and more dependent upon his union and governmental agencies. The world, he says, owes him a living. What is more natural for him to turn to his surgeon's or employer's insurance company, which appears to be a limitless source of wealth. He rationalizes this by saying that it won't take anything out of an individual's pocket.

The increasing interest of the public in medicine, and a knowledge of medical facts, are factors which exert a profound influence upon the practice of surgery. Articles fill magazines and newspapers, and scenes of the operating room are as familiar as frontier saloons on television screens. The general effect of public interest and knowledge of medicine has been good but often the popular presentation of a surgical procedure has been exaggerated to make it effective to the layman. The result may be that the reader, or viewer, who is not too discerning at best, may be misled to anticipate a more favorable outcome of an illness, or injury, than even the best surgeon or the best operation can deliver. Weekly picture magazines vividly portray the surgical anatomy, pathology and operative steps in the treatment of heart disease, or low back ailments — so clearly, in fact, that patients may regard their surgeon as slightly mentally retarded, if he expresses a reservation.

There is no justification for the surgeon who releases an announcement of the results of his experimental or clinical investigations, or an impending new operation, to the press prior to presentation before a scientific society of his peers. He is helpless to stop the press from reporting upon his presentation but, with the cooperation of his colleagues in the society, he can attempt to influence a reasonably factual report upon his experiences. However, regardless of all efforts, the headlines which cover the story are neither under the control of the writer, the surgeon or the society. They are written for the single purpose to sell newspapers and can, therefore, be entirely misleading to patients.

SOCIAL, ECONOMIC AND EDUCATIONAL FACTORS IN THE PRACTICE OF SURGERY

The practice of surgery is being influenced by social, economic and educational factors far more strongly than at any other time.

The United States is experiencing the trials, tribulations, and penalties of an era of the half-done job. To put it another way, this is an era in which there are constant attempts to legislate all facets of enterprise to the level of mediocrity. It is the age of plumbers who may come to fix a leaky faucet some day, maybe; of salesmen and salesladies who at their pleasure respond to inquiries about their merchandise; of teachers who demand a single salary schedule so that achievement cannot be rewarded; of students who take cinch courses; and of doctors who sponsor

fee schedules which reward the unqualified surgeon equally with the educated and trained surgeon. There appears to be a stampede away from the goal of first-rateness and responsibility.

With the basic tenets of democracy that all men are born free and equal and are entitled to life, liberty, and the pursuit of happiness, no one can take issue. It is manifestly absurd, however, to maintain that a physician with no education and training in surgery, who calls himself a surgeon and has the legal right to operate upon a patient without restriction, is the equal of the surgeon who has voluntarily spent many years in formal education and training to become qualified to express an authoritative opinion, which he can implement with skill and talent. Yet a study of specific categories of the most commonly performed surgical operations in hospitals of varying bed capacities in the United States showed that 50 per cent of these operations are performed by doctors who have sought the short cut, those who have not been willing to pursue the hard path toward the goal of first-rateness in surgery.

Self-declared surgeons have attempted to establish certifying boards by edict, with standards below the accepted minimum. Failing to receive acceptance, they used the goon tactics of labor union leaders in an attempt to force their will upon men who strive to maintain the first-rate in the care of surgical patients.

To strive for the first-rate in surgery entails the willingness to listen to the suggestions of the young, to modify and adopt them if possible in education, training and practice. It does not mean, however, the abandonment of experience and tradition, or substitution of the mediocre for the excellent. This pursuit of the first rate often encounters a philosophy that what is right is not as important as what is momentarily beneficial to the individual or the organization.

There is reason to have knowledge of and respect for orthodoxy in the education, training and practice of surgeons. This means the holding of the correct views which are in the best interests of the public, and the care of the surgical patient is a matter of public interest. The difficulty is to prevent orthodoxy from passing into stagnation, or assuming prerogatives which do not permit discarding theories and practices which have ceased to be commonly accepted or have no further value.

Gradually, medical school faculties and

universities have relinquished what little influence they have had in the determination of the character and maintenance of the quality of surgical education to groups which should function only as completely independent and unprejudiced examiners. These examining bodies should not be accountable for the review, approval or disapproval of the requirements and conduct of graduate study in surgery. The surgical faculty of the medical school should state that the candidate has fulfilled its prescribed course of graduate study in a satisfactory manner, and that he has been granted an advanced degree, which indicates that it believes him to be a properly educated surgeon. The faculty should state that the candidate is prepared for an examination of his qualifications as a surgeon. The faculty should publish the contents of its course of study in postgraduate surgical education just as is done in other fields of postgraduate study.

The existing Boards of surgery and the surgical specialties should examine the products of these university-directed programs of education in surgery. The method and scope of examination should be determined independently by each board of examiners. The quality of the product of graduate programs in surgical education may be judged by the results of the examination.

In recognition of completing the course of graduate surgical study and successfully passing the board examination, fellowship in the American College of Surgeons should be granted after a satisfactory demonstration of adherence to, and support of, the principles of ethical and professional practices and conduct promulgated by that College and the American Medical Association.

There can be no question about the important influence the Committee on Graduate Training in Surgery of the American College of Surgeons, the Council on Medical Education and Hospitals, the Advisory Board for Medical Specialties and the Boards of surgery and the surgical specialties have had upon raising the standards of education for surgeons, thus elevating the care of surgical patients. It is time, however, that universities and their medical school faculties played a more dominant and direct role in the postgraduate education of surgeons.

It is doubtful if a young man completing a surgical educational program can be examined properly by any method, or by any group of men, and graded justly or accurately. His chief and his associates are the ones who can judge most fairly and completely the breadth of his surgical knowledge, his integrity and his search for the first-rate in his surgical performances without thought of monthly remuneration or hours off duty.

The surgeon must learn to analyze himself and establish his highest level of performance and integrity. The initiative and responsibility for becoming first-rate rest with the individual. These qualities of the resident in surgery can be recognized and encouraged by his teachers but they cannot be measured and graded. They are the elements which finally distinguish the surgeon whose greatest reward is his own satisfaction with his individual performance.

Education in surgery is a continuing process. What will result from the shortening of the education process of a doctor to have him begin his surgical educational and training program at an earlier age? Is there an hour of a day in a certain month of a specific year when the surgical student can say, "Now I am a surgeon," and stop his learning process? Does it matter what name is given the year following graduation from medical school? Is it not a time for study and teaching, experience, and self-analysis just as is the tenth or twentieth postcommencement year?

There is a preoccupation with the problems of teaching students how to be good surgeons and care for patients by a group who have never practiced surgery competitively, or have found it beyond their talents. Thus, these men, in their own opinions, qualify to establish dicta and introduce the schism-producing phrase, "academic surgeon." Does this mean that he is the one who does not operate upon patients, but is academically or theoretically a surgeon? Does it mean that the surgeon who operates upon and cares for patients is not a scholar, cannot teach, and cannot investigate? Does it mean that the practicing surgeon who voluntarily gives his time, thought, and energy to teaching students and residents is not a good teacher because he receives no money for his teaching duties because his medical school does not have sufficient financial support to remunerate him?

There is an obligation to understand the privileges and responsibilities inherent in becoming a surgeon. He must be dedicated to keeping his own score in the pursuit of the first-rate. This involves his own code of personal and professional ethics, a feeling of obligation to contribute to the best of his ability and talents to the improvement of the care of surgical patients, a duty to uphold the values in education and training for which he will have sacrificed so much, a feeling for taste and style, and the capacity to recognize and enjoy the first-rate.

Guy de Chauliac (1300-1370) wrote a prescription for a surgeon to which little has been added or subtracted:

"Let the surgeon be bold in all sure things, and fearful in dangerous things; let him avoid all faulty treatments and practices. He ought to be gracious to the sick, considerate to his associates, cautious in his prognostications. Let him be modest, dignified, gentle, pitiful and merciful; not covetous nor an extortionist of money; but rather let his reward be according to his work, to the means of the patient, to the quality of the issue, and to his own dignity."

Chapter *40*

SURGICAL JUDGMENT

by
HAROLD LAUFMAN, M.D.

HAROLD LAUFMAN also contributed to the chapter on the Vascular System for this textbook. He has succeeded in expressing clearly a surgical philosophy and in stating his definition of a term that is in common use, but rarely defined.

If surgery were an exact science in the strictest sense of the word, the concept of surgical judgment would never have come into being. Facts could be collated to list all possible deviations from the healthy human state and universally applicable formulas could be devised to describe accurately and unerringly the exact procedures for their correction. Programmed instruction by an electronic console is being used experimentally in a number of fields to provide part of the input of factual information. Programmed instruction is defined as the construction of carefully arranged sequences of contingencies leading to the terminal performance. If this were the only requirement in surgical education, the student of surgery need but memorize a list of facts and develop through usage a high degree of mechanical skill to achieve pre-eminence in his field. He would never be faced with a host of conflicting variables requiring appraisal and interpretation; he would not need to make a separate decision upon each patient; he would not have to deal with his patients as people. He would be, in fact, no more than a superbly functioning machine.

Surgery is not, however, "exact" in that narrow sense. Insofar as the discipline of surgery is based on certain universally applicable principles of anatomy, bacteriology, physiology and related disciplines, it is a science. Insofar as it must apply these principles to the specific needs of an individual patient under particular circumstances at a given time, surgery is also an art.

Sound training in the fundamentals of surgery and a high degree of technical competence are the basic equipment of the surgeon; they are taken for granted. If he has nothing more, a surgeon may be adequate in ordinary situations. If, however, he is to translate his knowledge and apply his skills into their highest potential of healing for each individual, the surgeon must enter into the infinitely complex series of mental, moral and physical acts which for working purposes is called surgical judgment.

Since it is so complex, both as a concept and as a working process, a completely adequate consideration of surgical judgment would have to deal with virtually every aspect of a surgeon's life and the whole of his psychologic structure. Yet surgical judgment is said to be something that a surgeon either has or does not have. It is perennially offered to medical students as a distinguishing excellence they may one day hope to achieve.

Because of the comprehensive nature of surgical judgment, authoritative criteria for it cannot be codified. On the other hand, since it does exist as a therapeutic tool or as a catalyst for all other therapeutic tools, it warrants a more orderly and systematic consideration than has so far been accorded it. It should not remain forever in the realm of a mystique, implicitly acknowledged but always undefined.

Judgment, in general, is not just a static condition or quality, though it is regarded as something one "has." It is actually a mental process in which man is always consciously or unconsciously engaged. Daily, a number of trivial or important decisions are made based on momentary or prior evaluations. Daily, evaluations of one sort or another are made, on which future decisions will be based. Most of the time this process is not

1459

recognized and requires little conscious attention. An effort to define it would necessitate looking back on the decisions made over a time. A certain pattern of choices would emerge, a pattern of a fairly consistent nature; the nature of this pattern would serve to define the quality of judgment. Judgment can thus be defined as a series of mental acts involving an appraisal of factors leading to decision in the service of a goal.

Surgical judgment is a specialized application of this process requiring greater awareness and subject to more stringent criteria, since the attainment of such important goals depends on it. The goals of surgical judgment upon which all decisions are based and toward which all evaluations are oriented consist in the perennial aims of all therapy: prolongation of life and alleviation of suffering. The manner in which a surgeon employs his personal endowments, his education and his experience in the service of these ends will define him as a surgeon.

MOTIVATIONS IN SURGERY

A patient comes to a surgeon because either he or his referring physician thinks he may need surgery. The referral, strictly speaking, is for purposes of a surgical opinion rather than for surgery per se. Even if a given pathologic state is ordinarily amenable to surgery, the decision for or against surgical intervention in a particular instance must be made. Such a decision involves first the accumulation of pertinent data through the indispensable classic sources: a careful history, a thorough physical examination, diagnostic laboratory findings and the surgeon's general or clinical impression of the case. Each factor in the data accruing from these sources must be assessed first individually for its own implications and then in relation to all other factors. This appraisal is made to answer three prime questions: Is a surgical operation advisable at all? If it is advisable, is it also feasible in terms of risk to the patient and in terms of the anticipated result? And, third, how might the operation have to be modified to fit a specific set of circumstances?

Often the highest product of seasoned and responsible surgical judgment is the decision not to operate. A number of influences irrelevant to the patient's welfare may be brought to bear upon the surgeon in the formation of this important decision. The surgeon may be eager for experience; he may be influenced consciously or unconsciously by his own psychologic or financial needs; the referring physician may indicate a subtle but influencing preference; or the patient himself, for tangential reasons, may urge surgery. Sometimes a patient has a vague disorder which he hopes may be magically defined and cured; sometimes he has lived with a fear of surgery long enough that he "wants to get it over with"; sometimes he is just surgery prone. Without playing psychiatrist, a surgeon must remain alert to such distortions if he is effectively to resist them.

The most dangerous artifacts introduced into the area of surgical motivation are, of course, those which may occasionally arise out of the surgeon's own distortions or self-interest. No matter how well it can be rationalized, any motive that is not based exclusively on a concern for the patient's welfare is an artifact which violates the basic principles of surgical judgment. It is in this area of mixed motives that we encounter such aberrations of surgical behavior as fee splitting, ghost surgery, irresponsible timing of operations and unjustified surgery.

Equally dangerous distortions of clinical conduct can be made in the name of academia. Immaterial quantifying investigations which will not further knowledge or contribute to prognosis or treatment, and only cause anguish to a dying patient, must be considered either frivolous or vicious, but in either case, poor judgment.

If surgery is feasible at all, the only allowable motivation for it is a conclusion that it is necessary to the patient's welfare. There are, of course, different kinds and degrees of necessity. Surgery may be deemed necessary if the available information indicates that the patient's condition cannot improve in a reasonable time without surgery, if the condition may lead to complications or death without surgery or if accurate diagnosis leading to more accurate therapy depends upon surgical intervention.

When, according to the valid criteria, it does seem advisable to operate, all factors must be weighed to estimate the extent and nature of risk for the particular patient involved, since the next complexus of decisions is made with a view of minimizing, insofar as possible, the attendant risks. This consideration governs the selection of an optimal time, the most adequate available place, the course of preoperative care, the type of anesthesia, the best anatomic approach and the extent of permissible radicality. Estimation of risk also involves some knowledge of the possible complications and a reasonably close prediction of probable outcome, based on the nature and urgency of the case in light of the best results to be hoped for. It requires knowledge of the current statistics on morbidity, complications and mortality, based not only upon the literature, but upon the surgeon's own experience in comparable instances.

If his experience is sparse, a surgeon's use of the literature can help him in his estimates, but only up to a point. Results obtained by one surgeon do not necessarily reveal what another surgeon may expect. In order to make a cogent comparison one would need to presume approximate equality of experience, ability, facilities and judgment between the surgeons, as well as comparable lesions and risk components in the patients. A surgeon's use of the literature, therefore, must be discriminating and selective when he attempts to apply what he reads to his own practice. Although knowledge of current statistics may serve as a guiding factor to the surgeon's judgment, it cannot substitute for judgment nor even dominate it. The surgeon cannot operate on a statistical basis alone, for although it will certainly yield numbers, it cannot dependably yield meanings and interpretations.

RAPPORT

Once these preparatory preoperative judgments have been made by the surgeon, at least tentatively, he must inform and prepare the patient and responsible members of the patient's family. A good personal rapport with them will depend on two cardinal qualities in the surgeon, which may at first seem to conflict: honesty and tact. A patient is entitled to know everything pertinent both to his condition and to the probable course of his treatment which he is capable of understanding intellectually and able to accept emotionally. His questions must be respected and answered fully but simply, without recourse to unnecessarily technical language. Professional jargon has no place in talking with a patient; it is designed to impress rather than to inform. Oversimplification is equally out of taste; it is a condescension the patient is quick to sense and which he may justifiably resent. Needless to say, the abrupt dismissal,

"Let me worry about that," to which an earlier generation of surgeons was prone, insults the patient and argues an insufficiency in the surgeon.

Even as a patient must be respected intellectually, respect must also be accorded his particular emotional system. His tensions and anxieties must be accepted as natural. It is particularly difficult to do so when they are exaggerated or neurotic. A patient comes for help, not for censure; he needs assurance and perhaps the support of an authoritative figure, but the surgeon's authority must not be misused to reduce the patient's self-respect and dignity. The patient who is treated as an equal and cooperative adult will tend to be one.

STEREOTYPY AND ROUTINE

The dangers of stereotypy in general are among the most pervasive and pernicious of therapeutic fallacies. The organization of knowledge is part of the business of science: to define separate entities and classify them according to general type is a legitimate intellectual act. Except in rare instances, almost any condition in almost any patient can be placed, for the purposes of classification, into conformance with a familiar disease entity described previously in the literature or familiar to the physician. To establish this is only the first part of the surgeon's obligation. A second, sometimes larger, and equally cogent part is to know that there is no such thing as an average patient. Even the most ordinary patient with the simplest lesion has certain sensitivities, stresses, patterns peculiarly his own, requiring the surgeon's individual attention to his particular problem. A surgeon who works in the climate of this basic attitude will be swiftly and sensitively respondent to unexpected reactions and events for which surgeons who think in stereotypes may be unprepared.

Does a usual procedure need to be modified in its nature or degree for a particular patient? This question, again, must be answered by balancing the nature of the disease against a series of factors peculiar to a given patient. Among other things, these include: expected longevity in relation to existing pathology; the presence and severity of associated but not necessarily related infirmities; the degree of urgency deemed essential for preservation of health or life; the success of the physiologic preparation for surgery; an appraisal of the patient's tolerance for the several variations of the available procedural plans, and knowledge of the choice of goals to be sought.

Even as a patient must not be regarded as average, so the tendency to regard procedures as routine must be avoided. The word is often used to indicate a tested and reliable method of approach, or to describe a pattern of procedural steps which has proved dependable throughout the years in thousands of individual instances. The word routine is allowable, in this context, on practical and pragmatic grounds.

But when dealing, as here, with more precise meanings of concepts in terms of their ultimate implications for intellectual and clinical behavior, the word routine is best avoided. It suggests an unthinking, undifferentiating stereotypy in the surgeon's attitude which will, if adopted, obviate any real potential for what is called surgical judgment.

Flexibility must be preserved in even the most ordinary and familiar circumstance: new knowledges, insights and techniques must be correlated; unexpected variants of familiar surgical situations must be differentiated from their individual application.

In the well-disciplined surgeon who knows he will not violate basic surgical principles, and has no impulse to do so, there is no need for undeviating adherence to a rigid routine. Such a surgeon will, of course, make use of his experience, but he does not make a fetish of it. He will be able to respond to the specific needs of the moment, whether ordinary or deviant, within the principles of sound surgical practice.

FEAR

There are, generally speaking, two kinds of fear common to surgeons: rational fears which are a necessary tool of responsible surgery, and irrational fears which are an unnecessary and sometimes dangerous burden.

Rational fear recognizes realistically all potential danger to the patient; it keeps the surgeon alert to physiologic changes before, during and after surgery; it makes him respectful of tissue, attentive to detail, swiftly responsive to subtle changes, careful to avoid complications. He uses rational fear to quicken his purposeful responses and sharpen his skills so that he may avoid catastrophe and meet new problems flexibly when they arise.

Irrational fears are those germane not to the patient, but to the surgeon. They may immobilize him into a repetition of familiar and safe routines insufficient to or irrelevant to the problem at hand. They may spur him to irresponsible innovations or deviations from sound surgical principles. The surgeon may suffer from fears based on an insufficient knowledge of the kind of problem he is dealing with, or an insufficient experience with it. In such instance, he would do well to obtain assistance from a surgeon better versed in the problem or to refer the patient.

There are a host of other fears arising out of threats to the surgeon's own professional or personal welfare, but having no real pertinence to the condition of the patient; fear of criticism, fear because the patient is important, fear of extensive surgical procedures, fear conditioned by interpersonal difficulties with colleagues. The presence of any such irrational fear may distort the surgeon's motives, presence of mind and coordination to such a degree that his best surgical judgment is impossible. When fear of this sort is a major motivating force, it threatens the logical performance of what otherwise might be acceptable surgery.

TECHNICAL SKILL

A surgeon's confidence with tissue comes out of his basic physical coordination, his training and his experience. It is developed by work done in the experimental laboratory, at the autopsy table and in the operating room. Within the limits set by his manual dexterity, muscular coordination and total integration as an individual, each surgeon learns when to be gentle, how to be strong; he knows, or senses, the balance of strength and delicacy to be applied in a given instance. The sum of his relationship to tissue may be called a surgeon's technique. There are, of course, different technical styles having equal effectiveness and validity. It is interesting to observe two skilled surgeons, one with a slow, plodding manner, the other with spectacular rapidity of motion. Whatever their differences, they will have in common respect for tissue, meticulous attention to detail and a subordination of their physical procedures to the demands of their surgical judgment.

Although technique is of the greatest importance, it is not an end in itself, but only a highly developed instrument of the surgeon's intention. During the war, it became evident that technical skill at the operating table can be acquired rather easily by well-coordinated individuals. Often, outstanding surgical assistance was rendered by medical technicians who had been stockbrokers, saloon keepers or salesmen in civilian life. But without a surgeon's education and experience, even these especially skilled people could not be expected to estimate operative risk, to prepare a patient physiologically or psychologically for surgery, to know when or when not to operate, to adapt their skills to unfamiliar situations or to carry a patient through a stormy postoperative course.

Surgical judgment and surgical skill are interdependent but not identical qualities. The best surgical results are the product of sure surgical technique combined with sound preoperative diagnosis and preparation. They reflect planning, knowledge of risk factors, and ability to recognize and cope with postoperative problems. They are also irrefutable evidence of education and experience put to best use.

SURGICAL MANAGEMENT

Experienced surgeons are aware of their responsibility in managing certain aspects of surgical care which may appear less consequential than in fact they are. Other aspects merge into related or allied disciplines and are, therefore, often left to the responsibility of colleagues or house staff. Whatever the necessary and desirable collaboration with such colleagues as the anesthetist, the internist or members of the house staff, the surgeon must regard himself as the fulcrum of responsibility to the patient in a surgical situation.

Decisions about mode and type of anesthesia, for example, cannot be left entirely to the anesthetist; ultimately the surgeon must decide. Unusual reactions to the induction of anesthesia demand the surgeon's decision whether to proceed or to send the patient back to his bed without surgery. Certainly, many types of surgery can be postponed advantageously under these conditions.

Problems in judgment associated with so-called standard operative procedures are not necessarily inherent in application of the procedure, but in encountering, recognizing and acting upon unexpected findings necessitating change from the planned attack.

Such postoperative measures as bandaging, splinting and grading of motion may make the difference between success and failure.

In many instances, the most trying days for both the patient and the surgeon only begin with the day of surgery. It is in the postoperative period that some of the most perplexing problems in judgment arise. Since the surgeon assumes the responsibility for the patient's welfare by subjecting him to surgery, he must, by the same token, see the patient through the subsequent period. Nor should discharge from the hospital necessarily be the end of patient-surgeon relations.

In the immediate postoperative period the surgeon must cope with the intricacies of fluid and electrolyte balance; precautions against complications arising either from surgery or from unrelated infirmities by keeping in constant touch with the status of all the vital functions of the body through appropriate physical and laboratory examinations; the judicious employment of medications; the timing and grading of alimentation and ambulation; and not least, the encouragement of the patient to cooperate properly. All require judgment.

In the late postoperative period, it is the surgeon's obligation to the patient, to himself and to his profession to obtain follow-up information, especially for types of surgery in which such information is not well known or in which it may possibly alter his future surgical approach to comparable problems. Much of the present-day knowledge of what to expect from surgery has come from careful judgment exercised in appraisal of results. In turn, such information is bound to affect the judgment of other surgeons.

NEWNESS

The concept of newness often is confused with one of unfamiliarity. One need only reflect on how often rediscoveries are made. Yet the rediscovery is new to the rediscoverer. Familiarity by association constitutes a foundation of experience each surgeon must acquire for himself. Every skill grasped by the young surgeon in his graded program of training is, in a sense, a rediscovery. For the young man it is a discovery for himself, a realization that he is capable of doing something he was not sure he could do the day before.

One type of newness has to do with novel situations confronting a surgeon, perhaps unexpectedly, which may require a novel approach to be accomplished by variations of old and established techniques. Occasionally, discoveries are made by chance rather than by sagacity, but such advances ordinarily require a background of experience, ability to recognize and utilize a new turn and the skill to employ the discovery to advantage. Chance discovery and pragmatism have their place in surgery as they do in other fields, but they merely complement and do not replace sound judgment.

Most surgical advances employ standard techniques with some variations but are made possible by advances in sister fields of physiologic knowledge. Surgeons readily acknowledge the debt owed to other sciences for surgical advances. The gamut spans scientific fields from physiology to physics, from immunology to electronics, from chemistry to metallurgy.

A second variety of newness is seen in certain procedures which have proved satisfactory in the originator's hands but nonetheless require a fresh experimental and experiential background by every new team of surgeons, no matter how experienced they may be in other types of surgery. Such is the case, for example, in the use of oxygenators in open heart surgery.

Experimental types of surgery undertaken under carefully controlled conditions are often reported from large university centers. The surgeon who reads reports of this kind of work can easily become overstimulated and overenthused. Despite warnings by the reporting surgeons on the experimental nature of the work, the reader may tend to accept the new procedure too readily.

It is often difficult to distinguish newness, bigness or firstness from betterness. Also, it is important to realize that certain types of surgery cannot easily be done except within certain well-controlled surroundings. To proceed with new surgery on the basis of the printed word alone is injudicious. One cannot expect to acquire from the printed word every detail of technical know-how and every nuance of each phase of judgment. Only by a sensible use of skepticism and by his own observations, experimental work and experience with problems and pitfalls can the surgeon arrive at a surgical philosophy acceptable to himself. Nor is experience with numbers alone a guarantee of correctness. A numerically large experience will have been qualitatively small unless it yields changes for the better by the incorporation of changing concepts, aims toward simplification, safety precautions and advancement of knowledge.

A third type of newness involves the planned employment of an operative procedure for which there is no precedent. It is assumed that any planned operation which is to be undertaken as an experimental procedure upon a human being is preceded by its performance over and over again in animals or at the autopsy table. To undertake a life-endangering new procedure without a background of experimental work could be considered an unprincipled act. But once all phases of the technique, timing, use of special equipment and teamwork are mastered in experimental trials, and once "dry-runs" in the operating room run smoothly, a new procedure may be considered for application to a human being. It goes without saying that the patient or legal guardian must be apprised of the experimental nature of the procedure and must agree to its performance.

The odds for success based on the life-improving prospects of the proposed surgery, the surgeon's confidence in himself, his team, and his equipment, an estimate of the patient's chances of withstanding the surgery and the physiologic soundness of the procedure must all be assured within reasonable limits of expectancy. Even after successful performance, new procedures must be considered experimental until long term follow-up studies have proved their value.

CONFLICTING GOALS

Although there are rewarding advances in surgery, some defeating or essentially insoluble problems must be faced. Ordinarily, therapeutic goals such as the prolongation of life and the alleviation of suffering are adequate criteria, and we need only concern ourselves with how best to meet them. However, it is often necessary to make decisions when these two goals are not confluent at all, but antithetical.

If the only known method of alleviating pain involves a radical alteration or destruction of the personality, is it justifiable to act to alleviate it?

If it is known that death can only be postponed in the face of unalterable, intractable pain, is it justifiable to act only to postpone it?

These are among the gravest decisions surgeons are called upon to make. They are not properly matters for surgical judgment so much as they are matters for the judgment of the surgeon. Such problems will remain in the province of philosophy until better tools are developed—mechanical, chemical or intellectual—with which to solve them. Until then surgeons can only hope for a leavening of human wisdom with which to season their surgical judgment.

Surgical judgment is a distillate of physical, emotional, intellectual and moral capacities; of the training and experience which informed and disciplined them; of an individual's potential to grow, learn and create; of the capacity to apply known principles to new specific situations; and of dedication of the welfare of the patient.

No one can lay claim to superlatives in these things: one may hope to have some of each and to maintain an effectively productive balance among them. If one recognizes with rigorous honesty his own special abilities and limitations, if he remains sensitive to the needs of patients and the demands of the profession, he may lay some claim to participation in the development and understanding of his own surgical judgment.

Index